W9-BYI-835

Langenscheidt's
Pocket
Merriam-Webster

Medical
Dictionary

Langenscheidt's
Pocket
Merriam-Webster

Medical
Dictionary

LANGENSCHEIDT
NEW YORK • BERLIN • MUNICH • VIENNA • ZURICH

Contents

Preface

MERRIAM-WEBSTER'S MEDICAL DICTIONARY is a concise guide to the essential language of medicine. It is an abridged version of *Merriam-Webster's Medical Desk Dictionary*, and it shares many of the features of its parent volume. These are features that are standard for most desk dictionaries of the English language but are often missing from medical dictionaries. For example, users of this book will find how to pronounce *CABG*, *NSAID*, and *RU 486;* how to spell and pronounce the plurals of *arthritis*, *chlamydia*, and *uterus;* where to divide *arteriosclerosis* and *thrombolytic* at the end of a line; and the part-of-speech labels of *spermicide*, *spermicidal*, and *spermicidally.*

The 35,000 vocabulary entries include the most frequently used words of human and veterinary medicine. The reader will find entries not only for human diseases such as *AIDS*, *Lyme disease*, and *chronic fatigue syndrome* but also for those of domestic animals such as *heartworm* of dogs, *panleukopenia* of cats, and *foot-and-mouth disease* of cattle. In addition this dictionary includes the scientific and medically related words that are essential to understanding the definitions of the core vocabulary. Every word used in a definition in this book appears as a boldface vocabulary entry either in this dictionary or in its companion general paperback, *The Merriam-Webster Dictionary.*

This dictionary is designed to serve as an interface between the language of doctor and the language of patient, between sports medicine and the sports page, between the technical New Latin names of plants and animals and their common names, and between the old and the new in medical terminology. The user of this dictionary will find, for example, that the *abs, delts*, *glutes*, *lats*, and *pecs* of the physical fitness enthusiast are the *abdominal muscles*, *deltoidei*, *glutei*, *latissimi dorsi*, and *pectorales* of the anatomist. Both medicine and science sometimes give the impression that the latest technical terminology has no antecedents. There may be no clue on the medical page of the reader's daily newspaper that the bacteria referred to as *Gardnerella* and *Helicobacter* were formerly classified as *Haemophilus* and *Campylobacter*. Medical writers may neglect to mention that the *auditory tube* and *uterine tubes* of formal anatomy are still widely known as the *eustachian tube* and *fallopian tubes*. All of these words are entered and defined in this dictionary with mention of synonymous or former terminology when appropriate.

Entries known to be trademarks or service marks are so labeled and are treated in accordance with a formula approved by the United States Trademark Association. No entry in this dictionary, however, should be regarded as affecting the validity of any trademark or service mark.

When a trademark or service mark for a drug is entered in this dictionary, it is also mentioned in a cross-reference following the definition of its generic equivalent, so that, for example, from either of the entries for *diazepam* or *Valium*, *fluoxetine* or *Prozac*, *finasteride* or *Proscar*, the reader can determine which is a generic name and which a proprietary name for the same drug.

This dictionary contains material from its parent work supplemented by new material from the research files in the Merriam-Webster editorial offices which now include more than 14,500,000 citations (examples of English words used in context). Of these, a ten-year sample of approximately 1,300,000 citations containing about 20,000,000 words of text is available on-line for search and retrieval. The editors frequently consulted these sources in abridging the parent work as well as in evaluating new words for entry.

The language of medicine is vast, and as a result, infrequently used medical terms must be excluded from a book of this size. However, many of the excluded terms are compound words and this book compensates in large part for their omission by generous coverage of the prefixes, suffixes, and combining forms that are used in creating medical vocabulary. The entries for these forms can often be used to determine the meaning of words that are not common enough to warrant entry in this dictionary. For example, from the combining form *hemo-* and the noun *transfusion*, it can be determined that *hemotransfusion* means a blood transfusion.

Another important feature of this book is that words occurring only as part of compound terms are entered at their own place in alphabetical sequence with a cross-reference to the compound terms themselves. Thus, *herpetiformis* has a cross-reference to *dermatitis herpetiformis*, and *longus* is followed by a list of eleven compound terms of which it is part. These lists may help the reader unfamiliar with medical terminology to find the place of definition of compound terms.

The biographical information following words derived from the names of persons has been limited to the person's name, birth and death dates, nationality, and occupation or status. Such information is entered only for historical figures, not for fictional or mythical characters.

It is the intent of the editors that this dictionary serve the purposes of all those who seek information about medical English as it is currently spoken and written, whether in the context of a clinical setting, in correctly rendering spoken and written text, or from the perspective of lexicography as an art and science.

Merriam-Webster's Medical Dictionary is the result of a collective effort by the staff of Merriam-Webster Incorporated. The editor was assisted by Joan I. Narmontas, Assistant Editor, in preparing the basic text. Stephen J. Perrault, Senior Editor, copyedited the entire manuscript and identified areas where technical material needed to be clarified. Brian M. Sietsema, Ph.D., Associate Editor, prepared the pronunciations. The cross-referencing was done by Maria A. Sansalone, Assistant Editor, and Donna L. Rickerby, Assistant Editor, with the help of Adrienne M. Scholz. Robert D. Copeland, Senior Editor, adapted typesetting tapes for use on the personal computers in the editorial offices and wrote computer programs to facilitate specific cross-reference tasks. Other specialized editorial assistance was provided by Michael G. Belanger, Paul F. Cappellano, Jennifer N. Cislo, Jill J. Cooney, Peter D. Haraty, Amy K. Harris, Brett P. Palmer, James L. Rader, and Katherine C. Sietsema. Joan I. Narmontas supervised proofreading by Deanna Chiasson, Jennifer N. Cislo, Jill J. Cooney, Michael G. Guzzi, Amy K. Harris, Thomas F. Pitoniak, Ph.D., James L. Rader, Donna L. Rickerby, and Maria A. Sansalone. Ruth W. Gaines, Senior General Clerk, kept track of the copy as it moved about the editorial office and was assisted in the final stages by Carol A. Fugiel. Madeline L. Novak, Senior Editor, coordinated production. John M. Morse, Executive Editor, made numerous suggestions for improving the book and gave encouragement and moral support throughout.

Roger W. Pease, Jr., Ph.D.
Editor

Explanatory Notes

Entries

Main Entries

A boldface letter or a combination of such letters, including punctuation marks and diacritics where needed, that is set flush with the left-hand margin of each column of type is a main entry or entry word. The main entry may consist of letters set solid, of letters joined by a hyphen, or of letters separated by one or more spaces:

> **al·ler·gy** . . . *n*
>
> **¹an·ti–in·flam·ma·to·ry** . . . *adj*
>
> **blood vessel** *n*
>
> **non–A, non–B hepatitis** . . . *n*

The material in lightface type that follows each main entry explains and justifies its inclusion in the dictionary.

Variation in the styling of compound words in English is frequent and widespread. It is often completely acceptable to choose freely among open, hyphenated, and closed alternatives. To save space for other information, this dictionary usually limits itself to a single styling for a compound. When a compound is widely used and one styling predominates, that styling is shown. When a compound is uncommon or when the evidence indicates that two or three stylings are approximately equal in frequency, the styling shown is based on the analogy of parallel compounds.

Order of Main Entries

The main entries follow one another in alphabetical order letter by letter without regard to intervening spaces or hyphens: *elastic stocking* follows *elasticity* and *right-handed* follows *right hand*. Words that often begin with the abbreviation *St.* in common usage have the abbreviation spelled out: *Saint Anthony's fire, Saint Vitus' dance.*

Full words come before parts of words made up of the same letters. Parts of words with no hyphen in front but followed by a hyphen come before parts of words preceded by a hyphen. Solid words come first and are followed by hyphenated compounds and then by open compounds. Lowercase entries come before entries that begin with a capital letter:

> ²**path** *abbr*
>
> **path-** . . . *comb form*
>
> **-path** . . . *n comb form*
>
> **workup** . . . *n*
>
> **work up** . . . *vb*
>
> **tri•chi•na** . . . *n*
>
> **Trichina** . . . *n*

Entries containing an Arabic numeral within or at the end of the word are alphabetized as if the number were spelled out: *glucose phosphate* comes after *glucose-1-phosphate* and before *glucose= 6-phosphate* while *LD50* is between *LD* and *LDH*. Some chemical terms are preceded by one or more Arabic numerals or by a chemical prefix abbreviated to a Roman or Greek letter or by a combination of the two usually set off by a hyphen. In general the numerical or abbreviated prefix is ignored in determining the word's alphabetical place: *N-allylnormorphine* is entered in the letter *a*, *5-hydroxy-tryptamine* in the letter *h*, and *β₂-microglobulin* in the letter *m*. However, if the prefix is spelled out, it is used in alphabetizing the word: *beta globulin* is entered in the letter *b*, and *levo-dihydroxy-phenylalanine* in the letter *l*. In a few cases, entries have been made at more than one place to assist the reader in finding the place of definition, especially when the prefix has variants: *gamma= aminobutyric acid*, defined in the letter *g*, is often written with a Greek letter as *γ-aminobutyric acid*, and an entry has been made in the letter *a* to direct the reader to the place of definition.

If the names of two chemical substances differ only in their prefixes, the terms are alphabetized first by the main part of the word and then in relation to each other according to the prefix: *L-PAM* immediately precedes *2-PAM* in the letter *p*.

Guide Words

A pair of guide words is printed at the top of each page. The entries that fall alphabetically between the guide words are found on that page.

It is important to remember that alphabetical order rather than position of an entry on the page determines the selection of guide words. The first guide word is the alphabetically first entry on the page. The second guide word is usually the alphabetically last entry on the page:

acyanotic • adductor pollicis

The entry need not be a main entry. Another boldface word — a variant, an inflected form, or a defined or undefined run-on — may be selected as a guide word. For this reason the last main entry on a page is not always the last entry alphabetically.

All guide words must themselves be in alphabetical order from page to page throughout the dictionary; thus, the alphabetically last entry on a page is not used if it follows alphabetically the first guide word on the next page.

Homographs

When main entries are spelled alike, they are distinguished by superscript numerals preceding each word:

[1]ano·rex·ic . . . *adj*   [1]se·rum . . . *n*

[2]anorexic *n*   [2]serum *adj*

Although homographs are spelled alike, they may differ in pronunciation, derivation, or functional classification (as part of speech). The order of homographs is historical: the one first used in English is entered first with the exception that abbreviations and symbols are listed last in a series of homographs. Abbreviations appear before symbols when both are present.

End-of-Line Division

The centered dots within entry words indicate division points at which a hyphen may be put at the end of a line of print or writing. Centered dots are not shown after a single initial letter or before a single terminal letter because printers seldom cut off a single letter:

abort . . . *vb*

body . . . *n*

Nor are they shown at second and succeeding homographs unless these differ among themselves in division or pronunciation:

[1]mu·tant . . . *adj*   [1]pre·cip·i·tate . . . *vb*

[2]mutant . . . *n*   [2]pre·cip·i·tate . . . *n*

There are acceptable alternative end-of-line divisions just as there are acceptable variant spellings and pronunciations. No more than one division is, however, shown for an entry in this dictionary.

Many words have two or more common pronunciation variants, and the same end-of-line division is not always appropriate for each of them. The division *ho·me·op·a·thy*, for example, best fits the variant \ˌhō-mē-ˈä-pə-thē\ whereas the division *hom·e·op·a·thy* best fits the variant \ˌhä-mē-ˈä-pə-thē\. In instances like this, the division falling farther to the left is used, regardless of the order of the pronunciations:

ho•me•op•a•thy \ˌhō-mē-'ä-pə-thē, ˌhä-\

A double hyphen at the end of a line in this dictionary stands for a hyphen that belongs at that point in a hyphenated word and that is retained when the word is written as a unit on one line.

Variants

When a main entry is followed by the word *or* and another spelling, the two spellings are equal variants.

> ¹**neu•tro•phil** . . . *or* **neu•tro•phil•ic**

If two variants joined by *or* are out of alphabetical order, they remain equal variants. The one printed first is, however, slightly more common than the second:

> **phys•i•o•log•i•cal** . . . *or* **phys•i•o•log•ic**

When another spelling is joined to the main entry by the word *also*, the spelling after *also* is a secondary variant and occurs less frequently than the first:

> **lip•id** *also* **lip•ide**

If there are two secondary variants, the second is joined to the first by *or*. Once the word *also* is used to signal a secondary variant, all following variants are joined by *or:*

> **taen-** *or* **taeni-** *also* **ten-** *or* **teni-**

A variant whose own alphabetical place is at some distance from the main entry is entered at its own place with a cross‑reference to the main entry. Such variants at consecutive or nearly consecutive entries are listed together.

> **tendonitis** *var of* TENDINITIS
>
> **anchylose, anchylosis** *var of* ANKYLOSE, ANKYLOSIS

Variants having a usage label (as *Brit* or *chiefly Brit*) appear only at their own alphabetical places:

> **-aemia** *also* **-haemia** *chiefly Brit var of* -EMIA
>
> **anae•mia** *chiefly Brit var of* ANEMIA
>
> **haem-** *or* **haemo-** *chiefly Brit var of* HEM-
>
> **hae•mo•glo•bin** *chiefly Brit var of* HEMOGLOBIN

When long lists of such variants would be generated by entering all those at consecutive entries, only one or a few are given. The rest can be deduced by analogy with those which are entered. For example, the chiefly British variant *haemoglobinaemia* is formed analogously with *haemoglobin* and *anaemia* (it might also be recognized from the combining forms *-aemia* and *haem-* or *haemo-*).

Run-on Entries

A main entry may be followed by one or more derivatives or by a homograph with a different functional label. These are run-on entries. Each is introduced by a boldface dash and each has a functional label. They are not defined, however, since their meanings can readily be derived from the meaning of the root word:

> **healthy** . . . *adj* . . . — **health·i·ly** . . . *adv* — **health·i·ness** . . . *n*
> **drift** . . . *n* . . . — **drift** *vb*

A main entry may be followed by one or more phrases containing the entry word. These are also run-on entries. Each is introduced by a boldface dash but there is no functional label. They are, however, defined since their meanings are more than the sum of the meanings of their elements:

> ²**couch** *n* . . . — **on the couch** : . . .
> **risk** . . . *n* . . . — **at risk** : . . .

A run-on entry is an independent entry with respect to function and status. Labels at the main entry do not apply unless they are repeated.

Pronunciation

The matter between a pair of reversed virgules \ \ following the entry word indicates the pronunciation. The symbols used are listed in the chart printed on the page facing the first page of the dictionary proper and on the inside of the back cover.

Syllables

A hyphen is used in the pronunciation to show syllabic division. These hyphens sometimes coincide with the centered dots in the entry word that indicate end-of-line division; sometimes they do not:

> **ab·scess** \\'ab-ˌses\
> **met·ric** \\'me-trik\

Stress

A high-set mark \\'\\ indicates primary (strongest) stress or accent; a low-set mark \\ₗ\\ indicates secondary (medium) stress or accent:

ear·ache \\'ir-ₗāk\\

The stress mark stands at the beginning of the syllable that receives the stress.

Variant Pronunciations

The presence of variant pronunciations indicates that not all educated speakers pronounce words the same way. A second-place variant is not to be regarded as less acceptable than the pronunciation that is given first. It may, in fact, be used by as many educated speakers as the first variant, but the requirements of the printed page are such that one must precede the other:

oral \\'ōr-əl, 'är-\\
um·bi·li·cus \\ₗəm-bə-'lī-kəs, ₗəm-'bi-li-\\

Parentheses in Pronunciations

Low-set stress marks enclosed in parentheses indicate that the following syllable may be pronounced with secondary stress or with no stress:

de·sen·si·tize \\(ₗ)dē-'sen-sə-ₗtīz\\
RNA \\ₗär-(ₗ)en-'ā\\

Partial and Absent Pronunciations

When a main entry has less than a full pronunciation, the missing part is to be supplied from a pronunciation in a preceding entry or within the same pair of reversed virgules:

psy·cho·sur·gery \\-'sər-jə-rē\\
vit·i·li·go \\ₗvi-tə-'lī-gō, -'lē-\\

The pronunciation of the first two syllables of *psychosurgery* is found at the main entry *psychosurgeon:*

psy·cho·sur·geon \\ₗsī-kō-'sər-jən\\

Explanatory Notes

The hyphens before and after \-ˈlē-\ in the pronunciation of *vitiligo* indicate that both the first and the last parts of the pronunciation are to be taken from the immediately preceding pronunciation.

When a variation of stress is involved, a partial pronunciation may be terminated at the stress mark which stands at the beginning of a syllable not shown:

li·gate \ˈlī-ˌgāt, lī-ˈ\

In general, no pronunciation is indicated for open compounds consisting of two or more English words that have own-place entry:

lateral collateral ligament *n*

A pronunciation is shown, however, for any unentered element of an open compound:

Meiss·ner's corpuscle \ˈmīs-nərz-\

Only the first entry in a sequence of numbered homographs is given a pronunciation if their pronunciations are the same:

¹**sig·moid** \ˈsig-ˌmȯid\ *adj*
²**sigmoid** *n*

The pronunciation of unpronounced derivatives run on at a main entry is a combination of the pronunciation at the main entry and the pronunciation of the suffix or final element.

Abbreviations, Acronyms, and Symbols

Pronunciations are not usually shown for entries with the functional labels *abbr* or *symbol* since they are usually spoken by saying the individual letters in sequence or by giving the expansion. The pronunciation is given only if there is an unusual and unexpected way of saying the abbreviation or symbol:

ICU *abbr* intensive care unit
Al *symbol* aluminum
CABG \ˈka-bij\ *abbr* coronary artery bypass graft

Acronyms (as *DNA* and *NSAID*) and compounds (as *ACE inhibitor*) consisting of an acronym and a word element which have one of the traditional parts of speech labels (usually *n, adj, adv,* or *vb* in this book) are given a pronunciation even when the word is spoken by pronouncing the letters in sequence:

DNA \ˌdē-(ˌ)en-ˈā\ *n*
ACE inhibitor \ˈās-, ˌā-(ˌ)sē-ˈē-\ *n*
NSAID \ˈen-ˌsed, -ˌsād\ *n*

Functional Labels

An italic label indicating a part of speech or some other functional classification follows the pronunciation or, if no pronunciation is given, the main entry. Of the eight traditional parts of speech, five appear in this dictionary as follows:

healthy. . . *adj*

psy·cho·log·i·cal·ly . . . *adv*

hos·pi·tal . . . *n*

per . . . *prep*

pre·scribe . . . *vb*

Other italic labels used to indicate functional classifications that are not traditional parts of speech include:

tid *abbr*

pleur- *or* **pleuro-** *comb form*

-poi·e·sis . . . *n comb form*

-poi·et·ic . . . *adj comb form*

dys- *prefix*

-lyt·ic . . . *adj suffix*

-i·a·sis . . . *n suffix*

Rolf·ing . . . *service mark*

Ca *symbol*

Val·ium . . . *trademark*

Functional labels are sometimes combined:

sap·phic . . . *adj or n*

cold turkey *n* : . . . — **cold turkey** *adv or adj or vb*

Inflected Forms

The inflected forms recorded in this dictionary include the plurals of nouns; the past tense, the past participle when it differs from the past tense, and the present participle of verbs; and the comparative and superlative forms of adjectives and adverbs. When these inflected forms are created in a manner considered regular in English (as by adding -*s* or -*es* to nouns, -*ed* and -*ing* to verbs, and -*er* and -*est* to adjectives and adverbs) and when it seems that there is nothing about the formation to give the dictionary user doubts, the inflected form is not shown in order to save space for information more likely to be sought.

If the inflected form is created in an irregular way or if the dictionary user is likely to have doubts about it (even if it is formed regularly), the inflected form is shown in boldface either in full or, especially when the word has three or more syllables, cut back to a convenient and easily recognizable point.

The inflected forms of nouns, verbs, adjectives, and adverbs are shown in this dictionary when suffixation brings about a change in final *y* to *i*, when the word ends in *-ey*, when there are variant inflected forms, and when the dictionary user might have doubts about the spelling of the inflected form:

> **scaly** . . . *adj* **scal·i·er; -est**
>
> ²**atrophy** . . . *vb* **-phied; -phy·ing**
>
> **kid·ney** . . . *n, pl* **kid·neys**
>
> **sar·co·ma** . . . *n, pl* **-mas** *also* **-ma·ta**
>
> ¹**burn** . . . *vb* **burned** . . . *or* **burnt** . . . **burn·ing**
>
> **sta·tus** . . . *n, pl* **sta·tus·es**

A plural is also shown for a noun when it ends in a consonant plus *o* or in a double *oo*, and when its plural is identical with the singular. Many nouns in medical English have highly irregular plurals modeled after their language of origin. Sometimes more than one element of a compound term is pluralized:

> **ego** . . . *n, pl* **egos**
>
> **HMO** . . . *n, pl* **HMOs**
>
> **tattoo** *n, pl* **tattoos**
>
> ¹**pu·bes** . . . *n, pl* **pubes**
>
> **en·ceph·a·li·tis** . . . *n, pl* **-lit·i·des**
>
> **cor pul·mo·na·le** . . . *n, pl* **cor·dia pul·mo·na·lia**

Nouns that are plural in form and that are regularly used with a plural verb are labeled *n pl*:

> **in·nards** . . . *n pl*

If nouns that are plural in form are regularly used with a singular verb, they are labeled *n* or if they are used with either a singular or plural verb, they are labeled *n sing or pl*:

> **rick·ets** . . . *n*
>
> **blind stag·gers** . . . *n sing or pl*

The inflected forms of verbs, adjectives, and adverbs are also shown whenever suffixation brings about a doubling of a final consonant, elision of a final *e*, or a radical change in the base word itself. The principal parts of a verb are shown when a final *-c* changes to *-ck* in suffixation:

re·fer . . . *vb* re·ferred; re·fer·ring

hot . . . *adj* hot·ter; hot·test

op·er·ate . . . *vb* -at·ed; -at·ing

sane . . . *adj* san·er; san·est

¹break . . . *vb* broke . . . bro·ken . . . break·ing

¹ill . . . *adj* worse . . . worst

²physic *vb* phys·icked; phys·ick·ing

Inflected forms are not shown at undefined run-ons.

Capitalization

Most entries in this dictionary begin with a lowercase letter, indicating that the word is not ordinarily capitalized. A few entries have an italic label *often cap*, indicating that the word is as likely to begin with a capital letter as not and is equally acceptable either way. Some entries begin with an uppercase letter, which indicates that the word is usually capitalized.

pan·cre·as . . . *n*

braille . . . *n, often cap*

Gol·gi . . . *adj*

The capitalization of entries that are open or hyphenated compounds is similarly indicated by the form of the entry or by an italic label:

heart attack *n*

¹neo–Freud·ian . . . *adj, often cap N*

Agent Orange . . . *n*

Many acronyms are written entirely or partly in capitals, and this fact is shown by the form of the entry or by an italic label:

DNA . . . *n*

cgs *adj, often cap C&G&S*

A word that is capitalized in some senses and lowercase in others shows variations from the form of the main entry by the use of italic labels at the appropriate senses:

strep·to·coc·cus . . . *n* **1** *cap*

pill . . . *n* . . . **2** *often cap*

Attributive Nouns

The italicized label *often attrib* placed after the functional label *n* indicates that the noun is often used as an adjective equivalent in attributive position before another noun:

> **blood** . . . *n, often attrib*
>
> **hos·pi·tal** . . . *n, often attrib*

Examples of the attributive use of these nouns are *blood clot* and *hospital ward*.

While any noun may occasionally be used in attribution, the label *often attrib* is limited to those having broad attributive use. This label is not used when an adjective homograph (as *serum*) is entered. And it is not used at open compounds that are used in attribution with an inserted hyphen.

Etymology

Etymologies showing the origin of particular words are given in this dictionary only for some abbreviations and for all eponyms.

If any entry for an abbreviation is followed by the expansion from which it is derived, no etymology is given. However, if the abbreviation is derived from a phrase in a foreign language or in English that is not mentioned elsewhere in the entry, that phrase and its language of origin (if other than English) are given in square brackets following the functional label:

> **IFN** *abbr* interferon
>
> **bid** *abbr* [Latin *bis in die*] twice a day

Words derived from the names of persons are called eponyms. Eponymous entries in this dictionary that are derived from the names of one or more real persons are followed by the last name, personal name, birth and death dates where known, nationality, and occupation or status of the person (or persons) from whose name the term is derived:

> **pas·teu·rel·la** . . . *n* . . .
>
> **Pas·teur** . . . , **Louis (1822–1895),** French chemist and bacteriologist.

Doubtful dates are followed by a question mark, and approximate dates are preceded by *ca* (circa). In some instances only the years of principal activity are given, preceded by the abbreviation *fl* (flourished):

> **sap·phic** . . . *adj or n*
>
> **Sap·pho** . . . (*fl ca* 610 BC–*ca* 580 BC), Greek lyric poet.

If a series of main entries is derived from the name of one person, the data usually follow the first entry. The dictionary user who turns, for example, to *pasteurellosis, pasteurization,* or *Pasteur treatment* and seeks biographical information is expected to glance back to the first entry in the sequence, *pasteurella*.

If an eponymous entry is defined by a synonymous cross-reference to the entry where the biographical data appear, no other cross-reference is made. However, if the definition of an eponymous entry contains no clue as to the location of the data, the name of the individual is given following the entry and a directional cross-reference is made to the appropriate entry:

> **gland of Bartholin** *n* : BARTHOLIN'S GLAND
>
> **gland of Bow·man** . . . *n* : any of the tubular and often branched glands occurring beneath the olfactory epithelium of the nose . . .
> **W. Bowman** — see BOWMAN'S CAPSULE

The data for C. T. Bartholin can be found at *Bartholin's gland* and that for William Bowman at *Bowman's capsule*.

Usage

Usage Labels

Status labels are used in this dictionary to signal that a word or a sense of a word is restricted in usage.

A word or sense limited in use to a specific region of the English-speaking world has an appropriate label. The adverb *chiefly* precedes a label when the word has some currency outside the specified region, and a double label is used to indicate currency in each of two specific regions:

> **red bug** . . . *n, Southern & Midland*
>
> **ap·pen·di·cec·to·my** . . . *n* . . . *Brit*
>
> **fru·se·mide** . . . *n, chiefly Brit*

The stylistic label *slang* is used with words or senses that are especially appropriate in contexts of extreme informality, that usually have a currency not limited to a particular region or area of interest, and that are composed typically of shortened forms or extravagant or facetious figures of speech. Words with the label *slang* are entered if they have been or in the opinion of the editors are likely to be encountered in communicating with patients especially in emergencies. A few words from the huge informal argot of medicine are entered with the label *med slang* because they have appeared in general context or have been the subject of discussion in medical journals:

> **ben·ny** . . . *n* . . . *slang*
>
> **go·mer** . . . *n, med slang*

Subject orientation is generally given in the definition; however, a guide phrase is sometimes used to indicate a specific application of a word or sense:

> **¹drug** . . . *n* **1** . . . **b** *according to the Food, Drug, and Cosmetic Act*
>
> **erupt** . . . *vb* **1** *of a tooth*

Illustrations of Usage

Definitions are sometimes followed by verbal illustrations that show a typical use of the word in context. These illustrations are enclosed in angle brackets, and the word being illustrated is usually replaced by a lightface swung dash. The swung dash stands for the boldface entry word, and it may be followed by an italicized suffix:

> **ab·er·rant** . . . *adj* . . . **2** . . . ⟨∼ salivary tissue⟩
>
> **treat** . . . *vb* . . . ⟨∼*ed* their diseases⟩ ⟨∼*s* a patient⟩

The swung dash is not used when the form of the boldface entry word is changed in suffixation, and it is not used for open compounds:

> **ab·nor·mal·i·ty** . . . *n* . . . **2** . . . ⟨brain-wave *abnormalities*⟩
>
> **work up** . . . *vb* . . . ⟨*work up* a patient⟩

Usage Notes

Definitions are sometimes followed by usage notes that give supplementary information about such matters as idiom, syntax, semantic relationship, and status. For trademarks and service marks, a usage note is used in place of a definition. A usage note is introduced by a lightface dash:

> **pill** . . . *n* . . . **2** . . . : . . . — usu. used with *the*
>
> **bug** . . . *n* **1 a** : . . . — not used technically
>
> **hs** *abbr* . . . — used esp. in writing prescriptions
>
> **pec** . . . *n* . . . — usu. used in pl.
>
> **Val·ium** . . . *trademark* — used for a preparation of diazepam

Sometimes a usage note calls attention to one or more terms that mean the same thing as the main entry:

> **lep·ro·sy** . . . *n* . . . : a chronic disease caused by infection with an acid-fast bacillus of the genus *Mycobacterium* (*M. leprae*) . . . — called also *Hansen's disease, lepra*

The called-also terms are shown in italic type. If the called-also term falls alphabetically at some distance from the principal entry, the called-also term is entered in alphabetical sequence with the

sole definition being a synonymous cross-reference to the entry where
it appears in the usage note:

> **Hansen's disease** *n* : LEPROSY
>
> **lep·ra** . . . *n* : LEPROSY

Two or more usage notes are separated by a semicolon.

> **can·tha·ris** . . . *n* . . . **2 cantharides** . . . : a preparation of dried
> beetles . . . — used with a sing. or pl. verb; called also *Spanish
> fly*

Sense Division

A boldface colon is used in this dictionary to introduce a definition:

> **pul·mo·nary** . . . *adj* : relating to, functioning like, associated with,
> or carried on by the lungs

It is also used to separate two or more definitions of a single sense:

> **quack** . . . . *n* : a pretender to medical skill : an ignorant or dishonest
> practitioner

Boldface Arabic numerals separate the senses of a word that has
more than one sense:

> **nerve** . . . *n* **1** : any of the filamentous bands of nervous tissue that
> connect parts of the nervous system with other organs . . . **2** *pl*
> : a state or condition of nervous agitation or irritability **3** : the
> sensitive pulp of a tooth

Boldface lowercase letters separate the subsenses of a word:

> **¹dose** . . . *n* **1 a** : the measured quantity of a therapeutic agent to
> be taken at one time **b** : the quantity of radiation administered
> or absorbed **2** : a gonorrheal infection

Lightface numerals in parentheses indicate a further division of
subsenses:

> **ra·di·a·tion** . . . *n* . . . **2 a** : . . . **b** (1) : the process of emitting radiant
> energy . . . (2) : the combined processes of emission, transmission,
> and absorption of radiant energy

A lightface colon following a definition and immediately preceding
two or more subsenses indicates that the subsenses are subsumed by
the preceding definition:

> **mac·u·la** . . . *n* . . . **2** : an anatomical structure having the form of
> a spot differentiated from surrounding tissue: as **a** : MACULA ACUSTICA
> **b** : MACULA LUTEA

> **extensor ret·i·nac·u·lum** . . . *n* **1** : either of two fibrous bands of fascia crossing the front of the ankle: **a** : a lower band . . . **b** : an upper band . . .

The word *as* may or may not follow the lightface colon. Its presence (as at *macula*) indicates that the following subsenses are typical or significant examples. Its absence (as at *extensor retinaculum*) indicates that the subsenses which follow are exhaustive.

Sometimes a particular semantic relationship between senses is suggested by the use of one of four italic sense dividers: *esp, specif, also,* or *broadly.* The sense divider *esp* (for *especially*) is used to introduce the most common meaning subsumed in the more general preceding definition. The sense divider *specif* (for *specifically*) is used to introduce a common but highly restricted meaning subsumed in the more general preceding definition. The sense divider *also* is used to introduce a meaning that is closely related to but may be considered less important than the preceding sense. The sense divider *broadly* is used to introduce an extended or wider meaning of the preceding definition.

The order of senses within an entry is historical: the sense known to have been first used in English is entered first. This is not to be taken to mean, however, that each sense of a multisense word developed from the immediately preceding sense. It is altogether possible that sense 1 of a word has given rise to sense 2 and sense 2 to sense 3, but frequently sense 2 and sense 3 may have arisen independently of one another from sense 1.

Information coming between the entry word and the first definition of a multisense word applies to all senses and subsenses. Information applicable only to some senses or subsenses is given between the appropriate boldface numeral or letter and the symbolic colon.

> **bur** . . . *n* **1** *usu* **burr**
>
> **chla·myd·ia** . . . *n* **1** *cap* . . . **2** *pl* **-iae** *also* **-ias**

Names of Plants & Animals

The entries in this dictionary that define the names of plants and animals include common or vernacular names (as *mosquito* and *poison ivy*) and names of genera (as *Ctenocephalides* and *Rhus*) from the formal, codified, New Latin vocabulary of biological systematics. The vocabulary of biological nomenclature has been developed and used in accordance with international codes for the purpose of identifying and indicating the relationships of plants and animals. Organisms are classified into a hierarchy of groups — taxa — with each kind of organism having one — and only one — correct name and belonging to one — and only one — taxon at each level of classification in the hierarchy.

The fundamental taxon is the genus, which includes a group of closely related species of organisms and of which the name is a capitalized singular noun:

Cteno·ce·phal·i·des . . . *n* : a genus of fleas (family Pulicidae) including the dog flea (*C. canis*) and cat flea (*C. felis*)

rhus . . . *n* 1 *cap* : a genus of shrubs and trees of the cashew family (Anacardiaceae) that . . . include some (as poison ivy, poison oak, and poison sumac) producing irritating oils that cause dermatitis

Names of taxa higher than the genus (as family, order, class, and phylum) are not given main-entry status in this dictionary but may be used in parentheses within definitions (as the family names *Pulicidae* and *Anacardiaceae* at *Ctenocephalides* and *Rhus*, above).

The unique name of each kind of organism or species — the binomial or species name — consists of a singular capitalized genus name combined with an uncapitalized specific epithet. The name for a variety or subspecies — the trinomial, variety name, or subspecies name — adds a similar varietal or subspecific epithet. The head louse (*Pediculus humanus capitis*) is a subspecies of the species (*Pediculus humanus*) to which the body louse belongs.

If the name of a genus from biological nomenclature is used outside of parentheses as part of a definition, it appears in this dictionary as a vocabulary entry at its own place. If such a name is used inside parentheses in a definition, it may or may not appear as an entry. No binomial, specific, subspecific, or varietal name appears as a vocabulary entry (although common names derived from such names may be entered). In contrast, every common or vernacular name which is used in a definition whether inside or outside of parentheses is entered in this dictionary or in its companion volume, The Merriam-Webster Dictionary.

Many common names are derived directly from the names of taxa and especially genera with little or no modification. The genus name (as *Chlamydia* or *Giardia*) is capitalized and italicized but never takes a plural. In contrast the common name (as chlamydia or giardia) is not usually capitalized or italicized but does take a plural (as chlamydiae or giardias). In many cases both the systematic taxonomic name and the common name derived from it are entered in this dictionary.

chla·myd·ia . . . *n* 1 *cap* : a genus of coccoid to spherical gram≠ negative intracellular bacteria (family Chlamydiaceae) . . . 2 *pl* -iae *also* -ias a : a bacterium of the genus *Chlamydia*

giar·dia . . . *n* 1 *cap* : a genus of flagellate protozoans inhabiting the intestines of various mammals and including one (*G. lamblia*) that is associated with diarrhea in humans 2 : any flagellate of the genus *Giardia*

The entries defining the names of plants and animals are usually oriented to a taxon higher in the systematic hierarchy by a systematic name of higher rank (as *Chlamydiaceae* at *Chlamydia*), by a common name (as *mosquito* at *Anopheles* or *carrot family* at *hemlock*), or by a technical adjective (as *digenetic* at *fluke* or *dipteran* at *mosquito*) so that the systematic name of a higher, more inclusive taxon can usually be found by consulting another entry if it is not explicitly mentioned at the entry itself.

A genus name may be abbreviated to its initial letter when it is used as part of a binomial or trinomial name in the definition of the genus itself or when it is listed more than once in senses not separated by a boldface number.

A capitalized entry for a systematic taxonomic name of the form **X** *n, syn of* Y means that *X* has the same taxonomic rank and meaning as *Y* but that it is technically inferior to and less valid than *Y*. In a few cases a widely used synonym may be added after the currently recognized systematic name in some definitions:

> **Piro•plas•ma** . . . *n, syn of* BABESIA

> **plague** . . . *n* . . . **2** : a virulent contagious febrile disease that is caused by a bacterium of the genus *Yersinia* (*Y. pestis* syn. *Pasteurella pestis*)

Cross-Reference

Four different kinds of cross-references are used in this dictionary: directional, synonymous, cognate, and inflectional. In each instance the cross-reference is readily recognized by the lightface small capitals in which it is printed.

A cross-reference usually following a lightface dash and beginning with *see* or *compare* is a directional cross-reference. It directs the dictionary user to look elsewhere for further information. A *compare* cross-reference is regularly appended to a definition; a *see* cross-reference may stand alone:

> **can•cer** . . . *n* **1** . . . — compare CARCINOMA. SARCOMA: NEOPLASM. TUMOR

> **iron** . . . *n* **1** . . . — symbol *Fe;* see ELEMENT table

> **mammary artery** — see INTERNAL THORACIC ARTERY

A *see* cross-reference may be used to indicate the place of definition of an entry containing one or more Arabic numerals or abbreviated chemical prefixes that might cause doubt. Examples of chemical names are given above at "Order of Main Entries." The entry below follows the entry for the abbreviation *GP:*

> **G₁ phase, G₂ phase** — see entries alphabetized as G ONE PHASE. G TWO PHASE

A *see* cross-reference may follow a main entry that consists of a single word which does not stand alone but appears only in a compound term or terms; the *see* cross-reference at such entries indicates the compound term or terms in which the single word appears:

> **herpetiformis** — see DERMATITIS HERPETIFORMIS

> **dorsi** — see ILIOCOSTALIS DORSI. LATISSIMUS DORSI. LONGISSIMUS DORSI

A *see* cross-reference may appear after the definition of the name of a generic drug to refer the reader to a trademark used for a preparation of the drug:

di·az·e·pam . . . *n* . . . — see VALIUM

A cross-reference immediately following a boldface colon is a synonymous cross-reference. It may stand alone as the only definitional matter, it may follow an analytical definition, or it may be one of two synonymous cross-references separated by a comma:

serum hepatitis *n* : HEPATITIS b

liv·id . . . *adj* : discolored by bruising : BLACK-AND-BLUE

af·fec·tion . . . *n* . . . 2 . . . b : DISEASE, MALADY

A synonymous cross-reference indicates that a definition at the entry cross-referred to can be substituted as a definition for the entry or the sense or subsense in which the cross-reference appears.

A cross-reference following an italic *var of* is a cognate cross-reference:

pro·cary·ote *var of* PROKARYOTE

manoeuvre *Brit var of* MANEUVER

A cross-reference following an italic label that identifies an entry as an inflected form is an inflectional cross-reference. Inflectional cross-references appear only when the inflected form falls alphabetically at some distance from the main entry.

corpora *pl of* CORPUS

broke *past of* BREAK

When guidance seems needed as to which one of several homographs or which sense of a multisense word is being referred to, a superscript numeral may precede the cross-reference or a sense number may follow it or both:

ossa *pl of* [1]OS

lateral cuneiform bone *n* : CUNEIFORM BONE 1c

Combining Forms, Prefixes & Suffixes

An entry that begins or ends with a hyphen is a word element that forms part of an English compound:

pharmaco- *comb form* . . . ⟨*pharmaco*logy⟩

dys- *prefix* . . . ⟨*dys*plasia⟩

-i·a·sis *n suffix, pl* **-i·a·ses** . . . ⟨ancylostom*iasis*⟩

Combining forms, prefixes, and suffixes are entered in this dictionary for two reasons: to make understandable the meaning of many undefined run-ons and to make recognizable the meaningful elements of words that are not entered in the dictionary.

Abbreviations & Symbols

Abbreviations and symbols for chemical elements are included as main entries in the vocabulary:

RQ *abbr* respiratory quotient

Al *symbol* aluminum

Abbreviations are entered without periods and have been normalized to one form of capitalization. In practice, however, there is considerable variation, and stylings other than those given in this dictionary are often acceptable.

The more common abbreviations and the symbols of chemical elements also appear after the definition at the entries for the terms they represent:

respiratory quotient *n* : . . . abbr. *RQ*

Symbols that are not capable of being alphabetized are included in a separate section in the back of this book headed "Signs and Symbols."

Abbreviations Used in This Work

abbr	abbreviation	*n pl*	noun plural
adj	adjective	*occas*	occasionally
adv	adverb	*orig*	originally
attrib	attributive	*part*	participle
b	born	*pl*	plural
B.C.	before Christ	*pres*	present
Brit	British	*prob*	probably
C	Celsius	*sing*	singular
ca	circa	*So*	South
Canad	Canadian	*SoAfr*	South African
cap	capitalized	*specif*	specifically
comb	combining	*spp*	species (*pl*)
d	died	*syn*	synonym
esp	especially	*U.S.*	United States
F	Fahrenheit	*usu*	usually
fl	flourished	*var*	variant
n	noun	*vb*	verb
No	North		

PRONUNCIATION SYMBOLS

ə .... **a**but, c**o**llect, s**u**ppose

'ə, ˌə hum**dru**m

ᵊ .... (in ᵊl, ᵊn) batt**le**, cott**on**; (in lᵊ, mᵊ, rᵊ) French ta**ble**, pris**me**, tit**re**

ər ... op**er**ation, furth**er**

a .... m**a**p, p**a**tch

ā .... d**ay**, f**a**te

ä .... b**o**ther, c**o**t, f**a**ther

ȧ .... a sound between \a\ and \ä\, as in an Eastern New England pronunciation of **au**nt, **a**sk

au̇ ... n**ow**, **ou**t

b .... **b**a**b**y, ri**b**

ch ... **ch**in, cat**ch**

d .... **d**i**d**, a**dd**er

e .... s**e**t, r**e**d

ē .... b**ea**t, **ea**sy

f .... **f**i**f**ty, cu**ff**

g .... **g**o, bi**g**

h .... **h**at, a**h**ead

hw ... **wh**ale

i .... t**i**p, ban**i**sh

ī .... s**i**te, b**uy**

j ... **j**ob, e**dge**

k .... **k**in, coo**k**

k̲ .... German Ba**ch**, Scots lo**ch**

l .... **l**i**l**y, coo**l**

m ... **m**ur**m**ur, di**m**

n .... **n**i**n**e, ow**n**

ⁿ .... indicates that a preceding vowel is pronounced through both nose and mouth, as in French bon \bōⁿ\

ŋ .... si**ng**, si**ng**er, fi**ng**er, i**nk**

ō .... b**o**ne, holl**ow**

ȯ .... s**aw**

œ ... French b**œu**f, German H**ö**lle

œ̄ ... French f**eu**, German H**öh**le

ȯi ... t**oy**

p .... **p**e**pp**er, li**p**

r .... **r**a**r**ity

s .... **s**ource, le**ss**

sh ... **sh**y, mi**ss**ion

t .... **t**ie, a**tt**ack

th ... **th**in, e**th**er

th̲ ... **th**en, ei**th**er

ü .... b**oo**t, few \'fyü\

u̇ .... p**u**t, pure \'pyu̇r\

ue ... German f**ü**llen

ūe ... French r**u**e, German f**üh**len

v .... **v**i**v**id, gi**v**e

w ... **w**e, a**w**ay

y .... **y**ard, cue \'kyü\

ʸ .... indicates that a preceding \l\, \n\, or \w\ is modified by having the tongue approximate the position for \y\, as in French digne \dēnʸ\

z .... **z**one, rai**s**e

zh ... vi**s**ion, plea**s**ure

\ .... slant line used in pairs to mark the beginning and end of a transcription: \'pen\

' .... mark at the beginning of a syllable that has primary (strongest) stress: \'shə-fəl-ˌbōrd\

ˌ .... mark at the beginning of a syllable that has secondary (next-strongest) stress: \'shə-fəl-ˌbōrd\

- .... mark of a syllable division in pronunciations (the mark of end-of-line division in boldface entries is a centered dot ·)

() ... indicate that what is symbolized between sometimes occurs and sometimes does not occur in the pronunciation of the word: **bakery** \'bā-k(ə-)rē\ = \'bā-kə-rē, 'bā-krē\

A

A *abbr* **1** adenine **2** ampere

Å *symbol* angstrom unit

a- *or* **an-** *prefix* : not : without ⟨*asexual*⟩ — *a-* before consonants other than *h* and sometimes even before *h*, *an-* before vowels and usu. before *h* ⟨*achromatic*⟩ ⟨*anhydrous*⟩

aa *also* **aa** *abbr* [Latin *ana*] of each — used at the end of a list of two or more substances in a prescription to indicate that equal quantities of each are to be taken

AA *abbr* Alcoholics Anonymous

ab \'ab\ *n* : an abdominal muscle — usu. used in pl.

ab- *prefix* : from : away : off ⟨*aboral*⟩

abac·te·ri·al \ˌā-(ˌ)bak-'tir-ē-əl\ *adj* : not caused by or characterized by the presence of bacteria ⟨~ prostatitis⟩

A band *n* : one of the cross striations in striated muscle that contains myosin filaments and appears dark under the light microscope and light in polarized light

aba·sia \ə-'bā-zhə, -zhē-ə\ *n* : inability to walk caused by a defect in muscular coordination — compare ASTASIA

Ab·be–Est·lan·der operation \'a-bē-'äst-ˌlän-dər-, -'est-ˌlan-\ *n* : the grafting of a flap of tissue from one lip of the oral cavity to the other lip to correct a defect using a pedicle with an arterial supply

> **Abbe, Robert (1851–1928),** American surgeon.
> **Estlander, Jakob August (1831–1881),** Finnish surgeon.

abdom *abbr* abdomen; abdominal

ab·do·men \'ab-də-mən, (ˌ)ab-'dō-\ *n* **1 a** : the part of the body between the thorax and the pelvis — called also *belly* **b** : the cavity of this part of the trunk lined by the peritoneum, enclosed by the body walls, the diaphragm, and the pelvic floor, and containing the visceral organs (as the stomach, intestines, and liver) **c** : the portion of this cavity between the diaphragm and the brim of the pelvis — compare PELVIC CAVITY 2 **2** : the posterior often elongated region of the body behind the thorax in arthropods — **ab·dom·i·nal** \ab-'dä-mən-ᵊl\ *adj* — **ab·dom·i·nal·ly** *adv*

abdomin- *or* **abdomino-** *comb form* **1** : abdomen ⟨*abdomino*plasty⟩ **2** : abdominal and ⟨*abdomino*perineal⟩

abdominal aorta *n* : the portion of the aorta between the diaphragm and the bifurcation into the right and left common iliac arteries

abdominal cavity *n* : ABDOMEN 1b

abdominal reflex *n* : contraction of the muscles of the abdominal wall in response to stimulation of the overlying skin

abdominal region *n* : any of the nine areas into which the abdomen is divided by four imaginary planes of which two are vertical passing through the middle of the inguinal ligament on each side and two are horizontal passing respectively through the junction of the ninth rib and costal cartilage and through the top of the iliac crest — see EPIGASTRIC 2b, HYPOCHONDRIAC 2b, HYPOGASTRIC 1, ILIAC 2, LUMBAR 2, UMBILICAL 2

abdominis — see OBLIQUUS EXTERNUS ABDOMINIS, OBLIQUUS INTERNUS ABDOMINIS, RECTUS ABDOMINIS, TRANSVERSUS ABDOMINIS

ab·dom·i·no·pel·vic \(ˌ)ab-ˌdä-mə-nō-'pel-vik\ *adj* : relating to or being the abdominal and pelvic cavities of the body

ab·dom·i·no·per·i·ne·al \-ˌper-ə-'nē-əl\ *adj* : relating to the abdominal and perineal regions

abdominoperineal resection *n* : resection of a part of the lower bowel together with adjacent lymph nodes through abdominal and perineal incisions

ab·dom·i·no·plas·ty \ab-'dä-mə-nō-ˌplas-tē\ *n, pl* **-ties** : cosmetic surgery of the abdomen (as for removing wrinkles and tightening the skin over the stomach)

ab·du·cens nerve \ab-'dü-ˌsenz-, -'dyü-\ *n* : either of the 6th pair of cranial nerves which are motor nerves, arise beneath the floor of the fourth ventricle, and supply the lateral rectus muscle of each eye — called also *abdu ens, sixth cranial nerve*

ab·du·cent nerve \-sənt-\ *n* : ABDUCENS NERVE

ab·duct \ab-'dəkt *also* 'ab-ˌ\ *vb* : to draw or spread away (as a limb or the fingers) from a position near or parallel to the median axis of the body or from the axis of a limb — **ab·duc·tion** \ab-'dək-shən\ *n*

ab·duc·tor \ab-'dək-tər\ *n, pl* **ab·duc·to·res** \ˌab-ˌdək-'tōr-(ˌ)ēz\ *or* **abductors** : a muscle that draws a part away from the median line of the body or from the axis of an extremity

abductor di·gi·ti min·i·mi \-'di-jə-(ˌ)tē-'mi-nə-(ˌ)mē\ *n* **1** : a muscle of the hand that abducts the little finger and flexes the phalanx nearest the hand **2** : a muscle of the foot that abducts the little toe

abductor hal·lu·cis \-'hal-yə-səs; -'ha-lə-səs, -kəs\ *n* : a muscle of the foot that abducts the big toe

abductor pol·li·cis brev·is \-'pä-lə-səs-'bre-vəs, -lə-kəs\ *n* : a thin flat muscle of the hand that abducts the thumb at right angles to the plane of the palm

abductor pollicis lon·gus \-ˈlȯŋ-gəs\ *n* : a muscle of the forearm that abducts the thumb and wrist

ab·er·rant \a-ˈber-ənt; ˈa-bə-rənt, -₁ber-ənt\ *adj* **1** : straying from the right or normal way (∼ behavior) **2** : deviating from the usual or natural type : ATYPICAL (∼ salivary tissue)

ab·er·ra·tion \₁a-bə-ˈrā-shən\ *n* **1** : failure of a mirror, refracting surface, or lens to produce exact point-to-point correspondence between an object and its image **2** : unsoundness or disorder of the mind **3** : an aberrant organ or individual — **ab·er·ra·tion·al** \-sh(ə-)nəl\ *adj*

abey·ance \ə-ˈbā-əns\ *n* : temporary inactivity or suspension (as of function or a symptom)

ab·i·ence \ˈa-bē-əns\ *n* : a tendency to withdraw from a stimulus object or situation — compare ADIENCE — **abi·ent** \-ənt\ *adj*

abi·ot·ro·phy \₁ā-(₁)bī-ˈä-trə-fē\ *n, pl* **-phies** : degeneration or loss of function or vitality in an organism or in cells or tissues not due to any apparent injury

ab·late \a-ˈblāt\ *vb* **ab·lat·ed; ab·lat·ing** : to remove esp. by cutting

ab·la·tion \a-ˈblā-shən\ *n* : the process of ablating; *esp* : surgical removal

ab·la·tio pla·cen·tae \a-ˈblā-shē-ō-plə-ˈsen-(₁)tē\ *n* : ABRUPTIO PLACENTAE

¹ab·nor·mal \(₁)ab-ˈnȯr-məl\ *adj* : deviating from the normal or average; *esp* : departing from the usual or accepted standards of social behavior — **ab·nor·mal·ly** *adv*

²abnormal *n* : an abnormal person

ab·nor·mal·i·ty \₁ab-nȯr-ˈma-lə-tē\ *n, pl* **-ties 1** : the quality or state of being abnormal **2** : something abnormal (brain-wave abnormalities)

abnormal psychology *n* : a branch of psychology concerned with mental and emotional disorders (as neuroses and psychoses) and with certain incompletely understood normal phenomena (as dreams)

ABO blood group \₁ā-(₁)bē-ˈō-\ *n* : one of the four blood groups A, B, AB, or O comprising the ABO system

ab·oma·sum \₁a-bō-ˈmā-səm\ *n, pl* **-sa** \-sə\ : the fourth compartment of the ruminant stomach that follows the omasum and has a true digestive function — compare RUMEN, RETICULUM — **ab·oma·sal** \-səl\ *adj*

ab·oral \(₁)a-ˈbȯr-əl, -ˈbȯr-\ *adj* : situated opposite to or away from the mouth

abort \ə-ˈbȯrt\ *vb* **1** : to cause or undergo abortion **2** : to stop in the early stages (∼ a disease) — **abort·er** *n*

¹abor·ti·fa·cient \ə-₁bȯr-tə-ˈfā-shənt\ *adj* : inducing abortion

²abortifacient *n* : an agent (as a drug) that induces abortion

abor·tion \ə-ˈbȯr-shən\ *n* **1** : the termination of a pregnancy after, accompanied by, resulting in, or closely followed by the death of the embryo or fetus: **a** : spontaneous expulsion of a human fetus during the first 12 weeks of gestation — compare MISCARRIAGE **b** : induced expulsion of a human fetus **c** : expulsion of a fetus by a domestic animal often due to infection at any time before completion of pregnancy — see CONTAGIOUS ABORTION **2** : arrest of development of an organ so that it remains imperfect or is absorbed **3** : the arrest of a disease in its earliest stage

abor·tion·ist \-sh(ə-)nist\ *n* : one who induces abortion

abor·tive \ə-ˈbȯr-tiv\ *adj* **1** : imperfectly formed or developed : RUDIMENTARY **2 a** : ABORTIFACIENT **b** : cutting short (∼ treatment of pneumonia) **c** : failing to develop completely or typically

abor·tus \ə-ˈbȯr-təs\ *n* : an aborted fetus; *specif* : a human fetus less than 12 weeks old or weighing at birth less than 17 ounces

ABO system \₁ā-(₁)bē-ˈō-\ *n* : the basic system of antigens of human blood behaving in heredity as an allelic unit to produce any of the ABO blood groups

abou·lia *var of* ABULIA

abrade \ə-ˈbrād\ *vb* **abrad·ed; abrad·ing** : to irritate or roughen by rubbing : CHAFE

abra·sion \ə-ˈbrā-zhən\ *n* **1** : wearing, grinding, or rubbing away by friction **2 a** : the rubbing or scraping of the surface layer of cells or tissue from an area of the skin or mucous membrane; *also* : a place so abraded **b** : the mechanical wearing away of the tooth surfaces by chewing

¹abra·sive \ə-ˈbrā-siv, -ziv\ *adj* : tending to abrade — **abra·sive·ness** *n*

²abrasive *n* : a substance used for abrading, smoothing, or polishing

ab·re·ac·tion \₁a-brē-ˈak-shən\ *n* : the expression and emotional discharge of unconscious material (as a repressed idea or emotion) by verbalization esp. in the presence of a therapist — compare CATHARSIS 2 — **ab·re·act** \-ˈakt\ *vb* — **ab·re·ac·tive** \-ˈak-tiv\ *adj*

ab·rup·tio pla·cen·tae \ə-ˈbrəp-shē-ō-plə-ˈsen-(₁)tē, -tē-₁ō-\ *n* : premature detachment of the placenta from the wall of the uterus — called also *ablatio placentae*

abs \ˈabz\ *pl of* AB

ab·scess \ˈab-₁ses\ *n, pl* **ab·scess·es** \ˈab-sə-₁sēz, -(₁)se-səz\ : a localized collection of pus surrounded by inflamed tissue — **ab·scessed** \-₁sest\ *adj*

ab·scis·sion \ab-ˈsi-zhən\ *n* : the act or process of cutting off : ABLATION

ab·sco·pal \ab-ˈskō-pəl\ *adj* : relating to or being an effect on a nonirradiated part of the body that results from radiation of another part

ab·sence \'ab-səns\ n : a transient loss or impairment of consciousness beginning and ending abruptly, unremembered afterward, and seen chiefly in mild types of epilepsy

ab·so·lute \ab-sə-'lüt\ adj : pure or relatively free from mixture

absolute alcohol n : ethyl alcohol that contains no more than one percent by weight of water — called also *dehydrated alcohol*

absolute humidity n : the amount of water vapor present in a unit volume of air — compare RELATIVE HUMIDITY

absolute refractory period n : the period immediately following the firing of a nerve fiber when it cannot be stimulated no matter how great a stimulus is applied — called also *absolute refractory phase*; compare RELATIVE REFRACTORY PERIOD

absolute temperature n : temperature measured on a scale based on absolute zero

absolute zero n : a theoretical temperature characterized by complete absence of heat and exactly equal to −273.15°C or −459.67°F

ab·sorb \ab-'sorb, -'zorb\ vb 1 : to take up esp. by capillary, osmotic, solvent, or chemical action 2 : to transform (radiant energy) into a different form usu. with a resulting rise in temperature — **ab·sorb·able** \ab-'sor-bə-bəl, -'zor-\ adj — **ab·sorb·er** n

ab·sor·bent also **ab·sor·bant** \-bənt\ adj : able to absorb — **ab·sor·ben·cy** \-bən-sē\ n — **absorbent** also **absorbant** n

absorbent cotton n : cotton made absorbent by chemically freeing it from its fatty matter

ab·sorp·tion \ab-'sorp-shən, -'zorp-\ n : the process of absorbing or of being absorbed — compare ADSORPTION — **ab·sorp·tive** \-tiv\ adj

ab·stain \ab-'stān\ vb : to refrain deliberately and often with an effort of self-denial from an action or practice — **ab·stain·er** n

ab·sti·nence \'ab-stə-nəns\ n 1 : voluntary forbearance esp. from indulgence of an appetite or craving or from eating some foods 2 : habitual abstaining from intoxicating beverages — **ab·sti·nent** \-nənt\ adj

ab·stract \'ab-ˌstrakt\ n : a pharmaceutical preparation made by mixing a powdered solid extract of a vegetable substance with lactose in such proportions that one part of the final product represents two parts of the original drug from which the extract was made — **ab·stract** \'ab-ˌstrakt, ab-'\ vb

abu·lia \ā-'bü-lē-ə, ə-, -'byü-\ n : abnormal lack of ability to act or to make decisions characteristic of certain psychotic and neurotic conditions — **abu·lic** \-lik\ adj

¹**abuse** \ə-'byüs\ n 1 : improper or excessive use or treatment ⟨drug ∼⟩ — see SUBSTANCE ABUSE 2 : physical maltreatment: as **a** : the act of violating sexually : RAPE **b** *under some statutes* : rape or indecent assault not amounting to rape

²**abuse** \ə-'byüz\ vb **abused; abus·ing 1** : to put to a wrong or improper use ⟨∼ drugs⟩ 2 : to treat so as to injure or damage ⟨∼ a child⟩ **3 a** : MASTURBATE **b** : to subject to abuse and esp. to rape or indecent assault — **abus·able** \-'byü-zə-bəl\ adj — **abus·er** n

abut·ment \ə-'bət-mənt\ n : a tooth to which a prosthetic appliance (as a denture) is attached for support

ac abbr **1** acute **2** [Latin *ante cibum*] before meals — used in writing prescriptions

Ac symbol actinium

aca·cia \ə-'kā-shə\ n : GUM ARABIC

acal·cu·lia \ā-kal-'kyü-lē-ə\ n : lack or loss of the ability to perform simple arithmetic tasks

acanth- or **acantho-** comb form : spine : prickle : projection ⟨acanthoma⟩ ⟨acanthocyte⟩

acan·tho·ceph·a·lan \ə-ˌkan-thə-'se-fə-lan\ n : any of a group of elongated parasitic intestinal worms with a hooked proboscis that as adults lack a digestive tract and absorb food through the body wall and that are usu. considered a separate phylum (Acanthocephala) related to the flatworms — **acanthocephalan** adj

acan·tho·cyte \ə-'kan-thə-ˌsīt\ n : an abnormal red blood cell characterized by variously shaped protoplasmic projections

acan·tho·ma \ˌa-(ˌ)kan-'thō-mə, ˌā-\ n, pl **-mas** \-məz\ or **-ma·ta** \-mə-tə\ : a neoplasm originating in the skin and developing through excessive growth of skin cells esp. of the stratum spinosum

acan·tho·sis \-'thō-səs\ n, pl **-tho·ses** \-ˌsēz\ : a benign overgrowth of the stratum spinosum of the skin — **acan·thot·ic** \-'thä-tik\ adj

acanthosis ni·gri·cans \-'ni-grə-ˌkanz, -'nī-\ n : a skin disease characterized by gray-black warty patches usu. situated in the axilla or groin or on elbows or knees and sometimes associated with cancer of abdominal viscera

acap·nia \ə-'kap-nē-ə, (ˌ)ā-\ n : a condition of carbon dioxide deficiency in blood and tissues

acar- or **acari-** or **acaro-** comb form : mite ⟨acariasis⟩ ⟨acaricide⟩

ac·a·ri·a·sis \ˌa-kə-'rī-ə-səs\ n, pl **-a·ses** \-ˌsēz\ : infestation with or disease caused by mites

acar·i·cide \ə-'kar-ə-ˌsīd\ n : a pesticide that kills mites and ticks — **acar·i·cid·al** \ə-ˌkar-ə-'sīd-ᵊl\ adj

ac·a·rid \'a-kə-rəd\ n : any of an order (Acarina) of arachnids comprising the mites and ticks of which many are parasites of plants, animals, or humans; *esp* : any of a family (Acaridae) of mites that feed on organic substances and are sometimes responsible for dermatitis in persons exposed to repeated contacts with infested products — compare GROCER'S ITCH — **acarid** *adj*

ac·a·rine \'a-kə-ˌrīn, -ˌrēn, -rən\ *adj* : of, relating to, or caused by mites or ticks (∼ dermatitis) — **acarine** *n*

ac·a·rus \'a-kə-rəs\ *n, pl* **-ri** \-ˌrī, -ˌrē\ : MITE; *esp* : one of a formerly extensive genus (*Acarus*)

ac·cel·er·ate \ik-'se-lə-ˌrāt, ak-\ *vb* **-at·ed; -at·ing** : to speed up; *also* : to undergo or cause to undergo acceleration

ac·cel·er·a·tion \ik-ˌse-lə-'rā-shən, ak-\ *n* **1** : the act or process of accelerating : the state of being accelerated **2** : change of velocity; *also* : the rate of this change **3** : advancement in mental growth or achievement beyond the average for one's age

acceleration of gravity *n* : the acceleration of a body in free fall under the influence of the earth's gravity that has a standard value of 980.665 centimeters per second per second — abbr. **g**

ac·cel·er·a·tor \ik-'se-lə-ˌrā-tər, ak-\ *n* : a muscle or nerve that speeds the performance of an action (a cardiac ∼)

accelerator globulin *n* : FACTOR V

accelerator nerve *n* : a nerve whose impulses increase the rate of the heart

ac·cel·er·om·e·ter \ik-ˌse-lə-'rä-mə-tər, ak-\ *n* : an instrument for measuring acceleration or for detecting and measuring vibrations

ac·cep·tor \ik-'sep-tər, ak-\ *n* : a compound, atom, or elementary particle capable of receiving another entity (as an atom, radical, or elementary particle) to form a compound — compare DONOR 2

ac·ces·so·ry \ik-'se-sə-rē, ak-, -'ses-rē\ *adj* **1** : aiding, contributing, or associated in a secondary way: as **a** : being or functioning as a vitamin **b** : associated in position or function with something (as an organ or lesion) usu. of more importance **2** : SUPERNUMERARY (∼ spleens)

accessory hemiazygos vein *n* : a vein that drains the upper left side of the thoracic wall, descends along the left side of the spinal column, and empties into the azygos or hemiazygos veins near the middle of the thorax

accessory nerve *n* : either of a pair of motor nerves that are the 11th cranial nerves, arise from the medulla and the upper part of the spinal cord, and supply chiefly the pharynx and muscles of the upper chest, back, and shoulders — called also *accessory, spinal accessory nerve*

accessory olivary nucleus *n* : any of

several small masses or layers of gray matter that are situated adjacent to the inferior olive and of which there are typically two on each side

accessory pancreatic duct *n* : a duct of the pancreas that branches from the chief pancreatic duct and opens into the duodenum above it — called also *duct of Santorini*

ac·ci·dent \'ak-sə-dənt, -ˌdent\ *n* **1** : an unfortunate event resulting from carelessness, unawareness, ignorance, or a combination of causes **2** : an unexpected and medically important bodily event esp. when injurious (a cerebral vascular ∼) **3** : an unexpected happening causing loss or injury which is not due to any fault or misconduct on the part of the person injured but for which legal relief may be sought — **ac·ci·den·tal** \ˌak-sə-'dent-ᵊl\ *adj* — **ac·ci·den·tal·ly** \-'dent-lē, -ᵊl-ē\ *also* **ac·ci·dent·ly** \-'dent-lē\ *adv*

accident–prone *adj* **1** : having a greater than average number of accidents **2** : having personality traits that predispose to accidents

ac·cli·mate \'a-klə-ˌmāt; ə-'klī-mət, -ˌmāt\ *vb* **-mat·ed; -mat·ing** : ACCLIMATIZE

ac·cli·ma·tion \ˌa-klə-'mā-shən, -ˌklī-\ *n* : acclimatization esp. by physiological adjustment of an organism to environmental change

ac·cli·ma·tize \ə-'klī-mə-ˌtīz\ *vb* **-tized; -tiz·ing** : to adapt to a new temperature, altitude, climate, environment, or situation — **ac·cli·ma·ti·za·tion** \ə-ˌklī-mə-tə-'zā-shən\ *n*

ac·com·mo·date \ə-'kä-mə-ˌdāt\ *vb* **-dat·ed; -dat·ing** : to adapt oneself; *also* : to undergo visual accommodation — **ac·com·mo·da·tive** \-ˌdā-tiv\ *adj*

ac·com·mo·da·tion \ə-ˌkä-mə-'dā-shən\ *n* : an adaptation or adjustment esp. of a bodily part (as an organ): as **a** : the automatic adjustment of the eye for seeing at different distances effected chiefly by changes in the convexity of the crystalline lens **b** : the range over which such adjustment is possible

ac·couche·ment \ˌa-küsh-'mäⁿ, ə-'küsh-\ *n* : the time or act of giving birth

ac·cou·cheur \ˌa-ˌkü-'shər\ *n* : one that assists at a birth; *esp* : OBSTETRICIAN

ac·cou·cheuse \ˌa-ˌkü-'shərz, -'shüz\ *n* : MIDWIFE

ac·cre·tio cor·dis \ə-'krē-shē-ō-'kór-dəs\ *n* : adhesive pericarditis in which there are adhesions extending from the pericardium to the mediastinum, diaphragm, and chest wall

ac·cre·tion \ə-'krē-shən\ *n* : the process of growth or enlargement; *esp* : increase by external addition or accumulation — compare APPOSITION 1 — **ac·cre·tion·ary** \-shə-ˌner-ē\ *adj*

accumbens — see NUCLEUS ACCUMBENS

Ac·cu·tane \'a-kyù-₁tān\ *trademark* — used for a preparation of isotretinoin

Ace \'ās\ *trademark* — used for a bandage with elastic properties

ACE inhibitor \'ās-, ₁ā-(₁)sē-'ē-\ *n* : any of a group of antihypertensive drugs (as captopril) that relax arteries and promote renal excretion of salt and water by inhibiting the activity of angiotensin converting enzyme

acel·lu·lar \(₁)ā-'sel-yə-lər\ *adj* **1** : containing no cells (~ vaccines) **2** : not divided into cells : consisting of a single complex cell — used esp. of protozoa and ciliates

acen·tric \(₁)ā-'sen-trik\ *adj* : lacking a centromere (~ chromosomes)

acetabular notch \-'näch\ *n* : a notch in the rim of the acetabulum through which blood vessels and nerves pass

ac·e·tab·u·lo·plas·ty \₁a-sə-'ta-byə-(₁)lō-₁plas-tē\ *n, pl* **-ties** : a plastic operation on the acetabulum intended to restore its normal state

ac·e·tab·u·lum \-'ta-byə-ləm\ *n, pl* **-lums** *or* **-la** \-lə\ : the cup-shaped socket in the hipbone — **ac·e·tab·u·lar** \-lər\ *adj*

ac·et·al·de·hyde \₁a-sə-'tal-də-₁hīd\ *n* : a colorless volatile water-soluble liquid aldehyde C_2H_4O used chiefly in organic synthesis that can cause irritation to mucous membranes

acet·amin·o·phen \ə-₁sē-tə-'mi-nə-fən, -₁set-, -'mē-, ₁a-sə-tə-\ *n* : a crystalline compound $C_8H_9NO_2$ used in medicine instead of aspirin to relieve pain and fever — called also *paracetamol;* see TYLENOL

ac·et·an·i·lide *or* **ac·et·an·i·lid** \₁a-sə-'tan-əl-₁id, -əd\ *n* : a white crystalline compound C_8H_9NO used to relieve pain or fever

ac·e·tate \'a-sə-₁tāt\ *n* : a salt or ester of acetic acid

ac·et·azol·amide \₁a-sə-tə-'zō-lə-₁mīd, -'zä-, -₁məd\ *n* : a diuretic drug $C_4H_6N_4O_3S_2$ used esp. in the treatment of edema associated with congestive heart failure and of glaucoma

ace·tic acid \ə-'sē-tik-\ *n* : a colorless pungent acid $C_2H_4O_2$ that is the chief acid of vinegar and is used occas. in medicine as an astringent and styptic

ace·to·ac·e·tate \₁a-sə-tō-'a-sə-₁tāt, ə-₁sē-tō-\ *n* : a salt or ester of acetoacetic acid

ace·to·ace·tic acid \₁a-sə-(₁)tō-ə-₁sē-tik-, ə-₁sē-tō-\ *n* : an unstable acid $C_4H_6O_3$ that is one of the ketone bodies found in abnormal amounts in the blood and urine in certain conditions of impaired metabolism (as in starvation and diabetes mellitus) — called also *diacetic acid*

ace·to·hex·amide \-'hek-sə-₁mīd, ə-₁sē-tō-, -₁mid\ *n* : a sulfonylurea drug $C_{15}H_{20}N_2O_4S$ used in the oral treatment of some of the milder

forms of diabetes in adults to lower the level of glucose in the blood

ace·to·me·roc·tol \₁a-sə-(₁)tō-mə-'räk-₁tol, ə-₁sē-tō-, -'tōl\ *n* : a white crystalline mercury derivative $C_{16}H_{24}$-HgO_3 of phenol used in solution as a topical antiseptic

ace·ton·ae·mia *chiefly Brit var of* ACETONEMIA

ac·e·tone \'a-sə-₁tōn\ *n* : a volatile fragrant flammable liquid ketone C_3H_6O found in abnormal quantities in diabetic urine

acetone body *n* : KETONE BODY

ace·ton·emia \₁a-sə-tō-'nē-mē-ə\ *n* : KETOSIS 2; *also* : KETONEMIA 1

acetonide — see FLUOCINOLONE ACETONIDE

ace·ton·uria \₁a-sə-tō-'nùr-ē-ə, -'nyùr-\ *n* : KETONURIA

ace·to·phe·net·i·din \₁a-sə-(₁)tō-fə-'net-ə-dən, ə-₁sē-tō-\ *n* : PHENACETIN

ace·tyl \ə-'sēt-əl, 'a-sət-; 'a-sə-₁tēl\ *n* : the radical CH_3CO of acetic acid

acet·y·lase \ə-'set-əl-₁ās\ *n* : any of a class of enzymes that accelerate the synthesis of esters of acetic acid

acet·y·late \ə-'set-əl-₁āt\ *vb* **-lat·ed; -lat·ing** : to introduce the acetyl radical into (a compound) — **acet·y·la·tion** \-₁set-əl-'ā-shən\ *n*

ace·tyl·cho·line \ə-₁set-əl-'kō-₁lēn, -₁sēt-; ₁a-sə-tēl-\ *n* : a neurotransmitter $C_7H_{17}NO_3$ released at autonomic synapses and neuromuscular junctions, active in the transmission of nerve impulse, and formed enzymatically in the tissues from choline

ace·tyl·cho·lin·es·ter·ase \-₁kō-lə-'nes-tə-₁rās, -₁rāz\ *n* : an enzyme that occurs esp. in some nerve endings and in the blood and promotes the hydrolysis of acetylcholine

acetyl CoA \-₁kō-'ā\ *n* : ACETYL COENZYME A

acetyl coenzyme A *n* : a compound $C_{25}H_{38}N_7O_{17}P_3S$ formed as an intermediate in metabolism and active as a coenzyme in biological acetylations

ace·tyl·cys·te·ine \ə-₁set-əl-'sis-tə-₁ēn, -₁set-; ₁a-sə-tēl-, ₁a-sət-əl-\ *n* : a mucolytic agent $C_5H_9NO_3S$ used esp. to reduce the viscosity of abnormally viscid respiratory tract secretions — see MUCOMYST

ace·tyl·phen·yl·hy·dra·zine \-₁fen-əl-'hī-drə-₁zēn, -₁fēn-\ *n* : a white crystalline compound $C_8H_{10}ON_2$ used in the symptomatic treatment of polycythemia

ace·tyl·sa·lic·y·late \ə-₁sēt-əl-sə-'li-sə-₁lāt\ *n* : a salt or ester of acetylsalicylic acid

ace·tyl·sal·i·cyl·ic acid \ə-'sēt-əl-₁sa-lə-₁si-lik-\ *n* : ASPIRIN 1

AcG *abbr* [accelerator globulin] factor V

ACh *abbr* acetylcholine

acha·la·sia \₁a-kə-'lā-zhē-ə, -zhə\ *n* : failure of a ring of muscle (as a

sphincter) to relax — compare CAR-
DIOSPASM

¹ache \'āk\ vb ached; ach·ing : to suffer a usu. dull persistent pain

²ache n 1 : a usu. dull persistent pain 2 : a condition marked by aching

achieve·ment age \ə-'chēv-mənt-\ n : the level of an individual's educational achievement as measured by a standardized test and expressed as the age for which the test score would be the average score — compare CHRONOLOGICAL AGE

achievement test n : a standardized test for measuring the skill or knowledge attained by an individual in one or more fields of work or study

Achil·les reflex \ə-'ki-lēz-\ n : ANKLE JERK

Achilles tendon n : the strong tendon joining the muscles in the calf of the leg to the bone of the heel — called also tendon of Achilles

achlor·hyd·ria \ā-ä-₁klōr-'hi-drē-ə\ n : absence of hydrochloric acid from the gastric juice — compare HYPER-CHLORHYDRIA, HYPOCHLORHYDRIA — achlor·hy·dric \-'hi-drik, -'hī-\ adj

acho·lia \(₁)ā-'kō-lē-ə, -'kä-\ n : deficiency or absence of bile

achol·ic \(₁)ā-'kä-lik\ adj : exhibiting deficiency of bile (~ stools)

achol·uria \ā-kō-'lur-ē-ə, -kä-, -lyur-\ n : absence of bile pigment from the urine — achol·uric \-'lur-ik, -'lyur-\ adj

achon·dro·pla·sia \ā-₁kän-drə-'plā-zhē-ə, -zhə\ n : a genetic disorder disturbing normal growth of cartilage, resulting in a form of dwarfism characterized by a usu. normal torso and shortened limbs, and usu. inherited as an autosomal dominant — compare ATELIOSIS — achon·dro·plas·tic \-'plas-tik\ adj

achromat- or achromato- comb form : uncolored except for shades of black, gray, and white (achromatopsia)

ach·ro·mat·ic \ā-krə-'ma-tik\ adj 1 : not readily colored by the usual staining agents 2 : possessing or involving no hue : being or involving only black, gray, or white (~ visual sensations) — ach·ro·mat·i·cal·ly \-ti-k(ə-)lē\ adv — ach·ro·mat·ism \(₁)ā-'krō-mə-₁ti-zəm, a-\ n

achro·ma·top·sia \ā-₁krō-mə-'täp-sē-ə\ n : a visual defect marked by total color blindness in which the colors of the spectrum are seen as tones of white-gray-black

achro·mia \(₁)ā-'krō-mē-ə\ n : absence of normal pigmentation esp. in red blood cells and skin

achy \'ā-kē\ adj ach·i·er; ach·i·est : afflicted with aches — ach·i·ness n

achy·lia \(₁)ā-'kī-lē-ə\ n : ACHYLIA GASTRICA — achy·lous \(₁)ā-'kī-ləs\ adj

achylia gas·tri·ca \-'gas-tri-kə\ n 1 : partial or complete absence of gastric juice 2 : ACHLORHYDRIA

¹ac·id \'a-səd\ adj 1 : sour, sharp, or biting to the taste 2 a : of, relating to, or being an acid; also : having the reactions or characteristics of an acid b of salts and esters : derived by partial exchange of replaceable hydrogen (~ sodium carbonate NaHCO₃) c : marked by or resulting from an abnormally high concentration of acid (~ indigestion) — not used technically

²acid n 1 : a sour substance; specif : any of various typically water-soluble and sour compounds that in solution are capable of reacting with a base to form a salt, redden litmus, and have a pH less than 7, that are hydrogen-containing molecules or ions able to give up a proton to a base, or that are substances able to accept a pair of electrons from a base 2 : LSD

ac·i·dae·mia chiefly Brit var of ACIDE-MIA

acid–base balance \'a-səd-'bās-\ n : the state of equilibrium between proton donors and proton acceptors in the buffering system of the blood that is maintained at approximately pH 7.35 to 7.45 under normal conditions in arterial blood

ac·i·de·mia \₁a-sə-'dē-mē-ə\ n : a condition in which the hydrogen-ion concentration in the blood is increased

acid–fast \'a-səd-₁fast\ adj : not easily decolorized by acids (as when stained) — used esp. of bacteria and tissues

acid·ic \ə-'si-dik, a-\ adj 1 : acid-forming 2 : ACID

acid·i·fy \ə-'si-də-₁fī\ vb -fied; -fy·ing 1 : to make acid 2 : to convert into an acid — acid·i·fi·ca·tion \ə-₁si-də-fə-'kā-shən, a-\ n — acid·i·fi·er \ə-'si-də-₁fī-ər, a-\ n

acid·i·ty \ə-'si-də-tē, a-\ n, pl -ties 1 : the quality, state, or degree of being sour or chemically acid 2 : the quality or state of being excessively or abnormally acid : HYPERACIDITY

acid maltase deficiency n : POMPE'S DISEASE

acid·o·gen·ic \ə-₁si-də-'je-nik, ₁a-sə-dō-\ adj : acid-forming

¹acid·o·phil \ə-'si-də-₁fil, a-\ also acid·o·phile \-₁fil\ adj : ACIDOPHILIC 1

²acidophil also acidophile n : a substance, tissue, or organism that stains readily with acid stains

acid·o·phil·ic \-'fi-lik\ adj 1 : staining readily with acid stains 2 : preferring or thriving in a relatively acid environment (~ bacteria)

ac·i·doph·i·lus milk \₁a-sə-'dä-fə-ləs-\ n : milk fermented by any of several bacteria and used therapeutically to change the intestinal flora

ac·i·do·sis \₁a-sə-'dō-səs\ n, pl -do·ses \-₁sēz\ : a condition of decreased alkalinity of the blood and tissues marked by sickly sweet breath, headache, nausea and vomiting, and visual disturbances and usu. a result of excessive acid production — compare ALKALOSIS, KETOSIS 1 — **ac·i·dot·ic** \-ˈdä-tik\ *adj*

acid phosphatase *n* : a phosphatase (as the phosphomonoesterase from the prostate gland) active in acid medium

acid·u·late \ə-ˈsi-jə-ˌlāt\ *vb* **-lat·ed; -lat·ing** : to make acid or slightly acid — **acid·u·la·tion** \-ˌsi-jə-ˈlā-shən\ *n*

ac·id·uria \ˌa-sə-ˈdu̇r-ē-ə, -ˈdyu̇r-\ *n* : the condition of having acid in the urine esp. in abnormal amounts — see AMINOACIDURIA

ac·id·uric \ˌa-sə-ˈdu̇r-ik, -ˈdyu̇r-\ *adj* : tolerating a highly acid environment; *also* : ACIDOPHILIC 2

ac·i·nar \ˈa-sə-nər, -ˌnär\ *adj* : of, relating to, or comprising an acinus

acin·ic \ə-ˈsi-nik\ *adj* : ACINAR ⟨∼ and follicular carcinoma⟩

ac·i·nous \ˈa-sə-nəs, ə-ˈsī-nəs\ *adj* : consisting of or containing acini

aci·nus \ˈa-sə-nəs, ə-ˈsī-\ *n, pl* **aci·ni** \-ˌnī\ : any of the small sacs terminating the ducts of some exocrine glands and lined with secretory cells

ack·ee *var of* AKEE

ac·ne \ˈak-nē\ *n* : a disorder of the skin caused by inflammation of the skin glands and hair follicles; *specif* : a form found chiefly in adolescents and marked by pimples esp. on the face — **ac·ned** \-nēd\ *adj*

ac·ne·form \ˈak-nē-ˌform\ *or* **ac·nei·form** \ˈak-nē-ə-ˌform, ak-ˈnē-\ *adj* : resembling acne ⟨an ∼ eruption⟩

ac·ne·gen·ic \ˌak-ni-ˈje-nik\ *adj* : producing or increasing the severity of acne ⟨the ∼ effect of some hormones⟩

ac·ne ro·sa·cea \ˌak-nē-rō-ˈzā-shē-ə, -shə\ *n, pl* **ac·nae ro·sa·ce·ae** \ˌak-nē-rō-ˈzā-shē-ˌē\ : acne involving the skin of the nose, forehead, and cheeks that is common in middle age and characterized by congestion, flushing, telangiectasia, and marked nodular swelling of tissues esp. of the nose — called also *rosacea*

acne ur·ti·ca·ta \-ˌər-tə-ˈkä-tə\ *n* : an acneform eruption of the skin characterized by itching papular wheals

acne vul·gar·is \-ˌvəl-ˈgar-əs\ *n, pl* **ac·nae vul·gar·es** \-ˈgar-ˌēz\ : a chronic acne involving mainly the face, chest, and shoulders that is common in adolescent humans and various domestic animals and characterized by the intermittent formation of discrete papular or pustular lesions often resulting in considerable scarring

ACNM *abbr* American College of Nurse-Midwives

acous·tic \ə-ˈkü-stik\ *or* **acous·ti·cal** \-sti-kəl\ *adj* : of or relating to the sense or organs of hearing, to sound, or to the science of sounds — **acous·ti·cal·ly** \-k(ə-)lē\ *adv*

acoustic meatus *n* : AUDITORY CANAL

acoustic nerve *n* : AUDITORY NERVE

acoustic tubercle *n* : a pear-shaped prominence on the inferior cerebellar peduncle including the dorsal nucleus of the cochlear nerve

ac·quired \ə-ˈkwīrd\ *adj* **1** : arising in response to the action of the environment on the organism (as in the use or disuse of an organ) — compare GENIC, HEREDITARY **2** : developed after birth — compare CONGENITAL, FAMILIAL, HEREDITARY

acquired immune deficiency syndrome *n* : AIDS

acquired immunity *n* : immunity that develops after exposure to a suitable agent (as by an attack of a disease or by injection of antigens) — compare ACTIVE IMMUNITY, NATURAL IMMUNITY, PASSIVE IMMUNITY

acquired immunodeficiency syndrome *n* : AIDS

acr- *or* **acro-** *comb form* **1** : top : peak : summit ⟨*acro*cephaly⟩ **2** : height ⟨*acro*phobia⟩ **3** : extremity of the body ⟨*acro*cyanosis⟩

ac·rid \ˈa-krəd\ *adj* : irritatingly sharp and harsh or unpleasantly pungent in taste or odor — **ac·rid·ly** *adv*

ac·ri·dine \ˈa-krə-ˌdēn\ *n* : a colorless crystalline compound $C_{13}H_9N$ occurring in coal tar and important as the parent compound of dyes and pharmaceuticals

ac·ri·fla·vine \ˌa-krə-ˈflā-ˌvēn, -vən\ *n* : a yellow acridine dye $C_{14}H_{14}N_3Cl$ obtained by methylation of proflavine as red crystals or usu. in admixture with proflavine as a deep orange powder and used often in the form of its reddish brown hydrochloride as an antiseptic esp. for wounds

ac·ro·cen·tric \ˌa-krō-ˈsen-trik\ *adj* : having the centromere situated so that one chromosomal arm is much shorter than the other — compare METACENTRIC, TELOCENTRIC — **acrocentric** *n*

ac·ro·ceph·a·lo·syn·dac·ty·ly \-ˌse-fə-(ˌ)lō-sin-ˈdak-tə-lē\ *n, pl* **-lies** : a congenital syndrome characterized by a peaked head and webbed or fused fingers and toes

ac·ro·ceph·a·ly \ˌa-krə-ˈse-fə-lē\ *n, pl* **-lies** *also* **-lias** : OXYCEPHALY

ac·ro·chor·don \ˌa-krə-ˈkor-ˌdän\ *n* : SKIN TAG

ac·ro·cy·a·no·sis \ˌa-krō-ˌsī-ə-ˈnō-səs\ *n, pl* **-no·ses** \-ˌsēz\ : a disorder of the arterioles of the exposed parts of the hands and feet involving abnormal contraction of the arteriolar walls intensified by exposure to cold and resulting in bluish mottled skin, chilling, and sweating of the affected parts — **ac·ro·cy·a·not·ic** \-ˈnä-tik\ *adj*

ac·ro·der·ma·ti·tis \ˌa-krō-ˌdər-mə-ˈtī-təs\ *n* : inflammation of the skin of the extremities

acrodermatitis chron·i·ca atroph·i·cans

\-ıkrä-ni-kə-ə-¹trä-fi-ıkanz\ *n* : a skin condition of the extremities related to Lyme disease and characterized by erythematous and edematous lesions which tend to become atrophic giving the skin the appearance of wrinkled tissue paper

acrodermatitis en•tero•path•i•ca \-ıen-tə-rō-¹pa-thi-kə\ *n* : a severe human skin and gastrointestinal disease inherited as a recessive autosomal trait that is characterized by the symptoms of zinc deficiency and clears up when zinc is added to the diet

ac•ro•dyn•ia \ıa-krō-¹di-nē-ə\ *n* : a disease of infants and young children that is an allergic reaction to mercury, is characterized by dusky pink discoloration of hands and feet with local swelling and intense itching, and is accompanied by insomnia, irritability, and sensitivity to light — called also *erythredema, pink disease, Swift's disease* — **ac•ro•dyn•ic** \-¹di-nik\ *adj*

¹**ac•ro•meg•al•ic** \ıa-krō-mə-¹ga-lik\ *adj* : exhibiting acromegaly

²**acromegalic** *n* : one affected with acromegaly

ac•ro•meg•a•ly \ıa-krō-¹me-gə-lē\ *n, pl* **-lies** : chronic hyperpituitarism that is characterized by a gradual and permanent enlargement of the flat bones (as the lower jaw) and of the hands and feet, abdominal organs, nose, lips, and tongue and that develops after ossification is complete — compare GIGANTISM

acro•mi•al \ə-¹krō-mē-əl\ *adj* : of, relating to, or situated near the acromion

acromial process *n* : ACROMION

ac•ro•mi•cria \ıa-krō-¹mi-krē-ə, -¹mī-\ *n* : abnormal smallness of the extremities

acromio- *comb form* : acromial and ⟨*acromio*clavicular⟩

acro•mio•cla•vic•u•lar \ə-ıkrō-mē-(ı)ō-klə-¹vi-kyə-lər\ *adj* : relating to, being, or affecting the joint connecting the acromion and the clavicle

acro•mi•on \ə-¹krō-mē-ıän, -ən\ *n* : the outer end of the spine of the scapula that protects the glenoid cavity, forms the outer angle of the shoulder, and articulates with the clavicle — called also *acromial process, acromion process*

acro•mi•on•ec•to•my \ə-ıkrō-mē-ıän-¹ek-tə-mē, -mē-ə-¹nek-\ *n, pl* **-mies** : partial or total surgical excision of the acromion

acro•pa•chy \¹a-krō-ıpa-kē, ə-¹krä-pə-kē\ *n, pl* **-pa•chies** : OSTEOARTHROPATHY

ac•ro•par•es•the•sia \ıa-krō-ıpar-əs-¹thē-zhē-ə, -zhə\ *n* : a condition of burning, tingling, or pricking sensations or numbness in the extremities present on awaking and of unknown cause or produced by compression of nerves during sleep

acrop•a•thy \ə-¹krä-pə-thē\ *n, pl* **-thies** : a disease affecting the extremities

ac•ro•phobe \¹a-krə-ıfōb\ *n* : a person affected with acrophobia

ac•ro•pho•bia \ıa-krə-¹fō-bē-ə\ *n* : abnormal or pathological fear of being at a great height

ac•ro•sclero•der•ma \ıa-krō-ıskler-ə-¹dər-mə\ *n* : scleroderma affecting the extremities, face, and chest

ac•ro•scle•ro•sis \ıa-krō-sklə-¹rō-səs\ *n, pl* **-ro•ses** \-ısēz\ : ACROSCLERODERMA

ac•ro•some \¹a-krə-ısōm\ *n* : an anterior prolongation of a spermatozoon that releases egg-penetrating enzymes — **ac•ro•so•mal** \ıa-krə-¹sō-məl\ *adj*

ac•ry•late \¹ak-rə-ılāt\ *n* : a salt or ester of acrylic acid

¹**acryl•ic** \ə-¹kri-lik\ *adj* : of or relating to acrylic acid or its derivatives

²**acrylic** *n* : ACRYLIC RESIN

acrylic acid *n* : an unsaturated liquid acid $C_3H_4O_2$ that is obtained by synthesis and that polymerizes readily

acrylic resin *n* : a glassy acrylic thermoplastic used for cast and molded parts (as of medical prostheses and dental appliances) or as coatings and adhesives

ACSW *abbr* Academy of Certified Social Workers

ACTH \ıā-ısē-(ı)tē-¹āch\ *n* : a protein hormone of the anterior lobe of the pituitary gland that stimulates the adrenal cortex — called also *adrenocorticotropic hormone*

ac•tin \¹ak-tən\ *n* : a cellular protein found esp. in microfilaments (as those comprising myofibrils) and active in muscular contraction, cellular movement, and maintenance of cell shape — see F-ACTIN, G-ACTIN

actin- *or* **actini-** *or* **actino-** *comb form* : of, utilizing, or caused by actinic radiation (as X rays) ⟨*actino*therapy⟩

ac•tin•ic \ak-¹ti-nik\ *adj* : of, relating to, resulting from, or exhibiting chemical changes produced by radiant energy esp. in the visible and ultraviolet parts of the spectrum ⟨~ keratosis⟩ ⟨~ injury⟩

ac•tin•i•um \ak-¹ti-nē-əm\ *n* : a radioactive trivalent metallic element — symbol *Ac*; see ELEMENT table

ac•ti•no•bac•il•lo•sis \ıak-tə-(ı)nō-ıba-sə-¹lō-səs, ak-ıti-nō-\ *n, pl* **-lo•ses** \-ısēz\ : a disease that affects domestic animals and sometimes humans, resembles actinomycosis, and is caused by a bacterium of the genus *Actinobacillus* (A. *lignieresi*) — see WOODEN TONGUE

ac•ti•no•ba•cil•lus \-bə-¹si-ləs\ *n* 1 *cap* : a genus of aerobic gram-negative parasitic bacteria (family Pasturellaceae) forming filaments resembling streptobacilli — see ACTINOBACILLOSIS 2 *pl* **-li** \-ılī\ : a bacterium of the genus *Actinobacillus*

ac•ti•no•my•ces \ıak-tə-(ı)nō-¹mī-ısēz, ak-ıti-nō-\ *n* 1 *cap* : a genus of filamentous or rod-shaped gram-positive bacteria (family Actinomycetaceae) that includes usu. commensal and sometimes pathogenic forms inhabiting mucosal surfaces esp. of the oral cavity — compare ACTINOMYCOSIS 2 *pl* **actinomyces** : a bacterium of the genus *Actinomyces*

ac·ti·no·my·cete \-ˈmī-ˌsēt, -mī-ˈsēt\ *n* : any of an order (Actinomycetales) of filamentous or rod-shaped bacteria (as the actinomyces or streptomyces)

ac·ti·no·my·cin \-ˈmīs-ᵊn\ *n* : any of various red or yellow-red mostly toxic polypeptide antibiotics isolated from soil bacteria (esp. *Streptomyces antibioticus*)

actinomycin D *n* : DACTINOMYCIN

ac·ti·no·my·co·sis \ˌak-tə-nō-ˌmī-ˈkō-səs\ *n, pl* **-co·ses** \-ˌsēz\ : infection with or disease caused by actinomycetes

ac·ti·no·spec·ta·cin \ˌak-tə-(ˌ)nō-ˈspek-tə-sən, ak-ˌti-nō-\ *n* : SPECTINOMYCIN

ac·ti·no·ther·a·py \-ˈther-ə-pē\ *n, pl* **-pies** : application for therapeutic purposes of the chemically active rays of the spectrum (as ultraviolet light or X rays)

ac·tion \ˈak-shən\ *n* **1** : the process of exerting a force or bringing about an effect that results from the inherent capacity of an agent **2** : a function or the performance of a function of the body (as defecation) or of one of its parts ⟨heart ~⟩ **3** : an act of will **4** *pl* : BEHAVIOR ⟨aggressive ~s⟩

action potential *n* : a momentary change in electrical potential (as between the inside of a nerve cell and the extracellular medium) that occurs when a cell or tissue has been activated by a stimulus — compare RESTING POTENTIAL

ac·ti·vat·ed charcoal *n* : a highly absorptive, fine, black, odorless, and tasteless powdered charcoal used in medicine esp. as an antidote in many forms of poisoning and as an antiflatulent

ac·ti·va·tor \ˈak-tə-ˌvā-tər\ *n* **1** : a substance (as a chloride ion) that increases the activity of an enzyme — compare COENZYME **2** : a substance given off by developing tissue that stimulates differentiation of adjacent tissue; *also* : a structure giving off such a stimulant

ac·tive \ˈak-tiv\ *adj* **1** : capable of acting or reacting esp. in some specific way ⟨an ~ enzyme⟩ **2** : tending to progress or to cause degeneration ⟨~ tuberculosis⟩ **3** : exhibiting optical activity **4** : requiring the expenditure of energy — **ac·tive·ly** *adv*

active immunity *n* : usu. long-lasting immunity that is acquired through production of antibodies within the organism in response to the presence of antigens — compare ACQUIRED IM-

MUNITY, NATURAL IMMUNITY, PASSIVE IMMUNITY

active site *n* : a region esp. of a biologically active protein (as an enzyme or an antibody) where catalytic activity takes place and whose shape permits the binding only of a specific reactant molecule

active transport *n* : movement of a chemical substance by the expenditure of energy through a gradient (as across a cell membrane) in concentration or electrical potential and opposite to the direction of normal diffusion

ac·tiv·i·ty \ak-ˈti-və-tē\ *n, pl* **-ties 1** : natural or normal function ⟨digestive ~⟩ **2** : the characteristic of acting chemically or of promoting a chemical reaction ⟨the ~ of a catalyst⟩

ac·to·my·o·sin \ˌak-tə-ˈmī-ə-sən\ *n* : a viscous contractile complex of actin and myosin concerned together with ATP in muscular contraction

act out *vb* : to express (as an impulse or a fantasy) directly in overt behavior without modification to comply with social norms

acu- *comb form* : performed with a needle ⟨*acu*puncture⟩

acu·ity \ə-ˈkyü-ə-tē\ *n, pl* **-ities** : keenness of sense perception ⟨~ of hearing⟩ — see VISUAL ACUITY

acuminata — see CONDYLOMA ACUMINATUM, VERRUCA ACUMINATA

acuminatum — see CONDYLOMA ACUMINATUM

acu·pres·sure \ˈa-kyü-ˌpre-shər\ *n* : SHIATSU — **acu·pres·sur·ist** \-ˌpre-shə-rist\ *n*

acu·punc·ture \-ˌpəŋk-chər\ *n* : an orig. Chinese practice of puncturing the body (as with needles) at specific points to cure disease or relieve pain (as in surgery) — **acu·punc·tur·ist** \-chə-rist\ *n*

-acusis *n comb form* : hearing ⟨diplac*usis*⟩ ⟨hyperac*usis*⟩

acustica — see MACULA ACUSTICA

acusticus — see MEATUS ACUSTICUS EXTERNUS, MEATUS ACUSTICUS INTERNUS

acuta — see PITYRIASIS LICHENOIDES ET VARIOLIFORMIS ACUTA

acute \ə-ˈkyüt\ *adj* **1** : sensing or perceiving accurately, clearly, effectively, or sensitively ⟨~ vision⟩ **2 a** : characterized by sharpness or severity ⟨~ pain⟩ ⟨~ infection⟩ **b** : having a sudden onset, sharp rise, and short course ⟨~ disease⟩ — compare CHRONIC — **acute·ly** *adv* — **acute·ness** *n*

acute abdomen *n* : an acute internal abdominal condition requiring immediate operation

acute care *n* : short-term medical care in a hospital or emergency room esp. for serious acute disease or trauma

acute febrile neutrophilic dermatosis *n* : SWEET'S SYNDROME

acy·a·not·ic \ā-ˌsī-ə-ˈnä-tik\ *adj* : characterized by the absence of cyanosis ⟨∼ patients⟩ ⟨∼ heart disease⟩

acy·clo·vir \ā-ˈsī-klō-ˌvir\ *n* : a cyclic nucleoside $C_8H_{11}N_5O_3$ used esp. to treat the symptoms of the genital form of herpes simplex — see ZOVIRAX

ac·yl \ˈa-səl, -ˌsēl; ˈā-səl\ *n* : a radical derived usu. from an organic acid by removal of the hydroxyl from all acid groups

ADA *abbr* 1 adenosine deaminase 2 American Dietetic Association

adac·ty·lia \ˌā-ˌdak-ˈti-lē-ə\ *n* : congenital lack of fingers or toes

ad·a·man·ti·no·ma \ˌa-də-ˌmant-ᵊn-ˈō-mə\ *n, pl* **-mas** *also* **-ma·ta** \-mə-tə\ : AMELOBLASTOMA

Ad·am's ap·ple \ˈa-dəmz-ˈa-pəl\ *n* : the projection in the front of the neck that is formed by the thyroid cartilage and is particularly prominent in males

ad·am·site \ˈa-dəm-ˌzīt\ *n* : a yellow crystalline arsenical $C_{12}H_9AsClN$ used as a respiratory irritant in some forms of tear gas

Adams, Roger (1889–1971), American chemist.

Adams–Stokes syndrome *n* : STOKES-ADAMS SYNDROME

R. Adams — see STOKES-ADAMS SYNDROME

J. Stokes — see CHEYNE-STOKES RESPIRATION

adapt \ə-ˈdapt\ *vb* : to make or become fit often by modification

ad·ap·ta·tion \ˌa-ˌdap-ˈtā-shən\ *n* 1 : the act or process of adapting : the state of being adapted 2 : adjustment to environmental conditions — **adap·tive** \ə-ˈdap-tiv\ *adj*

ad·der \ˈa-dər\ *n* 1 : the common venomous European viper of the genus *Vipera* (*V. berus*); *broadly* : a terrestrial viper (family Viperidae) 2 : any of several No. American snakes that are harmless but are popularly believed to be venomous

¹ad·dict \ə-ˈdikt\ *vb* : to cause (a person) to become physiologically dependent upon a substance

²ad·dict \ˈa-(ˌ)dikt\ *n* : one who is addicted to a substance

ad·dic·tion \ə-ˈdik-shən\ *n* : compulsive need for and use of a habit-forming substance (as heroin, nicotine, or alcohol) characterized by tolerance and by well-defined physiological symptoms upon withdrawal; *broadly* : persistent compulsive use of a substance known by the user to be physically, psychologically, or socially harmful — compare HABITUATION, SUBSTANCE ABUSE — **ad·dic·tive** \-ˈdik-tiv\ *adj*

Ad·dis count \ˈa-dis-ˌkau̇nt\ *n* : a technique for the quantitative determination of cells, casts, and protein in a 12-hour urine sample used in the diagnosis and treatment of kidney disease

Addis, Thomas (1881–1949), American physician.

Ad·di·so·ni·an \ˌa-də-ˈsō-nē-ən, -nyən\ *adj* : of, relating to, or affected with Addison's disease ⟨∼ crisis⟩

Addison, Thomas (1793–1860), English physician.

addisonian anemia *n, often cap 1st A* : PERNICIOUS ANEMIA

Addison's disease *n* : a destructive disease marked by deficient adrenocortical secretion and characterized by extreme weakness, loss of weight, low blood pressure, gastrointestinal disturbances, and brownish pigmentation of the skin and mucous membranes

¹ad·di·tive \ˈa-də-tiv\ *adj* : characterized by, being, or producing effects (as drug responses or gene products) that when the causative factors act together are the sum of their individual effects — **ad·di·tive·ly** *adv* — **ad·di·tiv·i·ty** \ˌa-də-ˈti-və-tē\ *n*

²additive *n* : a substance added to another in relatively small amounts to impart or improve desirable properties or suppress undesirable properties ⟨food ∼s⟩

ad·duct \ə-ˈdəkt, a-\ *vb* : to draw (as a limb) toward or past the median axis of the body; *also* : to bring together (similar parts) ⟨∼ the fingers⟩ — **ad·duc·tion** \-ˈdək-shən, a-\ *n*

ad·duc·tor \-ˈdək-tər\ *n* 1 : any of three powerful triangular muscles that contribute to the adduction of the human thigh: **a** : one arising from the superior ramus of the pubis and inserted into the middle third of the linea aspera — called also *adductor longus* **b** : one arising from the inferior ramus of the pubis and inserted into the iliopectineal line and the upper part of the linea aspera — called also *adductor brevis* **c** : one arising from the inferior ramus of the pubis and the ischium and inserted behind the first two into the linea aspera — called also *adductor magnus* 2 : any of several muscles other than the adductors of the thigh that draw a part toward the median line of the body or toward the axis of an extremity

adductor brev·is \-ˈbre-vəs\ *n* : ADDUCTOR 1b

adductor hal·lu·cis \-ˈhal-yə-sis; -ˈha-lə-səs, -kəs\ *n* : a muscle of the foot that adducts and flexes the big toe and helps to support the arch of the foot — called also *adductor hallucis muscle*

adductor lon·gus \-ˈlȯŋ-gəs\ *n* : ADDUCTOR 1a

adductor mag·nus \-ˈmag-nəs\ *n* : ADDUCTOR 1c

adductor pol·li·cis \-ˈpä-lə-səs, -kəs\ *n* : a muscle of the hand with two heads that adducts the thumb by bringing it toward the palm — called also *adductor pollicis muscle*

ad•duc•tor tubercle *n* : a tubercle on the proximal part of the medial epicondyle of the femur that is the site of insertion of the adductor magnus

aden- *or* **adeno-** *comb form* : gland : glandular ⟨*adenitis*⟩ ⟨*adeno*carcinoma⟩

ad•e•nine \'ad-ᵊn-,ēn\ *n* : a purine base C₅H₅N₅ that codes hereditary information in the genetic code in DNA and RNA — compare CYTOSINE, GUANINE, THYMINE, URACIL

adenine arabinoside *n* : VIDARABINE

ad•e•ni•tis \,ad-ᵊn-'ī-təs\ *n* : inflammation of a gland; *esp* : LYMPHADENITIS

ad•e•no•ac•an•tho•ma \,ad-ᵊn-(,)ō-,a-,kan-'thō-mə\ *n, pl* **-mas** *or* **-ma•ta** \-mə-tə\ : an adenocarcinoma with epithelial cells differentiated and proliferated into squamous cells

ad•e•no•car•ci•no•ma \-,kärs-ᵊn-'ō-mə\ *n, pl* **-mas** *or* **-ma•ta** \-mə-tə\ : a malignant tumor originating in glandular epithelium — **ad•e•no•car•ci•no•ma•tous** \-mə-təs\ *adj*

ad•e•no•fi•bro•ma \-fī-'brō-mə\ *n, pl* **-mas** *or* **-ma•ta** \-mə-tə\ : a benign tumor of glandular and fibrous tissue

ad•e•no•hy•poph•y•sis \-hī-'pä-fə-səs\ *n, pl* **-y•ses** \-,sēz\ : the anterior part of the pituitary gland that is derived from the embryonic pharynx and is primarily glandular in nature — called also *anterior lobe*; compare NEUROHYPOPHYSIS — **ad•e•no•hy•poph•y•se•al** \-(,)hī-,pä-fə-'sē-əl\ *or* **ad•e•no•hy•po•phys•i•al** \-,hī-pə-'fi-zē-əl\ *adj*

¹**ad•e•noid** \'ad-ᵊn-,ȯid, 'ad-,nȯid\ *adj* **1** : of, like, or relating to glands or glandular tissue; *esp* : like or belonging to lymphoid tissue **2** : of or relating to the adenoids **3 a** : of, relating to, or affected with abnormally enlarged adenoids **b** : characteristic of one affected with abnormally enlarged adenoids ⟨∼ facies⟩

²**adenoid** *n* **1** : an abnormally enlarged mass of lymphoid tissue at the back of the pharynx characteristically obstructing the nasal and ear passages and inducing mouth breathing, a nasal voice, postnasal discharge, and dullness of facial expression — usu. used in pl. **2** : PHARYNGEAL TONSIL

ad•e•noi•dal \,ad-ᵊn-'ȯid-ᵊl\ *adj* : exhibiting the characteristics (as snoring, mouth breathing, and a nasal voice) of one affected with abnormally enlarged adenoids : ADENOID — not usu. used technically

ad•e•noid•ec•to•my \,ad-ᵊn-,ȯi-'dek-tə-mē\ *n, pl* **-mies** : surgical removal of the adenoids

ad•e•noid•itis \,ad-ᵊn-,ȯi-'dī-təs\ *n* : inflammation of the adenoids

ad•e•no•ma \,ad-ᵊn-'ō-mə\ *n, pl* **-mas** *also* **-ma•ta** \-mə-tə\ : a benign tumor of a glandular structure or of glandular origin — **ad•e•no•ma•tous** \-mə-təs\ *adj*

ad•e•no•ma•toid \,ad-ᵊn-'ō-mə-,tȯid\ *adj* : relating to or resembling an adenoma

ad•e•no•ma•to•sis \,ad-ᵊn-,ō-mə-'tō-səs\ *n, pl* **-to•ses** \-,sēz\ : a condition marked by multiple growths consisting of glandular tissue

ad•e•no•my•o•ma \,ad-ᵊn-(,)ō-,mī-'ō-mə\ *n, pl* **-mas** *or* **-ma•ta** \-mə-tə\ : a benign tumor composed of muscular and glandular elements

ad•e•no•my•o•sis \-,mī-'ō-səs\ *n, pl* **-o•ses** \-,sēz\ : endometriosis esp. when the endometrial tissue invades the myometrium

ad•e•nop•a•thy \,ad-ᵊn-'ä-pə-thē\ *n, pl* **-thies** : any disease or enlargement involving glandular tissue; *esp* : one involving lymph nodes

aden•o•sine \ə-'de-nə-,sēn, -sən\ *n* : a nucleoside C₁₀H₁₃N₅O₄ that is a constituent of RNA yielding adenine and ribose on hydrolysis

adenosine deaminase *n* : an enzyme which catalyzes the conversion of AMP, ADP, and ATP to inosine, whose deficiency causes a severe immunodeficiency disease by inhibiting DNA replication in lymphocytes, and whose marked increase is associated with a mild chronic hemolytic anemia — abbr. *ADA*

adenosine diphosphate *n* : ADP

adenosine mo•no•phos•phate \-,mä-nə-'fäs-,fāt, -mō-\ *n* : AMP

adenosine phosphate *n* : any of three phosphates of adenosine: **a** : AMP **b** : ADP **c** : ATP

adenosine 3′,5′-monophosphate \-'thrē-'fiv-\ *n* : CYCLIC AMP

adenosine tri•phos•pha•tase \-trī-'fäs-fə-,tās, -,tāz\ *n* : ATPASE

adenosine tri•phos•phate \-trī-'fäs-,fāt\ *n* : ATP

ad•e•no•sis \,ad-ᵊn-'ō-səs\ *n, pl* **-no•ses** \-,sēz\ : a disease of glandular tissue; *esp* : one involving abnormal proliferation or occurrence of glandular tissue ⟨vaginal ∼⟩

ad•e•not•o•my \,ad-ᵊn-'ä-tə-mē\ *n, pl* **-mies** : the operation of dissecting, incising, or removing a gland and esp. the adenoids

ad•e•no•vi•rus \,ad-ᵊn-ō-'vī-rəs\ *n* : any of a group of DNA-containing viruses shaped like a 20-sided polyhedron and orig. identified in human adenoid tissue, causing respiratory diseases (as catarrh), and including some capable of inducing malignant tumors in experimental animals — **ad•e•no•vi•ral** \-rəl\ *adj*

ad•e•nyl•ic acid \,ad-ᵊn-'i-lik-\ *n* : AMP

ADH *abbr* antidiuretic hormone

ADHD *abbr* attention-deficit hyperactivity disorder

ad•here \ad-'hir\ *vb* **ad•hered; ad•her•ing 1** : to hold fast or stick by or as if by gluing, suction, grasping, or fusing **2** : to become joined (as in pathological adhesion) — **ad·her·ence** \-'hir-əns\ n

ad·he·sion \ad-'hē-zhən\ n 1 : the action or state of adhering; *specif* : the abnormal union of surfaces normally separated by the formation of new fibrous tissue resulting from an inflammatory process; *also* : the newly formed uniting tissue (pleural ∼s) **b** : the union of wound edges esp. by first intention

¹**ad·he·sive** \-'hē-siv, -ziv\ *adj* **1 a** : relating to or having the ability to stick things together **b** : prepared for adhering **2** : characterized by adhesions — **ad·he·sive·ly** *adv*

²**adhesive** n **1** : a substance that bonds two materials together by adhering to the surface of each **2** : ADHESIVE TAPE

adhesive pericarditis n : pericarditis in which adhesions form between the two layers of pericardium — see ACCRETIO CORDIS

adhesive tape n : tape coated on one side with an adhesive mixture; *esp* : one used for covering wounds

adi·a·do·ko·ki·ne·sis \ˌa-dē-ˌa-də-ˌkō-kə-'nē-səs, ə-ˌdī-ə-ˌdō-(ˌ)kō-, -ki-'nē-, -kē-\ *n, pl* **-ses** \-ˌsēz\ : inability to make movements exhibiting a rapid change of motion (as in quickly rotating the wrist one way and then the other) due to cerebellar dysfunction — compare DYSDIADOCHOKINESIS

ad·i·ence \'a-dē-əns\ n : a tendency to approach or accept a stimulus object or situation — compare ABIENCE — **ad·i·ent** \-ənt\ *adj*

Ad·ie's syndrome \'a-dēz-\ *or* **Ad·ie syndrome** \-dē-\ n : a neurologic syndrome that affects esp. women between 20 and 40 and is characterized by an abnormally dilated pupil, absent or diminished light reflexes of the eye, abnormal accommodation, and lack of ankle-jerk and knee-jerk reflexes

Adie \'ā-dē\, **William John (1886–1935)**, British neurologist.

adip- *or* **adipo-** *comb form* : fat : fatty tissue ⟨adipocyte⟩

ad·i·phen·ine \ˌa-di-'fe-ˌnēn\ n : an antispasmodic drug $C_{20}H_{25}NO_2$ administered in the form of the hydrochloride — see TRASENTINE

ad·i·po·cere \'a-də-pə-ˌsir\ n : a waxy or unctuous brownish substance consisting chiefly of fatty acids and calcium soaps produced by chemical changes affecting dead body fat and muscle long buried or immersed in moisture

ad·i·po·cyte \'a-də-pə-ˌsīt\ n : FAT CELL

ad·i·pose \'a-də-ˌpōs\ *adj* : of or relating to fat; *broadly* : FAT

adipose tissue n : connective tissue in which fat is stored and which has the cells distended by droplets of fat

ad·i·pos·i·ty \ˌa-də-'pä-sə-tē\ n, pl **-ties**

: the quality or state of being fat : OBESITY

ad·i·po·so·gen·i·tal dystrophy \ˌa-də-ˌpō-sō-'je-nət-ᵊl-\ n : FRÖHLICH'S SYNDROME

adiposus — see PANNICULUS ADIPOSUS

adip·sia \ā-'dip-sē-ə, ə-\ n : loss of thirst; *also* : abnormal and esp. prolonged abstinence from the intake of fluids

ad·i·tus \'a-də-təs\ n, pl **aditus** *or* **ad·i·tus·es** : a passage or opening for entrance

ad·junct \'a-ˌjəŋkt\ n : ADJUVANT b

ad·junc·tive \ə-'jəŋk-tiv, a-\ *adj* : involving the medical use of an adjunct ⟨∼ therapy⟩ — **ad·junc·tive·ly** *adv*

ad·just \ə-'jəst\ *vb* **1** : to bring about orientation or adaptation of (oneself) **2** : to achieve mental and behavioral balance between one's own needs and the demands of others — **ad·just·ment** \-mənt\ n

ad·just·ed *adj* : having achieved an often specified and usu. harmonious relationship with the environment or with other individuals

¹**ad·ju·vant** \'a-jə-vənt\ *adj* **1** : serving to aid or contribute **2** : assisting in the prevention, amelioration, or cure of disease ⟨∼ chemotherapy following surgery⟩

²**adjuvant** n : one that helps or facilitates: as **a** : an ingredient (as in a prescription) that facilitates or modifies the action of the principal ingredient **b** : something (as a drug or method) that enhances the effectiveness of a medical treatment **c** : a substance enhancing the immune response to an antigen

ADL *abbr* activities of daily living

Ad·le·ri·an \ad-'lir-ē-ən, äd-\ *adj* : of, relating to, or being a theory and technique of psychotherapy emphasizing the importance of feelings of inferiority, a will to power, and overcompensation in neurotic processes

Ad·ler \'äd-lər\, **Alfred (1870–1937)**, Austrian psychiatrist.

ad lib \(ˌ)ad-'lib\ *adv* : without restraint or imposed limit : as much or as often as is wanted — often used in writing prescriptions

ad li·bi·tum \(ˌ)ad-'li-bə-təm\ *adv* : AD LIB ⟨rats fed *ad libitum*⟩

ad·min·is·ter \əd-'mi-nə-stər\ *vb* **ad·min·is·tered; ad·min·is·ter·ing** : to give remedially (as medicine) — **ad·min·is·tra·tion** \əd-ˌmi-nə-'strā-shən\ n

ad·nexa \ad-'nek-sə\ n pl : conjoined, subordinate, or associated anatomic parts ⟨the uterine ∼ include the ovaries and fallopian tubes⟩ — **ad·nex·al** \-səl\ *adj*

ad·nex·itis \ˌad-ˌnek-'sī-təs\ n : inflammation of adnexa (as of the uterus)

ad·o·les·cence \ˌad-ᵊl-'es-ᵊns\ n **1** : the state or process of growing up **2** : the period of life from puberty to maturity terminating legally at the age of majority

ad·o·les·cent \-ənt\ *n* : one in the state of adolescence — **adolescent** *adj* — **ad·o·les·cent·ly** *adv*

ADP \ā-(ˌ)dē-ˈpē\ *n* : an ester of adenosine that is reversibly converted to ATP for the storing of energy by the addition of a high-energy phosphate group — called also *adenosine diphosphate, adenosine phosphate*

adren- *or* **adreno-** *comb form* **1 a** : adrenal glands ⟨*adrenocortical*⟩ **b** : adrenal and ⟨*adrenogenital*⟩ **2** : adrenaline ⟨*adrenergic*⟩

¹ad·re·nal \ə-ˈdrēn-əl\ *adj* : of, relating to, or derived from the adrenal glands or their secretion — **ad·re·nal·ly** *adv*

²adrenal *n* : ADRENAL GLAND

ad·re·nal·ec·to·my \ə-ˌdrēn-əl-ˈek-tə-mē\ *n, pl* **-mies** : surgical removal of one or both adrenal glands

adrenal gland *n* : either of a pair of complex endocrine organs near the anterior medial border of the kidney consisting of a mesodermal cortex that produces glucocorticoid, mineralocorticoid, and androgenic hormones and an ectodermal medulla that produces epinephrine and norepinephrine — called also *adrenal, suprarenal gland*

Adren·a·lin \ə-ˈdren-əl-ən\ *trademark* — used for a preparation of levorotatory epinephrine

adren·a·line \ə-ˈdren-əl-ən\ *n* : EPINEPHRINE

adren·er·gic \ˌa-drə-ˈnər-jik\ *adj* **1** : liberating or activated by adrenaline or a substance like adrenaline — compare CHOLINERGIC 1, NORADRENERGIC **2** : resembling adrenaline esp. in physiological action — **ad·ren·er·gi·cal·ly** \-ji-k(ə-)lē\ *adv*

adreno- — see ADREN-

ad·re·no·cor·ti·cal \ə-ˌdrē-nō-ˈkȯr-ti-kəl\ *adj* : of, relating to, or derived from the cortex of the adrenal glands

ad·re·no·cor·ti·coid \-ˈkȯid\ *n* : a hormone secreted by the adrenal cortex — **adrenocorticoid** *adj*

ad·re·no·cor·ti·co·ste·roid \-ˈstir-ˌȯid, -ˈster-\ *n* : a steroid (as cortisone or hydrocortisone) obtained from, resembling, or having physiological effects like those of the adrenal cortex

ad·re·no·cor·ti·co·tro·pic \-ˈtrō-pik, -ˈträ-\ *also* **ad·re·no·cor·ti·co·tro·phic** \-ˈtrō-fik, -ˈträ-\ *adj* : acting on or stimulating the adrenal cortex

adrenocorticotropic hormone *n* : ACTH

ad·re·no·cor·ti·co·tro·pin \-ˈtrō-pən\ *also* **ad·re·no·cor·ti·co·tro·phin** \-fən\ *n* : ACTH

adre·no·gen·i·tal syndrome \ə-ˌdrē-nō-ˈje-nət-əl-, -ˌdren-\ *n* : CUSHING'S SYNDROME

adre·no·leu·ko·dys·tro·phy \-ˌlü-kō-ˈdis-trə-fē\ *n, pl* **-phies** : SCHILDER'S DISEASE

adre·no·lyt·ic \ə-ˌdren-əl-ˈi-tik, -ˌdren-\

adj : blocking the release or action of adrenaline at nerve endings

adre·no·med·ul·lary \ə-ˌdrē-nō-ˈmed-əl-ˌer-ē, -ˌdre-, -ˈme-jə-ˌler-; -mə-ˈdə-lə-rē\ *adj* : relating to or derived from the medulla of the adrenal glands ⟨∼ extracts⟩

adre·no·re·cep·tor \ə-ˌdrē-nō-ri-ˈsep-tər, -ˌdre-\ *n* : an adrenergic receptor

adre·no·ste·rone \ə-ˌdrē-nō-stə-ˈrōn, -ˌdre-; ˌa-drə-ˈnäs-tə-ˌ\ *n* : a crystalline steroid $C_{19}N_{24}O_3$ obtained from the adrenal cortex and having androgenic activity

Adria·my·cin \ˌā-drē-ə-ˈmīs-ən, ˌa-\ *trademark* — used for a preparation of the hydrochloride of doxorubicin

ad·sorb \ad-ˈsȯrb, -ˈzȯrb\ *vb* : to take up and hold by adsorption — **ad·sorb·able** \-ˈsȯr-bə-bəl, -ˈzȯr-\ *adj*

ad·sor·bent \-bənt\ *adj* : having the capacity or tendency to adsorb — **adsorbent** *n*

ad·sorp·tion \ad-ˈsȯrp-shən, -ˈzȯrp-\ *n* : the adhesion in an extremely thin layer of molecules (as of gases) to the surfaces of solid bodies or liquids with which they are in contact — compare ABSORPTION — **ad·sorp·tive** \-ˈsȯrp-tiv, -ˈzȯrp-\ *adj*

adult \ə-ˈdəlt, ˈa-ˌdəlt\ *n* **1** : one that has arrived at full development or maturity esp. in size, strength, or intellectual capacity **2** : a human male or female after a specific age (as 21) — **adult** *adj*

adul·ter·ate \ə-ˈdəl-tə-ˌrāt\ *vb* **-at·ed; -at·ing** : to corrupt, debase, or make impure by the addition of a foreign or inferior substance — **adul·ter·ant** \-rənt\ *n or adj* — **adul·ter·a·tion** \-ˈrā-shən\ *n*

adult·hood \ə-ˈdəlt-ˌhu̇d\ *n* : the state or time of being an adult

adult–onset diabetes *n* : NON-INSULIN= DEPENDENT DIABETES MELLITUS

adult respiratory distress syndrome *n* : respiratory failure in adults or children that results from diffuse injury to the endothelium of the lung (as in sepsis, chest trauma, massive blood transfusion, aspiration of the gastric contents, or diffuse pneumonia) and is characterized by pulmonary edema with an abnormally high amount of protein in the edematous fluid, and by respiratory distress, and hypoxemia — abbr. *ARDS*

ad·vance·ment \ad-ˈvans-mənt\ *n* : detachment of a muscle or tendon from its insertion and reattachment (as in the surgical correction of strabismus) at a more advanced point from its insertion (flexor tendon ∼)

advancement flap *n* : a flap of tissue stretched and sutured in place to cover a defect at a nearby position

ad·ven·ti·tia \ˌad-vən-ˈti-shə, -ˌven-\ *n* : the outer layer that makes up a tubular organ or structure and esp. a blood vessel, is composed of collagenous and elastic fibers, and is not covered with peritoneum — called also *tunica adventitia* — **ad·ven·ti·tial** \-shəl\ *adj*

ad·ven·ti·tious \-shəs\ *adj* : arising sporadically or in other than the usual location (an ∼ part in embryonic development)

ady·na·mia \ˌā-dī-ˈna-mē-ə, ˌa-də-, -ˈnā-\ *n* : asthenia caused by disease

ady·nam·ic \ˌā-(ˌ)dī-ˈna-mik, ˌa-də-\ *adj* : characterized by or causing a loss of strength or function (∼ ileus)

ae·des \ā-ˈē-(ˌ)dēz\ *n* 1 *cap* : a large cosmopolitan genus of mosquitoes that includes vectors of some diseases (as yellow fever and dengue) 2 *pl* **aedes** : any mosquito of the genus *Ae·des* — **ae·dine** \-ˌdīn, -ˌdēn\ *adj*

ae·goph·o·ny *chiefly Brit var of* EGOPHONY

ae·lu·ro·phobe, ae·lu·ro·pho·bia *var of* AILUROPHOBE, AILUROPHOBIA

-aemia *also* **-haemia** *chiefly Brit var of* -EMIA

aer- *or* **aero-** *comb form* 1 : air : atmosphere ⟨aerate⟩ ⟨aerobic⟩ 2 : gas ⟨aerosol⟩ 3 : aviation ⟨aeromedicine⟩

aer·ate \ˈar-ˌāt, ˈa-ər-\ *vb* **aer·at·ed; aer·at·ing** 1 : to supply (the blood) with oxygen by respiration 2 : to supply or impregnate (as a liquid) with air 3 : to combine or charge with a gas (as carbon dioxide) — **aer·a·tion** \ˌar-ˈā-shən, ˌa-ər-\ *n*

aer·obe \ˈar-ˌōb, ˈa-ər-\ *n* : an organism (as a bacterium) that lives only in the presence of oxygen

aer·o·bic \ˌar-ˈō-bik, ˌa-ər-\ *adj* 1 : living, active, or occurring only in the presence of oxygen ⟨∼ respiration⟩ 2 : of, relating to, or induced by aerobes 3 : involving or utilizing aerobics ⟨∼ exercises⟩ — **aer·o·bi·cal·ly** \-bi-k(ə-)lē\ *adv*

aer·o·bics \-biks\ *n pl* 1 : a system of physical conditioning involving exercises (as running, walking, swimming, or calisthenics) strenuously performed so as to cause marked temporary increase in respiration and heart rate — used with a sing. or pl. verb 2 : aerobic exercises

aer·o·bi·ol·o·gy \ˌar-ō-bī-ˈä-lə-jē\ *n, pl* **-gies** : the science dealing with the occurrence, transportation, and effects of airborne materials or microorganisms (as viruses or pollen)

aer·odon·tal·gia \ˌar-ō-dän-ˈtal-jē-ə, -jə\ *n* : toothache resulting from atmospheric decompression

aer·o·em·bo·lism \-ˈem-bə-ˌli-zəm\ *n* : decompression sickness caused by rapid ascent to high altitudes and resulting exposure to rapidly lowered air pressure — called also *air bends*

aer·o·med·i·cine \ˌar-ō-ˈme-də-sən\ *n* : a branch of medicine that deals with the diseases and disturbances arising from flying and the associated physiological and psychological problems

aero·med·i·cal \-ˈme-di-kəl\ *adj*

aer·o·oti·tis \ˌar-ə-wō-ˈtī-təs\ *n* : AEROOTITIS MEDIA

aero–otitis me·dia \-ˈmē-dē-ə\ *n* : the traumatic inflammation of the middle ear resulting from differences between atmospheric pressure and pressure in the middle ear

aero·pha·gia \ˌar-ō-ˈfā-jē-ə, -jə\ *also* **aer·oph·a·gy** \ˌar-ˈä-fə-jē, ˌa-ər-\ *n, pl* **-gias** *also* **-gies** : the swallowing of air esp. in hysteria

aero·pho·bia \ˌar-ō-ˈfō-bē-ə\ *n* : abnormal or excessive fear of drafts or of fresh air — **aero·pho·bic** \-bik\ *adj*

aero·sol \ˈar-ə-ˌsäl, -ˌsȯl\ *n* 1 : a suspension of fine solid or liquid particles in gas ⟨smoke and mist are ∼s⟩ 2 : a substance (as a medicine) dispensed from a pressurized container as an aerosol; *also* : the container for this

aero·sol·i·za·tion \ˌar-ə-ˌsä-lə-ˈzā-shən, -ˌsȯ-\ *n* : dispersal (as of a medicine) in the form of an aerosol — **aero·sol·ize** \ˈar-ə-sä-ˌlīz, -ˌsȯ-\ *vb* — **aero·sol·iz·er** *n*

aero·space medicine \ˈar-ō-ˌspās-\ *n* : a medical specialty concerned with the health and medical problems of flight personnel both in the earth's atmosphere and in space

aer·oti·tis \ˌar-ō-ˈtī-təs\ *n* : AEROOTITIS MEDIA

Aes·cu·la·pi·an staff \ˌes-kyə-ˈlā-pē-ən-\ *n* : STAFF OF AESCULAPIUS

aetio- *chiefly Brit var of* ETIO-

ae·ti·o·log·ic, ae·ti·ol·o·gy, ae·ti·o·patho·gen·e·sis *chiefly Brit var of* ETIOLOGIC, ETIOLOGY, ETIOPATHOGENESIS

afe·brile \(ˌ)ā-ˈfe-ˌbrīl *also* -ˈfē-\ *adj* : free from fever : not marked by fever

¹**af·fect** \ˈa-ˌfekt\ *n* : the conscious subjective aspect of an emotion considered apart from bodily changes

²**af·fect** \ə-ˈfekt, a-\ *vb* : to produce an effect upon; *esp* : to produce a material influence upon or alteration in

af·fec·tion \ə-ˈfek-shən\ *n* 1 : the action of affecting : the state of being affected 2 **a** : a bodily condition **b** : DISEASE, MALADY ⟨a pulmonary ∼⟩

af·fec·tive \a-ˈfek-tiv\ *adj* : relating to, arising from, or influencing feelings or emotions : EMOTIONAL ⟨∼ disorders⟩ — **af·fec·tive·ly** *adv* — **af·fec·tiv·i·ty** \ˌa-ˌfek-ˈti-və-tē\ *n*

¹**af·fer·ent** \ˈa-fə-rənt, -ˌfer-ənt\ *adj* : bearing or conducting inward; *specif* : conveying impulses to a nerve center (as the brain or spinal cord) — compare EFFERENT — **af·fer·ent·ly** *adv*

²**afferent** *n* : an afferent anatomical part (as a nerve)

af·fin·i·ty \ə-ˈfin-ət-ē\ *n, pl* **-ties** : an attractive force between substances or particles that causes them to enter into and remain in chemical combination

afi·brin·o·gen·emia \ā-(ı)fī-ıbri-nə-jə-ˈnē-mē-ə\ *n* : an abnormality of blood clotting caused by usu. congenital absence of fibrinogen in the blood

af·la·tox·in \ıa-flə-ˈtäk-sən\ *n* : any of several carcinogenic mycotoxins that are produced esp. in stored agricultural crops (as peanuts) by molds (as *Aspergillus flavus*)

AFP *abbr* alpha-fetoprotein

Af·ri·can·ized bee \ˈa-fri-kə-ınīzd-\ *n* : a honeybee that originated in Brazil as an accidental hybrid between an aggressive African subspecies (*Apis mellifera scutellata*) and previously established European honeybees and has spread to Mexico and the southernmost U.S. by breeding with local bees producing populations retaining most of the African bee's traits — called also *Africanized honeybee, killer bee*

African sleeping sickness *n* : SLEEPING SICKNESS 1

African trypanosomiasis *n* : any of several trypanosomiases caused by African trypanosomes; *esp* : SLEEPING SICKNESS 1

af·ter·birth \ˈaf-tər-ıbərth\ *n* : the placenta and fetal membranes that are expelled after delivery — called also *secundines*

af·ter·care \-ıkar\ *n* : the care, treatment, help, or supervision given to persons discharged from an institution (as a hospital or prison)

af·ter·ef·fect \ˈaf-tər-i-ıfekt\ *n* 1 : an effect that follows its cause after an interval 2 : a secondary result esp. in the action of a drug coming on after the subsidence of the first effect

af·ter·im·age \-i-mij\ *n* : a usu. visual sensation occurring after stimulation by its external cause has ceased — called also *aftersensation, aftervision*

af·ter·load \ˈaf-tər-ılōd\ *n* : the force against which a ventricle contracts that is contributed to by the vascular resistance esp. of the arteries and by the physical characteristics (as mass and viscosity) of the blood

af·ter·pain \-ıpān\ *n* : pain that follows its cause only after a distinct interval (the ∼ of a tooth extraction)

af·ter·taste \-ıtāst\ *n* : persistence of a sensation (as of flavor or an emotion) after the stimulating agent or experience has gone

af·to·sa \af-ˈtō-sə, -zə\ *n* : FOOT-AND= MOUTH DISEASE

Ag *symbol* [Latin *argentum*] silver

aga·lac·tia \ıā-gə-ˈlak-shē-ə, -shə, -tē-ə\ *n* : the failure of the secretion of milk from any cause other than the normal ending of the lactation period — **aga·lac·tic** \-ˈlak-tik\ *adj*

agam·ma·glob·u·lin·emia \(ı)ā-ıga-mə-ıglä-byə-lə-ˈnē-mē-ə\ *n* : a pathological condition in which the body forms few or no gamma globulins or anti-

bodies — compare DYSGAMMAGLOBU-LINEMIA

agan·gli·on·ic \(ı)ā-ıgaŋ-glē-ˈä-nik\ *adj* : lacking ganglia

agar \ˈä-gər\ *n* 1 : a gelatinous colloidal extractive of a red alga (as of the genera *Gelidium, Gracilaria,* and *Eucheuma*) used esp. in culture media or as a gelling and stabilizing agent in foods 2 : a culture medium containing agar

agar–agar \ıä-gər-ˈä-gər\ *n* : AGAR

aga·rose \ˈa-gə-ırōs, ˈä-, -ırōz\ *n* : a polysaccharide obtained from agar that is used esp. as a supporting medium in gel electrophoresis

¹age \ˈāj\ *n* 1 **a** : the part of life from birth to a given time (a child 10 years of ∼) **b** : the time or part of life at which some particular event, qualification, or capacity arises, occurs, or is lost (of reproductive ∼) — see MIDDLE AGE **c** : an advanced stage of life 2 : an individual's development measured in terms of the years requisite for like development of an average individual — see BINET AGE, MENTAL AGE

²age *vb* **aged; ag·ing** *or* **age·ing** : to grow old or cause to grow old

agen·e·sis \(ı)ā-ˈje-nə-səs\ *n, pl* **-e·ses** \-ısēz\ : lack or failure of development (as of a body part)

agent \ˈā-jənt\ *n* 1 : something that produces or is capable of producing an effect 2 : a chemically, physically, or biologically active principle — see OXIDIZING AGENT, REDUCING AGENT

Agent Orange \-ˈör-inj\ *n* : an herbicide widely used as a defoliant in the Vietnam War that is composed of 2,4-D and 2,4,5-T and contains dioxin as a contaminant

ageu·sia \ə-ˈgyü-zē-ə, (ı)ā-, -ˈjü-, -sē-ə\ *n* : the absence or impairment of the sense of taste — **ageu·sic** \-zik, -sik\ *adj*

ag·glu·ti·na·bil·i·ty \ə-ıglüt-ⁿn-ə-ˈbi-lə-tē\ *n, pl* **-ties** : capacity to be agglutinated — **ag·glu·ti·na·ble** \-ˈglüt-ⁿn-ə-bəl\ *adj*

¹ag·glu·ti·nate \ə-ˈglüt-ⁿn-ıāt\ *vb* **-nat·ed; -nat·ing** : to undergo or cause to undergo agglutination

²ag·glu·ti·nate \-ⁿn-ət, -ⁿn-ıāt\ *n* : a clump of agglutinated material (as blood cells or bacteria)

ag·glu·ti·na·tion \ə-ıglüt-ⁿn-ˈā-shən\ *n* : a reaction in which particles (as red blood cells or bacteria) suspended in a liquid collect into clumps and which occurs esp. as a serological response to a specific antibody — **ag·glu·ti·na·tive** \ə-ˈglüt-ⁿn-ıā-tiv, -ə-tiv\ *adj*

agglutination test *n* : any of several tests based on the ability of a specific serum to cause agglutination of a suitable system and used in the diagnosis of infections, the identification of microorganisms, and in blood typing — compare WIDAL TEST

ag·glu·ti·nin \ə-ˈglüt-ᵊn-ən\ *n* : a substance (as an antibody) producing agglutination

ag·glu·ti·no·gen \ə-ˈglüt-ᵊn-ə-jən\ *n* : an antigen whose presence results in the formation of an agglutinin — **ag·glu·ti·no·gen·ic** \-ˌglüt-ᵊn-ə-ˈje-nik\ *adj*

ag·gre·gate \ˈa-gri-gät\ *vb* **-gat·ed; -gat·ing** : to collect or gather into a mass or whole — **ag·gre·gate** \-gət\ *adj or n*

ag·gres·sion \ə-ˈgre-shən\ *n* : hostile, injurious, or destructive behavior or outlook esp. when caused by frustration

ag·gres·sive \ə-ˈgre-siv\ *adj* **1** : tending toward or exhibiting aggression 〈~ behavior〉 **2** : more severe, intensive, or comprehensive than usual esp. in dosage or extent 〈~ chemotherapy〉 — **ag·gres·sive·ly** *adv* — **ag·gres·sive·ness** *n* — **ag·gres·siv·i·ty** \ˌa-ˌgre-ˈsi-və-tē\ *n*

agitans — see PARALYSIS AGITANS

agly·cone \ˌa-ˈglī-ˌkōn\ *also* **agly·con** \-ˌkän\ *n* : an organic compound (as a phenol or alcohol) combined with the sugar portion of a glycoside

ag·na·thia \ag-ˈnä-thē-ə, (ˌ)äg-, -ˈnä-thē-\ *n* : the congenital complete or partial absence of one or both jaws

ag·no·gen·ic \ag-nō-ˈje-nik\ *adj* : of unknown cause 〈~ metaplasia〉

ag·no·sia \ag-ˈnō-zhə, -shə\ *n* : loss or diminution of the ability to recognize familiar objects or stimuli usu. as a result of brain damage

-agogue *n comb form* : substance that promotes the secretion or expulsion of 〈cholagogue〉 〈emmenagogue〉

ag·o·nal \ˈa-gən-ᵊl\ *adj* : of, relating to, or associated with agony and esp. the death agony — **ag·o·nal·ly** *adv*

ag·o·nist \ˈa-gə-nist\ *n* **1** : a muscle on contracting is automatically checked and controlled by the opposing simultaneous contraction of another muscle — called also *agonist muscle, prime mover;* compare ANTAGONIST a, SYNERGIST **2** : a chemical substance (as a drug) capable of combining with a receptor on a cell and initiating a reaction or activity 〈binding of adrenergic ~s〉 — compare ANTAGONIST b

ag·o·ny \ˈa-gə-nē\ *n, pl* **-nies 1** : intense pain of mind or body **2** : the struggle that precedes death

ag·o·ra·pho·bia \ˌa-gə-rə-ˈfō-bē-ə\ *n* : abnormal fear of being helpless in a situation from which escape may be difficult or embarrassing that is characterized initially often by panic or anticipatory anxiety and finally by avoidance of open or public places

¹**ag·o·ra·pho·bic** \-ˈfō-bik\ *adj* : of, relating to, or affected with agoraphobia

²**agoraphobic** *or* **ag·o·ra·phobe** \ˈa-gə-rə-ˌfōb\ *also* **ag·o·ra·pho·bi·ac** \ˌa-gə-rə-ˈfō-bē-ˌak\ *n* : a person affected with agoraphobia

-agra *n comb form* : seizure of pain 〈pellagra〉 〈podagra〉

agram·ma·tism \(ˌ)ā-ˈgra-mə-ˌti-zəm\ *n* : the pathological inability to use words in grammatical sequence

agran·u·lo·cyte \(ˌ)ā-ˈgran-yə-lō-ˌsīt\ *n* : a leukocyte without cytoplasmic granules — compare GRANULOCYTE

agran·u·lo·cyt·ic angina \ˌā-ˌgran-yə-lō-ˈsi-tik-\ *n* : AGRANULOCYTOSIS

agran·u·lo·cy·to·sis \ˌā-ˌgran-yə-lō-ˌsi-ˈtō-səs\ *n, pl* **-to·ses** \-ˌsēz\ : an acute febrile condition marked by severe depression of the granulocyte-producing bone marrow and by prostration, chills, swollen neck, and sore throat sometimes with local ulceration and believed to be basically a response to the side effects of certain drugs of the coal-tar series (as aminopyrine) — called also *agranulocytic angina, granulocytopenia*

agraph·ia \(ˌ)ā-ˈgra-fē-ə\ *n* : the pathological loss of the ability to write — **agraph·ic** \-fik\ *adj*

ague \ˈā-(ˌ)gyü\ *n* **1** : a fever (as malaria) marked by paroxysms of chills, fever, and sweating that recur at regular intervals **2** : a fit of shivering : CHILL

AHF *abbr* **1** antihemophilic factor **2** [*antihemophilic factor*] factor VIII

AHG *abbr* antihemophilic globulin

AI *abbr* artificial insemination

aid \ˈād\ *n* **1** : the act of helping or treating; *also* : the help or treatment given **2** : an assisting person or group 〈a laboratory ~〉 — compare AIDE **3** : something by which assistance is given : an assisting device; *esp* : HEARING AID

AID *abbr* artificial insemination by donor

aide \ˈād\ *n* : a person who acts as an assistant 〈volunteer ~s〉 〈psychiatric ~s〉 — see NURSE'S AIDE

AIDS \ˈādz\ *n* : a disease of the human immune system that is caused by infection with HIV, that is characterized cytologically esp. by reduction in the numbers of CD4-bearing helper T cells to 20 percent or less of normal, that in modern industrialized nations occurs esp. in homosexual and bisexual men and in intravenous users of illicit drugs, that is commonly transmitted in blood and bodily secretions (as semen), and that renders the subject highly vulnerable to life-threatening conditions (as Pneumocystis carinii pneumonia) and to some that become life-threatening (as Kaposi's sarcoma) — called also *acquired immune deficiency syndrome, acquired immunodeficiency syndrome*

AIDS–related complex *n* : a group of symptoms (as fever, weight loss, and lymphadenopathy) that is associated with the presence of antibodies to HIV and is followed by the development of AIDS in a certain proportion of cases — abbr. ARC

AIDS virus n : HIV

AIH abbr artificial insemination by husband

ail *āl\ vb **1** : to affect with an unnamed disease or physical or emotional pain or discomfort — used only of unspecified causes **2** : to be or become affected with pain or discomfort

ail·ment *āl-mənt\ n : a bodily disorder or chronic disease

ai·lu·ro·phobe \ī-*lúr-ə-ˌfōb, ā-\ n : a person who hates or fears cats

ai·lu·ro·pho·bia \-*fō-bē-ə\ n : abnormal fear of cats

air *ar\ n : a mixture of invisible odorless tasteless sound-transmitting gases that is composed by volume chiefly of 78 percent nitrogen, 21 percent oxygen, 0.9 percent argon, 0.03 percent carbon dioxide, varying amounts of water vapor, and minute amounts of rare gases (as helium), that surrounds the earth with half its mass within four miles of the earth's surface, that has a pressure at sea level of about 14.7 pounds per square inch, and that has a density of 1.293 grams per liter at 0°C and 760 mm. pressure

air bends n pl : AEROEMBOLISM

air·borne *ar-ˌbōrn\ adj : carried or transported by the air 〈~ allergens〉 〈~ bacteria〉

air embolism n : obstruction of the circulation by air that has gained entrance to veins usu. through wounds — compare AEROEMBOLISM

air hunger n : deep labored breathing at an increased or decreased rate

air sac n : ALVEOLUS b

air·sick *ar-ˌsik\ adj : affected with motion sickness associated with flying — **air·sick·ness** n

air·way \-ˌwā\ n : a passageway for air into or out of the lungs; specif : a device passed into the trachea by way of the mouth or nose or through an incision to maintain a clear respiratory passageway (as during anesthesia or convulsions)

aka·thi·sia \ˌä-kə-*thi-zhē-ə, -zhə, ˌa-, -*thē-\ n : a condition characterized by uncontrollable motor restlessness

ak·ee *a-kē, a-*kē\ n : the fruit of an African tree (Blighia sapida of the family Sapindaceae) that has edible flesh when ripe but is poisonous when immature or overripe; also : the tree

aki·ne·sia \ˌä-kī-*nē-zhē-ə, -zhə\ n : loss or impairment of voluntary activity (as of a muscle) — **aki·net·ic** \ˌä-kə-*ne-tik, -kī-\ adj

Al symbol aluminum

ala *ā-lə\ n, pl **alae** \-ˌlē\ : a wing or a winglike anatomic process or part; esp : ALA NASI

alaeque — see LEVATOR LABII SUPERIORIS ALAEQUE NASI

ala na·si \-*nā-ˌsī, -ˌzī\ n, pl **alae na·si** \-ˌsī, -ˌzī\: the expanded outer wall of cartilage on each side of the nose

al·a·nine *a-lə-ˌnēn\ n : a simple nonessential crystalline amino acid $C_3H_7NO_2$ formed esp. by the hydrolysis of proteins

alar cartilage *ā-lar-\ n : one of the pair of lower lateral cartilages of the nose

alar ligament n : either of a pair of strong rounded fibrous cords of which one arises on each side of the cranial part of the odontoid process, passes obliquely and laterally upward, and inserts on the medial side of a condyle of the occipital bone — called also check ligament

alarm reaction n : the initial reaction of an organism (as increased hormonal activity) to stress

alas·trim *a-lə-ˌstrim, ˌa-lə-*; ə-*las-trəm\ n : VARIOLA MINOR

alba — see LINEA ALBA, MATERIA ALBA, PHLEGMASIA ALBA DOLENS

Al·bers–Schön·berg disease *al-bərz-*shərn-ˌbərg-, -*shōn-\ n : OSTEOPETROSIS

  Albers–Schönberg, Heinrich Ernst (1865–1921), German roentgenologist.

albicans, albicantia — see CORPUS ALBICANS

albicantes — see LINEAE ALBICANTES

al·bi·nism *al-bə-ˌni-zəm, al-*bī-\ n : the condition of an albino — **al·bi·nis·tic** \ˌal-bə-*nis-tik\ adj

al·bi·no \al-*bī-(ˌ)nō\ n, pl **-nos** : an organism exhibiting deficient pigmentation; esp : a human being who is congenitally deficient in pigment and usu. has a milky or translucent skin, white or colorless hair, and eyes with pink or blue iris and deep-red pupil — **al·bin·ic** \-*bi-nik\ adj

al·bi·not·ic \ˌal-bə-*nä-tik\ adj **1** : of, relating to, or affected with albinism **2** : tending toward albinism

albuginea — see TUNICA ALBUGINEA

al·bu·men \al-*byü-mən; *al-ˌbyü-, -byə-\ n **1** : the white of an egg **2** : ALBUMIN

al·bu·min \al-*byü-mən; *al-ˌbyü-, -byə-\ n : any of numerous simple heat-coagulable water-soluble proteins that occur in blood plasma or serum, muscle, the whites of eggs, milk, and other animal substances and in many plant tissues and fluid

[1]al·bu·min·oid \-mə-ˌnöid\ adj : resembling albumin

[2]albuminoid n **1** : PROTEIN 1 2 : SCLEROPROTEIN

al·bu·min·uria \al-ˌbyü-mə-*nùr-ē-ə, -*nyùr-\ n : the presence of albumin in the urine that is usu. a symptom of disease of the kidneys but sometimes a response to other diseases or physiological disturbances of benign nature — **al·bu·min·uric** \-'nùr-ik, -'nyùr-\ adj

al·cap·ton·uria var of ALKAPTONURIA

al·co·hol \'al-kə-ˌhòl\ n **1 a** : ethanol esp. when considered as the intoxicating agent in fermented and distilled liquors **b** : drink (as whiskey or beer) containing ethanol **c** : a mixture of ethanol and water that is usu. 95 percent ethanol **2** : any of various compounds that are analogous to ethanol in constitution and that are hydroxyl derivatives of hydrocarbons

¹al·co·hol·ic \ˌal-kə-'hò-lik, -'hä-\ adj **1 a** : of, relating to, or caused by alcohol (~ hepatitis) **b** : containing alcohol **2** : affected with alcoholism — **al·co·hol·i·cal·ly** \-li-k(ə-)lē\ adv

²alcoholic n : one affected with alcoholism

al·co·hol·ism \'al-kə-ˌhò-ˌli-zəm, -kə-hə-\ n **1** : continued excessive or compulsive use of alcoholic drinks **2 a** : poisoning by alcohol **b** : a chronic, progressive, potentially fatal, psychological and nutritional disorder associated with excessive and usu. compulsive drinking of ethanol and characterized by frequent intoxication leading to dependence on or addiction to the substance, impairment of the ability to work and socialize, destructive behaviors (as drunken driving), tissue damage (as cirrhosis of the liver), and severe withdrawal symptoms upon detoxification

al·de·hyde \'al-də-ˌhīd\ n : ACETALDEHYDE; broadly : any of various highly reactive compounds typified by acetaldehyde and characterized by the group CHO — **al·de·hy·dic** \ˌal-də-'hī-dik\ adj

al·do·hex·ose \ˌal-dō-'hek-ˌsōs, -ˌsōz\ n : a hexose (as glucose or mannose) of an aldehyde nature

al·dose \'al-ˌdōs, -ˌdōz\ n : a sugar containing one aldehyde group per molecule

al·do·ste·rone \al-'däs-tə-ˌrōn; ˌal-dō-'stir-ˌōn, -stə-'rōn\ n : a steroid hormone $C_{13}H_{16}N_2O$ of the adrenal cortex that functions in the regulation of the salt and water balance of the body

al·do·ste·ron·ism \al-'däs-tə-ˌrō-ˌni-zəm, ˌal-dō-stə-'rō-\ n : a condition that is characterized by excessive secretion of aldosterone and typically by loss of body potassium, muscular weakness, and elevated blood pressure — called also hyperaldosteronism

al·drin \'òl-drən, 'al-\ n : an exceedingly poisonous insecticide $C_{12}H_8Cl_6$
    K. Alder — see DIELDRIN

aleu·ke·mia \ˌā-lü-'kē-mē-ə\ n : leukemia in which the circulating leukocytes are normal or decreased in number; esp : ALEUKEMIC LEUKEMIA

aleu·ke·mic \-'kē-mik\ adj : not marked by increase in circulating white blood cells

aleukemic leukemia n : leukemia resulting from changes in the leukocyte-forming tissues and characterized by a normal or decreased number of leukocytes in the circulating blood — called also aleukemic myelosis

alex·ia \ə-'lek-sē-ə\ n : aphasia characterized by loss of ability to read — **alex·ic** \-'lek-sik\ adj

alex·in \ə-'lek-sən\ n : COMPLEMENT 2 — **al·ex·in·ic** \ˌa-ˌlek-'si-nik\ adj

ALG abbr antilymphocyte globulin; antilymphocytic globulin

alg- or **algo-** comb form : pain ⟨algolagnia⟩

al·ga \'al-gə\ n, pl **al·gae** \'al-(ˌ)jē\ also **algas** : a plant or plantlike organism (as a seaweed) of any of several phyla, divisions, or classes of chiefly aquatic usu. chlorophyll-containing nonvascular organisms including green, yellow-green, brown, and red forms — see BROWN ALGA, RED ALGA — **al·gal** \-gəl\ adj

al·ge·sia \al-'jē-zē-ə, -'jē-zhə\ n : sensitivity to pain — **al·ge·sic** \-'jē-zik, -sik\ adj

-al·gia \'al-jə, -jē-ə\ n comb form : pain ⟨neuralgia⟩

al·gi·cide or **al·gae·cide** \'al-jə-ˌsīd\ n : an agent used to kill algae — **al·gi·cid·al** \ˌal-jə-'sīd-ᵊl\ adj

al·gin \'al-jən\ n : any of various colloidal substances (as an alginate or alginic acid) derived from marine brown algae and used esp. as emulsifiers or thickeners

al·gi·nate \'al-jə-ˌnāt\ n : a salt of alginic acid

al·gin·ic acid \(ˌ)al-'ji-nik-\ n : an insoluble colloidal acid $(C_6H_8O_6)_n$ that is used in making dental preparations and in preparing pharmaceuticals

algo- — see ALG-

al·go·gen·ic \ˌal-gō-'je-nik\ adj : producing pain

al·go·lag·nia \ˌal-gō-'lag-nē-ə\ n : a perversion (as masochism or sadism) in which pleasure and esp. sexual gratification is obtained by inflicting or suffering pain — **al·go·lag·nic** \-nik\ adj

al·gor mor·tis \'al-ˌgòr-'mòr-təs\ n : the gradual cooling of the body following death

ali- comb form : wing or winglike part ⟨alisphenoid⟩

alien·ate \'ā-lē-ə-ˌnāt, 'āl-yə-\ vb **-at·ed; -at·ing** : to make unfriendly, hostile, or indifferent where attachment formerly existed

alien·ation \ˌā-lē-ə-'nā-shən, ˌāl-yə-\ n **1** : a withdrawing or separation of a person or a person's affections from an object or position of former attachment **2** : a state of abnormal function; esp : mental derangement : INSANITY

alien·ist \'ā-lē-ə-nist, 'āl-yə-\ n : PSYCHIATRIST

al·i·men·ta·ry \ˌa-lə-ˈmen-tə-rē, ˈmen-trē\ *adj* : of, concerned with, or relating to nourishment or to the function of nutrition : NUTRITIVE

alimentary canal *n* : the tubular passage that extends from mouth to anus, functions in digestion and absorption of food and elimination of residual waste, and includes the mouth, pharynx, esophagus, stomach, small intestine, and large intestine

alimentary system *n* : the organ system devoted to the ingestion, digestion, and assimilation of food and the discharge of residual wastes and consisting of the alimentary canal and those glands or parts of complex glands that secrete digestive enzymes

al·i·men·ta·tion \ˌa-lə-mən-ˈtā-shən, -ˌmen-\ *n* : the act or process of affording nutriment or nourishment

al·i·phat·ic \ˌa-lə-ˈfa-tik\ *adj* : of, relating to, or being an organic compound having an open-chain structure (as an alkane)

¹**al·i·quot** \ˈa-lə-ˌkwät\ *adj* : being an equal fractional part (as of a solution) — **aliquot** *n*

²**aliquot** *vb* : to divide (as a solution) into equal parts

¹**ali·sphe·noid** \ˌa-ləs-ˈfē-ˌnoid, ˌa-\ *adj* : belonging or relating to or forming the wings of the sphenoid or the pair of bones that fuse with other sphenoidal elements to form the greater wings of the sphenoid in the adult

²**alisphenoid** *n* : an alisphenoid bone; *esp* : GREATER WING

alive \ə-ˈliv\ *adj* : having life : not dead or inanimate

al·ka·lae·mia *chiefly Brit var of* ALKALEMIA

al·ka·le·mia \ˌal-kə-ˈlē-mē-ə\ *n* : a condition in which the hydrogen ion concentration in the blood is decreased

al·ka·li \ˈal-kə-ˌlī\ *n, pl* **-lies** *or* **-lis** : a substance having marked basic properties — compare BASE

alkali disease *n* : SELENOSIS

al·ka·line \ˈal-kə-lən, -ˌlīn\ *adj* : of, relating to, containing, or having the properties of an alkali or alkali metal : BASIC; *esp, of a solution* : having a pH of more than 7 — **al·ka·lin·i·ty** \ˌal-kə-ˈli-nə-tē\ *n*

alkaline phosphatase *n* : any of the phosphatases optimally active in alkaline medium and occurring in esp. high concentrations in bone, the liver, the kidneys, and the placenta

al·ka·lin·ize \ˈal-kə-lə-ˌnīz\ *vb* **-ized; -iz·ing** : to make alkaline — **al·ka·lin·i·za·tion** \ˌal-kə-ˌli-nə-ˈzā-shən, -lə-\ *n*

al·ka·lize \ˈal-kə-ˌlīz\ *vb* **-lized; -liz·ing** : ALKALINIZE — **al·ka·li·za·tion** \ˌal-kə-lə-ˈzā-shən\ *n*

alkali reserve *n* : the concentration of one or more basic ions or substances in a fluid medium that buffer its pH by neutralizing acid; *esp* : the concentration of bicarbonate in the blood

al·ka·liz·er \ˈal-kə-ˌlī-zər\ *n* : an alkalinizing agent

al·ka·loid \ˈal-kə-ˌloid\ *n* : any of numerous usu. colorless, complex, and bitter organic bases (as morphine or codeine) containing nitrogen and usu. oxygen that occur esp. in seed plants — **al·ka·loi·dal** \ˌal-kə-ˈloid-əl\ *adj*

al·ka·lo·sis \ˌal-kə-ˈlō-səs\ *n, pl* **-lo·ses** \-ˌsēz\ : an abnormal condition of increased alkalinity of the blood and tissues — compare ACIDOSIS — **al·ka·lot·ic** \ˌal-kə-ˈlä-tik\ *adj*

al·kane \ˈal-ˌkān\ *n* : any of a series of aliphatic hydrocarbons C_nH_{2n+2} (as methane) in which each carbon is bonded to four other atoms — called also *paraffin*

al·kap·ton·uria \(ˌ)al-ˌkap-tə-ˈnùr-ē-ə, -ˈnyùr-\ *n* : a rare recessive metabolic anomaly marked by inability to complete the degradation of tyrosine and phenylalanine resulting in the presence of homogentisic acid in the urine — **al·kap·ton·uric** \-ˈnùr-ik, -ˈnyùr-\ *n or adj*

al·kene \ˈal-ˌkēn\ *n* : any of numerous unsaturated hydrocarbons having one double bond; *specif* : any of a series of open-chain hydrocarbons C_nH_{2n} (as ethylene)

¹**al·kyl** \ˈal-kəl\ *adj* : having an organic group with a chemical valence of one and esp. one C_nH_{2n+1} (as methyl) derived from an alkane (as methane)

²**alkyl** *n* : a compound of one or more alkyl groups with a metal

al·kyl·ate \ˈal-kə-ˌlāt\ *vb* **-at·ed; -at·ing** : to introduce one or more alkyl groups into (a compound) — **al·kyl·a·tion** \ˌal-kə-ˈlā-shən\ *n*

alkylating agent *n* : a substance that causes replacement of hydrogen by an alkyl group esp. in a biologically important molecule; *specif* : one with mutagenic activity that inhibits cell division and growth and is used to treat some cancers

ALL *abbr* acute lymphoblastic leukemia

all- *or* **allo-** *comb form* **1** : other : different : atypical ⟨allergy⟩ ⟨allopathy⟩ **2** *allo-* : isomeric form or variety of (a specified chemical compound) ⟨allopurinol⟩

al·lan·to·ic \ˌa-lən-ˈtō-ik, -ˌlan-\ *adj* : relating to, contained in, or characterized by an allantois

al·lan·to·in \ə-ˈlan-tə-wən\ *n* : a crystalline oxidation product $C_4H_6N_4O_3$ of uric acid used to promote healing of local wounds and infections

al·lan·to·is \ə-ˈlan-tə-wəs\ *n, pl* **al·lan·to·ides** \ˌa-lan-ˈtō-ə-ˌdēz, -ˌlan-\ : a vascular fetal membrane that is formed as a pouch from the hindgut and that in placental mammals is intimately associated with the chorion in formation of the placenta

al·lele \ə-ˈlēl\ *n* **1** : any of the alternative forms of a gene that may occur at a given locus **2** : either of a pair of alternative Mendelian characters (as ability versus inability to taste the chemical phenylthiocarbamide) — **al·le·lic** \ə-ˈlē-lik, -ˈle-\ *adj* — **al·lel·ism** \-ˈlē-ˌli-zəm, -ˈle-\ *n*

allele- *comb form* : alternative ⟨allelomorph⟩

al·le·lo·morph \ə-ˈlē-lə-ˌmȯrf, -ˈlē-\ *n* : ALLELE — **al·le·lo·mor·phic** \ə-ˌlē-lə-ˈmȯr-fik, -ˌlē-\ *adj* — **al·le·lo·mor·phism** \ə-ˈlē-lə-ˌmȯr-ˌfi-zəm, -ˈlē-\ *n*

al·ler·gen \ˈa-lər-jən\ *n* : a substance that induces allergy

al·ler·gen·ic \ˌa-lər-ˈje-nik\ *adj* : having the capacity to induce allergy ⟨∼ plants⟩ — **al·ler·ge·nic·i·ty** \-jə-ˈni-sə-tē\ *n*

al·ler·gic \ə-ˈlər-jik\ *adj* **1** : of, relating to, or characterized by allergy ⟨an ∼ reaction⟩ **2** : affected with allergy : subject to an allergic reaction

allergic encephalomyelitis *n* : encephalomyelitis produced by an allergic response following the introduction of an antigenic substance into the body

al·ler·gist \-jist\ *n* : a specialist in allergy

al·ler·gol·o·gy \ˌa-lər-ˈjä-lə-jē\ *n*, *pl* **-gies** : a branch of medicine concerned with allergy

al·ler·gy \ˈa-lər-jē\ *n*, *pl* **-gies 1** : altered bodily reactivity (as hypersensitivity) to an antigen in response to a first exposure **2** : exaggerated or pathological reaction (as by sneezing, respiratory embarrassment, itching, or skin rashes) to substances, situations, or physical states that are without comparable effect on the average individual **3** : medical practice concerned with allergies

al·le·thrin \ˈa-lə-thrən\ *n* : a light yellow oily synthetic insecticide $C_{19}H_{26}O_3$ used esp. in household aerosols

al·le·vi·ate \ə-ˈlē-vē-ˌāt\ *vb* **-at·ed; -at·ing** : to make (as symptoms) less severe or more bearable — **al·le·vi·a·tion** \-ˌlē-vē-ˈā-shən\ *n*

al·le·vi·a·tive \ə-ˈlē-vē-ˌā-tiv\ *adj* : tending to alleviate : PALLIATIVE ⟨a medicine that is ∼ but not curative⟩

al·li·cin \ˈa-lə-sən\ *n* : a liquid compound $C_6H_{10}OS_2$ with a garlic odor and antibacterial properties

allo- — see ALL-

al·lo·an·ti·body \ˌa-lō-ˈan-ti-ˌbä-dē\ *n*, *pl* **-bod·ies** : an antibody produced following introduction of an alloantigen into the system of an individual of a species lacking that particular antigen — called also *isoantibody*

al·lo·an·ti·gen \ˌa-lō-ˈan-tə-jən\ *n* : a genetically determined antigen present in some but not all individuals of a species (as those of a particular blood group) and capable of inducing the production of an alloantibody by individuals which lack it — called also *isoantigen* — **al·lo·an·ti·gen·ic** \-ˌan-tə-ˈje-nik\ *adj*

al·lo·bar·bi·tal \ˌa-lə-ˈbär-bə-ˌtȯl\ *n* : a white crystalline barbiturate $C_{10}H_{12}N_2O_3$ used as a sedative and hypnotic

al·lo·bar·bi·tone \-ˌtōn\ *n*, *chiefly Brit* : ALLOBARBITAL

al·lo·cor·tex \-ˈkȯr-ˌteks\ *n* : ARCHIPALLIUM

Al·lo·der·ma·nys·sus \-ˌdər-mə-ˈni-səs\ *n* : a genus of bloodsucking mites parasitic on rodents including one (*A. sanguineus*) implicated as a vector of rickettsialpox in humans

al·lo·ge·ne·ic \ˌa-lō-jə-ˈnē-ik\ *also* **al·lo·gen·ic** \-ˈje-nik\ *adj* : involving, derived from, or being individuals of the same species that are sufficiently unlike genetically to interact antigenically ⟨∼ skin grafts⟩ — compare SYNGENEIC, XENOGENEIC

al·lo·graft \ˈa-lə-ˌgraft\ *n* : a homograft between allogeneic individuals — **allograft** *vb*

al·lo·iso·leu·cine \ˌa-lō-ˌī-sə-ˈlü-ˌsēn\ *n* : either of two stereoisomers of isoleucine of which one is present in bodily fluids of individuals affected with maple syrup urine disease

al·lo·path \ˈa-lə-ˌpath\ *n* : one who practices allopathy

al·lop·a·thy \ə-ˈlä-pə-thē, a-\ *n*, *pl* **-thies 1** : a system of medical practice that aims to combat disease by use of remedies producing effects different from those produced by the special disease treated **2** : a system of medical practice making use of all measures that have proved of value in treatment of disease — compare HOMEOPATHY — **al·lo·path·ic** \ˌa-lə-ˈpa-thik\ *adj* — **al·lo·path·i·cal·ly** \-thi-k(ə-)lē\ *adv*

al·lo·pu·ri·nol \ˌa-lō-ˈpyu̇r-ə-ˌnȯl, -ˌnōl\ *n* : a drug $C_5H_4N_4O$ used to promote excretion of uric acid esp. in the treatment of gout

all—or—none *adj* : marked either by complete operation or effect or by none at all ⟨∼ response of a nerve cell⟩

all—or—none law *n* : a principle in physiology: in any single nerve or muscle fiber the response to a stimulus above threshold level is maximal and independent of the intensity of the stimulus

all—or—noth·ing *adj* : ALL-OR-NONE

al·lo·ste·ric \ˌa-lō-ˈster-ik, -ˈstir-\ *adj* : of, relating to, or being a change in the shape and activity of a protein (as an enzyme) that results from combination with another substance at a point other than the chemically active site — **al·lo·ste·ri·cal·ly** \-i-k(ə-)lē\ *adv*

al·lo·trans·plant \ˌa-lō-trans-ˈplant\ *vb* : to transplant between genetically different individuals — **al·lo·trans·plant** \-ˈtrans-\ *n* — **al·lo·trans·plan·ta·tion** \-ˌtrans-ˌplan-ˈtā-shən\ *n*

al·lo·type \ˈa-lə-ˌtip\ *n* : an alloantigen

that is part of a plasma protein (as an antibody) — compare IDIOTYPE, ISO-TYPE — **al·lo·typ·ic** \,a-lə-'ti-pik\ adj — **al·lo·typ·i·cal·ly** \-pi-k(ə-)lē\ adv — **al·lo·typy** \'a-lə-,tī-pē\ n

al·lox·an \ə-'läk-sən\ n : a crystalline compound $C_4H_2N_2O_4$ causing diabetes mellitus when injected into experimental animals — called also *mesoxalylurea*

al·loy \'a-,lòi, ə-'lòi\ n : a substance composed of two or more metals or of a metal and a nonmetal intimately united usu. by being fused together and dissolving in each other when molten; *also* : the state of union of the components — **al·loy** \ə-'lòi, 'a-,lòi\ vb

al·lo·zyme \'a-lə-,zīm\ n : any of the variants of an enzyme that are determined by alleles at a single genetic locus — **al·lo·zy·mic** \,a-lə-'zī-mik\ adj

al·lyl \'a-lēl\ n : an unsaturated radical C_3H_5 compounds of which are found in the oils of garlic and mustard — **al·lyl·ic** \ə-'li-lik, a-\ adj

allyl iso·thio·cy·a·nate \-,ī-sō-,thī-ə-'sī-ə-,nāt, -nət\ n : a colorless pungent irritating liquid ester C_4H_5NS that is the chief constituent of mustard oil used in medicine and is used as a medical counterirritant

N–al·lyl·nor·mor·phine \,en-,al-əl-,nòr-'mòr-,fēn\ n : NALORPHINE

al·oe \'a-(,)lō\ n 1 cap : a large genus of succulent chiefly southern African plants of the lily family (Liliaceae) 2 : a plant of the genus *Aloe* 3 : the dried juice of the leaves of various aloes used esp. formerly as a purgative and tonic — usu. used in pl. with a sing. verb

aloe vera \-'ver-ə, -'vir-\ n : an aloe (*Aloe barbadensis*) whose leaves furnish an emollient extract used esp. in cosmetics and skin creams; *also* : such a preparation

al·o·in \'a-lə-wən\ n : a bitter yellow crystalline cathartic obtained from the aloe and containing one or more glycosides

al·o·pe·cia \,a-lə-'pē-shē-ə, -shə\ n : loss of hair, wool, or feathers : BALDNESS — **al·o·pe·cic** \-'pē-sik\ adj

alopecia ar·e·a·ta \-,ar-ē-'ā-tə, -'ä-\ n : sudden loss of hair in circumscribed patches with little or no inflammation

¹**al·pha** \'al-fə\ n 1 : the 1st letter of the Greek alphabet — symbol A or α 2 : ALPHA RAY

²**alpha** or **al-** adj 1 : of or relating to one of two or more closely related chemical substances (the *alpha* chain of hemoglobin) — used somewhat arbitrarily to specify ordinal relationship or a particular physical form 2 : closest in position in the structure of an organic molecule to a particular group or atom; *also* : of, relating to, or having a structure characterized by such a position (α-substitution)

al·pha–ad·ren·er·gic \'al-fə-,a-drə-'nər-jik\ adj : of, relating to, or being an alpha-receptor (~ blocking action)

al·pha–ad·re·no·cep·tor \-ə-'drē-nə-,sep-tər\ *also* **al·pha–ad·re·no·cep·tor** \-ri-,sep-tər\ n : ALPHA-RECEPTOR

al·pha–ami·no acid or **α–ami·no acid** \-ə-'mē-nō-\ n : any of the more than 20 amino acids that have an amino group in the alpha position with most having the general formula $RCH-(NH_2)COOH$, that are synthesized in plant and animal tissues, that are considered the building blocks of proteins from which they can be obtained by hydrolysis, and that play an important role in metabolism, growth, maintenance, and repair of tissue

alpha cell n : an acidophilic glandular cell (as of the pancreas or the adenohypophysis) — compare BETA CELL

alpha–fetoprotein or **α–fetoprotein** n : a fetal blood protein present abnormally in adults with some forms of cancer (as of the liver) and normally in the amniotic fluid of pregnant women with very low levels tending to be associated with Down's syndrome in the fetus and very high levels with neural tube defects (as spina bifida) in which the tube remains open

alpha globulin n : any of several globulins of plasma or serum that have at alkaline pH the greatest electrophoretic mobility next to albumin — compare BETA GLOBULIN, GAMMA GLOBULIN

al·pha–he·lix or **α–he·lix** \,al-fə-'hē-liks\ n : the coiled structural arrangement of many proteins consisting of a single chain of amino acids stabilized by hydrogen bonds — compare DOUBLE HELIX — **al·pha–he·li·cal** \-'he-li-kəl, -'hē-\ adj

al·pha–ke·to·glu·tar·ic acid \-,kē-tō-glü-'tar-ik-\ n : the alpha keto isomer of ketoglutaric acid formed in various metabolic processes (as the Krebs cycle)

alpha–lipoprotein or **α–lipoprotein** n : HDL

al·pha–1–an·ti·tryp·sin \-,wən-,an-ti-'trip-sən, -,tī-\ n : a trypsin-inhibiting serum protein whose deficiency has been implicated as a factor in emphysema

alpha particle n : a positively charged nuclear particle identical with the nucleus of a helium atom that consists of two protons and two neutrons and is ejected at high speed in certain radioactive transformations

alpha ray n 1 : an alpha particle moving at high speed (as in radioactive emission) 2 : a stream of alpha particles — called also *alpha radiation*

al·pha–re·cep·tor \'al-fə-ri-,sep-tər\ n : any of a group of receptors postulated to exist on nerve cell membranes of the sympathetic nervous system to explain the specificity of certain adrenergic agents in affecting only some sympathetic activities (as vasoconstriction, relaxation of intestinal muscle, and contraction of most smooth muscle) — compare BETA-RECEPTOR

al·pha–to·coph·er·ol \al-fə-tō-ˈkä-fə-ˌrȯl, -ˌrōl\ n : a tocopherol $C_{29}H_{50}O_2$ with high vitamin E potency — called also *vitamin E*

alpha wave n : an electrical rhythm of the brain with a frequency of 8 to 13 cycles per second that is often associated with a state of wakeful relaxation — called also *alpha rhythm*

al·praz·o·lam \al-ˈpraz-ə-ˌlam\ n : a benzodiazepine tranquilizer $C_{17}H_{13}$-ClN_4 used esp. in the treatment of mild to moderate anxiety — see XANAX

al·pren·o·lol \al-ˈpre-nə-ˌlȯl, -ˌlōl\ n : a beta-adrenergic blocking agent $C_{15}H_{23}NO_2$ that has been used as the hydrochloride in the treatment of cardiac arrhythmias

ALS abbr **1** amyotrophic lateral sclerosis **2** antilymphocyte serum; antilymphocytic serum

al·ser·ox·y·lon \ˌal-sə-ˈräk-sə-ˌlän\ n : a complex extract from a rauwolfia (*Rauwolfia serpentina*) that has a physiological action resembling but milder than that of reserpine

al·ter \ˈȯl-tər\ vb **al·tered; al·ter·ing** : CASTRATE, SPAY

al·ter·a·tive \ˈȯl-tə-ˌrā-tiv, -rə-\ n : a drug used empirically to alter favorably the course of an ailment

altered state of consciousness n : any of various states of awareness that deviate from and are usu. clearly demarcated from ordinary waking consciousness

alternans — see PULSUS ALTERNANS

al·ter·nate host \ˈȯl-tər-nət-\ n : INTERMEDIATE HOST 1

alternating personality n : MULTIPLE PERSONALITY

alternation of generations n : the occurrence of two or more forms differently produced in the life cycle of a plant or animal usu. involving the regular alternation of a sexual with an asexual generation

altitude sickness n : the effects (as nosebleed or nausea) of oxygen deficiency in the blood and tissues developed in rarefied air at high altitudes

al·um \ˈa-ləm\ n : a potassium aluminum sulfate $KAl(SO_4)_2 \cdot 12H_2O$ or an ammonium aluminum sulfate NH_4-$Al(SO_4)_2 \cdot 12H_2O$ used esp. as an emetic and as an astringent and styptic

alu·mi·na \ə-ˈlü-mə-nə\ n : an oxide of aluminum Al_2O_3 that occurs native as corundum and in hydrated forms and is used in antacids — called also *aluminum oxide*

al·u·min·i·um \ˌal-yü-ˈmi-nē-əm\ n, chiefly Brit : ALUMINUM

alu·mi·num \ə-ˈlü-mə-nəm\ n, often attrib : a bluish silver-white malleable ductile light trivalent metallic element — symbol Al; see ELEMENT table

aluminum chloride n : a deliquescent compound $AlCl_3$ or Al_2Cl_3 that is used as a topical astringent and antiseptic on the skin, in some deodorants to control sweating, and in the anhydrous form as a catalyst

aluminum hydroxide n : any of several white gelatinous or crystalline hydrates $Al_2O_3 \cdot nH_2O$ of alumina; esp : one $Al_2O_3 \cdot 3H_2O$ or $Al(OH)_3$ used in medicine as an antacid

aluminum oxide n : ALUMINA

aluminum sulfate n : a colorless salt $Al_2(SO_4)_3$ that is a powerful astringent and is used as a local antiperspirant and in water purification

Al·u·pent \ˈa-lü-ˌpent\ trademark — used for a preparation of the sulfate of metaproterenol

alvei pl of ALVEUS

alveol- or **alveolo-** comb form : alveolus 〈alveolectomy〉

al·ve·o·lar \al-ˈvē-ə-lər\ adj : of, relating to, resembling, or having alveoli; esp : of, relating to, or constituting the part of the jaws where the teeth arise, the air-containing cells of the lungs, or glands with secretory cells about a central space

alveolar arch n : the arch of the upper or lower jaw formed by the alveolar processes

alveolar artery n : any of several arteries supplying the teeth; esp : POSTERIOR SUPERIOR ALVEOLAR ARTERY — compare INFERIOR ALVEOLAR ARTERY

alveolar canals n pl : the canals in the jawbones for the passage of the dental nerves and associated vessels

alveolar ducts n pl : the somewhat enlarged terminal sections of the bronchioles that branch into the terminal alveoli

alveolar process n : the bony ridge or raised thickened border on each side of the upper or lower jaw that contains the sockets of the teeth — called also *alveolar ridge*

al·ve·o·lec·to·my \al-ˌvē-ə-ˈlek-tə-mē, ˌal-vē-\ n, pl **-mies** : surgical excision of a portion of an alveolar process usu. as an aid in fitting dentures

al·ve·o·li·tis \al-ˌvē-ə-ˈlī-təs, ˌal-vē-\ n : inflammation of one or more alveoli esp. of the lung

al·ve·o·lo·plas·ty \al-ˈvē-ə-(ˌ)lō-ˌplas-tē\ or **al·veo·plas·ty** \ˈal-vē-ō-\ n, pl **-ties** : surgical shaping of the dental alveoli and alveolar processes esp. after extraction of several teeth or in preparation for dentures

al·ve·o·lus \al-ˈvē-ə-ləs\ n, pl **-li** \-ˌlī, -(ˌ)lē\ : a small cavity or pit: as a : a socket for a tooth b : an air cell of the lungs c : an acinus of a compound gland **d** : any of the pits in the wall of the stomach into which the glands open

al·ve·us \\'al-vē-əs\ *n, pl* **al·vei** \-vē-ı̄, -ē\ : a thin layer of medullary nerve fibers on the ventricular surface of the hippocampus

Alz·hei·mer's disease \\'älts-ı̄-hī-mərz-, 'alts-\ *n* : a degenerative disease of the central nervous system characterized esp. by premature senile mental deterioration — called also *Alzheimer's;* see NEUROFIBRILLARY TANGLE; compare PRESENILE DEMENTIA

Alzheimer, Alois (1864–1915), German neurologist.

Am *symbol* americium

AMA *abbr* **1** against medical advice **2** American Medical Association

am·a·crine cell \\'a-mə-krın-, (ı)ā-'ma-ı̄krin-\ *n* : a unipolar nerve cell found in the retina, in the olfactory bulb, and in close connection with the Purkinje cells of the cerebellum

amal·gam \ə-'mal-gəm\ *n* : an alloy of mercury with another metal that is solid or liquid at room temperature according to the proportion of mercury present and is used esp. in making tooth cements

am·a·ni·ta \ua-mə-'nī-tə, -'nē-\ *n* **1** *cap* : a genus of widely distributed whitespored basidiomycetous fungi that includes some deadly poisonous forms (as the death cap) **2** : a fungus of the genus *Amanita*

am·a·ni·tin \-'nit-ᵊn, -'nēt-\ *n* : a highly toxic cyclic peptide produced by the death cap (*Amanita phalloides*) that selectively inhibits mammalian RNA polymerase

aman·ta·dine \ə-'man-tə-ıdēn\ *n* : a drug used esp. as the hydrochloride $C_{10}H_{17}N \cdot HCl$ to prevent infection (as by an influenza virus) by interfering with virus penetration into host cells and in the treatment of Parkinson's disease — see SYMMETREL

Am·a·ran·thus \ıa-mə-'ran-thəs\ *n* : a large genus of coarse herbs (family Amaranthaceae including some which produce pollen that is an important hay fever allergen

amas·tia \(ı)ā-'mas-tē-ə\ *n* : the absence or underdevelopment of the mammary glands

am·au·ro·sis \ıa-mȯ-'rō-səs\ *n, pl* **-ro·ses** \-ısēz\ : partial or complete loss of sight occurring esp. without an externally perceptible change in the eye — **am·au·rot·ic** \-'rä-tik\ *adj*

amaurosis fu·gax \\'fü-ıgaks, -'fyü-\ *n* : temporary partial or complete loss of sight esp. from the effects of excessive acceleration (as in flight)

amaurotic idiocy *n* : any of several recessive genetic conditions characterized by the accumulation of lipidcontaining cells in the viscera and nervous system, mental retardation,

and impaired vision or blindness; *esp* : TAY-SACHS DISEASE

ambi- *prefix* : both ⟨*ambi*valence⟩ ⟨*ambi*sexuality⟩

am·bi·dex·ter·i·ty \ıam-bi-(ı)dek-'ster-ə-tē\ *n, pl* **-ties** : the quality or state of being ambidextrous

am·bi·dex·trous \ıam-bi-'dek-strəs\ *adj* : using both hands with equal ease — **am·bi·dex·trous·ly** *adv*

am·bi·ent \\'am-bē-ənt\ *adj* : surrounding on all sides ⟨∼ air pollution⟩

ambiguus — see NUCLEUS AMBIGUUS

am·bi·sex·u·al \ıam-bi-'sek-shə-wəl\ *adj* : BISEXUAL — **ambisexual** *n* — **am·bi·sex·u·al·i·ty** \-ısek-shə-'wa-lə-tē\ *n*

am·biv·a·lence \am-'bi-və-ləns\ *also* **am·biv·a·len·cy** \-lən-sē\ *n, pl* **-ces** *also* **-cies** : simultaneous and contradictory attitudes or feelings (as attraction and repulsion) toward an object, person, or action — **am·biv·a·lent** \-lənt\ *adj* — **am·biv·a·lent·ly** *adv*

am·bi·ver·sion \ıam-bi-'vər-zhən, -shən\ *n* : the personality configuration of an ambivert — **am·bi·ver·sive** \-'vər-siv, -ziv\ *adj*

am·bi·vert \\'am-bi-ıvərt\ *n* : a person having characteristics of both extrovert and introvert

ambly- *or* **amblyo-** *comb form* : connected with amblyopia ⟨*amblyo*scope⟩

Am·bly·om·ma \ıam-blē-'ä-mə\ *n* : a genus of ixodid ticks including the lone star tick (*A. americanum*) of the southern U.S. and the African bont tick (*A. hebraeum*)

am·bly·ope \\'am-blē-ıōp\ *n* : an individual affected with amblyopia

am·bly·opia \ıam-blē-'ō-pē-ə\ *n* : dimness of sight esp. in one eye without apparent change in the eye structures — called also *lazy eye, lazy-eye blindness* — **am·bly·opic** \-'ō-pik, -'ä-\ *adj*

am·bly·o·scope \\'am-blē-ə-ıskōp\ *n* : an instrument for training amblyopic eyes to function properly

Am·bro·sia \am-'brō-zhə, -zhē-ə\ *n* : a genus of mostly American composite herbs that includes the ragweeds

am·bu·lance \\'am-byə-ləns\ *n* : a vehicle equipped for transporting the injured or sick

am·bu·lant \\'am-byə-lənt\ *adj* : walking or in a walking position; *specif* : AMBULATORY ⟨an ∼ patient⟩

am·bu·late \-ılāt\ *vb* **-lat·ed; -lat·ing** : to move from place to place — **am·bu·la·tion** \ıam-byə-'lā-shən\ *n*

am·bu·la·to·ry \\'am-byə-lə-ıtȯr-ē\ *adj* **1** : of, relating to, or adapted to walking **2 a** : able to walk about and not bedridden ⟨an ∼ patient⟩ **b** : performed on or involving an ambulatory patient or an outpatient ⟨an ∼ electrocardiogram⟩ ⟨∼ medical care⟩ — **am·bu·la·to·ri·ly** \ıam-byə-lə-'tȯr-ə-lē\ *adv*

ame·ba \ə-'mē-bə\ *n, pl* **-bas** *or* **-bae** \-(ı)bē\ : a protozoan of the genus

Amoeba; broadly : an ameboid protozoan (as a naked rhizopod) — **ame·bic** \-bik\ *adj*

am·e·bi·a·sis \₁a-mi-'bī-ə-səs\ *n, pl* **-a·ses** \-₁sēz\ : infection with or disease caused by amebas

amebic abscess *n* : a specific purulent invasive lesion commonly of the liver caused by parasitic amebas (esp. *Entamoeba histolytica*)

amebic dysentery *n* : acute human intestinal amebiasis caused by a common ameba of the genus *Entamoeba* (*E. histolytica*) and marked by dysentery, griping, and erosion of the intestinal wall

ame·bi·cide \ə-'mē-bə-₁sīd\ *n* : a substance used to kill or capable of killing amebas and esp. parasitic amebas — **ame·bi·cid·al** \ə-₁mē-bə-'sīd-ᵊl\ *adj*

ame·bo·cyte \ə-'mē-bə-₁sīt\ *n* : a cell (as a phagocyte) having ameboid form or movements

ame·boid \-₁bȯid\ *adj* : resembling an ameba specif. in moving or changing shape by means of protoplasmic flow

amel·a·not·ic \₁ā-₁mel-ə-'nä-tik\ *adj* : containing little or no melanin (∼ melanocytes)

ame·lia \ə-'mē-lē-ə, (₁)ā-\ *n* : congenital absence of one or more limbs

am·e·lo·blast \'a-mə-lō-₁blast\ *n* : any of a group of columnar cells that produce and deposit enamel on the surface of a developing tooth — **ame·lo·blas·tic** \₁a-mə-lō-'blas-tik\ *adj*

am·e·lo·blas·to·ma \₁a-mə-lō-blas-'tō-mə\ *n, pl* **-mas** *or* **-ma·ta** \-mə-tə\ : a tumor of the jaw derived from remnants of the embryonic rudiment of tooth enamel — called also *adamantinoma*

am·e·lo·den·tin·al \-'den-₁tēn-ᵊl, -den-'tēn-\ *adj* : of or relating to enamel and dentin

am·e·lo·gen·e·sis \-'je-nə-səs\ *n, pl* **-e·ses** \-₁sēz\ : the process of forming tooth enamel

amelogenesis im·per·fec·ta \-₁im-(₁)pər-'fek-tə\ *n* : faulty development of tooth enamel that is genetically determined

amen·or·rhea \₁ā-₁me-nə-'rē-ə, ₁ā-\ *n* : abnormal absence or suppression of menstruation — **amen·or·rhe·ic** \-'rē-ik\ *adj*

amen·tia \(₁)ā-'men-chē-ə, -chə, -₁chä-\ *n* : MENTAL RETARDATION; *specif* : a condition of lack of development of intellectual capacity — compare DEMENTIA

American cockroach *n* : a free-flying cockroach (*Periplaneta americana*) that is a common domestic pest infesting ships or buildings in the northern hemisphere

American dog tick *n* : a common No. American ixodid tick of the genus *Dermacentor* (*D. variabilis*) esp. of dogs and humans that is an important vector of Rocky Mountain spotted fever and tularemia — called also *dog tick*

am·er·i·ci·um \₁a-mə-'ri-shē-əm, -sē-\ *n* : a radioactive metallic element produced by bombardment of plutonium with high-energy neutrons — symbol *Am*; see ELEMENT table

Ames test \'āmz-\ *n* : a test for identifying potential carcinogens by studying the frequency with which they cause histidine-producing genetic mutants in bacterial colonies of the genus *Salmonella* (*S. typhimurium*) initially lacking the ability to synthesize histidine

   Ames, Bruce Nathan (*b* 1928), American biochemist.

ameth·o·caine \ə-'me-thə-₁kān\ *n* : TETRACAINE

am·e·thop·ter·in \₁a-mə-'thäp-tə-rən\ *n* : METHOTREXATE

am·e·tro·pia \₁a-mə-'trō-pē-ə\ *n* : an abnormal refractive eye condition (as myopia, hyperopia, or astigmatism) in which images fail to focus upon the retina — **am·e·tro·pic** \-'trō-pik, -'trä-\ *adj*

AMI *abbr* acute myocardial infarction

am·ide \'am-₁īd, -əd\ *n* : a compound resulting from replacement of an atom of hydrogen in ammonia by an element or radical or of one or more atoms of hydrogen in ammonia by acid radicals having a chemical valence of one

am·i·done \'a-mə-₁dōn\ *n* : METHADONE

amil·o·ride \ə-'mil-ə-₁rīd\ *n* : a diuretic $C_6H_8ClN_7O$ that promotes sodium excretion and potassium retention

amine \ə-'mēn, 'a-₁mēn\ *n* : any of a class of organic compounds derived from ammonia by replacement of hydrogen by one or more alkyl groups

ami·no \ə-'mē-(₁)nō\ *adj* : relating to, being, or containing the amine group NH_2 or a substituted group NHR or NR_2 united to a radical other than an acid radical — often used in combination

amino acid *n* : an amphoteric organic acid containing the amino group NH_2; *esp* : ALPHA-AMINO ACID

ami·no·ac·i·de·mia \ə-₁mē-nō-₁a-sə-'dē-mē-ə\ *n* : a condition in which the concentration of amino acids in the blood is abnormally increased

ami·no·ac·id·uria \-₁a-sə-'dùr-ē-ə, -'dyùr-\ *n* : a condition in which one or more amino acids are excreted in excessive amounts

ami·no·ben·zo·ic acid \-₁mē-nō-ben-'zō-ik-\ *n* : any of three crystalline derivatives $C_7H_7NO_2$ of benzoic acid; *esp* : PARA-AMINOBENZOIC ACID

γ-aminobutyric acid *var of* GAMMA-AMINOBUTYRIC ACID

ami·no·glu·teth·i·mide \-glü-'te-thə-₁mīd\ *n* : a glutethimide derivative $C_{13}H_{16}N_2O_2$ used esp. as an anticonvulsant

ami·no·gly·co·side \-'glī-kə-₁sīd\ *n* : any

of a group of antibiotics (as strepto-mycin and neomycin) that inhibit bacterial protein synthesis and are active esp. against gram-negative bacteria

ami·no·pep·ti·dase \ə-ˌmē-nō-ˈpep-tə-ˌdās, -ˌdāz\ n : an enzyme (as one found in the duodenum) that hydro-lyzes peptides

am·i·noph·yl·line \ˌa-mə-ˈnä-fə-lən\ n : a theophylline derivative $C_{16}H_{24}$-$N_{10}O_4$ used esp. to stimulate the heart in congestive heart failure and to dilate the air passages in respirato-ry disorders — called also *theophyl-line ethylenediamine*

β–ami·no·pro·pio·ni·trile \ˌbā-tə-ə-ˌmē-nō-ˌprō-pē-ō-ˈnī-trəl, -ˌtril\ n : a potent lathyrogen $C_3H_6N_2$

ami·nop·ter·in \ˌa-mə-ˈnäp-tə-rən\ n : a derivative of glutamic acid C_{19}-$H_{20}N_8O_5$ used esp. as a rodenticide

ami·no·py·rine \ə-ˌmē-nō-ˈpir-ˌēn\ n : a white crystalline compound $C_{13}H_{17}$-N_3O formerly used to relieve pain and fever but now largely abandoned for this purpose because of the occur-rence of fatal agranulocytosis as a side effect in some users

ami·no·sal·i·cyl·ic acid \ə-ˌmē-nō-ˌsa-lə-ˈsi-lik-\ n : any of four isomeric deriv-atives $C_7H_8O_3N$ of salicylic acid that have a single amino group; *esp* : PARA-AMINOSALICYLIC ACID

ami·no·thi·a·zole \ə-ˌmē-nō-ˈthī-ə-ˌzōl\ n : a light yellow crystalline heterocy-clic amine $C_3H_4N_2S$ that has been used as a thyroid inhibitor in the treatment of hyperthyroidism

ami·no·trans·fer·ase \-ˈtrans-fə-ˌrās, -ˌrāz\ n : TRANSAMINASE

am·i·trip·ty·line \ˌa-mə-ˈtrip-tə-ˌlēn\ n : a tricyclic antidepressant drug $C_{20}H_{23}N$ administered as the hydro-chloride salt

am·mo·nia \ə-ˈmō-nyə\ n 1 : a pungent colorless gaseous alkaline compound of nitrogen and hydrogen NH_3 that is very soluble in water and can easily be condensed to a liquid by cold and pressure 2 : AMMONIA WATER

am·mo·ni·a·cal \ˌa-mə-ˈnī-ə-kəl\ *also* **am·mo·ni·ac** \ə-ˈmō-nē-ˌak\ *adj* : of, relating to, containing, or having the properties of ammonia

ammonia water n : a water solution of ammonia — called also *spirit of hartshorn*

am·mo·ni·um \ə-ˈmō-nē-əm\ n : an ion NH_4^+ derived from ammonia by combination with a hydrogen ion

ammonium carbonate n : a carbonate of ammonium; *specif* : the commer-cial mixture of the bicarbonate and carbamate used esp. in smelling salts

ammonium chloride n : a white crystal-line volatile salt NH_4Cl that is used in dry cells and as an expectorant — called also *sal ammoniac*

ammonium nitrate n : a colorless crys-talline salt $N_2H_4NO_3$ used in veteri-nary medicine as an expectorant and urinary acidifier

ammonium sulfate n : a colorless crys-talline salt $(NH_4)_2SO_4$ used in medi-cine as a local analgesic

am·ne·sia \am-ˈnē-zhə\ n 1 : loss of memory sometimes including the memory of personal identity due to brain injury, shock, fatigue, repres-sion, or illness or sometimes induced by anesthesia 2 : a gap in one's mem-ory

am·ne·si·ac \am-ˈnē-zhē-ˌak, -zē-\ *also* **am·ne·sic** \-zik, -sik\ n : a person af-fected with amnesia

am·ne·sic \am-ˈnē-zik, -sik\ *also* **am·ne·si·ac** \-zhē-ˌak, -zē-\ *adj* : of or re-lating to amnesia : affected with or caused by amnesia ⟨an ~ patient⟩

am·nes·tic \am-ˈnes-tik\ *adj* : AMNESI-AC; *also* : causing amnesia ⟨~ agents⟩

amnii — see LIQUOR AMNII

amnio- *comb form* : amnion ⟨*amnio-centesis*⟩

am·nio·cen·te·sis \ˌam-nē-ō-(ˌ)sen-ˈtē-səs\ n, pl **-te·ses** \-ˌsēz\ : the surgical insertion of a hollow needle through the abdominal wall and into the uter-us of a pregnant female to obtain am-niotic fluid esp. to examine the fetal chromosomes for an abnormality and for the determination of sex

am·ni·og·ra·phy \ˌam-nē-ˈä-grə-fē\ n, pl **-phies** : radiographic visualization of the outlines of the uterine cavity, pla-centa, and fetus after injection of a ra-diopaque substance into the amnion

am·ni·on \ˈam-nē-ˌän, -ən\ n, pl **amni-ons** *or* **am·nia** \-nē-ə\ : a thin mem-brane forming a closed sac about the embryos of reptiles, birds, and mam-mals and containing a serous fluid in which the embryo is immersed

am·nio·scope \ˈam-nē-ə-ˌskōp\ n : an endoscope for observation of the am-nion and its contents

am·ni·os·co·py \ˌam-nē-ˈäs-kə-pē\ n, pl **-pies** : visual observation of the amni-on and its contents by means of an endoscope

am·ni·ote \ˈam-nē-ˌōt\ n : any of a group (Amniota) of vertebrates that undergo embryonic development within an amnion and include the birds, reptiles, and mammals — **amniote** *adj*

am·ni·ot·ic \ˌam-nē-ˈä-tik\ *adj* 1 : of or relating to the amnion 2 : character-ized by the development of an amni-on

amniotic band n : a band of fibrous tis-sue extending between the embryo and amnion and often associated with faulty development of the fetus

amniotic cavity n : the fluid-filled space between the amnion and the fetus

amniotic fluid n : the serous fluid in which the embryo is suspended with-in the amnion

amniotic sac n : AMNION

am·ni·ot·o·my \ˌam-nē-ˈä-tə-mē\ n, pl

-mies : intentional rupture of the fetal membranes to induce or facilitate labor

amo·bar·bi·tal \ˌa-mō-ˈbär-bə-ˌtòl\ n : a barbiturate $C_{11}H_{18}N_2O_3$ used as a hypnotic and sedative; also : its sodium salt — called also *amylobarbitone*; see AMYTAL, TUINAL

amo·di·a·quine \ˌa-mə-ˈdī-ə-ˌkwin, -ˌkwēn\ or **amo·di·a·quin** \-ˌkwin\ n : a compound $C_{20}H_{22}ClN_3O$ derived from quinoline and used in the form of its dihydrochloride as an antimalarial

amoe·ba *chiefly Brit var of* AMEBA

Amoe·ba \ə-ˈmē-bə\ n : a large genus of naked rhizopod protozoans that have lobed and never anastomosing pseudopodia and are widely distributed in fresh and salt water and moist terrestrial environments

amoe·bi·a·sis, amoe·bi·cide, amoe·bo·cyte, amoe·boid *chiefly Brit var of* AMEBIASIS, AMEBICIDE, AMEBOCYTE, AMEBOID

Amoe·bo·tae·nia \ə-ˌmē-(ˌ)bō-ˈtē-nē-ə\ n : a genus of tapeworms (family Dilepididae) parasitic in the intestines of poultry

amor·phous \ə-ˈmòr-fəs\ adj 1 : having no apparent shape or organization 2 : having no real or apparent crystalline form

amox·a·pine \ə-ˈmäk-sə-ˌpēn\ n : an antidepressant drug $C_{17}H_{16}ClN_3O$

amox·i·cil·lin \ə-ˌmäk-si-ˈsi-lən\ n : a semisynthetic penicillin $C_{16}H_{19}N_3$ O_5S derived from ampicillin — see LAROTID

amox·y·cil·lin \ə-ˌmäk-sē-ˈsi-lən\ Brit var of AMOXICILLIN

AMP \ˌā-(ˌ)em-ˈpē\ n : a mononucleotide of adenine $C_{10}H_{12}N_5O_3H_2PO_4$ that was orig. isolated from mammalian muscle and is reversibly convertible to ADP and ATP in metabolic reactions — called also *adenosine monophosphate, adenosine phosphate;* compare CYCLIC AMP

am·pere \ˈam-ˌpir, -ˌper\ n : a unit of electric current equivalent to a steady current produced by one volt applied across a resistance of one ohm

am·phet·amine \am-ˈfe-tə-ˌmēn, -mən\ n : a racemic sympathomimetic amine $C_9H_{13}N$ or one of its derivatives (as dextroamphetamine or methamphetamine) frequently abused as a stimulant of the central nervous system but used clinically esp. as the sulfate or hydrochloride salt to treat hyperactive children and the symptoms of narcolepsy and as a short-term appetite suppressant in dieting — compare BENZEDRINE

amphi- *or* **amph-** *prefix* : on both sides : of both kinds : both ⟨*amphi*mixis⟩

am·phi·ar·thro·sis \ˌam-fē-(ˌ)är-ˈthrō-səs\ n, pl **-thro·ses** \-ˌsēz\ : a slightly movable articulation (as a symphysis)

am·phi·bol·ic \ˌam-fə-ˈbä-lik\ adj : having an uncertain or irregular outcome — used of stages in fevers or the critical period of disease when prognosis is uncertain

am·phi·mix·is \ˌam-fə-ˈmik-səs\ n, pl **-mix·es** \-ˌsēz\ : the union of gametes in sexual reproduction

am·phi·path·ic \ˌam-fə-ˈpa-thik\ adj : AMPHIPHILIC — **am·phi·path** \ˈam-fə-ˌpath\ n

am·phi·phil·ic \ˌam-fə-ˈfi-lik\ adj : of, relating to, consisting of, or being one or more molecules (as of a glycolipid or sphingolipid in a biological membrane) having a polar water-soluble terminal group attached to a water-insoluble hydrocarbon chain — **am·phi·phile** \ˈam-fə-ˌfil\ n

am·phi·stome \ˈam-fi-ˌstōm\ n : any of a suborder (Amphistomata) of digenetic trematodes — compare GASTRODISCOIDES — **amphistome** adj

am·phor·ic \am-ˈfor-ik\ adj : resembling the sound made by blowing across the mouth of an empty bottle ⟨∼ breathing⟩ ⟨∼ sounds⟩

am·pho·ter·ic \ˌam-fə-ˈter-ik\ adj : partly one and partly the other; specif : capable of reacting chemically either as an acid or as a base — **am·pho·ter·ism** \-ˈter-i-ˌzəm\ n

am·pho·ter·i·cin B \ˌam-fə-ˈter-ə-sən\ n : an antifungal antibiotic obtained from a soil actinomycete (*Streptomyces nodosus*) and used esp. to treat systemic fungal infections

am·pi·cil·lin \ˌam-pə-ˈsi-lən\ n : a penicillin $C_{16}H_{19}N_3O_4S$ that is effective against gram-negative and gram-positive bacteria and is used to treat various infections of the urinary, respiratory, and intestinal tracts — see PENBRITIN

am·pli·fi·ca·tion \ˌam-plə-fə-ˈkā-shən\ n 1 : an act, example, or product of amplifying 2 : a usu. massive replication esp. of a gene or DNA sequence (as in a polymerase chain reaction)

am·pli·fy \ˈam-plə-ˌfī\ vb **-fied; -fy·ing** 1 : to make larger or greater (as in amount or intensity) 2 : to cause (a gene or DNA sequence) to undergo amplification

am·pule *or* **am·poule** *also* **am·pul** \ˈam-ˌpyūl, -ˌpūl\ n 1 : a hermetically sealed small bulbous glass vessel that is used to hold a solution for esp. hypodermic injection 2 : a vial resembling an ampule

am·pul·la \am-ˈpu̇-lə, ˈam-ˌpyü-lə\ n, pl **-lae** \-ˌlē\ : a saccular anatomic swelling or pouch: as **a** : the dilatation containing a patch of sensory epithelium at one end of each semicircular canal of the ear **b** : one of the dilatations of the milk-carrying tubules of the mammary glands that serve as reservoirs for milk **c** (1) : the middle portion of the fallopian tube (2) : the distal dilatation of a vas deferens near the opening of the duct leading from the seminal vesicle **d** : a terminal dilatation of the rectum just before it joins the anal canal

ampulla of Va·ter \-'fä-tər\ *n* : a trumpet-mouthed dilatation of the duodenal wall at the opening of the fused pancreatic and common bile ducts — called also *papilla of Vater*

Vater, Abraham (1684–1751), German anatomist.

am·pul·la·ry \am-'pu̇-lə-rē\ *also* **am·pul·lar** \-'pu̇-lər\ *adj* : resembling or relating to an ampulla

am·pu·tate \'am-pyə-ˌtāt\ *vb* **-tat·ed; -tat·ing** : to cut (as a limb) from the body — **am·pu·ta·tion** \ˌam-pyə-'tā-shən\ *n*

amputation neuroma *n* : NEUROMA 2

am·pu·tee \ˌam-pyə-'tē\ *n* : one that has had a limb amputated

amygdal- *or* **amygdalo-** *comb form* **1** : almond ⟨amygdalin⟩ **2** : amygdala ⟨amygdalectomy⟩ ⟨amygdalotomy⟩

amyg·da·la \ə-'mig-də-lə\ *n, pl* **-lae** \-ˌlē, -ˌlī\ : the one of the four basal ganglia in each cerebral hemisphere that is part of the limbic system and consists of an almond-shaped mass of gray matter in the roof of the lateral ventricle — called also *amygdaloid body, amygdaloid nucleus*

amyg·da·lec·to·my \ə-ˌmig-də-'lek-tə-mē\ *n, pl* **-mies** : surgical removal of the amygdala — **amyg·da·lec·to·mized** \-tə-ˌmīzd\ *adj*

amyg·da·lin \ə-'mig-də-lən\ *n* : a white crystalline cyanogenetic glucoside $C_{20}H_{27}NO_{11}$ found esp. in the seeds of the apricot (*Prunus armeniaca*), peach (*Prunus persica*), and bitter almond

amyg·da·loid \-ˌloid\ *adj* **1** : almond-shaped **2** : of, relating to, or affecting an amygdala ⟨∼ lesions⟩

amygdaloid body *n* : AMYGDALA

amygdaloid nucleus *n* : AMYGDALA

amyg·da·lot·o·my \ə-ˌmig-də-'lä-tə-mē\ *n, pl* **-mies** : destruction of part of the amygdala of the brain (as for the control of epilepsy) esp. by surgical incision

amyl- *or* **amylo-** *comb form* : starch ⟨amylase⟩

am·y·lase \'a-mə-ˌlās, -ˌlāz\ *n* : any of a group of enzymes (as amylopsin) that catalyze the hydrolysis of starch and glycogen or their intermediate hydrolysis products

am·yl nitrite \'a-məl-\ *n* : a pale yellow pungent flammable liquid ester $C_5H_{11}NO_2$ that is used chiefly in medicine as a vasodilator esp. in angina pectoris and illicitly as an aphrodisiac — called also *isoamyl nitrite;* compare POPPER

am·y·lo·bar·bi·tone \ˌa-mə-lō-'bär-bə-ˌtōn\ *n, Brit* : AMOBARBITAL

¹**am·y·loid** \'a-mə-ˌloid\ *adj* : resembling or containing starch

²**amyloid** *n* : a waxy translucent substance consisting of protein in combination with polysaccharides that is deposited in some animal organs and tissue under abnormal conditions (as in Alzheimer's disease)

am·y·loid·osis \ˌa-mə-ˌloi-'dō-səs\ *n, pl* **-o·ses** \-ˌsēz\ : a disorder characterized by the deposition of amyloid in organs or tissues of the animal body — see PARAMYLOIDOSIS

am·y·lop·sin \ˌa-mə-'läp-sən\ *n* : the amylase of the pancreatic juice

am·y·lum \'a-mə-ləm\ *n* : STARCH

amyo·to·nia \ˌā-ˌmī-ə-'tō-nē-ə\ *n* : deficiency of muscle tone

amyotonia con·gen·i·ta \-kən-'je-nə-tə\ *n* : a congenital disease of infants characterized by the flaccidity of the skeletal muscles

amyo·tro·phia \ˌā-ˌmī-ə-'trō-fē-ə\ *or* **amy·ot·ro·phy** \-'mī-'ä-trə-fē\ *n, pl* **-phi·as** *or* **-phies** : atrophy of a muscle — **amyo·tro·phic** \-ˌmī-ə-'trä-fik, -'trō-\ *adj*

amyotrophic lateral sclerosis *n* : a rare fatal progressive degenerative disease that affects pyramidal motor neurons, usu. begins in middle age, and is characterized esp. by increasing and spreading muscular weakness — called also *Lou Gehrig's disease;* abbr. ALS

Am·y·tal \'a-mə-ˌtol\ *trademark* — used for a preparation of amobarbital

an- — see A-

ana \'a-nə\ *adv* : of each an equal quantity — used in prescriptions

ana- *or* **an-** *prefix* : up : upward ⟨anabolism⟩

ANA *abbr* American Nurses Association

anabolic steroid *n* : any of a group of usu. synthetic hormones that increase constructive metabolism and are sometimes abused by athletes in training to increase temporarily the size of their muscles

anab·o·lism \ə-'na-bə-ˌli-zəm\ *n* : the constructive part of metabolism concerned esp. with macromolecular synthesis — compare CATABOLISM — **an·a·bol·ic** \ˌa-nə-'bä-lik\ *adj*

an·ac·id·i·ty \ˌa-nə-'si-də-tē\ *n, pl* **-ties** : ACHLORHYDRIA

an·a·clit·ic \ˌa-nə-'kli-tik\ *adj* : of, relating to, or characterized by the direction of love toward an object (as the mother) that satisfies nonsexual needs (as hunger)

anaclitic depression *n* : impaired development of an infant resulting from separation from its mother

anac·ro·tism \ə-'na-krə-ˌti-zəm\ *n* : an abnormality of the blood circulation characterized by a secondary notch in the ascending part of a sphygmographic tracing of the pulse — **an·a·crot·ic** \ˌa-nə-'krä-tik\ *adj*

anae·mia *chiefly Brit var of* ANEMIA

an·aer·obe \'a-nə-ˌrōb, (ˌ)a-'nar-ˌōb\ : an anaerobic organism

an·aer·o·bic \ˌa-nə-ˈrō-bik, ˌa-ˌnar-ˈō-\ *adj* **1 a** : living, active, or occurring in the absence of free oxygen (~ respiration) **b** : of, relating to, or being activity in which the body incurs an oxygen debt (~ exercise) **2** : relating to or induced by anaerobes — **an·aer·o·bi·cal·ly** \-bi-k(ə-)lē\ *adv*

an·aes·the·sia, an·aes·the·si·ol·o·gist, an·aes·the·si·ol·o·gy, an·aes·thet·ic, an·aes·the·tist, an·aes·the·tize *chiefly Brit var of* ANESTHESIA, ANESTHESIOLOGIST, ANESTHESIOLOGY, ANESTHETIC, ANESTHETIST, ANESTHETIZE

an·a·gen \ˈa-nə-ˌjen\ *n* : the active phase of the hair growth cycle preceding telogen

anal \ˈān-ᵊl\ *adj* **1** : of, relating to, or situated near the anus **2 a** : of, relating to, or characterized by the stage of psychosexual development in psychoanalytic theory during which the child is concerned esp. with its feces **b** : of, relating to, or characterized by personality traits (as parsimony, meticulousness, and ill humor) considered typical of fixation at the anal stage of development — compare GENITAL 3, ORAL 2, PHALLIC 2 — **anal·ly** *adv*

anal *abbr* **1** analysis **2** analytic **3** analyze

anal canal *n* : the terminal section of the rectum

¹an·a·lep·tic \ˌa-nə-ˈlep-tik\ *adj* : of, relating to, or acting as an analeptic

²analeptic *n* : a restorative agent; *esp* : a drug that acts as a stimulant on the central nervous system

anal eroticism *n* : the experiencing of pleasurable sensations or sexual excitement associated with or symbolic of stimulation of the anus — called also *anal erotism* — **anal erotic** *adj*

an·al·ge·sia \ˌan-ᵊl-ˈjēzhə, -zhē-ə, -zē-\ *n* : insensibility to pain without loss of consciousness

¹an·al·ge·sic \-ˈjē-zik, -sik\ *adj* : relating to, characterized by, or producing analgesia

²analgesic *n* : an agent for producing analgesia

an·al·get·ic \-ˈje-tik\ *n or adj* : ANALGESIC

anal·i·ty \ā-ˈna-lə-tē\ *n, pl* **-ties** : an anal psychological state, stage, or quality

anal·o·gous \ə-ˈna-lə-gəs\ *adj* : having similar function but a different structure and origin (~ organs)

an·a·logue *or* **an·a·log** \ˈan-ᵊl-ˌȯg, -ˌäg\ *n* **1** : an organ similar in function to an organ of another animal or plant but different in structure and origin **2** *usu* *analog* : a chemical compound that is structurally similar to another but differs slightly in composition (as in the replacement of one atom by an atom of a different element or in the presence of a particular functional group)

anal·o·gy \ə-ˈna-lə-jē\ *n, pl* **-gies** : functional similarity between anatomical parts without similarity of structure and origin — compare HOMOLOGY 1

anal–re·ten·tive \ˈän-ᵊl-ri-ˈten-tiv\ *adj* : characterized by personality traits (as frugality and obstinacy) held to be psychological sequelae of toilet training — compare ANAL 2b — **anal retentive** *n* — **anal retentiveness** *n*

anal sadism *n* : the cluster of personality traits (as aggressiveness, negativism, destructiveness, and outwardly directed rage) typical of the anal stage of development — **anal–sa·dis·tic** \ˌän-ᵊl-sə-ˈdis-tik\ *adj*

anal sphincter *n* : either of two sphincters controlling the closing of the anus: **a** : an outer sphincter of striated muscle surrounding the anus immediately beneath the skin — called also *external anal sphincter, sphincter ani externus* **b** : an inner sphincter formed by thickening of the circular smooth muscle of the rectum — called also *internal anal sphincter, sphincter ani internus*

anal verge \-ˈvərj\ *n* : the distal margin of the anal canal comprising the muscular rim of the anus

anal·y·sand \ə-ˈna-lə-ˌsand\ *n* : one who is undergoing psychoanalysis

anal·y·sis \ə-ˈna-lə-səs\ *n, pl* **-y·ses** \-ˌsēz\ **1** : separation of a whole into its component parts **2 a** : the identification or separation of ingredients of a substance **b** : a statement of the constituents of a mixture **3** : PSYCHOANALYSIS

an·a·lyst \ˈan-ᵊl-ist\ *n* : PSYCHOANALYST

an·a·lyt·ic \ˌan-ᵊl-ˈi-tik\ *or* **an·a·lyt·i·cal** \-ti-kəl\ *adj* **1** : of or relating to analysis; *esp* : separating something into component parts or constituent elements **2** : PSYCHOANALYTIC — **an·a·lyt·i·cal·ly** \-ti-k(ə-)lē\ *adv*

analytic psychology *n* : a modification of psychoanalysis due to C. G. Jung that adds to the concept of the personal unconscious a racial or collective unconscious and advocates that psychotherapy be conducted in terms of the patient's present-day conflicts and maladjustments

an·a·lyze \ˈan-ᵊl-ˌīz\ *vb* **-lyzed; -lyz·ing 1** : to study or determine the nature and relationship of the parts of by analysis; *esp* : to examine by chemical analysis **2** : PSYCHOANALYZE

an·am·ne·sis \ˌa-ˌnam-ˈnē-səs\ *n, pl* **-ne·ses** \-ˌsēz\ **1** : a recalling to mind **2** : a preliminary case history of a medical or psychiatric patient — **an·am·nes·tic** \-ˈnes-tik\ *adj*

ana·phase \ˈa-nə-ˌfāz\ *n* : the stage of mitosis and meiosis in which the chromosomes move toward the poles of the spindle — **ana·pha·sic** \ˌa-nə-ˈfā-zik\ *adj*

an·aph·ro·dis·i·ac \-ˌde-zē-ˌak, -ˈdi-\ *adj* : of, relating to, or causing absence or impairment of sexual desire — **anaphrodisiac** *n*

ana·phy·lac·tic \ˌa-nə-fə-ˈlak-tik\ *adj* : of, relating to, affected by, or causing anaphylaxis or anaphylactic shock — **ana·phy·lac·ti·cal·ly** \-ti-k(ə-)lē\ *adv*

anaphylactic shock *n* : an often severe and sometimes fatal systemic reaction in a susceptible individual upon a second exposure to a specific antigen (as wasp venom or penicillin) after previous sensitization that is characterized esp. by respiratory symptoms, fainting, itching, and hives

ana·phy·lac·toid \ˌa-nə-fə-ˈlak-ˌtoid\ *adj* : resembling anaphylaxis or anaphylactic shock

ana·phy·lax·is \ˌa-nə-fə-ˈlak-səs\ *n, pl* **-lax·es** \-ˌsēz\ **1** : hypersensitivity (as to foreign proteins or drugs) resulting from sensitization following prior contact with the causative agent **2** : ANAPHYLACTIC SHOCK

an·a·pla·sia \ˌa-nə-ˈplā-zhē-ə, -zē-\ *n* : reversion of cells to a more primitive or undifferentiated form

an·a·plas·ma \ˌa-nə-ˈplaz-mə\ *n* **1** *cap* : a genus of bacteria (family Anaplasmataceae) that are found in the red blood cells of ruminants, are transmitted by biting arthropods, and cause anaplasmosis **2** *pl* **-ma·ta** \-mə-tə\ *or* **-mas** : any bacterium of the genus *Anaplasma*

an·a·plas·mo·sis \-ˌplaz-ˈmō-səs\ *n, pl* **-mo·ses** \-ˌsēz\ : a tick-borne disease of cattle, sheep, and deer caused by a bacterium of the genus *Anaplasma* (*A. marginale*) and characterized esp. by anemia and by jaundice

an·a·plas·tic \ˌa-nə-ˈplas-tik\ *adj* : characterized by, composed of, or being cells which have reverted to a relatively undifferentiated state

an·a·plas·tol·o·gy \-ˌplas-ˈtä-lə-jē\ *n, pl* **-gies** : a branch of medical technology concerned with the preparation and fitting of prosthetic devices (as artificial eyes and surgical implants) to individual specifications and with the study of the materials from which they are fabricated — **an·a·plas·tol·o·gist** \-jist\ *n*

an·ar·thria \a-ˈnär-thrē-ə\ *n* : inability to articulate remembered words as a result of a brain lesion — compare APHASIA

an·a·sar·ca \ˌa-nə-ˈsär-kə\ *n* : generalized edema with accumulation of serum in the connective tissue

an·a·stal·sis \ˌa-nə-ˈstol-səs, -ˈstäl-, -ˈstal-\ *n, pl* **-stal·ses** \-ˌsēz\ : ANTIPERISTALSIS

anas·to·mose \ə-ˈnas-tə-ˌmōz, -ˌmōs\ *vb* **-mosed; -mos·ing** : to connect, join, or communicate by anastomosis

anas·to·mo·sis \ə-ˌnas-tə-ˈmō-səs, ˌa-nəs-\ *n, pl* **-mo·ses** \-ˌsēz\ **1 a** : a communication between or coalescence of blood vessels **b** : the surgical union of parts and esp. hollow tubular parts **2** : a product of anastomosis; *esp* : a

network (as of channels or branches) produced by anastomosis — **anas·to·mot·ic** \-ˈmä-tik\ *adj*

anat *abbr* anatomic; anatomical; anatomy

an·a·tom·ic \ˌa-nə-ˈtä-mik\ *or* **an·a·tom·i·cal** \-mi-kəl\ *adj* **1** : of or relating to anatomy **2** : STRUCTURAL **1** ⟨an ∼ obstruction⟩ — **an·a·tom·i·cal·ly** \-mi-k(ə-)lē\ *adv*

Anatomica — see BASLE NOMINA ANATOMICA, NOMINA ANATOMICA

anatomical dead space *n* : the dead space in that portion of the respiratory system which is external to the alveoli and includes the air-conveying ducts from the nostrils to the terminal bronchioles — compare PHYSIOLOGICAL DEAD SPACE

anatomical position *n* : the normal position of the human body when active

anat·o·mist \ə-ˈna-tə-mist\ *n* : a student of anatomy; *esp* : one skilled in dissection

anat·o·my \ə-ˈna-tə-mē\ *n, pl* **-mies 1** : a branch of morphology that deals with the structure of organisms — compare PHYSIOLOGY **1 2** : a treatise on anatomic science or art **3** : the art of separating the parts of an organism in order to ascertain their position, relations, structure, and function : DISSECTION **4** : structural makeup esp. of an organism or any of its parts

ana·tox·in \ˌa-nə-ˈtäk-sən\ *n* : TOXOID

anchyl- *or* **anchylo-** — see ANKYL-

an·chy·lose, an·chy·lo·sis *var of* ANKYLOSE, ANKYLOSIS

an·cil·lary \ˈan-sə-ˌler-ē\ *adj* : being auxiliary or supplementary

an·co·ne·us \aŋ-ˈkō-nē-əs\ *n, pl* **-nei** \-nē-ˌī\ : a small triangular extensor muscle that is superficially situated behind and below the elbow joint and that extends the forearm — called also *anconeus muscle*

An·cy·los·to·ma \ˌaŋ-ki-ˈläs-tə-mə, ˌan-sə-\ *n* : a genus of hookworms (family Ancylostomatidae) that are intestinal parasites of mammals including humans — compare NECATOR

an·cy·lo·stome \aŋ-ˈki-lə-ˌstōm, -ˈsi-\ *n* : any of the genus *Ancylostoma* of hookworms

an·cy·lo·sto·mi·a·sis \ˌaŋ-ki-lō-stə-ˈmī-ə-səs, ˌan-sə-\ *n, pl* **-a·ses** \-ˌsēz\ : infestation with or disease caused by hookworms; *esp* : a lethargic anemic state due to blood loss through the feeding of hookworms in the small intestine — called also *hookworm disease*

andr- *or* **andro-** *comb form* **1** : male ⟨*andro*gen⟩ **2** : male and ⟨*andro*gynous⟩

an·dro·gen \ˈan-drə-jən\ *n* : a male sex hormone (as testosterone) — **an·dro·gen·ic** \ˌan-drə-ˈje-nik\ *adj*

an·drog·e·nize \an-ˈdrä-jə-ˌnīz\ *vb* **-nized; -niz·ing** : to treat or influence with male sex hormone esp. in excessive amounts

an·drog·y·nous \an-'drä-jə-nəs\ *adj* : having the characteristics or nature of both male and female — **an·drog·y·ny** \-nē\ *n*

an·droid \'an-ˌdrȯid\ *adj, of the pelvis* : having the angular form and narrow outlet typical of the human male — compare ANTHROPOID, GYNECOID, PLATYPELLOID

an·drom·e·do·tox·in \an-ˌdrä-mə-dō-'täk-sən\ *n* : a toxic compound $C_{31}H_{50}O_{10}$ found in various plants of the heath family (Ericaceae)

an·dro·stene·di·one \ˌan-drə-ˌstēn-'dī-ˌōn, -'stēn-dē-ˌōn\ *n* : a steroid sex hormone that is secreted by the testis, ovary, and adrenal cortex and acts more strongly in the production of male characteristics than testosterone

an·dros·ter·one \an-'dräs-tə-ˌrōn\ *n* : an androgenic hormone that is a hydroxy ketone $C_{19}H_{30}O_2$ found in human urine

Anec·tine \ə-'nek-tən\ *trademark* — used for a preparation of succinylcholine

an·elec·trot·o·nus \ˌan-ə-l-ˌek-'trät-ᵊn-əs\ *n* : the decreased irritability of a nerve in the region of a positive electrode or anode on the passage of a current of electricity through it

ane·mia \ə-'nē-mē-ə\ *n* 1 : a condition in which the blood is deficient in red blood cells, in hemoglobin, or in total volume — see APLASTIC ANEMIA, HYPERCHROMIC ANEMIA, HYPOCHROMIC ANEMIA, MEGALOBLASTIC ANEMIA, MICROCYTIC ANEMIA, PERNICIOUS ANEMIA, SICKLE-CELL ANEMIA 2 : ISCHEMIA — **ane·mic** \ə-'nē-mik\ *adj* — **ane·mi·cal·ly** \-mi-k(ə-)lē\ *adv*

an·en·ceph·a·lus \ˌan-(ˌ)en-'se-fə-ləs\ *n, pl* **-li** \-ˌlī\ : ANENCEPHALY

an·en·ceph·a·ly \ˌan-(ˌ)en-'se-fə-lē\ *n, pl* **-lies** : congenital absence of all or a major part of the brain — **an·en·ceph·al·ic** \-ˌen-sə-'fa-lik\ *adj or n*

aneph·ric \(ˌ)ā-'ne-frik, (ˌ)ā-\ *adj* : being without functioning kidneys

an·er·gy \'a-(ˌ)nər-jē\ *n, pl* **-gies** : a condition in which the body fails to react to an injected allergen or antigen (as tuberculin) — **an·er·gic** \-jik\ *adj*

an·es·the·sia \ˌa-nəs-'thē-zhə\ *n* 1 : loss of sensation esp. to touch usu. resulting from a lesion in the nervous system or from some other abnormality 2 : loss of sensation and usu. of consciousness without loss of vital functions artificially produced by the administration of one or more agents that block the passage of pain impulses along nerve pathways to the brain

Anes·the·sin \ə-'nes-thə-sən\ *trademark* — used for a preparation of benzocaine

an·es·the·si·ol·o·gist \ˌa-nəs-ˌthē-zē-'ä-lə-jist\ *n* : ANESTHETIST; *specif* : a physician specializing in anesthesiology

an·es·the·si·ol·o·gy \-jē\ *n, pl* **-gies** : a branch of medical science dealing with anesthesia and anesthetics

¹**an·es·thet·ic** \ˌa-nəs-'the-tik\ *adj* 1 : capable of producing anesthesia (~ agents) 2 : of, relating to, or caused by anesthesia (~ effect) (~ symptoms) — **an·es·thet·i·cal·ly** \-ti-k(ə-)lē\ *adv*

²**anesthetic** *n* : a substance that produces anesthesia

anes·the·tist \ə-'nes-thə-tist\ *n* : one who administers anesthetics — compare ANESTHESIOLOGIST

anes·the·tize \-ˌtīz\ *vb* **-tized; -tiz·ing** : to subject to anesthesia — **anes·the·ti·za·tion** \ə-ˌnes-thə-tə-'zā-shən\ *n*

an·es·trous \(ˌ)a-'nes-trəs\ *adj* 1 : not exhibiting estrus 2 : of or relating to anestrus

an·es·trus \-trəs\ *n* : the period of sexual quiescence between two periods of sexual activity in cyclically breeding mammals — compare ESTRUS

an·eu·ploid \'an-yü-ˌplȯid\ *adj* : having or being a chromosome number that is not an exact multiple of the usu. haploid number — **aneuploid** *n* — **an·eu·ploi·dy** \-ˌplȯi-dē\ *n*

an·eu·rine \'an-yə-ˌrēn, (ˌ)ā-'nyur-ˌēn\ *n* : THIAMINE

an·eu·rysm *also* **an·eu·rism** \'an-yə-ˌri-zəm\ *n* : an abnormal blood-filled dilatation of a blood vessel and esp. an artery resulting from disease of the vessel wall — **an·eu·rys·mal** *also* **an·eu·ris·mal** \ˌan-yə-'riz-məl\ *adj* — **an·eu·rys·mal·ly** *adv*

angel dust *n* : PHENCYCLIDINE

An·gel·man syndrome \'aŋ-jəl-mən-\ *also* **An·gel·man's syndrome** \-mənz-\ *n* : a genetic disorder characterized by severe mental retardation, hyperactivity, seizures, hypotonia, jerky movements, lack of speech, and frequent smiling and laughter

   Angelman, Harry (*fl* 1965), British physician.

angi- *or* **angio-** *comb form* 1 : blood or lymph vessel (*angioma*) (*angiogenesis*) 2 : blood vessels and (*angiocardiography*)

-angia *pl of* -ANGIUM

an·gi·i·tis \ˌan-jē-'ī-təs\ *n, pl* **-it·i·des** \-'i-tə-ˌdēz\ : inflammation of a blood or lymph vessel or duct

an·gi·na \an-'jī-nə, 'an-jə-\ *n* : a disease marked by spasmodic attacks of intense suffocative pain: as **a** : a severe inflammatory or ulcerated condition of the mouth or throat (diphtheritic ~) — see LUDWIG'S ANGINA, VINCENT'S ANGINA **b** : ANGINA PECTORIS — **an·gi·nal** \an-'jīn-ᵊl, 'an-jən-\ *adj*

angina pec·to·ris \-'pek-tə-rəs\ *n* : a disease marked by brief paroxysmal attacks of chest pain precipitated by deficient oxygenation of the heart muscles — see UNSTABLE ANGINA;

compare CORONARY INSUFFICIENCY, HEART FAILURE, MYOCARDIAL INFARCTION

an·gi·nose \'an-jə-ˌnōs, an-'jī-\ *or* **an·gi·nous** \(ˌ)an-'jī-nəs, 'an-jə-\ *adj* : relating to angina or angina pectoris

an·gio·car·dio·gram \ˌan-jē-ō-'kär-dē-ə-ˌgram\ *n* : a roentgenogram of the heart and its blood vessels prepared by angiocardiography

an·gio·car·di·og·ra·phy \-ˌkär-dē-'ä-grə-fē\ *n, pl* **-phies** : the roentgenographic visualization of the heart and its blood vessels after injection of a radiopaque substance — **an·gio·car·dio·graph·ic** \-dē-ə-'gra-fik\ *adj*

an·gio·ede·ma \ˌan-jē-ō-i-'dē-mə\ *n, pl* **-mas** *or* **-ma·ta** \-mə-tə\ : an allergic skin disease characterized by patches of circumscribed swelling involving the skin and its subcutaneous layers, the mucous membranes, and sometimes the viscera — called also *angioneurotic edema, giant urticaria, Quincke's disease, Quincke's edema*

an·gio·gen·e·sis \-'je-nə-səs\ *n, pl* **-e·ses** \-ˌsēz\ : the formation and differentiation of blood vessels

an·gio·gram \'an-jē-ə-ˌgram\ *n* : a roentgenogram made by angiography

an·gi·og·ra·phy \ˌan-jē-'ä-grə-fē\ *n, pl* **-phies** : the roentgenographic visualization of the blood vessels after injection of a radiopaque substance — **an·gio·graph·ic** \ˌan-jē-ə-'gra-fik\ *adj* — **an·gio·graph·i·cal·ly** \-fi-k(ə-)lē\ *adv*

an·gio·ker·a·to·ma \ˌan-jē-ō-ˌker-ə-'tō-mə\ *n, pl* **-mas** *or* **-ma·ta** \-mə-tə\ : a skin disease characterized by small warty elevations or telangiectasias and epidermal thickening

an·gi·ol·o·gy \ˌan-jē-'ä-lə-jē\ *n, pl* **-gies** : the study of blood vessels and lymphatics

an·gi·o·ma \ˌan-jē-'ō-mə\ *n, pl* **-mas** *or* **-ma·ta** \-mə-tə\ : a tumor (as a hemangioma) composed chiefly of blood vessels or lymphatic vessels — **an·gi·o·ma·tous** \-mə-təs\ *adj*

an·gi·o·ma·to·sis \ˌan-jē-(ˌ)ō-mə-'tō-səs\ *n, pl* **-to·ses** \-ˌsēz\ : a condition characterized by the formation of multiple angiomas

an·gio·neu·rot·ic edema \-nū-ˌrä-tik, -nyū-\ *n* : ANGIOEDEMA

an·gi·op·a·thy \ˌan-jē-'ä-pə-thē\ *n, pl* **-thies** : a disease of the blood or lymph vessels

an·gio·plas·ty \'an-jē-ə-ˌplas-tē\ *n, pl* **-ties** : surgical repair of a blood vessel; *esp* : BALLOON ANGIOPLASTY

an·gio·sar·co·ma \ˌan-jē-ō-sär-'kō-mə\ *n, pl* **-mas** *or* **-ma·ta** \-mə-tə\ : a rare malignant tumor affecting esp. the liver

an·gio·spasm \'an-jē-ō-ˌspa-zəm\ *n* : spasmodic contraction of the blood vessels with increase in blood pressure — **an·gio·spas·tic** \ˌan-jē-ō-'spas-tik\ *adj*

an·gio·ten·sin \ˌan-jē-ō-'ten-sən\ *n* **1** : either of two forms of a kinin of which one has marked physiological activity; *esp* : ANGIOTENSIN II **2** : a synthetic amide derivative of angiotensin II used to treat some forms of hypotension

an·gio·ten·sin·ase \ˌan-jē-ō-'ten-sə-ˌnās, -ˌnāz\ *n* : any of several enzymes in the blood that hydrolyze angiotensin — called also *hypertensinase*

angiotensin converting enzyme *n* : a proteolytic enzyme that converts angiotensin I to angiotensin II — see ACE INHIBITOR

an·gio·ten·sin·o·gen \-ten-'si-nə-jən\ *n* : a serum globulin formed by the liver that is cleaved by renin to produce angiotensin I — called also *hypertensinogen*

angiotensin I \-'wən\ *n* : the physiologically inactive form of angiotensin that is composed of 10 amino-acid residues and is a precursor of angiotensin II

angiotensin II \-'tü\ *n* : a protein with vasoconstrictive activity that is composed of eight amino-acid residues and is the physiologically active form of angiotensin

an·gio·to·nin \-'tō-nən\ *n* : ANGIOTENSIN

-angium *n comb form, pl* **-angia** : vessel : receptacle (mes*angium*)

an·gle \'aŋ-gəl\ *n* **1** : a corner whether constituting a projecting part or a partially enclosed space **2** : the figure formed by two lines extending from the same point

an·gle·ber·ry \'aŋ-gəl-ˌber-ē\ *n, pl* **-ries** : a papilloma or warty growth of the skin or mucous membranes of cattle and sometimes horses often occurring in great numbers

angle of the jaw *n* : GONIAL ANGLE

angle of the mandible *n* : GONIAL ANGLE

ang·strom \'aŋ-strəm\ *n* : a unit of length equal to one ten-billionth of a meter — used esp. for wavelengths of light

Ångström, Anders Jonas (1814–1874), Swedish astronomer and physicist.

angstrom unit *n* : ANGSTROM

an·gu·lar \'aŋ-gyə-lər\ *adj* **1 a** : having an angle or angles **b** : forming an angle or corner : sharp-cornered **2** : relating to or situated near an anatomical angle; *specif* : relating to or situated near the inner angle of the eye — **an·gu·lar·i·ty** \ˌaŋ-gyü-'lar-ə-tē\ *n* — **an·gu·lar·ly** *adv*

angular artery *n* : the terminal part of the facial artery that passes up alongside the nose to the inner angle of the orbit

angular gyrus *n* : the cerebral gyrus of the posterior part of the external surface of the parietal lobe that arches over the posterior end of the sulcus between the superior and middle gyri of the temporal lobe — called also *angular convolution*

angularis — see INCISURA ANGULARIS

angular vein *n* : a vein that comprises the first part of the facial vein and runs obliquely down at the side of the upper part of the nose

an·gu·la·tion \ˌaŋ-gyə-ˈlā-shən\ *n* : an angular position, formation or shape; *esp* : an abnormal bend or curve in an organ — **an·gu·late** \ˈaŋ-gyə-ˌlāt\ *vb*

anguli — see LEVATOR ANGULI ORIS

an·gu·lus \ˈaŋ-gyə-ləs\ *n, pl* **an·gu·li** \-ˌlī, -ˌlē\ : an anatomical angle; *also* : an angular part or relationship

an·he·do·nia \ˌan-hē-ˈdō-nē-ə\ *n* : a psychological condition characterized by inability to experience pleasure in normally pleasurable acts — compare ANALGESIA — **an·he·don·ic** \-ˈdä-nik\ *adj*

an·hi·dro·sis \ˌan-hi-ˈdrō-səs, -hī-\ *n, pl* **-dro·ses** \-ˌsēz\ : abnormal deficiency or absence of sweating

¹**an·hi·drot·ic** \-ˈdrä-tik\ *adj* : tending to check sweating

²**anhidrotic** *n* : an anhidrotic agent

anhydr- *or* **anhydro-** *comb form* : lacking water (*anhydremia*)

an·hy·drase \an-ˈhī-ˌdrās, -ˌdrāz\ *n* : an enzyme (as carbonic anhydrase) promoting a specific dehydration reaction and the reverse hydration reaction

an·hy·dre·mia \ˌan-(ˌ)hī-ˈdrē-mē-ə\ *n* : an abnormal reduction of water in the blood

an·hy·dride \(ˌ)an-ˈhī-ˌdrīd\ *n* : a compound derived from another (as an acid) by removal of the elements of water

an·hy·dro·hy·droxy·pro·ges·ter·one \an-ˌhī-drō-ˌhī-ˌdräk-sē-prō-ˈjes-tə-ˌrōn\ *n* : ETHISTERONE

an·hy·dro·sis, an·hy·drot·ic *var of* AN-HIDROSIS, ANHIDROTIC

an·hy·drous \(ˌ)an-ˈhī-drəs\ *adj* : free from water and esp. water that is chemically combined in a crystalline substance (∼ ammonia)

ani — see LEVATOR ANI, PRURITUS ANI

an·ic·ter·ic \ˌa-(ˌ)nik-ˈter-ik\ *adj* : not accompanied or characterized by jaundice (∼ hepatitis)

an·i·line \ˈan-əl-ən\ *n* : an oily liquid poisonous amine $C_6H_5NH_2$ used chiefly in organic synthesis (as of dyes and pharmaceuticals) — **aniline** *adj*

ani·lin·gus \ˌā-ni-ˈliŋ-gəs\ *or* **ani·linc·tus** \-ˈliŋk-təs\ *n* : erotic stimulation achieved by contact between mouth and anus

an·i·ma \ˈa-nə-mə\ *n* : an individual's true inner self that in the analytic psychology of C. G. Jung reflects archetypal ideals of conduct; *also* : an inner feminine part of the male personality — compare ANIMUS, PERSONA

animal heat *n* : heat produced in the body of a living animal by functional chemical and physical activities — called also *body heat*

animal model *n* : an animal sufficiently like humans in its anatomy, physiology, or response to a pathogen to be used in medical research in order to obtain results that can be extrapolated to human medicine

animal starch *n* : GLYCOGEN

an·i·mate \ˈa-nə-mət\ *adj* **1** : possessing or characterized by life **2** : of or relating to animal life as opposed to plant life

an·i·mus \ˈa-nə-məs\ *n* : an inner masculine part of the female personality in the analytic psychology of C. G. Jung — compare ANIMA

an·ion \ˈa-ˌnī-ən\ *n* : the ion in an electrolyzed solution that migrates to the anode; *broadly* : a negatively charged ion — **an·ion·ic** \ˌa-(ˌ)nī-ˈä-nik\ *adj* — **an·ion·i·cal·ly** \-ni-k(ə-)lē\ *adv*

an·irid·ia \ˌa-ˌnī-ˈri-dē-ə\ *n* : congenital or traumatically induced absence or defect of the iris

anis- *or* **aniso-** *comb form* : unequal (*aniseikonia*) (*anisocytosis*)

an·is·ei·ko·nia \ˌa-ˌnī-ˌsī-ˈkō-nē-ə\ *n* : a defect of binocular vision in which the two retinal images of an object differ in size — **an·is·ei·kon·ic** \-ˈkä-nik\ *adj*

an·iso·co·ria \ˌa-ˌnī-sō-ˈkōr-ē-ə\ *n* : inequality in the size of the pupils of the eyes

an·iso·cy·to·sis \-ˌsī-ˈtō-səs\ *n, pl* **-to·ses** \-ˌsēz\ : variation in size of cells and esp. of the red blood cells (as in pernicious anemia) — **an·iso·cy·tot·ic** \-ˈtä-tik\ *adj*

an·iso·me·tro·pia \ˌa-ˌnī-sə-mə-ˈtrō-pē-ə\ *n* : unequal refractive power in the two eyes — **an·iso·me·tro·pic** \-ˈträ-pik, -ˈtrō-\ *adj*

an·kle \ˈaŋ-kəl\ *n* **1** : the joint between the foot and the leg that constitutes in humans a ginglymus joint between the tibia and fibula above and the talus below — called also *ankle joint* **2** : the region of the ankle joint

an·kle·bone \-ˌbōn\ *n* : TALUS 1

ankle jerk *n* : a reflex downward movement of the foot produced by a spasmodic contraction of the muscles of the calf in response to sudden extension of the leg or the striking of the Achilles tendon above the heel — called also *Achilles reflex*

ankle joint *n* : ANKLE 1

ankyl- *or* **ankylo-** *also* **anchyl-** *or* **anchylo-** *comb form* : stiffness : immobility (*ankylosis*)

an·ky·lose \ˈaŋ-ki-ˌlōs, -ˌlōz\ *vb* **-losed; -los·ing 1** : to unite or stiffen by ankylosis **2** : to undergo ankylosis

ankylosing spondylitis *n* : rheumatoid arthritis of the spine — called also *Marie-Strümpell disease, rheumatoid spondylitis*

an·ky·lo·sis \ˌaṇ-ki-ˈlō-səs\ *n*, *pl* **-lo·ses** \-ˌsēz\ : stiffness or fixation of a joint by disease or surgery — **an·ky·lot·ic** \-ˈlä-tik\ *adj*

an·ky·lo·stome, an·ky·lo·sto·mi·a·sis *var of* ANCYLOSTOME, ANCYLOSTOMIASIS

an·la·ge \ˈän-ˌlä-gə\ *n*, *pl* **-gen** \-gən\ *also* **-ges** \-əz\ : the foundation of a subsequent development; *esp* : PRIMORDIUM

an·neal \ə-ˈnēl\ *vb* **1** : to heat and then cool (nucleic acid) in order to separate strands and induce combination at lower temperatures esp. with complementary strands of a different species **2** : to be capable of combining with complementary nucleic acid by a process of heating and cooling

an·ne·lid \ˈan-ᵊl-əd\ *n* : any of a phylum (Annelida) of usu. elongated segmented invertebrates (as earthworms and leeches) — **annelid** *adj*

annexa *var of* ADNEXA

an·nu·lar \ˈan-yə-lər\ *adj* : of, relating to, or forming a ring

annulare — *see* GRANULOMA ANNULARE

annular ligament *n* : a ringlike ligament or band of fibrous tissue encircling a part: as **a** : a strong band of fibers surrounding the head of the radius and retaining it in the radial notch of the ulna **b** : a ring attaching the base of the stapes to the oval window

an·nu·lus \ˈan-yə-ləs\ *n*, *pl* **-li** \-ˌlī\ *also* **-lus·es** : a ringlike part, structure, or marking; *esp* : any of various ringlike anatomical parts (as the inguinal ring)

annulus fi·bro·sus \-fī-ˈbrō-səs, -fi-\ *n* : a ring of fibrous or fibrocartilaginous tissue (as of an intervertebral disk)

¹ano- *prefix* : upward 〈*anoopsia*〉

²ano- *comb form* **1** : anus 〈*anoscope*〉 **2** : anus and 〈*anorectal*〉

ano·ci·as·so·ci·a·tion \ə-ˌnō-sē-ə-ˌsō-sē-ˈā-shən, a-, -ˌsō-shē-\ *n* : a method of preventing shock and exhaustion incident to surgical operations by preventing communication between the area of operation and the nervous system esp. by means of a local anesthetic or sharp dissection

an·odon·tia \ˌa-nō-ˈdän-chə, -chē-ə\ *n* : an esp. congenital absence of teeth

¹an·o·dyne \ˈa-nə-ˌdīn\ *adj* : serving to ease pain

²anodyne *n* : a drug that allays pain

ano·gen·i·tal \ˌā-nō-ˈje-nə-tᵊl\ *adj* : of, relating to, or involving the genital organs and the anus 〈an ~ infection〉

anom·a·lo·scope \ə-ˈnä-mə-lə-ˌskōp\ *n* : an optical device designed to test color vision

anom·a·lous \ə-ˈnä-mə-ləs\ *adj* : deviating from normal; *specif* : having abnormal vision with respect to a particular color but not color-blind

anom·a·ly \ə-ˈnä-mə-lē\ *n*, *pl* **-lies** : a deviation from normal esp. of a bodily part

ano·mia \ə-ˈnä-mē-ə, -ˈnō-\ *n* : ANOMIC APHASIA

ano·mic \ə-ˈnä-mik, ä-, -ˈnō-\ *adj* : relating to or characterized by anomie

anomic aphasia *n* : loss of the power to use or understand words denoting objects

an·o·mie *also* **an·o·my** \ˈa-nə-mē\ *n* : personal unrest, alienation, and anxiety that comes from a lack of purpose or ideals

an·onych·ia \ˌa-nə-ˈni-kē-ə\ *n* : congenital absence of the nails

ano·op·sia \ˌa-nō-ˈäp-sē-ə\ *n* : upward strabismus

anoph·e·les \ə-ˈnä-fə-ˌlēz\ *n* **1** *cap* : a genus of mosquitoes that includes all mosquitoes that transmit malaria to humans **2** : any mosquito of the genus *Anopheles* — **anopheles** *adj* — **an·oph·e·line** \-ˌlīn\ *adj or n*

an·oph·thal·mia \ˌa-ˌnäf-ˈthal-mē-ə, -ˌäp-\ *n* : congenital absence of the eyes — **an·oph·thal·mic** \-ˈthal-mik\ *adj*

an·oph·thal·mos \-ˈthal-məs\ *n* **1** : ANOPHTHALMIA **2** : an individual born without eyes

an·opia \ə-ˈnō-pē-ə, a-\ *n* : a defect of vision; *esp* : HEMIANOPIA

ano·plas·ty \ˈā-nə-ˌplas-tē, ˈa-\ *n*, *pl* **-ties** : a plastic operation on the anus (as for stricture)

An·op·lo·ceph·a·la \ˌa-nə-(ˌ)plō-ˈse-fə-lə\ *n* : a genus of taenioid tapeworms including some parasites of horses

an·op·sia \ə-ˈnäp-sē-ə, a-, -ˈnōp-\ *var of* ANOOPSIA

an·or·chid·ism \ə-ˈnȯr-ki-ˌdi-zəm, a-\ *n* : congenital absence of one or both testes

ano·rec·tal \ˌā-nō-ˈrekt-ᵊl, ˌa-nə-\ *adj* : of, relating to, or involving both the anus and rectum 〈~ surgery〉

¹ano·rec·tic \ˌā-nə-ˈrek-tik\ *also* **an·o·ret·ic** \-ˈre-tik\ *adj* **1 a** : lacking appetite **b** : ANOREXIC **2** **2** : causing loss of appetite 〈~ drugs〉

²anorectic *also* **anoretic** *n* **1** : an anorectic agent : ANOREXIC **2** : ANOREXIC

an·orex·ia \ˌa-nə-ˈrek-sē-ə, -ˈrek-shə\ *n* **1** : loss of appetite esp. when prolonged **2** : ANOREXIA NERVOSA

anorexia ner·vo·sa \-(ˌ)nər-ˈvō-sə, -zə\ *n* : a serious eating disorder primarily of young women in their teens and early twenties that is characterized esp. by a pathological fear of weight gain leading to faulty eating patterns, malnutrition, and usu. excessive weight loss

¹an·orex·i·ant \ˌa-nə-ˈrek-sē-ənt, -ˈrek-shənt\ *n* : a drug that suppresses appetite

²anorexiant *adj* : ANORECTIC 2

¹an·orex·ic \-ˈrek-sik\ *adj* **1** : ANORECTIC 1a, 2 **2** : affected with anorexia nervosa

²anorexic *n* : a person affected with anorexia nervosa

ano·rex·i·gen·ic \-\-ˈrek-sə-ˈje-nik\ *adj* : ANORECTIC 2

an·or·gas·mia \ˌa-nȯr-ˈgaz-mē-ə\ *n* : sexual dysfunction characterized by failure to achieve orgasm — **an·or·gas·mic** \-mik\ *adj*

ano·scope \ˈā-nə-ˌskōp\ *n* : an instrument for facilitating visual examination of the anal canal

ano·sco·py \ā-ˈnäs-kə-pē, ə-\ *n, pl* **-pies** : visual examination of the anal canal with an anoscope — **ano·scop·ic** \ˌā-nə-ˈskä-pik\ *adj*

an·os·mia \a-ˈnäz-mē-ə\ *n* : loss or impairment of the sense of smell — **an·os·mic** \-mik\ *adj*

ano·vag·i·nal \ˌā-nō-ˈva-jən-ᵊl\ *adj* : connecting the anal canal and the vagina ⟨a congenital ~ fistula⟩

an·ovu·la·tion \ˌa-ˌnä-vyə-ˈlā-shən, -ˌnō-\ *n* : failure or absence of ovulation

an·ovu·la·to·ry \(ˌ)a-ˈnä-vyə-lə-ˌtōr-ē, -ˈnō\ *adj* **1** : not involving or associated with ovulation ⟨~ bleeding⟩ **2** : suppressing ovulation ⟨~ drugs⟩

an·ox·emia \ˌa-ˌnäk-ˈsē-mē-ə\ *n* : a condition of subnormal oxygenation of the arterial blood — **an·ox·emic** \-mik\ *adj*

an·ox·ia \ə-ˈnäk-sē-ə, a-\ *n* : hypoxia esp. of such severity as to result in permanent damage — **an·ox·ic** \-sik\ *adj*

ANS *abbr* autonomic nervous system

an·sa \ˈan-sə\ *n, pl* **an·sae** \-ˌsē\ : a loop-shaped anatomical structure

ansa cer·vi·ca·lis \-ˌsər-və-ˈka-ləs, -ˈkä-\ *n* : a nerve loop from the upper cervical nerves that accompanies the hypoglossal nerve and innervates the infrahyoid muscles

ansa hy·po·glos·si \-ˌhī-pə-ˈglä-ˌsī, -ˈglō-, -(ˌ)sē\ *n* : ANSA CERVICALIS

ansa sub·cla·via \-ˌsəb-ˈklā-vē-ə\ *n* : a nerve loop of sympathetic fibers passing around the subclavian artery

anserinus — see PES ANSERINUS

ant- — see ANTI-

Ant·a·buse \ˈan-tə-ˌbyüs\ *trademark* — used for a preparation of disulfiram

¹**ant·ac·id** \(ˌ)ant-ˈa-səd\ *also* **an·ti·ac·id** \ˌan-tē-ˈa-səd, -ˌtī-\ *adj* : tending to counteract acidity

²**antacid** *also* **antiacid** *n* : an agent (as an alkali or absorbent) that counteracts or neutralizes acidity

an·tag·o·nism \an-ˈta-gə-ˌni-zəm\ *n* : opposition in physiological action: **a** : contrariety in the effect of contraction of muscles **b** : interaction of two or more substances such that the action of any one of them on living cells or tissues is lessened — compare SYNERGISM — **an·tag·o·nize** \an-ˈta-gə-ˌnīz\ *vb*

an·tag·o·nist \-nist\ *n* : an agent that acts in physiological opposition: as **a** : a muscle that contracts with and limits the action of an agonist with which it is paired — called also *an-*

tagonistic muscle; compare AGONIST 1, SYNERGIST 2 **b** : a chemical substance that opposes the action on the nervous system of a drug or a substance occurring naturally in the body by combining with and blocking its nervous receptor — compare AGONIST 2

an·tag·o·nis·tic \(ˌ)an-ˌta-gə-ˈnis-tik\ *adj* **1** : characterized by or resulting from antagonism **2** : relating to or being muscles that are antagonists — **an·tag·o·nis·ti·cal·ly** \-ti-k(ə-)lē\ *adv*

ante- *prefix* **1** : anterior : forward ⟨*an*tehypophysis⟩ **2 a** : prior to : earlier than ⟨*ante*partum⟩ **b** : in front of ⟨*ante*brachium⟩

an·te·bra·chi·um \ˌan-ti-ˈbrā-kē-əm\ *n, pl* **-chia** \-kē-ə\ : the part of the arm or forelimb between the brachium and the carpus : FOREARM

an·te·cu·bi·tal \ˌan-ti-ˈkyü-bət-ᵊl\ *adj* : of or relating to the inner or front surface of the forearm

antecubital fossa *n* : a triangular cavity of the elbow joint that contains a tendon of the biceps, the median nerve, and the brachial artery

an·te·flex·ion \ˌan-ti-ˈflek-shən\ *n* : a displacement forward of an organ (as the uterus) so that its axis is bent upon itself

an·te·grade \ˈan-ti-ˌgrād\ *adj* : occurring or performed in the usual direction of conduction or flow

an·te·hy·poph·y·sis \-hī-ˈpä-fə-səs\ *n, pl* **-y·ses** \-ˌsēz\ : the anterior lobe of the pituitary gland

an·te·mor·tem \-ˈmȯr-təm\ *adj* : preceding death

an·te·na·tal \-ˈnāt-ᵊl\ *adj* : PRENATAL ⟨~ diagnosis of birth defects⟩ — **an·te·na·tal·ly** *adv*

an·te·par·tum \-ˈpär-təm\ *adj* : relating to the period before parturition : before childbirth ⟨~ infection⟩ ⟨~ care⟩

an·te·ri·or \an-ˈtir-ē-ər\ *adj* **1** : relating to or situated near or toward the head or toward the part in headless animals most nearly corresponding to the head **2** : situated toward the front of the body : VENTRAL — used in human anatomy because of the upright posture of humans — **an·te·ri·or·ly** *adv*

anterior cerebral artery *n* : CEREBRAL ARTERY a

anterior chamber *n* : a space in the eye bounded in front by the cornea and in back by the iris and middle part of the lens — compare POSTERIOR CHAMBER

anterior column *n* : VENTRAL HORN

anterior commissure *n* : a band of nerve fibers crossing from one side of the brain to the other just anterior to the third ventricle

anterior communicating artery *n* : COMMUNICATING ARTERY a

anterior corticospinal tract *n* : VENTRAL CORTICOSPINAL TRACT

anterior cruciate ligament *n* : CRUCIATE LIGAMENT a(1)

anterior facial vein *n* : FACIAL VEIN

anterior fontanel *or* **anterior fontanelle** *n* : the fontanel occurring at the meeting point of the coronal and sagittal sutures

anterior funiculus *n* : a longitudinal division on each side of the spinal cord comprising white matter between the anterior median fissure and the ventral root — called also *ventral funiculus;* compare LATERAL FUNICULUS, POSTERIOR FUNICULUS

anterior gray column *n* : VENTRAL HORN

anterior horn *n* **1** : VENTRAL HORN **2** : the cornu of the lateral ventricle of each cerebral hemisphere that curves outward and forward into the frontal lobe — compare INFERIOR HORN, POSTERIOR HORN 2

anterior humeral circumflex artery *n* : an artery that branches from the axillary artery in the shoulder, curves around the front of the humerus, and is distributed esp. to the shoulder joint, head of the humerus, biceps brachii, and deltoid muscle — compare POSTERIOR HUMERAL CIRCUMFLEX ARTERY

anterior inferior cerebellar artery *n* : a artery that arises from the basilar artery and divides into branches distributed to the anterior parts of the inferior surface of the cerebellum

anterior inferior iliac spine *n* : a projection on the anterior margin of the ilium that is situated below the anterior superior iliac spine and is separated from it by a notch — called also *anterior inferior iliac spine*

anterior intercostal artery *n* : INTERCOSTAL ARTERY a

anterior jugular vein *n* : JUGULAR VEIN c

anterior lingual gland *n* : either of two mucus-secreting glands of the tip of the tongue

anterior lobe *n* : ADENOHYPOPHYSIS

anterior median fissure *n* : a groove along the anterior midline of the spinal cord that incompletely divides it into symmetrical halves — called also *ventral median fissure*

anterior nasal spine *n* : the nasal spine that is formed by the union of processes of the two premaxillae

anterior pillar of the fauces *n* : PALATOGLOSSAL ARCH

anterior root *n* : VENTRAL ROOT

anterior sacrococcygeal muscle *n* : SACROCOCCYGEUS VENTRALIS

anterior spinal artery *n* : SPINAL ARTERY a

anterior spinothalamic tract *n* : SPINOTHALAMIC TRACT a

anterior superior iliac spine *n* : a projection at the anterior end of the iliac crest — called also *anterior superior spine*

anterior synechia *n* : SYNECHIA a

anterior temporal artery *n* : TEMPORAL ARTERY 3a

anterior tibial artery *n* : TIBIAL ARTERY b

anterior tibial nerve *n* : DEEP PERONEAL NERVE

anterior tibial vein *n* : TIBIAL VEIN b

anterior triangle *n* : a triangular region that is a landmark in the neck and has its apex at the sternum pointing downward — compare POSTERIOR TRIANGLE

anterior ulnar recurrent artery *n* : ULNAR RECURRENT ARTERY a

antero- *comb form* : anterior and : extending from front to ⟨anterolateral⟩ ⟨anteroposterior⟩

an·tero·grade \ˈan-tə-ˌrō-ˌgrād\ *adj* **1** : effective for a period immediately following a shock or seizure; *specif* : effective for and in effect during the period from the time of seizure to the present ⟨∼ amnesia⟩ **2** : occurring along nerve cell processes away from the cell body ⟨∼ axonal transport⟩ — compare RETROGRADE 3

an·tero·in·fe·ri·or \ˌan-tə-ˌrō-in-ˈfir-ē-ər\ *adj* : located in front and below ⟨the ∼ aspect of the femur⟩ — **an·tero·in·fe·ri·or·ly** *adv*

an·tero·lat·er·al \-ˈla-tə-rəl, -trəl\ *adj* : situated or occurring in front and to the side — **an·tero·lat·er·al·ly** *adv*

an·tero·me·di·al \-ˈmē-dē-əl\ *adj* : located in front and toward the middle

an·tero·pos·te·ri·or \-pō-ˈstir-ē-ər, -pä-\ *adj* : concerned with or extending along a direction or axis from front to back or from anterior to posterior — **an·tero·pos·te·ri·or·ly** *adv*

an·tero·su·pe·ri·or \-ˈsu-ˈpir-ē-ər\ *adj* : located in front and above — **an·tero·su·pe·ri·or·ly** *adv*

an·te·ver·sion \ˌan-ti-ˈvər-zhən, -shən\ *n* : a condition of being anteverted — used esp. of the uterus

an·te·vert \ˈan-ti-ˌvərt, ˌan-ti-ˈ\ *vb* : to displace (a body organ) so that the whole axis is directed farther forward than normal

anth- — see ANTI-

anthelix *var of* ANTIHELIX

¹**an·thel·min·tic** \ˌant-ˌhel-ˈmin-tik, ˌan-ˌthel-\ *also* **an·thel·min·thic** \-ˈmin-thik\ *adj* : expelling or destroying parasitic worms (as tapeworms) esp. of the intestine

²**anthelmintic** *also* **anthelminthic** *n* : an anthelmintic drug

-anthem *or* **-anthema** *n comb form, pl* **-anthems** *or* **-anthemata** : eruption : rash ⟨enanthem⟩ ⟨exanthema⟩

anthrac- *or* **anthraco-** *comb form* : carbon : coal ⟨anthracosis⟩ ⟨anthracosilicosis⟩

an·thra·co·sil·i·co·sis \ˌan-thrə-(ˌ)kō-ˌsi-lə-ˈkō-səs\ *n, pl* **-co·ses** \-ˌsēz\ : massive fibrosis of the lungs resulting from inhalation of carbon and quartz dusts and marked by shortness of breath

an·thra·co·sis \ an-thrə-'kō-səs\ n, pl **-co·ses** \-ˌsēz\ : a benign deposition of coal dust within the lungs from inhalation of sooty air — compare ANTHRACOSILICOSIS — **an·thra·cot·ic** \-'kä-tik\ adj

an·thra·cy·cline \ an-thrə-'sī-ˌklēn\ n : any of a class of antineoplastic drugs (as doxorubicin) derived from an actionmycete of the genus *Streptomyces* (esp. *S. peucetius*)

an·thra·lin \'an-thrə-lən\ n : a yellowish brown crystalline compound $C_{14}H_{10}O_3$ used in the treatment of skin diseases (as psoriasis) — called also *dithranol*

an·thra·sil·i·co·sis \ an-thrə-ˌsi-lə-'kō-səs\ var of ANTHRACOSILICOSIS

an·thrax \'an-ˌthraks\ n, pl **-thra·ces** \-thrə-ˌsēz\ : an infectious disease of warm-blooded animals (as cattle and sheep) caused by a spore-forming bacterium (*Bacillus anthracis*), transmissible to humans esp. by the handling of infected products (as wool), and characterized by external ulcerating nodules or by lesions in the lungs

anthrop- or **anthropo-** comb form : human being ⟨*anthropo*philic⟩

an·thro·poid \'an-thrə-ˌpoid\ adj, of the pelvis : having a relatively great anteroposterior dimension — compare ANDROID, GYNECOID, PLATYPELLOID

an·thro·pom·e·try \ an-thrə-'pä-mə-trē\ n, pl **-tries** : the study of human body measurements esp. on a comparative basis — **an·thro·po·met·ric** \-pə-'metrik\ adj

an·thro·po·phil·ic \ an-thrə-(ˌ)pō-'fi-lik\ also **an·thro·poph·i·lous** \-'pä-fə-ləs\ adj : attracted to humans esp. as a source of food ⟨~ mosquitoes⟩

anti- or **ant-** or **anth-** prefix **1** : opposing in effect or activity : inhibiting ⟨*antac*-id⟩ ⟨*anth*elmintic⟩ ⟨*anti*histamine⟩ **2** : serving to prevent, cure, or alleviate ⟨*anti*anxiety⟩

an·ti·abor·tion \ an-tē-ə-'bôr-shən, -ˌtī-\ adj : opposed to abortion — **an·ti·abor·tion·ist** \-shə-nist\ n

antiacid var of ANTACID

an·ti·ac·ne \-'ak-nē\ adj : alleviating the symptoms of acne ⟨an ~ ointment⟩

an·ti-AIDS \-'ādz\ adj : used to treat or delay the development of AIDS ⟨the ~ drug AZT⟩

¹**an·ti·al·ler·gic** \-ə-'lər-jik\ also **an·ti·al·ler·gen·ic** \-ˌa-lər-'je-nik\ adj : tending to relieve or control allergic symptoms

²**antiallergic** also **antiallergenic** n : an antiallergic agent

an·ti·ana·phy·lax·is \-ˌa-nə-fə-'lak-səs\ n, pl **-lax·es** \-ˌsēz\ : the state of desensitization to an antigen

an·ti·an·dro·gen \-'an-drə-jən\ n : a sub-

stance that tends to inhibit the production, activity, or effects of a male sex hormone — **an·ti·an·dro·gen·ic** \-ˌan-drə-'je-nik\ adj

an·ti·ane·mic \-ə-'nē-mik\ adj : effective in or relating to the prevention or correction of anemia

an·ti·an·gi·nal \-'jin-əl, -'an-jən-ᵊl\ adj : used or tending to prevent or relieve angina pectoris ⟨~ drugs⟩

an·ti·an·ti·body \ an-tē-'an-ti-ˌbä-dē, ˌan-ˌtī-\ n, pl **-bod·ies** : an antibody with specific immunologic activity against another antibody

an·ti·anx·i·ety \-(ˌ)aŋ-'zī-ə-tē\ adj : tending to prevent or relieve anxiety

¹**an·ti·ar·rhyth·mic** \-(ˌ)ā-'rith-mik\ adj : counteracting or preventing cardiac arrhythmia ⟨an ~ agent⟩

²**antiarrhythmic** n : an antiarrhythmic agent

¹**an·ti·ar·thrit·ic** \-är-'thri-tik\ or **an·ti·ar·thri·tis** \-'thri-təs\ adj : tending to relieve or prevent arthritic symptoms

²**antiarthritic** n : an antiarthritic agent

an·ti·asth·ma \-'az-mə\ adj : used to relieve the symptoms of asthma ⟨~ drugs⟩

¹**an·ti·bac·te·ri·al** \ an-ti-bak-'tir-ē-əl, ˌan-ˌtī-\ adj : directed or effective against bacteria

²**antibacterial** n : an antibacterial agent

an·ti·bi·o·sis \ an-ti-bī-'ō-səs, ˌan-ˌtī-; an-ti-bē-\ n, pl **-oses** \-ˌsēz\ : antagonistic association between organisms to the detriment of one of them or between one organism and a metabolic product of another

¹**an·ti·bi·ot·ic** \-bī-'ä-tik, -bē-\ adj **1** : tending to prevent, inhibit, or destroy life **2** : of or relating to antibiotics or to antibiosis — **an·ti·bi·ot·i·cal·ly** \-ti-k(ə-)lē\ adv

²**antibiotic** n : a substance produced by or a semisynthetic substance derived from a microorganism and able in dilute solution to inhibit or kill another microorganism

an·ti·body \'an-ti-ˌbä-dē\ n, pl **-bod·ies** : any of a large number of proteins of high molecular weight that are produced normally by specialized B cells after stimulation by an antigen and act specifically against the antigen in an immune response, that are produced abnormally by some cancer cells, and that typically consist of four subunits including two heavy chains and two light chains — called also *immunoglobulin*

an·ti·bra·chi·um var of ANTEBRACHIUM

an·ti·can·cer \ an-ti-'kan-sər, ˌan-ˌtī-\ adj : used against or tending to arrest cancer ⟨~ drugs⟩ ⟨~ activity⟩

an·ti·car·cin·o·gen \-kär-'si-nə-jən, -ˌkärs-ᵊn-ə-ˌjen\ n : an anticarcinogenic agent

an·ti·car·ci·no·gen·ic \-ˌkärs-ᵊn-ō-'je-nik\ adj : tending to inhibit or prevent the activity of a carcinogen or the development of carcinoma

an·ti·car·ies \\,an-ti-'kar-ēz, ,an-,tī-\ *adj* : tending to inhibit the formation of caries

¹an·ti·cho·lin·er·gic \-,kō-lə-'nər-jik\ *adj* : opposing or blocking the physiological action of acetylcholine

²anticholinergic *n* : a substance having an anticholinergic action

an·ti·cho·lin·es·ter·ase \-'nes-tə-,rās, -,rāz\ *n* : any substance (as neostigmine) that inhibits a cholinesterase by combination with it

an·tic·i·pa·tion \(,)an-,ti-sə-'pā-shən\ *n* **1** : occurrence (as of a symptom) before the normal or expected time **2** : mental attitude that influences a later response — **an·tic·i·pate** \an-'ti-sə-,pāt\ *vb*

an·ti·clot·ting \,an-ti-'klä-tiŋ, ,an-,tī-\ *adj* : inhibiting the clotting of blood ⟨~ factors⟩

¹an·ti·co·ag·u·lant \-kō-'a-gyə-lənt\ *adj* : of, relating to, or utilizing anticoagulants ⟨~ therapy⟩

²anticoagulant *n* : a substance (as a drug) that hinders coagulation and esp. coagulation of the blood

an·ti·co·ag·u·la·tion \-kō-,a-gyə-'lā-shən\ *n* : the process of hindering the clotting of blood esp. by treatment with an anticoagulant — **an·ti·co·ag·u·late** \-kō-'a-gyə-,lāt\ *vb* — **an·ti·co·ag·u·la·to·ry** \-lə-,tōr-ē\ *adj*

an·ti·co·ag·u·la·tive \-'a-gyə-,lā-tiv\ *adj* : ANTICOAGULANT ⟨~ activity⟩

an·ti·co·ag·u·lin \-gyə-lən\ *n* : a substance (as one in snake venom) that retards clotting of vertebrate blood

an·ti·co·don \,an-ti-'kō-,dän\ *n* : a triplet of nucleotide bases in transfer RNA that identifies the amino acid carried and binds to a complementary codon in messenger RNA during protein synthesis at a ribosome

an·ti·com·ple·ment \-'käm-plə-mənt\ *n* : a substance that interferes with the activity of complement — **an·ti·com·ple·men·ta·ry** \-,käm-plə-'men-tə-rē, -men-trē\ *adj*

¹an·ti·con·vul·sant \-kən-'vəl-sənt\ *also* **an·ti·con·vul·sive** \-siv\ *n* : an anticonvulsant drug

²anticonvulsant *also* **anticonvulsive** *adj* : used or tending to control or prevent convulsions (as in epilepsy)

anticus — see SCALENUS ANTICUS, SCALENUS ANTICUS SYNDROME, TIBIALIS ANTICUS

an·ti·dan·druff \-'dan-drəf\ *adj* : tending to remove or prevent dandruff ⟨an ~ shampoo⟩

¹an·ti·de·pres·sant \-di-'pres-³nt\ *also* **an·ti·de·pres·sive** \-'pre-siv\ *adj* : used or tending to relieve or prevent psychic depression

²antidepressant *also* **antidepressive** *n* : an antidepressant drug — called *also* *energizer, psychic energizer;* compare TRICYCLIC ANTIDEPRESSANT

¹an·ti·di·a·bet·ic \-,dī-ə-'be-tik\ *n* : an antidiabetic drug

²antidiabetic *adj* : tending to relieve diabetes ⟨~ drugs⟩

¹an·ti·di·ar·rhe·al \-,dī-ə-'rē-əl\ *adj* : tending to prevent or relieve diarrhea

²antidiarrheal *n* : an antidiarrheal agent

an·ti·di·ure·sis \-,dī-yū-'rē-səs\ *n, pl* **-ure·ses** \-,sēz\ : reduction in or suppression of the excretion of urine

¹an·ti·di·uret·ic \-'re-tik\ *adj* : tending to oppose or check excretion of urine

²antidiuretic *n* : an antidiuretic substance

antidiuretic hormone *n* : VASOPRESSIN

an·ti·dote \'an-ti-,dōt\ *n* : a remedy that counteracts the effects of poison — **an·ti·dot·al** \,an-ti-'dōt-³l\ *adj* — **an·ti·dot·al·ly** *adv*

an·ti·dro·mic \,an-ti-'drä-mik, -'drō-\ *adj* : proceeding or conducting in a direction opposite to the usual one — used esp. of a nerve impulse or fiber ⟨~ action potentials⟩ — **an·ti·dro·mi·cal·ly** \-mi-k(ə-)lē\ *adv*

¹an·ti·dys·en·ter·ic \,an-ti-,dis-³n-'ter-ik, ,an-,tī-\ *adj* : tending to relieve or prevent dysentery

²antidysenteric *n* : an antidysenteric agent

¹an·ti·emet·ic \-ə-'me-tik\ *adj* : used or tending to prevent or check vomiting ⟨~ drugs⟩

²antiemetic *n* : an antiemetic agent

¹an·ti·ep·i·lep·tic \-,e-pə-'lep-tik\ *adj* : tending to suppress or prevent epilepsy ⟨~ treatment⟩

²antiepileptic *n* : an antiepileptic drug

an·ti·es·tro·gen \-'es-trə-jən\ *n* : a substance that inhibits the physiological action of an estrogen — **an·ti·es·tro·gen·ic** \-,es-trə-'je-nik\ *adj*

an·ti·fer·til·i·ty \-(,)fər-'ti-lə-tē\ *adj* : having the capacity or tending to reduce or destroy fertility : CONTRACEPTIVE ⟨~ agents⟩

an·ti·fi·bril·la·to·ry \-'fi-brə-lə-,tōr-ē, -'fī-\ *adj* : tending to suppress or prevent cardiac fibrillation

an·ti·fi·bri·no·ly·sin \-,fī-brən-³l-'īs-³n\ *n* : an antibody that acts specifically against fibrinolysins of hemolytic streptococci and that is used chiefly in some diagnostic tests — called also *antistreptokinase* — **an·ti·fi·bri·no·ly·sis** \-'ī-səs\ *n* — **an·ti·fi·bri·no·lyt·ic** \-'it-ik\ *adj*

¹an·ti·flat·u·lent \-'fla-chə-lənt\ *adj* : preventing or relieving flatulence

²antiflatulent *n* : an antiflatulent agent

an·ti·flu \-'flü\ *adj* : used to prevent infection by the myxovirus causing influenza ⟨an ~ drug⟩

¹an·ti·fun·gal \,an-ti-'fəŋ-gəl, ,an-,tī-\ *adj* : destroying fungi; *also* : inhibiting the growth of fungi

²antifungal *n* : an antifungal agent

an·ti·gen \'an-ti-jən\ *n* : a usu. protein or carbohydrate substance (as a toxin or enzyme) capable of stimulating an immune response — **an·ti·gen·ic** \,anti-ᵗje-nik\ *adj* — **an·ti·gen·i·cal·ly** \-ni-k(ə-)lē\ *adv*

an·ti·gen·emia \an-ti-jə-ᵗnē-mē-ə\ *n* : the condition of having an antigen in the blood

antigenic determinant *n* : EPITOPE

an·ti·gen·ic·i·ty \-ᵗni-sə-tē\ *n, pl* **-ties** : the capacity to act as an antigen

an·ti·glob·u·lin \an-ti-ᵗglä-byə-lən, ᵢan-ᵗtī-\ *n* : an antibody that combines with and precipitates globulin

an·ti·go·nad·o·trop·ic \-ᵢgō-ᵢna-də-ᵗträ-pik\ *adj* : tending to inhibit the physiological activity of gonadotropic hormones

an·ti·go·nad·o·tro·pin \-ᵗtrō-pən\ *n* : an antigonadotropic substance

an·ti·he·lix \ᵗhē-liks\ *n, pl* **-li·ces** \ᵗhe-lə-ᵢsēz, -ᵗhē-\ *or* **-lix·es** \ᵗhē-lik-səz\ : the curved elevation of cartilage within or in front of the helix

an·ti·he·mo·phil·ic factor \-ᵢhē-mə-ᵗfi-lik-\ *n* : FACTOR VIII — called also *antihemophilic globulin*

an·ti·hem·or·rhag·ic \-ᵢhe-mə-ᵗra-jik\ *adj* : tending to prevent or arrest hemorrhage

an·ti·her·pes \-ᵗhər-(ᵢ)pēz\ *adj* : acting against a herpesvirus or the symptoms caused by infection with it ⟨the ~ drug acyclovir⟩

an·ti·hi·drot·ic \-hi-ᵗdrä-tik, -hī-\ *adj* : tending to reduce or prevent sweat secretion

¹an·ti·his·ta·mine \-ᵗhis-tə-ᵢmēn, -mən\ *adj* : tending to block or counteract the physiological action of histamine

²antihistamine *n* : any of various compounds that oppose the actions of histamine and are used esp. for treating allergic reactions (as hay fever), cold symptoms, and motion sickness

an·ti·his·ta·min·ic \-ᵢhis-tə-ᵗmi-nik\ *adj or n* : ANTIHISTAMINE

an·ti·hu·man \-ᵗhyü-mən, -ᵗyü-\ *adj* : reacting strongly with human antigens ⟨~ antibodies⟩

an·ti·hy·per·lip·id·emic \-ᵢhī-pər-ᵢli-pə-ᵗdē-mik\ *adj* : acting to prevent or counteract the accumulation of lipids in the blood ⟨an ~ drug⟩

¹an·ti·hy·per·ten·sive \-ᵢhī-pər-ᵗten-siv\ *also* **an·ti·hy·per·ten·sion** \-ᵢhī-pər-ᵗten-chən\ *adj* : used or effective against high blood pressure ⟨~ drugs⟩

²antihypertensive *n* : an antihypertensive agent (as a drug)

an·ti·id·io·type \ᵢan-ti-ᵗi-dē-ə-ᵢtīp\ *n* : an antibody that treats another antibody as an antigen and suppresses its immunoreactivity — **an·ti·id·io·typ·ic** \-ᵢi-dē-ə-ᵗti-pik\ *adj*

¹an·ti·im·mu·no·glob·u·lin \ᵢan-tē-i-ᵢmyə-nō-ᵗglä-byə-lən, ᵢan-ᵢtī-, -ᵢi-ᵢmyü-nō-\ *adj* : acting against specific antibodies ⟨~ antibodies⟩ ⟨~ sera⟩

²anti–immunoglobulin *n* : an anti-immunoglobulin agent

¹an·ti–in·fec·tive \-in-ᵗfek-tiv\ *adj* : used against or tending to counteract or prevent infection ⟨~ agents⟩

²anti–infective *n* : an anti-infective agent

¹an·ti–in·flam·ma·to·ry \-in-ᵗfla-mə-ᵢtōr-ē\ *adj* : counteracting inflammation

²anti–inflammatory *n, pl* **-ries** : an anti-inflammatory agent (as a drug)

¹an·ti–in·su·lin \-ᵗin-sə-lən\ *adj* : tending to counteract the physiological action of insulin

²anti–insulin *n* : an anti-insulin substance

an·ti·ke·to·gen·ic \-ᵗje-nik\ *adj* : tending to prevent or counteract ketosis

an·ti·leu·ke·mic \-lü-ᵗkē-mik\ *also* **an·ti·leu·ke·mia** \-mē-ə\ *adj* : counteracting the effects of leukemia

an·ti·lu·et·ic \-lü-ᵗe-tik\ *n* : ANTISYPHILITIC

an·ti·lym·pho·cyte globulin \-ᵗlim-fə-ᵢsit-\ *n* : serum globulin containing antibodies against lymphocytes that is used similarly to antilymphocyte serum

antilymphocyte serum *n* : a serum containing antibodies against lymphocytes that is used for suppressing graft rejection

an·ti·lym·pho·cyt·ic globulin \-ᵢlim-fə-ᵗsi-tik-\ *n* : ANTILYMPHOCYTE GLOBULIN

antilymphocytic serum *n* : ANTILYMPHOCYTE SERUM

¹an·ti·ma·lar·i·al \-mə-ᵗler-ē-əl\ *or* **an·ti·ma·lar·ia** \-ə\ *adj* : serving to prevent, check, or cure malaria

²antimalarial *n* : an antimalarial drug

an·ti·me·tab·o·lite \-mə-ᵗta-bə-ᵢlīt\ *n* : a substance (as a sulfa drug) that replaces or inhibits the utilization of a metabolite

¹an·ti·mi·cro·bi·al \-ᵢmī-ᵗkrō-bē-əl\ *also* **an·ti·mi·cro·bic** \-ᵗkrō-bik\ *adj* : destroying or inhibiting the growth of microorganisms ⟨~ drugs⟩

²antimicrobial *also* **antimicrobic** *n* : an antimicrobial substance

¹an·ti·mi·tot·ic \-mī-ᵗtä-tik\ *adj* : inhibiting or disrupting mitosis ⟨~ agents⟩ ⟨~ activity⟩

²antimitotic *n* : an antimitotic substance

an·ti·mo·ny \ᵗan-tə-ᵢmō-nē\ *n, pl* **-nies** : a metalloid element that is commonly silvery white, crystalline, and brittle and is used in medicine as a constituent of various antiprotozoal agents (as tartar emetic) — symbol *Sb*; see ELEMENT TABLE

antimonyltartrate — see POTASSIUM ANTIMONYLTARTRATE

antimony potassium tartrate *n* : TARTAR EMETIC

an·ti·mus·ca·rin·ic \-ᵢməs-kə-ᵗri-nik\ *adj* : inhibiting muscarinic physiological effects ⟨an ~ agent⟩

an·ti·mu·ta·gen·ic \-ᵢmyü-tə-ᵗje-nik\ *adj* : reducing the rate of mutation ⟨~ substances⟩

an·ti·my·cin A \ᵢan-ti-ᵢmīs-ᵊn-ᵗā\ *n* : a crystalline antibiotic $C_{28}H_{40}N_2O_9$ used esp. as a fungicide, insecticide, and miticide — called also *antimycin*

an·ti·my·cot·ic \ˌan-ti-mī-ˈkä-tik, ˌan-ˌtī-\ *adj or n* : ANTIFUNGAL

an·ti·nau·sea \-ˈnȯ-zē-ə, -sē-; -ˈnȯ-zhə, -shə\ *also* **an·ti·nau·se·ant** \-ˈnȯ-zē-ənt, -zhē-, -sē-, -shē-\ *adj* : preventing or counteracting nausea ⟨∼ drugs⟩

an·ti·nau·se·ant \-ˈnȯ-zē-ənt, -zhē-, -sē-, -shē-\ *n* : an antinausea agent

¹**an·ti·neo·plas·tic** \-ˌnē-ə-ˈplas-tik\ *adj* : inhibiting or preventing the growth and spread of neoplasms or malignant cells ⟨∼ drugs⟩

²**antineoplastic** *n* : an antineoplastic agent

an·ti·neu·rit·ic \-nu̇-ˈri-tik, -nyu̇-\ *adj* : preventing or relieving neuritis

an·ti·no·ci·cep·tive \ˌan-ti-nō-si-ˈsep-tiv, ˌan-ˌtī-\ *adj* : ANALGESIC

an·ti·nu·cle·ar \-ˈnü-klē-ər, -ˈnyü-\ *adj* : tending to react with cell nuclei or their components (as DNA)

an·ti·ox·i·dant \-ˈäk-sə-dənt\ *n* : a substance (as beta-carotene or alpha‑tocopherol) that inhibits oxidation or reactions promoted by oxygen or peroxides — **antioxidant** *adj*

an·ti·par·a·sit·ic \-ˌpar-ə-ˈsi-tik\ *adj* : acting against parasites

an·ti·par·kin·so·nian \-ˌpär-kən-ˈsō-nē-ən, -nyən\ *also* **an·ti·par·kin·son** \-ˈpär-kən-sən\ *adj* : tending to relieve parkinsonism ⟨∼ drugs⟩

¹**an·ti·pe·ri·od·ic** \-ˌpir-ē-ˈä-dik\ *adj* : preventing periodic returns of disease

²**antiperiodic** *n* : an antiperiodic agent

an·ti·peri·stal·sis \-ˌper-ə-ˈstȯl-səs, -ˈstäl-, -ˈstal-\ *n, pl* **-stal·ses** \-ˌsēz\ : reversed peristalsis

an·ti·peri·stal·tic \-tik\ *adj* **1** : opposed to or checking peristaltic motion **2** : relating to antiperistalsis

an·ti·per·spi·rant \-ˈpər-spə-rənt\ *n* : a preparation used to check perspiration

an·ti·phlo·gis·tic \-flə-ˈjis-tik\ *adj or n* : ANTI-INFLAMMATORY

an·ti·plas·min \-ˈplaz-mən\ *n* : a substance (as an antifibrinolysin) that inhibits the action of plasmin

an·ti·plate·let \-ˈplāt-lət\ *adj* : acting against or destroying blood platelets

an·ti·pneu·mo·coc·cal \-ˌnü-mə-ˈkä-kəl, -ˌnyü-\ *or* **an·ti·pneu·mo·coc·cic** \-ˈkäk-(ˌ)sik\ *or* **an·ti·pneu·mo·coc·cus** \-ˈkä-kəs\ *adj* : destroying or inhibiting pneumococci

an·ti·pro·lif·er·a·tive \-prə-ˈli-fə-ˌrā-tiv\ *adj* : used or tending to inhibit cell growth ⟨∼ effects on tumor cells⟩

an·ti·pro·te·ase \-ˈprō-tē-ˌās, -ˌāz\ *n* : a substance that inhibits the enzymatic activity of a protease

an·ti·pro·throm·bin \-(ˌ)prō-ˈthräm-bən\ *n* : a substance that interferes with the conversion of prothrombin to thrombin — compare ANTITHROM-BIN, HEPARIN

¹**an·ti·pro·to·zo·al** \-ˌprō-tə-ˈzō-əl\ *adj* : tending to destroy or inhibit the growth of protozoa

²**antiprotozoal** *n* : an antiprotozoal agent

¹**an·ti·pru·rit·ic** \-ˈprü-ri-tik\ *adj* : tending to check or relieve itching

²**antipruritic** *n* : an antipruritic agent

an·ti·pseu·do·mo·nal \-ˌsü-də-ˈmōn-ᵊl, -ˌsü-ˈdä-mən-ᵊl\ *adj* : tending to destroy bacteria of the genus *Pseudomonas* ⟨∼ activity⟩

an·ti·psy·chot·ic \-si-ˈkä-tik\ *n or adj* : NEUROLEPTIC

an·ti·py·re·sis \-ˌpī-ˈrē-səs, -ˌsēz\ *n, pl* **-re·ses** \-ˌsēz\ : treatment of fever by use of antipyretics

¹**an·ti·py·ret·ic** \-ˈpī-ˈre-tik\ *n* : an antipyretic agent — called also *febrifuge*

²**antipyretic** *adj* : preventing, removing, or allaying fever

an·ti·py·rine \-ˈpīr-ˌēn\ *also* **an·ti·py·rin** \-ən\ *n* : an analgesic and antipyretic $C_{11}H_{12}N_2O$ formerly widely used but now largely replaced in oral use by less toxic drugs (as aspirin) — called also *phenazone*

¹**an·ti·ra·chit·ic** \-rə-ˈki-tik\ *adj* : used or tending to prevent the development of rickets ⟨an ∼ vitamin⟩

²**antirachitic** *n* : an antirachitic agent

an·ti·re·jec·tion \-ri-ˈjek-shən\ *adj* : used or tending to prevent organ transplant rejection ⟨∼ drugs⟩

an·ti·ret·ro·vi·ral \-ˈre-trō-ˌvī-rəl\ *adj* : acting, used, or effective against retroviruses ⟨∼ drugs⟩ ⟨∼ therapy⟩

¹**an·ti·rheu·mat·ic** \-ru̇-ˈma-tik\ *adj* : alleviating or preventing rheumatism

²**antirheumatic** *n* : an antirheumatic agent

an·ti·schis·to·so·mal \-ˌshis-tə-ˈsō-məl\ *adj* : tending to destroy or inhibit the development and reproduction of schistosomes

an·ti·schizo·phren·ic \-ˌskit-sə-ˈfre-nik\ *adj* : tending to relieve or suppress the symptoms of schizophrenia

¹**an·ti·scor·bu·tic** \-skȯr-ˈbyü-tik\ *adj* : counteracting scurvy ⟨the ∼ vitamin is vitamin C⟩

²**antiscorbutic** *n* : a remedy for scurvy

an·ti·se·cre·to·ry \-ˈsē-krə-ˌtōr-ē\ *adj* : tending to inhibit secretion

an·ti·sei·zure \-ˈsē-zhər\ *adj* : preventing or counteracting seizures ⟨∼ drugs⟩

an·ti·sense \ˈan-ˌtī-ˌsens, ˈan-ˌti-\ *adj* : having a complementary sequence to a segment of genetic material (as mRNA) and serving to inhibit gene function ⟨∼ nucleotides⟩ — compare MISSENSE, NONSENSE

an·ti·sep·sis \ˌan-tə-ˈsep-səs\ *n, pl* **-ses** \-ˌsēz\ : the inhibiting of the growth and multiplication of microorganisms by antiseptic means

¹**an·ti·sep·tic** \ˌan-tə-ˈsep-tik\ *adj* **1 a** : opposing sepsis, putrefaction, or decay; *esp* : preventing or arresting the growth of microorganisms (as on living tissue) **b** : acting or protecting like an antiseptic **2** : relating to or characterized by the use of antiseptics **3** : free of living microorganisms : scru-

pulously clean : ASEPTIC — **an·ti·sep·ti·cal·ly** \-ti-k(ə-)lē\ *adv*

²**antiseptic** *n* : a substance that checks the growth or action of microorganisms esp. in or on living tissue; *also* : GERMICIDE

an·ti·se·rum \'an-ti-ˌsir-əm, ˌan-ˌtī-, -ˌser-\ *n* : a serum containing antibodies — called also *immune serum*

an·ti·so·cial \-'sō-shəl\ *adj* : hostile or harmful to organized society: as **a** : being or marked by behavior deviating sharply from the social norm **b** : PSYCHOPATHIC (~ personality disorder)

¹**an·ti·spas·mod·ic** \-spaz-'mä-dik\ *n* : an antispasmodic agent

²**antispasmodic** *adj* : capable of preventing or relieving spasms or convulsions

an·ti·sperm \-'spərm\ *adj* : destroying or inactivating sperm (~ pills)

an·ti·strep·to·coc·cal \-ˌstrep-tə-'kä-kəl\ *or* **an·ti·strep·to·coc·cic** \-'kä-kik, -'käk-sik\ *adj* : tending to destroy or inhibit the growth and reproduction of streptococci (~ antibodies)

an·ti·strep·to·ki·nase \-ˌstrep-tō-'kī-ˌnās, -'nāz\ *n* : ANTIFIBRINOLYSIN

an·ti·strep·to·ly·sin \-ˌstrep-tə-'lis-ᵊn\ *n* : an antibody against a streptolysin produced by an individual injected with a streptolysin-forming streptococcus

¹**an·ti·syph·i·lit·ic** \-ˌsi-fə-'li-tik\ *adj* : effective against syphilis (~ treatment)

²**antisyphilitic** *n* : an antisyphilitic agent

an·ti·throm·bin \-'thräm-bən\ *n* : any of a group of substances in blood that inhibit blood clotting by inactivating thrombin — compare ANTIPROTHROMBIN, HEPARIN

an·ti·throm·bo·plas·tin \-ˌthräm-bə-'plas-tən\ *n* : an anticoagulant substance that counteracts the effects of thromboplastin

an·ti·throm·bot·ic \-thräm-'bä-tik\ *adj* : used against or tending to prevent thrombosis (~ agents) (~ therapy)

an·ti·thy·roid \-'thī-ˌroid\ *adj* : able to counteract excessive thyroid activity (~ drugs)

an·ti·tox·ic \-'täk-sik\ *adj* 1 : counteracting toxins 2 : being or containing antitoxins (~ serum)

an·ti·tox·in \ˌan-ti-'täk-sən\ *n* : an antibody that is capable of neutralizing the specific toxin (as a specific causative agent of disease) that stimulated its production in the body and is produced in animals for medical purposes by injection of a toxin or toxoid with the resulting serum being used to counteract the toxin in other individuals; *also* : an antiserum containing antitoxins

an·ti·trag·i·cus \ˌan-ti-'tra-jə-kəs\ *n, pl* **-i·ci** \-jə-ˌsī, -ˌsē\ : a small muscle arising from the outer part of the antitragus and inserted into the antihelix

an·ti·tra·gus \-'trā-gəs\ *n, pl* **-gi** \-ˌjī, -ˌgī\ : a prominence on the lower posterior portion of the concha of the external ear opposite the tragus

an·ti·try·pano·so·mal \-tri-ˌpa-nə-'sō-məl\ *or* **an·ti·try·pano·some** \-tri-'pa-nə-ˌsōm\ *adj* : TRYPANOCIDAL

an·ti·tryp·sin \'an-ti-'trip-sən, ˌan-ˌtī-\ *n* : a substance that inhibits the action of trypsin — see ALPHA-1-ANTITRYPSIN — **an·ti·tryp·tic** \-'trip-tik\ *adj*

an·ti·tu·ber·cu·lous \ˌan-ti-tù-'bər-kyə-ləs, ˌan-ˌtī-, -tyù-\ *or* **an·ti·tu·ber·cu·lo·sis** \-ˌbər-kyə-'lō-səs\ *also* **an·ti·tu·ber·cu·lar** \-'bər-kyə-lər\ *adj* : used or effective against tuberculosis

an·ti·tu·mor \'an-ti-ˌtü-mər, 'an-ˌtī-, -ˌtyü-\ *also* **an·ti·tu·mor·al** \-mə-rəl\ *adj* : ANTICANCER (~ agents)

¹**an·ti·tus·sive** \ˌan-ti-'tə-siv, ˌan-ˌtī-\ *adj* : tending or having the power to act as a cough suppressant (~ action)

²**antitussive** *n* : a cough suppressant

an·ti·ty·phoid \-'tī-ˌfoid, -tī-'foid\ *adj* : tending to prevent or cure typhoid

an·ti·ul·cer \-'əl-sər\ *adj* : tending to prevent or heal ulcers (~ drugs)

an·ti·ven·in \-'ve-nən\ *n* : an antitoxin to a venom; *also* : an antiserum containing such an antitoxin

An·ti·vert \'an-ti-ˌvərt, -ˌtī-\ *trademark* — used for a preparation of the hydrochloride of meclizine

an·ti·vi·ral \ˌan-ti-'vī-rəl, ˌan-ˌtī-\ *also* **an·ti·vi·rus** \-'vī-rəs\ *adj* : acting, effective, or directed against viruses (~ drugs)

an·ti·vi·ta·min \'an-ti-ˌvī-tə-mən, 'an-ˌtī-\ *n* : a substance that makes a vitamin metabolically ineffective

antr- *or* **antro-** *comb form* : antrum (*antrostomy*)

an·tral \'an-trəl\ *adj* : of or relating to an antrum

an·trec·to·my \an-'trek-tə-mē\ *n, pl* **-mies** : excision of an antrum (as of the stomach or mastoid)

an·tros·to·my \an-'träs-tə-mē\ *n, pl* **-mies** : the operation of opening an antrum (as for drainage); *also* : the opening made in such an operation

an·trot·o·my \an-'trä-tə-mē\ *n, pl* **-mies** : incision of an antrum; *also* : ANTROSTOMY

an·trum \'an-trəm\ *n, pl* **an·tra** \-trə\ : the cavity of a hollow organ or a sinus (the ~ of the Graafian follicle)

antrum of High·more \-'hī-ˌmor\ *n* : MAXILLARY SINUS
    Highmore, Nathaniel (1613–1685), British surgeon.

anu·cle·ate \(ˌ)ā-'nü-klē-ət, -'nyü-\ *or* **anu·cle·at·ed** \-klē-ˌā-təd\ *adj* : lacking a cell nucleus

an·u·lus fibrosus *var of* ANNULUS FIBROSUS

an·uria \ə-'nùr-ē-ə, a-, -'nyùr-\ *n* : absence of or defective urine excretion — **an·uric** \-'nùr-ik, -'nyùr-\ *adj*

anus \'ā-nəs\ *n, pl* **anus·es** *or* **ani** \'ā-

(ₗ)nī\ : the posterior opening of the alimentary canal

an·vil \'an-vəl\ n : INCUS

anx·i·e·ty \aŋ-'zī-ə-tē\ n, pl **-eties 1 a** : a painful or apprehensive uneasiness of mind usu. over an impending or anticipated ill **b** : a cause of anxiety **2** : an abnormal and overwhelming sense of apprehension and fear often marked by physiological signs (as sweating, tension, and increased pulse), by doubt concerning the reality and nature of the threat, and by self-doubt about one's capacity to cope with it

anxiety neurosis n : a psychoneurotic disorder characterized by anxiety unattached to any obvious source and often accompanied by physiological manifestations of fear (as sweating, cardiac disturbances, diarrhea, or vertigo) — called also *anxiety reaction, anxiety state*

¹**anx·io·lyt·ic** \aŋ-zē-ō-'li-tik, aŋ-sē-\ n : a drug that relieves anxiety

²**anxiolytic** adj : relieving anxiety

anx·ious \'aŋk-shəs\ adj **1** : characterized by extreme uneasiness of mind or brooding fear about some contingency **2** : characterized by, resulting from, or causing anxiety

AOB abbr alcohol on breath

aort- or **aorto-** comb form **1** : aorta ⟨aortitis⟩ **2** : aortic and ⟨aortocoronary⟩

aor·ta \ā-'ór-tə\ n, pl **-tas** or **-tae** \-tē\ : the large arterial trunk that carries blood from the heart to be distributed by branch arteries through the body

aor·tic \ā-'ór-tik\ also **aor·tal** \-'órt-əl\ adj : of, relating to, or affecting an aorta ⟨an ~ aneurysm⟩

aortic arch n : ARCH OF THE AORTA

aortic hiatus n : an opening in the diaphragm through which the aorta passes

aortic incompetence n : AORTIC REGURGITATION

aortic insufficiency n : AORTIC REGURGITATION

aor·ti·co·pul·mo·nary \ā-órt-ə-kō-'púl-mə-ner-ē, -'pàl-\ adj : relating to or joining the aorta and the pulmonary artery

aor·ti·co·re·nal \-'rēn-əl\ adj : relating to or situated near the aorta and the kidney

aortic regurgitation n : leakage of blood from the aorta back into the left ventricle during diastole because of failure of an aortic valve to close properly — called also *aortic incompetence, aortic insufficiency, Corrigan's disease*

aortic sinus n : SINUS OF VALSALVA

aortic stenosis n : a condition usu. the result of disease in which the aorta esp. its orifice is abnormally narrow

aortic valve n : the semilunar valve separating the aorta from the left ventricle that prevents blood from flowing back into the left ventricle

aor·ti·tis \ā-ór-'tī-təs\ n : inflammation of the aorta

aor·to·cor·o·nary \ā-ór-tō-'kòr-ə-ner-ē, -'kär-\ adj : of, relating to, or joining the aorta and the coronary arteries ⟨~ bypass surgery⟩

aor·to·fem·o·ral \-'fe-mə-rəl\ adj : of, relating to, or joining the abdominal aorta and the femoral arteries ⟨~ bypass graft⟩

aor·to·gram \ā-'ór-tə-gram\ n : an X-ray picture of the aorta made by arteriography

aor·tog·ra·phy \ā-ór-'tä-grə-fē\ n, pl **-phies** : arteriography of the aorta — **aor·to·graph·ic** \(ₗ)ā-ór-tə-'gra-fik\ adj

aor·to·il·i·ac \ā-ór-tō-'i-lē-ak\ adj : of, relating to, or joining the abdominal aorta and the iliac arteries

aor·to·pul·mo·nary window \ā-ór-tō-'púl-mə-ner-ē, -'pàl-\ n : a congenital circulatory defect in which there is direct communication between the aorta and the pulmonary artery — called also *aortopulmonary fenestration*

aor·to·sub·cla·vi·an \-səb-'klā-vē-ən\ adj : relating to or joining the aorta and the subclavian arteries

AOTA abbr American Occupational Therapy Association

ap- — see APO-

apar·a·lyt·ic \ā-par-ə-'li-tik\ adj : not characterized by paralysis

ap·a·thet·ic \a-pə-'the-tik\ adj : having or showing little or no feeling or emotion — **ap·a·thet·i·cal·ly** \-ti-k(ə-)lē\ adv

ap·a·thy \'a-pə-thē\ n, pl **-thies** : lack of feeling or emotion

ap·a·tite \'a-pə-tīt\ n : any of a group of calcium phosphate minerals comprising the chief constituent of bones and teeth; specif : calcium phosphate fluoride $Ca_5F(PO_4)_3$

APC abbr aspirin, phenacetin, and caffeine

¹**ap·er·i·ent** \ə-'pir-ē-ənt\ adj : gently causing the bowels to move : LAXATIVE

²**aperient** n : an aperient agent

ape·ri·od·ic \ā-pir-ē-'ä-dik\ adj : of irregular occurrence

aperi·stal·sis \ā-per-ə-'stòl-səs, -'stäl-, -'stal-\ n, pl **-stal·ses** \-sēz\ : absence of peristalsis

apex \'ā-peks\ n, pl **apex·es** or **api·ces** \'ā-pə-sēz\ : a narrowed or pointed end of an anatomical structure: as **a** : the narrow somewhat conical upper part of a lung extending into the root **b** : the lower pointed end of the heart situated in humans opposite the space between the cartilages of the fifth and sixth ribs on the left side **c** : the extremity of the root of a tooth

apex·car·di·og·ra·phy \ā-peks-kär-dē-'ä-grə-fē\ n, pl **-phies** : a procedure for measuring the beat in the apex region of the heart by recording movements in the nearby wall of the chest

Ap·gar score \'ap-ˌgär-\ n : an index used to evaluate the condition of a newborn infant based on a rating of 0, 1, or 2 for each of the five characteristics of color, heart rate, response to stimulation of the sole of the foot, muscle tone, and respiration with 10 being a perfect score

   Apgar, Virginia (1909–1974), American physician.

aph- — see APO-

apha·gia \ə-'fā-jə, a-, -jē-ə\ n : loss of the ability to swallow

apha·kia \ə-'fā-kē-ə, a-\ n : absence of the crystalline lens of the eye; *also* : the resulting anomalous state of refraction

¹**apha·kic** \ə-'fā-kik, a-\ adj : of, relating to, or affected with aphakia

²**aphakic** n : an individual who has had the lens of an eye removed

apha·sia \ə-'fā-zhə, -zhē-ə\ n : loss or impairment of the power to use or comprehend words usu. resulting from brain damage — compare ANARTHRIA; see MOTOR APHASIA

¹**apha·sic** \ə-'fā-zik\ adj : of, relating to, or affected with aphasia

²**aphasic** or **apha·si·ac** \ə-'fā-zē-ˌak, -zhē-\ : an individual affected with aphasia

apha·si·ol·o·gy \ə-ˌfā-zē-'ä-lə-jē, -zhē-\ n, pl **-gies** : the study of aphasia — **apha·si·ol·o·gist** \-jist\ n

apher·e·sis \ˌā-fə-'rē-səs, n, pl **-re·ses** \-ˌsēz\ : PHERESIS

apho·nia \(ˌ)ā-'fō-nē-ə\ n : loss of voice and of all but whispered speech — **apho·nic** \-'fä-nik, -'fō-\ adj

aphos·pho·ro·sis \ˌā-ˌfäs-fə-'rō-səs\ n, pl **-ro·ses** \-ˌsēz\ : a deficiency disease esp. of domestic cattle caused by inadequate intake of dietary phosphorus

¹**aph·ro·di·si·ac** \ˌa-frə-'dē-zē-ˌak, -'di-\ *also* **aph·ro·di·si·a·cal** \ˌa-frə-də-'zī-ə-kəl, -'sī-\ adj : exciting sexual desire

²**aphrodisiac** n : an aphrodisiac agent

aph·tha \'af-thə\ n, pl **aph·thae** \-ˌthē\ : a speck, flake, or blister on the mucous membranes (as of the mouth, gastrointestinal tract, or lips) — **aph·thous** \-thəs\ adj

aph·thoid \'af-ˌthȯid\ adj : having the characteristics of aphthae; *specif* : resembling thrush

aphthous fever n : FOOT-AND-MOUTH DISEASE

aphthous stomatitis n : a very common disorder of the oral mucosa that is characterized by the formation of canker sores on movable mucous membranes and that has a multiple etiology but is not caused by the virus causing herpes simplex

apic- or **apici-** or **apico-** *comb form* : apex : tip esp. of an organ ⟨*apic*ectomy⟩

api·cal \'ā-pi-kəl, 'a-\ adj : of, relating to, or situated at an apex — **api·cal·ly** \-k(ə-)lē\ adv

apical foramen n : the opening of the pulp canal in the root of a tooth

apic·ec·to·my \ˌā-pə-'sek-tə-mē\ n, pl **-mies** : surgical removal of an anatomical apex (as of the root of a tooth)

apices pl of APEX

api·co·ec·to·my \ˌā-pi-(ˌ)kō-'ek-tə-mē, ˌa-\ n, pl **-mies** : excision of the root tip of a tooth

apla·sia \(ˌ)ā-'plā-zhə, -zhē-ə, ə-\ n : incomplete or faulty development of an organ or part — **aplas·tic** \-'plas-tik-\ adj

aplastic anemia n : anemia that is characterized by defective function of the blood-forming organs (as the bone marrow) and is caused by toxic agents (as chemicals or X rays) or is idiopathic in origin — called also *hypoplastic anemia*

ap·nea \'ap-nē-ə, ap-'nē-\ n 1 : transient cessation of respiration 2 : ASPHYXIA — **ap·ne·ic** \ap-'nē-ik\ adj

ap·neu·sis \ap-'nü-səs, -'nyü-\ n, pl **ap·neu·ses** \-ˌsēz\ : sustained tonic contraction of the respiratory muscles resulting in prolonged inspiration — **ap·neus·tic** \-'nü-stik, -'nyü-\ adj

ap·noea \ap-'nē-ə, 'ap-nē-\ *chiefly Brit* var of APNEA

apo- or **ap-** or **aph-** *prefix* : formed from : related to ⟨*apo*morphine⟩

apo·crine \'a-pə-krən, -ˌkrīn, -ˌkrēn\ adj : producing a fluid secretion by pinching off one end of the secreting cells which then reform and repeat the process; *also* : produced by an apocrine gland — compare ECCRINE, HOLOCRINE, MEROCRINE

apo·en·zyme \ˌa-pō-'en-ˌzīm\ n : a protein that forms an active enzyme system by combination with a coenzyme and determines the specificity of this system for a substrate

ap·o·fer·ri·tin \ˌa-pə-'fer-ət-ᵊn\ n : a colorless crystalline protein capable of storing iron in bodily cells esp. of the liver

apo·li·po·pro·tein \ˌa-pə-ˌlī-pō-'prō-ˌtēn, -ˌlī-\ n : a protein that combines with a lipid to form a lipoprotein

apo·mor·phine \ˌa-pə-'mȯr-ˌfēn\ n : a crystalline morphine derivative $C_{17}H_{17}NO_2$ that is a dopamine agonist and is administered as the hydrochloride for its powerful emetic action

apo·neu·ro·sis \ˌa-pə-nu̇-'rō-səs, -nyu̇-\ n, pl **-ro·ses** \-ˌsēz\ : any of the broad flat sheets of dense fibrous collagenous connective tissue that cover, invest, and form the terminations and attachments of various muscles — **apo·neu·rot·ic** \-'rä-tik\ adj

aponeurotica — see GALEA APONEUROTICA

apoph·y·sis \ə-'pä-fə-səs\ n, pl **-y·ses** \-ˌsēz\ : an expanded or projecting part esp. of an organism — **apoph·y·se·al** \-ˌpä-fə-ˈsē-əl\ *adj*

ap·o·plec·tic \ˌa-pə-ˈplek-tik\ *adj* **1** : of, relating to, or causing stroke **2** : affected with, inclined to, or showing symptoms of stroke — **ap·o·plec·ti·cal·ly** \-ti-k(ə-)lē\ *adv*

ap·o·plexy \ˈa-pə-ˌplek-sē\ *n, pl* **-plex·ies 1** : STROKE **2** : copious hemorrhage into a cavity or into the substance of an organ ⟨abdominal ∼⟩ ⟨adrenal ∼⟩

apo·pro·tein \ˌa-pə-ˈprō-ˌtēn\ *n* : a protein that combines with a prosthetic group to form a conjugated protein

apothecaries' measure *n* : a system of liquid units of measure used in compounding medical prescriptions that include the gallon, pint, fluid ounce, fluid dram, and minim

apothecaries' weight *n* : a system of weights used chiefly by pharmacists in compounding medical prescriptions that include the pound of 12 ounces, the dram of 60 grains, and the scruple

apoth·e·cary \ə-ˈpä-thə-ˌker-ē\ *n, pl* **-car·ies 1** : a person who prepares and sells drugs or compounds for medicinal purposes : DRUGGIST, PHARMACIST **2** : PHARMACY 2a

ap·pa·ra·tus \ˌa-pə-ˈra-təs, -ˈrä-\ *n, pl* **-tus·es** *or* **-tus** : a group of anatomical or cytological parts functioning together — see GOLGI APPARATUS

append- *or* **appendo-** *or* **appendic-** *or* **appendico-** *comb form* : vermiform appendix ⟨append ectomy⟩ ⟨appendicitis⟩

ap·pend·age \ə-ˈpen-dij\ *n* : a subordinate or derivative body part; *esp* : a limb or analogous part

ap·pen·dec·to·my \ˌa-pən-ˈdek-tə-mē\ *n, pl* **-mies** : surgical removal of the vermiform appendix

ap·pen·di·ceal \ə-ˌpen-də-ˈsē-əl\ *also* **ap·pen·di·cal** \ə-ˈpen-di-kəl\ *adj* : of, relating to, or involving the vermiform appendix ⟨∼ inflammation⟩

ap·pen·di·cec·to·my \ə-ˌpen-də-ˈsek-tə-mē\ *n, pl* **-mies** *Brit* : APPENDECTOMY

ap·pen·di·ces epi·ploi·cae \ə-ˈpen-də-ˌsēz-ˌe-pi-ˈploi-sē\ *n pl* : small peritoneal pouches filled with fat that are situated along the large intestine

ap·pen·di·ci·tis \ə-ˌpen-də-ˈsī-təs\ *n* : inflammation of the vermiform appendix

ap·pen·dic·u·lar \ˌa-pən-ˈdi-kyə-lər\ *adj* : of or relating to an appendage: **a** : of or relating to a limb or limbs ⟨the ∼ skeleton⟩ **b** : APPENDICEAL

ap·pen·dix \ə-ˈpen-diks\ *n, pl* **-dix·es** *or* **-di·ces** \-də-ˌsēz\ : a bodily outgrowth or process; *specif* : VERMIFORM APPENDIX

ap·per·ceive \ˌa-pər-ˈsēv\ *vb* **-ceived; -ceiv·ing** : to have apperception of

ap·per·cep·tion \ˌa-pər-ˈsep-shən\ *n* : mental perception; *esp* : the process of understanding something perceived in terms of previous experience — compare ASSIMILATION 3 — **ap·per·cep·tive** \-ˈsep-tiv\ *adj*

ap·pe·stat \ˈa-pə-ˌstat\ *n* : the neural center in the brain that regulates appetite and is thought to be in the hypothalamus

ap·pe·tite \ˈa-pə-ˌtīt\ *n* : any of the instinctive desires necessary to keep up organic life; *esp* : the desire to eat — **ap·pe·ti·tive** \-ˌtī-tiv\ *adj*

ap·pla·na·tion \ˌa-plə-ˈnā-shən\ *n* : abnormal flattening of a convex surface (as of the cornea of the eye)

applanation tonometer *n* : an ophthalmologic instrument used to determine pressure within the eye by measuring the force necessary to flatten an area of the cornea with a small disk

ap·pli·ance \ə-ˈplī-əns\ *n* : an instrument or device designed for a particular use ⟨prosthetic ∼s⟩

ap·pli·ca·tion \ˌa-plə-ˈkā-shən\ *n* **1** : an act of applying **2** : a medicated or protective layer or material

ap·pli·ca·tor \ˈa-plə-ˌkā-tər\ *n* : one that applies; *specif* : a device for applying a substance (as medicine)

ap·ply \ə-ˈplī\ *vb* **ap·plied; ap·ply·ing** : to lay or spread on

ap·po·si·tion \ˌa-pə-ˈzi-shən\ *n* **1** : the placing of things in juxtaposition or proximity; *specif* : deposition of successive layers upon those already present (as in cell walls) — compare ACCRETION **2** : the state of being in juxtaposition or proximity (as in the drawing together of cut edges of tissue in healing) — **ap·pose** \a-ˈpōz\ *vb* — **ap·po·si·tion·al** \ˌa-pə-ˈzi-shə-nəl\ *adj*

ap·proach \ə-ˈprōch\ *n* : the surgical procedure by which access is gained to a bodily part

approach–approach conflict *n* : psychological conflict that results when a choice must be made between two desirable alternatives — compare APPROACH-AVOIDANCE CONFLICT, AVOIDANCE-AVOIDANCE CONFLICT

approach–avoidance conflict *n* : psychological conflict that results when a goal is both desirable and undesirable — compare APPROACH-APPROACH CONFLICT, AVOIDANCE-AVOIDANCE CONFLICT

ap·prox·i·mate \ə-ˈpräk-sə-ˌmāt\ *vb* **-mat·ed; -mat·ing** : to bring together ⟨∼ cut edges of tissue⟩

aprax·ia \(ˌ)ā-ˈprak-sē-ə\ *n* : loss or impairment of the ability to execute complex coordinated movements without impairment of the muscles or senses — **aprac·tic** \-ˈprak-tik\ *or* **aprax·ic** \-ˈprak-sik\ *adj*

apro·ti·nin \ā-ˈprō-tə-nin\ *n* : a polypeptide used for its proteinase-inhibiting properties esp. in the treatment of pancreatitis — see TRASYLOL

aptha *var of* APHTHA

ap·ti·tude \ˈap-tə-ˌtüd, -ˌtyüd\ *n* : a natural or acquired capacity or ability; *esp* : a tendency, capacity, or inclination to learn or understand

aptitude test *n* : a standardized test designed to predict an individual's ability to learn certain skills — compare INTELLIGENCE TEST

apy•rex•ia \ˌa-ˌpī-ˈrek-sē-ə, ˌa-pə-ˈrek-\ *n* : absence or intermission of fever

aqua \ˈa-kwə, ˈä-\ *n, pl* **aquae** \ˈa-(ˌ)kwē, ˈä-ˌkwī\ *or* **aquas** : WATER; *esp* : an aqueous solution

aq•ue•duct \ˈa-kwə-ˌdəkt\ *n* : a canal or passage in a part or organ

aqueduct of Syl•vi•us \-ˈsil-vē-əs\ *n* : a channel connecting the third and fourth ventricles of the brain — called also *cerebral aqueduct*
   Du•bois \dü̟-ˈbwä, dü-, dyü-\, **Jacques** (Latin, **Jacobus Sylvius**) (1478–1555), French anatomist.

¹**aque•ous** \ˈā-kwē-əs, ˈa-\ *adj* **1 a** : of, relating to, or resembling water (an ∼ vapor) **b** : made from, with, or by water (an ∼ solution) **2** : of or relating to the aqueous humor

²**aqueous** *n* : AQUEOUS HUMOR

aqueous flare *n* : FLARE 3

aqueous humor *n* : a transparent fluid occupying the space between the crystalline lens and the cornea of the eye

Ar *symbol* argon

ara–A \ˌar-ə-ˈā\ *n* : VIDARABINE

arab•i•nose \ə-ˈra-bə-ˌnōs, -ˌnōz\ *n* : a white crystalline aldose sugar $C_5H_{10}O_5$ occurring esp. in vegetable gums

ara•bi•no•side \ˌar-ə-ˈbi-nə-ˌsīd, ə-ˈra-bə-nō-ˌsīd\ *n* : a glycoside that yields arabinose on hydrolysis

ar•a•chi•don•ic acid \ˌar-ə-kə-ˈdä-nik-\ *n* : a liquid unsaturated fatty acid $C_{20}H_{32}O_2$ that occurs in most animal fats, is a precursor of prostaglandins, and is considered essential in animal nutrition

arachn- *or* **arachno-** *comb form* : spider ⟨*arachno*dactyly⟩

arach•nid \ə-ˈrak-nəd\ *n* : any of a large class of arthropods (Arachnida) comprising mostly air-breathing invertebrates, including the spiders and scorpions, mites, and ticks, and having a segmented body divided into two regions of which the anterior bears four pairs of legs but no antennae — **arach•nid** *adj*

arach•nid•ism \-nə-ˌdi-zəm\ *n* : poisoning caused by the bite or sting of an arachnid (as a spider, tick, or scorpion); *esp* : a syndrome marked by extreme pain and muscular rigidity due to the bite of a black widow spider

arach•no•dac•ty•ly \ə-ˌrak-nō-ˈdak-tə-lē\ *n, pl* **-lies** : a hereditary condition characterized esp. by excessive length of the fingers and toes

arach•noid \ə-ˈrak-ˌnȯid\ *n* : a thin membrane of the brain and spinal cord that lies between the dura mater

and the pia mater — **arachnoid** *also* **arach•noi•dal** \ə-ˌrak-ˈnȯid-ᵊl\ *adj*

arachnoid granulation *n* : any of the small whitish processes that are enlarged villi of the arachnoid membrane of the brain which protrude into the superior sagittal sinus and into depressions in the neighboring bone — called also *arachnoid villus*, *pacchionian body*

arach•noid•itis \ə-ˌrak-ˌnȯi-ˈdī-təs\ *n* : inflammation of the arachnoid membrane

ar•bor \ˈär-bər\ *n* : a branching anatomical structure resembling a tree

ar•bo•ri•za•tion \ˌär-bə-rə-ˈzā-shən\ *n* : a treelike figure or arrangement of branching parts; *esp* : a treelike part or process (as a dendrite) of a nerve cell

ar•bo•rize \ˈär-bə-ˌrīz\ *vb* **-rized; -riz•ing** : to branch freely and repeatedly

ar•bo•vi•rus \ˈär-bə-ˈvī-rəs\ *n* : any of a group of RNA viruses (as the causative agents of encephalitis, yellow fever, and dengue) transmitted by arthropods

ARC *abbr* **1** AIDS-related complex **2** American Red Cross

ar•cade \är-ˈkād\ *n* **1** : an anatomical structure comprising a series of arches **2** : DENTAL ARCH

arch \ˈärch\ *n* **1** : an anatomical structure that resembles an arch in form or function: as **a** : either of two vaulted portions of the bony structure of the foot that impart elasticity to it **b** : ARCH OF THE AORTA **2** : a fingerprint in which all the ridges run from side to side and make no backward turn

arch- *or* **archi-** *prefix* : primitive : original : primary ⟨*arch*enteron⟩

arch•en•ter•on \är-ˈken-tə-ˌrän, -rən\ *n, pl* **-tera** \-tə-rə\ : the cavity of the gastrula of an embryo forming a primitive gut

ar•che•type \ˈär-ki-ˌtīp\ *n* : an inherited idea or mode of thought in the psychology of C. G. Jung that is derived from the experience of the race and is present in the unconscious of the individual — **ar•che•typ•al** \ˌär-ki-ˈtī-pəl\ *adj*

ar•chi•pal•li•um \ˌär-ki-ˈpa-lē-əm\ *n* : the olfactory part of the cerebral cortex comprising the hippocampus and the part of the hippocampal gyrus — compare NEOPALLIUM

ar•chi•tec•ton•ics \-tek-ˈtä-niks\ *n sing or pl* : the structural arrangement or makeup of an anatomical part or system — **ar•chi•tec•ton•ic** \-nik\ *adj*

ar•chi•tec•ture \ˈär-kə-ˌtek-chər\ *n* : the basic structural form esp. of a bodily part or of a large molecule — **ar•chi•tec•tur•al** \ˌär-kə-ˈtek-chə-rəl, -ˈtek-shrəl\ *adj* — **ar•chi•tec•tur•al•ly** *adv*

arch of the aorta *n* : the curved transverse part of the aorta that connects the ascending aorta with the descending aorta — called also *aortic arch*

ar·cu·ate \'är-kyə-wət, -ˌwāt\ *adj* : curved like a bow

arcuate artery *n* : any of the branches of the interlobar arteries of the kidney that form arches over the base of the pyramids

arcuate ligament — see LATERAL ARCUATE LIGAMENT, MEDIAL ARCUATE LIGAMENT, MEDIAN ARCUATE LIGAMENT

arcuate nucleus *n* : any of several cellular masses in the thalamus, hypothalamus, or medulla oblongata

arcuate popliteal ligament *n* : a triangular ligamentous band in the posterior part of the knee that passes medially downward from the lateral condyle of the femur to the area between the condyles of the tibia and to the head of the fibula — compare OBLIQUE POPLITEAL LIGAMENT

arcuate vein *n* : any of the veins of the kidney that accompany the arcuate arteries, drain blood from the interlobular veins, and empty into the interlobar veins

ar·cus \'är-kəs\ *n, pl* **arcus** : an anatomical arch

arcus se·nil·is \-sə-'ni-ləs\ *n* : a whitish ring-shaped or bow-shaped deposit in the cornea that frequently occurs in old age

ARDS *abbr* adult respiratory distress syndrome

ar·ea \'ar-ē-ə\ *n* : a part of the cerebral cortex having a particular function — see ASSOCIATION AREA, MOTOR AREA, SENSORY AREA

area po·stre·ma \-pōs-'trē-mə, -päs-\ *n* : a tongue-shaped structure in the caudal region of the fourth ventricle of the brain

areata — see ALOPECIA AREATA

arec·o·line \ə-'re-kə-ˌlēn\ *n* : a toxic parasympathomimetic alkaloid $C_8H_{13}NO_2$ that is used as a veterinary anthelmintic and occurs naturally in betel nuts

are·flex·ia \ˌā-ri-'flek-sē-ə\ *n* : absence of reflexes — **are·flex·ic** \-'flek-sik\ *adj*

are·na·vi·rus \ˌar-ə-nə-'vī-rəs\ *n* : any of a group of viruses containing a single strand of RNA, having a grainy appearance due to the presence of ribosomes in the virion, and including the Machupo virus and the causative agents of lymphocytic choriomeningitis and Lassa fever

are·o·la \ə-'rē-ə-lə\ *n, pl* **-lae** \-ˌlē\ *or* **-las** 1 : the colored ring around the nipple or around a vesicle or pustule 2 : the portion of the iris that borders the pupil of the eye

are·o·lar \-lər\ *adj* 1 : of, relating to, or like an areola 2 : of, relating to, or consisting of areolar tissue

areolar tissue *n* : fibrous connective tissue having the fibers loosely arranged in a net or meshwork

Ar·gas \'är-gəs, -ˌgas\ *n* : a genus of ticks (family Argasidae) including the fowl ticks (as *A. persicus*)

argent- *or* **argenti-** *or* **argento-** *comb form* : silver (*argento*phil)

ar·gen·taf·fin cell *or* **ar·gen·taf·fine cell** \-fən-, -ˌfēn-\ *n* : one of the specialized epithelial cells of the gastrointestinal tract that stain readily with silver salts

ar·gen·to·phil \är-'jen-tə-ˌfil\ *or* **ar·gen·to·phile** \-ˌfil\ *or* **ar·gen·to·phil·ic** \-ˌjen-tə-'fi-lik\ *adj* : having an affinity for silver — used of certain cells, structures, or tissues

ar·gi·nine \'är-jə-ˌnēn\ *n* : a crystalline basic amino acid $C_6H_{14}N_4O_2$ derived from guanidine

ar·gon \'är-ˌgän\ *n* : a colorless odorless inert gaseous element — symbol *Ar*; see ELEMENT table

Ar·gyll Rob·ert·son pupil \'är-ˌgil-'rä-bərt-sən-, är-ˌ'gil-\ *n* : a pupil characteristic of neurosyphilis that fails to react to light but still reacts in accommodation to distance

   Robertson, Douglas Argyll (1837–1909), British ophthalmologist.

argyr- *or* **argyro-** *comb form* : silver (*argyria*)

ar·gyr·ia \är-'jir-ē-ə\ *n* : permanent dark discoloration of skin caused by overuse of medicinal silver preparations

Ar·gy·rol \'är-jə-ˌról, -ˌrōl\ *trademark* — used for a silver-protein compound whose aqueous solution is used as a local antiseptic esp. for mucous membranes

ar·gyr·o·phil \'är-jə-(ˌ)rō-ˌfil, -rə-\ *or* **ar·gyr·o·phile** \-ˌfil\ *or* **ar·gyr·o·phil·ic** \ˌär-jə-(ˌ)rō-'fi-lik, -rə-\ *adj* : ARGENTOPHIL (∼ cytoplasmic inclusions)

ari·bo·fla·vin·osis \ˌā-ˌrī-bə-ˌflā-və-'nō-səs\ *n, pl* **-oses** \-ˌsēz\ : a deficiency disease due to inadequate intake of riboflavin and characterized by sores on the mouth

arith·mo·ma·nia \ə-ˌrith-mō-'mā-nē-ə, -nyə\ *n* : a morbid compulsion to count objects

-ar·i·um \'ar-ē-əm\ *n suffix, pl* **-ariums** *or* **-ar·ia** \-ē-ə\ : thing or place belonging to or connected with (sanit*arium*)

arm \'ärm\ *n* **1** : a human upper limb; *esp* : the part between the shoulder and the wrist **2 a** : the forelimb of a vertebrate other than a human being **b** : a limb of an invertebrate animal **c** : any of the usu. two parts of a chromosome lateral to the centromere — **armed** \'ärmd\ *adj*

ar·ma·men·tar·i·um \ˌär-mə-ˌmen-'ter-ē-əm, -mən-\ *n, pl* **-tar·ia** \-ē-ə\ : the equipment and methods used esp. in medicine

arm·pit \'ärm-ˌpit\ *n* : the hollow beneath the junction of the arm and shoulder : AXILLA

aro·ma·ther·a·py \ə-ˌrō-mə-'ther-ə-pē\ *n, pl* **-pies** : massage of the body and esp. of the face with a preparation of fragrant essential oils extracted from herbs, flowers, and fruits — **aro·ma·ther·a·pist** \-¡pist\ *n*

aromatic ammonia spirit *n* : a solution of ammonia and ammonium carbonate in alcohol and distilled water used as a stimulant, carminative, and antacid — called also *aromatic spirit of ammonia*

arous·al \ə-'raú-zəl\ *n* : the act of arousing : state of being aroused (sexual ~); *specif* : responsiveness to stimuli

arouse \ə-'raúz\ *vb* **aroused; arous·ing** : to rouse or stimulate to action or to physiological readiness for activity

ar·rec·tor pi·li muscle \ə-'rek-tər-¡pi-¡li-, -'pi-lē-\ *n* : one of the small fan-shaped smooth muscles associated with the base of each hair that contract when the body surface is chilled and erect the hairs, compress an oil gland above each muscle, and produce the appearance of goose bumps

¹ar·rest \ə-'rest\ *vb* : to bring to a standstill or state of inactivity

²arrest *n* : the condition of being stopped — see CARDIAC ARREST

ar·rhe·no·blas·to·ma \¡ar-ə-¡nō-¡bla-'stō-mə, ə-¡rē-¡nō-\ *n, pl* **-mas** *also* **-ma·ta** \-mə-tə\ : a sometimes malignant tumor of the ovary that by the secretion of male hormone induces development of secondary male characteristics — compare GYNANDROBLASTOMA

ar·rhyth·mia \ā-'rith-mē-ə\ *n* : an alteration in rhythm of the heartbeat either in time or force

ar·rhyth·mic \-mik\ *adj* : lacking rhythm or regularity

ar·row·root \'ar-ō-¡rüt, -¡rút\ *n* : an easily digested starch obtained from the rootstock of a tropical American plant (esp. *Maranta arundinacea* of the family Marantaceae)

ARRT *abbr* **1** American registered respiratory therapist **2** American Registry of Radiologic Technologists

ars- *comb form* : arsenic ⟨*arsine*⟩ ⟨*arsphenamine*⟩

ars·en·ate \'är-sə-nət, -¡nāt\ *n* : a salt or ester of an arsenic acid

¹ar·se·nic \-nik\ *n* **1** : a solid poisonous element that is commonly metallic steel-gray, crystalline, and brittle — symbol *As*; see ELEMENT table **2** : ARSENIC TRIOXIDE

²ar·sen·ic \är-'se-nik\ *adj* : of, relating to, or containing arsenic esp. with a valence of five

ar·sen·ic acid \är-'se-nik-\ *n* : any of three arsenic-containing acids that are analogous to the phosphoric acids

¹ar·sen·i·cal \är-'se-ni-kəl\ *adj* : of, relating to, containing, or caused by arsenic (~ poisoning)

²arsenical *n* : a compound or preparation containing arsenic

ar·se·nic trioxide \'är-sə-nik-\ *n* : a poisonous trioxide As_2O_3 or As_4O_6 of arsenic that was formerly used in medicine and dentistry and is now used esp. as an insecticide and weed killer — called also *arsenic*

ar·sine \är-'sēn, 'är-¡\ *n* : a colorless flammable extremely poisonous gas AsH_3 with an odor like garlic

ars·phen·a·mine \ärs-'fe-nə-¡mēn, -mən\ *n* : a toxic powder $C_{12}H_{14}As_2N_2O_2 \cdot 2H_2O$ formerly used in the treatment esp. of syphilis and yaws — called also *salvarsan, six-o-six*

ART *abbr* accredited record technician

ar·te·ria \är-'tir-ē-ə\ *n, pl* **-ri·ae** \-ē-¡ē\ : ARTERY

arteri- *or* **arterio-** *comb form* **1** : artery ⟨*arteri*ography⟩ **2** : arterial and ⟨*arteriovenous*⟩

ar·te·ri·al \är-'tir-ē-əl\ *adj* **1** : of or relating to an artery **2** : relating to or being the bright red blood present in most arteries that has been oxygenated in lungs or gills — compare VENOUS 3 — **ar·te·ri·al·ly** *adv*

ar·te·rio·gram \är-'tir-ē-ə-¡gram\ *n* : a roentgenogram of an artery made by arteriography

ar·te·ri·og·ra·phy \är-¡tir-ē-'ä-grə-fē\ *n, pl* **-phies** : the roentgenographic visualization of an artery after injection of a radiopaque substance — **ar·te·rio·graph·ic** \-ē-ə-'gra-fik\ *adj* — **ar·te·rio·graph·i·cal·ly** \-fi-k(ə-)lē\ *adv*

ar·te·ri·o·la \är-¡tir-ē-'ō-lə\ *n, pl* **-lae** \-¡lē\ : ARTERIOLE

ar·te·ri·ole \är-'tir-ē-¡ōl\ *n* : any of the small terminal twigs of an artery that ends in capillaries — **ar·te·ri·o·lar** \-¡tir-ē-'ō-¡lär, -lər\ *adj*

ar·te·ri·o·li·tis \är-¡tir-ē-ō-'lī-təs\ *n* : inflammation of the arterioles

ar·te·ri·o·lu·mi·nal \är-¡tir-ē-ō-'lü-mən-³l\ *adj* : relating to or being the small vessels that branch from the arterioles of the heart and empty directly into its lumen

ar·te·ri·op·a·thy \är-¡tir-ē-'ä-pə-thē\ *n, pl* **-thies** : a disease of the arteries

ar·te·ri·or·rha·phy \är-¡tir-ē-'ór-ə-fē\ *n, pl* **-phies** : a surgical operation of suturing an artery

ar·te·rio·scle·ro·sis \är-¡tir-ē-ō-sklə-'rō-səs\ *n, pl* **-ro·ses** \-¡sēz\ : a chronic disease characterized by abnormal thickening and hardening of the arterial walls with resulting loss of elasticity

arteriosclerosis ob·lit·er·ans \-ä-'bli-tə-¡ranz\ *n* : chronic arteriosclerosis marked by occlusion of arteries and esp. those supplying the extremities

¹ar·te·rio·scle·rot·ic \-'rä-tik\ *adj* : of, relating to, or affected with arteriosclerosis

²arteriosclerotic *n* : an arteriosclerotic individual

arteriosi — see CONUS ARTERIOSUS

ar·te·rio·si·nu·soi·dal \är-¡tir-ē-ō-¡sī-nyə-'sóid-³l, -nə-\ *adj* : relating to or being the vessels that connect the arterioles and sinusoids of the heart

ar·te·rio·spasm \är-ˈtir-ē-ō-ˌspa-zəm\ *n* : spasm of an artery — **ar·te·rio·spas·tic** \-ˌtir-ē-ō-ˈspas-tik\ *adj*

arteriosum — see LIGAMENTUM ARTERIOSUM

arteriosus — see CONUS ARTERIOSUS, DUCTUS ARTERIOSUS, PATENT DUCTUS ARTERIOSUS

ar·te·ri·ot·o·my \är-ˌtir-ē-ˈä-tə-mē\ *n, pl* **-mies** : the surgical incision of an artery

ar·te·rio·ve·nous \ˌär-ˌtir-ē-ō-ˈvē-nəs\ *adj* : of, relating to, or connecting the arteries and veins ⟨∼ anastomoses⟩

ar·ter·itis \ˌär-tə-ˈrī-təs\ *n* : arterial inflammation — see GIANT CELL ARTERITIS — **ar·ter·it·ic** \-ˈri-tik\ *adj*

ar·tery \ˈär-tə-rē\ *n, pl* **-ter·ies** : any of the tubular branching muscular- and elastic-walled vessels that carry blood from the heart through the body

arthr- *or* **arthro-** *comb form* : joint ⟨*arthr*algia⟩ ⟨*arthro*pathy⟩

ar·thral·gia \är-ˈthral-jə, -jē-ə\ *n* : pain in one or more joints — **ar·thral·gic** \-jik\ *adj*

ar·threc·to·my \är-ˈthrek-tə-mē\ *n, pl* **-mies** : surgical excision of a joint

¹**ar·thrit·ic** \är-ˈthri-tik\ *adj* : of, relating to, or affected with arthritis — **arthrit·i·cal·ly** \-ti-k(ə-)lē\ *adv*

²**arthritic** *n* : a person affected with arthritis

ar·thri·tis \är-ˈthrī-təs\ *n, pl* **-thrit·i·des** \-ˈthri-tə-ˌdēz\ : inflammation of joints due to infectious, metabolic, or constitutional causes; *also* : a specific arthritic condition ⟨the gonococcal and pneumococcal *arthritides*⟩

arthritis de·for·mans \-dē-ˈfor-ˌmanz\ *n* : a chronic arthritis marked by deformation of affected joints

ar·thro·cen·te·sis \ˌär-(ˌ)thrō-sen-ˈtē-səs\ *n, pl* **-te·ses** \-ˌsēz\ : surgical puncture of a joint

ar·throd·e·sis \är-ˈthrä-də-səs\ *n, pl* **-e·ses** \-ˌsēz\ : the surgical immobilization of a joint so that the bones grow solidly together : artificial ankylosis

ar·thro·dia \är-ˈthrō-dē-ə\ *n, pl* **-di·ae** \-dē-ˌē\ : GLIDING JOINT

ar·thro·dys·pla·sia \ˌär-(ˌ)thrō-dis-ˈplā-zhə, zhē-ə, -zē-ə\ *n* : abnormal development of a joint

ar·thro·gram \ˈär-thrō-ˌgram\ *n* : a roentgenogram of a joint made by arthrography

ar·throg·ra·phy \är-ˈthrä-grə-fē\ *n, pl* **-phies** : the roentgenographic visualization of a joint after the injection of a radiopaque substance — **ar·thro·graph·ic** \ˌär-thrə-ˈgra-fik\ *adj*

ar·thro·gry·po·sis \ˌär-(ˌ)thrō-gri-ˈpō-səs\ *n* : permanent flexure of a joint

arthrogryposis mul·ti·plex con·gen·i·ta \-ˈməl-tə-ˌpleks-kən-ˈje-nə-tə\ *n* : a congenital syndrome characterized by deformed joints with limited movement, atrophy of muscles, and contractures

ar·throl·o·gy \är-ˈthrä-lə-jē\ *n, pl* **-gies** : a science concerned with the study of joints

ar·throp·a·thy \är-ˈthrä-pə-thē\ *n, pl* **-thies** : a disease of a joint

ar·thro·plas·ty \ˈär-thrə-ˌplas-tē\ *n, pl* **-ties** : plastic surgery of a joint : the operative formation or restoration of a joint

ar·thro·pod \ˈär-thrə-ˌpäd\ *n* : any of a phylum (Arthropoda) of invertebrate animals (as insects, arachnids, and crustaceans) having a segmented body and jointed appendages, usu. a shell of chitin molted at intervals, and an anterior brain dorsal to the alimentary canal and connected with a ventral chain of ganglia — **arthropod** *adj* — **ar·throp·o·dan** \är-ˈthrä-pəd-ᵊn\ *adj*

ar·thro·scope \ˈär-thrə-ˌskōp\ *n* : a surgical instrument for the visual examination of the interior of a joint (as the knee)

ar·thros·co·py \är-ˈthrä-skə-pē\ *n, pl* **-pies** : examination of a joint with an arthroscope; *also* : joint surgery using an arthroscope — **ar·thro·scop·ic** \ˌär-thrə-ˈskä-pik\ *adj*

ar·thro·sis \är-ˈthrō-səs\ *n, pl* **-thro·ses** \-ˌsēz\ **1** : an articulation or line of juncture between bones **2** : a degenerative disease of a joint

ar·throt·o·my \är-ˈthrä-tə-mē\ *n, pl* **-mies** : incision into a joint

Ar·thus reaction \ˈär-thəs-, är-ˈtües-\ *n* : a reaction that follows injection of an antigen into an animal in which hypersensitivity has been previously established and that involves infiltrations, edema, sterile abscesses, and in severe cases gangrene — called also *Arthus phenomenon*

Arthus, Nicolas Maurice (1862–1945), French bacteriologist and physiologist.

ar·tic·u·lar \är-ˈti-kyə-lər\ *adj* : of or relating to a joint

articular capsule *n* : a ligamentous sac that surrounds the articular cavity of a freely movable joint, is attached to the bones, completely encloses the joint, and is composed of an outer fibrous membrane and an inner synovial membrane — called also *joint capsule*

articular cartilage *n* : cartilage that covers the articular surfaces of bones

articular disc *n* : a cartilage interposed between two articular surfaces and partially or completely separating the joint cavity into two compartments

articular process *n* : either of two processes on each side of a vertebra that articulate with adjoining vertebrae: **a** : one on each side of the neural arch that projects upward and articulates with an inferior articular process of the next more cranial vertebra —

called also *superior articular process* **b** : one on each side of the neural arch that projects downward and articulates with a superior articular process of the next more caudal vertebra — called also *inferior articular process*

ar·tic·u·late \är-'ti-kyə-ˌlāt\ *vb* **-lat·ed; -lat·ing 1** : to unite or be united by means of a joint (bones that ~ with each other) **2** : to arrange (artificial teeth) on an articulator

ar·tic·u·la·tion \är-ˌti-kyə-'lā-shən\ *n* **1** : the action or manner in which the parts come together at a joint **2 a** : a joint between bones or cartilages in the vertebrate skeleton that is immovable when the bones are directly united, slightly movable when they are united by an intervening substance, or more or less freely movable when the articular surfaces are covered with smooth cartilage and surrounded by an articular capsule — see AMPHIARTHROSIS, DIARTHROSIS, SYNARTHROSIS **b** : a movable joint between rigid parts of any animal (as between the segments of an insect appendage) **3 a** (1) : the act of properly arranging artificial teeth (2) : an arrangement of artificial teeth **b** : OCCLUSION 2a

ar·tic·u·la·tor \är-'ti-kyə-ˌlā-tər\ *n* : an apparatus used in dentistry for obtaining correct articulation of artificial teeth

ar·tic·u·la·to·ry \är-'ti-kyə-lə-ˌtōr-ē\ *adj* : of or relating to articulation

ar·ti·fact \'är-tə-ˌfakt\ *n* **1** : a product of artificial character due to usu. extraneous (as human) agency; *specif* : a product or formation in a microscopic preparation of a fixed tissue or cell that is caused by manipulation or reagents and is not indicative of actual structural relationships **2** : an electrocardiographic and electroencephalographic wave that arises from sources other than the heart or brain — **ar·ti·fac·tu·al** \ˌär-tə-'fak-chə-wəl, -shə-wəl\ *adj*

ar·ti·fi·cial \ˌär-tə-'fi-shəl\ *adj* : humanly contrived often on a natural model (an ~ limb) (an ~ eye) — **ar·ti·fi·cial·ly** *adv*

artificial insemination *n* : introduction of semen into the uterus or oviduct by other than natural means

artificial kidney *n* : an apparatus designed to do the work of the kidney during temporary stoppage of kidney function — called also *hemodialyzer*

artificial respiration *n* : the process of restoring or initiating breathing by forcing air into and out of the lungs to establish the rhythm of inspiration and expiration — see MOUTH-TO-MOUTH

ary·ep·i·glot·tic \ˌar-ē-ˌe-pə-'glä-tik\ *adj* : relating to or linking the arytenoid cartilage and the epiglottis (~ folds)

¹**ary·te·noid** \ˌar-ə-'tē-ˌnoid, ə-'rit-ᵊn-ˌoid\ *adj* **1** : relating to or being either of two small cartilages to which the vocal cords are attached and which are situated at the upper back part of the larynx **2** : relating to or being either of a pair of small muscles or an unpaired muscle of the larynx

²**arytenoid** *n* : an arytenoid cartilage or muscle

ary·te·noi·dec·to·my \ˌar-ə-ˌtē-ˌnoi-'dek-tə-mē, ə-ˌrit-ᵊn-ˌoi-\ *n, pl* **-mies** : surgical excision of an arytenoid cartilage

ary·te·noi·do·pexy \ˌar-ə-tə-'noi-də-ˌpek-sē, ə-ˌrit-ᵊn-'oid-\ *n, pl* **-pex·ies** : surgical fixation of arytenoid muscles or cartilages

As *symbol* arsenic

AS *abbr* **1** aortic stenosis **2** arteriosclerosis

ASA *abbr* [acetylsalicylic acid] aspirin

asa·fet·i·da or **asa·foet·i·da** \ˌa-sə-'fi-tə-dē, -'fe-tə-də\ *n* : the fetid gum resin of various Asian plants (genus *Ferula*) of the carrot family (Umbelliferae) that was formerly used in medicine as an antispasmodic and in folk medicine as a general prophylactic against disease

as·bes·tos \as-'bes-təs, az-\ *n* : any of several minerals that readily separate into long flexible fibers, that have been implicated as causes of certain cancers, and that have been used esp. formerly as fireproof insulating materials

as·bes·to·sis \ˌas-ˌbes-'tō-səs, ˌaz-\ *n, pl* **-to·ses** \-ˌsēz\ : a pneumoconiosis due to asbestos particles

as·car·i·a·sis \ˌas-kə-'rī-ə-səs\ *n, pl* **-a·ses** \-ˌsēz\ : infestation with or disease caused by ascarids

as·car·i·cid·al \ə-ˌskar-ə-'sīd-ᵊl\ *adj* : capable of destroying ascarids

as·car·i·cide \ə-'skar-ə-ˌsīd\ *n* : an agent destructive of ascarids

as·ca·rid \'as-kə-rəd\ *n* : any of a family (Ascaridae) of nematode worms that are usu. parasitic in the intestines of vertebrates — see ASCARIDIA, ASCARIS — **ascarid** *adj*

As·ca·rid·ia \ˌas-kə-'ri-dē-ə\ *n* : a genus of ascarid nematode worms that include an important intestinal parasite (*A. galli*) of some domestic fowl

as·car·i·di·a·sis \ə-ˌskar-ə-'dī-ə-səs\ *n, pl* **-a·ses** : ASCARIASIS

as·car·i·do·sis \ə-ˌskar-ə-'dō-səs\ *n, pl* **-do·ses** \-ˌsēz\ : ASCARIASIS

as·ca·ris \'as-kə-rəs\ *n* **1** *cap* : a genus of ascarid nematode worms that resemble earthworms in size and superficial appearance and include one (*A. lumbricoides*) parasitic in the human intestine **2** *pl* **as·car·i·des** \ə-'skar-ə-ˌdēz\ : ASCARID

As·ca·rops \'as-kə-ˌräps\ *n* : a genus of nematode worms (family Spiruridae) including a common reddish stomach worm (*A. strongylina*) of wild and domestic swine

as·cend \ə-'send\ *vb* : to move upward: as **a** : to conduct nerve impulses toward or to the brain **b** : to affect the extremities and esp. the lower limbs first and then the central nervous system

ascending aorta *n* : the part of the aorta from its origin to the beginning of the arch

ascending colon *n* : the part of the large intestine that extends from the cecum to the bend on the right side below the liver — compare DESCENDING COLON, TRANSVERSE COLON

ascending lumbar vein *n* : a longitudinal vein on each side that connects the lumbar veins and is frequently the origin of the azygos vein on the right side and of the hemiazygos vein on the left

ascending palatine artery *n* : PALATINE ARTERY 1a

Asch·heim–Zon·dek test \'äsh-ˌhīm-'zän-dik-, -'tsän-\ *n* : a test formerly used esp. to determine human pregnancy in its early stages on the basis of the effect of a subcutaneous injection of the patient's urine on the ovaries of an immature female mouse

Asch·heim \'äsh-ˌhīm\, **Selmor Samuel (1878–1965)**, and **Zon·dek** \'tson-ˌdek\, **Bernhard (1891–1966)**, German obstetrician-gynecologists.

Asch·off body \'ä-ˌshof-\ *n* : one of the tiny lumps in heart muscle typical of rheumatic heart disease; *also* : one of the similar but larger lumps found under the skin esp. in rheumatic fever or polyarthritis — called also *Aschoff nodule*

Aschoff, Karl Albert Ludwig (1866–1942), German pathologist.

as·ci·tes \ə-'sī-tēz\ *n, pl* **ascites** : accumulation of serous fluid in the spaces between tissues and organs in the cavity of the abdomen — **as·cit·ic** \-'sit-ik\ *adj*

as·co·my·cete \ˌas-kō-'mī-ˌsēt, -ˌmī-'sēt\ *n* : any of a class (Ascomycetes) or subdivision (Ascomycotina) of fungi (as yeasts or molds) with spores formed in asci — **as·co·my·ce·tous** \-ˌmī-'sē-təs\ *adj*

ascor·bate \ə-'skor-ˌbāt, -bət\ *n* : a salt of ascorbic acid

ascor·bic acid \ə-'skor-bik-\ *n* : VITAMIN C

ASCP *abbr* American Society of Clinical Pathologists

as·cus \'as-kəs\ *n, pl* **asci** \'as-ˌkī, -ˌkē; 'a-ˌsī\ : the membranous oval or tubular spore case of an ascomycete

ASCVD *abbr* arteriosclerotic cardiovascular disease

-ase *n suffix* : enzyme ⟨prote*ase*⟩ ⟨ure*ase*⟩

asep·sis \(ˌ)ā-'sep-səs, ə-\ *n, pl* **asep·ses** \-ˌsēz\ **1** : the condition of being aseptic **2** : the methods of producing

or maintaining an aseptic condition

asep·tic \-'sep-tik\ *adj* **1** : preventing infection ⟨∼ techniques⟩ **2** : free or freed from pathogenic microorganisms ⟨an ∼ operating room⟩ — **asep·ti·cal·ly** \-ti-k(ə-)lē\ *adv*

asex·u·al \(ˌ)ā-'sek-shə-wəl\ *adj* **1** : lacking sex or functional sexual organs **2** : produced without sexual action or differentiation ⟨∼ spores⟩ — **asex·u·al·ly** *adv*

asexual generation *n* : a generation that reproduces only by asexual processes — used of organisms exhibiting alternation of generations

asexual reproduction *n* : reproduction (as spore formation, fission, or budding) without union of individuals or germ cells

ASHD *abbr* arteriosclerotic heart disease

Asian influenza *n* : influenza caused by a mutant strain of the influenza virus isolated during the 1957 epidemic in Asia — called also *Asian flu*

Asi·at·ic cholera \ˌā-zhē-'a-tik-, -zē-\ *n* : cholera of Asian origin that is produced by virulent strains of the causative vibrio (*Vibrio cholerae*)

aso·cial \(ˌ)ā-'sō-shəl\ *adj* : not social: as **a** : rejecting or lacking the capacity for social interaction **b** : ANTISOCIAL

as·pa·rag·i·nase \as-pə-'ra-jə-ˌnās, -ˌnāz\ *n* : an enzyme that hydrolyzes asparagine to aspartic acid and ammonia

L–asparaginase — see entry alphabetized as L-ASPARAGINASE

as·par·a·gine \ə-'spar-ə-ˌjēn\ *n* : a white crystalline amino acid $C_4H_8N_2$-O_3 that is an amide of aspartic acid

as·par·tame \'as-pər-ˌtām, ə-'spär-\ *n* : a crystalline protein $C_{14}H_{18}N_2O_5$ that is derived from the amino acids phenylalanine and aspartic acid and is used as a low-calorie sweetener — see NUTRASWEET

as·par·tate \-ˌtāt\ *n* : a salt or ester of aspartic acid

as·par·tic acid \ə-'spär-tik-\ *n* : a crystalline amino acid $C_4H_7NO_4$ that is obtained from many proteins by hydrolysis

as·par·tyl \ə-'spär-təl, a-, -ˌtēl\ *n* : the bivalent radical –OCCH$_2$CH(NH$_2$)-CO– of aspartic acid

as·pect \'as-ˌpekt\ *n* : the part of an object (as an organ) in a particular position

aspera — see LINEA ASPERA

as·per·gil·lin \as-pər-'ji-lən\ *n* : an antibacterial substance isolated from two molds of the genus *Aspergillus* (*A. flavus* and *A. fumigatus*)

as·per·gil·lo·sis \ˌas-pər-(ˌ)ji-'lō-səs\ *n, pl* **-lo·ses** \-ˌsēz\ : infection with or disease caused (as in poultry) by molds of the genus *Aspergillus*

as·per·gil·lus \-'ji-ləs\ *n* **1** *cap* : a genus of ascomycetous fungi that include many common molds **2** *pl* **-gil·li** \-'ji-**

.lī, -(,)lē\ : any fungus of the genus *Aspergillus*

asper·mia \-'spər-mē-ə\ *n* : inability to produce or ejaculate semen — compare AZOOSPERMIA — **asper·mic** \-mik\ *adj*

as·phyx·ia \as-'fik-sē-ə, əs-\ *n* : a lack of oxygen or excess of carbon dioxide in the body that is usu. caused by interruption of breathing and that causes unconsciousness — **as·phyx·i·al** \-sē-əl\ *adj*

as·phyx·i·ant \-sē-ənt\ *n* : an agent (as a gas) capable of causing asphyxia

as·phyx·i·ate \-,āt\ *vb* **-at·ed; -at·ing 1** : to cause asphyxia in; *also* : to kill or make unconscious by inadequate oxygen, presence of noxious agents, or other obstruction to normal breathing **2** : to become asphyxiated — **as·phyx·i·a·tion** \-,fik-sē-'ā-shən\ *n* — **as·phyx·i·a·tor** \-'fik-sē-,ā-tər\ *n*

¹**as·pi·rate** \'as-pə-,rāt\ *vb* **-rat·ed; -rat·ing 1** : to draw by suction **2** : to remove (as blood) by aspiration **3** : to take into the lungs by aspiration

²**as·pi·rate** \-rət\ *n* : material removed by aspiration

as·pi·ra·tion \,as-pə-'rā-shən\ *n* **1** : the act of breathing and esp. of breathing in **2** : the withdrawal of fluid or friable tissue from the body **3** : the taking of foreign matter into the lungs with the respiratory current — **as·pi·ra·tion·al** \-sh(ə-)nəl\ *adj*

as·pi·ra·tor \'as-pə-,rā-tər\ *n* : an apparatus for producing suction or moving or collecting materials by suction; *esp* : a hollow tubular instrument connected with a partial vacuum and used to remove fluid or tissue or foreign bodies from the body

as·pi·rin \'as-prən, -pə-rən\ *n, pl* **aspirin** *or* **aspirins 1** : a white crystalline derivative C₉H₈O₄ of salicylic acid used for relief of pain and fever **2** : a tablet of aspirin

as·say \'a-,sā, a-'sā\ *n* **1** : examination and determination as to characteristics (as weight, measure, or quality) **2** : analysis (as of a drug) to determine the presence, absence, or quantity of one or more components — compare BIOASSAY **3** : a substance to be assayed; *also* : the tabulated result of assaying — **as·say** \a-'sā, 'a-,sā\ *vb*

as·sim·i·la·ble \ə-'si-mə-lə-bəl\ *adj* : capable of being assimilated

¹**as·sim·i·late** \ə-'si-mə-,lāt\ *vb* **-lat·ed; -lat·ing 1** : to take in and appropriate as nourishment : absorb into the system **2** : to become absorbed or incorporated into the system

²**as·sim·i·late** \-lət, -,lāt\ *n* : something that is assimilated

as·sim·i·la·tion \ə-,si-mə-'lā-shən\ *n* **1 a** : an act, process, or instance of assimilating **b** : the state of being assimilated **2** : the incorporation or conversion of nutrients into protoplasm

that in animals follows digestion and absorption **3** : the process of receiving new facts or of responding to new situations in conformity with what is already available to consciousness — compare APPERCEPTION

as·so·ci·a·tion \ə-,sō-sē-'ā-shən, -shē-\ *n* **1** : something linked in memory or imagination with a thing or person **2** : the process of forming mental connections or bonds between sensations, ideas, or memories **3** : the aggregation of chemical species to form (as with hydrogen bonds) loosely bound chemical complexes — compare POLYMERIZATION — **as·so·ci·a·tion·al** \-sh(ə-)nəl\ *adj*

association area *n* : an area of the cerebral cortex considered to function in linking and coordinating the sensory and motor areas

association fiber *n* : a nerve fiber connecting different parts of the brain; *esp* : any of the fibers connecting different areas within the cortex of each cerebral hemisphere — compare PROJECTION FIBER

as·so·cia·tive \ə-'sō-shē-,ā-tiv, -sē-; -shə-tiv\ *adj* **1** : of or relating to association esp. of ideas or images **2 a** : dependent on or characterized by association (an ~ reaction) **b** : acquired by a process of learning (an ~ reflex)

associative learning *n* : a learning process in which discrete ideas and percepts which are experienced together become linked to one another — compare PAIRED-ASSOCIATE LEARNING

associative neuron *n* : a neuron that conveys nerve impulses from one neuron to another — compare MOTONEURON, SENSORY NEURON

as·sort·ment \ə-'sort-mənt\ — see INDEPENDENT ASSORTMENT

asta·sia \ə-'stā-zhə, -zhē-ə\ *n* : muscular incoordination in standing — compare ABASIA — **astat·ic** \ə-'sta-tik\ *adj*

as·ta·tine \'as-tə-,tēn\ *n* : a radioactive halogen element discovered by bombarding bismuth with helium nuclei and also formed by radioactive decay — symbol *At*; see ELEMENT table

as·ter \'as-tər\ *n* : a system of microtubules arranged radially about a centriole at either end of the mitotic or meiotic spindle

aster·eog·no·sis \(,)ā-,ster-ē-äg-'nō-səs, -,stir-\ *n, pl* **-no·ses** \-,sēz\ : loss of the ability to recognize the shapes of objects by handling them

as·te·rix·is \,as-tə-'rik-sis\ *n* : a motor disorder characterized by jerking movements (as of the outstretched hands) and associated with various encephalopathies due esp. to faulty metabolism

asthen- *or* **astheno-** *comb form* : weak ⟨*asthen*opia⟩

as·the·nia \as-ˈthē-nē-ə\ *n* : lack or loss of strength : DEBILITY

as·then·ic \as-ˈthe-nik\ *adj* **1** : of, relating to, or exhibiting asthenia : DEBILITATED **2** : characterized by slender build and slight muscular development : ECTOMORPHIC

as·the·no·pia \ˌas-thə-ˈnō-pē-ə\ *n* : weakness or rapid fatigue of the eyes often accompanied by pain and headache — **as·the·no·pic** \-ˈnä-pik, -ˈnō-\ *adj*

asth·ma \ˈaz-mə\ *n* : a condition often of allergic origin that is marked by continuous or paroxysmal labored breathing accompanied by wheezing, by a sense of constriction in the chest, and often by attacks of coughing or gasping

¹**asth·mat·ic** \az-ˈma-tik\ *adj* : of, relating to, or affected with asthma ⟨an ~ attack⟩ — **asth·mat·i·cal·ly** \-ti-k(ə-)lē\ *adv*

²**asthmatic** *n* : a person affected with asthma

asthmaticus — see STATUS ASTHMATICUS

asth·mo·gen·ic \ˌaz-mə-ˈje-nik\ *adj* : causing asthmatic attacks

¹**astig·mat·ic** \ˌas-tig-ˈma-tik\ *adj* : affected with, relating to, or correcting astigmatism

²**astigmatic** *n* : a person affected with astigmatism

astig·ma·tism \ə-ˈstig-mə-ˌti-zəm\ *n* **1** : a defect of an optical system (as a lens) causing rays from a point to fail to meet in a focal point resulting in a blurred and imperfect image **2** : a defect of vision due to astigmatism of the refractive system of the eye and esp. to corneal irregularity — compare EMMETROPIA, MYOPIA

as tol *abbr* as tolerated

astr- *or* **astro-** *comb form* **1** : star ⟨*astrocyte*⟩ **2** : astrocyte ⟨*astroblastoma*⟩ ⟨*astroglia*⟩

astragal- *or* **astragalo-** *comb form* : astragalus ⟨*astragalectomy*⟩

astrag·a·lec·to·my \ə-ˌstra-gə-ˈlek-tə-mē\ *n, pl* **-mies** : surgical removal of the astragalus

as·trag·a·lus \ə-ˈstra-gə-ləs\ *n, pl* **-li** \-ˌlī, -ˌlē\ : one of the proximal bones of the tarsus of the higher vertebrates — see TALUS 1

astral ray *n* : one of the thin fibrils that make up the mitotic or meiotic aster

¹**as·trin·gent** \ə-ˈstrin-jənt\ *adj* : having the property of drawing together the soft organic tissues ⟨~ cosmetic lotions⟩: **a** : tending to shrink mucous membranes or raw or exposed tissues : checking discharge (as of serum or mucus) : STYPTIC **b** : tending to pucker the tissues of the mouth — **as·trin·gen·cy** \-jən-sē\ *n*

²**astringent** *n* : an astringent agent or substance

as·tro·blas·to·ma \ˌas-trə-(ˌ)blas-ˈtō-mə\ *n, pl* **-mas** *or* **-ma·ta** \-mə-tə\ : an

astrocytoma of moderate malignancy

as·tro·cyte \ˈas-trə-ˌsīt\ *n* : a star-shaped cell; *esp* : any comparatively large much-branched neuroglial cell — **as·tro·cyt·ic** \ˌas-trə-ˈsi-tik\ *adj*

as·tro·cy·to·ma \ˌas-trə-sī-ˈtō-mə\ *n, pl* **-mas** *or* **-ma·ta** \-mə-tə\ : a nerve-tissue tumor composed of astrocytes

as·tro·glia \ə-ˈsträ-glē-ə, ˌas-trə-ˈglī-ə\ *n* : neuroglia tissue composed of astrocytes — **as·tro·gli·al** \-əl\ *adj*

asy·lum \ə-ˈsī-ləm\ *n* : an institution for the relief or care of the destitute or sick and esp. the insane

asym·bo·lia \ˌā-(ˌ)sim-ˈbō-lē-ə\ *n* : loss of the power to understand previously familiar symbols and signs

asym·met·ri·cal \ˌā-sə-ˈme-tri-kəl\ *or* **asym·met·ric** \-ˈtrik\ *adj* **1** : not symmetrical **2** : characterized by bonding to different atoms or groups — **asym·met·ri·cal·ly** \-tri-k(ə-)lē\ *adv*

asym·me·try \(ˌ)ā-ˈsi-mə-trē\ *n, pl* **-tries** **1** : lack or absence of symmetry: as **a** : lack of proportion between the parts of a thing; *esp* : want of bilateral symmetry ⟨~ in the development of the two sides of the brain⟩ **b** : lack of coordination of two parts acting in connection with one another ⟨~ of convergence of the eyes⟩ **2** : lack of symmetry in spatial arrangement of atoms and groups in a molecule

asymp·tom·at·ic \ˌā-ˌsimp-tə-ˈma-tik\ *adj* : presenting no symptoms of disease — **asymp·tom·at·i·cal·ly** \-ti-k(ə-)lē\ *adv*

asyn·ap·sis \ˌā-sə-ˈnap-səs\ *n, pl* **-ap·ses** \-ˌsēz\ : failure of pairing of homologous chromosomes in meiosis

asyn·cli·tism \(ˌ)ā-ˈsin-klə-ˌti-zəm, -ˈsin-\ *n* : presentation of the fetal head during childbirth with the axis oriented obliquely to the axial planes of the pelvis

asy·ner·gia \ˌā-sə-ˈnər-jē-ə, -jə\ *or* **asyn·er·gy** \(ˌ)ā-ˈsi-nər-jē\ *n, pl* **-gi·as** *or* **-gies** : lack of coordination (as of muscles) — **asy·ner·gic** \ˌā-sə-ˈnər-jik\ *adj*

asys·to·le \(ˌ)ā-ˈsis-tə-(ˌ)lē\ *n* : a condition of weakening or cessation of systole — **asys·tol·ic** \ˌā-sis-ˈtä-lik\ *adj*

At *symbol* astatine

Ata·brine \ˈa-tə-brən\ *trademark* — used for a preparation of quinacrine

¹**at·a·rac·tic** \ˌa-tə-ˈrak-tik\ *or* **at·a·rax·ic** \-ˈrak-sik\ *adj* : tending to tranquilize ⟨~ drugs⟩

²**ataractic** *or* **ataraxic** *n* : TRANQUILIZER

at·a·rax·ia \ˌa-tə-ˈrak-sē-ə\ *or* **at·a·raxy** \ˈa-tə-ˌrak-sē\ *n, pl* **-rax·ias** *or* **-rax·ies** : calmness untroubled by mental or emotional disquiet

at·a·vism \ˈa-tə-ˌvi-zəm\ *n* : recurrence in an organism of a trait or character typical of an ancestral form and usu. due to genetic recombination **2** : an individual or character manifesting atavism : THROWBACK — **at·a·vis·tic** \ˌa-tə-ˈvis-tik\ *adj*

atax·ia \ə-ˈtak-sē-ə, (ˌ)ā-\ *n* : an inability to coordinate voluntary muscular movements that is symptomatic of some nervous disorders — **atax·ic** \-sik\ *adj*

atel- *or* **atelo-** *comb form* : defective ⟨**atel**ectasis⟩

at·el·ec·ta·sis \ˌat-əl-'ek-tə-səs\ *n, pl* **-ses** \-ˌsēz\ : collapse of the expanded lung; *also* : defective expansion of the pulmonary alveoli at birth — **at·el·ec·tat·ic** \-ek-'ta-tik\ *adj*

ate·li·o·sis \ə-ˌte-lē-'ō-səs, -ˌtē-\ *n, pl* **-oses** \-ˌsēz\ : incomplete development; *esp* : dwarfism associated with anterior pituitary deficiencies and marked by essentially normal intelligence and proportions — compare ACHONDROPLASIA

¹**ate·li·ot·ic** \-'ä-tik\ *adj* : of, relating to, or affected with ateliosis

²**ateliotic** *n* : a person affected with ateliosis

aten·o·lol \ə-'te-nə-ˌlȯl, -ˌlōl\ *n* : a beta-blocker $C_{14}H_{22}N_2O_3$ used in the treatment of hypertension

athero- *comb form* : atheroma ⟨**athero**genic⟩

ath·er·o·gen·e·sis \ˌa-thə-rō-'je-nə-səs, *n, pl* **-eses** \-ˌsēz\ : the process of developing atheroma

ath·er·o·gen·ic \-'je-nik\ *adj* : relating to or producing degenerative changes in arterial walls ⟨∼ diet⟩ — **ath·ero·ge·nic·i·ty** \-jə-'ni-sə-tē\ *n*

ath·er·o·ma \ˌa-thə-'rō-mə\ *n, pl* **-mas** *also* **-ma·ta** \-mə-tə\ **1** : fatty degeneration of the inner coat of the arteries **2** : an abnormal fatty deposit in an artery — **ath·er·o·ma·tous** \-'rō-mə-təs\ *adj*

ath·er·o·ma·to·sis \ˌa-thə-rō-mə-'tō-səs, *n, pl* **-toses** \-ˌsēz\ : a disease characterized by atheromatous degeneration of the arteries

ath·er·o·scle·ro·sis \ˌa-thə-rō-sklə-'rō-səs, *n, pl* **-roses** \-ˌsēz\ : an arteriosclerosis characterized by atheromatous deposits in and fibrosis of the inner layer of the arteries — **ath·ero·scle·rot·ic** \-sklə-'rä-tik\ *adj* — **ath·ero·scle·rot·i·cal·ly** \-i-k(ə-)lē\ *adv*

¹**ath·e·toid** \'a-thə-ˌtȯid\ *adj* : exhibiting or characteristic of athetosis

²**athetoid** *n* : an athetoid individual

ath·e·to·sis \ˌa-thə-'tō-səs, *n, pl* **-toses** \-ˌsēz\ : a nervous disorder that is marked by continual slow movements esp. of the extremities and is usu. due to a brain lesion

athlete's foot *n* : ringworm of the feet — called also *tinea pedis*

ath·let·ic \ath-'le-tik\ *adj* : characterized by heavy frame, large chest, and powerful muscular development : MESOMORPHIC

athletic supporter *n* : a supporter for the genitals worn by men participating in sports or strenuous activities — called also *jockstrap*; see CUP 1

ath·ro·cyte \'a-thrə-ˌsīt\ *n* : a cell capable of athrocytosis — **ath·ro·cyt·ic** \ˌa-thrə-'si-tik\ *adj*

ath·ro·cy·to·sis \ˌa-thrə-sī-'tō-səs, *n, pl* **-toses** \-ˌsēz\ : the capacity of some cells (as of the proximal convoluted tubule of the kidney) to pick up foreign material and store it in granular form in the cytoplasm

athy·mic \(ˌ)ā-'thī-mik\ *adj* : lacking a thymus

At·i·van \'at-i-ˌvan\ *trademark* — used for a preparation of lorazepam

atlant- *or* **atlanto-** *comb form* **1** : atlas ⟨**atlant**al⟩ **2** : atlantal and ⟨**atlant**ooccipital⟩

at·lan·tal \-'lant-əl\ *adj* **1** : of or relating to the atlas **2** : ANTERIOR 1, CEPHALIC

at·lan·to·ax·i·al \ət-ˌlan-tō-'ak-sē-əl, at-\ *adj* : relating to or being anatomical structures that connect the atlas and the axis

at·lan·to·oc·cip·i·tal \-äk-'si-pət-əl\ *adj* : relating to or being structures (as a joint or ligament) joining the atlas and the occipital bone

at·las \'at-ləs\ *n* : the first vertebra of the neck

at·mo·sphere \'at-mə-ˌsfir\ *n* **1** : the whole mass of air surrounding the earth **2** : the air of a locality **3** : a unit of pressure equal to the pressure of the air at sea level or approximately 14.7 pounds per square inch (101,000 newtons per square meter) — **at·mo·spher·ic** \ˌat-mə-'sfir-ik, -'sfer-\ *adj*

atmospheric pressure *n* : the pressure exerted in every direction at any given point by the weight of the atmosphere

at·om \'a-təm\ *n* : the smallest particle of an element that can exist either alone or in combination — **atom·ic** \ə-'tä-mik\ *adj*

atomic cocktail *n* : a radioactive substance (as iodide of sodium) dissolved in water and administered orally to patients with cancer

atomic energy *n* : energy that can be liberated by changes in the nucleus of an atom (as by fission of a heavy nucleus or fusion of light nuclei into heavier ones with accompanying loss of mass)

atomic number *n* : the number of protons in the nucleus of an element — see ELEMENT table

atomic weight *n* : the average relative mass of one atom of an element usu. with carbon of atomic weight 12 being taken as the standard — see ELEMENT table

at·om·ize \'a-tə-ˌmīz\ *vb* **-ized; -iz·ing** : to convert to minute particles or to a fine spray — **at·om·i·za·tion** \ˌa-tə-mə-'zā-shən\ *n*

at·om·iz·er \'a-tə-ˌmī-zər\ *n* : an instrument for atomizing usu. a perfume, disinfectant, or medicament

aton·ic \(ˌ)ā-'tä-nik, (ˌ)a-\ *adj* : characterized by atony

at·o·ny \'at-ᵊn-ē\ *or* **ato·nia** \(ˌ)ā-'tō-nē-**

ə\ *n, pl* **-nies** *or* **-ni·as** : lack of physiological tone esp. of a contractile organ

at·o·py \'a-tə-pē\ *n, pl* **-pies** : a probably hereditary allergy characterized by symptoms (as asthma, hay fever, or hives) produced upon exposure to the exciting antigen without inoculation — **ato·pic** \(ı)ā-'tä-pik. -'tō-\ *adj*

ATP \aā-(ı)tē-'pē\ *n* : a phosphorylated nucleoside $C_{10}H_{16}N_5O_{13}P_3$ of adenine that when reversibly converted esp. to ADP releases energy in the cell for many metabolic reactions (as protein synthesis) — called also *adenosine triphosphate*

ATPase \ā-(ı)tē-'pē-ıās. -ıāz\ *n* : an enzyme that hydrolyzes ATP; *esp* : one that hydrolyzes ATP to ADP and inorganic phosphate — called also *adenosine triphosphatase*

atre·sia \ə-'trē-zhə\ *n* 1 : absence or closure of a natural passage of the body ⟨∼ of the small intestine⟩ 2 : absence or disappearance of an anatomical part (as an ovarian follicle) by degeneration — **atret·ic** \ə-'tre-tik\ *adj*

atri- *or* **atrio-** *comb form* 1 : atrium ⟨*atrial*⟩ 2 : atrial and ⟨*atrioventricular*⟩

atria *pl of* ATRIUM

atri·al \'ā-trē-əl\ *adj* : of, relating to, or affecting an atrium ⟨∼ disorder⟩

atrial fibrillation *n* : very rapid uncoordinated contractions of the atria of the heart resulting in a lack of synchronism between heartbeat and pulse beat — called also *auricular fibrillation*

atrial flutter *n* : an irregularity of the heartbeat in which the contractions of the atria exceed in number those of the ventricle — called also *auricular flutter*

atrial natriuretic factor *n* : a peptide hormone secreted by the cardiac atria that stimulates natriuresis and diuresis and helps regulate blood pressure

atrial septum *n* : INTERATRIAL SEPTUM

atrich·ia \ā-'tri-kē-ə, ə-\ *n* : congenital or acquired baldness : ALOPECIA

atrio·ven·tric·u·lar \ıā-trē-(ı)ō-ven-'tri-kyə-lər\ *adj* 1 : of, relating to, or situated between an atrium and ventricle 2 : of, involving, or being the atrioventricular node

atrioventricular bundle *n* : BUNDLE OF HIS

atrioventricular canal *n* : the canal joining the atrium and ventricle in the tubular embryonic heart

atrioventricular node *n* : a small mass of tissue that is situated in the wall of the right atrium adjacent to the septum between the atria and passes impulses received from the sinoatrial node to the ventricles by way of the bundle of His

atrioventricular valve *n* : a valve between an atrium and ventricle of the heart: **a** : BICUSPID VALVE **b** : TRICUSPID VALVE

atri·um \'ā-trē-əm\ *n, pl* **atria** \-trē-ə\ *also* **atri·ums** : an anatomical cavity or passage; *esp* : a chamber of the heart that receives blood from the veins and forces it into a ventricle or ventricles

At·ro·pa \'a-trə-pə\ *n* : a genus of Eurasian and African herbs (as belladonna) of the nightshade family (Solanaceae) that are a source of medicinal alkaloids (as atropine and scopolamine)

atro·phic \(ı)ā-'trō-fik, ə-, -'trä-\ *adj* : relating to or characterized by atrophy ⟨an ∼ jaw⟩

atrophicans — see ACRODERMATITIS CHRONICA ATROPHICANS

atrophic rhinitis *n* 1 : a disease of swine that is characterized by purulent inflammation of the nasal mucosa, atrophy of the nasal conchae, and abnormal swelling of the face 2 : OZENA

atrophicus — see LICHEN SCLEROSUS ET ATROPHICUS

atrophic vaginitis *n* : inflammation of the vagina with thinning of the epithelial lining that occurs following menopause

¹**at·ro·phy** \'a-trə-fē\ *n, pl* **-phies** : decrease in size or wasting away of a body part or tissue; *also* : arrested development or loss of a part or organ incidental to the normal development or life of an animal or plant — **atro·phic** \ā-'trō-fik\ *adj*

²**atrophy** \'a-trə-fē, -ıfī\ *vb* **-phied; -phy·ing** : to undergo or cause to undergo atrophy

at·ro·pine \'a-trə-ıpēn\ *n* : a racemic mixture of hyoscyamine obtained from belladonna and related plants (family Solanaceae) and used esp. in the form of its sulfate for its anticholinergic effects (as relief of smooth muscle spasms or dilation of the pupil of the eye)

at·ro·pin·ism \-ıpē-ıni-zəm\ *n* : poisoning by atropine

at·ro·pin·i·za·tion \ıa-trə-ıpē-nə-'zā-shən\ *n* : the physiological condition of being under the influence of atropine — **at·ro·pin·ize** \'a-trə-pə-ınīz\ *vb*

at·ro·scine \'a-trə-ısēn, -sən\ *n* : racemic scopolamine

at·tach·ment \ə-'tach-mənt\ *n* : the physical connection by which one thing is attached to another — **at·tach** \ə-'tach\ *vb*

¹**at·tack** \ə-'tak\ *vb* : to begin to affect or to act on injuriously

²**attack** *n* : a fit of sickness; *esp* : an active episode of a chronic or recurrent disease

at·tend \ə-'tend\ *vb* : to visit or stay with professionally as a physician or nurse

¹**at·tend·ing** \ə-'ten-diŋ\ *adj* : serving as a physician or surgeon on the staff of a hospital, regularly visiting and

treating patients, and often supervising students, fellows, and the house staff

²**attending** *n* : an attending physician or surgeon

at·ten·tion \ə-'ten-chən\ *n* **1** : the act or state of attending : the application of the mind to any object of sense or thought **2 a** : an organismic condition of selective awareness or perceptual receptivity **b** : the process of focusing consciousness to produce greater vividness and clarity of certain of its contents relative to others — **at·ten·tion·al** \-'ten-chə-nəl\ *adj*

attention deficit disorder *n* : a syndrome of learning and behavioral problems that is not caused by any serious underlying physical or mental disorder and is characterized esp. by difficulty in sustaining attention, by impulsive behavior (as in speaking out of turn), and usu. by excessive activity — called also *minimal brain dysfunction*

attention–deficit hyperactivity disorder *n* : ATTENTION DEFICIT DISORDER

at·ten·u·ate \ə-'ten-yə-ˌwāt\ *vb* **-at·ed; -at·ing** : to reduce the severity of (a disease) or virulence or vitality of (a pathogenic agent) ⟨a procedure to ∼ severe diabetes⟩ ⟨attenuated bacilli⟩

at·ten·u·a·tion \ə-ˌten-yə-'wā-shən\ *n* : a decrease in the pathogenicity or vitality of a microorganism or in the severity of a disease

at·tic \'a-tik\ *n* : the small upper space of the middle ear — called also *epitympanic recess*

at·ti·co·to·my \ˌa-tə-'kä-tə-mē\ *n, pl* **-mies** : surgical incision of the tympanic attic

at·ti·tude \'a-tə-ˌtüd, -ˌtyüd\ *n* **1** : the arrangement of the parts of the body : POSTURE **2 a** : a mental position with regard to a fact or state **b** : a feeling or emotion toward a fact or state **3** : an organismic state of readiness to respond in a characteristic way to a stimulus (as an object, concept, or situation)

at·ti·tu·di·nal \ˌa-tə-'tüd-ᵊn-əl, -'tyüd-\ *adj* : relating to, based on, or expressive of personal attitudes or feelings

at·tri·tion \ə-'tri-shən\ *n* : the act of rubbing together; *also* : the wearing or grinding down by friction ⟨∼ of teeth⟩

atyp·ia \ˌ(ˌ)ā-'ti-pē-ə\ *n* : ATYPISM

atyp·i·cal \ˌ(ˌ)ā-'ti-pi-kəl\ *adj* : not typical : not like the usual or normal type — **atyp·i·cal·ly** \-pi-k(ə-)lē\ *adv*

atypical pneumonia *n* : PRIMARY ATYPICAL PNEUMONIA

atyp·ism \ˌ(ˌ)ā-'ti-ˌpi-zəm\ *n* : the condition of being uncharacteristic or lacking uniformity

Au *symbol* [L *aurum*] gold

au·di·ble \'ȯ-də-bəl\ *adj* : heard or capable of being heard — **au·di·bil·i·ty** \ˌȯ-də-'bi-lə-tē\ *n* — **au·di·bly** \'ȯ-də-blē\ *adv*

¹**au·dile** \'ȯ-ˌdīl\ *n* : a person whose mental imagery is auditory rather than visual or motor — compare TACTILE, VISUALIZER

²**audile** *adj* **1** : of or relating to hearing : AUDITORY **2** : of, relating to, or being an audile

audio- *comb form* **1** : hearing ⟨*audiol*ogy⟩ **2** : sound ⟨*audio*genic⟩

au·dio·gen·ic \ˌȯ-dē-ō-'je-nik\ *adj* : produced by frequencies corresponding to sound waves — used esp. of epileptoid responses ⟨∼ seizures⟩

au·dio·gram \'ȯ-dē-ə-ˌgram\ *n* : a graphic representation of the relation of vibration frequency and the minimum sound intensity for hearing

au·di·ol·o·gist \ˌȯ-dē-'ä-lə-jist\ *n* : a specialist in audiology

au·di·ol·o·gy \ˌȯ-dē-'ä-lə-jē\ *n, pl* **-gies** : a branch of science dealing with hearing; *specif* : therapy of individuals having impaired hearing — **au·dio·log·i·cal** \-dē-ə-'lä-ji-kəl\ *also* **au·dio·log·ic** \-dē-ə-'lä-jik\ *adj*

au·di·om·e·ter \ˌȯ-dē-'ä-mə-tər\ *n* : an instrument used in measuring the acuity of hearing

au·di·om·e·try \ˌȯ-dē-'ä-mə-trē\ *n, pl* **-tries** : the testing and measurement of hearing acuity for variations in sound intensity and pitch and for tonal purity — **au·dio·met·ric** \-ō-'me-trik\ *adj* — **au·di·om·e·trist** \-'ä-mə-trist\ *n*

au·di·to·ry \'ȯ-də-ˌtōr-ē\ *adj* **1** : of or relating to hearing **2** : attained, experienced, or produced through or as if through hearing ⟨∼ images⟩ ⟨∼ hallucinations⟩ **3** : marked by great susceptibility to impressions and reactions produced by acoustic stimuli

auditory area *n* : a sensory area in the temporal cortex associated with the organ of hearing — called also *auditory center, auditory cortex*

auditory canal *n* : either of two passages of the ear — called also *acoustic meatus, auditory meatus*; compare EXTERNAL AUDITORY MEATUS, INTERNAL AUDITORY MEATUS

auditory cortex *n* : AUDITORY AREA

auditory nerve *n* : either of the 8th pair of cranial nerves connecting the inner ear with the brain, transmitting impulses concerned with hearing and balance, and composed of the cochlear nerve and the vestibular nerve — called also *acoustic nerve, auditory, eighth cranial nerve, vestibulocochlear nerve*

auditory tube *n* : EUSTACHIAN TUBE

Auer·bach's plexus \'au̇-ər-ˌbäks-, -ˌbäks-\ *n* : MYENTERIC PLEXUS
Auer·bach \'au̇-ər-ˌbäk, -ˌbäk\ , **Le·opold (1828–1897)**, German anatomist.

aug·ment \ȯg-'ment, 'ȯg-ˌment\ *vb* : to increase in size, amount, degree, or severity — **aug·men·ta·tion** \óg-mən-'tā-shən, -ˌmen-\ *n*

aur- *or* **auri-** *comb form* : ear ⟨aural⟩

au·ra \'ȯr-ə\ *n, pl* **auras** *also* **au·rae** \-ē\ : a subjective sensation (as of voices or colored lights) experienced before an attack of some disorders (as epilepsy or migraine)

au·ral \'ȯr-əl\ *adj* : of or relating to the ear or to the sense of hearing — **au·ral·ly** *adv*

Au·reo·my·cin \ˌȯr-ē-ō-'mī-sən\ *trademark* — used for a preparation of the hydrochloride of chlortetracycline

au·ri·cle \'ȯr-i-kəl\ *n* **1 a** : PINNA **b** : an atrium of the heart **2** : an angular or ear-shaped anatomical lobe or process

au·ric·u·la \ȯ-'ri-kyu̇-lə\ *n, pl* **-lae** \-ˌlē\ : AURICLE; *esp* : AURICULAR APPENDAGE

au·ric·u·lar \ȯ-'ri-kyu̇-lər\ *adj* **1** : of, relating to, or using the ear or the sense of hearing **2** : understood or recognized by the sense of hearing **3** : of or relating to an auricle or auricular appendage ⟨∼ fibrillation⟩

auricular appendage *n* : an ear-shaped pouch projecting from each atrium of the heart — called also *auricular appendix*

auricular artery — see POSTERIOR AURICULAR ARTERY

auricular fibrillation *n* : ATRIAL FIBRILLATION

auricular flutter *n* : ATRIAL FLUTTER

au·ric·u·lar·is \ȯ-ˌri-kyu̇-'lar-əs, -'lär-\ *n, pl* **-lar·es** \-ˌēz\ : any of three muscles attached to the cartilage of the external ear that assist in moving the scalp and in some individuals the external ear itself and that consist of one that is anterior, one superior, and one posterior in position — called also respectively *auricularis anterior*, *auricularis superior*, and *auricularis posterior*

auricular tubercle of Darwin *n* : DARWIN'S TUBERCLE

auricular vein — see POSTERIOR AURICULAR VEIN

auriculo- *comb form* : of or belonging to an auricle of the heart and ⟨auriculoventricular⟩

au·ric·u·lo·tem·po·ral nerve \ȯ-ˌri-kyu̇-(ˌ)lō-'tem-pə-rəl-\ *n* : the branch of the mandibular nerve that supplies sensory fibers to the skin of the external ear and temporal region and autonomic fibers from the otic ganglion to the parotid gland

au·ric·u·lo·ven·tric·u·lar \-ven-'tri-kyu̇-lər,-vən-\ *adj* : ATRIOVENTRICULAR

au·ro·thio·glu·cose \ˌȯr-ō-ˌthī-ō-'glü-ˌkōs, -ˌkōz\ *n* : GOLD THIOGLUCOSE

aus·cul·ta·tion \ˌȯ-skəl-'tā-shən\ *n* : the act of listening to sounds arising within organs (as the lungs or heart) as an aid to diagnosis and treatment — **aus·cul·tate** \'ȯ-skəl-ˌtāt\ *vb* — **aus·cul·ta·to·ry** \ȯ-'skəl-tə-ˌtȯr-ē\ *adj*

Aus·tra·lia antigen \ȯ-'strāl-yə-\ *also* **Aus·tra·lian antigen** \-yən-\ *n* : HEPATITIS B SURFACE ANTIGEN

aut- *or* **auto-** *comb form* : self : same one ⟨autism⟩: **a** : of, by, affecting, from, or for the same individual ⟨autograft⟩ ⟨autotransfusion⟩ ⟨autovaccination⟩ **b** : arising or produced within the individual and acting or directed toward or against the individual or the individual's own body, tissues, or molecules ⟨autoimmunity⟩ ⟨autosuggestion⟩ ⟨autoerotism⟩

au·ta·coid \'ȯ-tə-ˌkȯid\ *n* : a physiologically active substance (as serotonin, bradykinin, or angiotensin) produced by and acting within the body

au·tism \'ȯ-ˌti-zəm\ *n* **1** : absorption in self-centered subjective mental activity (as daydreams, fantasies, delusions, and hallucinations) esp. when accompanied by marked withdrawal from reality **2** : a mental disorder originating in infancy that is characterized by self-absorption, inability to interact socially, repetitive behavior, and language dysfunction (as echolalia)

¹au·tis·tic \ȯ-'tis-tik\ *adj* : of, relating to, or marked by autism ⟨∼ behavior⟩ ⟨∼ children⟩

²autistic *n* : a person affected with autism

au·to·ag·glu·ti·na·tion \ˌȯ-tō-ə-ˌglüt-ᵊn-'ā-shən\ *n* : agglutination of red blood cells by cold agglutinins in an individual's own serum usu. at lower than body temperature

au·to·ag·glu·ti·nin \ˌȯ-tō-ə-'glüt-ᵊn-ən\ *n* : an antibody that agglutinates the red blood cells of the individual producing it — compare COLD AGGLUTININ

Au·to·an·a·lyz·er \ˌȯ-tō-'an-ᵊl-ˌī-zər\ *trademark* — used for an instrument designed for automatic chemical analysis (as of blood glucose level)

au·to·an·ti·body \ˌȯ-tō-(ˌ)tō-'an-ti-ˌbä-dē\ *n, pl* **-bod·ies** : an antibody active against a tissue constituent of the individual producing it

au·to·an·ti·gen \ˌȯ-tō-'an-ti-jen\ *n* : an antigen that is a normal bodily constituent and against which the immune system produces autoantibodies

au·toch·tho·nous \(ˌ)ȯ-'täk-thə-nəs\ *adj* **1 a** : indigenous or endemic to a region ⟨∼ malaria⟩ **b** : contracted in the area where reported **2** : originated in that part of the body where found — used chiefly of pathological conditions — **au·toch·tho·nous·ly** *adv*

au·to·clav·able \'ȯ-tə-ˌklā-və-bəl\ *adj* : able to withstand the action of an autoclave — **au·to·clav·abil·i·ty** \ˌȯ-tə-ˌklā-və-'bi-lə-tē\ *n*

au·to·clave \'ȯ-tō-ˌklāv\ *n* : an apparatus (as for sterilizing) using superheated steam under pressure — **autoclave** *vb*

au·to·er·o·tism \ˌȯ-tō-'er-ə-ˌti-zəm\ *or*

au·to·erot·i·cism \-i-'rä-tə-ˌsi-zəm\ *n* **1** : sexual gratification obtained solely through stimulation by oneself of one's own body **2** : sexual feeling arising without known external stimulation — **au·to·erot·ic** \-i-'rä-tik\ *adj* — **au·to·erot·i·cal·ly** \-ti-k(ə-)lē\ *adv*

au·to·gen·ic \ˌȯ-tə-'je-nik\ *adj* **1** : AUTOGENOUS **2** : of or relating to any of several relaxation techniques that actively involve the patient (as by meditation or biofeedback) in attempts to control physiological variables (as blood pressure)

au·tog·e·nous \ȯ-'tä-jə-nəs\ *adj* **1** : produced independently of external influence or aid : ENDOGENOUS **2** : originating or derived from sources within the same individual ⟨an ∼ graft⟩ ⟨∼ vaccine⟩

au·to·graft \'ȯ-tō-ˌgraft\ *n* : a tissue or organ that is transplanted from one part to another part of the same body — **autograft** *vb*

au·to·he·mo·ly·sin \ˌȯ-tō-ˌhē-mə-'līs-ᵊn\ *n* : a hemolysin that acts on the red blood cells of the individual in whose blood it is found

au·to·he·mol·y·sis \-hi-'mä-lə-səs, -ˌhē-mə-'lī-səs\ *n, pl* **-ly·ses** \-ˌsēz\ : hemolysis of red blood cells by factors in the serum of the person from whom the blood is taken

au·to·ther·a·py \-ˌhē-mō-'ther-ə-pē\ *n, pl* **-pies** : treatment of disease by modification (as by irradiation) of the patient's own blood or by its introduction (as by intramuscular injection) outside the bloodstream

au·to·hyp·no·sis \ˌȯ-tō-hip-'nō-səs\ *n, pl* **-no·ses** \-ˌsēz\ : self-induced and usu. automatic hypnosis — **au·to·hyp·not·ic** \-'nä-tik\ *adj*

au·to·im·mune \-i-'myün\ *adj* : of, relating to, or caused by antibodies or T cells that attack molecules, cells, or tissues of the organism producing them ⟨∼ diseases⟩

au·to·im·mu·ni·ty \ˌȯ-tō-i-'myü-nə-tē\ *n, pl* **-ties** : a condition in which the body produces an immune response against its own tissue constituents — **au·to·im·mu·ni·za·tion** \-i-myə-nə-'zā-shən *also* -ˌī-myə-nə-\ *n* — **au·to·im·mu·nize** \-'i-myə-ˌnīz\ *vb*

au·to·in·fec·tion \-in-'fek-shən\ *n* : reinfection with larvae produced by parasitic worms already in the body — compare HYPERINFECTION

au·to·in·oc·u·la·tion \-i-ˌnä-kyə-'lā-shən\ *n* **1** : inoculation with vaccine prepared from material from one's own body **2** : spread of infection from one part to other parts of the same body — **au·to·in·oc·u·la·ble** \ȯ-tō-i-'nä-kyə-lə-bəl\ *adj*

au·to·ki·ne·sis \ˌȯ-tō-kə-'nē-səs, -kī-\ *n, pl* **-ne·ses** \-ˌsēz\ : spontaneous or voluntary movement

au·tol·o·gous \ȯ-'tä-lə-gəs\ *adj* **1** : derived from the same individual ⟨∼

grafts⟩ — compare HETEROLOGOUS 1, HOMOLOGOUS 2 **2** : involving one individual as both donor and recipient (as of blood) ⟨∼ transfusion⟩

au·tol·y·sate \ȯ-'tä-lə-ˌsāt, -ˌzāt\ *also* **au·tol·y·zate** \-ˌzāt\ *n* : a product of autolysis

au·tol·y·sin \-lə-sən\ *n* : a substance that produces autolysis

au·tol·y·sis \-lə-səs\ *n, pl* **-y·ses** \-lə-ˌsēz\ : breakdown of all or part of a cell or tissue by self-produced enzymes — **au·to·lyt·ic** \ˌȯt-ᵊl-'i-tik\ *adj* — **au·to·lyze** \'ȯt-ᵊl-ˌīz\ *vb*

au·tom·a·tism \ȯ-'tä-mə-ˌti-zəm\ *n* **1** : an automatic action; *esp* : any action performed without the doer's intention or awareness **2** : the power or fact of moving or functioning without conscious control either independently of external stimulation (as in the beating of the heart) or more or less directly under the influence of external stimuli (as in the dilating or contracting of the pupil of the eye)

au·to·nom·ic \ˌȯ-tə-'nä-mik\ *adj* **1 a** : acting or occurring involuntarily ⟨∼ reflexes⟩ **b** : relating to, affecting, or controlled by the autonomic nervous system ⟨∼ ganglia⟩ **2** : having an effect upon tissue supplied by the autonomic nervous system ⟨∼ drugs⟩ — **au·to·nom·i·cal·ly** \-mi-k(ə-)lē\ *adv*

autonomic nervous system *n* : a part of the vertebrate nervous system that innervates smooth and cardiac muscle and glandular tissues and governs involuntary actions (as secretion, vasoconstriction, or peristalsis) and that consists of the sympathetic nervous system and the parasympathetic nervous system — compare CENTRAL NERVOUS SYSTEM, PERIPHERAL NERVOUS SYSTEM

au·ton·o·my \ȯ-'tä-nə-mē\ *n, pl* **-mies 1** : the quality or state of being independent, free, and self-directing **2** : independence from the organism as a whole in the capacity of a part for growth, reactivity, or responsiveness — **au·ton·o·mous** \-məs\ *adj* — **au·ton·o·mous·ly** *adv*

au·to·pro·throm·bin \ˌȯ-tō-prō-'thräm-bən\ *n* : any of several blood factors formed in the conversion of prothrombin to thrombin: as **a** : FACTOR VII — called also *autoprothrombin I* **b** : FACTOR IX — called also *autoprothrombin II*

¹**au·top·sy** \'ȯ-ˌtäp-sē, -təp-\ *n, pl* **-sies** : an examination of the body after death usu. with such dissection as will expose the vital organs for determining the cause of death or the character and extent of changes produced by disease — called also *necropsy, postmortem, postmortem examination*

²**autopsy** *vb* **-sied; -sy·ing** : to perform an autopsy on

au·to·ra·dio·gram \ȯ-tō-ˈrā-dē-ə-ˌgram\ *n* : AUTORADIOGRAPH

au·to·ra·dio·graph \-ˌgraf\ *n* : an image produced on a photographic film or plate by the radiations from a radioactive substance in an object which is in close contact with the emulsion — called also *radioautogram, radioautograph* — **autoradiograph** *vb* — **au·to·ra·dio·graph·ic** \-ˌrā-dē-ə-ˈgra-fik\ *adj* — **au·to·ra·di·og·ra·phy** \-ˈrā-dē-ˈä-grə-fē\ *n*

au·to·reg·u·la·tion \ˌȯ-tō-ˌre-gyə-ˈlā-shən\ *n* : the maintenance of relative constancy of a physiological process by a bodily part or system under varying conditions; *esp* : the maintenance of a constant supply of blood to an organ in spite of varying arterial pressure — **au·to·reg·u·late** \-ˈre-gyə-ˌlāt\ *vb* — **au·to·reg·u·la·to·ry** \-ˈre-gyə-lə-ˌtȯr-ē\ *adj*

au·to·sen·si·ti·za·tion \ˌȯ-tō-ˌsen-sə-tə-ˈzā-shən\ *n* : AUTOIMMUNIZATION

au·to·some \ˈȯ-tə-ˌsōm\ *n* : a chromosome other than a sex chromosome — **au·to·so·mal** \ˌȯ-tə-ˈsō-məl\ *adj* — **au·to·so·mal·ly** *adv*

au·to·sug·ges·tion \-səg-ˈjes-chən, -ˈjesh-\ *n* : an influencing of one's own attitudes, behavior, or physical condition by mental processes other than conscious thought : SELF-HYPNOSIS — **au·to·sug·gest** \-səg-ˈjest\ *vb*

au·to·ther·a·py \ˈȯ-tō-ˌther-ə-pē\ *n, pl* **-pies** : SELF-TREATMENT

au·to·top·ag·no·sia \ˌȯ-tō-ˌtä-pig-ˈnō-zhə\ *n* : loss of the power to recognize or orient a bodily part due to a brain lesion

autotoxicus — see HORROR AUTOTOXICUS

au·to·trans·fu·sion \-trans-ˈfyü-zhən\ *n* : return of autologous blood to the patient's own circulatory system — **au·to·trans·fuse** \-trans-ˈfyüz\ *vb*

au·to·trans·plant \-ˈtrans-ˌplant\ *n* : AUTOGRAFT — **au·to·trans·plant** \-trans-ˈ\ *vb* — **au·to·trans·plan·ta·tion** \-ˌtrans-ˌplan-ˈtä-shən\ *n*

au·to·troph \ˈȯ-tə-ˌtrȯf, -ˌträf\ *n* : an autotrophic organism

au·to·tro·phic \ˌȯ-tə-ˈtrō-fik\ *adj* 1 : needing only carbon dioxide or carbonates as a source of carbon and a simple inorganic nitrogen compound for metabolic synthesis 2 : not requiring a specified exogenous factor for normal metabolism — **au·to·tro·phi·cal·ly** \-fi-k(ə-)lē\ *adv* — **au·to·tro·phy** \ˈȯ-tə-ˌtrō-fē, ȯ-ˈtä-trə-fē\ *n*

au·to·vac·ci·na·tion \ˌȯ-tō-ˌvak-sə-ˈnā-shən\ *n* : vaccination of an individual by material from the individual's own body or with a vaccine prepared from such material

au·tumn cro·cus \ˌȯ-təm-ˈkrō-kəs\ *n* : an autumn-blooming herb (*Colchicum autumnale*) of the lily family (Liliaceae) that is the source of medicinal colchicum

¹aux·il·ia·ry \ȯg-ˈzil-yə-rē, -ˈzi-lə-rē, -ˈzil-rē\ *adj* : serving to supplement or assist (∼ springs in a dental appliance)

²auxiliary *n* 1 : one who assists or serves another person esp. in dentistry 2 : an organization that assists (as by donations or volunteer services) the work esp. of a hospital

auxo·troph \ˈȯk-sə-ˌtrȯf, -ˌträf\ *n* : an auxotrophic strain or individual

auxo·tro·phic \ˌȯk-sə-ˈtrō-fik\ *adj* : requiring a specific growth substance beyond the minimum required for normal metabolism and reproduction of the parental or wild-type strain (∼ mutants of bacteria) — **aux·ot·ro·phy** \ȯk-ˈsä-trə-fē\ *n*

AV *abbr* 1 arteriovenous 2 atrioventricular

avas·cu·lar \(ˌ)ā-ˈvas-kyə-lər\ *adj* : having few or no blood vessels (∼ necrosis) — **avas·cu·lar·i·ty** \-ˌvas-kyə-ˈlar-ə-tē\ *n*

Aven·tyl \ˈa-vən-ˌtil\ *trademark* — used for a preparation of nortriptyline

aver·sion \ə-ˈvər-zhən, -shən\ *n* 1 : a feeling of repugnance toward something with a desire to avoid or turn from it 2 : a tendency to extinguish a behavior or to avoid a thing or situation and esp. a usu. pleasurable one because it is or has been associated with a noxious stimulus

aversion therapy *n* : therapy intended to change habits or antisocial behavior by inducing a dislike for them through association with a noxious stimulus

aver·sive \ə-ˈvər-siv, -ziv\ *adj* : tending to avoid or causing avoidance of a noxious or punishing stimulus (behavior modification by ∼ conditioning) — **aver·sive·ly** *adv* — **aver·sive·ness** *n*

avi·an influenza \ˈā-vē-ən-\ *n* : any of several highly variable diseases of domestic and wild birds that are caused by orthomyxoviruses and characterized usu. by respiratory symptoms but sometimes by gastrointestinal, integumentary, and urogenital symptoms — called also *fowl plague*

avian tuberculosis *n* : tuberculosis of birds usu. caused by a bacterium of the genus *Mycobacterium* (*M. avium*); *also* : infection of mammals (as swine) by the same bacterium

avi·din \ˈa-və-din\ *n* : a protein found in egg white that inactivates biotin by combining with it

avir·u·lent \(ˌ)ā-ˈvir-ə-lənt, -ˈvir-yə-\ *adj* : not virulent (an ∼ tubercle bacillus) — compare NONPATHOGENIC

avis — see CALCAR AVIS

avi·ta·min·o·sis \ˌā-ˌvī-tə-mə-ˈnō-səs\ *n, pl* **-o·ses** \-ˌsēz\ : disease (as pellagra) resulting from a deficiency of one or more vitamins — called also *hypovi-*

taminosis — **avi·ta·min·ot·ic** \-mə-'nä-tik\ *adj*

A–V node *or* **AV node** \ä-'vē-\ *n* : ATRIOVENTRICULAR NODE

avoid·ance \ə-'void-ᵊns\ *n, often attrib* : the act or practice of keeping away from or withdrawing from something undesirable; *esp* : an anticipatory response undertaken to avoid a noxious stimulus

avoidance–avoidance conflict *n* : psychological conflict that results when a choice must be made between two undesirable alternatives — compare APPROACH-APPROACH CONFLICT, APPROACH-AVOIDANCE CONFLICT

avoid·ant \ə-'void-ᵊnt\ *adj* : characterized by turning away or by withdrawal or defensive behavior ⟨an ~ personality⟩

av·oir·du·pois \ˌa-vər-də-'poiz, -'pwä\ *adj* : expressed in avoirdupois weight ⟨~ units⟩ ⟨5 ounces ~⟩

avoirdupois pound *n* : POUND b

avoirdupois weight *n* : a system of weights based on a pound of 16 ounces and an ounce of 437.5 grains (28.350 grams) and in general use in the U.S. except for precious metals, gems, and drugs

avul·sion \ə-'vəl-shən\ *n* : a tearing away of a body part accidentally or surgically — **avulse** \ə-'vəls\ *vb*

ax- *or* **axo-** *comb form* : axon ⟨*axo*dendritic⟩

axe·nic \(ˌ)ā-'ze-nik, -'zē-\ *adj* : free from other living organisms ⟨an ~ culture of bacteria⟩ — **axe·ni·cal·ly** \-ni-k(ə)lē\ *adv*

ax·i·al \'ak-sē-əl\ *adj* **1** : of, relating to, or having the characteristics of an axis **2** : situated around, in the direction of, on, or along an axis

axial skeleton *n* : the skeleton of the trunk and head

ax·il·la \ag-'zi-lə, ak-'si-\ *n, pl* **-lae** \-(ˌ)lē, -ˌlī\ *or* **-las** : the cavity beneath the junction of the arm or anterior appendage and shoulder or pectoral girdle containing the axillary artery and vein, a part of the brachial plexus of nerves, many lymph nodes, and fat and areolar tissue; *esp* : ARMPIT

ax·il·lary \'ak-sə-ˌler-ē\ *adj* : of, relating to, or located near the axilla ⟨~ lymph nodes⟩

axillary artery *n* : the part of the main artery of the arm that lies in the axilla and that is continuous with the subclavian artery above and the brachial artery below

axillary nerve *n* : a large nerve arising from the posterior cord of the brachial plexus and supplying the deltoid and teres minor muscles and the skin of the shoulder

axillary node *n* : any of the lymph nodes of the axilla

axillary vein *n* : the large vein passing through the axilla continuous with the basilic vein below and the subclavian vein above

ax·is \'ak-səs\ *n, pl* **ax·es** \-ˌsēz\ **1 a** : a straight line about which a body or a geometric figure rotates or may be thought of as rotating **b** : a straight line with respect to which a body, organ, or figure is symmetrical **2 a** : the second vertebra of the neck of the higher vertebrates that is prolonged anteriorly within the foramen of the first vertebra and united with the odontoid process which serves as a pivot for the atlas and head to turn upon — called also *epistropheus* **b** : any of various central, fundamental, or axial parts ⟨the cerebrospinal ~⟩ ⟨the skeletal ~⟩ **c** : AXILLA

axis cylinder *n* : AXON; *esp* : the axon of a myelinated neuron

axo- — see AX-

axo·ax·o·nal \ˌak-sō-'ak-sən-ᵊl, -ak-'sän-, -'sōn-\ *or* **axo·ax·on·ic** \-ak-'sä-nik\ *adj* : relating to or being a synapse between an axon of one neuron and an axon of another

axo·den·drit·ic \ˌak-sō-den-'dri-tik\ *adj* : relating to or being a nerve synapse between an axon of one neuron and a dendrite of another

axo·lem·ma \'ak-sə-ˌle-mə\ *n* : the plasma membrane of an axon

ax·on \'ak-ˌsän\ *also* **ax·one** \-ˌsōn\ *n* : a usu. long and single nerve-cell process that usu. conducts impulses away from the cell body — **ax·o·nal** \'ak-sən-ᵊl; ak-'sän-, -'sōn-\ *adj*

ax·on·o·tme·sis \ˌak-sə-nət-'mē-səs\ *n, pl* **-me·ses** \-ˌsēz\ : axonal nerve damage that does not completely sever the surrounding endoneurial sheath so that regeneration can take place

axo·plasm \'ak-sə-ˌpla-zəm\ *n* : the protoplasm of an axon — **axo·plas·mic** \ˌak-sə-'plaz-mik\ *adj*

axo·so·mat·ic \ˌak-sō-sō-'ma-tik\ *adj* : relating to or being a nerve synapse between the cell body of one neuron and an axon of another

Ayer·za's disease \ə-'yər-zəz-\ *n* : a complex of symptoms marked esp. by cyanosis, dyspnea, polycythemia, and sclerosis of the pulmonary artery

Ayerza, Abel (1861–1918), Argentinean physician.

az- *or* **azo-** *comb form* : containing ⟨*azo*temia⟩

aza·thio·prine \ˌa-zə-'thī-ə-ˌprēn\ *n* : a purine antimetabolite $C_9H_7N_7O_2S$ that is used esp. as an immunosuppressant — see IMURAN

az·i·do·thy·mi·dine \ˌa-zi-dō-'thī-mə-ˌdēn\ *n* : an antiviral drug $C_{10}H_{13}$-N_5O_4 that inhibits replication of some retroviruses (as HIV) and is used to treat AIDS — called also *AZT, zidovudine;* see RETROVIR

azo \'ā-(ˌ)zō, 'a-\ *adj* : relating to or containing the bivalent group N=N united at both ends to carbon

azo dye *n* : any of numerous dyes containing azo groups

azo·osper·mia \ˌā-ˌzō-ə-ˈspər-mē-ə, ə-ˌzō-\ *n* : absence of spermatozoa from the seminal fluid — compare ASPERMIA — **azo·osper·mic** \-ˈspər-mik\ *adj*

azo·sul·fa·mide \ˌā-zō-ˈsəl-fə-ˌmīd\ *n* : a dark red crystalline azo compound $C_{18}H_{14}N_4Na_2O_{10}S_3$ of the sulfa class having antibacterial effect similar to that of sulfanilamide — called also *prontosil*

azo·te·mia \ˌā-zō-ˈtē-mē-ə\ *n* : an excess of nitrogenous bodies in the blood as a result of kidney insufficiency — compare UREMIA — **azo·te·mic** \-ˈtē-mik\ *adj*

azo·tu·ria \ˌā-zō-ˈtùr-ē-ə, -ˈtyùr-\ *n* : an abnormal condition of horses characterized by an excess of urea or other nitrogenous substances in the urine and by muscle damage esp. to the hindquarters

AZT \ˌā-(ˌ)zē-ˈtē\ *n* : AZIDOTHYMIDINE

azygo- *comb form* : azygos ⟨*azygo*graphy⟩

azy·gog·ra·phy \ˌā-zī-ˈgä-grə-fē\ *n, pl* **-phies** : roentgenographic visualization of the azygos system of veins after injection of a radiopaque medium

[1]**azy·gos** \ā-ˈzī-gəs\ *n* : an azygos anatomical part

[2]**azy·gos** *also* **azy·gous** \(ˌ)ā-ˈzī-gəs\ *adj* : not being one of a pair ⟨the ~ muscle of the uvula⟩

azygos vein *n* : any of a system of three veins which drain the thoracic and much of the abdominal wall and which form a collateral circulation when either the inferior or superior vena cava is obstructed; *esp* : a vein that receives blood from the right half of the thoracic and abdominal walls, ascends along the right side of the vertebral column, and empties into the superior vena cava — compare ACCESSORY HEMIAZYGOS VEIN, HEMIAZYGOS VEIN

B

b *abbr* bicuspid
B *symbol* boron
Ba *symbol* barium
ba·be·sia \bə-ˈbē-zhə, -zhē-ə\ *n* 1 *cap* : a genus of sporozoans (family Babesiidae) parasitic in mammalian red blood cells (as in Texas fever) and transmitted by the bite of a tick 2 : any sporozoan of the genus *Babesia* or sometimes the family (Babesiidae) to which it belongs — called also *piroplasm*

   Babès, Victor (1854–1926), Romanian bacteriologist.

babe·si·a·sis \ˌba-bə-ˈsī-ə-səs\ *n, pl* **-ases** \-ˌsēz\ : BABESIOSIS

ba·be·si·o·sis \ˌba-bə-ˈsī-ə-səs, bə-ˌbē-zē-ˈō-səs\ *n, pl* **-oses** \-ˌsēz\ : infection with or disease caused by babesias — called also *babesiasis*

Ba·bin·ski reflex \bə-ˈbin-skē-\ *also* **Ba·bin·ski's reflex** \-ˈskēz-\ *n* : a reflex movement in which when the sole is tickled the great toe turns upward instead of downward and which is normal in infancy but indicates damage to the central nervous system (as in the pyramidal tracts) when occurring later in life — called also *Babinski sign, Babinski's sign*; compare PLANTAR REFLEX

   Babinski, Joseph–François–Felix (1857–1932), French neurologist.

ba·by \ˈbā-bē\ *n, pl* **babies** : an extremely young child or animal; *esp* : INFANT — see BLUE BABY

baby talk *n* 1 : the imperfect speech or modified forms used by small children learning to talk 2 : the consciously imperfect or altered speech often used by adults in speaking to small children

baby tooth *n* : MILK TOOTH

bacill- *or* **bacilli-** *or* **bacillo-** *comb form* : bacillus ⟨*bacill*osis⟩

ba·cil·lary \ˈba-sə-ˌler-ē, bə-ˈsi-lə-rē\ *also* **ba·cil·lar** \bə-ˈsi-lər, ˈba-sə-lər\ *adj* : shaped like a rod; *also* : consisting of small rods 2 : of, relating to, or caused by bacilli ⟨~ meningitis⟩

bac·il·le·mia \ˌba-sə-ˈlē-mē-ə\ *n* : BACTEREMIA

bac·il·lo·sis \ˌba-sə-ˈlō-səs\ *n, pl* **-lo·ses** \-ˌsēz\ : infection with bacilli

bac·il·lu·ria \ˌba-sə-ˈlùr-ē-ə, -ˈlyùr-\ *n* : the passage of bacilli with the urine — **bac·il·lu·ric** \-ik\ *adj*

ba·cil·lus \bə-ˈsi-ləs\ *n, pl* **-li** \-ˌlī *also* -ˌlē\ 1 *cap* : a genus of aerobic rod≠ shaped gram-positive bacteria (family Bacillaceae) that include many saprophytes and some parasites (as *B. anthracis* of anthrax) **b** : any bacterium of the genus *Bacillus; broadly* : a straight rod-shaped bacterium 2 : BACTERIUM; *esp* : a disease≠ producing bacterium

bacillus Cal·mette–Gué·rin \-ˌkal-ˈmet-(ˌ)gä-ˈraⁿ, -ˈran\ *n* : an attenuated strain of tubercle bacillus developed by repeated culture on a medium containing bile and used in preparation of tuberculosis vaccines — compare BCG VACCINE

   Calmette, Albert Léon Charles (1863–1933), French bacteriologist, and **Guérin, Camille (1872–1961)**, French veterinarian.

bac·i·tra·cin \ˌba-sə-ˈtrās-ᵊn\ *n* : a toxic polypeptide antibiotic isolated from a bacillus (*Bacillus subtilis*) and usu. used topically esp. against gram-positive bacteria

Tra·cy \'trā-sē\, **Margaret,** American hospital patient.

back \'bak\ *n* **1 a** : the rear part of the human body esp. from the neck to the end of the spine **b** : the corresponding part of a lower animal (as a quadruped) **c** : SPINAL COLUMN **2** : the part of the upper surface of the tongue behind the front and lying opposite the soft palate when the tongue is at rest

back·ache \'bak-ˌāk\ *n* : a pain in the lower back

back·bone \-ˌbōn\ *n* : SPINAL COLUMN, SPINE

¹back·cross \'bak-ˌkrós\ *vb* : to cross (a first-generation hybrid) with one of the parental types

²backcross *n* : a mating that involves backcrossing; *also* : an individual produced by backcrossing

back·ing \'ba-kiŋ\ *n* : the metal portion of a dental crown, bridge, or similar structure to which a porcelain or plastic tooth facing is attached

back·rest \'bak-ˌrest\ *n* : a rest for the back

back·side \-'sīd\ *n* : BUTTOCKS — often used in pl.

bac·lo·fen \'ba-klō-ˌfen\ *n* : a gamma-aminobutyric acid analogue $C_{10}H_{12}ClNO_2$ used as a relaxant of skeletal muscle esp. in treating spasticity (as in multiple sclerosis)

bact *abbr* **1** bacteria; bacterial **2** bacteriological; bacteriology **3** bacterium

bac·ter·emia \ˌbak-tə-'rē-mē-ə\ *n* : the usu. transient presence of bacteria in the blood — **bac·ter·emic** \-mik\ *adj*

bacteri- *or* **bacterio-** *comb form* : bacteria : bacterial (*bacteri*olysis)

¹bacteria *pl of* BACTERIUM

²bacteria *n* : BACTERIUM — not usu. used technically

bac·te·ri·al \bak-'tir-ē-əl\ *adj* : of, relating to, or caused by bacteria (a ~ chromosome) (~ infection) — **bac·te·ri·al·ly** *adv*

bac·te·ri·cid·al \bak-ˌtir-ə-'sīd-³l\ *also* **bac·te·ri·o·cid·al** \-ˌtir-ē-ə-'sīd-\ *adj* : destroying bacteria — **bac·te·ri·cid·al·ly** *adv* — **bac·te·ri·cide** \-'tir-ə-ˌsīd\ *n*

bac·te·ri·o·cin \bak-'tir-ē-ə-'sīd-³n\ *or* **bac·te·ri·o·cid·in** \-ˌtir-ē-ə-'sīd-\ *n* : a bactericidal antibody

bac·ter·in \'bak-tə-rən\ *n* : a suspension of killed or attenuated bacteria for use as a vaccine

bac·te·rio·cin \bak-'tir-ē-ə-sən\ *n* : an antibiotic (as colicin) produced by bacteria

bac·te·ri·ol·o·gist \(ˌ)bak-ˌtir-ē-'ä-lə-jist\ *n* : a specialist in bacteriology

bac·te·ri·ol·o·gy \(ˌ)bak-ˌtir-ē-'ä-lə-jē\ *n, pl* **-gies 1** : a science that deals with bacteria and their relations to medicine, industry, and agriculture **2** : bacterial life and phenomena — **bac-**

te·ri·o·log·ic \bak-ˌtir-ē-ə-'lä-jik\ *or* **bac·te·ri·o·log·i·cal** \-'lä-ji-kəl\ *adj* — **bac·te·ri·o·log·i·cal·ly** \-ji-k(ə-)lē\ *adv*

bac·te·rio·ly·sin \bak-ˌtir-ē-ə-'līs-³n\ *n* : an antibody that acts to destroy a bacterium

bac·te·ri·ol·y·sis \(ˌ)bak-ˌtir-ē-'ä-lə-səs\ *n, pl* **-ly·ses** \-ˌsēz\ : destruction or dissolution of bacterial cells — **bac·te·ri·o·lyt·ic** \bak-ˌtir-ē-ə-'lit-ik\ *adj*

bac·te·rio·phage \bak-'tir-ē-ə-ˌfāj, -ˌfäzh\ *n* : a virus that infects bacteria — called also *phage*

bacteriophage lambda *n* : PHAGE LAMBDA

bac·te·rio·sta·sis \bak-ˌtir-ē-ō-'stā-səs\ *n, pl* **-sta·ses** \-ˌsēz\ : inhibition of the growth of bacteria without destruction

bac·te·rio·stat \-'tir-ē-ō-ˌstat\ *also* **bac·te·rio·stat·ic** \-ˌtir-ē-ō-'sta-tik\ *n* : an agent that causes bacteriostasis

bac·te·rio·stat·ic \-ˌtir-ē-ō-'sta-tik\ *adj* : causing bacteriostasis (a ~ agent) — **bac·te·rio·stat·i·cal·ly** \-ti-k(ə-)lē\ *adv*

bac·te·ri·um \bak-'tir-ē-əm\ *n, pl* **-ria** \-ē-ə\ : any of a group (as Kingdom Procaryotae or Kingdom Monera) of prokaryotic unicellular round, spiral, or rod-shaped single-celled microorganisms that are often aggregated into colonies or motile by means of flagella, that live in soil, water, organic matter, or the bodies of plants and animals, and that are autotrophic, saprophytic, or parasitic in nutrition and important because of their biochemical effects and pathogenicity

bac·te·ri·uria \bak-ˌtir-ē-'ur-ē-ə, -'yur-\ *n* : the presence of bacteria in the urine — **bac·te·ri·uric** \-ik\ *adj*

bac·te·roi·des \-'rói-(ˌ)dēz\ *n* **1** *cap* : a genus of gram-negative anaerobic bacteria (family Bacteroidaceae) that have rounded ends and occur usu. in the normal intestinal flora **2** *pl* **-roides** : a bacterium of the genus *Bacteroides* or of a closely related genus

Bac·trim \'bak-trim\ *trademark* — used for a preparation of sulfamethoxazole and trimethoprim

bag \'bag\ *n* : a pouched or pendulous bodily part or organ

ba·gasse \bə-'gas\ *n* : plant residue (as of sugarcane or grapes) left after a product (as juice) has been extracted

bag·as·so·sis \ˌba-gə-'sō-səs\ *n, pl* **-so·ses** \-ˌsēz\ : an industrial disease characterized by cough, difficult breathing, chills, fever, and prolonged weakness and caused by the inhalation of the dust of bagasse — called also *bagasse disease*

bag of waters *n* : the double-walled fluid-filled sac that encloses and protects the fetus in the mother's womb and that breaks releasing its fluid during the birth process

Bain·bridge reflex \'bān-(ˌ)brij\ *n* : a homeostatic reflex mechanism that causes acceleration of heartbeat following the stimulation of local muscle spindles when blood pressure in the venae cavae and right atrium is increased

Bainbridge, Francis Arthur (1874–1921), British physiologist.

Ba·ker's cyst \'bā-kərz\ *n* : a swelling behind the knee that is composed of a membrane-lined sac filled with synovial fluid and is associated with certain joint disorders (as arthritis)

Baker, William Morrant (1839–1896), British surgeon.

bak·er's itch \-bā-kərz-\ *n* : GROCER'S ITCH

bak·ing soda \'bā-kiŋ-\ *n* : SODIUM BICARBONATE

BAL \ˌbē-(ˌ)ā-'el\ *n* : DIMERCAPROL

balan- *or* **balano-** *comb form* : glans penis ⟨*balanitis*⟩ ⟨*balano*posthitis⟩

bal·ance \'ba-ləns\ *n* **1** : an instrument for weighing **2** : mental and emotional steadiness **3** : the relation in physiology between the intake of a particular nutrient and its excretion — see NITROGEN BALANCE, WATER BALANCE

bal·anced \-lənst\ *adj* **1** : having the physiologically active elements mutually counteracting ⟨a ∼ solution⟩ **2** *of a diet or ration* : furnishing all needed nutrients in the amount, form, and proportions needed to support healthy growth and productivity

bal·a·ni·tis \ˌba-lə-'nī-təs\ *n* : inflammation of the glans penis

bal·a·no·pos·thi·tis \ˌba-lə-(ˌ)nō-päs-'thī-təs\ *n* : inflammation of the glans penis and of the prepuce

bal·an·ti·di·a·sis \ˌba-lən-tə-'dī-ə-səs, bə-ˌlan-\ *also* **bal·an·tid·i·o·sis** \ˌba-lən-ˌti-dē-'ō-səs\ *n, pl* **-a·ses** *also* **-o·ses** \-ˌsēz\ : infection with or disease caused by protozoans of the genus *Balantidium*

bal·an·tid·i·um \ˌba-lən-'ti-dē-əm\ *n* **1** *cap* : a genus of large parasitic ciliate protozoans (order Heterotricha) including one (*B. coli*) that infests the intestines of some mammals and esp. swine and may cause a chronic ulcerative dysentery in humans **2** *pl* **-ia** \-dē-ə\ : a protozoan of the genus *Balantidium* — **bal·an·tid·i·al** \-dē-əl\ *adj*

bald \'bȯld\ *adj* : lacking all or a significant part of the hair on the head or sometimes on other parts of the body — **bald** *vb*

bald·ness *n* : the state of being bald — see MALE-PATTERN BALDNESS

Bal·kan frame \'bȯl-kən-\ *n* : a frame employed in the treatment of fractured bones of the leg or arm that provides overhead weights and pulleys for suspension, traction, and continuous extension of the splinted fractured limb

ball \'bȯl\ *n* **1** : a roundish protuberant part of the body: as **a** : the rounded eminence by which the base of the thumb is continuous with the palm of the hand **b** : the rounded broad part of the sole of the human foot between toes and arch and on which the main weight of the body first rests in normal walking **2** : EYEBALL **3** : TESTIS — usu. considered vulgar

ball–and–socket joint *n* : an articulation (as the hip joint) in which the rounded head of one bone fits into a cuplike cavity of the other and admits movement in any direction — called also *enarthrosis*

bal·lism \'ba-ˌli-zəm\ *or* **bal·lis·mus** \ba-'liz-məs\ *n, pl* **-isms** *or* **-is·mus·es** : the abnormal swinging jerking movements sometimes seen in chorea

bal·lis·to·car·dio·gram \ˌba-lis-tō-'kär-dē-ə-ˌgram\ *n* : the record made by a ballistocardiograph

bal·lis·to·car·dio·graph \-ˌgraf\ *n* : a device for measuring the amount of blood passing through the heart in a specified time by recording the recoil movements of the body that result from contraction of the heart muscle in ejecting blood from the ventricles — **bal·lis·to·car·dio·graph·ic** \-ˌkär-dē-ə-'gra-fik\ *adj* — **bal·lis·to·car·di·og·ra·phy** \-ē-'ä-grə-fē\ *n*

¹bal·loon \bə-'lün\ *n* : a nonporous bag of tough light material that can be inflated (as in a bodily cavity) with air or gas

²balloon *vb* : to inflate, swell, or puff out like a balloon

balloon angioplasty *n* : dilatation of an atherosclerotically obstructed artery by the passage of a balloon catheter through the vessel to the area of disease where inflation of the catheter compresses the plaque against the vessel wall

balloon catheter *n* : a catheter that has two lumens and an inflatable tip which can be expanded by the passage of gas, water, or a radiopaque medium through one of the lumens and that is used esp. to measure blood pressure in a blood vessel or to expand a partly closed or obstructed bodily passage or tube (as a coronary artery) — see PERCUTANEOUS TRANSLUMINAL ANGIOPLASTY, SWAN-GANZ CATHETER

bal·lotte·ment \bə-'lät-mənt\ *n* : a sharp upward pushing against the uterine wall with a finger inserted into the vagina for diagnosing pregnancy by feeling the return impact of the displaced fetus; *also* : a similar procedure for detecting a floating kidney

balm \'bäm, 'bȧlm, 'bȯm\ *n* **1** : an aromatic preparation (as a healing ointment) **2** : a soothing restorative agency

balne- *or* **balneo-** *comb form* : bath : bathing ⟨*balneo*therapy⟩

bal·ne·ol·o·gy \ˌbal-nē-'ä-lə-jē\ *n, pl* **-gies** : the science of the therapeutic use of baths

bal·neo·ther·a·py \ˌbal-nē-ō-'ther-ə-pē\

n, pl **-pies** : the treatment of disease by baths

bal·sam \'bȯl-səm\ *n* **1** : any of several resinous substances used esp. in medicine **2** : BALM 2 — **bal·sam·ic** \bȯl-'sa-mik\ *adj*

balsam of Pe·ru \-pə-'rü\ *n* : a leguminous balsam from a tropical American tree (*Myroxylon pereirae*) used esp. as an irritant and to promote wound healing — called also *Peru balsam, Peruvian balsam*

balsam of To·lu \-tə-'lü\ *n* : a balsam from a tropical American leguminous tree (*Myroxylon balsamum*) used esp. as an expectorant and as a flavoring for cough syrups — called also *tolu, tolu balsam*

bam·boo spine \(ˌ)bam-'bü-\ *n* : a spinal column in the advanced stage of ankylosing spondylitis esp. as observed in an X ray with ossified layers at the margins of the vertebrae giving the whole an appearance of a stick of bamboo

Ban·croft·i·an filariasis \'ban-ˌkrȯf-tē-ən-, 'baŋ-\ *or* **Ban·croft's filariasis** \-ˌkrȯfts-\ *n* : filariasis caused by a slender white filaria of the genus *Wuchereria* (*W. bancrofti*) that is transmitted in larval form by mosquitoes, lives in lymph vessels and lymphoid tissues, and often causes elephantiasis by blocking lymphatic drainage

Ban·croft \'ban-ˌkrȯft, 'baŋ-\, **Joseph** (1836–1894), British physician.

band \'band\ *n* **1** : a thin flat encircling strip esp. for binding: as **a** : a strip of cloth used to protect a newborn baby's navel — called also *bellyband* **b** : a thin flat strip of metal that encircles a tooth ⟨orthodontic ~s⟩ **2** : a strip separated by some characteristic color or texture or considered apart from what is adjacent: as **a** : a line or streak of differentiated cells **b** : one of the alternating dark and light segments of skeletal muscle fibers **c** : a strip of abnormal tissue either congenital or acquired; *esp* : a strip of connective tissue that causes obstruction of the bowel

¹ban·dage \'ban-dij\ *n* : a strip of fabric used to cover a wound, hold a dressing in place, immobilize an injured part, or apply pressure — see CAPELINE, ESMARCH BANDAGE, PRESSURE BANDAGE, SPICA, VELPEAU BANDAGE

²bandage *vb* **ban·daged; ban·dag·ing** : to bind, dress, or cover with a bandage ⟨~ a wound⟩ ⟨~ a sprained ankle⟩

Band–Aid \'ban-ˌdād\ *trademark* — used for a small adhesive strip with a gauze pad for covering minor wounds

band form *n* : a young neutrophil in the stage of development following a metamyelocyte and having an elongated nucleus that has not yet become lobed as in a mature neutrophil — called also *band cell, stab cell*

band keratopathy *n* : calcium deposition in Bowman's membrane and the stroma of the cornea that appears as an opaque gray streak and occurs in hypercalcemia and various chronic inflammatory conditions of the eye

bane·ber·ry \'bān-ˌber-ē, -bə-rē, -brē\ *n, pl* **-ries** : the acid poisonous berry of any plant of a genus (*Actaea*) of the buttercup family (Ranunculaceae); *also* : one of these plants

bang \'baŋ\ *var of* BHANG

Bang's disease \'baŋz-\ *n* : BRUCELLOSIS; *specif* : contagious abortion of cattle caused by a bacterium of the genus *Brucella* (*B. abortus*) — called also *Bang's*

Bang \'baŋ\, **Bernhard Lauritz Frederik** (1848–1932), Danish veterinarian.

bank \'baŋk\ *n* : a depot for the collection and storage of a biological product of human origin for medical use ⟨bone ~⟩ — see BLOOD BANK

Ban·thine \'ban-ˌthīn\ *trademark* — used for a preparation of methanthe line

Ban·ti's disease \'ban-tēz-\ *n* : a disorder characterized by congestion and great enlargement of the spleen usu. accompanied by anemia, leukopenia, and cirrhosis of the liver — called also *Banti's syndrome*

Ban·ti \'ban-tē\, **Guido** (1852–1925), Italian physician.

¹bar \'bär\ *n, often attrib* **1** : a piece of metal that connects parts of a removable partial denture **2** : a straight stripe, band, or line much longer than it is wide **3** : the space in front of the molar teeth of a horse in which the bit is placed

²bar *vb* **barred; bar·ring** : to cut free and ligate (a vein in a horse's leg) above and below the site of a projected operative procedure

³bar *n* : a unit of pressure equal to one million dynes per square centimeter

bar- *or* **baro-** *comb form* : weight : pressure ⟨bariatrics⟩ ⟨barotrauma⟩

Bá·rá·ny chair \bə-'rän-(y)ē-ˌcha(ə)r, -ˌche(ə)r\ *n* : a chair for testing the effects of circular motion esp. on airplane pilots

Bá·rá·ny \'bä-ˌränᵞ\, **Robert** (1876–1936), Austrian otologist.

barb \'bärb\ *n, slang* : BARBITURATE

barbae *see* SYCOSIS BARBAE

bar·ber's itch \ˌbär-bərz-\ *n* : ringworm of the face and neck

bar·bi·tal \'bär-bə-ˌtȯl\ *n* : a white crystalline addictive hypnotic C_8H_{12}-N_2O_3 often administered in the form of its soluble sodium salt — see MEDINAL, VERONAL

bar·bi·tone \'bär-bə-ˌtōn\ *n, Brit* : BARBITAL

bar·bi·tu·rate \bär-'bi-chə-rət\ *n* **1** : a salt or ester of barbituric acid **2** : any of various derivatives of barbituric acid used esp. as sedatives, hypnotics, and antispasmodics

bar·bi·tu·ric acid \ˌbär-bə-ˈtür-ik, -ˈtyür-\ n : a synthetic crystalline acid $C_4H_4N_2O_3$ that is a derivative of pyrimidine; also : any of its acid derivatives of which some are used as hypnotics

bar·bi·tur·ism \bär-ˈbi-chə-ˌri-zəm, ˈbär-bi-\ n : a condition characterized by deleterious effects on the mind or body by excess use of barbiturates

barefoot doctor n : an auxiliary medical worker trained to provide health care in rural areas of China

bar·ia·tri·cian \ˌbar-ē-ə-ˈtri-shən\ n : a specialist in bariatrics

bar·iat·rics \ˌbar-ē-ˈa-triks\ n : a branch of medicine that deals with the treatment of obesity — **bar·iat·ric** \-trik\ adj

bar·i·to·sis \ˌbar-ə-ˈtō-səs\ n, pl **-to·ses** \-ˌsēz\ : pneumoconiosis caused by inhalation of dust composed of barium or its compounds

bar·i·um \ˈbar-ē-əm\ n : a silver-white malleable toxic bivalent metallic element — symbol Ba; see ELEMENT table

barium chloride n : a water-soluble toxic salt $BaCl_2 \cdot 2H_2O$ used as a reagent in analysis and as a cardiac stimulant

barium enema n : a suspension of barium sulfate injected into the lower bowel to render it radiopaque, usu. followed by injection of air to inflate the bowel and increase definition, and used in the roentgenographic diagnosis of intestinal lesions

barium meal n : a solution of barium sulfate that is swallowed by a patient to facilitate fluoroscopic or roentgenographic diagnosis

barium sulfate n : a colorless crystalline insoluble salt $BaSO_4$ used medically chiefly as a radiopaque substance

Bar·low's disease \ˈbär-ˌlōz-\ n : INFANTILE SCURVY

    Barlow, Sir Thomas (1845–1945), British physician.

baro- — see BAR-

baro·re·cep·tor \ˌbar-ō-ri-ˈsep-tər\ also **baro·cep·tor** \-ō-ˈsep-\ n : a neural receptor (as of the carotid sinus) sensitive to changes in pressure

baro·trau·ma \ˈtrau-mə, -ˈtrȯ-\ n, pl **-ma·ta** \-mə-tə\ : injury of a part or organ as a result of changes in barometric pressure; specif : AERO-OTITIS MEDIA

Barr body \ˈbär-\ n : material of the inactivated X chromosome present in each somatic cell of most female mammals that is used as a test of genetic femaleness (as in a fetus or an athlete) — called also sex chromatin

    Barr, Murray Llewellyn (b 1908), Canadian anatomist.

bar·rel chest \ˈbar-əl-\ n : the enlarged chest with a rounded cross section and fixed horizontal position of the ribs that occurs in chronic pulmonary emphysema

bar·ren \ˈbar-ən\ adj : incapable of producing offspring — used esp. of females or matings — **bar·ren·ness** \-ən-nəs\ n

bar·ri·er \ˈbar-ē-ər\ n : a material object or set of objects that separates, demarcates, or serves as a barricade — see BLOOD-BRAIN BARRIER, PLACENTAL BARRIER

bar·tho·lin·itis \ˌbär-ˌtō-lə-ˈnī-təs\ n, pl **-lin·ites** \-ˌtēz\ : inflammation of the Bartholin's glands

Bar·tho·lin's gland \ˈbärt-ᵊl-ənz-, ˈbär-thə-lənz-\ n : either of two oval racemose glands lying one to each side of the lower part of the vagina and secreting a lubricating mucus — called also gland of Bartholin, greater vestibular gland; compare COWPER'S GLAND

    Bar·tho·lin \ˈbär-ˈtü-lin\, **Caspar Thomèson (1655–1738),** Danish anatomist.

bar·ton·el·la \ˌbärt-ᵊn-ˈe-lə\ n 1 cap : a genus of gram-negative bacteria (family Bartonellaceae) that include the causative agent (B. bacilliformis) of bartonellosis 2 : any bacterium of the genus Bartonella

    Bar·ton \ˈbär-ˌtōn\, **Alberto L. (b 1874),** Peruvian physician.

bar·ton·el·lo·sis \ˌbärt-ᵊn-ˌe-ˈlō-səs\ n, pl **-lo·ses** \-ˌsēz\ : a disease that occurs in So. America, is characterized by severe anemia and high fever followed by an eruption like warts on the skin, and is caused by a bacterium of the genus Bartonella (B. bacilliformis) that invades the red blood cells and is transmitted by sand flies (genus Phlebotomus) — called also Carrión's disease

ba·sal \ˈbā-səl, -zəl\ adj 1 : relating to, situated at, or forming the base 2 : of, relating to, or essential for maintaining the fundamental vital activities of an organism (as respiration, heartbeat, or excretion) ⟨∼ diet⟩ 3 : serving as or serving to induce an initial comatose or unconscious state that forms a basis for further anesthetization ⟨∼ narcosis⟩ ⟨∼ anesthetic⟩ — **ba·sal·ly** adv

basal cell n : one of the innermost cells of the deeper epidermis of the skin

basal–cell carcinoma n : a skin cancer derived from and preserving the form of the basal cells of the skin

basal ganglion n : any of four deeply placed masses of gray matter within each cerebral hemisphere comprising the caudate nucleus, the lentiform nucleus, the amygdala, and the claustrum — usu. used in pl.; called also basal nucleus

basale, basalia — see STRATUM BASALE

basalis — see DECIDUA BASALIS

basal lamina *n* : the part of the gray matter of the embryonic neural tube from which the motor nerve roots arise

basal metabolic rate *n* : the rate at which heat is given off by an organism at complete rest

basal metabolism *n* : the turnover of energy in a fasting and resting organism using energy solely to maintain vital cellular activity, respiration, and circulation as measured by the basal metabolic rate

basal plate *n* : an underlying structure: as **a** : the ventral portion of the neural tube **b** : the part of the decidua of a placental mammal that is intimately fused with the placenta

base \'bās\ *n*, *pl* **bas·es** \'bā-səz\ **1** : that portion of a bodily organ or part by which it is attached to another more central structure of the organism (the ∼ of the thumb) **2 a** : the usu. inactive ingredient of a preparation serving as the vehicle for the active medicinal preparation **b** : the chief active ingredient of a preparation — called also *basis* **3 a** : any of various typically water-soluble and bitter tasting compounds that in solution have a pH greater than 7, are capable of reacting with an acid to form a salt, are molecules or ions able to take up a proton from an acid or are substances able to give up a pair of electrons to an acid — compare ALKALI **b** : any of the five purine or pyrimidine bases of DNA and RNA that include cytosine, guanine, adenine, thymine, and uracil — **based** \'bāst\ *adj*

Base·dow's disease \'bä-zə-ˌdōz-\ *n* : GRAVES' DISEASE
Base·dow \'bä-zə-ˌdō\, **Karl Adolph von** (1799–1854), German physician.

base·line \'bās-ˌlīn\ *n* : a set of critical observations or data used for comparison or a control

base·ment membrane \'bā-smənt-\ *n* : a thin membranous layer of connective tissue that separates a layer of epithelial cells from the underlying lamina propria

base pair *n* : one of the pairs of chemical bases composed of a purine on one strand of DNA joined by hydrogen bonds to a pyrimidine on the other that hold together the two complementary strands much like the rungs of a ladder and include adenine linked to thymine or sometimes to uracil and guanine linked to cytosine

base·plate \'bās-ˌplāt\ *n* **1** : the portion of an artificial denture in contact with the jaw **2** : the sheet of plastic material used in the making of trial denture plates

basi- *also* **baso-** *comb form* **1** : of or belonging to the base or lower part of ⟨*basi*cranial⟩ **2** : chemical base ⟨*baso*philic⟩

ba·sic \'bā-sik, -zik\ *adj* **1** : of, relating to, or forming the base or essence **2 a** : of, relating to, containing, or having the character of a base **b** : having an alkaline reaction

ba·si·cra·ni·al \ˌbā-si-'krā-nē-əl\ *adj* : of or relating to the base of the skull

ba·sid·io·my·cete \bə-ˌsi-dē-ō-'mī-ˌsēt\ *n* : any of a large class (Basidiomycetes) or subdivision (Basidiomycotina) of higher fungi that include rusts (order Uredinales), smuts (order Ustilaginales), and numerous edible forms (as many mushrooms) — **ba·sid·io·my·ce·tous** \-mī-'sē-təs\ *adj*

bas·i·lar \'ba-zə-lər, -sə- *also* 'bā-\ *adj* : of, relating to, or situated at the base

basilar artery *n* : an unpaired artery that is formed by the union of the two vertebral arteries, runs forward within the skull just under the pons, divides into the two posterior cerebral arteries, and supplies the pons, cerebellum, posterior part of the cerebrum, and the internal ear

basilar membrane *n* : a membrane that extends from the margin of the bony shelf of the cochlea to the outer wall and that supports the organ of Corti

basilar process *n* : an anterior median projection of the occipital bone in front of the foramen magnum articulating in front with the body of the sphenoid by the basilar suture

basilic vein *n* : a vein of the upper arm lying along the inner border of the biceps muscle, draining the whole limb, and opening into the axillary vein

¹ba·si·oc·cip·i·tal \ˌbā-sē-äk-'sip-ət-ᵊl\ *adj* : relating to or being a bone in the base of the cranium immediately in front of the foramen magnum that is represented in humans by the basilar process of the occipital bone

²basioccipital *n* : the basioccipital bone

ba·si·on \'bā-sē-ˌän, -zē-\ *n* : the midpoint of the anterior margin of the foramen magnum

ba·sis \'bā-səs\ *n*, *pl* **ba·ses** \-ˌsēz\ **1** : any of various anatomical parts that function as a foundation **2** : BASE 2b

ba·si·sphe·noid \ˌbā-səs-'fē-ˌnoid\ *also* **ba·si·sphe·noi·dal** \-səs-fi-'noid-ᵊl\ *adj* : relating to or being the part of the base of the cranium that lies between the basioccipital and the presphenoid bones and that usu. ossifies separately and becomes a part of the sphenoid bone only in the adult — **basisphenoid** *n*

basket cell *n* : any of the cells in the molecular layer of the cerebellum whose axons pass inward and end in a basketlike network around the Purkinje cells

Basle Nom·i·na An·a·tom·i·ca \'bä-zəl-ˌnä-mə-nə-ˌa-nə-'tä-mi-kə\ *n* : the anatomical nomenclature adopted at the 1895 meeting of the German Anatomical Society at Basel, Switzerland, and superseded by the Nomina Anatomica adopted at the Sixth International Congress of Anatomists in 1955 — abbr. *BNA*

baso- — see BASI-

ba·so·phil \'bā-sə-ˌfil, -zə-\ or **ba·so·phile** \-ˌfīl\ *n* : a basophilic substance or structure; *esp* : a white blood cell with basophilic granules that is similar in function to a mast cell

ba·so·phil·ia \ˌbā-sə-'fil-ē-ə, -zə-\ *n* **1** : tendency to stain with basic dyes **2** : an abnormal condition in which some tissue element has increased basophilia

ba·so·phil·ic \-'fil-ik\ *also* **ba·so·phil** \'bā-sə-ˌfil, -zə-\ or **ba·so·phile** \-ˌfīl\ *adj* : staining readily with or being a basic stain

bath \'bath, 'bàth\ *n, pl* **baths** \'bathz, 'baths, 'bàthz, 'bàths\ **1** : a washing or soaking (as in water) of all or part of the body — see MUD BATH, SITZ BATH **2** : water used for bathing **3** : a place resorted to esp. for medical treatment by bathing : SPA — usu. used in pl.

bathe \'bāth\ *vb* **bathed; bath·ing 1** : to wash in a liquid (as water) **2** : to apply water or a liquid medicament to

Bath·i·nette \ˌba-thə-'net, ˌbā-\ *trademark* — used for a portable bathtub for babies

ba·tra·cho·tox·in \bə-ˌtra-kə-'täk-sən, ˌba-trə-kō-\ *n* : a very powerful steroid venom $C_{31}H_{42}N_2O_6$ extracted from the skin of a So. American frog (*Phyllobates aurotaenia*)

battered child syndrome *n* : the complex of physical injuries (as fractures, hematomas, and contusions) that results from gross abuse (as by a parent) of a young child

bat·tery \'ba-tə-rē\ *n, pl* **-ter·ies** : a group or series of tests; *esp* : a group of intelligence or personality tests given to a subject as an aid in psychological analysis

battle fatigue *n* : COMBAT FATIGUE — **bat·tle-fa·tigued** *adj*

Bau·hin's valve \'bō-ˌanz-, bō-'aⁿz-\ : ILEOCECAL VALVE

Bauhin, Gaspard *or* **Caspar** (1560–1624), Swiss anatomist and botanist.

B cell *n* : any of the lymphocytes that have antibody molecules on the surface and comprise the antibody-secreting plasma cells when mature — called also *B lymphocyte;* compare T CELL

BCG *abbr* bacillus Calmette-Guérin

BCG vaccine \ˌbē-(ˌ)sē-'jē-\ *n* : a vaccine prepared from a living attenuated strain of tubercle bacilli and used to vaccinate human beings against tuberculosis

A. L. C. Calmette and **C. Guérin** — see BACILLUS CALMETTE-GUÉRIN

BCNU \ˌbē-(ˌ)sē-(ˌ)en-'yü\ *n* : a nitrosourea $C_5H_9Cl_2N_3O_2$ used as an antineoplastic drug — called also *carmustine*

B complex *n* : VITAMIN B COMPLEX

b.d. *abbr* [Latin *bis die*] twice a day — used in writing prescriptions

Bdel·lo·nys·sus \ˌde-lə-'ni-səs\ *n* : a genus of mites (family Dermanyssidae) that are parasitic on vertebrates and include the rat mite (*B. bacoti*) and serious pests (as *B. bursa* and *B. sylviarum*) of domestic fowl

Be *symbol* beryllium

bead·ing \'bē-diŋ\ *n* : the beadlike nodules occurring in rickets at the junction of the ribs with their cartilages — called also *rachitic rosary*

bear down *vb* : to contract the abdominal muscles and the diaphragm during childbirth

¹**beat** \'bēt\ *vb* **beat; beat·en** \'bēt-ᵊn\ *or* **beat; beat·ing** : PULSATE, THROB

²**beat** *n* : a single stroke or pulsation (as of the heart) (ectopic ~s) — see EXTRASYSTOLE

Be symbol beryllium

bec·lo·meth·a·sone \ˌbe-klə-'me-thə-ˌzōn, -sōn\ *n* : a steroid anti-inflammatory drug administered in the form of its dipropionate $C_{28}H_{37}ClO_7$ as an inhalant in the treatment of asthma

Bec·que·rel ray \be-'krel-, ˌbe-kə-'rel-\ *n* : a ray emitted by a radioactive substance — used before adoption of the terms *alpha ray, beta ray, gamma ray*

Becquerel, Antoine–Henri (1852–1908), French physicist.

bed \'bed\ *n* **1 a** : a piece of furniture on or in which one may lie and sleep — see HOSPITAL BED **b** : the equipment and services needed to care for one hospitalized patient **2** : a layer of specialized or altered tissue esp. when separating dissimilar structures — see NAIL BED, VASCULAR BED

bed·bug \'bed-ˌbəg\ *n* : a wingless bloodsucking bug (*Cimex lectularius*) sometimes infesting houses and esp. beds and feeding on human blood — called also *chinch*

bed·pan \'bed-ˌpan\ *n* : a shallow vessel used by a bedridden person for urination or defecation

bed rest *n* : confinement of a sick person to bed

bed·rid·den \'bed-ˌrid-ᵊn\ *or* **bed·rid** \-ˌrid\ *adj* : confined to bed (as by illness)

¹**bed·side** \'bed-ˌsīd\ *n* : a place beside a bed esp. of a bedridden person

²**bedside** *adj* **1** : of, relating to, or conducted at the bedside of a bedridden patient ⟨a ~ diagnosis⟩ **2** : suitable for a bedridden person

bedside manner *n* : the manner that a physician assumes toward a patient

bed·so·nia \bed-'sō-nē-ə\ *n, pl* **-ni·ae** \-nē-ˌē, -ˌī\ : CHLAMYDIA 2a

Bedson, 'bed-sᵊn\ Sir Samuel Phillips (1886–1969), English bacteriologist.

bed·sore \'bed-ˌsōr\ *n* : an ulceration of tissue deprived of adequate blood supply by prolonged pressure —

called also *decubitus, decubitus ulcer;* compare PRESSURE POINT

bed–wet·ting \-ˌwe-tiŋ\ *n* : enuresis esp. when occurring in bed during sleep — **bed–wet·ter** \-ˌwe-tər\ *n*

bee \'bē\ *n* : HONEYBEE; *broadly* : any of numerous hymenopterous insects (superfamily Apoidea) that differ from the related wasps esp. in the heavier hairier body and in having sucking as well as chewing mouthparts — see AFRICANIZED BEE

beef measles *n sing or pl* : the infestation of beef muscle by cysticerci of the beef tapeworm which make oval white vesicles giving a measly appearance to beef

beef tapeworm *n* : a tapeworm of the genus *Taenia* (*T. saginata*) that infests the human intestine as an adult, has a cysticercus larva that develops in cattle, and is contracted through ingestion of the larva in raw or rare beef

bees·wax \'bēz-ˌwaks\ *n* 1 : WAX 1 2 : YELLOW WAX

be·hav·ior \bi-'hā-vyər\ *n* 1 : the manner of conducting oneself 2 a : anything that an organism does involving action and response to stimulation b : the response of an individual, group, or species to its environment — **be·hav·ior·al** \-vyə-rəl\ *adj* — **be·hav·ior·al·ly** *adv*

behavioral science *n* : a science (as psychology, sociology, or anthropology) that deals with human action and seeks to generalize about human behavior in society — **behavioral scientist** *n*

be·hav·ior·ism \bi-'hā-vyə-ˌri-zəm\ *n* : a school of psychology that takes the objective evidence of behavior (as measured responses to stimuli) as the only concern of its research and the only basis of its theory without reference to conscious experience — **be·hav·ior·ist** \-rist\ *n or adj* — **be·hav·ior·is·tic** \-ˌhā-vyə-'ris-tik\ *adj*

behavior therapist *n* : a specialist in behavior therapy

behavior therapy *n* : psychotherapy that emphasizes the application of the principles of learning to substitute desirable responses and behavior patterns for undesirable ones — called also *behavior modification;* compare COGNITIVE THERAPY

be·hav·iour, be·hav·iour·ism *chiefly Brit var of* BEHAVIOR, BEHAVIORISM

Beh·cet's syndrome \bə-'chets-\ *n* : a group of symptoms of unknown etiology that occur esp. in young men and include esp. ulcerative lesions of the mouth and genitalia and inflammation of the eye (as uveitis and iridocyclitis) — called also *Behcet's disease*

Behçet, Hulusi (1889–1948), Turkish dermatologist.

bej·el \'be-jəl\ *n* : a disease that is chiefly endemic in children in northern Africa and Asia Minor, is marked by bone and skin lesions, and is caused by a spirochete of the genus *Treponema* very similar to the causative agent of syphilis

bel \'bel\ *n* : ten decibels

Bell \'bel\, **Alexander Graham** (1847–1922), American inventor.

¹**belch** \'belch\ *vb* : to expel gas from the stomach suddenly : ERUCT

²**belch** *n* : an act or instance of belching : ERUCTATION

bel·la·don·na \ˌbe-lə-'dä-nə\ *n* 1 : an Old World poisonous plant of the genus *Atropa* (*A. belladonna*) having purple or green flowers, glossy black berries, and a root and leaves that yield atropine — called also *deadly nightshade* 2 : a medicinal extract (as atropine) from the belladonna plant

Bell–Ma·gen·die law \'bel-mä-zhan-'dē-\ *n* : BELL'S LAW

Bell, Sir Charles (1774–1842), British anatomist.

Magendie, François (1783–1855), French physiologist.

bel·lows \'be-(ˌ)lōz\ *n sing or pl* : LUNGS

Bell's law \'belz-\ *n* : a statement in physiology: the roots of the spinal nerves coming from the ventral portion of the spinal cord are motor in function and those coming from the dorsal portion are sensory — called also *Bell–Magendie law*

Bell's palsy *n* : paralysis of the facial nerve producing distortion on one side of the face

bel·ly \'be-lē\ *n, pl* **bellies** 1 a : ABDOMEN 1a b : the undersurface of an animal's body c : the stomach and its adjuncts 2 : the enlarged fleshy body of a muscle

bel·ly·ache \'be-lē-ˌāk\ *n* : pain in the abdomen and esp. in the bowels : COLIC

bel·ly·band \-ˌband\ *n* : a band around or across the belly; *esp* : BAND 1a

belly button *n* : the human navel

be·me·gride \'be-mə-ˌgrīd, 'bē-\ *n* : an analeptic drug $C_8H_{13}NO_2$ used esp. to counteract the effects of barbiturates — see MEGIMIDE

Ben·a·dryl \'be-nə-ˌdril\ *trademark* — used for a preparation of the hydrochloride of diphenhydramine

Bence–Jones protein \'bens-'jōnz-\ *n* : a polypeptide composed of one or two antibody light chains that is found esp. in the urine of persons affected with multiple myeloma

Bence–Jones, Henry (1814–1873), British physician.

Ben·der Gestalt test \'ben-dər-\ *n* : a test in which the subject copies geometric figures and which is used esp. to assess organic brain damage and degree of nervous system maturation

Bender, Lauretta (*b* 1897), American psychiatrist.

bends \'bendz\ *n sing or pl* : the painful

manifestations (as joint pain) of decompression sickness; *also* : DECOMPRESSION SICKNESS — usu. used with preceding *the* ⟨a case of the ∼⟩

Ben·e·dict's solution \'be-nə-ˌdikts-\ *n* : a blue solution that contains sodium carbonate, sodium citrate, and copper sulfate $CuSO_4$ and is used to test for reducing sugars in Benedict's test

Ben·e·dict \'be-nə-ˌdikt\, **Stanley Rossiter (1884–1936),** American chemist.

Benedict's test *n* : a test for the presence of a reducing sugar (as in urine) by heating the solution to be tested with Benedict's solution which yields a red, yellow, or orange precipitate upon warming with a reducing sugar (as glucose or maltose)

be·nign \bi-'nīn\ *adj* **1** : of a mild type or character that does not threaten health or life ⟨∼ malaria⟩ ⟨a ∼ tumor⟩ — compare MALIGNANT **1 2** : having a good prognosis : responding favorably to treatment ⟨a ∼ psychosis⟩ — **be·nig·ni·ty** \bi-'nig-nə-tē\ *n*

ben·ny \'be-nē\ *n, pl* **bennies** *slang* : a tablet of amphetamine taken as a stimulant

ben·ton·ite \'bent-ᵊn-ˌīt\ *n* : an absorptive and colloidal clay used in pharmacy esp. to stabilize suspensions

benz- *or* **benzo-** *comb form* **1** : related to benzene or benzoic acid ⟨*benz*oate⟩ **2** : containing a benzene ring fused on one side to one side of another ring ⟨*benz*imidazole⟩

benz·al·ko·ni·um chloride \ˌben-zal-'kō-nē-əm-\ *n* : a white or yellowish white mixture of chloride salts used as an antiseptic and germicide — see ZEPHIRAN

ben·za·thine penicillin G \'ben-zə-ˌthēn-, -thən-\ *n* : a long-acting relatively insoluble salt of penicillin G

Ben·ze·drine \'ben-zə-ˌdrēn\ *trademark* — used for a preparation of the sulfate of amphetamine

ben·zene \'ben-ˌzēn, ben-'\ *n* : a colorless volatile flammable toxic liquid aromatic hydrocarbon C_6H_6 used in organic synthesis, as a solvent, and as a motor fuel

benzene hexa·chlor·ide \-ˌhek-sə-'klōr-ˌīd\ *n* : a compound $C_6H_6Cl_6$ occurring in several stereoisomeric forms : BHC; *esp* : GAMMA BENZENE HEXACHLORIDE — see LINDANE

benzene ring *n* : a ring of six carbon atoms linked by alternate single and double bonds in a plane symmetrical hexagon that occurs in benzene and related compounds

ben·zes·trol \ben-'zes-ˌtrōl, -ˌtrōl\ *n* : a crystalline estrogenic compound $C_{20}H_{26}O_2$

ben·zi·dine \'ben-zə-ˌdēn\ *n* : a crystalline base $C_{12}H_{12}N_2$ used esp. in making dyes and in a test for blood

benzidine test *n* : a test for blood (as in feces) based on its production of a

blue color in a solution containing benzidine

benzilate — see QUINUCLIDINYL BENZILATE

benz·imid·azole \ˌben-ˌzi-mə-'da-ˌzōl, ˌben-zə-'mi-də-ˌzōl\ *n* : a crystalline base $C_7H_6N_2$ used esp. to inhibit the growth of various viruses, parasitic worms, and fungi; *also* : one of its derivatives

benzo- — see BENZ-

ben·zo·[a]·py·rene \ˌben-zō-ˌā-'pīr-ˌēn, -zō-ˌal-fə-, -ˌpī-'rēn\ *also* **3,4-benzpyrene** \-benz-'pīr-ˌēn, -ˌbenz-pī-'rēn\ *n* : the yellow crystalline highly carcinogenic isomer of the benzopyrene mixture that is formed esp. in the burning of cigarettes, coal, and gasoline

ben·zo·ate \'ben-zə-ˌwāt\ *n* : a salt or ester of benzoic acid

ben·zo·caine \'ben-zə-ˌkān\ *n* : a crystalline ester $C_9H_{11}NO_2$ used as a local anesthetic — called also *ethyl aminobenzoate*

ben·zo·di·az·e·pine \ˌben-zō-dī-'a-zə-ˌpēn\ *n* : any of a group of aromatic lipophilic amines (as diazepam and chlordiazepoxide) used esp. as tranquilizers

ben·zo·ic acid \ben-'zō-ik-\ *n* : a white crystalline acid $C_6H_6O_2$ used as a preservative of foods and in medicine

ben·zo·in \'ben-zō-wən, -ˌwēn, -ˌzōin\ *n* **1** : a yellowish balsamic resin from trees (genus *Styrax* of the family styracaceae) of southeastern Asia used esp. as an expectorant and topically to relieve skin irritations **2** : a white crystalline hydroxy ketone $C_{14}H_{12}O_2$

ben·zo·mor·phan \ˌben-zō-'mor-ˌfan\ *n* : any of a group of synthetic compounds whose best-known members are analgesics (as phenazocine or pentazocine)

ben·zo·phe·none \ˌben-zō-fi-'nōn, -'fē-ˌnōn\ *n* : a colorless crystalline ketone $C_{13}H_{10}O$ used in sunscreens

ben·zo·py·rene \ben-zō-'pīr-ˌēn, -ˌpī-'rēn\ *or* **benz·py·rene** \benz-'pīr-ˌēn, ˌbenz-pī-'rēn\ *n* : a mixture of two isomeric hydrocarbons $C_{20}H_{12}$ of which one is highly carcinogenic — see BENZO[A]PYRENE

ben·zo·yl \'ben-ˌzōil, 'ben-zə-ˌwil\ *n* : the radical C_6H_5CO of benzoic acid

benzoyl peroxide *n* : a white crystalline flammable compound $C_{14}H_{10}O_4$ used in medicine esp. in the treatment of acne

benz·pyr·in·i·um bromide \ˌbenz-pə-'ri-nē-əm-\ *n* : a cholinergic drug $C_{15}H_{17}BrN_2O_2$ that has actions and uses similar to those of neostigmine and has been used esp. to relieve postoperative urinary retention — called also *benzpyrinium*

benz·tro·pine \benz-'trō-ˌpēn, -pən\ *n* : a parasympatholytic drug used in the form of one of its salts $C_{21}H_{25}NO\cdot$

CH_4O_3S esp. in the treatment of Parkinson's disease

ben·zyl \'ben-₁zēl. -zəl\ *n* : the radical $C_6H_5CH_2$ having a chemical valence of one

benzyl benzoate *n* : a colorless oily ester $C_{14}H_{12}O_2$ used esp. as a scabicide

ben·zyl·pen·i·cil·lin \₁ben-zēl-(₁)pe-nə-'si-lən, -zēl-\ *n* : PENICILLIN G

beri·beri \₁ber-ē-'ber-ē\ *n* : a deficiency disease marked by inflammatory or degenerative changes of the nerves, digestive system, and heart and caused by a lack of or inability to assimilate thiamine

berke·li·um \'bər-klē-əm\ *n* : a radioactive metallic element — symbol *Bk*; see ELEMENT table

ber·lock dermatitis \'bər-₁läk-\ *n* : a brownish discoloration of the skin that develops on exposure to sunlight after the use of perfume containing certain essential oils

Ber·tin's column \ber-'taⁿz-\ *n* : RENAL COLUMN

> **Ber·tin** \ber- taⁿ\, **Exupère Joseph (1712–1781)**, French anatomist.

be·ryl·li·o·sis \bə-₁ri-lē-'ō-səs\ *also* **ber·yl·lo·sis** \-ber-ə-'lō-\ *n, pl* **-li·o·ses** \-₁sēz\ *or* **-lo·ses** \-₁sēz\ : poisoning resulting from exposure to fumes and dusts of beryllium compounds or alloys and occurring chiefly as an acute pneumonitis or as a granulomatosis involving esp. the lungs

be·ryl·li·um \bə-'ri-lē-əm\ *n* : a steel-gray light strong brittle toxic bivalent metallic element — symbol *Be*; see ELEMENT table

bes·ti·al·i·ty \₁bes-chē-'a-lə-tē, ₁bēs-\ *n, pl* **-ties** : sexual relations between a human being and a lower animal

¹**be·ta** \'bā-tə\ *n* **1** : the second letter of the Greek alphabet — B or β **2** : BETA PARTICLE **3** : BETA WAVE

²**beta** *or* **β-** *adj* **1** : of or relating to one of two or more closely related chemical substances (the *beta* chain of hemoglobin) — used somewhat arbitrarily to specify ordinal relationship or a particular physical form **2** : second in position in the structure of an organic molecule from a particular group or atom; *also* : of, relating to, or having a structure characterized by such a position (β–substitution) **3** : producing a zone of decolorization when grown on blood media — used of some hemolytic streptococci or of the hemolysis they cause

be·ta–ad·ren·er·gic \-₁a-drə-'nər-jik\ *adj* : of, relating to, or being a beta-receptor (~ blocking action)

beta–adrenergic receptor *n* : BETA–RECEPTOR

be·ta–ad·re·no·cep·tor \-ə-'drē-nə-₁sep-tər\ *also* **be·ta–ad·re·no·re·cep·tor** \-ri-₁sep-tər\ *n* : BETA–RECEPTOR

be·ta–block·er \-'blä-kər\ *n* : any of a class of heart drugs (as propranolol) that combine with and block the activity of a beta-receptor

be·ta–block·ing \-'blä-kiŋ\ *adj* : blocking or relating to the blocking of beta-receptor activity (~ drugs)

be·ta–car·o·tene *or* **β-carotene** \-'kar-ə-₁tēn\ *n* : an isomer of carotene that is found in dark green and dark yellow vegetables and fruits

beta cell *n* : any of various secretory cells distinguished by their basophilic staining characters: as **a** : a pituitary basophil **b** : an insulin-secreting cell of the islets of Langerhans — compare ALPHA CELL

Be·ta·dine \'bā-tə-₁dīn\ *trademark* — used for a preparation of povidone-iodine

be·ta–en·dor·phin *or* **β-endorphin** \₁bā-tə-en-'dor-fən\ *n* : an endorphin of the pituitary gland with much greater analgesic potency than morphine — see BETA-LIPOPROTEIN

beta globulin *n* : any of several globulins of plasma or serum that have at alkaline pH electrophoretic mobilities intermediate between those of the alpha globulins and gamma globulins

beta hemolysis *n* : a sharply defined clear colorless zone of hemolysis surrounding colonies of certain streptococci on blood agar plates — **be·ta–he·mo·lyt·ic** \₁bā-tə-₁hē-mə-'li-tik\ *adj*

be·ta–lac·tam *or* **β-lactam** \₁bā-tə-'lak-₁tam\ *n* : any of a large class of antibiotics (as the penicillins and cephalosporins) with a lactam ring

be·ta–lac·ta·mase *or* **β-lactamase** \-'lak-tə-₁mās, -₁māz\ *n* : PENICILLINASE

beta–lipoprotein *or* **β-lipoprotein** *n* : LDL

be·ta–li·po·tro·pin \₁bā-tə-₁li-pə-'trō-pən, -₁li-\ *n* : a lipotropin of the anterior pituitary that contains beta-endorphin as the terminal sequence of 31 amino acids in its polypeptide chain

be·ta–meth·a·sone \₁bā-tə-'me-thə-₁zōn, -₁sōn\ *n* : a potent glucocorticoid $C_{22}H_{29}FO_5$ that is isomeric with dexamethasone and has potent antiinflammatory activity

beta particle *n* : an electron or positron ejected from the nucleus of an atom during radioactive decay; *also* : a high-speed electron or positron

beta ray *n* **1** : BETA PARTICLE **2** : a stream of beta particles

be·ta–re·cep·tor \₁bā-tə-ri-'sep-tər\ *n* : any of a group of receptors postulated to exist on nerve cell membranes of the sympathetic nervous system to explain the specificity of certain adrenergic agents in affecting only some sympathetic activities (as vasodilation, increase in muscular contraction and beat of the heart, and relaxation of smooth muscle in the bronchi and intestine) — called also *beta-adren-*

ergic receptor, beta-adrenoceptor; compare ALPHA-RECEPTOR

beta–thalassemia *or* **β-thalassemia** *n* : thalassemia in which the hemoglobin chain designated beta is affected and which comprises Cooley's anemia in the homozygous condition and thalassemia minor in the heterozygous condition

beta wave *n* : an electrical rhythm of the brain with a frequency of 13 to 30 cycles per second that is associated with normal conscious waking experience — called also *beta, beta rhythm*

betel nut *n* : the astringent seed of an Asian palm (*Areca catechu*) that is a source of arecoline

be·tha·ne·chol \bə-'thā-nə-ˌkȯl, -'tha-, -ˌkōl\ *n* : a parasympathomimetic agent administered in the form of its chloride $C_7H_{17}ClN_2O_2$ and used esp. to treat gastric and urinary retention — see URECHOLINE

be·tween·brain \bi-'twēn-ˌbrān\ *n* : DIENCEPHALON

Betz cell \'bets-\ *n* : a very large pyramidal nerve cell of the motor area of the cerebral cortex

Betz, Vladimir Aleksandrovich (1834–1894), Russian anatomist.

be·zoar \'bē-ˌzȯr\ *n* : any of various calculi found in the gastrointestinal organs esp. of ruminants — called also *bezoar stone*

BFP *abbr* biologic false-positive

BHA \ˌbē-(ˌ)āch-'ā\ *n* : a phenolic antioxidant $C_{11}H_{16}O_2$ used esp. to preserve fats and oils in food — called also *butylated hydroxyanisole*

bhang \'bäŋ, 'bȯŋ, 'baŋ\ *n* **1 a** : HEMP 1 b : the leaves and flowering tops of uncultivated hemp : CANNABIS — compare MARIJUANA 2 : an intoxicant product obtained from bhang — compare HASHISH

BHC \ˌbē-(ˌ)āch-'sē\ *n* **1** : BENZENE HEXACHLORIDE **2** : LINDANE

BHT \ˌbē-(ˌ)āch-'tē\ *n* : a phenolic antioxidant $C_{15}H_{24}O$ used esp. to preserve fats and oils in food, cosmetics, and pharmaceuticals — called also *butylated hydroxytoluene*

Bi *symbol* bismuth

¹bi- *prefix* **1 a** : two (*bi*lateral) **b** : into two parts (*bi*furcate) **2** : twice : doubly : on both sides (*bi*convex) **3** : between, involving, or affecting two (specified) symmetrical parts (*bi*labial) **4 a** : containing one (specified) constituent in double the proportion of the other constituent or in double the ordinary proportion (*bi*carbonate) **b** : DI- (*bi*phenyl)

²bi- *or* **bio-** *comb form* : life : living organisms or tissue (*bio*chemistry)

bib·li·o·ther·a·py \ˌbi-blē-ō-'ther-ə-pē\ *n, pl* **-pies** : the use of selected reading materials as therapeutic adjuvants in medicine and in psychiatry; *also* : guidance in the solution of personal

problems through directed reading — **bib·li·o·ther·a·peu·tic** \-ther-ə-'pyüt-ik\ *adj* — **bib·li·o·ther·a·pist** \-'ther-ə-pist\ *n*

bi·carb \'bī-ˌkärb, bī-'\ *n* : SODIUM BICARBONATE

bi·car·bon·ate \(ˌ)bī-'kär-bə-ˌnāt, -nət\ *n* : an acid carbonate

bicarbonate of soda *n* : SODIUM BICARBONATE

bi·ceps \'bī-ˌseps\ *n, pl* **biceps** *also* **bi·cepses** : a muscle having two heads: as **a** : the large flexor muscle of the front of the upper arm **b** : the large flexor muscle of the back of the upper leg

biceps bra·chii \-'brā-kē-ˌē, -ˌī\ *n* : BICEPS a

biceps fem·o·ris \-'fē-mə-rəs, -'fe-\ *n* : BICEPS b

biceps flex·or cu·bi·ti \-'flek-ˌsȯr-'kyü-bə-ˌtī, -ˌtē\ *n* : BICEPS a

bi·chlo·ride of mercury \(ˌ)bī-ˌklȯr-ˌīd-\ *n* : MERCURIC CHLORIDE

bi·cip·i·tal \(ˌ)bī-'si-pət-ᵊl\ *adj* **1** *of muscles* : having two heads or origins **2** : of or relating to a biceps muscle

bicipital aponeurosis *n* : an aponeurosis given off from the tendon of the biceps of the arm and continuous with the deep fascia of the forearm

bicipital groove *n* : a furrow on the upper part of the humerus occupied by the long head of the biceps — called also *intertubercular groove*

bicipital tuberosity *n* : the rough eminence which is on the anterior inner aspect of the neck of the radius and into which the tendon of the biceps is inserted

bi·con·cave \ˌbī-(ˌ)kän-'kāv, (ˌ)bī-'kän-ˌ\ *adj* : concave on both sides — **bi·con·cav·i·ty** \ˌbī-(ˌ)kän-'ka-və-tē\ *n*

bi·con·vex \ˌbī-(ˌ)kän-'veks, (ˌ)bī-'kän-ˌ, ˌbī-kən-'\ *adj* : convex on both sides — **bi·con·vex·i·ty** \ˌbī-kən-'vek-sə-tē, -(ˌ)kän-'\ *n*

bi·cor·nu·ate \(ˌ)bī-'kȯrn-yə-ˌwāt, -wət\ *also* **bi·cor·nate** \-'kȯr-ˌnāt, -nət\ *adj* : having two horns or horn-shaped processes (a ~ uterus)

bi·cu·cul·line \bī-'kü-kyə-ˌlēn, -lən\ *n* : a convulsant alkaloid $C_{20}H_{17}NO_6$ obtained from plants (family Fumariaceae) and having the capacity to antagonize the action of gamma-aminobutyric acid in the central nervous system

¹bi·cus·pid \(ˌ)bī-'kəs-pəd\ *adj* : having or ending in two points (~ teeth)

²bicuspid *n* : either of the two double-pointed teeth that in humans are situated between the canines and the molars on each side of each jaw : PREMOLAR

bicuspid valve *n* : a valve in the heart consisting of two triangular flaps which allow only unidirectional flow from the left atrium to the ventricle — called also *left atrioventricular valve, mitral valve*

bi·cy·clic \(ˌ)bī-ˈsī-klik, -ˈsi-\ *adj* : containing two usu. fused rings in the structure of a molecule

bid *abbr* [Latin *bis in die*] twice a day — used in writing prescriptions

bi·det \bi-ˈdā\ *n* : a bathroom fixture used esp. for bathing the external genitals and the posterior parts of the body

bi·di·rec·tion·al \ˌbī-də-ˈrek-sh(ə-)nəl, -dī-\ *adj* : involving, moving, or taking place in two usu. opposite directions 〈∼ flow of materials in axons〉 — **bi·di·rec·tion·al·ly** *adv*

bi·fid \ˈbī-ˌfid, -fəd\ *adj* : divided into two equal lobes or parts by a median cleft (repair of a ∼ digit)

bifida — see SPINA BIFIDA, SPINA BIFIDA OCCULTA

¹bi·fo·cal \(ˌ)bī-ˈfō-kəl\ *adj* **1** : having two focal lengths **2** : having one part that corrects for near vision and one for distant vision 〈a ∼ eyeglass lens〉

²bifocal *n* **1** : a bifocal glass or lens **2** *pl* : eyeglasses with bifocal lenses

bi·func·tion·al \ˌbī-ˈfəŋk-sh(ə-)nəl\ *adj* : having two functions 〈∼ neurons〉

bi·fur·cate \ˈbī-(ˌ)fər-ˌkāt, bī-ˈfər-\ *vb* **-cat·ed; -cat·ing** : to divide into two branches or parts — **bi·fur·cate** \(ˌ)bī-ˈfər-kət, -ˌkāt; ˈbī-(ˌ)fər-ˌkāt *or* bī-fur·cat·ed \-ˌkā-təd\ *adj* — **bi·fur·ca·tion** \ˌbī-(ˌ)fər-ˈkā-shən\ *n*

bi·gem·i·ny \bī-ˈje-mə-nē\ *n, pl* **-nies** : the state of having a pulse characterized by two beats close together with a pause following each pair of beats — **bi·gem·i·nal** \-nəl\ *adj*

big·head \ˈbig-ˌhed\ *n* : any of several diseases of animals: as **a** : equine osteoporosis **b** : an acute photosensitization of sheep and goats that follows the ingestion of various plants — compare FAGOPYRISM

big toe *n* : the innermost and largest digit of the foot — called also *great toe*

bi·gua·nide \(ˌ)bī-ˈgwä-ˌnīd, -nəd\ *n* : any of a group of hypoglycemia-inducing drugs (as phenformin) used esp. in the treatment of diabetes — see PALUDRINE

bi·la·bi·al \(ˌ)bī-ˈlā-bē-əl\ *adj* : of or relating to both lips

bi·lat·er·al \(ˌ)bī-ˈla-tə-rəl, -ˈla-trəl\ *adj* **1** : of, relating to, or affecting the right and left sides of the body or the right and left members of paired organs 〈∼ nephrectomy〉 **2** : having bilateral symmetry — **bi·lat·er·al·i·ty** \(ˌ)bī-ˌla-tə-ˈra-lə-tē\ *n* — **bi·lat·er·al·ly** *adv*

bilateral symmetry *n* : symmetry in which similar anatomical parts are arranged on opposite sides of a median axis so that one and only one plane can divide the individual into essentially identical halves

bi·lay·er \ˈbī-ˌlā-ər\ *n* : a film or membrane with two molecular layers — **bilayer** *adj*

bile \ˈbīl\ *n* : a yellow or greenish viscid alkaline fluid secreted by the liver and passed into the duodenum where it aids esp. in the emulsification and absorption of fats

bile acid *n* : any of several steroid acids (as cholic acid) that occur in bile usu. in the form of sodium salts conjugated with glycine or taurine

bile duct *n* : a duct by which bile passes from the liver or gallbladder to the duodenum

bile fluke *n* : CHINESE LIVER FLUKE

bile pigment *n* : any of several coloring matters (as bilirubin or biliverdin) in bile

bile salt *n* **1** : a salt of bile acid **2** **bile salts** *pl* : a dry mixture of the salts of the gall of the ox used as a liver stimulant and as a laxative

bil·har·zia \bil-ˈhär-zē-ə, -ˈhärt-sē-ə\ *n* **1** : SCHISTOSOME **2** : SCHISTOSOMIASIS — **bil·har·zi·al** \-zē-əl, -sē-\ *adj*

Bil·harz \ˈbil-ˌhärts\, **Theodor Maximilian (1825–1862),** German anatomist and helminthologist.

bil·har·zi·a·sis \ˌbil-ˌhär-ˈzī-ə-səs, -ˌhärt-ˈsī-\ *n, pl* **-a·ses** \-ˌsēz\ : SCHISTOSOMIASIS

bili- *comb form* **1** : bile 〈*bili*ary〉 **2** : derived from bile 〈*bili*rubin〉

bil·i·ary \ˈbi-lē-ˌer-ē\ *adj* **1** : of, relating to, or conveying bile **2** : affecting the bile-conveying structures

biliary cirrhosis *n* : cirrhosis of the liver due to inflammation or obstruction of the bile ducts resulting in the accumulation of bile in and functional impairment of the liver

biliary dyskinesia *n* : pain or discomfort in the epigastric region resulting from spasm esp. of the sphincter of Oddi following cholecystectomy

biliary fever *n* : piroplasmosis esp. of dogs and horses

biliary tree *n* : the bile ducts and gallbladder

bil·ious \ˈbil-yəs\ *adj* **1** : of or relating to bile **2** : marked by or affected with disordered liver function and esp. excessive secretion of bile — **bil·ious·ness** *n*

bil·i·ru·bin \ˌbi-li-ˈrü-bən, ˈbi-li-ˌ\ *n* : a reddish yellow pigment $C_{33}H_{36}N_4O_6$ that occurs esp. in bile and blood and causes jaundice if accumulated in excess

bil·i·ru·bi·nae·mia \ˌbi-li-ˌrü-bə-ˈnē-mē-ə\ *chiefly Brit var of* BILIRUBINEMIA

bil·i·ru·bi·ne·mia \-ˈnē-mē-ə\ *n* : HYPERBILIRUBINEMIA

bil·i·ru·bi·nu·ria \-ˈnúr-ē-ə, -nyúr-\ *n* : excretion of bilirubin in the urine

bil·i·ver·din \ˌbi-li-ˈvərd-ən, ˈbi-li-ˌ\ *n* : a green pigment $C_{33}H_{34}N_4O_6$ that occurs in bile and is an intermediate in the degradation of hemoglobin heme groups to bilirubin

bi·lobed \(ˌ)bī-ˈlōbd\ *adj* : divided into two lobes 〈a ∼ organ〉

Bil·tri·cide \'bil-trə-₁sīd\ *trademark* — used for a preparation of praziquantel

bi·man·u·al \(₁)bī-'man-yə-wəl\ *adj* : done with or requiring the use of both hands (~ pelvic examination)

bin- *comb form* : two : two by two : two at a time (*binaural*)

bi·na·ry \'bī-nə-rē\ *adj* 1 : compounded or consisting of or marked by two things or parts 2 : composed of two chemical elements, an element and a radical that acts as an element, or two such radicals

binary fission *n* : reproduction of a cell by division into two approximately equal parts

bin·au·ral \(₁)bī-'nȯr-əl, (₁)bi-\ *adj* : of, relating to, or involving two or both ears — **bin·au·ral·ly** \-ē\ *adv*

bind \'bīnd\ *vb* **bound** \'baùnd\; **bind·ing** 1 : to wrap up (an injury) with a cloth : BANDAGE 2 : to take up and hold usu. by chemical forces : combine with (cellulose ~s water) 3 : to combine or be taken up esp. by chemical action (an antibody *bound* to a specific antigen) 4 : to make costive : CONSTIPATE

bind·er \'bīn-dər\ *n* 1 : a broad bandage applied (as about the chest) for support 2 : a substance (as glucose or acacia) used in pharmacy to hold together the ingredients of a compressed tablet

Bi·net age \bē-'nā-, bi-\ *n* : mental age as determined by the Binet-Simon scale

   Bi·net \bē-nā\, **Alfred (1857–1911)**, French psychologist, and **Si·mon** \sē-mōⁿ\, **Théodore (1873–1961)**, French physician.

Bi·net-Si·mon scale \bi-'nā-sē-'mōⁿ-\ *n* : an intelligence test consisting orig. of tasks graded from the level of the average 3-year-old to that of the average 12-year-old but later extended in range — called also *Binet-Simon test, Binet test*; see STANFORD-BINET TEST

binge \'binj\ *vb* **binged**; **binge·ing** *or* **bing·ing** : to eat compulsively or greedily esp. as a symptom of bulimia — **bing·er** \'bin-jər\ *n*

bin·oc·u·lar \bī-'nä-kyə-lər, bə-\ *adj* : of, relating to, using, or adapted to the use of both eyes (a ~ infection) (~ vision) — **bin·oc·u·lar·ly** *adv*

bi·no·mi·al \bī-'nō-mē-əl\ *n* : a biological species name consisting of two terms — **binomial** *adj*

binomial nomenclature *n* : a system of nomenclature in which each species of animal or plant receives a name of two terms of which the first identifies the genus to which it belongs and the second the species itself

bin·ovu·lar \(₁)bī-'nä-vyə-lər, -'nō-\ *adj* : BIOVULAR (~ twinning)

bi·nu·cle·ate \(₁)bī-'nü-klē-ət, -'nyü-\ *also* **bi·nu·cle·at·ed** \-klē-₁ā-təd\ *adj* : having two nuclei (~ lymphocytes)

bio- — see BI-

bio·ac·cu·mu·la·tion \₁bī-ō-ə-₁kyü-myə-'lā-shən\ *n* : the accumulation of a substance (as a pesticide) in a living organism

bio·ac·tive \₁bī-ō-'ak-tiv\ *adj* : having an effect on a living organism (~ pharmaceuticals and pesticides) — **bio·ac·tiv·i·ty** \-ak-'ti-və-tē\ *n*

bio·as·say \₁bī-(₁)ō-'a-₁sā, -a-'sā\ *n* : determination of the relative strength of a substance (as a drug) by comparing its effect on a test organism with that of a standard preparation — **bio·as·say** \-a-'sā, -₁a-₁sā\ *vb*

bio·avail·abil·i·ty \₁bī-(₁)ō-ə-₁vā-lə-'bi-lə-tē\ *n, pl* **-ties** : the degree and rate at which a substance (as a drug) is absorbed into a living system or is made available at the site of physiological activity — **bio·avail·able** \-'vā-lə-bəl\ *adj*

bio·cat·a·lyst \₁bī-ō-'kat-əl-əst\ *n* : ENZYME

bio·chem·i·cal \₁bī-ō-'ke-mi-kəl\ *adj* 1 : of or relating to biochemistry 2 : characterized by, produced by, or involving chemical reactions in living organisms (~ derangements) — **bio·chemical** *n* — **bio·chem·i·cal·ly** \-k(ə-)lē\ *adv*

bio·chem·is·try \₁bī-ō-'ke-mə-strē\ *n, pl* **-tries** 1 : chemistry that deals with the chemical compounds and processes occurring in organisms 2 : the chemical characteristics and reactions of a particular living system or biological substance — **bio·chem·ist** \-'ke-mist\ *n*

bio·cide \'bī-ə-₁sīd\ *n* : a substance (as DDT) that is destructive to many different organisms — **bio·cid·al** \₁bī-ə-'sīd-əl\ *adj*

bio·com·pat·i·bil·i·ty \₁bī-ō-kəm-₁pa-tə-'bi-lə-tē\ *n, pl* **-ties** : the condition of being compatible with living tissue or a living system by not being toxic or injurious and not causing immunological rejection — **bio·com·pat·i·ble** \-kəm-'pa-tə-bəl\ *adj*

bio·de·grad·able \₁bī-(₁)ō-di-'grā-də-bəl\ *adj* : capable of being broken down esp. into innocuous products by the action of living things (as microorganisms) — **bio·de·grad·abil·i·ty** \-₁grā-də-'bi-lə-tē\ *n* — **bio·deg·ra·da·tion** \-₁de-grə-'dā-shən\ *n* — **bio·de·grade** \-di-'grād\ *vb*

bio·elec·tri·cal \-i-'lek-tri-kəl\ *also* **bio·elec·tric** \-trik\ *adj* : of or relating to electric phenomena in living organisms (human cortical ~ activity) — **bio·elec·tric·i·ty** \-₁lek-'tri-sə-tē\ *n*

bio·elec·tron·ics \-i-(₁)lek-'trä-niks\ *n* 1 : a branch of the life sciences that deals with electronic control of physiological function 2 : a branch of science that deals with the role of electron transfer in biological processes

bio·en·er·get·ics \-₁e-nər-'je-tiks\ *n* : a

system of therapy that combines breathing and body exercises, psychological therapy, and the free expression of impulses and emotions and that is held to increase well-being by releasing blocked physical and psychic energy — **bio·en·er·get·ic** \-tik\ *adj*

bio·en·gi·neer·ing \-,en-jə-'nir-iŋ\ *n* : biological or medical application of engineering principles or engineering equipment; *broadly* : BIOTECHNOLOGY — **bio·en·gi·neer** \-'nir\ *n or vb*

bio·equiv·a·lence \-i-'kwi-və-ləns\ *n* : the property that two drugs or dosage forms have when they have the same bioavailability and produce the same effect at the site of physiological activity — **bio·equiv·a·lent** \-lənt\ *adj*

bio·equiv·a·len·cy \-lən-sē\ *n, pl* -cies : BIOEQUIVALENCE

bio·eth·i·cist \-'e-thə-sist\ *n* : an expert in bioethics

bio·eth·ics \-'e-thiks\ *n* : the discipline dealing with the ethical implications of biological research and applications esp. in medicine — **bio·ethic** \-thik\ *n* — **bio·ethical** \-thi-kəl\ *adj*

bio·feed·back \-'fēd-,bak\ *n* : the technique of making unconscious or involuntary bodily processes (as heartbeat or brain waves) perceptible to the senses (as by the use of an oscilloscope) in order to manipulate them by conscious mental control

bio·fla·vo·noid \-'flā-və-,noid\ *n* : biologically active flavonoid

bio·gen·ic \-'je-nik\ *adj* : produced by living organisms (~ amines)

bio·haz·ard \'bī-ō-,ha-zərd\ *n* : a biological agent or condition (as an infectious organism or insecure laboratory procedures) that constitutes a hazard to humans or the environment; *also* : a hazard posed by such an agent or condition — **bio·haz·ard·ous** \,bī-ō-'ha-zər-dəs\ *adj*

biol *abbr* biologic; biological; biologist; biology

bio·log·ic \,bī-ə-'lä-jik\ *or* **bio·log·i·cal** \-ji-kəl\ *n* : a biological product (as a globulin, serum, vaccine, antitoxin, or antigen) used in the prevention or treatment of disease

biological *also* **biologic** *adj* **1** : of or relating to biology or to life and living processes **2** : used in or produced by applied biology **3** : related by direct genetic relationship rather than by adoption or marriage (~ parents) — **bio·log·i·cal·ly** \-ji-k(ə-)lē\ *adv*

biological clock *n* : an inherent timing mechanism that is inferred to exist in some living systems (as a cell) in order to explain various cyclical behaviors and physiological processes

biological control *n* : reduction in numbers or elimination of pest organisms by interference with their ecology

biological half–life *or* **biologic half–life** *n*

: the time that a living body requires to eliminate one half the quantity of an administered substance (as a radioisotope) through its normal channels of elimination

biological warfare *n* : warfare involving the use of living organisms (as disease germs) or their toxic products as weapons; *also* : warfare involving the use of herbicides

biologic false–positive *n* : a positive serological reaction for syphilis given by blood of a person who does not have syphilis

bi·ol·o·gist \bī-'ä-lə-jist\ *n* : a specialist in biology

bi·ol·o·gy \bī-'ä-lə-jē\ *n, pl* -gies **1** : a branch of science that deals with living organisms and vital processes **2** : the laws and phenomena relating to an organism or group

bio·ma·te·ri·al \,bī-ō-mə-'tir-ē-əl\ *n* : material used for or suitable for use in prostheses that come in direct contact with living tissues

bio·me·chan·ics \,bī-ō-mi-'ka-niks\ *n sing or pl* : the mechanical bases of biological, esp. muscular, activity; *also* : the study of the principles and relations involved — **bio·me·chan·i·cal** \-ni-kəl\ *adj*

bio·med·i·cal \-'me-di-kəl\ *adj* **1** : of or relating to biomedicine (~ studies) **2** : of, relating to, or involving biological, medical, and physical science — **bio·med·i·cal·ly** \-k(ə-)lē\ *adv*

biomedical engineering *n* : BIOENGINEERING

bio·med·i·cine \-'me-də-sən\ *n* : medicine based on the application of the principles of the natural sciences and esp. biology and biochemistry

bio·met·rics \-'me-triks\ *n sing or pl* : BIOMETRY

bi·om·e·try \bī-'ä-mə-trē\ *n, pl* -tries : the statistical analysis of biological observations and phenomena — **bio·met·ric** \,bī-ō-'me-trik\ *or* **bio·met·ri·cal** \-tri-kəl\ *adj* — **bio·me·tri·cian** \-me-'tri-shən\ *n*

bio·mi·cro·scope \,bī-ō-'mī-krə-,skōp\ *n* : a binocular microscope used for examination of the anterior part of the eye

bio·mi·cros·co·py \-mī-'kräs-kə-pē\ *n, pl* -pies : the microscopic examination and study of living cells and tissues; *specif* : examination of the living eye with the biomicroscope

bio·mol·e·cule \,bī-ō-'mä-li-,kyül\ *n* : an organic molecule and esp. a macromolecule (as a protein or nucleic acid) in living organisms — **bio·mo·lec·u·lar** \-mə-'le-kyə-lər\ *adj*

bi·on·ic \bī-'ä-nik\ *adj* **1** : of or relating to bionics **2** : having natural biological capability or performance enhanced by or as if by electronic or electrically actuated mechanical devices

bi·on·ics \bī-'ä-niks\ *n sing or pl* : a science concerned with the application of data about the functioning of biological systems to the solution of engineering problems

bio·phar·ma·ceu·tics \ˌbī-ō-ˌfär-mə-ˈsü-tiks\ *n* : the study of the relationships between the physical and chemical properties, dosage, and form of administration of a drug and its activity in the living body — **bio·phar·ma·ceu·ti·cal** \-ti-kəl\ *adj*

bio·phys·i·cist \-ˈfi-zə-sist\ *n* : a specialist in biophysics

bio·phys·ics \ˌbī-ō-ˈfi-ziks\ *n* : a branch of knowledge concerned with the application of physical principles and methods to biological problems — **bio·phys·i·cal** \-zi-kəl\ *adj*

bio·poly·mer \ˌbī-ō-ˈpä-lə-mər\ *n* : a polymeric substance (as a protein or polysaccharide) formed in a biological system

bi·op·sy \ˈbī-ˌäp-sē\ *n, pl* **-sies** : the removal and examination of tissue, cells, or fluids from the living body — **biopsy** *vb*

bio·psy·chol·o·gy \ˌbī-ō-sī-ˈkä-lə-jē\ *n, pl* **-gies** : psychology as related to biology or as a part of the vital processes — **bio·psy·chol·o·gist** \-jist\ *n*

bio·re·ac·tor \-rē-ˈak-tər\ *n* : a device or apparatus in which living organisms and esp. bacteria synthesize useful substances (as interferon) or break down harmful ones (as in sewage)

bio·rhythm \ˈbī-ō-ˌri-thəm\ *n* : an innately determined rhythmic biological process or function (as sleep behavior); *also* : an innate rhythmic determiner of such a process or function — **bio·rhyth·mic** \ˌbī-ō-ˈrith-mik\ *adj*

bio·sci·ence \ˈbī-ō-ˌsī-əns\ *n* : BIOLOGY; *also* : LIFE SCIENCE — **bio·sci·en·tist** \ˌbī-ō-ˈsī-ən-tist\ *n*

bio·sen·sor \ˈbī-ō-ˌsen-ˌsȯr, -sər\ *n* : a device that is sensitive to a physical or chemical stimulus (as heat or an ion) and transmits information about a life process

-bi·o·sis \(ˌ)bī-ˈō-səs, bē-ˈ\ *n comb form, pl* **-bi·o·ses** \-ˌsēz\ : mode of life ⟨para*biosis*⟩ ⟨sym*biosis*⟩

bio·sta·tis·tics \ˌbī-ō-stə-ˈtis-tiks\ *n* : statistical processes and methods applied to the analysis of biological phenomena — **bio·stat·is·ti·cian** \-ˌsta-tə-ˈsti-shən\ *n*

bio·syn·the·sis \ˌbī-ō-ˈsin-thə-səs\ *n, pl* **-the·ses** : production of a chemical compound by a living organism — **bio·syn·the·size** \-ˌsin-thə-ˌsīz\ *vb* — **bio·syn·thet·ic** \-sin-ˈthe-tik\ *adj* — **bio·syn·thet·i·cal·ly** \-i-k(ə-)lē\ *adv*

bio·tech·ni·cal \-ˈtek-ni-kəl\ *adj* : of or relating to biotechnology

bio·tech·nol·o·gy \ˌbī-ō-tek-ˈnä-lə-jē\ *n, pl* **-gies** 1 : applied biological science (as bioengineering or recombinant DNA technology) 2 : ERGONOMICS —

bio·tech·no·log·i·cal \-ˌtek-nə-ˈlä-ji-kəl\ *adj*

bio·te·lem·e·try \-tə-ˈle-mə-trē\ *n, pl* **-tries** : remote detection and measurement of a human or animal condition, activity, or function (as heartbeat or body temperature) — **bio·tel·e·met·ric** \-ˌte-lə-ˈme-trik\ *adj*

bi·ot·ic \bī-ˈä-tik\ *adj* : of or relating to life; *esp* : caused or produced by living beings

-bi·ot·ic \bī-ˈä-tik\ *adj comb form* 1 : relating to life ⟨anti*biotic*⟩ 2 : having a (specified) mode of life ⟨necro*biotic*⟩

bio·tin \ˈbī-ə-tən\ *n* : a colorless crystalline growth vitamin $C_{10}H_{16}N_2O_3S$ of the vitamin B complex found esp. in yeast, liver, and egg yolk — called also *vitamin H*

bio·trans·for·ma·tion \ˈbī-ō-ˌtrans-fər-ˈmä-shən, -ˌfȯr-\ *n* : the transformation of chemical compounds within a living system

bi·o·vu·lar \(ˌ)bī-ˈä-vyə-lər, -ˈō-\ *adj, of fraternal twins* : derived from two ova

bi·pa·ri·etal \ˌbī-pə-ˈrī-ət-əl\ *adj* : of or relating to the parietal bones; *specif* : being a measurement between the most distant opposite points of the two parietal bones

bi·ped \ˈbī-ˌped\ *n* : a two-footed animal — **biped** or **bi·ped·al** \(ˌ)bī-ˈped-əl\ *adj*

bi·pen·nate \(ˌ)bī-ˈpe-ˌnāt\ *adj* : BIPENNIFORM

bi·pen·ni·form \-ˈpe-ni-ˌfȯrm\ *adj* : resembling a feather barbed on both sides — used of muscles

bi·per·i·den \bī-ˈper-ə-dən\ *n* : a white crystalline muscle relaxant $C_{21}H_{29}$-NO used esp. to reduce the symptoms (as tremors, akinesia, and muscle rigidity) associated with Parkinson's disease

bi·phe·nyl \(ˌ)bī-ˈfen-əl, -ˈfēn-\ *n* : a white crystalline hydrocarbon C_6H_5-C_6H_5

bi·po·lar \(ˌ)bī-ˈpō-lər\ *adj* 1 : having or involving the use of two poles ⟨∼ encephalograph leads⟩ 2 *of a neuron* : having an efferent and an afferent process 3 : characterized by the alternation of manic and depressive states ⟨a ∼ affective disorder⟩

bird louse *n* : BITING LOUSE

bi·re·frin·gence \ˌbī-ri-ˈfrin-jəns\ *n* : the refraction of light in two slightly different directions to form two rays — **bi·re·frin·gent** \-jənt\ *adj*

birth \ˈbərth\ *n, often attrib* 1 : the emergence of a new individual from the body of its parent 2 : the act or process of bringing forth young from the womb — **birth** *vb*

birth canal *n* : the channel formed by the cervix, vagina, and vulva through which the fetus is expelled during birth

birth certificate *n* : a copy of an official

record of a person's date and place of birth and parentage

birth control n : control of the number of children born esp. by preventing or lessening the frequency of conception — compare CONTRACEPTION

birth defect n : a physical or biochemical defect (as cleft palate, phenylketonuria, or Down's syndrome) that is present at birth and may be inherited or environmentally induced

birthing center n : a facility usu. staffed by nurse-midwives that provides a less institutionalized setting than a hospital for women who wish to deliver by natural childbirth

birthing room n : a comfortably furnished hospital room where both labor and delivery take place and in which the baby usu. remains during the hospital stay

birth·mark \'bərth-ˌmärk\ n : an unusual mark or blemish on the skin at birth : NEVUS — **birthmark** vb

birth pang n : one of the regularly recurrent pains that are characteristic of childbirth — usu. used in pl.

birth·rate \'bərth-ˌrāt\ n : the ratio between births and individuals in a specified population and time often expressed as number of live births per hundred or per thousand population per year — called also *natality*

birth trauma n : the physical injury or emotional shock sustained by an infant in the process of birth

bis·a·co·dyl \ˌbi-sə-'kō-(ˌ)dil\ n : a white crystalline laxative $C_{22}H_{19}NO_4$ administered orally or as a suppository

¹**bi·sex·u·al** \(ˌ)bī-'sek-shə-wəl\ adj **1 a** : possessing characters of both sexes : HERMAPHRODITIC **b** : sexually oriented toward both sexes (a ~ person who engages in both heterosexual and homosexual practices) **2** : of, relating to, or involving two sexes — **bi·sex·u·al·i·ty** \ˌbī-ˌsek-shə-'wa-lə-tē\ n — **bi·sex·u·al·ly** adv

²**bisexual** n : a bisexual individual

bis·hy·droxy·cou·ma·rin \ˌbis-(ˌ)hī-ˌdräk-sē-'kü-mə-rən\ n : DICUMAROL

bis·muth \'biz-məth\ n : a brittle grayish white chiefly trivalent metallic element — symbol Bi; see ELEMENT table

bismuth sub·car·bon·ate \-ˌsəb-'kär-bə-ˌnāt, -ˌnət\ n : a white or pale yellowish white powder used chiefly in treating gastrointestinal disorders, topically as a protective in lotions and ointments, and in cosmetics

bismuth sub·ni·trate \-ˌsəb-'nī-ˌtrāt\ n : a white powder $Bi_5O(OH)_9(NO_3)_4$ that is used in medicine similarly to bismuth subcarbonate

bis·tou·ry \'bis-tə-rē\ n, pl **-ries** : a small slender straight or curved surgical knife that is sharp-pointed or probe-pointed

¹**bite** \'bīt\ vb **bit** \'bit\; **bit·ten** \'bit-ᵊn\

also **bit; bit·ing 1** : to seize esp. with teeth or jaws so as to enter, grip, or wound **2** : to wound, pierce, or sting esp. with a fang or a proboscis

²**bite** n **1** : the act or manner of biting; esp : OCCLUSION 2a **2** : a wound made by biting

bite block n : a device used in dentistry for recording the spatial relation of the jaws esp. in respect to the occlusion of the teeth

bi·tem·po·ral \(ˌ)bī-'tem-pə-rəl\ adj : relating to, involving, or joining the two temporal bones or the areas that they occupy

bite plane n : a removable dental appliance used to cover the occlusal surfaces of the teeth so that they cannot be brought into contact

bite plate n : a dental appliance used in orthodontics and prosthodontics that is usu. made of plastic and wire and is worn in the palate or sometimes on the lower jaw

bite·wing \'bīt-ˌwiŋ\ n : dental X-ray film designed to show the crowns of the upper and lower teeth simultaneously

biting fly n : a dipteran fly (as a mosquito, midge, or horsefly) having mouthparts adapted for piercing and biting

biting louse n : any of numerous wingless insects (order Mallophaga) parasitic esp. on birds — called also *bird louse*

biting midge n : any of a large family (Ceratopogonidae) of tiny dipteran flies of which some are vectors of filarial worms

Bi·tot's spots \bē-'tōz-\ n : shiny pearly spots of triangular shape occurring on the conjunctiva in severe vitamin A deficiency esp. in children

Bi·tot \bē-'tō\, **Pierre A. (1822–1888)**, French physician.

bit·ter \'bi-tər\ adj : being or inducing the one of the four basic taste sensations that is peculiarly acrid, astringent, or disagreeable — compare SALT, SOUR, SWEET — **bit·ter·ness** n

bitter almond n : an almond with a bitter taste that contains amygdalin; *also* : a tree (*Prunus dulcis amara*) of the rose family (Rosaceae) producing bitter almonds

bi·uret \'bī-yə-ˌret\ n : a white crystalline compound $N_3H_5C_2O_2$ formed by heating urea

biuret reaction n : a reaction that is shown by biuret, proteins, and most peptides on treatment in alkaline solution with copper sulfate and that results in a violet color

biuret test n : a test esp. for proteins using the biuret reaction

¹**bi·va·lent** \(ˌ)bī-'vā-lᵊnt\ adj : associated in pairs in synapsis

²**bivalent** n : a pair of synaptic chromosomes

bi·valve \'bī-ˌvalv\ vb **bi·valved; bi-**

valv·ing : to split (a cast) along one or two sides (as to renew surgical dressings or to restore circulation)

Bk *symbol* berkelium

BK *abbr* below left knee

black–and–blue \blak-ᵊn-'blü\ *adj* : darkly discolored from blood effused by bruising

black damp *n* : a nonexplosive mine gas that is a mixture containing carbon dioxide and is incapable of supporting life or flame — compare FIREDAMP

black death *n, often cap B&D* **1** : PLAGUE 2 **2** : a severe epidemic of plague and esp. bubonic plague that occurred in Asia and Europe in the 14th century

black disease *n* : a fatal toxemia of sheep associated with simultaneous infection by liver flukes (*Fasciola hepatica*) and an anaerobic toxin-producing clostridium (*Clostridium novyi*) and characterized by liver necrosis and subcutaneous hemorrhage — compare BLACKLEG, BRAXY, LIVER ROT, MALIGNANT EDEMA

black eye *n* : a discoloration of the skin around the eye from bruising

black·fly \'blak-ₐflī\ *n, pl* **-flies** : any of a family (Simuliidae) and esp. genus *Simulium* of bloodsucking dipteran flies

black hairy tongue *n* : BLACKTONGUE 1

black·head \'blak-ₐhed\ *n* **1** : a small plug of sebum blocking the duct of a sebaceous gland esp. on the face — compare MILIUM 2 **2** : a destructive disease of turkeys and related birds caused by a protozoan of the genus *Histomonas* (*H. meleagridis*) that invades the intestinal ceca and liver — called also *enterohepatitis, histomoniasis, infectious enterohepatitis*

black henbane *n* : HENBANE

black·leg \'blak-ₐleg\ *n* : a usu. fatal toxemia esp. of young cattle caused by toxins produced by an anaerobic soil bacterium of the genus *Clostridium* (*C. chauvoei*) — compare BLACK DISEASE, MALIGNANT EDEMA

black lung *n* : pneumoconiosis caused by habitual inhalation of coal dust — called also *black lung disease*

black·out \'blak-ₐau̇t\ *n* : a transient dulling or loss of vision, consciousness, or memory (as from temporary impairment of cerebral circulation, retinal anoxia, a traumatic emotional blow, or an alcoholic binge) — compare GRAYOUT, REDOUT — **black out** *vb*

black quarter *n* : BLACKLEG

black rat *n* : a rat of the genus *Rattus* (*R. rattus*) that infests houses and has been the chief vector of bubonic plague

black·tongue \'blak-ₐtᵊng\ *n* **1** : a dark furry or hairy discoloration of the tongue that is due to hyperplasia of the filiform papillae with an over-growth of microorganisms and is often associated with prolonged use of antibiotics — called also *black hairy tongue* **2** : a disease of dogs that is caused by a deficient diet and that is identical with pellagra in humans

black·wa·ter \'blak-ₐwȯ-tər, -ₐwä-\ *n* : any of several diseases (as blackwater fever or Texas fever) characterized by dark-colored urine

blackwater fever *n* : a rare febrile complication of repeated malarial attacks that is marked by destruction of blood cells with hemoglobinuria and extensive kidney damage

black widow *n* : a venomous New World spider of the genus *Latrodectus* (*L. mactans*) the female of which is black with an hourglass-shaped red mark on the abdominal underside

blad·der \'bla-dər\ *n* **1** : a membranous sac in animals that serves as the receptacle of a liquid or contains gas; *esp* : URINARY BLADDER **2** : a vesicle or pouch forming part of an animal body (the ∼ of a tapeworm larva)

bladder worm *n* : CYSTICERCUS

blade \'blād\ *n* **1** : a broad flat body part (as the shoulder blade) **2** : the flat portion of the tongue immediately behind the tip; *also* : this portion together with the tip **3** : a flat working and esp. cutting part of an implement (as a scalpel)

blain \'blān\ *n* : an inflammatory swelling or sore

Bla·lock–Taus·sig operation \'blā-ₐläk-'tau̇-sig-\ *n* : surgical correction of the tetralogy of Fallot — called also *blue baby operation*

Blalock, **Alfred (1899–1964),** and Taussig, **Helen B. (1898–1986),** American physicians.

blast \'blast\ *n* : an immature or imperfectly developed cell (leukemic ∼s) — **blas·tic** \'blas-tik\ *also* **blast** *adj*

blast- *or* **blasto-** *comb form* : bud : budding : germ (*blasto*disc) (*blas*tula)

-blast \ₐblast\ *n comb form* : formative unit esp. of living matter : germ : cell layer (epi*blast*)

blast cell *n* : a blood cell precursor that is in the earliest stage of development in which it is recognizably committed to development along a particular cell lineage

blas·te·ma \bla-'stē-mə\ *n, pl* **-mas** *or* **-ma·ta** \-mə-tə\ : a mass of living substance capable of growth and differentiation

-blas·tic \'blas-tik\ *adj comb form* : sprouting or germinating (in a specified way) (hemocyto*blastic*) : having (such or so many) sprouts, buds, or germ layers (meso*blastic*)

blas·to·coel *or* **blas·to·coele** \'blas-tə-ₐsēl\ *n* : the cavity of a blastula — **blas·to·coe·lic** \ₐblas-tə-¹sē-lik\ *adj*

blas·to·cyst \'blas-tə-ₐsist\ *n* : the modified blastula of a placental mammal

blas·to·derm \-ₐdərm\ *n* : a blastodisc

after completion of cleavage and formation of the blastocoel

blas·to·derm·ic vesicle \,blas-tə-'dər-mik-\ n : BLASTOCYST

blas·to·disc or **blas·to·disk** \'blas-tə-,disk\ n : the embryo-forming portion of an egg with discoidal cleavage usu. appearing as a small disc on the upper surface of the yolk mass

blas·to·gen·e·sis \,blas-tə-'je-nə-səs\ n, pl **-e·ses** \-,sēz\ : the transformation of lymphocytes into larger cells capable of undergoing mitosis — **blas·to·gen·ic** \-'je-nik\ adj

blas·to·mere \'blas-tə-,mir\ n : a cell produced during cleavage of a fertilized egg — called also cleavage cell

Blas·to·my·ces \,blas-tə-'mī-,sēz\ n, in some classifications : a genus of yeastlike fungi to which the causative agents of blastomycosis are sometimes assigned

blas·to·my·cin \-'mīs-ᵊn\ n : a preparation of growth products of the causative agent of North American blastomycosis that is used esp. to test for this disease

blas·to·my·co·sis \-,mī-'kō-səs\ n, pl **-co·ses** \-,sēz\ : either of two infectious diseases caused by yeastlike fungi — see BLASTOMYCES; NORTH AMERICAN BLASTOMYCOSIS, SOUTH AMERICAN BLASTOMYCOSIS — **blas·to·my·cot·ic** \-'kä-tik\ adj

blas·to·pore \'blas-tə-,pō(ə)r, -,pȯ(ə)r\ n : the opening of the archenteron

blas·tu·la \'blas-chə-lə\ n, pl **-las** or **-lae** \-,lē\ : an early metazoan embryo typically having the form of a hollow fluid-filled rounded cavity bounded by a single layer of cells — compare GASTRULA, MORULA — **blas·tu·lar** \-lər\ adj — **blas·tu·la·tion** \,blas-chə-'lā-shən\ n

Blat·ta \'bla-tə\ n : a genus (family Blattidae) of cockroaches including the common oriental cockroach (B. orientalis) that infests buildings in America and most other parts of the world

Blat·tel·la \blə-'te-lə\ n : a genus of cockroaches including the abundant small domestic German cockroach (B. germanica)

bleb \'bleb\ n : a small blister — compare BULLA 2

bleed \'blēd\ vb \'bled\ \'bled\; **bleed·ing 1:** to emit or lose blood **2 :** to escape by oozing or flowing (as from a wound); also : to remove or draw blood from

bleed·er \'blē-dər\ n **1 :** one that draws blood; esp : a person who draws blood for medical reasons : BLOODLETTER **2 :** one that gives up blood: **a :** HEMOPHILIAC **b :** a large blood vessel divided during surgery

bleed·ing n : an act, instance, or result of being bled or the process by which something is bled: as **a :** the escape of blood from vessels : HEMORRHAGE **b**

: the operation of bleeding a person medically : PHLEBOTOMY

bleeding time n : a period of time of usu. about two and a half minutes during which a small wound (as a pin-prick) continues to bleed

blem·ish \'ble-mish\ n : a mark of physical deformity or injury; esp : any small mark on the skin (as a pimple or birthmark)

blen·nor·rha·gia \,ble-nə-'rā-jē-ə, -jə\ n **1 :** BLENNORRHEA **2 :** GONORRHEA

blennorrhagica — see KERATOSIS BLENNORRHAGICA

blennorrhagicum — see KERATODERMA BLENNORRHAGICUM

blen·nor·rhea \,ble-nə-'rē-ə\ n : an excessive secretion and discharge of mucus — **blen·nor·rheal** \-'rē-əl\ adj

blen·nor·rhoea chiefly Brit var of BLENNORRHEA

bleo·my·cin \,blē-ə-'mīs-ᵊn\ n : a mixture of glycoprotein antibiotics derived from a streptomyces (Streptomyces verticillus) and used in the form of the sulfates as an antineoplastic agent

blephar- or **blepharo-** comb form : eyelid (blepharospasm)

bleph·a·ri·tis \,ble-fə-'rī-təs\ n, pl **-rit·i·des** \-'ri-tə-,dēz\ : inflammation esp. of the margins of the eyelids

bleph·a·ro·con·junc·ti·vi·tis \,ble-fə-(,)rō-kən-,jəŋk-tə-'vī-təs\ n : inflammation of the eyelid and conjunctiva

bleph·a·ro·plas·ty \'ble-fə-rō-,plas-tē\ n, pl **-ties** : plastic surgery on an eyelid esp. to remove fatty or excess tissue

bleph·a·rop·to·sis \,ble-fə-rəp-'tō-səs\ n, pl **-to·ses** \-,sēz\ : a drooping or abnormal relaxation of the upper eyelid

bleph·a·ro·spasm \'ble-fə-rō-,spa-zəm, -rə-\ n : spasmodic winking from involuntary contraction of the orbicularis oculi muscle of the eyelids

bleph·a·rot·o·my \,ble-fə-'rä-tə-mē\ n, pl **-mies** : surgical incision of an eyelid

blind \'blīnd\ adj **1 a :** lacking or deficient in sight; esp : having less than ¹/₁₀ of normal vision in the more efficient eye when refractive defects are fully corrected by lenses **b :** of or relating to sightless persons ⟨~ care⟩ **2 :** made or done without sight of certain objects or knowledge of certain facts by the participants that could serve for guidance ⟨a ~ test⟩ — see DOUBLE-BLIND, SINGLE-BLIND **3 :** having but one opening or outlet ⟨the cecum is a ~ pouch⟩ — **blind** vb — **blind·ly** adv — **blind·ness** n

blind gut n : the cecum of the large intestine

blind spot n : the point in the retina where the optic nerve enters that is not sensitive to light — called also optic disk

blind stag·gers \-'sta-gərz\ n sing or pl : a severe form of selenosis characterized esp. by impairment of vision and an unsteady gait; *also* : a similar condition not caused by selenium poisoning

blink \'bliŋk\ *vb* **1** : to close and open the eye involuntarily **2** : to remove (as tears) from the eye by blinking — **blink** *n*

blis·ter \'blis-tər\ *n* **1** : an elevation of the epidermis containing watery liquid **2** : an agent that causes blistering — **blister** *vb* — **blis·tery** \-tə-rē\ *adj*

¹bloat \'blōt\ *vb* : to make or become turgid: **a** : to produce edema in **b** : to cause or result in accumulation of gas in the digestive tract of

²bloat *n* : a flatulent digestive disturbance of domestic animals and esp. cattle marked by abdominal bloating

¹block \'bläk\ *n, often attrib* **1** : interruption of normal physiological function of a tissue or organ; *esp* : HEART BLOCK **2 a** : BLOCK ANESTHESIA **b** : NERVE BLOCK **1 3** : interruption of a train of thought by competing thoughts or psychological suppression

²block *vb* **1** : to prevent normal functioning of (a bodily element); *also* : to experience or exhibit psychological blocking or blockage **2** : to obstruct the effect of

block·ade \blä-'kād\ *n* : interruption of normal physiological function (as transmission of nerve impulses) of a tissue or organ — **blockade** *vb*

block·age \'blä-kij\ *n* **1** : the action of blocking or the state of being blocked **2** : internal resistance to understanding a communicated idea, to learning new material, or to adopting a new mode of response because of existing habitual ways of thinking, perceiving, and acting — compare BLOCKING

block anesthesia *n* : local anesthesia (as by injection) produced by interruption of the flow of impulses along a nerve trunk — compare REGIONAL ANESTHESIA

block·er \'blä-kər\ *n* : one that blocks — see BETA-BLOCKER, CALCIUM CHANNEL BLOCKER

block·ing \'blä-kiŋ\ *n* : interruption of a trend of associative thought by the arousal of an opposing trend or through the welling up into consciousness of a complex of unpleasant ideas — compare BLOCKAGE 2

blocking antibody *n* : an antibody that combines with an antigen without visible reaction but prevents another antibody from later combining with or producing its usual effect on that antigen

blood \'bləd\ *n, often attrib* **1** : the fluid that circulates in the heart, arteries, capillaries, and veins of a vertebrate animal carrying nourishment and oxygen to and bringing away waste products from all parts of the body **2** : a fluid of an invertebrate comparable to blood

blood bank *n* : a place for storage of or an institution storing blood or plasma; *also* : blood so stored

blood banking *n* : the activity of administering or working in a blood bank

blood–brain barrier *n* : a barrier created by the modification of brain capillaries (as by reduction in fenestration and formation of tight cell-to-cell contacts) that prevents many substances from leaving the blood and crossing the capillary walls into the brain tissues

blood cell *n* : a cell normally present in blood — see RED BLOOD CELL, WHITE BLOOD CELL

blood count *n* : the determination of the blood cells in a definite volume of blood; *also* : the number of cells so determined — see COMPLETE BLOOD COUNT, DIFFERENTIAL BLOOD COUNT

blood doping *n* : a technique for temporarily improving athletic performance in which oxygen-carrying red blood cells from blood previously withdrawn from an athlete are injected back just before an event — called also *blood packing*

blood fluke *n* : SCHISTOSOME

blood group *n* : one of the classes (as A, B, AB, or O) into which individual vertebrates and esp. human beings or their blood can be separated on the basis of the presence or absence of specific antigens in the blood — called also *blood type*

blood grouping *n* : BLOOD TYPING

blood island *n* : any of the reddish areas in the extraembryonic mesoblast of developing vertebrate eggs where blood cells and vessels are forming — called also *blood islet*

blood·less \'bləd-ləs\ *adj* : free from or lacking blood (a ~ surgical field)

blood·let·ter \'bləd-ˌle-tər\ *n* : a practitioner of phlebotomy

blood·let·ting \-ˌle-tiŋ\ *n* : PHLEBOTOMY

blood·mo·bile \-mō-ˌbēl\ *n* : a motor vehicle staffed and equipped for collecting blood from donors

blood platelet *n* : one of the minute protoplasmic disks of vertebrate blood that assist in blood clotting — called also *platelet, thrombocyte*

blood poisoning *n* : SEPTICEMIA

blood pressure *n* : pressure exerted by the blood upon the walls of the blood vessels and esp. arteries, usu. measured on the radial artery by means of a sphygmomanometer, and expressed in millimeters of mercury either as a fraction having as numerator the maximum pressure that follows systole of the left ventricle of the heart and as denominator the minimum pressure that accompanies cardiac diastole or as a whole number representing the first value only (a *blood pressure* of 120/80) (a *blood pressure* of 120) — abbr. *BP*

blood serum *n* : SERUM a (1)

blood·shot \'bləd-ˌshät\ *adj, of an eye* : inflamed to redness

blood·stain \-ˌstān\ *n* : a discoloration caused by blood — **blood·stained** \-ˌstānd\ *adj*

blood·stream \-ˌstrēm\ *n* : the flowing blood in a circulatory system

blood·suck·er \-ˌsə-kər\ *n* : an animal that sucks blood; *esp* : LEECH — **blood·suck·ing** \-kiŋ\ *adj*

blood sugar *n* : the glucose in the blood; *also* : its concentration (as in milligrams per 100 milliliters)

blood test *n* : a test of the blood; *esp* : a serological test for syphilis

blood type *n* : BLOOD GROUP

blood typ·ing \-ˌtī-piŋ\ *n* : the action or process of determining an individual's blood group

blood vessel *n* : any of the vessels through which blood circulates in the body

blood·worm \'bləd-ˌwərm\ *n* : any of several nematode worms of the genus *Strongylus* that are parasitic in the large intestine of horses — called also *palisade worm, red worm*

bloody \'blə-dē\ *adj* **blood·i·er; -est 1 a** : containing or made up of blood **b** : of or contained in the blood **2 a** : smeared or stained with blood **b** : dripping blood : BLEEDING (a ∼ nose)

blot \'blät\ *n* : a sheet usu. of a cellulose derivative that contains spots of immobilized macromolecules (as of DNA, RNA, or protein) or their fragments and that is used to identify specific components of the spots by applying a suitable molecular probe (as a complementary nucleic acid or a radioactively labeled antibody) — see NORTHERN BLOT, SOUTHERN BLOT, WESTERN BLOT — **blot** *vb*

blotch \'bläch\ *n* : a blemished patch on the skin (a face covered with ∼*es*) — **blotch** *vb* — **blotchy** \'blä-chē\ *adj*

blow·fish \-ˌfish\ *n* : PUFFER

blow·fly \-ˌflī\ *n, pl* **-flies** : any of a family (Calliphoridae) of dipteran flies (as a bluebottle or screwworm)

blue baby *n* : an infant with a bluish tint usu. from a congenital heart defect marked by mingling of venous and arterial blood

blue–baby operation *n* : BLALOCK-TAUSSIG OPERATION

blue bag *n* : gangrenous mastitis of sheep

blue·bot·tle \'blü-ˌbät-ᵊl\ *n* : any of several blowflies (genus *Calliphora*) that have the abdomen or the whole body iridescent blue in color and that make a loud buzzing noise in flight

blue comb *n* : a severe avian disease esp. of domestic fowl caused by a coronavirus

blue heaven *n, slang* : amobarbital or its sodium derivative in a blue tablet or capsule

blue nevus *n* : a small blue or bluish

black spot on the skin that is sharply circumscribed, rounded, and flat or slightly raised and is usu. benign but often mistaken for a melanoma

blue·tongue \'blü-ˌtəŋ\ *n* : a virus disease esp. of sheep marked by hyperemia, cyanosis, and by swelling and sloughing of the epithelium esp. about the mouth and tongue and caused by an orbivirus

blunt dissection *n* : surgical separation of tissue layers by means of an instrument without a cutting edge or by the fingers

blunt trauma *n* : an injury caused by a blunt object

B lym·pho·cyte \'bē-ˈlim-fə-ˌsīt\ *n* : B CELL

BM *abbr* **1** Bachelor of Medicine **2** bowel movement

BMR *abbr* basal metabolic rate

BNA *abbr* Basle Nomina Anatomica

BO *abbr* body odor

board \'bōrd\ *n* **1** : a group of persons having supervisory, managerial, investigative, or advisory powers (medical licensing ∼*s*) (a ∼ of health) **2** : an examination given by an examining board — often used in pl.

board–certified *adj* : being a physician who has graduated from medical school, completed residency, trained under supervision in a specialty, and passed a qualifying exam given by a medical specialty board

Bo·dan·sky unit \bə-ˈdan-skē-, -ˈdän-\ *n* : a unit that is used as a measure of phosphatase concentration (as in the blood) esp. in the diagnosis of various pathological conditions and that has a normal value for the blood averaging about 7 for children and about 4 for adults

Bodansky, Aaron (1887–1960), American biochemist.

bod·i·ly \'bäd-ᵊl-ē\ *adj* : of or relating to the body (∼ organs)

body \'bä-dē\ *n, pl* **bod·ies 1 a** (1) : the material part or nature of a human being (2) : the dead organism : CORPSE **b** : a human being **2 a** : the main part of a plant or animal body esp. as distinguished from limbs and head : TRUNK **b** : the main part of an organ (as the uterus) **3** : a kind or form of matter : a material substance — see KETONE BODY

body bag *n* : a large zippered usu. rubber bag in which a human corpse is placed esp. for transportation

body–build \-ˌbild\ *n* : the distinctive physical makeup of a human being

body cavity *n* : a cavity within an animal body; *specif* : COELOM

body heat *n* : ANIMAL HEAT

body image *n* : a subjective picture of one's own physical appearance established both by self-observation and by noting the reactions of others

body louse *n* : a louse feeding primarily on the body; *esp* : a sucking louse of the genus *Pediculus* (*P. humanus humanus*) feeding on the human body and living in clothing — called also *cootie*

body odor *n* : an unpleasant odor from a perspiring or unclean person

body stalk *n* : the mesodermal cord that contains the umbilical vessels and that connects a fetus with its chorion

Boeck's sarcoid \'beks-\ *n* : SARCOIDOSIS

　Boeck \'bek\, **Caesar Peter Moeller (1845–1917),** Norwegian dermatologist.

Bohr effect \'bōər-\ *n* : the decrease in oxygen affinity of a respiratory pigment (as hemoglobin) in response to decreased blood pH resulting from increased carbon dioxide concentration

　Bohr, Christian (1855–1911), Danish physiologist.

boil \'bȯil\ *n* : a localized swelling and inflammation of the skin resulting from bacterial infection in a skin gland, having a hard central core, and forming pus — called also *furuncle*

boiling point *n* : the temperature at which a liquid boils

bo·lus \'bō-ləs\ *n* : a rounded mass: as **a** : a large pill **b** : a soft mass of chewed food

bombé — see IRIS BOMBÉ

bom·be·sin \'bäm-bə-sin\ *n* : a polypeptide that is found in the brain and gastrointestinal tract and has been shown experimentally to cause the secretion of various substances (as gastrin and cholecystokinin) and to inhibit intestinal motility

bond \'bänd\ *n* : an attractive force that holds together atoms, ions, or groups of atoms in a molecule or crystal — usu. represented in formulas by a line or dot — **bond** *vb*

bond·ing *n* **1** : the formation of a close personal relationship (as between a mother and child) esp. through frequent or constant association — see MALE BONDING **2** : a dental technique in which a material and esp. plastic or porcelain is attached to a tooth surface to correct minor defects (as for chipped or discolored teeth) esp. for cosmetic purposes

bone \'bōn\ *n, often attrib* **1** : one of the hard parts of the skeleton of a vertebrate (the ∼s of the arm) **2** : the hard largely calcareous connective tissue of which the adult skeleton of most vertebrates is chiefly composed (cancellous ∼) (compact ∼) — compare CARTILAGE 1

bone marrow *n* : MARROW

bont tick \'bänt-\ *n* : a southern African tick of the genus *Amblyomma* (*A. hebraeum*) that attacks livestock, birds, and sometimes humans and transmits heartwater of sheep, goats, and cattle; *broadly* : any African tick of the genus *Amblyomma*

bony *also* **bon·ey** \'bō-nē\ *adj* **bon·i·**

er; -est : consisting of or resembling bone (∼ prominences of the skull)

bony labyrinth *n* : the cavity in the petrous portion of the temporal bone that contains the membranous labyrinth of the inner ear — called also *osseous labyrinth*

Bo·oph·i·lus \bō-'ä-fə-ləs\ *n* : a genus of ticks some of which are pests esp. of cattle and vectors of disease — see CATTLE TICK

boost·er \'bü-stər\ *n* : a substance that increases the effectiveness of a medicament; *esp* : BOOSTER SHOT

booster shot *n* : a supplementary dose of an immunizing agent — called also *booster, booster dose*

bo·rac·ic acid \bə-'ra-sik-\ *n* : BORIC ACID

bo·rate \'bȯr-ˌāt\ *n* : a salt or ester of a boric acid

bor·bo·ryg·mus \ˌbȯr-bə-'rig-məs\ *n, pl* **-mi** \-ˌmī\ : a rumbling sound made by the movement of gas in the intestine — **bor·bo·ryg·mic** \-mik\ *adj*

bor·der·line \'bȯr-dər-ˌlīn\ *adj* **1** : being in an intermediate position or state : not fully classifiable as one thing or its opposite; *esp* : not quite up to what is usual, standard, or expected (∼ intelligence) **2** : exhibiting typical but not altogether conclusive symptoms **3** : characterized by psychological instability in several areas (as interpersonal relations, behavior, mood, and identity) often with impaired social and vocational functioning but with brief or no psychotic episodes (a ∼ personality disorder)

Bor·de·tel·la \ˌbȯr-də-'te-lə\ *n* : a genus of bacteria comprising minute and very short gram-negative strictly aerobic coccuslike bacilli and including the causative agent (*B. pertussis*) of whooping cough

　J.–J.–B.–V. Bordet — see BORDET≠GENGOU BACILLUS

Bor·det–Gen·gou bacillus \bȯr-'dā-zhä⁻-'gü-\ *n* : a small ovoid bacillus of the genus *Bordetella* (*B. pertussis*) that is the causative agent of whooping cough

　Bordet, Jules–Jean–Baptiste–Vincent (1870–1961), Belgian bacteriologist, and **Gengou, Octave (1875–1957),** French bacteriologist.

bo·ric acid \'bȯr-ik-\ *n* : a white crystalline acid H₃BO₃ used esp. as a weak antiseptic — called also *boracic acid*

Born·holm disease \'bȯrn-ˌhōlm-\ *n* : EPIDEMIC PLEURODYNIA

bo·ron \'bȯr-ˌän\ *n* : a trivalent metalloid element found in nature only in combination — symbol *B*; see ELEMENT table

bor·re·lia \bə-'re-lē-ə, -'rē-\ *n* *cap* : a genus of small spirochetes (family Spirochaetaceae) that are parasites of humans and warm-blooded animals and include the causative agents of septicemia in chickens (*B. recur-*

rentis), relapsing fever in Africa (*B. duttoni*), and Lyme disease in the U.S. (*B. burgdorferi*) **2** : a spirochete of the genus *Borrelia*

bos·se·lat·ed \'bä-sə-ˌlā-təd, 'bȯ-\ *adj* : marked or covered with protuberances ⟨a ~ tumor⟩

bot *also* **bott** \'bät\ *n* : the larva of a botfly; *esp* : one infesting the horse

bo·tan·i·cal \bə-'ta-ni-kəl\ *n* : a vegetable drug esp. in the crude state

bot·fly \'bät-ˌflī\ *n, pl* **-flies** : any of various stout dipteran flies (family Oestridae) with larvae parasitic in cavities or tissues of various mammals including humans

botry- *or* **botryo-** *comb form* **1** : bunch of grapes ⟨*botry*oid⟩ **2** : botryoid ⟨*botry*omycosis⟩

bot·ry·oid \'bä-trē-ˌȯid\ *adj* : having the form of a bunch of grapes ⟨~ sarcoma⟩

botryoides — see SARCOMA BOTRYOIDES

bot·ry·o·my·co·sis \ˌbä-trē-(ˌ)ō-mī-'kō-səs\ *n, pl* **-co·ses** \-ˌsēz\ : a bacterial infection of domestic animals and humans marked by the formation of usu. superficial vascular granulomatous masses, associated esp. with wounds, and sometimes followed by metastatic visceral tumors — **bot·ry·o·my·cot·ic** \-'kä-tik\ *adj*

bot·tle \'bät-əl\ *n, often attrib* **1** : a container typically of glass or plastic having a comparatively narrow neck or mouth and usu. no handle **2** : liquid food usu. consisting of milk and supplements that is fed from a bottle (as to an infant) in place of mother's milk

bottle baby *n* : a baby fed chiefly or wholly on the bottle as contrasted with a baby that is chiefly or wholly breast-fed

bot·tle-feed \'bät-əl-ˌfēd\ *vb* **-fed; -feeding** : to feed (an infant) from a bottle rather than by breast-feeding

bottle jaw *n* : a pendulous edematous condition of the tissues under the lower jaw in cattle and sheep resulting from infestation with bloodsucking gastrointestinal parasites (as of the genus *Haemonchus*)

bot·u·lin \'bä-chə-lən\ *n* : a neurotoxin formed by botulinum and causing botulism

bot·u·li·num \ˌbä-chə-'lī-nəm\ *also* **bot·u·li·nus** \-nəs\ *n* : a spore-forming bacterium of the genus *Clostridium* (*C. botulinum*) that secretes botulin — **bot·u·li·nal** \-'lī-nᵊl\ *adj*

bot·u·lism \'bä-chə-ˌli-zəm\ *n* : acute food poisoning caused by a toxic product produced in food by a bacterium of the genus *Clostridium* (*C. botulinum*) and characterized by muscle weakness and paralysis, disturbances of vision, swallowing, and speech, and a high mortality rate — compare BOTULIN

bou·gie \'bü-ˌzhē, -ˌjē\ *n* **1** : a tapering cylindrical instrument for introduction into a tubular passage of the body **2** : SUPPOSITORY

bou·gie·nage *or* **bou·gi·nage** \ˌbü-zhē-'näzh\ *n* : the dilation of a tubular cavity (as a constricted esophagus) with a bougie

-boulia — see -BULIA

bound \'baund\ *adj* **1** : made costive : CONSTIPATED **2** : held in chemical or physical combination

bou·ton \bü-'tōⁿ\ *n* : a terminal club-shaped enlargement of a nerve fiber at a synapse with another neuron

bou·ton·neuse fever \ˌbü-tȯ-'nüz-, -'nœz-\ *n* : a disease of the Mediterranean area that is characterized by headache, pain in muscles and joints, and an eruption over the body and is caused by a tick-borne rickettsia (*Rickettsia conorii*) — called also *fièvre boutonneuse, Marseilles fever;* see TICK TYPHUS

Bo·vic·o·la \bō-'vi-kə-lə\ *n* : a genus of biting lice (order Mallophaga) including several that infest the hair of domestic mammals

bo·vine \'bō-ˌvīn, -ˌvēn\ *n* : an ox (genus *Bos*) or a closely related animal — **bovine** *adj*

bovine mastitis *n* : inflammation of the udder of a cow resulting from injury or more commonly from bacterial infection

bovinum — see COR BOVINUM

bow \'bō\ *n* : a frame for the lenses of eyeglasses; *also* : the curved sidepiece of the frame passing over the ear

bow·el \'baül\ *n* : INTESTINE, GUT; *also* : one of the divisions of the intestines — usu. used in pl. except in medical use ⟨move your ~s⟩ ⟨surgery of the involved ~⟩

bowel worm *n* : a common strongylid nematode worm of the genus *Chabertia* (*C. ovina*) infesting the colon of sheep and feeding on blood and tissue

Bow·en's disease \'bō-ənz-\ *n* : a precancerous lesion of the skin or mucous membranes characterized by small solid elevations covered by thickened horny tissue

Bow·en \'bō-ən\, **John Templeton (1857–1941),** American dermatologist.

bow·leg \'bō-ˌleg\ *n* : a leg bowed outward at or below the knee — called also *genu varum*

bow·legged \'bō-ˌle-gəd, -ˌlegd\ *adj* : having bowlegs

Bow·man's capsule \'bō-mənz-\ *n* : a thin membranous double-walled capsule surrounding the glomerulus of a vertebrate nephron — called also *capsule of Bowman, glomerular capsule*

Bow·man \'bō-mən\, **Sir William (1816–1892),** British ophthalmologist, anatomist, and physiologist.

Bowman's gland *n* : GLAND OF BOWMAN

Bowman's membrane *n* : the thin outer layer of the substantia propria of the cornea immediately underlying the epithelium

box·ing \'bäk-siŋ\ *n* : construction of the base of a dental cast by building up the walls of an impression while preserving important landmarks

bp *abbr* base pair

BP *abbr* blood pressure

Br *symbol* bromine

¹**brace** \'brās\ *n, pl* **brac·es 1** : an appliance that gives support to movable parts (as a joint), to weak muscles (as in paralysis), or to strained ligaments (as of the lower back) **2** *pl* : dental appliances used to exert pressure to straighten misaligned teeth

²**brace** *vb* **braced; brac·ing** : to furnish or support with a brace

brachi- *or* **brachio-** *comb form* **1** : arm ⟨*brachio*radialis⟩ **2** : brachial and ⟨*brachio*cephalic artery⟩

bra·chi·al \'brā-kē-əl\ *adj* : of or relating to the arm

brachial artery *n* : the chief artery of the upper arm that is a direct continuation of the axillary artery and divides into the radial and ulnar arteries just below the elbow — see DEEP BRACHIAL ARTERY

bra·chi·a·lis \‚brā-kē-'a-ləs, -'ā-, -'ä-\ *n* : a flexor that lies in front of the lower part of the humerus whence it arises and is inserted into the ulna

brachial plexus *n* : a complex network of nerves that is formed chiefly by the lower four cervical nerves and the first thoracic nerve and supplies nerves to the chest, shoulder, and arm

brachial vein *n* : one of a pair of veins accompanying the brachial artery and uniting with each other and with the basilic vein to form the axillary vein

brachii — see BICEPS BRACHII, TRICEPS BRACHII

bra·chio·ce·phal·ic artery \‚brā-kē-(‚)ō-sə-'fa-lik-\ *n* : a short artery that arises from the arch of the aorta and divides into the carotid and subclavian arteries of the right side — called also *innominate artery*

brachiocephalicus — see TRUNCUS BRACHIOCEPHALICUS

brachiocephalic vein *n* : either of two large veins that occur one on each side of the neck, receive blood from the head and neck, are formed by the union of the internal jugular and the subclavian veins, and unite to form the superior vena cava — called also *innominate vein*

bra·chio·ra·di·a·lis \‚brā-kē-ō-‚rā-dē-'a-ləs, -'ä-, -'ä-\ *n, pl* **-a·les** \‚lēz\ : a flexor of the radial side of the forearm arising from the lateral supracondylar ridge of the humerus and inserted into the styloid process of the radius

bra·chi·um \'brā-kē-əm\ *n, pl* **-chia** \-kē-ə\ : the upper segment of the arm extending from the shoulder to the elbow

brachium con·junc·ti·vum \-‚kän-(‚)jəŋk-'tī-vəm\ *n* : CEREBELLAR PEDUNCLE a

brachium pon·tis \-'pän-təs\ *n* : CEREBELLAR PEDUNCLE b

brachy- *comb form* : short ⟨*brachy*cephalic⟩ ⟨*brachy*dactylous⟩

brachy·ce·phal·ic \‚bra-ki-sə-'fa-lik\ *adj* : short-headed or broad-headed with a cephalic index of over 80 — **brachy·ceph·a·ly** \-'se-fə-lē\ *n*

brachy·dac·ty·lous \‚bra-ki-'dak-tə-ləs\ *adj* : having abnormally short digits — **brachy·dac·ty·ly** \-lē\ *n*

brachy·ther·a·py \-'ther-ə-pē\ *n, pl* **-pies** : radiotherapy in which the source of radiation is close to the area being treated

Brad·ford frame \'brad-fərd-\ *n* : a frame used to support a patient with disease or fractures of the spine, hip, or pelvis

Bradford, Edward Hickling (1848–1926), American orthopedist.

brad·sot \'brad-sot\ *n* : BRAXY

brady- *comb form* : slow ⟨*brady*cardia⟩

brady·car·dia \‚brā-di-'kär-dē-ə *also* ‚bra-\ *n* : relatively slow heart action whether physiological or pathological — compare TACHYCARDIA

brady·ki·ne·sia \-ki-'nē-zhē-ə, -zhə, -zē-ə\ *n* : extreme slowness of movements and reflexes (as in catatonic schizophrenia)

brady·ki·nin \-'kī-nən\ *n* : a kinin that is formed locally in injured tissue, acts in vasodilation of small arterioles, is considered to play a part in inflammatory processes, and is composed of a chain of nine amino-acid residues

brady·pnea \‚brā-dəp-'nē-ə, ‚bra-\ *n* : abnormally slow breathing

brady·pnoea *chiefly Brit var of* BRADYPNEA

braille \'brāl\ *n, often cap* : a system of writing for the blind that uses characters made up of raised dots — **braille** *vb*

Braille \'brī, 'brāl\, **Louis (1809–1852),** French inventor and teacher.

brain \'brān\ *n* : the portion of the vertebrate central nervous system that constitutes the organ of thought and neural coordination, includes all the higher nervous centers receiving stimuli from the sense organs and interpreting and correlating them to formulate the motor impulses, is made up of neurons and supporting and nutritive structures, is enclosed within the skull, and is continuous with the spinal cord through the foramen magnum

brain·case \-‚kās\ *n* : the part of the skull that encloses the brain — see CRANIUM

brain death *n* : final cessation of activity in the central nervous system esp. as indicated by a flat electroencephalogram for a predetermined length of time — **brain–dead** *adj*

brain stem *n* : the part of the brain composed of the midbrain, pons, and medulla oblongata and connecting the spinal cord with the forebrain and cerebrum

brain vesicle *n* : any of the divisions into which the developing embryonic brain of vertebrates is marked off by incomplete transverse constrictions

brain·wash·ing \'brān-ˌwȯ-shiŋ, -ˌwä-\ *n* : a forcible indoctrination to induce someone to give up basic political, social, or religious beliefs and attitudes and to accept contrasting regimented ideas — **brain·wash** *vb*

brain wave *n* 1 : rhythmic fluctuations of voltage between parts of the brain resulting in the flow of an electric current 2 : a current produced by brain waves — compare ALPHA WAVE, BETA WAVE

bran \'bran\ *n* : the edible broken seed coats of cereal grain separated from the flour or meal by sifting

branch \'branch\ *n* : something that extends from or enters into a main body or source ⟨a ~ of an artery⟩ — **branch** *vb*

bran·chi·al \'bran-kē-əl\ *adj* : of or relating to the parts of the body derived from the embryonic branchial arches and clefts

branchial arch *n* : one of a series of bony or cartilaginous arches that develop in the walls of the mouth cavity and pharynx of a vertebrate embryo and correspond to the gill arches of fishes and amphibians — called also *pharyngeal arch, visceral arch*

branchial cleft *n* : one of the open or potentially open clefts that occur on each side of the neck region of a vertebrate embryo between the branchial arches and correspond to the gill slits of fishes and amphibians — called also *pharyngeal cleft*

brash \'brash\ *n* : WATER BRASH

Brax·ton–Hicks contractions \'brak-stən-'hiks-\ *n pl* : relatively painless nonrhythmic contractions of the uterus that occur during pregnancy with increasing frequency over time but are not associated with labor

Hicks, John Braxton (1823–1897), British gynecologist.

braxy \'brak-sē\ *n, pl* **brax·ies** : a malignant edema of sheep that involves gastrointestinal invasion by a bacterium of the genus *Clostridium* (*C. septicum*) — compare BLACK DISEASE

¹**break** \'brāk\ *vb* **broke** \'brōk\; **broken** \'brō-kən\ **break·ing** 1 a : to snap into pieces : FRACTURE ⟨~ a bone⟩ **b** : to fracture the bone of (a bodily part) ⟨the blow *broke* her arm⟩ **c** : DISLOCATE ⟨~ing his neck⟩ **2 a** : to cause an open wound in : RUPTURE ⟨~ the

skin⟩ **b** : to rupture the surface of and permit flowing out or effusing ⟨~ an artery⟩ **3** : to fail in strength or resistance **4** : to suffer complete or marked loss of resistance, composure, resolution, morale, or command of a situation — often used with *down*

²**break** *n* **1** : an act or action of breaking : FRACTURE **2** : a condition produced by breaking ⟨gave him something to relieve the pain of the ~ in his leg⟩

break·bone fever \'brāk-ˌbōn-\ *n* : DENGUE

¹**break·down** \'brāk-ˌdau̇n\ *n* **1** : a failure to function **2** : a physical, mental, or nervous collapse **3** : the process of decomposing ⟨~ of food during digestion⟩ — **break down** *vb*

²**breakdown** *adj* : obtained or resulting from disintegration or decomposition of a substance ⟨a ~ product of hemoglobin⟩

break out *vb* **1** : to become affected with a skin eruption **2** of a disease : to manifest itself by skin eruptions **3** : to become covered with ⟨*break out* in a sweat⟩

break·through bleeding \ˌbrāk-ˌthrü-\ *n* : prolonged bleeding due to irregular sloughing of the endometrium in the menstrual cycle in women on contraceptive hormones

breast \'brest\ *n* **1** : either of the pair of mammary glands extending from the front of the chest in pubescent and adult females; *also* : either of the analogous but rudimentary organs of the male chest esp. when enlarged **2** : the fore or ventral part of the body between the neck and the abdomen

breast·bone \'brest-ˌbōn\ *n* : STERNUM

breast–feed \'brest-ˌfēd\ *vb* : to feed (an infant) from a mother's breast rather than from a bottle

breath \'breth\ *n* **1 a** : the faculty of breathing **b** : an act or an instance of breathing or inhaling ⟨fought to his last ~⟩ **2 a** : air inhaled and exhaled in breathing ⟨bad ~⟩ **b** : something (as moisture on a cold surface) produced by breath or breathing — **out of breath** : breathing very rapidly

Breath·a·lyz·er \'bre-thə-ˌlī-zər\ *trademark* — used for a device that is used to determine the alcohol content of a breath sample

breathe \'brēth\ *vb* **breathed; breathing 1** : to draw air into and expel it from the lungs : RESPIRE; *broadly* : to take in oxygen and give out carbon dioxide through natural processes **2** : to inhale and exhale freely

breath·er \'brē-thər\ *n* : one that breathes usu. in a specified way — SEE MOUTH BREATHER

breath·less \'breth-ləs\ *adj* **1** : panting or gasping for breath **2** : suffering from dyspnea

breech \'brēch\ *n* **1** : the hind end of the body : BUTTOCKS **2** : BREECH PRESEN-

TATION; *also* : a fetus that is presented breech first

breech delivery *n* : delivery of a fetus by breech presentation

breech presentation *n* : presentation of the fetus in which the breech is the first part to appear at the uterine cervix

breg·ma \'breg-mə\ *n*, *pl* **-ma·ta** \-mə-tə\ : the point of junction of the coronal and sagittal sutures of the skull — **breg·mat·ic** \breg-'ma-tik\ *adj*

bre·tyl·i·um \brə-'ti-lē-əm\ *n* : an antiarrhythmic drug administered in the form of its tosylate $C_{18}H_{24}BrNO_3S$ in the treatment of ventricular fibrillation and tachycardia and formerly used as an antihypertensive

brevis — see ABDUCTOR POLLICIS BREVIS, ADDUCTOR BREVIS, EXTENSOR CARPI RADIALIS BREVIS, EXTENSOR DIGITORUM BREVIS, EXTENSOR HALLUCIS BREVIS, EXTENSOR POLLICIS BREVIS, FLEXOR DIGITI MINIMI BREVIS, FLEXOR DIGITORUM BREVIS, FLEXOR HALLUCIS BREVIS, FLEXOR POLLICIS BREVIS, PALMARIS BREVIS, PERONEUS BREVIS

brewer's yeast *n* : the dried pulverized cells of a yeast of the genus *Saccharomyces* (*S. cerevisiae*) used as a source of B-complex vitamins

bridge \'brij\ *n* **1 a** : the upper bony part of the nose **b** : the curved part of a pair of glasses that rests upon this part of the nose **2 a** : PONS **b** : a strand of protoplasm extending between two cells **c** : a partial denture held in place by anchorage to adjacent teeth

bridge·work \-ˌwərk\ *n* : dental bridges; *also* : prosthodontics concerned with their construction

bright·ness \'brīt-nəs\ *n* : the one of the three psychological dimensions of color perception by which visual stimuli are ordered continuously from light to dark and which is correlated with light intensity — compare HUE, SATURATION

Bright's disease \'brīts-\ *n* : any of several kidney diseases marked esp. by albumin in the urine

  Bright \'brīt\, **Richard** (1789–1858), British internist and pathologist.

Brill's disease \'brilz-\ *n* : an acute infectious disease milder than epidemic typhus but caused by the same rickettsia

  Brill \'bril\, **Nathan Edwin** (1860–1925), American physician.

bring up *vt* : VOMIT

British an·ti·lew·is·ite \-ˌan-tē-'lü-ə-ˌsīt, -ˌan-ˌtī-\ *n* : DIMERCAPROL

  W. L. Lewis — see LEWISITE

brit·tle \'brit-ᵊl\ *adj* : affected with or being a form of insulin-dependent diabetes mellitus characterized by large and unpredictable fluctuations in blood glucose level (~ diabetes)

broach \'brōch\ *n* : a fine tapered flexible instrument used in dentistry in

removing the dental pulp and in dressing a root canal

broad bean *n* : the large flat edible seed of an Old World upright vetch (*Vicia faba*); *also* : the plant itself — see FAVISM

broad ligament *n* : either of the two lateral ligaments of the uterus composed of a double sheet of peritoneum and bearing the ovary supended from the dorsal surface

broad–spectrum *adj* : effective against a wide range of organisms (as insects or bacteria) — compare NARROW-SPECTRUM

Bro·ca's aphasia \'brō-ˌkəz-\ *n* : MOTOR APHASIA

  Bro·ca \brō-'kä\, **Pierre–Paul** (1824–1880), French surgeon and anthropologist.

Broca's area *n* : a brain center associated with the motor control of speech and usu. located in the left but sometimes in the right inferior frontal gyrus — called also *Broca's convolution, Broca's gyrus, convolution of Broca*

Brod·mann area \'bräd-mən-\ *or* **Brodmann's area** \-mənz-\ *n* : one of the several structurally distinguishable and presumably functionally distinct regions into which the cortex of each cerebral hemisphere can be divided

  Brod·mann \'brōt-ˌmän, 'bräd-mən\, **Korbinian** (1868–1918), German neurologist.

broke *past of* BREAK

bro·ken \'brō-kən\ *adj* : having undergone or been subjected to fracture

broken wind *n* : HEAVES **1** — **bro·ken–wind·ed** \-ˌwind-əd\ *adj*

brom- *or* **bromo-** *comb form* **1** : bromine (*bromide*) **2** *now usu* **bromo-** : containing bromine in place of hydrogen — in names of organic compounds (*bromo*uracil)

bro·me·lain *also* **bro·me·lin** \'brō-mə-lən\ *n* : a protease obtained from the juice of the pineapple (*Ananas comosus* of the family Bromeliaceae)

bro·mide \'brō-ˌmīd\ *n* **1** : a binary compound of bromine with another element or a radical including some (as potassium bromide) used as sedatives **2** : a dose of bromide taken usu. as a sedative

brom·hi·dro·sis \ˌbrō-mə-'drō-səs *also* ˌbrōm-hə-\ *also* **bro·mi·dro·sis** \ˌbrō-mə-\ *n*, *pl* **-dro·ses** \-ˌsēz\ : foul-smelling sweat

bro·mine \'brō-ˌmēn\ *n* : a nonmetallic element that is normally a red corrosive toxic liquid — symbol *Br*; see ELEMENT table

bro·mism \'brō-ˌmi-zəm\ *n* : an abnormal state due to excessive or prolonged use of bromides

bro·mo \'brō-(ˌ)mō\ *n*, *pl* **bromos** : a proprietary effervescent mixture used as a headache remedy, sedative, and alkalinizing agent; *also* : a dose of such a mixture

bro·mo·crip·tine \ˌbrō-mō-ˈkrip-ˌtēn\ *n* : a polypeptide alkaloid $C_{32}H_{40}$-BrN_5O_5 that is a derivative of ergot and mimics the activity of dopamine in selectively inhibiting prolactin secretion

bro·mo·de·oxy·ur·i·dine \ˌbrō-mō-ˌdē-ˌäk-sē-ˈyur-ə-ˌdēn, -dən\ *or* **5-bro-mo·de·oxy·ur·i·dine** \ˈfiv-\ *n* : a mutagenic analog $C_9H_{11}O_5NBr$ of thymidine that induces chromosomal breakage esp. in heterochromatic regions — abbr. *BUdR*

bro·mo·der·ma \ˈbrō-mə-ˌdər-mə\ *n* : a skin eruption caused in susceptible persons by the use of bromides

bro·mo·ura·cil \ˌbrō-mō-ˈyur-ə-ˌsil, -səl\ *n* : a mutagenic uracil derivative $C_4H_3N_2O_2Br$ that is an analog of thymine and pairs readily with adenine and sometimes with guanine

Brom·sul·pha·lein \ˌbrōm-(ˌ)səl-ˈfa-lē-ən, -ˈfā-\ *trademark* — used for a dye derived from phenolphthalein that is used in the form of its disodium salt in a liver function test

bronch- *or* **broncho-** *comb form* : bronchial tube : bronchial (*bronchitis*)

bronchi *pl of* BRONCHUS

bronchi- *or* **bronchio-** *comb form* : bronchial tubes (*bronchiectasis*)

bron·chi·al \ˈbräŋ-kē-əl\ *adj* : of or relating to the bronchi or their ramifications in the lungs — **bron·chi·al·ly** *adv*

bronchial artery *n* : any branch of the descending aorta or first intercostal artery that accompanies the bronchi

bronchial asthma *n* : asthma resulting from spasmodic contraction of bronchial muscles

bronchial pneumonia *n* : BRONCHO-PNEUMONIA

bronchial tree *n* : the bronchi together with their branches

bronchial tube *n* : a primary bronchus; *also* : any of its branches

bronchial vein *n* : any vein accompanying the bronchi and their branches and emptying into the azygos and superior intercostal veins

bron·chi·ec·ta·sis \ˌbräŋ-kē-ˈek-tə-səs\ *also* **bron·chi·ec·ta·sia** \-ek-ˈtā-zhə, -zhē-ə\ *n*, *pl* **-ta·ses** \-ˌsēz\ *also* **-ta·sias** \-zhəz, -zhē-əz\ : a chronic inflammatory or degenerative condition of one or more bronchi or bronchioles marked by dilatation and loss of elasticity of the walls — **bron·chi·ec·tat·ic** \-ek-ˈta-tik\ *adj*

bron·chio·gen·ic \ˌbräŋ-kē-ō-ˈje-nik\ *adj* : BRONCHOGENIC

bron·chi·ole \ˈbräŋ-kē-ˌōl\ *n* : a minute thin-walled branch of a bronchus — **bron·chi·o·lar** \ˌbräŋ-kē-ˈō-lər\ *adj*

bron·chi·ol·itis \ˌbräŋ-kē-ō-ˈlī-təs\ *n* : inflammation of the bronchioles

bron·chi·o·lus \ˌbräŋ-ˈkī-ə-ləs\ *n*, *pl* **-o·li** \-ˌlī\ : BRONCHIOLE

bron·chi·tis \brän-ˈkī-təs, bräŋ-\ *n*

: acute or chronic inflammation of the bronchial tubes; *also* : a disease marked by this — **bron·chit·ic** \-ˈki-tik\ *adj*

broncho- — see BRONCH-

bron·cho·al·ve·o·lar \ˌbräŋ-kō-al-ˈvē-ə-lər\ *adj* : of, relating to, or involving the bronchioles and alveoli of the lungs ⟨~ lavage as a diagnostic technique⟩

bron·cho·con·stric·tion \-kən-ˈstrik-shən\ *n* : constriction of the bronchial air passages — **bron·cho·con·stric·tor** \-ˈstrik-tər\ *adj*

bron·cho·di·la·ta·tion \-ˌdi-lə-ˈtā-shən, -ˌdī-\ *n* : BRONCHODILATION

bron·cho·di·la·tion \-ˈlā-shən\ *n* : expansion of the bronchial air passages

¹bron·cho·di·la·tor \-dī-ˈlā-tər, -ˈdī-ˌlā-\ *also* **bron·cho·di·la·to·ry** \-dī-ˈlā-tə-rē\ *adj* : relating to or causing expansion of the bronchial air passages ⟨~ activity⟩ ⟨~ drugs⟩

²bronchodilator *n* : a drug that relaxes bronchial muscle resulting in expansion of the bronchial air passages

bron·cho·gen·ic \ˌbräŋ-kə-ˈje-nik\ *adj* : of, relating to, or arising in or by way of the air passages of the lungs ⟨~ carcinoma⟩

bron·cho·gram \ˈbräŋ-kə-ˌgram, -kō-\ *n* : a roentgenogram of the bronchial tree after injection of a radiopaque substance

bron·chog·ra·phy \bräŋ-ˈkä-grə-fē, brän-\ *n*, *pl* **-phies** : the roentgenographic visualization of the bronchi and their branches after injection of a radiopaque substance — **bron·cho·graph·ic** \ˌbräŋ-kə-ˈgra-fik\ *adj*

bron·choph·o·ny \brän-ˈkä-fə-nē\ *n*, *pl* **-nies** : the sound of the voice heard through the stethoscope over a healthy bronchus and over other portions of the chest in cases of consolidation of the lung tissue — compare PECTORILOQUY

bron·cho·plas·ty \ˈbräŋ-kə-ˌplas-tē\ *n*, *pl* **-ties** : surgical repair of a bronchial defect

bron·cho·pleu·ral \ˌbräŋ-kō-ˈplur-əl\ *adj* : joining a bronchus and the pleural cavity ⟨a ~ fistula⟩

bron·cho·pneu·mo·nia \ˌbräŋ-(ˌ)kō-nu̇-ˈmō-nyə, -nyu̇-\ *n* : pneumonia involving many relatively small areas of lung tissue — called also *bronchial pneumonia* — **bron·cho·pneu·mon·ic** \-ˈmä-nik\ *adj*

bron·cho·pul·mo·nary \ˌbräŋ-kō-ˈpul-mə-ˌner-ē, -ˈpəl-\ *adj* : of, relating to, or affecting the bronchi and the lungs

bron·cho·scope \ˈbräŋ-kə-ˌskōp\ *n* : a tubular illuminated instrument used for inspecting or passing instruments into the bronchi — **bron·cho·scop·ic** \ˌbräŋ-kə-ˈskä-pik\ *adj* — **bron·chos·co·pist** \bräŋ-ˈkäs-kə-pist\ *n* — **bron·chos·co·py** \brän-ˈkäs-kə-pē\ *n*

bron·cho·spasm \ˈbräŋ-kə-ˌspa-zəm\ *n* : constriction of the air passages of the lung (as in asthma) by spasmodic contraction of the bronchial muscles — **bron·cho·spas·tic** \ˌbräŋ-kə-ˈspas-tik\ adj

bron·cho·spi·rom·e·try \ˌbräŋ-kō-spī-ˈrä-mə-trē\ n, pl **-tries** : independent measurement of the vital capacity of each lung by means of a spirometer in direct continuity with one of the primary bronchi — **bron·cho·spi·rom·e·ter** \-ˈrä-mə-tər\ n

bron·cho·ste·no·sis \ˌbräŋ-kō-stə-ˈnō-səs\ n, pl **-no·ses** \-ˌsēz\ : stenosis of a bronchus

bron·chus \ˈbräŋ-kəs\ n, pl **bron·chi** \ˈbräŋ-ˌkī, -ˌkē\ : either of the two primary divisions of the trachea that lead respectively into the right and the left lung; broadly : BRONCHIAL TUBE

broth \ˈbroth\ n, pl **broths** \ˈbroths, ˈброthz\ **1** : liquid in which meat or sometimes vegetable food has been cooked **2** : a fluid culture medium

brow \ˈbrau̇\ n **1** : EYEBROW **2** : either of the lateral prominences of the forehead **3** : FOREHEAD

brown alga n : any of a major taxonomic group (Phaeophyta) of variable mostly marine algae with chlorophyll masked by brown pigment — see ALGIN

brown dog tick n : a widely distributed reddish brown tick of the genus *Rhipicephalus* (*R. sanguineus*) that occurs esp. on dogs and that transmits canine babesiosis

brown fat n : a mammalian heat-producing tissue occurring esp. in human newborn infants — called also *brown adipose fat*

brown lung disease n : BYSSINOSIS

brown rat n : a common domestic rat of the genus *Rattus* (*R. norvegicus*) that has been introduced worldwide — called also *Norway rat*

brown recluse spider n : a venomous spider of the genus *Loxosceles* (*L. reclusa*) introduced into the southern U.S. that produces a dangerous cytotoxin — called also *brown recluse*

brown snake n : any of several Australian venomous elapid snakes (genus *Demansia*); esp : a widely distributed brownish or blackish snake (*D. textilis*)

brow·ridge \ˈbrau̇-ˌrij\ n : SUPERCILIARY RIDGE

BRP abbr bathroom privileges

bru·cel·la \brü-ˈse-lə\ n **1** cap : a genus of nonmotile capsulated bacteria (family Brucellaceae) that cause disease in humans and domestic animals **2** pl **-cel·lae** \-ˈse-(ˌ)lē\ or **-cel·las** : any bacterium of the genus *Brucella*

Bruce \ˈbrüs\, **Sir David (1855–1931)**, British bacteriologist.

bru·cel·lo·sis \ˌbrü-sə-ˈlō-səs\ n, pl **-lo·ses** \-ˌsēz\ : a disease caused by bacteria of the genus *Brucella*: **a** : a dis-

ease of humans caused by any of four organisms (*Brucella melitensis* of goats, *B. suis* of hogs, *B. abortus* of cattle, and *B. canis* of dogs), characterized by weakness, extreme exhaustion on slight effort, night sweats, chills, remittent fever, and generalized aches and pains, and acquired through direct contact with infected animals or animal products or from the consumption of milk, dairy products, or meat from infected animals — called also *Malta fever, undulant fever* **b** : CONTAGIOUS ABORTION

bru·cine \ˈbrü-ˌsēn\ n : a poisonous alkaloid $C_{23}H_{26}N_2O_4$ found with strychnine esp. in nux vomica

Bruce \ˈbrüs\, **James (1730–1794)**, British explorer.

Brud·zin·ski sign \brü-ˈjin-skē-, brüd-ˈzin-\ or **Brud·zin·ski's sign** \-skēz-\ n : any of several symptoms of meningeal irritation occurring esp. in meningitis: as **a** : flexion of the lower limbs induced by passive flexion of the head on the chest **b** : flexion of one lower limb following passive flexion of the other

Brudzinski, Josef (1874–1917), Polish physician.

¹bruise \ˈbrüz\ vb **bruised; bruis·ing 1** : to inflict a bruise on : CONTUSE **2** : WOUND, INJURE; esp : to inflict psychological hurt on **3** : to become bruised

²bruise n **1** : an injury transmitted through unbroken skin to underlying tissue causing rupture of small blood vessels and escape of blood into the tissue with resulting discoloration : CONTUSION **2** : an injury or hurt (as to the feelings or the pride)

bruit \ˈbrü-ē\ n : any of several generally abnormal sounds heard on auscultation

Brun·ner's gland \ˈbrü-nərz-\ n : any of the compound racemose glands in the submucous layer of the duodenum that secrete alkaline mucus and a potent proteolytic enzyme — called also *gland of Brunner*

Brun·ner \ˈbrü-nər\, **Johann Conrad (1653–1727)**, Swiss anatomist.

brush border n : a stria of microvilli on the plasma membrane of an epithelial cell (as in a kidney tubule) that is specialized for absorption

brux·ism \ˈbrək-ˌsi-zəm\ n : the habit of unconsciously gritting or grinding the teeth esp. in situations of stress or during sleep

BS abbr **1** bowel sounds **2** breath sounds

BSN abbr bachelor of science in nursing

BST abbr blood serological test

bu·bo \ˈbü-(ˌ)bō, ˈbyü-\ n, pl **buboes** : an inflammatory swelling of a lymph node esp. in the groin — **bu·bon·ic** \bü-ˈbä-nik, byü-\ adj

bubonic plague *n* : plague caused by a bacterium of the genus *Yersinia* (*Y. pestis* syn. *Pasteurella pestis*) and characterized esp. by the formation of buboes — compare PNEUMONIC PLAGUE

buc·cal \'bə-kəl\ *adj* **1** : of, relating to, near, involving, or supplying a cheek (the ~ surface of a tooth) **2** : of, relating to, involving, or lying in the mouth — **buc·cal·ly** *adv*

buccal gland *n* : any of the small racemose mucous glands in the mucous membrane lining the cheeks

buc·ci·na·tor \'bək-sə-ˌnā-tər\ *n* : a thin broad muscle forming the wall of the cheek and serving to compress the cheek against the teeth — called also *buccinator muscle*

bucco- *comb form* : buccal and ⟨bucco-lingual⟩

buc·co·lin·gual \ˌbə-kō-'liŋ-gwəl, -gyə-wəl\ *adj* **1** : relating to or affecting the cheek and the tongue **2** : of or relating to the buccal and lingual aspects of a tooth (the ~ width of a molar) — **buc·co·lin·gual·ly** *adv*

buc·co·pha·ryn·geal \-ˌfar-ən-'jē-əl, -fə-'rin-jəl, -jē-əl\ *adj* : relating to or near the cheek and the pharynx

buck·thorn \'bək-ˌthȯrn\ *n* : any of a genus (*Rhamnus* of the family Rhamnaceae) of shrubs and trees some of which yield purgative principles in their bark or sap

buck·tooth \-'tüth\ *n* : a large projecting front tooth — **buck-toothed** \-'tütht\ *adj*

¹bud \'bəd\ *n* **1 a** : an asexual reproductive structure **b** : a primordium having potentialities for growth and development into a definitive structure ⟨an embryonic limb ~⟩ **2** : an anatomical structure (as a tactile corpuscle) resembling a bud

²bud *vb* **bud·ded; bud·ding** : to reproduce asexually esp. by the pinching off of a small part of the parent

BUdR *abbr* bromodeoxyuridine

Buer·ger's disease \'bər-gərz-, 'bur-\ *n* : THROMBOANGIITIS OBLITERANS

Buer·ger \'bər-gər, 'bur-\. **Leo** (1879–1943), American pathologist.

¹buff·er \'bə-fər\ *n* : a substance or mixture of substances (as bicarbonates) that in solution tends to stabilize the hydrogen-ion concentration by neutralizing within limits both acids and bases

²buffer *vb* : to treat (as a solution or its acidity) with a buffer; *also* : to prepare (aspirin) with an antacid

buffy coat \'bə-fē-\ *n* : the superficial layer of yellowish or buff coagulated plasma from which the red corpuscles have settled out in slowly coagulated blood

bu·fo·ten·ine \ˌbyü-fə-'te-ˌnēn, -nən\ *or* **bu·fo·ten·in** \-nən\ *n* : a toxic hallucinogenic alkaloid $C_{12}H_{16}N_2O$ that is obtained esp. from poisonous secretions of toads (order Anura and esp. family Bufonidae) and from some mushrooms and has hypertensive and vasoconstrictor activity

bug \'bəg\ *n* **1 a** : an insect or other creeping or crawling invertebrate animal (as a spider) — not used technically **b** : any of various insects commonly considered esp. obnoxious: as (1) : BEDBUG (2) : COCKROACH (3) : HEAD LOUSE **c** : any of an order (Hemiptera and esp. its suborder Heteroptera) of insects that have sucking mouthparts and forewings thickened at the base and that lack a pupal stage between the immature stages and the adult — called also *true bug* **2 a** : a disease-producing microorganism and esp. a germ **b** : a disease caused by such microorganisms; *esp* : any of various respiratory conditions (as influenza or grippe) of virus origin

bulb \'bəlb\ *n* **1** : a protuberance resembling a plant bulb: as **a** : a rounded dilatation or expansion of something cylindrical (the ~ of a thermometer); *esp* : a rounded or pear-shaped enlargement on a small base (the ~ of an eyedropper) **2** : a rounded part: as **a** : a rounded enlargement of one end of a part — see BULB OF THE PENIS, BULB OF THE VESTIBULE, END BULB, OLFACTORY BULB **b** : MEDULLA OBLONGATA; *broadly* : the hindbrain exclusive of the cerebellum

bulb- *or* **bulbo-** *comb form* **1** : bulb ⟨bulbar⟩ **2** : bulbar and ⟨bulbospinal⟩ ⟨bulbourethral gland⟩

bul·bar \'bəl-bər, -ˌbär\ *adj* : of or relating to a bulb; *specif* : involving the medulla oblongata

bulbar paralysis *n* : destruction of nerve centers of the medulla oblongata and paralysis of the parts innervated from the medulla with interruption of their functions (as swallowing or speech)

bulbi — see PHTHISIS BULBI

bul·bo·caver·no·sus \ˌbəl-(ˌ)bō-ˌka-vər-'nō-səs\ *n, pl* **-no·si** \-ˌsī\ : a muscle that in the male surrounds and compresses the bulb of the penis and the bulbar portion of the urethra and in the female serves to compress the vagina — see SPHINCTER VAGINAE

bulb of the penis *n* : the proximal expanded part of the corpus cavernosum of the male urethra

bulb of the vestibule *n* : a structure in the female vulva that is homologous to the bulb of the penis and the adjoining corpus spongiosum in the male and that consists of an elongated mass of erectile tissue on each side of the vaginal opening united anteriorly to the contralateral mass by a narrow median band passing along the lower surface of the clitoris

bul·bo·spi·nal \ˌbəl-bō-'spīn-əl\ *adj* : of,

relating to, or connecting the medulla oblongata and the spinal cord

bul·bo·spon·gi·o·sus muscle \ˌbəl-(ˌ)bō-ˌspän-jē-ˈō-səs-\ *n* : BULBOCAVERNOSUS

bul·bo·ure·thral gland \-yù-ˈrē-thrəl-\ *n* : COWPER'S GLAND

bul·bous \ˈbəl-bəs\ *adj* : resembling a bulb esp. in roundness or the gross enlargement of a part

bul·bus \ˈbəl-bəs\ *n, pl* **bul·bi** \-ˌbī, -ˌbē\ : a bulb-shaped anatomical part

-bulia *also* **-boulia** *n comb form* : condition of having (such) will ⟨abulia⟩

-bulic *adj comb form* : of, relating to, or characterized by a (specified) state of will ⟨abulic⟩

bu·lim·a·rex·ia \bü-ˌli-mə-ˈrek-sē-ə, byü-, -ˌlē-\ *n* : BULIMIA 2 — **bu·lim·a·rex·ic** \-sik\ *n or adj*

bu·lim·ia \bü-ˈli-mē-ə, byü-, -ˈlē-\ *n* 1 : an abnormal and constant craving for food 2 : a serious eating disorder that occurs chiefly in females, is characterized by compulsive overeating usu. followed by self-induced vomiting or laxative or diuretic abuse, and is often accompanied by guilt and depression

bulimia ner·vo·sa \-(ˌ)nər-ˈvō-sə, -zə\ *n* : BULIMIA 2

¹**bu·lim·ic** \-mik\ *adj* : of, relating to, or affected with bulimia

²**bulimic** *n* : a person affected with bulimia

bulk \ˈbəlk\ *n* : material (as indigestible fibrous residues of food) that forms a mass in the intestine; *esp* : FIBER 2

bul·la \ˈbù-lə\ *n, pl* **bul·lae** \ˈbù-ˌlē, -ˌlī\ 1 : a hollow thin-walled rounded bony prominence 2 : a large vesicle or blister — compare BLEB

bull·nose \ˈbùl-ˌnōz\ *n* : a necrobacillosis arising in facial wounds of swine

bul·lous \ˈbù-ləs\ *adj* : resembling or characterized by bullae : VESICULAR ⟨~ lesions⟩

bullous pemphigoid *n* : a chronic skin disease affecting esp. elderly persons that is characterized by the formation of numerous hard blisters over a widespread area

BUN \ˌbē-(ˌ)yü-ˈen\ *n* : the concentration of nitrogen in the form of urea in the blood

bun·dle \ˈbənd-ᵊl\ *n* : a small band of mostly parallel fibers (as of nerve or muscle) : FASCICULUS, TRACT

bundle branch *n* : either of the parts of the bundle of His passing respectively to the right and left ventricles

bundle branch block *n* : heart block due to a lesion in one of the bundle branches

bundle of His \-ˈhis\ *n* : a slender bundle of modified cardiac muscle that passes from the atrioventricular node in the right atrium to the right and left ventricles by way of the septum and that maintains the normal sequence

of the heartbeat — called also *atrioventricular bundle, His bundle*

His, Wilhelm (1863–1934), German physician.

bun·ga·ro·tox·in \ˈbəŋ-gə-rō-ˌtäk-sən\ *n* : a potent neurotoxin obtained from the venom of an Asian elapid snake (genus *Bungarus*)

bun·ion \ˈbən-yən\ *n* : an inflamed swelling of the small sac on the first joint of the big toe — compare HALLUX VALGUS

bun·io·nec·to·my \ˌbən-yə-ˈnek-tə-mē\ *n, pl* **-mies** : surgical excision of a bunion

Bu·nos·to·mum \byü-ˈnäs-tə-məm\ *n* : a genus of nematode worms including the hookworms of sheep and cattle

buph·thal·mos \büf-ˈthal-məs, byüf-, ˌbəf-, -ˌmäs\ *also* **buph·thal·mia** \-mē-ə\ *n, pl* **-mos·es** *also* **-mias** : marked enlargement of the eye that is usu. congenital and attended by symptoms of glaucoma

bu·piv·a·caine \byü-ˈpi-və-ˌkān\ *n* : a local anesthetic $C_{18}H_{28}N_2O$ that is like lidocaine in its action but is longer acting

¹**bur** \ˈbər\ *n* 1 *usu* **burr** : a small surgical cutting tool (as for making an opening in bone) 2 : a bit used on a dental drill

bur·den \ˈbər-dən\ *n* : the amount of a deleterious parasite, growth, or substance present in the body ⟨worm ~⟩ ⟨cancer ~⟩ — called also *load*

Bur·kitt's lymphoma \ˈbər-kəts-\ *also* **Burkitt lymphoma** \-kət-\ *n* : a malignant lymphoma that occurs esp. in children of central Africa and is associated with Epstein-Barr virus

Bur·kitt \ˈbər-kət\, **Denis Parsons** (1911–1993), British surgeon.

Burkitt's tumor *also* **Burkitt tumor** *n* : BURKITT'S LYMPHOMA

¹**burn** \ˈbərn\ *vb* **burned** \ˈbərnd, ˈbərnt\ *or* **burnt** \ˈbərnt\; **burn·ing** 1 : to produce or undergo discomfort or pain ⟨iodine ~s so⟩; *also* : to injure or damage by exposure to fire, heat, or radiation ⟨~ed his hand⟩ 2 : to receive sunburn

²**burn** *n* 1 : bodily injury resulting from exposure to heat, caustics, electricity, or some radiations, marked by varying degrees of skin destruction and hyperemia often with the formation of watery blisters and in severe cases by charring of the tissues, and classified according to the extent and degree of the injury — see FIRST-DEGREE BURN, SECOND-DEGREE BURN, THIRD-DEGREE BURN 2 : an abrasion having the appearance of a burn ⟨friction ~s⟩ 3 : a burning sensation ⟨the ~ of iodine applied to a cut⟩

¹**burn·ing** \ˈbər-niŋ\ *adj* 1 : affecting with or as if with heat ⟨a ~ fever⟩ 2 : resembling that produced by a burn

²**burning** *n* : a sensation of being on fire or excessively heated ⟨gastric ~⟩

burn·out \'bərn-₁aút\ *n* **1 a** : exhaustion of physical or emotional strength usu. as a result of prolonged stress or frustration **b** : a person affected with burnout **b** : a person showing the effects of drug abuse

Bu·row's solution \'bü-(₁)rōz-\ *n* : a solution of the acetate of aluminum used as an antiseptic and astringent

Bu·row \'bü-(₁)rō\, **Karl August von (1809–1874),** German military surgeon and anatomist.

¹**burp** \'bərp\ *n* : BELCH

²**burp** *vb* **1** : BELCH **2** : to help (a baby) expel gas from the stomach esp. by patting or rubbing the back

burr *var of* BUR

bur·row \'bər-₁ō\ *n* : a passage or gallery formed in or under the skin by the wandering of a parasite (as the mite of scabies or a foreign hookworm) — **burrow** *vb*

bur·sa \'bər-sə\ *n, pl* **bur·sas** \-səz\ *or* **bur·sae** \-₁sē, -₁sī\ : a bodily pouch or sac: as **a** : a small serous sac between a tendon and a bone **b** : BURSA OF FABRICIUS — **bur·sal** \-səl\ *adj*

bursa of Fa·bri·cius \-fə-'bri-shəs, -shē-əs\ *n* : a blind glandular sac that opens into the cloaca of birds and functions in B cell production

Fabricius, Johann Christian (1745–1808), Danish entomologist.

bur·si·tis \(₁)bər-'sī-təs\ *n* : inflammation of a bursa esp. of the shoulder or elbow

bush·mas·ter \'bush-₁mas-tər\ *n* : a tropical American pit viper (*Lachesis mutus*)

Bu·Spar \'byü-₁spär\ *trademark* — used for a preparation of the hydrochloride of buspirone

bu·spi·rone \byü-'spi-₁rōn\ *n* : a mild antianxiety tranquilizer $C_{21}H_{31}N_5O_2$ that is used in the form of its hydrochloride and does not induce significant tolerance or psychological dependence — see BUSPAR

bu·sul·fan \byü-'səl-fən\ *n* : an antineoplastic agent $C_6H_{14}O_6S_2$ used in the treatment of chronic myelogenous leukemia — see MYLERAN

bu·ta·bar·bi·tal \₁byü-tə-'bär-bə-₁tal\ *n* : a synthetic barbiturate used esp. in the form of its sodium salt $C_{10}H_{15}N_2NaO_3$ as a sedative and hypnotic

bu·ta·caine \'byü-tə-₁kān\ *n* : a local anesthetic that is an ester of para-aminobenzoic acid and is applied in the form of its sulfate $(C_{18}H_{30}N_2O_2)_2 \cdot H_2SO_4$ to mucous membranes

Bu·ta·zol·i·din \₁byü-tə-'zä-lə-dən\ *trademark* — used for a preparation of phenylbutazone

bute \'byüt\ *n* : PHENYLBUTAZONE

butoxide — see PIPERONYL BUTOXIDE

¹**but·ter·fly** \'bə-tər-₁flī\ *n, pl* **-flies 1 a** : a feeling of hollowness or queasiness caused esp. by emotional or nervous tension or anxious anticipation **2** : a bandage with wing-shaped extensions

²**butterfly** *adj* : being, relating to, or affecting the area of the face including both cheeks connected by a band across the nose (the typical ∼ lesion of lupus erythematosus)

but·tock \'bə-tək\ *n* **1** : the back of a hip that forms one of the fleshy parts on which a person sits **2** *pl* : the seat of the body; *also* : the corresponding part of a quadruped : RUMP

but·ton \'bət-ᵊn\ *n* : something that resembles a small knob or disk: as **a** : the terminal segment of a rattlesnake's rattle **b** : COTYLEDON 1

bu·tyl·at·ed hy·droxy·an·i·sole \byüt-ᵊl-₁ā-təd-₁hī-₁dräk-sē-'a-nə-₁sōl\ *n* : BHA

butylated hy·droxy·tol·u·ene \-(₁)hī-₁dräk-sē-'täl-yə-₁wēn\ *n* : BHT

bu·tyl nitrite \'byüt-ᵊl-\ *n* : ISOBUTYL NITRITE

bu·ty·rate \'byü-tə-₁rāt\ *n* : a salt or ester of butyric acid

bu·tyr·ic acid \byü-'tir-ik-\ *n* : either of two isomeric fatty acids $C_4H_8O_2$; *esp* : a normal acid of unpleasant odor found in rancid butter and in perspiration

bu·ty·ro·phe·none \₁byü-tə-(₁)rō-fə-'nōn\ *n* : any of a class of neuroleptic drugs (as haloperidol) used esp. in the treatment of schizophrenia

Bx [by analogy with *Rx*] *abbr* biopsy

by·pass \'bī-₁pas\ *n* : a surgically established shunt; *also* : a surgical procedure for the establishment of a shunt (have a coronary ∼) — **bypass** *vb*

bys·si·no·sis \₁bi-sə-'nō-səs\ *n, pl* **-no·ses** \-₁sēz\ : an occupational respiratory disease asssociated with inhalation of cotton, flax, or hemp dust and characterized initially by chest tightness, shortness of breath, and cough, and eventually by irreversible lung disease — called also *brown lung, brown lung disease*

BZ \bē-'zē\ *n* : a gas $C_{21}H_{23}NO_3$ that when breathed produces incapacitating physical and mental effects — called also *quinuclidinyl benzilate*

C

c *abbr* **1** canine **2** centimeter **3** curie **4** *or* **c̄** [Latin *cum*] with — used in writing prescriptions

¹C *abbr* **1** Celsius **2** centigrade **3** cervical — used esp. with a number from 1 to 7 to indicate a vertebra or segment of the spinal cord **4** cocaine **5** [Latin *congius*] gallon **6** cytosine

²C *symbol* carbon

Ca *symbol* calcium

CA *abbr* chronological age

CABG \ˈka-bij\ *abbr* coronary artery bypass graft

cacao butter *var of* COCOA BUTTER

ca·chec·tic \kə-ˈkek-tik, ka-\ *adj* : relating to or affected by cachexia

ca·chet \ka-ˈshā\ *n* : a medicinal preparation for swallowing consisting of a case usu. of rice-flour paste containing an unpleasant-tasting medicine

ca·chex·ia \kə-ˈkek-sē-ə, ka-\ *n* : general physical wasting and malnutrition usu. associated with chronic disease

cac·o·dyl·ic acid \ˌka-kə-ˈdil-ik-\ *n* : a toxic crystalline compound of arsenic $C_2H_7AsO_2$ used esp. as an herbicide

ca·cos·mia \kə-ˈkäs-mē-ə, ka-,-ˈkäz-\ *n* : a hallucination of a disagreeable odor

CAD *abbr* coronary artery disease

ca·dav·er \kə-ˈda-vər\ *n* : a dead body; *specif* : one intended for dissection — **ca·dav·er·ic** \-və-rik\ *adj*

ca·dav·er·ous \kə-ˈda-və-rəs\ *adj* **1** : of or relating to a corpse **2** of a *complexion* : being pallid or livid like a corpse

cade oil *n* : JUNIPER TAR

cad·mi·um \ˈkad-mē-əm\ *n* : a bluish white malleable ductile toxic bivalent metallic element — symbol Cd; see ELEMENT table

cadmium sulfide *n* : a yellow-brown poisonous salt CdS used esp. in the treatment of seborrheic dermatitis of the scalp

ca·du·ceus \kə-ˈdü-sē-əs, -ˈdyü-,-shəs\ *n, pl* **-cei** \-sē-ˌī\ : a medical insignia bearing a representation of a staff with two entwined snakes and two wings at the top — compare STAFF OF AESCULAPIUS

caec- *or* **caeci-** *or* **caeco-** *chiefly Brit var of* CEC-

cae·sar·ean *also* **cae·sar·ian** *var of* CESAREAN

cae·si·um *chiefly Brit var of* CESIUM

ca·fé au lait spot \kä-ˌfā-ō-ˈlā-\ *n* : any of the medium brown spots usu. on the trunk, pelvis, and creases of the elbow and knees that are often numerous in neurofibromatosis — usu. used in pl.

caf·fe·ine \ka-ˈfēn, ˈka-ˌ\ *n* : a bitter alkaloid $C_8H_{10}N_4O_2$ found esp. in coffee and tea and used medicinally as a stimulant and diuretic — **caf·fein·ic** \ka-ˈfē-nik\ *adj*

caf·fein·ism \-ˌni-zəm\ *n* : a morbid condition caused by caffeine (as from excessive consumption of coffee)

-caine *n comb form* : synthetic alkaloid anesthetic (pro*caine*) (lido*caine*)

cais·son disease \ˈkā-ˌsän-, ˈkäs-ˀn-\ *n* : DECOMPRESSION SICKNESS

caj·e·put·ol *or* **caj·u·put·ol** \ˈka-jə-pə-ˌtȯl, -ˌtōl\ *n* : EUCALYPTOL

caked breast \ˈkākt-\ *n* : a localized hardening in one or more segments of a lactating breast caused by accumulation of blood in dilated veins and milk in obstructed ducts

cal *abbr* small calorie

Cal *abbr* large calorie

Cal·a·bar swelling \ˈka-lə-ˌbär-\ *n* : a transient subcutaneous swelling marking the migratory course through the tissues of the adult filarial eye worm of the genus *Loa* (*L. loa*) — compare LOAIASIS

cal·a·mine \ˈka-lə-ˌmīn, -mən\ *n* : a mixture of zinc oxide or zinc carbonate with a small amount of ferric oxide that is used in lotions, liniments, and ointments

cal·ca·ne·al \kal-ˈkā-nē-əl\ *adj* **1** : relating to the heel **2** : relating to the calcaneus

calcaneal tendon *n* : ACHILLES TENDON

calcaneo- *comb form* : calcaneal and (*calcaneo*cuboid)

cal·ca·neo·cu·boid \(ˌ)kal-ˌkā-nē-ō-ˈkyü-ˌbȯid\ *adj* : of or relating to the calcaneus and the cuboid bone

cal·ca·ne·um \kal-ˈkā-nē-əm\ *n, pl* **-nea** \-nē-ə\ : CALCANEUS

cal·ca·ne·us \-nē-əs\ *n, pl* **-nei** \-nē-ˌī\ : a tarsal bone that in humans is the large bone of the heel — called also *heel bone, os calcis*

cal·car \ˈkal-ˌkär\ *n, pl* **cal·car·ia** \kal-ˈkar-ē-ə\ : a spurred anatomical prominence

calcar avis \-ˈā-vəs, -ˈä-\ *n, pl* **calcaria avium** \-vē-əm\ : a curved ridge on the medial wall of the posterior horn of each lateral ventricle of the brain opposite the calcarine sulcus

cal·car·e·ous \kal-ˈkar-ē-əs\ *adj* : resembling, consisting of, or containing calcium carbonate; *also* : containing calcium

cal·ca·rine sulcus \ˈkal-kə-ˌrīn-\ *n* : a sulcus on the mesial surface of the occipital lobe of the cerebrum — called also *calcarine fissure*

cal·cif·er·ol \kal-ˈsi-fə-ˌrȯl, -ˌrōl\ *n* : an alcohol $C_{28}H_{43}OH$ usu. prepared by irradiation of ergosterol and used as a dietary supplement in nutrition and medicinally esp. in the control of rickets — called also *ergocalciferol, viosterol, vitamin D, vitamin D₂*; see DRISDOL

cal·cif·ic \kal-ˈsi-fik\ *adj* : involving or

caused by calcification ⟨∼ lesions⟩

cal·ci·fi·ca·tion \ˌkal-sə-fə-ˈkā-shən\ n **1** : impregnation with calcareous matter: as **a** : deposition of calcium salts within the matrix of cartilage often as the preliminary step in the formation of bone — compare OSSIFICATION 1a **b** : abnormal deposition of calcium salts within tissue **2** : a calcified structure or part — **cal·ci·fy** \ˈkal-sə-ˌfī\ vb

cal·ci·no·sis \ˌkal-sə-ˈnō-səs\ n, pl **-no·ses** \-ˌsēz\ : the abnormal deposition of calcium salts in a part or tissue of the body

calcis — see OS CALCIS

cal·ci·to·nin \ˌkal-sə-ˈtō-nən\ n : a polypeptide hormone esp. from the thyroid gland that tends to lower the level of calcium in the blood plasma — called also thyrocalcitonin

cal·ci·um \ˈkal-sē-əm\ n, often attrib : a silver-white bivalent metal that is an essential constituent of most plants and animals — symbol Ca; see ELEMENT table

calcium blocker n : CALCIUM CHANNEL BLOCKER

calcium carbonate n : a calcium salt $CaCO_3$ that is found in limestone, chalk, and bones and that is used in dentifrices and in pharmaceuticals as an antacid and to supplement bodily calcium stores

calcium channel blocker n : any of a class of drugs (as verapamil) that prevent or slow the influx of calcium ions into smooth muscle cells esp. of the heart and that are used to treat some forms of angina pectoris and some cardiac arrhythmias — called also calcium blocker

calcium chloride n : a salt $CaCl_2$ used in medicine as a source of calcium and as a diuretic

calcium gluconate n : a white crystalline or granular powdery salt $C_{12}H_{22}CaO_{14}$ used to supplement bodily calcium stores

calcium hydroxide n : a strong alkali $Ca(OH)_2$ — see SODA LIME

calcium lactate n : a white almost tasteless crystalline salt $C_6H_{10}CaO_6·5H_2O$ used chiefly in medicine as a source of calcium and in foods (as in baking powder)

calcium levulinate n : a white powdery salt $C_{10}H_{14}CaO_6·H_2O$ used in medicine as a source of calcium

calcium oxalate n : a crystalline salt $CaC_2O_4·H_2O$ that is noted for its insolubility in urine and is sometimes excreted in or retained in the form of urinary calculi

calcium pantothenate n : a white powdery salt $C_{18}H_{32}CaN_2O_{10}$ made synthetically and used as a source of pantothenic acid

calcium phosphate n **1** : a phosphate of calcium $CaHPO_4$ used in pharmaceutical preparations and animal feeds **2** : a naturally occurring phosphate of

calcium $Ca_5(F,Cl,OH,½CO_3)(PO_4)_3$ that contains other elements or radicals and is the chief constituent of bones and teeth

calcium propionate n : a mold-inhibiting salt $(CH_3CH_2COO)_2Ca$ used chiefly as a food preservative

calcium stearate n : a white powder consisting essentially of calcium salts of stearic acid and palmitic acid and used as a conditioning agent in food and pharmaceuticals

calcium sulfate n : a white calcium salt $CaSO_4$ used esp. as a diluent in tablets and in hydrated form as plaster of paris

cal·co·sphe·rite \ˌkal-kō-ˈsfir-ˌīt\ n : a granular or laminated deposit of calcium salts in the body

cal·cu·lo·sis \ˌkal-kyə-ˈlō-səs\ n, pl **-lo·ses** \-ˌsēz\ : the formation of or the condition of having a calculus or calculi

cal·cu·lous \ˈkal-kyə-ləs\ adj : caused or characterized by a calculus or calculi

cal·cu·lus \-ləs\ n, pl **-li** \-ˌlī, -ˌlē\ also **-lus·es 1** : a concretion usu. of mineral salts around organic material found esp. in hollow organs or ducts **2** : a concretion on teeth : TARTAR

Cald·well–Luc operation \ˈkōld-ˌwel-ˈlük-, ˈkäld-, -ˈlüek-\ n : a surgical procedure used esp. for clearing a blocked or infected maxillary sinus that involves entering the sinus through the mouth by way of an incision into the canine fossa above a canine tooth, cleaning the sinus, and creating a new and enlarged opening for drainage through the nose

Caldwell, George Walter (1866–1946), American surgeon.

Luc \lük\. **Henri (1855–1925)**, French laryngologist.

calf \ˈkaf, ˈkaf\ n, pl **calves** \ˈkavz, ˈkävz\ : the fleshy back part of the leg below the knee

calf bone n : FIBULA

calf diphtheria n : an infectious disease of the mouth and pharynx of calves and young cattle associated with the presence of large numbers of a bacterium of the genus Fusobacterium (F. necrophorum) and commonly passing into pneumonia or generalized septicemia if untreated

cal·i·ber \ˈka-lə-bər\ n : the diameter of a round body; esp : the internal diameter of a hollow cylinder

cal·i·bre chiefly Brit var of CALIBER

cal·i·ce·al var of CALYCEAL

cal·i·for·ni·um \ˌka-lə-ˈfor-nē-əm\ n : an artificially prepared radioactive element — symbol Cf; see ELEMENT table

cal·i·per splint \ˈka-lə-pər-\ n : a support for the leg consisting of two metal rods extending between a foot plate and a padded thigh band and worn so that the weight is borne mainly by the hipbone — called also *caliper*

cal·is·then·ics \ˌka-ləs-'the-niks\ *n sing or pl* **1** : systematic rhythmic bodily exercises performed usu. without apparatus **2** *usu sing* : the art or practice of calisthenics — **cal·is·then·ic** \-nik\ *adj*

ca·lix *n, pl* **ca·lices** *var of* CALYX

cal·li·per splint *chiefly Brit var of* CALIPER SPLINT

cal·is·then·ics *Brit var of* CALISTHENICS

cal·lo·sal \ka-'lō-səl\ *adj* : of, relating to, or adjoining the corpus callosum

cal·los·i·ty \ka-'lä-sə-tē\ *n, pl* **-ties** : the quality or state of being callous; *esp* : marked or abnormal hardness and thickness (as of the skin)

callosum — see CORPUS CALLOSUM

cal·lous \'ka-ləs\ *adj* **1** : being hardened and thickened **2** : having calluses

cal·loused *or* **cal·lused** \'ka-ləst\ *adj* : CALLOUS 2 (~ hands)

cal·lus \'ka-ləs\ *n* **1** : a thickening of or a hard thickened area on skin **2** : a mass of exudate and connective tissue that forms around a break in a bone and is converted into bone in the healing of the break

calm·ant \'kä-mənt, 'kälm-\ *n* : SEDATIVE

calm·ative \'kä-mə-tiv, 'kälm-ə-\ *n or adj* : SEDATIVE

cal·mod·u·lin \ˌkal-'mä-jə-lən\ *n* : a calcium-binding protein that regulates cellular metabolic processes (as muscle-fiber contraction) by modifying the activity of specific calcium-sensitive enzymes

cal·o·mel \'ka-lə-məl, -ˌmel\ *n* : a white tasteless compound Hg_2Cl_2 used esp. as a fungicide and insecticide and occas. in medicine as a purgative — called also *mercurous chloride*

cal·or \'ka-ˌlȯr\ *n* : bodily heat that is a sign of inflammation

calori- *comb form* : heat (*calorigenic*) (*calorimeter*)

ca·lor·ic \kə-'lȯr-ik, -'lär-; ˌka-lə-'rik\ *adj* **1** : of or relating to heat **2** : of or relating to calories — **ca·lor·i·cal·ly** \kə-'lȯr-i-k(ə-)lē, -'lär-\ *adv*

cal·o·rie *also* **cal·o·ry** \'ka-lə-rē\ *n, pl* **-ries 1 a** : the amount of heat required at a pressure of one atmosphere to raise the temperature of one gram of water one degree centigrade — called also *gram calorie, small calorie*; abbr. *cal* **b** : the amount of heat required to raise the temperature of one kilogram of water one degree centigrade : 1000 gram calories — called also *kilocalorie, kilogram calorie, large calorie*; abbr. *Cal* **2 a** : a unit equivalent to the large calorie expressing heat-producing or energy-producing value in food when oxidized in the body **b** : an amount of food having an energy-producing value of one large calorie

cal·o·rif·ic \ˌka-lə-'ri-fik\ *adj* **1** : CALOR-

IC **2** : of or relating to the production of heat

ca·lor·i·gen·ic \kə-ˌlȯr-ə-'je-nik, -ˌlär-; ˌka-lə-rə-\ *adj* : generating heat or energy (~foodstuffs)

cal·o·rim·e·ter \ˌka-lə-'ri-mə-tər\ *n* : any of several apparatuses for measuring quantities of absorbed or evolved heat or for determining specific heats — **ca·lo·ri·met·ric** \ˌka-lə-rə-'me-trik; kə-ˌlȯr-ə-, -ˌlär-\ *adj* — **ca·lo·rim·e·try** \ˌka-lə-'ri-mə-trē\ *n*

cal·va \'kal-və\ *n, pl* **calvas** *or* **cal·vae** \-ˌvē, -ˌvī\ : the upper part of the human cranium — compare CALVARIUM

cal·var·ia \kal-'var-ē-ə\ *n, pl* **-i·ae** \-ē-ˌē, -ē-ˌī\ : CALVARIUM

cal·var·i·um \-ē-əm\ *n, pl* **-ia** \-ē-ə\ : an incomplete skull; *esp* : the portion of a skull including the braincase and excluding the lower jaw or lower jaw and facial portion — **cal·var·i·al** \-ē-əl\ *adj*

calves *pl of* CALF

cal·vi·ties \kal-'vi-shē-ˌēz, -(ˌ)shēz\ *n, pl* **calvities** : the condition of being bald : BALDNESS

calx \'kalks\ *n, pl* **cal·ces** \'kal-ˌsēz\ : HEEL

ca·ly·ce·al \ˌka-lə-'sē-əl, ˌkā-\ *adj* : of or relating to a calyx

calyces *pl of* CALYX

Ca·lym·ma·to·bac·te·ri·um \kə-ˌli-mə-tō-bak-'tir-ē-əm\ *n* : a genus of pleomorphic nonmotile rod bacteria (family Brucellaceae) including only the causative agent (*C. granulomatis*) of granuloma inguinale — see DONOVAN BODY

ca·lyx \'ka-liks, 'kā-\ *n, pl* **ca·lyx·es** *or* **ca·ly·ces** \'kā-lə-ˌsēz, 'ka-\ : a cuplike division of the renal pelvis surrounding one or more renal papillae

cam·i·sole \'ka-mə-ˌsōl\ *n* : a long-sleeved straitjacket

cAMP *abbr* cyclic AMP

cam·phor \'kam-fər\ *n* : a tough gummy volatile aromatic crystalline compound $C_{10}H_{16}O$ that is obtained esp. from the wood and bark of a large evergreen tree (*Cinnamomum camphora*) of the laurel family (Lauraceae) and is used esp. as a liniment and mild topical analgesic and as an insect repellent

cam·phor·at·ed \'kam-fə-ˌrā-təd\ *adj* : impregnated or treated with camphor

cam·phor·ic acid \kam-'fȯr-ik-, -'fär-\ *n* : the dextrorotatory form of a white crystalline acid $C_{10}H_{16}O_2$ that is used in pharmaceuticals

cam·pim·e·ter \kam-'pi-mə-tər\ *n* : an instrument for testing indirect or peripheral visual perception of form and color — **cam·pim·e·try** \-trē\ *n*

camp·to·cor·mia \ˌkam-tə-'kȯr-mē-ə\ *n* : an hysterical condition marked by forward bending of the trunk and sometimes accompanied by lumbar pain

camp·to·dac·ty·ly \ˌkam-tə-ˈdak-tə-lē\ *n, pl* **-lies** : permanent flexion of one or more finger joints

camp·to·the·cin \ˌkamp-tə-ˈthē-sən\ *n* : an alkaloid $C_{20}H_{16}N_2O_4$ from the wood of a Chinese tree (*Camptotheca acuminata* of the family Nyssaceae) that has shown some antileukemic and antitumor activity

cam·py·lo·bac·ter \ˈkam-pə-lō-ˌbak-tər\ *n* **1** *cap* : a genus of slender spirally curved rod bacteria (family Spirillaceae) that include some forms pathogenic for domestic animals or humans — see HELICOBACTER **2** : any bacterium of the genus *Campylobacter*

ca·nal \kə-ˈnal\ *n* : a tubular anatomical passage or channel : DUCT — see ALIMENTARY CANAL, HAVERSIAN CANAL, INGUINAL CANAL

can·a·lic·u·lus \ˌkan-ᵊl-ˈi-kyə-ləs\ *n, pl* **-li** \-ˌlī, -ˌlē\ : a minute canal in a bodily structure — **can·a·lic·u·lar** \-lər\ *adj*

ca·na·lis \kə-ˈna-ləs, -ˈnä-\ *n, pl* **ca·na·les** \-ˈna-(ˌ)lēz, -ˈnä-(ˌ)lās\ : CANAL

ca·na·li·za·tion \ˌkan-ᵊl-ə-ˈzā-shən\ *n* **1** : surgical formation of holes or canals for drainage without tubes **2** : natural formation of new channels in tissue (as formation of new blood vessels through a blood clot) **3** : establishment of new pathways in the central nervous system by repeated passage of nerve impulses

can·a·lize \ˈkan-ᵊl-ˌīz\ *vb* **-lized; -lizing 1** : to drain (a wound) by forming channels without the use of tubes **2** : to develop new channels (as new capillaries in a blood clot)

canal of Schlemm \-ˈshlem\ *n* : a circular canal lying in the substance of the sclerocorneal junction of the eye and draining the aqueous humor from the anterior chamber into the veins draining the eyeball — called also *Schlemm's canal, sinus venosus sclerae*

    Schlemm, Friedrich S. (1795–1858), German anatomist.

can·cel·lous \ˈkan-ˈse-ləs, ˈkan-sə-\ *adj* : having a porous structure made up of intersecting plates and bars that form small cavities or cells (~bone) — compare COMPACT

can·cer \ˈkan-sər\ *n* **1** : a malignant tumor of potentially unlimited growth that expands locally by invasion and systemically by metastasis — compare CARCINOMA, SARCOMA, NEOPLASM, TUMOR **2** : an abnormal state marked by a cancer — **can·cer·ous** \-sə-rəs\ *adj*

can·cer·i·ci·dal or **can·cer·o·ci·dal** \ˌkan-sə-rə-ˈsīd-ᵊl\ *adj* : destructive of cancer cells

can·cer·i·za·tion \-ˈzā-shən\ *n* : transformation into cancer or from a normal to a cancerous state

can·cer·o·gen·ic \ˈje-nik, -ˌrō-\ *or* **can·cer·i·gen·ic** \-rə-\ *adj* : CARCINOGENIC

can·cer·ol·o·gist \-ˈrä-lə-jist\ *n* : a cancer specialist

can·cer·ol·o·gy \-lə-jē\ *n, pl* **-gies** : the study of cancer

can·cer·pho·bia \ˌkan-sər-ˈfō-bē-ə\ *or* **can·cer·o·pho·bia** \-sər-ō-ˈfō-\ *n* : an abnormal dread of cancer

can·crum oris \ˌkaŋ-krəm-ˈōr-əs, -ˈär-\ *n, pl* **can·cra oris** \-krə-\ : noma of the oral tissues — called also *gangrenous stomatitis*

can·de·la \kan-ˈdē-lə, -ˈde-\ *n* : CANDLE 2

can·di·ci·din \ˌkan-də-ˈsīd-ᵊn\ *n* : an antibiotic obtained from a streptomyces (*Streptomyces griseus*) and active against some fungi of the genus *Candida*

can·di·da \ˈkan-də-də\ *n* **1** *cap* : a genus of parasitic imperfect fungi (order Moniliales) that resemble yeasts, occur esp. in the mouth, vagina, and intestinal tract, are usu. benign but can become pathogenic, and include the causative agent (*C. albicans*) of thrush **2** : any fungus of the genus *Candida* — **can·di·dal** \-dəd-ᵊl\ *adj*

can·di·di·a·sis \ˌkan-də-ˈdī-ə-səs\ *n, pl* **-a·ses** \-ˌsēz\ : infection with or disease caused by a fungus of the genus *Candida* — called also *monilia, moniliasis*

can·dle \ˈkand-ᵊl\ *n* **1** : a medicated candle or lozenge used for fumigation **2** : a unit of luminous intensity — called also *candela, new candle*

candy striper *n* : a volunteer nurse's aide

ca·nic·o·la fever \kə-ˈni-kə-lə-\ *n* : an acute disease of humans and dogs characterized by gastroenteritis and mild jaundice and caused by a spirochete of the genus *Leptospira* (*L. canicola*)

¹ca·nine \ˈkā-ˌnīn\ *n* **1** : a conical pointed tooth; *esp* : one situated between the lateral incisor and the first premolar **2** : a canine mammal : DOG

²canine *adj* : of or relating to dogs or to the family (Canidae) to which they belong

canine fossa *n* : a depression external to and somewhat above the prominence on the surface of the superior maxillary bone caused by the socket of the canine tooth

ca·ni·nus \kā-ˈnī-nəs, kə-\ *n, pl* **ca·ni·ni** \-ˈnī-ˌnī\ : LEVATOR ANGULI ORIS

ca·ni·ties \kə-ˈni-shē-ˌēz\ *n* : grayness or whiteness of the hair

can·ker \ˈkaŋ-kər\ *n* **1 a** : an erosive or spreading sore **b** : CANKER SORE **2 a** : chronic inflammation of the ear in dogs, cats, or rabbits; *esp* : a localized form of mange **b** : a chronic and progressive inflammation of the hooves of horses resulting in softening and destruction of the horny layers — **can·kered** \-kərd\ *adj*

canker sore *n* : a painful shallow ulceration of the oral mucous membranes that has a grayish-white base surrounded by a reddish inflamed area and is characteristic of aphthous stomatitis — compare COLD SORE

can·na·bi·noid \'ka-nə-bə-ˌnȯid, kə-'na-\ *n* : any of various chemical constituents (as THC) of cannabis or marijuana

can·na·bis \'ka-nə-bəs\ *n* **1 a** *cap* : a genus of annual herbs (family Moraceae) that have leaves with three to seven elongate leaflets and pistillate flowers in spikes along the leafy erect stems and that include the hemp (*C. sativa*) **b** : HEMP 1 **2** : any of the preparations (as marijuana or hashish) or chemicals (as THC) that are derived from the hemp and are psychoactive — **cannabis in·di·ca** \-'in-di-kə\ *n*, *pl* **can·na·bes in·di·cae** \'ka-nə-ˌbēz-'in-də-ˌsē, -ˌbās-'in-di-ˌki\ : cannabis of a variety obtained in India

can·ni·bal·ism \'ka-nə-bi-ˌzəm\ *n* **1** : habituation to the use of cannabis **2** : chronic poisoning from excessive smoking or chewing of cannabis

can·ni·bal \'ka-nə-bəl\ *n* : one that eats the flesh of its own kind — **cannibal** *adj*

can·ni·bal·ism \-bə-ˌli-zəm\ *n* **1** : the usu. ritualistic eating of human flesh by a human being **2** : the eating of the flesh or the eggs of any animal by its own kind

can·non \'ka-nən\ *n* : the part of the leg in which the cannon bone is found

cannon bone *n* : a bone in hoofed mammals that supports the leg from the hock joint to the fetlock

can·nu·la *also* **can·u·la** \'kan-yə-lə\ *n*, *pl* **-las** *or* **-lae** \-ˌlē, -ˌlī\ : a small tube for insertion into a body cavity, duct, or vessel

can·nu·late \-ˌlāt\ *vb* **-lat·ed -lat·ing** : to insert a cannula into — **can·nu·la·tion** \ˌkan-yə-'lā-shən\ *n*

can·nu·lize \'kan-yə-ˌlīz\ *vb* **-lized; -liz·ing** : CANNULATE — **can·nu·li·za·tion** \ˌkan-yə-lə-'zā-shən\ *n*

ca·no·la \kə-'nō-lə\ *n* **1** : a rape plant (*Brassica napus*) of the mustard family of an improved variety with seeds that are low in erucic acid and are the source of canola oil **2** : CANOLA OIL

canola oil *n* : an edible vegetable oil obtained from the seeds of canola that is high in monounsaturated fatty acids

can·thar·i·din \kan-'thar-əd-ən\ *n* : a bitter crystalline compound $C_{10}H_{12}O_4$ that is the active blister-producing ingredient of cantharides

can·thar·is \'kan-thə-rəs\ *n*, *pl* **can·thar·i·des** \kan-'thar-ə-ˌdēz\ **1** : SPANISH FLY 1 **2** *cantharides* : a preparation of dried beetles and esp. Spanish flies that contains cantharidin and is used in medicine as a blister-pro-

ducing agent and formerly as an aphrodisiac — used with a sing. or pl. verb; called also *Spanish fly*

can·tha·xan·thin \ˌkan-thə-'zan-ˌthin\ *n* : a carotenoid $C_{40}H_{52}O_2$ used esp. as a color additive in food

can·thus \'kan-thəs\ *n*, *pl* **can·thi** \'kan-ˌthī, -ˌthē\ : either of the angles formed by the meeting of the upper and lower eyelids

¹cap \'kap\ *n*, *often attrib* **1** : something that serves as a cover or protection esp. for a tip, knob, or end (as of a tooth) **2** : PATELLA, KNEECAP **3** *Brit* : CERVICAL CAP

²cap *vb* **capped; cap·ping 1** : to invest (a student nurse) with a cap as an indication of completion of a probationary period of study **2** : to cover (a diseased or exposed part of a tooth) with a protective substance

³cap *abbr* capsule

ca·pac·i·ta·tion \kə-ˌpa-sə-'tā-shən\ *n* : the change undergone by sperm in the female reproductive tract that enables them to penetrate and fertilize an egg — **ca·pac·i·tate** \-ˌtāt\ *vb*

ca·pac·i·ty \kə-'pa-sə-tē, -'pas-tē\ *n*, *pl* **-ties 1** : a measure of content : VOLUME — see VITAL CAPACITY **2** : legal qualification, competency, power, or fitness

cap·e·line \'ka-pə-ˌlēn, -lən\ *n* : a cup-shaped bandage for the head, the shoulder, or the stump of an amputated limb

cap·il·lar·ia \ˌka-pə-'lar-ē-ə\ *n* **1** *cap* : a genus of slender white nematode worms (family Trichuridae) that include serious pathogens of the alimentary tract of fowls and some tissue and organ parasites of mammals including one (*C. hepatica*) which is common in rodents and occas. invades the human liver sometimes with fatal results **2** : a nematode worm of the genus *Capillaria* — **cap·il·lar·id** \-'lar-əd, kə-'pi-lə-rəd\ *n*

ca·pil·la·ri·a·sis \kə-ˌpi-lə-'rī-ə-səs\ *also* **cap·il·lar·i·o·sis** \ˌka-pə-ˌler-ē-'ō-səs\ *n*, *pl* **-a·ses** \-'rī-ə-ˌsēz\ *also* **-o·ses** \-'ō-ˌsēz\ : infestation with or disease caused by nematode worms of the genus *Capillaria*

cap·il·lar·o·scope \ˌka-pə-'lar-ə-ˌskōp\ *n* : a microscope that permits visual examination of the living capillaries in nail beds, skin, and conjunctiva — **cap·il·la·ros·co·py** \ˌka-pə-lə-'räs-kə-pē\ *n*

¹cap·il·lary \'ka-pə-ˌler-ē\ *adj* **1 a** : resembling a hair esp. in slender elongated form **b** : having a very small bore (a ~ tube) **2** : of or relating to capillaries

²capillary *n*, *pl* **-lar·ies** : a capillary tube; *esp* : any of the smallest blood vessels connecting arterioles with venules and forming networks throughout the body

capillary bed *n* : the whole system of

capillaries of a body, part, or organ

capita *pl of* CAPUT

¹cap·i·tate \'ka-pə-₁tāt\ *adj* : abruptly enlarged and globe-shaped

²capitate *n* : the largest bone of the wrist that is situated between the hamate and the trapezoid in the distal row of carpal bones and that articulates with the third metacarpal

cap·i·ta·tum \₁ka-pə-'tā-təm, -'tä-\ *n, pl* **cap·i·ta·ta** \-tə\ : CAPITATE

cap·i·tel·lum \₁ka-pə-'te-ləm\ *n, pl* **-tel·la** \-lə\ : a knoblike protuberance esp. at the end of a bone (as the humerus)

capitis — see LONGISSIMUS CAPITIS, LONGUS CAPITIS, OBLIQUUS CAPITIS INFERIOR, OBLIQUUS CAPITIS SUPERIOR, PEDICULOSIS CAPITIS, RECTUS CAPITIS POSTERIOR MAJOR, RECTUS CAPITIS POSTERIOR MINOR, SEMISPINALIS CAPITIS, SPINALIS CAPITIS, SPLENIUS CAPITIS, TINEA CAPITIS

ca·pit·u·lum \kə-'pi-chə-ləm\ *n, pl* **-la** \-lə\ : a rounded protuberance of an anatomical part — **ca·pit·u·lar** \-lər, -₁lär\ *adj*

Cap·lets \'ka-pləts\ *trademark* — used for capsule-shaped medicinal tablets

-capnia *n comb form* : carbon dioxide in the blood 〈hyper*capnia*〉 〈hypo*capnia*〉

Cap·o·ten \'ka-pō-₁ten\ *trademark* — used for a preparation of captopril

cap·re·o·my·cin \₁ka-prē-ō-'mis-ᵊn\ *n* : an antibiotic obtained from a bacterium of the genus *Streptomyces* (*S. capreolus*) that is used to treat tuberculosis

ca·pro·ic acid \kə-₁prō-ik-\ *n* : a liquid fatty acid $C_6H_{12}O_2$ that is found as a glycerol ester in fats and oils and is used in pharmaceuticals and flavors

cap·ry·late \'ka-prə-₁lāt\ *n* : a salt or ester of caprylic acid — see SODIUM CAPRYLATE

ca·pryl·ic acid \kə-'pri-lik-\ *n* : a fatty acid $C_8H_{16}O_2$ of rancid odor occurring in fats and oils

cap·sa·i·cin \kap-'sā-ə-sən\ *n* : a colorless irritant substance $C_{18}H_{27}NO_3$ obtained from various capsicums

cap·si·cum \'kap-si-kəm\ *n* **1** : any of a genus (*Capsicum*) of tropical plants of the nightshade family (Solanaceae) that are widely cultivated for their many-seeded usu. fleshy-walled berries **2** : the dried ripe fruit of some capsicums (as *C. frutescens*) used as a gastric and intestinal stimulant

cap·sid \'kap-səd\ *n* : the outer protein shell of a virus particle

cap·so·mer \'kap-sə-mər\ *or* **cap·so·mere** \'kap-sə-₁mir\ *n* : one of the subunits making up a viral capsid

capsul- *or* **capsuli-** *or* **capsulo-** *comb form* : capsule 〈*capsul*itis〉 〈*capsulec*-tomy〉

cap·su·la \'kap-sə-lə\ *n, pl* **cap·su·lae** \-₁lē, -₁lī\ : CAPSULE

cap·su·lar \'kap-sə-lər\ *adj* : of, relating to, affecting, or resembling a capsule

capsularis — see DECIDUA CAPSULARIS

cap·su·lat·ed \-lā-təd\ *also* **cap·su·late** \-₁lāt, -lət\ *adj* : enclosed in a capsule

cap·su·la·tion \₁kap-sə-'lā-shən\ *n* : enclosure in a capsule

cap·sule \'kap-səl, -(₁)sül\ *n* **1 a** : a membrane or saclike structure enclosing a part or organ 〈the ～ of the kidney〉 **b** : either of two layers or laminae of white matter in the cerebrum: (1) : a layer that consists largely of fibers passing to and from the cerebral cortex and that lies internal to the lentiform nucleus — called also *internal capsule* (2) : one that lies between the lentiform nucleus and the claustrum — called also *external capsule* **2** : a shell usu. of gelatin for packaging something (as a drug or vitamins); *also* : a usu. medicinal or nutritional preparation for oral use consisting of the shell and its contents **3** : a viscous or gelatinous often polysaccharide envelope surrounding certain microscopic organisms (as the pneumococcus)

cap·su·lec·to·my \₁kap-sə-'lek-tə-mē\ *n, pl* **-mies** : excision of a capsule (as of a joint, kidney, or lens)

capsule of Bow·man \'bō-mən\ *n* : BOWMAN'S CAPSULE

capsule of Te·non \-tə-'nōⁿ\ *n* : TENON'S CAPSULE

cap·su·li·tis \₁kap-sə-'lī-təs\ *n* : inflammation of a capsule (as that of the crystalline lens)

cap·su·lor·rha·phy \₁kap-sə-'lȯr-ə-fē\ *n, pl* **-phies** : suture of a cut or wounded capsule (as of the knee joint)

cap·su·lot·o·my \-'lä-tə-mē\ *n, pl* **-mies** : incision of a capsule esp. of the crystalline lens (as in a cataract operation)

cap·to·pril \'kap-tə-₁pril\ *n* : an antihypertensive drug $C_9H_{15}NO_3S$ that is an ACE inhibitor — see CAPOTEN

ca·put \'kä-₁put, -pət\ *n, pl* **ca·pi·ta** \'kä-pə-₁tä, 'ka-pə-tə\ **1** : a knoblike protuberance (as of a bone or muscle) **2** : CAPUT SUCCEDANEUM

caput suc·ce·da·ne·um \₁sək-sə-'dā-nē-əm\ *n, pl* **capita suc·ce·da·nea** \-ə\ : a swelling formed upon the presenting part of the fetus during labor

ca·ra·te \kə-'rä-tē\ *n* : PINTA

car·a·way oil \'kar-ə-₁wā-\ *n* : an essential oil obtained from the seeds of caraway (*Carum carvi*) of the carrot family (Umbelliferae) and used in pharmaceuticals and as a flavoring agent

car·ba·chol \'kär-bə-₁kȯl, -₁kōl\ *n* : a synthetic parasympathomimetic drug $C_6H_{15}ClN_2O_2$ that is used in veterinary medicine and topically in glaucoma

car·ba·mate \'kär-bə-₁māt, kär-'ba-₁māt\ *n* : a salt or ester of carbamic acid — see URETHANE

car·ba·maz·e·pine \₁kär-bə-'ma-zə-₁pēn\ *n* : a tricyclic anticonvulsant and analgesic $C_{15}H_{12}N_2O$ used in the treatment of trigeminal neuralgia and epilepsy — see TEGRETOL

car·bam·ic acid \(ˌ)kär-ˈba-mik-\ n : an acid CH_3NO_2 known in the form of salts and esters

carb·ami·no·he·mo·glo·bin \ˌkär-bə-ˌmē-(ˌ)nō-ˈhē-mə-ˌglō-bən\ n : CARB-HEMOGLOBIN

car·bar·sone \kär-ˈbär-ˌsōn\ n : a white powder $C_7H_9N_2O_4As$ used esp. in treating intestinal amebiasis

car·ba·zole \ˈkär-bə-ˌzōl\ n : a crystalline slightly basic cyclic compound $C_{12}H_9N$ used in testing for carbohydrates (as sugars)

car·ben·i·cil·lin \ˌkär-ˌbe-nə-ˈsi-lən\ : a broad-spectrum semisynthetic penicillin that is used esp. against gram-negative bacteria (as pseudomonas)

carb·he·mo·glo·bin \(ˌ)kärb-ˈhē-mə-ˌglō-bən\ n : a compound of hemoglobin with carbon dioxide

car·bo·hy·drase \ˌkär-bō-ˈhī-ˌdrās, -bə-, -ˌdrāz\ n : any of a group of enzymes (as amylase) that promote hydrolysis or synthesis of a carbohydrate (as a disaccharide)

car·bo·hy·drate \-ˌdrāt, -drət\ n : any of various neutral compounds of carbon, hydrogen, and oxygen (as sugars, starches, and celluloses) most of which are formed by green plants and which constitute a major class of animal foods

car·bol·fuch·sin paint \ˈkär-(ˌ)bäl-ˈfyük-sən, -(ˌ)bōl-\ n : a solution containing boric acid, phenol, resorcinol, and fuchsin in acetone, alcohol, and water that is applied externally in the treatment of fungal infections of the skin — called also *Castellani's paint*

car·bol·ic \kär-ˈbä-lik\ n : PHENOL 1

carbolic acid n : PHENOL 1

car·bo·my·cin \ˌkär-bə-ˈmīs-ᵊn\ n : a colorless crystalline basic macrolide antibiotic $C_{42}H_{67}NO_{16}$ produced by a bacterium of the genus *Streptomyces* (*S. halstedii*) and active esp. in inhibiting the growth of gram-positive bacteria — see MAGNAMYCIN

car·bon \ˈkär-bən\ n, often attrib : a nonmetallic element found native (as in diamonds and graphite) or as a constituent of coal, petroleum, asphalt, limestone, and organic compounds or obtained artificially (as in activated charcoal) — symbol *C*; see ELEMENT table

car·bon·ate \ˈkär-bə-ˌnāt, -nət\ n : a salt or ester of carbonic acid

carbon dioxide n : a heavy colorless gas CO_2 that does not support combustion, dissolves in water to form carbonic acid and is formed esp. in animal respiration and in the decay or combustion of animal and vegetable matter

carbon 14 n : a heavy radioactive isotope of carbon of mass number 14 used esp. in tracer studies

car·bon·ic acid \bä-ˈnik-\ n : a weak acid H_2CO_3 known only in solution that reacts with bases to form carbonates

carbonic anhydrase n : a zinc-containing enzyme that occurs in living tissues (as red blood cells) and aids carbon-dioxide transport from the tissues and its release from the blood in the lungs by catalyzing the reversible hydration of carbon dioxide to carbonic acid

carbon monoxide n : a colorless odorless very toxic gas CO that is formed as a product of the incomplete combustion of carbon

carbon tetrachloride n : a colorless nonflammable toxic carcinogenic liquid CCl_4 that has an odor resembling that of chloroform and is used as a solvent and a refrigerant

car·boxy·he·mo·glo·bin \(ˌ)kär-ˌbäk-sē-ˈhē-mə-ˌglō-bən\ n : a very stable combination of hemoglobin and carbon monoxide formed in the blood when carbon monoxide is inhaled with resulting loss of ability of the blood to combine with oxygen

car·box·yl \kär-ˈbäk-səl\ n : a univalent group –COOH typical of organic acids — called also *carboxyl group* — **car·box·yl·ic** \ˌkär-(ˌ)bäk-ˈsi-lik\ adj

car·box·yl·ase \kär-ˈbäk-sə-ˌlās, -ˌlāz\ n : an enzyme that catalyzes decarboxylation or carboxylation

car·box·yl·ate \-ˌlāt, -lət\ n : a salt or ester of a carboxylic acid — **car·box·yl·ate** \-ˌlāt\ vb — **car·box·yl·ation** \(ˌ)kär-ˌbäk-sə-ˈlā-shən\ n

carboxylic acid n : an organic acid (as an acetic acid) containing one or more carboxyl groups

car·boxy·meth·yl·cel·lu·lose \(ˌ)kär-ˌbäk-sē-ˌme-thəl-ˈsel-yə-ˌlōs, -ˌlōz\ n : a derivative of cellulose that in the form of its sodium salt is used as a bulk laxative in medicine

car·boxy·pep·ti·dase \ˈpep-tə-ˌdās, -ˌdāz\ n : an enzyme that hydrolyzes peptides and esp. polypeptides by splitting off sequentially the amino acids at the end of the peptide chain which contain free carboxyl groups

car·bun·cle \ˈkär-ˌbəŋ-kəl\ n : a painful local purulent inflammation of the skin and deeper tissues with multiple openings for the discharge of pus and usu. necrosis and sloughing of dead tissue — **car·bun·cu·lar** \kär-ˈbəŋ-kyə-lər\ adj

car·bun·cu·lo·sis \ˌkär-bən-kyə-ˈlō-səs\ n, pl **-lo·ses** \-ˌsēz\ : a condition marked by the formation of many carbuncles simultaneously or in rapid succession

carcin- or **carcino-** comb form : tumor : cancer (*carcinogenic*)

car·ci·no·em·bry·on·ic antigen \ˌkärs-ᵊn-ō-ˌem-brē-ˈä-nik-\ n : a glycoprotein present in fetal gut tissues during the first two trimesters of pregnancy and in peripheral blood of patients with cancer of the digestive system — abbr. *CEA*

car·cin·o·gen \kär-'si-nə-jən, 'kärs-ən-ə-jen\ *n* : a substance or agent causing cancer

car·ci·no·gen·e·sis \ˌkärs-ən-ō-'je-nə-səs\ *n, pl* **-eses** \-ˌsēz\ : the production of cancer

car·ci·no·gen·ic \ˌkärs-ən-ō-'je-nik\ *adj* : producing or tending to produce cancer — **car·ci·no·gen·i·cal·ly** \-ni-k(ə-)lē\ *adv* — **car·ci·no·ge·nic·i·ty** \-jə-'ni-sə-tē\ *n*

car·ci·noid \'kärs-ən-ˌoid\ *n* : a benign or malignant tumor arising esp. from the mucosa of the gastrointestinal tract (as in the stomach or appendix)

carcinoid syndrome *n* : a syndrome that is caused by vasoactive substances secreted by carcinoid tumors and is characterized by flushing, cyanosis, abdominal cramps, diarrhea, and valvular heart disease

car·ci·no·ma \ˌkärs-ən-'ō-mə\ *n, pl* **-mas** *or* **-ma·ta** \-mə-tə\ : a malignant tumor of epithelial origin — compare CANCER 1, SARCOMA — **car·ci·no·ma·tous** \-mə-təs\ *adj*

carcinoma in situ *n* : carcinoma in the stage of development when the cancer cells are still within their site of origin (as the mouth or uterine cervix)

car·ci·no·ma·to·sis \-ˌō-mə-'tō-səs\ *n, pl* **-to·ses** \-ˌsēz\ : a condition in which multiple carcinomas develop simultaneously usu. after dissemination from a primary source

car·ci·no·sar·co·ma \ˌkärs-ən-ō-(ˌ)sär-'kō-mə\ *n, pl* **-mas** *or* **-ma·ta** \-mə-tə\ : a malignant tumor combining elements of carcinoma and sarcoma

cardi- *or* **cardio-** *comb form* : heart : cardiac : cardiac and (*cardio*gram) (*cardio*vascular)

car·dia \'kär-dē-ə\ *n, pl* **car·di·ae** \-ē\ *or* **cardias** **1** : the opening of the esophagus into the stomach **2** : the part of the stomach adjoining the cardia

¹-car·dia \'kär-dē-ə\ *n comb form* : heart action or location (of a specified type) (dextro*cardia*) (tachy*cardia*)

²-cardia *pl of* -CARDIUM

¹car·di·ac \'kär-dē-ˌak\ *adj* **1 a** : of, relating to, situated near, or acting on the heart **b** : of or relating to the cardia of the stomach **2** : of, relating to, or affected with heart disease

²cardiac *n* : a person with heart disease

cardiac arrest *n* : temporary or permanent cessation of the heartbeat

cardiac asthma *n* : asthma due to heart disease (as heart failure) that occurs in paroxysms usu. at night and is characterized by difficult wheezing respiration, pallor, and anxiety — called also *paroxysmal dyspnea*

cardiac cycle *n* : the complete sequence of events in the heart from the beginning of one beat to the beginning of the following beat : a complete heartbeat including systole and diastole

cardiac failure *n* : HEART FAILURE

cardiac gland *n* : any of the branched tubular mucus-secreting glands of the cardia of the stomach; *also* : one of the similar glands of the esophagus

cardiac muscle *n* : the principal muscle tissue of the vertebrate heart made up of striated fibers that appear to be separated from each other under the electron microscope but that function in long-term rhythmic contraction as if in protoplasmic continuity — compare SMOOTH MUSCLE, STRIATED MUSCLE

cardiac nerve *n* : any of the three nerves connecting the cervical ganglia of the sympathetic nervous system with the cardiac plexus

cardiac neurosis *n* : NEUROCIRCULATORY ASTHENIA

cardiac output *n* : the volume of blood ejected from the left side of the heart in one minute — called also *minute volume*

cardiac plexus *n* : a nerve plexus of the autonomic nervous system supplying the heart and neighboring structures and situated near the heart and the arch and ascending part of the aorta

cardiac reserve *n* : the difference between the rate at which a heart pumps blood at a particular time and its maximum capacity for pumping blood

cardiac sphincter *n* : the somewhat thickened muscular ring surrounding the opening between the esophagus and the stomach

cardiac tamponade *n* : mechanical compression of the heart by large amounts of fluid or blood within the pericardial space that limits the normal range of motion and function of the heart

cardiac vein *n* : any of the veins returning the blood from the tissues of the heart that open into the right atrium either directly or through the coronary sinus

car·di·al·gia \ˌkär-dē-'al-jə, -jē-ə\ *n* **1** : HEARTBURN **2** : pain in the heart

car·di·ec·to·my \ˌkär-dē-'ek-tə-mē\ *n, pl* **-mies** : excision of the cardiac portion of the stomach

cardinal vein *n* : any of four longitudinal veins of the vertebrate embryo running anteriorly and posteriorly along each side of the spinal column with the pair on each side meeting at and discharging blood to the heart through a large venous sinus — called also *cardinal sinus, Cuvierian vein*

cardio- — see CARDI-

car·dio·ac·cel·er·a·tor \ˌkär-dē-(ˌ)ō-ik-'se-lə-ˌrā-tər, -ak-\ *adj* : speeding up the action of the heart — **car·dio·ac·cel·er·a·tion** \-ˌse-lə-ˈrā-shən\ n

car·dio·ac·tive \-ˈak-tiv\ adj : having an influence on the heart ⟨∼ drugs⟩

car·dio·cir·cu·la·to·ry \ˈsər-kyə-lə-ˌtōr-ē\ adj : of or relating to the heart and circulatory system ⟨temporary ∼ assist⟩

car·dio·dy·nam·ics \-dī-ˈna-miks\ n sing or pl : the dynamics of the heart's action in pumping blood — **car·dio·dy·nam·ic** \-mik\ adj

car·dio·gen·ic \-ˈje-nik\ adj : originating in the heart : caused by a cardiac condition ⟨∼ shock⟩

car·dio·gram \ˈkär-dē-ə-ˌgram\ n : the curve or tracing made by a cardiograph

car·dio·graph \-ˌgraf\ n : an instrument that registers graphically movements of the heart — **car·dio·graph·ic** \ˌkär-dē-ə-ˈgra-fik\ adj — **car·di·og·ra·phy** \ˌkär-dē-ˈä-grə-fē\ n

car·dio·in·hib·i·to·ry \ˌkär-dē-(ˌ)ō-in-ˈhi-bə-ˌtōr-ē\ adj : interfering with or slowing the normal sequence of events in the cardiac cycle ⟨the ∼ center of the medulla⟩

car·dio·lip·in \ˌkär-dē-ō-ˈli-pən\ n : a phospholipid used in combination with lecithin and cholesterol as an antigen in diagnostic blood tests for syphilis

car·di·ol·o·gy \ˌkär-dē-ˈä-lə-jē\ n, pl -gies : the study of the heart and its action and diseases — **car·di·o·log·i·cal** \-ə-ˈlä-ji-kəl\ adj — **car·di·ol·o·gist** \-ˈä-lə-jist\ n

car·dio·meg·a·ly \ˌkär-dē-ō-ˈme-gə-lē\ n, pl -lies : enlargement of the heart

car·dio·my·op·a·thy \ˈkär-dē-ō-(ˌ)mī-ˈä-pə-thē\ n, pl -thies : a typically chronic disorder of heart muscle that may involve hypertrophy and obstructive damage to the heart

car·dio·path·y \ˌkär-dē-ˈä-pə-thē\ n, pl -thies : any disease of the heart

car·dio·plas·ty \ˈkär-dē-ō-ˌplas-tē\ n, pl -ties : a plastic operation performed on the gastric cardiac sphincter

car·dio·ple·gia \ˌkär-dē-ō-ˈplē-jə, -jē-ə\ n : temporary cardiac arrest induced (as by drugs) during heart surgery — **car·dio·ple·gic** \-jik\ adj

car·dio·pul·mo·nary \ˌkär-dē-ō-ˈpúl-mə-ˌner-ē, -ˈpəl-\ adj : of or relating to the heart and lungs ⟨a ∼ bypass⟩

cardiopulmonary resuscitation n : a procedure designed to restore normal breathing after cardiac arrest that includes the clearance of air passages to the lungs, the mouth-to-mouth method of artificial respiration, and heart massage by the exertion of pressure on the chest — abbr. **CPR**

car·dio·re·nal \-ˈrēn-əl\ adj : of or relating to the heart and the kidneys ⟨∼ disorders⟩

car·dio·re·spi·ra·to·ry \ˌkär-dē-ō-ˈres-pə-rə-ˌtōr-ē, -ri-ˈspi-rə-\ adj : of or relating to the heart and the respiratory

system ⟨∼ CARDIOPULMONARY ⟨∼ ailments⟩ ⟨∼ responses⟩

car·dio·scle·ro·sis \ˌkär-dē-(ˌ)ō-sklə-ˈrō-səs\ n, pl -ro·ses \-ˌsēz\ : induration of the heart caused by formation of fibrous tissue in the cardiac muscle

car·dio·spasm \ˈkär-dē-ō-ˌspa-zəm\ n : failure of the cardiac sphincter to relax during swallowing with resultant esophageal obstruction — compare ACHALASIA

car·dio·ta·chom·e·ter \ˌkär-dē-ō-ta-ˈkä-mə-tər\ n : a device for prolonged graphic recording of the heartbeat

car·dio·tho·ra·cic \-thə-ˈra-sik\ adj : relating to, involving, or specializing in the heart and chest ⟨∼ surgeon⟩ ⟨∼ surgery⟩

car·di·ot·o·my \ˌkär-dē-ˈä-tə-mē\ n, pl -mies 1 : surgical incision of the heart 2 : surgical incision of the stomach cardia

¹**car·dio·ton·ic** \ˌkär-dē-ō-ˈtä-nik\ adj : tending to increase the tonus of heart muscle ⟨∼ steroids⟩

²**cardiotonic** n : a cardiotonic substance

car·dio·tox·ic \-ˈtäk-sik\ adj : having a toxic effect on the heart — **car·dio·tox·ic·i·ty** \-täk-ˈsi-sə-tē\ n

¹**car·dio·vas·cu·lar** \-ˈvas-kyə-lər\ adj : of, relating to, or involving the heart and blood vessels ⟨∼ disease⟩

²**cardiovascular** n : a substance (as a drug) that affects the heart or blood vessels

car·dio·ver·sion \-ˈvər-zhən, -shən\ n : application of an electric shock in order to restore normal heartbeat

car·dio·ver·ter \ˈkär-dē-ō-ˌvər-tər\ n : a device for the administration of an electric shock in cardioversion

car·di·tis \kär-ˈdī-təs\ n, pl **car·dit·i·des** \-ˈdi-tə-ˌdēz\ : inflammation of the heart muscle : MYOCARDITIS

-car·di·um \ˈkär-dē-əm\ n comb form, pl **-car·dia** \-ē-ə\ : heart ⟨epicardium⟩

care \ˈker, ˈkar\ n : responsibility for or attention to health, well-being, and safety — see HEALTH CARE, INTENSIVE CARE, PRIMARY CARE, TERTIARY CARE — **care** vb

care·giv·er \-ˌgi-vər\ n : a person who provides direct care (as for children or the chronically ill); esp : one who has primary responsibility for a child — **care·giv·ing** \-ˌgi-viŋ\ n

car·ies \ˈkar-ēz, ˈker-\ n, pl **caries** : a progressive destruction of bone or tooth; esp : tooth decay

ca·ri·na \kə-ˈrī-nə, -ˈrē-\ n, pl **carinas** or **ca·ri·nae** \ˈrī-ˌnē, -ˈrē-ˌnī\ : any of various keel-shaped anatomical structures, ridges, or processes

carinii — see PNEUMOCYSTIS CARINII PNEUMONIA

car·io·gen·ic \ˌkar-ē-ō-ˈje-nik\ adj : producing or promoting the development of tooth decay ⟨∼ foods⟩

car·io·stat·ic \-ˈsta-tik\ adj : tending to

car·i·ous \'kar-ē-əs, 'ker-\ *adj* : affected with caries ⟨~ teeth⟩

ca·ri·so·pro·dol \kə-₁rī-sə-'prō-₁dol, -zə-, -₁dȯl\ *n* : a drug $C_{12}H_{24}N_2O_4$ related to meprobamate that is used to relax muscle and relieve pain

¹car·min·a·tive \kär-'mi-nə-tiv, 'kär-mə-nā-\ *adj* : expelling or causing the expulsion of gas from the alimentary canal so as to relieve colic or griping

²carminative *n* : a carminative agent

car·mus·tine \'kär-mə-₁stēn\ *n* : BCNU

car·ni·tine \'kär-nə-₁tēn\ *n* : a quaternary ammonium compound $C_7H_{15}N$ O_3 present esp. in vertebrate muscle and involved in the transfer of fatty acids across mitochondrial membranes

car·o·ten·ae·mia *chiefly Brit var of* CAROTENEMIA

car·o·tene \'kar-ə-₁tēn\ *n* : any of several orange or red hydrocarbon pigments (as $C_{40}H_{56}$) that occur in plants and plant-eating animals and are convertible to vitamin A — see BETA-CAROTENE

car·o·ten·emia \₁kar-ə-tə-'nē-mē-ə\ *n* : the presence in the circulating blood of carotene which may cause a yellowing of the skin resembling jaundice

ca·rot·en·oid \kə-'rät-ᵊn-₁ȯid\ *n* : any of various usu. yellow to red pigments (as carotenes) found widely in plants and animals — **carotenoid** *adj*

caroticum — see GLOMUS CAROTICUM

ca·rot·id \kə-'rä-təd\ *adj* : of, situated near, or involving a carotid artery

carotid artery *n* : either of the two main arteries that supply blood to the head of which the left in humans arises from the arch of the aorta and the right by bifurcation of the brachiocephalic artery — called also *carotid*; see COMMON CAROTID ARTERY, EXTERNAL CAROTID ARTERY, INTERNAL CAROTID ARTERY

carotid body *n* : a small body of vascular tissue that adjoins the carotid sinus, functions as a chemoreceptor sensitive to change in the oxygen content of blood, and mediates reflex changes in respiratory activity — called also *carotid gland, glomus caroticum*

carotid canal *n* : the canal by which the internal carotid artery enters the skull — called also *carotid foramen*

carotid plexus *n* : a network of nerves of the sympathetic nervous system surrounding the internal carotid artery

carotid sinus *n* : a small but richly innervated arterial enlargement that is located near the point in the neck where the common carotid artery divides into the internal and the external carotid arteries and that functions in the regulation of heart rate and blood pressure

carp- *or* **carpo-** *comb form* **1** : carpus ⟨*carpectomy*⟩ **2** : carpal and ⟨*carpometacarpal*⟩

¹car·pal \'kär-pəl\ *adj* : relating to the carpus

²carpal *n* : a carpal element : CARPALE

car·pa·le \kär-'pa-(₁)lē, -'pä-, -'pä-\ *n*, *pl* **-lia** \-lē-ə\ : a carpal bone : *esp* : one of the distal series articulating with the metacarpals

carpal tunnel *n* : a passage between the flexor retinaculum of the hand and the carpal bones that is sometimes a site of compression of the median nerve

carpal tunnel syndrome *n* : a condition caused by compression of the median nerve in the carpal tunnel and characterized esp. by weakness, pain, and disturbances of sensation in the hand

car·pec·to·my \kär-'pek-tə-mē\ *n*, *pl* **-mies** : excision of a carpal bone

carpi — see EXTENSOR CARPI RADIALIS BREVIS, EXTENSOR CARPI RADIALIS LONGUS, EXTENSOR CARPI ULNARIS, FLEXOR CARPI RADIALIS, FLEXOR CARPI ULNARIS

carpo- — see CARP-

car·po·meta·car·pal \₁kär-pō-'me-tə-₁kär-pəl\ *adj* : relating to, situated between, or joining a carpus and metacarpus ⟨a ~ joint⟩

car·po·ped·al spasm \₁kär-pə-'ped-ᵊl-, -'pēd-\ *n* : a spasmodic contraction of the muscles of the hands and feet or esp. of the wrists and ankles in disorders such as alkalosis and tetany

car·pus \'kär-pəs\ *n*, *pl* **car·pi** \-₁pī, -₁pē\ **1** : WRIST **2** : the group of bones supporting the wrist comprising in humans a proximal row which contains the scaphoid, lunate, triquetrum, and pisiform that articulate with the radius and a distal row which contains the trapezium, trapezoid, capitate, and hamate that articulate with the metacarpals

car·ri·er \'kar-ē-ər\ *n* **1 a** : a person, animal, or plant that harbors and disseminates the specific agent (as a microorganism) causing an infectious disease from which it has recovered or to which it is immune ⟨~ of typhoid fever⟩ — compare RESERVOIR 2, VECTOR **1 b** : an individual possessing a specified gene and capable of transmitting it to offspring but not of showing its typical expression; *esp* : one that is heterozygous for a recessive factor **2** : a vehicle serving esp. as a diluent (as for a drug)

Car·ri·ón's disease \₁kar-ē-'ȯnz-\ *n* : BARTONELLOSIS

Carrión, Daniel A. (1850–1885), Peruvian medical student.

car·sick \'kär-₁sik\ *adj* : affected with motion sickness esp. in an automobile — **car sickness** *n*

car·ti·lage \\'kärt-ᵊl-ij, 'kärt-lij\ *n* **1** : a usu. translucent somewhat elastic tissue that composes most of the skeleton of vertebrate embryos and except for a small number of structures (as some joints, respiratory passages, and the external ear) is replaced by bone during ossification in the higher vertebrates **2** : a part or structure composed of cartilage

car·ti·lag·i·nous \\,kärt-ᵊl-'a-jə-nəs\ *adj* : composed of, relating to, or resembling cartilage

car·un·cle \\'kar-əŋ-kəl, kə-'rəŋ-\ *n* : a small fleshy growth; *specif* : a reddish growth situated at the urethral meatus in women causing pain and bleeding — see LACRIMAL CARUNCLE

ca·run·cu·la \kə-'rəŋ-kyə-lə\ *n, pl* **-lae** \-ₗlē, -ₗlī\ : CARUNCLE

cary- *or* **caryo-** — see KARY

cas·cade \\(ₗ)kas-'kād\ *n* : a molecular, biochemical, or physiological process occurring in a succession of stages each of which is closely related to or depends on the output of the previous stage ⟨a ∼ of enzymatic reactions⟩ ⟨the ∼ of events comprising the immune response⟩

cas·cara sa·gra·da \kas-'kar-ə-sə-'grä-də, -'kär-; 'kas-kə-rə-\ *n* : the dried bark of a buckthorn (*Rhamnus purshiana*) of the Pacific coast of the U.S. that is used as a mild laxative — called also *cascara*

case \\'kās\ *n* **1** : the circumstances and situation of a particular person or group **2 a** : an instance of disease or injury ⟨10 ∼*s* of pneumonia⟩ **b** : PATIENT **1**

ca·se·ation \\,kā-sē-'ā-shən\ *n* : necrosis with conversion of damaged tissue into a soft cheesy substance — **ca·se·ate** \\'kā-sē-ₗāt\ *vb*

case·book \\'kās-ₗbůk\ *n* : a book containing medical records of illustrative cases that is used for reference and instruction

case history *n* : a record of an individual's personal or family history and environment for use in analysis or instructive illustration

ca·sein \kā-'sēn, 'kā-sē-ən\ *n* : any of several phosphoproteins of milk

case load *n* : the number of cases handled in a particular period (as by a clinic)

caseosa — see VERNIX CASEOSA

ca·se·ous \\'kā-sē-əs\ *adj* : marked by caseation

caseous lymphadenitis *n* : a chronic infectious disease of sheep and goats characterized by caseation of the lymph glands and occas. of parts of the lungs, liver, spleen, and kidneys that is caused by a bacterium of the genus *Corynebacterium* (*C. pseudotuberculosis*) — called also *pseudotuberculosis*

case·work \\'kās-ₗwərk\ *n* : social work involving direct consideration of the problems, needs, and adjustments of the individual case (as a person or family in need of psychiatric aid) — **case·work·er** \-ₗwər-kər\ *n*

cas·sette *also* **ca·sette** \kə-'set, ka-\ *n* : a lightproof magazine for holding the intensifying screens and film in X-ray photography

cassia oil *n* : CINNAMON OIL

cast \\'kast\ *n* **1** : a slight strabismus **2** : a rigid dressing of gauze impregnated with plaster of paris for immobilizing a diseased or broken part **3** : a mass of plastic matter formed in cavities of diseased organs (as the kidneys) and discharged from the body

Cas·tel·la·ni's paint \ₗkas-tə-'lä-nēz-\ *n* : CARBOLFUCHSIN PAINT

Cas·tel·la·ni \ₗkäs-tə-'lä-nē\, **Aldo (1878–1971),** Italian physician.

cas·tor bean \\'kas-tər-\ *n* : the very poisonous seed of the castor-oil plant; *also* : CASTOR-OIL PLANT

castor oil *n* : a pale viscous fatty oil from castor beans used esp. as a cathartic

castor–oil plant *n* : a tropical Old World herb (*Ricinus communis*) of the spurge family (Euphorbiaceae) widely grown as an ornamental or for its oil-rich castor beans that are a source of castor oil

¹cas·trate \\'kas-ₗtrāt\ *vb* **cas·trat·ed; cas·trat·ing 1 a** : to deprive of the testes : GELD **b** : to deprive of the ovaries : SPAY **2** : to render impotent or deprive of vitality esp. by psychological means — **cas·trat·er** *or* **cas·tra·tor** \-'trā-tər\ *n* — **cas·tra·tion** \kas-'trā-shən\ *n*

²castrate *n* : a castrated individual

castration complex *n* : a child's fear or delusion of genital injury at the hands of the parent of the same sex as punishment for unconscious guilt over oedipal strivings; *broadly* : the often unconscious fear or feeling of bodily injury or loss of power at the hands of authority

ca·su·al·ty \\'ka-zhəl-tē, 'ka-zhə-wəl-\ *n, pl* **-ties 1** : a serious or fatal accident **2** : a military person lost through death, wounds, injury, sickness, internment, or capture or through being missing in action **3 a** : injury or death from accident **b** : one injured or killed (as by accident)

ca·su·is·tic \ₗka-zhə-'wis-tik\ *adj* : of or based on the study of actual cases or case histories

cat \\'kat\ *n, often attrib* **1** : a carnivorous mammal (*Felis catus*) long domesticated and kept as a pet or for catching rats and mice **2** : any of a family (Felidae) of mammals including the domestic cat, lion (*Panthera leo*), tiger (*Panthera tigris*), leopard (*Panthera pardus*), cougar (*Felis concolor*), and their relatives

CAT *abbr* computed axial tomography; computerized axial tomography

cata- *or* **cat-** *or* **cath-** *prefix* : down ⟨*cat-amnesis*⟩ ⟨*cataplexy*⟩

ca·tab·o·lism \kə-ˈta-bə-ˌli-zəm\ *n* : destructive metabolism involving the release of energy and resulting in the breakdown of complex materials within the organism — compare AN-ABOLISM — **cat·a·bol·ic** \ˌka-tə-ˈbä-lik\ *adj* — **cat·a·bol·i·cal·ly** \-li-k(ə-)lē\ *adv*

ca·tab·o·lite \-ˌlīt\ *n* : a product of catabolism

ca·tab·o·lize \-ˌlīz\ *vb* **-lized; -liz·ing** : to subject to or undergo catabolism

cat·a·lase \ˈkat-ᵊl-ˌās, -ˌāz\ *n* : an enzyme that consists of a protein complex with hematin groups and catalyzes the decomposition of hydrogen peroxide into water and oxygen

cat·a·lep·sy \ˈkat-ᵊl-ˌep-sē\ *n, pl* **-sies** : a condition of suspended animation and loss of voluntary motion associated with hysteria and schizophrenia in humans and with organic nervous disease in animals and characterized by a trancelike state of consciousness and a posture in which the limbs hold any position they are placed in — compare WAXY FLEXIBILITY

¹**cat·a·lep·tic** \ˌkat-ᵊl-ˈep-tik\ *adj* : of, having the characteristics of, or affected with catalepsy ⟨a ∼ state⟩

²**cataleptic** *n* : one affected with catalepsy

ca·tal·y·sis \kə-ˈta-lə-səs\ *n, pl* **-y·ses** \-ˌsēz\ : a change and esp. increase in the rate of a chemical reaction brought about by a substance (**cat·a·lyst** \ˈkat-ᵊl-ˌist\) that is itself unchanged at the end of the reaction — **cat·a·lyt·ic** \ˌkat-ᵊl-ˈi-tik\ *adj* — **cat·a·lyt·i·cal·ly** \-i-k(ə-)lē\ *adv*

cat·a·lyze \ˈkat-ᵊl-ˌīz\ *vb* **-lyzed; -lyz·ing** : to bring about the catalysis of (a chemical reaction) — **cat·a·lyz·er** *n*

cat·a·me·nia \ˌka-tə-ˈmē-nē-ə\ *n pl* : MENSES — **cat·a·me·ni·al** \-nē-əl\ *adj*

cat·am·ne·sis \ˌkat-ˌam-ˈnē-səs\ *n, pl* **-ne·ses** \-ˌsēz\ : the follow-up medical history of a patient — **cat·am·nes·tic** \-ˈnes-tik\ *adj*

cat·a·plasm \ˈka-tə-ˌpla-zəm\ *n* : POULTICE

cat·a·plexy \ˈka-tə-ˌplek-sē\ *n, pl* **-plex·ies** \-ˌsēz\ : sudden loss of muscle power with retention of consciousness following a strong emotional stimulus (as fright, anger, or shock)

cat·a·ract \ˈka-tə-ˌrakt\ *n* : a clouding of the lens of the eye or its surrounding transparent membrane that obstructs the passage of light

cat·a·ract·ous \ˌka-tə-ˌrak-təs\ *adj* : of, relating to, or affected with an eye cataract

ca·tarrh \kə-ˈtär\ *n* : inflammation of a mucous membrane in humans or animals; *esp* : one chronically affecting the human nose and air passages — **ca·tarrh·al** \-əl\ *adj*

catarrhal fever *n* : MALIGNANT CATARRHAL FEVER

cata·to·nia \ˌka-tə-ˈtō-nē-ə\ *n* : catatonic schizophrenia

¹**cata·ton·ic** \ˌka-tə-ˈtä-nik\ *adj* : of, relating to, being, or affected by schizophrenia characterized esp. by a marked psychomotor disturbance that may involve stupor or mutism, negativism, rigidity, purposeless excitement, and inappropriate or bizarre posturing — **cata·ton·i·cal·ly** \-ni-k(ə-)lē\ *adv*

²**catatonic** *n* : a catatonic person

catch·ment area \ˈkach-mənt-\ *n* : the geographical area served by an institution

cat cry syndrome *n* : CRI DU CHAT SYNDROME

cat distemper *n* : PANLEUKOPENIA

cat·e·chol·amine \ˌka-tə-ˈkō-lə-ˌmēn, -ˈkō-\ *n* : any of various substances (as epinephrine, norepinephrine, and dopamine) that function as hormones or neurotransmitters or both

cat·e·chol·amin·er·gic \-ˌkō-lə-mē-ˈnər-jik\ *adj* : involving, liberating, or mediated by catecholamine ⟨∼ transmission in the nervous system⟩

cat fever *n* : PANLEUKOPENIA

cat flea *n* : a common often pestiferous flea of the genus *Ctenocephalides* (*C. felis*) that breeds chiefly on cats, dogs, and rats

cat·gut \ˈkat-ˌgət\ *n* : a tough cord made usu. from sheep intestines and used esp. for sutures in closing wounds

cath *abbr* 1 cathartic 2 catheter

cath- — see CATA-

ca·thar·sis \kə-ˈthär-səs\ *n, pl* **ca·thar·ses** \-ˌsēz\ 1 : PURGATION 2 : elimination of a complex by bringing it to consciousness and affording it expression

¹**ca·thar·tic** \kə-ˈthär-tik\ *adj* : of, relating to, or producing catharsis

²**cathartic** *n* : a cathartic medicine : PURGATIVE

ca·thect \kə-ˈthekt, ka-\ *vb* : to invest with mental or emotional energy

ca·thec·tic \kə-ˈthek-tik, ka-\ *adj* : of, relating to, or invested with mental or emotional energy

cath·e·ter \ˈka-thə-tər, ˈkath-tər\ *n* : a tubular medical device for insertion into canals, vessels, passageways, or body cavities usu. to permit injection or withdrawal of fluids or to keep a passage open

cath·e·ter·iza·tion \ˌka-thə-tə-rə-ˈzā-shən, ˌkath-tə-rə-\ *n* : the use of or insertion of a catheter (as in or into the bladder, trachea, or heart) — **cath·e·ter·ize** \ˈka-thə-tə-ˌrīz, ˈkath-tə-\ *vb*

cath·e·ter·ized *adj* : obtained by catheterization ⟨∼ urine specimens⟩

ca·thex·is \kə-ˈthek-səs, ka-\ *n, pl* **ca·thex·es** \-ˌsēz\ 1 : investment of mental or emotional energy in a person, object, or idea 2 : libidinal energy that is either invested or being invested

cath•ode–ray oscilloscope \'ka-ˌthōd-\ *n* : OSCILLOSCOPE

cathode–ray tube *n* : a vacuum tube in which a beam of electrons is projected on a fluorescent screen to produce a luminous spot

cat•ion \'kat-ˌī-ən, 'ka-(ˌ)tī-ən\ *n* : the ion in an electrolyte that migrates to the cathode; *also* : a positively charged ion — **cat•ion•ic** \ˌkat-(ˌ)ī-'ä-nik, ˌka-(ˌ)tī-\ *adj* — **cat•ion•i•cal•ly** *adv*

cat louse *n* : a biting louse (*Felicola subrostratus* of the family Trichodectidae) common on cats esp. in warm regions

CAT scan \'kat-\ *n* : a sectional view of the body constructed by computed tomography — **CAT scanning** *n*

CAT scanner *n* : a medical instrument consisting of integrated X-ray and computing equipment and used for computed tomography

cat scratch disease *n* : an illness that is characterized by chills, slight fever, and swelling of the lymph glands and is caused by a gram-negative bacillus (*Afipia felis*) transmitted esp. by a cat scratch — called also *cat scratch fever*

cat tapeworm *n* : a common tapeworm of the genus *Taenia* (*T. taeniaeformis*) of cats who ingest cysticercus-infected livers of various rodents

cattle grub *n* : either of two warble flies of the genus *Hypoderma* esp. in the larval stage: **a** : COMMON CATTLE GRUB **b** : NORTHERN CATTLE GRUB

cattle louse *n* : a louse infesting cattle — see LONG-NOSED CATTLE LOUSE, SHORT-NOSED CATTLE LOUSE

cattle tick *n* : either of two ixodid ticks of the genus *Boophilus* (*B. annulatus* and *B. microplus*) that infest cattle and transmit the protozoan which causes Texas fever

cau•dad \'kȯ-ˌdad\ *adv* : toward the tail or posterior end

cau•da equi•na \ˌkau̇-də-ə-'kwē-nə, 'kȯ-də-, -ˌkwī-\ *n, pl* **caudae equi•nae** \ˌkau̇-ˌdī-ē-'kwē-ˌnī, 'kȯ-ˌdē-ē-'kwī-ˌnē\ : the roots of the upper sacral nerves that extend beyond the termination of the spinal cord at the first lumbar vertebra in the form of a bundle of filaments within the spinal canal resembling a horse's tail

cau•dal \'kȯd-ᵊl\ *adj* : of, relating to, or being a tail **2** : situated in or directed toward the hind part of the body — **cau•dal•ly** *adv*

caudal anesthesia *n* : loss of pain sensation below the umbilicus produced by injection of an anesthetic into the caudal portion of the spinal canal — called also *caudal analgesia*

cau•date lobe \'kȯ-ˌdāt-\ *n* : a lobe of the liver bounded on the right by the inferior vena cava, on the left by the fissure of the ductus venosus, and

connected with the right lobe by a narrow prolongation

caudate nucleus *n* : the one of the four basal ganglia in each cerebral hemisphere that comprises a mass of gray matter in the corpus striatum, forms part of the floor of the lateral ventricle, and is separated from the lentiform nucleus by the internal capsule — called also *caudate*

caul \'kȯl\ *n* **1** : GREATER OMENTUM **2** : the inner embryonic membrane of higher vertebrates esp. when covering the head at birth

cauliflower ear *n* : an ear deformed from injury and excessive growth of reparative tissue

cau•sal•gia \kȯ-'zal-jə, -'sal-, -jē-ə\ *n* : a constant usu. burning pain resulting from injury to a peripheral nerve — **cau•sal•gic** \-jik\ *adj*

¹caus•tic \'kȯ-stik\ *adj* : capable of destroying or eating away organic tissue and esp. animal tissue by chemical action

²caustic *n* : a caustic agent; *esp* : a substance or means that can burn, corrode, or destroy animal or other organic tissue by chemical action : ESCHAROTIC

cau•ter•ize \'kȯ-tə-ˌrīz\ *vb* **-ized; -izing** : to sear with a cautery or caustic — **cau•ter•i•za•tion** \ˌkȯ-tə-rə-'zā-shən\ *n*

cau•tery \'kȯ-tə-rē\ *n, pl* **-ter•ies 1** : the act or effect of cauterizing : CAUTERIZATION **2** : an agent (as a hot iron or caustic) used to burn, sear, or destroy tissue

¹ca•va \'kä-və, 'kā-\ *n, pl* **ca•vae** \'kä-ˌvē, -ˌvī; 'kä-ˌvē\ : VENA CAVA — **ca•val** \-vəl\ *adj*

²cava *pl of* CAVUM

cavernosum, cavernosa — see CORPUS CAVERNOSUM

cav•ern•ous \'ka-vər-nəs\ *adj* **1** : having caverns or cavities **2** : of tissue : composed largely of vascular sinuses and capable of dilating with blood to bring about the erection of a body part

cavernous sinus *n* : either of a pair of large venous sinuses situated in a groove at the side of the body of the sphenoid bone in the cranial cavity and opening behind into the petrosal sinuses

cav•i•tary \'ka-və-ˌter-ē\ *adj* : of, relating to, or characterized by bodily cavitation ⟨∼ tuberculosis⟩ ⟨∼ lesions⟩

cav•i•ta•tion \ˌka-və-'tā-shən\ *n* **1** : the process of cavitating; *esp* : the formation of cavities in an organ or tissue esp. in disease **2** : a cavity formed by cavitation — **cav•i•tate** \'ka-və-ˌtāt\ *vb*

cav•i•ty \'ka-və-tē\ *n, pl* **-ties 1** : an unfilled space within a mass — see PELVIC CAVITY **2** : an area of decay in a tooth : CARIES

ca·vum \\'kä-vəm, 'kā-\\ *n, pl* **ca·va** \\-və\\ : an anatomical recess or hollow

cavus — see PES CAVUS

Cb *symbol* columbium

CB *abbr* [Latin *Chirurgiae Baccalaureus*] bachelor of surgery

CBC *abbr* complete blood count

CBW *abbr* chemical and biological warfare

cc *abbr* cubic centimeter

CC *abbr* **1** chief complaint **2** current complaint

CCK *abbr* cholecystokinin

CCU *abbr* **1** cardiac care unit **2** coronary care unit **3** critical care unit

Cd *symbol* cadmium

CD *abbr* cluster of differentiation — used with an integer to denote any of numerous antigenic proteins on the surface of thymocytes and esp. T cells; see CD4

CDC *abbr* Centers for Disease Control

CD4 \\ˌsē-(ˌ)dē-'fôr\\ *n* : a large glycoprotein esp. on the surface of helper T cells that is the receptor for HIV; *also* : a cell and esp. a helper T cell bearing the CD4 receptor

cDNA \\ˌsē-(ˌ)dē-(ˌ)en-'ā\\ *n* : DNA that is complementary to a given messenger RNA and that serves as a template for production of the messenger RNA in the presence of a reverse transcriptase — called also *complementary DNA*

Ce *symbol* cerium

CEA *abbr* carcinoembryonic antigen

cec- *or* **ceci-** *or* **ceco-** *comb form* : cecum ⟨*cecitis*⟩ ⟨*cecostomy*⟩

ce·cal \\'sē-kəl\\ *adj* : of or like a cecum — **ce·cal·ly** *adv*

ce·ci·tis \\sē-'sī-təs\\ *n* : inflammation of the cecum

ce·co·pexy \\'sē-kə-ˌpek-sē\\ *n, pl* **-pex·ies** : a surgical operation to fix the cecum to the abdominal wall

ce·cos·to·my \\sē-'käs-tə-mē\\ *n, pl* **-mies** : the surgical formation of an opening into the cecum to serve as an artificial anus

ce·cum \\'sē-kəm\\ *n, pl* **ce·ca** \\-kə\\ : the blind pouch at the beginning of the large intestine into which the ileum opens from one side and which is continuous with the colon

¹-cele *n comb form* : tumor : hernia ⟨cystocele⟩

²-cele — see -COELE

celi- *or* **celio-** *comb form* : belly : abdomen ⟨*celioscopy*⟩ ⟨*celiotomy*⟩

¹ce·li·ac \\'sē-lē-ˌak\\ *adj* **1** : of or relating to the abdominal cavity **2** : belonging to or prescribed for celiac disease ⟨the ~ syndrome⟩ ⟨a ~ diet⟩

²celiac *n* : a celiac part (as a nerve)

celiac artery *n* : a short thick artery arising from the aorta just below the diaphragm and dividing almost immediately into the gastric, hepatic, and splenic arteries — called also *celiac axis, truncus celiacus*

celiac disease *n* : a chronic nutritional disorder esp. in young children that is characterized by defective digestion and utilization of fats and often by abdominal distension, diarrhea, and fatty stools — called also *nontropical sprue*

celiac ganglion *n* : either of a pair of collateral sympathetic ganglia that are the largest of the autonomic nervous system and lie one on each side of the celiac artery near the adrenal gland on the same side

celiac plexus *n* : a nerve plexus that is situated in the abdomen behind the stomach and in front of the aorta and the crura of the diaphragm, surrounds the celiac artery and the root of the superior mesenteric artery, contains several ganglia of which the most important are the celiac ganglia, and distributes nerve fibers to all the abdominal viscera — called also *solar plexus*

celiacus — see TRUNCUS CELIACUS

ce·li·os·co·py \\ˌsē-lē-'äs-kə-pē\\ *n, pl* **-pies** : examination of the abdominal cavity by surgical insertion of an endoscope through the abdominal wall

ce·li·ot·o·my \\ˌsē-lē-'ä-tə-mē\\ *n, pl* **-mies** : surgical incision of the abdomen

cell \\'sel\\ *n* : a small usu. microscopic mass of protoplasm bounded externally by a semipermeable membrane, usu. including one or more nuclei and various nonliving products, capable alone or interacting with other cells of performing all the fundamental functions of life, and forming the smallest structural unit of living matter capable of functioning independently

cell body *n* : the nucleus-containing central part of a neuron exclusive of its axons and dendrites that is the major structural element of the gray matter of the brain and spinal cord, the ganglia, and the retina — called also *soma*

cell count *n* : a count of cells esp. of the blood or other body fluid in a standard volume (as a cubic millimeter)

cell cycle *n* : the complete series of events from one cell division to the next — see G₁ PHASE, G₂ PHASE, M PHASE, S PHASE

cell division *n* : the process by which cells multiply involving both nuclear and cytoplasmic division — compare MEIOSIS, MITOSIS

celled \\'seld\\ *adj* : having (such or so many) cells — used in combination ⟨single-*celled* organisms⟩

cell line *n* : a cell culture selected for uniformity from a cell population derived from a usu. homogeneous tissue source (as an organ) ⟨a *cell line* derived from a malignant tumor⟩

cell–me·di·at·ed \\'sel-'mē-dē-ˌā-təd\\ *adj* : relating to or being the part of immunity or the immune response that is mediated primarily by T cells and esp. cytotoxic T cells rather than by antibodies secreted by B cells 〈~ immunity〉 — compare HUMORAL 2

cell membrane *n* **1** : PLASMA MEMBRANE **2** : CELL WALL

cell of Ley·dig \-'lī-dig\ *n* : LEYDIG CELL

cell plate *n* : a disk formed in a dividing plant cell that eventually forms the middle lamella of the wall between the daughter cells

cell sap *n* **1** : the liquid contents of a plant cell vacuole **2** : CYTOSOL

cell theory *n* : a theory in biology that includes one or both of the statements that the cell is the fundamental structural and functional unit of living matter and that the organism is composed of autonomous cells with its properties being the sum of those of its cells

cel·lu·lar \'sel-yə-lər\ *adj* **1** : of, relating to, or consisting of cells **2** : CELL-MEDIATED — **cel·lu·lar·i·ty** \₁sel-yə-'lar-ə-tē\ *n*

cel·lu·lite \'sel-yə-₁līt, -₁lēt\ *n* : lumpy fat found in the thighs, hips, and buttocks of some women

cel·lu·li·tis \₁sel-yə-'lī-təs\ *n* : diffuse and esp. subcutaneous inflammation of connective tissue

cel·lu·lose \'sel-yə-₁lōs, -₁lōz\ *n* : a polysaccharide $(C_6H_{10}O_5)_x$ of glucose units that constitutes the chief part of the cell walls of plants — **cel·lu·los·ic** \₁sel-yə-'lō-sik, -zik\ *adj*

cellulose acetate phthal·ate \-'ta-₁lāt\ *n* : a derivative of cellulose used as a coating for enteric tablets

cell wall *n* : the usu. rigid nonliving permeable wall that surrounds the plasma membrane and encloses and supports the cells of most plants, bacteria, fungi, and algae

Cel·si·us \'sel-sē-əs, -shəs\ *adj* : relating to or having a scale for measuring temperature on which the interval between the triple point and the boiling point of water is divided into 99.99 degrees with 0.01° being the triple point and 100.00° the boiling point — abbr. *C*; compare CENTIGRADE

Celsius, Anders (1701–1744), Swedish astronomer.

ce·ment \si-'ment\ *n* **1** : CEMENTUM **2** : a plastic composition made esp. of zinc or silica for filling dental cavities

ce·men·ta·tion \₁sē-₁men-'tā-shən\ *n* : the act or process of attaching (as a dental restoration to a natural tooth) by means of cement

ce·men·ti·cle \si-'men-ti-kəl\ *n* : a calcified body formed in the periodontal membrane of a tooth

ce·men·to·enam·el \si-₁men-tō-i-'na-məl\ *adj* : of, relating to, or joining the cementum and enamel of a tooth 〈the ~ junction〉

ce·men·to·ma \₁sē-₁men-'tō-mə\ *n, pl* **-mas** *or* **-ma·ta** \-mə-tə\ : a tumor resembling cementum in structure

ce·men·tum \si-'men-təm\ *n* : a specialized external bony layer covering the dentin of the part of a tooth normally within the gum — called also *cement;* compare DENTIN, ENAMEL

cen·sor \'sen-sər\ *n* : a hypothetical psychic agency that represses unacceptable notions before they reach consciousness — **cen·so·ri·al** \sen-'sōr-ē-əl\ *adj*

cen·sor·ship \'sen-sər-₁ship\ *n* : exclusion from consciousness by the psychic censor

cen·ter \'sen-tər\ *n* : a group of nerve cells having a common function 〈respiratory ~〉 — called also *nerve center*

cen·te·sis \sen-'tē-səs\ *n, pl* **cen·te·ses** \-₁sēz\ : surgical puncture (as of a tumor or membrane) — usu. used in compounds 〈para*centesis*〉

cen·ti·grade \'sen-tə-₁grād, 'sän-\ *adj* : relating to, conforming to, or having a thermometer scale on which the interval between the freezing and boiling points of water is divided into 100 degrees with 0° representing the freezing point and 100° the boiling point $(10° \sim)$ — abbr. *C*; compare CELSIUS

cen·ti·gram \-₁gram\ *n* : a unit of mass and weight equal to ¹⁄₁₀₀ gram

cen·ti·li·ter \-₁lē-tər\ *n* : a unit of liquid capacity equal to ¹⁄₁₀₀ liter

cen·ti·me·ter \-₁mē-tər\ *n* : a unit of length equal to ¹⁄₁₀₀ meter

centimeter–gram–second *adj* : CGS

cen·ti·pede \'sen-tə-pēd\ *n* : any of a class (Chilopoda) of long flattened many-segmented predaceous arthropods with each segment bearing one pair of legs of which the foremost pair is modified into poison fangs

centra *pl of* CENTRUM

cen·tral \'sen-trəl\ *adj* **1** : of or concerning the centrum of a vertebra **2** : of, relating to, or comprising the brain and spinal cord; *also* : originating within the central nervous system — **cen·tral·ly** *adv*

central artery *n* : a branch of the ophthalmic artery or the lacrimal artery that enters the substance of the optic nerve and supplies the nerve

central artery of the retina *n* : a branch of the ophthalmic artery that passes to the retina in the middle of the optic nerve and branches to form the arterioles of the retina — called also *central retinal artery*

central canal *n* : a minute canal running through the gray matter of the whole length of the spinal cord and continuous anteriorly with the ventricles of the brain

central deafness *n* : hearing loss or impairment resulting from defects in the central nervous system (as in the auditory area) rather than in the ear itself or the auditory nerve — compare CONDUCTION DEAFNESS, NERVE DEAFNESS

centralis — see FOVEA CENTRALIS
central lobe n : INSULA
central nervous system n : the part of the nervous system which in vertebrates consists of the brain and spinal cord, to which sensory impulses are transmitted and from which motor impulses pass out, and which supervises and coordinates the activity of the entire nervous system — compare AUTONOMIC NERVOUS SYSTEM, PERIPHERAL NERVOUS SYSTEM
central pontine myelinolysis n : disintegration of the myelin sheaths in the pons that is associated with malnutrition and esp. with alcoholism
central retinal artery n : CENTRAL ARTERY OF THE RETINA
central retinal vein n : CENTRAL VEIN OF THE RETINA
central sulcus n : the sulcus separating the frontal lobe of the cerebral cortex from the parietal lobe — called also *fissure of Rolando*
central tendon n : a 3-lobed aponeurosis located near the central portion of the diaphragm caudal to the pericardium and composed of intersecting planes of collagenous fibers
central vein n : any of the veins in the lobules of the liver that occur one in each lobule running from the apex to the base, receive blood from the sinusoids, and empty into the sublobular veins — called also *intralobular vein*
central vein of the retina n : a vein that is formed by union of the veins draining the retina, passes with the central artery of the retina in the optic nerve, and empties into the superior ophthalmic vein — called also *central retinal vein*
central venous pressure n : the venous pressure of the right atrium of the heart obtained by inserting a catheter into the median cubital vein and advancing it to right atrium through the superior vena cava — abbr. *CVP*
centre chiefly Brit var of CENTER
cen·tric \'sen-trik\ adj **1** : of or relating to a nerve center **2** of dental occlusion : involving spatial relationships such that all teeth of both jaws meet in a normal manner and forces exerted by the lower on the upper jaw are perfectly distributed in the dental arch
cen·trif·u·gal \sen-'tri-fyə-gəl, -fi-\ adj : passing outward (as from a nerve center to a muscle or gland) : EFFERENT — **cen·trif·u·gal·ly** adv
cen·trif·u·ga·tion \₁sen-trə-fyü-'gā-shən\ n : the process of centrifuging
¹cen·tri·fuge \'sen-trə-₁fyüj\ n : a machine using centrifugal force for separating substances of different densities, for removing moisture, or for simulating gravitational effects
²centrifuge vb **-fuged; -fug·ing** : to subject to centrifugal action esp. in a centrifuge
cen·tri·lob·u·lar \₁sen-trə-'lä-byə-lər\

adj : relating to or affecting the center of a lobule ⟨∼ necrosis in the liver⟩; also : affecting the central parts of the lobules containing clusters of branching functional and anatomical units of the lung ⟨∼ emphysema⟩
cen·tri·ole \'sen-trē-₁ōl\ n : one of a pair of cellular organelles that occur esp. in animals, are adjacent to the nucleus, function in the formation of the spindle apparatus during cell division, and consist of a cylinder with nine microtubules arranged peripherally in a circle
cen·trip·e·tal \sen-'tri-pət-ᵊl\ adj : passing inward (as from a sense organ to the brain or spinal cord) : AFFERENT — **cen·trip·e·tal·ly** adv
cen·tro·mere \'sen-trə-₁mir\ n : the point or region on a chromosome to which the spindle attaches during mitosis and meiosis — called also *kinetochore* — **cen·tro·mer·ic** \₁sen-trə-'mer-ik, -'mir-\ adj
cen·tro·some \'sen-trə-₁sōm\ n : the centriole-containing region of clear cytoplasm adjacent to the cell nucleus
cen·trum \'sen-trəm\ n, pl **centrums** or **cen·tra** \-trə\ **1** : the center esp. of an anatomical part **2** : the body of a vertebra ventral to the neural arch
Cen·tru·roi·des \₁sen-trə-'roi-(₁)dēz\ n : a genus of scorpions containing the only U.S. forms dangerous to humans
cephal- or **cephalo-** comb form **1** : head ⟨*cephal*algia⟩ ⟨*cephalo*metry⟩ **2** : cephalic and ⟨*cephalo*pelvic⟩
ceph·a·lad \'se-fə-₁lad\ adv : toward the head or anterior end of the body
ceph·a·lal·gia \₁se-fə-'lal-jə, -jē-ə\ n : HEADACHE
ceph·a·lex·in \₁se-fə-'lek-sən\ n : a semisynthetic cephalosporin $C_{16}H_{17}$-N_3O_4S with a spectrum of antibiotic activity similar to the penicillins
ce·phal·gia \se-'fal-jə, -jē-ə\ n : HEADACHE
ceph·al·he·ma·to·ma \₁se-fəl-₁hē-mə-'tō-mə\ n, pl **-mas** or **-ma·ta** \-mə-tə\ : a blood-filled tumor or swelling beneath the pericardium that occurs frequently in newborn infants as a result of injury (as by forceps) during birth
-cephali pl of -CEPHALUS
ce·phal·ic \sə-'fa-lik\ adj **1** : of or relating to the head **2** : directed toward or situated on or in or near the head — **ce·phal·i·cal·ly** \-li-k(ə-)lē\ adv
cephalic flexure n : the middle of the three anterior flexures of an embryo in which the front part of the brain bends downward in an angle of 90 degrees
cephalic index n : the ratio multiplied by 100 of the maximum breadth of the head to its maximum length — compare CRANIAL INDEX
cephalic vein n : any of various superficial veins of the arm ; specif : a large vein of the upper arm lying along the

outer edge of the biceps muscle and emptying into the axillary vein

ceph·a·lin \\'ke-fə-lən, 'se-\ *n* : PHOSPHATIDYLETHANOLAMINE

cephalo- — see CEPHAL-

ceph·a·lo·cau·dal \,se-fə-lō-'kȯd-ᵊl\ *adj* : proceeding or occurring in the long axis of the body esp. in the direction from head to tail — **ceph·a·lo·cau·dal·ly** *adv*

ceph·a·lom·e·ter \,se-fə-'lä-mə-tər\ *n* : an instrument for measuring the head

ceph·a·lom·e·try \,se-fə-'lä-mə-trē\ *n*, *pl* **-tries** : the science of measuring the head in living individuals — **ceph·a·lo·met·ric** \-lō-'me-trik\ *adj*

ceph·a·lo·pel·vic disproportion \,se-fə-lō-'pel-vik-\ *n* : a condition in which a maternal pelvis is small in relation to the size of the fetal head

ceph·a·lor·i·dine \,se-fə-'lȯr-ə-,dēn, -'lär-\ *n* : a semisynthetic broadspectrum antibiotic $C_{19}H_{17}N_3O_4S_2$ derived from cephalosporin

ceph·a·lo·spo·rin \,se-fə-lə-'spȯr-ən\ *n* : any of several antibiotics produced by an imperfect fungus (genus *Cephalosporium*)

ceph·a·lo·thin \'se-fə-lə-(,)thin\ *n* : a semisynthetic broad-spectrum antibiotic $C_{16}H_{15}N_2NaO_6S_2$ that is an analog of a cephalosporin and is effective against penicillin-resistant staphylococci

ceph·a·lo·tho·ra·cop·a·gus \,se-fə-,lō-,thȯr-ə-'kä-pə-gəs\ *n*, *pl* **-agi** \-,gī, -,gē\ : teratological twin fetuses joined at the head, neck, and thorax

-cephalus *n comb form*, *pl* **-cephali** : cephalic abnormality (of a specified type) ⟨hydro*cephalus*⟩ ⟨micro*cephalus*⟩

cer·amide \'sir-ə-,mid\ *n* : any of a group of amides formed by linking a fatty acid to sphingosine and found widely but in small amounts in plant and animal tissue

cer·amide·tri·hex·o·si·dase \,sir-ə-,mīd-,trī-,hek-sə-'si-,dās, -,dāz\ *n* : an enzyme that breaks down ceramidetrihexoside and is deficient in individuals affected with Fabry's disease

cer·amide·tri·hex·o·side \-(,)trī-'hek-sə-,sīd\ *n* : a lipid that accumulates in body tissues of individuals affected with Fabry's disease

ce·rate \'sir-,āt\ *n* : an unctuous preparation for external use consisting of wax or resin mixed with oil, lard, and medicinal ingredients

cer·a·to·hy·al \,ser-ə-(,)tō-'hī-əl\ *or* **cer·a·to·hy·oid** \-'hī-,oid\ *n* : the smaller inner projection of the two lateral hyoid bone on each side of the human hyoid bone — called also *lesser cornu*; compare THYROHYAL

cer·car·ia \(,)sər-'kar-ē-ə, -'ker-\ *n*, *pl* **-i·ae** \-ē-,ē\ : a usu. tadpole-shaped larval trematode worm that develops

in a molluscan host from a redia — **cer·car·i·al** \-əl\ *adj*

cer·clage \ser-'kläzh, (,)sər-\ *n* : any of several procedures for increasing tissue resistance in a functionally incompetent uterine cervix that usu. involve reinforcement with an inert substance esp. in the form of sutures near the internal opening

ce·rea flex·i·bil·i·tas \,sir-ē-ə-,flek-sə-'bi-lə-,tas, -,täs\ *n* : the capacity (as in catalepsy) to maintain the limbs or other bodily parts in whatever position they have been placed

cerebell- *or* **cerebelli-** *or* **cerebello-** *comb form* : cerebellum ⟨*cerebell*itis⟩

cerebella *pl of* CEREBELLUM

cerebellar artery *n* : any of several branches of the basilar and vertebral arteries that supply the cerebellum

cerebellaris — see PEDUNCULUS CEREBELLARIS INFERIOR, PEDUNCULUS CEREBELLARIS MEDIUS, PEDUNCULUS CEREBELLARIS SUPERIOR

cerebellar peduncle *n* : any of three large bands of nerve fibers that join each hemisphere of the cerebellum with the parts of the brain below and in front: **a** : one connecting the cerebellum with the midbrain — called also *brachium conjunctivum, pedunculus cerebellaris superior, superior cerebellar peduncle* **b** : one connecting the cerebellum with the pons — called also *brachium pontis, middle cerebellar peduncle, middle peduncle, pedunculus cerebellaris medius* **c** : one that connects the cerebellum with the medulla oblongata and the spinal cord — called also *inferior cerebellar peduncle, pedunculus cerebellaris inferior, restiform body*

cerebelli — see FALX CEREBELLI, TENTORIUM CEREBELLI

cer·e·bel·li·tis \,ser-ə-bə-'lī-təs, -be-\ *n* : inflammation of the cerebellum

cer·e·bel·lo·pon·tine angle \,ser-ə-,be-lō-,pän-,tēn-, -,tin-\ *n* : a region of the brain at the junction of the pons and cerebellum that is a frequent site of tumor formation

cer·e·bel·lum \,ser-ə-'be-ləm\ *n*, *pl* **-bellums** *or* **-bel·la** \-lə\ : a large dorsally projecting part of the brain concerned esp. with the coordination of muscles and the maintenance of bodily equilibrium, situated between the brain stem and the back of the cerebrum and formed in humans of two lateral lobes and a median lobe — **cer·e·bel·lar** \-lər\ *adj*

cerebr- *or* **cerebro-** *comb form* **1** : brain : cerebrum ⟨*cerebr*ation⟩ **2** : cerebral and ⟨*cerebro*spinal⟩

cerebra *pl of* CEREBRUM

ce·re·bral \sə-'rē-brəl, 'ser-ə-\ *adj* **1** : of or relating to the brain or the intellect **2** : of, relating to, or being the cerebrum

cerebral accident *n* : an occurrence of sudden damage (as by hemorrhage) to the cerebral vascular system — compare STROKE

cerebral aqueduct *n* : AQUEDUCT OF SYLVIUS

cerebral artery *n* : any of the arteries supplying the cerebral cortex: **a** : an artery that arises from the internal carotid artery, forms the anterior portion of the circle of Willis where it is linked to the artery on the opposite side by the anterior communicating artery, and passes on to supply the medial surfaces of the cerebrum — called also *anterior cerebral artery* **b** : an artery that arises from the internal carotid artery, passes along the lateral fissure, and supplies the lateral surfaces of the cerebral cortex — called also *middle cerebral artery* **c** : an artery that arises by the terminal forking of the basilar artery where it forms the posterior portion of the circle of Willis and passes on to supply the lower surfaces of the temporal and occipital lobes — called also *posterior cerebral artery*

cerebral cortex *n* : the surface layer of gray matter of the cerebrum that functions chiefly in coordination of sensory and motor information — called also *pallium*

cerebral dominance *n* : dominance in development and functioning of one of the cerebral hemispheres

cerebral hemisphere *n* : either of the two hollow convoluted lateral halves of the cerebrum

cerebral hemorrhage *n* : the bleeding into the tissue of the brain and esp. of the cerebrum from a ruptured blood vessel

cerebral palsy *n* : a disability resulting from damage to the brain before, during, or shortly after birth and outwardly manifested by muscular incoordination and speech disturbances — compare SPASTIC PARALYSIS — **cerebral palsied** *adj*

cerebral peduncle *n* : either of two large bundles of nerve fibers passing from the pons forward and outward to form the main connection between the cerebral hemispheres and the spinal cord

cerebral vein *n* : any of various veins that drain the surface and inner tissues of the cerebral hemispheres — see GALEN'S VEIN, GREAT CEREBRAL VEIN

cer·e·brate \'ser-ə-₁brāt\ *vb* **-brat·ed; -brat·ing** : to use the mind — **cere·bra·tion** \₁ser-ə-'brā-shən\ *n*

cerebri — see CRURA CEREBRI, FALX CEREBRI, HYPOPHYSIS CEREBRI, PSEUDOTUMOR CEREBRI

cerebro- — see CEREBR-

ce·re·bro·side \sə-'rē-brə-₁sīd, 'ser-ə-\ *n* : any of various lipids composed of ceramide and a monosaccharide and found esp. in the myelin sheath of nerves

ce·re·bro·spi·nal \sə-₁rē-brō-'spīn-ᵊl, ₁ser-ə-\ *adj* : of or relating to the brain and spinal cord or to these together with the cranial and spinal nerves that innervate voluntary muscles

cerebrospinal fluid *n* : a liquid that is comparable to serum but contains less dissolved material, that is secreted from the blood into the lateral ventricles of the brain, about that serves chiefly to maintain uniform pressure within the brain and spinal cord — called also *spinal fluid*

cerebrospinal meningitis *n* : inflammation of the meninges of both brain and spinal cord; *specif* : an infectious epidemic and often fatal meningitis caused by the meningococcus

ce·re·bro·vas·cu·lar \sə-₁rē-brō-'vas-kyə-lər, ₁ser-ə-\ *adj* : of or involving the cerebrum and the blood vessels supplying it (~ disease)

ce·re·brum \sə-'rē-brəm, 'ser-ə-\ *n, pl* **-brums** *or* **-bra** \-brə\ : the expanded anterior portion of the brain that overlies the rest of the brain, consists of cerebral hemispheres and connecting structures, and is considered to be the seat of conscious mental processes — see TELENCEPHALON

cer·e·sin \'ser-ə-sən\ *n* : a white or yellow hard brittle wax used as a substitute for beeswax

ce·ri·um \'sir-ē-əm\ *n* : a malleable ductile metallic element — symbol *Ce*; see ELEMENT table

ce·roid \'sir-₁öid\ *n* : a yellow to brown pigment found esp. in the liver in cirrhosis

cert *abbr* certificate; certification; certified; certify

cer·ti·fy \'sər-tə-₁fī\ *vb* **-fied; -fy·ing 1** : to attest officially to the insanity of **2** : to designate as having met the requirements to practice medicine or a particular medical specialty — **cer·ti·fi·able** \₁sər-tə-'fī-ə-bəl\ *adj* — **cer·ti·fi·ably** \-blē\ *adv* — **cer·ti·fi·ca·tion** \-fə-'kā-shən\ *n*

cerulea — see PHLEGMASIA CERULEA DOLENS

ceruleus, cerulei — see LOCUS COERULEUS

ce·ru·lo·plas·min \sə-₁rü-lō-'plaz-mən\ *n* : a blue alpha globulin active in the biological storage and transport of copper

ce·ru·men \sə-'rü-mən\ *n* : EARWAX

ce·ru·mi·nous gland \sə-'rü-mə-nəs-\ *n* : one of the modified sweat glands of the ear that produce earwax

cervic- *or* **cervici-** *or* **cervico-** *comb form* **1** : neck : cervix of an organ (*cervicitis*) **2** : cervical and (*cervicovaginal*) (*cervicothoracic*)

cer·vi·cal \'sər-vi-kəl\ *adj* : of or relating to a neck or cervix (~ cancer)

cervical canal *n* : the passage through the cervix uteri

cervical cap *n* : a usu. rubber or plastic contraceptive device in the form of a thimble-shaped molded cap that fits snugly over the uterine cervix and blocks sperm from entering the uterus — called also *Dutch cap*

cervical flexure *n* : a ventral bend in the neural tube of the embryo marking the point of transition from brain to spinal cord

cervical ganglion *n* : any of three sympathetic ganglia on each side of the neck

cervicalis — see ANSA CERVICALIS

cervical nerve *n* : one of the spinal nerves of the cervical region of which there are eight on each side in most mammals including humans

cervical plexus *n* : a plexus formed by the anterior divisions of the four upper cervical nerves

cervical plug *n* : a mass of tenacious secretion by glands of the uterine cervix present during pregnancy and tending to close the uterine orifice

cervical rib *n* : a supernumerary rib sometimes found in the neck above the usual first rib

cervical vertebra *n* : any of the seven vertebrae of the neck

cer·vi·cec·to·my \ˌsər-və-'sek-tə-mē\ *n, pl* **-mies** : surgical excision of the uterine cervix — called also *trachelectomy*

cervici- *or* **cervico-** — see CERVIC-

cervicis — see ILIOCOSTALIS CERVICIS, LONGISSIMUS CERVICIS, SEMISPINALIS CERVICIS, SPINALIS CERVICIS, SPLENIUS CERVICIS, TRANSVERSALIS CERVICIS

cer·vi·ci·tis \ˌsər-və-'sī-təs\ *n* : inflammation of the uterine cervix

cer·vi·co·fa·cial nerve \ˌsər-və-(ˌ)kō-'fā-shəl-\ *n* : a branch of the facial nerve supplying the lower part of the face and upper part of the neck

cer·vi·co·tho·rac·ic \ˌsər-vi-(ˌ)kō-thə-'ra-sik, -thō-\ *adj* : of or relating to the neck and thorax ⟨∼ sympathectomy⟩

cer·vi·co·vag·i·nal \-'va-jən-əl\ *adj* : of or relating to the uterine cervix and the vagina ⟨∼ flora⟩ ⟨∼ carcinoma⟩

cer·vix \'sər-viks\ *n, pl* **cer·vi·ces** \-və-ˌsēz, ˌsər-'vī-(ˌ)sēz\ *or* **cervixes** *n* 1 : NECK 1a; *esp* : the back part of the neck 2 : a constricted portion of an organ or part: as **a** : the narrow lower or outer end of the uterus **b** : the constricted cementoenamel junction on a tooth

cervix uteri \-'yü-tə-ˌrī\ *n* : CERVIX 2a

¹**ce·sar·e·an** *also* **ce·sar·i·an** \si-'zar-ē-ən\ *adj* : of, relating to, or being a cesarean section ⟨a ∼ birth⟩

²**cesarean** *also* **cesarian** *n* : CESAREAN SECTION

Cae·sar \'sē-zər\, **Gaius Julius (100–44 B.C.)**, Roman general and statesman.

cesarean section *n* : surgical incision of the walls of the abdomen and uterus for delivery of offspring

ce·si·um \'sē-zē-əm\ *n* : a silver-white

soft ductile element — symbol *Cs*; see ELEMENT table

ces·tode \'ses-ˌtōd\ *n* : TAPEWORM — **cestode** *adj*

cet·ri·mide \'se-trə-ˌmīd\ *n* : a mixture of bromides of ammonium used esp. as a detergent and antiseptic

ce·tyl alcohol \'sēt-əl-\ *n* : a waxy crystalline alcohol $C_{16}H_{34}O$ used in pharmaceutical and cosmetic preparations

ce·tyl·py·ri·din·i·um chloride \ˌsēt-əl-ˌpī-rə-'di-nē-əm-\ *n* : a white powder consisting of a quaternary ammonium salt $C_{21}H_{38}ClN \cdot H_2O$ and used as a detergent and antiseptic

Cf *symbol* californium

CF *abbr* cystic fibrosis

CG *abbr* chorionic gonadotropin

cgs *adj, often cap C&G&S* : of, relating to, or being a system of units based on the centimeter as the unit of length, the gram as the unit of mass, and the second as the unit of time ⟨∼ system⟩ ⟨∼ units⟩

Cha·ber·tia \shə-'bər-tē-ə, -'bər-\ *n* : a genus of strongylid nematode worms including one (*C. ovina*) that infests the colon esp. of sheep and causes a bloody diarrhea

Cha·bert \shä-'ber\, **Philibert (1737–1814)**, French veterinarian.

chafe \'chāf\ *n* : injury caused by friction — **chafe** *vb*

Cha·gas' disease \'shä-gəs, -gə-səz-\ *n* : a tropical American disease that is caused by a flagellate of the genus *Trypanosoma* (*T. cruzi*) and is marked by prolonged high fever, edema, and enlargement of the spleen, liver, and lymph nodes

Chagas, Carlos Ribeiro Justiniano (1879–1934), Brazilian physician.

cha·go·ma \shə-'gō-mə\ *n, pl* **-mas** *or* **-ma·ta** \-tə\ : a swelling resembling a tumor that appears at the site of infection in Chagas' disease

κ-chain \'ka-pə-\ *var of* KAPPA CHAIN

chain reflex *n* : a series of responses each serving as a stimulus that evokes the next response

chair·side \'char-ˌsīd\ *adj* : relating to, performed in the vicinity of, or assisting in the work done on a patient in a dentist's chair ⟨a dental ∼ assistant⟩ ⟨a good ∼ manner⟩

chair time *n* : the time that a dental patient spends in the dentist's chair

cha·la·sia \kə-'lā-zhə, ka-\ *n* : the relaxation of a ring of muscle (as the cardiac sphincter of the esophagus) surrounding a bodily opening

cha·la·zi·on \kə-'lā-zē-ən, -ˌän\ *n, pl* **-zia** \-zē-ə\ : a small circumscribed tumor of the eyelid formed by retention of secretions of the meibomian gland and sometimes accompanied by inflammation

chal·i·co·sis \ˌka-li-'kō-səs\ *n, pl* **-co·ses** \-ˌsēz\ : a pulmonary affection occurring among stone cutters that is caused by inhalation of stone dust

chalk \'chȯk\ *n* : a soft white, gray, or buff limestone sometimes used medicinally as a source of calcium carbonate — see PRECIPITATED CHALK, PREPARED CHALK — **chalky** \'chȯ-kē\ *adj*

chal·lenge \'cha-lənj\ *n* : the process of provoking or testing physiological activity by exposure to a specific substance; *esp* : a test of immunity by exposure to an antigen after immunization against it — **challenge** *vb*

cha·lone \'kā-ˌlōn, 'ka-\ *n* : an endogenous secretion that is held to inhibit mitosis in a specific tissue

cham·ber \'chām-bər\ *n* : an enclosed space within the body of an animal — see ANTERIOR CHAMBER, POSTERIOR CHAMBER

chamber pot *n* : a bedroom vessel for urination and defecation

chan·cre \'shaŋ-kər\ *n* : a primary sore or ulcer at the site of entry of a pathogen (as in tularemia); *esp* : the initial lesion of syphilis

chan·croid \'shaŋ-ˌkrȯid\ *n* : a venereal disease caused by a hemophilic bacterium of the genus *Haemophilus* (*H. ducreyi*) and characterized by chancres that unlike those of syphilis lack firm indurated margins — called also *soft chancre*; see DUCREY'S BACILLUS

change of life *n* : CLIMACTERIC

chan·nel \'chan-əl\ *n* **1** : a usu. tubular enclosed passage **2** : a passage created in a selectively permeable membrane by a conformational change in membrane proteins

chap \'chap\ *n* : a crack in or a sore roughening of the skin caused by exposure to wind or cold — **chap** *vb*

Chap Stick \'chap-ˌstik\ *trademark* — used for a lip balm in stick form

char·ac·ter \'kar-ik-tər\ *n* **1** : one of the attributes or features that make up and distinguish the individual **2** : the detectable expression of the action of a gene or group of genes **3** : the complex of mental and ethical traits marking and often individualizing a person, group, or nation

¹char·ac·ter·is·tic \ˌkar-ik-tə-ˈris-tik\ *adj* : serving to reveal and distinguish the individual character — **char·ac·ter·is·ti·cal·ly** \-ti-k(ə-)lē\ *adv*

²characteristic *n* : a distinguishing trait, quality, or property

cha·ras \'chär-əs\ *n* : HASHISH

char·coal \'chär-ˌkōl\ *n* : a dark or black porous carbon prepared from vegetable or animal substances — see ACTIVATED CHARCOAL

Char·cot–Ley·den crystals \ˌshär-kō-ˈli-dᵊn-\ *n pl* : minute colorless crystals that occur in various pathological discharges and esp. in the sputum following an asthmatic attack and that

are thought to be formed by the disintegration of eosinophils

Char·cot \shär-ˈkō\, **Jean–Martin (1825–1893),** French neurologist.

Leyden, Ernst Viktor von (1832–1910), German physician.

Char·cot–Ma·rie–Tooth disease \(ˌ)shär-ˈkō-mə-ˈrē-ˈtüth-\ *n* : PERONEAL MUSCULAR ATROPHY

P. Marie — see MARIE-STRÜMPELL DISEASE

Tooth, Howard Henry (1856–1925), British physician.

Char·cot's joint \(ˌ)shär-ˈkōz-\ *or* **Char·cot joint** \-ˈkō-\ *n* : a destructive condition affecting one or more joints, occurring in diseases of the spinal cord, and ultimately resulting in a flail joint — called also *Charcot's disease*

charge \'chärj\ *n* **1** : a plaster or ointment used on a domestic animal **2** : CATHEXIS 2

charge nurse *n* : a nurse who is in charge of a health-care unit (as a hospital ward, emergency room, or nursing home)

char·la·tan \'shär-lə-tən\ *n* : QUACK

char·ley horse \'chär-lē-ˌhȯrs\ *n* : a muscular pain, cramping, or stiffness esp. of the quadriceps that results from a strain or bruise

chart \'chärt\ *n* : a record of medical information for a patient

Chas·tek paralysis \'chas-ˌtek-\ *n* : a fatal paralytic vitamin deficiency of foxes and minks that are bred in captivity and fed raw fish and that is caused by enzymatic inactivation of thiamine by thiaminase present in the fish

Chastek, John Simeon (1886–1954), American breeder of fur-bearing animals.

CHD *abbr* coronary heart disease

check·bite \'chek-ˌbīt\ *n* **1 a** : an act of biting into a sheet of material (as wax) to record the relation between the opposing surfaces of upper and lower teeth **b** : the record obtained **2** : the material for checkbites

check ligament *n* **1** : ALAR LIGAMENT **2** : either of two expansions of the sheaths of rectus muscles of the eye each of which prob. restrains the activity of the muscle with which it is associated

check·up \'chek-ˌəp\ *n* : EXAMINATION; *esp* : a general physical examination

Che·di·ak–Hi·ga·shi syndrome \shād-ˈyäk-hē-ˈgä-shē-\ *n* : a genetic disorder inherited as an autosomal recessive and characterized by partial albinism, abnormal granules in the white blood cells, and marked susceptibility to bacterial infections

Che·di·ak \shād-ˈyäk\, **Moises (*fl* 1952),** French physician.

Hi·ga·shi \hē-ˈgä-shē\, **Ototaka (*fl* 1954),** Japanese physician.

cheek \'chēk\ *n* **1** : the fleshy side of the

face below the eye and above and to the side of the mouth; *broadly* : the lateral aspect of the head **2** : BUTTOCK 1

cheek·bone \'chēk-,bōn\ *n* : the prominence below the eye that is formed by the zygomatic bone; *also* : ZYGOMATIC BONE

cheek tooth *n* : any of the molar or premolar teeth

cheese skipper *n* : a dipteran fly (*Piophila casei*) whose larva lives in cheese and cured meats and is a cause of intestinal myiasis

cheesy \'chē-zē\ *adj* **chees·i·er; -est** : resembling cheese in consistency ⟨~ lesions⟩ ⟨a ~ discharge⟩

cheil- *or* **cheilo-** *also* **chil-** *or* **chilo-** *comb form* : lip ⟨*cheilitis*⟩ ⟨*cheiloplasty*⟩

cheil·i·tis \kī-'lī-təs\ *n* : inflammation of the lip

cheil·o·plas·ty \'kī-lō-,plas-tē\ *n, pl* **-ties** : plastic surgery to repair lip defects

cheil·os·chi·sis \kī-'läs-kə-səs\ *n, pl* **-chi·ses** \-,sēz\ : CLEFT LIP

cheil·o·sis \kī-'lō-səs\ *n, pl* **-lo·ses** \-,sēz\ : an abnormal condition of the lips characterized by scaling of the surface and by the formation of fissures in the corners of the mouth

cheir- *or* **cheiro-** — see CHIR-

chei·ro·pom·pho·lyx \kī-rō-'päm-fə-,liks\ *n* : a skin disease characterized by itching vesicles or blebs occurring in groups on the hands or feet

che·late \'kē-,lāt\ *n* : a compound having a ring structure that usu. contains a metal ion held by coordinate bonds — **chelate** *adj or vb* — **che·la·tion** \kē-'lā-shən\ *n*

che·lat·ing agent \'kē-,lā-tiŋ-\ *n* : any of various compounds that combine with metals to form chelates and that include some used medically in the treatment of metal poisoning (as by lead)

che·la·tion therapy \kē-'lā-shən-\ *n* : the use of a chelating agent to bind with a metal in the body to form a chelate so that the metal loses its toxic effect or physiological activity

che·la·tor \'kē-,lā-tər\ *n* : CHELATING AGENT

chem *abbr* chemical; chemist; chemistry

chem- *or* **chemo-** *also* **chemi-** *comb form* : chemical; chemistry ⟨*chemotherapy*⟩

¹chem·i·cal \'ke-mi-kəl\ *adj* **1** : of, relating to, used in, or produced by chemistry **2** : acting or operated or produced by chemicals — **chem·i·cal·ly** \-mi-k(ə-)lē\ *adv*

²chemical *n* : a substance obtained by a chemical process or used for producing a chemical effect

chemical peel *n* : PEEL

chemical warfare *n* : warfare using incendiary mixtures, smokes, or irritant, burning, poisonous, or asphyxiating gases

chem·ist \'ke-məst\ *n* **1** : one trained in chemistry **2** *Brit* : PHARMACIST

chem·is·try \'ke-mə-strē\ *n, pl* **-tries 1** : a science that deals with the composition, structure, and properties of substances and of the transformations that they undergo **2 a** : the composition and chemical properties of a substance ⟨the ~ of hemoglobin⟩ **b** : chemical processes and phenomena (as of an organism) ⟨blood ~⟩

chemist's shop *n, Brit* : a place where medicines are sold

chemo \'kē-,mō\ *n* : CHEMOTHERAPY

chemo- — see CHEM-

che·mo·dec·to·ma \,kē-mō-'dek-tə-mə, ,ke-\ *n, pl* **-mas** *or* **-ma·ta** \-mə-tə\ : a tumor that affects tissue (as of the carotid body) populated with chemoreceptors

che·mo·nu·cle·ol·y·sis \-,nü-klē-'ä-lə-səs, -,nyü-\ *n, pl* **-y·ses** \-,sēz\ : treatment of a slipped disk by the injection of chymopapain to dissolve the displaced nucleus pulposus

che·mo·pal·li·dec·to·my \-,pa-lə-'dek-tə-mē\ *n, pl* **-mies** : destruction of the globus pallidus by the injection of a chemical agent (as ethyl alcohol) esp. for the relief of parkinsonian tremors

che·mo·pro·phy·lax·is \-,prō-fə-'lak-səs, -,prä-\ *n, pl* **-lax·es** \-,sēz\ : the prevention of infectious disease by the use of chemical agents — **che·mo·pro·phy·lac·tic** \-'lak-tik\ *adj*

che·mo·re·cep·tion \-ri-'sep-shən\ *n* : the physiological reception of chemical stimuli — **che·mo·re·cep·tive** \-'tiv\ *adj*

che·mo·re·cep·tor \-ri-'sep-tər\ *n* : a sense organ (as a taste bud) responding to chemical stimuli

che·mo·re·flex \,kē-mō-'rē-,fleks *also* -ke-\ *n* : a physiological reflex initiated by a chemical stimulus or in a chemoreceptor — **chemoreflex** *adj*

che·mo·re·sis·tance \-ri-'zis-təns\ *n* : the quality or state of being resistant to a chemical (as a drug) — **che·mo·re·sis·tant** \-tənt\ *adj*

che·mo·sen·si·tive \-'sen-sə-tiv\ *adj* : susceptible to the action of a (particular) chemical — used esp. of strains of bacteria — **che·mo·sen·si·tiv·i·ty** \-,sen-sə-'ti-və-tē\ *n*

che·mo·sis \kə-'mō-səs\ *n, pl* **-mo·ses** \-,sēz\ : swelling of the conjunctival tissue around the cornea

che·mo·sur·gery \,kē-mō-'sər-jə-rē\ *n, pl* **-ger·ies** : removal by chemical means of diseased or unwanted tissue — **che·mo·sur·gi·cal** \-'sər-ji-kəl\ *adj*

che·mo·tac·tic \-'tak-tik\ *adj* : involving, inducing, or exhibiting chemotaxis — **che·mo·tac·ti·cal·ly** \-ti-k(ə-)lē\ *adv*

che·mo·tax·is \-'tak-səs\ *n, pl* **-tax·es** \-,sēz\ : orientation or movement of an organism or cell in relation to chemical agents

¹che·mo·ther·a·peu·tic \-,ther-ə-'pyü-tik\

adj : of, relating to, or used in chemotherapy — **che·mo·ther·a·peu·ti·cal·ly** \-ti-k(ə-)lē\ *adv*

²**chemotherapeutic** *n* : an agent used in chemotherapy

che·mo·ther·a·py \-ᵀther-ə-pē\ *n, pl* **-pies** : the use of chemical agents in the treatment or control of disease or mental illness — **che·mo·ther·a·pist** \-pist\ *n*

che·mot·ic \ki-ᵀmä-tik\ *adj* : marked by or belonging to chemosis

che·mot·ro·pism \ki-ᵀmä-trə-ₚpi-zəm, ke-\ *n* : orientation of cells or organisms in relation to chemical stimuli

che·no·de·oxy·cho·lic acid \ₚkē-(ₚ)nō-ₚdē-ₚäk-si-ᵀkō-lik-, -ᵀkä-\ *n* : a bile acid $C_{24}H_{40}O_4$

cher·ub·ism \ᵀcher-ù-ₚbi-zəm\ *n* : a hereditary condition characterized by swelling of the jawbones and esp. in young children by a characteristic facies marked by protuberant cheeks and upturned eyes

chest \ᵀchest\ *n* 1 : a cupboard used esp. for storing medicines or first-aid supplies — called also *medicine cabinet, medicine chest* 2 : the part of the body enclosed by the ribs and sternum

chest·nut \ᵀches-(ₚ)nət\ *n* : a callosity on the inner side of the leg of the horse

chesty \ᵀches-tē\ *adj* : of, relating to, or affected with disease of the chest — not used technically

Cheyne–Stokes respiration \ᵀchān-ᵀstōks-\ *n* : cyclic breathing marked by a gradual increase in the rapidity of respiration followed by a gradual decrease and total cessation for from 5 to 50 seconds and found esp. in advanced kidney and heart disease, asthma, and increased intracranial pressure — called also *Cheyne=Stokes breathing*

   Cheyne \ᵀchān, ᵀchā-nē\, **John (1777–1836),** British physician.
   Stokes \ᵀstōks\, **William (1804–1878),** British physician.

CHF *abbr* congestive heart failure

Chi·ari–From·mel syndrome \kē-ᵀär-ē-ᵀfrō-məl-, -ᵀfrä-\ *n* : a condition usu. occurring postpartum and characterized by amenorrhea, galactorrhea, obesity, and atrophy of the uterus and ovaries

   Chiari, Johann Baptist (1817–1854), German surgeon.
   Frommel, Richard Julius Ernst (1854–1912), German gynecologist.

chi·asm \ᵀkī-ₚa-zəm, ᵀkē-\ *n* : CHIASMA 1

chi·as·ma \kī-ᵀaz-mə, kē-\ *n, pl* **-ma·ta** \-mə-tə\ 1 : an anatomical intersection or decussation — see OPTIC CHIASMA 2 : a cross-shaped configuration of paired chromatids visible in the diplotene of meiotic prophase and considered the cytological equivalent of genetic crossing-over — **chi·as·mat·ic** \ₚkī-əz-ᵀma-tik, ₚkē-\ *adj*

chiasmatic groove *n* : a narrow transverse groove that lies near the front of the superior surface of the sphenoid bone, is continuous with the optic foramen, and houses the optic chiasma

chicken mite *n* : a small mite of the genus *Dermanyssus* (*D. gallinae*) that infests poultry esp. in warm regions

chicken pox *n* : an acute contagious disease esp. of children marked by low-grade fever and formation of vesicles and caused by a herpes virus — called also *varicella*; compare SHINGLES

chief cell *n* 1 : one of the cells that line the lumen of the fundic glands of the stomach; *esp* : a small cell with granular cytoplasm that secretes pepsin — compare PARIETAL CELL 2 : one of the secretory cells of the parathyroid glands

chig·ger \ᵀchi-gər, ᵀji-\ *n* : CHIGOE 1 2 : a 6-legged mite larva (family Trombiculidae) that sucks the blood and causes intense irritation

chi·goe \ᵀchi-(ₚ)gō, ᵀchē-\ *n* : a tropical flea belonging to the genus *Tunga* (*T. penetrans*) of which the fertile female causes great discomfort by burrowing under the skin — called also *chigger, sand flea* 2 : CHIGGER 2

chil- *or* **chilo-** — see CHEIL-

chil·blain \ᵀchil-ₚblān\ *n* : an inflammatory swelling or sore caused by exposure (as of the feet or hands) to cold — called also *pernio*

child \ᵀchild\ *n, pl* **chil·dren** \ᵀchil-drən, -dərn\ 1 : an unborn or recently born person 2 : a young person esp. between infancy and youth — **with child** : PREGNANT

child·bear·ing \ᵀchild-ₚbar-iŋ\ *n* : the act of bringing forth children : PARTURITION — **childbearing** *adj*

child·bed \-ₚbed\ *n* : the condition of a woman in childbirth

childbed fever *n* : PUERPERAL FEVER

child·birth \-ₚbərth\ *n* : PARTURITION

child guidance *n* : the clinical study and treatment of the personality and behavior problems of esp. maladjusted and delinquent children by a staff of specialists usu. comprising a physician or psychiatrist, a clinical psychologist, and a psychiatric social worker

child·hood \ᵀchild-ₚhùd\ *n* : the state or period of being a child

child psychiatry *n* : psychiatry applied to the treatment of children

child psychology *n* : the study of the psychological characteristics of infants and children and the application of general psychological principles to infancy and childhood

¹**chill** \ᵀchil\ *n* 1 : a sensation of cold accompanied by shivering 2 : a disagreeable sensation of coldness

²**chill** *vb* 1 **a** : to make or become cold **b** : to shiver or quake with or as if with

cold 2 : to become affected with a chill

chill factor *n* : WINDCHILL

chi·me·ra *or* **chi·mae·ra** \kī-ˈmir-ə, kə-\ *n* : an individual, organ, or part consisting of tissues of diverse genetic constitution — **chi·me·ric** \-ˈmir-ik, -ˈmer-\ *adj* — **chi·me·rism** \-ˈmir-ˌi-zəm, kə-; ˈkī-mə-ˌri-z\ *n*

chin \ˈchin\ *n* : the lower portion of the face lying below the lower lip and including the prominence of the lower jaw — called also *mentum* — **chin·less** \-ləs\ *adj*

chin·bone \ˈchin-ˌbōn\ *n* : JAW 1b; *esp* : the median anterior part of the bone of the lower jaw

chinch \ˈchinch\ *n* : BEDBUG

Chinese liver fluke *n* : a common and destructive Asian liver fluke of the genus *Clonorchis* (*C. sinensis*) that invades the human liver causing clonorchiasis

Chinese restaurant syndrome *n* : a group of symptoms (as numbness of the neck, arms, and back with headache, dizziness, and palpitations) that is held to affect susceptible persons eating food and esp. Chinese food heavily seasoned with monosodium glutamate

chip–blow·er \ˈchip-ˌblō-ər\ *n* : a dental instrument typically consisting of a rubber bulb with a long metal tube that is used to blow drilling debris from a cavity being prepared for filling

chir- *or* **chiro-** *also* **cheir-** *or* **cheiro-** *comb form* : hand ⟨*chiro*practic⟩

chi·rop·o·dy \kə-ˈrä-pə-dē, shə-, kī-\ *n*, *pl* **-dies** : PODIATRY — **chi·ro·po·di·al** \ˌkī-rə-ˈpō-dē-əl\ *adj* — **chi·rop·o·dist** \kə-ˈrä-pə-dist, shə-, kī-\ *n*

chi·ro·prac·tic \ˈkī-rə-ˌprak-tik\ *n* : a system of therapy which holds that disease results from a lack of normal nerve function and which employs manipulation and specific adjustment of body structures (as the spinal column) — **chi·ro·prac·tor** \-tər\ *n*

chi·rur·gi·cal \kī-ˈrər-ji-kəl\ *adj*, *archaic* : of or relating to surgery : SURGICAL

chis·el \ˈchi-zəl\ *n* : a metal tool with a cutting edge at the end of a blade; *esp* : one used in dentistry (as for shaping enamel)

chi·tin \ˈkīt-ᵊn\ *n* : a horny polysaccharide that forms part of the hard outer integument esp. of insects, arachnids, and crustaceans — **chi·tin·ous** \ˈkītᵊn-əs\ *adj*

chla·myd·ia \klə-ˈmi-dē-ə\ *n* **1** *cap* : a genus of coccoid to spherical gram-negative intracellular bacteria (family Chlamydiaceae) including one (*C. trachomatis*) that causes or is associated with various diseases of the eye and genitourinary tract including trachoma, lymphogranuloma venereum,

cervicitis, and some forms of non-gonococcal urethritis **2** *pl* **-iae** *also* **-ias a** : a bacterium of the genus *Chlamydia* **b** : an infection or disease caused by chlamydiae — **chla·myd·ial** \-əl\ *adj*

chlo·as·ma \klō-ˈaz-mə\ *n*, *pl* **-ma·ta** \-mə-tə\ : irregular brownish or blackish spots esp. on the face that occur sometimes in pregnancy and in disorders of or functional changes in the uterus and ovaries — see LIVER SPOTS

chlor- *or* **chloro-** *comb form* **1** : green ⟨*chlor*ine⟩ ⟨*chlor*osis⟩ **2** : containing or caused by chlorine ⟨*chlor*acne⟩ ⟨*chlor*dane⟩

chloracetophenone *var of* CHLOROACETOPHENONE

chlor·ac·ne \(ˌ)klōr-ˈak-nē\ *n* : a skin eruption resembling acne and resulting from exposure to chlorine or its compounds

chlo·ral \ˈklōr-əl\ *n* : CHLORAL HYDRATE

chloral hydrate *n* : a bitter white crystalline drug $C_2H_3Cl_3O_2$ used as a hypnotic and sedative

chlo·ral·ose \ˈklōr-ə-ˌlōs, -ˌlōz\ *n* : a bitter crystalline compound $C_8H_{11}Cl_3$-O_6 used esp. to anesthetize animals — **chlo·ral·osed** \-ˌlōst, -ˌlōzd\ *adj*

chlo·ram·bu·cil \klōr-ˈam-byə-ˌsil\ *n* : an anticancer drug $C_{14}H_{19}Cl_2NO_2$ used esp. to treat leukemias, multiple myeloma, some lymphomas, and Hodgkin's disease

chlo·ra·mine \ˈklōr-ə-ˌmēn\ *n* : any of various organic compounds containing nitrogen and chlorine; *esp* : CHLORAMINE-T

chloramine–T \-ˈtē\ *n* : a white or faintly yellow crystalline compound C_7-$H_7ClNNaO_2S·3H_2O$ used as an antiseptic (as in treating wounds)

chlor·am·phen·i·col \ˌklōr-ˌam-ˈfe-ni-kȯl, -ˌkōl\ *n* : a broad-spectrum antibiotic $C_{11}H_{12}Cl_2N_2O_5$ isolated from cultures of a soil actinomycete of the genus *Streptomyces* (*S. venezuelae*) or prepared synthetically — see CHLOROMYCETIN

chlor·bu·tol \ˈklōr-byə-ˌtȯl\ *n*, *chiefly Brit* : CHLOROBUTANOL

chlor·cy·cli·zine \klōr-ˈsī-klə-ˌzēn\ *n* : a cyclic antihistamine $C_{18}H_{21}ClN_2$ administered as the hydrochloride

chlor·dane \ˈklōr-ˌdān\ *n* : a highly chlorinated viscous volatile liquid insecticide $C_{10}H_6Cl_8$

chlor·di·az·epox·ide \ˌklōr-dī-ˌa-zə-ˈpäk-ˌsīd\ *n* : a benzodiazepine $C_{16}H_{14}ClN_3O$ structurally and pharmacologically related to diazepam that is used in the form of its hydrochloride esp. as a tranquilizer and to treat the withdrawal symptoms of alcoholism — see LIBRIUM

chlor·hex·i·dine \klōr-ˈhek-sə-ˌdīn, -ˌdēn\ *n* : a biguanide derivative $C_{22}H_{30}Cl_2N_{10}$ used as a local antiseptic esp. in the form of its hydrochloride or acetate

chlo·ride \'klōr-₁īd\ n : a compound of chlorine with another element or radical; *esp* : a salt or ester of hydrochloric acid

chloride shift n : the passage of chloride ions from the plasma into the red blood cells when carbon dioxide enters the plasma from the tissues and their return to the plasma when the carbon dioxide is discharged in the lungs that is a major factor both in maintenance of blood pH and in transport of carbon dioxide

chlo·ri·nate \'klōr-ə-₁nāt\ vb **-nat·ed; -nat·ing** : to treat or cause to combine with chlorine or a chlorine compound — **chlo·ri·na·tion** \₁klōr-ə-'nā-shən\ n

chlo·rine \'klōr-₁ēn, -ən\ n : a halogen element that is isolated as a heavy greenish yellow gas of pungent odor and is used esp. as a bleach, oxidizing agent, and disinfectant in water purification — symbol *Cl*; see ELEMENT table

chlor·mer·o·drin \klōr-'mer-ə-drən\ n : a mercurial diuretic $C_5H_{11}ClHgN_2O_2$ used in the treatment of some forms of edema, ascites, and nephritis

chloro- — see CHLOR-

chlo·ro·ace·to·phe·none \₁klōr-ō-₁a-sə-(₁)tō-fə-'nōn, -ə-₁sē-\ n : a chlorine-containing compound C_8H_7ClO used esp. as a tear gas

chlo·ro·az·o·din \₁klōr-ō-'a-zəd-ᵊn\ n : a yellow crystalline compound $C_2H_4Cl_2N_6$ used in solution as a surgical antiseptic

chlo·ro·bu·ta·nol \-'byüt-ᵊn-₁ol, -₁ōl\ n : a white crystalline alcohol $C_4H_7Cl_3O$ with an odor and taste like camphor that is used as a local anesthetic, sedative, and preservative (as for hypodermic solutions)

chlo·ro·cre·sol \-'krē-₁sol, -₁sōl\ n : a chlorine derivative C_7H_7ClO of cresol used as an antiseptic and preservative

¹chlo·ro·form \'klōr-ə-₁form\ n : a colorless volatile heavy toxic liquid $CHCl_3$ with an ether odor that is used esp. as a solvent or as a veterinary anesthetic — called also *trichloromethane*

²chloroform vb : to treat with chloroform esp. so as to produce anesthesia or death

chlo·ro·gua·nide \₁klōr-ō-'gwä-₁nīd, -nəd\ n : an antimalarial drug $C_{11}H_{16}N_5Cl$ administered as the bitter crystalline hydrochloride — called also *proguanil*

chlo·ro·leu·ke·mia \-lü-'kē-mē-ə\ n : CHLOROMA 1

chlo·ro·ma \klə-'rō-mə\ n, pl **-mas** or **-ma·ta** \-mə-tə\ 1 : leukemia originating in the bone marrow and marked by the formation of growths of myeloid tissue resembling tumors beneath

the periosteum of flat bones (as the skull, ribs, or pelvis) 2 : one of the tumorous growths characteristic of chloroma

Chlo·ro·my·ce·tin \₁klōr-ō-mī-'sēt-ᵊn\ *trademark* — used for chloramphenicol

chlo·ro·phyll \'klōr-ə-₁fil, -fəl\ n 1 : the green photosynthetic coloring matter of plants 2 : a waxy green chlorophyll-containing substance extracted from green plants and used as a coloring agent or deodorant

chlo·ro·pic·rin \₁klōr-ə-'pik-rən\ n : a heavy colorless liquid CCl_3NO_2 that causes tears and vomiting and is used esp. as a soil fumigant

chlo·ro·pro·caine \₁klōr-ō-'prō-₁kān\ n : a local anesthetic $C_{13}H_{19}ClN_2O_2$ — see NESACAINE

chlo·ro·quine \'klōr-ə-₁kwēn\ n : an antimalarial drug $C_{18}H_{26}ClN_3$ administered as the bitter crystalline diphosphate

chlo·ro·sis \klə-'rō-səs\ n, pl **-ro·ses** \-₁sēz\ : an iron-deficiency anemia esp. of adolescent girls that may impart a greenish tint to the skin — called also *greensickness* — **chlo·rot·ic** \-'rä-tik\ adj

chlo·ro·thi·a·zide \₁klōr-ə-'thī-ə-₁zīd, -zəd\ n : a thiazide diuretic $C_7H_6ClN_3O_4S_2$ used esp. in the treatment of edema and hypertension — see DIURIL

chlo·ro·tri·an·i·sene \-₁trī-'a-nə-₁sēn\ n : a synthetic estrogen $C_{23}H_{21}ClO_3$ used to treat menopausal symptoms

chlor·phen·e·sin carbamate \(₁)klōr-'fen-ə-sin-\ n : a drug $C_{10}H_{12}ClNO_4$ used to relax skeletal muscle — see MAOLATE

chlor·prom·a·zine \klōr-'prä-mə-₁zēn\ n : a phenothiazine $C_{17}H_{19}ClN_2S$ used as a tranquilizer esp. in the form of its hydrochloride to suppress the more flagrant symptoms of psychotic disorders (as in schizophrenia) — see LARGACTIL, THORAZINE

chlor·prop·amide \-'prä-pə-₁mīd, -'prō-\ n : a sulfonylurea drug $C_{10}H_{13}ClN_2O_3S$ used orally to reduce blood sugar in the treatment of mild diabetes

chlor·tet·ra·cy·cline \₁klōr-₁te-trə-'sī-₁klēn\ n : a yellow crystalline broad-spectrum antibiotic $C_{22}H_{23}ClN_2O_8$ produced by a soil actinomycete of the genus *Streptomyces* (*S. aureofaciens*) and sometimes used in animal feeds to stimulate growth — see AUREOMYCIN

chlor·thal·i·done \klōr-'tha-lə-₁dōn\ n : a diuretic sulfonamide $C_{14}H_{11}ClN_2O_4S$ used esp. in the treatment of edema and hypertension — see HYGROTON

cho·a·nae \'kō-ə-₁nē\ n pl : the pair of posterior apertures of the nasal cavity that open into the nasopharynx —

called also *posterior nares* — **cho·a·nal** \-nəl\ *adj*

Cho·a·no·tae·nia \ˌkō-ə-(ˌ)nō-ˈtē-nē-ə\ *n* : a genus of tapeworms including one (*C. infundibulum*) which is an intestinal parasite of birds

¹**choke** \ˈchōk\ *vb* **choked; chok·ing 1** : to keep from breathing in a normal way by compressing or obstructing the windpipe or by poisoning or adulterating available air **2** : to have the windpipe blocked entirely or partly

²**choke** *n* **1** : the act of choking **2 chokes** *pl* : decompression sickness when marked by suffocation — used with *the*

choked disk *n* : PAPILLEDEMA

chol- *or* **chole** *or* **cholo-** *comb form* : bile : gall ⟨*cholate*⟩ ⟨*cholelith*⟩ ⟨*cholorrhea*⟩

cho·lae·mia *chiefly Brit var of* CHOLEMIA

cho·la·gogue \ˈkä-lə-ˌgäg, ˈkō-\ *n* : an agent that promotes an increased flow of bile — **cho·la·gog·ic** \ˌkä-lə-ˈgä-jik, ˌkō-\ *adj*

chol·an·gio·gram \kə-ˈlan-jē-ə-ˌgram, kō-\ *n* : a roentgenogram of the bile ducts made after the ingestion or injection of a radiopaque substance

chol·an·gi·og·ra·phy \kə-ˌlan-jē-ˈä-grə-fē, (ˌ)kō-\ *n, pl* **-phies** : radiographic visualization of the bile ducts after ingestion or injection of a radiopaque substance — **chol·an·gio·graph·ic** \-jē-ə-ˈgra-fik\ *adj*

chol·an·gi·o·li·tis \-ə-ˈlī-təs, (ˌ)kō-\ *n, pl* **-lit·i·des** \-ˈli-tə-ˌdēz\ : inflammation of bile capillaries — **chol·an·gi·o·lit·ic** \-ˈli-tik\ *adj*

chol·an·gi·tis \ˌkō-ˌlan-ˈjī-təs\ *n, pl* **-git·i·des** \-ˈji-tə-ˌdēz\ : inflammation of one or more bile ducts

cho·late \ˈkō-ˌlāt\ *n* : a salt or ester of cholic acid

chole- *see* CHOL-

cho·le·cal·cif·er·ol \ˌkō-lə-(ˌ)kal-ˈsi-fə-ˌrōl, -ˌrōl\ *n* : a sterol $C_{27}H_{43}OH$ that is a natural form of vitamin D found esp. in fish, egg yolks, and fish-liver oils and is formed in the skin on exposure to sunlight or ultraviolet rays — called also *vitamin D, vitamin D_3*

cho·le·cys·tec·to·my \ˌkō-lə-(ˌ)sis-ˈtek-tə-mē\ *n, pl* **-mies** : surgical excision of the gallbladder — **cho·le·cys·tec·to·mized** \-ˌmīzd\ *adj*

cho·le·cys·ti·tis \-(ˌ)sis-ˈtī-təs, -(ˌ)sis-\ *n, pl* **-tit·i·des** \-ˈti-tə-ˌdēz\ : inflammation of the gallbladder

cho·le·cys·to·en·ter·os·to·my \-ˌsis-tō-ˌen-tə-ˈräs-tə-mē\ *n, pl* **-mies** : surgical union of and creation of a passage between the gallbladder and the intestine

cho·le·cys·to·gram \-ˈsis-tə-ˌgram\ *n* : a roentgenogram of the gallbladder made after ingestion or injection of a radiopaque substance

cho·le·cys·tog·ra·phy \-(ˌ)sis-ˈtä-grə-fē\ *n, pl* **-phies** : the roentgenographic visualization of the gallbladder after ingestion or injection of a radiopaque substance — **cho·le·cys·to·graph·ic** \-ˌsis-tə-ˈgra-fik\ *adj*

cho·le·cys·to·ki·net·ic \-ˌsis-tə-kə-ˈne-tik, -kī-\ *adj* : tending to cause the gallbladder to contract and discharge bile

cho·le·cys·to·ki·nin \-ˌsis-tə-ˈkī-nən\ *n* : a hormone secreted esp. by the duodenal mucosa that regulates the emptying of the gallbladder and secretion of enzymes by the pancreas and that has been found in the brain — called also *cholecystokinin-pancreozymin, pancreozymin*

cho·le·cys·tor·rha·phy \-(ˌ)sis-ˈtȯr-ə-fē\ *n, pl* **-phies** : repair of the gallbladder by suturing

cho·le·cys·tos·to·my \-(ˌ)sis-ˈtäs-tə-mē\ *n, pl* **-mies** : surgical incision of the gallbladder usu. to effect drainage

cho·le·cys·tot·o·my \-ˈtä-tə-mē\ *n, pl* **-mies** : surgical incision of the gallbladder esp. for exploration or to remove a gallstone

cho·le·doch·al \ˈkō-lə-ˌdä-kəl, kə-ˈle-də-kəl\ *adj* : relating to, being, or occurring in the common bile duct

cho·le·do·chi·tis \kə-ˌle-də-ˈkī-təs, ˌkō-lə-\ *n* : inflammation of the common bile duct

cho·led·o·cho·je·ju·nos·to·my \kə-ˌle-də-(ˌ)kō-ji-(ˌ)jü-ˈnäs-tə-mē\ *n, pl* **-mies** : surgical creation of a passage uniting the common bile duct and the jejunum

cho·led·o·cho·li·thi·a·sis \-li-ˈthī-ə-səs\ *n, pl* **-a·ses** \-ˌsēz\ : a condition marked by presence of calculi in the gallbladder and common bile duct

cho·led·o·cho·li·thot·o·my \-li-ˈthä-tə-mē\ *n, pl* **-mies** : surgical incision of the common bile duct for removal of a gallstone

cho·led·o·chor·ra·phy \kə-ˌle-də-ˈkȯr-ə-fē\ *n, pl* **-ra·phies** : surgical union of the separated ends of the common bile duct by suturing

cho·led·o·chos·to·my \-ˈkäs-tə-mē\ *n, pl* **-mies** : surgical incision of the common bile duct usu. to effect drainage

cho·led·o·chot·o·my \-ˈkä-tə-mē\ *n, pl* **-mies** : surgical incision of the common bile duct

cho·led·o·chus \kə-ˈle-də-kəs\ *n, pl* **-o·chi** \-ˌkī, -ˌkē\ : COMMON BILE DUCT

cho·le·glo·bin \ˈkō-lə-ˌglō-bən, ˈkä-\ *n* : a green pigment that occurs in bile and is formed by breakdown of hemoglobin

cho·le·lith \ˈkō-li-ˌlith, ˈkä-\ *n* : GALLSTONE

cho·le·li·thi·a·sis \ˌkō-li-li-ˈthī-ə-səs\ *n, pl* **-a·ses** \-ˌsēz\ : production of gallstones ; *also* : the resulting abnormal condition

cho·le·mia \kō-ˈlē-mē-ə\ *n* : the presence of excess bile in the blood usu. indicative of liver disease — **cho·le·mic** \-mik\ *adj*

cho·le·poi·e·sis \ˌkō-lə-ˌpȯi-ˈē-səs, ˌkä-\ n, pl **-e·ses** \-ˌsēz\ : production of bile — compare CHOLERESIS — **cho·le·poi·et·ic** \-ˈe-tik\ adj

chol·era \ˈkä-lə-rə\ n : any of several diseases of humans and domestic animals usu. marked by severe gastrointestinal symptoms: as **a** : an acute diarrheal disease caused by an enterotoxin produced by a comma-shaped gram-negative bacillus of the genus *Vibrio* (*V. cholerae* syn. *V. comma*) when it is present in large numbers in the proximal part of the human small intestine — see ASIATIC CHOLERA **b** : FOWL CHOLERA **c** : HOG CHOLERA — **chol·e·ra·ic** \ˌkä-lə-ˈrā-ik\ adj

cholera mor·bus \-ˈmȯr-bəs\ n : a gastrointestinal disturbance characterized by griping, diarrhea, and sometimes vomiting — not used technically

cho·le·re·sis \ˌkō-lə-ˈrē-səs, ˌkä-\ n, pl **-re·ses** \-ˌsēz\ : the flow of bile from the liver esp. when increased above a previous or normal level — compare CHOLAGOGUE, CHOLEPOIESIS, HYDROCHOLERESIS

¹**cho·le·ret·ic** \ˌkō-lə-ˈre-tik, ˌkä-\ adj : promoting bile secretion by the liver (~ action of bile salts)

²**choleretic** n : a choleretic agent

cho·le·sta·sis \ˌkō-lə-ˈstā-səs, ˌkä-\ n, pl **-sta·ses** \-ˈstā-ˌsēz\ : a checking or failure of bile flow — **cho·le·stat·ic** \-ˈsta-tik\ adj

cho·les·te·a·to·ma \kə-ˌles-tē-ə-ˈtō-mə, ˌkō-lə-ˌstē-, ˌkä-lə-\ n, pl **-mas** or **-ma·ta** \-mə-tə\ **1** : an epidermoid cyst usu. in the brain appearing as a compact shiny flaky mass **2** : a tumor usu. growing in a confined space (as the middle ear) and frequently constituting a sequel to chronic otitis media — **cho·les·te·a·to·ma·tous** \-mə-təs\ adj

cho·les·ter·ol \kə-ˈles-tə-ˌrȯl, -ˌrōl\ n : a steroid alcohol $C_{27}H_{45}OH$ present in animal cells and body fluids that regulates membrane fluidity, functions as a precursor molecule in various metabolic pathways, and as a constituent of LDL may cause arteriosclerosis — **cho·les·ter·ic** \ˈles-tə-rik; ˌkō-lə-ˈster-ik, ˌkä-\ adj

cho·les·ter·ol·ae·mia also **cho·les·te·rae·mia** chiefly Brit var of CHOLESTEROLEMIA

cho·les·ter·ol·emia \kə-ˌles-tə-rə-ˈlē-mē-ə\ also **cho·les·ter·emia** \-ˈrē-mē-ə\ n : the presence of cholesterol in the blood

cho·les·ter·ol·osis \kə-ˌles-tə-rə-ˈlō-səs\ or **cho·les·ter·osis** \kə-ˌles-tə-ˈrō-səs\ n, pl **-oses** \-ˌsēz\ : abnormal deposition of cholesterol (as in blood vessels)

cho·les·tyr·amine \kō-ˈles-tir-ə-ˌmēn\ n : a strongly basic synthetic resin used to lower cholesterol levels in hypercholesterolemic patients

cho·lic acid \ˈkō-lik-\ n : a crystalline bile acid $C_{24}H_{40}O_5$

cho·line \ˈkō-ˌlēn\ n : a base $C_5H_{15}NO_2$ that occurs as a component of phospholipids esp. in animals, is a precursor of acetylcholine, and is essential to liver function

cho·lin·er·gic \ˌkō-lə-ˈnər-jik\ adj **1** of autonomic nerve fibers : liberating, activated by, or involving acetylcholine — compare ADRENERGIC 1, NORADRENERGIC **2** : resembling acetylcholine esp. in physiologic action — **cho·lin·er·gi·cal·ly** \-ji-k(ə-)lē\ adv

cho·lin·es·ter·ase \ˌkō-lə-ˈnes-tə-ˌrās, -ˌrāz\ n **1** : ACETYLCHOLINESTERASE **2** : an enzyme that hydrolyzes choline esters and that is found esp. in blood plasma — called also *pseudocholinesterase*

¹**cho·li·no·lyt·ic** \ˌkō-lə-nō-ˈli-tik\ adj : interfering with the action of acetylcholine or cholinergic agents

²**cholinolytic** n : a cholinolytic substance

¹**cho·li·no·mi·met·ic** \ˌkō-lə-nō-mə-ˈme-tik, -ˌkä-, -mī-\ adj : resembling acetylcholine or simulating its physiologic action

²**cholinomimetic** n : a cholinomimetic substance

cholo- — see CHOL-

cho·lor·rhea \ˌkä-lə-ˈrē-ə, ˌkō-\ n : excessive secretion of bile

cho·lor·rhoea chiefly Brit var of CHOLORRHEA

chol·uria \kō-ˈlu̇r-ē-ə, kōl-ˈyu̇r-\ n : presence of bile in urine

chondr- or **chondri-** or **chondro-** comb form : cartilage (*chondral*) (*chondrodysplasia*)

chon·dral \ˈkän-drəl\ adj : of or relating to cartilage

chon·dri·tis \kän-ˈdrī-təs\ n : inflammation of cartilage

chon·dro·blast \ˈkän-drə-ˌblast, -drō-\ n : a cell that produces cartilage — **chon·dro·blas·tic** \ˌkän-drə-ˈblas-tik, -drō-\ adj

chon·dro·clast \ˈkän-drə-ˌklast, -drō-\ n : a cell that absorbs cartilage — compare OSTEOCLAST 1

chon·dro·cos·tal \ˌkän-drə-ˈkäst-ᵊl, -drō-\ adj : of or relating to the costal cartilages and the ribs

chon·dro·cyte \ˈkän-drə-ˌsīt, -drō-\ n : a cartilage cell

chon·dro·dys·pla·sia \ˌkän-drə-dis-ˈplā-zhə, -drō-, -zhē-ə\ n : a hereditary skeletal disorder characterized by the formation of exostoses at the epiphyses and resulting in arrested development and deformity — called also *dyschondroplasia*

chon·dro·dys·tro·phia \-dis-ˈtrō-fē-ə\ n : ACHONDROPLASIA

chon·dro·dys·tro·phy \-ˈdis-trə-fē\ n, pl **-phies** : ACHONDROPLASIA — **chon·dro·dys·tro·phic** \-dis-ˈtrō-fik\ adj

chon·dro·gen·e·sis \-ˈje-nə-səs\ n, pl **-e·ses** \-ˌsēz\ : the development of cartilage — **chon·dro·gen·ic** \-ˈje-nik\ adj

chon·droid \'kän-ˌdrȯid\ *adj* : resembling cartilage

chon·droi·tin \kän-'drȯit-ᵊn, -'drō-ət-ᵊn\ *n* : any of several glycosaminoglycans occurring in sulfated form in various tissues (as cartilage and tendons)

chon·drol·o·gy \kän-'drä-lə-jē\ *n, pl* **-gies** : a branch of anatomy concerned with cartilage

chon·dro·ma \kän-'drō-mə\ *n, pl* **-mas** \-məz\ *also* **-ma·ta** \-mə-tə\ : a benign tumor containing the structural elements of cartilage — compare CHONDROSARCOMA — **chon·dro·ma·tous** \(')kän-'drä-mə-təs, -'drō-\ *adj*

chon·dro·ma·la·cia \ˌkän-drō-mə-'lā-shə, -shē-ə\ *n* : abnormal softness of cartilage

chon·dro·os·teo·dys·tro·phy \-ˌäs-tē-ō-'dis-trə-fē\ *n, pl* **-phies** : any of several mucopolysaccharidoses (as Hurler's syndrome) characterized esp. by disorders of bone and cartilage

chon·dro·phyte \'kän-drō-ˌfīt\ *n* : an outgrowth or spur of cartilage

chon·dro·sar·co·ma \ˌkän-drō-sär-'kō-mə\ *n, pl* **-mas** *or* **-ma·ta** \-mə-tə\ : a sarcoma containing cartilage cells

chon·dro·ster·nal \ˌkän-drō-'stərn-ᵊl\ *adj* : of or relating to the costal cartilages and sternum

Cho·part's joint \(ˌ)shō-'pärz-\ *n* : the tarsal joint that comprises the talonavicular and calcaneocuboid articulations

    Cho·part \shō-pár\, **François (1743–1795)**, French surgeon.

chor·da ten·din·ea \ˌkȯr-də-ˌten-'di-nē-ə\ *n, pl* **chor·dae ten·din·e·ae** \-nē-ˌē\ : any of the delicate tendinous cords that are attached to the edges of the atrioventricular valves of the heart and to the papillary muscles and serve to prevent the valves from being pushed into the atrium during the ventricular contraction

chorda tym·pa·ni \-'tim-pə-ˌnī\ *n* : a branch of the facial nerve that traverses the middle ear cavity and the inframpetoral fossa and supplies autonomic fibers to the sublingual and submandibular glands and sensory fibers to the anterior part of the tongue

chor·dee \'kȯr-ˌdē, -ˌdā, ˌkȯr-'\ *n* : painful erection of the penis often with a downward curvature that may be present in a congenital condition (as hypospadias) or accompany gonorrhea

chor·do·ma \kȯr-'dō-mə\ *n, pl* **-mas** *or* **-ma·ta** \-mə-tə\ : a malignant tumor that is derived from remnants of the embryonic notochord and occurs along the spine

chor·dot·o·my *var of* CORDOTOMY

cho·rea \kə-'rē-ə\ *n* : any of various nervous disorders of infectious or organic origin marked by spasmodic movements of the limbs and facial muscles and by incoordination —

called also *Saint Vitus' dance*; see HUNTINGTON'S DISEASE, SYDENHAM'S CHOREA — **cho·re·at·ic** \ˌkȯr-ē-'a-tik\ *adj* — **cho·re·ic** \kə-'rē-ik\ *adj*

cho·re·i·form \kə-'rē-ə-ˌfȯrm\ *adj* : resembling chorea (∼ convulsions)

cho·reo·ath·e·to·sis \-ˌa-thə-'tō-səs\ *n, pl* **-to·ses** \-ˌsēz\ : a nervous disturbance marked by the involuntary movements characteristic of chorea and athetosis

cho·rio·al·lan·to·is \ˌkȯr-ē-ō-ə-'lan-tə-wəs\ *n, pl* **-to·ides** \-ō-ˌa-lən-'tō-ə-ˌdēz, -ˌlan-\ : a vascular fetal membrane composed of the fused chorion and adjacent wall of the allantois — called also *chorioallantoic membrane* — **cho·rio·al·lan·to·ic** \-ˌa-lən-'tō-ik\ *adj*

cho·rio·am·ni·o·ni·tis \-ˌam-nē-ō-'nī-təs\ *n* : inflammation of the fetal membranes

cho·rio·cap·il·lar·is \-ˌka-pə-'lar-əs\ *n* : the inner of the two vascular layers of the choroid of the eye that is composed largely of capillaries

cho·rio·car·ci·no·ma \-ˌkärs-ᵊn-'ō-mə\ *n, pl* **-mas** *or* **-ma·ta** \-mə-tə\ : a malignant tumor developing in the uterus from the trophoblast and rarely in the testes from a neoplasm

cho·rio·ep·i·the·li·o·ma \-ˌe-pə-ˌthē-lē-'ō-mə\ *n, pl* **-mas** *or* **-ma·ta** \-mə-tə\ : CHORIOCARCINOMA

cho·rio·id·itis \ˌkȯr-ē-ˌȯi-'dī-təs\ *var of* CHOROIDITIS

cho·ri·o·ma \ˌkȯr-ē-'ō-mə\ *n, pl* **-mas** *or* **-ma·ta** \-mə-tə\ : a tumor formed of chorionic tissue

cho·rio·men·in·gi·tis \ˌkȯr-ē-(ˌ)ō-ˌme-nən-'ji-təs\ *n, pl* **-git·i·des** \-'ji-tə-ˌdēz\ : cerebral meningitis; *specif* : LYMPHOCYTIC CHORIOMENINGITIS

cho·ri·on \'kȯr-ē-ˌän\ *n* : the highly vascular outer embryonic membrane that is associated with the allantois in the formation of the placenta

cho·ri·on·ep·i·the·li·o·ma \ˌkȯr-ē-ˌä-ne-pə-ˌthē-lē-'ō-mə\ *n, pl* **-omas** *or* **-o·ma·ta** \-mə-tə\ : CHORIOCARCINOMA

chorion fron·do·sum \-frän-'dō-səm\ *n* : the part of the chorion that has persistent villi and that with the decidua basalis forms the placenta — see CHORIONIC VILLUS SAMPLING

cho·ri·on·ic \ˌkȯr-ē-'ä-nik\ *adj* **1** : of, relating to, or being part of the chorion ⟨∼ villi⟩ **2** : secreted or produced by chorionic or a related tissue (as in the placenta or a choriocarcinoma) ⟨human ∼ gonadotropin⟩

chorionic villus sampling *also* **chorionic villi sampling** *n* : biopsy of the chorion frondosum through the abdominal wall or by way of the vagina and uterine cervix at nine to 12 weeks of gestation to obtain fetal cells for the prenatal diagnosis of genetic disorder — abbr. *CVS*

Cho·ri·op·tes \ˌkȯr-ē-'äp-ˌtēz\ *n* : a genus of small parasitic mites infesting domestic animals — **cho·ri·op·tic** \-'äp-tik\ *adj*

chorioptic mange *n* : mange caused by mites of the genus *Chorioptes* that usu. attack only the surface of the skin — compare DEMODECTIC MANGE, SARCOPTIC MANGE

cho·rio·ret·i·nal \ˌkōr-ē-ō-'ret-ᵊn-əl\ *adj* : of, relating to, or affecting the choroid and the retina of the eye (∼ burns) (∼ lesions)

cho·rio·ret·i·ni·tis \-ˌret-ᵊn-'ī-təs\ *n, pl* **-nit·i·des** \-'i-tə-ˌdēz\ : inflammation of the retina and choroid of the eye

cho·roid \'kōr-ˌoid\ *n* : a vascular membrane containing large branched pigment cells that lies between the retina and the sclera of the eye — called also *choroid coat* — **choroid** or **cho·roi·dal** \kə-'roid-ᵊl\ *adj*

choroidea — see TELA CHOROIDEA

cho·roi·de·re·mia \ˌkōr-ˌoi-də-'rē-mē-ə\ *n* : progressive degeneration of the choroid

cho·roid·i·tis \ˌkōr-ˌoi-'dī-təs\ *n* : inflammation of the choroid of the eye

cho·roi·do·iri·tis \kə-ˌroi-dō-ī-'rī-təs\ : inflammation of the choroid and iris of the eye

cho·roid·op·a·thy \ˌkōr-ˌoi-'dä-pə-thē\ *n, pl* **-thies** : a diseased condition affecting the choroid of the eye

cho·roi·do·ret·i·ni·tis \kə-ˌroi-dō-ˌret-ᵊn-'ī-təs\ *var of* CHORIORETINITIS

choroid plexus *n* : a highly vascular portion of the pia mater that projects into the ventricles of the brain and is thought to secrete the cerebrospinal fluid

Christ·mas disease \'kris-məs-\ *n* : a hereditary sex-linked hemorrhagic disease involving absence of a coagulation factor in the blood and failure of the clotting mechanism — called also *hemophilia B;* compare HEMOPHILIA

Christmas, Stephen, British child patient.

Christmas factor *n* : FACTOR IX

chrom·aes·the·sia *chiefly Brit var of* CHROMESTHESIA

chro·maf·fin \'krō-mə-fən\ *adj* : staining deeply with chromium salts

chro·maf·fi·no·ma \ˌkrō-mə-fə-'nō-mə, krō-ˌma-\ *n, pl* **-mas** *or* **-ma·ta** \-mə-tə\ : a tumor containing chromaffin cells; *esp* : PHEOCHROMOCYTOMA

chro·ma·phil \'krō-mə-ˌfil\ *adj* : CHROMAFFIN (∼ tissue)

chromat- *or* **chromato-** *comb form* **1** : color (*chromat*id) **2** : chromatin (*chromato*lysis)

chro·mat·ic \krō-'ma-tik\ *adj* **1** : of, relating to, or characterized by color or color phenomena or sensations (∼ stimuli) **2** : capable of being colored by staining agents (∼ substances)

chromatic vision *n* **1** : normal color vision in which the colors of the spectrum are distinguished and evaluated **2** : CHROMATOPSIA

chro·ma·tid \'krō-mə-təd\ *n* : one of the usu. paired and parallel strands of a duplicated chromosome joined by a single centromere — see CHROMONEMA

chro·ma·tin \'krō-mə-tən\ *n* : a complex of a nucleic acid with basic proteins (as histone) in eukaryotic cells that is usu. dispersed in the interphase nucleus and condensed into chromosomes in mitosis and meiosis — **chro·ma·tin·ic** \ˌkrō-mə-'tin-ik\ *adj*

chro·ma·tism \'krō-mə-ˌti-zəm\ *n* : CHROMESTHESIA

chromato- — see CHROMAT-

chro·ma·to·gram \krō-'ma-tə-ˌgram, krə-\ *n* : the pattern formed on the adsorbent medium by the layers of components separated by chromatography

chro·ma·to·graph \krō-'ma-tə-ˌgraf, krə-\ *n* : an instrument for producing chromatograms — **chromatograph** *vb*

chro·ma·tog·ra·phy \ˌkrō-mə-'tä-grə-fē\ *n, pl* **-phies** : a process in which a chemical mixture carried by a liquid or gas is separated into components as a result of differential distribution of the solutes as they flow around or over a stationary liquid or solid phase — **chro·ma·to·graph·ic** \krō-ˌma-tə-'gra-fik, krə-\ *adj* — **chro·ma·to·graph·i·cal·ly** \-fi-k(ə-)lē\ *adv*

chro·ma·tol·y·sis \ˌkrō-mə-'tä-lə-səs\ *n, pl* **-y·ses** \-ˌsēz\ : the dissolution and breaking up of chromophil material (as chromatin) of a cell — **chro·ma·to·lyt·ic** \krō-ˌmat-ᵊl-'i-tik, krə-\ *adj*

chro·ma·to·phore \krō-'mat-ə-ˌfōr, krə-\ *n* : a pigment-bearing cell esp. in the skin

chro·ma·top·sia \ˌkrō-mə-'täp-sē-ə\ *n* : a disturbance of vision which is sometimes caused by drugs and in which colorless objects appear colored

chro·ma·to·sis \ˌkrō-mə-'tō-səs\ *n, pl* **-to·ses** \-ˌsēz\ : PIGMENTATION; *specif* : deposit of pigment in a normally unpigmented area or excessive pigmentation in a normally pigmented site

chrom·es·the·sia \ˌkrō-mes-'thē-zhə, -zhē-ə\ *n* : synesthesia in which color is perceived in response to stimuli (as words or numbers) that contain no element of color — called also *chromatism*

chrom·hi·dro·sis \ˌkrōm-hī-'drō-səs\ *var of* CHROMIDROSIS

chro·mid·i·al substance \krō-'mi-dē-əl-\ *n* : NISSL STANCE

chro·mi·dro·sis \ˌkrō-mə-'drō-səs\ *n, pl* **-dro·ses** \-ˌsēz\ : secretion of colored sweat

chro·mi·um \'krō-mē-əm\ *n* : a blue= white metallic element found naturally only in combination — symbol *Cr;* see ELEMENT table

chro·mo·blas·to·my·co·sis \ˌkrō-mə-ˌblas-tə-ˌmī-'kō-səs\ *n, pl* **-co·ses** \-ˌsēz\ : a skin disease that is caused by any of several pigmented fungi (esp. genera *Phialophora*, *Cladosporium*, and *Fonsecaea*) and is marked by the formation of warty colored nodules usu. on the legs — called also *chromomycosis*

¹**chro·mo·mere** \'krō-mə-₁mir\ *n* : the highly refractile portion of a thrombocyte or blood platelet — compare HYALOMERE

²**chromomere** *n* : one of the small bead= shaped and heavily staining concentrations of chromatin that are linearly arranged along the chromosome —
chro·mo·mer·ic \₁krō-mə-'mer-ik, -'mir-\ *adj*

chro·mo·my·co·sis \₁krō-mə-₁mī-'kō-səs\, *n, pl* **-co·ses** \-₁sēz\ : CHROMOBLASTOMYCOSIS

chro·mo·ne·ma \₁krō-mə-'nē-mə\ *n, pl* **-ne·ma·ta** \-'nē-mə-tə\ : the coiled filamentous core of a chromatid — **chro·mo·ne·mat·ic** \-ni-'ma-tik\ *adj*

chro·mo·phil \'krō-mə-₁fil\ *adj* : staining readily with dyes

¹**chro·mo·phobe** \'krō-mə-₁fōb\ *adj* : not readily absorbing stains : difficult to stain ⟨~ tumors⟩

²**chromophobe** *n* : a chromophobe cell esp. of the pituitary gland

chro·mo·pro·tein \₁kro-mə-'prō-₁tēn\ *n* : any of various proteins (as hemoglobins, carotenoids, or flavoproteins) having a pigment as a prosthetic group

chro·mo·some \'krō-mə-₁sōm, -₁zōm\ *n* : one of the linear or sometimes circular basophilic bodies of viruses, prokaryotic organisms, and the cell nucleus of eukaryotic organisms that contain most or all of the genes of the individual — **chro·mo·som·al** \₁krō-mə-'sō-məl, -'zō-\ *adj* — **chro·mo·som·al·ly** *adv*

chromosome complement *n* : the entire group of chromosomes in a nucleus

chromosome number *n* : the usu. constant number of chromosomes characteristic of a particular kind of animal or plant

chron·ax·ie *or* **chron·axy** \'krō-₁nak-sē, 'krä-\ *n, pl* **-ax·ies** : the minimum time required for excitation of a structure (as a nerve cell) by a constant electric current of twice the threshold voltage

¹**chron·ic** \'krä-nik\ *also* **chron·i·cal** \-ni-kəl\ *adj* **1 a** : marked by long duration, by frequent recurrence over a long time, and often by slowly progressing seriousness : not acute ⟨~ indigestion⟩ **b** : suffering from a disease or ailment of long duration or frequent recurrence ⟨~ arthritic⟩ **2** : having a slow progressive course of indefinite duration — used esp. of degenerative invasive diseases, some infections, psychoses, inflammations, and the carrier state ⟨~ heart disease⟩ ⟨~ arthritis⟩ — compare ACUTE 2b — **chron·i·cal·ly** \-ni-k(ə-)lē\ *adv* — **chro·nic·i·ty** \krä-'ni-sə-tē, krō-\ *n*

²**chronic** *n* : one that suffers from a chronic disease

chronica — see ACRODERMATITIS CHRONICA ATROPHICANS

chronic alcoholism *n* : ALCOHOLISM 2b

chronic fatigue syndrome *n* : a group of symptoms of unknown cause including fatigue, cognitive dysfunction, and sometimes fever and lymphadenopathy that affect esp. young adults between the ages of 20 and 40 — called also *yuppie flu*

chronicum — see ERYTHEMA CHRONICUM MIGRANS

chronicus — see LICHEN SIMPLEX CHRONICUS

chro·no·bi·ol·o·gy \₁krä-nə-bī-'ä-lə-jē, ₁krō-\ *n, pl* **-gies** : the study of biological rhythms — **chro·no·bi·o·log·ic** \-₁bī-ə-'lä-jik\ *or* **chro·no·bi·o·log·i·cal** \-ji-kəl\ *adj* — **chro·no·bi·ol·o·gist** \-'ä-lə-jist\ *n*

chro·no·log·i·cal age \₁krän-ᵊl-'ä-ji-kəl-, ₁krōn-\ *n* : the age of a person as measured from birth to a given date — compare ACHIEVEMENT AGE

chro·no·ther·a·py \₁krä-nə-'ther-ə-pē, ₁krō-\ *n, pl* **-pies** : treatment of a sleep disorder (as insomnia) by changing sleeping and waking times in an attempt to reset the patient's biological clock

chro·no·trop·ic \-'trä-pik\ *adj* : influencing the rate esp. of the heartbeat

chro·not·ro·pism \krə-'nä-trə-₁pi-zəm\ *n* : interference with the rate of the heartbeat

chrys·a·ro·bin \₁kri-sə-'rō-bən\ *n* : a powder derived from the wood of a tropical tree (*Andira araroba*) of the legume family (Leguminosae) that is used to treat skin diseases

chrys·i·a·sis \krə-'sī-ə-səs\ *n, pl* **-a·ses** \-₁sēz\ : an ash-gray or mauve pigmentation of the skin due to deposition of gold in the tissues

Chrys·ops \'kri-₁säps\ *n* : a genus of small horseflies (family Tabanidae) of which the American deerflies in certain areas transmit tularemia while the African mango flies are vectors of the eye worm (*Loa loa*)

chrys·o·ther·a·py \₁kri-sə-'ther-ə-pē\ *n, pl* **-pies** : treatment (as of arthritis) by injection of gold salts

Chvos·tek's sign \'vȯs-₁teks-, 'kvȯs-\ *or* **Chvos·tek sign** \-₁tek-\ *n* : a twitch of the facial muscles following gentle tapping over the facial nerve in front of the ear that indicates hyperirritability of the facial nerve

Chvostek, Franz (1835–1884), Austrian surgeon.

chyl- *or* **chyli-** *or* **chylo-** *comb form* : chyle ⟨*chyluria*⟩ ⟨*chylothorax*⟩

chyle \'kīl\ *n* : lymph that is milky from emulsified fats, is characteristically present in the lacteals, and is most apparent during intestinal absorption of fats

chyli — see CISTERNA CHYLI

-chylia *n comb form* : condition of having (such) chyle ⟨a*chylia*⟩

chy·lo·mi·cron \ˌkī-lō-ˈmī-ˌkrän\ *n* : a microscopic lipid particle common in the blood during fat digestion and assimilation

chy·lo·mi·cro·nae·mia *chiefly Brit var of* CHYLOMICRONEMIA

chy·lo·mi·cro·ne·mia \-ˌmī-krə-ˈnē-mē-ə\ *n* : an excessive number of chylomicrons in the blood ⟨postprandial ∼⟩

chy·lo·tho·rax \-ˈthōr-ˌaks\ *n, pl* **-rax·es** *or* **-ra·ces** \-ˈthōr-ə-ˌsēz\ : an effusion of chyle or chylous fluid into the thoracic cavity

chy·lous \ˈkī-ləs\ *adj* : consisting of or like chyle ⟨∼ ascites⟩

chy·lu·ria \kī-ˈlür-ē-ə, kīl-ˈyür-\ *n* : the presence of chyle in the urine as a result of organic disease (as of the kidney) or of mechanical lymphatic esp. parasitic obstruction

chyme \ˈkīm\ *n* : the semifluid mass of partly digested food expelled by the stomach into the duodenum — **chy·mous** \ˈkī-məs\ *adj*

chy·mo·pa·pa·in \ˌkī-mō-pə-ˈpā-ən, -ˈpī-ən\ *n* : a proteolytic enzyme from the latex of the papaya that is used in meat tenderizer and has been used medically in chemonucleolysis

chy·mo·tryp·sin \ˌkī-mō-ˈtrip-sən\ *n* : a protease that hydrolyzes peptide bonds and is formed in the intestine from chymotrypsinogen — **chy·mo·tryp·tic** \-ˈtrip-tik\ *adj*

chy·mo·tryp·sin·o·gen \-ˌtrip-ˈsi-nə-jən\ *n* : a zymogen that is secreted by the pancreas and is converted by trypsin to chymotrypsin

ci·ca·trix \ˈsi-kə-ˌtriks, sə-ˈkā-triks\ *n, pl* **ci·ca·tri·ces** \ˌsi-kə-ˈtrī-(ˌ)sēz, sə-ˈkā-trə-ˌsēz\ : a scar resulting from formation and contraction of fibrous tissue in a flesh wound — **ci·ca·tri·cial** \ˌsi-kə-ˈtri-shəl\ *adj*

cic·a·tri·zant \ˌsi-kə-ˈtrīz-ᵊnt\ *adj* : promoting the healing of a wound or the formation of a cicatrix

cic·a·tri·za·tion \ˌsi-kə-trə-ˈzā-shən\ *n* : scar formation at the site of a healing wound — **cic·a·trize** \ˈsi-kə-ˌtrīz\ *vb*

CICU *abbr* coronary intensive care unit

cic·u·tox·in \ˌsi-kyə-ˈtäk-sən, ˈsi-kyə-ˌ\ *n* : an amorphous poisonous principle $C_{19}H_{26}O_3$ in water hemlock, spotted cowbane, and related plants (genus *Cicuta*)

cigarette drain *n* : a cigarette-shaped gauze wick enclosed in rubber dam tissue or rubber tubing for draining wounds — called also *Penrose drain*

ci·gua·te·ra \ˌsē-gwə-ˈter-ə, ˌsi-\ *n* : poisoning caused by the ingestion of various normally edible tropical fish in whose flesh a toxic substance has accumulated

ci·gua·tox·in \ˈsē-gwə-ˌtäk-sən, ˈsi-\ *n* : a potent lipid neurotoxin associated

with ciguatera that has been found widely in normally edible fish

cil·ia *pl of* CILIUM

ciliaris — *see* ORBICULARIS CILIARIS, ZONULA CILIARIS

cil·i·ary \ˈsi-lē-ˌer-ē\ *adj* **1** : of or relating to cilia **2** : of, relating to, or being the annular suspension of the lens of the eye

ciliary artery *n* : any of several arteries that arise from the ophthalmic artery or its branches and supply various parts of the eye — *see* LONG POSTERIOR CILIARY ARTERY, SHORT POSTERIOR CILIARY ARTERY

ciliary body *n* : an annular structure on the inner surface of the anterior wall of the eyeball composed largely of the ciliary muscle and bearing the ciliary processes

ciliary ganglion *n* : a small autonomic ganglion on the nasociliary branch of the ophthalmic nerve receiving preganglionic fibers from the oculomotor nerve and sending postganglionic fibers to the ciliary muscle and to the sphincter pupillae

ciliary muscle *n* : a circular band of smooth muscle fibers situated in the ciliary body and serving as the chief agent in accommodation when it contracts by drawing the ciliary processes centripetally and relaxing the suspensory ligament of the lens so that the lens is permitted to become more convex

ciliary nerve — *see* LONG CILIARY NERVE, SHORT CILIARY NERVE

ciliary process *n* : any of the vascular folds on the inner surface of the ciliary body that give attachment to the suspensory ligament of the lens

ciliary ring *n* : ORBICULUS CILIARIS

cil·i·ate \ˈsi-lē-ət, -ˌāt\ *n* : any of a phylum or subphylum (Ciliophora) of ciliate protozoans

cil·i·at·ed \ˈsi-lē-ˌā-təd\ *or* **ciliate** *adj* : provided with cilia ⟨*ciliated* epithelium⟩ ⟨the *ciliate* protozoans⟩

cil·io·ret·i·nal \ˌsi-lē-ō-ˈret-ᵊn-əl\ *adj* : of, relating to, or supplying the part of the eye including the ciliary body and the retina

cil·i·um \ˈsi-lē-əm\ *n, pl* **-ia** \-ə\ **1** : EYELASH **2** : a minute short hairlike process often forming part of a fringe; *esp* : one of a cell that in free unicellular organisms produces locomotion or in higher forms a current of fluid

ci·met·i·dine \sī-ˈme-tə-ˌdēn\ *n* : a histamine analog $C_{10}H_{16}N_6S$ used in the treatment of duodenal ulcers and pathological hypersecretory disorders — *see* TAGAMET

ci·mex \ˈsī-ˌmeks\ *n* **1** *pl* **ci·mi·ces** \ˈsī-mə-ˌsēz, ˈsi-\ : BEDBUG **2** *cap* : a genus of bloodsucking bugs (family Cimicidae) that includes the common bedbug

cin- *or* **cino-** — *see* KIN-

cin·cho·caine \'siŋ-kə-ˌkān, 'sin-\ *n*, *chiefly Brit* : DIBUCAINE

cin·cho·na \siŋ-'kō-nə, sin-'chō-\ *n* : the dried bark of any of several trees (genus *Cinchona* of the family Rubiaceae and esp. *C. ledgeriana* and *C. succirubra*) containing alkaloids (as quinine) used esp. formerly as a specific in malaria, an antipyretic in other fevers, and a tonic and stomachic — called also *cinchona bark*

Chin·chón \chin-'chōn\, **Countess of (Doña Francisca Henriquez de Ribera),** Peruvian noblewoman.

cin·cho·nism \'siŋ-kə-ˌni-zəm, 'sin-chə-\ *n* : a disorder due to excessive or prolonged use of cinchona or its alkaloids and marked by temporary deafness, ringing in the ears, headache, dizziness, and rash

cine·an·gio·car·di·og·ra·phy \ˌsi-nē-ˌan-jē-ō-ˌkär-dē-'ä-grə-fē\ *n*, *pl* **-phies** : motion-picture photography of a fluoroscopic screen recording passage of a contrasting medium through the chambers of the heart and large blood vessels — **cine·an·gio·car·di·o·graph·ic** \-ˌkär-dē-ə-'gra-fik\ *adj*

cine·an·gi·og·ra·phy \-ˌan-jē-'ä-grə-fē\ *n*, *pl* **-phies** : motion-picture photography of a fluorescent screen recording passage of a contrasting medium through the blood vessels — **cine·an·gio·graph·ic** \-jē-ō-'gra-fik\ *adj*

cine·flu·o·rog·ra·phy \-ˌflur-'ä-grə-fē\ *n*, *pl* **-phies** : the process of making motion pictures of images of objects by means of X rays with the aid of a fluorescent screen (as for revealing the motions of organs in the body) — compare CINERADIOGRAPHY — **cine·flu·o·ro·graph·ic** \-ˌflur-ə-'gra-fik\ *adj*

cin·e·ole \'si-nē-ˌōl\ *n* : EUCALYPTOL

cin·e·plas·ty \'si-nə-ˌplas-tē\ *n*, *pl* **-ties 1** : surgical fitting of a lever to a muscle in an amputation stump to facilitate the operation of an artificial hand **2** : surgical isolation of a loop of muscle of chest or arm, covering it with skin, and attaching to it a prosthetic device to be operated by contraction of the muscle in the loop — **cin·e·plas·tic** \ˌsi-nə-'plas-tik\ *adj*

cine·ra·di·og·ra·phy \ˌsi-nē-ˌrā-dē-'ä-grə-fē\ *n*, *pl* **-phies** : the process of making radiographs of moving objects (as the heart or joints) in sufficiently rapid sequence so that the radiographs or copies made from them may be projected as motion pictures — compare CINEFLUOROGRAPHY — **cine·ra·dio·graph·ic** \-ˌrä-dē-ō-'gra-fik\ *adj*

ci·ne·rea \sə-'nir-ē-ə\ *n* : the gray matter of nerve tissue

cinereum — see TUBER CINEREUM

cine·roent·gen·og·ra·phy \ˌsi-nē-ˌrent-gən-'ä-grə-fē\ *n*, *pl* **-phies** : CINERADIOGRAPHY

cin·gu·late gyrus \'siŋ-gyə-lət-, -ˌlāt-\ *n* : a medial gyrus of each cerebral hemisphere that partly surrounds the corpus callosum

cin·gu·lot·o·my \ˌsiŋ-gyə-'lä-tə-mē\ *n*, *pl* **-mies** : surgical destruction of all or part (as the cingulum) of the cingulate gyrus

cin·gu·lum \'siŋ-gyə-ləm\ *n*, *pl* **cin·gu·la** \-lə\ **1** : a ridge about the base of the crown of a tooth **2** : a tract of association fibers lying within the cingulate gyrus and connecting the callosal and hippocampal convolutions of the brain

cin·na·mon \'si-nə-mən\ *n*, *often attrib* **1** : any of several Asian trees (genus *Cinnamomum*) of the laurel family (Lauraceae) **2** : an aromatic spice prepared from the dried inner bark of a cinnamon (esp. *C. zeylanicum*); *also* : the bark

cinnamon oil *n* : a yellowish or brownish essential oil obtained from the leaves and young twigs of a cinnamon tree (*Cinnamomum cassia*) and used chiefly as a flavoring — called also *cassia oil*

cino- — see KIN-

cir·ca·di·an \(ˌ)sər-'ka-dē-ən, -'kā-; ˌsər-kə-'dī-ən, -'dē-\ *adj* : being, having, characterized by, or occurring in approximately 24-hour periods or cycles (as of biological activity or function) (∼ rhythms in behavior)

cir·ci·nate \'sərs-ᵊn-ˌāt\ *adj*, *of lesions* : having a sharply circumscribed and somewhat circular margin

circle of Wil·lis \-'wi-ləs\ *n* : a complete ring of arteries at the base of the brain that is formed by the cerebral and communicating arteries and is a site of aneurysms

Willis, Thomas (1621–1675), British physician.

circling disease *n* : listeriosis of sheep or cattle

cir·cu·lar \'sər-kyə-lər\ *adj* : MANIC-DEPRESSIVE; *esp* : BIPOLAR 3

circulares — see PLICAE CIRCULARES

circular sinus *n* : a circular venous channel around the pituitary gland formed by the cavernous and intercavernous sinuses

cir·cu·late \'sər-kyə-ˌlāt\ *vb* **-lat·ed; -lat·ing** : to flow or be propelled naturally through a closed system of channels (as blood vessels)

cir·cu·la·tion \ˌsər-kyə-'lā-shən\ *n* : the movement of blood through the vessels of the body that is induced by the pumping action of the heart and serves to distribute nutrients and oxygen to and remove waste products from all parts of the body — see PULMONARY CIRCULATION, SYSTEMIC CIRCULATION

cir·cu·la·to·ry \'sər-kyə-lə-ˌtōr-ē\ *adj* : of or relating to circulation or the circulatory system (∼ failure)

circulatory system *n* : the system of blood, blood vessels, lymphatics, and heart concerned with the circulation of the blood and lymph

cir·cu·lus \'sər-kyə-ləs\ n, pl **-li** \-ˌlī\ : an anatomical circle or ring esp. of veins or arteries

cir·cum·cise \'sər-kəm-ˌsīz\ vb **-cised; -cis·ing** : to cut off the prepuce of (a male) or the clitoris of (a female) — **cir·cum·cis·er** n

cir·cum·ci·sion \ˌsər-kəm-'si-zhən\ n **1** : the act of circumcising; esp : the cutting off of the prepuce of males that is practiced as a religious rite by Jews and Muslims and as a sanitary measure in modern surgery **2** : the condition of being circumcised

cir·cum·cor·ne·al injection \ˌsir-kəm-'kȯr-nē-əl-\ n : enlargement of the ciliary and conjunctival blood vessels near the margin of the cornea with reduction in size peripherally

cir·cum·duc·tion \ˌsər-kəm-'dək-shən\ n : movement of a limb or extremity so that the distal end describes a circle while the proximal end remains fixed — **cir·cum·duct** \-'dəkt\ vb

cir·cum·flex \'sər-kəm-ˌfleks\ adj, of nerves and blood vessels : bending around

circumflex artery n : any of several paired curving arteries: as **a** : either of two arteries that branch from the deep femoral artery or from the femoral artery itself: (1) : LATERAL FEMORAL CIRCUMFLEX ARTERY (2) : MEDIAL FEMORAL CIRCUMFLEX ARTERY **b** : either of two branches of the axillary artery that wind around the neck of the humerus: (1) : ANTERIOR HUMERAL CIRCUMFLEX ARTERY (2) : POSTERIOR HUMERAL CIRCUMFLEX ARTERY **c** : CIRCUMFLEX ILIAC ARTERY **d** : a branch of the subscapular artery supplying the muscles of the shoulder

circumflex iliac artery n : either of two arteries arching anteriorly near the inguinal ligament: **a** : an artery lying internal to the iliac crest and arising from the external iliac artery **b** : a more superficially located artery that is a branch of the femoral artery

circumflex nerve n : AXILLARY NERVE

cir·cum·oral \ˌsər-kəm-'ȯr-əl, -'är-\ adj : surrounding the mouth ⟨∼ pallor⟩

cir·cum·scribed \'sər-kəm-ˌskrībd\ adj : confined to a limited area ⟨a ∼ neurosis⟩ ⟨∼ loss of hair⟩

cir·cum·stan·ti·al·i·ty \ˌsər-kəm-ˌstan-chē-'a-lə-tē\ n, pl **-ties** : a conversational pattern (as in some manic states) exhibiting excessive attention to irrelevant and digressive details

cir·cum·val·late \ˌsər-kəm-'va-ˌlāt, -lət\ adj : enclosed by a ridge of tissue

circumvallate papilla n : any of approximately 12 large papillae near the back of the tongue each of which is surrounded with a marginal sulcus and supplied with taste buds responsive esp. to bitter flavors — called also vallate papilla

cir·rho·sis \sə-'rō-səs\ n, pl **-rho·ses** \-ˌsēz\ : widespread disruption of normal liver structure by fibrosis and the formation of regenerative nodules that is caused by any of various chronic progressive conditions affecting the liver (as long-term alcohol abuse or hepatitis) — see BILIARY CIRRHOSIS

¹cir·rhot·ic \sə-'rä-tik\ adj : of, relating to, caused by, or affected with cirrhosis ⟨∼ degeneration⟩ ⟨a ∼ liver⟩

²cirrhotic n : an individual affected with cirrhosis

cirs- or **cirso-** comb form : swollen vein : varix ⟨cirsoid⟩

cir·soid \'sər-ˌsȯid\ adj : resembling a dilated tortuous vein ⟨a ∼ aneurysm of the scalp⟩

cis·plat·in \'sis-ˌplat-ⁿn\ n : a platinum–containing antineoplastic drug PtN₂H₆Cl₂ used esp. as a palliative therapy in testicular and ovarian tumors and in advanced bladder cancer — see PLATINOL

cis–platinum \-'plat-ⁿn-əm\ n : CISPLATIN

cis·ter·na \sis-'tər-nə\ n, pl **-nae** \-ˌnē\ : a fluid-containing sac or cavity in an organism : as **a** : CISTERNA MAGNA **b** : CISTERNA CHYLI

cisterna chy·li \-'kī-ˌlī\ n, pl cisternae chyli : a dilated lymph channel usu. opposite the 1st and 2d lumbar vertebrae and marking the beginning of the thoracic duct

cis·ter·nal \(ˌ)sis-'tərn-əl\ adj : of or relating to a cisterna and esp. the cisterna magna ⟨∼ puncture⟩ — **cis·ter·nal·ly** adv

cisterna mag·na \-'mag-nə\ n, pl cisternae mag·nae \-ˌnē\ : a large subarachnoid space between the caudal part of the cerebellum and the medulla oblongata

cis·ter·nog·ra·phy \ˌsis-(ˌ)tər-'nä-grə-fē\ n, pl **-phies** : roentgenographic visualization of the subarachnoid spaces containing cerebrospinal fluid following injection of an opaque contrast medium

cis·tron \'sis-ˌträn\ n : a segment of DNA that is equivalent to a gene and that specifies a single functional unit (as a protein or enzyme) — **cis·tron·ic** \sis-'trä-nik\ adj

cit·rate \'si-ˌtrāt\ n : a salt or ester of citric acid

cit·rat·ed \'si-ˌtrā-təd\ adj : treated with a citrate esp. of sodium or potassium to prevent coagulation ⟨∼ blood⟩

cit·ric acid \'si-trik-\ n : a sour organic acid C₆H₈O₇ occurring in cellular metabolism, obtained esp. from lemon and lime juices or by fermentation of sugars, and used as a flavoring

citric acid cycle n : KREBS CYCLE

cit·ri·nin \si-'trī-nən\ n : a toxic antibiotic C₁₃H₁₄O₅ that is produced esp. by two molds of the genus Penicillium

(*P. citrinum*) and the genus *Aspergillus* (*A. niveus*) and is effective against some gram-positive bacteria

cit·rov·o·rum factor \sə-'trä-və-rəm-\ *n* : a metabolically active form of folic acid that has been used in cancer therapy to protect normal cells against methotrexate — called also *folinic acid, leucovorin*

cit·ru·line \'si-trə-ˌlēn, si-'trə-ˌlēn, -lən\ *n* : a crystalline amino acid $C_6H_{13}N_3O_3$ formed esp. as an intermediate in the conversion of ornithine to arginine in the living system

cit·rul·lin·ae·mia *chiefly Brit var of* CIT-RULLINEMIA

cit·rul·lin·emia \ˌsi-trə-lə-'nē-mē-ə, si-ˌtrə-lə-'nē-\ *n* : an inherited disorder of amino acid metabolism accompanied by excess amounts of citrulline in the blood, urine, and cerebrospinal fluid and ammonia intoxication

cit·rus \'si-trəs\ *n, often attrib* : any plant or fruit of a genus (*Citrus*) of the rue family (Rutaceae) of often thorny trees and shrubs that are grown in warm regions and include the oranges (esp. *C. sinensis*), lemon (*C. limon*), lime (*C. aurantifolia*), and related plants

CK *abbr* creatine kinase

cl *abbr* centiliter

Cl *symbol* chlorine

CLA *abbr* certified laboratory assistant

clair·voy·ance \klar-'vȯi-əns, kler-\ *n* : the power or faculty of discerning objects or matters not present to the senses — **clair·voy·ant** \-ənt\ *adj*

clam·my \'kla-mē\ *adj* **clam·mi·er; -est** : being moist and sticky (~ hands) (~ sweating)

clamp \'klamp\ *n* : any of various instruments or appliances having parts brought together for holding or compressing something; *esp* : an instrument used to hold, compress, or crush vessels and hollow organs and to aid in surgical excision of parts — **clamp** *vb*

clang association *n* : word association (as in a psychological test) based on sound rather than meaning

clap \'klap\ *n* : GONORRHEA — often used with *the*

clasp \'klasp\ *n* : a device designed to encircle a tooth to hold a denture in place

class \'klas\ *n* : a major category in biological taxonomy ranking above the order and below the phylum

clas·sic \'kla-sik\ *or* **clas·si·cal** \-si-kəl\ *adj* : standard or recognized esp. because of great frequency or consistency or occurrence (the ~ symptoms of a disease)

classical conditioning *n* : conditioning in which the conditioned stimulus (as the sound of a bell) is paired with and precedes the unconditioned stimulus (as the sight of food) until the conditioned stimulus alone is sufficient to elicit the response (as in salivation in a dog) — compare OPERANT CONDITIONING

clau·di·ca·tion \ˌklȯ-də-'kā-shən\ *n* **1** : the quality or state of being lame **2** : INTERMITTENT CLAUDICATION

claus·tro·phobe \'klȯ-strə-ˌfōb\ *n* : one affected with claustrophobia

claus·tro·pho·bia \ˌklȯ-strə-'fō-bē-ə\ *n* : abnormal dread of being in closed or narrow spaces

¹claus·tro·pho·bic \ˌklȯ-strə-'fō-bik\ *adj* **1** : suffering from or inclined to claustrophobia **2** : inducing or suggesting claustrophobia — **claus·tro·pho·bi·cal·ly** \-bi-k(ə-)lē\ *adv*

²claustrophobic *n* : CLAUSTROPHOBE

claus·trum \'klȯ-strəm, 'klau-\ *n, pl* **claus·tra** \-strə\ : the one of the four basal ganglia in each cerebral hemisphere that consists of a thin lamina of gray matter between the lentiform nucleus and the insula

clav·i·cle \'kla-vi-kəl\ *n* : a bone of the pectoral girdle that links the scapula and sternum, is situated just above the first rib on either side of the neck, and has the form of a narrow elongated S — called also *collarbone* — **cla·vic·u·lar** \kla-'vi-kyə-lər, klə-\ *adj*

clavicular notch *n* : a notch on each side of the upper part of the manubrium that is the site of articulation with a clavicle

cla·vic·u·lec·to·my \kla-ˌvi-kyə-'lek-tə-mē, klə-\ *n, pl* **-mies** : surgical removal of all or part of a clavicle

cla·vus \'klā-vəs, 'klä-\ *n, pl* **cla·vi** \'klā-ˌvī, 'klä-ˌvē\ : CORN

claw foot *n* : a deformity of the foot characterized by an exaggerated curvature of the longitudinal arch

claw hand *n* : a deformity of the hand characterized by extreme extension of the wrist and the first phalanges and extreme flexion of the other phalanges

claw toe *n* : HAMMERTOE

¹clean \'klēn\ *adj* **1 a** : free from dirt or pollution **b** : free from disease or infectious agents **2** : free from drug addiction

²clean *vb* **1** : to brush (the teeth) with a cleanser (as a dentifrice) **2** : to perform dental prophylaxis on (the teeth)

¹clear \'klir\ *adj* **1** *of the skin or complexion* : good in texture and color and without blemish or discoloration **2** : free from abnormal sounds on auscultation

²clear *vb* : to rid (the throat) of phlegm or of something that makes the voice indistinct or husky

clear·ance \'klir-əns\ *n* : the volume of blood or plasma that could be freed of a specified constituent in a specified time (usu. one minute) by excretion of the constituent into the urine through the kidneys — called also *renal clearance*

cleavage • clitoris   122

cleav·age \\'klē-vij\\ *n* **1** : the series of synchronized mitotic cell divisions of the fertilized egg that results in the formation of the blastomeres and changes the single-celled zygote into a multicellular embryo; *also* : one of these cell divisions **2** : the splitting of a molecule into simpler molecules — **cleave** \\'klēv\\ *vb*

cleavage cell *n* : BLASTOMERE

cleft \\'kleft\\ *n* **1** : a usu. abnormal fissure or opening esp. when resulting from failure of parts to fuse during embryonic development **2** : a usu. V-shaped indented formation : a hollow between ridges or protuberances **3** : SYNAPTIC CLEFT

cleft lip *n* : a birth defect characterized by one or more clefts in the upper lip resulting from failure of the embryonic parts of the lip to unite — called also *cheiloschisis, harelip*

cleft palate *n* : congenital fissure of the roof of the mouth produced by failure of the two maxillae to unite during embryonic development and often associated with cleft lip

cleid- *or* **cleido-** *comb form* : clavicular : clavicular and ⟨*cleido*cranial⟩

clei·do·cra·ni·al dysostosis \\'klī-dō-'krā-nē-əl-\\ *n* : a rare condition inherited as an autosomal dominant and characterized esp. by partial or complete absence of the clavicles, defective ossification of the skull, and faulty occlusion due to missing, misplaced, or supernumerary teeth

cle·oid \\'klē-ˌoid\\ *n* : a dental excavator with a claw-shaped working point

click \\'klik\\ *n* : a short sharp sound heard in auscultation and associated with various abnormalities of the heart

cli·mac·ter·ic \\klī-'mak-tə-rik, ˌklī-ˌmak-'ter-ik\\ *n* **1** : MENOPAUSE **2** : a period in the life of a male corresponding to female menopause and usu. occurring with less well-defined physiological and psychological changes — **climacteric** *adj*

cli·mac·te·ri·um \\ˌklī-ˌmak-'tir-ē-əm\\ *n, pl* **-ria** \\-ē-ə\\ : the bodily and psychic involutional changes accompanying the transition from middle life to old age; *specif* : menopause and the bodily and mental changes that accompany it

cli·mac·tic \\klī-'mak-tik\\ *adj* : of, relating to, or constituting a climax

cli·ma·to·ther·a·py \\ˌklī-mə-tō-'ther-ə-pē\\ *n, pl* **-pies** : treatment of disease by means of residence in a suitable climate

cli·max \\'klī-ˌmaks\\ *n* **1** : the highest or most intense point **2** : ORGASM **3** : MENOPAUSE

clin *abbr* clinical

clin·da·my·cin \\ˌklin-də-'mī-sən\\ *n* : an antibiotic C₁₈H₃₃ClN₂O₅S derived from and used similarly to lincomycin

clin·ic \\'kli-nik\\ *n* **1 a** : a session or class

of medical instruction in a hospital held at the bedside of patients serving as case studies **b** : a group of selected patients presented with discussion before doctors for purposes of instruction **2 a** : an institution connected with a hospital or medical school where diagnosis and treatment are made available to outpatients **b** : a form of group practice in which several physicians work in cooperative association

clin·i·cal \\'kli-ni-kəl\\ *adj* : of, relating to, or conducted in or as if in a clinic: as **a** : involving or depending on direct observation of the living patient ⟨~ diagnosis⟩ **b** : observable or diagnosable by clinical inspection ⟨~ tuberculosis⟩ **c** : based on clinical observation ⟨~ treatment⟩ **d** : applying objective or standardized methods (as interviews and personality tests) to the description, evaluation, and modification of human behavior ⟨~ psychology⟩ — **clin·i·cal·ly** \\-k(ə-)lē\\ *adv*

clinical crown *n* : the part of a tooth that projects above the gums

clinical thermometer *n* : a thermometer for measuring body temperature that has a constriction in the tube where the column of liquid breaks when the temperature drops from its maximum and that continues to indicate the maximum temperature by the part of the column above the constriction until reset by shaking — called also *fever thermometer*

cli·ni·cian \\kli-'ni-shən\\ *n* : one qualified in the clinical practice of medicine, psychiatry, or psychology

clinico- *comb form* : clinical : clinical and ⟨*clinico*pathologic⟩

clin·i·co·path·o·log·ic \\ˌkli-ni-(ˌ)kō-ˌpa-thə-'lä-jik\\ *or* **clin·i·co·path·o·log·i·cal** \\-'lä-ji-kəl\\ *adj* : relating to or concerned both with the signs and symptoms directly observable by the physician and with the results of laboratory examination ⟨a ~ study of the patient⟩ — **clin·i·co·path·o·log·i·cal·ly** \\-ji-k(ə-)lē\\ *adv*

cli·no·dac·ty·ly \\ˌklī-nō-'dak-tə-lē\\ *n, pl* **-ty·lies** : a deformity of the hand marked by deviation or deflection of the fingers

cli·noid process \\'klī-ˌnoid-\\ *n* : any of several processes of the sphenoid bone

clip \\'klip\\ *n* : a device used to arrest bleeding from vessels or tissues during surgical operations

clitorid- *or* **clitorido-** *comb form* : clitoris ⟨*clitorid*ectomy⟩

clit·o·ri·dec·to·my \\ˌkli-tə-rə-'dek-tə-mē\\ *also* **clit·o·rec·to·my** \\-'rek-tə-mē\\ *n, pl* **-mies** : excision of all or part of the clitoris

clitoridis — see PREPUTIUM CLITORIDIS

cli·to·ris \\'kli-tə-rəs, kli-'tor-əs\\ *n, pl* **cli·to·ri·des** \\kli-'tor-ə-ˌdēz\\ : a small erectile organ at the anterior or ventral part of the vulva homologous to the penis — **cli·to·ral** \ˈkli-tə-rəl\ *also* **cli·tor·ic** \kli-ˈtȯr-ik, -ˈtär-\ *adj*

cli·vus \ˈklī-vəs\ *n, pl* **cli·vi** \-ˌvī\ : the smooth sloping surface on the upper posterior part of the body of the sphenoid bone supporting the pons and the basilar artery

CLL *abbr* chronic lymphocytic leukemia

clo·aca \klō-ˈā-kə\ *n, pl* **-acae** \-ˌkē, -ˌsē\ **1** : the terminal part of the embryonic hindgut of a mammal before it divides into rectum, bladder, and genital precursors **2** : a passage in a bone leading to a cavity containing a sequestrum — **clo·acal** \-kəl\ *adj*

cloacal membrane *n* : a plate of fused embryonic ectoderm and endoderm closing the fetal anus

clo·a·ci·tis \ˌklō-ə-ˈsī-təs\ *n* : a chronic inflammatory process of the cloaca of the domestic chicken that is of undetermined cause but is apparently transmitted by copulation — called also *vent gleet*

clock \ˈkläk\ *n* : BIOLOGICAL CLOCK

clo·fi·brate \klō-ˈfī-ˌbrāt, -ˈfi-\ *n* : a synthetic drug $C_{12}H_{15}ClO_3$ used esp. to lower abnormally high concentrations of fats and cholesterol in the blood

clo·mi·phene \ˈklä-mə-ˌfēn, ˈklō-\ *n* : a synthetic drug $C_{26}H_{28}ClNO$ used in the form of its citrate to induce ovulation

clo·mip·ra·mine \klō-ˈmi-prə-ˌmēn\ *n* : a tricyclic antidepressant $C_{19}H_{23}-ClN_2$ used in the form of its hydrochloride to treat obsessive-compulsive disorder

clo·naz·e·pam \(ˌ)klō-ˈna-zə-ˌpam\ *n* : a benzodiazepine $C_{15}H_{10}ClN_3O_3$ used as an anticonvulsant in the treatment of epilepsy

clone \ˈklōn\ *n* **1** : the aggregate of the asexually produced progeny of an individual **2** : an individual grown from a single somatic cell of its parent and genetically identical to it — **clon·al** \ˈklōn-əl\ *adj* — **clon·al·ly** *adv* — **clone** *vb*

clon·ic \ˈklä-nik\ *adj* : exhibiting, relating to, or involving clonus (~ contraction) (~ spasm) — **clo·nic·i·ty** \klō-ˈni-sə-tē, klä-\ *n*

clo·ni·dine \ˈklä-nə-ˌdēn, ˈklō-, -ˌdīn\ *n* : an antihypertensive drug $C_9H_9-Cl_2N_3$ used esp. to treat essential hypertension, to prevent migraine headache, and to diminish opiate withdrawal symptoms

clo·nor·chi·a·sis \ˌklō-nȯr-ˈkī-ə-səs\ *n, pl* **-a·ses** \-ˌsēz\ : infestation with or disease caused by the Chinese liver fluke (*Clonorchis sinensis*) that invades bile ducts of the liver after ingestion in uncooked fish and when present in numbers causes severe systemic reactions including edema, liver enlargement, and diarrhea

Clo·nor·chis \klō-ˈnȯr-kəs\ *n* : a genus of trematode worms (family Opisthorchiidae) that includes the Chinese liver fluke (*C. sinensis*)

clo·nus \ˈklō-nəs\ *n* : a series of alternating contractions and partial relaxations of a muscle that in some nervous diseases occurs in the form of convulsive spasms — compare TONUS 2

closed \ˈklōzd\ *adj* **1** : covered by unbroken skin (~ fracture) **2** : not discharging pathogenic organisms to the outside (a case of ~ tuberculosis) — compare OPEN 1c

closed–angle glaucoma *n* : glaucoma in which the drainage channel for the aqueous humor composed of the attachment at the edge of the iris and the junction of the sclera and cornea is blocked by the iris — called also *narrow-angle glaucoma*; compare OPEN-ANGLE GLAUCOMA

closed reduction *n* : the reduction of a displaced part (as a fractured bone) by manipulation without incision — compare OPEN REDUCTION

clos·trid·i·um \kläs-ˈtri-dē-əm\ *n* **1** *cap* : a genus of saprophytic anaerobic bacteria (family Bacillaceae) that are commonly found in soil and in the intestinal tracts of humans and animals and that include important pathogens — see BLACKLEG, BOTULISM, GAS GANGRENE, TETANUS BACILLUS; compare LIMBERNECK **2** *pl* **clos·trid·ia** \-dē-ə\ **a** : any bacterium of the genus *Clostridium* **b** : a spindle-shaped or ovoid bacterial cell; *esp* : one swollen at the center by an endospore — **clos·trid·i·al** \-dē-əl\ *adj*

clo·sure \ˈklō-zhər\ *n* **1 a** : an act of closing up or condition of being closed up **b** : a drawing together of edges or parts to form a united integument (wound ~ by suture) **2** : the perception of incomplete figures or situations as though complete by ignoring the missing parts or by compensating for them by projection based on past experience

¹clot \ˈklät\ *n* : a coagulated mass produced by clotting of blood

²clot *vb* **clot·ted; clot·ting** : to undergo a sequence of reactions that results in conversion of fluid blood into a coagulum and that involves shedding of blood, release of thromboplastin, inactivation of heparin, conversion of prothrombin to thrombin, interaction of thrombin with fibrinogen to form an insoluble fibrin network, and contraction of the network to squeeze out excess fluid : COAGULATE

clot·bust·er \ˈklät-ˌbəs-tər\ *n* : a drug (as streptokinase or tissue plasminogen activator) used to dissolve blood clots — **clot·bust·ing** \-tiŋ\ *adj*

clot retraction *n* : the process by which

a blood clot becomes smaller and draws the edges of a broken blood vessel together and which involves the shortening of fibrin threads and the squeezing out of excess serum

clo·tri·ma·zole \klō-ˈtrī-mə-ˌzōl, -ˌzól\ n : an antifungal agent $C_{22}H_{17}ClN_2$ used to treat candida infections, tinea, and ringworm — see LOTRIMIN

clotting factor n : any of several plasma components (as fibrinogen, prothrombin, and thromboplastin) that are involved in the clotting of blood — see TRANSGLUTAMINASE: compare FACTOR V, FACTOR VII, FACTOR VIII, FACTOR IX, FACTOR X, FACTOR XII, FACTOR XIII

clove \ˈklōv\ n : the fragrant dried aromatic flower bud of a tropical tree (Syzygium aromaticum) of the myrtle family (Myrtaceae) that yields a colorless to pale yellow essential oil (**clove oil**) which is a source of eugenol, has a powerful germicidal action, and is used topically to relieve toothache

cloverleaf skull n : a birth defect in which some or all of the usu. separate bones of the skull have grown together resulting in a 3-lobed skull with associated deformities of the features and skeleton

clox·a·cil·lin \ˌkläk-sə-ˈsi-lən\ n : a semisynthetic oral penicillin $C_{19}H_{17}$-ClN_3NaO_5S effective esp. against staphylococci which secrete penicillinase — see TEGOPEN

clo·za·pine \ˈklō-zə-ˌpēn\ n : an antipsychotic drug $C_{18}H_{19}ClN_4$ with serious side effects that is used in the management of severe schizophrenia — see CLOZARIL

Clo·za·ril \ˈklō-zə-ril\ trademark — used for a preparation of clozapine

clubbed \ˈkləbd\ adj 1 : having a bulbous enlargement of the tip with convex overhanging nail (a ~ finger) 2 : affected with clubfoot — **club·bing** \ˈklə-biŋ\ n

club·foot \ˈkləb-ˌfút\ n, pl **club·feet** \-ˌfēt\ 1 : any of numerous congenital deformities of the foot in which it is twisted out of position or shape — called also talipes; compare TALIPES EQUINOVARUS, TALIPES EQUINUS, TALIPES VALGUS, TALIPES VARUS 2 : a foot affected with clubfoot — **club·foot·ed** \-ˌfú-təd\ adj

club·hand \ˌkləb-ˌhand\ n 1 : a congenital deformity in which the hand is short and distorted 2 : a hand affected with clubhand

clump \ˈkləmp\ n : a clustered mass of particles (as bacteria or blood cells) — compare AGGLUTINATION — **clump** vb

cluster headache n : a headache that is characterized by severe unilateral pain in the eye or temple, affects primarily men, and tends to recur in a series of attacks

clut·ter·ing \ˈklə-tə-riŋ\ n : a speech defect in which phonetic units are dropped, condensed, or otherwise distorted as a result of overly rapid agitated utterance

Clut·ton's joints \ˈklət-ᵊnz-\ n pl : symmetrical hydrarthrosis esp. of the knees or elbows that occurs in congenital syphilis

Clut·ton \ˈklət-ᵊn\, **Henry Hugh** (1850–1909), British surgeon.

cly·sis \ˈklī-səs\ n, pl **cly·ses** \-ˌsēz\ : the introduction of large amounts of fluid into the body usu. by parenteral injection to replace that lost (as from hemorrhage or in dysentery or burns), to provide nutrients, or to maintain blood pressure — see HYPODERMOCLYSIS, PROCTOCLYSIS

clys·ter \ˈklis-tər\ n : ENEMA

cm abbr centimeter

Cm symbol curium

CMA abbr certified medical assistant

CMHC abbr Community Mental Health Center

CMV abbr cytomegalovirus

cne·mi·al \ˈnē-mē-əl\ adj : relating to the shin or shinbone

cne·mis \ˈnē-məs\ n, pl **cnem·i·des** \ˈne-mə-ˌdēz\ : SHIN, TIBIA

cni·dar·i·an \nī-ˈdar-ē-ən\ n : COELENTERATE — **cnidarian** adj

CNM abbr certified nurse-midwife

CNS abbr central nervous system

Co symbol cobalt

c/o abbr complains of

co·ag·u·lant \kō-ˈa-gyə-lənt\ n : something that produces coagulation

co·ag·u·lase \kō-ˈa-gyə-ˌlās, -ˌlāz\ n : any of several enzymes that cause coagulation (as of blood)

¹co·ag·u·late \kō-ˈa-gyə-ˌlāt\ vb -lat·ed; -lat·ing : to become or cause to become viscous or thickened into a coherent mass : CLOT — **co·ag·u·la·bil·i·ty** \kō-ˌa-gyə-lə-ˈbi-lə-tē\ n — **co·ag·u·la·ble** \-ˈa-gyə-lə-bəl\ adj

²co·ag·u·late \-lət, -ˌlāt\ n : COAGULUM

co·ag·u·la·tion \kō-ˌa-gyə-ˈlā-shən\ n 1 a : the process of becoming viscous, jellylike, or solid; esp : the change from a liquid to a thickened curdlike state not by evaporation but by chemical reaction b : the process by which such change of state takes place consisting of the alteration of a soluble substance (as protein) into an insoluble form or of the flocculation or separation of colloidal or suspended matter 2 : a substance or body formed by coagulation : COAGULUM

coagulation time n : the time required by shed blood to clot that is a measure of the normality of the blood

co·ag·u·lop·a·thy \kō-ˌa-gyə-ˈlä-pə-thē\ n, pl -thies : a disease affecting blood coagulation

co·ag·u·lum \kō-ˈa-gyə-ləm\ n, pl -u·la \-lə\ or -u·lums : a coagulated mass or substance : CLOT

coal tar n : tar obtained by distillation

of bituminous coal and used in the treatment of some skin diseases by direct local application to the skin

co·apt \kō-'apt\ *vb* : to close or fasten together : cause to adhere — **co·ap·ta·tion** \(ˌ)kō-ˌap-'tā-shən\ *n*

co·arct \kō-'ärkt\ *vb* : to cause (the aorta) to become narrow or (the heart) to constrict

co·arc·ta·tion \(ˌ)kō-ˌärk-'tā-shən\ *n* : a stricture or narrowing esp. of a canal or vessel (as the aorta)

coarse \'kȯrs\ *adj* **1** : visible to the naked eye or by means of a compound microscope **2** *of a tremor* : of wide excursion **3** : harsh, raucous, or rough in tone — used of some sounds heard in auscultation in pathological states of the chest ⟨∼ rales⟩

coat \'kōt\ *n* **1** : the external growth on an animal **2** : a layer of one substance covering or lining another; *esp* : one covering or lining an organ (the ∼ of the eyeball)

coat·ed \'kō-təd\ *adj*, *of the tongue* : covered with a yellowish white deposit of desquamated cells, bacteria, and debris usu. as an accompaniment of digestive disorder

Coats's disease \'kōts, 'kōt-səz-\ *n* : a chronic inflammatory disease of the eye that is characterized by white or yellow areas around the optic disk due to edematous accumulation under the retina and that leads to destruction of the macula and to blindness

Coats \'kōts\, **George (1876–1915),** British ophthalmologist.

co·bal·a·min \kō-'ba-lə-mən\ *n* : VITAMIN B₁₂

co·balt \'kō-ˌbȯlt\ *n* : a tough lustrous silver-white magnetic metallic element — symbol *Co*; see ELEMENT table

cobalt 60 *n* : a heavy radioactive isotope of cobalt having the mass number 60 and used as a source of gamma rays esp. in place of radium (as in the treatment of cancer and in radiography) — called also *radio-cobalt*

co·bra \'kō-brə\ *n* **1** : any of several very venomous Asian and African elapid snakes (genera *Naja* and *Ophiophagus*) **2** : RINGHALS **3** : MAMBA

co·ca \'kō-kə\ *n* **1** : any of several So. American shrubs (genus *Erythroxylon* of the family Erythroxylaceae); *esp* : one (*E. coca*) that is the primary source of cocaine **2** : dried leaves of a coca (esp. *E. coca*) containing alkaloids including cocaine

co·caine \kō-'kān, 'kō-ˌ\ *n* : a bitter crystalline alkaloid $C_{17}H_{21}NO_4$ obtained from coca leaves that is used medically esp. in the form of its hydrochloride as a topical anesthetic and illicitly for its euphoric effects and that may result in a compulsive psychological need

co·cain·ize \kō-'kā-ˌnīz\ *vb* **-ized; -izing** : to treat or anesthetize with cocaine — **co·cain·iza·tion** \-ˌkā-nə-'zā-shən\ *n*

co·car·cin·o·gen \kō-kär-'si-nə-jən, kō-'kärs-ᵊn-ə-ˌjen\ *n* : an agent that aggravates the carcinogenic effects of another substance — **co·car·cin·o·gen·ic** \ˌkō-ˌkärs-ᵊn-ō-'je-nik\ *adj*

coc·cal \'kä-kəl\ *adj* : of or relating to a coccus

cocci *pl of* COCCUS

coc·cid·ia \käk-'si-dē-ə\ *n pl* : a sporozoans of an order (Coccidia) parasitic in the digestive epithelium of vertebrates and higher invertebrates and including several forms of economic importance — compare CRYPTOSPORIDIUM, EIMERIA, ISOSPORA — **coc·cid·i·an** \-dē-ən\ *adj or n*

Coc·cid·i·oi·des \käk-ˌsi-dē-'ȯi-ˌdēz\ *n* : a genus of imperfect fungi including one (*C. immitis*) causing coccidioidomycosis

coc·cid·i·oi·din \-'ȯid-ᵊn, -'ȯi-ˌdin\ *n* : an antigen prepared from a fungus of the genus *Coccidioides* (*C. immitis*) and used to detect skin sensitivity to and, by inference, infection with this organism

coc·cid·i·oi·do·my·co·sis \-ˌȯi-dō-(ˌ)mī-'kō-səs\ *n, pl* **-co·ses** \-ˌsēz\ : a disease of humans and domestic animals caused by a fungus of the genus *Coccidioides* (*C. immitis*) and marked esp. by fever and localized pulmonary symptoms — called also *San Joaquin fever, San Joaquin valley fever, valley fever*

coc·cid·io·my·co·sis \(ˌ)käk-ˌsi-dē-ō-(ˌ)mī-'kō-səs\ *n, pl* **-co·ses** \-ˌsēz\ : COCCIDIOIDOMYCOSIS

coc·cid·io·sis \(ˌ)käk-ˌsi-dē-'ō-səs\ *n, pl* **-o·ses** \-ˌsēz\ : infestation with or disease caused by coccidia

coc·cid·io·stat \(ˌ)käk-'si-dē-ō-ˌstat\ *n* : a chemical agent added to animal feed (as for poultry) that serves to retard the life cycle or reduce the population of a pathogenic coccidium to the point that disease is minimized and the host develops immunity

coc·co·ba·cil·lus \ˌkä-(ˌ)kō-bə-'si-ləs\ *n, pl* **-li** \-ˌlī, -ˌlē\ : a very short bacillus esp. of the genus *Pasteurella* — **coc·co·ba·cil·la·ry** \-'ba-sə-ˌler-ē, -bə-'si-lə-rē\ *adj*

coc·coid \'kä-ˌkȯid\ *adj* : of, related to, or resembling a coccus — **coccoid** *n*

coc·cus \'kä-kəs\ *n, pl* **coc·ci** \'kä-ˌkī, -ˌkē; 'käk-ˌsī, -ˌsē\ : a spherical bacterium

coccyg- *or* **coccygo-** *comb form* : coccyx ⟨*coccygectomy*⟩

coc·cy·ge·al \käk-'si-jəl, -jē-əl\ *adj* : of, relating to, or affecting the coccyx

coccygeal body *n* : GLOMUS COCCYGEUM

coccygeal gland *n* : GLOMUS COCCYGEUM

coccygeal nerve *n* : either of the 31st or lowest pair of spinal nerves

coc·cy·gec·to·my \ˌkäk-sə-ˈjek-tə-mē\ *n*, *pl* **-mies** : the surgical removal of the coccyx

coccygeum — see GLOMUS COCCYGEUM

coc·cyg·e·us \käk-ˈsij-ē-əs\ *n*, *pl* **coc·cyg·ei** \-jē-ˌī\ : a muscle arising from the ischium and sacrospinous ligament and inserted into the coccyx and sacrum — called also *coccygeus muscle, ischiococcygeus*

coc·cy·go·dyn·ia \ˌkäk-sə-(ˌ)gō-ˈdi-nē-ə\ *n* : pain in the coccyx and adjacent regions

coc·cyx \ˈkäk-siks\ *n*, *pl* **coc·cy·ges** \-ˌsə-ˌjēz\ *also* **coc·cyx·es** \-sik-səz\ : a small bone that articulates with the sacrum and that usu. consists of four fused vertebrae which form the terminus of the spinal column

co·chlea \ˈkō-klē-ə, ˈkä-\ *n*, *pl* **co·chleas** *or* **co·chle·ae** \-ē, -ˌī\ : a division of the bony labyrinth of the inner ear coiled into the form of a snail shell and consisting of a spiral canal in the petrous part of the temporal bone in which lies a smaller membranous spiral passage that communicates with the saccule at the base of the spiral, ends blindly near its apex, and contains the organ of Corti — **co·chle·ar** \-ər\ *adj*

cochlear canal *n* : SCALA MEDIA

cochlear duct *n* : SCALA MEDIA

cochlear nerve *n* : a branch of the auditory nerve that arises in the spiral ganglion of the cochlea and conducts sensory stimuli from the organ of hearing to the brain — called also *cochlear, cochlear branch, cochlear division*

cochlear nucleus *n* : the nucleus of the cochlear nerve situated in the caudal part of the pons and consisting of dorsal and ventral parts which are continuous and lie on the dorsal and lateral aspects of the inferior cerebellar peduncle

co·chleo·ves·tib·u·lar \ˌkō-klē-(ˌ)ō-ve-ˈsti-byə-lər, ˌkä-\ *adj* : relating to or affecting the cochlea and vestibule of the ear

Coch·lio·my·ia \ˌkä-klē-ə-ˈmī-ə\ *n* : a genus of No. American blowflies that includes the screwworms (*C. hominivorax* and *C. macellaria*)

cock·roach \ˈkäk-ˌrōch\ *n* : any of an order or suborder (Blattodea) of chiefly nocturnal insects including some that are domestic pests — see BLATTA, BLATTELLA

cock·tail \ˈkäk-ˌtāl\ *n* : a solution of agents taken or used together esp. for medical treatment or diagnosis

cocoa butter *n* : a pale vegetable fat obtained from cacao beans that is used in the manufacture of chocolate candy, in cosmetics as an emollient, and in pharmacy for making suppositories — called also *theobroma oil*

co·con·scious \(ˌ)kō-ˈkän-chəs\ *n* : mental processes outside the main stream

of consciousness but sometimes available to it — **coconscious** *adj*

co·con·scious·ness *n* : COCONSCIOUS

¹**code** \ˈkōd\ *n* : GENETIC CODE

²**code** *vb* **cod·ed; cod·ing** : to specify the genetic code ⟨a gene that ~s for a protein⟩

co·deine \ˈkō-ˌdēn, ˈkō-dē-ən\ *n* : a morphine derivative $C_{18}H_{21}NO_3 \cdot H_2O$ that is found in opium, is weaker in action than morphine, and is used esp. in cough remedies

co·de·pen·dence \ˌkō-di-ˈpen-dəns\ *n* : CODEPENDENCY

co·de·pen·den·cy \-dən-sē\ *n*, *pl* **-cies** : a psychological condition or a relationship in which a person is controlled or manipulated by another who is affected with a pathological condition (as an addiction to alcohol or heroin)

¹**co·de·pen·dent** \-dənt\ *n* : a codependent person

²**codependent** *adj* : participating in or exhibiting codependency

co·dex \ˈkō-ˌdeks\ *n*, *pl* **co·di·ces** \ˈkō-də-ˌsēz, ˈkä-\ : an official or standard collection of drug formulas and descriptions ⟨the British Pharmaceutical Codex⟩

cod–liver oil *n* : a pale yellow fatty oil obtained from the liver of the cod (*Gadus morrhua* of the family Gadidae) and related fishes and used in medicine chiefly as a source of vitamins A and D in conditions (as rickets) due to abnormal calcium and phosphorus metabolism

co·dom·i·nant \(ˌ)kō-ˈdä-mə-nənt\ *adj* : being fully expressed in the heterozygous condition — **codominant** *n*

co·don \ˈkō-ˌdän\ *n* : a specific sequence of three consecutive nucleotides that is part of the genetic code and that specifies a particular amino acid in a protein or starts or stops protein synthesis — called also *triplet*

co·ef·fi·cient \ˌkō-ə-ˈfi-shənt\ *n* : a number that serves as a measure of some property (as of a substance) or characteristic (as of a device or process)

-coele *or* **-coel** *also* **-cele** *n comb form* : cavity : chamber : ventricle ⟨blastocoel⟩

coe·len·ter·ate \si-ˈlen-tə-ˌrāt, -rət\ *n* : any of a phylum (Cnidaria syn. Coelenterata) of invertebrate animals with radial symmetry including some forms (as the jellyfishes) with tentacles studded with stinging cells — called also *cnidarian* — **coelenterate** *adj*

coeli- *or* **coelio-** *chiefly Brit var of* CELI-

coe·li·ac, coe·li·os·co·py, coe·li·ot·o·my *chiefly Brit var of* CELIAC, CELIOSCOPY, CELIOTOMY

coe·lom \ˈsē-ləm\ *n*, *pl* **coeloms** *or* **coe·lo·ma·ta** \si-ˈlō-mə-tə\ : the usu. epithelium-lined body cavity of metazoans above the lower worms that forms a large space when well developed between the alimentary viscera and the body walls — **coe·lo·mate** \\'sē-lə-ˌmāt\ *adj or n* — **coe·lo·mic** \si-'lä-mik, -'lō-\ *adj*

coe·nu·ro·sis \ˌsēn-yə-'rō-səs, ˌsen-\ *or* **coe·nu·ri·a·sis** \-'rī-ə-səs\ *n, pl* **-oses** \-ˌsēz\ *or* **-a·ses** \-ˌsēz\ : infestation with or disease caused by coenuri (as gid of sheep)

coe·nu·rus \sə-'nur-əs, sē-, -'nyur-\ *n, pl* **-nu·ri** \-'nur-ˌī, -'nyur-\ : a complex tapeworm larva growing interstitially in vertebrate tissues and consisting of a large fluid-filled sac from the inner wall of which numerous scolices develop — see GID, MULTICEPS

co·en·zyme \(ˌ)kō-'en-ˌzīm\ *n* : a thermostable nonprotein compound that forms the active portion of an enzyme system after combination with an apoenzyme — compare ACTIVATOR 1 — **co·en·zy·mat·ic** \-ˌen-zə-'ma-tik, -(ˌ)zī-\ *adj* — **co·en·zy·mat·i·cal·ly** \-ti-k(ə-)lē\ *adv*

coenzyme A *n* : a coenzyme $C_{21}H_{36}$-$N_7O_{16}P_3S$ that occurs in all living cells and is essential to the metabolism of carbohydrates, fats, and some amino acids

coenzyme Q *n* : UBIQUINONE

coeruleus, coerulei — see LOCUS COERULEUS

co·fac·tor \\'kō-ˌfak-tər\ *n* : a substance that acts with another substance to bring about certain effects; *esp* : COENZYME

co·ge·ner *var of* CONGENER

Cog·gins test \\'kä-gənz-\ *n* : a serological immunodiffusion test for the diagnosis of equine infectious anemia esp. in horses by the presence of antibodies to the causative virus — called also *Coggins* — **Coggins test** *vb* **Coggins, Leroy (1932–)**, American veterinary virologist.

cog·ni·tion \käg-'ni-shən\ *n* 1 : cognitive mental processes 2 : a conscious intellectual act (conflict between ∼ s)

cog·ni·tive \\'käg-nə-tiv\ *adj* : of, relating to, or being conscious intellectual activity (as thinking, reasoning, remembering, imagining, or learning words) — **cog·ni·tive·ly** *adv*

cognitive dissonance *n* : psychological conflict resulting from simultaneously held incongruous beliefs and attitudes

cognitive therapy *n* : psychotherapy esp. for depression that emphasizes the substitution of desirable patterns of thinking for undesirable ones — compare BEHAVIOR THERAPY, CHEMOTHERAPY

co·he·sion \kō-'hē-zhən\ *n* 1 : the act or process of sticking together tightly 2 : the molecular attraction by which the particles of a body are united throughout the mass — **co·he·sive** \kō-'hē-siv, -ziv\ *adj* — **co·he·sive·ly** *adv* — **co·he·sive·ness** *n*

coin lesion *n* : a round well-circum-scribed nodule in a lung that is seen in an X-ray photograph as a shadow the size and shape of a coin

coital exanthema *n* : a highly contagious disease of horses that is caused by a herpesvirus transmitted chiefly by copulation

co·ition \kō-'i-shən\ *n* : COITUS — **co·ition·al** \-'ish-nəl, -'i-shən-ᵊl\ *adj*

co·itus \\'kō-ə-təs, kō-'ē-; 'koi-təs\ *n* : physical union of male and female genitalia accompanied by rhythmic movements leading to the ejaculation of semen from the penis into the female reproductive tract; *also* : INTERCOURSE — compare ORGASM — **co·ital** \-ət-ᵊl, -'ēt-\ *adj* — **co·ital·ly** \-ᵊl-ē\ *adv*

coitus in·ter·rup·tus \-ˌin-tə-'rəp-təs\ *n* : coitus in which the penis is withdrawn prior to ejaculation to prevent the deposit of sperm in the vagina

coitus res·er·va·tus \-ˌre-zər-'vä-təs\ *n* : prolonged coitus in which ejaculation of sperm is deliberately withheld

col- *or* **coli-** *or* **colo-** *comb form* 1 : colon ⟨*colitis*⟩ ⟨*colostomy*⟩ 2 : colon bacillus ⟨*coliform*⟩

cola *pl of* COLON

col·chi·cine \\'käl-chə-ˌsēn, 'käl-kə-\ *n* : a poisonous alkaloid $C_{22}H_{25}NO_6$ that inhibits mitosis, is extracted from the corms or seeds of the autumn crocus, and is used in the treatment of gout and acute attacks of gouty arthritis

col·chi·cum \-kəm\ *n* : the dried corm or dried ripe seeds of the autumn crocus containing the alkaloid colchicine

¹**cold** \\'kōld\ *adj* 1 a : having or being a temperature that is noticeably lower than body temperature and esp. that is uncomfortable for humans **b** : having a relatively low temperature or one that is lower than normal or expected **c** : receptive to the sensation of coldness : stimulated by cold 2 : marked by the loss of normal body heat (∼ hands) 3 : DEAD 4 : exhibiting little or no radioactivity when subjected to radionuclide scanning — **cold·ness** *n*

²**cold** *n* 1 : bodily sensation produced by loss or lack of heat 2 : a bodily disorder popularly associated with chilling: **a** *in humans* : COMMON COLD **b** *in domestic animals* : CORYZA

COLD *abbr* chronic obstructive lung disease

cold agglutinin *n* : any of several agglutinins sometimes present in the blood (as that of many patients with primary atypical pneumonia) that at low temperatures agglutinate compatible as well as incompatible erythrocytes, including the patient's own — compare AUTOAGGLUTININ

cold–blood·ed \\'kōld-'blə-dəd\ *adj* : having a body temperature not internally regulated but approximating that of the environment : POIKILO-THERMIC — **cold–blood·ed·ness** *n*

cold cream *n* : a soothing and cleansing cosmetic basically consisting of a perfumed emulsion of a bland vegetable oil or heavy mineral oil

cold pack *n* : a sheet or blanket wrung out of cold water, wrapped around the patient's body, and covered with dry blankets — compare HOT PACK

cold sore *n* : a group of blisters appearing about or within the mouth and caused by a herpes simplex virus — called also *fever blister;* compare CANKER SORE

cold sweat *n* : perspiration accompanied by feelings of chill or cold and usu. induced or accompanied by dread, fear, or shock

cold turkey *n* : abrupt complete cessation of the use of an addictive drug; *also* : the symptoms experienced by one undergoing withdrawal from a drug — **cold turkey** *adv or adj or vb*

col·ec·to·my \kə-ˈlek-tə-mē, kō-\ *n, pl* **-mies** : excision of a portion or all of the colon

co·les·ti·pol \kə-ˈles-tə-ˌpōl\ *n* : a strongly basic resin with an affinity for bile acids that is used in the form of its hydrochloride to treat hypercholesterolemia and disorders associated with the accumulation of bile acids

co·li \ˈkō-ˌlī\ *adj* : of or relating to bacteria normally inhabiting the intestine or colon and esp. those of the genus *Escherichia* (as *E. coli*) — **coli** *n*

coli— see COL-

co·li·ba·cil·lo·sis \ˌkō-lə-ˌba-sə-ˈlō-səs\ *n, pl* **-loses** \-ˌsēz\ : infection with or disease caused by colon bacilli (esp. *Escherichia coli*)

¹col·ic \ˈkä-lik\ *n* : a paroxysm of acute abdominal pain localized in a hollow organ and often caused by spasm, obstruction, or twisting

²colic *adj* : of or relating to colic : COL-ICKY ⟨∼ crying⟩

³co·lic \ˈkō-lik, ˈkä-\ *adj* : of or relating to the colon

colic artery *n* : any of three arteries that branch from the mesenteric arteries and supply the large intestine

co·li·cin \ˈkä-lə-sən\ *also* **co·li·cine** \-ˌsēn\ *n* : any of various antibacterial proteins that are produced by strains of intestinal bacteria (as *Escherichia coli*) and that often act to inhibit macromolecular synthesis in related strains

col·icky \ˈkä-li-kē\ *adj* **1** : relating to or associated with colic ⟨∼ pain⟩ **2** : suffering from colic ⟨∼ babies⟩

co·li·form \ˈkō-lə-ˌform, ˈkä-\ *adj* : relating to, resembling, or being colon bacilli — **coliform** *n*

co·li·phage \ˈkō-lə-ˌfāj, -ˌfāzh\ *n* : a bacteriophage active against colon bacilli

co·lis·tin \kə-ˈlis-tən, kō-\ *n* : a poly-

myxin produced by a bacterium of the genus *Bacillus* (*B. polymyxa* var. *colistinus*)

co·li·tis \kō-ˈlī-təs, kə-\ *n* : inflammation of the colon — see ULCERATIVE COLITIS

colla *pl of* COLLUM

col·la·gen \ˈkä-lə-jən\ *n* : an insoluble fibrous protein of vertebrates that is the chief constituent of the fibrils of connective tissue (as in skin and tendons) and of the organic substance of bones and yields gelatin and glue on prolonged heating with water — **col·lag·e·nous** \kə-ˈla-jə-nəs\ *adj*

col·la·ge·nase \kə-ˈla-jə-ˌnās, ˈkä-lə-, -ˌnāz\ *n* : any of a group of proteolytic enzymes that decompose collagen and gelatin

collagen disease *n* : CONNECTIVE TISSUE DISEASE

col·la·gen·o·lyt·ic \ˌkä-lə-jə-nə-ˈli-tik, -ˌje-\ *adj* : relating to or having the capacity to break down collagen

col·la·ge·no·sis \ˌkä-lə-jə-ˈnō-səs\ *n, pl* **-noses** \-ˌsēz\ : CONNECTIVE TISSUE DISEASE

collagen vascular disease *n* : CONNECTIVE TISSUE DISEASE

¹col·lapse \kə-ˈlaps\ *vb* **col·lapsed; col·laps·ing 1** : to fall or shrink together abruptly and completely : fall into a jumbled or flattened mass through the force of external pressure ⟨a blood vessel that *collapsed*⟩ **2** : to break down in vital energy, stamina, or self-control through exhaustion or disease; *esp* : to fall helpless or unconscious — **col·laps·ibil·i·ty** \-ˌlap-sə-ˈbi-lə-tē\ *n* — **col·laps·ible** \-ˈlap-sə-bəl\ *adj*

²collapse *n* **1** : a breakdown in vital energy, strength, or stamina : complete sudden enervation **2** : a state of extreme prostration and physical depression resulting from circulatory failure, great loss of body fluids, or heart disease and occurring terminally in diseases such as cholera, typhoid fever, and pneumonia **3** : an airless state of a lung of spontaneous origin or induced surgically — see ATELECTASIS **4** : an abnormal falling together of the walls of an organ ⟨∼ of blood vessels⟩

col·lar \ˈkä-lər\ *n* : a band (as of cotton) worn around the neck for therapeutic purposes (as support or retention of body heat)

col·lar·bone \ˈkä-lər-ˌbōn\ *n* : CLAVICLE

¹col·lat·er·al \kə-ˈla-tə-rəl, -trəl\ *adj* **1** : relating to or being branches of a bodily part ⟨∼ sprouting of nerves⟩ **2** : relating to or being part of the collateral circulation

²collateral *n* **1** : a branch esp. of a blood vessel, nerve, or the axon of a nerve cell **2** : a bodily part that is lateral in position

collateral circulation *n* : circulation of blood established through enlargement of minor vessels and anastomosis of vessels with those of adjacent parts when a major vein or artery is functionally impaired (as by obstruction); *also* : the modified vessels through which such circulation occurs

collateral ligament *n* : any of various ligaments on one or the other side of a hinge joint (as the knee, elbow, or the joints between the phalanges of the toes and fingers): as **a** : LATERAL COLLATERAL LIGAMENT **b** : MEDIAL COLLATERAL LIGAMENT

collateral sulcus *n* : a sulcus of the tentorial surface of the cerebrum lying below and external to the calcarine sulcus and causing an elevation on the floor of the lateral ventricle between the hippocampi — called also *collateral fissure*

collecting tubule *n* : a nonsecretory tubule that receives urine from several nephrons and discharges it into the pelvis of the kidney — called also *collecting duct*

collective unconscious *n* : the genetically determined part of the unconscious that esp. in the psychoanalytic theory of C. G. Jung occurs in all the members of a people or race

Col·les' fracture \\'kä-ləs-, -ˌlēz-\ *n* : a fracture of the lower end of the radius with backward displacement of the lower fragment and radial deviation of the hand at the wrist that produces a characteristic deformity — compare SMITH FRACTURE

Col·les \\'kä-ləs\, **Abraham** (1773–1843), British surgeon.

col·lic·u·lus \kə-'li-kyə-ləs\ *n, pl* **-u·li** \-ˌlī, -ˌlē\ : an anatomical prominence; *esp* : any of the four prominences constituting the corpora quadrigemina — see INFERIOR COLLICULUS, SUPERIOR COLLICULUS

col·li·ma·tor \\'kä-lə-ˌmā-tər\ *n* : a device for obtaining a beam of radiation (as X rays) of limited cross section

col·li·qua·tion \ˌkä-lə-'kwā-zhən, -shən\ *n* : the breakdown and liquefaction of tissue — **col·li·qua·tive** \\'kä-li-ˌkwā-tiv, kə-'li-kwə-\ *adj*

col·lo·di·on \kə-'lō-dē-ən\ *n* : a viscous solution of pyroxylin used as a coating for wounds

col·loid \\'kä-ˌloid\ *n* **1** : a gelatinous or mucinous substance found in tissues in disease or normally (as in the thyroid) **2 a** : a substance that consists of particles dispersed throughout another substance which are too small for resolution with an ordinary light microscope but are incapable of passing through a semipermeable membrane **b** : a mixture (as smoke) consisting of a colloid together with the medium in which it is dispersed — **col·loi·dal** \kə-'loid-əl, kä-\ *adj* — **col·loi·dal·ly** *adv*

col·lum \\'kä-ləm\ *n, pl* **col·la** \-lə\ : an

anatomical neck or neckline part or process

col·lu·to·ri·um \ˌkä-lə-'tōr-ē-əm\ *n, pl* **-to·ria** \-ē-ə\ : MOUTHWASH

col·lyr·i·um \kə-'lir-ē-əm\ *n, pl* **-ia** \-ē-ə\ *or* **-i·ums** : an eye lotion : EYEWASH

colo- — see COL-

col·o·bo·ma \ˌkä-lə-'bō-mə\ *n, pl* **-ma·ta** \-mə-tə\ : a fissure of the eye usu. of congenital origin

co·lon \\'kō-lən\ *n, pl* **colons** *or* **co·la** \-lə\ : the part of the large intestine that extends from the cecum to the rectum

colon bacillus *n* : any of several bacilli esp. of the genus *Escherichia* that are normally commensal in vertebrate intestines; *esp* : one (*E. coli*) used extensively in genetic research

¹co·lon·ic \kō-'lä-nik, kə-\ *adj* : of or relating to the colon

²colonic *n* : irrigation of the colon : ENEMA — see HIGH COLONIC

col·o·nize \\'kä-lə-ˌnīz\ *vb* **-nized; -nizing** : to establish a colony in or on — **col·o·ni·za·tion** \ˌkä-lə-nə-'zā-shən\ *n*

col·o·no·scope \kō-'lä-nə-ˌskōp\ *n* : a flexible tube containing a fiberscope for visual inspection of the colon and apparatus for taking tissue samples

co·lo·nos·co·py \ˌkō-lə-'näs-kə-pē, ˌkä-\ *n, pl* **-pies** : endoscopic examination of the colon — **col·o·no·scop·ic** \kō-ˌlä-nə-'skä-pik\ *adj*

col·o·ny \\'kä-lə-nē\ *n, pl* **-nies** : a circumscribed mass of microorganisms usu. growing in or on a solid medium

colony-stimulating factor *n* : any of several glycoproteins that promote the differentiation of stem cells esp. into blood granulocytes and macrophages and that stimulate their proliferation into colonies in culture

co·lo·proc·tos·to·my \ˌkō-lō-ˌpräk-'täs-tə-mē, ˌkä-\ *n, pl* **-mies** : surgical formation of an artificial passage between the colon and the rectum

col·or \\'kə-lər\ *n, often attrib* **1 a** : a phenomenon of light (as red, brown, pink, or gray) or visual perception that enables one to differentiate otherwise identical objects **b** : the aspect of objects and light sources that may be described in terms of hue, lightness, and saturation for objects and hue, brightness, and saturation for light sources **c** : a hue as contrasted with black, white, or gray **2** : complexion tint; *esp* : the tint characteristic of good health

Colorado tick fever *n* : a mild disease of the western U.S. and western Canada that is characterized by the absence of a rash, intermittent fever, malaise, headaches, and myalgia and is caused by an orbivirus transmitted by the Rocky Mountain wood tick

col·or–blind \-ˌblind\ *adj* : affected with partial or total inability to distinguish one or more chromatic colors — **color blindness** *n*

co·lo·rec·tal \ˌkō-lə-'rekt-əl, ˌkä-\ *adj*

: relating to or affecting the colon and the rectum ⟨~ cancer⟩ ⟨~ surgery⟩

col·or·im·e·ter \ˌkə-lə-ˈri-mə-tər\ *n* : any of various instruments used to objectively determine the color of a solution — **col·or·i·met·ric** \ˌkə-lə-rə-ˈme-trik\ *adj* — **col·or·i·met·ri·cal·ly** \-tri-k(ə-)lē\ *adv* — **col·or·im·e·try** \ˌkə-lə-ˈri-mə-trē\ *n*

color index *n* : a figure that represents the ratio of the amount of hemoglobin to the number of red cells in a given volume of blood and that is a measure of the normality of the hemoglobin content of the individual cells

color vision *n* : perception of and ability to distinguish colors

co·los·to·mize \kə-ˈläs-tə-ˌmīz\ *vb* **-mized; -miz·ing** : to perform a colostomy on

co·los·to·my \kə-ˈläs-tə-mē\ *n, pl* **-mies** : surgical formation of an artificial anus by connecting the colon to an opening in the abdominal wall

colostomy bag *n* : a container kept constantly in position to receive feces discharged through a colostomy

co·los·trum \kə-ˈläs-trəm\ *n* : milk secreted for a few days after parturition and characterized by high protein and antibody content — **co·los·tral** \-trəl\ *adj*

col·our *chiefly Brit var of* COLOR

colp- *or* **colpo-** *comb form* : vagina ⟨*colpitis*⟩ ⟨*colposcope*⟩

col·pec·to·my \ˌkäl-ˈpek-tə-mē\ *n, pl* **-mies** : partial or complete surgical excision of the vagina — called also *vaginectomy*

col·pi·tis \käl-ˈpī-təs\ *n* : VAGINITIS

col·po·cen·te·sis \ˌkäl-(ˌ)pō-sen-ˈtē-səs\ *n, pl* **-te·ses** \-ˌsēz\ : surgical puncture of the vagina

col·po·cle·i·sis \ˌkäl-pō-ˈklī-səs\ *n, pl* **-cle·i·ses** \-ˌsēz\ : the suturing of posterior and anterior walls of the vagina to prevent uterine prolapse

col·po·per·i·ne·or·rha·phy \ˌkäl-pō-ˌper-ə-(ˌ)nē-ˈor-ə-fē\ *n, pl* **-phies** : the suturing of an injury to the vagina and the perineum

col·po·pexy \ˈkäl-pə-ˌpek-sē\ *n, pl* **-pex·ies** : fixation of the vagina by suturing it to the adjacent abdominal wall

col·por·rha·phy \käl-ˈpor-ə-fē\ *n, pl* **-phies** : surgical repair of the vaginal wall

-colpos *n comb form* : vaginal disorder (of a specified type) ⟨hydrometro*colpos*⟩

col·po·scope \ˈkäl-pə-ˌskōp\ *n* : an instrument designed to facilitate visual inspection of the vagina — **col·po·scop·ic** \ˌkäl-pə-ˈskä-pik\ *adj* — **col·po·scop·i·cal·ly** \-pi-k(ə-)lē\ *adv* — **col·pos·co·py** \käl-ˈpäs-kə-pē\ *n*

col·pot·o·my \käl-ˈpä-tə-mē\ *n, pl* **-mies** : surgical incision of the vagina

co·lum·bi·um \kə-ˈləm-bē-əm\ *n* : NIOBIUM

col·u·mel·la \ˌkä-lə-ˈme-lə, ˌkäl-yə-\ *n,*

pl **-mel·lae** \-ˈme-(ˌ)lē, -ˌlī\ : any of various anatomical parts likened to a column: **a** : the bony central axis of the cochlea **b** : the lower part of the nasal septum — **col·u·mel·lar** \-lər\ *adj*

col·umn \ˈkä-ləm\ *n* : a longitudinal subdivision of the spinal cord that resembles a column or pillar: as **a** : any of the principal longitudinal subdivisions of gray matter or white matter in each lateral half of the spinal cord — see DORSAL HORN, GRAY COLUMN, LATERAL COLUMN 1, VENTRAL HORN; compare FUNICULUS a **b** : any of a number of smaller bundles of spinal nerve fibers : FASCICULUS

co·lum·nar \kə-ˈləm-nər\ *adj* : of, relating to, being, or composed of tall narrow somewhat cylindrical epithelial cells

column chromatography *n* : chromatography in which the substances to be separated are introduced onto the top of a column packed with an adsorbent (as silica gel or alumina), pass through the column at different rates that depend on the affinity of each substance for the adsorbent and for the solvent or solvent mixture, and are usu. collected in solution as they pass from the column at different times — compare PAPER CHROMATOGRAPHY, THIN-LAYER CHROMATOGRAPHY

column of Ber·tin \-ber-ˈtaⁿ\ *n* : RENAL COLUMN

E. J. Bertin — see BERTIN'S COLUMN

column of Bur·dach \-ˈbər-dək, -ˈbür-, -ˌdäk\ *n* : FASCICULUS CUNEATUS

Bur·dach \ˈbür-däk\, **Karl Friedrich** (1776–1847), German anatomist.

co·ma \ˈkō-mə\ *n* : a state of profound unconsciousness caused by disease, injury, or poison

co·ma·tose \ˈkō-mə-ˌtōs, ˈkä-\ *adj* : of, resembling, or affected with coma ⟨a ~ patient⟩ ⟨a ~ condition⟩

combat fatigue *n* : a traumatic psychoneurotic reaction or an acute psychotic reaction occurring under conditions (as wartime combat) that cause intense stress — called also *battle fatigue*; compare POSTTRAUMATIC STRESS DISORDER

com·e·do \ˈkä-mə-ˌdō\ *n, pl* **com·e·do·nes** \ˌkä-mə-ˈdō-(ˌ)nēz\ : BLACKHEAD 1

com·e·do·car·ci·no·ma \ˌkä-mə-ˌdō-ˌkärs-ən-ˈō-mə\ *n, pl* **-mas** *or* **-ma·ta** \-mə-tə\ : a breast cancer that arises in the larger ducts and is characterized by slow growth, late metastasis, and the accumulation of solid plugs of atypical and degenerating cells in the ducts

come to *vb* : to recover consciousness

comitans — see VENA COMITANS

com·men·sal·ism \kə-ˈmen-sə-ˌli-zəm\ *n* : a relation between two kinds of organisms in which one obtains food or other benefits from the other without damaging or benefiting it — **com·men·sal** \-səl\ *adj or n* — **com·men·sal·ly** *adv*

com·mi·nut·ed \ˈkä-mə-ˌnü-təd, -ˈnyü-\ *adj* : being a fracture in which the bone is splintered or crushed into numerous pieces

com·mis·su·ra \ˌkä-mə-ˈshùr-ə\ *n, pl* **-rae** \-ˈshùr-ē\ : COMMISSURE

com·mis·sure \ˈkä-mə-ˌshùr\ *n* **1** : a point or line of union or junction between two anatomical parts (as the lips at their angles or adjacent heart valves) **2** : a connecting band of nerve tissue in the brain or spinal cord — see ANTERIOR COMMISSURE, GRAY COMMISSURE, HABENULAR COMMISSURE, HIPPOCAMPAL COMMISSURE, POSTERIOR COMMISSURE; compare CORPUS CALLOSUM, MASSA INTERMEDIA — **com·mis·su·ral** \ˌkä-mə-ˈshùr-əl\ *adj*

com·mis·sur·ot·o·my \ˌkä-mə-ˌshùr-ˈä-tə-mē, -shə-ˈrä-\ *n, pl* **-mies** : the operation of cutting through a band of muscle or nerve fibers; *specif* : separation of the flaps of a bicuspid valve to relieve mitral stenosis : VALVULOTOMY

com·mit \kə-ˈmit\ *vb* **com·mit·ted; com·mit·ting** : to place in a prison or mental institution — **com·mit·ment** \kə-ˈmit-mənt\ *n* — **com·mit·ta·ble** \-ˈmi-tə-bəl\ *adj*

com·mon \ˈkä-mən\ *adj* : formed of or dividing into two or more branches (the ∼ facial vein) (∼ iliac vessels)

common bile duct *n* : the duct formed by the union of the hepatic and cystic ducts and opening into the duodenum

common carotid artery *n* : the part of either carotid artery between its point of origin and its division into the internal and external carotid arteries — called also *common carotid*

common cattle grub *n* : a cattle grub of the genus *Hypoderma* (*H. lineatum*) which is found throughout the U.S. and whose larva is particularly destructive to cattle

common cold *n* : an acute contagious disease of the upper respiratory tract caused by a virus and characterized by inflammation of the mucous membranes of the nose, throat, eyes, and eustachian tubes with a watery then purulent discharge

common iliac artery *n* : ILIAC ARTERY 1

common iliac vein *n* : ILIAC VEIN a

common interosseous artery *n* : a short thick artery that arises from the ulnar artery near the proximal end of the radius and that divides into anterior and posterior branches which pass down the forearm toward the wrist

common peroneal nerve *n* : the smaller of the branches into which the sciatic nerve divides passing outward and downward from the popliteal space and to the neck of the fibula where it divides into the deep peroneal nerve

and the superficial peroneal nerve — called also *lateral popliteal nerve*, *peroneal nerve*

com·mu·ni·ca·ble \kə-ˈmyü-ni-kə-bəl\ *adj* : capable of being transmitted from person to person, animal to person, animal to human, or human to animal : TRANSMISSIBLE — **com·mu·ni·ca·bil·i·ty** \-ˌmyü-ni-kə-ˈbi-lə-tē\ *n*

communicable disease *n* : an infectious disease transmissible (as from person to person) by direct contact with an affected individual or the individual's discharges or by indirect means (as by a vector) — compare CONTAGIOUS DISEASE

communicans — see RAMUS COMMUNICANS, WHITE RAMUS COMMUNICANS

communicantes — see RAMUS COMMUNICANS

communicating artery *n* : any of three arteries in the brain that form parts of the circle of Willis: **a** : one connecting the anterior cerebral arteries — called also *anterior communicating artery* **b** : either of two arteries that occur one on each side of the circle of Willis and connect an internal carotid artery with a posterior cerebral artery — called also *posterior communicating artery*

com·mu·ni·ca·tion \kə-ˌmyü-nə-ˈkā-shən\ *n* **1** : the act or process of transmitting information (as about ideas, attitudes, emotions, or objective behavior) (nonverbal interpersonal ∼) **2** : information communicated **3** : a connection between bodily parts (an artificial ∼ between the esophagus and the stomach)

communis — see EXTENSOR DIGITORUM COMMUNIS

com·pact \kəm-ˈpakt, käm-ˈ, ˈkäm-ˌ\ *adj* : having a dense structure without small cavities or cells (∼ bone) — compare CANCELLOUS

compacta — see PARS COMPACTA

compactum — see STRATUM COMPACTUM

com·par·a·tive \kəm-ˈpar-ə-tiv\ *adj* : characterized by the systematic comparison of phenomena and esp. of likenesses and dissimilarities (∼ anatomy)

com·pat·i·ble \kəm-ˈpa-tə-bəl\ *adj* **1** : capable of existing together in a satisfactory relationship (as marriage) **2** : capable of being used in transfusion or grafting without immunological reaction (as agglutination or tissue rejection) **3** *of medications* : capable of being administered jointly without interacting to produce deleterious effects or impairing their respective actions — **com·pat·i·bil·i·ty** \-ˌpa-tə-ˈbi-lə-tē\ *n*

Com·pa·zine \ˈkäm-pə-ˌzēn\ *trademark* — used for a preparation of prochlorperazine

com·pen·sate \ˈkäm-pən-ˌsāt, -ˌpen-\ *vb* **-sat·ed; -sat·ing 1** : to subject to or remedy by physiological compensation 2 : to undergo or engage in psychic or physiological compensation

com·pen·sat·ed *adj* : buffered so that there is no change in the pH of the blood ⟨∼ acidosis⟩ — compare UNCOMPENSATED

com·pen·sa·tion \ˌkäm-pən-ˈsā-shən, -ˌpen-\ *n* 1 : correction of an organic defect by excessive development or by increased functioning of another organ or unimpaired parts of the same organ ⟨cardiac ∼⟩ — see DECOMPENSATION 2 : a psychological mechanism by which feelings of inferiority, frustration, or failure in one field are counterbalanced by achievement in another

com·pen·sa·to·ry \kəm-ˈpen-sə-ˌtōr-ē\ *adj* : making up for a loss: *esp* : serving as psychic or physiological compensation

com·pe·tence \ˈkäm-pə-təns\ *n* : the quality or state of being functionally adequate ⟨drugs that improve the ∼ of a failing heart⟩

com·pe·ten·cy \-tən-sē\ *n, pl* **-cies** : COMPETENCE

com·pe·tent \ˈkäm-pə-tənt\ *adj* : having the capacity to function or develop in a particular way

com·pet·i·tive \kəm-ˈpe-tə-tiv\ *adj* : depending for effectiveness on the relative concentration of two or more substances ⟨∼ inhibition of an enzyme⟩ ⟨∼ protein binding⟩

com·plain \kəm-ˈplān\ *vb* : to speak of one's illness or symptoms ⟨the patient visited the office ∼ing of jaundice⟩

com·plaint \kəm-ˈplānt\ *n* : a bodily ailment or disease

com·ple·ment \ˈkäm-plə-mənt\ *n* 1 : a group or set (as of chromosomes) that is typical of the complete organism or one of its parts — see CHROMOSOME COMPLEMENT 2 : the thermolabile group of proteins in normal blood serum and plasma that in combination with antibodies causes the destruction *esp.* of particulate antigens

com·ple·men·tar·i·ty \ˌkäm-plə-(ˌ)men-ˈtar-ə-tē, -mən-\ *n, pl* **-ties** : correspondence in reverse of part of one molecule to part of another: as **a** : the arrangement of chemical groups and electric charges that enables a combining group of an antibody to combine with a specific determinant group of an antigen or hapten **b** : the correspondence between strands or nucleotides of DNA or sometimes RNA that permits their precise pairing

com·ple·men·ta·ry \ˌkäm-plə-ˈmen-tə-rē, -trē\ *adj* : characterized by molecular complementarity; *esp* : characterized by the capacity for precise pairing of purine and pyrimidine bases between strands of DNA and sometimes RNA such that the structure of one strand determines the other — **com·ple·men·ta·ri·ly** \-ˈmen-trə-lē, -(ˌ)men-ˈter-ə-lē, -ˈmen-tə-rə-lē\ *adv* — **com·ple·men·ta·ri·ness** \-ˈmen-tə-rē-nəs, -ˈmen-trē-\ *n*

complementary DNA *n* : CDNA

complement fixation *n* : the process of binding serum complement to the product formed by the union of an antibody and the antigen for which it is specific that occurs when complement is added to a mixture (in proper proportion) of such an antibody and antigen

complement–fixation test *n* : a diagnostic test for the presence of a particular antibody in the serum of a patient that involves inactivation of the complement in the serum, addition of measured amounts of the antigen for which the antibody is specific and of foreign complement, and detection of the presence or absence of complement fixation by the addition of a suitable indicator system — see WASSERMAN TEST

com·plete \kəm-ˈplēt\ *adj* 1 *of insect metamorphosis* : having a pupal stage intercalated between the motile immature stages and the adult — compare INCOMPLETE 1 2 *of a bone fracture* : characterized by a break passing entirely across the bone — compare INCOMPLETE 2

complete blood count *n* : a blood count that includes separate counts for red and white blood cells — called also *complete blood cell count;* compare DIFFERENTIAL BLOOD COUNT

¹com·plex \käm-ˈpleks, kəm-ˈ, ˈkäm-ˌ\ *adj* : formed by the union of simpler chemical substances ⟨∼ proteins⟩

²com·plex \ˈkäm-ˌpleks\ *n* 1 : a group of repressed memories, desires, and ideas that exert a dominant influence on the personality and behavior ⟨a guilt ∼⟩ — see CASTRATION COMPLEX, ELECTRA COMPLEX, INFERIORITY COMPLEX, OEDIPUS COMPLEX, PERSECUTION COMPLEX, SUPERIORITY COMPLEX 2 : a group of chromosomes arranged or behaving in a particular way — see GENE COMPLEX 3 : a complex chemical substance ⟨molecular ∼es⟩ 4 : the sum of the factors (as symptoms and lesions) characterizing a disease ⟨primary tuberculous ∼⟩

³com·plex \käm-ˈpleks, kəm-ˈ, ˈkäm-ˌ\ *vb* : to form or cause to form into a complex ⟨RNA ∼ed with protein⟩

com·plex·ion \kəm-ˈplek-shən\ *n* : the hue or appearance of the skin and esp. of the face ⟨a dark ∼⟩ — **com·plex·ioned** \-shənd\ *adj*

com·plex·us \kəm-ˈplek-səs, käm-\ *n* : SEMISPINALIS CAPITIS — called also *complexus muscle*

com·pli·ance \kəm-ˈplī-əns\ *n* 1 : the ability or process of yielding to changes in pressure without disruption of structure or function ⟨a study of pulmonary ∼⟩ 2 : the process of complying with a regimen of treatment

com·pli·cate \'käm-plə-ˌkāt\ vb **-cated; -cat·ing :** to cause to be more complex or severe (a virus disease *complicated* by bacterial infection)

com·pli·cat·ed adj, of a bone fracture **:** characterized by injury to nearby parts

com·pli·ca·tion \ˌkäm-plə-'kā-shən\ n **:** a secondary disease or condition that develops in the course of a primary disease or condition and arises either as a result of it or from independent causes

com·pos men·tis \ˌkäm-pəs-'men-təs\ adj **:** of sound mind, memory, and understanding

¹**com·pound** \käm-'paúnd, kəm-', 'käm-ˌ\ vb **:** to form by combining parts (~ a medicine)

²**com·pound** \'käm-ˌpaúnd, käm-', kəm-'\ adj **:** composed of or resulting from union of separate elements, ingredients, or parts (a ~ substance) (~ glands)

³**com·pound** \'käm-ˌpaúnd\ n **:** something formed by a union of elements or parts; *specif* **:** a distinct substance formed by chemical union of two or more ingredients in definite proportion by weight

compound benzoin tincture n **:** FRIAR'S BALSAM

compound fracture n **:** a bone fracture resulting in an open wound through which bone fragments usu. protrude — compare SIMPLE FRACTURE

compound microscope n **:** a microscope consisting of an objective and an eyepiece mounted in a telescoping tube

¹**com·press** \kəm-'pres\ vb **:** to press or squeeze together

²**com·press** \'käm-ˌpres\ n **1 :** a covering consisting usu. of a folded cloth that is applied and held firmly by the aid of a bandage over a wound dressing to prevent oozing **2 :** a folded wet or dry cloth applied firmly to a part (as to allay inflammation)

compressed–air illness n **:** DECOMPRESSION SICKNESS

com·pres·sion \kəm-'pre-shən\ n **:** the act, process, or result of compressing esp. when involving a compressing force on a bodily part (~ of an artery by forceps)

compression fracture n **:** fracture (as of a vertebra) caused by compression of one bone against another

com·pro·mise \'käm-prə-ˌmīz\ vb **-mised; -mis·ing :** to cause the impairment of (a *compromised* immune system) (a seriously *compromised* patient)

com·pul·sion \kəm-'pəl-shən\ n **:** an irresistible impulse to perform an irrational act — compare OBSESSION, PHOBIA

¹**com·pul·sive** \-siv\ adj **:** of, relating to, caused by, or suggestive of psycho-

logical compulsion or obsession (repetitive and ~ behavior) (a ~ gambler) — **com·pul·sive·ly** adv — **com·pul·sive·ness** n — **com·pul·siv·i·ty** \ˌkäm-ˌpəl-'si-və-tē, ˌkäm-ˌ\ n

²**compulsive** n **:** one who is subject to a psychological compulsion

com·put·ed axial tomography \kəm-'pyü-təd-\ n **:** COMPUTED TOMOGRAPHY — abbr. CAT

computed tomography n **:** radiography in which a three-dimensional image of a body structure is constructed by computer from a series of plane cross-sectional images made along an axis — abbr. CT

com·pu·ter·ized axial tomography \kəm-'pyü-tə-ˌrīzd-\ n **:** COMPUTED TOMOGRAPHY — abbr. CAT

computerized tomography n **:** COMPUTED TOMOGRAPHY — abbr. CT

co·na·tion \kō-'nā-shən\ n **:** an inclination (as an instinct, a drive, a wish, or a craving) to act purposefully **:** IMPULSE 2 — **co·na·tive** \'kō-nə-tiv, -ˌnā-; 'kä-\ adj

conc abbr concentrated; concentration

con·ca·nav·a·lin \ˌkän-kə-'na-və-lən\ n **:** either of two crystalline globulins occurring esp. in the seeds of a tropical American leguminous plant (*Canavalia ensiformis*); *esp* **:** one that is a potent hemagglutinin

con·ceive \kən-'sēv\ vb **con·ceived; con·ceiv·ing :** to become pregnant

con·cen·trate \'kän-sən-ˌtrāt, -ˌsen-\ vb **-trat·ed; -trat·ing 1 a :** to bring or direct toward a common center or objective **b :** to accumulate (a toxic substance) in bodily tissues (fish ~ mercury) **2 :** to make less dilute **3 :** to fix one's powers, efforts, or attention on one thing

con·cen·tra·tion \ˌkän-sən-'trā-shən, -ˌsen-\ n **1 :** the act or action of concentrating: as **a :** a directing of the attention or of the mental faculties toward a single object **b :** an increasing of strength (as of a solute) by partial or total removal of diluents **2 :** a crude active principle of a vegetable esp. for pharmaceutical use in the form of a powder or resin **3 :** the relative content of a component (as dissolved or dispersed material) of a solution, mixture, or dispersion that may be expressed in percentage by weight or by volume, in parts per million, or in grams per liter

con·cep·tion \kən-'sep-shən\ n **1 a :** the process of becoming pregnant involving fertilization or implantation or both **b :** EMBRYO, FETUS **2 a :** the capacity, function, or process of forming or understanding ideas or abstractions or their symbols **b :** a general idea

con·cep·tive \kən-'sep-tiv\ adj **:** capable of or relating to conceiving

con·cep·tus \kən-'sep-təs\ n **:** a fertilized egg, embryo, or fetus

conch \'käŋk, 'känch, 'koŋk\ *n, pl* **conchs** \'käŋks, 'koŋks\ *or* **conch·es** \'kän-chəz\ : CONCHA 1

con·cha \'käŋ-kə, 'koŋ-\ *n, pl* **con·chae** \-ˌkē, -ˌkī\ **1** : the largest and deepest concavity of the external ear **2** : NASAL CONCHA — **con·chal** \-kəl\ *adj*

con·cor·dant \kən-'kord-ənt\ *adj, of twins* : similar with respect to one or more discordant characters — compare DISCORDANT — **con·cor·dance** \-ən(t)s\ *n*

con·cre·ment \'käŋ-krə-mənt, 'kän-\ *n* : CONCRETION

con·cre·tion \kän-'krē-shən, kən-\ *n* : a hard usu. inorganic mass (as a bezoar or tophus) formed in a living body

con·cuss \kən-'kəs\ *vb* : to affect with concussion

con·cus·sion \kən-'kə-shən\ *n* **1** : a hard blow or collision **2** : a condition resulting from the effects of a hard blow; *esp* : a jarring injury of the brain resulting in disturbance of cerebral function — **con·cus·sive** \-'kə-siv\ *adj*

con·den·sa·tion \ˌkän-ˌden-'sā-shən, -dən-\ *n* **1** : the act or process of condensing: as **a** : a chemical reaction involving union between molecules often with elimination of a simple molecule (as water) or a reduction to a denser form (as from steam to water) **2** : representation of several apparently discrete ideas by a single symbol esp. in dreams **3** : an abnormal hardening of an organ or tissue ⟨connective tissue ∼s⟩

con·dense \kən-'den(t)s\ *vb* **con·densed; con·dens·ing** : to make denser or more compact; *esp* : to subject to or undergo condensation

¹con·di·tion \kən-'di-shən\ *n* **1** : something essential to the appearance or occurrence of something else; *esp* : an environmental requirement **2 a** : a usu. defective state of health ⟨a serious heart ∼⟩ **b** : a state of physical fitness

²condition *vb* **con·di·tioned; con·di·tion·ing** : to cause to undergo a change so that an act or response previously associated with another — **con·di·tion·able** \kən-'di-sh(ə-)nə-bəl\ *adj*

con·di·tion·al \kən-'dish-nəl, -'dish-ən-ᵊl\ *adj* **1** : CONDITIONED ⟨∼ reflex⟩ **2** : eliciting a conditional response ⟨a ∼ stimulus⟩ — **con·di·tion·al·ly** \-'dish-nə-lē, -'di-shən-ᵊl-ē\ *adv*

con·di·tioned *adj* : determined or established by conditioning

con·dom \'kän-dəm\ *n* **1** : a sheath commonly of rubber worn over the penis (as to prevent conception or venereal infection during coitus) — called also *sheath* **2** : a device inserted into the vagina that is similar to a condom

con·duct \kən-'dəkt, 'kän-ˌdəkt\ *vb* **1** : to act as a medium for conveying **2** : to have the quality of transmitting

something — **con·duc·tance** \kən-'dək-təns\ *n*

con·duc·tion \kən-'dək-shən\ *n* **1** : transmission through or by means of something (as a conductor) **2** : the transmission of excitation through living tissue and esp. nervous tissue

conduction deafness *n* : hearing loss or impairment resulting from interference with the transmission of sound waves to the organ of Corti — called also *conductive deafness, transmission deafness*; compare CENTRAL DEAFNESS, NERVE DEAFNESS

con·duc·tive \-'dək-tiv\ *adj* **1** : having the power to conduct **2** : caused by failure in the mechanisms for sound transmission in the external or middle ear ⟨∼ hearing loss⟩ — **con·duc·tiv·i·ty** \ˌkän-ˌdək-'ti-və-tē, kən-\ *n*

con·duc·tor \kən-'dək-tər\ *n* **1** : a substance or body capable of transmitting electricity, heat, or sound **2** : a bodily part (as a nerve fiber) that transmits excitation

condyl- *or* **condylo-** *comb form* : joint : condyle ⟨condylectomy⟩ ⟨condyloid joint⟩

con·dy·lar·thro·sis \ˌkän-də-lär-'thrō-səs\ *n, pl* **-thro·ses** \-ˌsēz\ : articulation by means of a condyle

con·dyle \'kän-ˌdil, 'känd-ᵊl\ *n* : an articular prominence of a bone — used chiefly of such as occur in pairs resembling a pair of knuckles (as those of the occipital bone for articulation with the atlas, those at the distal end of the humerus and femur, and those of the lower jaw); see LATERAL CONDYLE, MEDIAL CONDYLE — **con·dy·lar** \'kän-də-lər\ *adj* — **con·dy·loid** \'kän-də-ˌloid\ *adj*

con·dyl·ec·to·my \ˌkän-ˌdī-'lek-tə-mē, ˌkänd-ᵊl-'ek-\ *n, pl* **-mies** : surgical removal of a condyle

con·dy·loid joint \'kän-də-ˌloid-\ *n* : an articulation in which an ovoid head is received into an elliptical cavity permitting all movements except axial rotation

condyloid process *n* : the rounded process by which the ramus of the mandible articulates with the temporal bone

con·dy·lo·ma \ˌkän-də-'lō-mə\ *n, pl* **-ma·ta** \-mə-tə\ *also* **-mas** : CONDYLOMA ACUMINATUM — **con·dy·lo·ma·tous** \-mə-təs\ *adj*

condyloma acu·mi·na·tum \-ə-ˌkyü-mə-'nā-təm\ *n, pl* **condylomata acu·mi·na·ta** \-'nä-tə\ : a warty growth on the skin or adjoining mucous membrane usu. near the anus and genital organs — called also *genital wart, venereal wart*

condyloma la·tum \-'lä-təm\ *n, pl* **condylomata la·ta** \-tə\ : a highly infectious flattened often hypertrophic papule of secondary syphilis that forms in moist areas of skin and at mucocutaneous junctions

cone \'kōn\ *n* **1** : any of the conical photosensitive receptor cells of the retina that function in color vision — compare ROD 1 **2** : any of a family (Conidae) of numerous somewhat conical tropical gastropod mollusks that include a few highly poisonous forms **3** : a cusp of a tooth esp. in the upper jaw

cone-nose \'kōn-,nōz\ *n* : any of various large bloodsucking bugs esp. of the genus *Triatoma* including some capable of inflicting painful bites — called also *kissing bug*

con·fab·u·la·tion \kən-,fa-byə-'lā-shən, ,kän-\ *n* : a filling in of gaps in memory by unconstrained fabrication — **con·fab·u·late** \kən-'fa-byə-,lāt\ *vb*

con·fec·tion \kən-'fek-shən\ *n* : a medicinal preparation usu. made with sugar, syrup, or honey — called also *electuary*

con·fine \kən-'fīn\ *vb* **con·fined; con·fin·ing** : to keep from leaving accustomed quarters (as one's room or bed) under pressure of infirmity, childbirth, or detention

con·fined \kən-'fīnd\ *adj* : undergoing childbirth

con·fine·ment \kən-'fīn-mənt\ *n* : an act of confining : the state of being confined; esp : LYING-IN

con·flict \'kän-,flikt\ *n* : mental struggle resulting from incompatible or opposing needs, drives, wishes, or external or internal demands — **con·flict·ful** \'kän-,flikt-fəl\ *adj* — **con·flic·tu·al** \kän-'flik-chə-wəl, kən-\ *adj*

con·flict·ed \kən-'flik-təd\ *adj* : having or expressing emotional conflict ⟨~ about one's sexual identity⟩

con·flu·ence of sinuses \'kän-,flü-ənts-, kən-'flü-\ *n* : the junction of several of the sinuses of the dura mater in the internal occipital region — called also *confluence of the sinuses*

con·flu·ent \'kän-,flü-ənt, kən-'\ *adj* **1** : flowing or coming together; *also* : run together ⟨~ pustules⟩ **2** : characterized by confluent lesions ⟨~ smallpox⟩ — compare DISCRETE

con·for·ma·tion \,kän-(,)for-'mā-shən, -fər-\ *n* : any of the spatial arrangements of a molecule that can be obtained by rotation of the atoms about a single bond — **con·for·ma·tion·al·ly** \-shnəl, -shən-ᵊl\ *adj* — **con·for·ma·tion·al·ly** *adv*

con·form·er \kən-'for-mər\ *n* : a mold (as of plastic) used to prevent collapse or closing of a cavity, vessel, or opening during surgical repair

con·fu·sion \kən-'fyü-zhən\ *n* : disturbance of consciousness characterized by inability to engage in orderly thought or by lack of power to distinguish, choose, or act decisively — **con·fused** \-'fyüzd\ *adj* — **con·fu·sion·al** \-zhnəl, -zhən-ᵊl\ *adj*

con·geal \kən-'jēl\ *vb* **1** : to change from

a fluid to a solid state by or as if by cold **2** : to make viscid or curdled : COAGULATE

con·ge·ner \'kän-jə-nər, kən-'jē-\ *n* **1** : a member of the same taxonomic genus as another plant or animal **2** : a chemical substance related to another (tetracycline and its ~s) — **con·ge·ner·ic** \,kän-jə-'ner-ik\ *adj*

congenita — see AMYOTONIA CONGENITA, ARTHROGRYPOSIS MULTIPLEX CONGENITA, MYOTONIA CONGENITA, OSTEOGENESIS IMPERFECTA CONGENITA

con·gen·i·tal \kän-'je-nət-ᵊl\ *adj* **1** : existing at or dating from birth ⟨~ deafness⟩ **2** : acquired during development in the uterus and not through heredity ⟨~ syphilis⟩ — compare ACQUIRED 2, FAMILIAL, HEREDITARY — **con·gen·i·tal·ly** *adv*

congenital megacolon *n* : HIRSCHSPRUNG'S DISEASE

con·gest·ed \kən-'jes-təd\ *adj* : containing an excessive accumulation of blood : HYPEREMIC ⟨~ mucous membranes⟩

con·ges·tion \kən-'jes-chən, -'jesh-\ *n* : an excessive accumulation esp. of blood in the blood vessels of an organ or part whether natural or artificially induced (as for therapeutic purposes) — **con·ges·tive** \-'jes-tiv\ *adj*

congestive heart failure *n* : heart failure in which the heart is unable to maintain adequate circulation of blood in the tissues of the body or to pump out the venous blood returned to it by the venous circulation

con·glu·ti·nate \kən-'glüt-ᵊn-,āt, kän-\ *vb* **-nat·ed; -nat·ing** : to unite or become united by or as if by a glutinous substance (blood platelets ~ in blood clotting) — **con·glu·ti·na·tion** \-,glüt-ᵊn-'ā-shən\ *n*

Congo red \'käŋ-(,)gō-\ *n* : an azo dye $C_{32}H_{22}N_6Na_2O_6S_2$ used in a number of diagnostic tests and esp. for the detection of amyloidosis since the injected dye tends to be retained by abnormal amyloid deposits

con·gress \'käŋ-grəs, -rəs\ *n* : COITUS

coni *pl of* CONUS

con·iza·tion \,kō-nə-'zā-shən, ,kä-\ *n* : the electrosurgical excision of a cone of tissue from a diseased uterine cervix

con·ju·ga·ta \,kän-jə-'gā-tə\ *n*, *pl* **-ga·tae** \-'gā-,tē\ : CONJUGATE DIAMETER

¹con·ju·gate \'kän-ji-gət, -jə-,gāt\ *adj* **1** : functioning or operating simultaneously as if joined **2** *of an acid or base* : related by the difference of a proton — **con·ju·gate·ly** *adv*

²con·ju·gate \-jə-,gāt\ *vb* **-gat·ed; -gat·ing** **1** : to unite (as with the elimination of water) so that the product is easily broken down (as by hydrolysis) into the original compounds **2** : to pair and fuse in conjugation **3** : to pair in synapsis

³con·ju·gate \-ji-gət, -jə-,gāt\ *n* : a chemical compound formed by the union of two compounds or united with another compound — **con·ju·gat·ed** \'kän-jə-ˌgā-təd\ *adj*

conjugate diameter *n* : the anteroposterior diameter of the human pelvis measured from the sacral promontory to the pubic symphysis — called also *conjugata, true conjugate*

conjugated protein *n* : a compound of a protein with a nonprotein ⟨hemoglobin is a *conjugated protein* of heme and globin⟩

con·ju·ga·tion \ˌkän-jə-'gā-shən\ *n* **1** : the act of conjugating : the state of being conjugated **2 a** : temporary cytoplasmic union with exchange of nuclear material that is the usual sexual process in ciliated protozoans **b** : the one-way transfer of DNA between bacteria in cellular contact — **con·ju·ga·tion·al** \-shnəl, -shən-ᵊl\ *adj*

con·junc·ti·va \ˌkän-ˌjəŋk-'tī-və, kən-\ *n, pl* **-vas** *or* **-vae** \-(ˌ)vē\ : the mucous membrane that lines the inner surface of the eyelids and is continued over the forepart of the eyeball — **con·junc·ti·val** \-vəl\ *adj*

con·junc·ti·vi·tis \kən-ˌjəŋk-ti-'vī-təs\ *n* : inflammation of the conjunctiva

con·junc·ti·vo·plas·ty \kən-'jəŋk-ti-(ˌ)vō-ˌplas-tē\ *n, pl* **-plas·ties** : plastic repair of a defect in the conjunctiva

con·junc·ti·vo·rhi·nos·to·my \kən-ˌjəŋk-ti-(ˌ)vō-ˌrī-'näs-tə-mē\ *n, pl* **-to·mies** : surgical creation of a passage through the conjunctiva to the nasal cavity

conjunctivum — see BRACHIUM CONJUNCTIVUM

connective tissue *n* : a tissue of mesodermal origin rich in intercellular substance or interlacing processes with little tendency for the cells to come together in sheets or masses; *specif* : connective tissue of stellate or spindle-shaped cells with interlacing processes that pervades, supports, and binds together other tissues and forms ligaments, tendons, and aponeuroses

connective tissue disease *n* : any of various diseases or abnormal states (as rheumatoid arthritis, systemic lupus erythematosus, polyarteritis nodosa, rheumatic fever, and dermatomyositis) characterized by inflammatory or degenerative changes in connective tissue — called also *collagen disease, collagenolysis, collagen vascular disease*

con·nec·tor \kə-'nek-tər\ *n* : a part of a partial denture which joins its components

conniventes — see VALVULAE CONNIVENTES

Conn's syndrome \'känz-\ *n* : PRIMARY ALDOSTERONISM

Conn, Jerome W. (*b* 1907), American physician.

con·san·guine \kän-'saŋ-gwən, kən-\ *adj* : CONSANGUINEOUS

con·san·guin·e·ous \ˌkän-ˌsan-'gwi-nē-əs, -ˌsaŋ-\ *adj* : of the same blood or origin; *specif* : relating to or involving persons (as first cousins) that are relatively closely related ⟨∼ marriages⟩ — **con·san·guin·i·ty** \-nə-tē\ *n*

con·science \'kän-chəns\ *n* : the part of the superego in psychoanalysis that transmits commands and admonitions to the ego

¹con·scious \'kän-chəs\ *adj* **1** : capable of or marked by thought, will, design, or perception : relating to, being, or being part of consciousness ⟨the ∼ mind⟩ **2** : having mental faculties undulled by sleep, faintness, or stupor — **con·scious·ly** *adv*

²conscious *n* : CONSCIOUSNESS 3

con·scious·ness \-nəs\ *n* **1** : the totality in psychology of sensations, perceptions, ideas, attitudes, and feelings of which an individual or a group is aware at any given time or within a given time span **2** : waking life (as that to which one returns after sleep, trance, or fever) in which one's normal mental powers are present **3** : the upper part of mental life of which the person is aware as contrasted with unconscious processes

con·sen·su·al \kən-'sen-chə-wəl\ *adj* **1** : existing or made by mutual consent ⟨∼ sexual behavior⟩ **2** : relating to or being the constrictive pupillary response of an eye that is covered when the other eye is exposed to light — **con·sen·su·al·ly** *adv*

con·ser·va·tive \kən-'sər-və-tiv\ *adj* : designed to preserve parts or restore function ⟨∼ surgery⟩ — compare RADICAL — **con·ser·va·tive·ly** *adv*

con·serve \kən-'sərv\ *vb* **con·served; con·serv·ing** : to maintain (a quantity) constant during a process of chemical, physical, or evolutionary change

con·sol·i·da·tion \kən-ˌsä-lə-'dā-shən\ *n* : the process by which an infected lung passes from an aerated collapsible condition to one of airless solid consistency through the accumulation of exudate in the alveoli and adjoining ducts; *also* : tissue that has undergone consolidation

con·spe·cif·ic \ˌkän-spi-'si-fik\ *adj* : of the same species — **conspecific** *n*

constant region *n* : the part of the polypeptide chain of a light or heavy chain of an antibody that ends in a free carboxyl group –COOH and that is relatively constant in its sequence of amino-acid residues from one antibody to another — called also *constant domain;* compare VARIABLE REGION

con·stel·la·tion \ˌkän-stə-'lā-shən\ *n* : a set of ideas, conditions, symptoms, or traits that fall into or appear to fall into a pattern

con·sti·pa·tion \ˌkän-stə-ˈpā-shən\ n : abnormally delayed or infrequent passage of usu. dry hardened feces — **con·sti·pate** \ˈkän-stə-ˌpāt\ vb — **con·sti·pat·ed** \-ˌpā-təd\ adj

con·sti·tu·tion \ˌkän-stə-ˈtü-shən, -ˈtyü-\ n : the physical makeup of the individual comprising inherited qualities modified by environment — **con·sti·tu·tion·al** \-shnəl, -shən-ᵊl\ adj

con·sti·tu·tion·al \-shnəl, -shən-ᵊl\ n : a walk taken for one's health

con·strict \kən-ˈstrikt\ vb 1 : to make narrow or draw together 2 : to subject (as a body part) to compression ⟨∼ a nerve⟩ — **con·stric·tion** \-ˈstrik-shən\ n — **con·stric·tive** \-ˈstrik-tiv\ adj

con·stric·tor \-ˈstrik-tər\ n : a muscle that contracts a cavity or orifice or compresses an organ — see INFERIOR CONSTRICTOR, MIDDLE CONSTRICTOR, SUPERIOR CONSTRICTOR

constrictor pha·ryn·gis inferior \-fə-ˈrin-jəs-\ n : INFERIOR CONSTRICTOR

constrictor pharyngis me·di·us \-ˈmē-dē-əs\ n : MIDDLE CONSTRICTOR

constrictor pharyngis superior n : SUPERIOR CONSTRICTOR

con·struct \ˈkän-ˌstrəkt\ n : something constructed esp. by mental synthesis (form a ∼ of a physical object)

con·sult \kən-ˈsəlt\ vb : to ask the advice or opinion of ⟨∼ a doctor⟩

con·sul·tant \kən-ˈsəlt-ᵊnt\ n : a physician and esp. a specialist called in for professional advice or services usu. at the request of another physician — called also *consulting physician*

con·sul·ta·tion \ˌkän-səl-ˈtā-shən\ n : a deliberation between physicians on a case or its treatment — **con·sul·ta·tive** \kən-ˈsəl-tə-tiv, ˈkän-səl-ˌtā-tiv\ adj

con·sum·ma·to·ry \kən-ˈsə-mə-ˌtōr-ē\ adj : of, relating to, or being a response or act (as eating or copulating) that terminates a period of usu. goal-directed behavior

con·sump·tion \kən-ˈsəmp-shən\ n 1 : a progressive wasting away of the body esp. from pulmonary tuberculosis : TUBERCULOSIS

¹**con·sump·tive** \-ˈsəmp-tiv\ adj : of, relating to, or affected with consumption ⟨a ∼ cough⟩

²**consumptive** n : a person affected with consumption

¹**con·tact** \ˈkän-ˌtakt\ n 1 : union or junction of body surfaces ⟨sexual ∼⟩ 2 : direct experience through the senses 3 : CONTACT LENS

²**contact** adj : caused or transmitted by direct or indirect contact (as with an allergen or a contagious disease)

contact lens n : a thin lens designed to fit over the cornea and usu. worn to correct defects in vision

con·ta·gion \kən-ˈtā-jən\ n 1 : the transmission of a disease by direct or indirect contact 2 : CONTAGIOUS DISEASE 3 : a disease-producing agent (as a virus)

contagiosa — see IMPETIGO CONTAGIOSA, MOLLUSCUM CONTAGIOSUM

contagiosum — see MOLLUSCUM CONTAGIOSUM

con·ta·gious \-jəs\ adj 1 : communicable by contact — compare INFECTIOUS 2 2 : bearing contagion 3 : used for contagious diseases ⟨a ∼ ward⟩ — **con·ta·gious·ly** adv — **con·ta·gious·ness** n

contagious abortion n 1 : brucellosis in domestic animals characterized by abortion; *esp* : a disease affecting esp. cattle that is caused by a brucella (*Brucella abortus*), that is contracted by ingestion, by copulation, or possibly by wound infection, and that is characterized by proliferation of the causative organism in the fetal membranes inducing abortion 2 : any of several contagious or infectious diseases of domestic animals marked by abortion (as vibrionic abortion of sheep) — called also *infectious abortion*

contagious disease n : an infectious disease communicable by contact with one suffering from it, with a bodily discharge of such a patient, or with an object touched by such a patient or by bodily discharges — compare COMMUNICABLE DISEASE

con·ta·gium \kən-ˈtā-jəm, -jē-əm\ n, pl **-gia** \-jə, -jē-ə\ : a virus or living organism capable of causing a communicable disease

con·tam·i·nant \kən-ˈta-mə-nənt\ n : something that contaminates

con·tam·i·nate \kən-ˈta-mə-ˌnāt\ vb **-nat·ed; -nat·ing** 1 : to soil, stain, or infect by contact or association (bacteria *contaminated* the wound) 2 : to make inferior or impure by admixture ⟨air *contaminated* by sulfur dioxide⟩ — **con·tam·i·na·tion** \kən-ˌta-mə-ˈnā-shən\ n

con·tent \ˈkän-ˌtent\ n : the subject matter or symbolic significance of something — see LATENT CONTENT, MANIFEST CONTENT

con·ti·nence \ˈkänt-ᵊn-əns\ n 1 : self-restraint in refraining from sexual intercourse 2 : the ability to retain a bodily discharge voluntarily ⟨fecal ∼⟩ — **con·ti·nent** \-ənt\ adj — **con·ti·nent·ly** adv

continuous positive airway pressure n : a technique of assisting breathing by maintaining the air pressure in the lungs and air passages constant and above atmospheric pressure throughout the breathing cycle — abbr. CPAP

con·tra·cep·tion \ˌkän-trə-ˈsep-shən\ n : deliberate prevention of conception or impregnation — **con·tra·cep·tive** \-ˈsep-tiv\ adj or n

con·tract \kən-ˈtrakt, ˈkän-ˌtrakt\ vb 1 : to become affected with ⟨∼ pneumonia⟩ 2 : to draw together so as to become diminished in size; *also* : to shorten and broaden ⟨muscle ~s in tetanus⟩

con·trac·tile \kən-'trakt-ᵊl, -'trak-ˌtīl\ *adj* : having or concerned with the power or property of contracting

con·trac·til·i·ty \ˌkän-ˌtrak-'ti-lə-tē\ *n, pl* **-ties** : the capability or quality of shrinking or contracting; *esp* : the power of muscle fibers of shortening into a more compact form

con·trac·tion \kən-'trak-shən\ *n* **1** : the action or process of contracting : the state of being contracted **2** : the shortening and thickening of a functioning muscle or muscle fiber

con·trac·tor \'kän-ˌtrak-tər, kən-'\ *n* : something (as a muscle) that contracts or shortens

con·trac·ture \kən-'trak-chər\ *n* : a permanent shortening (as of muscle or scar tissue) producing deformity or distortion — see DUPUYTREN'S CONTRACTURE

con·tra·in·di·ca·tion \ˌkän-trə-ˌin-də-'kā-shən\ *n* : something (as a symptom or condition) that makes a particular treatment or procedure inadvisable — **con·tra·in·di·cate** \-'in-də-ˌkāt\ *vb*

con·tra·lat·er·al \-'la-tə-rəl, -'la-trəl\ *adj* : occurring on or acting in conjunction with a part on the opposite side of the body — compare IPSILATERAL

contrast bath *n* : a therapeutic immersion of a part of the body (as an extremity) alternately in hot and cold water

contrast medium *n* : a material comparatively opaque to X rays that is injected into a hollow organ to provide a contrast with the surrounding tissue and make possible radiographic and fluoroscopic examination

con·tre·coup \'kōn-trə-ˌkü, 'kän-\ *n* : injury occurring on one side of an organ (as the brain) when it recoils against a hard surface (as of the skull) following a blow on the opposite side

¹con·trol \kən-'trōl\ *vb* **con·trolled; con·trol·ling 1 a** : to check, test, or verify by evidence or experiments **b** : to incorporate suitable controls in ⟨a *controlled* experiment⟩ **2** : to reduce the incidence or severity of esp. to innocuous levels ⟨~ outbreaks of cholera⟩

²control *n* **1** : an act or instance of controlling something ⟨~ of acute intermittent porphyria⟩ **2** : one that is used in controlling something: as **a** : an experiment in which the subjects are treated as in a parallel experiment except for omission of the procedure or agent under test and which is used as a standard of comparison in judging experimental effects — called also *control experiment* **b** : one (as an organism) that is part of a control

con·trolled \kən-'trōld\ *adj* : regulated by law with regard to possession and use ⟨~ drugs⟩

controlled hypotension *n* : low blood pressure induced and maintained to reduce blood loss or to provide a bloodless field during surgery

con·tu·sion \kən-'tü-zhən, -'tyü-\ *n* : injury to tissue usu. without laceration : BRUISE 1 — **con·tuse** \-'tüz, -'tyüz\ *vb*

co·nus \'kō-nəs\ *n, pl* **co·ni** \-ˌnī, -(ˌ)nē\ : CONUS ARTERIOSUS

co·nus ar·te·ri·o·sus \'kō-nəs-är-ˌtir-ē-'ō-səs\ *n, pl* **co·ni ar·te·ri·o·si** \-ˌnī-är-ˌtir-ē-'ō-ˌsī, -(ˌ)nē-\ : a conical prolongation of the right ventricle from which the pulmonary arteries emerge — called also *conus*

conus med·ul·lar·is \-ˌmed-ᵊl-'er-əs, -ˌme-jə-'ler-\ *n* : a tapering lower part of the spinal cord at the level of the first lumbar segment

con·va·les·cence \ˌkän-və-'les-ᵊns\ *n* **1** : gradual recovery of health and strength after disease **2** : the time between the subsidence of a disease and complete restoration to health — **con·va·lesce** \ˌkän-və-'les\ *vb*

¹con·va·les·cent \ˌkän-və-'les-ᵊnt\ *adj* **1** : recovering from sickness or debility : partially restored to health or strength **2** : of, for, or relating to convalescence or convalescents ⟨a ~ ward⟩

²convalescent *n* : one recovering from sickness

convalescent home *n* : an institution for the care of convalescent patients

con·ver·gence \kən-'vər-jəns\ *n* **1** : movement of the two eyes so coordinated that the images of a single point fall on corresponding points of the two retinas **2** : overlapping synaptic innervation of a single cell by more than one nerve fiber — compare DIVERGENCE **2** — **con·verge** \-'vərj\ *vb* — **con·ver·gent** \-'vər-jənt\ *adj*

con·ver·sion \kən-'vər-zhən, -shən\ *n* : the transformation of an unconscious mental conflict into a symbolically equivalent bodily symptom

conversion reaction *n* : a psychoneurosis in which bodily symptoms (as paralysis of the limbs) appear without physical basis — called also *conversion hysteria*

con·vo·lut·ed \'kän-və-ˌlü-təd\ *adj* : folded in curved or tortuous windings; *specif* : having convolutions

convoluted tubule *n* **1** : PROXIMAL CONVOLUTED TUBULE **2** : DISTAL CONVOLUTED TUBULE

con·vo·lu·tion \ˌkän-və-'lü-shən\ *n* : any of the irregular ridges on the surface of the brain and esp. of the cerebrum — called also *gyrus;* compare SULCUS

convolution of Broca *n* : BROCA'S AREA

¹con·vul·sant \kən-'vəl-sənt\ *adj* : causing convulsions : CONVULSIVE

²convulsant *n* : an agent and esp. a drug that produces convulsions

con·vulse \kən-'vəls\ *vb* **con·vulsed; con·vuls·ing 1** : to shake or agitate violently; *esp* : to shake or cause to shake with or as if with irregular spasms **2** : to become affected with convulsions

con·vul·sion \kən-'vəl-shən\ *n* : an abnormal violent and involuntary contraction or series of contractions of the muscles — often used in pl. ⟨a patient suffering from ∼*s*⟩ — **con·vul·sive** \-siv\ *adj* — **con·vul·sive·ly** *adv*

convulsive therapy *n* : SHOCK THERAPY

Coo·ley's anemia \'kü-lēz-\ *n* : a severe thalassemia anemia that is associated with the presence of microcytes, enlargement of the liver and spleen, increase in the erythroid bone marrow, and jaundice and that occurs esp. in children of Mediterranean parents — called also *thalassemia major*

    Coo·ley \'kü-lē\, **Thomas Benton (1871–1945),** American pediatrician.

Coo·mas·sie blue \kü-'ma-sē-, -'mä-\ *n* : a bright blue acid dye used as a biological stain esp. for proteins in gel electrophoresis

Coombs test \'kümz-\ *n* : an agglutination test used to detect proteins and esp. antibodies on the surface of red blood cells

    Coombs, Robert Royston Amos (*b* 1921), British immunologist.

Coo·pe·ria \kü-'pir-ē-ə\ *n* : a genus of small reddish brown nematode worms (family Trichostrongylidae) including several species infesting the small intestine of sheep, goats, and cattle

    Curtice, Cooper (1856–1939), American veterinarian.

coordinate bond *n* : a covalent bond that consists of a pair of electrons supplied by only one of the two atoms it joins

co·or·di·na·tion \(ˌ)kō-ˌȯrd-ᵊn-'ā-shən\ *n* **1** : the act or action of bringing into a common action, movement, or condition **2** : the harmonious functioning of parts (as muscle and nerves) for most effective results — **co·or·di·nate** \kō-'ȯrd-ᵊn-ˌāt\ *vb* — **co·or·di·nat·ed** \-ˌā-təd\ *adj*

coo·tie \'kü-tē\ *n* : BODY LOUSE

co–pay·ment \(ˌ)kō-'pā-mənt\ *n* : a relatively small fixed fee required by a health insurer (as an HMO) to be paid by the patient at the time of each office visit, outpatient service, or filling of a prescription

COPD *abbr* chronic obstructive pulmonary disease

cope \'kōp\ *vb* **coped; cop·ing** : to deal with and attempt to overcome problems and difficulties — usu. used with *with* ⟨teachers *coping* with violence in schools⟩

COPE *abbr* chronic obstructive pulmonary emphysema

cop·per \'kä-pər\ *n, often attrib* : a common reddish metallic element that is ductile and malleable — symbol *Cu*; see ELEMENT table

cop·per·head \'kä-pər-ˌhed\ *n* : a pit viper (*Agkistrodon contortrix*) widely distributed in upland areas of the eastern U.S. that attains a length of three feet or 0.9 meter, is coppery brown above with dark transverse blotches that render it inconspicuous among fallen leaves, and is usu. regarded as much less dangerous than a rattlesnake of comparable size

copper sulfate *n* : a sulfate of copper; *esp* : the sulfate of copper that is most familiar in its blue hydrous crystalline form $CuSO_4 \cdot 5H_2O$, is used as an algicide and fungicide, and has been used medicinally in solution as an emetic but is not now recommended for such use because of its potential toxicity

copr- *or* **copro-** *comb form* **1** : dung : feces ⟨*copr*ophagy⟩ **2** : obscenity ⟨*copro*lalia⟩

cop·ro·an·ti·body \ˌkä-prō-'an-ti-ˌbä-dē\ *n, pl* **-bod·ies** : an antibody whose presence in the intestinal tract is demonstrated by examination of an extract of the feces

cop·ro·la·lia \ˌkä-prə-'lā-lē-ə\ *n* **1** : obsessive or uncontrollable use of obscene language **2** : the use of obscene (as scatological) language as sexual gratification — **cop·ro·la·lic** \-'la-lik\ *adj*

cop·ro·pha·gia \ˌkä-prə-'fā-jə, -jē-ə\ *n* : COPROPHAGY

co·proph·a·gy \kə-'prä-fə-jē\ *n, pl* **-gies** : the eating of excrement that is normal behavior among many esp. young animals but in humans is a symptom of some forms of insanity — **co·proph·a·gous** \-gəs\ *adj*

cop·ro·phil·ia \ˌkä-prə-'fi-lē-ə\ *n* : marked interest in excrement; *esp* : the use of feces or filth for sexual excitement — **cop·ro·phil·i·ac** \-ˌak\ *n*

cop·ro·por·phy·rin \ˌkä-prə-'pȯr-fə-rən\ *n* : any of four isomeric porphyrins $C_{36}H_{38}N_4O_8$ of which types I and III are found in feces and urine esp. in certain pathological conditions

cop·u·late \'kä-pyə-ˌlāt\ *vb* **-lat·ed; -lat·ing** : to engage in sexual intercourse — **cop·u·la·tion** \ˌkä-pyə-'lā-shən\ *n* — **cop·u·la·to·ry** \'kä-pyə-lə-ˌtȯr-ē\ *adj*

coraco- *comb form* : coracoid and ⟨*coraco*humeral⟩

cor·a·co·acro·mi·al \ˌkȯr-ə-(ˌ)kō-ə-'krō-mē-əl\ *adj* : relating to or connecting the acromion and the coracoid process

cor·a·co·bra·chi·a·lis \ˌkȯr-ə-(ˌ)kō-ˌbrā-kē-'ā-ləs\ *n, pl* **-a·les** \-ˌlēz\ : a muscle extending between the coracoid process and the middle of the medial surface of the humerus — called also *coracobrachialis muscle*

cor·a·co·cla·vic·u·lar ligament \-klə-ˌvi-kyə-lər-, -kla-\ *n* : a ligament that joins the clavicle and the coracoid process of the scapula

cor·a·co·hu·mer·al \-'hyü-mə-rəl\ *adj*

: relating to or connecting the coracoid process and the humerus

¹cor·a·coid \'kor-ə-,koid, 'kär-\ adj : of, relating to, or being a process of the scapula in most mammals or a well-developed cartilage-bone of many lower vertebrates that extends from the scapula to or toward the sternum

²coracoid n : a coracoid bone or process

coracoid process n : a process of the scapula in most mammals representing the remnant of the coracoid bone of lower vertebrates that has become fused with the scapula and in humans is situated on its superior border and serves for the attachment of various muscles

coral snake \'kor-əl-, 'kär-\ n : any of several venomous chiefly tropical New World elapid snakes of the genus *Micrurus* that are brilliantly banded in red, black, and yellow or white and include two (M. *fulvius* and M. *euryxanthus*) ranging northward into the southern U.S.

cor bo·vi·num \'kor-bō-'vī-nəm\ n : a greatly enlarged heart

cord \'kord\ n : a slender flexible anatomical structure (as a nerve) — see SPERMATIC CORD, SPINAL CORD, UMBILICAL CORD, VOCAL CORD 1

cord blood n : blood from the umbilical cord of a fetus or newborn

cor·dec·to·my \kor-'dek-tə-mē\ n, pl -mies : surgical removal of one or more vocal cords

cordia pulmonalia pl of COR PULMONALE

cordis — see ACCRETIO CORDIS, VENAE CORDIS MINIMAE

cor·dot·o·my \kor-'dä-tə-mē\ n, pl -mies : surgical division of a tract of the spinal cord for relief of severe intractable pain

core \'kor\ n : the central part of a body, mass, or part

co·re·pres·sor \kō-ri-'pres-ər\ n : a substance that activates or inactivates a particular genetic repressor by combining with it

core temperature n : the temperature deep within a living body (as in the viscera)

Cori cycle \'kor-ē-\ n : the cycle in carbohydrate metabolism consisting of the conversion of glycogen to lactic acid in muscle, diffusion of the lactic acid into the bloodstream which carries it to the liver where it is converted into glycogen, and the breakdown of liver glycogen to glucose which is transported to muscle by the bloodstream and reconverted into glycogen

Cori, Carl Ferdinand (1896–1984) and Gerty Theresa (1896–1957), American biochemists.

co·ri·um \'kor-ē-əm\ n, pl co·ria \-ē-ə\ : DERMIS

corn \'korn\ n : a local hardening and thickening of epidermis (as on a toe)

corne- or **corneo-** comb form : cornea : corneal and ⟨*corneo*scleral⟩

cor·nea \'kor-nē-ə\ n : the transparent part of the coat of the eyeball that covers the iris and pupil and admits light to the interior — **cor·ne·al** \-əl\ adj

cor·neo·scler·al \,kor-nē-ə-'skler-əl\ adj : of, relating to, or affecting both the cornea and the sclera (the ~ junction)

cor·ner \'kor(r)-nər\ n : CORNER TOOTH

corner tooth n : one of the third or outer pair of incisor teeth of each jaw of a horse — compare DIVIDER, NIPPER

cor·ne·um \'kor-nē-əm\ n, pl cor·nea \-nē-ə\ : STRATUM CORNEUM

cor·nic·u·late cartilage \kor-'ni-kyə-lət-\ n : either of two small nodules of yellow elastic cartilage articulating with the apex of the arytenoid

cor·ni·fi·ca·tion \,kor-nə-fə-'kā-shən\ n 1 : conversion into horn or a horny substance or tissue 2 : the conversion of the vaginal epithelium from the columnar to the squamous type — **cor·ni·fy** \'kor-nə-fī\ vb

corn oil n : a yellow fatty oil obtained from the germ of Indian corn kernels that is used in medicine as a solvent and as a vehicle for injections

cor·nu \'kor-(,)nü, -(,)nyü\ n, pl **cornua** \-nü-ə, -nyü-\ : a horn-shaped anatomical structure (as either of the lateral divisions of a bicornuate uterus or one of the lateral processes of the hyoid bone) — **cor·nu·al** \-nü-əl, -nyü-\ adj

co·ro·na \kə-'rō-nə\ n : the upper portion of a bodily part

co·ro·nal \'kor-ən-əl, 'kär-; kə-'rōn-\ adj 1 : of, relating to, or being a corona 2 : lying in the direction of the coronal suture 3 : of or relating to the frontal plane that passes through the long axis of the body

coronal suture n : a suture extending across the skull between the parietal and frontal bones — called also *frontoparietal suture*

co·ro·na ra·di·a·ta \kə-'rō-nə-,rā-dē-'ā-tə, -'ä-\ n, pl **co·ro·nae ra·di·a·tae** \-(,)nē-,rā-dē-'ā-(,)tē, -'ä-\ 1 : the zone of small follicular cells immediately surrounding the ovum in the graafian follicle and accompanying the ovum on its discharge from the follicle 2 : a large mass of myelinated nerve fibers radiating from the internal capsule to the cerebral cortex

¹cor·o·nary \'kor-ə-,ner-ē, 'kär-\ adj 1 : of, relating to, affecting, or being the coronary arteries or veins of the heart ⟨~ bypass⟩ ⟨~ sclerosis⟩; *broadly* : of or relating to the heart 2 : of, relating to, or affected with coronary heart disease ⟨~ care unit⟩

²coronary n, pl -nar·ies 1 a : CORONARY ARTERY b : CORONARY VEIN 2 : CORONARY THROMBOSIS; *broadly* : HEART ATTACK

coronary artery *n* : either of two arteries that arise one from the left and one from the right side of the aorta immediately above the semilunar valves and supply the tissues of the heart itself

coronary band *n* : a thickened band of extremely vascular tissue that lies at the upper border of the wall of the hoof of the horse and related animals and that plays an important part in the secretion of the horny walls — called also *coronary cushion*

coronary failure *n* : heart failure in which the heart muscle is deprived of the blood necessary to meet its functional needs as a result of narrowing or blocking of one or more of the coronary arteries — compare CONGESTIVE HEART FAILURE

coronary heart disease *n* : a condition (as sclerosis or thrombosis) that reduces the blood flow through the coronary arteries to the heart muscle — called also *coronary artery disease, coronary disease*

coronary insufficiency *n* : cardiac insufficiency of relatively mild degree — compare ANGINA PECTORIS, HEART FAILURE 1, MYOCARDIAL INFARCTION

coronary ligament *n* **1** : the folds of peritoneum connecting the posterior surface of the liver and the diaphragm **2** : a part of the articular capsule of the knee connecting each semilunar cartilage with the margin of the head of the tibia

coronary occlusion *n* : the partial or complete blocking (as by a thrombus or by sclerosis) of a coronary artery

coronary plexus *n* : one of two nerve plexuses that are extensions of the cardiac plexus along the coronary arteries

coronary sinus *n* : a venous channel that is derived from the sinus venosus, is continuous with the largest of the cardiac veins, receives most of the blood from the walls of the heart, and empties into the right atrium

coronary thrombosis *n* : the blocking of a coronary artery of the heart by a thrombus

coronary vein *n* **1 a** : any of several veins that drain the tissues of the heart and empty into the coronary sinus **b** : CARDIAC VEIN — not used technically **2** : a vein draining the lesser curvature of the stomach and emptying into the portal vein

co·ro·na·vi·rus \kə-ˈrō-nə-ˌvī-rəs\ *n* : any of a group of viruses that resemble myxoviruses and include some causing respiratory symptoms in humans

cor·o·ner \ˈkȯr-ə-nər, ˈkär-\ *n* : a public officer whose principal duty is to inquire by an inquest into the cause of any death which there is reason to suppose is not due to natural causes

cor·o·net \ˌkȯr-ə-ˈnet, ˌkär-\ *n* : the lower part of a horse's pastern where the horn terminates in skin

cor·o·noid·ec·to·my \ˌkȯr-ə-ˌnȯi-ˈdek-tə-mē\ *n, pl* **-mies** : surgical removal of the mandibular coronoid process

coronoid fossa *n* : a depression of the humerus into which the coronoid process fits when the arm is flexed — compare OLECRANON FOSSA

coronoid process *n* **1** : the anterior process of the superior border of the ramus of the mandible **2** : a flared process of the upper anterior part of the upper articular surface of the ulna fitting into the coronoid fossa when the arm is flexed

corpora *pl of* CORPUS

cor·po·ral \ˈkȯr-pə-rəl, -prəl\ *adj* : of, relating to, or affecting the body ⟨∼ punishment⟩

cor·po·ra quad·ri·gem·i·na \ˌkȯr-pə-rə-ˌkwä-drə-ˈje-mə-nə, ˌkȯr-prə-\ *n pl* : two pairs of colliculi on the dorsal surface of the midbrain composed of white matter externally and gray matter within, the superior pair containing correlation centers for optic reflexes and the inferior pair containing correlation centers for auditory reflexes

cor·po·re·al \kȯr-ˈpȯr-ē-əl\ *adj* : having, consisting of, or relating to a physical material body

corporis — see PEDICULOSIS CORPORIS, TINEA CORPORIS

corpse \ˈkȯrps\ *n* : a dead body esp. of a human being

corps·man \ˈkȯr-mən, ˈkȯrz-\ *n, pl* **corps·men** \-mən\ : an enlisted man trained to give first aid and minor medical treatment

cor pul·mo·na·le \ˌkȯr-ˌpu̇l-mə-ˈnä-lē, -ˌpäl-, -ˈna-\ *n, pl* **cor·dia pul·mo·na·lia** \ˈkȯr-dē-ə-ˌpu̇l-mə-ˈnä-lē-ə, -ˌpäl-, -ˈna-\ : disease of the heart characterized by hypertrophy and dilatation of the right ventricle and secondary to disease of the lungs or their blood vessels

cor·pus \ˈkȯr-pəs\ *n, pl* **cor·po·ra** \-pə-rə, -prə\ **1** : the human or animal body esp. when dead **2** : the main part or body of a bodily structure or organ

corpus al·bi·cans \-ˈal-bə-ˌkanz\ *n, pl* **corpora al·bi·can·tia** \-ˌal-bə-ˈkan-chē-ə\ **1** : MAMMILLARY BODY **2** : the white fibrous scar that remains in the ovary after resorption of the corpus luteum and replaces a discharged graafian follicle

corpus cal·lo·sum \-ka-ˈlō-səm\ *n, pl* **corpora cal·lo·sa** \-sə\ : the great band of commissural fibers uniting the cerebral hemispheres

corpus ca·ver·no·sum \-ˌka-vər-ˈnō-səm\ *n, pl* **corpora ca·ver·no·sa** \-sə\ : a mass of erectile tissue with large interspaces capable of being distended with blood; *esp* : one of those that form the bulk of the body of the penis or of the clitoris

cor·pus·cle \'kȯr-(ˌ)pə-səl\ *n* **1** : a living cell; *esp* : one (as a red or white blood cell or a cell in cartilage or bone) not aggregated into continuous tissues **2** : any of various small circumscribed multicellular bodies — usu. used with a qualifying term ⟨Malpighian ∼s⟩ — **cor·pus·cu·lar** \kȯr-'pəs-kyə-lər\ *adj*

corpuscle of Krause *n* : KRAUSE'S COR-PUSCLE

corpus he·mor·rhag·i·cum \-ˌhe-mə-'ra-ji-kəm\ *n* : a ruptured graafian follicle containing a blood clot that is absorbed as the cells lining the follicle form the corpus luteum

corpus lu·te·um \-'lü-tē-əm, -lü-'tē-əm\ *n*, *pl* **corpora lu·tea** \-ə\ : a yellowish mass of progesterone-secreting endocrine tissue that consists of pale secretory cells derived from granulosa cells, that forms immediately after ovulation from the ruptured graafian follicle in the mammalian ovary, and that regresses rather quickly if the ovum is not fertilized but persists throughout the ensuing pregnancy if it is fertilized

corpus spon·gi·o·sum \-ˌspən-jē-'ō-səm, -ˌspän-\ *n* : the median longitudinal column of erectile tissue of the penis that contains the urethra and is ventral to the two corpora cavernosa

corpus stri·a·tum \-strī-'ā-təm\ *n*, *pl* **corpora stri·a·ta** \-'ā-tə\ : either of a pair of masses of nerve tissue which lie beneath and external to the anterior cornua of the lateral ventricles of the brain and form part of their floor and each of which contains a caudate nucleus and a lentiform nucleus separated by sheets of white matter to give the mass a striated appearance in section

corpus ute·ri \-'yü-tə-ˌrī\ *n* : the main body of the uterus above the constriction behind the cervix and below the openings of the fallopian tubes

¹cor·rec·tive \kə-'rek-tiv\ *adj* : intended to correct ⟨∼ lenses⟩ ⟨∼ surgery⟩ — **cor·rec·tive·ly** *adv*

²corrective *n* : a medication that removes undesirable or unpleasant side effects of other medication

corresponding points *n pl* : points on the retinas of the two eyes which when simultaneously stimulated normally produce a single visual impression

Cor·ri·gan's disease \'kȯr-i-gənz-\ *n* : AORTIC REGURGITATION

Cor·ri·gan \'kȯr-i-gən\, **Sir Dominic John (1802–1880),** British pathologist.

Corrigan's pulse *or* **Corrigan pulse** *n* : a pulse characterized by a sharp rise to full expansion followed by immediate collapse that is seen in aortic insufficiency — called also *water-hammer pulse*

cor·rode \kə-'rōd\ *vb* **cor·rod·ed; cor·rod·ing** : to eat or be eaten away gradually (as by chemcial action) — **cor·ro·sion** \kə-'rō-zhən\ *n*

¹cor·ro·sive \-'rō-siv, -ziv\ *adj* : tending or having the power to corrode ⟨∼ acids⟩ — **cor·ro·sive·ness** *n*

²corrosive *n* : a substance that corrodes : CAUSTIC

corrosive sublimate *n* : MERCURIC CHLORIDE

cor·ru·ga·tor \'kȯr-ə-ˌgā-tər\ *n* : a muscle that contracts the skin into wrinkles; *esp* : one that draws the eyebrows together and wrinkles the brow in frowning

cor·tex \'kȯr-ˌteks\ *n*, *pl* **cor·ti·ces** \'kȯr-tə-ˌsēz\ *or* **cor·tex·es** : the outer or superficial part of an organ or body structure (as the kidney, adrenal gland, or a hair); *esp* : the outer layer of gray matter of the cerebrum and cerebellum

cor·ti·cal \'kȯr-ti-kəl\ *adj* **1** : of, relating to, or consisting of cortex ⟨∼ tissue⟩ **2** : involving or resulting from the action or condition of the cerebral cortex — **cor·ti·cal·ly** *adv*

cortico- *comb form* **1** : cortex ⟨*cortico*tropin⟩ **2** : cortical and ⟨*cortico*spinal⟩

cor·ti·co·ad·re·nal \ˌkȯr-ti-kō-ə-'drēn-ᵊl\ *adj* : of or relating to the cortex of the adrenal gland ⟨∼ hormones⟩ ⟨∼ insufficiency⟩

cor·ti·co·bul·bar \-'bəl-bər, -ˌbär\ *adj* : relating to or connecting the cerebral cortex and the medulla oblongata

cor·ti·coid \'kȯr-ti-ˌkȯid\ *n* : CORTICO-STEROID — **corticoid** *adj*

cor·ti·co·pon·tine \ˌkȯr-ti-kō-'pän-ˌtīn\ *adj* : relating to or connecting the cerebral cortex and the pons

cor·ti·co·pon·to·cer·e·bel·lar \-ˌpän-tō-ˌser-ə-'be-lər\ *adj* : of, relating to, or being a tract of nerve fibers or a path for nervous impulses that passes from the cerebral cortex through the internal capsule to the pons to the white matter and cortex of the cerebellum

cor·ti·co·spi·nal \-'spin-ᵊl\ *adj* : of or relating to the cerebral cortex and spinal cord or to the corticospinal tract

corticospinal tract *n* : any of four columns of motor fibers of which two run on each side of the spinal cord and which are continuations of the pyramids of the medulla oblongata: **a** : LATERAL CORTICOSPINAL TRACT **b** : VENTRAL CORTICOSPINAL TRACT

cor·ti·co·ste·roid \ˌkȯr-ti-kō-'stir-ˌȯid, -'ster-\ *n* : any of various adrenal-cortex steroids (as corticosterone, cortisone, and aldosterone) used medically esp. as anti-inflammatory agents

cor·ti·co·ste·rone \ˌkȯr-tə-'käs-tə-ˌrōn, -kō-stə-'; ˌkȯr-ti-kō-'stir-ˌōn, -'ster-\ *n* : a colorless crystalline corticosteroid $C_{21}H_{30}O_4$ of the adrenal cortex that is important in protein and carbohydrate metabolism

cor·ti·co·tro·pic \ˌkȯr-ti-kō-ˈtrō-pik\ *also* **cor·ti·co·tro·phic** \-fik\ *adj* : influencing or stimulating the adrenal cortex

cor·ti·co·tro·pin \-ˈtrō-pən\ *also* **cor·ti·co·tro·phin** \-fən\ *n* : ACTH; *also* : a preparation of ACTH that is used esp. in the treatment of rheumatoid arthritis and rheumatic fever

corticotropin–releasing factor *or* **corticotrophin–releasing factor** *n* : a substance secreted by the median eminence of the hypothalamus that regulates the release of ACTH by the anterior lobe of the pituitary gland

cor·tin \ˈkȯrt-ᵊn\ *n* : the active principle of the adrenal cortex now known to consist of several hormones

cor·ti·sol \ˈkȯrt-ə-ˌsȯl, -ˌzȯl, -ˌsōl, -ˌzōl\ *n* : HYDROCORTISONE

cor·ti·sone \-ˌsōn, -ˌzōn\ *n* : a glucocorticoid $C_{21}H_{28}O_5$ of the adrenal cortex used esp. in the treatment of rheumatoid arthritis — compare *11-DEHYDROCORTICOSTERONE*

cor·y·ne·bac·te·ri·um \kȯr-ə-(ˌ)nē-bak-ˈtir-ē-əm\ *n* **1** *cap* : a large genus (family Corynebacteriaceae) of usu. gram-positive nonmotile bacteria that occur as irregular or branching rods and include a number of important parasites — see DIPHTHERIA 2 *pl* **-ria** \-ē-ə\ : any bacterium of the genus *Corynebacterium*

co·ryne·form \kə-ˈri-nə-ˌfȯrm\ *adj* : being or resembling bacteria of the genus *Corynebacterium*

co·ry·za \kə-ˈrī-zə\ *n* : an acute inflammatory contagious disease involving the upper respiratory tract: **a** : COMMON COLD **b** : any of several diseases of domestic animals characterized by inflammation and discharge from the mucous membranes of the upper respiratory tract, sinuses, and eyes; *esp* : INFECTIOUS CORYZA — **co·ry·zal** \-zəl\ *adj*

¹**cos·met·ic** \käz-ˈme-tik\ *n* : a cosmetic preparation for external use

²**cosmetic** *adj* **1** : of, relating to, or making for beauty esp. of the complexion ⟨∼ salves⟩ **2** : correcting defects esp. of the face ⟨∼ surgery⟩ — **cos·met·i·cal·ly** *adv*

cos·mid \ˈkäz-məd\ *n* : a plasmid whose original genome has been altered so that a large segment of DNA can be inserted for cloning purposes

cost- *or* **costi-** *or* **costo-** *comb form* : rib ⟨*costal* and ⟨*costochondral*⟩

cos·ta \ˈkäs-tə\ *n, pl* **cos·tae** \-(ˌ)tē, -ˌtī\ : RIB

cos·tal \ˈkäst-ᵊl\ *adj* : of, relating to, involving, or situated near a rib

costal breathing *n* : inspiration and expiration produced chiefly by movements of the ribs

costal cartilage *n* : any of the cartilages that connect the distal ends of the ribs with the sternum and by their elastic-ity permit movement of the chest in respiration

costarum — see LEVATORES COSTARUM

cos·tive \ˈkäs-tiv, ˈkȯs-\ *adj* **1** : affected with constipation **2** : causing constipation — **cos·tive·ness** *n*

cos·to·cer·vi·cal trunk \ˌkäs-tə-ˈsər-və-kəl-, -tō-\ *n* : a branch of the subclavian artery that divides to supply the first or first two intercostal spaces and the deep structures of the neck — see INTERCOSTAL ARTERY b

cos·to·chon·dral \-ˈkän-drəl\ *adj* : relating to or joining a rib and costal cartilage ⟨a ∼ junction⟩

cos·to·chon·dri·tis \-kän-ˈdrī-təs\ *n* : TIETZE'S SYNDROME

cos·to·di·a·phrag·mat·ic \ˌkäs-tə-ˌdī-ə-fra-ˈma-tik, ˌkäs-tō-, -ˌfrag-, -ˌfrag-\ *adj* : relating to or involving the ribs and diaphragm

cos·to·phren·ic \ˌkäs-tə-ˈfre-nik, -tō-\ *adj* : of or relating to the ribs and the diaphragm

cos·to·trans·verse \ˌkäs-tə-trans-ˈvərs, -tō-, -tranz-, -ˈtrans-ˌ, -ˈtranz-ˌ\ *adj* : relating to or connecting a rib and the transverse process of a vertebra ⟨a ∼ joint⟩

cos·to·trans·ver·sec·to·my \-ˌtrans-(ˌ)vər-ˈsek-tə-mē, -ˌtranz-\ *n, pl* **-mies** : surgical excision of part of a rib and the transverse process of the adjoining vertebra

cos·to·ver·te·bral \-(ˌ)vər-ˈtē-brəl, -ˈvər-tə-\ *adj* : of or relating to a rib and its adjoining vertebra ⟨∼ pain⟩

¹**cot** \ˈkät\ *n* : a protective cover for a finger — called also *fingerstall*

²**cot** *n* : a wheeled stretcher for hospital, mortuary, or ambulance service

COTA *abbr* certified occupational therapy assistant

cot death *n, chiefly Brit* : SUDDEN INFANT DEATH SYNDROME

co·throm·bo·plas·tin \(ˌ)kō-ˌthräm-bō-ˈplas-tən\ *n* : FACTOR VII

co·tri·mox·a·zole \ˌkō-trī-ˈmäk-sə-ˌzōl\ *n* : a bactericidal combination of trimethoprim and sulfamethoxazole in the ratio of one to five used esp. for chronic urinary tract infections

cot·ton·mouth \ˈkät-ᵊn-ˌmau̇th\ *n* : WATER MOCCASIN

cottonmouth moccasin *n* : WATER MOCCASIN

cotton–wool *n, Brit* : ABSORBENT COTTON

cot·y·le·don \ˌkät-ᵊl-ˈēd-ᵊn\ *n* : a lobule of a mammalian placenta — **cot·y·le·don·ary** \-ˈēd-ᵊn-ˌer-ē\ *adj*

¹**couch** \ˈkau̇ch\ *vb* : to treat (a cataract or a person having a cataract) by displacing the lens of the eye into the vitreous humor

²**couch** *n* : an article of furniture used (as by a patient undergoing psychoanalysis) for sitting or reclining — **on the couch** : receiving psychiatric treatment

¹**cough** \ˈkȯf\ *vb* **1** : to expel air from the

lungs suddenly with an explosive noise usu. in a series of efforts **2** : to expel by coughing — often used with *up* ⟨~ up mucus⟩

²**cough** *n* **1** : an ailment manifesting itself by frequent coughing ⟨he has a bad ~⟩ **2** : an explosive expulsion of air from the lungs acting as a protective mechanism to clear the air passages or as a symptom of pulmonary disturbance

cough drop *n* : a lozenge used to relieve coughing

cough syrup *n* : any of various sweet usu. medicated liquids used to relieve coughing

cou·lomb \'kü-₁läm, -₁lōm, kü-'\ *n* : the practical mks unit of electric charge equal to the quantity of electricity transferred by a current of one ampere in one second

Coulomb, Charles–Augustin de (1736–1806), French physicist.

Cou·ma·din \'kü-mə-dən\ *trademark* — used for a preparation of warfarin

cou·ma·phos \'kü-mə-₁fäs\ *n* : an organophosphorus systemic insecticide $C_{14}H_{16}ClO_5PS$ administered esp. to cattle and poultry as a feed additive

cou·ma·rin \'kü-mə-rən\ *n* : a toxic white crystalline lactone $C_9H_6O_2$ found in plants or made synthetically and used as the parent compound in various anticoagulant agents (as warfarin)

coun·sel·ing \'kaún-s(ə-)liŋ\ *n* : professional guidance of the individual by utilizing psychological methods

coun·sel·or *or* **coun·sel·lor** \'kaún-s(ə-)lər\ *n* : a person engaged in counseling

¹**count** \'kaúnt\ *vb* : to indicate or name by units or groups so as to find the total number of units involved

²**count** *n* : the total number of individual things in a given unit or sample (as of blood) obtained by counting all or a subsample of them

¹**count·er** \'kaún-tər\ *n* : a level surface over which transactions are conducted or food is served or on which goods are displayed or work is conducted — **over the counter** : without a prescription ⟨drugs available *over the counter*⟩

²**counter** *n* : a device for indicating a number or amount — see GEIGER COUNTER

coun·ter·act \₁kaún-tər-'akt\ *vb* : to make ineffective or restrain or neutralize the usu. ill effects of by an opposite force — **coun·ter·ac·tion** \-'ak-shən\ *n*

coun·ter·con·di·tion·ing \-kən-'di-shə-niŋ\ *n* : conditioning in order to replace an undesirable response (as fear) to a stimulus (as an engagement in public speaking) by a favorable one

coun·ter·cur·rent \₁kaún-tər-'kər-ənt, -'kə-rənt\ *adj* **1** : flowing in an opposite direction **2** : involving flow of materials in opposite directions ⟨~ dialysis⟩

coun·ter·elec·tro·pho·re·sis \-i-₁lek-trə-fə-'rē-səs\ *n, pl* **-re·ses** \-₁sēz\ : an electrophoretic method of testing blood esp. for hepatitis antigens

coun·ter·im·mu·no·elec·tro·pho·re·sis \-₁im-yə-nō-i-₁lek-trō-fə-'rē-səs\ *n, pl* **-re·ses** : COUNTERELECTROPHORESIS

coun·ter·ir·ri·tant \-'ir-ə-tənt\ *n* : an agent applied locally to produce superficial inflammation with the object of reducing inflammation in deeper adjacent structures — **counterirritant** *adj*

coun·ter·ir·ri·ta·tion \-₁tā-shən\ *n* : the reaction produced by treatment with a counterirritant; *also* : the treatment itself

coun·ter·pho·bic \-₁fō-bik\ *adj* : relating to or characterized by a preference for or the seeking out of a situation that is feared ⟨~ reaction patterns⟩

coun·ter·pul·sa·tion \-₁pəl-₁sā-shən\ *n* : a technique for reducing the work load on the heart by lowering systemic blood pressure just before or during expulsion of blood from the ventricle and by raising blood pressure during diastole — see INTRA-AORTIC BALLOON COUNTERPULSATION

coun·ter·shock \-₁shäk\ *n* : therapeutic electric shock applied to a heart for the purpose of altering a disturbed rhythm

coun·ter·stain \-₁stān\ *n* : a stain used to color parts of a microscopy specimen not affected by another stain; *esp* : a cytoplasmic stain used to contrast with or enhance a nuclear stain — **counterstain** *vb*

coun·ter·trac·tion \'kaún-tər-₁trak-shən\ *n* : a traction opposed to another traction used in reducing fractures

coun·ter·trans·fer·ence \₁kaún-tər-trans-'fər-əns, -'trans-(₁)\ *n* **1** : psychological transference esp. by a psychotherapist during the course of treatment; *esp* : the psychotherapist's reactions to the patient's transference **2** : the complex of feelings of a psychotherapist toward the patient

cou·pling \'kə-pliŋ, -pə-liŋ\ *n* : the joining of or the part of the body that joins the hindquarters to the forequarters of a quadruped

course \'kōrs\ *n* : an ordered process or succession; *esp* : a series of doses or medications administered over a designated period

court plaster \'kōrt-\ *n* : an adhesive plaster esp. of silk coated with isinglass and glycerin

cou·vade \kü-'väd\ *n* : a custom in some cultures in which when a child is born the father takes to bed as if bearing the child and submits himself to fasting, purification, or taboos

Cou·ve·laire uterus \₁kü-və-'ler-\ *n* : a pregnant uterus in which the placenta has detached prematurely with extravasation of blood into the uterine musculature

Couvelaire, Alexandre (1873–1948), French obstetrician.

co·va·lent bond \(\)kō-'vā-lənt-\ n : a chemical bond that is not ionic and is formed by one or more shared pairs of electrons

cover glass n : a piece of very thin glass used to cover material on a glass microscope slide

cover·slip \'kə-vər-ˌslip\ n : COVER GLASS

Cow·dria \'kaü-drē-ə\ n : a genus of small pleomorphic intracellular rickettsial bacteria known chiefly from ticks but including the causative organism (*C. ruminantium*) of heartwater of ruminants

Cow·dry \'kaü-drē\, **Edmund Vincent (1888–1975),** American anatomist.

cow·hage also **cow·age** \'kaü-ij\ n : a tropical leguminous woody vine (*Mucuna pruriens*) with crooked pods covered with barbed hairs that cause severe itching; also : these hairs formerly used as a vermifuge

Cow·per's gland \'kaü-pərz-, 'kü-, 'kü-\ n : either of two small glands of which one lies on each side of the male urethra below the prostate gland and discharges a secretion into the semen — called also *bulbourethral gland*; compare BARTHOLIN'S GLAND

Cow·per \'kaü-pər, 'kü-, 'kü-\, **William (1666–1709),** British anatomist.

cow·pox \'kaü-ˌpäks\ n : a mild eruptive disease of the cow that is caused by a poxvirus and when communicated to humans protects against smallpox — called also *variola vaccinia*

cox- or **coxo-** comb form : hip : thigh : of the hip and (*coxofemoral*)

coxa \'käk-sə\ n, pl **coxae** \-ˌsē, -ˌsī\ : HIP JOINT, HIP

coxa vara \ˌkäk-sə-'var-ə\ n : a deformed hip joint in which the neck of the femur is bent downward

Cox·i·el·la \ˌkäk-sē-'e-lə\ n : a genus of small pleomorphic rickettsial bacteria occurring intercellularly in ticks and intracellularly in the cytoplasm of vertebrates and including the causative organism (*C. burnetii*) of Q fever

Cox \'käks\, **Herald Rea (b 1907),** American bacteriologist.

coxo·fem·o·ral \ˌkäk-sō-'fe-mə-rəl\ adj : of or relating to the hip and thigh

cox·sack·ie·vi·rus \(ˌ)käk-ˌsa-kē-'vī-rəs\ n : any of several enteroviruses associated with human diseases (as meningitis) — see EPIDEMIC PLEURODYNIA

CP abbr cerebral palsy

CPAP abbr continuous positive airway pressure

CPB abbr competitive protein binding

C–pep·tide \'sē-'pep-ˌtid\ n : a protein fragment 35 amino-acid residues long produced by enzymatic cleavage of proinsulin in the formation of insulin

CPK abbr creatine phosphokinase

CPR abbr cardiopulmonary resuscitation

Cr symbol chromium

CR abbr conditioned response

crab louse n, pl **crab lice** : a sucking louse of the genus *Phthirius* (*P. pubis*) infesting the pubic region of the human body

crabs \'krabz\ n pl : infestation with crab lice

crack \'krak\ n, often attrib : potent highly purified cocaine in the free-based form of small chips used illicitly usu. for smoking

cra·dle \'krād-ᵊl\ n : a frame to keep the bedding from contact with an injured part of the body

cradle cap n : a seborrheic condition in infants that usu. affects the scalp and is characterized by greasy gray or dark brown adherent scaly crusts

¹cramp \'kramp\ n 1 : a painful involuntary spasmodic contraction of a muscle ⟨a ∼ in the leg⟩ 2 : a temporary paralysis of muscles from overuse — see WRITER'S CRAMP 3 a : sharp abdominal pain — usu. used in pl. **b** : persistent and often intense though dull lower abdominal pain associated with dysmenorrhea — usu. used in pl.

²cramp vb : to affect with or be affected with a cramp or cramps

crani- or **cranio-** comb form 1 : cranium ⟨*cranio*synostosis⟩ 2 : cranial and ⟨*cranio*sacral⟩

-crania n comb form : condition of the skull or head ⟨hemi*crania*⟩

cra·ni·ad \'krā-nē-ˌad\ adv : toward the head or anterior end

cra·ni·al \'krā-nē-əl\ adj 1 : of or relating to the skull or cranium 2 : CEPHALIC — **cra·ni·al·ly** adv

cranial arteritis n : GIANT CELL ARTERITIS

cranial fossa n : any of the three large depressions in the posterior, middle, and anterior aspects of the floor of the cranial cavity

cranial index n : the ratio multiplied by 100 of the maximum breadth of the bare skull to its maximum length from front to back — compare CEPHALIC INDEX

cranial nerve n : any of the 12 paired nerves that arise from the lower surface of the brain with one of each pair on each side and pass through openings in the skull to the periphery of the body — see ABDUCENS NERVE, ACCESSORY NERVE, AUDITORY NERVE, FACIAL NERVE, GLOSSOPHARYNGEAL NERVE, HYPOGLOSSAL NERVE, OCULOMOTOR NERVE, OLFACTORY NERVE, OPTIC NERVE, TRIGEMINAL NERVE, TROCHLEAR NERVE, VAGUS NERVE

cra·ni·ec·to·my \ˌkrā-nē-'ek-tə-mē\ n, pl **-mies** : the surgical removal of a portion of the skull

cra·nio·ce·re·bral \ˌkrā-nē-ō-sə-'rē-brəl, -'ser-ə-\ adj : involving both cranium and brain 〈~ injury〉

cra·nio·fa·cial \ˌkrā-nē-ō-'fā-shəl\ adj : of, relating to, or involving both the cranium and the face

cra·ni·ol·o·gy \ˌkrā-nē-'ä-lə-jē\ n, pl **-gies** : a science dealing with variations in size, shape, and proportions of skulls among human races

cra·ni·om·e·try \-'ä-mə-trē\ n, pl **-tries** : a science dealing with cranial measurement

cra·ni·op·a·gus \ˌkrā-nē-'ä-pə-gəs\ n, pl **-agi** \-pə-ˌjē, -ˌjī\ : a pair of twins joined at the heads

cra·nio·pha·ryn·geal \ˌkrā-nē-ō-ˌfar-ən-'jē-əl, -fə-'rin-jəl, -jē-əl\ adj : relating to or connecting the cavity of the skull and the pharynx

cra·nio·pha·ryn·gi·o·ma \-ˌfar-ən-jē-'ō-mə, -fə-ˌrin-jē-'ō-mə\ n, pl **-mas** or **-ma·ta** \-mə-tə\ : a tumor of the brain near the pituitary gland that develops esp. in children or young adults from epithelium derived from the embryonic craniopharyngeal canal and that is often associated with increased intracranial pressure

cra·nio·plas·ty \'krā-nē-ō-ˌplas-tē\ n, pl **-ties** : the surgical correction of skull defects

cra·nio·ra·chis·chi·sis \ˌkrā-nē-(ˌ)ō-rə-'kis-kə-səs\ n, pl **-chi·ses** \-ˌsēz\ : a congenital fissure of the skull and spine

cra·nio·sa·cral \ˌkrā-nē-ō-'sa-krəl, -'sā-\ adj 1 : of or relating to the cranium and the sacrum 2 : PARASYMPATHETIC

cra·nio·os·chi·sis \ˌkrā-nē-'äs-kə-səs\ n, pl **-chi·ses** \-ˌsēz\ : a congenital fissure of the skull

cra·nio·ste·no·sis \ˌkrā-nē-(ˌ)ō-stə-'nō-səs\ n, pl **-no·ses** \-ˌsēz\ : malformation of the skull caused by premature closure of the cranial sutures

cra·nio·syn·os·to·sis \-ˌsi-ˌnäs-'tō-səs\ n, pl **-to·ses** \-ˌsēz\ or **-to·sis·es** : premature fusion of the sutures of the skull

cra·nio·ta·bes \ˌkrā-nē-ə-'tā-(ˌ)bēz\ n, pl **craniotabes** : a thinning and softening of the infantile skull in spots usu. due to rickets or syphilis

cra·ni·ot·o·my \ˌkrā-nē-'ä-tə-mē\ n, pl **-mies** 1 : the operation of cutting or crushing the fetal head to effect delivery 2 : surgical opening of the skull

cra·ni·um \'krā-nē-əm\ n, pl **-ni·ums** or **-nia** \-nē-ə\ : SKULL; specif : BRAINCASE

crank \'kraŋk\ n : CRYSTAL 2

cra·ter \'krā-tər\ n : an eroded lesion of a wall or surface 〈ulcer ~s〉

cra·ter·iza·tion \ˌkrā-tər-ə-'zā-shən\ n : surgical excision of a crater-shaped piece of bone

craz·ing \'krāz-iŋ\ n : the formation of minute cracks (as in acrylic resin teeth) usu. attributed to shrinkage or to moisture

cra·zy \'krā-zē\ adj **craz·i·er; -est** : MAD 1, INSANE — **cra·zi·ly** \-zə-lē\ adv — **cra·zi·ness** \-zē-nəs\ n

crazy bone n : FUNNY BONE

CRD abbr chronic respiratory disease

C—re·ac·tive protein \'sē-rē-'ak-tiv-\ n : a protein present in blood serum in various abnormal states (as inflammation)

cream \'krēm\ n 1 : the yellowish part of milk containing from 18 to about 40 percent butterfat 2 : something having the consistency of cream; esp : a usu. emulsified medicinal or cosmetic preparation — **creamy** \'krē-mē\ adj

crease \'krēs\ n : a line or mark made by or as if by folding a pliable substance (as the skin) — **crease** vb

cre·a·tine \'krē-ə-ˌtēn, -ət-ən\ n : a nitrogenous substance $C_4H_9N_3O_2$ found esp. in vertebrate muscles either free or as phosphocreatine

creatine kinase n : an enzyme of vertebrate skeletal and myocardial muscle that catalyzes the transfer of a high-energy phosphate group from phosphocreatine to ADP with the formation of ATP and creatine

creatine phosphate n : PHOSPHOCREATINE

creatine phosphokinase n : CREATINE KINASE

cre·a·ti·nine \krē-'at-ə̇n-ˌēn, -ə̇n-ən\ n : a white crystalline strongly basic compound $C_4H_7N_3O$ formed from creatine and found esp. in muscle, blood, and urine

cre·a·tin·uria \ˌkrē-ə-tə-'nu̇r-ē-ə, -'nyu̇r-\ n : the presence of creatine in urine; esp : an increased or abnormal amount in the urine

creeping eruption n : a human skin disorder that is characterized by a red line of eruption which fades at one end as it progresses at the other and that is usu. caused by insect or worm larvae and esp. those of the dog hookworm burrowing in the deeper layers of the skin — called also larval migrans, larva migrans

creeps \'krēps\ n pl : a deficiency disease esp. of sheep and cattle associated with an abnormal dietary calcium-phosphorus ratio

cre·mas·ter \krē-'mas-tər, krə-\ n : a thin muscle consisting of loops of fibers derived from the internal oblique muscle and descending upon the spermatic cord to surround and suspend the testicle — called also cremaster muscle — **cre·mas·ter·ic** \ˌkrē-mə-'ster-ik\ adj

crème \'krem, 'krēm\ n, pl **crèmes** \'krem, 'kremz, 'krēmz\ : CREAM 2

cre·nat·ed \'krē-ˌnā-təd\ also **cre·nate** \-ˌnāt\ adj : having the margin or surface cut into rounded scallops 〈~ red blood cells〉

cre·na·tion \kri-'nā-shən\ n : shrinkage of red blood cells resulting in crenated margins

cre·o·sote \'krē-ə-ˌsōt\ *n* **1** : an oily liquid mixture of phenolic compounds obtained by the distillation of wood tar and used esp. as a disinfectant and as an expectorant in chronic bronchitis **2** : a brownish oily liquid consisting chiefly of aromatic hydrocarbons obtained by distillation of coal tar and used esp. as a wood preservative

crep·i·tant rale \'kre-pə-tənt-\ *n* : a peculiar crackling sound associated with inspiration in pneumonia and other lung diseases

crep·i·ta·tion \ˌkre-pə-'tā-shən\ *n* : a grating or crackling sound or sensation (as that produced by the fractured ends of a bone moving against each other) ⟨~ in the arthritic knee⟩

crep·i·tus \'kre-pə-təs\ *n, pl* **crepitus** : CREPITATION

crescent of Gian·nuz·zi *or* **crescent of Gia·nuz·zi** \-jə-'nüt-sē\ *n* : DEMILUNE

G. Giannuzzi — see DEMILUNE OF GIANNUZZI

cre·sol \'krē-ˌsȯl, -ˌsōl\ *n* : any of three poisonous colorless crystalline or liquid isomeric phenols C_7H_8O that are used as disinfectants, in making phenolic resins, and in organic synthesis — see METACRESOL

crest \'krest\ *n* : a ridge esp. on a bone ⟨the ~ of the tibia⟩ — see OCCIPITAL CREST

cre·tin \'krēt-ᵊn\ *n* : one affected with cretinism — **cre·tin·ous** \-ᵊn-əs\ *adj*

cre·tin·ism \-ᵊn-ˌi-zəm\ *n* : a usu. congenital abnormal condition marked by physical stunting and mental deficiency and caused by severe thyroid deficiency

Creutz·feldt–Ja·kob disease *also* **Creutz·feld–Ja·cob disease** \'krȯits-ˌfelt-'yä-(ˌ)kōb-, -(ˌ)kȯp-\ *n* : a rare progressive fatal encephalopathy caused by a slow virus and marked by development of porous brain tissue, premature dementia in middle age, and gradual loss of muscular coordination — called also *Jakob-Creutzfeldt disease*

Creutzfeldt, Hans Gerhard (1885–1964) *and* **Jakob, Alfons Maria (1884–1931),** German psychiatrists.

crev·ice \'kre-vəs\ *n* : a narrow fissure or cleft — see GINGIVAL CREVICE

cre·vic·u·lar \krə-'vi-kyə-lər\ *adj* : of, relating to, or involving a crevice and esp. the gingival crevice ⟨gingival ~ fluid⟩

crib·bing \'kri-biŋ\ *n* : a vice of horses characterized by gnawing (as at a manger) while slobbering and salivating

crib biting *n* : CRIBBING

crib death *n* : SUDDEN INFANT DEATH SYNDROME

crib·ri·form plate \'kri-brə-ˌfȯrm-\ *n* **1** : the horizontal plate of the ethmoid bone perforated with numerous foramina for the passage of the olfactory nerve filaments from the nasal

cavity — called also *lamina cribrosa* **2** : LAMINA DURA

cribrosa — see LAMINA CRIBROSA

crick \'krik\ *n* : a painful spasmodic condition of muscles (as of the neck or back) — **crick** *vb*

crico- *comb form* **1** : cricoid cartilage and ⟨cricothyroid⟩ **2** : cricoid cartilage and ⟨cricopharyngeal⟩

cri·co·ar·y·te·noid \ˌkrī-kō-ˌar-ə-'tē-ˌnȯid, -kō-ə-'rit-ᵊn-ˌȯid\ *n* : a muscle of the larynx that arises from the upper margin of the arch of the cricoid cartilage, inserts into the front of the process of the arytenoid cartilage, and helps to narrow the opening of the vocal cords — called also *lateral cricoarytenoid* **2** : a muscle of the larynx that arises from the posterior surface of the lamina of the cricoid cartilage, inserts into the posterior of the process of the arytenoid cartilage, and widens the opening of the vocal cords — called also *posterior cricoarytenoid*

cri·coid cartilage \'krī-ˌkȯid-\ *n* : a cartilage of the larynx which articulates with the lower cornua of the thyroid cartilage and with which the arytenoid cartilages articulate — called also *cricoid*

cri·co·pha·ryn·geal \ˌkrī-kō-ˌfar-ən-'jē-əl, -fə-'rin-jəl, -jē-əl\ *adj* : of or relating to the cricoid cartilage and the pharynx

¹cri·co·thy·roid \-'thī-ˌrȯid\ *adj* : relating to or connecting the cricoid cartilage and the thyroid cartilage

²cricothyroid *n* : a triangular muscle of the larynx that is attached to the cricoid and thyroid cartilages and is the principal tensor of the vocal cords — called also *cricothyroid muscle*

cri·co·thy·roi·de·us \ˌkrī-kō-thī-'rȯi-dē-əs\ *n, pl* **-dei** \-dē-ˌī\ : CRICOTHYROID

cri du chat syndrome \ˌkrē-dü-'shä-, -də-\ *n* : an inherited condition characterized by a mewing cry, mental retardation, physical anomalies, and the absence of part of a chromosome — called also *cat cry syndrome*

¹crip·ple \'kri-pəl\ *n* : a lame or partly disabled individual — sometimes taken to be offensive

²cripple *vb* **crip·pled; crip·pling** \-p(ə-)liŋ\ : to deprive of the use of a limb and esp. a leg ⟨*crippled* by arthritis⟩

crip·pler \-p(ə-)lər\ *n* : a disease that results in crippling

cri·sis \'krī-səs\ *n, pl* **cri·ses** \-ˌsēz\ **1** : the turning point for better or worse in an acute disease or fever; *esp* : a sudden turn for the better (as sudden abatement in severity of symptoms or abrupt drop in temperature) — compare LYSIS **2** : a paroxysmal attack of pain, distress, or disordered function ⟨tabetic ~⟩ ⟨cardiac ~⟩ **3** : an emotionally significant event or radical change of status in a person's life **4** : a psychological or social condition characterized by unusual instability caused by excessive stress and either endangering or felt to endanger the continuity of an individual or group; *esp* : such a social condition requiring the transformation of cultural patterns and values

crisis center *n* : a facility run usu. by nonprofessionals who counsel those who telephone for help in a personal crisis

cris·ta \'kris-tə\ *n, pl* **cris·tae** \-ₜtē, -ₜtī\ **1** : one of the areas of specialized sensory epithelium in the ampullae of the semicircular canals of the ear serving as end organs for the labyrinthine sense **2** : an elevation of the surface of a bone for the attachment of a muscle or tendon **3** : any of the inwardly projecting folds of the inner membrane of a mitochondrion

crista gal·li \-'ga-lē, -'gȯ-\ *n* : an upright process on the anterior portion of the cribriform plate to which the anterior part of the falx cerebri is attached

crit·i·cal \'kri-ti-kəl\ *adj* **1** : relating to, indicating, or being the stage of a disease at which an abrupt change for better or worse may be anticipated with reasonable certainty (the ∼ phase of a fever) **2** : being or relating to an illness or condition involving danger of death (∼ care) (a ∼ head injury) — **crit·i·cal·ly** \-k(ə-)lē\ *adv*

CRNA *abbr* certified registered nurse anesthetist

crock \'kräk\ *n* : a complaining medical patient whose illness is largely imaginary or psychosomatic

Crohn's disease \'krōnz-\ *n* : ileitis that typically involves the distal portion of the ileum, often spreads to the colon, and is characterized by diarrhea, cramping, and loss of appetite and weight with local abscesses and scarring — called also *regional enteritis, regional ileitis*

Crohn \'krōn\, Burrill Bernard (1884–1983), American physician.

cro·mo·gly·cate \ₜkrō-mō-'gli-ₜkāt\ — see CROMOLYN SODIUM

cro·mo·lyn sodium \'krō-mə-lən-\ *n* : a drug $C_{23}H_{14}Na_2O_{11}$ that inhibits the release of histamine from mast cells and is used usu. as an inhalant to prevent the onset of bronchial asthma attacks — called also *cromolyn, disodium cromoglycate, sodium cromoglycate*

¹cross \'krȯs\ *n* **1** : an act of crossing dissimilar individuals **2** : a crossbred individual or kind

²cross *vb* : to interbreed or cause (an animal or plant) to interbreed with one of a different kind : HYBRIDIZE

³cross *adj* : CROSSBRED, HYBRID

cross·bred \'krȯs-'bred\ *adj* : produced by crossbreeding : HYBRID — **cross·bred** \-ₜbred\ *n*

¹cross·breed \'krȯs-ₜbrēd, -'brēd\ *vb* **-bred** \-ₜbred, -'bred\; **-breed·ing** : HYBRIDIZE, CROSS; *esp* : to cross (two varieties or breeds) within the same species

²cross·breed \-ₜbrēd\ *n* : HYBRID

cross·bridge \'krȯs-ₜbrij\ *n* : the globular head of a myosin molecule that projects from a myosin filament in muscle and in the sliding filament hypothesis of muscle contraction is held to attach temporarily to an adjacent actin filament and draw it into the A band of a sarcomere between the myosin filaments

crossed \'krȯst\ *adj* : forming a decussation (a ∼ tract of nerve fibers)

cross–eye \'krȯs-ₜī\ *n* **1** : squint in which the eye turns inward toward the nose — called also *esotropia;* compare WALLEYE 2a **2 cross–eyes** \-ₜīz\ *pl* : eyes affected with cross-eye — **cross–eyed** \-ₜīd\ *adj*

cross·ing–over \ₜkrȯs-siŋ-'ō-vər\ *n* : an interchange of genes or segments between homologous chromosomes

cross·match·ing \'krȯs-'ma-chiŋ\ *or* **cross·match** \-'mach\ *n* : the testing of the compatibility of the bloods of a transfusion donor and a recipient by mixing the serum of each with the red cells of the other to determine the absence of agglutination reactions — **crossmatch** *vb*

¹cross·over \'krȯs-ₜō-vər\ *n* **1** : an instance or product of genetic crossing-over **2** : a crossover interchange in an experiment

²crossover *adj* : involving or using interchange of the control group and the experimental group during the course of an experiment

cross–re·ac·tion \ₜkrȯs-rē-'ak-shən\ *n* : reaction of one antigen with antibodies developed against another antigen — **cross–re·act** \-'akt\ *vb* — **cross–re·ac·tive** \-rē-'ak-tiv\ *adj* — **cross–re·ac·tiv·i·ty** \-(ₜ)rē-ₜak-'ti-və-tē\ *n*

cross section *n* : a cutting or piece of something cut off at right angles to an axis; *also* : a representation of such a cutting — **cross–sec·tion·al** \ₜkrȯs-'sek-shə-nəl\ *adj*

cross–tol·er·ance \'krȯs-'tä-lə-rəns\ *n* : tolerance or resistance to a drug that develops through continued use of another drug with similar pharmacological action

cro·ta·lar·ia \ₜkrō-tə-'lar-ē-ə, ₜkrä-\ *n* **1** *cap* : a large genus of usu. tropical and subtropical plants (family Leguminosae) with yellow flowers and inflated pods including some containing toxic alkaloids esp. in the seeds that are poisonous to farm animals and humans **2** : any plant of the genus *Crotalaria* — called also *rattlebox*

Cro·ta·lus \'krōt-əl-əs, 'krät-\ *n* : a genus of American pit vipers including many of the rattlesnakes

crotch \'kräch\ *n* : an angle formed by

the parting of two legs, branches, or members

-crotic *adj comb form* : having (such) a heartbeat or pulse ⟨di*crotic*⟩

-crotism *n comb form* : condition of having (such) a heartbeat or pulse ⟨di*crotism*⟩

Cro·ton bug \'krōt-ᵊn-\ *n* : GERMAN COCKROACH

cro·ton oil \'krōt-ᵊn-\ *n* : a viscid acrid fixed oil from an Asian plant (*Croton tiglium* of the family Euphorbiaceae) that was formerly used as a drastic cathartic but is now used esp. in pharmacological experiments as an irritant

croup \'krüp\ *n* : a spasmodic laryngitis esp. of infants marked by episodes of difficult breathing, stridor, and a hoarse grating cough — **croup·ous** \'krü-pəs\ *adj* — **croup·y** \-pē\ *adj*

¹crown \'kraůn\ *n* **1** : the topmost part of the skull or head **2** : the part of a tooth external to the gum or an artificial substitute for this

²crown *vb* **1** : to put an artificial crown on (a tooth) **2** *in childbirth* : to appear at the vaginal opening — used of the first part (as the crown of the head) of the infant to appear ⟨the head ∼ed⟩

crow's-foot \'krōz-ˌfůt\ *n*, *pl* **crow's-feet** \-ˌfēt\ : a wrinkle extending from the outer corner of the eye — usu. used in pl.

CRT \ˌsē-(ˌ)är-'tē\ *n*, *pl* **CRTs** or **CRT's** : CATHODE-RAY TUBE; *also* : a display device incorporating a cathode-ray tube

CRTT *abbr* certified respiratory therapy technician

cru·ci·ate \'krü-shē-ˌāt\ *adj* : shaped like a cross

cruciate ligament *n* : any of several more or less cross-shaped ligaments: as **a** : either of two ligaments in the knee joint which cross each other from femur to tibia: (1) : an anterior one that limits extension and rotation — called also *anterior cruciate ligament* (2) : a posterior one that prevents dislocation of the femur in a forward direction — called also *posterior cruciate ligament* **b** : a complex ligament made up of the transverse ligament of the atlas and vertical fibrocartilage extending from the odontoid process to the border of the foramen magnum

crude protein *n* : the approximate amount of protein in foods that is calculated from the determined nitrogen content by multiplying by a factor (as 6.25 for many foods and 5.7 for wheat) derived from the average percentage of nitrogen in the food proteins and that may contain an appreciable error if the nitrogen is derived from nonprotein material or from a protein of unusual composition

crura *pl of* CRUS

cru·ra ce·re·bri \ˌkrůr-ə-'ser-ə-ˌbī, -'ker-ə-ˌbrē\ *n pl* : CRUS 2c

crura for·ni·cis \-'fòr-nə-ˌsis, -ə-ˌkis\ *n pl* : CRUS 2e

cru·ral \'krůr-əl\ *adj* : of or relating to the thigh or leg; *specif* : FEMORAL

cruris — see TINEA CRURIS

crus \'krüs, 'krəs\ *n*, *pl* **cru·ra** \'krůr-ə\ **1** : the part of the hind limb between the femur or thigh and the ankle or tarsus : SHANK **2** : any of various anatomical parts likened to a leg or to a pair of legs: as **a** : either of the diverging proximal ends of the corpora cavernosa **b** : the tendinous attachments of the diaphragm to the bodies of the lumbar vertebrae forming the sides of the aortic opening — often used in pl. **c** *pl* : the peduncles of the cerebrum — called also *crura cerebri* **d** *pl* : the peduncles of the cerebellum **e** *pl* : the posterior pillars of the fornix — called also *crura fornicis* **f** (1) : a long bony process of the incus that articulates with the stapes; *also* : a shorter one projecting from the body of the incus perpendicular to this (2) : either of the two bony processes forming the sides of the arch of the stapes

crush syndrome *n* : the physical responses to severe crushing injury of muscle tissue involving esp. shock and partial or complete renal failure; *also* : the renal failure associated with such responses

crust \'krəst\ *n* **1** : SCAB 2 **2** : an encrusting deposit of serum, cellular debris, and bacteria present over or about lesions in some skin diseases (as impetigo or eczema) — **crust** *vb*

crutch \'krəch\ *n* **1** : a support typically fitting under the armpit for use as an aid in walking **2** : the crotch esp. of an animal

cry- or **cryo-** *comb form* : cold : freezing ⟨*cryo*surgery⟩

cryo·bi·ol·o·gy \ˌkrī-ō-bī-'ä-lə-jē\ *n*, *pl* **-gies** : the study of the effects of extremely low temperature on biological systems (as cells or organisms) — **cryo·bi·o·log·i·cal** \-ˌbī-ə-'lä-ji-kəl\ *adj* — **cryo·bi·ol·o·gist** \-ō-bī-'ä-lə-jist\ *n*

cryo·cau·tery \-'kò-tə-rē\ *n*, *pl* **-ter·ies** : destruction of tissue by use of extreme cold

cryo·ex·trac·tion \-ik-'strak-shən\ *n* : extraction of a cataract through use of a cryoprobe whose refrigerated tip adheres to and freezes tissue of the lens permitting its removal

cryo·ex·trac·tor \-ik-'strak-tər, -'ek-ˌ\ *n* : a cryoprobe used for removal of cataracts

cryo·fi·brin·o·gen \-fī-'bri-nə-jən\ *n* : fibrinogen that precipitates upon cooling to 4° C (39° F) and redissolves at 37° C (98.6° F)

cryo·gen·ic \ˌkrī-ə-'je-nik\ *adj* **1 a** : of or relating to the production of very low temperatures **b** : being or relating to very low temperatures **2** : requiring or involving the use of a cryogenic temperature (∼ surgery) — **cryo·gen·i·cal·ly** \-ni-k(ə-)lē\ *adv*

cryo·gen·ics \-niks\ *n* : a branch of physics that deals with the production and effects of very low temperatures

cryo·glob·u·lin \ˌkrī-ō-ˈglä-byə-lən\ *n* : any of several proteins similar to gamma globulins (as in molecular weight) that precipitate when in the cold from blood serum esp. in pathological conditions (as multiple myeloma)

cryo·glob·u·lin·emia \-ˌglä-byə-lə-ˈnē-mē-ə\ *n* : the condition of having abnormal quantities of cryoglobulins in the blood

cry·on·ics \krī-ˈä-niks\ *n* : the practice of freezing the body of a person who has died from a disease in hopes of restoring life at some future time when a cure for the disease has been developed — **cry·on·ic** \-nik\ *adj*

cryo·pexy \ˈkrī-ō-ˌpek-sē\ *n, pl* **-pex·ies** : cryosurgery for fixation of the retina in retinal detachment or for repair of a retinal tear or hole

cryo·pre·cip·i·tate \ˌkrī-ō-pri-ˈsi-pə-tət, -ˌtāt\ *n* : a precipitate that is formed by cooling a solution — **cryo·pre·cip·i·ta·tion** \-ˌsi-pə-ˈtā-shən\ *n*

cryo·pres·er·va·tion \-ˌpre-zər-ˈvā-shən\ *n* : preservation (as of sperm or eggs) by subjection to extremely low temperatures — **cryo·pre·serve** \-pri-ˈzərv\ *vb*

cryo·probe \ˈkrī-ə-ˌprōb\ *n* : a blunt chilled instrument used to freeze tissues in cryosurgery

cryo·pro·tec·tive \ˌkrī-ō-prə-ˈtek-tiv\ *adj* : serving to protect against the deleterious effects of subjection to freezing temperatures (a ∼ agent) — **cryo·pro·tec·tant** \-tənt\ *n or adj*

cryo·stat \ˈkrī-ə-ˌstat\ *n* : an apparatus for maintaining a constant low temperature esp. below 0°C or 32°F (as by means of liquid helium); *esp* : one containing a microtome for obtaining sections of frozen tissue — **cryo·stat·ic** \ˌkrī-ə-ˈsta-tik\ *adj*

cryo·sur·gery \ˌkrī-ō-ˈsərj-rē, -ˈsər-jə-rē\ *n, pl* **-ger·ies** : surgery in which the tissue to be treated or operated on is frozen (as by liquid nitrogen) — **cryo·sur·geon** \-ˈsər-jən\ *n* — **cryo·sur·gi·cal** \-ˈsər-ji-kəl\ *adj*

cryo·ther·a·py \-ˈther-ə-pē\ *n, pl* **-pies** : the therapeutic use of cold

crypt \ˈkript\ *n* **1** : an anatomical pit or depression **2** : a simple tubular gland (as a crypt of Lieberkühn)

crypt- *or* **crypto-** *comb form* : hidden : covered (*cryptogenic*)

crypt·ec·to·my \krip-ˈtek-tə-mē\ *n, pl* **-mies** : surgical removal or destruction of a crypt

cryp·tic \ˈkrip-tik\ *adj* : not recognized (a ∼ infection)

cryp·ti·tis \krip-ˈtī-təs\ *n* : inflammation of a crypt (as an anal crypt)

cryp·to·coc·co·sis \ˌkrip-tə-(ˌ)kä-ˈkō-səs\ *n, pl* **-co·ses** \-(ˌ)sēz\ : an infectious disease that is caused by a fungus of the genus *Cryptococcus* (*C. neoformans*) and is characterized by the production of nodular lesions or abscesses in the lungs, subcutaneous tissues, joints, and esp. the brain and meninges — called also *torulosis*

cryp·to·coc·cus \-ˈkä-kəs\ *n* **1** *cap* : a genus of imperfect fungi (family Cryptococcaceae) that resemble yeasts and include a number of saprophytes and a few serious pathogens **2** *pl* **-coc·ci** \-ˈkäk-ˌsī, -ˌsē; -ˈkäk-ˌkī, -ˌkē\ : any fungus of the genus *Cryptococcus* — **cryp·to·coc·cal** \-ˈkä-kəl\ *adj*

crypt of Lie·ber·kühn \-ˈlē-bər-ˌkün, -ˌkyün, -ˌkün-\ *n* : any of the tubular glands of the intestinal mucous membrane — called also *intestinal gland*

Lieberkühn, **Johannes Nathanael** (1711–1756), German anatomist.

crypt of Mor·ga·gni \-mȯr-ˈgän-yē\ *n* : any of the pouched cavities of the rectal mucosa immediately above the anorectal junction, intervening between vertical folds of the rectal mucosa

Morgagni, Giovanni Battista (1682–1771), Italian anatomist and pathologist.

cryp·to·ge·net·ic \ˌkrip-tō-jə-ˈne-tik\ *adj* : CRYPTOGENIC

cryp·to·gen·ic \ˌkrip-tə-ˈje-nik\ *adj* : of obscure or unknown origin (∼ epilepsy)

crypt·or·chid \krip-ˈtȯr-kəd\ *n* : one affected with cryptorchidism — compare MONORCHID — **cryptorchid** *adj*

crypt·or·chi·dism \-kə-ˌdi-zəm\ *also* **crypt·or·chism** \-ki-zəm\ *n* : a condition in which one or both testes fail to descend normally — compare MONORCHIDISM

cryp·to·spo·rid·i·o·sis \ˌkrip-tō-spȯr-ˌi-dē-ˈō-səs\ *n, pl* **-o·ses** \-ˌsēz\ : a disease caused by cryptosporidia

cryp·to·spo·rid·i·um \ˌkrip-tō-spȯr-ˈi-dē-əm\ *n* **1** *cap* : a genus of coccidian protozoans parasitic in the gut of many vertebrates including humans and sometimes causing diarrhea esp. in individuals who are immunocompromised (as in AIDS) **2** *pl* **-rid·ia** \-dē-ə\ : any protozoan of the genus *Cryptosporidium*

cryp·to·xan·thin \ˌkrip-tə-ˈzan-thən\ *n* : a red crystalline carotenoid alcohol $C_{40}H_{55}OH$ that occurs in many plants, in blood serum, and in some animal products (as butter and egg yolk) and that is a precursor of vitamin A

cryp·to·zo·ite \-ˈzō-ˌīt\ *n* : a malaria parasite that develops in tissue cells and gives rise to the forms that invade blood cells — compare METACRYPTO-ZOITE

crys·tal \'krist-ᵊl\ n 1 : a body that is formed by the solidification of a chemical element, a compound, or a mixture and has a regularly repeating internal arrangement of its atoms and often external plane faces 2 : powdered methamphetamine — **crystal** adj — **crys·tal·line** \'kris-tə-lən, -ₗlin, -ₗlēn\ adj

crys·tal·lin \'kris-tə-lən\ n : either of two globulins in the crystalline lens

crystallina — see MILIARIA CRYSTALLI-NA

crystalline lens n : the lens of the eye

crys·tal·lize also **crys·tal·ize** \'kris-tə-ₗlīz\ vb **-lized** also **-ized; -liz·ing** also **-iz·ing** : to cause to form crystals or assume crystalline form — **crys·tal·liz·able** \ₗkris-tə-'lī-zə-bəl\ adj — **crys·tal·li·za·tion** \ₗkris-tə-lə-'zā-shən\ n

crys·tal·lu·ria \ₗkris-tə-'lür-ē-ə, -təl-'yür-\ n : the presence of crystals in the urine indicating renal irritation

cs abbr conditioned stimulus

Cs symbol cesium

CS \ₗsē-'es\ n : a potent lacrimatory and nausea-producing gas $C_{10}H_5ClN_2$ used in riot control and chemical warfare

C–sec·tion \'sē-ₗsek-shən\ n : CESARE-AN

CSF \ₗsē-(ₗ)es-'ef\ n : COLONY-STIMU-LATING FACTOR

CSF abbr cerebrospinal fluid

CT abbr computed tomography; computerized tomography

Cte·no·ce·phal·i·des \ₗte-nō-sə-'fa-lə-ₗdēz\ n : a genus of fleas (family Pulicidae) including the dog flea (C. canis) and cat flea (C. felis)

CT scan \'sē-'tē-\ n : CAT SCAN — **CT scanning** n

CT scanner n : CAT SCANNER

C–type \'sē-ₗtīp\ adj : TYPE C

Cu symbol copper

¹**cu·bi·tal** \'kyü-bət-ᵊl\ adj : of or relating to a cubitus

²**cubital** n : CUBITUS

cubiti — see BICEPS FLEXOR CUBITI

cu·bi·tus \'kyü-bə-təs\ n, pl **cu·bi·ti** \-ₗtī\ 1 : FOREARM, ANTEBRACHIUM 2 : ULNA

cubitus valgus n : a condition of the arm in which the forearm deviates away from the midline of the body when extended

cubitus varus n : a condition of the arm in which the forearm deviates toward the midline of the body when extended

¹**cu·boid** \'kyü-ₗbȯid\ adj 1 : relating to or being the cuboid (the ~ bone) 2 : shaped approximately like a cube

²**cuboid** n : the outermost bone in the distal row of tarsal bones of the foot that supports the fourth and fifth metatarsals

cu·boi·dal \kyü-'bȯid-ᵊl\ adj 1 : CUBOID

2 2 : composed of nearly cubical elements (~ epithelium)

cud \'kəd\ n : food brought up into the mouth by a ruminating animal from its first stomach to be chewed again

cue \'kyü\ n : a minor stimulus acting as an indication of the nature of the perceived object or situation

cuff \'kəf\ n 1 : an inflatable band that is wrapped around an extremity to control the flow of blood through the part when recording blood pressure with a sphygmomanometer 2 : an anatomical structure shaped like a cuff; esp : ROTATOR CUFF

cui·rass \kwi-'ras, kyū-\ n 1 : a plaster cast for the trunk and neck 2 : a respirator that covers the chest or the chest and abdomen and provides artificial respiration by means of an electric pump

cul–de–sac \ₗkəl-di-'sak, ₗkül-\ n, pl **culs–de–sac** \same or ₗkəlz-, ₗkülz-\ also **cul–de–sacs** \-'saks\ 1 : a blind diverticulum or pouch; also : the closed end of such a pouch 2 : POUCH OF DOUGLAS

cul–de–sac of Douglas n : POUCH OF DOUGLAS

culdo- comb form : pouch of Douglas (culdoscopy)

cul·do·cen·te·sis \ₗkəl-dō-ₗsen-'tē-səs, ₗkül-\ n, pl **-te·ses** \-ₗsēz\ : removal of material from the pouch of Douglas by means of puncture of the vaginal wall

cul·dos·co·py \kəl-'däs-kə-pē, ₗkül-\ n, pl **-pies** : a technique for endoscopic visualization and minor operative procedures on the female pelvic organs in which the instrument is introduced through a puncture in the wall of the pouch of Douglas — **cul·do·scop·ic** \ₗkəl-də-'skä-pik, ₗkül-\ adj

cul·dot·o·my \kəl-'dä-tə-mē, ₗkül-\ n, pl **-mies** : surgical incision of the pouch of Douglas

cu·lex \'kyü-ₗleks\ n 1 cap : a large cosmopolitan genus of mosquitoes (family Culicidae) that includes the common house mosquito (C. pipiens) of Europe and No. America, a widespread tropical mosquito (C. quinquefasciatus syn. C. fatigans) which transmits some filarial worms parasitic in humans, and other mosquitoes which have been implicated as vectors of virus encephalitides and possibly of other diseases — compare ANOPHELES 2 : a mosquito of the genus Culex — **cu·li·cine** \'kyü-lə-ₗsin\ adj or n

cu·li·cide \'kyü-lə-ₗsīd\ n : an insecticide that destroys mosquitoes

Cu·li·coi·des \ₗkyü-lə-'kȯi-ₗdēz\ n : a genus of bloodsucking midges (family Ceratopogonidae) of which some are intermediate hosts of filarial parasites

cul·men \'kəl-mən\ n : a lobe of the cerebellum lying in the superior vermis just in front of the primary fissure

cul·ti·vate \'kəl-tə-ˌvāt\ vb **-vat·ed; -vat·ing** : CULTURE 1

cul·ti·va·tion \ˌkəl-tə-'vā-shən\ n : CULTURE 2

¹**cul·ture** \'kəl-chər\ n 1 a : the integrated pattern of human behavior that includes thought, speech, action, and artifacts and depends upon the human capacity for learning and transmitting knowledge to succeeding generations b : the customary beliefs, social forms, and material traits of a racial, religious, or social group 2 a : the act or process of growing living material (as bacteria or viruses) in prepared nutrient media b : a product of cultivation in nutrient media — **cul·tur·al** \'kəl-chə-rəl\ adj — **cul·tur·al·ly** adv

²**culture** vb **cul·tured; cul·tur·ing** 1 : to grow (as microorganisms or tissues) in a prepared medium 2 : to start a culture from; also : to make a culture of 〈~ milk〉

culture shock n : a sense of confusion and uncertainty sometimes with feelings of anxiety that may affect people exposed to an alien culture or environment without adequate preparation

cu·mu·la·tive \'kyü-myə-lə-tiv, -ˌlā-\ adj : increasing in effect by successive doses (as of a drug or poison) — **cu·mu·la·tive·ly** adv

cu·mu·lus \'kyü-myə-ləs\ n, pl **cu·mu·li** \-ˌlī, -ˌlē\ : the projecting mass of granulosa cells that bears the developing ovum in a graafian follicle — called also **discus proligerus**

cumulus ooph·o·rus \-ō-'ä-fə-rəs\ n : CUMULUS

cu·ne·ate fasciculus \'kyü-nē-ˌāt-, -ət-\ n, pl **cuneate fasciculi** : FASCICULUS CUNEATUS

cuneate nucleus n : NUCLEUS CUNEATUS

cuneatus — see FASCICULUS CUNEATUS, NUCLEUS CUNEATUS

¹**cu·ne·i·form** \kyü-'nē-ə-ˌform, 'kyü-; 'kyü-nə-\ adj 1 : of, relating to, or being a cuneiform bone or cartilage 2 of a human skull : wedge-shaped as viewed from above

²**cuneiform** n : a cuneiform bone or cartilage

cuneiform bone n 1 : any of three small bones of the tarsus situated between the navicular and the first three metatarsals: a : one on the medial side of the foot that is just proximal to the first metatarsal bone and is the largest of the three bones — called also **medial cuneiform, medial cuneiform bone** b : one that is situated between the other two bones proximal to the second metatarsal bone and is the smallest of the three bones — called also **intermediate cuneiform, intermediate cuneiform bone** c : one that is situated proximal to the third metatarsal bone and that lies between the intermediate cuneiform bone and the

cuboid — called also **lateral cuneiform bone** 2 : TRIQUETRAL BONE

cuneiform cartilage n : either of a pair of rods of yellow elastic cartilage of which each lies on one side of the larynx in an aryepiglottic fold just below the arytenoid cartilage

cu·ne·us \'kyü-nē-əs\ n, pl **cu·nei** \-nē-ˌī\ : a convolution of the mesial surface of the occipital lobe of the brain above the calcarine sulcus that forms a part of the visual area

cun·ni·lin·gus \ˌkə-ni-'liŋ-gəs\ also **cun·ni·linc·tus** \-'liŋk-təs\ n : oral stimulation of the vulva or clitoris

¹**cup** \'kəp\ n 1 : an athletic supporter reinforced for providing extra protection to the wearer in certain strenuous sports (as boxing, hockey, football) 2 : a cap of metal shaped like the femoral head and used in plastic reconstruction of the hip joint

²**cup** vb **cupped; cup·ping** 1 : to treat by cupping 2 : to undergo or perform cupping

cup·ping n : a technique formerly employed for drawing blood to the surface of the body by application of a glass vessel from which air had been evacuated by heat to form a partial vacuum

cu·pu·la \'kyü-pyü-lə, -pü-\ n, pl **cu·pu·lae** \-ˌlē\ 1 : the bony apex of the cochlea 2 : the peak of the pleural sac covering the apex of the lung

cur·able \'kyür-ə-bəl\ adj : capable of being cured

cu·ra·re also **cu·ra·ri** \kyù-'rär-ē, kù-\ n : a dried aqueous extract esp. of a vine (as **Strychnos toxifera** of the family Loganiaceae or **Chondodendron tomentosum** of the family Menispermaceae) used in arrow poisons by So. American Indians and in medicine to produce muscular relaxation

cu·ra·ri·form \kyü-'rär-ə-ˌform, kù-\ adj : producing or characterized by the muscular relaxation typical of curare 〈~ drugs〉

cu·ra·rize \-'rär-ˌīz\ vb **-rized; -riz·ing** : to treat with curare — **cu·ra·ri·za·tion** \-ˌrär-ə-'zā-shən\ n

cu·ra·tive \'kyür-ə-tiv\ adj : relating to or used in the cure of diseases — **curative** n — **cu·ra·tive·ly** adv

curb \'kərb\ n : a swelling on the back of the hind leg of a horse just behind the lowest part of the hock joint that is due to strain or rupture of the ligament and generally causes lameness

¹**cure** \'kyür\ n 1 : recovery from a disease 〈his ~ was complete〉; also : remission of signs or symptoms of a disease esp. during a prolonged period of observation 〈clinical ~〉 — compare ARREST, REMISSION 2 : a drug, treatment, regimen, or other agency that cures a disease 3 : a course or period of treatment; esp : one designed to interrupt an addic-

tion or compulsive habit or to improve general health **4** : SPA

²cure *vb* **cured; cur·ing 1 a** : to make or become healthy, sound, or normal again ⟨*curing* his patients rapidly by new procedures⟩ **b** : to bring about recovery from ⟨antibiotics ∼ many formerly intractable infections⟩ **2** : to take a cure (as in a sanatorium or at a spa) — **cur·er** *n*

cu·ret·tage \ˌkyu̇r-ə-ˈtäzh\ *n* : a surgical scraping or cleaning by means of a curette

¹cu·rette *also* **cu·ret** \kyu̇-ˈret\ *n* : a surgical instrument that has a scoop, loop, or ring at its tip and is used in performing curettage

²curette *also* **curet** *vb* **cu·rett·ed; cu·rett·ing** : to perform curettage on — **cu·rette·ment** \kyu̇-ˈret-mənt\ *n*

cu·rie \ˈkyu̇r-(ˌ)ē, kyu̇-ˈrē\ *n* **1** : a unit quantity of any radioactive nuclide in which 3.7×10^{10} disintegrations occur per second **2** : a unit of radioactivity equal to 3.7×10^{10} disintegrations per second

Curie, Pierre (1859–1906), and Marie Sklodowska (1867–1934), French chemists and physicists.

cu·ri·um \ˈkyu̇r-ē-əm\ *n* : a metallic radioactive trivalent element artificially produced — symbol *Cm*; see ELEMENT table

Cur·ling's ulcer \ˈkər-liŋz-\ *n* : acute gastroduodenal ulceration following severe skin burns

Cur·ling \ˈkər-liŋ\, Thomas Blizard (1811–1888), British surgeon.

cur·rent \ˈkər-ənt\ *n* : a flow of electric charge; *also* : the rate of such flow

cur·va·ture \ˈkər-və-ˌchu̇r, -chər, -ˌtyu̇r\ *n* **1** : an abnormal curving (as of the spine) — see KYPHOSIS, SCOLIOSIS **2** : a curved surface of an organ (as the stomach) — see GREATER CURVATURE, LESSER CURVATURE

cush·ing·oid \ˈku̇-shiŋ-ˌȯid\ *adj, often cap* : resembling Cushing's disease esp. in facies or habitus

Cushing's disease \ˈku̇-shiŋz-\ *n* : Cushing's syndrome esp. when caused by excessive production of ACTH by the pituitary gland

Cushing, Harvey Williams (1869–1939), American neurosurgeon.

Cushing's syndrome *n* : an abnormal bodily condition characterized by obesity and muscular weakness due to excess corticosteroids and esp. hydrocortisone from adrenal or pituitary hyperfunction — called also *adrenogenital syndrome*

cush·ion \ˈku̇-shən\ *n* **1** : a bodily part resembling a pad **2** : a medical procedure or drug that eases discomfort without necessarily affecting the basic condition of the patient

cusp \ˈkəsp\ *n* **1** : a point on the grinding surface of a tooth **2** : a fold or flap of a cardiac valve

cus·pid \ˈkəs-pəd\ *n* : a canine tooth

cus·pi·date \ˈkəs-pə-ˌdāt\ *adj* : having a cusp : terminating in a point ⟨∼ molars⟩

cus·to·di·al \ˌkəs-ˈtō-dē-əl\ *adj* : marked by or given to watching and protecting rather than seeking to cure ⟨∼ care⟩

¹cut \ˈkət\ *vb* **cut; cut·ting 1 a** : to penetrate with or as if with an edged instrument **b** : to cut or operate on in surgery: as (1) : to subject (a domestic animal) to castration (2) : to perform lithotomy on **c** : to experience the emergence of (a tooth) through the gum **2** : to function as or in the manner of an edged tool ⟨a knife that ∼s well⟩ **3** : to subject to trimming or paring ⟨∼ one's nails⟩

²cut *n* **1 a** : an opening made with an edged instrument **b** : a wound made by something sharp **2** : a stroke or blow with the edge of a sharp implement (as a knife)

cu·ta·ne·ous \kyu̇-ˈtā-nē-əs\ *adj* : of, relating to, or affecting the skin ⟨a ∼ infection⟩ — **cu·ta·ne·ous·ly** *adv*

cut·down \ˈkət-ˌdau̇n\ *n* : incision of a superficial blood vessel (as a vein) to facilitate insertion of a catheter (as for administration of fluids)

Cu·te·re·bra \ˌkyu̇-tə-ˈrē-brə, kyu̇-ˈter-ə-brə\ *n* : a genus of large usu. darkcolored botflies (family Cuterebridae) with larvae that form tumors under the skin of rodents, cats, and other small mammals

cu·ti·cle \ˈkyu̇-ti-kəl\ *n* **1 a** : the outermost layer of integument composed of epidermis **b** : the outermost membranous layer of a hair consisting of cornified epithelial cells **2** : dead or horny epidermis (as that surrounding the base and sides of a fingernail or toenail) — **cu·tic·u·lar** \kyu̇-ˈti-kyə-lər\ *adj*

cu·ti·re·ac·tion \ˌkyu̇-ti-rē-ˈak-shən, ˈkyu̇-ti-rē-ˌ\ *n* : a local inflammatory reaction of the skin that occurs in certain infectious diseases following the application to or injection into the skin of a preparation of organisms producing the disease

cu·tis \ˈkyu̇-təs\ *n, pl* **cu·tes** \-ˌtēz\ *or* **cu·tis·es** : DERMIS

cu·vette \kyu̇-ˈvet\ *n* : a small often transparent laboratory vessel (as a tube)

Cu·vie·ri·an vein \(ˌ)kyu̇-ˈvir-ē-ən-, ˌkyu̇-vē-ˈir-\ *n* : CARDINAL VEIN

Cu·vier \ˈkü-vē-ā, ˈkyü-; kǖ-ˈvyä\, Georges (*orig.* Jean-Léopold-Nicolas-Frédéric) **(1769–1832),** French naturalist.

CVA *abbr* cerebrovascular accident

CVP *abbr* central venous pressure

CVS *abbr* chorionic villus sampling

cyan- *or* **cyano-** *comb form* **1** : blue ⟨cyanosis⟩ **2** : cyanide ⟨cyanogenetic⟩

cy·a·nide \ˈsī-ə-ˌnīd, -nəd\ *n* : any of several compounds (as potassium cyanide) that contain the radical CN having a chemical valence of one, re-act with and inactivate respiratory enzymes, and are rapidly lethal producing drowsiness, tachycardia, coma, and finally death

cy·a·no·ac·ry·late \ˌsī-ə-nō-ˈa-krə-ˌlāt, si-ˌa-nō-ə-\ *n* : any of several liquid acrylate monomers used as adhesives in medicine on living tissue to close wounds in surgery

cy·a·no·co·bal·a·min \-kō-ˈba-lə-mən\ *also* **cy·a·no·co·bal·a·mine** \-ˌmēn\ *n* : VITAMIN B₁₂

cy·a·no·ge·net·ic \ˌsī-ə-nō-jə-ˈne-tik, si-ˌa-nō-\ *or* **cy·a·no·gen·ic** \-ˈje-nik\ *adj* : capable of producing cyanide (as hydrogen cyanide) ⟨a ~ plant that is dangerous to livestock⟩ — **cy·a·no·gen·e·sis** \-ˈje-nə-səs\ *n*

cy·a·no·met·he·mo·glo·bin \ˌsī-ə-nō-(ˌ)met-ˈhē-mə-ˌglō-bən\ *or* **cy·an·met·he·mo·glo·bin** \ˌsī-ˌan-(ˌ)met-, ˌsī-ˌən-\ *n* : a bright red crystalline compound formed by the action of hydrogen cyanide on methemoglobin in the cold or on oxyhemoglobin at body temperature

cy·a·nosed \ˈsī-ə-ˌnōst, -ˌnōzd\ *adj* : affected with cyanosis

cy·a·no·sis \ˌsī-ə-ˈnō-səs\ *n, pl* **-no·ses** \-ˌsēz\ : a bluish or purplish discoloration (as of skin) due to deficient oxygenation of the blood — **cy·a·not·ic** \-ˈnä-tik\ *adj*

cycl- *or* **cyclo-** *comb form* : ciliary body (of the eye) ⟨*cycl*itis⟩ ⟨*cyclo*dialysis⟩

cy·cla·mate \ˈsī-klə-ˌmāt, -mət\ *n* : an artificially prepared salt of sodium or calcium used esp. formerly as a sweetener but now largely discontinued because of the possibly harmful effects of its metabolic breakdown product cyclohexylamine

cy·clan·de·late \ˌsī-ˈkland-ᵊl-ˌāt\ *n* : an antispasmodic drug C₁₇H₂₄O₃ used esp. as a vasodilator in the treatment of diseased arteries

cy·claz·o·cine \ˌsī-ˈkla-zə-ˌsēn, -sən\ *n* : an analgesic drug C₁₈H₂₅NO that inhibits the effects of morphine and related addictive drugs and is used in the treatment of drug addiction

¹**cy·cle** \ˈsī-kəl\ *n* : a recurring series of events: as **a** (1) : a series of stages through which an organism tends to pass once in a fixed order; *also* : a series of stages through which a population of organisms tends to pass more or less together — see LIFE CYCLE (2) : a series of physiological, biochemical, or psychological stages that recur in the same individual — see CARDIAC CYCLE, MENSTRUAL CYCLE; KREBS CYCLE **b** : one complete performance of a vibration, electric oscillation, current alternation, or other periodic process — **cy·clic** \ˈsī-klik, ˈsi-\ *or* **cy·cli·cal** \ˈsī-kli-kəl, ˈsi-\ *adj* — **cy·cli·cal·ly** *also* **cy·clic·ly** *adv*

²**cycle** *vb* **cycled; cycling** : to undergo the estrous cycle

cy·clec·to·my \sī-ˈklek-tə-mē, si-\ *n, pl* **-mies** : surgical removal of part of the ciliary muscle or body

cyclic adenosine monophosphate *n* : CYCLIC AMP

cyclic AMP *n* : a cyclic mononucleotide of adenosine that is formed from ATP and is responsible for the intracellular mediation of hormonal effects on various cellular processes — abbr. *CAMP*

cyclic GMP \-ˌjē-(ˌ)em-ˈpē\ *n* : a cyclic mononucleotide of guanosine that acts similarly to cyclic AMP as a secondary messenger in response to hormones

cyclic guanosine monophosphate *n* : CYCLIC GMP

cy·clic·i·ty \sī-ˈkli-sə-tē, si-\ *n, pl* **-ties** : the quality or state of being cyclic ⟨estrous ~⟩

cy·cli·tis \sə-ˈklī-təs, sī-\ *n* : inflammation of the ciliary body

cy·cli·zine \ˈsī-klə-ˌzēn\ *n* : an antiemetic drug C₁₈H₂₂N₂ used esp. in the form of its hydrochloride in the treatment of motion sickness — see MAREZINE

cyclo- — see CYCL-

cy·clo·di·al·y·sis \ˌsī-klō-dī-ˈa-lə-səs\ *n, pl* **-y·ses** \-ˌsēz\ : surgical detachment of the ciliary body from the sclera to reduce tension in the eyeball in some cases of glaucoma

cy·clo·dia·ther·my \-ˈdī-ə-ˌthər-mē\ *n, pl* **-mies** : partial or complete destruction of the ciliary body by diathermy to relieve some conditions (as glaucoma) characterized by increased tension within the eyeball

Cy·clo·gyl \ˈsī-klō-ˌgil\ *trademark* — used for a preparation of the hydrochloride of cyclopentolate

cy·clo·hex·ane \ˌsī-klō-ˈhek-ˌsān\ *n* : a pungent saturated hydrocarbon C₆H₁₂ found in petroleum or made synthetically

cy·clo·hex·yl·a·mine \-hek-ˈsi-lə-ˌmēn\ *n* : a colorless liquid amine C₆H₁₁N-H₂ of cyclohexane that is believed to be harmful as a metabolic breakdown product of cyclamate

¹**cy·cloid** \ˈsī-ˌkloid\ *n* : a cycloid individual

²**cycloid** *adj* : relating to or being a personality characterized by alternating high and low moods — compare CYCLOTHYMIC

cy·clo·ox·y·gen·ase \ˌsī-klō-ˈäk-si-jə-ˌnās, -äk-ˈsi-jə-, -ˌnāz\ *n* : an enzyme that catalyzes the conversion of arachidonic acid into prostaglandins of which some are associated with arthritic inflammation and that is held to be inactivated by aspirin with temporary partial relief of arthritic symptoms

cy·clo·pen·to·late \ˌsī-klō-ˈpen-tə-ˌlāt, ˌsi-\ *n* : an anticholinergic drug used esp. in the form of its hydrochloride

$C_{17}H_{25}NO_3 \cdot HCl$ to dilate the pupil of the eye for ophthalmologic examination — see CYCLOGYL

cy·clo·phos·pha·mide \-'fäs-fə-ˌmīd\ *n* : an immunosuppressive and antineoplastic drug $C_7H_{15}Cl_2N_2O_2P$ used in the treatment of lymphomas and some leukemias — see CYTOXAN

cy·clo·pia \sī-'klō-pē-ə\ *n* : a developmental anomaly characterized by the presence of a single median eye

cy·clo·ple·gia \ˌsī-klō-'plē-jə, ˌsī-, -jē-ə\ *n* : paralysis of the ciliary muscle of the eye

¹**cy·clo·ple·gic** \-'plē-jik\ *adj* : producing, involving, or characterized by cycloplegia (~ agents) (~ refraction)

²**cycloplegic** *n* : a cycloplegic agent

cy·clo·pro·pane \-'prō-ˌpān\ *n* : a flammable gaseous saturated cyclic hydrocarbon C_3H_6 sometimes used as a general anesthetic

cy·clops \'sī-ˌkläps\ *n, pl* **cy·clo·pes** \sī-'klō-(ˌ)pēz\ : an individual or fetus abnormal in having a single eye or the usual two orbits fused

cy·clo·ser·ine \ˌsī-klō-'ser-ˌēn, ˌsi-\ *n* : an amino antibiotic $C_3H_6N_2O_2$ produced by an actinomycete or the genus *Streptomyces* (*S. orchidaceus*) and used esp. in the treatment of tuberculosis

cy·clo·spor·in \ˌsī-klə-'spȯr-ᵊn\ *n* : any of a group of polypeptides obtained as metabolites from various imperfect fungi (as *Tolypocladium inflatum Gams* syn. *Trichoderma polysporum*); *esp* : CYCLOSPORINE

cyclosporin A \-'ā\ : CYCLOSPORINE

cy·clo·spor·ine \ˌsī-klə-'spȯr-ᵊn, -ˌēn\ *n* : a cyclosporin $C_{62}H_{111}N_{11}O_{12}$ used as an immunosuppressive drug esp. to prevent rejection of transplanted organs

cy·clo·thyme \'sī-klə-ˌthīm\ *n* : a cyclothymic individual

cy·clo·thy·mia \ˌsī-klə-'thī-mē-ə\ *n* : a cyclothymic affective disorder

¹**cy·clo·thy·mic** \-'thī-mik\ *adj* : relating to or being an affective disorder characterized by the alternation of depressed moods with elevated, expansive, or irritable moods without psychotic features (as hallucinations or delusions) — compare CYCLOID

²**cyclothymic** *n* : a cyclothymic individual

cy·clo·tome \'sī-klə-ˌtōm\ *n* : a knife used in cyclotomy

cy·clot·o·my \sī-'klä-tə-mē\ *n, pl* **-mies** : incision or division of the ciliary body

cy·clo·tro·pia \ˌsī-klə-'trō-pē-ə\ *n* : squint in which the eye rolls outward or inward around its front-to-back axis

cy·e·sis \sī-'ē-səs\ *n, pl* **cy·e·ses** \-ˌsēz\ : PREGNANCY

cyl·in·droid \'si-lən-ˌdrȯid, sə-'lin-\ *n* : a spurious or mucous urinary cast

that resembles a hyaline cast but has one tapered, stringy, twisted end

cyl·in·dro·ma \ˌsi-lən-'drō-mə\ *n, pl* **-mas** *or* **-ma·ta** \-mə-tə\ : a tumor characterized by cylindrical masses consisting of epithelial cells and hyalinized stroma: **a** : a malignant tumor esp. of the respiratory tract or salivary glands **b** : a benign tumor of the skin and esp. the scalp

cyl·in·dru·ria \ˌsi-lən-'drür-ē-ə\ *n* : the presence of casts in the urine

cy·no·mol·gus monkey \ˌsī-nə-'mäl-gəs-\ *n* : a macaque (*Macaca fascicularis* syn. *M. cynomolgus*) of southeastern Asia, Borneo, and the Philippines that is often used in medical research

cy·no·pho·bia \-'fō-bē-ə\ *n* : a morbid fear of dogs

cy·pro·hep·ta·dine \ˌsī-prō-'hep-tə-ˌdēn\ *n* : a drug $C_{21}H_{21}N$ that acts antagonistically to histamine and serotonin and is used esp. in the treatment of asthma

cy·prot·er·one \sī-'prä-tə-ˌrōn\ *n* : a synthetic steroid $C_{22}H_{27}ClO_3$ used in the form of its acetate to inhibit androgenic secretions (as testosterone)

cyst \'sist\ *n* **1** : a closed sac having a distinct membrane and developing abnormally in a body cavity or structure **2** : a body resembling a cyst: as **a** : a capsule formed about a minute organism going into a resting or spore stage; *also* : this capsule with its contents **b** : a resistant cover about a parasite produced by the parasite or the host — compare HYDATID 2a

cyst- *or* **cysti-** *or* **cysto-** *comb form* **1** : bladder (*cystitis*) (*cysto*plasty) **2** : cyst (*cysto*gastrostomy)

-cyst \ˌsist\ *n comb form* : bladder : sac (blasto*cyst*)

cyst·ad·e·no·ma \ˌsis-ˌtad-ᵊn-'ō-mə\ *n, pl* **-mas** *or* **-ma·ta** \-mə-tə\ : an adenoma marked by a cystic structure — **cyst·ad·e·no·ma·tous** \-mə-təs\ *adj*

cys·te·amine \sis-'tē-ə-mən\ *n* : a cysteine derivative C_2H_7NS that has been used experimentally in the prevention of radiation sickness (as in cancer patients)

cys·tec·to·my \sis-'tek-tə-mē\ *n, pl* **-mies** **1** : the surgical excision of a cyst (ovarian ~) **2** : the removal of all or a portion of the urinary bladder

cys·te·ine \'sis-tə-ˌēn\ *n* : a sulfur-containing amino acid $C_3H_7NO_2S$ occurring in many proteins and glutathione and readily oxidizable to cystine

cysti- — see CYST-

cys·tic \'sis-tik\ *adj* **1** : relating to, composed of, or containing cysts (a ~ tumor) **2** : of or relating to the urinary bladder or the gallbladder **3** : enclosed in a cyst (a ~ worm larva)

cystica — see OSTEITIS FIBROSA CYSTICA, OSTEITIS FIBROSA CYSTICA GENERALISTA

cystic duct *n* : the duct from the gallbladder that unites with the hepatic duct to form the common bile duct

cys·ti·cer·coid \,sis-tə-'sər-,kȯid\ *n* : a tapeworm larva having an invaginated scolex and solid hind part

cys·ti·cer·co·sis \-(,)sər-'kō-səs\ *n*, *pl* **-co·ses** \-,sēz\ : infestation with or disease caused by cysticerci

cys·ti·cer·cus \-'sər-kəs\ *n*, *pl* **-cer·ci** \-'sər-,sī, -,kī\ : a tapeworm larva that consists of a fluid-filled sac containing an invaginated scolex, is situated in the tissues of an intermediate host, and is capable of developing into an adult tapeworm when eaten by a suitable definitive host — called also *bladder worm*, *measle* — **cys·ti·cer·cal** \-'sər-kəl\ *adj*

cystic fibrosis *n* : a common hereditary disease esp. in Caucasian populations that appears usu. in early childhood, involves functional disorder of the exocrine glands, and is marked esp. by faulty digestion due to a deficiency of pancreatic enzymes, by difficulty in breathing due to mucus accumulation in airways, and by excessive loss of salt in the sweat — called also *fibrocystic disease of the pancreas*, *mucoviscidosis*

cys·tine \'sis-,tēn\ *n* : a crystalline amino acid $C_6H_{12}N_2O_4S_2$ that is widespread in proteins (as keratins) and is a major metabolic sulfur source

cys·ti·no·sis \,sis-tə-'nō-səs\ *n*, *pl* **-no·ses** \-,sēz\ : a recessive autosomally inherited disease characterized esp. by cystinuria and deposits of cystine throughout the body — **cys·ti·not·ic** \-'nä-tik\ *adj*

cys·tin·uria \,sis-tə-'nȯr-ē-ə, -'nyu̇r-\ *n* : a metabolic defect characterized by excretion of excessive amounts of cystine in the urine and sometimes by the formation of stones in the urinary tract and inherited as an autosomal recessive trait — **cys·tin·uric** \-'nu̇r-ik, -'nyu̇r-\ *adj*

cys·ti·tis \sis-'tī-təs\ *n*, *pl* **cys·tit·i·des** \-'ti-tə-,dēz\ : inflammation of the urinary bladder — **cys·tit·ic** \(')sis-'ti-tik\ *adj*

cysto- — see CYST-

cys·to·cele \'sis-tə-,sēl\ *n* : hernia of a bladder and esp. the urinary bladder : vesical hernia

cys·to·gas·tros·to·my \,sis-tō-(,)gas-'träs-tə-mē\ *n*, *pl* **-mies** : creation of a surgical opening between the stomach and a nearby cyst for drainage

cys·to·gram \'sis-tə-,gram\ *n* : a roentgenogram made by cystography

cys·tog·ra·phy \sis-'tä-grə-fē\ *n*, *pl* **-phies** : X-ray photography of the urinary bladder after injection of a contrast medium — **cys·to·graph·ic** \-tə-'gra-fik\ *adj*

cys·toid \'sis-,tȯid\ *adj* : resembling a bladder

cys·to·lith \'sis-tə-,lith\ *n* : a urinary calculus

cys·to·li·thi·a·sis \,sis-tō-li-'thī-ə-səs\ *n*, *pl* **-a·ses** \-,sēz\ : the presence of calculi in the urinary bladder

cys·to·li·thot·o·my \-li-'thä-tə-mē\ *n*, *pl* **-mies** : surgical removal of a calculus from the urinary bladder

cys·tom·e·ter \sis-'tä-mə-tər\ *n* : an instrument designed to measure pressure within the urinary bladder in relation to its capacity — **cys·to·met·ric** \,sis-tə-'me-trik\ *adj* — **cys·tom·e·try** \sis-'tä-mə-trē\ *n*

cys·to·met·ro·gram \,sis-tə-'me-trə-,gram, -'mē-\ *n* : a graphic recording of a cystometric measurement

cys·to·me·trog·ra·phy \-mə-'trä-grə-fē\ *n*, *pl* **-phies** : the process of making a cystometrogram

cys·to·plas·ty \'sis-tə-,plas-tē\ *n*, *pl* **-ties** : a plastic operation upon the urinary bladder

cys·to·py·eli·tis \,sis-tə-,pī-ə-'lī-təs\ *n* : inflammation of the urinary bladder and of the pelvis of one or both kidneys

cys·tor·rha·phy \sis-'tȯr-ə-fē\ *n*, *pl* **-phies** : suture of a wound, injury, or rupture in the urinary bladder

cys·to·sar·co·ma phyl·lodes \,sis-tō-sär-'kō-mə-fi-,lōdz\ *n* : a slow-growing tumor of the breast that resembles a fibroadenoma

cys·to·scope \'sis-tə-,skōp\ *n* : a medical instrument for the visual examination of the urinary bladder and the passage of instruments under visual control — **cys·to·scop·ic** \,sis-tə-'skä-pik\ *adj* — **cys·tos·co·pist** \sis-'täs-kə-pist\ *n*

cys·tos·co·py \sis-'täs-kə-pē\ *n*, *pl* **-pies** : the use of a cystoscope to examine the bladder

cys·tos·to·my \sis-'täs-tə-mē\ *n*, *pl* **-mies** : formation of an opening into the urinary bladder by surgical incision

cys·tot·o·my \sis-'tä-tə-mē\ *n*, *pl* **-mies** : surgical incision of the urinary bladder

cys·to·ure·ter·itis \,sis-tō-yu̇r-ə-tə-'rī-təs\ *n* : combined inflammation of the urinary bladder and ureters

cys·to·ure·thro·cele \,sis-tō-yu̇-'rē-thrə-,sēl\ *n* : herniation of the neck of the female bladder and associated urethra into the vagina

cys·to·ure·thro·gram \-yu̇-'rē-thrə-,gram\ *n* : an X-ray photograph of the urinary bladder and urethra made after injection of these organs with a contrast medium — **cys·to·ure·throg·ra·phy** \-,yu̇r-i-'thrä-grə-fē\ *n*

cys·to·ure·thro·scope \,sis-tō-yu̇-'rē-thrə-,skōp\ *n* : an instrument used for the examination of the posterior urethra and bladder — **cys·to·ure·thros·co·py** \-,yu̇r-i-'thräs-kə-pē\ *n*

cyt- *or* **cyto-** *comb form* **1** : cell ⟨*cytol*-ogy⟩ **2** : cytoplasm ⟨*cytokinesis*⟩

cyt·ar·a·bine \sī-'tar-ə-ˌbēn\ n : CYTOSINE ARABINOSIDE

-cyte \ˌsīt\ n comb form : cell ⟨leukocyte⟩

cy·to·ar·chi·tec·ton·ics \ˌsī-tō-ˌär-kə-(ˌ)tek-'tä-niks\ n sing or pl : CYTOARCHITECTURE — **cy·to·ar·chi·tec·ton·ic** \-nik\ adj

cy·to·ar·chi·tec·ture \ˌsī-tō-'är-kə-ˌtek-chər\ n : the cellular makeup of a bodily tissue or structure — **cy·to·ar·chi·tec·tur·al** \-ˌär-kə-'tek-chə-rəl\ adj — **cy·to·ar·chi·tec·tur·al·ly** adv

cy·to·chem·is·try \-'ke-mə-strē\ n, pl **-tries 1** : microscopic biochemistry **2** : the chemistry of cells — **cy·to·chem·i·cal** \-'ke-mi-kəl\ adj — **cy·to·chem·i·cal·ly** \-mi-k(ə-)lē\ adv — **cy·to·chem·ist** \-'ke-mist\ n

cy·to·chrome \'sī-tə-ˌkrōm\ n : any of several intracellular hemoprotein respiratory pigments that are enzymes functioning in electron transport as carriers of electrons

cytochrome c n, often italicized 3d c : the most abundant and stable of the cytochromes

cytochrome oxidase n : an iron-porphyrin enzyme important in cell respiration because of its ability to catalyze the oxidation of reduced cytochrome c in the presence of oxygen

cy·to·cid·al \ˌsī-tə-'sīd-ə\l adj : killing or tending to kill individual cells ⟨∼ RNA-containing viruses⟩

cy·to·di·ag·no·sis \ˌsī-tō-ˌdī-ig-'nō-səs, -əg-\ n, pl **-no·ses** \-ˌsēz\ : diagnosis based upon the examination of cells found in the tissues or fluids of the body — **cy·to·di·ag·nos·tic** \-'näs-tik\ adj

cy·to·dif·fer·en·ti·a·tion \ˌsī-tō-ˌdi-fə-ˌren-chē-'ā-shən\ n : the development of specialized cells (as muscle, blood, or nerve cells) from undifferentiated precursors

cy·to·ge·net·ics \-jə-'ne-tiks\ n sing or pl : a branch of biology that deals with the study of heredity and variation by the methods of both cytology and genetics — **cy·to·ge·net·ic** \-'ne-tik\ or **cy·to·ge·net·i·cal** \-ti-kəl\ adj — **cy·to·ge·net·i·cal·ly** \-ti-k(ə-)lē\ adv — **cy·to·ge·net·i·cist** \-'ne-tə-sist\ n

cy·toid body \'sī-ˌtóid-\ n : one of the white globular masses resembling cells that are found in the retina in some abnormal conditions

cy·to·kine \'sī-tə-ˌkīn\ n : any of a class of immunoregulatory substances (as lymphokines) that are secreted by cells of the immune system

cy·to·ki·ne·sis \ˌsī-tō-kə-'nē-səs, -kī-\ n, pl **-ne·ses** \-ˌsēz\ **1** : the cytoplasmic changes accompanying mitosis **2** : cleavage of the cytoplasm into daughter cells following nuclear division — compare KARYOKINESIS — **cy·to·ki·net·ic** \-'ne-tik\ adj

cytol abbr cytological; cytology

cy·tol·o·gy \sī-'tä-lə-jē\ n, pl **-gies 1** : a branch of biology dealing with the structure, function, multiplication, pathology, and life history of cells **2** : the cytological aspects of a process or structure — **cy·to·log·i·cal** \ˌsit-ə-'lä-ji-kəl\ or **cy·to·log·ic** \-'lä-jik\ adj — **cy·to·log·i·cal·ly** \-'lä-ji-k(ə-)lē\ adv — **cy·tol·o·gist** \sī-'tä-lə-jist\ n

cy·to·ly·sin \ˌsī-tə-'līs-ᵊn\ n : a substance (as an antibody that lyses bacteria) producing cytolysis

cy·tol·y·sis \sī-'tä-lə-səs\ n, pl **-y·ses** \-ˌsēz\ : the usu. pathologic dissolution or disintegration of cells — **cy·to·lyt·ic** \ˌsīt-ə-'li-tik\ adj

cytomegalic inclusion disease n : a severe disease esp. of newborns that is caused by a cytomegalovirus and usu. affects the salivary glands, brain, kidneys, liver, and lungs — called also inclusion disease

cy·to·meg·a·lo·vi·rus \ˌsī-tə-ˌme-gə-lō-'vī-rəs\ n : any of several herpesviruses that cause cellular enlargement and formation of eosinophilic inclusion bodies esp. in the nucleus and include some acting as opportunistic infectious agents in immunosuppressed conditions (as AIDS)

cy·tom·e·ter \sī-'tä-mə-tər\ n : an apparatus for counting and measuring cells

cy·tom·e·try \sī-'tä-mə-trē\ n, pl **-tries** : a technical specialty concerned with the counting of cells and esp. blood cells — **cy·to·met·ric** \ˌsī-tə-'me-trik\ adj

cy·to·mor·phol·o·gy \ˌsī-tə-mór-'fä-lə-jē\ n, pl **-gies** : the morphology of cells — **cy·to·mor·pho·log·i·cal** \-ˌmór-fə-'lä-ji-kəl\ adj

cy·to·path·ic \ˌsī-tə-'pa-thik\ adj : of, relating to, characterized by, or producing pathological changes in cells

cy·to·patho·gen·ic \-ˌpa-thə-'je-nik\ adj : pathologic for or destructive to cells — **cy·to·patho·ge·nic·i·ty** \-jə-'ni-sə-tē\ n

cy·to·pa·thol·o·gy \-pə-'thä-lə-jē, -pa-\ n, pl **-gies** : a branch of pathology that deals with manifestations of disease at the cellular level — **cy·to·patho·log·ic** \-ˌpa-thə-'lä-jik\ also **cy·to·patho·log·i·cal** \-ji-kəl\ adj — **cy·to·pa·thol·o·gist** \-pə-'thä-lə-jist, -pa-\ n

cy·to·pe·nia \-'pē-nē-ə\ n : a deficiency of cellular elements of the blood; esp : deficiency of a specific element (as granulocytes in granulocytopenia) — **cy·to·pe·nic** \-'pē-nik\ adj

cy·to·phil·ic \ˌsī-tə-'fi-lik\ adj : having an affinity for cells

cy·to·pho·tom·e·ter \ˌsī-tō-fō-'tä-mə-tər\ n : a photometer for use in cytophotometry

cy·to·pho·tom·e·try \-(ˌ)fō-'tä-mə-trē\ n, pl **-tries** : photometry applied to the study of the cell or its constituents — **cy·to·pho·to·met·ric** \-₁fō-tə-¹me-trik\ *adj* — **cy·to·pho·to·met·ri·cal·ly** \-tri-k(ə-)lē\ *adv*

cy·to·phys·i·ol·o·gy \-₁fi-zē-¹ä-lə-jē\ *n, pl* **-gies** : the physiology of cells — **cy·to·phys·i·o·log·i·cal** \-zē-ə-¹lä-ji-kəl\ *adj*

cy·to·pi·pette \₁sī-tō-pī-¹pet\ *n* : a pipette with a bulb that contains a fluid which is released into the vagina and then sucked back with a sample of cells for a vaginal smear

cy·to·plasm \¹sī-tə-₁pla-zəm\ *n* : the organized complex of inorganic and organic substances external to the nuclear membrane of a cell and including the cytosol and membrane-bound organelles (as mitochondria) — **cy·to·plas·mic** \₁sī-tə-¹plaz-mik\ *adj* — **cy·to·plas·mi·cal·ly** \-mi-k(ə-)lē\ *adv*

cy·to·sine \¹sī-tə-₁sēn\ *n* : a pyrimidine base $C_4H_5N_3O$ that codes genetic information in the polynucleotide chain of DNA or RNA — compare ADENINE, GUANINE, THYMINE, URACIL

cytosine arabinoside *n* : a cytotoxic antineoplastic agent $C_9H_{13}N_3O_5$ that is a synthetic isomer of the naturally occurring nucleoside of cytosine and arabinose and is used esp. in the treatment of acute myelogenous leukemia in adults

cy·to·skel·e·ton \₁sī-tō-¹ske-lət-ᵊn\ *n* : the network of protein filaments and microtubules in the cytoplasm that controls cell shape, maintains intracellular organization, and is involved

in cell movement — **cy·to·skel·e·tal** \-ᵊl\ *adj*

cy·to·sol \¹sī-tə-₁säl, -₁sȯl\ *n* : the fluid portion of the cytoplasm exclusive of organelles and membranes — called also *hyaloplasm, ground substance* — **cy·to·sol·ic** \₁sī-tə-¹sä-lik, -¹sȯ-\ *adj*

¹cy·to·stat·ic \₁sī-tə-¹sta-tik\ *adj* : tending to retard cellular activity and multiplication (~ treatment of tumors) — **cy·to·stat·i·cal·ly** \-ti-k(ə-)lē\ *adv*

²cytostatic *n* : a cytostatic agent

cy·to·tech·ni·cian \₁sī-tō-(₁)tek-¹ni-shən\ *n* : CYTOTECHNOLOGIST

cy·to·tech·nol·o·gist \-¹nä-lə-jist\ *n* : a medical technician trained in cytotechnology

cy·to·tech·nol·o·gy \-¹nä-lə-jē\ *n, pl* **-gies** : a specialty in medical technology concerned with the identification of cells and cellular abnormalities (as in cancer)

cy·to·tox·ic \₁sī-tə-¹täk-sik\ *adj* : toxic to cells (~ lymphocytes) (~ drugs) — **cy·to·tox·ic·i·ty** \-(₁)täk-¹si-sə-tē\ *n*

cy·to·tox·in \-¹täk-sən\ *n* : a substance (as a toxin or antibody) having a toxic effect on cells

cy·to·tro·pho·blast \₁sī-tə-¹trō-fə-₁blast\ *n* : the inner cellular layer of the trophoblast of an embryonic placenta forming mammal that gives rise to the plasmodial syncytiotrophoblast covering the placental villi — **cy·to·tro·pho·blas·tic** \-₁trō-fə-¹blas-tik\ *adj*

Cy·tox·an \sī-¹täk-sən\ *trademark* — used for a preparation of cyclophosphamide

D

d *abbr* 1 died 2 diopter 3 disease

d- \₁dē, ¹dē\ *prefix* 1 : dextrorotatory — usu. printed in italic (*d*-tartaric acid) 2 : having a similar configuration at a selected carbon atom to the configuration of dextrorotatory glyceraldehyde — usu. printed as a small capital (D-fructose)

2,4-D — see entry alphabetized as TWO,FOUR-D in the letter *t*

da·car·ba·zine \də-¹kär-bə-₁zēn\ *n* : an antineoplastic agent $C_6H_{10}N_6O$ used to treat esp. metastatic malignant melanoma, tumors of adult soft tissue, and Hodgkin's disease

dacry- *or* **dacryo-** *comb form* : lacrimal (*dacryocystitis*)

dac·ryo·ad·e·nec·to·my \₁da-krē-(₁)ō-₁ad-ᵊn-¹ek-tə-mē\ *n, pl* **-mies** : excision of a lacrimal gland

dac·ryo·cyst \¹da-krē-ə-₁sist\ *n* : LACRIMAL SAC

dac·ryo·cys·tec·to·my \₁da-krē-(₁)ō-sis-¹tek-tə-mē\ *n, pl* **-mies** : excision of a lacrimal sac

dac·ryo·cys·ti·tis \-sis-¹tī-təs\ *n* : inflammation of the lacrimal sac

dac·ryo·cys·tog·ra·phy \-sis-¹tä-grə-fē\

n, pl **-phies** : radiographic visualization of the lacrimal sacs and associated structures after injection of a contrast medium

dac·ryo·cys·to·rhi·nos·to·my \-₁sis-tə-₁rī-¹näs-tə-mē\ *n, pl* **-mies** : surgical creation of a passage for drainage between the lacrimal sac and the nasal cavity

dac·ryo·cys·tos·to·my \-sis-¹täs-tə-mē\ *n, pl* **-mies** : an operation on a lacrimal sac to form a new opening (as for drainage)

dac·ryo·cys·tot·o·my \-sis-¹tä-tə-mē\ *n, pl* **-mies** : incision (as for drainage) of a lacrimal sac

dac·ryo·lith \¹da-krē-ə-₁lith\ *n* : a concretion formed in a lacrimal passage

dac·ryo·ste·no·sis \₁da-krē-(₁)ō-sti-¹nō-səs\ *n, pl* **-o·ses** \-₁sēz\ : a narrowing of the lacrimal duct

dac·ti·no·my·cin \₁dak-tə-nō-¹mīs-ᵊn\ *n* : a toxic antineoplastic drug $C_{62}H_{86}N_{12}O_{16}$ of the actinomycin group — called also *actinomycin D*

dactyl- *or* **dactylo-** *comb form* : finger : toe : digit (*dactylology*)

-dactylia *n comb form* : -DACTYLY ⟨a*dactylia*⟩

-dactylism *n comb form* : -DACTYLY ⟨oligo*dactylism*⟩

dac·ty·lol·o·gy \ˌdak-tə-ˈlä-lə-jē\ *n, pl* **-gies** : the art of communicating ideas by signs made with the fingers

-dactylous *adj comb form* : having (such or so many) fingers or toes ⟨brachy*dactylous*⟩

-dactyly *n comb form* : condition of having (such or so many) fingers or toes ⟨poly*dactyly*⟩ ⟨syn*dactyly*⟩

dag·ga \ˈda-gə, ˈdä-\ *n, chiefly SoAfr* : MARIJUANA

DAH *abbr* disordered action of the heart

Dal·mane \ˈdal-ˌmān\ *trademark* — used for a preparation of flurazepam hydrochloride

Dal·ton·ism \ˈdȯlt-ᵊn-ˌi-zəm\ *n* : red-green blindness occurring as a recessive sex-linked genetic trait; *broadly* : any form of color blindness

Dalton, John (1766–1844), British chemist and physicist.

¹**dam** \ˈdam\ *n* : a female parent — used esp. of a domestic animal

²**dam** *n* : RUBBER DAM — see DENTAL DAM

³**dam** *abbr* dekameter

damp \ˈdamp\ *n* : a noxious or stifling gas or vapor; *esp* : one occuring in coal mines — usu. used in pl.; see BLACK DAMP, FIREDAMP

da·na·zol \ˈdä-nə-ˌzȯl, ˈda-, -ˌzōl\ *n* : a synthetic androgenic derivative $C_{22}H_{27}NO_2$ of ethisterone that suppresses hormone secretion by the adenohypophysis and is used esp. in the treatment of endometriosis

D&C *abbr* dilation and curettage

D&E *abbr* dilation and evacuation

dan·der \ˈdan-dər\ *n* : DANDRUFF; *specif* : minute scales from hair, feathers, or skin that may act as allergens

dan·druff \ˈdan-drəf\ *n* : a scurf that forms on the skin esp. of the scalp and comes off in small white or grayish scales — **dan·druffy** \-drə-fē\ *adj*

dan·dy fever \ˈdan-dē-\ *n* : DENGUE

Dane particle \ˈdān-\ *n* : a spherical particle found in the serum in hepatitis B that is the virion of the causative virus

Dane, David Maurice Surrey (*b* **1923),** British pathologist.

Da·nysz phenomenon \ˈdä-nish-\ *n* : the exhibition of residual toxicity by a mixture of toxin and antitoxin in which the toxin has been added in several increments to an amount of antitoxin sufficient to completely neutralize it if it had been added as a single increment — called also *Danysz effect*

Danysz, Jean (1860–1928), Polish-French pathologist.

dap·pen dish \ˈda-pən-\ *n* : a small heavy 10-sided piece of glass each

end of which is ground into a small cup for mixing dental medicaments or fillings — called also *dappen glass*

dap·sone \ˈdap-ˌsōn, -ˌzōn\ *n* : an antimicrobial agent $C_{12}H_{12}N_2O_2S$ used esp. against leprosy and sometimes against malaria — called also *diaminodiphenyl sulfone*

Da·ri·er's disease \dar-ˈyāz-\ *n* : a genetically determined skin condition characterized by patches of keratotic papules — called also *keratosis follicularis*

Darier, Ferdinand-Jean (1856–1938), French dermatologist.

dark adaptation *n* : the phenomena including dilation of the pupil, increase in retinal sensitivity, shift of the region of maximum luminosity toward the blue, and regeneration of rhodopsin by which the eye adapts to conditions of reduced illumination — compare LIGHT ADAPTATION — **dark–adapted** *adj*

dark field *n* : the dark area that serves as the background for objects viewed in an ultramicroscope — **dark–field** *adj*

dark–field microscope *n* : ULTRAMICROSCOPE — **dark–field microscopy** *n*

dar·tos \ˈdär-ˌtäs, -təs\ *n* : a thin layer of vascular contractile tissue that contains smooth muscle fibers but no fat and is situated beneath the skin of the scrotum or beneath that of the labia majora

Dar·von \ˈdär-ˌvän\ *trademark* — used for a preparation of the hydrochloride of propoxyphene

Dar·win·ism \ˈdär-wə-ˌni-zəm\ *n* : a theory of the origin and perpetuation of new species of animals and plants that offspring of a given organism vary, that natural selection favors the survival of some of these variations over others, that new these species have arisen and may continue to arise by these processes, and that widely divergent groups of plants and animals have arisen from the same ancestors; *broadly* : a theory of biological evolution — **Dar·win·ist** \-nist\ *n or adj*

Dar·win \ˈdär-wən\, **Charles Robert (1809–1882),** British naturalist.

Darwin's tubercle *n* : the slight projection occas. present on the edge of the external human ear and assumed by some scientists to represent the pointed part of the ear of quadrupeds — called also *auricular tubercle of Darwin*

da·ta \ˈdä-tə, ˈda-, ˈdä-\ *n sing or pl* : factual information (as measurements or statistics) used as a basis for reasoning, discussion, or calculation ⟨comprehensive ~ on the incidence of sexually transmitted diseases⟩

da·tu·ra \də-ˈtur-ə, -ˈtyur-\ *n* **1** *cap* : a genus of widely distributed strong-scented herbs, shrubs, or trees (family Solanaceae) related to the potato and tomato and including some used as sources of medicinal alkaloids (as stramonium from jimsonweed) or in folk rites or illicitly for their poisonous, narcotic, or hallucinogenic properties **2** : any plant or flower of the genus *Datura*

dau *abbr* daughter

¹daugh·ter \'do-tər\ *n* **1 a** : a human female having the relation of child to a parent **b** : a female offspring of an animal **2** : an atomic species that is the immediate product of the radioactive decay of a given element (radon, the ∼ of radium)

²daughter *adj* **1** : having the characteristics or relationship of a daughter **2** : belonging to the first generation of offspring, organelles, or molecules produced by reproduction, division, or replication (∼ cell) (∼ chromosomes) (∼ DNA molecules)

dau·no·my·cin \ˌdȯ-nə-ˈmīs-ᵊn, ˌdaù-\ *n* : DAUNORUBICIN

dau·no·ru·bi·cin \-ˈrü-bə-sən\ *n* : an antibiotic nitrogenous glycoside used in the form of its hydrochloride $C_{27}H_{29}NO_{10}$·HCl esp. in the treatment of some leukemias

day·dream \'dā-ˌdrēm\ *n* : a visionary creation of the imagination experienced while awake; *esp* : a gratifying reverie usu. of wish fulfillment — **daydream** *vb* — **day·dream·er** *n*

day·mare \'dā-ˌmar\ *n* : a nightmarish fantasy experienced while awake

day nursery *n* : a public center for the care and training of young children

DBCP \ˌdē-(ˌ)bē-(ˌ)sē-ˈpē\ *n* : an agricultural pesticide $C_3H_5Br_2Cl$ that is a suspected carcinogen and cause of sterility in human males

DBP *abbr* diastolic blood pressure

DC *abbr* doctor of chiropractic

DD *abbr* developmentally disabled

DDC *or* **ddC** \ˌdē-(ˌ)dē-ˈsē\ *n* : an antiviral drug $C_{10}H_{13}N_3O_3$ used to reduce virus growth and reproduction in AIDS and HIV infection — called also *dideoxycytidine, zalcitabine*

DDD \-ˈdē\ *n* : an insecticide $C_{14}H_{10}Cl_4$ closely related chemically and similar in properties to DDT

DDE \-ˈē\ *n* : a persistent organochlorine $C_{15}H_8Cl_4$ that is produced by the metabolic breakdown of DDT

DDI *or* **ddI** \-ˈī\ *n* : an antiviral drug $C_{10}H_{12}N_4O_3$ used to reduce virus growth and reproduction in AIDS and HIV infection — called also *didanosine, dideoxyinosine*; see VIDEX

DDS *abbr* doctor of dental surgery

DDT \ˌdēd-(ˌ)ē-ˈtē\ *n* : a colorless odorless water-insoluble crystalline insecticide $C_{14}H_9Cl_5$ that tends to accumulate in ecosystems and has toxic effects on many vertebrates

DDVP \ˌdē-(ˌ)dē-(ˌ)vē-ˈpē\ *n* : DICHLORVOS

¹dead \'ded\ *adj* **1** : deprived of life

: having died **2** : lacking power to move, feel, or respond : NUMB

²dead *n, pl* **dead** : one that is dead — usu. used collectively

dead·ly \'ded-lē\ *adj* **dead·li·er; -est** : likely to cause or capable of causing death (a ∼ disease) (a ∼ poison) — **dead·li·ness** \-nəs\ *n*

deadly nightshade *n* : BELLADONNA 1

dead space *n* **1** : space in the respiratory system in which air does not undergo significant gaseous exchange — see ANATOMICAL DEAD SPACE, PHYSIOLOGICAL DEAD SPACE **2** : a space (as that in the chest following excision of a lung) left in the body as the result of a surgical procedure

deaf \'def\ *adj* : lacking or deficient in the sense of hearing — **deaf·ness** *n*

deaf–aid \'def-ˌād\ *n, chiefly Brit* : HEARING AID

deaf·en \'de-fən\ *vb* **deaf·ened; deaf·en·ing 1** : to make deaf **2** : to cause deafness or stun one with noise — **deaf·en·ing·ly** \-f(ə-)niŋ-lē\ *adv*

de·af·fer·en·ta·tion \ˌdē-ˌa-fə-ˌren-ˈtā-shən\ *n* : the freeing of a motor nerve from sensory components by severing the dorsal root central to the dorsal ganglion

¹deaf–mute \'def-ˈmyüt\ *adj* : lacking the sense of hearing and the ability to speak — **deaf–mute·ness** *n* — **deaf–mut·ism** \-ˈmyü-ˌti-zəm\ *n*

²deaf–mute *n* : a person who is deaf-mute

de·am·i·nase \(ˌ)dē-ˈa-mə-ˌnās, -ˌnāz\ *also* **des·am·i·nase** \(ˌ)des-\ *n* : an enzyme that hydrolyzes amino compounds (as amino acids) with removal of the amino group

de·am·i·nate \-ˌnāt\ *vb* **-nat·ed; -nat·ing** : to remove the amino group from (a compound) — **de·am·i·na·tion** \(ˌ)dē-ˌa-mə-ˈnā-shən\ *n*

death \'deth\ *n* **1** : the irreversible cessation of all vital functions esp. as indicated by permanent stoppage of the heart, respiration, and brain activity : the end of life — see BRAIN DEATH **2** : the cause or occasion of loss of life (drinking was the ∼ of him) **3** : the state of being dead (in ∼ as in life)

death·bed \'deth-ˌbed\ *n* **1** : the bed in which a person dies **2** : the last hours of life — **on one's deathbed** : near the point of death

death cap *n* : a very poisonous mushroom of the genus *Amanita* (*A. phalloides*) of deciduous woods of No. America and Europe that varies in color from pure white to olive or yellow and has a prominent cup at the base of the stem — called also *death cup*; see THIOCTIC ACID

death instinct *n* : an innate and unconscious tendency toward self-destruction postulated in psychoanalytic theory to explain aggressive and destructure behavior not satisfactorily explained by the pleasure principle — called also *Thanatos*; compare EROS

death rate *n* : the ratio of deaths to number of individuals in a population usu. expressed as number of deaths per hundred or per thousand population for a given time

death rattle *n* : a rattling or gurgling sound produced by air passing through mucus in the lungs and air passages of a dying person

death wish *n* : the conscious or unconscious desire for the death of another or of oneself

de·bil·i·tate \di-ˈbi-lə-ˌtāt\ *vb* **-tat·ed;** **-tat·ing** : to impair the strength of (a body *debilitated* by disease) — **de·bil·i·ta·tion** \-ˌbi-lə-ˈtā-shən\ *n*

de·bil·i·ty \di-ˈbi-lə-tē\ *n, pl* **-ties** : the quality or state of being weak, feeble, or infirm; *esp* : physical weakness

de·bride·ment \di-ˈbrēd-mənt, dā-, -ˌmänt, -ˌmäⁿ\ *n* : the surgical removal of lacerated, devitalized, or contaminated tissue — **de·bride** \də-ˈbrēd, dā-\ *vb*

de·bris \də-ˈbrē, dā-ˈ, ˈdā-ˌ\ *n, pl* **debris** : organic waste from dead or damaged tissue

de·bris·o·quin \də-ˈbri-sō-ˌkwin\ *or* **de·bris·o·quine** \-ˌkwīn\ *n* : an antihypertensive drug $C_{10}H_{13}N_3$ used esp. in the form of the sulfate

dec *abbr* deceased

Dec·a·dron \ˈde-kə-ˌdrän\ *trademark* — used for a preparation of dexamethasone

de·cal·ci·fi·ca·tion \(ˌ)dē-ˌkal-sə-fə-ˈkā-shən\ *n* : the removal or loss of calcium or calcium compounds (as from bones) — **de·cal·ci·fy** \-ˈkal-sə-ˌfī\ *vb*

deca·me·tho·ni·um \ˌde-kə-mə-ˈthō-nē-əm\ *n* : a synthetic ion used in the form of either its bromide or iodide salts ($C_{16}H_{38}Br_2N_2$ *or* $C_{16}H_{38}I_2N_2$) as a skeletal muscle relaxant; *also* : either of these salts

¹**de·cap·i·tate** \di-ˈka-pə-ˌtāt\ *vb* **-tat·ed;** **-tat·ing** : to cut off the head of — **de·cap·i·ta·tion** \-ˌka-pə-ˈtā-shən\ *n*

²**de·cap·i·tate** \-ˌtāt, -tət\ *adj* : relating to or being a decapitated experimental animal

de·cap·su·late \(ˌ)dē-ˈkap-sə-ˌlāt\ *vb* **-lat·ed; -lat·ing** : to remove the capsule from (∼ a kidney) — **de·cap·su·la·tion** \-ˌkap-sə-ˈlā-shən\ *n*

de·car·box·yl·ase \ˌdē-kär-ˈbäk-sə-ˌlās, -ˌlāz\ *n* : any of a group of enzymes that accelerate decarboxylation esp. of amino acids

de·car·box·yl·ate \-sə-ˌlāt\ *vb* **-lat·ed; -lat·ing** : to remove carboxyl from — **de·car·box·yl·ation** \-ˌbäk-sə-ˈlā-shən\ *n*

de·cay \di-ˈkā\ *n* **1 a** : ROT 1; *specif* : aerobic decomposition of proteins chiefly by bacteria **b** : the product of decay **2 a** : spontaneous decrease in the number of radioactive atoms in radioactive material **b** : spontaneous disintegration (as of an atom or a nuclear particle) — **decay** *vb*

decay constant *n* : the constant ratio of the number of radioactive atoms disintegrating in any specified short unit interval of time to the total number of atoms of the same kind still intact at the beginning of that interval

de·cer·e·brate \(ˌ)dē-ˈser-ə-brət, -ˌbrāt; -dē-sə-ˈrē-brət\ *also* **de·cer·e·brat·ed** \-ˈser-ə-ˌbrā-təd\ *adj* : having the cerebrum removed or made inactive; *also* : characteristic of the resulting condition (∼ rigidity) — **de·cer·e·bra·tion** \-ˌser-ə-ˈbrā-shən\ *n*

deci·bel \ˈde-sə-ˌbel, -bəl\ *n* : a unit for expressing the relative intensity of sounds on a scale from zero for the average least perceptible sound to about 130 for the average pain level

de·cid·ua \di-ˈsi-jə-wə\ *n, pl* **-uae** \-ˌwē\ **1** : the part of the mucous membrane lining the uterus that in higher placental mammals undergoes special modifications in preparation for and during pregnancy and is cast off at parturition, being made up in the human of a part lining the uterus, a part enveloping the embryo, and a part participating with the chorion in the formation of the placenta — see DECIDUA BASALIS, DECIDUA CAPSULARIS, DECIDUA PARIETALIS **2** : the mucous membrane of the uterus cast off in the ordinary process of menstruation — **de·cid·u·al** \-wəl\ *adj*

decidua ba·sa·lis \-bə-ˈsā-ləs\ *n* : the part of the endometrium in the pregnant human female that participates with the chorion in the formation of the placenta

decidua cap·su·lar·is \-ˌkap-sə-ˈlar-əs\ *n* : the part of the decidua in the pregnant human female that envelops the embryo

decidua pa·ri·etal·is \-ˌpa-rī-ə-ˈta-ləs\ *n* : the part of the decidua in the pregnant human female lining the uterus

decidua pla·cen·tal·is \-ˌplā-sən-ˈta-ləs, -sen-\ *n* : DECIDUA BASALIS

de·cid·u·ate \di-ˈsi-jə-wət\ *adj* : having the fetal and maternal tissues firmly interlocked so that a layer of maternal tissue is torn away at parturition and forms a part of the afterbirth

decidua ve·ra \-ˈvir-ə, -ˈver-\ *n* : DECIDUA PARIETALIS

de·cid·u·oma \di-ˌsi-jə-ˈwō-mə\ *n, pl* **-mas** *or* **-ma·ta** \-mə-tə\ **1** : a mass of tissue formed in the uterus following pregnancy that contains remnants of chorionic or decidual tissue **2** : decidual tissue induced in the uterus (as by trauma) in the absence of pregnancy

de·cid·u·ous \di-ˈsi-jə-wəs\ *adj* **1** : falling off or shed at a certain stage in the life cycle (a ∼ dentition) **2** : having deciduous parts

deciduous tooth *n* : MILK TOOTH

deci·gram \ˈde-sə-ˌgram\ *n* : a metric

unit of mass and weight equal to ¹/₁₀ gram

deci·li·ter \'de-sə-ˌlē-tər\ n : a metric unit of capacity equal to ¹/₁₀ liter

deci·me·ter \'de-sə-ˌmē-tər\ n : a metric unit of length equal to ¹/₁₀ meter

de·cline \di-'klīn, 'de-ˌklīn\ n **1** : a gradual physical or mental sinking and wasting away **2** : the period during which the end of life is approaching **3** : a wasting disease; esp : pulmonary tuberculosis — **de·cline** \di-'klīn\ vb

de·clive \di-'klīv\ n : a part of the monticulus of the cerebellum that is dorsal to the culmen

de·clot \(ˌ)dē-'klät\ vb **de·clot·ted; de·clot·ting** : to remove blood clots from

de·coc·tion \di-'käk-shən\ n **1** : the act or process of boiling usu. in water so as to extract the flavor or active principle — compare INFUSION 2a **2** : an extract or liquid preparation obtained by decoction esp. of a medicinal plant — **de·coct** \-'käkt\ vb

de·col·or·ize \(ˌ)dē-'kə-lə-ˌrīz\ vb **-or·ized; -or·iz·ing** : to remove color from — **de·col·or·iza·tion** \-ˌkə-lə-rə-'zā-shən\ n

de·com·pen·sa·tion \(ˌ)dē-ˌkäm-pən-'sā-shən, -pen-\ n : loss of physiological compensation or psychological balance; esp : inability of the heart to maintain adequate circulation — **de·com·pen·sate** \-'käm-pə-ˌsāt, -ˌpen-\ vb — **de·com·pen·sa·to·ry** \-de-kəm-'pen-sə-ˌtōr-ē\ adj

de·com·pose \ˌdē-kəm-'pōz\ vb **-posed; -pos·ing 1** : to separate into constituent parts or elements or into simpler compounds **2** : to undergo chemical breakdown : DECAY, ROT — **de·com·pos·able** \-'pō-zə-bəl\ adj — **de·com·po·si·tion** \(ˌ)dē-ˌkäm-pə-'zi-shən\ n

de·com·pres·sion \ˌdē-kəm-'pre-shən\ n **1 a** : the decrease of ambient pressure experienced in an air lock on return to atmospheric pressure after a period of breathing compressed air (as in a diving apparatus or caisson) or experienced in ascent to a great altitude without a pressure suit or pressurized cabin **b** : the decrease of water pressure experienced by a diver when ascending rapidly **2** : an operation or technique used to relieve pressure upon an organ (as in fractures of the skull or spine) or within a hollow organ (as in intestinal obstruction) — **de·com·press** \-'pres\ vb

decompression chamber n **1** : a chamber in which excessive pressure can be reduced gradually to atmospheric pressure **2** : a chamber in which an individual can be gradually subjected to decreased atmospheric pressure (as in simulating conditions at high altitudes)

decompression sickness n : a sometimes fatal disorder that is marked by neuralgic pains and paralysis, distress in

breathing, and often collapse and that is caused by the release of gas bubbles (as of nitrogen) in tissue upon too rapid decrease in air pressure after a stay in a compressed atmosphere — called also bends, caisson disease; see AEROEMBOLISM

de·com·pres·sive \ˌdē-kəm-'pre-siv\ adj : tending to relieve or reduce pressure ⟨a ∼ operation in obstruction of the large bowel⟩

de·con·di·tion \ˌdē-kən-'di-shən\ vb **1** : to cause to lose physical fitness **2** : to cause extinction of (a conditioned response)

de·con·di·tion·ing \-'di-shə-niŋ\ n : a decrease in the responsiveness of heart muscle that sometimes occurs after long periods of weightlessness and may be marked by decrease in blood volume and pooling of the blood in the legs upon return to normal conditions

¹de·con·ges·tant \ˌdē-kən-'jes-tənt\ n : an agent that relieves congestion (as of mucous membranes)

²decongestant adj : relieving or tending to relieve congestion

de·con·ges·tion \-'jes-chən\ n : the process of relieving congestion — **de·con·ges·tive** \-'jes-tiv\ adj

de·con·tam·i·nate \ˌdē-kən-'ta-mə-ˌnāt\ vb **-nat·ed; -nat·ing** : to rid of contamination (as radioactive material) — **de·con·tam·i·na·tion** \-ˌta-mə-'nā-shən\ n

¹de·cor·ti·cate \(ˌ)dē-'kòr-tə-ˌkāt\ vb **-cat·ed; -cat·ing** : to remove all or part of the cortex from (as the brain)

²de·cor·ti·cate \-ˌkāt, -kət\ adj : lacking a cortex and esp. the cerebral cortex

de·cor·ti·ca·tion \-ˌkòr-ti-'kā-shən\ n : the surgical removal of the cortex of an organ, an enveloping membrane, or a constrictive fibrinous covering ⟨the ∼ of a lung⟩

de·cu·bi·tal \di-'kyü-bət-ᵊl\ adj **1** : relating to or resulting from lying down ⟨a ∼ sore⟩ **2** : relating to or resembling a decubitus

de·cu·bi·tus \-bə-təs\ n, pl **-bi·ti** \-ˌtī, -ˌtē\ **1** : a position assumed in lying down ⟨the dorsal ∼⟩ **2 a** : ULCER **b** : BEDSORE **3** : prolonged lying down (as in bed)

decubitus ulcer n : BEDSORE

de·cus·sa·tion \ˌdē-(ˌ)kə-'sā-shən\ n **1** : the action of intersecting or crossing (as of nerve fibers) esp. in the form of an X — see DECUSSATION OF PYRAMIDS **2 a** : a band of nerve fibers that connects unlike centers on opposite sides of the nervous system **b** : a crossed tract of nerve fibers passing between centers on opposite sides of the central nervous system : COMMISSURE — **de·cus·sate** \'de-kə-ˌsāt, di-'kə-ˌsāt\ vb

decussation of pyramids n : the crossing of the fibers of the corticospinal tracts from one side of the central nervous system to the other near the junction of the medulla and the spinal cord

de·dif·fer·en·ti·a·tion \(ˌ)dē-ˌdi-fə-ˌren-chē-ˈā-shən\ *n* : reversion of specialized structures (as cells) to a more generalized or primitive condition often as a preliminary to major change — **de·dif·fer·en·ti·ate** \-ˈren-chē-ˌāt\ *vb*

deep \ˈdēp\ *adj* **1 a** : extending well inward from an outer surface (a ∼ gash) **b** (1) : not located superficially within the body or one of its parts (∼ veins) (2) : resulting from or involving stimulation of deep structures (∼ pain) (∼ reflexes) **2** : being below the level of the conscious (∼ neuroses) — **deep·ly** *adv*

deep brachial artery *n* : the largest branch of the brachial artery in the upper part of the arm

deep external pudendal artery *n* : EXTERNAL PUDENDAL ARTERY b

deep facial vein *n* : a tributary of the facial vein draining part of the pterygoid plexus and nearby structures

deep fascia *n* : a firm fascia that ensheathes and binds together muscles and other internal structures — compare SUPERFICIAL FASCIA

deep femoral artery *n* : the large deep branch of the femoral artery formed where it divides about two inches (five centimeters) below the inguinal ligament

deep inguinal ring *n* : the internal opening of the inguinal canal — called also *internal inguinal ring;* compare SUPERFICIAL INGUINAL RING, INGUINAL RING

deep palmar arch *n* : PALMAR ARCH a

deep peroneal nerve *n* : a nerve that arises as a branch of the common peroneal nerve and that innervates or gives off branches innervating the muscles of the anterior part of the leg, the extensor digitorum brevis of the foot, and the skin between the big toe and the second toe — compare SUPERFICIAL PERONEAL NERVE

deep petrosal nerve *n* : a sympathetic nerve that originates in the carotid plexus, passes through the cartilage of the Eustachian tube, joins with the greater petrosal nerve to form the Vidian nerve, and as part of this nerve is distributed to the mucous membranes of the nasal cavity and palate

deep temporal artery *n* : TEMPORAL ARTERY 1

deep temporal nerve *n* : either of two motor branches of the mandibular nerve on each side of the head that are distributed to the temporalis

deep temporal vein *n* : TEMPORAL VEIN b

deer·fly \ˈdir-ˌflī\ *n* : any of numerous small horseflies esp. of the genus *Chrysops* that include important vectors of tularemia

deer tick *n* : a tick of the genus *Ixodes* (*I. dammini*) that transmits the bacterium causing Lyme disease

def·e·cate \ˈde-fi-ˌkāt\ *vb* **-cat·ed; -cat·ing 1** : to discharge from the anus **2** : to discharge feces from the bowels — **def·e·ca·tion** \ˌde-fi-ˈkā-shən\ *n*

de·fect \ˈdē-ˌfekt, di-ˈ\ *n* : a lack or deficiency of something necessary for adequacy in form or function

¹de·fec·tive \di-ˈfek-tiv\ *adj* : falling below the norm in structure or in mental or physical function (∼ eyesight) — **de·fec·tive·ness** \-nəs\ *n*

²defective *n* : one that is subnormal physically or mentally

de·fem·i·nize \(ˌ)dē-ˈfe-mə-ˌnīz\ *vb* **-nized; -niz·ing** : to divest of feminine qualities or physical characteristics : MASCULINIZE — **de·fem·i·ni·za·tion** \-fe-mə-nə-ˈzā-shən\ *n*

de·fense \di-ˈfens\ *n* : a means or method of protecting the physical or functional integrity of body or mind (a ∼ against anxiety)

defense mechanism *n* : an often unconscious mental process (as repression, projection, or sublimation) that makes possible compromise solutions to personal problems

de·fen·sive \di-ˈfen-siv, ˈdē-ˌ\ *adj* **1** : serving to defend or protect (as the ego) **2** : devoted to resisting or preventing aggression or attack (∼ behavior) — **de·fen·sive·ly** *adv* — **de·fen·sive·ness** *n*

deferens — see DUCTUS DEFERENS, VAS DEFERENS

deferentes — see DUCTUS DEFERENS

deferentia — see VAS DEFERENS

de·fer·ves·cence \ˌdē-(ˌ)fər-ˈves-ᵊns, ˌde-fər-\ *n* : the subsidence of a fever

de·fi·bril·la·tion \(ˌ)dē-ˌfi-brə-ˈlā-shən, -ˌfī-\ *n* : restoration of the rhythm of a fibrillating heart — **de·fi·bril·late** \(ˌ)dē-ˈfi-brə-ˌlāt, -ˈfī-\ *vb*

de·fi·bril·la·tor \-ˈfi-brə-ˌlā-tər, -ˈfī-\ *n* : an electronic device used to defibrillate a heart by applying an electric shock to it

de·fi·bri·nate \-ˈfi-brə-ˌnāt, -ˈfī-\ *vb* **-at·ed; -at·ing** : to remove fibrin from (blood) — **de·fi·bri·na·tion** \-ˌfi-brə-ˈnā-shən, -ˌfī-\ *n*

de·fi·cien·cy \di-ˈfi-shən-sē\ *n, pl* **-cies 1** : a shortage of substances (as vitamins) necessary to health **2** : DELETION

deficiency anemia *n* : NUTRITIONAL ANEMIA

deficiency disease *n* : a disease (as scurvy) caused by a lack of essential dietary elements and esp. a vitamin or mineral

¹de·fi·cient \di-ˈfi-shənt\ *adj* **1** : lacking in some necessary quality or element (a ∼ diet) **2** : not up to a normal standard or complement (∼ strength)

²deficient *n* : one that is deficient

de·fi·cit \'de-fə-sət\ n : a deficiency of a substance; *also* : a lack or impairment of a functional capacity ⟨cognitive ∼s⟩

de·fin·i·tive \di-'fi-nə-tiv\ *adj* : fully differentiated or developed ⟨a ∼ organ⟩

definitive host n : the host in which the sexual reproduction of a parasite takes place — compare INTERMEDIATE HOST 1

de·flo·ra·tion \,de-flə-'rā-shən, ,dē-\ n : rupture of the hymen — **de·flo·rate** \'de-flə-,rāt, 'dē-\ *vb*

de·flu·vi·um \dē-'flü-vē-əm\ n : the pathological loss of a part (as hair or nails)

de·fo·cus \(,)dē-'fō-kəs\ *vb* **de·fo·cused; de·fo·cus·ing** : to cause to be out of focus ⟨∼ed his eye⟩ ⟨a ∼ed image⟩

deformans — see ARTHRITIS DEFORMANS, DYSTONIA MUSCULORUM DEFORMANS, OSTEITIS DEFORMANS

de·formed \di-'formd, dē-\ *adj* : misshapen esp. in body or limbs

de·for·mi·ty \di-'for-mə-tē\ n, pl **-ties 1** : the state of being deformed **2** : a physical blemish or distortion

deg *abbr* degree

de·gen·er·a·cy \di-'je-nə-rə-sē\ n, pl **-cies 1** : sexual perversion **2** : the coding of an amino acid by more than one codon of the genetic code

¹de·gen·er·ate \-rət\ *adj* **1 a** : having declined (as in nature, character, structure, or function) from an ancestral or former state; *esp* : having deteriorated progressively (as in the process of evolution) esp. through loss of structure and function **b** : having sunk to a lower and usu. corrupt and vicious state **2** : having more than one codon representing an amino acid; *also* : being such a codon

²degenerate n : one that is degenerate

de·gen·er·a·tion \di-,je-nə-'rā-shən, ,dē-\ n **1** : progressive deterioration of physical characters from a level representing the norm of earlier generations or forms : regression of the morphology of a group or kind of organism toward a simpler less highly organized state ⟨parasitism leads to ∼⟩ **2** : deterioration of a tissue or an organ in which its vitality is diminished or its structure impaired; *esp* : deterioration in which specialized cells are replaced by less specialized cells (as in fibrosis or in malignancies) or in which cells are functionally impaired (as by deposition of abnormal matter in the tissue) — **de·gen·er·ate** \-'je-nə-,rāt\ *vb* — **de·gen·er·a·tive** \di-'je-nə-,rā-tiv, -rə-\ *adj*

degenerative arthritis n : OSTEOARTHRITIS

degenerative disease n : a disease (as arteriosclerosis, diabetes mellitus, or osteoarthritis) characterized by progressive degenerative changes in tissue

degenerative joint disease n : OSTEOARTHRITIS

de·germ \(,)dē-'jərm\ *vb* : to remove germs from (as the skin) — **de·germ·ation** \-,jər-'mā-shən\ n

de·glu·ti·tion \,dē-,glü-'ti-shən, ,de-\ n : the act, power, or process of swallowing

deg·ra·da·tion \,de-grə-'dā-shən\ n : change of a chemical compound to a less complex compound — **deg·ra·da·tive** \'de-grə-,dā-tiv\ *adj*

de·grade \di-'grād\ *vb* **1** : to reduce the complexity of (a chemical compound) by splitting off one or more groups or larger components : DECOMPOSE **2** : to undergo chemical degradation — **de·grad·able** \-'grā-də-bəl\ *adj*

de·gran·u·la·tion \(,)dē-,gran-yə-'lā-shən\ n : the process of losing granules ⟨∼ of leukocytes⟩ — **de·gran·u·late** \-'gran-yə-,lāt\ *vb*

de·gree \di-'grē\ n **1** : a measure of damage to tissue caused by injury or disease — see FIRST-DEGREE BURN, SECOND-DEGREE BURN, THIRD-DEGREE BURN **2** : one of the divisions or intervals marked on a scale of a measuring instrument; *specif* : any of various units for measuring temperature

de·his·cence \di-'his-əns\ n : the parting of the sutured lips of a surgical wound — **de·hisce** \-'his\ *vb*

de·hu·mid·i·fy \,dē-hyü-'mi-də-,fī, ,dē-yü-\ *vb* **-fied; -fy·ing** : to remove moisture from (as air) — **de·hu·mid·i·fi·ca·tion** \-,mi-də-fə-'kā-shən\ n — **de·hu·mid·i·fi·er** \-'mi-də-,fī-ər\ n

de·hy·drate \(,)dē-'hī-,drāt\ *vb* **-drat·ed; -drat·ing 1** : to remove bound water or hydrogen and oxygen from (a chemical compound) in the proportion in which they form water **2** : to remove water from (as foods) **3** : to lose water or body fluids — **de·hy·dra·tor** \-,drā-tər\ n

dehydrated alcohol n : ABSOLUTE ALCOHOL

de·hy·dra·tion \,dē-hī-'drā-shən\ n : the process of dehydrating; *esp* : an abnormal depletion of body fluids

de·hy·dro·as·cor·bic acid \(,)dē-,hī-drō-ə-'skor-bik-\ n : a crystalline oxidation product $C_6H_6O_6$ of vitamin C

de·hy·dro·cho·late \(,)dē-'hī-drō-'kō-,lāt\ n : a salt of dehydrocholic acid

7–de·hy·dro·cho·les·ter·ol \'se-vən-(,)dē-,hī-drō-kə-'les-tə-,rol, -,rōl\ n : a crystalline steroid alcohol $C_{27}H_{43}$-OH that occurs (as in the skin) chiefly in higher animals and humans and that yields vitamin D_3 on irradiation with ultraviolet light

de·hy·dro·cho·lic acid \(')dē-,hī-drə-'kō-lik-\ n : a colorless crystalline acid $C_{23}H_{33}O_3COOH$ used often in the form of its sodium salt esp. as a laxative and choleretic

11–de·hy·dro·cor·ti·co·ste·rone \i-'le-vən-(,)dē-,hī-drō-,kor-tə-'käs-tə-,rōn, -,kō-stə-'rōn, -kō-'stir-,ōn\ n : a steroid $C_{21}H_{28}O_4$ extracted from the adrenal cortex and also made synthetically — compare CORTISONE

de·hy·dro·epi·an·dros·ter·one \(₁)dē-₁hī-drō-₁e-pē-an-'dräs-tə-₁rōn\ n : an androgenic ketosteroid $C_{19}H_{28}O_2$ found in human urine and the adrenal cortex that is thought to be an intermediate in the biosynthesis of testosterone

de·hy·dro·ge·nase \dē-(₁)hī-'drä-jə-₁nās, -'hī-drə-jə-, -₁nāz\ n : an enzyme that accelerates the removal of hydrogen from metabolites and its transfer to other substances

de·hy·dro·ge·nate \dē-(₁)hī-'drä-jə-₁nāt, -'hī-drə-jə-\ vb **-nat·ed; -nat·ing** : to remove hydrogen from — **de·hy·dro·ge·na·tion** \-(₁)hī-drä-jə-'nā-shən, -₁hī-drə-jə-\ n

de·hy·dro·ge·nize \(₁)dē-'hī-drə-jə-₁nīz\ vb **-ized; -iz·ing** : DEHYDROGENATE

de·in·sti·tu·tion·al·iza·tion \₁dē-₁in-stə-₁tü-shə-nə-lə-'zā-shən, -₁tyü-\ n : the release of institutionalized individuals (as mental patients) from institutional care to care in the community — **de·in·sti·tu·tion·al·ize** \-'tü-shə-nə-₁līz, -'tyü-\ vb

de·ion·ize \(₁)dē-'ī-ə-₁nīz\ vb **-ized; -iz·ing** : to remove ions from (∼ water) — **de·ion·iza·tion** \-₁ī-ə-nə-'zā-shən\ n — **de·ion·iz·er** \-'ī-ə-₁nī-zər\ n

Dei·ters' nucleus \'dī-tərz-\ n : LATERAL VESTIBULAR NUCLEUS

dé·jà vu \dā-₁zhä-'vü\ n : PARAMNESIA b

delayed–stress disorder n : POST= TRAUMATIC STRESS DISORDER

delayed–stress syndrome n : POST-TRAUMATIC STRESS SYNDROME

de·lead \(₁)dē-'led\ vb : to remove lead from (∼ a chemical)

del·e·te·ri·ous \₁de-lə-'tir-ē-əs\ adj : harmful often in a subtle or an unexpected way (∼ genes)

de·le·tion \di-'lē-shən\ n 1 : the absence of a section of genetic material from a chromosome 2 : the mutational process that results in a deletion

de·lin·quen·cy \di-'liŋ-kwən-sē, -'lin-\ n, pl **-cies** : conduct that is out of accord with accepted behavior or the law; esp : JUVENILE DELINQUENCY

¹**de·lin·quent** \-kwənt\ n : a transgressor against duty or the law esp. in a degree not constituting crime; specif : one whose behavior has been labeled juvenile delinquency

²**delinquent** adj 1 : offending by neglect or violation of duty or of law 2 : of, relating to, or characteristic of delinquents : marked by delinquency — **de·lin·quent·ly** adv

de·lir·i·um \di-'lir-ē-əm\ n : a mental disturbance characterized by confusion, disordered speech, and hallucinations — **de·lir·i·ous** \-ē-əs\ adj — **de·lir·i·ous·ly** adv

delirium tre·mens \-'trē-mənz, -'tre-\ n : a violent delirium with tremors that

is induced by excessive and prolonged use of alcoholic liquors — called also d.t.'s \₁dē-'tēz\

de·liv·er \di-'li-vər\ vb **de·liv·ered; de·liv·er·ing 1 a** : to assist (a parturient female) in giving birth (she was ∼ed of a fine boy) **b** : to aid in the birth of (∼ a child with forceps) **2** : to give birth to (she ∼ed a pair of healthy twins)

de·liv·ery \di-'li-və-rē\ n, pl **-er·ies 1** : the act of giving birth : the expulsion or extraction of a fetus and its membranes : PARTURITION **2** : the procedure of delivering the fetus and placenta by manual, instrumental, or surgical means

delivery room n : a hospital room esp. equipped for the delivery of pregnant women

de·louse \(₁)dē-'laús, -'laúz\ vb **de·loused; de·lous·ing** : to remove lice from

del·phin·i·um \del-'fin-ē-əm\ n 1 cap : a large genus of the buttercup family (Ranunculaceae) comprising chiefly perennial branching herbs with divided leaves and showy flowers and including several esp. of the western U.S. that are toxic to grazing animals and esp. cattle **2** : any plant of the genus Delphinium

delt \'delt\ n : DELTOID — usu. used in pl.

¹**del·ta** \'del-tə\ n 1 : the fourth letter of the Greek alphabet — symbol Δ or δ **2** : DELTA WAVE

²**delta** or δ- adj : of or relating to one of four or more closely related chemical substances (the delta chain of hemoglobin) — used somewhat arbitrarily to specify ordinal relationship or a particular physical form

delta wave n : a high amplitude electrical rhythm of the brain with a frequency of less than 6 cycles per second that occurs esp. in deep sleep, in infancy, and in many diseased conditions of the brain — called also delta, delta rhythm

¹**del·toid** \'del-₁tóid\ n : a large triangular muscle that covers the shoulder joint, serves to raise the arm laterally, arises from the upper anterior part of the outer third of the clavicle and from the acromion and spine of the scapula, and is inserted into the outer side of the middle of the shaft of the humerus — called also deltoid muscle; see DELTOID TUBEROSITY

²**deltoid** adj : relating to, associated with, or supplying the deltoid

del·toi·de·us \del-'tói-dē-əs\ n, pl **-dei** \-dē-ē, -₁ī\ : DELTOID

deltoid ligament n : a strong radiating ligament of the inner aspect of the ankle that binds the base of the tibia to the bones of the foot

deltoid tuberosity n : a rough triangular bump on the outer side of the middle of the humerus that is the site of insertion of the deltoid

delts \'delts\ *pl of* DELT

de·lude \di-'lüd\ *vb* **de·lud·ed; de·lud·ing** : to mislead the mind or judgment of

de·lu·sion \di-'lü-zhən\ *n* **1 a** : the act of deluding : the state of being deluded **b** : an abnormal mental state characterized by the occurrence of psychotic delusions **2** : a false belief regarding the self or persons or objects outside the self that persists despite the facts and occurs in some psychotic states — **de·lu·sion·al** \-'lü-zhən-ᵊl\ *adj*

delusion of reference *n* : IDEA OF REFERENCE

de·mas·cu·lin·ize \(₁)dē-'mas-kyə-lə-₁nīz, di-\ *vb* **-ized; -iz·ing** : to remove the masculine character or qualities of — **de·mas·cu·lin·iza·tion** \-₁mas-kyə-lə-nə-'zā-shən, -₁ni-\ *n*

dem·e·car·i·um \₁de-mi-'kar-ē-əm, -'ker-\ *n* : a long-acting cholinesterase-inhibiting ammonium compound that is used as the bromide $C_{32}H_{52}Br_2N_4O_4$ in an ophthalmic solution esp. in the treatment of glaucoma and esotropia

de·ment·ed \di-'men-təd\ *adj* : MAD, INSANE — **de·ment·ed·ly** *adv* — **de·ment·ed·ness** *n*

de·men·tia \di-'men-chə\ *n* : a condition of deteriorated mentality that is characterized by marked decline from the individual's former intellectual level and often by emotional apathy — compare AMENTIA — **de·men·tial** \-chəl\ *adj*

dementia par·a·lyt·i·ca \-₁par-ə-'li-ti-kə\ *n, pl* **de·men·ti·ae par·a·lyt·i·cae** \di-'men-chē-₁ē-₁par-ə-'li-ti-₁sē\ : GENERAL PARESIS

dementia prae·cox \-'prē-₁käks\ *n* : SCHIZOPHRENIA

de·ment·ing \di-'men-tiŋ\ *adj* : causing or characterized by dementia ⟨a ~ illness⟩

Dem·er·ol \'de-mə-₁rȯl, -₁rōl\ *trademark* — used for meperidine

demi·lune \'de-mē-₁lün\ *n* : one of the small crescentic groups of granular deeply staining zymogen-secreting cells lying between the clearer mucus-producing cells and the basement membrane in the alveoli of mixed salivary glands — called also *crescent of Giannuzzi*

demilune of Gian·nuz·zi *also* **demilune of Gia·nuz·zi** \-jä-'nüt-sē\ *n* : DEMILUNE

Giannuzzi, Giuseppe (1839–1876), Italian anatomist.

de·min·er·al·iza·tion \(₁)dē-₁mi-nə-rə-lə-'zā-shən\ *n* **1** : loss of minerals (as salts of calcium) from the body esp. in disease **2** : the process of removing mineral matter or salts (as from water) — **de·min·er·al·ize** \-'mi-nə-rə-₁līz\ *vb*

dem·o·dec·tic mange \₁de-mə-'dek-tik-\

n : mange caused by mites of the genus *Demodex* that burrow in the hair follicles esp. of dogs — compare CHORIOPTIC MANGE, SARCOPTIC MANGE

de·mo·dex \'de-mə-₁deks, 'dē-\ *n* **1** *cap* : a genus (family Demodicidae) of minute mites that live in the hair follicles esp. about the face of humans and various furred mammals and in the latter often cause demodectic mange **2** : any mite of the genus *Demodex* : FOLLICLE MITE

de·mog·ra·phy \di-'mä-grə-fē\ *n, pl* **-phies** : the statistical study of human populations esp. with reference to size and density, distribution, and vital statistics — **de·mog·ra·pher** \-fər\ *n* — **de·mo·graph·ic** \₁de-mə-'gra-fik, ₁dē-\ *adj* — **de·mo·graph·i·cal·ly** \-fi-k(ə-)lē\ *adv*

¹de·mul·cent \di-'məl-sᵊnt\ *adj* : tending to sooth or soften ⟨~ expectorants⟩

²demulcent *n* : a usu. mucilaginous or oily substance that can soothe or protect an abraded mucous membrane

de·my·elin·at·ing \(₁)dē-'mī-ə-lə-₁nā-tiŋ\ *adj* : causing or characterized by the loss or destruction of myelin

de·my·eli·na·tion \-₁mī-ə-lə-'nā-shən\ *n* : the state resulting from the loss or destruction of myelin; *also* : the process of such loss or destruction

de·my·elin·iza·tion \-lə-nə-'zā-shən\ *n* : DEMYELINATION

de·na·tur·ant \(₁)dē-'nā-chər-ənt\ *n* : a denaturing agent

de·na·ture \-'nā-chər\ *vb* **de·na·tured; de·na·tur·ing** : to deprive or become deprived of natural qualities: as **a** : to make (alcohol) unfit for drinking (as by adding an obnoxious substance) without impairing usefulness for other purposes **b** : to modify the molecular structure of (as a protein or DNA) esp. by heat, acid, alkali, or ultraviolet radiation so as to destroy or diminish some of the original properties and esp. the specific biological activity — **de·na·tur·ation** \-₁nā-chə-'rā-shən\ *n*

den·drite \'den-₁drīt\ *n* : any of the usu. branching protoplasmic processes that conduct impulses toward the body of a nerve cell — **den·drit·ic** \den-'dri-tik\ *adj*

den·dro·den·drit·ic \₁den-drō-₁den-'dri-tik\ *adj* : relating to or being a nerve synapse between a dendrite of one cell and a dendrite of another

de·ner·vate \'dē-(₁)nər-₁vāt\ *vb* **-vat·ed; -vat·ing** : to deprive of a nerve supply (as by cutting a nerve) — **de·ner·va·tion** \₁dē-(₁)nər-'vā-shən\ *n*

den·gue \'deŋ-gē, -₁gā\ *n* : an acute infectious disease caused by an arbovirus, transmitted by aedes mosquitoes, and characterized by headache, severe joint pain, and a rash — called also *breakbone fever, dengue fever*

de·ni·al \di-'nī-əl\ *n* : a psychological defense mechanism in which confrontation with a personal problem or with reality is avoided by denying the existence of the problem or reality

den·i·da·tion \ˌde-nə-ˈdā-shən\ n : the sloughing of the endometrium of the uterus esp. during menstruation

de·ni·trog·e·nate \(ˌ)dē-ˌnī-ˈträ-jə-ˌnāt\ vb **-nat·ed; -nat·ing** : to reduce the stored nitrogen in the body of by forced breathing of pure oxygen for a period of time esp. as a measure designed to prevent development of decompression sickness — **de·ni·trog·e·na·tion** \-ˌträ-jə-ˈnā-shən\ n

dens \ˈdenz\ n, pl **den·tes** \ˈden-ˌtēz\ : ODONTOID PROCESS

densa — see MACULA DENSA

den·si·tom·e·ter \ˌden-sə-ˈtä-mə-tər\ n : an instrument for determining optical or photographic density — **den·si·to·met·ric** \ˌden-sə-tə-ˈme-trik\ adj — **den·si·tom·e·try** \ˌden-sə-ˈtä-mə-trē\ n

den·si·ty \ˈden-sə-tē\ n, pl **-ties 1** : the quantity per unit volume, unit area, or unit length: as **a** : the mass of a substance per unit volume **b** : the distribution of a quantity (as mass, electricity, or energy) per unit usu. of space **c** : the average number of individuals or units per space unit **2** : the degree of opacity of a translucent medium

dent- or **denti-** or **dento-** comb form **1** : tooth : teeth ⟨dental⟩ **2** : dental and ⟨dentofacial⟩

den·tal \ˈdent-ᵊl\ adj **1** : relating to, specializing in, or used in dentistry **2** : relating to or used on the teeth ⟨∼ paste⟩ — **den·tal·ly** adv

dental arch n : the curve of the row of teeth in each jaw — called also arcade

dental dam n : a rubber dam used in dentistry

dental floss n : a thread used to clean between the teeth

dental formula n : an abridged expression for the number and kind of teeth of mammals in which the kind of teeth are represented by i (incisor), c (canine), pm (premolar) or b (bicuspid), and m (molar) and the number in each jaw is written like a fraction with the figures above the horizontal line showing the number in the upper jaw and those below the number in the lower jaw and with a dash separating the figures representing the teeth on each side of the jaw ⟨the dental formula of a human adult is

$$i\,\frac{2\text{-}2}{2\text{-}2},\ \ c\,\frac{1\text{-}1}{1\text{-}1},\ b\text{ or }pm\,\frac{2\text{-}2}{2\text{-}2},$$

$$m\,\frac{3\text{-}3}{3\text{-}3}\ =\ 32⟩$$

dental hygienist n : one who assists a dentist esp. in cleaning teeth

dental lamina n : a linear zone of epithelial cells of the covering of each embryonic jaw that gives rise to the enamel organs of the teeth — called also dental ridge

dental nerve n — see INFERIOR ALVEOLAR NERVE

dental papilla n : the mass of mesenchyme that gives rise to the dentin and the pulp of the tooth

dental plate n : DENTURE 2

dental pulp n : the highly vascular sensitive tissue occupying the central cavity of a tooth

dental surgeon n : DENTIST; esp : one engaging in oral surgery

dental technician n : a technician who makes dental appliances

den·tate \ˈden-ˌtāt\ adj : having teeth or pointed conical projections ⟨the ∼ border of the retina⟩

dentate gyrus n : a narrow strip of cortex associated with the hippocampal sulcus that continues forward to the uncus

dentate nucleus n : a large laminar nucleus of gray matter forming an incomplete capsule within the white matter of each cerebellar hemisphere

dentes pl of DENS

denti- — see DENT-

den·ti·cle \ˈden-ti-kəl\ n : PULP STONE

den·tic·u·late ligament \den-ˈti-kyə-lət-\ n : a band of fibrous pia mater extending along the spinal cord on each side between the dorsal and ventral roots

den·ti·frice \ˈden-tə-frəs\ n : a powder, paste, or liquid for cleaning the teeth

den·tig·er·ous cyst \den-ˈti-jə-rəs\ n : an epithelial cyst containing fluid and one or more imperfect teeth

den·tin \ˈdent-ᵊn\ or **den·tine** \ˈden-ˌtēn, den-ˈtēn\ n : a calcareous material similar to bone but harder and denser that composes the principal mass of a tooth and is formed by the odontoblasts — compare CEMENTUM, ENAMEL — **den·ti·nal** \ˈdent-ᵊn-əl; ˈden-ˌtēn-ᵊl, den-ˈ\ adj

dentinal tubule n : one of the minute parallel tubules of the dentin of a tooth that communicate with the dental pulp

den·tino·enam·el \den-ˌtē-nō-i-ˈna-məl\ n : relating to or connecting the dentin and enamel of a tooth ⟨the ∼ junction⟩

den·tino·gen·e·sis \den-ˌtē-nə-ˈje-nə-səs\ n, pl **-e·ses** \-ˌsēz\ : the formation of dentin

den·tist \ˈden-tist\ n : one who is skilled in and licensed to practice the prevention, diagnosis, and treatment of diseases, injuries, and malformations of the teeth, jaws, and mouth and who makes and inserts false teeth — **den·tist·ry** \ˈden-tə-strē\ n

den·ti·tion \den-ˈti-shən\ n **1** : the development and cutting of teeth **2** : the character of a set of teeth esp. with regard to their number, kind, and arrangement **3** : TEETH

dento- — see DENT-

den·to·al·ve·o·lar \den-tō-al-'vē-ə-lər\ *adj* : of, relating to, or involving the teeth and their sockets ⟨∼ structures⟩

den·to·fa·cial \den-tə-'fā-shəl\ *adj* : of or relating to the dentition and face

den·to·gin·gi·val \den-tō-'jin-jə-vəl\ *adj* : of, relating to, or connecting the teeth and the gums ⟨the ∼ junction⟩

den·tu·lous \'den-chə-ləs\ *adj* : having teeth

den·ture \'den-chər\ *n* **1** : a set of teeth **2** : an artificial replacement for one or more teeth; *esp* : a set of false teeth

den·tur·ist \-chə-rist\ *n* : a dental technician who makes, fits, and repairs dentures directly for the public

de·nu·da·tion \dē-nü-'dā-shən, de-, -nyü-\ *n* : the act or process of removing surface layers (as of skin) or an outer covering (as of myelin); *also* : the condition that results from this — **de·nude** \di-'nüd, -'nyüd\ *vb*

¹de·odor·ant \dē-'ō-də-rənt\ *adj* : destroying or masking offensive odors

²deodorant *n* : any of various preparations or solutions (as a soap or disinfectant) that destroy or mask unpleasant odors; *esp* : a cosmetic that neutralizes perspiration odors

de·odor·ize \dē-'ō-də-ˌrīz\ *vb* **-ized; -iz·ing** : to eliminate or prevent the offensive odor of — **de·odor·iza·tion** \-ˌō-də-rə-'zā-shən\ *n* — **de·odor·iz·er** *n*

de·oxy \dē-'äk-sē\ *also* **des·oxy** \dez-\ *adj* : containing less oxygen per molecule than the compound from which it is derived ⟨∼ sugars⟩ — usu. used in combination ⟨deoxyribonucleic acid⟩ ⟨desoxycorticosterone⟩

de·oxy·cho·late \ˌdē-ˌäk-sē-'kō-ˌlāt\ *n* : a salt or ester of deoxycholic acid

de·oxy·cho·lic acid \-'kō-lik-\ *n* : a crystalline acid $C_{24}H_{40}O_4$ found esp. in bile

de·oxy·cor·ti·co·ste·rone *var of* DESOXYCORTICOSTERONE

de·oxy·cor·tone *chiefly Brit var of* DESOXYCORTONE

de·oxy·gen·ate \ˌdē-'äk-si-jə-ˌnāt, ˌdē-äk-'si-jə-\ *vb* **-at·ed; -at·ing** : to remove oxygen from — **de·oxy·gen·ation** \-ˌäk-si-jə-'nā-shən, -ˌdē-äk-ˌsi-jə-\ *n*

de·oxy·gen·at·ed *adj* : having the hemoglobin in the reduced state

de·oxy·ri·bo·nu·cle·ase \ˌdē-ˌäk-si-ˌrī-bō-'nü-klē-ˌās, -'nyü-, -ˌāz\ *n* : an enzyme that hydrolyzes DNA to nucleotides — called also *DNase*

de·oxy·ri·bo·nu·cle·ic acid \ˌdē-ˌäk-si-ˌrī-bō-nü-'klē-ik-, -ˌnyü-, -'klā-\ *n* : DNA

de·oxy·ri·bo·nu·cle·o·tide \-'nü-klē-ə-ˌtīd, -'nyü-\ *n* : a nucleotide that contains deoxyribose and is a constituent of DNA

de·oxy·ri·bose \ˌdē-ˌäk-si-ˌrī-ˌbōs,

-ˌbōz\ *n* : a pentose sugar $C_5H_{10}O_4$ that is a structural element of DNA

de·pen·dence \di-'pen-dəns\ *n* **1** : the quality or state of being dependent upon or unduly subject to the influence of another **2 a** : drug addiction **b** : HABITUATION 2b

de·pen·den·cy \-dən-sē\ *n, pl* **-cies** : DEPENDENCE

de·pen·dent \di-'pen-dənt\ *adj* **1** : unable to exist, sustain oneself, or act appropriately or normally without the assistance or direction of another **2** : affected with a drug dependence — **de·pen·dent·ly** *adv*

de·per·son·al·iza·tion \(ˌ)dē-ˌpər-sə-nə-lə-'zā-shən\ *n* : the act or process of causing or the state resulting from loss of the sense of personal identity; *esp* : a psychopathological syndrome characterized by loss of identity and feelings of unreality or strangeness about one's own behavior — **de·per·son·al·ize** \(')dē-'pər-sə-nə-ˌlīz\ *vb*

de·phos·phor·y·la·tion \(ˌ)dē-ˌfäs-ˌfor-ə-'lā-shən\ *n* : the process of removing phosphate groups from an organic compound (as ATP) by hydrolysis; *also* : the resulting state — **de·phos·phor·y·late** \-'fäs-'for-ə-ˌlāt\ *vb*

dep·i·la·tion \ˌdep-ə-'lā-shən\ *n* : removal of hair, wool, or bristles by chemical or mechanical methods — **dep·i·late** \'de-pə-ˌlāt\ *vb*

¹de·pil·a·to·ry \di-'pi-lə-ˌtōr-ē\ *adj* : having the power to remove hair

²depilatory *n* : a cosmetic for the temporary removal of undesired hair

de·plete \di-'plēt\ *vb* **de·plet·ed; de·plet·ing** : to empty of a principal substance ⟨tissues *depleted* of vitamins⟩

de·ple·tion \di-'plē-shən\ *n* : the act or process of depleting or the state of being depleted: as **a** : the reduction or loss of blood, body fluids, chemical constituents, or stored materials from the body (as by hemorrhage or malnutrition) **b** : a debilitated state caused by excessive loss of body fluids or other constituents

de·po·lar·iza·tion \(ˌ)dē-ˌpō-lə-rə-'zā-shən\ *n* : loss of polarization; *esp* : loss of the difference in charge between the inside and outside of the plasma membrane of a muscle or nerve cell due to a change in permeability and migration of sodium ions to the interior — **de·po·lar·ize** \-'pō-lə-ˌrīz\ *vb*

Depo–Pro·ve·ra \ˌde-pō-prō-'ver-ə\ *trademark* — used for an aqueous suspension of medroxyprogesterone acetate

de·pos·it \də-'pä-zət\ *n* : something laid down; *esp* : matter deposited by a natural process — **deposit** *vb*

¹de·pot \'de-(ˌ)pō, 'dē-\ *n* : a bodily location where a substance is stored usu. for later utilization

²**depot** *adj* : being in storage ⟨~ fat⟩; *also* : acting over a prolonged period ⟨~ insulin⟩

de·press \di-ˈpres\ *vb* **1** : to diminish the activity, strength, or yield of **2** : to lower in spirit or mood

¹**de·pres·sant** \-ᵊnt\ *adj* : tending to depress; *esp* : lowering or tending to lower functional or vital activity ⟨a drug with a ~ effect on heart rate⟩

²**depressant** *n* : one that depresses; *specif* : an agent that reduces bodily functional activity or an instinctive desire (as appetite)

de·pressed \di-ˈprest\ *adj* **1** : low in spirits; *specif* : affected by psychological depression ⟨a severely ~ patient⟩ **2** : having the central part lower than the margin

depressed fracture *n* : a fracture esp. of the skull in which the fragment is depressed below the normal surface

de·pres·sion \di-ˈpre-shən\ *n* **1** : a placement downward or inward ⟨~ of the jaw⟩ **2** : an act of depressing or a state of being depressed: as **a** (1) : a state of feeling sad ⟨a psychoneurotic or psychotic disorder marked esp. by sadness, inactivity, difficulty with thinking and concentration, a significant increase or decrease in appetite and time spent sleeping, feelings of dejection and hopelessness, and sometimes suicidal thoughts or an attempt to commit suicide **b** : a reduction in functional activity, amount, quality, or force ⟨~ of autonomic function⟩

¹**de·pres·sive** \di-ˈpre-siv\ *adj* **1** : tending to depress **2** : of, relating to, marked by, or affected by psychological depression

²**depressive** *n* : one who is affected with or prone to psychological depression

de·pres·sor \di-ˈpre-sər\ *n* : one that depresses: as **a** : a muscle that draws down a part — compare LEVATOR **b** : a device for pressing a part down or aside — see TONGUE DEPRESSOR **c** : a nerve or nerve fiber that decreases the activity or the tone of the organ or part it innervates

depressor sep·ti \-ˈsep-ˌtī\ *n* : a small muscle of each side of the upper lip that is inserted into the nasal septum and wing of the nose on each side and constricts the nasal opening by drawing the wing downward

de·pri·va·tion \ˌde-prə-ˈvā-shən, ˌdē-ˌprī-\ *n* : the act or process of removing or the condition resulting from removal of something normally present and usu. essential for mental or physical well-being ⟨emotional ~ in childhood⟩ ⟨sensory ~⟩ — **de·prive** \di-ˈpriv\ *vb*

de·pro·tein·ate \(ˌ)dē-ˈprō-ˌtē-ˌnāt, -ˈprō-tē-ə-ˌnāt\ *vb* **-at·ed; -at·ing** : DE-

PROTEINIZE — **de·pro·tein·ation** \(ˌ)dē-ˌprō-ˌtē-ˈnā-shən, -ˌprō-tē-ə-\ *n*

de·pro·tein·iza·tion \(ˌ)dē-ˌprō-ˌtē-nə-ˈzā-shən, -ˌprō-tē-ə-nə-\ *n* : the process of removing protein

de·pro·tein·ize \(ˌ)dē-ˈprō-tē-ˌnīz, -ˈprō-tē-ə-ˌnīz\ *vb* **-ized; -iz·ing** : to subject to deproteinization

depth \ˈdepth\ *n, pl* **depths 1** : the distance between upper and lower or between dorsal and ventral points of a body **2** : the quality of a state of consciousness, a bodily state, or a physiological function of being intense or complete ⟨the ~ of anesthesia⟩

depth perception *n* : the ability to judge the distance of objects and the spatial relationship of objects at different distances

depth psychology *n* : PSYCHOANALYSIS; *also* : psychology concerned esp. with the unconscious mind

de·Quer·vain's disease \də-(ˌ)kər-ˈvaⁿz-\ *n* : inflammation of tendons and their sheaths at the styloid process of the radius that often causes pain in the thumb side of the wrist **Quer·vain** \ker-ˈvaⁿ\, **Fritz de** (1868–1940), Swiss physician.

de·range·ment \di-ˈrānj-mənt\ *n* **1** : a disturbance of normal bodily functioning or operation **2** : INSANITY — **de·range** \di-ˈrānj\ *vb*

de·re·al·iza·tion \(ˌ)dē-ˌrē-ə-lə-ˈzā-shən\ *n* : a feeling of altered reality that occurs often in schizophrenia and in some drug reactions

de·re·press \ˌdē-ri-ˈpres\ *vb* : to activate (a gene or enzyme) by releasing from a blocked state — **de·re·pres·sion** \-ˈpre-shən\ *n*

¹**de·riv·a·tive** \di-ˈri-və-tiv\ *adj* **1** : formed by derivation **2** : made up of or marked by derived elements

²**derivative** *n* **1** : something that is obtained from, grows out of, or results from an earlier or more fundamental state or condition **2 a** : a chemical substance related structurally to another substance and theoretically derivable from it **b** : a substance that can be made from another substance in one or more steps

de·rive \di-ˈriv\ *vb* **de·rived; de·riv·ing** : to take, receive, or obtain esp. from a specified source; *specif* : to obtain (a chemical substance) actually or theoretically from a parent substance — **der·i·va·tion** \ˌder-ə-ˈvā-shən\ *n*

derm- *or* **derma-** *or* **dermo-** *comb form* : skin ⟨*derm*al⟩ ⟨*dermo*pathy⟩

-derm \ˌdərm\ *n comb form* : skin : covering ⟨ecto*derm*⟩

-der·ma \ˈdər-mə\ *n comb form, pl* **-dermas** *or* **-der·ma·ta** \-mə-tə\ : skin or skin ailment of a (specified) type ⟨sclero*derma*⟩

derm·abra·sion \ˌdər-mə-ˈbrā-zhən\ *n* : surgical removal of skin blemishes or imperfections (as scars or tattoos) by abrasion

Der·ma·cen·tor \\ˈdər-mə-ˌsen-tər\ *n* : a large widely distributed genus of ornate ixodid ticks including several vectors of important diseases (as Rocky Mountain spotted fever)

der·mal \ˈdər-məl\ *adj* **1** : of or relating to skin and esp. to the dermis : CUTANEOUS **2** : EPIDERMAL

Der·ma·nys·sus \ˌdər-mə-ˈni-səs\ *n* : a genus (family Dermanyssidae) of blood-sucking mites that are parasitic on birds — see CHICKEN MITE

dermat- or **dermato-** *comb form* : skin 〈*dermatitis*〉 〈*dermatology*〉

der·ma·ti·tis \ˌdər-mə-ˈtī-təs\ *n*, *pl* **-ti·tis·es** or **-tit·i·des** \-ˈti-tə-ˌdēz\ : inflammation of the skin — **der·ma·tit·ic** \-ˈti-tik\ *adj*

dermatitis her·pe·ti·for·mis \-ˌhər-pə-tə-ˈfor-məs\ *n* : chronic dermatitis characterized by eruption of itching papules, vesicles, and lesions resembling hives typically in clusters

Der·ma·to·bia \ˌdər-mə-ˈtō-bē-ə\ *n* : a genus of botflies including one (*D. hominis*) whose larvae live under the skin of domestic mammals and sometimes of humans in tropical America

der·ma·to·fi·bro·ma \ˌdər-mə-tō-fī-ˈbrō-mə\ *n*, *pl* **-mas** *also* **-ma·ta** \-mə-tə\ : a benign chiefly fibroblastic nodule of the skin found esp. on the extremities of adults

der·ma·to·fi·bro·sar·co·ma \-ˌfī-brō-sär-ˈkō-mə\ *n*, *pl* **-mas** or **-ma·ta** \-mə-tə\ : a fibrosarcoma affecting the skin

dermatofibrosarcoma pro·tu·ber·ans \-prō-ˈtü-bə-ˌranz, -ˈtyü-\ *n* : a dermal fibroblastic neoplasm composed of firm nodular masses that usu. do not metastasize

der·ma·to·glyph·ics \ˌdər-mə-tə-ˈgli-fiks\ *n* **1** : skin patterns; *esp* : patterns of the specialized skin of the inferior surfaces of the hands and feet **2** : the science of the study of skin patterns — **der·ma·to·glyph·ic** \-fik\ *adj*

der·ma·to·graph·ia \-ˈgra-fē-ə\ *n* : DERMOGRAPHISM

der·ma·to·graph·ism \-ˈgra-fi-zəm\ *n* : DERMOGRAPHISM

der·ma·to·log·ic \ˌdər-mət-əl-ˈä-jik\ or **der·ma·to·log·i·cal** \-ji-kəl\ *adj* : of or relating to dermatology

der·ma·to·log·i·cal \-ji-kəl\ *n* : a medicinal agent for application to the skin

der·ma·tol·o·gy \ˌdər-mə-ˈtä-lə-jē\ *n*, *pl* **-gies** : a branch of science dealing with the skin, its structure, functions, and diseases — **der·ma·tol·o·gist** \-mə-ˈtä-lə-jist\ *n*

der·ma·tome \ˈdər-mə-ˌtōm\ *n* **1** : an instrument for cutting skin for use in grafting **2** : the lateral wall of a somite from which the dermis is produced — **der·ma·to·mal** \ˌdər-mə-ˈtō-məl\ or **der·ma·to·mic** \-mik\ *adj*

der·ma·to·my·co·sis \ˌdər-mə-tō-ˌmī-ˈkō-səs, ˌ)dər-ma-\ *n*, *pl* **-co·ses** \-ˌsēz\ : a disease (as ringworm) of the skin caused by infection with a fungus

der·ma·to·my·o·si·tis \-ˌmī-ə-ˈsī-təs\ *n*, *pl* **-si·tis·es** or **-sit·i·des** \-ˈsi-tə-ˌdēz\ : a chronic inflammation of the skin, subcutaneous tissue, and skeletal muscles of unknown cause

der·ma·to·pa·thol·o·gy \-pə-ˈthä-lə-jē, -pa-\ *n*, *pl* **-gies** : pathology of the skin — **der·ma·to·pa·thol·o·gist** \-jist\ *n*

der·ma·to·phyte \(ˌ)dər-ˈma-tə-ˌfīt, ˈdər-mə-tə-\ *n* : a fungus parasitic upon the skin or skin derivatives (as hair or nails) — compare DERMATOMYCOSIS

der·ma·to·phy·tid \(ˌ)dər-ˌma-tə-ˈfī-təd, ˌdər-mə-\ *n* : a skin eruption associated with a fungus infection; *esp* : one considered to be due to allergic reaction

der·ma·to·phy·to·sis \-ˌfī-ˈtō-səs\ *n*, *pl* **-to·ses** \-ˌsēz\ : a disease (as athlete's foot) of the skin or skin derivatives that is caused by a dermatophyte

der·ma·to·plas·ty \(ˌ)dər-ˈma-tə-ˌplas-tē, ˈdər-mə-\ *n*, *pl* **-ties** : plastic surgery of the skin

der·ma·to·sis \ˌdər-mə-ˈtō-səs\ *n*, *pl* **-to·ses** \-ˌsēz\ : a disease of the skin

-der·ma·tous \ˈdər-mə-təs\ *adj comb form* : having a (specified) type of skin 〈*sclero*dermatous〉

-der·mia \ˈdər-mē-ə\ *n comb form* : skin or skin ailment of a (specified) type 〈kerato*dermia*〉

der·mis \ˈdər-məs\ *n* : the sensitive vascular inner mesodermic layer of the skin — called also *corium*, *cutis*

-der·mis \ˈdər-məs\ *n comb form* : layer of skin or tissue 〈epi*dermis*〉

dermo- — see DERM-

der·mo·graph·ia \ˌdər-mə-ˈgra-fē-ə\ *n* : DERMOGRAPHISM

der·mog·ra·phism \(ˌ)dər-ˈmä-grə-ˌfi-zəm\ *n* : a condition in which pressure or friction on the skin gives rise to a transient raised usu. reddish mark so that a word traced on the skin becomes visible — called also *dermatographia*, *dermatographism*

der·moid \ˈdər-ˌmoid\ *also* **der·moi·dal** \(ˌ)dər-ˈmoid-əl\ *adj* **1** : made up of cutaneous elements and esp. ectodermal derivatives 〈a ~ tumor〉 **2** : resembling skin

dermoid cyst *n* : a cystic tumor often of the ovary that contains skin and skin derivatives (as hair or teeth) — called also *dermoid*

der·mo·ne·crot·ic \ˌdər-mō-ni-ˈkrä-tik\ *adj* : relating to or causing necrosis of the skin 〈a ~ toxin〉 〈~ effects〉

der·mop·a·thy \(ˌ)dər-ˈmä-pə-thē\ *n*, *pl* **-thies** : a disease of the skin

DES \ˌdē-(ˌ)ē-ˈes\ *n* : DIETHYLSTILBESTROL

des·am·i·nase \de-ˈza-mə-ˌnās, -ˌnāz\ *var of* DEAMINASE

des·ce·met·o·cele \ˌde-sə-ˈme-tə-ˌsēl\ *n* : protrusion of Descemet's membrane through the cornea

Des·ce·met's membrane \de-sə-'māz-, des-'māz-\ *n* : a transparent highly elastic apparently structureless membrane that covers the inner surface of the cornea and is lined with endothelium — called also *membrane of Descemet, posterior elastic lamina*
Des·ce·met \des-'mā\, **Jean (1732–1810),** French physician.

descending *adj* **1** : moving or directed downward **2** : being a nerve, nerve fiber, or nerve tract that carries nerve impulses in a direction away from the central nervous system : EFFERENT, MOTOR

descending aorta *n* : the part of the aorta from the arch to its bifurcation into the two common iliac arteries that passes downward in the thoracic and abdominal cavities

descending colon *n* : the part of the large intestine on the left side that extends from the bend below the spleen to the sigmoid flexure — compare ASCENDING COLON, TRANSVERSE COLON

de·scen·sus \di-'sen-səs\ *n* : the process of descending or prolapsing

de·sen·si·tize \(ˌ)dē-'sen-sə-ˌtīz\ *vb* **-tized; -tiz·ing 1** : to make (a sensitized or hypersensitive individual) insensitive or nonreactive to a sensitizing agent **2** : to extinguish an emotional response (as of fear, anxiety, or guilt) to stimuli which formerly induced it : make emotionally insensitive — **de·sen·si·ti·za·tion** \-ˌsen-sə-tə-'zā-shən\ *n*

de·sen·si·tiz·er \-'sen-sə-ˌtī-zər\ *n* : a desensitizing agent; *esp* : a drug that reduces sensitivity to pain

de·sex \(ˌ)dē-'seks\ *vb* : CASTRATE, SPAY

¹des·ic·cant \'de-si-kənt\ *adj* : tending to dry or desiccate

²desiccant *n* : a drying agent (as calcium chloride)

des·ic·cate \'de-si-ˌkāt\ *vb* **-cat·ed; -cat·ing** : to dry up or cause to dry up : deprive or exhaust of moisture; *esp* : to dry thoroughly

des·ic·ca·tion \ˌde-si-'kā-shən\ *n* : the act or process of desiccating or the state of being or becoming desiccated; *esp* : a complete or nearly complete deprivation of moisture or of water not chemically combined : DEHYDRATION

designer drug *n* : a synthetic version of a controlled substance (as heroin) that is produced with a slightly altered molecular structure to avoid classification as an illicit drug

de·si·pra·mine \ˌde-zə-'pra-mən, də-'zi-prə-ˌmēn\ *n* : a tricyclic antidepressant $C_{18}H_{22}N_2$ administered as the hydrochloride esp. in the treatment of endogenous depressions (as a manic-depressive psychosis) — see PERTOFRANE

-de·sis \də-səs\ *n comb form, pl* **-de-**

ses \-ˌsēz\ : binding or fixation ⟨arthro*desis*⟩

desm- *or* **desmo-** *comb form* : connective tissue ⟨*desmo*plasia⟩

des·meth·yl·imip·ra·mine \ˌdes-ˌme-thəl-im-'i-prə-ˌmēn\ *n* : DESIPRAMINE

des·moid \'dez-ˌmȯid\ *n* : a dense benign connective-tissue tumor

des·mo·pla·sia \ˌdez-mə-'plā-zhə, -zhē-ə\ *n* : formation of fibrous connective tissue by proliferation of fibroblasts

des·mo·plas·tic \-'plas-tik\ *adj* : characterized by the formation of fibrous tissue ⟨~ fibromas⟩

des·mo·some \'dez-mə-ˌsōm\ *n* : a specialized local thickening of the cell membrane of an epithelial cell that serves to anchor contiguous cells together — **des·mo·som·al** \-ˌsō-məl\ *adj*

des·oxy \de-'zäk-sē\ *var of* DEOXY

des·oxy·ri·bo·nu·cle·ic acid *var of* DEOXYRIBONUCLEIC ACID

des·oxy·cor·ti·co·ste·rone \ˌdez-ˌäk-si-ˌkȯr-ti-'käs-tə-ˌrōn, -ˌkō-stə-'rōn\ *n* : a steroid hormone $C_{21}H_{30}O_3$ of the adrenal cortex

des·oxy·cor·tone \ˌdez-ˌäk-si-'kȯr-ˌtōn\ *n* : DESOXYCORTICOSTERONE

des·qua·mate \'des-kwə-ˌmāt\ *vb* **-mat·ed; -mat·ing** : to peel off in the form of scales : scale off ⟨*desquamated* epithelial cells⟩ — **des·qua·ma·tion** \ˌdes-kwə-'mā-shən\ *n* — **des·qua·ma·tive** \'des-kwə-ˌmā-tiv, di-'skwa-mə-\ *adj*

destroying angel *n* : DEATH CAP; *also* : a mushroom of the genus *Amanita* (*A. verna*) closely related to the death cap

detached retina *n* : RETINAL DETACHMENT

detachment of the retina *n* : RETINAL DETACHMENT

detail man *n* : a representative of a drug manufacturer who introduces new drugs esp. to physicians and pharmacists

¹de·ter·gent \di-'tər-jənt\ *adj* : having a cleansing action

²detergent *n* : a cleansing agent (as a soap)

de·te·ri·o·rate \di-'tir-ē-ə-ˌrāt\ *vb* **-rat·ed; -rat·ing** : to become impaired in quality, functioning, or condition : DEGENERATE — **de·te·ri·o·ra·tion** \di-ˌtir-ē-ə-'rā-shən\ *n*

de·ter·mi·nant \di-'tər-mə-nənt\ *n* **1** : GENE **2** : EPITOPE

de·ter·mi·nate \di-'tər-mə-nət\ *adj* : relating to, being, or undergoing determinate cleavage

determinate cleavage *n* : cleavage of an egg in which each division irreversibly separates portions of the zygote with specific potencies for further development — compare INDETERMINATE CLEAVAGE

de·ter·min·er \-'tər-mə-nər\ *n* : GENE

de·tick \dē-'tik\ *vb* : to remove ticks from ⟨~ dogs⟩

¹de·tox \(ˌ)dē-'täks\ *vb* : DETOXIFY 2

²de·tox \'dē-ˌtäks\ *n, often attrib* : detoxification from an intoxicating or an addictive substance ⟨an alcohol ∼ clinic⟩

de·tox·i·cant \(ˌ)dē-ˈtäk-si-kənt\ *n* : a detoxicating agent

de·tox·i·cate \-ˈtäk-sə-ˌkāt\ *vb* **-cat·ed; -cat·ing** : DETOXIFY — **de·tox·i·ca·tion** \-ˌtäk-sə-ˈkā-shən\ *n*

de·tox·i·fy \-ˈtäk-sə-ˌfī\ *vb* **-fied; -fy·ing 1 a** : to remove a poison or toxin or the effect of such from **b** : to render (a harmful substance) harmless **2** : to free (as a drug user or an alcoholic) from an intoxicating or an addictive substance in the body or from dependence on or addiction to such a substance — **de·tox·i·fi·ca·tion** \-ˌtäk-sə-fə-ˈkā-shən\ *n*

de·tru·sor \di-ˈtrü-zər, -sər\ *n* : the outer largely longitudinally arranged musculature of the bladder wall — called also *detrusor muscle*

detrusor uri·nae \-yə-ˈrī-(ˌ)nē\ *n* : the external longitudinal musculature of the urinary bladder

de·tu·mes·cence \ˌdē-tü-ˈmes-ᵊns, -tyü-\ *n* : subsidence or diminution of swelling or erection — **de·tu·mes·cent** \-ᵊnt\ *adj*

deu·ter·anom·a·lous \ˌdü-tə-rə-ˈnä-mə-ləs, ˌdyü-\ *adj* : exhibiting partial loss of green color vision so that an increased intensity of this color is required in a mixture of red and green to match a given yellow

deu·ter·anom·a·ly \-mə-lē\ *n, pl* **-lies** : the condition of being deuteranomalous — compare PROTANOMALY, TRICHROMATISM

deu·ter·an·ope \ˈdü-tə-rə-ˌnōp, ˈdyü-\ *n* : an individual affected with deuteranopia

deu·ter·an·opia \ˌdü-tə-rə-ˈnō-pē-ə, ˌdyü-\ *n* : color blindness marked by confusion of purplish red and green — **deu·ter·an·opic** \-ˈnō-pik, -ˈnä-\ *adj*

deux — see FOLIE À DEUX

de·vas·cu·lar·iza·tion \(ˌ)dē-ˌvas-kyə-lə-rə-ˈzā-shən\ *n* : loss of the blood supply to a bodily part due to obstruction or obstruction of blood vessels — **de·vas·cu·lar·ized** \ˈvas-kyə-lə-ˌrīzd\ *adj*

de·vel·op \di-ˈve-ləp\ *vb* **1 a** : to expand by a process of growth **b** : to go through a process of natural growth, differentiation, or evolution by successive stages **2** : to have (something) unfold or differentiate within one — used esp. of diseases and abnormalities ⟨∼ed tuberculosis⟩ **3** : to acquire secondary sex characters

de·vel·op·ment \di-ˈve-ləp-mənt\ *n* **1** : the action or process of developing: as **a** : the process of growth and differentiation by which the potentialities of a zygote, spore, or embryo are realized **b** : the gradual advance through evolutionary stages : EVOLUTION **2** : the state of being developed — **de·vel·op·men·tal** \-ˌve-ləp-ˈment-ᵊl\ *adj* — **de·vel·op·men·tal·ly** *adv*

developmentally disabled *adj* : having a physical or mental handicap (as mental retardation) that impedes or prevents normal development — abbr. *DD*

developmental quotient *n* : a number expressing the development of a child determined by dividing the age of the group into which test scores place the child by the child's chronological age and multiplying by 100

de·vi·ance \ˈdē-vē-əns\ *n* : deviant quality, state, or behavior

¹de·vi·ant \-ənt\ *adj* **1** : deviating esp. from some accepted norm **2** : characterized by deviation (as from a standard of conduct) ⟨∼ children⟩

²deviant *n* : something that deviates from a norm; *esp* : a person who differs markedly (as in intelligence, social adjustment, or sexual behavior) from what is considered normal for a group

¹de·vi·ate \ˈdē-vē-ət, -vē-ˌāt\ *adj* : characterized by or given to significant departure from the behavioral norms of a particular society

²deviate *n* : one that deviates from a norm; *esp* : a person who differs markedly from a group norm

de·vi·a·tion \ˌdē-vē-ˈā-shən\ *n* : an act or instance of diverging (as in growth or behavior) from an established way or in a new direction

de·vi·tal·iza·tion \(ˌ)dē-ˌvīt-ᵊl-ə-ˈzā-shən\ *n* : destruction and usu. removal of the pulp from a tooth — **de·vi·tal·ize** \-ˈvīt-ᵊl-ˌīz\ *vb*

dew·claw \ˈdü-ˌklȯ, ˈdyü-\ *n* : a vestigial digit not reaching to the ground on the foot of a mammal; *also* : a claw or hoof terminating such a digit — **dew·clawed** \-ˌklȯd\ *adj*

dew·lap \-ˌlap\ *n* : loose skin hanging under the neck esp. of a bovine animal — **dew·lapped** \-ˌlapt\ *adj*

de·worm \(ˌ)dē-ˈwərm\ *vb* : to rid (as a dog) of worms : WORM

de·worm·er \-ˈwər-mər\ *n* : WORMER 1

dex \ˈdeks\ *n* : the sulfate of dextroamphetamine

dexa·meth·a·sone \ˌdek-sə-ˈme-thə-ˌsōn, -ˌzōn\ *n* : a synthetic glucocorticoid $C_{22}H_{29}FO_5$ used esp. as an anti-inflammatory and antiallergic agent — see DECADRON

Dex·e·drine \ˈdek-sə-ˌdrēn, -drən\ *trademark* — used for a preparation of the sulfate of dextroamphetamine

dex·ies \ˈdek-sēz\ *n pl* : tablets or capsules of the sulfate of dextroamphetamine

dextr- *or* **dextro-** *comb form* **1** : right : on or toward the right ⟨*dextro*cardia⟩ **2** *usu* **dextro-** : dextrorotatory ⟨*dex*troamphetamine⟩

¹dex·tral \ˈdek-strəl\ *adj* : of or relating to the right; *esp* : RIGHT-HANDED — **dex·tral·ly** *adv*

²**dextral** *n* : a person exhibiting dominance of the right hand and eye

dex·tral·i·ty \dek-ˈstra-lə-tē\ *n, pl* **-ties** : the quality or state of having the right side or some parts (as the hand or eye) different from and usu. more efficient than the left or corresponding parts; *also* : RIGHT-HANDEDNESS

dex·tran \ˈdek-ˌstran, -strən\ *n* : any of numerous glucose biopolymers $(C_6H_{10}O_5)_n$ of variable molecular weight that are produced esp. by the fermentation of sucrose by bacteria (genus *Leuconostoc*), are found in dental plaque, and are used esp. to increase the volume of blood plasma

dex·tran·ase \-strə-ˌnās, -ˌnāz\ *n* : a hydrolase that prevents tooth decay by breaking down dextran and eliminating plaque

dex·trin \ˈdek-strən\ *n* : any of various soluble gummy polysaccharides $(C_6H_{10}O_5)_n$ obtained from starch by the action of heat, acids, or enzymes

dex·tro \ˈdek-(ˌ)strō\ *adj* : DEXTROROTATORY

dex·tro·am·phet·amine \ˌdek-(ˌ)strō-am-ˈfe-tə-ˌmēn, -mən\ *n* : a drug consisting of dextrorotatory amphetamine that is usu. administered as the sulfate $(C_9H_{13}N)_2 \cdot H_2SO_4$, is a strong stimulant of the central nervous system, is a common drug of abuse, and is used medicinally esp. in the treatment of narcolepsy and attention deficit disorder — see DEXEDRINE

dex·tro·car·dia \ˌdek-strō-ˈkär-dē-ə\ *n* : an abnormal condition in which the heart is situated on the right side and the great blood vessels of the right and left sides are reversed — **dex·tro·car·di·al** \-dē-əl\ *adj*

dex·tro·pro·poxy·phene \ˌdek-strə-prō-ˈpäk-sə-ˌfēn\ *n* : PROPOXYPHENE

dex·tro·ro·ta·to·ry \-ˈrō-tə-ˌtōr-ē\ *also* **dex·tro·ro·ta·ry** \-ˈrō-tə-rē\ *adj* : turning clockwise or toward the right; *esp* : rotating the plane of polarization of light toward the right (∼ crystals) — compare LEVOROTATORY

dex·trose \ˈdek-ˌstrōs, -ˌstrōz\ *n* : dextrorotatory glucose — called also *grape sugar*

DFP \ˌdē-(ˌ)ef-ˈpē\ *n* : ISOFLUROPHATE

DHPG \ˌdē-(ˌ)āch-(ˌ)pē-ˈjē\ *n* : GANCICLOVIR

di- *comb form* **1** : twice : twofold : double ⟨*diphasic*⟩ ⟨*dizygotic*⟩ **2** : containing two atoms, radicals, or groups ⟨*dioxide*⟩

di·a·be·tes \ˌdī-ə-ˈbē-tēz, -təs\ *n, pl* **diabetes** : any of various abnormal conditions characterized by the secretion and excretion of excessive amounts of urine; *esp* : DIABETES MELLITUS

diabetes in·sip·i·dus \-in-ˈsi-pə-dəs\ *n* : a disorder of the pituitary gland characterized by intense thirst and by the excretion of large amounts of urine

diabetes mel·li·tus \-ˈme-lə-təs\ *n* : a variable disorder of carbohydrate metabolism caused by a combination of hereditary and environmental factors and usu. characterized by inadequate secretion or utilization of insulin, by excessive urine production, by excessive amounts of sugar in the blood and urine, and by thirst, hunger, and loss of weight — see INSULIN-DEPENDENT DIABETES MELLITUS, NON-INSULIN-DEPENDENT DIABETES MELLITUS

¹**di·a·bet·ic** \ˌdī-ə-ˈbe-tik\ *adj* **1** : of or relating to diabetes or diabetics **2** : affected with diabetes **3** : occurring in or caused by diabetes ⟨∼ coma⟩ **4** : suitable for diabetics ⟨∼ food⟩

²**diabetic** *n* : a person affected with diabetes

diabeticorum — see NECROBIOSIS LIPOIDICA DIABETICORUM

di·a·be·to·gen·ic \ˌdī-ə-ˌbē-tə-ˈje-nik\ *adj* : producing diabetes ⟨∼ drugs⟩ ⟨a ∼ diet⟩

di·a·be·tol·o·gist \ˌdī-ə-bə-ˈtä-lə-jist\ *n* : a specialist in diabetes

di·ace·tic acid \ˌdī-ə-ˌsēt-ik-\ *n* : ACETOACETIC ACID

di·ace·tyl·mor·phine \ˌdī-ə-ˌsēt-ᵊl-ˈmór-ˌfēn, dī-ˌa-sət-ᵊl-\ *n* : HEROIN

di·ag·nose \ˈdī-ig-ˌnōs, -ˌnōz, ˌdī-ig-ˈ, -əg-\ *vb* **-nosed; -nos·ing 1** : to recognize (as a disease) by signs and symptoms **2** : to diagnose a disease or condition in ⟨*diagnosed* the patient⟩ — **di·ag·nos·able** *also* **di·ag·nose·able** \ˌdī-ig-ˈnō-sə-bəl, -əg-, -zə-\ *adj*

di·ag·no·sis \ˌdī-ig-ˈnō-səs, -əg-\ *n, pl* **-no·ses** \-ˌsēz\ **1** : the art or act of identifying a disease from its signs and symptoms **2** : the decision reached by diagnosis

diagnosis related group *n* : DRG

di·ag·nos·tic \-ˈnäs-tik\ *also* **di·ag·nos·ti·cal** \-ti-kəl\ *adj* **1** : of, relating to, or used in diagnosis **2** : using the methods of or yielding a diagnosis — **di·ag·nos·ti·cal·ly** \-ti-k(ə-)lē\ *adv*

²**diagnostic** *n* : the art or practice of diagnosis — often used in pl.

di·ag·nos·ti·cian \-(ˌ)näs-ˈti-shən\ *n* : a specialist in medical diagnostics

dia·ki·ne·sis \ˌdī-ə-kə-ˈnē-səs, -(ˌ)kī-\ *n, pl* **-ne·ses** \-ˌsēz\ : the final stage of the meiotic prophase marked by contraction of each chromosome pair — **dia·ki·net·ic** \-ˈne-tik\ *adj*

di·al·y·sance \dī-ˈa-lə-səns\ *n* : blood volume in milliliters per unit time cleared of a substance by dialysis (as by an artificial kidney)

di·al·y·sate \dī-ˈa-lə-ˌzāt, -ˌsāt\ *also* **di·al·y·zate** \-ˌzāt\ *n* **1** : the material that passes through the membrane in dialysis **2** : the liquid into which material passes by way of the membrane in dialysis

di·al·y·sis \dī-ˈa-lə-səs\ *n, pl* **-y·ses** \-ˌsēz\ **1** : the separation of substances in solution by means of their unequal diffusion through semipermeable membranes; *esp* : such a separation of colloids from soluble substances **2** : HEMODIALYSIS — **di·a·lyt·ic** \ˌdī-ə-ˈli-tik\ *adj*

di·a·lyze \ˈdī-ə-ˌlīz\ *vb* **-lyzed; -lyz·ing 1** : to subject to or undergo dialysis **2** : to separate or obtain by dialysis — **di·a·lyz·abil·i·ty** \ˌdī-ə-ˌlī-zə-ˈbi-lə-tē\ *n* — **di·a·lyz·able** \-ˈlī-zə-bəl\ *adj*

di·a·lyz·er \-ˌlī-zər\ *n* : an apparatus in which dialysis is carried out consisting essentially of one or more containers for liquids separated into compartments by membranes

di·am·e·ter \dī-ˈa-mə-tər\ *n* **1** : a unit of magnification of a magnifying device equal to the number of times the linear dimensions of the object are increased (a microscope magnifying 60 ∼*s*) **2** : one of the maximal breadths of a part of the body (the transverse ∼ of the inlet of the pelvis)

di·ami·no·di·phe·nyl sul·fone \ˌdī-ə-ˌmē-(ˌ)nō-dī-ˈfen-əl-ˈsəl-ˌfōn, -ˈfēn-\ *n* : DAPSONE

di·a·mond·back rattlesnake \ˈdī-mənd-ˌbak-, ˈdī-ə-\ *n* : either of two large and deadly rattlesnakes of the genus *Crotalus* (*C. adamanteus* of the southeastern U.S. and *C. atrox* of the south central and southwestern U.S. and Mexico) — called also *diamondback, diamondback rattler*

di·a·mor·phine \ˌdī-ə-ˈmȯr-ˌfēn\ *n* : HEROIN

di·a·pe·de·sis \ˌdī-ə-pə-ˈdē-səs\ *n, pl* **-de·ses** \-ˌsēz\ : the passage of blood cells through capillary walls into the tissues — **di·a·pe·det·ic** \-ˈde-tik\ *adj*

¹**di·a·per** \ˈdī-pər, ˈdī-ə-\ *n* : a basic garment esp. for infants consisting of a folded cloth or other absorbent material drawn up between the legs and fastened about the waist

²**diaper** *vb* **di·a·pered; di·a·per·ing** : to put on or change the diaper of (an infant)

diaper rash *n* : skin irritation of the diaper-covered area and usu. the buttocks of an infant esp. from exposure to feces and urinary ammonia

di·a·pho·re·sis \ˌdī-ə-fə-ˈrē-səs, (ˌ)dī-ˌa-fə-\ *n, pl* **-re·ses** \-ˌsēz\ : PERSPIRATION; *esp* : profuse perspiration artificially induced

¹**di·a·pho·ret·ic** \-ˈre-tik\ *adj* : having the power to increase sweating

²**diaphoretic** *n* : an agent capable of inducing sweating

di·a·phragm \ˈdī-ə-ˌfram\ *n* **1** : a body partition of muscle and connective tissue; *specif* : the partition separating the chest and abdominal cavities in mammals — compare PELVIC DIAPHRAGM, UROGENITAL DIAPHRAGM **2** : a device that limits the aperture of a lens or optical system **3** : a molded cap usu. of thin rubber fitted over the uterine cervix to act as a mechanical contraceptive barrier

di·a·phrag·ma sel·lae \ˌdī-ə-ˈfrag-mə-

ˈse-ˌlī, -ˌlē\ *n, pl* : a small horizontal fold of the dura mater that roofs over the sella turcica and is pierced by a small opening for the infundibulum

di·a·phrag·mat·ic \ˌdī-ə-frə-ˈma-tik, -ˌfrag-\ *adj* : of, involving, or resembling a diaphragm (∼ hernia)

di·aph·y·se·al \ˌdī-ˌa-fə-ˈsē-əl, -ˈzē-\ *or* **di·a·phys·i·al** \ˌdī-ə-ˈfi-zē-əl\ *adj* : of, relating to, or involving a diaphysis

di·a·phy·sec·to·my \ˌdī-ə-fə-ˈzek-tə-mē, -ˈsek-\ *n, pl* **-mies** : surgical excision of all or part of a diaphysis (as of the femur)

di·aph·y·sis \dī-ˈa-fə-səs\ *n, pl* **-y·ses** \-ˌsēz\ : the shaft of a long bone

di·ar·rhea \ˌdī-ə-ˈrē-ə\ *n* : abnormally frequent intestinal evacuations with more or less fluid stools

di·ar·rhe·al \-ˈrē-əl\ *adj* : DIARRHEIC

di·ar·rhe·ic \-ˈrē-ik\ *adj* : of or relating to diarrhea

di·ar·rhet·ic \-ˈre-tik\ *adj* : DIARRHEIC

di·ar·rhoea, di·ar·rhoe·al, di·ar·rhoe·ic, di·ar·rhoet·ic *chiefly Brit var of* DIARRHEA, DIARRHEAL, DIARRHEIC, DIARRHETIC

di·ar·thro·sis \ˌdī-är-ˈthrō-səs\ *n, pl* **-thro·ses** \-ˌsēz\ **1** : articulation that permits free movement **2** : a freely movable joint — called also *synovial joint* — **di·ar·thro·di·al** \ˌdī-är-ˈthrō-dē-əl\ *adj*

di·a·stase \ˈdī-ə-ˌstās, -ˌstāz\ *n* **1** : AMYLASE; *esp* : a mixture of amylases from malt **2** : ENZYME

di·a·sta·sis \dī-ˈas-tə-səs\ *n, pl* **-ta·ses** \-ˌsēz\ **1** : an abnormal separation of parts normally joined together **2** : the rest phase of cardiac diastole occurring between filling of the ventricle and the start of atrial contraction

di·a·stat·ic \ˌdī-ə-ˈsta-tik\ *adj* : relating to or having the properties of diastase; *esp* : converting starch into sugar

di·a·ste·ma \ˌdī-ə-ˈstē-mə\ *n, pl* **-ma·ta** \-mə-tə\ : a space between teeth in a jaw

di·a·ste·ma·to·my·e·lia \ˌdī-ə-ˌstē-mə-tō-mī-ˈē-lē-ə, -ˌste-\ *n* : congenital division of all or part of the spinal cord

di·as·to·le \dī-ˈas-tə-(ˌ)lē\ *n* : the passive rhythmical expansion or dilation of the cavities of the heart during which they fill with blood — compare SYSTOLE — **di·a·stol·ic** \ˌdī-ə-ˈstä-lik\ *adj*

diastolic pressure *n* : the lowest arterial blood pressure of a cardiac cycle occurring during diastole of the heart — compare SYSTOLIC PRESSURE

di·a·stroph·ic dwarfism \ˌdī-ə-ˈsträ-fik-\ *n* : an inherited dysplasia affecting bones and joints and characterized esp. by clubfoot, deformities of the digits of the hand, malformed pinnae, and cleft palate

dia·ther·my \ˈdī-ə-ˌthər-mē\ *n, pl* **-mies** : the generation of heat in tissue by electric currents for medical or surgical purposes — see ELECTROCOAG- ULATION — **dia·ther·mic** \ˌdī-ə-ˈthər-mik\ *adj*

di·ath·e·sis \dī-ˈa-thə-səs\ *n, pl* **-e·ses** \-ˌsēz\ : a constitutional predisposition toward a particular state or condition and esp. one that is abnormal or diseased

dia·tri·zo·ate \ˌdī-ə-ˌtrī-ˈzō-ˌāt\ *n* : either of two salts of the acid $C_{11}H_9$-$I_3N_2O_4$ administered in solution as a radiopaque medium for various forms of radiographic diagnosis — see HYPAQUE

di·az·e·pam \dī-ˈa-zə-ˌpam\ *n* : a synthetic tranquilizer $C_{16}H_{13}ClN_2O$ used esp. to relieve anxiety and tension and as a muscle relaxant — see VALIUM

Di·az·i·non \dī-ˈa-zə-ˌnän\ *trademark* — used for an organophosphate insecticide $C_{12}H_{21}N_2O_3PS$ that is a cholinesterase inhibitor dangerous to humans if ingested

di·az·ox·ide \ˌdī-ˌa-ˈzäk-ˌsīd\ *n* : an antihypertensive drug $C_8H_7ClN_2O_2S$ that has a structure similar to chlorothiazide but no diuretic activity

di·benz·an·thra·cene *or* **1,2:5,6-di·benz·an·thra·cene** \ˌwən-ˌtü-ˌfīv-ˌsiks-)dī-ˌben-ˈzan-thrə-ˌsēn\ *n* : a carcinogenic cyclic hydrocarbon $C_{22}H_{14}$ found in trace amounts in coal tar

di·ben·zo·fu·ran \ˈdī-ˌben-zō-ˈfyü-ˌran, -fyə-ˈran\ *n* : a highly toxic chemical compound $C_{12}H_8O$ that is used in chemical synthesis and as an insecticide and is a hazardous pollutant in its chlorinated form

di·bu·caine \ˈdī-ˌbyü-ˌkān, ˈdī-ˈ\ *n* : a local anesthetic $C_{20}H_{29}N_3O_2$ used for temporary relief of pain and itching esp. from burns, sunburn, insect bites, or hemorrhoids — called also *cinchocaine*; see NUPERCAINE

dibucaine number *n* : a number expressing the percentage by which cholinesterase activity in a serum sample is inhibited by dibucaine

di·cen·tric \(ˌ)dī-ˈsen-trik\ *adj* : having two centromeres ⟨a ∼ chromosome⟩ — **dicentric** *n*

dich- *or* **dicho-** *comb form* : apart : separate ⟨*dich*otic⟩

di·chlor·a·mine-T \ˌdī-ˌklōr-ə-ˌmēn-ˈtē\ *n* : a yellow crystalline compound $C_7H_7Cl_2NO_2S$ used esp. formerly as an antiseptic — compare CHLORAMINE-T

p–di·chlo·ro·ben·zene *var of* PARADICHLOROBENZENE

2,4–di·chlo·ro·phen·oxy·ace·tic acid *also* **di·chlo·ro·phen·oxy·ace·tic acid** \(ˌtü-ˌfōr-)di-ˌklōr-ō-(ˌ)phe-ˌnäk-sē-ə-ˈsē-tik-\ *n* : 2,4-D

di·chlor·vos \(ˌ)dī-ˈklōr-ˌväs, -vəs\ *n* : an organophosphorus insecticide and anthelmintic $C_4H_7Cl_2O_4P$ used esp. in veterinary medicine — called also *DDVP*

dich·otic \(ˌ)dī-ˈkō-tik\ *adj* : relating to

or involving the presentation of a stimulus to one ear that differs in some respect (as pitch, loudness, frequency, or energy) from that presented to the other ear ⟨∼ listening⟩ — **dich·ot·i·cal·ly** \-ti-k(ə-)lē\ *adv*

di·chot·o·my \dī-ˈkä-tə-mē\ *n, pl* **-mies** : a division or forking into branches; *esp* : repeated bifurcation — **di·chot·o·mous** \dī-ˈkä-tə-məs\ *adj*

di·chro·mat \ˈdī-krō-ˌmat, (ˌ)dī-ˈ\ *n* : one affected with dichromatism

di·chro·ma·tism \ˈdī-ˈkrō-mə-ˌti-zəm\ *n* : partial color blindness in which only two colors are perceptible — **di·chro·mat·ic** \ˌdī-krō-ˈma-tik\ *adj*

Dick test \ˈdik-\ *n* : a test to determine susceptibility or immunity to scarlet fever by an injection of scarlet fever toxin

Dick, George Frederick (1881–1967) and Gladys Henry (1881–1963), American physicians.

di·clox·a·cil·lin \(ˌ)dī-ˌkläk-sə-ˈsi-lən\ *n* : a semisynthetic penicillin used in the form of its sodium salt $C_{19}H_{16}Cl_2N_3$-$NaO_5S·H_2O$ esp. against penicillinase-producing staphylococci

di·cou·ma·rin \(ˌ)dī-ˈkü-mə-rən\ *n* : DICUMAROL

Di·cro·coe·li·um \ˌdī-krə-ˈsē-lē-əm\ *n* : a widely distributed genus (family Dicrocoeliidae) that includes small digenetic trematodes infesting the livers of ruminants or occas. other mammals including humans — see LANCET FLUKE

di·crot·ic \(ˌ)dī-ˈkrä-tik\ *adj* **1** *of the pulse* : having a double beat (as in certain febrile states in which the heart is overactive and the arterial walls are lacking in tone) — compare MONOCROTIC **2** : being or relating to the second part of the arterial pulse occurring during diastole of the heart or of an arterial pressure recording made during the same period — **di·cro·tism** \ˈdī-krə-ˌti-zəm\ *n*

dicrotic notch *n* : a secondary upstroke in the descending part of a pulse tracing corresponding to the transient increase in aortic pressure upon closure of the aortic valve

Dic·ty·o·cau·lus \ˌdik-tē-ə-ˈkȯ-ləs\ *n* : a genus (family Metastrongylidae) of small slender lungworms infesting mammals (as ruminants) and often causing severe bronchial symptoms or even pneumonia in young animals

dic·tyo·some \ˈdik-tē-ə-ˌsōm\ *n* : any of the membranous or vesicular structures making up the Golgi apparatus

di·cu·ma·rol *also* **di·cou·ma·rol** \dī-ˈkü-mə-ˌrȯl, -ˈkyü-, -ˌrōl\ *n* : a crystalline compound $C_{19}H_{12}O_6$ used to delay clotting of blood esp. in preventing and treating thromboembolic disease

di·cy·clo·mine \(ˌ)dī-ˈsī-klə-ˌmēn, -ˈsi-\ *n* : an anticholinergic drug used in the form of its hydrochloride salt C_{19}-$H_{35}NO_2·HCl$ for its antispasmodic effect on smooth muscle in gastrointestinal functional disorders

di·dan·o·sine \dī-'da-nə-₁sēn\ n : DDI

di·de·oxy·cy·ti·dine \₁dī-(₁)dē-₁äk-sē-'si-tə-₁dēn, -'sī-\ n : DDC

di·de·oxy·ino·sine \-'i-nə-₁sēn, -'ī-, -₁sən\ n : DDI

die \'dī\ vb **died; dy·ing** \'dī-iŋ\ **1** : to suffer total and irreversible loss of the bodily attributes and functions that constitute life **2** : to suffer or face the pains of death

diel·drin \'dēl-drən\ n : a white crystalline persistent chlorinated hydrocarbon insecticide $C_{12}H_8Cl_6O$

Diels \'dēls\, **Otto Paul Hermann (1876–1954)**, and **Al·der**, **Kurt (1902–1958)**, German chemists.

di·en·ceph·a·lon \₁dī-ən-'se-fə-₁län, ₁dī-(₁)en-, -₁lən\ n : the posterior subdivision of the forebrain — called also **betweenbrain** — **di·en·ce·phal·ic** \-sə-'fa-lik\ adj

die·ner \'dē-nər\ n : a laboratory helper esp. in a medical school

di·en·es·trol \₁dī-ə-'nes-₁tról, -₁tról\ n : a white crystalline estrogenic compound $C_{18}H_{18}O_2$ structurally related to diethylstilbestrol and used topically to treat atrophic vaginitis and kraurosis vulvae

di·en·oes·trol \₁dī-ə-'nēs-₁tról, -₁tról\ chiefly Brit var of DIENESTROL

Di·ent·amoe·ba \₁dī-₁en-tə-'mē-bə\ n : a genus of amebic protozoans parasitic in the intestines of humans and monkeys that include one (*D. fragilis*) known to cause abdominal pain, anorexia, and loose stools in humans

di·es·trus \(₁)dī-'es-trəs\ n : a period of sexual quiescence that intervenes between two periods of estrus — **di·es·trous** \-trəs\ adj

¹di·et \'dī-ət\ n **1** : food and drink regularly provided or consumed **2** : habitual nourishment **3** : the kind and amount of food prescribed for a person or animal for a special reason

²diet vb : to eat or cause to eat less or according to a prescribed rule

³diet adj : reduced in calories ⟨a ∼ soft drink⟩

¹di·etary \'dī-ə-₁ter-ē\ n, pl **di·etar·ies** : the kinds and amounts of food available to or eaten by an individual, group, or population

²dietary adj : of or relating to a diet or to the rules of a diet ⟨∼ habits⟩ — **di·etar·i·ly** \₁dī-ə-'ter-ə-lē\ adv

dietary fiber n : FIBER 2

di·et·er \'dī-ə-tər\ n : one that diets; esp : a person that consumes a reduced allowance of food in order to lose weight

di·etet·ic \₁dī-ə-'te-tik\ adj **1** : of or relating to diet **2** : adapted (as by the elimination of salt or sugar) for use in special diets — **di·etet·i·cal·ly** \-ti-k(ə-)lē\ adv

di·etet·ics \-'te-tiks\ n sing or pl : the

science or art of applying the principles of nutrition to feeding

diethylamide — see LYSERGIC ACID DIETHYLAMIDE

di·eth·yl·car·bam·azine \₁dī-₁e-thəl-kär-'ba-mə-₁zēn, -zən\ n : an anthelmintic derived from piperazine and administered in the form of its crystalline citrate $C_{10}H_{21}N_3O \cdot C_6H_8O_7$ esp. to control filariasis in humans and large roundworms in dogs and cats

di·eth·yl ether \(₁)dī-'e-thəl-\ n : ETHER 1

di·eth·yl·pro·pi·on \(₁)dī-₁e-thəl-'prō-pē-₁än\ n : a sympathomimetic amine related structurally to amphetamine and used esp. in the form of its hydrochloride $C_{13}H_{19}NO \cdot HCl$ as an appetite suppressant to promote weight loss — see TENUATE

di·eth·yl·stil·bes·trol \-stil-'bes-₁tról, -₁tról\ n : a colorless crystalline synthetic compound $C_{18}H_{20}O_2$ used as a potent estrogen but contraindicated in pregnancy for its tendency to cause cancer or birth defects in offspring — called also DES, stilbestrol

di·eth·yl·stil·boes·trol \-'bēs-₁tról, -₁tról\ chiefly Brit var of DIETHYLSTILBESTROL

di·eti·tian or **di·eti·cian** \₁dī-ə-'ti-shən\ n : a specialist in dietetics

Die·tl's crisis \'dēt-əlz-\ n : an attack of violent pain in the kidney region accompanied by chills, nausea, vomiting, and collapse that is caused by the formation of kinks in the ureter and is usu. associated with a floating kidney

Dietl \'dēt-əl\, **Josef (1804–1878)**, Polish physician.

differential blood count n : a blood count which includes separate counts for each kind of white blood cell — compare COMPLETE BLOOD COUNT

differential diagnosis n : the distinguishing of a disease or condition from others presenting similar symptoms

dif·fer·en·ti·ate \₁di-fə-'ren-chē-₁āt\ vb **-at·ed; -at·ing 1** : to constitute a difference that distinguishes **2 a** : to cause differentiation of in the course of development **b** : to undergo differentiation **3** : to sense, recognize, or give expression to a difference (as in stimuli) **4** : to cause differentiation in (a specimen for microscopic examination) by staining

dif·fer·en·ti·a·tion \-₁ren-chē-'ā-shən\ n **1 a** : the act or process of differentiating **b** : the enhancement of microscopically visible differences between tissue or cell parts by partial selective decolorization or removal of excess stain **2 a** : modification of different parts of the body for performance of particular functions; also : specialization of parts or organs in the course of evolution **b** : the sum of the developmental processes whereby apparently unspecialized cells, tissues, and structures attain their adult form and function

dif·flu·ent \'di-(₁)flü-ənt\ *adj* : soft like mush ⟨a ∼ spleen⟩

dif·fu·sate \di-'fyü-₁zāt\ *n* : DIALYSATE

¹dif·fuse \di-'fyüs\ *adj* : not concentrated or localized ⟨∼ sclerosis⟩

²dif·fuse \di-'fyüz\ *vb* **dif·fused; dif·fus·ing 1** : to subject to or undergo diffusion **2** : to break up and distribute (incident light) by reflection (as from a rough surface) — **dif·fus·ible** \di-'fyü-zə-bəl\ *adj* — **dif·fus·ibil·i·ty** \-₁fyü-zə-'bi-lə-tē\ *n*

dif·fu·sion \di-'fyü-zhən\ *n* **1** : the process whereby particles of liquids, gases, or solids intermingle as the result of their spontaneous movement caused by thermal agitation and in dissolved substances move from a region of higher to one of lower concentration **2 a** : reflection of light by a rough reflecting surface **b** : transmission of light through a translucent material — **dif·fu·sion·al** \-'fyü-zhə-nəl\ *adj*

di·flu·ni·sal \(₁)dī-'flü-nə-₁sal\ *n* : a nonsteroidal anti-inflammatory drug $C_{13}H_8F_2O_3$ related to aspirin that is used to relieve mild to moderately severe pain — see DOLOBID

di·gas·tric muscle \(₁)dī-'gas-trik-\ *n* : either of a pair of muscles having two bellies separated by a tendon that extend from the anterior inferior margin of the mandible and serve to open the jaw — called also *digastric*

di·gas·tri·cus \-tri-kəs\ *n* : DIGASTRIC MUSCLE

di·ge·net·ic \₁dī-jə-'ne-tik\ *adj* : of or relating to a subclass (Digenea) of trematode worms in which sexual reproduction as an internal parasite of a vertebrate alternates with asexual reproduction in a mollusk and which include a number of parasites (as the Chinese liver fluke) of humans

¹di·gest \'dī-₁jest\ *n* : a product of digestion

²di·gest \dī-'jest, də-\ *vb* **1** : to convert (food) into absorbable form **2 a** : to soften, decompose, or break down by heat and moisture or chemicals **b** : to extract soluble ingredients from by warming with a liquid — **di·gest·er** \-'jes-tər\ *n*

di·gest·ant \-'jes-tənt\ *n* : a substance that digests or aids in digestion — compare DIGESTIVE 1

di·gest·ibil·i·ty \-₁jes-tə-'bi-lə-tē\ *n, pl* **-ties 1** : the fitness of something for digestion **2** : the percentage of a foodstuff taken into the digestive tract that is absorbed into the body

di·gest·ible \-'jes-tə-bəl\ *adj* : capable of being digested

di·ges·tion \-'jes-chən\ *n* : the action, process, or power of digesting; *esp* : the process of making food absorb-

able by dissolving it and breaking it down into simpler chemical compounds that occurs in the living body chiefly through the action of enzymes secreted into the alimentary canal

¹di·ges·tive \-'jes-tiv\ *n* **1** : something that aids digestion esp. of food — compare DIGESTANT **2** : a substance which promotes suppuration

²digestive *adj* **1** : relating to or functioning in digestion ⟨the ∼ system⟩ **2** : having the power to cause or promote digestion ⟨∼ enzymes⟩

digestive gland *n* : a gland secreting digestive enzymes

dig·i·lan·id \₁di-jə-'la-nəd\ *or* **dig·i·lan·ide** \-₁nid, -nəd\ *n* : LANATOSIDE

digilanid A *or* **digilanide A** *n* : LANATOSIDE A

digilanid B *or* **digilanide B** *n* : LANATOSIDE B

digilanid C *or* **digilanide C** *n* : LANATOSIDE C

dig·it \'di-jət\ *n* : any of the divisions (as a finger or toe) in which the limbs of amphibians and all higher vertebrates terminate and which in humans are five in number on each limb

dig·i·tal \'di-jət-ᵊl\ *adj* **1** : of, relating to, or supplying one or more fingers or toes ⟨a ∼ branch of an artery⟩ **2** : done with a finger ⟨a ∼ examination⟩ — **dig·i·tal·ly** *adv*

dig·i·tal·in \₁di-jə-'ta-lən, -'tā-\ *n* **1** : a white crystalline steroid glycoside $C_{36}H_{56}O_{14}$ obtained from seeds esp. of the common foxglove **2** : a mixture of the glycosides of digitalis leaves or seeds

dig·i·tal·is \-ləs\ *n* **1 a** *cap* : a genus of Eurasian herbs (family Scrophulariaceae) that have alternate leaves and stalks of snowy bell-shaped flowers and comprise the foxgloves **b** : FOXGLOVE **2** : the dried leaf of the common European foxglove (*D. purpurea*) containing the active principles digitoxin and gitoxin, serving as a powerful cardiac stimulant and a diuretic, and used in standardized powdered form esp. in the treatment of congestive heart failure

dig·i·tal·i·za·tion \₁di-jət-ᵊl-ə-'zā-shən\ *n* : the administration of digitalis (as in heart disease) until the desired physiological adjustment is attained; *also* : the bodily state so produced — **dig·i·tal·ize** \di-jət-ᵊl-₁īz\ *vb*

digital nerve *n* **1** : any of several branches of the median nerve and the ulnar nerve supplying the fingers and thumb **2** : any of several branches of the medial plantar nerve supplying the toes

digiti — see ABDUCTOR DIGITI MINIMI, EXTENSOR DIGITI MINIMI, EXTENSOR DIGITI QUINTI PROPRIUS, FLEXOR DIGITI MINIMI BREVIS, OPPONENS DIGITI MINIMI

digitorum — see EXTENSOR DIGITORUM BREVIS, EXTENSOR DIGITORUM COM-

MUNIS, EXTENSOR DIGITORUM LON-GUS, FLEXOR DIGITORUM BREVIS, FLEXOR DIGITORUM LONGUS, FLEXOR DIGITORUM PROFUNDUS, FLEXOR DIGITORUM SUPERFICIALIS

dig·i·tox·in \ˌdi-jə-ˈtäk-sən\ n : a poisonous glycoside $C_{41}H_{64}O_{13}$ that is the most active constituent of digitalis; *also* : a mixture of digitalis glycosides consisting chiefly of digitoxin

di·glyc·er·ide \dī-ˈgli-sə-ˌrīd\ n : an ester of glycerol that contains two ester groups and involves one or two acids

di·gox·in \di-ˈjäk-sən, -ˈgäk-\ n : a poisonous cardiotonic glycoside $C_{41}H_{64}O_{14}$ obtained from the leaves of a foxglove (*Digitalis lanata*) and used similarly to digitalis — see LANOXIN

di·hy·dro·chlo·ride \(ˌ)dī-hī-drə-ˈklȯr-ˌid\ n : a chemical compound with two molecules of hydrochloric acid (quinine — $C_{20}H_{24}N_2O_2 \cdot 2HCl$)

di·hy·dro·co·de·inone \-kō-ˈdē-ə-ˌnōn\ n : a habit-forming codeine derivative $C_{18}H_{21}NO_3$ used as an analgesic and cough sedative — called also *hydrocodone*; see HYCODAN

di·hy·dro·er·got·a·mine \-ˌhī-drō-ˌər-ˈgä-tə-ˌmēn\ n : a hydrogenated derivative $C_{33}H_{37}N_5O_5$ of ergotamine that is used in the treatment of migraine

di·hy·dro·mor·phi·none \-ˈmȯr-fə-ˌnōn\ n : HYDROMORPHONE

di·hy·dro·strep·to·my·cin \-ˌstrep-tə-ˈmis-ᵊn\ n : a toxic antibiotic $C_{21}H_{41}N_7O_{12}$ formerly used but abandoned because of its tendency to impair hearing

di·hy·dro·tachy·ste·rol \-ˌta-ki-ˈster-ˌȯl, -ˈstir-, -ˌȯl\ n : an alcohol $C_{28}H_{45}OH$ used in the treatment of hypocalcemia

di·hy·dro·tes·tos·ter·one \-te-ˈstäs-tə-ˌrōn\ n : a derivative $C_{19}H_{30}O_2$ of testosterone with similar androgenic activity

di·hy·dro·the·elin \-ˈthē-ə-lən\ n : ESTRADIOL

di·hy·droxy·ac·e·tone \ˌdī-hī-ˌdräk-sē-ˈa-sə-ˌtōn\ n : a glyceraldehyde isomer $C_3H_6O_3$ that is used esp. to stain the skin to simulate a tan

1,25-di·hy·droxy·cho·le·cal·cif·er·ol\ˌwən-ˌtwen-tē-ˌfīv-ˌdī-hī-ˌdräk-sē-ˌkō-lə-(ˌ)kal-ˈsi-fə-ˌrȯl, -ˌrōl\ n : a physiologically active metabolic derivative $C_{27}H_{44}O_3$ of vitamin D that is synthesized in the kidney

di·hy·droxy·phe·nyl·al·a·nine \ˌdī-hī-ˌdräk-sē-ˌfen-ᵊl-ˈa-lə-ˌnēn, -ˌfēn-\ n 1 *or* **3,4-dihydroxyphenylalanine** \ˌthrē-ˌfȯr-\ : DOPA 2 *or* L**-3,4-dihydroxyphenylalanine** \ˌel-\ *or* L**-dihydroxyphenylalanine** : L-DOPA

di·io·do·hy·droxy·quin \ˌdī-ˌī-ə-dō-hī-ˈdräk-si-kwən\ n : IODOQUINOL

di·io·do·hy·droxy·quin·o·line \-hī-ˌdräk-si-ˈkwin-ᵊl-ˌēn\ n : IODOQUINOL

di·io·do·ty·ro·sine \-ˈtī-rə-ˌsēn\ n : a compound $C_9H_9I_2NO_3$ of tyrosine

and iodine that is produced in the thyroid gland from monoiodotyrosine and that combines with monoiodotyrosine to form triiodothyronine

di·iso·pro·pyl fluo·ro·phos·phate \ˌdī-ˌī-sə-ˈprō-pəl-ˌflür-ō-ˈfäs-ˌfāt\ n : ISO-FLUROPHATE

di·lac·er·a·tion \(ˌ)dī-ˌla-sə-ˈrā-shən\ n : injury (as partial fracture) to a developing tooth that results in a curve in the long axis as development continues — **di·lac·er·at·ed** \(ˌ)dī-ˈla-sə-ˌrā-təd\ adj

Di·lan·tin \dī-ˈlant-ᵊn, də-\ trademark — used for a preparation of phenytoin

di·la·ta·tion \ˌdi-lə-ˈtā-shən, ˌdī-\ n 1 : the condition of being stretched beyond normal dimensions esp. as a result of overwork or disease or of abnormal relaxation 2 : DILATION 2

di·la·ta·tor \ˈdi-lə-ˌtā-tər, ˈdī-\ n : DILATOR b

di·late \dī-ˈlāt, ˈdī-\ vb **di·lat·ed; di·lat·ing** 1 : to enlarge, stretch, or cause to expand 2 : to become expanded or swollen

di·la·tion \dī-ˈlā-shən\ n 1 : the state of being dilated : DILATATION 2 : the action of stretching or enlarging an organ or part of the body

di·la·tor \(ˌ)dī-ˈlā-tər, də-\ n : one that dilates: as **a** : an instrument for expanding a tube, duct, or cavity (a urethral ~) **b** : a muscle that dilates a part (: a drug (as a vasodilator) causing dilation

Di·lau·did \(ˌ)dī-ˈlȯ-did\ trademark — used for a preparation of hydromorphone

dil·do \ˈdil-(ˌ)dō\ n, pl **dildos** : an object serving as a penis substitute for vaginal insertion

dil·ti·a·zem \dil-ˈtī-ə-(ˌ)zem\ n : a calcium channel blocker $C_{22}H_{26}N_2O_4S$ used esp. in the form of its hydrochloride as a coronary vasodilator

¹**dil·u·ent** \ˈdil-yə-wənt\ n : a diluting agent (as the vehicle in a medicinal preparation)

²**diluent** adj : making thinner or less concentrated by admixture : DILUTING

¹**di·lute** \dī-ˈlüt, də-\ vb **di·lut·ed; di·lut·ing** : to make thinner or more liquid by admixture — **di·lut·or** *also* **di·lut·er** \-ˈlü-tər\ n

²**dilute** adj : of relatively low strength or concentration

di·lu·tion \dī-ˈlü-shən, də-\ n 1 : the action of diluting : the state of being diluted 2 : something (as a solution) that is diluted

di·men·hy·dri·nate \ˌdī-men-ˈhī-drə-ˌnāt\ n : a crystalline antihistaminic compound $C_{24}H_{28}ClN_5O_3$ used esp. to prevent nausea (as in motion sickness)

di·mer \ˈdī-mər\ n : a compound formed by the union of two radicals or two molecules of a simpler compound; *specif* : a polymer formed from two molecules of a monomer — **di·mer·ic** \(ˌ)dī-ˈmer-ik\ *adj*

di·mer·ca·prol \ˌdī-(ˌ)mər-ˈka-ˌpról, -ˌpról\ *n* : a colorless viscous oily compound $C_3H_8OS_2$ with an offensive odor used in treating arsenic, mercury, and gold poisoning — called also *BAL, British anti-lewisite*

di·meth·yl·ni·tros·amine \(ˌ)dī-ˌme-thəl-(ˌ)nī-ˈtrō-sə-ˌmēn\ *n* : a carcinogenic nitrosamine $C_2H_6N_2O$ that occurs esp. in tobacco smoke — called also *nitrosodimethylamine*

dimethyl sul·fox·ide \-səl-ˈfäk-ˌsīd\ *n* : an anti-inflammatory agent $(CH_3)_2SO$ used in the treatment of interstitial cystitis — called also *DMSO*

di·meth·yl·tryp·ta·mine \-ˈtrip-tə-ˌmēn\ *n* : a hallucinogenic drug $C_{12}H_{16}N_2$ that is chemically similar to but shorter acting than psilocybin — called also *DMT*

dim·ple \ˈdim-pəl\ *n* : a slight natural indentation or hollow in the surface of some part of the human body (as on a cheek or the chin) — **dimple** *vb*

dinitrate — see ISOSORBIDE DINITRATE

di·ni·tro·phe·nol \ˌdī-ˌnī-trō-ˈfē-ˌnól, -fi-ˈ\ *n* : any of six isomeric compounds $C_6H_4N_2O_5$ some of whose derivatives are pesticides; *esp* : a highly toxic compound formerly used in weight control

di·no·fla·gel·late \ˌdī-nō-ˈfla-jə-lət, -ˌlāt, -flə-ˈjə-lət\ *n* : any of an order (Dinoflagellata) of chiefly marine planktonic plantlike unicellular flagellates of which some cause red tide

Di·oc·to·phy·me \(ˌ)dī-ˌäk-tə-ˈfī-(ˌ)mē\ *n* : a genus (family Dioctophymidae) of nematode worms including a single species (*D. renale*) which is a destructive parasite of the kidney of dogs, minks, and sometimes humans

Di·o·drast \ˈdī-ə-ˌdrast\ *trademark* — used for a sterile solution of iodopyracet for injection

di·oes·trus *chiefly Brit var of* DIESTRUS

di·op·ter \dī-ˈäp-tər, ˈdī-ˌäp-\ *n* : a unit of measurement of the refractive power of a lens equal to the reciprocal of the focal length in meters

di·op·tric \(ˌ)dī-ˈäp-trik\ *adj* **1** : producing or serving in refraction of a beam of light : REFRACTIVE; *specif* : assisting vision by refracting and focusing light **2** : produced by means of refraction

di·ox·ide \(ˌ)dī-ˈäk-ˌsīd\ *n* : an oxide (as carbon dioxide) containing two atoms of oxygen in a molecule

di·ox·in \(ˌ)dī-ˈäk-sən\ *n* : any of several heterocyclic hydrocarbons that occur esp. as persistent toxic impurities in herbicides; *esp* : TCDD — see AGENT ORANGE

di·oxy·ben·zone \(ˌ)dī-ˌäk-sē-ˈben-ˌzōn, -ben-ˈ\ *n* : a sunscreen $C_{14}H_{12}O_4$ that absorbs throughout the ultraviolet spectrum

dip \ˈdip\ *n* : a liquid preparation of an insecticide or parasiticide which is applied to animals by immersing them in it — see SHEEP-DIP — **dip** *vb*

di·pep·ti·dase \dī-ˈpep-tə-ˌdās, -ˌdāz\ *n* : any of various enzymes that hydrolyze dipeptides but not polypeptides

di·pep·tide \(ˌ)dī-ˈpep-ˌtīd\ *n* : a peptide that yields two molecules of amino acid on hydrolysis

di·pha·sic \(ˌ)dī-ˈfā-zik\ *adj* : having two phases: as **a** : exhibiting a stage of stimulation followed by a stage of depression or vice versa ⟨the ~ action of certain drugs⟩ **b** : relating to or being a record of a nerve impulse that is negative and positive — compare MONOPHASIC 1, POLYPHASIC 1

di·phen·hy·dra·mine \ˌdī-ˌfen-ˈhī-drə-ˌmēn\ *n* : an antihistamine $C_{17}H_{21}NO$ used esp. in the form of its hydrochloride $C_{17}H_{21}NO\cdot HCl$ to treat allergy symptoms and motion sickness

di·phen·oxy·late \ˌdī-ˌfen-ˈäk-sə-ˌlāt\ *n* : an antidiarrheal agent chemically related to meperidine and used in the form of its hydrochloride $C_{30}H_{32}N_2O_2\cdot HCl$ — see LOMOTIL

di·phe·nyl·hy·dan·to·in \(ˌ)dī-ˌfen-əl-hī-ˈdan-tə-wən, -ˌfen-ˈl-hī-\ *n* : PHENYTOIN

di·phos·phate \(ˌ)dī-ˈfäs-ˌfāt\ *n* : a phosphate containing two phosphate groups

2,3–di·phos·pho·glyc·er·ate *also* **di·phos·pho·glyc·er·ate** \(ˌtü-ˌthrē-)dī-ˌfäs-fō-ˈgli-sə-ˌrāt\ *n* : a phosphate that occurs in human erythrocytes and facilitates release of oxygen by decreasing the oxygen affinity of hemoglobin

di·phos·pho·pyr·i·dine nucleotide \-ˌpir-ə-ˌdēn-\ *n* : NAD

diph·the·ria \dif-ˈthir-ē-ə, dip-\ *n* : an acute febrile contagious disease marked by the formation of a false membrane esp. in the throat and caused by a bacterium of the genus *Corynebacterium* (*C. diphtheriae*) which produces a toxin causing inflammation of the heart and nervous system — **diph·the·ri·al** \-ē-əl\ *adj*

diph·ther·it·ic \ˌdif-thə-ˈri-tik, ˌdip-\ *adj* : relating to, produced in, or affected with diphtheria; *also* : resembling diphtheria esp. in the formation of a false membrane ⟨~ dysentery⟩

¹diph·the·roid \ˈdif-thə-ˌróid\ *adj* : resembling diphtheria

²diphtheroid *n* : a bacterium (esp. genus *Corynebacterium*) that resembles the bacterium of diphtheria but does not produce diphtheria toxin

di·phyl·lo·both·ri·a·sis \(ˌ)dī-ˌfi-lō-bä-ˈthrī-ə-səs\ *n, pl* **-a·ses** \-ˌsēz\ : infestation with or disease caused by the fish tapeworm (*Diphyllobothrium latum*)

Di·phyl·lo·both·ri·um \-ˈbä-thrē-əm\ *n* : a large genus of tapeworms (family Diphyllobothriidae) that includes the common fish tapeworm (*D. latum*)

dipl- *or* **diplo-** *comb form* : double : twofold ⟨*diplococcus*⟩ ⟨*diplopia*⟩

dip·la·cu·sis \ˌdi-plə-ˈkyü-səs\ *n, pl* **-cu·ses** \-ˌsēz\ : the hearing of a single tone as if it were two tones of different pitch

di·ple·gia \dī-ˈplē-jə, -jē-ə\ *n* : paralysis of corresponding parts (as the legs) on both sides of the body

dip·lo·coc·cus \ˌdi-plō-ˈkä-kəs\ *n, pl* **-coc·ci** \-ˈkä-ˌkī, -ˌkē; ˈkäk-ˌsī, -ˌsē\ : any of various encapsulated bacteria (as the pneumococcus) that usu. occur in pairs and that were formerly grouped in a single taxon (genus *Diplococcus*) but are now all assigned to other genera — **di·plo·coc·cal** \-kəl\ *adj*

dip·loe \ˈdi-plə-ˌwē\ *n* : cancellous bony tissue between the external and internal layers of the skull — **di·plo·ic** \də-ˈplō-ik, dī-\ *adj*

diploic vein *n* : any of several veins situated in channels in the diploe

¹**dip·loid** \ˈdi-ˌploid\ *adj* : having the basic chromosome number doubled — **dip·loi·dy** \-ˌploi-dē\ *n*

²**diploid** *n* : a single cell, individual, or generation characterized by the diploid chromosome number

dip·lo·mate \ˈdi-plə-ˌmāt\ *n* : a physician qualified to practice in a medical specialty by advanced training and experience in the specialty followed by passing an intensive examination by a national board of senior specialists

dip·lo·pia \di-ˈplō-pē-ə\ *n* : a disorder of vision in which two images of a single object are seen because of unequal action of the eye muscles — called also *double vision* — **dip·lo·pic** \-ˈplō-pik, -ˈplä-\ *adj*

dip·lo·tene \ˈdi-plə-ˌtēn\ *n* : a stage of meiotic prophase which follows the pachytene and during which the paired homologous chromosomes begin to separate and chiasmata become visible — **diplotene** *adj*

di·pole \ˈdī-ˌpōl\ *n* 1 : a pair of equal and opposite electric charges or magnetic poles of opposite sign separated by a small distance 2 : a body or system (as a molecule) having such charges — **di·po·lar** \-ˌpō-lər, -ˈpō-\ *adj*

di·pro·pi·o·nate \(ˌ)dī-ˈprō-pē-ə-ˌnāt\ *n* : an ester containing two propionate groups

dip·so·ma·nia \ˌdip-sə-ˈmā-nē-ə, -nyə\ *n* : an uncontrollable craving for alcoholic liquors — **dip·so·ma·ni·ac** \-nē-ˌak\ *n* — **dip·so·ma·ni·a·cal** \ˌdip-sō-mə-ˈnī-ə-kəl\ *adj*

dip·stick \ˈdip-ˌstik\ *n* : a chemically sensitive strip of cellulose used to identify the constituents (as glucose) of urine by immersion

dip·ter·an \ˈdip-tə-rən\ *adj* : of, relating to, or being a fly (sense 2a) — **dipteran** *n* — **dip·ter·ous** \-rəs\ *adj*

Di·py·lid·i·um \ˌdī-pī-ˈli-dē-əm, -pə-\ *n* : a genus of taenioid tapeworms including the common dog tapeworm (*D. caninum*)

di·pyr·i·dam·ole \(ˌ)dī-pir-ə-ˈda-ˌmōl, -ˌmōl\ *n* : a drug $C_{24}H_{40}N_8O_4$ used as a coronary vasodilator — see PERSANTINE

di·rec·tive \də-ˈrek-tiv, dī-\ *adj* : of or relating to psychotherapy in which the therapist introduces information, content, or attitudes not previously expressed by the client

di·rec·tor \də-ˈrek-tər, dī-\ *n* : an instrument grooved to guide and limit the motion of a surgical knife

direct pyramidal tract *n* : VENTRAL CORTICOSPINAL TRACT

Di·ro·fi·lar·ia \ˌdī-(ˌ)rō-fə-ˈlar-ē-ə\ *n* : a genus of filarial worms (family Dipetalonematidae) that includes the heartworm (*D. immitis*) — **di·ro·fi·lar·i·al** \-ē-əl\ *adj*

di·ro·fi·la·ri·a·sis \-ˌfi-lə-ˈrī-ə-səs\ *n, pl* **-a·ses** \-ˌsēz\ : infestation with filarial worms of the genus *Dirofilaria* and esp. with the heartworm (*D. immitis*)

dirty \ˈdər-tē\ *adj* **dirt·i·er; -est** : contaminated with infecting organisms

dis·abil·i·ty \ˌdi-sə-ˈbi-lə-tē\ *n, pl* **-ties** 1 : the condition of being disabled 2 : inability to pursue an occupation because of physical or mental impairment

dis·able \di-ˈsā-bəl, -ˈzā-\ *vb* **dis·abled; dis·abling** : to deprive of a mental or physical capacity

dis·abled *adj* : incapacitated by illness, injury, or wounds; *broadly* : physically or mentally impaired

dis·able·ment \-mənt\ *n* : the act of becoming disabled to the extent that full wages cannot be earned; *also* : the state of being so disabled

di·sac·cha·ri·dase \(ˌ)dī-ˈsa-kə-rə-ˌdās, -ˌdāz\ *n* : an enzyme (as maltase) that hydrolyzes disaccharides

di·sac·cha·ride \(ˌ)dī-ˈsa-kə-ˌrīd\ *n* : any of a class of sugars (as sucrose) that on hydrolysis yields two monosaccharide molecules

dis·ar·tic·u·la·tion \ˌdi-sär-ˌti-kyə-ˈlā-shən\ *n* : separation or amputation of a body part at a joint (∼ of the shoulder) — **dis·ar·tic·u·late** \-ˈti-kyə-ˌlāt\ *vb*

disc *var of* DISK

disc- *or* **disci-** *or* **disco-** *comb form* : disk ⟨*disci*form⟩

¹**dis·charge** \dis-ˈchärj, ˈdis-\ *vb* **dis·charged; dis·charg·ing** 1 : to release from confinement, custody, or care (∼ a patient from the hospital) 2 a : to give outlet to or emit (a boil *discharging* pus) b : to release or give expression to

²**dis·charge** \ˈdis-ˌchärj, dis-ˈ\ *n* 1 : the act of relieving of something (∼ of a repressed impulse) 2 : release from confinement, custody, or care 3

: something that is emitted or evacuated ⟨a purulent ∼⟩

disci pl of DISCUS

dis·ci·form \'di-sə-ˌförm\ adj : round or oval in shape

dis·cis·sion \də-'si-shən, -zhən\ n : an incision (as in treating cataract) of the capsule of the lens of the eye

dis·clos·ing \dis-'klō-ziŋ\ adj : being or using an agent (as a tablet or liquid) that contains a usu. red dye that adheres to and stains dental plaque

disc·o·gram, dis·cog·ra·phy var of DISKOGRAM, DISKOGRAPHY

¹**dis·coid** \'dis-ˌköid\ adj 1 : resembling a disk : being flat and circular 2 : characterized by macules ⟨∼ lupus erythematosus⟩

²**discoid** n : an instrument with a disk-shaped blade used in dentistry for carving

dis·coi·dal \dis-'köid-ᵊl\ adj : of, resembling, or producing a disk; esp : having the villi restricted to one or more disklike areas

dis·cop·a·thy \dis-'kä-pə-thē\ n, pl **-thies** : any disease affecting an intervertebral disk

dis·cor·dant \dis-'kórd-ᵊnt\ adj, of twins : dissimilar with respect to one or more particular characters — compare CONCORDANT — **dis·cor·dance** \-ᵊns\ n

dis·crete \dis-'krēt, 'dis-ˌ\ adj : characterized by distinct unconnected lesions ⟨∼ smallpox⟩ — compare CONFLUENT 2

dis·crim·i·nate \dis-'kri-mə-ˌnāt\ vb **-nat·ed; -nat·ing** : to respond selectively to (a stimulus)

dis·crim·i·na·tion \dis-ˌkri-mə-'nā-shən\ n : the process by which two stimuli differing in some aspect are responded to differently

dis·cus \'dis-kəs\ n, pl **dis·ci** \-ˌkī, -kē\ : any of various rounded and flattened anatomical structures

discus pro·lig·er·us \-prō-'li-jə-rəs\ n : CUMULUS

dis·ease \di-'zēz\ n : an impairment of the normal state of the living body or one of its parts that interrupts or modifies the performance of the vital functions and is a response to environmental factors (as malnutrition), to specific infective agents (as viruses), to inherent defects of the organism (as genetic anomalies), or to combinations of these factors : SICKNESS, ILLNESS — **dis·eased** \-'zēzd\ adj

dis·equi·lib·ri·um \(ˌ)di-ˌsē-kwə-'li-brē-əm, -ˌse-\ n, pl **-ri·ums** or **-ria** : loss or lack of equilibrium

dis·func·tion var of DYSFUNCTION

dis·har·mo·ny \(ˌ)dis-'här-mə-nē\ n, pl **-nies** : lack of harmony — see OCCLUSAL DISHARMONY

dis·in·fect \ˌdis-ᵊn-'fekt\ vb : to free from infection esp. by destroying

harmful microorganisms — **dis·in·fec·tion** \-'fek-shən\ n

¹**dis·in·fec·tant** \-'fek-tənt\ n : an agent that frees from infection; esp : a chemical that destroys vegetative forms of harmful microorganisms but not ordinarily bacterial spores

²**disinfectant** adj : serving or tending to disinfect : suitable for use in disinfecting

dis·in·fest \ˌdis-ᵊn-'fest\ vb : to rid of small animal pests (as insects or rodents) — **dis·in·fes·ta·tion** \(ˌ)dis-ˌin-ˌfes-'tā-shən\ n

dis·in·fes·tant \ˌdis-ᵊn-'fes-tənt\ n : a disinfesting agent

dis·in·hi·bi·tion \(ˌ)di-ˌsin-hə-'bi-shən, -ˌsi-nə-\ n : loss or reduction of an inhibition (as by the action of interfering stimuli or events) ⟨∼ of a reflex⟩

dis·in·hib·i·to·ry \-in-'hi-bə-ˌtör-ē\ adj : tending to overcome psychological inhibition ⟨∼ drugs⟩

dis·in·ter \ˌdis-in-'tər\ vb : to take out of the grave or tomb — **dis·in·ter·ment** \-mənt\ n

dis·junc·tion \dis-'jəŋk-shən\ n : the separation of chromosomes or chromatids during anaphase of mitosis or meiosis

disk \'disk\ n : any of various rounded or flattened anatomical structures: as **a** : a mammalian blood cell **b** : BLIND SPOT **c** : INTERVERTEBRAL DISK — see SLIPPED DISK

disk·ec·to·my \dis-'kek-tə-mē\ n, pl **-mies** : surgical removal of an intervertebral disk

disk·o·gram \'dis-kə-ˌgram\ n : a roentgenogram of an intervertebral disk made after injection of a radiopaque substance

dis·kog·ra·phy \dis-'kä-grə-fē\ n, pl **-phies** : the process of making a diskogram

dis·lo·cate \'dis-lō-ˌkāt, -lə-; (ˌ)dis-'lō-ˌkāt\ vb **-cat·ed; -cat·ing** : to put (a body part) out of order by displacing a bone from its normal connections with another bone; also : to displace (a bone) from normal connections with another bone

dis·lo·ca·tion \ˌdis-(ˌ)lō-'kā-shən, -lə-\ n : displacement of one or more bones at a joint : LUXATION

dismutase — see SUPEROXIDE DISMUTASE

di·so·di·um \(ˌ)dī-'sō-dē-əm\ adj : containing two atoms of sodium in a molecule

disodium cromoglycate n : CROMOLYN SODIUM

disodium ed·e·tate \-'e-də-ˌtāt\ n : a hydrated disodium salt $C_{10}H_{14}N_2Na_2$-$O_8 \cdot 2H_2O$ of EDTA that has an affinity for calcium and is used to treat hypercalcemia and pathological calcification

di·so·pyr·a·mide \ˌdī-(ˌ)sō-'pir-ə-ˌmīd\ n : a cardiac depressant $C_{21}H_{29}N_3O$

used in the treatment of ventricular arrhythmias

¹dis·or·der \(ₗ)di-ˈsȯr-dər, -ˈzȯr-\ vb dis·or·dered; dis·or·der·ing : to disturb the regular or normal functions of

²disorder n : an abnormal physical or mental condition : AILMENT

dis·or·dered adj 1 : not functioning in a normal orderly healthy way ⟨∼ bodily functions⟩ 2 : mentally unbalanced ⟨a ∼ patient⟩

dis·or·ga·ni·za·tion \(ₗ)di-ₗsȯr-gə-nə-ˈzā-shən\ n : psychopathological inconsistency in personality, mental functions, or overt behavior — dis·or·ga·nize \(ₗ)di-ˈsȯr-gə-ₗnīz\ vb

dis·ori·ent \(ₗ)di-ˈsȯr-ē-ₗent\ vb : to produce a state of disorientation in : DISORIENTATE

dis·ori·en·ta·tion \(ₗ)di-ₗsȯr-ē-ən-ˈtā-shən, -ₗen-\ n : a usu. transient state of confusion esp. as to time, place, or identity often as a result of disease or drugs — dis·ori·en·tate \-ˈsȯr-ē-ən-ₗtāt, -ₗen-\ vb

dis·par·i·ty \di-ˈspar-ə-tē\ n, pl -ties : the state of being different or dissimilar (as in the sensory information received) — see RETINAL DISPARITY

dis·pen·sa·ry \di-ˈspen-sə-rē\ n, pl -ries : a place where medicine or medical or dental treatment is dispensed

dis·pen·sa·to·ry \di-ˈspen-sə-ₗtȯr-ē\ n, pl -ries 1 : a book or medicinal formulary containing a systematic description of the drugs and preparations used in medicine — compare PHARMACOPOEIA 2 : DISPENSARY

dis·pense \dis-ˈpens\ vb dis·pensed; dis·pens·ing 1 : to put up (a prescription or medicine) 2 : to prepare and distribute (medication) — dis·pen·sa·tion \ₗdis-pən-ˈsā-shən, -pen-\ n

dispensing optician n, Brit : a person qualified and licensed to fit and supply eyeglasses

dispersion medium n : the liquid, gaseous, or solid phase in a two-phase system in which the particles of the other phase are distributed

dis·place·ment \dis-ˈsplā-smənt\ n 1 : the act or process of removing something from its usual or proper place or the state resulting from this : DISLOCATION ⟨the ∼ of a knee joint⟩ 2 : the quantity in which or the degree to which something is displaced 3 a : the direction of an emotion or impulse away from its original object (as an idea or person) to something that is more acceptable b : SUBLIMATION c : the substitution of another form of behavior for what is usual or expected esp. when the usual response is nonadaptive — dis·place \-ˈsplās\ vb

dis·pro·por·tion \ₗdis-prə-ˈpȯr-shən\ n : absence of symmetry or the proper dimensional relationship — see CEPHALOPELVIC DISPROPORTION

dis·rup·tive \dis-ˈrəp-tiv\ adj : characterized by psychologically disorganized behavior ⟨a confused, incoherent, and ∼ patient in the manic phase⟩

dissecans — see OSTEOCHONDRITIS DISSECANS

dis·sect \di-ˈsekt, dī-; ˈdī-ₗ\ vb 1 : to cut so as to separate into pieces or to expose the several parts of (as an animal or a cadaver) for scientific examination; specif : to separate or follow along natural lines of cleavage (as through connective tissue) 2 : to make a medical dissection — dis·sec·tor \-ˈsek-tər, -ₗsek-\ n

dis·sec·tion \di-ˈsek-shən, dī-; ˈdī-ₗ\ n 1 : the act or process of dissecting or separating: as a : the surgical removal along natural lines of cleavage of tissues which are or might become diseased b : the digital separation of tissues (as in heart-valve operations) — compare FINGER FRACTURE 2 a : something (as a part or the whole of an animal) that has been dissected b : an anatomical specimen prepared in this way

dis·sem·i·nat·ed \di-ˈse-mə-ₗnā-təd\ adj : widely dispersed in a tissue, organ, or the entire body ⟨∼ gonococcal disease⟩ — dis·sem·i·na·tion \-ₗse-mə-ˈnā-shən\ n

dis·so·ci·a·tion \(ₗ)di-ₗsō-sē-ˈā-shən, -shē-\ n 1 : the process by which a chemical combination breaks up into simpler constituents 2 : the separation of whole segments of the personality (as in multiple personality) or of discrete mental processes (as in the schizophrenias) from the mainstream of consciousness or of behavior — dis·so·ci·ate \-ˈsō-sē-ₗāt, -shē-\ vb — dis·so·cia·tive \(ₗ)di-ˈsō-shē-ₗā-tiv, -sē-, -shə-tiv\ adj

dis·so·lu·tion \ₗdi-sə-ˈlü-shən\ n : the act or process of dissolving

dis·solve \di-ˈzälv, -ˈzȯlv\ vb dis·solved; dis·solv·ing 1 : to pass or cause to pass into solution 2 : to cause to melt or liquefy 3 : to become fluid — dis·solv·er n

dis·so·nance \ˈdi-sə-nəns\ n : inconsistency between the beliefs one holds or between one's actions and one's beliefs — see COGNITIVE DISSONANCE

dist- — see DISTO-

dis·tal \ˈdist-əl\ adj 1 : situated away from the point of attachment or origin or a central point: as a : located away from the center of the body ⟨the ∼ end of a bone⟩ — compare PROXIMAL 1a b : located away from the mesial plane of the body — compare MESIAL 2 c : of, relating to, or being the surface of a tooth that is next to the following tooth counting from the middle of the front of the upper or lower jaw or that faces the back of the mouth in the case of the last tooth on each side — compare MESIAL 3, PROXIMAL 1b 2 : physical or social rather than sensory — compare PROXIMAL 2 — **dis·tal·ly** *adv*

distal convoluted tubule *n* : the convoluted portion of the nephron lying between the loop of Henle and the nonsecretory part of the nephron and concerned esp. with the concentration of urine — called also *convoluted tubule, distal tubule*

distalis — see PARS DISTALIS

distal radioulnar joint *n* : a pivot joint between the lower end of the ulna and the ulnar notch on the lower end of the radius that permits rotation of the distal end of the radius around the longitudinal axis of the ulna — called also *inferior radioulnar joint*

dis·tem·per \dis-ˈtem-pər\ *n* : a disordered or abnormal bodily state esp. of quadruped mammals: as **a** : a highly contagious virus disease esp. of dogs that is marked by fever, leukopenia, and respiratory, gastrointestinal, and neurological symptoms and that is caused by a paramyxovirus **b** : STRANGLES **c** : PANLEUKOPENIA

dis·tend \di-ˈstend\ *vb* : to enlarge or stretch out (as from internal pressure)

dis·ten·si·ble \-ˈsten-sə-bəl\ *adj* : capable of being distended, extended, or dilated — **dis·ten·si·bil·i·ty** \-ˌsten-sə-ˈbi-lə-tē\ *n*

dis·ten·sion *or* **dis·ten·tion** \di-ˈstenchən\ *n* : the act of distending or the state of being distended esp. unduly or abnormally

disto- *also* **dist-** *or* **disti-** *comb form* : distal ⟨*disto*buccal⟩

dis·to·buc·cal \ˌdis-tō-ˈbə-kəl\ *adj* : relating to or located on the distal and buccal surfaces of a molar or premolar — **dis·to·buc·cal·ly** *adv*

dis·to·lin·gual \-ˈliŋ-gwel, -gyə-wəl\ *adj* : relating to or situated on the distal and lingual surfaces of a tooth

dis·to·ma·to·sis \ˌdī-stō-mə-ˈtō-səs\ *n, pl* **-to·ses** \-ˌsēz\ : infestation with or disease (as liver rot) caused by digenetic trematode worms

dis·to·mi·a·sis \ˌdī-stō-ˈmī-ə-səs\ *n, pl* **-a·ses** \-ˌsēz\ : DISTOMATOSIS

dis·tor·tion \di-ˈstor-shən\ *n* **1** : the censorship of unacceptable unconscious impulses so that they are unrecognizable to the ego in the manifest content of a dream **2** : a lack of correspondence of size or intensity in an image resulting from defects in an optical system

dis·tract·i·bil·i·ty \di-ˌstrak-tə-ˈbi-lə-tē\ *n, pl* **-ties** : a condition in which the attention of the mind is easily distracted by small and irrelevant stimuli — **dis·tract·i·ble** \-ˈstrak-tə-bəl\ *adj*

dis·trac·tion \di-ˈstrak-shən\ *n* **1 a** : diversion of the attention **b** : mental derangement **2** : excessive separation (as from improper traction) of fracture fragments — **dis·tract** \di-ˈstrakt\ *vb*

dis·tress \di-ˈstres\ *n* : pain or suffering affecting the body, a bodily part, or the mind ⟨gastric ∼⟩ ⟨respiratory ∼⟩

dis·tri·bu·tion \ˌdis-trə-ˈbyü-shən\ *n* : the pattern of branching and termination of a ramifying anatomical structure (as a nerve or artery)

district nurse *n, Brit* : a qualified nurse who is employed by a local authority to visit and treat patients in their own homes — compare VISITING NURSE

dis·turbed \di-ˈstərbd\ *adj* : showing symptoms of emotional illness ⟨∼ children⟩ — **dis·tur·bance** \-ˈstər-bəns\ *n*

di·sul·fi·ram \dī-ˈsəl-fə-ˌram\ *n* : a compound $C_{10}H_{20}N_2S_4$ that causes a severe physiological reaction to alcohol and is used esp. in the treatment of alcoholism — called also *tetraethylthiuram disulfide;* see ANTABUSE

di·sul·phi·ram *chiefly Brit var of* DISULFIRAM

di·thra·nol \ˈdī-thrə-ˌnȯl, ˈdi-, -ˌnōl\ *n, chiefly Brit* : ANTHRALIN

di·ure·sis \ˌdī-yə-ˈrē-səs\ *n, pl* **di·ure·ses** \-ˌsēz\ : an increased excretion of urine

di·uret·ic \ˌdī-yə-ˈre-tik\ *adj* : tending to increase the flow of urine — **di·uret·i·cal·ly** \-ti-k(ə-)lē\ *adv*

²diuretic *n* : an agent that increases the flow of urine

Di·ur·il \ˈdī-yur-il\ *trademark* — used for a preparation of chlorothiazide

di·ur·nal \dī-ˈərn-ᵊl\ *adj* **1** : having a daily cycle ⟨∼ rhythms⟩ **2** : of, relating to, or occurring in the daytime ⟨∼ activity⟩ — **di·ur·nal·ly** *adv*

di·ver·gence \də-ˈvər-jəns, dī-\ *n* **1** : a drawing apart **2** : dissemination of the effect of activity of a single nerve cell through multiple synaptic connections — compare CONVERGENCE 2 — **di·verge** \-ˈvərj\ *vb* — **di·ver·gent** \-ˈvər-jənt\ *adj*

di·ver·tic·u·lar \ˌdī-vər-ˈti-kyə-lər\ *adj* : consisting of or resembling a diverticulum

di·ver·tic·u·lec·to·my \ˌdī-vər-ˌti-kyə-ˈlek-tə-mē\ *n, pl* **-mies** : the surgical removal of a diverticulum

di·ver·tic·u·li·tis \-ˈlī-təs\ *n* : inflammation of a diverticulum — called also *diverticular disease*

di·ver·tic·u·lo·pexy \-ˈlä-pək-sē\ *n, pl* **-ex·ies** : surgical obliteration or fixation of a diverticulum

di·ver·tic·u·lo·sis \-ˈlō-səs\ *n, pl* **-lo·ses** \-ˌsēz\ : an intestinal disorder characterized by the presence of many diverticula

di·ver·tic·u·lum \ˌdī-vər-ˈti-kyə-ləm\ *n, pl* **-la** \-lə\ **1** : an abnormal pouch or sac opening from a hollow organ (as the intestine or bladder) **2** : a blind tube or sac branching off from a cavity or canal of the body

di·vide \də-ˈvīd\ *vb* **di·vid·ed; di·vid·ing 1** : to separate into two or more parts ⟨∼ a nerve surgically⟩ **2** : to undergo replication, multiplication, fission, or separation into parts ⟨actively *dividing* cells⟩

di·vid·er \də-'vī-dər\ *n* : the second incisor tooth of a horse situated between the center and corner incisors on each side — compare NIPPER

di·vi·sion \də-'vi-zhən\ *n* **1** : the act or process of dividing : the state of being divided — see CELL DIVISION **2** : a group of organisms forming part of a larger group; *specif* : a primary category of the plant kingdom that is equivalent to a phylum — **di·vi·sion·al** \-'vi-zhə-nəl\ *adj*

di·zy·got·ic \dī-zī-'gä-tik\ *adj, of twins* : FRATERNAL

di·zy·gous \(')dī-'zī-gəs\ *var of* DIZYGOTIC

diz·zi·ness \'di-zē-nəs\ *n* : the condition of being dizzy; *esp* : a sensation of unsteadiness accompanied by a feeling of movement within the head — compare VERTIGO 1

diz·zy \'di-zē\ *adj* **diz·zi·er; -est** **1** : having a whirling sensation in the head with a tendency to fall **2** : mentally confused — **diz·zi·ly** \'di-zə-lē\ *adv*

DJD *abbr* degenerative joint disease

DM *abbr* diabetes mellitus

DMD *abbr* [Latin *dentariae medicinae doctor*] doctor of dental medicine

DMF *abbr* decayed, missing, and filled teeth

DMSO \dē-(')em-(')es-'ō\ *n* : DIMETHYL SULFOXIDE

DMT \dē-(')em-'tē\ *n* : DIMETHYLTRYPTAMINE

DNA \dē-(')en-'ā\ *n* : any of various nucleic acids that are usu. the molecular basis of heredity, are localized esp. in cell nuclei, and are constructed of a double helix held together by hydrogen bonds between purine and pyrimidine bases which project inward from two chains containing alternate links of deoxyribose and phosphate — called also *deoxyribonucleic acid;* see RECOMBINANT DNA

DNA fingerprinting *n* : a method of identification (as for forensic purposes) by determining the sequence of base pairs in the DNA esp. of a person — **DNA fingerprint** *n*

DNA polymerase *n* : any of several polymerases that promote replication or repair of DNA usu. using single‡stranded DNA as a template

DN·ase \(')dē-'en-ˌās, -ˌāz\ *also* **DNA·ase** \(')dē-'en-'ā-ˌās, -ˌāz\ *n* : DEOXYRIBONUCLEASE

DNR *abbr* do not resuscitate

DO *abbr* doctor of osteopathy

DOA *abbr* dead on arrival

DOB *abbr* date of birth

do·bu·ta·mine \dō-'byü-tə-ˌmēn\ *n* : a strongly inotropic catecholamine used in the form of its hydrochloride $C_{18}H_{23}NO_3·HCl$ esp. to increase cardiac output and lower wedge pressure in heart failure and after cardiopulmonary bypass surgery

doc \'däk\ *n* : DOCTOR — used chiefly as a familiar term of address

¹doc·tor \'däk-tər\ *n* **1 a** : a person who has earned one of the highest academic degrees (as a PhD) conferred by a university **b** : a person awarded an honorary doctorate by a college or university **2** : one skilled or specializing in healing arts; *esp* : a physician, surgeon, dentist, or veterinarian licensed to practice his or her profession

²doctor *vb* **doc·tored; doc·tor·ing 1 a** : to give medical treatment to **b** : to practice medicine **2** : CASTRATE, SPAY

doc·u·sate \'dä-kyü-ˌsāt\ *n* : any of several laxative salts and esp. the sodium salt $C_{20}H_{37}NaO_7S$ used to soften stools

dog \'dog\ *n, often attrib* : a highly variable carnivorous domesticated mammal (*Canis familiaris*); *broadly* : any member of the family (Canidae) to which the dog belongs

dog flea *n* : a flea of the genus *Ctenocephalides* (*C. canis*) that feeds chiefly on dogs and cats

dog tapeworm *n* : a tapeworm of the genus *Dipylidium* (*D. caninum*) occurring in dogs and cats and sometimes in humans

dog tick *n* : AMERICAN DOG TICK

dolens — see PHLEGMASIA ALBA DOLENS, PHLEGMASIA CERULEA DOLENS

dolicho- *comb form* : long ⟨*dolichocephalic*⟩

dol·i·cho·ce·phal·ic \dä-li-kō-sə-'fa-lik\ *adj* : having a relatively long head with a cephalic index of less than 75 — **dol·i·cho·ceph·a·ly** \-'se-fə-lē\ *n*

Do·lo·bid \'dō-lə-ˌbid\ *trademark* — used for a preparation of diflunisal

do·lor \'dō-lər, 'dä-\ *n* **1** *obs* : physical pain — used in old medicine as one of five cardinal symptoms of inflammation **2** : mental suffering or anguish

DOM \dē-(')ō-'em\ *n* : STP

dome \'dōm\ *n* : a rounded-arch element in the wave tracing in an electroencephalogram

do·mi·cil·i·ary \dä-mə-'si-lē-ˌer-ē, ˌdō-\ *adj* **1** : provided or attended in the home rather than in an institution ⟨∼ midwifery⟩ **2** : providing, constituting, or provided by an institution for chronically ill or permanently disabled persons requiring minimal medical attention ⟨∼ care⟩

dom·i·nance \'dä-mə-nəns\ *n* : the fact or state of being dominant: as **a** : the property of one of a pair of alleles or traits that suppresses expression of the other in the heterozygous condition **b** : functional asymmetry between a pair of bodily structures (as the right and left hands)

¹dom·i·nant \-nənt\ *adj* **1** : exerting forcefulness or having dominance in a social hierarchy **2** : being the one of a pair of bodily structures that is the more effective or predominant in action (the $\sim$ eye) **3** : of, relating to, or exerting genetic dominance — **dom·i·nant·ly** adv

²dominant n **1** : a dominant genetic character or factor **2** : a dominant individual in a social hierarchy

do·nee \dō-'nē\ n : a recipient of biological material (as blood or a graft)

Don Juan·ism \'dän-'hwä-₁ni-zəm, -'wä-\ n, pl **Don Juanisms** : male sexual promiscuity that is motivated by impotence or feelings of inferiority or unconscious homosexual impulses

do·nor \'dō-nər, -₁nȯr\ n **1** : one used as a source of biological material (as blood or an organ) **2** : a compound capable of giving up a part (as an atom) for combination with an acceptor

Don·o·van body \'dä-nə-vən-, 'də-\ n : an encapsulated gram-negative bacterium of the genus *Calymmatobacterium* (*C. granulomatis*) that is the causative agent of granuloma inguinale and is characterized by one or two opposite polar chromatin masses — compare LEISHMAN-DONOVAN BODY

  C. Donovan — see LEISHMAN-DONOVAN BODY

do·pa \'dō-pə, -(₁)pä\ n : an amino acid $C_9H_{11}NO_4$ that in the levorotatory form is found in the broad bean and is used in the treatment of Parkinson's disease

L–dopa — see entry alphabetized in the letter *l*

do·pa·mine \'dō-pə-₁mēn\ n : a monoamine $C_8H_{11}NO_2$ that is a decarboxylated form of dopa and occurs esp. as a neurotransmitter in the brain and as an intermediate in the biosynthesis of epinephrine — see INTROPIN

do·pa·mi·ner·gic \₁dō-pə-ə-mē-'nər-jik\ adj : relating to, participating in, or activated by the neurotransmitter activity of dopamine or related substances ($\sim$ activity) ($\sim$ neurons)

dope \'dōp\ n **1** : a preparation of an illicit, habit-forming, or narcotic drug (as opium, heroin, or marijuana) **2** : a preparation given to a racehorse to help or hinder its performance — **dope** vb

Dopp·ler \'dä-plər\ adj : of, relating to, or utilizing a shift in frequency in accordance with the Doppler effect

  Doppler, Christian Johann (1803–1853), Austrian physicist and mathematician.

Doppler effect n : a change in the frequency with which waves (as sound or light) from a given source reach an observer when the source and the observer are in rapid motion with respect to each other so that the frequency increases or decreases according to the speed at which the distance is decreasing or increasing

dors- — see DORSO-

dorsa pl of DORSUM

¹dor·sal \'dȯr-səl\ adj **1** : being or located near, on, or toward the upper surface of an animal (as a quadruped) opposite the lower or ventral surface **2** : being or located near, on, or toward the back or posterior part of the human body — **dor·sal·ly** \-sə-lē\ adv

²dorsal n : a dorsally located part; esp : a thoracic vertebra

dorsal column n : DORSAL HORN

dorsal horn n : a longitudinal subdivision of gray matter in the dorsal part of each lateral half of the spinal cord that receives terminals from some afferent fibers of the dorsal roots of the spinal nerves — called also *dorsal column, posterior column, posterior gray column, posterior horn*; compare LATERAL COLUMN 1, VENTRAL HORN

dorsal interosseus n **1** : any of four small muscles of the hand that act to draw the fingers away from the long axis of the middle finger, flex the fingers at the metacarpophalangeal joints, and extend their distal two phalanges **2** : any of four small muscles of the foot that act to draw the toes away from the long axis of the second toe, flex their proximal phalanges, and extend the distal phalanges

dorsalis — see INTEROSSEUS DORSALIS, SACROCOCCYGEUS DORSALIS, TABES DORSALIS

dorsalis pe·dis \dȯr-'sa-ləs-'pe-dəs, -'sā-, -'sä-, -'pē-\ n : an artery of the upper surface of the foot that is a direct continuation of the anterior tibial artery — called also *dorsalis pedis artery*

dorsal lip n : the margin of the fold of blastula wall that delineates the dorsal limit of the blastopore

dorsal mesogastrium n : MESOGASTRIUM 2

dorsal root n : the one of the two roots of a spinal nerve that passes posteriorly to the spinal cord separating the posterior and lateral funiculi and that consists of sensory fibers — called also *posterior root*; compare VENTRAL ROOT

dorsal root ganglion n : SPINAL GANGLION

dorsal spinocerebellar tract n : SPINOCEREBELLAR TRACT A

dorsi — see ILIOCOSTALIS DORSI, LATISSIMUS DORSI, LONGISSIMUS DORSI

dor·si·flex·ion \₁dȯr-sə-'flek-shən\ n : flexion in a dorsal direction; esp : flexion of the foot in an upward direction — compare PLANTAR FLEXION — **dor·si·flex** \'dȯr-sə-₁fleks\ vb

dor·si·flex·or \'dȯr-sə-₁flek-sər\ n : a muscle causing flexion in a dorsal direction

dorso- or **dorsi-** also **dors-** comb form **1** : dorsal (*dorsi*flexion) **2** : dorsal and (*dorso*lateral)

dor·so·lat·er·al \₁dȯr-sō-'la-tə-rəl, -'la-trəl\ adj : of, relating to, or involving both the back and the sides (lesions of the $\sim$ hypothalamus⟩ — **dor·so·lat·er·al·ly** *adv*

dorsolateral tract *n* : a slender column of white matter between the dorsal gray column and the periphery of the spinal cord — called also *tract of Lissauer*

dor·so·me·di·al \-ˈmē-dē-əl\ *adj* : located toward the back and near the midline

dor·so·ven·tral \-ˈven-trəl\ *adj* : relating to, involving, or extending along the axis joining the dorsal and ventral sides — **dor·so·ven·tral·ly** *adv*

dor·sum \ˈdȯr-səm\ *n, pl* **dor·sa** \-sə\ **1** : the upper surface of an appendage or part **2** : BACK; *esp* : the entire dorsal surface of an animal

dos·age \ˈdō-sij\ *n* **1 a** : the addition of an ingredient or the application of an agent in a measured dose **b** : the presence and relative representation or strength of a factor or agent (as a gene) **2 a** : DOSE 1 **b** (1) : the giving of a dose (2) : regulation or determination of doses

¹**dose** \ˈdōs\ *n* **1 a** : the measured quantity of a therapeutic agent to be taken at one time **b** : the quantity of radiation administered or absorbed **2** : a gonorrheal infection

²**dose** *vb* **dosed; dos·ing 1** : to divide (as a medicine) into doses **2** : to give a dose to; *esp* : to give medicine to **3** : to take medicine **4** : to treat with an application or agent

do·sim·e·ter \dō-ˈsi-mə-tər\ *n* : a device for measuring doses of radiations (as X rays) — **do·si·met·ric** \ˌdō-sə-ˈme-trik\ *adj* — **do·sim·e·try** \dō-ˈsi-mə-trē\ *n*

double bind *n* : a psychological predicament in which a person receives from a single source conflicting messages that allow no appropriate response to be made

dou·ble–blind \ˌdə-bəl-ˈblīnd\ *adj* : of, relating to, or being an experimental procedure in which neither the subjects nor the experimenters know the identity of the individuals in the test and control groups during the actual course of the experiments — compare SINGLE-BLIND

double bond *n* : a chemical bond consisting of two covalent bonds between two atoms in a molecule — compare TRIPLE BOND; see UNSATURATED b

double chin *n* : a fleshy or fatty fold under the chin — **dou·ble–chinned** \-ˈchind\ *adj*

double helix *n* : the structural arrangement of DNA in space that consists of paired polynucleotide strands stabilized by chemical bonds between the chains linking purine and pyrimidine bases — compare ALPHA-HELIX, WATSON-CRICK MODEL — **dou·ble–he·li·cal** \-ˈhe-li-kəl, -ˈhē-\ *adj*

dou·ble–joint·ed \ˌdə-bəl-ˈjȯin-təd\ *adj*

: having a joint that permits an exceptional degree of freedom of motion of the parts joined

double pneumonia *n* : pneumonia affecting both lungs

double vision *n* : DIPLOPIA

douche \ˈdüsh\ *n* **1 a** : a jet or current esp. of water directed against a part or into a cavity of the body **b** : an act of cleansing with a douche **2** : a device for giving douches — **douche** *vb*

Doug·las bag \ˈdə-gləs-\ *n* : an inflatable bag used to collect expired air for the determination of oxygen consumption and basal metabolic rate

Douglas, Claude Gordon (1882–1963), British physiologist.

Douglas's cul·de·sac \ˈdə-glə-ˌsəz-\ *n* : POUCH OF DOUGLAS

Douglas's pouch *n* : POUCH OF DOUGLAS

douloureux — see TIC DOULOUREUX

dow·a·ger's hump \ˈdau̇-i-jərz-\ *n* : an abnormal outward curvature of the upper back with round shoulders and stooped posture caused esp. by bone loss and anterior compression of the vertebrae in osteoporosis

down·er \ˈdau̇-nər\ *n* : a depressant drug; *esp* : BARBITURATE

Down's syndrome \ˈdau̇nz-\ *or* **Down syndrome** \ˈdau̇n-\ *n* : a congenital condition characterized by moderate to severe mental retardation, slanting eyes, a broad short skull, broad hands with short fingers, and by trisomy of the human chromosome numbered 21 — called also *Down's, trisomy 21*

Down \ˈdau̇n\, John Langdon Haydon (1828–1896), British physician.

down·stream \ˈdau̇n-ˈstrēm\ *adv or adj* : in the same direction along a molecule of DNA or RNA as that in which transcription and translation take place and toward the end having a hydroxyl group attached to the position labeled 3′ in the terminal nucleotide — compare UPSTREAM

dox·e·pin \ˈdäk-sə-ˌpin, -pən\ *n* : a tricyclic antidepressant administered as the hydrochloride salt $C_9H_{21}NO·HCl$ — see SINEQUAN

doxo·ru·bi·cin \ˌdäk-sə-ˈrü-bə-sən\ *n* : an anthracycline antibiotic with broad antitumor activity that is obtained from a bacterium of the genus *Streptomyces* (*S. peucetius*) and is administered in the form of its hydrochloride $C_{27}H_{29}NO_{11}·HCl$ — see ADRIAMYCIN

doxy·cy·cline \ˌdäk-sə-ˈsī-ˌklēn\ *n* : a broad-spectrum tetracycline antibiotic $C_{22}H_{24}N_2O_8$ with potent antibacterial activity that is often taken orally by travelers as a prophylactic against diarrhea — see VIBRAMYCIN

dox·yl·amine \däk-ˈsi-lə-ˌmēn, -mən\ *n* : an antihistamine usu. used in the form of its succinate $C_{17}H_{22}N_2O·C_4H_6O_4$

DP *abbr* doctor of podiatry

DPH *abbr* **1** department of public health **2** doctor of public health

DPM *abbr* doctor of podiatric medicine

DPT *abbr* diphtheria-pertussis-tetanus (vaccines)

dr *abbr* dram

Dr *abbr* doctor

drac·on·ti·a·sis \ˌdra-ˌkän-ˈtī-ə-səs\ *n, pl* **-a·ses** \-ˌsēz\ : DRACUNCULIASIS

dra·cun·cu·li·a·sis \drə-ˌkəŋ-kyə-ˈlī-ə-səs\ *n, pl* **-a·ses** \-ˌsēz\ : infestation with or disease caused by the guinea worm

dra·cun·cu·lo·sis \-ˈlō-səs\ *n, pl* **-lo·ses** \-ˌsēz\ : DRACUNCULIASIS

Dra·cun·cu·lus \drə-ˈkəŋ-kyə-ləs\ *n* : a genus (family Dracunculidae) of greatly elongated nematode worms including the guinea worm

draft \ˈdraft, ˈdraft\ *n* **1** : a portion (as of medicine) poured out or mixed for drinking : DOSE **2** : a current of air in a closed-in space — **drafty** \ˈdraf-tē, ˈdraf-\ *adj*

¹**drain** \ˈdrān\ *vb* **1** : to draw off (liquid) gradually or completely ⟨~ pus from an abscess⟩ **2** : to carry away or give passage to a bodily fluid or a discharge from ⟨~ an abscess⟩

²**drain** *n* : a tube or cylinder usu. of absorbent material for drainage of a wound — see CIGARETTE DRAIN

drain·age \ˈdrā-nij\ *n* : the act or process of drawing off fluids from a cavity or wound by means of suction or gravity

Draize test \ˈdrāz-\ *n* : a test that is used as a criterion for harmfulness of chemicals to the human eye and that involves dropping the test substance into one eye of rabbits without anesthesia with the other eye used as a control — called also *Draize eye test*

Draize, John H. (b 1900), American pharmacologist.

dram \ˈdram\ *n* **1** : either of two units of weight: **a** : an avoirdupois unit equal to 1.772 grams or 27.344 grains **b** : a unit of apothecaries' weight equal to 3.888 grams or 60 grains **2** : FLUID DRAM

Dram·amine \ˈdra-mə-ˌmēn\ *trademark* — used for dimenhydrinate

drape *n* : a sterile covering used in an operating room — usu. used in pl. — **drape** *vb*

dras·tic \ˈdras-tik\ *adj* : acting rapidly or violently — used chiefly of purgatives — **dras·ti·cal·ly** \-ti-k(ə-)lē\ *adv*

draught *chiefly Brit var of* DRAFT

draw \ˈdrȯ\ *vb* **drew** \ˈdrü\; **drawn** \ˈdrȯn\; **draw·ing 1** : INHALE **2 a** : to localize in or cause to move toward a surface — used in the phrase *draw to a head* (using a poultice to ~ inflammation to a head) **b** : to cause local congestion : induce blood or other body fluid to localize at a particular point

draw·sheet \ˈdrȯ-ˌshēt\ *n* : a narrow

sheet used chiefly in hospitals and stretched across the bed lengthwise often over a rubber sheet underneath the patient's trunk

dream \ˈdrēm\ *n, often attrib* : a series of thoughts, images, or emotions occurring during sleep and esp. during REM sleep — compare DAYDREAM — **dream** *vb*

¹**drench** \ˈdrench\ *n* : a poisonous or medicinal drink; *specif* : a large dose of medicine mixed with liquid and put down the throat of an animal

²**drench** *vb* : to administer a drench to (an animal)

dress \ˈdres\ *vb* : to apply dressings or medicaments to

dress·ing *n* : a covering (as of ointment or gauze) applied to a lesion

DRG \ˌdē-(ˌ)är-ˈjē\ *n* : any of about 500 payment categories that are used to classify patients and esp. Medicare patients for the purpose of reimbursing hospitals for each case in a given category with a fixed fee regardless of the actual costs incurred and that are based esp. on the principal diagnosis, surgical procedure used, age of patient, and expected length of stay in the hospital — called also *diagnosis related group*

drier *comparative of* DRY

driest *superlative of* DRY

drift \ˈdrift\ *n* **1** : movement of a tooth in the dental arch **2** : GENETIC DRIFT — **drift** *vb*

drill *n* : an instrument with an edged or pointed end for making holes in hard substances (as teeth) by revolving — **drill** *vb*

Drink·er respirator \ˈdriŋ-kər-\ *n* : IRON LUNG

Drinker, Philip (1894–1972), American industrial hygienist.

drip \ˈdrip\ *n* **1 a** : a falling in drops **b** : liquid that falls, overflows, or is extruded in drops **2** : a device for the administration of a fluid at a slow rate esp. into a vein; *also* : a material so administered ⟨a glucose ~⟩ — **drip** *vb*

Dris·dol \ˈdris-ˌdȯl, -ˌdōl\ *trademark* — used for a preparation of calciferol

drive \ˈdrīv\ *n* : an urgent, basic, or instinctual need : a motivating physiological condition of the organism ⟨a sexual ~⟩

drool \ˈdrül\ *vb* **1** : to secrete saliva in anticipation of food **2** : to let saliva or some other substance flow from the mouth — **drool** *n*

¹**drop** \ˈdräp\ *n* **1 a** : the quantity of fluid that falls in one spherical mass **b** **drops** *pl* : a dose of medicine measured by drops; *specif* : a solution for dilating the pupil of the eye **2** : the smallest practical unit of liquid measure that varies in size according to the specific gravity and viscosity of the liquid and to the conditions under which it is formed — compare MINIM

²**drop** *vb* **dropped**; **drop·ping 1** : to fall in

drops **2** *of an animal* : to give birth to ⟨lambs *dropped* in June⟩ **3** : to take (a drug) orally ⟨~ acid⟩

drop·let \'dräp-lət\ *n* : a tiny drop (as of a liquid)

droplet infection *n* : infection transmitted by airborne droplets of sputum containing infectious organisms

drop·per \'drä-pər\ *n* : a short glass tube fitted with a rubber bulb and used to measure liquids by drops — called also *eyedropper, medicine dropper* — **drop·per·ful** \-ˌfúl\ *n*

drop·si·cal \'dräp-si-kəl\ *adj* : relating to or affected with edema

drop·sy \'dräp-sē\ *n, pl* **drop·sies** : EDEMA

drown \'draún\ *vb* **drowned** \'draúnd\; **drown·ing** \'draú-niṇ\ **1** : to suffocate in water or some other liquid **2** : to suffocate because of excess of body fluid that interferes with the passage of oxygen from the lungs to the body tissues (as in pulmonary edema)

DrPH *abbr* doctor of public health

¹**drug** \'drəg\ *n* **1 a** : a substance used as a medication or in the preparation of medication **b** *according to the Food, Drug, and Cosmetic Act* (1) : a substance recognized in an official pharmacopoeia or formulary (2) : a substance intended for use in the diagnosis, cure, mitigation, treatment, or prevention of disease (3) : a substance other than food intended to affect the structure or function of the body (4) : a substance intended for use as a component of a medicine but not a device or a component, part, or accessory of a device **2** : something and often an illicit substance that causes addiction, habituation, or a marked change in consciousness

²**drug** *vb* **drugged; drug·ging 1** : to affect with a drug; *esp* : to stupefy by a narcotic drug **2** : to administer a drug to **3** : to take drugs for narcotic effect

drug·gist \'drə-gist\ *n* : one who sells or dispenses drugs and medicines: **as a** : PHARMACIST **b** : one who owns or manages a drugstore

drug·mak·er \'drəg-ˌmā-kər\ *n* : one that manufactures pharmaceuticals

drug·store \-ˌstōr\ *n* : a retail store where medicines and miscellaneous articles (as food, cosmetics, and film) are sold — called also *pharmacy*

drum \'drəm\ *n* : TYMPANIC MEMBRANE

drum·head \-ˌhed\ *n* : TYMPANIC MEMBRANE

drum·stick \-ˌstik\ *n* : a small projection from the cell nucleus that occurs in a small percentage of the polymorphonuclear leukocytes in the normal human female

druse \'drüz, 'drüˈzə\ *n, pl* **dru·sen** \'drü-zən\ : one of the small hyaline usu. laminated bodies sometimes appearing behind the retina of the eye

dry \'drī\ *adj* **dri·er** \'drī-ər\; **dri·est** \-əst\ **1** : marked by the absence or

scantiness of secretions, effusions, or other forms of moisture **2** *of a cough* : not accompanied by the raising of mucus or phlegm

dry gangrene *n* : gangrene that develops in the presence of arterial obstruction, is sharply localized, and is characterized by dryness of the dead tissue which is distinguishable from adjacent tissue by a line of inflammation

dry mouth *n* : XEROSTOMIA

dry out *vb* : to undergo an extended period of withdrawal from alcohol or drug use esp. at a special clinic : DETOXIFY

dry socket *n* : a tooth socket in which after tooth extraction a blood clot fails to form or disintegrates without undergoing organization; *also* : a condition that is marked by the occurrence of such a socket or sockets and that is usu. accompanied by neuralgic pain but without suppuration

DSC *abbr* doctor of surgical chiropody

DT *abbr* delirium tremens

DTP *abbr* diphtheria, tetanus, pertussis (vaccines)

d.t.'s \ˌdē-'tēz\ *n pl, often cap D&T* : DELIRIUM TREMENS

Du·chenne \dü-'shen, də-\ *also* **Du·chenne's** \-'shenz\ *adj* : relating to or being a severe form of muscular dystrophy of males that affects the muscles of the pelvic and shoulder girdles and the pectoral muscles first and is inherited as a sex-linked recessive trait ⟨muscular dystrophy of the ~ type⟩

Du·chenne \dü-'shen\, **Guillaume–Benjamin–Amand (1806–1875),** French neurologist.

Du·crey's bacillus \dü-'krāz-\ *n* : a gram-negative bacillus of the genus *Haemophilus* (*H. ducreyi*) that is the causative agent of chancroid

Du·crey \dü-'krā\, **Augusto (1860–1940),** Italian dermatologist.

duct \'dəkt\ *n* : a bodily tube or vessel esp. when carrying the secretion of a gland

duc·tal \'dək-t²l\ *adj* : of or belonging to a duct : made up of ducts ⟨the biliary ~ system⟩

duc·tion \'dək-shən\ *n* : a turning or rotating movement of the eye

duct·less \'dəkt-ləs\ *adj* : being without a duct

ductless gland *n* : ENDOCRINE GLAND

duct of Bel·li·ni \-be-'lē-nē\ *n* : any of the large excretory ducts of the uriniferous tubules of the kidney that open on the free surface of the papillae

Bellini, Lorenzo (1643–1704), Italian anatomist and physiologist.

duct of Gart·ner \-'gärt-nər\ *n* : GARTNER'S DUCT

duct of Ri·vi·nus \-rə-'vē-nəs\ *n* : any of several small inconstant efferent ducts of the sublingual gland

Rivinus, Augustus Quirinus (1652–

1723), German anatomist and botanist.

duct of San·to·ri·ni \-ˌsan-tə-ˈrē-nē, -ˌsän-\ *n* : ACCESSORY PANCREATIC DUCT

Santorini, Giovanni Domenico (1681–1737), Italian anatomist.

duct of Wir·sung \-ˈvir-(ˌ)zùŋ, -zəŋ\ *n* : PANCREATIC DUCT a — compare ACCESSORY PANCREATIC DUCT

Wirsung, Johann Georg (1600–1643), German anatomist.

duct·ule \ˈdək-(ˌ)tyül\ *n* : a small duct

duc·tu·li ef·fe·ren·tes \ˈdək-tyü-ˌlī-ˌef-ə-ˈren-(ˌ)tēz, -tü-, -(ˌ)lē-\ *n pl* : a group of ducts that convey sperm from the testis to the epididymis

duc·tu·lus \ˈdək-tyü-ləs, -tü-\ *n, pl* **-li** \-ˌlī, -(ˌ)lē\ : DUCTULE

duc·tus \ˈdək-təs\ *n, pl* **ductus** : DUCT

ductus ar·te·ri·o·sus \-ˌär-ˌtir-ē-ˈō-səs\ *n* : a short broad vessel in the fetus that connects the pulmonary artery with the aorta and conducts most of the blood directly from the right ventricle to the aorta bypassing the lungs

ductus de·fer·ens \-ˈde-fə-ˌrenz, -rənz\ *n, pl* **ductus de·fer·en·tes** \-ˌde-fə-ˈren-ˌtēz\ : VAS DEFERENS

ductus re·uni·ens \-rē-ˈyü-nē-ˌenz, -ˈü-\ *n* : a passage in the ear that connects the cochlea and the saccule

ductus ve·no·sus \-vi-ˈnō-səs\ *n* : a vein passing through the liver and connecting the left umbilical vein with the inferior vena cava of the fetus, losing its circulatory function after birth, and persisting as the ligamentum venosum of the liver

Duf·fy \ˈdə-fē\ *adj* : relating to, characteristic of, or being a system of blood groups determined by the presence or absence of any of several antigens in red blood cells ⟨~ blood typing⟩

Duffy, Richard (1906–1956), British hemophiliac.

Dührs·sen's incisions \ˈdūēr-sənz-\ *n pl* : a set of three incisions in the cervix of the uterus to facilitate delivery if dilation is inadequate

Dührs·sen \ˈdūēr-sən\, **Alfred (1862–1933),** German obstetrician-gynecologist.

dull \ˈdəl\ *adj* **1** : mentally slow or stupid **2** : slow in perception or sensibility **3** : lacking sharpness or edge or point ⟨a ~ scalpel⟩ **4** : lacking in force, intensity, or acuteness ⟨a ~ pain⟩ — **dull** *vb* — **dull·ness** *or* **dul·ness** \ˈdəl-nəs\ *n* — **dul·ly** *adv*

dumb \ˈdəm\ *adj* : lacking the power of speech

dumb rabies *n* : PARALYTIC RABIES

dumb·dum fever \ˈdəm-ˌdəm-\ *n* : KALAAZAR

dum·my \ˈdə-mē\ *n, pl* **dummies** : PLACEBO

dump·ing syndrome \ˈdəm-piŋ-\ *n* : a condition characterized by weakness, dizziness, flushing and warmth, nausea, and palpitation immediately or shortly after eating and produced by abnormally rapid emptying of the stomach in persons who have had part of the stomach removed or in hypersensitive or neurotic individuals

duoden- *or* **duodeno-** *comb form* **1** : duodenum ⟨*duoden*itis⟩ **2** : duodenal and ⟨*duodeno*jejunal⟩

du·o·de·nal ulcer \ˌdü-ə-ˈdēn-ᵊl-, ˌdyü-\ *n* : a peptic ulcer situated in the duodenum

du·o·de·ni·tis \ˌdü-ˌäd-ᵊn-ˈī-təs, ˌdyü-\ *n* : inflammation of the duodenum

du·o·de·no·cho·led·o·chot·o·my \ˌdü-ˌäd-ᵊn-ō-kə-ˌle-də-ˈkä-tə-mē, ˌdyü-\ *n, pl* **-mies** : choledochotomy performed by approach through the duodenum by incision

du·o·de·nog·ra·phy \ˌdü-ˌäd-ᵊn-ˈä-grə-fē, ˌdyü-\ *n, pl* **-phies** : radiographic visualization of the duodenum with a contrast medium

du·o·de·no·je·ju·nal \ˌdü-ˌäd-ᵊn-ō-ji-ˈjün-ᵊl, ˌdyü-\ *adj* : of, relating to, or joining the duodenum and the jejunum

du·o·de·no·je·ju·nos·to·my \-ji-jü-ˈnäs-tə-mē\ *n, pl* **-mies** : a surgical operation that joins part of the duodenum and the jejunum with creation of an artificial opening between them

du·o·de·not·o·my \ˌdü-ˌäd-ᵊn-ˈä-tə-mē, ˌdyü-\ *n, pl* **-mies** : incision of the duodenum

du·o·de·num \ˌdü-ə-ˈdē-nəm, ˌdyü-; dù-ˈäd-ᵊn-əm, dyù-\ *n, pl* **-de·na** \-ˈdē-nə, -ᵊn-ə\ *or* **-de·nums** : the first, shortest, and widest part of the small intestine that in humans is about 10 inches (25 centimeters) long and that extends from the pylorus to the undersurface of the liver where it descends for a variable distance and receives the bile and pancreatic ducts and then bends to the left and finally upward to join the jejunum near the second lumbar vertebra — **du·o·de·nal** \-ˈdēn-ᵊl, -ᵊn-əl\ *adj*

¹du·plex \ˈdü-ˌpleks, ˈdyü\ *adj* : having complementary polynucleotide strands of DNA or of DNA and RNA

²duplex *n* : a duplex molecule of DNA or of DNA and RNA

du·pli·cate \ˈdü-pli-ˌkāt, ˈdyü\ *vb* **-cat·ed; -cat·ing** : to become duplicate : REPLICATE ⟨DNA in chromosomes ~ s⟩

du·pli·ca·tion \ˌdü-pli-ˈkā-shən, ˌdyü-\ *n* **1** : the act or process of duplicating : the quality or state of being duplicated **2** : a part of a chromosome in which the genetic material is repeated; *also* : the process of forming a duplication

Du·puy·tren's contracture \də-ˌpwē-ˈtraⁿz-, -ˈpwē-trənz-\ *n* : a condition marked by fibrosis with shortening and thickening of the palmar aponeurosis resulting in flexion contracture of the fingers into the palm of the hand

Du·puy·tren \də-pwē-'traⁿ\, **Guillaume** (1777–1835), French surgeon.

dura — see LAMINA DURA

du·ral \'dùr-əl, 'dyùr-\ *adj* : of or relating to the dura mater

dural sinus *n* : SINUS OF THE DURA MATER

du·ra ma·ter \'dùr-ə-,mā-tər, 'dyùr-, -,mä-\ *n* : the tough fibrous membrane lined with endothelium on the inner surface that envelops the brain and spinal cord external to the arachnoid and pia mater, that in the cranium closely lines the bone, does not dip down between the convolutions, and contains numerous blood vessels and venous sinuses, and that in the spinal cord is separated from the bone by a considerable space and contains no venous sinuses — called also *dura*

dust cell *n* : a pulmonary histiocyte that takes up and eliminates foreign particles introduced into the lung alveoli with inspired air

dust·ing powder \'dəs-tiŋ-\ *n* : a powder used on the skin or on wounds esp. for allaying irritation or absorbing moisture

Dutch cap *n* : CERVICAL CAP

DVM *abbr* doctor of veterinary medicine

¹**dwarf** \'dwórf\ *n, pl* **dwarfs** \'dwórfs\ *also* **dwarves** \'dwórvz\ *often attrib* **1** : a person of unusually small stature; *esp* : one whose bodily proportions are abnormal **2** : an animal much below normal size

²**dwarf** *vb* : to restrict the growth of

dwarf·ism \'dwór-,fi-zəm\ *n* : the condition of stunted growth

Dx *abbr* diagnosis

Dy *symbol* dysprosium

dy·ad \'dī-,ad, -əd\ *n* : a meiotic chromosome after separation of the two homologous members of a tetrad — **dy·ad·ic** \dī-'a-dik\ *adj*

dy·dro·ges·ter·one \,dī-drō-'jes-tə-,rōn\ *n* : a synthetic progestational agent $C_{21}H_{28}O_2$ — called also *isopregnenone*

dying *pres part of* DIE

-dynamia *n comb form* : strength : condition of having (such) strength ⟨adynamia⟩

dy·nam·ic \dī-'na-mik\ *also* **dy·nam·i·cal** \-mi-kəl\ *adj* **1 a** : of or relating to physical force or energy **b** : of or relating to dynamics **2** : FUNCTIONAL 1b ⟨a ~ disease⟩ **3 a** : marked by continuous usu. productive activity or change **b** : marked by energy ⟨a ~ personality⟩ — **dy·nam·i·cal·ly** \-mi-k(ə-)lē\ *adv*

dy·nam·ics \dī-'na-miks\ *n sing or pl* **1** : a branch of mechanics that deals with forces and their relation primarily to the motion but sometimes also to the equilibrium of bodies **2** : PSYCHODYNAMICS **3** : the pattern of change or growth of an object or phenomenon ⟨personality ~⟩ ⟨population ~⟩

dy·na·mom·e·ter \,dī-nə-'mä-mə-tər\ *n* : an instrument for measuring the force of muscular contraction esp. of the hand

dyne \'dīn\ *n* : the unit of force in the cgs system equal to the force that would give a free mass of one gram an acceleration of one centimeter per second per second

dy·nein \'dī-,nēn, -,nē-ən\ *n* : an ATPase that is associated esp. with microtubules involved in the ciliary and flagellar movement of cells

dy·nor·phin \dī-'nór-fən\ *n* : any of a group of potent opioid peptides found in the mammalian central nervous system that have a strong affinity for opiate receptors

dy·phyl·line \dī-'fi-,lēn\ *n* : a theophylline derivative $C_{10}H_{14}N_4O_4$ used as a diuretic and for its bronchodilator and peripheral vasodilator effects — see NEOTHYLLINE

dys- *prefix* **1** : abnormal ⟨dysplasia⟩ **2** : difficult ⟨dyspnea⟩ **3** : impaired ⟨dysfunction⟩

dys·aes·the·sia *chiefly Brit var of* DYSESTHESIA

dys·ar·thria \dis-'är-thrē-ə\ *n* : difficulty in articulating words due to disease of the central nervous system — compare DYSPHASIA — **dys·ar·thric** \-thrik\ *adj*

dys·ar·thro·sis \,dis-,är-'thrō-səs\ *n, pl* **-thro·ses** \-,sēz\ **1** : a condition of reduced joint motion due to deformity, dislocation, or disease **2** : DYSARTHRIA

dys·au·to·no·mia \,dis-,ò-tə-'nō-mē-ə\ *n* : a familial disorder of the nervous system characterized esp. by multiple sensory deficiency (as of taste and pain) and by excessive sweating and salivation — **dys·au·to·nom·ic** \-'nä-mik\ *adj*

dys·ba·rism \'dis-bə-,ri-zəm\ *n* : the complex of symptoms (as bends or headache) that accompanies exposure to excessively low or rapidly changing environmental air pressure

dys·cal·cu·lia \,dis-,kal-'kyü-lē-ə\ *n* : impairment of mathematical ability due to an organic condition of the brain

dys·che·zia \dis-'kē-zē-ə, -'ke-, -zhə, -zhē-ə\ *n* : constipation associated with a defective reflex for defecation — **dys·che·zic** \-'kē-zik, -'ke-\ *adj*

dys·chon·dro·pla·sia \dis-,kän-drō-'plā-zhə, -zhē-ə\ *n* : CHONDRODYSPLASIA

dys·cra·sia \dis-'krā-zhə, -zhē-ə\ *n* : an abnormal condition of the body; *esp* : an imbalance of components of the blood

dys·di·ad·o·cho·ki·ne·sia *or* **dys·di·ad·o·ko·ki·ne·sia** \,dis-,dī-,a-də-,kō-ki-'nē-zhə, -zhē-ə\ *n* : impairment of the ability to make movements exhibiting a rapid change of motion that is caused by cerebellar dysfunction — compare ADIADOKOKINESIS

dys·en·ter·ic \ˌdis-ᵊn-ˈter-ik\ *adj* : of or relating to dysentery

dys·en·tery \ˈdis-ᵊn-ˌter-ē\ *n, pl* **-ter·ies 1** : a disease characterized by severe diarrhea with passage of mucus and blood and usu. caused by infection **2** : DIARRHEA

dys·es·the·sia \ˌdi-ses-ˈthē-zhə, -zhē-ə\ *n* : impairment of sensitivity esp. to touch — **dys·es·thet·ic** \-ˈthe-tik\ *adj*

dys·func·tion \(ˈ)dis-ˈfəŋk-shən\ *n* : impaired or abnormal functioning (as of an organ of the body) — **dys·func·tion·al** \-shnəl, -shən-ᵊl\ *adj* — **dys·func·tion·ing** \-shə-niŋ\ *n*

dys·gam·ma·glob·u·li·ne·mia \ˌdis-ˌga-mə-ˌglä-byə-lə-ˈnē-mē-ə\ *n* : a disorder involving abnormality in structure or frequency of gamma globulins — compare AGAMMAGLOBULINEMIA

dys·gen·e·sis \(ˌ)dis-ˈje-nə-səs\ *n, pl* **-e·ses** \-ˌsēz\ : defective development esp. of the gonads (as in Klinefelter's syndrome or Turner's syndrome)

dys·ger·mi·no·ma \ˌdis-ˌjər-mə-ˈnō-mə\ *n, pl* **-mas** *or* **-ma·ta** \-mə-tə\ : a malignant tumor of the ovary arising from undifferentiated germinal epithelium

dys·geu·sia \(ˌ)dis-ˈgü-zē-ə, -ˈgyü-, -zhə, -zhē-ə\ *n* : dysfunction of the sense of taste

dys·graph·ia \(ˌ)dis-ˈgra-fē-ə\ *n* : impairment of the ability to write caused by brain damage

dys·hi·dro·sis \ˌdis-ˌhi-ˈdrō-səs, -hə-\ *n, pl* **-dro·ses** \-ˌsēz\ : POMPHOLYX 2

dys·kary·o·sis \ˌdis-kar-ē-ˈō-səs\ *n, pl* **-o·ses** \-ˌsēz\ *or* **-o·sis·es** : abnormality esp. of exfoliated cells (as from the uterine cervix) that affects the nucleus but not the cytoplasm

dys·ker·a·to·sis \ˌdis-ˌker-ə-ˈtō-səs\ *n, pl* **-to·ses** \-ˌsēz\ : faulty development of the epidermis with abnormal keratinization — **dys·ker·a·tot·ic** \-ˈtä-tik\ *adj*

dys·ki·ne·sia \ˌdis-kə-ˈnē-zhə, -kī-, -zhē-ə\ *n* : impairment of voluntary movements resulting in fragmented or jerky motions (as in Parkinson's disease) — see TARDIVE DYSKINESIA — **dys·ki·net·ic** \-ˈne-tik\ *adj*

dys·lec·tic \dis-ˈlek-tik\ *adj or n* : DYSLEXIC

dys·lex·ia \dis-ˈlek-sē-ə\ *n* : a disturbance of the ability to read; *broadly* : disturbance of the ability to use language

¹dys·lex·ic \-ˈlek-sik\ *adj* : affected with dyslexia

²dyslexic *n* : a dyslexic person

dys·men·or·rhea \(ˌ)dis-ˌme-nə-ˈrē-ə\ *n* : painful menstruation — **dys·men·or·rhe·ic** \-ˈrē-ik\ *adj*

dys·met·ria \dis-ˈme-trē-ə\ *n* : impaired ability to estimate distance in muscular action

dys·mor·phia \-ˈmor-fē-ə\ *n* : DYSMORPHISM — **dys·mor·phic** \-fik\ *adj*

dys·mor·phism \-ˈmor-ˌfi-zəm\ *n* : an anatomical malformation

dys·os·mia \di-ˈsäz-mē-ə, -ˈsäs-\ *n* : dysfunction of the sense of smell

dys·os·to·sis \ˌdi-ˌsäs-ˈtō-səs\ *n, pl* **-to·ses** \-ˌsēz\ : defective formation of bone — **dys·os·tot·ic** \-ˈtä-tik\ *adj*

dys·pa·reu·nia \ˌdis-pə-ˈrü-nē-ə, -nyə\ *n* : difficult or painful sexual intercourse

dys·pep·sia \dis-ˈpep-shə, -sē-ə\ *n* : INDIGESTION

¹dys·pep·tic \-ˈpep-tik\ *adj* : relating to or having dyspepsia

²dyspeptic *n* : person having dyspepsia

dys·pha·gia \dis-ˈfā-jə, -jē-ə\ *n* : difficulty in swallowing — **dys·phag·ic** \-ˈfa-jik\ *adj*

dys·pha·sia \dis-ˈfā-zhə, -zhē-ə\ *n* : loss of or deficiency in the power to use or understand language as a result of injury to or disease of the brain — compare DYSARTHRIA

¹dys·pha·sic \-ˈfā-zik\ *adj* : relating to or affected with dysphasia

²dysphasic *n* : a dysphasic person

dys·pho·nia \dis-ˈfō-nē-ə\ *n* : defective use of the voice

dys·pho·ria \dis-ˈfōr-ē-ə\ *n* : a state of feeling unwell or unhappy — compare EUPHORIA — **dys·phor·ic** \-ˈfor-ik, -ˈfär-\ *adj*

dys·pla·sia \dis-ˈplā-zhə, -zhē-ə\ *n* : abnormal growth or development (as of organs or cells); *broadly* : abnormal anatomic structure due to such growth — **dys·plas·tic** \-ˈplas-tik\ *adj*

dys·pnea \ˈdis-nē-ə, ˈdisp-\ *n* : difficult or labored respiration — compare EUPNEA — **dys·pne·ic** \-nē-ik\ *adj*

dys·pnoea *chiefly Brit var of* DYSPNEA

dys·prax·ia \dis-ˈprak-sē-ə, -ˈprak-shə, -shē-ə\ *n* : impairment of the ability to perform coordinated movements

dys·pro·si·um \dis-ˈprō-zē-əm, -zhəm, -zhē-əm\ *n* : an element that forms highly magnetic compounds — symbol *Dy*; see ELEMENT table

dys·pro·tein·ae·mia *chiefly Brit var of* DYSPROTEINEMIA

dys·pro·tein·emia \ˌdis-ˌprōt-ᵊn-ˈē-mē-ə, -ˌprō-ˌtē-ᵊn-ˈē-, -ˌprō-tē-ə-ˈnē-\ *n* : any abnormality of the protein content of the blood — **dys·pro·tein·emic** \-mik\ *adj*

dys·reg·u·la·tion \ˌdis-ˌre-gyə-ˈlā-shən\ *n* : impairment of regulatory mechanisms (as those governing concentration of a substance in the blood or the function of an organ)

dys·rhyth·mia \dis-ˈrith-mē-ə\ *n* **1** : an abnormal rhythm; *esp* : a disordered rhythm exhibited in a record of electrical activity of the brain or heart **2** : JET LAG — **dys·rhyth·mic** \-mik\ *adj*

dys·syn·er·gia \ˌdis-sə-ˈnər-jə, -jē-ə\ *n* : DYSKINESIA — **dys·syn·er·gic** \-ˈnər-jik\ *adj*

dys·thy·mia \dis-ˈthī-mē-ə\ *n* : an affective disorder characterized by chronic mildly depressed or irritable mood often accompanied by other symptoms (as eating and sleeping disturbances, fatigue, and poor self esteem) — **dysthymic** \-mik\ *adj*

dys•to•cia \dis-ˈtō-shə, -shē-ə\ *or* **dys•to•kia** \-ˈtō-kē-ə\ *n* : slow or difficult labor or delivery

dys•to•nia \dis-ˈtō-nē-ə\ *n* : a state of disordered tonicity of tissues (as of muscle) — **dys•ton•ic** \-ˈtä-nik\ *adj*

dystonia mus•cu•lo•rum de•for•mans \-ˌməs-kyə-ˈlȯr-əm-di-ˈfȯr-ˌmanz\ *n* : a rare inherited neurological disorder characterized by progressive muscular spasticity causing severe involuntary contortions esp. of the trunk and limbs — called also *torsion dystonia*

dys•tro•phic \dis-ˈtrō-fik\ *adj* **1** : relating to or caused by faulty nutrition **2** : relating to or affected with a dystrophy

dystrophica — see MYOTONIA DYSTROPHICA

dys•tro•phy \ˈdis-trə-fē\ *n, pl* **-phies 1** : a condition produced by faulty nutrition **2** : any myogenic atrophy: *esp* : MUSCULAR DYSTROPHY

dys•uria \dis-ˈyür-ē-ə\ *n* : difficult or painful discharge of urine — **dys•uric** \-ˈyür-ik\ *adj*

E

e- *prefix* : missing : absent ⟨*edentulous*⟩

ear \ˈir\ *n* **1** : the vertebrate organ of hearing and equilibrium consisting in the typical mammal of a sound-collecting outer ear separated by the tympanic membrane from a sound-transmitting middle ear that in turn is separated from a sensory inner ear by membranous fenestrae **2 a** : the external ear of humans and most mammals **b** : a human earlobe — **eared** \ˈird\ *adj*

ear•ache \ˈir-ˌāk\ *n* : an ache or pain in the ear — called also *otalgia*

ear•drum \-ˌdrəm\ *n* : TYMPANIC MEMBRANE

ear•lobe \ˈir-ˌlōb\ *n* : the pendent part of the ear esp. of humans

ear mange *n* : canker of the ear esp. in cats and dogs that is caused by mites; *esp* : OTODECTIC MANGE

ear mite *n* : any of various mites attacking the ears of mammals

ear pick *n* : a device for removing wax or foreign bodies from the ear

ear•piece \ˈir-ˌpēs\ *n* **1** : a part of an instrument (as a stethoscope or hearing aid) that is applied to the ear **2** : one of the two sidepieces that support eyeglasses by passing over or behind the ears

ear•plug \-ˌpləg\ *n* : a device of pliable material for insertion into the outer opening of the ear (as to keep out water or deaden sound)

ear tick *n* : any of several ticks infesting the ears of mammals; *esp* : SPINOSE EAR TICK

ear•wax \ˈir-ˌwaks\ *n* : the yellow waxy secretion from the glands of the external ear — called also *cerumen*

east coast fever *n* : an acute highly fatal febrile disease of cattle esp. of eastern and southern Africa that is caused by a protozoan of the genus *Theileria* (*T. parva*) transmitted by ticks esp. of the genera *Rhipicephalus* and *Hyalomma*

eastern equine encephalomyelitis *n* : EQUINE ENCEPHALOMYELITIS a

eating disorder *n* : any of several psychological disorders (as anorexia nervosa or bulimia) characterized by gross disturbances of eating behavior

Ea•ton agent \ˈēt-ᵊn-\ *n* : a microorganism of the genus *Mycoplasma* (*M. pneumoniae*) that is the causative agent of primary atypical pneumonia

Eaton, Monroe Davis (*b* 1904), American microbiologist.

eb•ur•nat•ed \ˈe-bər-ˌnā-təd, ˈē-\ *adj* : hard and dense like ivory ⟨~ cartilage⟩ ⟨~ bone⟩ — **eb•ur•na•tion** \ˌe-bər-ˈnā-shən, ˌē-\ *n*

EBV *abbr* Epstein-Barr virus

EB virus \ˌē-ˈbē-\ *n* : EPSTEIN-BARR VIRUS

ec- *prefix* : out of : outside of : outside ⟨*eccrine*⟩

eccentric hypertrophy *n* : hypertrophy of the wall of a hollow organ and esp. the heart with dilatation of its cavity

ec•chon•dro•ma \ˌe-kən-ˈdrō-mə\ *n, pl* **-ma•ta** \-mə-tə\ *or* **-mas** : a cartilaginous tumor projecting from bone or cartilage

ec•chy•mo•sis \ˌe-kə-ˈmō-səs\ *n, pl* **-mo•ses** \-ˌsēz\ : the escape of blood into the tissues from ruptured blood vessels marked by a livid black-and-blue or purple spot or area; *also* : the discoloration so caused — compare PETECHIA — **ec•chy•mosed** \ˈe-kə-ˌmōzd, -ˌmōst\ *adj* — **ec•chy•mot•ic** \ˌe-kə-ˈmä-tik\ *adj*

ec•crine \ˈe-krən, -ˌkrīn, -ˌkrēn\ *adj* : of, relating to, having, or being eccrine glands — compare APOCRINE, HOLOCRINE, MEROCRINE

eccrine gland *n* : any of the rather small sweat glands that produce a fluid secretion without removing cytoplasm from the secreting cells and that are restricted to the human skin — called also *eccrine sweat gland*

ECG *abbr* electrocardiogram

Echid•noph•a•ga \ˌek-(ˌ)id-ˈnä-fə-gə\ *n*

: a genus of fleas (family Pulicidae) including the sticktight flea (*E. gallinacea*

echi·no·coc·co·sis \i-ˌkī-nə-kä-ˈkō-səs\ *n, pl* **-co·ses** \-ˌsēz\ : infestation with or disease caused by a small tapeworm of the genus *Echinococcus* (*E. granulosus*); *esp* : HYDATID DISEASE

echi·no·coc·cus \-nə-ˈkä-kəs\ *n* **1** *cap* : a genus of taeniid tapeworms that alternate a minute adult living as a harmless commensal in the intestine of dogs and other carnivores with a hydatid larva invading tissues esp. of the liver of cattle, sheep, swine, and humans, and acting as a serious often fatal pathogen **2** *pl* **-coc·ci** \-ˈkä-ˌkī, -ˌkē: -ˈkäk-ˌsī, -ˌsē\ : any tapeworm of the genus *Echinococcus*; *also* : HYDATID

echo·car·dio·gram \e-kō-ˈkär-dē-ə-ˌgram\ *n* : a visual record made by echocardiography

echo·car·di·og·ra·phy \-ˌkär-dē-ˈä-grə-fē\ *n, pl* **-phies** : the use of ultrasound to examine and measure structure and functioning of the heart and to diagnose abnormalities and disease — **echo·car·dio·graph·er** \-grə-fər\ *n* — **echo·car·dio·graph·ic** \-dē-ə-ˈgra-fik\ *adj*

echo·en·ceph·a·lo·gram \e-kō-in-ˈse-fə-lə-ˌgram\ *n* : a visual record obtained by echoencephalography

echo·en·ceph·a·log·ra·phy \-in-ˌse-fə-ˈlä-grə-fē\ *n, pl* **-phies** : the use of ultrasound to examine and measure internal structures (as the ventricles) of the skull and to diagnose abnormalities and disease — **echo·en·ceph·a·lo·graph·ic** \-fə-lə-ˈgra-fik\ *adj*

echo·gram \ˈe-kō-ˌgram\ *n* : the record made by echography — called also *ultrasonogram*

echo·graph \-ˌgraf\ *n* : an instrument used for echography

echog·ra·phy \i-ˈkä-grə-fē\ *n, pl* **-phies** : ULTRASOUND 2 — **echo·graph·ic** \e-kō-ˈgra-fik\ *adj* — **echo·graph·i·cal·ly** \-fi-k(ə-)lē\ *adv*

echo·la·lia \e-kō-ˈlā-lē-ə\ *n* : the often pathological repetition of what is said by other people as if echoing them — **echo·lal·ic** \-ˈla-lik\ *adj*

echo·prax·ia \e-kō-ˈprak-sē-ə\ *n* : pathological repetition of the actions of other people as if echoing them

echo·thi·o·phate iodide \-ˈthī-ə-ˌfāt-\ *n* : a long-acting anticholinesterase C₉H₂₃INO₃PS used esp. to reduce intraocular pressure in the treatment of glaucoma — called also *echothiophate*

echo·vi·rus \ˈe-kō-ˌvī-rəs\ *n* : any of a group of picornaviruses that are found in the gastrointestinal tract, that cause cytopathic changes in cells in tissue culture, and that are sometimes associated with respiratory ailments and meningitis

ec·lamp·sia \i-ˈklamp-sē-ə, e-\ *n* : a convulsive state : an attack of convulsions: as **a** : toxemia of pregnancy esp. when severe and marked by convulsions and coma — compare PREECLAMPSIA **b** : a condition comparable to milk fever of cows occurring in domestic animals (as dogs and cats) — **ec·lamp·tic** \-tik\ *adj*

¹eclec·tic \e-ˈklek-tik, i-\ *adj* **1** : selecting what appears to be best in various doctrines or methods **2** : of, relating to, or practicing eclecticism — **eclec·ti·cal·ly** \-ti-k(ə-)lē\ *adv*

²eclectic *n* : one who uses an eclectic method or approach

eclec·ti·cism \-ˈklek-tə-ˌsi-zəm\ *n* **1** : a theory or practice (as of medicine or psychotherapy) that combines doctrines or methods (as therapeutic procedures) from diverse sources **2** : a system of medicine once popular in the U.S. that depended on plant remedies

ecol·o·gy \i-ˈkä-lə-jē, e-\ *n, pl* **-gies 1** : a branch of science concerned with the interrelationship of organisms and their environments **2** : the totality or pattern of relations between organisms and their environment **3** : HUMAN ECOLOGY — **eco·log·i·cal** \ˌē-kə-ˈlä-ji-kəl, ˌe-\ *also* **eco·log·ic** \-jik\ *adj* — **eco·log·i·cal·ly** \-ji-k(ə-)lē\ *adv* — **ecol·o·gist** \i-ˈkä-lə-jist, e-\ *n*

eco·sys·tem \ˈē-kō-ˌsis-təm, ˈe-\ *n* : the complex of a community and its environment functioning as an ecological unit in nature

écra·seur \ˌā-krä-ˈzər, ˌē-\ *n* : a surgical instrument used to encircle and sever a projecting mass of tissue

ec·sta·sy \ˈek-stə-sē\ *n, pl* **-sies 1** : a trance state in which intense absorption is accompanied by loss of sense perception and voluntary control **2** : a synthetic amphetamine analog C₁₁H₁₅NO₂ used illicitly for its mood≠enhancing and hallucinogenic properties — called also *MDMA* — **ec·stat·ic** \ek-ˈsta-tik\ *adj*

ECT *abbr* electroconvulsive therapy

ec·ta·sia \ek-ˈtā-zhē-ə, -zhə\ *n* : the expansion of a hollow or tubular organ — **ec·tat·ic** \ek-ˈta-tik\ *adj*

ec·ta·sis \ˈek-tə-səs\ *n, pl* **-ta·ses** \-ˌsēz\ : ECTASIA

ec·thy·ma \ek-ˈthī-mə\ *n* **1** : a cutaneous eruption marked by large flat pustules that have a hardened base surrounded by inflammation and occur esp. on the lower legs **2** : sore mouth of sheep — **ec·thy·ma·tous** \ek-ˈthi-mə-təs, -ˈthī-\ *adj*

ecto- *also* **ect-** *comb form* : outside : external ⟨*ecto*derm⟩ — compare END- 1, EXO-

ec·to·cyst \ˈek-tə-ˌsist\ *n* : the external layer of a hydatid cyst

ec·to·derm \-ˌdərm\ *n* **1** : the outermost of the three primary germ layers of an embryo **2** : a tissue (as neural tissue) derived from ectoderm — **ec·to·der·mal** \₁ek-tə-ˈdər-məl\ *adj*

ec·to·en·zyme \₁ek-tō-ˈen-₁zīm\ *n* : an enzyme acting outside the cell

ec·to·mor·phic \₁ek-tə-ˈmȯr-fik\ *adj* 1 : of or relating to the component in W. H. Sheldon's classification of body types that measures the body's degree of thinness, angularity, and fragility — compare ENDOMORPHIC 1, MESOMORPHIC 2 2 : having a light body build — **ec·to·morph** \ˈek-tə-₁mȯrf\ *n* — **ec·to·mor·phy** \ˈek-tə-₁mȯr-fē\ *n*

-ec·to·my \ˈek-tə-mē\ *n comb form, pl* **-ec·to·mies** : surgical removal (appendectomy)

ec·to·par·a·site \₁ek-tō-ˈpar-ə-₁sīt\ *n* : a parasite that lives on the exterior of its host — compare ENDOPARASITE — **ec·to·par·a·sit·ic** \-₁par-ə-ˈsi-tik\ *adj*

ec·to·pia \ek-ˈtō-pē-ə\ *n* : an abnormal congenital or acquired position of an organ or part (~ of the heart)

ec·top·ic \ek-ˈtä-pik\ *adj* 1 : occurring in an abnormal position (an ~ kidney) 2 : originating in an area of the heart other than the sinoatrial node (~ beats); *also* : initiating ectopic heartbeats — **ec·top·i·cal·ly** \-pi-k(ə-)lē\ *adv*

ectopic pregnancy *n* : gestation elsewhere than in the uterus (as in a fallopian tube or in the peritoneal cavity) — called also *ectopic gestation, extrauterine pregnancy*

ec·to·pla·cen·ta \₁ek-tō-plə-ˈsen-tə\ *n* : TROPHOBLAST — **ec·to·pla·cen·tal** \-ˈsent-ᵊl\ *adj*

ec·to·plasm \ˈek-tə-₁pla-zəm\ *n* : the outer relatively rigid granule-free layer of the cytoplasm — compare ENDOPLASM

ec·to·py \ˈek-tə-pē\ *n, pl* **-pies** : ECTOPIA

ectro- *comb form* : congenitally absent — usu. indicating absence of a particular limb or part (ectrodactyly)

ec·tro·dac·tyl·ia \₁ek-trō-dak-ˈti-lē-ə\ *n* : ECTRODACTYLY

ec·tro·dac·tyl·ism \-ˈdak-tə-₁li-zəm\ *n* : ECTRODACTYLY

ec·tro·dac·ty·ly \-ˈdak-tə-lē\ *n, pl* **-lies** : congenital complete or partial absence of one or more digits

ec·tro·me·lia \₁ek-trō-ˈmē-lē-ə\ *n* 1 : congenital absence or imperfection of one or more limbs 2 : MOUSEPOX

ec·tro·pi·on \ek-ˈtrō-pē-₁än, -ən\ *n* : an abnormal turning out of a part (as an eyelid)

ec·ze·ma \ig-ˈzē-mə, ˈeg-zə-mə, ˈek-sə-\ *n* : an inflammatory condition of the skin characterized by redness, itching, and oozing vesicular lesions which become scaly, crusted, or hardened — **ec·zem·a·tous** \ig-ˈze-mə-təs\ *adj*

ec·ze·ma·toid \ig-ˈzē-mə-₁tȯid, -ˈze-\ *adj* : resembling eczema

ED *abbr* effective dose

EDB *abbr* ethylene dibromide

ede·ma \i-ˈdē-mə\ *n* : an abnormal excess accumulation of serous fluid in connective tissue or in a serous cavity — called also *dropsy* — **edem·a·tous** \-ˈde-mə-təs\ *adj*

eden·tu·lous \(₁)ē-ˈden-chə-ləs\ *adj* : TOOTHLESS (an ~ upper jaw)

edetate — see DISODIUM EDETATE

Ed·ing·er–West·phal nucleus \ˈe-diŋ-ər-ˈwest-₁fäl-, -₁fȯl-\ *n* : the lateral portion of the group of nerve cells lying ventral to the aqueduct of Sylvius which give rise to autonomic fibers of the oculomotor nerve

Ed·ing·er \ˈe-diŋ-ər\, **Ludwig (1855–1918),** German neurologist.

West·phal \ˈwest-₁fäl, -₁fȯl\, **Carl Friedrich Otto (1833–1890),** German neurologist.

EDR *abbr* electrodermal response

ed·ro·pho·ni·um \₁e-drə-ˈfō-nē-əm\ *n* : an anticholinesterase $C_{10}H_{16}ClNO$ used esp. to stimulate skeletal muscle and in the diagnosis of myasthenia gravis — called also *edrophonium chloride*; see TENSILON

EDTA \₁e-(₁)dē-(₁)tē-ˈā\ *n* : a white crystalline acid $C_{10}H_{16}N_2O_8$ used in medicine as an anticoagulant and in the treatment of lead poisoning — called also *ethylenediaminetetraacetic acid*

ed·u·ca·ble \ˈe-jə-kə-bəl\ *adj* : affected with mild mental retardation and capable of developing academic, social, and occupational skills within the capabilities of one with a mental age between 9 and 12 years — compare TRAINABLE

EEE *abbr* eastern equine encephalomyelitis

EEG *abbr* electroencephalogram; electroencephalograph

EENT *abbr* eye, ear, nose, and throat

ef·face·ment \i-ˈfās-mənt, e-\ *n* : obliteration of the uterine cervix by shortening and softening during labor so that only the external orifice remains — **ef·face** \-ˈfās\ *vb*

ef·fect \i-ˈfekt\ *n* : something that is produced by an agent or cause

ef·fec·tive \i-ˈfek-tiv\ *adj* : producing a decided, decisive, claimed, or desired effect — **ef·fec·tive·ness** *n*

ef·fec·tor \i-ˈfek-tər, -₁tȯr\ *n* 1 : a bodily organ (as a gland or muscle) that becomes active in response to stimulation 2 : a substance (as an inducer or corepressor) that controls protein synthesis by combining allosterically with a genetic repressor

¹**ef·fer·ent** \ˈe-fə-rənt; ˈe-₁fer-ənt, ˈē-₁fer-\ *adj* : conducting outward from a part or organ; *specif* : conveying nervous impulses to an effector (~ neurons) — compare AFFERENT

²**efferent** *n* : an efferent part (as a blood vessel or nerve fiber)

efferentes — see DUCTULI EFFERENTES

efferentia — see VASA EFFERENTIA

ef·fleu·rage \₁e-flə-ˈräzh, -(₁)flü-\ *n* : a

light stroking movement used in massage

effort syndrome *n* : NEUROCIRCULATORY ASTHENIA

ef·fuse \i-ˈfyüs, e-\ *adj* : spread out flat without definite form

ef·fu·sion \i-ˈfyü-zhən, e-\ *n* **1** : the escape of a fluid from anatomical vessels by rupture or exudation **2** : the fluid that escapes by extravasation — see PLEURAL EFFUSION

eges·tion \i-ˈjes-chən\ *n* : the act or process of discharging undigested or waste material from a cell or organism; *specif* : DEFECATION — **egest** \i-ˈjest\ *vb*

EGF *abbr* epidermal growth factor

egg \ˈeg, ˈag\ *n* **1** : the hard-shelled reproductive body produced by a bird and esp. by the common domestic chicken (*Gallus gallus*) **2** : an animal reproductive body consisting of an ovum together with its nutritive and protective envelopes and having the capacity to develop into a new individual capable of independent existence **3** : OVUM

egg cell *n* : OVUM

ego \ˈē-(ˌ)gō\ *n, pl* **egos** **1** : the self esp. as contrasted with another self or the world **2** : the one of the three divisions of the psyche in psychoanalytic theory that serves as the organized conscious mediator between the person and reality esp. by functioning both in the perception of and adaptation to reality — compare [1]ID, SUPEREGO

[1]ego·cen·tric \ˌē-gō-ˈsen-trik\ *adj* **1** : limited in outlook or concern to one's own activities or needs **2** : being self-centered or selfish — **ego·cen·tri·cal·ly** \-tri-k(ə-)lē\ *adv* — **ego·cen·tric·i·ty** \ˌē-gō-(ˌ)sen-ˈtris-ət-ē, -sən-\ *n* — **ego·cen·trism** \-ˈsen-ˌtri-zəm\ *n*

[2]egocentric *n* : an egocentric person

ego–defense *n* : DEFENSE MECHANISM

ego–dys·ton·ic \-dis-ˈtä-nik\ *adj* : incompatible with or unacceptable to the ego — compare EGO-SYNTONIC

ego ideal *n* : the positive standards, ideals, and ambitions that according to psychoanalytic theory are assimilated from the superego

ego–involvement *n* : an involvement of one's self-esteem in the performance of a task or in an object — **ego–involve** *vb*

ego·ism \ˈē-gə-ˌwi-zəm\ *n* **1 a** : a doctrine that individual self-interest is the actual motive of all conscious action **b** : a doctrine that individual self-interest is the valid end of all actions **2** : excessive concern for oneself without exaggerated feelings of self-importance — compare EGOTISM — **ego·ist** \-wist\ *n* — **ego·is·tic** \ˌē-gə-ˈwis-tik\ *also* **ego·is·ti·cal** \-ti-kəl\ *adj* — **ego·is·ti·cal·ly** \-ti-k(ə-)lē\ *adv*

ego·ma·nia \ˌē-gō-ˈmā-nē-ə, -nyə\ *n* : the quality or state of being extremely egocentric — **ego·ma·ni·ac** \-nē-ˌak\ *n* — **ego·ma·ni·a·cal** \ˌē-gō-mə-ˈnī-ə-kəl\ *adj* — **ego·ma·ni·a·cal·ly** \-k(ə-)lē\ *adv*

egoph·o·ny \ē-ˈgä-fə-nē\ *n, pl* **-nies** : a modification of the voice resembling bleating heard on auscultation of the chest in some diseases (as in pleurisy with effusion)

ego–syn·ton·ic \ˌē-gō-sin-ˈtä-nik\ *adj* : compatible with or acceptable to the ego — compare EGO-DYSTONIC

ego·tism \ˈē-gə-ˌti-zəm\ *n* : an exaggerated sense of self-importance — compare EGOISM **2** — **ego·tist** \-tist\ *n* — **ego·tis·tic** \ˌē-gə-ˈtis-tik\ *or* **ego·tis·ti·cal** \-ˈtis-ti-kəl\ *adj* — **ego·tis·ti·cal·ly** \-ˈtis-ti-k(ə-)lē\ *adv*

Eh·lers–Dan·los syndrome \ˈā-lərz-ˈdan-(ˌ)läs-\ *n* : a rare inherited disorder of connective tissue characterized by extremely flexible joints and elastic skin

Eh·lers \ˈā-(ˌ)lerz\, **Edvard L. (1863–1937),** Danish dermatologist.

Dan·los \dän-lō\, **Henri–Alexandre (1844–1912),** French dermatologist.

Ehr·lich·ia \er-ˈli-kē-ə\ *n* : a genus of gram-negative nonmotile rickettsial bacteria that are intracellular parasites infecting the cytoplasm of reticuloendothelial cells and circulating leukocytes but not erythrocytes

Ehr·lich \ˈär-ˌlik\, **Paul (1854–1915),** German chemist and bacteriologist.

ehrlichiosis *n* : infection with or a disease caused by rickettsial bacteria of the genus *Ehrlichia*

ei·co·sa·noid \ī-ˈkō-sə-ˌnóid\ *n* : any of a class of compounds (as the prostaglandins, leukotrienes, and thromboxanes) derived from polyunsaturated fatty acids and involved in cellular activity

ei·det·ic \ī-ˈde-tik\ *adj* : marked by or involving extraordinarily accurate and vivid recall esp. of visual images — **ei·det·i·cal·ly** \-ti-k(ə-)lē\ *adv*

eighth cranial nerve *n* : AUDITORY NERVE

eighth nerve *n* : AUDITORY NERVE

ei·ko·nom·e·ter \ˌī-kə-ˈnä-mə-tər\ *n* : a device to detect aniseikonia or to test stereoscopic vision

Ei·me·ria \ī-ˈmir-ē-ə\ *n* : a genus of coccidian protozoans that invade the visceral epithelia and esp. the intestinal wall of many vertebrates and include serious pathogens

Ei·mer \ˈī-mər\, **Theodor Gustav Heinrich (1843–1898),** German zoologist.

ein·stei·ni·um \īn-ˈstī-nē-əm\ *n* : a radioactive element produced artificially — symbol *Es*; see ELEMENT table

Einstein \ˈīn-ˌstīn, -ˌshtīn\, **Albert (1879–1955),** German physicist.

[1]ejac·u·late \i-ˈja-kyə-ˌlāt\ *vb* **-lat·ed; -lat·ing** : to eject from a living body; *specif* : to eject (semen) in orgasm — **ejac·u·la·tor** \-ˌlā-tər\ *n*

²**ejac·u·late** \-lət\ n : the semen released by one ejaculation

ejac·u·la·tion \i-₁ja-kyə-ᵛlā-shən\ n : the act or process of ejaculating; *specif* : the sudden or spontaneous discharging of a fluid (as semen in orgasm) from a duct — see PREMATURE EJACULATION

ejac·u·la·tio prae·cox \-ᵛlā-shē-ō-ᵛprē-₁käks\ n : PREMATURE EJACULATION

ejac·u·la·to·ry \i-ᵛja-kyə-lə-₁tōr-ē\ adj : associated with or concerned in physiological ejaculation (∼ vessels)

ejaculatory duct n : either of the paired ducts in the human male that are formed by the junction of the duct from the seminal vesicle with the vas deferens, pass through the prostate, and open into or close to the prostatic utricle

ejection fraction n : the ratio of the volume of blood the heart empties during systole to the volume of blood in the heart at the end of diastole expressed as a percentage normally between 56 and 78 percent

ejec·tor \i-ᵛjek-tər\ n : something that ejects — see SALIVA EJECTOR

EKG \ᵛē-(₁)kā-ᵛjē\ n 1 : ELECTROCARDIOGRAM 2 : ELECTROCARDIOGRAPH

elab·o·rate \i-ᵛla-bə-₁rāt\ vb **-rat·ed; -rat·ing** *of a living organism* : to build up (complex organic compounds) from simple ingredients — **elab·o·ra·tion** \i-₁la-bə-ᵛrā-shən\ n

el·a·pid \ᵛe-lə-pəd\ n : any of a family (Elapidae) of venomous snakes with grooved fangs that include the cobras and mambas, the coral snakes of the New World, and the majority of Australian snakes — **elapid** adj

elast- or **elasto-** comb form : elasticity ⟨*elastosis*⟩

elas·tase \i-ᵛlas-₁tās, -₁tāz\ n : an enzyme esp. of pancreatic juice that digests elastin

¹**elas·tic** \i-ᵛlas-tik\ adj : capable of being easily stretched or expanded and resuming former shape — **elas·ti·cal·ly** \-ti-k(ə-)lē\ adv

²**elastic** n 1 a : easily stretched rubber usu. prepared in cords, strings, or bands b : a band of elastic used esp. in orthodontics; *also* : one placed around a tooth at the gum line in effecting its nonsurgical removal 2 a : an elastic fabric usu. made of yarns containing rubber b : something made from this fabric

elastic cartilage n : a yellowish flexible cartilage having the matrix infiltrated in all directions by a network of elastic fibers and occurring chiefly in the external ear, eustachian tube, and some cartilages of the larynx and epiglottis

elastic fiber n : a thick very elastic smooth yellowish anastomosing fiber of connective tissue that contains elastin

elas·tic·i·ty \i-₁las-ᵛti-sə-tē, ₁ē-\ n, pl **-ties** : the quality or state of being elastic

elastic stocking n : a stocking woven or knitted with an elastic material and used (as in the treatment of varicose veins) to provide support for the leg

elastic tissue n : tissue consisting chiefly of elastic fibers that is found esp. in some ligaments and tendons

elasticum — see PSEUDOXANTHOMA ELASTICUM

elas·tin \i-ᵛlas-tən\ n : a protein that is similar to collagen and is the chief constituent of elastic fibers

elas·to·sis \i-₁las-ᵛtō-səs\ n, pl **-to·ses** \-₁sēz\ : a condition marked by loss of elasticity of the skin in elderly people due to degeneration of connective tissue

El·a·vil \ᵛe-lə-₁vil\ *trademark* — used for a preparation of amitriptyline

el·bow \ᵛel-₁bō\ n : the joint between the human forearm and the upper arm that supports the outer curve of the arm when bent — called also *elbow joint*

elec·tive \i-ᵛlek-tiv\ adj : beneficial to the patient but not essential for survival (an ∼ appendectomy)

Elec·tra complex \i-ᵛlek-trə-\ n : the Oedipus complex when it occurs in a female

electrical potential or **electric potential** n : the potential energy measured in volts of a unit of positive charge in an electric field

electric eel n : a large eel-shaped bony fish (*Electrophorus electricus* of the family Electrophoridae) of the Orinoco and Amazon basins that is capable of giving a severe shock with electricity generated by a special tract of tissue

electric ray n : any of various round-bodied short-tailed rays (family Torpedinidae) of warm seas that have a pair of specialized tracts of tissue in which electricity is generated

electric shock n 1 : SHOCK 3 2 : ELECTROSHOCK THERAPY

electric shock therapy n : ELECTROSHOCK THERAPY

electric shock treatment n : ELECTROSHOCK THERAPY

elec·tro·car·dio·gram \-ᵛkär-dē-ə-₁gram\ n : the tracing made by an electrocardiograph

elec·tro·car·dio·graph \-₁graf\ n : an instrument for recording the changes of electrical potential occurring during the heartbeat used esp. in diagnosing abnormalities of heart action — **elec·tro·car·dio·graph·ic** \-₁kär-dē-ə-ᵛgra-fik\ adj — **elec·tro·car·dio·graph·i·cal·ly** \-fi-k(ə-)lē\ adv — **elec·tro·car·di·og·ra·phy** \-dē-ᵛä-grə-fē\ n

elec·tro·cau·tery \-ᵛkò-tə-rē\ n, pl **-ter·ies** 1 : a cautery operated by an electric current 2 : the cauterization of tissue by means of an electrocautery

elec·tro·co·ag·u·la·tion \-kō-₁a-gyə-ᵛlā-shən\ *n* : the surgical coagulation of tissue by diathermy — **elec·tro·co·ag·u·late** \-kō-ˈa-gyə-ˌlāt\ *vb*

elec·tro·con·vul·sive \i-ˌlek-trō-kən-ˈvəl-siv\ *adj* : of, relating to, or involving convulsive response to electroshock

electroconvulsive therapy *n* : ELECTRO-SHOCK THERAPY

elec·tro·cor·ti·cal \-ˈkòr-ti-kəl\ *adj* : of, relating to, or being the electrical activity occurring in the cerebral cortex

elec·tro·cor·ti·co·gram \-ˈkòr-ti-kə-ˌgram\ *n* : an electroencephalogram made with the electrodes in direct contact with the brain

elec·tro·cor·ti·cog·ra·phy \-ˌkòr-ti-ˈkä-grə-fē\ *n, pl* **-phies** : the process of recording electrical activity in the brain by placing electrodes in direct contact with the cerebral cortex — **elec·tro·cor·ti·co·graph·ic** \-kə-ˈgra-fik\ *adj* — **elec·tro·cor·ti·co·graph·i·cal·ly** \-fi-k(ə-)lē\ *adv*

elec·troc·u·lo·gram \i-ˌlek-ˈträ-kyə-lə-ˌgram\ *n* : a recording of the moving eye

elec·tro·cute \i-ˈlek-trə-ˌkyüt\ *vb* **-cut·ed; -cut·ing 1** : to execute (a criminal) by electricity **2** : to kill by electric shock — **elec·tro·cu·tion** \-ˌlek-trə-ˈkyü-shən\ *n*

elec·trode \i-ˈlek-ˌtrōd\ *n* : a conductor used to establish electrical contact with a nonmetallic part of a circuit

elec·tro·der·mal \i-ˌlek-trō-ˈdər-məl\ *adj* : of or relating to electrical activity in or electrical properties of the skin

elec·tro·des·ic·ca·tion \-ˌde-si-ˈkä-shən\ *n* : the drying of tissue by a high-frequency electric current applied with a needle-shaped electrode — called also *fulguration* — **elec·tro·des·ic·cate** \-ˈde-si-ˌkāt\ *vb*

elec·tro·di·ag·no·sis \-ˌdī-ig-ˈnō-səs\ *n, pl* **-no·ses** \-ˌsēz\ : diagnosis based on electrodiagnostic tests or procedures

elec·tro·di·ag·nos·tic \-ˌdī-ig-ˈnäs-tik\ *adj* : involving or obtained from the recording of responses to electrical stimulation or of spontaneous electrical activity (as in electromyography) for purposes of diagnosing a pathological condition (~ studies) — **elec·tro·di·ag·nos·ti·cal·ly** \-ti-k(ə-)lē\ *adv*

elec·tro·di·al·y·sis \i-ˌlek-trō-dī-ˈa-lə-səs\ *n, pl* **-y·ses** \-ˌsēz\ : dialysis accelerated by an electromotive force applied by electrodes adjacent to the membranes — **elec·tro·di·a·lyt·ic** \-ˈdī-ə-ˈlit-ik\ *adj* — **elec·tro·di·a·lyze** \-ˈdī-ə-ˌlīz\ *vb* — **elec·tro·di·a·lyz·er** *n*

elec·tro·en·ceph·a·lo·gram \-in-ˈse-fə-lə-ˌgram\ *n* : the tracing of brain waves made by an electroencephalograph

elec·tro·en·ceph·a·lo·graph \-ˌgraf\ *n* : an apparatus for detecting and recording brain waves — called also *encephalograph* — **elec·tro·en·ceph·a·lo·graph·ic** \-ˌse-fə-lə-ˈgra-fik\ *adj* —

\-fi-k(ə-)lē\ *adv* — **elec·tro·en·ceph·a·log·ra·phy** \-ˈlä-grə-fē\ *n*

elec·tro·en·ceph·a·log·ra·pher \-in-ˌse-fə-ˈlä-grə-fər\ *n* : a person who specializes in electroencephalography

elec·tro·gen·ic \-ˈje-nik\ *adj* : of or relating to the production of electrical activity in living tissue — **elec·tro·gen·e·sis** \i-ˌlek-trə-ˈje-nə-səs\ *n*

elec·tro·gram \i-ˈlek-trə-ˌgram\ *n* : a tracing of the electrical potentials of a tissue (as the brain or heart) made by means of electrodes placed directly in the tissue instead of on the surface of the body

elec·tro·graph·ic \i-ˌlek-trə-ˈgra-fik\ *adj* : relating to, involving, or produced by the use of electrodes implanted directly in living tissue (~ stimulation of the brain) — **elec·tro·graph·i·cal·ly** \-fi-k(ə-)lē\ *adv*

elec·tro·ky·mo·graph \-ˈkī-mə-ˌgraf\ *n* : an instrument for recording graphically the motion of the heart as seen in silhouette on a fluoroscopic screen — **elec·tro·ky·mog·ra·phy** \-kī-ˈmä-grə-fē\ *n*

elec·trol·o·gist \i-ˈlek-ˈträ-lə-jist\ *n* : a person who removes hair, warts, moles, and birthmarks by means of an electric current applied to the body with a needle-shaped electrode

elec·trol·y·sis \i-ˈträ-lə-səs\ *n, pl* **-y·ses** \-ˌsēz\ **1 a** : the producing of chemical changes by passage of an electric current through an electrolyte **b** : subjection to this action **2** : the destruction of hair roots with an electric current

elec·tro·lyte \i-ˈlek-trə-ˌlit\ *n* **1** : a nonmetallic electric conductor in which current is carried by the movement of ions **2** : a substance (as an acid or salt) that when dissolved in a suitable solvent (as water) or when fused becomes an ionic conductor

elec·tro·lyt·ic \i-ˌlek-trə-ˈli-tik\ *adj* : of or relating to electrolysis or an electrolyte; *also* : involving or produced by electrolysis — **elec·tro·lyt·i·cal·ly** \-ti-k(ə-)lē\ *adv*

elec·tro·mag·net·ic \-mag-ˈne-tik\ *adj* : of, relating to, or produced by electromagnetism

electromagnetic field *n* : a field (as around a working computer or a transmitting high voltage power line) that is made up of associated electric and magnetic components, that results from the motion of an electric charge, and that possesses a definite amount of electromagnetic energy (the purported effects of *electromagnetic fields* on human health)

electromagnetic radiation *n* : a series of electromagnetic waves

electromagnetic spectrum *n* : the entire range of wavelengths or frequencies of electromagnetic radiation extending from gamma rays to the longest radio waves and including visible light

electromagnetic wave *n* : one of the waves that are propagated by simultaneous periodic variations of electric and magnetic field intensity and that include radio waves, infrared, visible light, ultraviolet, X rays, and gamma rays

elec·tro·mag·ne·tism \i-ˌlek-trō-ˈmag-nə-ˌti-zəm\ *n* **1** : magnetism developed by a current of electricity **2** : physics dealing with the relations between electricity and magnetism

elec·tro·mo·tive force \i-ˌlek-trō-ˈmō-tiv-, -trə-\ *n* : something that moves or tends to move electricity : the amount of energy derived from an electrical source per unit quantity of electricity passing through the source (as a cell or generator)

elec·tro·myo·gram \i-ˌlek-trō-ˈmī-ə-ˌgram\ *n* : a tracing made with an electromyograph

elec·tro·myo·graph \-ˌgraf\ *n* : an instrument that converts the electrical activity associated with functioning skeletal muscle into a visual record or into sound and has been used to diagnose neuromuscular disorders and in biofeedback training — **elec·tro·myo·graph·ic** \-ˌmī-ə-ˈgra-fik\ *adj* — **elec·tro·myo·graph·i·cal·ly** \-fi-k(ə-)lē\ *adv* — **elec·tro·my·og·ra·phy** \-mī-ˈä-grə-fē\ *n*

elec·tron \i-ˈlek-ˌträn\ *n* : an elementary particle consisting of a charge of negative electricity equal to about 1.602×10^{-19} coulomb and having a mass when at rest of about 9.109534×10^{-28} gram or about $1/1836$ that of a proton

elec·tro·nar·co·sis \i-ˌlek-trō-när-ˈkō-səs\ *n, pl* **-co·ses** \-ˌsēz\ : unconsciousness induced by passing a weak electric current through the brain

elec·tron·ic \i-ˌlek-ˈträ-nik\ *adj* : of or relating to electrons or electronics — **elec·tron·i·cal·ly** \-ni-k(ə-)lē\ *adv*

elec·tron·ics \i-ˌlek-ˈträ-niks\ *n* **1** : the physics of electrons and electronic devices **2** : electronic devices or equipment

electron micrograph *n* : a micrograph made with an electron microscope

electron microscope *n* : an electron= optical instrument in which a beam of electrons is used to produce an enlarged image of a minute object on a fluorescent screen or photographic plate — **electron microscopist** *n* — **electron microscopy** *n*

electron transport *n* : the sequential transfer of electrons esp. by cytochromes in cellular respiration from an oxidizable substrate to molecular oxygen by a series of oxidation= reduction reactions

elec·tro·nys·tag·mog·ra·phy \i-ˌlek-trō-ˌnis-ˌtag-ˈmä-grə-fē\ *n, pl* **-phies** : the use of electrooculography to study

nystagmus — **elec·tro·nys·tag·mo·graph·ic** \-(ˌ)nis-ˌtag-mə-ˈgra-fik\ *adj*

elec·tro·oc·u·lo·gram \-ˈä-kyə-lə-ˌgram\ *n* : a record of the standing voltage between the front and back of the eye that is correlated with eyeball movement (as in REM sleep) and obtained by electrodes suitably placed on the skin near the eye

elec·tro·oc·u·log·ra·phy \-ˈä-kyə-ˈlä-grə-fē\ *n, pl* **-phies** : the preparation and study of electrooculograms — **elec·tro·oc·u·lo·graph·ic** \-lə-ˈgra-fik\ *adj*

elec·tro·phe·ro·gram \-trə-ˈfir-ə-ˌgram, -ˈfer-\ *n* : ELECTROPHORETOGRAM

elec·tro·pho·re·sis \-trə-fə-ˈrē-səs\ *n, pl* **-re·ses** \-ˈsēz\ : the movement of suspended particles through a fluid or gel under the action of an electromotive force applied to electrodes in contact with the suspension — **elec·tro·pho·rese** \-ˈrēs, -ˈrēz\ *vb* — **elec·tro·pho·ret·ic** \-ˈre-tik\ *adj* — **elec·tro·pho·ret·i·cal·ly** \-ti-k(ə-)lē\ *adv*

elec·tro·pho·reto·gram \-fə-ˈre-tə-ˌgram\ *n* : a record that consists of the separated components of a mixture (as of proteins) produced by electrophoresis in a supporting medium

elec·tro·phren·ic \i-ˌlek-trə-ˈfre-nik\ *adj* : relating to or induced by electrical stimulation of the phrenic nerve (~ respiration) (~ respirator)

elec·tro·phys·i·ol·o·gy \i-ˌlek-trō-ˌfi-zē-ˈä-lə-jē\ *n, pl* **-gies 1** : physiology that is concerned with the electrical aspects of physiological phenomena **2** : electrical phenomena associated with a physiological process (as the function of a body or bodily part) — **elec·tro·phys·i·o·log·i·cal** \-ə-ˈlä-ji-kəl\ *also* **elec·tro·phys·i·o·log·ic** \-jik\ *adj* — **elec·tro·phys·i·o·log·i·cal·ly** \-ji-k(ə-)lē\ *adv* — **elec·tro·phys·i·ol·o·gist** \-ˈä-lə-jist\ *n*

elec·tro·re·sec·tion \-rē-ˈsek-shən\ *n* : resection by electrosurgical means

elec·tro·ret·i·no·gram \-ˈret-ᵊn-ə-ˌgram\ *n* : a graphic record of electrical activity of the retina

elec·tro·ret·i·no·graph \-ˌgraf\ *n* : an instrument for recording electrical activity in the retina — **elec·tro·ret·i·no·graph·ic** \-ˌret-ᵊn-ə-ˈgra-fik\ *adj* — **elec·tro·ret·i·nog·ra·phy** \-ᵊn-ˈä-grə-fē\ *n*

elec·tro·shock \i-ˈlek-trō-ˌshäk\ *n* **1** : SHOCK 3 **2** : ELECTROSHOCK THERAPY

electroshock therapy *n* : the treatment of mental disorder and esp. depression by the induction of unconsciousness and convulsions through the use of an electric current now usu. on an anesthetized patient — called also *electric shock, electric shock therapy, electric shock treatment, electroconvulsive therapy*

elec·tro·sleep \-ˌslēp\ *n* : profound relaxation or a state of unconsciousness induced by the passage of a very low voltage electric current through the brain

elec·tro·stat·ic \i-ˌlek-trə-ˈsta-tik\ *adj* : of or relating to stationary electric charges or to the study of the forces of attraction and repulsion acting between such charges

elec·tro·stim·u·la·tion \i-ˌlek-trō-ˌstim-yə-ˈlā-shən\ *n* : electroshock administered in nonconvulsive doses

elec·tro·sur·gery \-ˈsər-jə-rē\ *n, pl* **-ger·ies** : surgery by means of diathermy — **elec·tro·sur·gi·cal** \-ji-kəl\ *adj*

elec·tro·ther·a·py \-ˈther-ə-pē\ *n, pl* **-pies** : treatment of disease by means of electricity (as in diathermy)

elec·tro·tome \i-ˈlek-trə-ˌtōm\ *n* : an electric cutting instrument used in electrosurgery

elec·tro·ton·ic \i-ˌlek-trə-ˈtä-nik\ *adj* **1** : of, induced by, relating to, or constituting electrotonus ⟨the ～ condition of a nerve⟩ **2** : of, relating to, or being the spread of electrical activity through living tissue or cells in the absence of repeated action potentials — **elec·tro·ton·i·cal·ly** \-ni-k(ə-)lē\ *adv*

elec·trot·o·nus \i-ˌlek-ˈträt-ᵊn-əs\ *n* : the altered sensitivity of a nerve when a constant current of electricity passes through any part of it

elec·tu·ary \i-ˈlek-chə-ˌwer-ē\ *n, pl* **-ar·ies** : CONFECTION; *esp* : a medicated paste prepared with a sweet (as honey) and used in veterinary practice

el·e·doi·sin \ˌe-lə-ˈdois-ᵊn\ *n* : a small protein $C_{54}H_{85}N_{13}O_{15}S$ from the salivary glands of several octopuses (genus *Eledone*) that is a powerful vasodilator and hypotensive agent

el·e·ment \ˈe-lə-mənt\ *n* **1** : any of more than 100 fundamental substances that consist of atoms of only one kind and that singly or in combination constitute all matter **2** : one of the basic constituent units (as a cell or fiber) of a tissue

CHEMICAL ELEMENTS

ELEMENT	SYMBOL	ATOMIC NUMBER	ATOMIC WEIGHT (C = 12)
actinium	Ac	89	227.0278
aluminum	Al	13	26.98154
americium	Am	95	
antimony	Sb	51	121.75
argon	Ar	18	39.948
arsenic	As	33	74.9216
astatine	At	85	
barium	Ba	56	137.33
berkelium	Bk	97	
beryllium	Be	4	9.01218
bismuth	Bi	83	208.9804
boron	B	5	10.81
bromine	Br	35	79.904
cadmium	Cd	48	112.41
calcium	Ca	20	40.08
californium	Cf	98	

ELEMENT	SYMBOL	ATOMIC NUMBER	ATOMIC WEIGHT (C = 12)
carbon	C	6	12.011
cerium	Ce	58	140.12
cesium	Cs	55	132.9054
chlorine	Cl	17	35.453
chromium	Cr	24	51.996
cobalt	Co	27	58.9332
copper	Cu	29	63.546
curium	Cm	96	
dysprosium	Dy	66	162.50
einsteinium	Es	99	
erbium	Er	68	167.26
europium	Eu	63	151.96
fermium	Fm	100	
fluorine	F	9	18.998403
francium	Fr	87	
gadolinium	Gd	64	157.25
gallium	Ga	31	69.72
germanium	Ge	32	72.59
gold	Au	79	196.9665
hafnium	Hf	72	178.49
helium	He	2	4.00260
holmium	Ho	67	164.9304
hydrogen	H	1	1.0079
indium	In	49	114.82
iodine	I	53	126.9045
iridium	Ir	77	192.22
iron	Fe	26	55.847
krypton	Kr	36	83.80
lanthanum	La	57	138.9055
lawrencium	Lr	103	
lead	Pb	82	207.2
lithium	Li	3	6.941
lutetium	Lu	71	174.967
magnesium	Mg	12	24.305
manganese	Mn	25	54.9380
mendelevium	Md	101	
mercury	Hg	80	200.59
molybdenum	Mo	42	95.94
neodymium	Nd	60	144.24
neon	Ne	10	20.179
neptunium	Np	93	237.0482
nickel	Ni	28	58.69
niobium	Nb	41	92.9064
nitrogen	N	7	14.0067
nobelium	No	102	
osmium	Os	76	190.2
oxygen	O	8	15.9994
palladium	Pd	46	106.42
phosphorus	P	15	30.97376
platinum	Pt	78	195.08
plutonium	Pu	94	
polonium	Po	84	
potassium	K	19	39.0983
praseodymium	Pr	59	140.9077
promethium	Pm	61	
protactinium	Pa	91	231.0359
radium	Ra	88	226.0254
radon	Rn	86	
rhenium	Re	75	186.207
rhodium	Rh	45	102.9055
rubidium	Rb	37	85.4678
ruthenium	Ru	44	101.07
samarium	Sm	62	150.36
scandium	Sc	21	44.9559
selenium	Se	34	78.96
silicon	Si	14	28.0855
silver	Ag	47	107.868

ELEMENT	SYMBOL	ATOMIC NUMBER	ATOMIC WEIGHT (C = 12)
sodium	Na	11	22.98977
strontium	Sr	38	87.62
sulfur	S	16	32.06
tantalum	Ta	73	180.9479
technetium	Tc	43	
tellurium	Te	52	127.60
terbium	Tb	65	158.9254
thallium	Tl	81	204.383
thorium	Th	90	232.0381
thulium	Tm	69	168.9342
tin	Sn	50	118.69
titanium	Ti	22	47.88
tungsten	W	74	183.85
unnilhexium	Unh	106	
unnilpentium	Unp	105	
unnilquadium	Unq	104	
uranium	U	92	238.0289
vanadium	V	23	50.9415
xenon	Xe	54	131.29
ytterbium	Yb	70	173.04
yttrium	Y	39	88.9059
zinc	Zn	30	65.38
zirconium	Zr	40	91.22

el·e·men·tal \ˌe-lə-ˈment-ᵊl\ *adj* : of, relating to, or being an element; *specif* : existing as an uncombined chemical element

elementary body *n* : an infectious particle of any of several microorganisms; *esp* : a chlamydial cell of an extracellular infectious form that attaches to receptors on the membrane of the host cell and is taken up by endocytosis — compare RETICULATE BODY

elementary particle *n* : any of the subatomic units of matter and energy (as the electron, neutrino, proton, or photon) that do not appear to be made up of other smaller particles

el·e·phan·ti·a·sis \ˌe-lə-fən-ˈtī-ə-səs, -ˌfan-\ *n, pl* **-a·ses** \-ˌsēz\ : enlargement and thickening of tissues; *specif* : the enormous enlargement of a limb or the scrotum caused by obstruction of lymphatics by filarial worms of the genus *Wuchereria* (*W. bancrofti*) or a related genus (*Brugia malayi*)

el·e·vat·ed \ˈe-lə-ˌvā-təd\ *adj* : increased esp. abnormally ⟨an ∼ pulse rate⟩

el·e·va·tion \ˌe-lə-ˈvā-shən\ *n* **1** : a swelling esp. on the skin **2** : a usu. abnormal increase (as in degree or amount) ⟨an ∼ of temperature⟩

el·e·va·tor \ˈe-lə-ˌvā-tər\ *n* **1** : a dental instrument that is used for removing teeth or the roots of teeth which cannot be gripped with a forceps **2** : a surgical instrument for raising a depressed part (as a bone) or for separating contiguous parts

eleventh cranial nerve *n* : ACCESSORY NERVE

elim·i·nate \i-ˈli-mə-ˌnāt\ *vb* **-nat·ed;** **-nat·ing** : to expel (as waste) from the living body

elim·i·na·tion \i-ˌli-mə-ˈnā-shən\ *n* **1** : the act of discharging or excreting waste products or foreign substances from the body **2** **eliminations** *pl* : bodily discharges including urine, feces, and vomit

ELISA \ē-ˈlī-sə, -zə\ *n* : ENZYME-LINKED IMMUNOSORBENT ASSAY

elix·ir \i-ˈlik-sər\ *n* : a sweetened liquid usu. containing alcohol that is used in medication either for its medicinal ingredients or as a flavoring

Eliz·a·be·than collar \i-ˌli-zə-ˈbē-thən-\ *n* : a broad circle of stiff cardboard or other material placed about the neck of a cat or dog to prevent it from licking or biting an injured part

el·lip·to·cyte \i-ˈlip-tə-ˌsīt\ *n* : an elliptical red blood cell

el·lip·to·cy·to·sis \i-ˌlip-tə-ˌsī-ˈtō-səs\ *n, pl* **-to·ses** \-ˌsēz\ : a human hereditary trait manifested by the presence in the blood of red blood cells which are oval in shape with rounded ends — compare SICKLE-CELL TRAIT

el·u·ant *or* **el·u·ent** \ˈel-yə-wənt\ *n* : a solvent used in eluting

el·u·ate \ˈel-yə-wət, -ˌwāt\ *n* : the washings obtained by eluting

elute \ē-ˈlüt\ *vb* **elut·ed; elut·ing** : to wash out or extract; *specif* : to remove (adsorbed material) from an adsorbent by means of a solvent — **elu·tion** \-ˈlü-shən\ *n*

ema·ci·ate \i-ˈmā-shē-ˌāt\ *vb* **-at·ed; -at·ing 1** : to cause to lose flesh so as to become very thin **2** : to waste away physically — **ema·ci·a·tion** \-ˌmā-shē-ˈā-shən, -sē-\ *n*

emas·cu·late \i-ˈmas-kyə-ˌlāt\ *vb* **-lat·ed; -lat·ing** : to deprive of virility or procreative power : CASTRATE — **emas·cu·la·tion** \-ˌmas-kyə-ˈlā-shən\ *n*

emas·cu·la·tor \i-ˈmas-kyə-ˌlā-tər\ *n* : an instrument often with a broad surface and a cutting edge used in castrating livestock

em·balm \im-ˈbäm, -ˈbälm\ *vb* : to treat (a dead body) so as to protect from decay — **em·balm·er** *n*

em·bar·rass \im-ˈbar-əs\ *vb* : to impair the activity of (a bodily function) or the function of (a bodily part)

em·bar·rass·ment \im-ˈbar-əs-mənt\ *n* : difficulty in functioning as a result of disease ⟨cardiac ∼⟩ ⟨respiratory ∼⟩

em·bed \im-ˈbed\ *vb* **em·bed·ded; em·bed·ding** : to prepare (a microscopy specimen) for sectioning by infiltrating with and enclosing in a supporting substance — **em·bed·ment** \-ˈbed-mənt\ *n*

embol- *comb form* : embolus ⟨*embolectomy*⟩

em·bo·lec·to·my \ˌem-bə-ˈlek-tə-mē\ *n, pl* **-mies** : surgical removal of an embolus

em·bol·ic \em-ˈbä-lik, im-\ *adj* : of or relating to an embolus or embolism

em·bo·lism \'em-bə-ıli-zəm\ n **1** : the sudden obstruction of a blood vessel by an embolus **2** : EMBOLUS

em·bo·li·za·tion \ıem-bə-lə-'zā-shən\ n : the process by which or state in which a blood vessel or organ is obstructed by the lodgment of a material mass (as an embolus) (pulmonary ~) ⟨~ of a thrombus⟩; *also* : an operation in which pellets are introduced into the circulatory system in order to induce embolization in specific abnormal blood vessels

em·bo·lize \'em-bə-ılīz\ vb **-lized; -liz·ing 1** *of an embolus* : to lodge in and obstruct (as a blood vessel or organ) **2** : to break up into emboli or become an embolus

em·bo·lus \'em-bə-ləs\ n, pl **-li** \-ılī\ : an abnormal particle (as an air bubble) circulating in the blood — compare THROMBUS

em·bra·sure \im-'brā-zhər\ n : the sloped valley between adjacent teeth

em·bro·ca·tion \ıem-brə-'kā-shən\ n : LINIMENT

embry- *or* **embryo-** *comb form* : embryo ⟨*embryonic*⟩ ⟨*embryogenesis*⟩

em·bryo \'em-brē-ıō\ n, pl **embry·os** : an animal in the early stages of growth and differentiation that are characterized by cleavage, the laying down of fundamental tissues, and the formation of primitive organs and organ systems; *esp* : the developing human individual from the time of implantation to the end of the eighth week after conception — compare FETUS

em·bryo·gen·e·sis \ıem-brē-ō-'je-nə-səs\ n, pl **-eses** \-ısēz\ : the formation and development of the embryo — **em·bryo·ge·net·ic** \-jə-'ne-tik\ adj

em·bryo·ge·ny \ıem-brē-'ä-jə-nē\ n, pl **-nies** : EMBRYOGENESIS — **em·bryo·gen·ic** \-brē-ō-'je-nik\ adj

em·bry·ol·o·gist \ıem-brē-'ä-lə-jist\ n : a specialist in embryology

em·bry·ol·o·gy \-jē\ n, pl **-gies 1** : a branch of biology dealing with embryos and their development **2** : the features and phenomena exhibited in the formation and development of an embryo — **em·bryo·log·i·cal** \-brē-ə-'lä-ji-kəl\ *also* **em·bryo·log·ic** \-jik\ adj — **em·bryo·log·i·cal·ly** \-ji-k(ə-)lē\ adv

em·bry·o·ma \ıem-brē-'ō-mə\ n, pl **-mas** *or* **-ma·ta** \-mə-tə\ : a tumor derived from embryonic structures : TERATOMA

embryon- *or* **embryoni-** *comb form* : embryo ⟨*embryonic*⟩

em·bry·o·nal \em-'brī-ən-ᵊl\ adj : EMBRYONIC 1

embryonal carcinoma n : a highly malignant cancer of the testis

em·bry·o·nate \'em-brē-ə-ınāt\ vb **-nat·ed; -nat·ing** *of an egg or zygote* : to produce or differentiate into an embryo

em·bry·o·nat·ed adj : having an embryo

em·bry·on·ic \ıem-brē-'ä-nik\ adj **1** : of or relating to an embryo **2** : being in an early stage of development : INCIPIENT, RUDIMENTARY — **em·bry·on·i·cal·ly** \-ni-k(ə-)lē\ adv

embryonic disk *or* **embryonic disc** n **1 a** : BLASTODISC **b** : BLASTODERM **2** : the part of the inner cell mass of a blastocyst from which the embryo of a placental mammal develops

embryonic membrane n : a structure (as the amnion) that derives from the fertilized ovum but does not form a part of the embryo

em·bry·op·a·thy \ıem-brē-'ä-pə-thē\ n, pl **-thies** : a developmental abnormality of an embryo or fetus esp. when caused by a disease (as German measles or mumps) in the mother

em·bryo·tox·ic·i·ty \ıem-brē-ō-ıtäk-'si-sə-tē\ n, pl **-ties** : the state of being toxic to embryos — **em·bryo·tox·ic** \-'täk-sik\ adj

embryo transfer n : a procedure used esp. in animal breeding in which an embryo from a superovulated female is removed and reimplanted in the uterus of another female — called also *embryo transplant*

emer·gence \i-'mər-jəns\ n : a recovering of consciousness (as from anesthesia)

emer·gen·cy \i-'mər-jən-sē\ n, pl **-cies** : an unforeseen combination of circumstances or the resulting state that calls for immediate action: as **a** : a sudden bodily alteration (as a ruptured appendix) such as is likely to require immediate medical attention **b** : a usu. distressing event or condition that can often be anticipated or prepared for but seldom exactly foreseen

emergency medical technician n : EMT

emergency room n : a hospital room or area staffed and equipped for the reception and treatment of persons with conditions (as illness or trauma) requiring immediate medical care

emer·gent \i-'mər-jənt\ adj : calling for prompt or urgent action

eme·sis \'e-mə-səs, i-'mē-\ n, pl **eme·ses** \-ısēz\ : VOMITING

¹emet·ic \i-'me-tik\ n : an agent that induces vomiting

²emetic adj : having the capacity to induce vomiting

em·e·tine \'e-mə-ıtēn\ n : an amorphous alkaloid $C_{29}H_{40}N_2O_4$ extracted from ipecac root and used as an emetic and expectorant

EMF abbr **1** electromotive force **2** electromagnetic field

EMG abbr electromyogram; electromyograph; electromyography

-emia \'ē-mē-ə\ *or* **-hemia** \'hē-\ comb form **1** : condition of having (such) blood ⟨leuk*emia*⟩ ⟨septic*emia*⟩ **2** : condition of having (a specified thing) in the blood ⟨chol*emia*⟩ ⟨ur*emia*⟩

em·i·nence \'e-mə-nəns\ n : a protuberance or projection on a bodily part and esp. a bone

emissary vein *n* : any of the veins that pass through apertures in the skull and connect the venous sinuses of the dura mater with veins external to the skull

emis·sion \ē-ˈmi-shən\ *n* **1** : a discharge of fluid from a living body; *esp* : EJACULATE — see NOCTURNAL EMISSION **2** : substances and esp. pollutants discharged into the air (as by a smokestack or an automobile gasoline engine)

em·men·a·gogue \ə-ˈme-nə-ˌgäg, e-\ *n* : an agent that promotes the menstrual discharge

em·me·tro·pia \ˌe-mə-ˈtrō-pē-ə\ *n* : the normal refractive condition of the eye in which with accommodation relaxed parallel rays of light are all brought accurately to a focus upon the retina — compare ASTIGMATISM, MYOPIA — **em·me·trop·ic** \-ˈträ-pik, -ˈtrō-\ *adj*

¹emol·lient \i-ˈmäl-yənt\ *adj* : making soft or supple; *also* : soothing esp. to the skin or mucous membrane

²emollient *n* : an emollient agent (an ∼ for the hands)

emo·tion \i-ˈmō-shən\ *n* : a psychic and physical reaction (as anger or fear) subjectively experienced as strong feeling and physiologically involving changes that prepare the body for immediate vigorous action — **emo·tion·al** \-shə-nəl\ *adj* — **emo·tion·al·i·ty** \-ˌmō-shə-ˈna-lə-tē\ *n* — **emo·tion·al·ly** *adv*

em·pa·thy \ˈem-pə-thē\ *n, pl* **-thies** : the action of understanding, being aware of, being sensitive to, and vicariously experiencing the feelings, thoughts, and experience of another of either the past or present without having the feelings, thoughts, and experience fully communicated in an objectively explicit manner; *also* : the capacity for empathy — **em·path·ic** \em-ˈpa-thik, im-\ *adj* — **em·path·i·cal·ly** *adv* — **em·pa·thize** \ˈem-pə-ˌthīz\ *vb*

em·phy·se·ma \ˌem-fə-ˈzē-mə, -ˈsē-\ *n* : a condition characterized by air-filled expansions like blisters in interstitial or subcutaneous tissues; *specif* : a local or generalized condition of the lung marked by distension, progressive loss of elasticity, and eventual rupture of the alveoli and accompanied by labored breathing, a husky cough, and frequently by impairment of heart action — **em·phy·se·ma·tous** \-ˈze-mə-təs, -ˈse-, -ˈzē-, -ˈsē-\ *adj* — **em·phy·se·mic** \-ˈzē-mik, -ˈsē-\ *adj*

em·pir·ic \im-ˈpir-ik, em-\ *n* : EMPIRICIST

em·pir·i·cal \-i-kəl\ *or* **em·pir·ic** \-ik\ *adj* **1** : originating in or based on observation or experiment **2** : capable of being confirmed, verified, or disproved by observation or experiment ⟨∼ statements or laws⟩ — **em·pir·i·cal·ly** \-i-k(ə-)lē\ *adv*

empirical formula *n* : a chemical formula showing the simplest ratio of elements in a compound rather than the total number of atoms in the molecule ⟨CH_2O is the *empirical formula* for glucose⟩

em·pir·i·cism \im-ˈpir-ə-ˌsi-zəm, em-\ *n* **1 a** : a former school of medical practice founded on experience without the aid of science or theory **b** : QUACKERY **2** : the practice of relying on observation and experiment esp. in the natural sciences

em·pir·i·cist \-sist\ *n* : one that advocates or practices empiricism

em·py·ema \ˌem-ˌpī-ˈē-mə\ *n, pl* **-ema·ta** \-mə-tə\ *or* **-emas** : the presence of pus in a bodily cavity (as the pleural cavity) — called also *pyothorax* — **em·py·emic** \-mik\ *adj*

EMT \ˌē-(ˌ)em-ˈtē\ *n* : a specially trained medical technician licensed to provide basic emergency services (as cardiopulmonary resuscitation) before and during transportation to a hospital — called also *emergency medical technician*; compare PARAMEDIC 2

emul·si·fi·er \i-ˈməl-sə-ˌfī-ər\ *n* : one that emulsifies; *esp* : a surface-active agent (as a soap) promoting the formation and stabilization of an emulsion

emul·si·fy \-ˌfī\ *vb* **-fied; -fy·ing** : to disperse (as an oil) in an emulsion — **emul·si·fi·ca·tion** \-ˌməl-sə-fə-ˈkā-shən\ *n*

emul·sion \i-ˈməl-shən\ *n* **1 a** : a system (as fat in milk) consisting of a liquid dispersed with or without an emulsifier in an immiscible liquid usu. in droplets of larger than colloidal size **b** : the state of such a system **2** : SUSPENSION 2

enal·a·pril \e-ˈna-lə-ˌpril\ *n* : an antihypertensive drug $C_{20}H_{28}N_2O_5$ that is an ACE inhibitor administered orally in the form of its maleate — see VASOTEC

enal·a·pril·at \e-ˈna-lə-ˌpri-lət\ *n* : the metabolically active form $C_{18}H_{24}$-$N_2O_5 \cdot 2H_2O$ of enalapril administered intravenously

enam·el \in-ˈa-məl\ *n* : the hard calcareous substance that forms a thin layer partly covering the teeth and consists of minute prisms secreted by ameloblasts, arranged at right angles to the surface, and bound together by a cement substance — compare CEMENTUM, DENTIN

enamel organ *n* : an ectodermal ingrowth from the dental lamina that forms a cap with two walls separated by a reticulum of stellate cells, encloses the anterior part of the developing dental papilla and the cells of the inner enamel layer adjacent to the papilla, and differentiates into colum-nar ameloblasts which lay down the enamel rods of the tooth

enamel rod *n* : one of the elongated prismatic bodies making up the enam-el of a tooth — called also *enamel prism*

enanthate — see TESTOSTERONE ENAN-THATE

en·an·them \i-ˈnan-thəm\ *or* **en·an·the·ma** \en-ˌan-ˈthē-mə\ *n, pl* **-thems** *or* **-the·ma·ta** \-mə-tə\ : an eruption on a mucous surface

en·an·tio·mer \i-ˈnan-tē-ə-mər\ *n* : ei-ther of a pair of chemical compounds whose molecular structures have a mirror-image relationship to each other — **en·an·tio·mer·ic** \-ˌnan-tē-ə-ˈmer-ik\ *adj* — **en·an·tio·mer·i·cal·ly** \-i-k(ə-)lē\ *adv*

en·an·tio·morph \i-ˈnan-tē-ə-ˌmorf\ *n* : ENANTIOMER

en·ar·thro·sis \ˌen-ˌär-ˈthrō-səs\ *n, pl* **-thro·ses** \-ˌsēz\ : BALL-AND-SOCKET JOINT

en·cap·su·late \in-ˈkap-sə-ˌlāt\ *vb* **-lat·ed; -lat·ing** : to encase or become en-cased in or as if in a capsule — **en·cap·su·la·tion** \-ˌkap-sə-ˈlā-shən\ *n*

en·cap·su·lat·ed *adj* : surrounded by a gelatinous or membranous envelope

en·ceinte \äⁿ-ˈsant\ *adj* : PREGNANT

encephal- *or* **encephalo-** *comb form* **1** : brain ⟨*encephalitis*⟩ ⟨*encephalocele*⟩ **2** : of, relating to, or affecting the brain and ⟨*encephalo*myelitis⟩

-encephali *pl of* -ENCEPHALUS

en·ceph·a·li·tis \in-ˌse-fə-ˈlī-təs\ *n, pl* **-lit·i·des** \-ˈli-tə-ˌdēz\ : inflammation of the brain — **en·ceph·a·lit·ic** \-ˈli-tik\ *adj*

encephalitis le·thar·gi·ca \-li-ˈthär-ji-kə, -le-\ *n* : epidemic virus encephalitis in which somnolence is marked

en·ceph·a·lit·o·gen \in-ˌse-fə-ˈli-tə-jən, -ˌjen\ *n* : an encephalitogenic agent (as a virus)

en·ceph·a·lit·o·gen·ic \-ˌse-fə-ˌli-tə-ˈje-nik\ *adj* : tending to cause enceph-alitis (an ~ strain of a virus)

en·ceph·a·lo·cele \in-ˈse-fə-lō-ˌsēl\ *n* : hernia of the brain that is either con-genital or due to trauma

en·ceph·a·lo·gram \in-ˈse-fə-lō-ˌgram\ *n* : an X-ray picture of the brain made by encephalography

en·ceph·a·lo·graph \-ˌgraf\ *n* **1** : EN-CEPHALOGRAM **2** : ELECTROENCEPHA-LOGRAPH

en·ceph·a·log·ra·phy \in-ˌse-fə-ˈlä-grə-fē\ *n, pl* **-phies** : roentgenography of the brain after the cerebrospinal fluid has been replaced by a gas (as air) — **en·ceph·a·lo·graph·ic** \-lə-ˈgra-fik\ *adj* — **en·ceph·a·lo·graph·i·cal·ly** \-fi-k(ə-)lē\ *adv*

en·ceph·a·lo·ma·la·cia \in-ˌse-fə-lō-mə-ˈlā-shē-ə, -shə\ *n* : softening of the brain due to degenerative changes in nervous tissue

en·ceph·a·lo·my·eli·tis \in-ˌse-fə-lō-ˌmī-

ə-ˈlī-təs\ *n, pl* **-elit·i·des** \-ə-ˈli-tə-ˌdēz\ : inflammation of the brain and spinal cord; *specif* : EQUINE ENCEPHALOMYELITIS — **en·ceph·a·lo·my·elit·ic** \-ə-ˈli-tik\ *adj*

en·ceph·a·lo·my·elop·a·thy \-ˌmī-ə-ˈlä-pə-thē\ *n, pl* **-thies** : any disease that affects the brain and spinal cord

en·ceph·a·lo·myo·car·di·tis \-ˌmī-ə-kär-ˈdī-təs\ *n* : an acute febrile virus dis-ease characterized by degeneration and inflammation of skeletal and car-diac muscle and lesions of the central nervous system

en·ceph·a·lop·a·thy \in-ˌse-fə-ˈlä-pə-thē\ *n, pl* **-thies** : a disease of the brain: *esp* : one involving alterations of brain structure — **en·ceph·a·lo·path·ic** \-lə-ˈpa-thik\ *adj*

-en·ceph·a·lus \in-ˈse-fə-ləs\ *n comb form, pl* **-en·ceph·a·li** \-ˌlī, -ˌlē\ **1** : fe-tus having (such) a brain ⟨in*iencephalus*⟩ **2** : condition of having (such) a brain ⟨hydr*encephalus*⟩

-en·ceph·a·ly \in-ˈse-fə-lē\ *n comb form, pl* **-en·ceph·a·lies** \in-ˈse-fə-lēz\ : condition of having (such) a brain ⟨micr*encephaly*⟩

en·chon·dral \(ˌ)en-ˈkän-drəl, (ˌ)eŋ-\ *adj* : ENDOCHONDRAL

en·chon·dro·ma \ˌen-ˌkän-ˈdrō-mə, ˌeŋ-\ *n, pl* **-mas** *or* **-ma·ta** \-mə-tə\ : a tumor consisting of cartilaginous tis-sue; *esp* : one arising where cartilage does not normally exist

en·code \in-ˈkōd, en-\ *vb* : to specify the genetic code for

en·co·pre·sis \ˌen-kä-ˈprē-səs, -kə-\ *n, pl* **-re·ses** \-ˌsēz\ : involuntary defeca-tion of psychic origin

encounter group *n* : a usu. unstructured group that seeks to develop the ca-pacity of the individual to express feelings and to form emotional ties by unrestrained confrontation of individ-uals — compare T-GROUP

en·crus·ta·tion \ˌin-ˌkrəs-ˈtā-shən, ˌen-\ *var of* INCRUSTATION

en·cyst \in-ˈsist, en-\ *vb* : to enclose in or become enclosed in a cyst (proto-zoans ~*ing* in order to resist desicca-tion) — **en·cyst·ment** *n*

end- *or* **endo-** *comb form* **1** : within : in-side ⟨*end*aural⟩ ⟨*endo*skeleton⟩ — compare ECT-, EXO- I **2** : taking in ⟨*en*docytosis⟩

end·ar·ter·ec·to·my \ˌen-ˌdär-tə-ˈrek-tə-mē\ *n, pl* **-mies** : surgical removal of the inner layer of an artery when thickened and atheromatous or oc-cluded (as by intimal plaques)

end·ar·te·ri·tis \ˌen-ˌdär-tə-ˈrī-təs\ *n* : inflammation of the intima of one or more arteries

endarteritis ob·lit·er·ans \-ə-ˈbli-tə-ˌranz, -ˌranz\ *n* : endarteritis in which the intimal tissue plugs the lumen of an affected artery — called also *oblit-erating endarteritis*

end artery *n* : a terminal artery (as a

coronary artery) supplying all or most of the blood to a body part

end·au·ral \(ˌ)en-ˈdȯr-əl\ *adj* : performed or applied within the ear ⟨∼ surgery⟩

end·brain \ˈend-ˌbrān\ *n* : TELENCEPHALON

end brush *n* : END PLATE

end bud *n* : TAIL BUD

end bulb *n* : a bulbous termination of a sensory nerve fiber (as in the skin) — compare KRAUSE'S CORPUSCLE

end–di·a·stol·ic \ˌen-ˌdī-ə-ˈstä-lik\ *adj* : relating to or occurring in the moment immediately preceding contraction of the heart ⟨∼ pressure⟩

¹**en·dem·ic** \en-ˈde-mik, in-\ *adj* : restricted or peculiar to a locality or region ⟨∼ diseases⟩ — compare EPIDEMIC 1, SPORADIC — **en·dem·i·cal·ly** \-mi-k(ə)lē\ *adv*

²**endemic** *n* **1** : an endemic disease or an instance of its occurrence **2** : an endemic organism

en·de·mic·i·ty \ˌen-ˌde-ˈmi-sə-tē, -də-\ *n, pl* **-ties** : the quality or state of being endemic

endemic typhus *n* : MURINE TYPHUS

en·de·mism \ˈen-də-ˌmi-zəm\ *n* : ENDEMICITY

end foot *n, pl* **end feet** : BOUTON

endo– see END-

en·do·ab·dom·i·nal \ˌen-dō-ab-ˈdä-mən-ᵊl\ *adj* : relating to or occurring in the interior of the abdomen

en·do·an·eu·rys·mor·rha·phy \ˌen-dō-ˌan-yə-ˌriz-ˈmȯr-ə-fē\ *n, pl* **-phies** : a surgical treatment of aneurysm that involves opening its sac and collapsing, folding, and suturing its walls

en·do·bron·chi·al \ˌen-dō-ˈbräŋ-kē-əl\ *adj* : located within a bronchus ⟨∼ tuberculosis⟩ — **en·do·bron·chi·al·ly** *adv*

en·do·car·di·al \-ˈkär-dē-əl\ *adj* **1** : situated within the heart **2** : of or relating to the endocardium ⟨∼ biopsy⟩

endocardial fibroelastosis *n* : a condition usu. associated with congestive heart failure and enlargement of the heart that is characterized by conversion of the endocardium to fibroelastic tissue

en·do·car·di·tis \-ˌkär-ˈdī-təs\ *n* : inflammation of the lining of the heart and its valves

en·do·car·di·um \-ˈkär-dē-əm\ *n, pl* **-dia** \-dē-ə\ : a thin serous membrane lining the cavities of the heart

en·do·cer·vi·cal \-ˈsər-vi-kəl\ *adj* : of, relating to, or affecting the endocervix

en·do·cer·vi·ci·tis \-ˌsər-və-ˈsī-təs\ *n* : inflammation of the lining of the uterine cervix

en·do·cer·vix \-ˈsər-viks\ *n, pl* **-vi·ces** \-və-ˌsēz\ : the epithelial and glandular lining of the uterine cervix

en·do·chon·dral \ˌen-də-ˈkän-drəl\ *adj* : relating to, formed by, or being ossification that takes place from centers arising in cartilage and involves deposition of lime salts in the carti-

lage matrix followed by secondary absorption and replacement by true bony tissue

¹**en·do·crine** \ˈen-də-krən, -ˌkrīn, -ˌkrēn\ *adj* **1** : secreting internally; *specif* : producing secretions that are distributed in the body by way of the bloodstream ⟨an ∼ system⟩ **2** : of, relating to, affecting, or resembling an endocrine gland or secretion

²**endocrine** *n* **1** : HORMONE **2** : ENDOCRINE GLAND

endocrine gland *n* : a gland (as the thyroid or the pituitary) that produces an endocrine secretion — called also *ductless gland, gland of internal secretion*

endocrine system *n* : the glands and parts of glands that produce endocrine secretions, help to integrate and control bodily metabolic activity, and include esp. the pituitary, thyroid, parathyroids, adrenals, islets of Langerhans, ovaries, and testes

en·do·cri·no·log·ic \ˌen-də-ˌkrin-əl-ˈä-jik, -ˌkrīn-, -ˌkrēn-\ *or* **en·do·cri·no·log·i·cal** \-ji-kəl\ *adj* : involving or relating to the endocrine glands or secretions or to endocrinology

en·do·cri·nol·o·gy \ˌen-də-krə-ˈnä-lə-jē, -ˌkrī-\ *n, pl* **-gies** : a science dealing with the endocrine glands — **en·do·cri·nol·o·gist** \-jist\ *n*

en·do·cri·nop·a·thy \-krə-ˈnä-pə-thē, -ˌkrī-, -ˌkrē-\ *n, pl* **-thies** : a disease marked by dysfunction of an endocrine gland — **en·do·crin·o·path·ic** \-ˌkri-nə-ˈpa-thik, -ˌkrī-, -ˌkrē-\ *adj*

en·do·cyt·ic \-ˈsi-tik\ *adj* : of or relating to endocytosis : ENDOCYTOTIC ⟨∼ vesicles⟩

en·do·cy·to·sis \-sī-ˈtō-səs\ *n, pl* **-to·ses** \-ˌsēz\ : incorporation of substances into a cell by phagocytosis or pinocytosis — **en·do·cy·tose** \-ˈsī-ˌtōs, -ˌtōz\ *vb* — **en·do·cy·tot·ic** \-sī-ˈtä-tik\ *adj*

en·do·derm \ˈen-də-ˌdərm\ *n* : the innermost of the germ layers of an embryo that is the source of the epithelium of the digestive tract and its derivatives; *also* : a tissue that is derived from this germ layer — **en·do·der·mal** \ˌen-də-ˈdər-məl\ *adj*

end·odon·tia \ˌen-də-ˈdän-chē-ə, -chə\ *n* : ENDODONTICS

end·odon·tics \-ˈdän-tiks\ *n* : a branch of dentistry concerned with diseases of the pulp — **end·odon·tic** \-tik\ *adj* — **end·odon·ti·cal·ly** \-ti-k(ə-)lē\ *adv*

end·odon·tist \-tist\ *n* : a specialist in endodontics

en·do·en·zyme \ˌen-dō-ˈen-ˌzīm\ *n* : an enzyme that functions inside the cell — compare EXOENZYME

en·dog·e·nous \en-ˈdä-jə-nəs\ *also* **en·do·gen·ic** \ˌen-də-ˈje-nik\ *adj* **1** : caused by factors within the body or mind or arising from internal structural or functional causes ⟨∼ malnutrition⟩ ⟨∼ psychic depression⟩ **2** : relating to or produced by metabolic synthesis in the body ⟨ ∼ opioids⟩ — compare EXOGENOUS — **en·dog·e·nous·ly** *adv*

en·do·lymph \'en-də-ˌlimf\ *n* : the watery fluid in the membranous labyrinth of the ear — **en·do·lym·phat·ic** \ˌen-də-lim-'fa-tik\ *adj*

en·do·me·ninx \ˌen-də-'mē-nis, -'me-\ *n, pl* **-nin·ges** \-mə-'nin-(ˌ)jēz\ : the layer of embryonic mesoderm from which the arachnoid coat and pia mater of the brain develop

en·do·me·tri·al \ˌen-də-'mē-trē-əl\ *adj* : of, belonging to, or consisting of endometrium

en·do·me·tri·o·ma \-ˌmē-trē-'ō-mə\ *n, pl* **-mas** *or* **-ma·ta** \-mə-tə\ **1** : a tumor containing endometrial tissue **2** : ENDOMETRIOSIS — used chiefly of isolated foci of endometrium outside the uterus

en·do·me·tri·osis \ˌen-dō-ˌmē-trē-'ō-səs\ *n, pl* **-oses** \-ˌsēz\ : the presence and growth of functioning endometrial tissue in places other than the uterus that often results in severe pain and infertility — see ADENOMYOSIS

en·do·me·tri·tis \-mə-'trī-təs\ *n* : inflammation of the endometrium

en·do·me·tri·um \-'mē-trē-əm\ *n, pl* **-tria** \-trē-ə\ : the mucous membrane lining the uterus

en·do·morph \'en-də-ˌmȯrf\ *n* : an endomorphic individual

en·do·mor·phic \ˌen-də-'mȯr-fik\ *adj* **1** : of or relating to the component in W. H. Sheldon's classification of body types that measures the degree to which the digestive viscera are massive and the body build rounded and soft — compare ECTOMORPHIC 1, MESOMORPHIC 2 **2** : having a heavy rounded body build often with a marked tendency to become fat — **en·do·mor·phy** \'en-də-ˌmȯr-fē\ *n*

en·do·myo·car·di·al \ˌen-dō-ˌmī-ə-'kär-dē-əl\ *adj* : of, relating to, or affecting the endocardium and the myocardium ⟨ ∼ fibrosis⟩ ⟨ ∼ biopsy⟩ — **en·do·myo·car·di·um** \-dē-əm\ *n*

en·do·my·si·um \ˌen-də-'mi-zē-əm, -zhē-əm, -zhəm\ *n, pl* **-sia** \-zē-ə, -zhē-ə, -zhə\ : the delicate connective tissue surrounding the individual muscular fibers — compare EPIMYSIUM

en·do·neu·ri·um \ˌen-dō-'nūr-ē-əm, -'nyur-\ *n, pl* **-ria** \-ē-ə\ : the delicate connective tissue network holding together the individual fibers of a nerve trunk — **en·do·neu·ri·al** \-ē-əl\ *adj*

en·do·nu·cle·ase \'en-dō-'nü-klē-ˌās, -'nyü-, -ˌāz\ *n* : an enzyme that breaks down a nucleotide chain into two or more shorter chains by breaking it at points not adjacent to the ends — see RESTRICTION ENZYME; compare EXONUCLEASE

en·do·nu·cleo·lyt·ic \-ˌnü-klē-ō-'li-tik, -ˌnyü-\ *adj* : breaking a nucleotide

chain into two parts at an internal point ⟨ ∼ nicks⟩

en·do·par·a·site \-'par-ə-ˌsīt\ *n* : a parasite that lives in the internal organs or tissues of its host — compare ECTOPARASITE — **en·do·par·a·sit·ic** \-ˌpar-ə-'si-tik\ *adj* — **en·do·par·a·sit·ism** \-'par-ə-sī-ˌtiz-əm, -sə-\ *n*

en·do·pep·ti·dase \-'pep-tə-ˌdās, -ˌdāz\ *n* : any of a group of enzymes that hydrolyze peptide bonds within the long chains of protein molecules : PROTEASE — compare EXOPEPTIDASE

en·do·per·ox·ide \-pə-'räk-ˌsīd\ *n* : any of various biosynthetic intermediates in the formation of prostaglandins

en·do·phle·bi·tis \ˌen-dō-fli-'bī-təs\ *n, pl* **-bi·tis·es** *or* **-bit·i·des** \-'bi-tə-ˌdēz\ : inflammation of the intima of a vein

en·doph·thal·mi·tis \ˌen-ˌdäf-thal-'mī-təs\ *n* : inflammation that affects the interior of the eyeball

en·do·phyt·ic \ˌen-dō-'fī-tik\ *adj* : tending to grow inward into tissues in fingerlike projections from a superficial site of origin — used of tumors; compare EXOPHYTIC

en·do·plasm \'en-də-ˌpla-zəm\ *n* : the inner relatively fluid part of the cytoplasm — compare ECTOPLASM — **en·do·plas·mic** \ˌen-də-'plaz-mik\ *adj*

endoplasmic reticulum *n* : a system of mutually connected vesicular and lamellar cytoplasmic membranes that functions esp. in the transport of materials within the cell and that is studded with ribosomes in some places

en·do·pros·the·sis \ˌen-dō-präs-'thē-səs\ *n, pl* **-the·ses** \-ˌsēz\ : an artificial device to replace a missing bodily part that is placed inside the body

end organ *n* : a structure forming the peripheral end of a path of nerve conduction and consisting of an effector or a receptor with its associated nerve terminations

en·dor·phin \en-'dȯr-fən\ *n* : any of a group of proteins with potent analgesic properties that occur naturally in the brain — see BETA-ENDORPHIN; compare ENKEPHALIN

β-endorphin *var of* BETA-ENDORPHIN

en·do·scope \'en-də-ˌskōp\ *n* : an instrument for visualizing the interior of a hollow organ (as the rectum or urethra) — **en·dos·co·py** \en-'däs-kə-pē\ *n*

en·do·scop·ic \ˌen-də-'skä-pik\ *adj* : of, relating to, or performed by means of an endoscope or endoscopy — **en·do·scop·i·cal·ly** \-pi-k(ə-)lē\ *adv*

en·dos·co·pist \en-'däs-kə-pist\ *n* : a person trained in the use of the endoscope

en·do·skel·e·ton \ˌen-dō-'skel-ət-ᵊn\ *n* : an internal skeleton or supporting framework in an animal — **en·do·skel·e·tal** \-ət-ᵊl\ *adj*

en·do·spore \-ˌspȯr\ *n* : an asexual spore developed within the cell esp. in bacteria

end·os·te·al \en-ˈdäs-tē-əl\ *adj* **1** : of or relating to the endosteum **2** : located within bone or cartilage — **end·os·te·al·ly** *adv*

end·os·te·um \en-ˈdäs-tē-əm\ *n, pl* **-tea** \-ə\ : the layer of vascular connective tissue lining the medullary cavities of bone

endotheli- *or* **endothelio-** *comb form* : endothelium ⟨*endothelioma*⟩

en·do·the·li·al \ˌen-də-ˈthē-lē-əl\ *adj* : of, relating to, or produced from endothelium

en·do·the·li·o·ma \-ˌthē-lē-ˈō-mə\ *n, pl* **-omas** *or* **-oma·ta** \-mə-tə\ : a tumor developing from endothelial tissue

en·do·the·li·um \ˌen-də-ˈthē-lē-əm\ *n, pl* **-lia** \-ə\ : an epithelium of mesoblastic origin composed of a single layer of thin flattened cells that lines internal body cavities (as the serous cavities or the interior of the heart)

en·do·tox·emia \ˌen-dō-täk-ˈsē-mē-ə\ *n* : the presence of endotoxins in the blood

en·do·tox·in \ˌen-dō-ˈtäk-sən\ *n* : a toxin of internal origin; *specif* : a poisonous substance present in bacteria but separable from the cell body only on its disintegration — compare EXOTOXIN — **en·do·tox·ic** \-sik\ *adj*

en·do·tra·che·al \-ˈtrā-kē-əl\ *adj* **1** : placed within the trachea (an ~ tube) **2** : applied or effected through the trachea

end plate *n* : a complex terminal arborization of a motor nerve fiber — called also *end brush*

en·e·ma \ˈe-nə-mə\ *n, pl* **enemas** *also* **ene·ma·ta** \ˌe-nə-ˈmä-tə, ˈe-nə-mə-tə\ : the injection of liquid into the intestine by way of the anus (as for cleansing); *also* : the liquid so injected

en·er·get·ic \ˌe-nər-ˈje-tik\ *adj* : of or relating to energy

en·er·get·ics \-tiks\ *n* **1** : a branch of physics that deals primarily with energy and its transformations **2** : the total energy relations and transformations of a physical, chemical, or biological system ⟨~ of muscular contraction⟩

en·er·giz·er \ˈe-nər-ˌjī-zər\ *n* : ANTIDEPRESSANT

en·er·gy \ˈe-nər-jē\ *n, pl* **-gies** **1** : the force driving and sustaining mental activity **2** : the capacity for doing work

en·er·vate \ˈe-nər-ˌvāt\ *vb* **-vat·ed; -vat·ing** : to lessen the vitality or strength of — **en·er·va·tion** \ˌe-nər-ˈvā-shən\ *n*

en·flur·ane \en-ˈflur-ˌān\ *n* : a liquid inhalational general anesthetic $C_3H_2ClF_5O$ prepared from methanol

en·gage·ment \in-ˈgāj-mənt\ *n* : the phase of parturition in which the fetal head passes into the cavity of the true pelvis

en·gi·neer \ˌen-jə-ˈnir\ *vb* : to modify or produce by genetic engineering

En·glish system \ˈiŋ-glish-, ˈiŋ-lish-\ *n* : the foot-pound-second system of units

en·gorge \in-ˈgȯrj\ *vb* **en·gorged; en·gorg·ing** **1** : to fill with blood to the point of congestion ⟨the gastric mucosa was greatly *engorged*⟩ **2** : to suck blood to the limit of body capacity ⟨a tick *engorging* on its host⟩ — **en·gorge·ment** *n*

en·graft \in-ˈgraft\ *vb* : GRAFT — **en·graft·ment** *n*

en·gram *also* **en·gramme** \ˈen-ˌgram\ *n* : a hypothetical change in neural tissue postulated in order to account for persistence of memory — called also *memory trace*

en·hanc·er \in-ˈhan-sər, en-\ *n* : a nucleotide sequence that increases the rate of genetic transcription by increasing the activity of the nearest promoter on the same DNA molecule

en·keph·a·lin \in-ˈke-fə-lən, -(ˌ)lin\ *n* : either of two pentapeptides with opiate and analgesic activity that occur naturally in the brain and have a marked affinity for opiate receptors: **a** : LEUCINE-ENKEPHALIN **b** : METHIONINE-ENKEPHALIN — compare ENDORPHIN

en·keph·a·lin·er·gic \-ˌke-fə-lə-ˈnər-jik\ *adj* : liberating or activated by enkephalins ⟨~ neurons⟩

eno·lase \ˈē-nə-ˌlās, -ˌlāz\ *n* : an enzyme that is found esp. in muscle and is important in the metabolism of carbohydrates

en·oph·thal·mos \ˌe-ˌnäf-ˈthal-məs, -ˌnäp-, -ˌmäs\ *also* **en·oph·thal·mus** \-məs\ *n* : a sinking of the eyeball into the orbital cavity

en·os·to·sis \ˌe-ˌnäs-ˈtō-səs\ *n, pl* **-to·ses** \-ˌsēz\ : a bony tumor arising within a bone

Eno·vid \e-ˈnō-vid\ *trademark* — used for an oral contraceptive containing norethynodrel and mestranol

en·sheathe \in-ˈshēth\ *vb* : to cover with or as if with a sheath

ensiform cartilage *n* : XIPHOID PROCESS

ensiform process *n* : XIPHOID PROCESS

ENT *abbr* ear, nose, and throat

ent- *or* **ento-** *comb form* : inner : within ⟨*entoptic*⟩ ⟨*entoderm*⟩

ent·ame·ba \ˌen-tə-ˈmē-bə\ *n, pl* **-bas** *or* **-bae** \-(ˌ)bē\ : any ameba of the genus *Entamoeba* — **ent·ame·bic** \-bik\ *adj*

ent·am·e·bi·a·sis \ˌen-ˌta-mi-ˈbī-ə-səs\ *n, pl* **-a·ses** \-ˌsēz\ : infection with or disease caused by a protozoan of the genus *Entamoeba* — called also AMEBIASIS

ent·amoe·ba *chiefly Brit var of* ENTAMEBA

Ent·amoe·ba \ˌen-tə-ˈmē-bə, ˈen-tə-\ *n* : a genus of ameboid protozoans (order Amoebida) that are parasitic in the alimentary canal and esp. in the intestines and that include the causative agent (*E. histolytica*) of amebic dysentery

enter- *or* **entero-** *comb form* **1** : intestine ⟨*enteritis*⟩ **2** : intestinal and ⟨*entero*hepatic⟩

en·ter·al \\'en-tə-rəl\\ *adj* : ENTERIC — **en·ter·al·ly** *adv*

en·ter·ec·to·my \\,en-tə-'rek-tə-mē\\ *n, pl* **-mies** : the surgical removal of a portion of the intestine

en·ter·ic \\en-'ter-ik, in-\\ *adj* **1** : of or relating to the intestines; *broadly* : ALIMENTARY **2** : of, relating to, or being a medicinal preparation treated to pass through the stomach unaltered and disintegrate in the intestines

enteric fever *n* : TYPHOID FEVER; *also* : PARATYPHOID

entericus — see SUCCUS ENTERICUS

en·ter·i·tis \\,en-tə-'rī-təs\\, *n, pl* **en·ter·it·i·des** \\-'ri-tə-,dēz\\ *or* **en·ter·i·tis·es 1** : inflammation of the intestines and esp. of the human ileum **2** : a disease of domestic animals (as panleukopenia of cats) marked by enteritis and diarrhea

En·te·ro·bac·ter \\'en-tə-rō-,bak-tər\\ *n* : a genus of enterobacteria that are widely distributed in nature (as in feces, soil, water, and the contents of human and animal intestines) and include some that may be pathogenic

en·tero·bac·te·ri·um \\,en-tə-rō-bak-'tir-ē-əm\\ *n, pl* **-ria** \\-ē-ə\\ : any of a family (Enterobacteriaceae) of gram-negative rod-shaped bacteria (as a salmonella or colon bacillus) that ferment glucose and include some serious animal pathogens — **en·tero·bac·te·ri·al** \\-ē-əl\\ *adj*

en·tero·bi·a·sis \\-'bī-ə-səs\\, *n, pl* **-a·ses** \\-,sēz\\ : infestation with or disease caused by pinworms of the genus *Enterobius* that occurs esp. in children

En·te·ro·bi·us \\,en-tə-'rō-bē-əs\\ *n* : a genus of small nematode worms (family Oxyuridae) that includes the common pinworm (*E. vermicularis*) of the human intestine

en·ter·o·cele \\'en-tə-rō-,sēl\\ *n* : a hernia containing a portion of the intestines

en·tero·chro·maf·fin \\,en-tə-rō-'krō-mə-fən\\ *adj* : of, relating to, or being epithelial cells of the intestinal mucosa that stain esp. with chromium salts and usu. contain serotonin

en·tero·coc·cus \\,en-tə-rō-'kä-kəs\\ *n, pl* **-coc·ci** \\-'käk-,sī, -,sē; -'käk-ī, -ē\\ : STREPTOCOCCUS **2**; *esp* : a streptococcus (as *Streptococcus faecalis*) normally present in the intestine — **en·tero·coc·cal** \\-'kä-kəl\\ *adj*

en·tero·co·li·tis \\,en-tə-rō-kə-'lī-təs\\ *n* : enteritis affecting both the large and small intestine

en·tero·en·ter·os·to·my \\-,en-tə-'räs-tə-mē\\ *n, pl* **-mies** : surgical anastomosis of two parts of the intestine with creation of an opening between them

en·tero·gas·tric reflex \\-,gas-trik-\\ *n* : reflex inhibition of the emptying of the stomach's contents through the pylorus that occurs when the duodenum is stimulated by the presence of irri-

tants, is overloaded, or is obstructed

en·tero·gas·trone \\-'gas-,trōn\\ *n* : a hormone that is held to be produced by the duodenal mucosa and to inhibit gastric motility and secretion — compare UROGASTRONE

en·tero·he·pat·ic \\-hi-'pa-tik\\ *adj* : of or involving the intestine and the liver ⟨∼ circulation of bile salts⟩

en·tero·hep·a·ti·tis \\-,he-pə-'tī-təs\\ *n* : BLACKHEAD **2**

en·tero·ki·nase \\-'kī-,nās, -,nāz\\ *n* : an enzyme that activates trypsinogen by converting it to trypsin

en·ter·o·lith \\en-tə-rō-,lith\\ *n* : an intestinal calculus

enteropathica — see ACRODERMATITIS ENTEROPATHICA

en·tero·patho·gen·ic \\,en-tə-rō-,pa-thə-'je-nik\\ *adj* : tending to produce disease in the intestinal tract ⟨∼ bacteria⟩ — **en·tero·patho·gen** \\-'pa-thə-jən\\ *n*

en·ter·op·a·thy \\,en-tə-'rä-pə-thē\\ *n, pl* **-thies** : a disease of the intestinal tract

en·ter·os·to·my \\,en-tə-'räs-tə-mē\\ *n, pl* **-mies** : a surgical formation of an opening into the intestine through the abdominal wall — **en·ter·os·to·mal** \\-tə-məl\\ *adj*

en·ter·ot·o·my \\,en-tə-'rä-tə-mē\\ *n, pl* **-mies** : incision into the intestines

en·tero·tox·emia \\,en-tə-rō-,täk-'sē-mē-ə\\ *n* : a disease (as pulpy kidney disease of lambs) attributed to absorption of a toxin from the intestine — called also *overeating disease*

en·tero·toxi·gen·ic \\-,täk-sə-'je-nik\\ *adj* : producing enterotoxin

en·tero·tox·in \\-'täk-sən\\ *n* : a toxin that is produced by microorganisms (as some staphylococci) and causes gastrointestinal symptoms

en·tero·vi·rus \\-'vī-rəs\\ *n* : any of a group of picornaviruses (as the poliomyelitis virus) that typically occur in the gastrointestinal tract but may be involved in respiratory ailments, meningitis, and neurological disorders — **en·tero·vi·ral** \\-rəl\\ *adj*

ento- — see ENT-

en·to·derm \\'en-tə-,dərm\\ *n* : ENDODERM

en·to·mo·pho·bia \\,en-tə-mō-'fō-bē-ə\\ *n* : fear of insects

ent·op·tic \\(,)en-'täp-tik\\ *adj* : lying or originating within the eyeball — used esp. of visual sensations due to the shadows of retinal blood vessels or of opaque particles in the vitreous humor falling upon the retina

en·tro·pi·on \\en-'trō-pē-,än, -ən\\ *n* : the inversion or turning inward of the border of the eyelid against the eyeball

¹enu·cle·ate \\(,)ē-'nü-klē-,āt, -'nyü-\\ *vb* **-at·ed; -at·ing 1** : to deprive of a nucleus **2** : to remove without cutting into ⟨∼ a tumor⟩ ⟨∼ the eyeball⟩ — **enu·cle·ation** \\(,)ē-,nü-klē-'ā-shən, -,nyü-\\

n — **enu·cle·a·tor** \-(₁)ē-'nü-klē-₁ā-tər, -'nyü-\ *n*

²**enu·cle·ate** \-klē-ət, -₁āt\ *adj* : lacking a nucleus ⟨~ cells⟩

en·ure·sis \₁en-yu̇-'rē-səs\ *n, pl* **-ure·ses** \-₁sēz\ : an involuntary discharge of urine : incontinence of urine — **enu·ret·ic** \-'re-tik\ *adj or n*

en·ve·lope \'en-və-₁lōp, 'än-\ *n* : a natural enclosing covering (as a membrane or integument)

en·ven·om·ation \in-₁ve-nə-'mā-shən\ *n* : an act or instance of impregnating with a venom (as of a snake or spider); *also* : ENVENOMIZATION

en·ven·om·iza·tion \-mə-'zā-shən\ *n* : a poisoning caused by a bite or sting

en·vi·ron·ment \in-'vī-rən-mənt, -'vī-ərn-\ *n* **1** : the complex of physical, chemical, and biotic factors (as climate, soil, and living things) that act upon an organism or an ecological community and ultimately determine its form and survival **2** : the aggregate of social and cultural conditions that influence the life of an individual or community — **en·vi·ron·men·tal** \-₁vī-rən-'men-t°l, -₁vī-ərn-\ *adj* — **en·vi·ron·men·tal·ly** *adv*

¹**en·zo·ot·ic** \₁en-zə-'wä-tik\ *adj, of animal diseases* : peculiar to or constantly present in a locality — **en·zo·ot·i·cal·ly** \-ti-k(ə-)lē\ *adv*

²**enzootic** *n* : an enzootic disease

en·zy·mat·ic \₁en-zə-'ma-tik\ *also* **en·zy·mic** \en-'zī-mik\ *adj* : of, relating to, or produced by an enzyme — **en·zy·mat·i·cal·ly** \-ti-k(ə-)lē\ *also* **en·zy·mi·cal·ly** \en-'zī-mi-k(ə-)lē\ *adv*

en·zyme \'en-₁zīm\ *n* : any of numerous complex proteins that are produced by living cells and catalyze specific biochemical reactions at body temperatures

enzyme–linked immunosorbent assay *n* : a quantitative *in vitro* test for an antibody or antigen in which the test material is adsorbed on a surface and exposed to a complex of an enzyme linked to an antibody specific for the suspected antibody or antigen being tested for with a positive result indicated by a treatment yielding a color in proportion to the amount of antigen or antibody in the test material — called also *ELISA*

en·zy·mol·o·gy \₁en-₁zī-'mä-lə-jē, -zə-\ *n, pl* **-gies** : a branch of biochemistry dealing with enzymes, their nature, activity, and significance — **en·zy·mo·log·i·cal** \-mə-'lä-ji-kəl\ *adj* — **en·zy·mol·o·gist** \₁en-₁zī-'mä-lə-jist\ *n*

EOG *abbr* electrooculogram

eon·ism \'ē-ə-₁ni-zəm\ *n* : TRANSVESTISM

Éon de Beau·mont \ā-ōⁿ-də-bō-mōⁿ\, **Charles (1728–1810),** French chevalier and adventurer.

eo·sin \'ē-ə-sən\ *also* **eo·sine** \-sən, -₁sēn\ *n* : a red fluorescent dye $C_{20}H_8Br_4O_5$; *also* : its red to brown sodium or potassium salt used esp. as a biological stain for cytoplasmic structures

eo·sin·o·pe·nia \₁ē-ə-₁si-nə-'pē-nē-ə, -nyə\ *n* : an abnormal decrease in the number of eosinophils in the blood — **eo·sin·o·pe·nic** \-'pē-nik\ *adj*

¹**eo·sin·o·phil** \₁ē-ə-'si-nə-₁fil\ *also* **eo·sin·o·phile** \-₁fīl\ *adj* : EOSINOPHILIC 1

²**eosinophil** *also* **eosinophile** *n* : a leukocyte or other granulocyte with cytoplasmic inclusions readily stained by eosin

eo·sin·o·phil·ia \-₁si-nə-'fi-lē-ə\ *n* : abnormal increase in the number of eosinophils in the blood that is characteristic of allergic states and various parasitic infections

eo·sin·o·phil·ic \-₁si-nə-'fi-lik\ *adj* **1** : staining readily with eosin **2** : of, relating to, or characterized by eosinophilia

eosinophilic granuloma *n* : a disease of adolescents and young adults marked by the formation of granulomas in bone and the presence in them of histiocytes and eosinophilic cells with secondary deposition of cholesterol

ep- — see EPI-

ep·ar·te·ri·al \₁e-pär-'tir-ē-əl\ *adj* : situated above an artery; *specif* : of or relating to the first branch of the right bronchus

ependym- *or* **ependymo-** *comb form* : ependyma ⟨*ependym*itis⟩

ep·en·dy·ma \e-'pen-də-mə\ *n* : an epithelial membrane lining the ventricles of the brain and the canal of the spinal cord — **ep·en·dy·mal** \(₁)e-'pen-də-məl\ *adj*

ep·en·dy·mi·tis \₁e-₁pen-də-'mī-təs\ *n, pl* **-mit·i·des** \-'mi-tə-₁dēz\ : inflammation of the ependyma

ep·en·dy·mo·ma \(₁)e-₁pen-də-'mō-mə\ *n, pl* **-mas** *also* **-ma·ta** \-mə-tə\ : a glioma arising in or near the ependyma

ep·eryth·ro·zo·on \₁e-pə-₁rith-rə-'zō-₁än\ *n* **1** *cap* : a genus of bacteria (family Anaplasmataceae) comprising blood parasites of vertebrates **2** *pl* **-zoa** \-'zō-ə\ : a bacterium of the genus *Eperythrozoon*

ep·eryth·ro·zo·on·o·sis \-₁zō-ə-'nō-səs\ *n, pl* **-oses** \-₁sēz\ : infection with or disease caused by bacteria of the genus *Eperythrozoon* that is esp. severe in young pigs

ephed·rine \i-'fe-drən\ *n* : a crystalline alkaloid $C_{10}H_{15}NO$ extracted from a Chinese shrub (*Ephedra sinica* of the family Gnetaceae) or synthesized that has the physiological action of epinephrine and is used in the form of a salt for relief of hay fever, asthma, and nasal congestion

ephe·lis \i-'fē-ləs\ *n, pl* **-li·des** \-'fē-lə-₁dēz, -'fe-\ : FRECKLE

ephem·er·al \i-'fe-mə-rəl\ *adj* : lasting a very short time

epi- *or* **ep-** *prefix* : upon ⟨*epi*cranial⟩

: besides ⟨*epi*phenomenon⟩ : attached to ⟨*epi*didymis⟩ : outer ⟨*epi*blast⟩

epi·an·dros·ter·one \ˌe-pē-ˌan-ˈdräs-tə-ˌrōn\ *n* : an androsterone derivative C₁₉H₃₀O₂ that occurs in normal human urine

epi·blast \ˈe-pə-ˌblast\ *n* : the outer layer of the blastoderm : ECTODERM — **epi·blas·tic** \ˌe-pə-ˈblas-tik\ *adj*

epi·can·thic fold \ˌe-pə-ˈkan-thik-\ *n* : a prolongation of a fold of the skin of the upper eyelid over the inner angle or both angles of the eye

epi·can·thus \-ˈkan-thəs\ *n* : EPICANTHIC FOLD

epi·car·di·um \ˌe-pi-ˈkär-dē-əm\ *n, pl* **-dia** \-ə\ : the visceral part of the pericardium that closely envelops the heart — called also *visceral pericardium;* compare PARIETAL PERICARDIUM — **epi·car·di·al** \-dē-əl\ *adj*

epi·con·dyle \ˌe-pi-ˈkän-ˌdīl, -dəl\ *n* : any of several prominences on the distal part of a long bone serving for the attachment of muscles and ligaments: **a** : one on the outer aspect of the distal part of the humerus or proximal to the lateral condyle of the femur — called also *lateral epicondyle* **b** : a larger and more prominent one on the inner aspect of the distal part of the humerus or proximal to the medial condyle of the femur — called also *medial epicondyle;* see EPITROCHLEA — **epi·con·dy·lar** \-də-lər\ *adj*

epi·con·dy·li·tis \-ˌkän-dī-ˈlī-təs, -də-\ *n* : inflammation of an epicondyle or of adjacent tissues — compare TENNIS ELBOW

epi·cra·ni·al \ˌe-pə-ˈkrā-nē-əl\ *adj* : situated on the cranium

epicranial aponeurosis *n* : GALEA APONEUROTICA

epi·cra·ni·um \-ˈkrā-nē-əm\ *n, pl* **-nia** \-nē-ə\ : the structures covering the vertebrate cranium

epi·cra·ni·us \ˌe-pə-ˈkrā-nē-əs\ *n, pl* **-cra·nii** \-nē-ˌī\ : OCCIPITOFRONTALIS

epi·crit·ic \-ˈkri-tik\ *adj* : of, relating to, being, or mediating cutaneous sensory reception that is marked by accurate discrimination between small degrees of sensation — compare PROTOPATHIC

¹**epi·dem·ic** \ˌe-pə-ˈde-mik\ *also* **epi·dem·i·cal** \-mi-kəl\ *adj* **1** : affecting or tending to affect an atypically large number of individuals within a population, community, or region at the same time (typhoid was ∼) — compare ENDEMIC, SPORADIC **2** : of, relating to, or constituting an epidemic — **epi·dem·i·cal·ly** \-mi-k(ə-)lē\ *adv*

²**epidemic** *n* : an outbreak of epidemic disease

epidemic hemorrhagic fever *n* : KOREAN HEMORRHAGIC FEVER

epi·de·mic·i·ty \ˌe-pə-ˌde-ˈmi-sə-tē, -də-\ *n, pl* **-ties** : the quality or state of being epidemic; *specif* : the relative

ability to spread from one host to others (∼ of typhoid bacteria)

epidemic keratoconjunctivitis *n* : an infectious often epidemic disease that is caused by an adenovirus and is marked by pain, by redness and swelling of the conjunctiva, by edema of the tissues around the eye, and by tenderness of the adjacent lymph nodes

epidemic parotitis *n* : MUMPS

epidemic pleurodynia *n* : an acute virus infection that is typically caused by a coxsackievirus and is characterized by sudden onset with fever, headache, and acute diaphragmatic pain

epidemic typhus *n* : TYPHUS a

epi·de·mi·ol·o·gist \ˌe-pə-ˌdē-mē-ˈä-lə-jist, -ˌde-\ *n* : a specialist in epidemiology

epi·de·mi·ol·o·gy \-jē\ *n, pl* **-gies 1** : a branch of medical science that deals with the incidence, distribution, and control of disease in a population **2** : the sum of the factors controlling the presence or absence of a disease or pathogen — **epi·de·mi·o·log·i·cal** \-ə-ˌläj-i-kəl\ *also* **epi·de·mi·o·log·ic** \-jik\ *adj* — **epi·de·mi·o·log·i·cal·ly** \-ji-k(ə-)lē\ *adv*

epiderm- *or* **epidermo-** *comb form* : epidermis ⟨*epidermitis*⟩ ⟨*epidermolysis*⟩

epi·derm \ˈe-pə-ˌdərm\ *n* : EPIDERMIS

epi·der·mal \ˌe-pə-ˈdər-məl\ *adj* : of, relating to, or arising from the epidermis

epidermal growth factor *n* : a polypeptide hormone that stimulates cell proliferation esp. of epithelial cells by binding to receptor proteins on the cell surface — abbr. *EGF*

epidermal necrolysis *n* : TOXIC EPIDERMAL NECROLYSIS

epi·der·mic \ˌe-pə-ˈdər-mik\ *adj* : EPIDERMAL

epi·der·mis \-məs\ *n* : the outer epithelial layer of the external integument of the animal body that is derived from the embryonic epiblast; *specif* : the outer nonsensitive and nonvascular layer of the skin that overlies the dermis

epi·der·mi·tis \-(ˌ)dər-ˈmī-təs\ *n, pl* **-mi·tis·es** *or* **-mit·i·des** \-ˈmi-tə-ˌdēz\ : inflammation of the epidermis

epidermo- — see EPIDERM-

epi·der·moid \-ˈdər-ˌmȯid\ *adj* : resembling epidermis or epidermal cells : made up of elements like those of epidermis ⟨∼ cancer of the lung⟩

epidermoid cyst *n* : a cystic tumor containing epidermal or similar tissue — called also *epidermoid;* see CHOLESTEATOMA

epi·der·mol·y·sis \ˌep-ə-(ˌ)dər-ˈmä-lə-səs\ *n, pl* **-y·ses** \-ˌsēz\ : a state of detachment or loosening of the epidermis

Epi·der·moph·y·ton \-(ˌ)dər-ˈmä-fə-ˌtän\ *n* : a genus of fungi that comprises dermatophytes causing disease (as athlete's foot and tinea cruris), that now usu. includes a single species (*E. floccosums* syn. *E. inguinale* and *E. cruris*), and that is sometimes considered a synonym of *Trichophyton*

ep·i·der·moph·y·to·sis \-₁mä-fə-'tō-səs\ *n, pl* **-to·ses** \-₁sēz\ : a disease (as athlete's foot) of the skin or nails caused by a dermatophyte

epididym- *or* **epididymo-** *comb form* **1** : epididymis 〈*epididym*ectomy〉 **2** : epididymis and 〈*epididymo*orchitis〉

ep·i·did·y·mec·to·my \-₁di-də-'mek-tə-mē\ *n, pl* **-mies** : excision of the epididymis

ep·i·did·y·mis \-'di-də-məs\ *n, pl* **-mi·des** \-mə-₁dēz\ : a system of ductules that emerges posteriorly from the testis, holds sperm during maturation, and forms a tangled mass before uniting into a single coiled duct which comprises the highly convoluted body and tail of the system and is continuous with the vas deferens — see VASA EFFERENTIA — **ep·i·did·y·mal** \-məl\ *adj*

ep·i·did·y·mi·tis \-₁di-də-'mī-təs\ *n* : inflammation of the epididymis

ep·i·did·y·mo-or·chi·tis \-₁di-də-₁mō-ȯr-'kī-təs\ *n* : combined inflammation of the epididymis and testis

ep·i·did·y·mo·vas·os·to·my \-va-'säs-tə-mē\ *n, pl* **-mies** : surgical severing of the vas deferens with anastomosis of the distal part to the epididymis esp. to circumvent an obstruction

¹epi·du·ral \₁ep-i-'dur-əl, -'dyur-\ *adj* : situated upon or administered outside the dura mater — **epi·du·ral·ly** *adv*

²epidural *n* : EPIDURAL ANESTHESIA

epidural anesthesia *n* : anesthesia produced by injection of a local anesthetic into the peridural space of the spinal cord beneath the ligamentum flavum — called also *peridural anesthesia*

epi·gas·tric \₁e-pə-'gas-trik\ *adj* **1** : lying upon or over the stomach **2 a** : of or relating to the anterior walls of the abdomen 〈~ veins〉 **b** : of or relating to the abdominal region lying between the hypochondriac regions and above the umbilical region

epigastric artery *n* : any of the three arteries supplying the anterior walls of the abdomen

epi·gas·tri·um \₁e-pə-'gas-trē-əm\ *n, pl* **-tria** \-trē-ə\ : the epigastric region

epi·glot·tic \₁e-pə-'glä-tik\ *or* **epi·glot·tal** \-'glät-ᵊl\ *adj* : of, relating to, or produced with the aid of the epiglottis

epi·glot·ti·dec·to·my \-₁glä-tə-'dek-tə-mē\ *n, pl* **-mies** : excision of all or part of the epiglottis

epi·glot·tis \-'glä-təs\ *n* : a thin lamella of yellow elastic cartilage that ordinarily projects upward behind the tongue and just in front of the glottis and that with the arytenoid cartilages

serves to cover the glottis during the act of swallowing

ep·i·glot·ti·tis \-glä-'tī-təs\ *n* : inflammation of the epiglottis

ep·i·la·tion \-'lā-shən\ *n* : the loss or removal of hair

ep·i·lep·sy \'e-pə-₁lep-sē\ *n, pl* **-sies** : any of various disorders marked by disturbed electrical rhythms of the central nervous system and typically manifested by convulsive attacks usu. with clouding of consciousness — called also *falling sickness*; see GRAND MAL, PETIT MAL; JACKSONIAN EPILEPSY

epilept- *or* **epilepti-** *or* **epilepto-** *comb form* : epilepsy 〈*epilept*oid〉 〈*epilepti*form〉 〈*epilepto*genic〉

ep·i·lep·tic \₁e-pə-'lep-tik\ *adj* : relating to, affected with, or having the characteristics of epilepsy — **epileptic** *n* — **ep·i·lep·ti·cal·ly** \-ti-k(ə-)lē\ *adv*

epilepticus — see STATUS EPILEPTICUS

ep·i·lep·ti·form \-'lep-tə-₁form\ *adj* : resembling that of epilepsy 〈an ~ convulsion〉

ep·i·lep·to·gen·ic \-₁lep-tə-'je-nik\ *adj* : inducing or tending to induce epilepsy 〈an ~ drug〉

ep·i·lep·toid \-'lep-₁tȯid\ *adj* **1** : EPILEPTIFORM **2** : exhibiting symptoms resembling those of epilepsy

ep·i·loia \₁e-pə-'lȯi-ə\ *n* : a deleterious dominant genetic trait marked by mental deficiency and multiple tumor formation of the skin and brain and maintained in human populations by a high mutation rate — called also *tuberous sclerosis*

epi·my·si·um \₁e-pə-'mizh-ē-əm, -zē-\ *n, pl* **-sia** \-zhē-ə, -zē-ə\ : the external connective-tissue sheath of a muscle — compare ENDOMYSIUM

epi·neph·rine *also* **epi·neph·rin** \₁e-pə-'ne-frən\ *n* : a crystalline feebly basic sympathomimetic hormone $C_9H_{13}N$-O_3 that is the principal blood-pressure-raising hormone secreted by the adrenal medulla, is prepared from adrenal extracts or made synthetically, and is used medicinally esp. as a heart stimulant, as a vasoconstrictor in controlling hemorrhages of the skin and in prolonging the effects of local anesthetics, and as a muscle relaxant in bronchial asthma — called also *adrenaline*

¹epi·neu·ral \₁e-pə-'nur-əl, -'nyur-\ *adj* : arising from the neural arch of a vertebra

²epineural *n* : a spine or process arising from the neural arch of a vertebra

epi·neu·ri·um \₁e-pə-'nur-ē-əm, -'nyur-\ *n* : the external connective-tissue sheath of a nerve trunk

epi·phe·nom·e·non \₁e-pi-fə-'nä-mə-₁nän, -nən\ *n* : an accidental or accessory event or process occurring in the course of a disease but not necessarily related to that disease

epiph·o·ra \i-'pi-fə-rə\ *n* : a watering of

the eyes due to excessive secretion of tears or to obstruction of the lacrimal passages

epiph·y·se·al \i-₁pi-fə-ˈsē-əl\ *also* **ep·i·phys·i·al** \₁e-pə-ˈfi-zē-əl\ *adj* : of or relating to an epiphysis

epiphyseal line *n* : the line marking the site of the epiphyseal plate

epiphyseal plate *n* : the cartilage that contains an epiphysis, unites it with the shaft, and is the site of longitudinal growth of the bone — called also *epiphyseal cartilage*

epiph·y·si·od·e·sis \i-₁pi-fə-sē-ˈä-də-səs, ₁e-pə-ˈfi-zē-\ *n, pl* **-e·ses** \-₁sēz\ : the surgical reattachment of a separated epiphysis to the shaft of its bone

epiph·y·sis \i-ˈpi-fə-səs\ *n, pl* **-y·ses** \-₁sēz\ **1** : a part or process of a bone that ossifies separately and later becomes ankylosed to the main part of the bone; *esp* : an end of a long bone — compare DIAPHYSIS **2** : PINEAL GLAND

epiph·y·si·tis \i-₁pi-fə-ˈsī-təs\ *n* : inflammation of an epiphysis

epi·plo·ec·to·my \₁e-pə-plō-ˈek-tə-mē\ *n, pl* **-mies** : OMENTECTOMY

ep·i·plo·ic \₁e-pə-ˈplō-ik\ *adj* : of or associated with an omentum : OMENTAL

epiploicae — see APPENDICES EPIPLOICAE

epiploic foramen *n* : the only opening between the omental bursa and the general peritoneal sac — called also *foramen of Winslow*

epi·plo·on \₁e-pə-ˈplō-₁än\ *n, pl* **-ploa** \-ˈplō-ə\ : OMENTUM; *specif* : GREATER OMENTUM

epi·pter·ic \₁ep-ip-ˈter-ik\ *adj* : relating to or being a small Wormian bone sometimes present in the human skull between the parietal and the greater wing of the sphenoid

epi·sclera \₁e-pə-ˈskler-ə\ *n* : the layer of connective tissue between the conjunctiva and the sclera of the eye

epi·scler·al \-ˈskler-əl\ *adj* **1** : situated upon the scleroic coat of the eye **2** : of or relating to the episclera

epi·scler·i·tis \-₁sklə-ˈrī-təs\ *n* : inflammation of the superficial layers of the sclera

episio- *comb form* **1** : vulva ⟨*episiotomy*⟩ **2** : vulva and ⟨*episioperineorrhaphy*⟩

epi·sio·per·i·ne·or·rha·phy \i-₁pi-zē-ō-₁per-ə-nē-ˈȯr-ə-fē, -₁pē-\ *n, pl* **-phies** : surgical repair of the vulva and perineum by suturing

epi·si·or·rha·phy \-zē-ˈȯr-ə-fē\ *n, pl* **-phies** : surgical repair of injury to the vulva by suturing

epi·si·ot·o·my \i-₁pi-zē-ˈä-tə-mē, -₁pē-\ *n, pl* **-mies** : surgical enlargement of the vulval orifice for obstetrical purposes during parturition

ep·i·sode \ˈe-pə-₁sōd, -₁zōd\ *n* : an event that is distinctive and separate although part of a larger series; *esp* : an occurrence of a usu. recurrent pathological abnormal condition —
ep·i·sod·ic \₁e-pə-ˈsä-dik, -ˈzä-\ *adj* —
ep·i·sod·i·cal·ly \-di-k(ə-)lē\ *adv*

epi·some \ˈe-pə-₁sōm, -₁zōm\ *n* : a genetic determinant (as the DNA of some bacteriophages) that can replicate either autonomously in bacterial cytoplasm or as an integral part of their chromosomes — compare PLASMID — **epi·som·al** \₁e-pə-ˈsō-məl, -ˈzō-\ *adj* — **epi·som·al·ly** \-mə-lē\ *adv*

ep·i·spa·di·as \₁e-pə-ˈspā-dē-əs\ *n* : a congenital defect in which the urethra opens upon the upper surface of the penis

epis·ta·sis \i-ˈpis-tə-səs\ *n, pl* **-ta·ses** \-₁sēz\ **1 a** : suppression of a secretion or discharge **b** : a scum on the surface of urine **2** : suppression of the effect of a gene by a nonallelic gene — **epi·stat·ic** \₁e-pə-ˈsta-tik\ *adj*

ep·i·stax·is \₁e-pə-ˈstak-səs\ *n, pl* **-stax·es** \-₁sēz\ : NOSEBLEED

ep·i·stro·phe·us \₁e-pə-ˈstrō-fē-əs\ *n* : AXIS 2a

ep·i·thal·a·mus \₁e-pə-ˈtha-lə-məs\ *n, pl* **-mi** \-₁mī\ : a dorsal segment of the diencephalon containing the habenula and the pineal gland

epithel- *comb form* : epithelium ⟨*epithelize*⟩

epitheli- *or* **epithelio-** *comb form* : epithelium ⟨*epithelioma*⟩

ep·i·the·li·al \₁e-pə-ˈthē-lē-əl\ *adj* : of or relating to epithelium ⟨~ cells⟩

ep·i·the·li·oid \-ˈthē-lē-₁ȯid\ *adj* : resembling epithelium

ep·i·the·li·o·ma \-₁thē-lē-ˈō-mə\ *n, pl* **-mas** *or* **-ma·ta** \-mə-tə\ : a tumor derived from epithelial tissue

ep·i·the·li·um \₁e-pə-ˈthē-lē-əm\ *n, pl* **-lia** \-lē-ə\ : a membranous cellular tissue that covers a free surface or lines a tube or cavity of an animal body and serves esp. to enclose and protect the other parts of the body, to produce secretions and excretions, and to function in assimilation

ep·i·the·li·za·tion \₁e-pə-₁thē-lə-ˈzā-shən\ *or* **ep·i·the·li·al·iza·tion** \-₁thē-lē-ə-lə-\ *n* : the process of becoming covered with or converted to epithelium — **ep·i·the·lize** \₁e-pə-ˈthē-₁līz\ *or* **ep·i·the·li·al·ize** \-ˈthē-lē-ə-₁līz\ *vb*

ep·i·thet \ˈe-pə-₁thet, -thət\ *n* : the part of a scientific name identifying the species, variety, or other subunit within a genus — see SPECIFIC EPITHET

epi·tope \ˈe-pə-₁tōp\ *n* : a molecular region on the surface of an antigen capable of eliciting an immune response and of combining with the specific antibody produced by such a response — called also *determinant, antigenic determinant*

epi·troch·lea \₁e-pi-ˈträ-klē-ə\ *n* : the medial epicondyle at the distal end of the humerus — **epi·troch·le·ar** \-klē-ər\ *adj*

epi·tym·pan·ic \-tim-ˈpa-nik\ *adj* : situated above the tympanic membrane

epitympanic recess n : ATTIC

epi·tym·pa·num \-'tim-pə-nəm\ n : the upper portion of the middle ear — compare HYPOTYMPANUM

epi·zo·ot·ic \ı·e-pə-zō-'wä-tik\ n : an outbreak of disease affecting many animals of one kind at the same time; also : the disease itself — **epizootic** adj

epizootic lymphangitis n : a chronic contagious inflammation that affects chiefly the superficial lymphatics and lymph nodes of horses, mules, and donkeys and is caused by a fungus of the genus Histoplasma (H. farciminosum)

epi·zo·ot·i·ol·o·gy \ı·e-pə-zō-ı·wä-tē-'ä-lə-jē\ also **epi·zo·otol·o·gy** \-ı·zō-ə-'tä-lə-jē\ n, pl **-gies** 1 : a science that deals with the character, ecology, and causes of outbreaks of animal diseases 2 : the sum of the factors controlling the occurrence of a disease or pathogen of animals — **epi·zo·oti·o·log·i·cal** \-ı·zō-ı·wō-tē-ə-'lä-ji-kəl, -ı·wä-\ also **epi·zo·oti·o·log·ic** \-jik\ adj

ep·o·nych·i·um \ı·e-pə-'ni-kē-əm\ n : the quick of a nail

ep·onym \'e-pə-ınim\ n 1 : the person for whom something (as a disease) is or is believed to be named 2 : a name (as of a drug or a disease) based on or derived from the name of a person — **epon·y·mous** \i-'pä-nə-məs, e-\ adj

ep·oopho·o·ron \ı·e-pō-'ä-fə-ı·rän\ n : a rudimentary organ homologous with the male epididymis that lies in the broad ligament of the uterus — called also **organ of Rosenmüller, parovarium**

Ep·som salt \'ep-səm-\ n : EPSOM SALTS

Epsom salts n : a bitter colorless or white crystalline salt MgSO₄·7H₂O that is a hydrated magnesium sulfate with cathartic properties

Ep·stein–Barr virus \'ep-ı·stīn-'bär-\ n : a herpesvirus that causes infectious mononucleosis and is associated with Burkitt's lymphoma and nasopharyngeal carcinoma — called also **EB virus**

Epstein, Michael Anthony (b 1921) and Barr, Y. M. (fl 1964), British virologists.

epu·lis \ə-'pyü-ləs\ n, pl **epu·li·des** \-lə-ıdēz\ : a tumor or tumorous growth of the gum

equa·tion·al \i-'kwā-zhə-nəl\ adj : dividing into two equal parts — used esp. of the mitotic cell division usu. following reduction in meiosis — **equa·tion·al·ly** adv

equa·tor \i-'kwā-tər, 'ē-ı\ n 1 : a circle dividing the surface of a body into two usu. equal and symmetrical parts esp. at the place of greatest width (the ~ of the lens of the eye) 2 : EQUATORIAL PLANE — **equa·to·ri·al** \ı·ē-kwə-'tōr-ē-əl, ı·e-\ adj

equatorial plane n : the plane perpendicular to the spindle of a dividing cell and midway between the poles

equatorial plate n 1 : METAPHASE PLATE 2 : EQUATORIAL PLANE

equi·an·al·ge·sic \ı·ē-kwi-ı·an-əl-'jē-zik, ı·e-, -sik\ adj : producing the same degree of analgesia

equi·len·in \ı·e-kwə-'le-nən, ə-'kwi-lə-nən\ n : a weakly estrogenic steroid hormone C₁₈H₁₈O₂ obtained from the urine of pregnant mares

equi·lib·ri·um \ı·ē-kwə-'li-brē-əm, ı·e-\ n, pl **-ri·ums** or **-ria** \-brē-ə\ 1 : a state of balance between opposing forces or actions that is either static (as in a body acted on by forces whose resultant is zero) or dynamic (as in a reversible chemical reaction when the velocities in both directions are equal) 2 : a state of intellectual or emotional balance

equina — see CAUDA EQUINA

equine \'ē-ı·kwīn, 'e-\ n : any of a family (Equidae) of hoofed mammals that include the horses, asses and zebras; esp : HORSE — **equine** adj

equine babesiosis n : a babesiosis that affects horses and related equines, is caused by two protozoans of the genus Babesia (B. caballi and B. equi), and is characterized esp. by fever, anemia, weakness, icterus, and sometimes hemoglobinuria and edema just below the skin around the head — called also **equine piroplasmosis**

equine encephalitis n : EQUINE ENCEPHALOMYELITIS

equine encephalomyelitis n : any of three encephalomyelitides that attack chiefly equines and humans and are caused by three related strains of arbovirus: **a** : one that occurs esp. in the eastern U.S. — called also **eastern equine encephalomyelitis b** : one that occurs esp. in the western U.S. — called also **western equine encephalomyelitis c** : one that occurs esp. from northern So. America to Mexico — called also **Venezuelan equine encephalitis, Venezuelan equine encephalomyelitis**

equine infectious anemia n : a serious sometimes fatal disease of horses that is caused by a lentivirus and is marked by intermittent fever, depression, weakness, anemia and anemia — called also **swamp fever**

equine piroplasmosis n : EQUINE BABESIOSIS

equinovarus — see TALIPES EQUINOVARUS

equinus — see TALIPES EQUINUS

equi·po·tent \ı·ē-kwə-'pōt-ənt, ı·e-\ adj : having equal effects or capacities (~ doses of different drugs)

Er symbol erbium

ER abbr emergency room

er·bi·um \'ər-bē-əm\ n : a metallic element that occurs with yttrium — symbol Er; see ELEMENT table

Erb's palsy \\'erbz-, 'erps-\ *n* : paralysis affecting the muscles of the upper arm and shoulder that is caused by an injury during birth to the upper part of the brachial plexus

erect \i 'rekt\ *adj* **1** : standing up or out from the body ⟨∼ hairs⟩ **2** : being in a state of physiological erection

erec·tile \i 'rekt-ᵊl, - 'rek-ₜtil\ *adj* : capable of being raised to an erect position; *esp* : CAVERNOUS 2 — **erec·til·i·ty** \ₜrek- 'til-ə-tē\ *n*

erec·tion \i- 'rek-shən\ *n* **1** : the state marked by firm turgid form and erect position of a previously flaccid bodily part containing cavernous tissue when that tissue becomes dilated with blood **2** : an occurrence of erection in the penis or clitoris

erec·tor \i- 'rek-tər\ *n* : a muscle that raises or keeps a part erect

erector spi·nae \- 'spī-ₜnē\ *n* : SACROSPINALIS

erep·sin \i- 'rep-sən\ *n* : a proteolytic fraction obtained esp. from the intestinal juice

er·e·thism \'er-ə- ₜthi-zəm\ *n* : abnormal irritability or responsiveness to stimulation

erg \'ərg\ *n* : a cgs unit of work equal to the work done by a force of one dyne acting through a distance of one centimeter

ERG *abbr* electroretinogram

erg- *or* **ergo-** *comb form* : work ⟨*ergo*meter⟩

-er·gic \'ər-jik\ *adj comb form* **1** : allergic ⟨hyper*ergic*⟩ **2** : exhibiting or stimulating activity esp. of (such) a neurotransmitter substance ⟨adren*ergic*⟩ ⟨dopamin*ergic*⟩

ergo- *comb form* : ergot ⟨*ergo*sterol⟩

er·go·cal·cif·er·ol \ₜər-(ₜ)gō-kal- 'si-fə-ₜrȯl, - ₜrōl\ *n* : CALCIFEROL

er·go·loid mesylates \'ər-gə-ₜlȯid-\ *n pl* : a combination of equal amounts of three ergot alkaloids used with varying success in the treatment of cognitive decline and dementia esp. in elderly patients — see HYDERGINE

er·gom·e·ter \(ₜ)ər- 'gä-mə-tər\ *n* : an apparatus for measuring the work performed (as by a person exercising); *also* : an exercise machine equipped with an ergometer — **er·go·met·ric** \ₜər-gə- 'me-trik\ *adj*

er·go·met·rine \ₜər-gə- 'me-ₜtrēn, -ₜtrən\ *n* : ERGONOVINE

er·go·nom·ics \ₜər-gə- 'nä-miks\ *n sing or pl* : an applied science concerned with the characteristics of people that need to be considered in designing and arranging things that they use in order that those things may be used most easily, effectively, and safely — called also *human engineering*, *human factors engineering* — **er·go·nom·ic** \-mik\ *adj* — **er·go·nom·i·cal·ly** \-mi-k(ə-)lē\ *adv* — **er·gon·o·mist** \(ₜ)ər- 'gä-nə-mist\ *n*

er·go·no·vine \ₜər-gə- 'nō-ₜvēn, -vən\ *n*

: an alkaloid $C_{19}H_{23}N_3O_2$ that is derived from ergot and is used esp. in the form of its maleate to prevent or treat postpartum bleeding

er·gos·ter·ol \(ₜ)ər- 'gäs-tə-ₜrȯl, - ₜrōl\ *n* : a crystalline steroid alcohol $C_{28}H_{44}O$ that occurs esp. in yeast, molds, and ergot and is converted by ultraviolet irradiation ultimately into vitamin D_2

er·got \'ər-gət, -ₜgät\ *n* **1** : the black or dark purple sclerotium of fungi of an ascomycetous genus (*Claviceps*); *also* : any fungus of this genus **2 a** : the dried sclerotial bodies of an ergot fungus grown on rye and containing several alkaloids (as ergonovine, ergotamine) **b** : any of such alkaloids used medicinally for their contractile effect on smooth muscle (as of the uterus) — see ERGOTISM

er·got·a·mine \(ₜ)ər- 'gä-tə-ₜmēn\ *n* : an alkaloid $C_{33}H_{35}N_5O_5$ that is derived from ergot and is used chiefly in the form of its tartrate esp. in treating migraine

er·got·ism \'ər-gə-ₜti-zəm\ *n* : a toxic condition produced by eating grain, grain products (as rye bread), or grasses infected with ergot fungus or by chronic excessive use of an ergot drug

er·got·ized \-ₜtīzd\ *adj* : infected with ergot ⟨∼ grain⟩; *also* : poisoned by ergot ⟨∼ cattle⟩

erigens, erigentes — see NERVUS ERIGENS

er·i·o·dic·ty·on \ₜer-ē-ə- 'dik-tē-ₜän\ *n* : the dried leaves of yerba santa used as a flavoring in medicine esp. to disguise the taste of quinine

erode \i- 'rōd\ *vb* **erod·ed; erod·ing 1** : to eat into or away by slow destruction of substance ⟨acids that ∼ the teeth⟩ ⟨bone *eroded* by cancer⟩ **2** : to remove with an abrasive

erog·e·nous \i- 'rä-jə-nəs\ *adj* **1** : producing sexual excitement or libidinal gratification when stimulated : sexually sensitive **2** : of, relating to, or arousing sexual feelings — **er·o·ge·ne·ity** \ₜer-ə-jə- 'nē-ə-tē\ *n*

Eros \'er-ₜäs, 'ir-\ *n* : the sum of life-preserving instincts that are manifested as impulses to gratify basic needs (as sex), as sublimated impulses motivated by the same needs, and as impulses to protect and preserve the body and mind — compare DEATH INSTINCT

ero·sion \i- 'rō-zhən\ *n* **1 a** : the superficial destruction of a surface area of tissue (as mucous membrane) by inflammation, ulceration, or trauma ⟨∼ of the uterine cervix⟩ **b** : progressive loss of the hard substance of a tooth **2** : an instance or product of erosion — **ero·sive** \i- 'rō-siv, -ziv\ *adj*

erot·ic \i- 'rä-tik\ *also* **erot·i·cal** \i- 'rä-ti-kəl\ *adj* **1** : of, devoted to, or tending to arouse sexual love or desire **2**

: strongly marked or affected by sexual desire — **erot·i·cal·ly** \-ti-k(ə-)lē\ *adv*

erot·i·ca \i-ˈrä-ti-kə\ *n sing or pl* : literary or artistic works having an erotic theme or quality

erot·i·cism \i-ˈrä-tə-ˌsi-zəm\ *n* 1 : a state of sexual arousal or anticipation 2 : insistent sexual impulse or desire

erot·i·cize \-ˌsīz\ *vb* **-cized; -ciz·ing** : to make erotic — **erot·i·ci·za·tion** \i-ˌrä-tə-sə-ˈzā-shən\ *n*

er·o·tism \ˈer-ə-ˌti-zəm\ *n* : EROTICISM

ero·tize \ˈer-ə-ˌtīz\ *vb* **-tized; -tiz·ing** : to invest with erotic significance or sexual feeling — **er·o·ti·za·tion** \ˌer-ə-tə-ˈzā-shən\ *n*

eroto- *comb form* : sexual desire ⟨*erotomania*⟩

ero·to·gen·ic \i-ˌrō-tə-ˈje-nik, -ˌrä-\ *adj* : EROGENOUS

ero·to·ma·nia \-ˈmā-nē-ə\ *n* : excessive sexual desire esp. as a symptom of mental disorder

ero·to·ma·ni·ac \-ˈmā-nē-ˌak\ *n* : one affected with erotomania

ero·to·pho·bia \-ˈfō-bē-ə\ *n* : a morbid aversion to sexual love or desire

eru·cic acid \i-ˈrü-sik-\ *n* : a crystalline fatty acid $C_{22}H_{42}O_2$ found in the form of glycerides esp. in an oil obtained from the seeds of the rape plant (*Brassica napus* of the mustard family)

eruct \i-ˈrəkt\ *vb* : BELCH

eruc·ta·tion \i-ˌrək-ˈtā-shən, ˌē-\ *n* : an act or instance of belching

erupt \i-ˈrəpt\ *vb* 1 *of a tooth* : to emerge through the gum 2 : to break out (as with a skin eruption) — **erup·tive** \-ˈrəp-tiv\ *adj*

erup·tion \i-ˈrəp-shən\ *n* 1 : an act, process, or instance of erupting; *specif* : the breaking out of an exanthem or enanthem on the skin or mucous membrane (as in measles) 2 : something produced by an act or process of erupting: as **a** : the condition of the skin or mucous membrane caused by erupting **b** : one of the lesions (as a pustule) constituting this condition

er·y·sip·e·las \ˌer-ə-ˈsi-pə-ləs, ˌir-\ *n* : an acute febrile disease that is associated with intense often vesicular and edematous local inflammation of the skin and subcutaneous tissues and that is caused by a hemolytic streptococcus 2 : SWINE ERYSIPELAS — used esp. when the disease affects other hosts than swine

er·y·sip·e·loid \ˌer-ə-ˈsi-pə-ˌlȯid, ˌir-\ *n* : a localized nonfebrile dermatitis resembling erysipelas, caused by the parasite of the genus *Erysipelothrix* (*E. rhusiopathiae*) that causes swine erysipelas, and occurring esp. about the hands of persons exposed to this organism (as by handling contaminated flesh) — **erysipeloid** *adj*

er·y·sip·e·lo·thrix \ˌer-ə-ˈsi-pə-lō-ˌthriks\ *n* 1 *cap* : a genus of gram-positive, rod-shaped bacteria (family Corynebacteriaceae) that are usu. considered to comprise a single form (*E. rhusiopathiae*) which is the causative agent of swine erysipelas, an arthritis of lambs, and erysipeloid of humans 2 : a bacterium of the genus *Erysipelothrix*

er·y·the·ma \ˌer-ə-ˈthē-mə\ *n* : abnormal redness of the skin due to capillary congestion (as in inflammation) — **er·y·the·mal** \-məl\ *adj*

erythema chron·i·cum mi·grans \-ˈkrä-nə-kəm-ˈmī-grənz\ *n* : a spreading annular erythematous skin lesion that is an early symptom of Lyme disease and that develops at the site of the bite of a tick (as the deer tick) infected with the causative spirochete

erythema in·fec·ti·o·sum \-ˌin-ˌfek-shē-ˈō-səm\ *n* : an acute eruptive disease esp. of children that is caused by a parvovirus and is first manifested by a blotchy maculopapular rash on the cheeks which gradually spreads to the extremities and that is usu. accompanied by fever and malaise — called also *fifth disease*

erythema mul·ti·for·me \-ˌməl-tə-ˈfȯr-mē\ *n* : a skin disease characterized by papular or vesicular lesions and reddening or discoloration of the skin often in concentric zones about the lesions

erythema no·do·sum \-nō-ˈdō-səm\ *n* : a skin condition characterized by small tender reddened nodules under the skin (as over the shin bones) often accompanied by fever and transitory arthritic pains

erythematosus — see LUPUS ERYTHEMATOSUS, LUPUS ERYTHEMATOSUS CELL, PEMPHIGUS ERYTHEMATOSUS, SYSTEMIC LUPUS ERYTHEMATOSUS

er·y·them·a·tous \ˌer-ə-ˈthe-mə-təs, -ˈthē-\ *adj* : relating to or marked by erythema

er·y·thor·bate \ˌer-ə-ˈthȯr-ˌbāt\ *n* : a salt of erythorbic acid that is used in foods as an antioxidant

erythorbic acid *n* : a stereoisomer of vitamin C

erythr- *or* **erythro-** *comb form* 1 : red ⟨*erythrocyte*⟩ 2 : erythrocyte ⟨*erythroid*⟩

er·y·thrae·mia *chiefly Brit var of* ERYTHREMIA

er·y·thras·ma \ˌer-ə-ˈthraz-mə\ *n* : a chronic contagious dermatitis that affects warm moist areas of the body (as the axilla and groin) and is caused by a bacterium of the genus *Corynebacterium* (*C. minutissimum*)

eryth·re·de·ma \i-ˌri-thrə-ˈdē-mə\ *n* : ACRODYNIA

er·y·thre·mia \ˌer-ə-ˈthrē-mē-ə\ *n* : POLYCYTHEMIA VERA

er·y·thrism \ˈer-ə-ˌthri-zəm\ *n* : a condition marked by exceptional prevalence of red pigmentation (as in skin or hair) — **er·y·thris·tic** \ˌer-ə-ˈthris-**

tik\ *also* **er·y·thris·mal** \-ˈthriz-məl\ *adj*

eryth·ri·tyl tet·ra·ni·trate \i-ˈri-thrə-ˌtil-ˌte-trə-ˈni-ˌtrāt\ *n* : a vasodilator $C_4H_{10}N_4O_{12}$ used to prevent angina pectoris — called also *erythritol tetranitrate*

erythro- — see ERYTHR-

eryth·ro·blast \i-ˈri-thrə-ˌblast\ *n* : a polychromatic nucleated cell of red marrow that synthesizes hemoglobin and that is an intermediate in the initial stage of red blood cell formation; *broadly* : a cell ancestral to red blood cells — compare NORMOBLAST — **eryth·ro·blas·tic** \-ˌri-thrə-ˈblas-tik\ *adj*

eryth·ro·blas·to·pe·nia \i-ˌri-thrə-ˌblas-tə-ˈpē-nē-ə\ *n* : a deficiency in bone marrow erythroblasts

eryth·ro·blas·to·sis \i-ˌblas-ˈtō-səs\ *n, pl* **-to·ses** \-ˌsēz\ : abnormal presence of erythroblasts in the circulating blood; *esp* : ERYTHROBLASTOSIS FETALIS

erythroblastosis fe·ta·lis \-fi-ˈta-ləs\ *n* : a hemolytic disease of the fetus and newborn that is characterized by an increase in circulating erythroblasts and by jaundice and that occurs when the system of an Rh-negative mother produces antibodies to an antigen in the blood of an Rh-positive fetus — called also *hemolytic disease of the newborn, Rh disease*

eryth·ro·blas·tot·ic \i-ˌri-thrə-blas-ˈtä-tik\ *adj* : of, relating to, or affected by erythroblastosis ⟨an ~ infant⟩

eryth·ro·cyte \i-ˈri-thrə-ˌsīt\ *n* : RED BLOOD CELL — **eryth·ro·cyt·ic** \-ˌri-thrə-ˈsi-tik\ *adj*

eryth·ro·cy·to·pe·nia \i-ˌri-thrə-ˌsī-tə-ˈpē-nē-ə\ *n* : red-blood-cell deficiency

eryth·ro·cy·tor·rhex·is \-ˈrek-səs\ *n, pl* **-rhex·es** \-ˈrek-ˌsēz\ : rupture of a red blood cell

eryth·ro·cy·to·sis \i-ˌri-thrə-ˌsī-ˈtō-səs\ *n, pl* **-to·ses** \-ˈtō-ˌsēz\ : an increase in the number of circulating red blood cells resulting from a known stimulus (as hypoxia) — compare POLYCYTHEMIA VERA

eryth·ro·der·ma \-ˈdər-mə\ *n, pl* **-mas** \-məz\ *or* **-ma·ta** \-mə-tə\ : ERYTHEMA

eryth·ro·der·mia \-ˈdər-mē-ə\ *n* : ERYTHEMA

eryth·ro·gen·ic \-ˈje-nik\ *adj* 1 : producing red blood cells : ERYTHROPOIETIC 2 : inducing reddening of the skin

ery·throid \i-ˈri-ˌthroid, ˈer-ə-\ *adj* : relating to erythrocytes or their precursors

eryth·ro·leu·ke·mia \i-ˌri-thrə-lü-ˈkē-mē-ə\ *n* : a malignant disorder that is marked by proliferation of erythroblastic and myeloblastic tissue and in later stages by leukemia — **eryth·ro·leu·ke·mic** \-mik\ *adj*

eryth·ro·mel·al·gia \-mə-ˈlal-jə\ *n* : a state of excessive dilation of the superficial blood vessels usu. of the feet accompanied by hyperemia, increased skin temperature, and burning pain

eryth·ro·my·cin \i-ˌri-thrə-ˈmīs-ᵊn\ *n* : a broad-spectrum antibiotic $C_{37}H_{67}NO_{13}$ produced by a bacterium of the genus *Streptomyces* (*S. erythreus*), resembling penicillin in antibacterial activity, and effective also against amebae, treponemata, and pinworms — see ILOSONE, ILOTYCIN

eryth·ro·phago·cy·to·sis \i-ˈri-thrə-ˌfa-gə-sə-ˈtō-səs, -ˌsī-\ *n, pl* **-to·ses** \-ˈtō-ˌsēz\ : consumption of red blood cells by histiocytes and sometimes other phagocytes

eryth·ro·pla·sia \-ˈplā-zhə, -zhē-ə\ *n* : a reddened patch with a velvety surface on the oral or genital mucosa that is considered to be a precancerous lesion

eryth·ro·poi·e·sis \i-ˌri-thrō-pȯi-ˈē-səs\ *n, pl* **-e·ses** \-ˌsēz\ : the production of red blood cells (as from the bone marrow) — **eryth·ro·poi·et·ic** \-ˈe-tik\ *adj*

erythropoietic protoporphyria *n* : a rare porphyria usu. appearing in young children and marked by excessive protoporphyrin in erythrocytes, blood plasma, and feces and by skin lesions resulting from photosensitivity

eryth·ro·poi·e·tin \-ˈpȯi-ət-ᵊn\ *n* : a hormonal substance that is formed esp. in the kidney and stimulates red blood cell formation

eryth·ro·sine \i-ˈri-thrə-sən, -ˌsēn\ *also* **eryth·ro·sin** \-sən\ *n* : a brick-red powdered xanthene dye $C_{20}H_6I_4Na_2O_5$ that is used as a biological stain and in dentistry as an agent to disclose plaque on teeth — called also *erythrosine sodium*

Es *symbol* einsteinium

ESB *abbr* electrical stimulation of the brain

es·cape \i-ˈskāp\ *n* 1 : evasion of something undesirable ⟨~ from pain and suffering⟩ 2 : distraction or relief from routine or reality; *esp* : mental distraction or relief by flight into idealizing fantasy or fiction — **escape** *vb* — **escape** *adj*

escape mechanism *n* : a mode of behavior or thinking adopted to evade unpleasant facts or responsibilities : DEFENSE MECHANISM

es·cap·ism \i-ˈskā-ˌpi-zəm\ *n* : habitual diversion of the mind to purely imaginative activity or entertainment as an escape from reality or routine — **es·cap·ist** \-pist\ *adj or n*

es·char \ˈes-ˌkär\ *n* : a scab formed esp. after a burn

¹**es·cha·rot·ic** \ˌes-kə-ˈrä-tik\ *adj* : producing an eschar

²**escharotic** *n* : an escharotic agent (as a drug)

Esch·e·rich·ia \ˌe-shə-ˈri-kē-ə\ *n* : a genus of aerobic gram-negative rod-shaped bacteria (family Enterobacteriaceae) that include occas. pathogenic forms (as some strains of *E. coli*) normally present in the human intestine and other forms which typically occur in soil and water

Esch•e•rich \'e-shə-ˌrik\, **Theodor** (1857–1911), German pediatrician.

es•cutch•eon \i-'skə-chən\ *n* : the configuration of adult pubic hair

es•er•ine \'e-sə-ˌrēn\ *n* : PHYSOSTIG-MINE

Es•march bandage \'es-ˌmärk, 'ez-\ or **Es•march's bandage** \-ˌmärks-\ *n* : a tight rubber bandage for driving the blood out of a limb

Esmarch, Johannes Friedrich August von (1823–1908), German surgeon.

eso- *prefix* : inner (*esotropia*)

esophag- or **esophago-** *comb form* **1** : esophagus (*esophagectomy*) (*esophagoplasty*) **2** : esophagus and (*esophagogastrectomy*)

esoph•a•ge•al \i-ˌsä-fə-'jē-əl\ *adj* : of or relating to the esophagus

esophageal artery *n* : any of several arteries that arise from the front of the aorta, anastomose along the esophagus, and terminate by anastomosis with adjacent arteries

esophageal gland *n* : one of the racemose glands in the walls of the esophagus that in humans are small and serve principally to lubricate the food but in some birds secrete a milky fluid on which the young are fed

esophageal hiatus *n* : the aperture in the diaphragm that gives passage to the esophagus — see HIATAL HERNIA

esophageal plexus *n* : a nerve plexus formed by the branches of the vagus nerve which surround and supply the esophagus

esophageal speech *n* : a method of speaking which is used by individuals whose larynx has been removed and in which phonation is achieved by expelling swallowed air from the esophagus

esoph•a•gec•to•my \i-ˌsä-fə-'jek-tə-mē\ *n, pl* **-mies** : excision of part of the esophagus

esophagi *pl of* ESOPHAGUS

esoph•a•gi•tis \i-ˌsä-fə-'jī-təs, -'gī-, (ˌ)ē-\ *n* : inflammation of the esophagus

esophago- — see ESOPHAG-

esoph•a•go•gas•trec•to•my \i-ˌsä-fə-gō-ˌgas-'trek-tə-mē\ *n, pl* **-mies** : excision of part of the esophagus (esp. the lower third) and the stomach

esoph•a•go•gas•tric \-'gas-trik\ *adj* : of, relating to, involving, or affecting the esophagus and the stomach (~ ulcers)

esoph•a•go•gas•tros•co•py \-ˌgas-'träs-kə-pē\ *n, pl* **-pies** : examination of the interior of the esophagus and stomach by means of an endoscope

esoph•a•go•gas•tros•to•my \-ˌgas-'träs-tə-mē\ *n, pl* **-mies** : the surgical formation of an artificial communication between the esophagus and the stomach

esoph•a•go•je•ju•nos•to•my \-ˌje-jə-'näs-tə-mē\ *n, pl* **-mies** : the surgical formation of an artificial communication between the esophagus and the jejunum

esoph•a•go•my•ot•o•my \-ˌmī-'ä-tə-mē\ *n, pl* **-mies** : incision through the musculature of the esophagus and esp. the distal part (as for the relief of esophageal achalasia)

esoph•a•go•plas•ty \i-'sä-fə-gə-ˌplas-tē\ *n, pl* **-ties** : plastic repair or reconstruction of the esophagus

esoph•a•go•scope \-ˌskōp\ *n* : an instrument for inspecting the interior of the esophagus

esoph•a•gos•co•py \i-ˌsä-fə-'gäs-kə-pē\ *n, pl* **-pies** : examination of the esophagus by means of an esophagoscope — **esoph•a•go•scop•ic** \i-ˌsä-fə-gə-'skä-pik\ *adj*

esoph•a•go•sto•mi•a•sis *var of* OESOPHA-GOSTOMIASIS

esoph•a•gos•to•my \i-ˌsä-fə-'gäs-tə-mē\ *n, pl* **-mies** : surgical creation of an artificial opening into the esophagus

esoph•a•got•o•my \-'gä-tə-mē\ *n, pl* **-mies** : incision of the esophagus (as for the removal of an obstruction or the relief of esophageal achalasia)

esoph•a•gus \i-'sä-fə-gəs\ *n, pl* **-gi** \-ˌgī, -ˌjī\ : a muscular tube that in humans is about nine inches (23 centimeters) long and passes from the pharynx down the neck between the trachea and the spinal column and behind the left bronchus where it pierces the diaphragm slightly to the left of the middle line and joins the cardiac end of the stomach

es•o•pho•ria \ˌe-sə-'fōr-ē-ə, *sometimes* ˌē-\ *n* : squint in which the eyes tend to turn inward toward the nose

es•o•tro•pia \ˌe-sə-'trō-pē-ə, ˌē-\ *n* : CROSS-EYE 1 — **es•o•trop•ic** \-'trä-pik\ *adj*

ESP \ˌē-(ˌ)es-'pē\ *n* : EXTRASENSORY PERCEPTION

es•pun•dia \is-'pün-dē-ə, -'pün-\ *n* : leishmaniasis of the mouth, pharynx, and nose that is prevalent in Central and So. America

ESR *abbr* erythrocyte sedimentation rate

es•sen•tial \i-'sen-chəl\ *adj* : having no obvious or known cause : IDIOPATHIC (~ disease)

essential amino acid *n* : any of various alpha-amino acids that are required for normal health and growth, are either not manufactured in the body or manufactured in insufficient quantities, are usu. supplied by dietary protein, and in humans include isoleucine, leucine, lysine, methionine, phenylalanine, threonine, tryptophan, and valine

essential hypertension *n* : abnormally high systolic and diastolic blood pressure occurring in the absence of any evident cause and resulting typically in marked hypertrophic and degenerative changes in small arteries, hypertrophy of the heart, and often more or less severe kidney damage — called also *primary hypertension;* see MALIGNANT HYPERTENSION

essential oil *n* : any of a large class of volatile oils of vegetable origin that give plants their characteristic odors and are used esp. in perfumes, flavorings, and pharmaceutical preparations — called also *volatile oil;* compare FATTY OIL, FIXED OIL

EST *abbr* electroshock therapy

es·ter \'es-tər\ *n* : any of a class of often fragrant compounds that can be represented by the formula RCOOR' and that are usu. formed by the reaction between an acid and an alcohol usu. with elimination of water

es·ter·ase \'es-tə-₁rās, -₁rāz\ *n* : an enzyme that accelerates the hydrolysis or synthesis of esters

es·ter·i·fy \e-'ster-ə-₁fī\ *vb* **-fied; -fy-ing** : to convert into an ester — **es·ter·i·fi·ca·tion** \e-₁ster-ə-fə-'kā-shən\ *n*

estr- *or* **estro-** *comb form* : estrus ⟨*estrogen*⟩

es·tra·di·ol \₁es-trə-'dī-₁ol, -₁ol\ *n* : an estrogenic hormone that is a phenolic steroid alcohol $C_{18}H_{24}O_2$ usu. made synthetically and that is often used combined as an ester esp. in treating menopausal symptoms — called also *dihydrotheelin*

es·tral cycle \'es-trəl-\ *n* : ESTROUS CYCLE

es·trin \'es-trən\ *n* : an estrogenic hormone; *esp* : ESTRONE

es·tri·ol \'es-trī-₁ol, e-'strī-, -₁ol\ *n* : a crystalline estrogenic hormone $C_{18}H_{24}O_3$ usu. obtained from the urine of pregnant women

estro- — see ESTR-

es·tro·gen \'es-trə-jən\ *n* : a substance (as a sex hormone) tending to promote estrus and stimulate the development of female secondary sex characteristics

es·tro·gen·ic \₁es-trə-'je-nik\ *adj* **1** : promoting estrus **2** : of, relating to, caused by, or being an estrogen — **es·tro·gen·i·cal·ly** \-ni-k(ə-)lē\ *adv* — **es·tro·gen·ic·i·ty** \-jə-'ni-sə-tē\ *n*

es·trone \'es-₁trōn\ *n* : an estrogenic hormone that is a ketone $C_{18}H_{22}O_2$, is usu. obtained from the urine of pregnant women, and is used similarly to estradiol — see THEELIN

es·trous \'es-trəs\ *adj* **1** : of, relating to, or characteristic of estrus **2** : being in heat

estrous cycle *n* : the correlated phenomena of the endocrine and generative systems of a female mammal from the beginning of one period of estrus to the beginning of the next — called also *estral cycle, estrus cycle*

es·tru·al \'es-trə-wəl\ *adj* : ESTROUS

es·trus \'es-trəs\ *n* : a regularly recurrent state of sexual excitability during

which the female of most mammals will accept the male and is capable of conceiving : HEAT; *also* : a single occurrence of this state

eth·a·cryn·ic acid \₁e-thə-'kri-nik-\ *n* : a potent synthetic diuretic $C_{13}H_{12}Cl_2$-O_4 used esp. in the treatment of edema

eth·am·bu·tol \e-'tham-byü-₁tȯl, -₁tōl\ *n* : a synthetic drug $C_{10}H_{24}N_2O_2$ used esp. in the treatment of tuberculosis — see MYAMBUTOL

etha·mi·van \e-'tha-mə-₁van, ₁e-thə-'mī-vən\ *n* : an analeptic drug and central nervous stimulant $C_{12}H_{17}NO_3$ used as a respiratory stimulant for intoxication with central nervous depressants (as barbiturates) and for chronic lung diseases

eth·a·nol \'e-thə-₁nȯl, -₁nōl\ *n* : a colorless volatile flammable liquid C_2H_5-OH that is the intoxicating agent in liquors and is also used as a solvent — called also *ethyl alcohol, grain alcohol;* see ALCOHOL 1

eth·chlor·vy·nol \₁eth-'klȯr-və-₁nȯl, -₁nōl\ *n* : a pungent liquid alcohol C_7H_9ClO derived from methanol and used esp. as a mild hypnotic — see PLACIDYL

eth·ene \'e-₁thēn\ *n* : ETHYLENE

ether \'ē-thər\ *n* **1** : a light volatile flammable liquid $C_4H_{10}O$ used esp. formerly as an anesthetic — called also *diethyl ether, ethyl ether* **2** : any of various organic compounds characterized by an oxygen atom attached to two carbon atoms

ether·ize \'ē-thə-₁rīz\ *vb* **-ized; -iz·ing** : to treat or anesthetize with ether

¹eth·i·cal \'e-thi-kəl\ *also* **eth·ic** \-thik\ *adj* **1** : conforming to accepted professional standards of conduct **2** *of a drug* : restricted to sale only on a doctor's prescription — **eth·i·cal·ly** \-thi-k(ə-)lē\ *adv*

²ethical *n* : an ethical drug

eth·ics \'e-thiks\ *n sing or pl* : the principles of conduct governing an individual or a group ⟨medical ∼⟩

ethid·i·um bromide \e-'thi-dē-əm-\ *n* : a biological dye used to block nucleic acid synthesis (as in mitochondria) and to destroy trypanosomes

ethi·nyl *var of* ETHYNYL — used esp. in pharmacology

ethi·nyl estradiol \'e-thə-ni-₁les-trə-'dī-₁ol, -₁ol\ *n* : a very potent synthetic estrogen $C_{20}H_{24}O_2$ used orally

eth·ion·amide \₁e-thē-'ä-nə-₁mid\ *n* : a compound $C_8H_{10}N_2S$ used against mycobacteria (as in tuberculosis and leprosy)

ethi·o·nine \e-'thī-ə-₁nēn\ *n* : an amino acid $C_6H_{13}NO_2S$ that is biologically antagonistic to methionine

ethis·ter·one \i-'this-tə-₁rōn\ *n* : a synthetic female sex hormone $C_{21}H_{28}O_2$ administered in cases of deficiency of progesterone — called also *anhydrohydroxyprogesterone*

ethmo- *comb form* : ethmoid and ⟨*ethmo*maxillary⟩

¹eth·moid \'eth-₁mȯid\ *or* **eth·moi·dal** \eth-'mȯid-ᵊl\ *adj* : of, relating to, adjoining, or being one or more bones of the walls and septum of the nasal cavity

²ethmoid *n* : ETHMOID BONE

ethmoidal air cells *n pl* : the cavities in the lateral masses of the ethmoid bone that are partly completed by adjoining bones and communicate with the nasal cavity

ethmoid bone *n* : a light spongy cubical bone forming much of the walls of the nasal cavity and part of those of the orbits

eth·moid·ec·to·my \₁eth-₁mȯi-'dek-tə-mē\ *n, pl* **-mies** : excision of all or some of the ethmoidal air cells or part of the ethmoid bone

eth·moid·itis \-'dī-təs\ *n* : inflammation of the ethmoid bone or its sinuses

ethmoid sinus *also* **ethmoidal sinus** *n* : either of two sinuses each of which is situated in a lateral part of the ethmoid bone alongside the nose and consists of ethmoidal air cells

eth·mo·max·il·lary \₁eth-(₁)mō-'mak-sə-₁ler-ē\ *adj* : of or relating to the ethmoid and maxillary bones

etho·sux·i·mide \₁e-(₁)thō-'sək-sə-₁mīd, -₁məd\ *n* : an antidepressant drug $C_7H_{11}NO_2$ used to treat epilepsy

eth·o·to·in \₁e-thə-'tō-ən\ *n* : an anticonvulsant drug $C_{11}H_{12}N_2O_2$ used in the treatment of epilepsy — see PEGANONE

eth·yl alcohol \'e-thəl-\ *n* : ETHANOL

ethyl aminobenzoate *n* : BENZOCAINE

ethyl bromide *n* : a volatile liquid compound C_2H_5Br used as an inhalation anesthetic

ethyl carbamate *n* : URETHANE

ethyl chloride *n* : a colorless pungent flammable gaseous or volatile liquid C_2H_5Cl used esp. as a local surface anesthetic

eth·yl·ene \'e-thə-₁lēn\ *n* : a colorless flammable gaseous unsaturated hydrocarbon C_2H_4 used in medicine as a general inhalation anesthetic and occurring in plants where it functions esp. as a natural growth regulator that promotes the ripening of fruit — called also *ethene*

ethylene bromide *n* : ETHYLENE DIBROMIDE

ethylene di·amine \-'dī-ə-₁mēn, -dī-'a-mən\ *n* : a colorless volatile liquid base $C_2H_8N_2$ used in medicine to stabilize aminophylline when used in injections

eth·yl·ene·di·amine·tetra·ac·e·tate \₁e-thə-₁lēn-₁dī-ə-₁mēn-₁te-trə-'a-sə-₁tāt, -dī-'a-mən-\ *n* : a salt of EDTA

eth·yl·ene·di·amine·tetra·ace·tic acid \-ə-'sē-tik-\ *n* : EDTA

ethylene dibromide *n* : a colorless toxic liquid compound $C_2H_4Br_2$ that has been shown by experiments with lab-

oratory animals to be strongly carcinogenic and that was used formerly in the U.S. as an agricultural pesticide — abbr. *EDB*; called also *ethylene bromide*

ethylene glycol *n* : a thick liquid alcohol $C_2H_6O_2$ used esp. as an antifreeze

ethylene oxide *n* : a colorless flammable toxic gaseous or liquid compound C_2H_4O used in fumigation and sterilization (as of medical instruments)

eth·yl·es·tren·ol \₁e-thəl-'es-trə-₁nȯl, -₁nōl\ *n* : an anabolic steroid $C_{20}H_{32}O$ having androgenic activity — see MAXIBOLIN

ethyl ether *n* : ETHER 1

eth·yl·mor·phine \₁e-thəl-'mȯr-₁fēn\ *n* : a synthetic toxic alkaloid $C_{19}H_{23}$-NO_3 used esp. in the form of its hydrochloride similarly to morphine and codeine

ethy·nyl \e-'thīn-ᵊl, 'e-thə-₁nil\ *n* : a monovalent unsaturated group $HC\equiv C-$

ethy·nyl·es·tra·di·ol *var of* ETHINYL ESTRADIOL

etio- *comb form* : cause ⟨*etio*logic⟩ ⟨*etio*pathogenesis⟩

etio·chol·an·ol·one \₁ē-tē-ō-₁kō-'la-nə-₁lōn, -e-\ *n* : a testosterone metabolite $C_{19}H_{30}O_2$ that occurs in urine

eti·o·log·ic \₁ē-tē-ə-'lä-jik\ *or* **eti·o·log·i·cal** \-ji-kəl\ *adj* 1 : of, relating to, or based on etiology ⟨~ investigations⟩ 2 : causing or contributing to the cause of a disease or condition — **eti·o·log·i·cal·ly** \-ji-k(ə-)lē\ *adv*

eti·ol·o·gy \₁ē-tē-'ä-lə-jē\ *n, pl* **-gies** 1 : all of the causes of a disease or abnormal condition 2 : a branch of medical science dealing with the causes and origin of diseases

etio·patho·gen·e·sis \₁ē-tē-ō-₁pa-thə-'je-nə-səs, ₁e-\ *n, pl* **-e·ses** \-₁sēz\ : the cause and development of a disease or abnormal condition

etor·phine \e-'tȯr-₁fēn, i-\ *n* : a synthetic narcotic drug $C_{25}H_{33}NO_4$ related to morphine but with more potent analgesic properties

eu- *comb form* 1 : good : normal ⟨*eu*thyroid⟩ 2 : true ⟨*eu*globulin⟩

Eu *symbol* europium

eu·ca·lyp·tol *also* **eu·ca·lyp·tole** \₁yü-kə-'lip-₁tȯl, -₁tōl\ *n* : a liquid $C_{10}H_{18}O$ with an odor of camphor that is contained in many essential oils (as of eucalyptus) and is used esp. as an expectorant — called also *cajeputol*, *cineole*

eu·ca·lyp·tus oil \₁yü-kə-'lip-təs-\ *n* : any of various essential oils obtained from the leaves of an Australian tree (genus *Eucalyptus* and esp. *E. globulus*) of the myrtle family (Myrtaceae) and used in pharmaceutical preparations (as antiseptics or cough drops)

eu·cary·ote *var of* EUKARYOTE

euc·at·ro·pine \yü-'ka-trə-₁pēn\ *n* : a synthetic alkaloid used in the form of its white crystalline hydrochloride $C_{17}H_{25}NO_3 \cdot HCl$ as a mydriatic

eu·chro·ma·tin \(ˌ)yü-ˈkrō-mə-tən\ *n* : the genetically active portion of chromatin that is largely composed of genes — **eu·chro·mat·ic** \ˌyü-krō-ˈma-tik\ *adj*

eu·gen·ics \yù-ˈje-niks\ *n* : a science that deals with the improvement (as by control of human mating) of hereditary qualities of a race or breed — **eu·gen·ic** \-nik\ *adj* — **eu·gen·i·cist** \-nə-sist\ *n* — **eu·gen·i·cal·ly** *adv*

eu·ge·nol \ˈyü-jə-ˌnōl, -ˌnȯl\ *n* : an aromatic liquid phenol $C_{10}H_{12}O_2$ found esp. in clove oil and used in dentistry as an analgesic

eu·glob·u·lin \yü-ˈglä-byə-lən\ *n* : a simple protein that does not dissolve in pure water

eu·gly·ce·mia \ˌyü-ˌglī-ˈsē-mē-ə\ *n* : a normal level of sugar in the blood

eu·kary·ote \(ˌ)yü-ˈkar-ē-ˌōt, -ē-ət\ *n* : an organism composed of one or more cells containing visibly evident nuclei and organelles — compare PROKARYOTE ; *also* **eu·cary·ot·ic** \-ˌkar-ē-ˈä-tik\ *adj*

eu·nuch \ˈyü-nək, -nik\ *n* : a man or boy deprived of the testes or external genitals — **eu·nuch·ism** \-nə-ˌki-zəm, -ni-\ *n*

¹**eu·nuch·oid** \ˈyü-nə-ˌkȯid\ *adj* : of, relating to, or characterized by eunuchoidism : resembling a eunuch

²**eunuchoid** *n* : a sexually deficient individual; *esp* : one lacking in sexual differentiation and tending toward the intersex state

eu·nuch·oid·ism \ˈyü-nə-ˌkȯi-ˌdi-zəm\ *n* : a state suggestive of that of a eunuch in being marked by deficiency of sexual development, by persistence of prepubertal characteristics, and often by the presence of characteristics typical of the opposite sex

eu·pep·sia \yü-ˈpep-shə, -sē-ə\ *n* : good digestion — **eu·pep·tic** \-ˈpep-tik\ *adj*

eu·phen·ics \yü-ˈfe-niks\ *n* : a science that deals with the biological improvement of human beings after birth — **eu·phen·ic** \-nik\ *adj*

eu·pho·ria \yù-ˈfȯr-ē-ə\ *n* : a feeling of well-being or elation; *esp* : one that is groundless, disproportionate to its cause, or inappropriate to one's life situation — compare DYSPHORIA — **eu·phor·ic** \-ˈfȯr-ik, -ˈfär-\ *adj* — **eu·phor·i·cal·ly** \-i-k(ə-)lē\ *adv*

¹**eu·pho·ri·ant** \yù-ˈfȯr-ē-ənt\ *n* : a drug that tends to induce euphoria

²**euphoriant** *adj* : tending to induce euphoria ⟨a ~ drug⟩

eu·phor·i·gen·ic \yü-ˌfȯr-ə-ˈje-nik\ *adj* : tending to cause euphoria

eup·nea \yüp-ˈnē-ə\ *n* : normal respiration — compare DYSPNEA — **eup·ne·ic** \-ˈnē-ik\ *adj*

eup·noea *chiefly Brit var of* EUPNEA

eu·ro·pi·um \yü-ˈrō-pē-əm\ *n* : a biva-

lent and trivalent metallic element — symbol *Eu*; see ELEMENT table

-eus \ē-əs\ *n comb form, pl* **-ei** \ē-ī\ *also* **-eus·es** \ē-ə-səz\ : muscle that constitutes, has the form of, or joins a (specified) part, thing, or structure ⟨glut*eus*⟩ ⟨rhomboid*eus*⟩ ⟨iliococcyg*eus*⟩

eu·sta·chian tube \yü-ˈstā-shən-, -shē-ən-, -kē-ən-\ *n, often cap E* : a bony and cartilaginous tube connecting the middle ear with the nasopharynx and equalizing air pressure on both sides of the tympanic membrane — called also *auditory tube, pharyngotympanic tube*

> **Eu·sta·chio** \äü-ˈstäk-yō\, **Bartolomeo** (ca 1520–1574), Italian anatomist.

eu·tha·na·sia \ˌyü-thə-ˈnā-zhə, -zhē-ə\ *n* : the act or practice of killing hopelessly sick or injured individuals (as persons or domestic animals) in a relatively painless way for reasons of mercy; *also* : the act or practice of allowing a hopelessly sick or injured patient to die by taking less than complete medical measures to prolong life — called also *mercy killing*

eu·than·a·tize \yü-ˈtha-nə-ˌtīz\ *also* **eu·tha·nize** \ˈyü-thə-ˌnīz\ *vb* **-tized** *also* **-nized; -tiz·ing** *also* **-niz·ing** : to subject to euthanasia

eu·then·ics \yù-ˈthe-niks\ *n sing or pl* : a science that deals with development of human well-being by improvement of living conditions — **eu·then·ist** \yù-ˈthe-nist, ˈyü-thə-\ *n*

eu·thy·roid \(ˌ)yü-ˈthī-ˌrȯid\ *adj* : characterized by normal thyroid function — **eu·thy·roid·ism** \-ˌrȯi-ˌdi-zəm\ *n*

¹**evac·u·ant** \i-ˈva-kyə-wənt\ *n* : an evacuant agent

²**evacuant** *adj* : EMETIC, DIURETIC, PURGATIVE, CATHARTIC

evac·u·ate \i-ˈva-kyə-ˌwāt\ *vb* **-at·ed; -at·ing** **1** : to remove the contents of ⟨~ an abscess⟩ **2** : to discharge (as urine or feces) from the body as waste : VOID — **evac·u·a·tive** \-ˌwā-tiv\ *adj*

evac·u·a·tion \i-ˌva-kyə-ˈwā-shən\ *n* **1** : the act or process of evacuating **2** : something evacuated or discharged

evag·i·na·tion \i-ˌva-jə-ˈnā-shən\ *n* **1** : a process of turning outward or inside out ⟨~ of a cell membrane⟩ **2** : a part or structure that is produced by evagination — called also *outpocketing, outpouching* — **evag·i·nate** \i-ˈva-jə-ˌnāt\ *vb*

ev·a·nes·cent \ˌe-və-ˈnes-ᵊnt\ *adj* : tending to disappear quickly : of relatively short duration ⟨an ~ rash⟩

Evans blue \ˈe-vənz-\ *n* : a dye $C_{34}H_{24}$-$N_6Na_4O_{14}S_4$ that on injection into the blood stream combines with serum albumin and is used to determine blood volume colorimetrically

> **Evans, Herbert McLean (1882–**

1971), American anatomist and physiologist.

even·tra·tion \ˌē-ˌven-ˈtrā-shən\ n : protrusion of abdominal organs through the abdominal wall

ever·sion \i-ˈvər-zhən, -shən\ n 1 : the act of turning inside out : the state of being turned inside out (∼ of the eyelid) 2 : the condition (as of the foot) of being turned or rotated outward — compare INVERSION 1b

evert \i-ˈvərt\ vb : to turn outward (∼ the foot); also : to turn inside out

evis·cer·ate \i-ˈvi-sə-ˌrāt\ vb -at·ed; -at·ing 1 a : to remove the viscera of b : to remove an organ from (a patient) or the contents of (an organ) 2 : to protrude through a surgical incision or suffer protrusion of a part through an incision — **evis·cer·a·tion** \i-ˌvi-sə-ˈrā-shən\ n

evo·ca·tion \ˌē-vō-ˈkā-shən, ˌe-\ n : INDUCTION 2b

evo·ca·tor \ˈē-vō-ˌkā-tər, ˈe-\ n : the specific chemical constituent responsible for the physiological effects of an organizer

evoked potential \ē-ˈvōkt-\ n : an electrical response esp. in the cerebral cortex as recorded following stimulation of a peripheral sense receptor

evo·lu·tion \ˌe-və-ˈlü-shən, ˌē-\ n 1 : a process of change in a certain direction 2 a : the historical development of a biological group (as a race or species) : PHYLOGENY b : a theory that the various types of animals and plants have their origin in other preexisting types and that the distinguishable differences are due to modifications in successive generations — **evo·lu·tion·ari·ly** \-shə-ˌner-ə-lē\ adv — **evo·lu·tion·ary** \-shə-ˌner-ē\ adj — **evo·lu·tio·nist** \-shə-nist\ n

evolve \i-ˈvälv, -ˈvȯlv\ vb evolved; evolv·ing : to produce or develop by natural evolutionary processes

evul·sion \i-ˈvəl-shən\ n : the act of extracting forcibly : EXTRACTION (∼ of a tooth) — **evulse** \i-ˈvəls\ vb

ewe-neck \ˈyü-ˈnek\ n : a thin neck with a concave arch occurring as a defect in dogs and horses — **ewe-necked** \-ˈnekt\ adj

Ew·ing's sarcoma \ˈyü-iŋz-\ n : a tumor that invades the shaft of a long bone and that tends to recur but rarely metastasizes — called also Ewing's tumor

Ewing, James (1866–1943), American pathologist.

ex- — see EXO-

ex·ac·er·bate \ig-ˈza-sər-ˌbāt\ vb -bat·ed; -bat·ing : to cause (a disease or its symptoms) to become more severe — **ex·ac·er·ba·tion** \-ˌza-sər-ˈbā-shən\ n

ex·al·ta·tion \ˌeg-ˌzȯl-ˈtā-shən, ˌek-ˌsȯl-\ n 1 : marked by excessive intensification of a mental state or of the activity of a bodily part or function 2 : an abnormal sense of personal well-

being, power, or importance : a delusional euphoria

ex·am \ig-ˈzam\ n : EXAMINATION

ex·am·i·na·tion \ig-ˌza-mə-ˈnā-shən\ n : the act or process of inspecting or testing for evidence of disease or abnormality — see PHYSICAL EXAMINATION — **ex·am·ine** \ig-ˈza-mən\ vb

ex·am·in·ee \ig-ˌza-mə-ˈnē\ n : a person who is examined

ex·am·in·er \ig-ˈza-mə-nər\ n : one that examines — see MEDICAL EXAMINER

ex·an·them \eg-ˈzan-thəm, ˈek-ˌsan-ˌthem\ also **ex·an·the·ma** \ˌeg-ˌzan-ˈthē-mə\ n, pl -thems also -them·a·ta \ˌeg-ˌzan-ˈthe-mə-tə\ or -themas : an eruptive disease (as measles) or its symptomatic eruption — **ex·an·them·a·tous** \ˌeg-ˌzan-ˈthe-mə-təs\ or **ex·an·the·mat·ic** \-ˌzan-thə-ˈma-tik\ adj

ex·ca·va·tion \ˌek-skə-ˈvā-shən\ n 1 : the action or process of forming or undergoing formation of a cavity or hole 2 : a cavity formed by or as if by cutting, digging, or scooping — **ex·ca·vate** vb \ˈek-skə-ˌvāt\

ex·ca·va·tor \ˈek-skə-ˌvā-tər\ n : an instrument used to open bodily cavities (as in the teeth) or remove material from them

excavatum — see PECTUS EXCAVATUM

ex·ce·men·to·sis \ˌeks-si-ˌmen-ˈtō-səs\ n, pl -to·ses \-ˌsēz\ or -to·sis·es : abnormal outgrowth of the cementum of the root of a tooth

ex·change transfusion \iks-ˈchānj-\ n : simultaneous withdrawal of the recipient's blood and transfusion with the donor's blood esp. in the treatment of erythroblastosis

ex·cip·i·ent \ik-ˈsi-pē-ənt\ n : a usu. inert substance (as gum arabic or starch) that forms a vehicle (as for a drug)

ex·ci·sion \ik-ˈsi-zhən\ n : surgical removal or resection (as of a diseased part) — **ex·cise** \-ˈsīz\ vb — **ex·ci·sion·al** \-ˈsi-zhə-nəl\ adj

ex·cit·able \ik-ˈsī-tə-bəl\ adj, of living tissue or an organism : capable of being activated by and reacting to stimuli : exhibiting irritability — **ex·cit·abil·i·ty** \-ˌsī-tə-ˈbi-lə-tē\ n

ex·ci·tant \ik-ˈsīt-ənt, ˈek-sə-tənt\ n : an agent that arouses or augments physiological activity (as of the nervous system) — **excitant** adj

ex·ci·ta·tion \ˌek-ˌsī-ˈtā-shən, -sə-\ n : EXCITEMENT: as a : the disturbed or altered condition resulting from arousal of activity (as by neural or electrical stimulation) in an individual organ or tissue b : the arousing of such activity

ex·cit·ato·ry \ik-ˈsī-tə-ˌtōr-ē\ adj 1 : tending to induce excitation (as of a neuron\} **2** : exhibiting, resulting from, related to, or produced by excitement or excitation

ex·cite \ik-ˈsīt\ *vb* **ex·cit·ed; ex·cit·ing** : to increase the activity of (as a living organism) : STIMULATE

ex·cite·ment \-ˈsīt-mənt\ *n* **1** : the act of exciting **2** : the state of being excited: as **a** : aroused, augmented, or abnormal activity of an organism or functioning of an organ or part **b** : extreme motor hyperactivity (as in catatonic schizophrenia)

ex·co·ri·a·tion \(ˌ)ek-ˌskōr-ē-ˈā-shən\ *n* **1** : the act of abrading or wearing off the skin **2** : a raw irritated lesion (as of the skin or a mucosal surface) — **ex·co·ri·ate** \ek-ˈskōr-ē-ˌāt\ *vb*

ex·cre·ment \ˈek-skrə-mənt\ *n* : waste matter discharged from the body; *esp* : waste (as feces) discharged from the alimentary canal — **ex·cre·men·tal** \ˌek-skrə-ˈment-ᵊl\ *adj*

ex·cres·cence \ik-ˈskres-ᵊns\ *n* : an outgrowth or enlargement: as **a** : a natural and normal appendage or development **b** : an abnormal outgrowth — **ex·cres·cent** \ik-ˈskres-ᵊnt\ *adj*

ex·cre·ta \ik-ˈskrē-tə\ *n pl* : waste matter eliminated or separated from an organism — compare EXCRETION 2 — **ex·cre·tal** \-ˈskrē-təl\ *adj*

ex·crete \ik-ˈskrēt\ *vb* **ex·cret·ed; ex·cret·ing** : to separate and eliminate or discharge (waste) from the blood or tissues or from the active protoplasm

ex·cret·er \-ˈskrē-tər\ *n* : one that excretes something *esp.* an atypical bodily product (as a pathogenic microorganism)

ex·cre·tion \ik-ˈskrē-shən\ *n* **1** : the act or process of excreting **2 a** : something eliminated by the process of excretion that is composed chiefly of urine or sweat in mammals including humans and in other animals, characteristically includes products of protein degradation (as urea or uric acid), usu. differs from ordinary bodily secretions by lacking any further utility to the organism that produces it, and is distinguished from waste materials (as feces) that have merely passed into or through the alimentary canal without being incorporated into the body proper **b** : a waste product (as urine, feces, or vomitus) eliminated from an animal body : EXCREMENT — not used technically

ex·cre·to·ry \ˈek-skrə-ˌtōr-ē\ *adj* : of, relating to, or functioning in excretion ⟨∼ ducts⟩

ex·cur·sion \ik-ˈskər-zhən\ *n* **1 a** : movement outward and back or from a mean position or axis **2** : one complete movement of expansion and contraction of the lungs and their membranes (as in breathing)

ex·cyst \ˌeks-ˈsist\ *vb* : to emerge from

a cyst — **ex·cys·ta·tion** \ˌeks-ˌsis-ˈtā-shən\ *n* — **ex·cyst·ment** \ˌeks-ˈsist-mənt\ *n*

ex·en·ter·a·tion \ig-ˌzen-tə-ˈrā-shən\ *n* : surgical removal of the contents of a bodily cavity (as the orbit, pelvis, or a sinus) — **ex·en·ter·ate** \ig-ˈzen-tə-ˌrāt\ *vb*

ex·er·cise \ˈek-sər-ˌsīz\ *n* **1** : regular or repeated use of a faculty or bodily organ **2** : bodily exertion for the sake of developing and maintaining physical fitness — **exercise** \"\ *vb*

ex·er·cis·er \ˈek-sər-ˌsī-zər\ *n* **1** : one that exercises **2** : an apparatus for use in physical exercise

Ex·er·cy·cle \ˈek-sər-ˌsī-kəl\ *trademark* — used for a stationary bicycle

ex·er·e·sis \ig-ˈzer-ə-səs\ *n, pl* **-e·ses** \-ˌsēz\ : surgical removal of a part or organ (as a nerve)

ex·flag·el·la·tion \(ˌ)eks-ˌfla·jə-ˈlā-shən\ *n* : the formation of microgametes in sporozoans (as the malaria parasite) by extrusion of nuclear material into peripheral processes resembling flagella — **ex·flag·el·late** \-ˈfla·jə-ˌlāt\ *vb*

ex·fo·li·ate \(ˌ)eks-ˈfō-lē-ˌāt\ *vb* **-at·ed; -at·ing** **1** : to cast or come off in scales or laminae **2** : to remove the surface of in scales or laminae **3** : to shed (teeth) by exfoliation

ex·fo·li·a·tion \(ˌ)eks-ˌfō-lē-ˈā-shən\ *n* : the action or process of exfoliating: as **a** : the peeling of the horny layer of the skin **b** : the shedding of surface components **c** : the shedding of a superficial layer of bone or of a tooth or part of a tooth — **ex·fo·li·a·tive** \eks-ˈfō-lē-ˌā-tiv\ *adj*

exfoliative cytology *n* : the study of cells shed from body surfaces esp. for determining the presence or absence of a cancerous condition

ex·ha·la·tion \ˌeks-hə-ˈlā-shən, ˌek-sə-ˈ\ *n* **1** : the action of forcing air out of the lungs **2** : something (as the breath) that is exhaled or given off — **ex·hale** \eks-ˈhāl, ek-ˈsāl\ *vb*

ex·haust \ig-ˈzȯst\ *vb* **1 a** : to draw off or let out completely **b** : to empty by drawing off the contents; *specif* : to create a vacuum in **2 a** : to use up : consume completely **b** : to tire extremely or completely (∼*ed* by overwork) **3** : to extract completely with a solvent

ex·haus·tion \ig-ˈzȯs-chən\ *n* **1** : the act or process of exhausting : the state of being exhausted **2** : neurosis following overstrain or overexertion esp. in military combat

ex·hib·it \ig-ˈzi-bət\ *vb* : to administer for medical purposes

ex·hi·bi·tion·ism \ˌek-sə-ˈbi-shə-ˌni-zəm\ *n* **1 a** : a perversion marked by a tendency to indecent exposure **b** : an act of such exposure **2** : the act or practice of behaving so as to attract attention to oneself — **ex·hi·bi·tion-**

ist \-nist\ *n* — **ex·hi·bi·tion·is·tic** \-₁bish-ə-'nis-tik\ *also* **exhibitionist** *adj* — **ex·hi·bi·tion·is·ti·cal·ly** \-ti-k(ə-)lē\ *adv*

ex·hume \ig-'züm, igz-'yüm; iks-'hyüm, -'yüm\ *vb* **ex·humed; ex·hum·ing** : DISINTER — **ex·hu·ma·tion** \₁eks-hyü-'mā-shən, ₁eks-yü-; ₁egz-yü-, ₁eg-zü-\ *n*

ex·i·tus \'ek-sə-təs\ *n, pl* **exitus** \-₁tüs, -₁tüs\ : DEATH; *esp* : fatal termination of a disease

exo- *or* **ex-** *comb form* : outside : outer ⟨*exo*enzyme⟩ — compare ECT-, END- 1

exo·crine \'ek-sə-krən, -₁krīn, -₁krēn\ *adj* : producing, being, or relating to a secretion that is released outside its source

exocrine gland *n* : a gland (as a salivary gland) that releases a secretion external to or at the surface of an organ by means of a canal or duct — called also *gland of external excretion*

exo·cri·nol·o·gy \₁ek-sə-kri-'nä-lə-jē, -₁krī-, -₁krē-\ *n, pl* **-gies** : the study of external secretions (as pheromones) that serve an integrative function

exo·cy·to·sis \₁ek-sō-sī-'tō-səs\ *n, pl* **-to·ses** \-₁sēz\ : the release of cellular substances (as secretory products) contained in cell vesicles by fusion of the vesicular membrane with the plasma membrane and subsequent release of the contents to the exterior of the cell — **exo·cy·tot·ic** \-'tä-tik\ *adj*

ex·odon·tia \₁ek-sə-'dän-chə, -chē-ə\ *n* : a branch of dentistry that deals with the extraction of teeth — **ex·odon·tist** \-'dän-tist\ *n*

exo·en·zyme \₁ek-sō-'en-₁zīm\ *n* : an extracellular enzyme

exo·eryth·ro·cyt·ic \₁ek-sō-i-₁ri-thrə-'si-tik\ *adj* : occurring outside the red blood cells — used of stages of malaria parasites

ex·og·e·nous \ek-'sä-jə-nəs\ *also* **ex·o·gen·ic** \₁ek-sō-'je-nik\ *adj* **1** : growing from or on the outside **2** : caused by factors (as food or a traumatic factor) or an agent (as a disease-producing organism) from outside the organism or system ⟨∼ obesity⟩ ⟨∼ psychic depression⟩ **3** : introduced from or produced outside the organism or system; *specif* : not synthesized within the organism or system — compare ENDOGENOUS — **ex·og·e·nous·ly** *adv*

ex·on \'ek-₁sän\ *n* : a polynucleotide sequence in a nucleic acid that codes information for protein synthesis and that is copied and spliced together with other such sequences to form messenger RNA — compare INTRON — **ex·on·ic** \ek-'sä-nik\ *adj*

exo·nu·cle·ase \₁ek-sō-'nü-klē-₁ās, -'nyü-, -₁āz\ *n* : an enzyme that breaks down a nucleic acid by removing nucleotides one by one from the end of a chain — compare ENDONUCLEASE

exo·nu·cleo·lyt·ic \₁ek-sō-₁nü-klē-ə-'li-tik, -₁nyü-\ *adj* : breaking a nucleotide chain into two parts at a point adjacent to one of its ends

exo·pep·ti·dase \-'pep-tə-₁dās, -₁dāz\ *n* : any of a group of enzymes that hydrolyze peptide bonds formed by the terminal amino acids of peptide chains : PEPTIDASE — compare ENDOPEPTIDASE

exo·pho·ria \₁ek-sə-'fōr-ē-ə\ *n* : latent strabismus in which the visual axes tend outward toward the temple — compare HETEROPHORIA

ex·oph·thal·mia \₁ek-₁säf-'thal-mē-ə\ *n* : EXOPHTHALMOS

ex·oph·thal·mic goiter \₁ek-säf-'thal-mik-\ *n* : GRAVES' DISEASE

ex·oph·thal·mos *also* **ex·oph·thal·mus** \₁ek-säf-'thal-məs, -səf-\ *n* : abnormal protrusion of the eyeball — **exophthalmic** *adj*

exo·phyt·ic \₁ek-sō-'fi-tik\ *adj* : tending to grow outward beyond the surface epithelium from which it originates — used of tumors; compare ENDOPHYTIC

ex·os·tec·to·my \₁ek-(₁)säs-'tek-tə-mē\ *n, pl* **-mies** : excision of an exostosis

ex·os·to·sis \₁ek-(₁)säs-'tō-səs\ *n, pl* **-to·ses** \-₁sēz\ : a spur or bony outgrowth from a bone or the root of a tooth — **ex·os·tot·ic** \-'tä-tik\ *adj*

exo·tox·in \₁ek-sō-'täk-sən\ *n* : a soluble poisonous substance produced during growth of a microorganism and released into the surrounding medium ⟨tetanus ∼⟩ — compare ENDOTOXIN

exo·tro·pia \₁ek-sə-'trō-pē-ə\ *n* : WALLEYE 2a

ex·pan·der \ik-'span-dər\ *n* : any of several colloidal substances (as dextran) of high molecular weight used as a blood or plasma substitute for increasing the blood volume — called also **extender**

ex·pect \ik-'spekt\ *vb* : to be pregnant : await the birth of one's child — used in progressive tenses ⟨she's ∼*ing* next month⟩

ex·pec·tan·cy \-'spek-tən-sē\ *n, pl* **-cies** : the expected amount (as of the number of years of life) based on statistical probability — see LIFE EXPECTANCY

ex·pec·tant \-'spek-tənt\ *adj* : expecting the birth of a child

ex·pec·to·rant \ik-'spek-tə-rənt\ *n* : an agent that promotes the discharge or expulsion of mucus from the respiratory tract; *broadly* : ANTITUSSIVE — **expectorant** *adj*

ex·pec·to·rate \-₁rāt\ *vb* **-rat·ed; -rat·ing 1** : to eject matter from the throat or lungs by coughing or hawking and spitting **2** : SPIT

ex·pec·to·ra·tion \ik-₁spek-tə-'rā-shən\ *n* **1** : the act or an instance of expectorating **2** : expectorated matter

ex·per·i·ment \ik-'sper-ə-mənt, -'spir-\ *n* **1** : a procedure carried out under controlled conditions in order to discover an unknown effect or law, to test or establish a hypothesis, or to illustrate a known law **2** : the process of testing — **experiment** vb — **ex·per·i·men·ta·tion** \ik-ˌsper-ə-mən-ˈtā-shən, -ˌspir-, -ˌmen-\ n — **ex·per·i·ment·er** \-ˈsper-ə-mən-tər, -ˈspir-\ n

ex·per·i·men·tal \ik-ˌsper-ə-ˈment-ᵊl, -ˌspir-\ adj **1** : of, relating to, or based on experience or experiment **2** : founded on or derived from experiment **3** of a disease : intentionally produced esp. in laboratory animals for the purpose of study ⟨∼ diabetes⟩ — **ex·per·i·men·tal·ly** adv

ex·pi·ra·tion \ˌek-spə-ˈrā-shən\ n **1 a** : the act or process of releasing air from the lungs through the nose or mouth **b** : the escape of carbon dioxide from the body protoplasm (as through the blood and lungs or by diffusion) **2** : something produced by breathing out

ex·pi·ra·to·ry \ik-ˈspī-rə-ˌtōr-ē, ek-; ˈek-spə-rə-\ adj : of, relating to, or employed in the expiration of air from the lungs ⟨∼ muscles⟩

expiratory reserve volume n : the additional amount of air that can be expired from the lungs by determined effort after normal expiration — compare INSPIRATORY RESERVE VOLUME

ex·pire \ik-ˈspīr, ek-\ vb **ex·pired; ex·pir·ing 1** : to breathe one's last breath : DIE **2 a** : to breathe out from or as if from the lungs **b** : to emit the breath

ex·plant \ˈek-ˌsplant\ n : living tissue removed from an organism and placed in a medium for tissue culture — **ex·plant** \(ˌ)ek-ˈsplant\ vb — **ex·plan·ta·tion** \ˌek-ˌsplan-ˈtā-shən\ n

ex·plor·a·to·ry \ik-ˈsplōr-ə-ˌtōr-ē\ adj : of, relating to, or being exploration ⟨∼ surgery⟩

ex·plore \ik-ˈsplōr\ vb **ex·plored; ex·plor·ing** : to examine minutely (as by surgery) esp. for diagnostic purposes — **ex·plo·ra·tion** \ˌek-splə-ˈrā-shən\ n

ex·plor·er \ik-ˈsplōr-ər\ n : an instrument for exploring cavities esp. in teeth : PROBE 1

ex·pose \ik-ˈspōz\ vb **ex·posed; ex·pos·ing 1** : to make liable to or accessible to something (as a disease or environmental conditions) that may have a detrimental effect ⟨children exposed to diphtheria⟩ **2** : to lay open to view: as **a** : to conduct (oneself) as an exhibitionist **b** : to reveal (a bodily part) esp. by dissection

ex·po·sure \ik-ˈspō-zhər\ n **1** : the act or an instance of exposing — see INDECENT EXPOSURE **2** : the condition of being exposed to severe weather conditions

ex·press \ik-ˈspres, ek-\ vb **1** : to make known or exhibit by an expression **2** : to cause (a gene) to manifest its effects in the phenotype

ex·pres·sion \ik-ˈspre-shən\ n **1 a** : something that manifests, represents, reflects, embodies, or symbolizes something else (the first clinical ∼ of a disease) **b** : the detectable effect of a gene; also : EXPRESSIVITY 2 : facial aspect or vocal intonation as indicative of feeling

ex·pres·siv·i·ty \ˌek-ˌspre-ˈsi-və-tē\ n, pl **-ties** : the relative capacity of a gene to affect the phenotype of the organism of which it is a part — compare PENETRANCE

ex·pul·sive \ik-ˈspəl-siv\ adj : serving to expel ⟨∼ efforts during labor⟩

ex·san·gui·na·tion \(ˌ)eks-ˌsaŋ-gwə-ˈnā-shən\ n : the action or process of draining or losing blood — **ex·san·gui·nate** \eks-ˈsaŋ-gwə-ˌnāt\ vb

ex·sic·co·sis \ˌek-si-ˈkō-səs\ n, pl **-co·ses** \-ˌsēz\ n : insufficient intake of fluids; also : the resulting condition of bodily dehydration

ex·stro·phy \ˈek-strə-fē\ n, pl **-phies** : eversion of a part or organ; specif : a congenital malformation of the bladder in which the normally internal mucosa of the organ lies exposed on the abdominal wall

ex·tend \ik-ˈstend\ vb : to straighten out (as an arm or leg)

extended family n : a family that includes in one household near relatives in addition to a nuclear family

ex·tend·er \ik-ˈsten-dər\ n **1** : a substance added to a product esp. in the capacity of a diluent, adulterant, or modifier **2** : EXPANDER

ex·ten·si·bil·i·ty \ik-ˌsten-sə-ˈbi-lə-tē\ n, pl **-ties** : the capability of being stretched ⟨∼ of muscle⟩ — **ex·ten·si·ble** \ik-ˈsten-sə-bəl\ adj

ex·ten·sion \ik-ˈsten-chən\ n **1** : the stretching of a fractured or dislocated limb so as to restore it to its natural position **2** : an unbending movement around a joint in a limb (as the knee or elbow) that increases the angle between the bones of the limb at the joint — compare FLEXION 1

ex·ten·sor \ik-ˈsten-sər, -sȯr\ n : a muscle serving to extend a bodily part (as a limb) — called also extensor muscle; compare FLEXOR

extensor car·pi ra·di·al·is brev·is \-ˈkär-ˌpī-ˌrā-dē-ˈā-ləs-ˈbre-vəs, -ˈkär-ˌpē-\ n : a short muscle on the radial side of the back of the forearm that extends and may abduct the hand

extensor carpi radialis lon·gus \-ˈlȯŋ-gəs\ n : a long muscle on the radial side of the back of the forearm that extends and abducts the hand

extensor carpi ul·na·ris \-ˌəl-ˈnar-əs\ n : a muscle on the ulnar side of the back of the forearm that extends and adducts the hand

extensor dig·i·ti min·i·mi \-ˈdi-jə-ˌtī-ˈmi-nə-ˌmī, -ˈdi-jə-ˌtē-ˈmi-nə-ˌmē\ n : a slender muscle on the medial side of the extensor digitorum communis that extends the little finger

extensor digiti quin·ti pro·pri·us \-ˈkwin-ˌtī-ˈprō-prē-əs, -ˈkwin-ˌtē-\ *n* : EXTENSOR DIGITI MINIMI

extensor dig·i·to·rum brev·is \-ˌdi-jə-ˈtōr-əm-ˈbre-vəs\ *n* : a muscle on the dorsum of the foot that extends the toes

extensor digitorum com·mu·nis \-kə-ˈmyü-nəs, -ˈkä-myə-\ *n* : a muscle on the back of the forearm that extends the fingers and wrist

extensor digitorum lon·gus \-ˈloṅ-gəs\ *n* : a pennate muscle on the lateral part of the front of the leg that extends the four small toes and dorsally flexes and pronates the foot

extensor hal·lu·cis brev·is \-ˈha-lü-səs-ˈbre-vəs, -lyü-, -ˈha-lə-kəs-\ *n* : the part of the extensor digitorum brevis that extends the big toe

extensor hallucis lon·gus \-ˈloṅ-gəs\ *n* : a long thin muscle situated on the shin that extends the big toe and dorsiflexes and supinates the foot

extensor in·di·cis \-ˈin-də-səs, -də-kəs\ *n* : a thin muscle that arises from the ulna in the more distal part of the forearm and extends the index finger

extensor indicis pro·pri·us \-ˈprō-prē-əs\ *n* : EXTENSOR INDICIS

extensor pol·li·cis brev·is \-ˈpä-lə-səs-ˈbre-vəs, -lə-kəs-\ *n* : a muscle that arises from the dorsal surface of the radius, extends the first phalanx of the thumb, and adducts the hand

extensor pollicis lon·gus \-ˈloṅ-gəs\ *n* : a muscle that arises dorsolaterally from the middle part of the ulna, extends the second phalanx of the thumb, and abducts the hand

extensor ret·i·nac·u·lum \-ˌret-ᵊn-ˈa-kyə-ləm\ *n* **1** : either of two fibrous bands of fascia crossing the front of the ankle: **a** : a lower band that is attached laterally to the superior aspect of the calcaneus and passes medially to divide in the shape of a Y and that passes over or both over and under the tendons of the extensor muscles at the ankle — called also *inferior extensor retinaculum* **b** : an upper band passing over and binding down the tendons of the tibialis anterior, extensor hallucis longus, extensor digitorum longus, and peroneus tertius just above the ankle joint — called also *superior extensor retinaculum, transverse crural ligament* **2** : a fibrous band of fascia crossing the back of the wrist and binding down the tendons of the extensor muscles

ex·te·ri·or·ize \ek-ˈstir-ē-ə-ˌrīz\ *vb* **-ized; -iz·ing 1** : EXTERNALIZE 2 **b** : to bring out of the body (as for surgery) ⟨the section of perforated colon was *exteriorized*⟩ — **ex·te·ri·or·iza·tion** \-ˌstir-ē-ə-rə-ˈzā-shən\ *n*

ex·tern \ˈek-ˌstərn\ *n* : a nonresident doctor or medical student at a hospital — **ex·tern·ship** \-ˌship\ *n*

externa — see MUSCULARIS EXTERNA, OTITIS EXTERNA, THECA EXTERNA

ex·ter·nal \ek-ˈstərn-ᵊl\ *adj* **1** : capable of being perceived outwardly : BODILY ⟨~ signs of a disease⟩ **2 a** : situated at, on, or near the outside ⟨an ~ muscle⟩ **b** : directed toward the outside : having an outside object ⟨~ perception⟩ **c** : used by applying to the outside ⟨an ~ lotion⟩ **3 a** (1) : situated near or toward the surface of the body; *also* : situated away from the mesial plane ⟨the ~ condyle of the humerus⟩ (2) : arising or acting from outside : having an outside origin ⟨~ stimuli⟩ **b** : of, relating to, or consisting of something outside the mind : having existence independent of the mind ⟨~ reality⟩ — **ex·ter·nal·ly** *adv*

external anal sphincter *n* : ANAL SPHINCTER a

external auditory meatus *n* : the passage leading from the opening of the external ear to the eardrum — called also *external acoustic meatus, external auditory canal, meatus acusticus externus*

external capsule *n* : CAPSULE 1b(2)

external carotid artery *n* : the outer branch of the carotid artery that supplies the face, tongue, and external parts of the head — called also *external carotid*

external ear *n* : the parts of the ear that are external to the eardrum; *also* : PINNA

external iliac artery *n* : ILIAC ARTERY 2

external iliac node *n* : any of the lymph nodes grouped around the external iliac artery and the external iliac vein — compare INTERNAL ILIAC NODE

external iliac vein *n* : ILIAC VEIN b

external inguinal ring *n* : SUPERFICIAL INGUINAL RING

external intercostal muscle *n* : INTERCOSTAL MUSCLE a — called also *external intercostal*

ex·ter·nal·ize \ek-ˈstern-ᵊl-ˌīz\ *vb* **-ized; -iz·ing 1 a** : to transform from a mental image into an apparently real object (as in hallucinations) : attribute (a mental image) to external causation **b** : to invent an explanation for by attributing to causes outside the self : RATIONALIZE, PROJECT **2** : to direct outward socially (*externalized* anger) — **ex·ter·nal·iza·tion** \-ˌstern-ᵊl-ə-ˈzā-shən\ *n*

external jugular vein *n* : JUGULAR VEIN b — called also *external jugular*

external malleolus *n* : MALLEOLUS a

external maxillary artery *n* : FACIAL ARTERY

external oblique *n* : OBLIQUE a (1)

external occipital crest *n* : OCCIPITAL CREST a

external occipital protuberance *n* : OCCIPITAL PROTUBERANCE a

external pterygoid muscle n : PTERY-GOID MUSCLE a

external pudendal artery n : either of two branches of the femoral artery: **a** : one that is distributed to the skin of the lower abdomen, to the penis and scrotum in the male, and to one of the labia majora in the female — called also *superficial external pudendal artery* **b** : one that follows a deeper course, that is distributed to the medial aspect of the thigh, to the skin of the scrotum and perineum in the male, and to one of the labia majora in the female — called also *deep external pudendal artery*

external respiration n : exchange of gases between the external environment and the lungs or between the alveoli of the lungs and the blood — compare INTERNAL RESPIRATION

ex·terne *var of* EXTERN

externus — see MEATUS ACUSTICUS EXTERNUS, OBLIQUUS EXTERNUS ABDOMINIS, OBTURATOR EXTERNUS, SPHINCTER ANI EXTERNUS

ex·tero·cep·tive \ˌek-stə-rō-ˈsep-tiv\ adj : activated by, relating to, or being stimuli received by an organism from outside

ex·tero·cep·tor \-ˈsep-tər\ n : a sense receptor (as of touch, temperature, smell, vision, or hearing) excited by exteroceptive stimuli — compare INTEROCEPTOR

ex·tinc·tion \ik-ˈstiŋk-shən\ n : the process of eliminating or reducing a conditioned response by not reinforcing it

ex·tin·guish \ik-ˈstiŋ-gwish\ vb : to cause extinction of (a conditioned response)

ex·tir·pa·tion \ˌek-stər-ˈpā-shən\ n : complete excision or surgical destruction of a body part — **ex·tir·pate** \ˈek-stər-ˌpāt\ vb

extra- prefix : outside : beyond ⟨extrauterine⟩

ex·tra·cap·su·lar \ˌek-strə-ˈkap-sə-lər, -ˌsyü-lər\ adj **1** : situated outside a capsule **2** of a cataract operation : involving removal of the front part of the capsule and the central part of the lens — compare INTRACAPSULAR 2

ex·tra·cel·lu·lar \ˈsel-yə-lər\ adj : situated or occurring outside a cell or the cells of the body ⟨~ digestion⟩ ⟨~ enzymes⟩ — **ex·tra·cel·lu·lar·ly** adv

ex·tra·chro·mo·som·al \ˌkrō-mə-ˈsō-məl, -ˈzō-\ adj : situated or controlled by factors outside the chromosome ⟨~ inheritance⟩ ⟨~ DNA⟩

ex·tra·cor·po·re·al \-kȯr-ˈpōr-ē-əl\ adj : occurring or based outside the living body ⟨heart surgery employing ~ circulation⟩ — **ex·tra·cor·po·re·al·ly** adv

ex·tra·cra·ni·al \-ˈkrā-nē-əl\ adj : situated or occurring outside the cranium

¹**ex·tract** \ik-ˈstrakt\ vb **1** : to pull or take out forcibly ⟨~ed a wisdom tooth⟩ **2** : to separate the medicinally-active components of a plant or animal tissue by the use of solvents — **ex·trac·tion** \-ˈstrak-shən\ n

²**ex·tract** \ˈek-ˌstrakt\ n : something prepared by extracting; *esp* : a medicinally-active pharmaceutical solution

¹**ex·trac·tive** \ik-ˈstrak-tiv, ˈek-ˌ\ adj : of, relating to, or involving the process of extracting

²**extractive** n : EXTRACT

ex·tra·du·ral \ˌek-strə-ˈdúr-əl, -dyúr-\ adj : situated or occurring outside the dura mater but within the skull ⟨an ~ hemorrhage⟩

ex·tra·em·bry·on·ic \-ˌem-brē-ˈä-nik\ adj : situated outside the embryo proper; *esp* : developed from the zygote but not part of the embryo ⟨~ membranes⟩

extraembryonic coelom n : the space between the chorion and amnion which in early stages is continuous with the coelom of the embryo proper

ex·tra·fu·sal \ˌek-strə-ˈfyü-zəl\ adj : situated outside a striated muscle spindle ⟨~ muscle fibers⟩ — compare INTRAFUSAL

ex·tra·gen·i·tal \-ˈje-nə-təl\ adj : situated or originating outside the genital region or organs

ex·tra·he·pat·ic \-hi-ˈpa-tik\ adj : situated or originating outside the liver

ex·tra·in·tes·ti·nal \-in-ˈtes-tə-nəl\ adj : situated or occurring outside the intestines ⟨~ infections⟩

ex·tra·mac·u·lar \-ˈma-kyə-lər\ adj : relating to or being the part of the retina other than the macula lutea

ex·tra·med·ul·lary \-ˈmed-əl-ˌer-ē, -ˈme-jə-ˌler-ē, -mə-ˈdə-lə-rē\ adj **1** : situated or occurring outside the spinal cord or the medulla oblongata **2** : located or taking place outside the bone marrow

ex·tra·mi·to·chon·dri·al \-ˌmī-tə-ˈkändrē-əl\ adj : situated or occurring in the cell outside the mitochondria

ex·tra·nu·cle·ar \-ˈnü-klē-ər, -ˈnyü-\ adj : situated in or affecting the parts of a cell external to the nucleus : CYTOPLASMIC

ex·tra·oc·u·lar muscle \-ˈä-kyə-lər-\ n : any of six small voluntary muscles that pass between the eyeball and the orbit and control the movement of the eyeball in relation to the orbit

ex·tra·oral \-ˈōr-əl, -ˈär-\ adj : situated or occurring outside the mouth ⟨an ~ abscess⟩

ex·tra·peri·to·ne·al \-ˌper-ət-ᵊn-ˈē-əl\ adj : located or taking place outside the peritoneal cavity

ex·tra·pi·tu·itary \-pə-ˈtü-ə-ˌter-ē, -ˈtyü-\ adj : situated or arising outside the pituitary gland

ex·tra·pla·cen·tal \-plə-ˈsent-ᵊl\ adj : being outside of or independent of the placenta

ex·tra·py·ra·mi·dal \-pə-ˈra-məd-əl, -ˌpir-ə-ˈmid-əl\ adj : situated outside of and esp. involving descending nerve tracts other than the pyramidal tracts (~ brain lesions)

ex·tra·re·nal \-'rēn-ə]\ *adj* : situated or occurring outside the kidneys

ex·tra·ret·i·nal \-'re-tə-nəl\ *adj* : situated or occurring outside the retina (~ photoreception)

ex·tra·sen·so·ry \ek-strə-'sen-sə-rē\ *adj* : residing beyond or outside the ordinary senses

extrasensory perception *n* : perception (as in telepathy, clairvoyance, and precognition) that involves awareness of information about events external to the self not gained through the senses and not deducible from previous experience — called also *ESP*

ex·tra·sys·to·le \-'sis-tə-(,)lē\ *n* : a prematurely occurring beat of one of the chambers of the heart that leads to momentary arrhythmia but leaves the fundamental rhythm unchanged — called also *premature beat* — **ex·tra·sys·tol·ic** \-sis-'tä-lik\ *adj*

ex·tra·uter·ine \-'yü-tə-rən, -,rīn\ *adj* : situated or occurring outside the uterus

extrauterine pregnancy *n* : ECTOPIC PREGNANCY

ex·trav·a·sate \ik-'stra-və-,sāt, -,zāt\ *vb* **-sat·ed; -sat·ing** : to force out, cause to escape, or pass by infiltration or effusion from a proper vessel or channel (as a blood vessel) into surrounding tissue

ex·trav·a·sa·tion \ik-,stra-və-'zā-shən, -'sā-\ *n* 1 : the action of extravasating 2 a : an extravasated fluid (as blood) (~s from the nose and mouth) b : a deposit formed by extravasation

ex·tra·vas·cu·lar \,ek-strə-'vas-kyə-lər\ *adj* : not occurring or contained in body vessels — **ex·tra·vas·cu·lar·ly** *adv*

ex·tra·ven·tric·u·lar \-ven-'tri-kyə-lər, -vən-\ *adj* : located or taking place outside a ventricle (~ lesions)

ex·tra·ver·sion, ex·tra·vert *var of* EXTROVERSION, EXTROVERT

ex·trem·i·ty \ik-'stre-mə-tē\ *n, pl* **-ties** 1 : the farthest or most remote part, section, or point 2 : a limb of the body; *esp* : a hand or foot

ex·trin·sic \ek-'strin-zik, -sik\ *adj* 1 : originating or due to causes or factors from or on the outside of a body, organ, or part 2 : originating outside a part and acting on the part as a whole — used esp. of certain muscles; compare INTRINSIC 2 — **ex·trin·si·cal·ly** \-zi-k(ə-)lē, -si-\ *adv*

extrinsic factor *n* : VITAMIN B₁₂

extro- *prefix* : outside : outward (*extro*vert) — compare INTRO-

ex·tro·ver·sion \,ek-strə-'vər-zhən, -shən\ *n* : the act, state, or habit of being predominantly concerned with and obtaining gratification from what is outside the self — compare INTROVERSION

ex·tro·vert \'ek-strə-,vərt\ *n* : one whose personality is characterized by extroversion; *broadly* : a gregarious and unreserved person — compare INTROVERT — **extrovert** *adj* — **ex·tro·vert·ed** \-,ver-təd\ *adj*

ex·trude \ik-'strüd\ *vb* **ex·trud·ed; ex·trud·ing** : to force, press, or push out; *also* : to become extruded (blood *extruding* through arteries) — **ex·tru·sion** \ik-'strü-zhən\ *n*

ex·tu·ba·tion \,ek-,stü-'bā-shən, -,styü-\ *n* : the removal of a tube esp. from the larynx after intubation — **ex·tu·bate** \ek-'stü-,bāt, -'styü-, 'ek-,stü-, -,styü-\ *vb*

ex·u·date \'ek-su̇-,dāt, -syu̇-, -shu̇-\ *n* : exuded matter; *esp* : the material composed of serum, fibrin, and white blood cells that escapes from blood vessels into a superficial lesion or area of inflammation

ex·u·da·tion \,ek-su̇-'dā-shən, -syu̇-, -shu̇-\ *n* 1 : the process of exuding 2 : EXUDATE — **ex·u·da·tive** \ig-'zü-də-tiv; 'ek-su̇-,dā-tiv, -syu̇-, -shu̇-\ *adj*

ex·ude \ig-'züd\ *vb* **ex·ud·ed; ex·ud·ing** 1 : to ooze or cause to ooze out 2 : to undergo diffusion

eye \'ī\ *n* 1 : a nearly spherical hollow organ that is lined with a sensitive retina, is lodged in a bony orbit in the skull, is the vertebrate organ of sight, and is normally paired 2 : all the visible structures within and surrounding the orbit and including eyelids, eyelashes, and eyebrows 3 : the faculty of seeing with eyes

eye·ball \'ī-,bȯl\ *n* : the more or less globular capsule of the vertebrate eye formed by the sclera and cornea together with their contained structures

eye bank *n* : a storage place for human corneas from the newly dead for transplanting to the eyes of those blind through corneal defects

eye·brow \'ī-,brau̇\ *n* : the ridge over the eye or hair growing on it — called also *brow*

eye chart *n* : a chart that is read at a fixed distance for purposes of testing sight; *esp* : one with rows of letters or objects of decreasing size

eye·cup \'ī-,kəp\ *n* 1 : a small oval cup with a rim curved to fit the orbit of the eye used for applying liquid remedies to the eyes 2 : OPTIC CUP

eyed \'īd\ *adj* : having an eye or eyes esp. of a specified kind or number — often used in combination (a blue= *eyed* patient)

eyed·ness \'īd-nəs\ *n* : preference for the use of one eye instead of the other

eye doctor *n* : a specialist (as an optometrist or ophthalmologist) in the examination, treatment, or care of the eyes

eye·drop·per \'ī-,drä-pər\ *n* : DROPPER

eye·drops \'ī-,dräps\ *n pl* : a medicated solution for the eyes that is applied in drops — **eye·drop** \-,dräp\ *adj*

227 eyeglass • facial vein

eye·glass \'ī-ˌglas\ *n* **1 a** : a lens worn to aid vision; *specif* : MONOCLE **b** *pl* : GLASSES, SPECTACLES **2** : EYECUP 1

eye gnat *n* : any of several small dipteran flies (genus *Hippelates* of the family Chloropidae and esp. *H. pusio*) including some that are held to be vectors of pinkeye and yaws — called also *eye fly*

eye·ground \'ī-ˌgraünd\ *n* : the fundus of the eye; *esp* : the retina as viewed through an ophthalmoscope

eye·lash \'ī-ˌlash\ *n* **1** : the fringe of hair edging the eyelid — usu. used in pl. **2** : a single hair of the eyelashes

eye·lid \'ī-ˌlid\ *n* : either of the movable lids of skin and muscle that can be closed over the eyeball — called also *palpebra*

eye·sight \'ī-ˌsīt\ *n* : SIGHT 2

eye socket *n* : ORBIT

eye·strain \'ī-ˌstrān\ *n* : weariness or a strained state of the eye

eye·tooth \'ī-ˌtüth\ *n, pl* **eye·teeth** \-ˌtēth\ : a canine tooth of the upper jaw

eye·wash \'ī-ˌwȯsh, -ˌwäsh\ *n* : an eye lotion

eye·wear \'ī-ˌwar, -ˌwer\ *n* : corrective or protective devices (as glasses or contact lenses) for the eyes

eye worm *n* **1** : either of two slender nematode worms of the genus *Oxyspirura* (*O. mansoni* and *O. petrowi*) living beneath the nictitating membrane of the eyes of birds and esp. chickens **2** : any member of the nematode genus *Thelazia* living in the tear duct and beneath the eyelid of dogs, cats, sheep, humans, and other mammals and sometimes causing blindness **3** : an African filarial worm of the genus *Loa* (*L. loa*) that migrates through the eyeball and subcutaneous tissues of humans — compare CALABAR SWELLING

F

f *symbol* focal length

¹F *abbr* Fahrenheit

²F *symbol* **1** filial generation — usu. used with a subscript F_1 for the first, F_2 for the second, etc. **2** fluorine

fab·ri·ca·tion \ˌfa-bri-'kā-shən\ *n* : CONFABULATION

Fa·bry's disease \'fä-brēz-\ *n* : a sex-linked inherited disorder of lipid catabolism characterized esp. by renal dysfunction, a rash in the inguinal, scrotal, and umbilical regions, and corneal defects

  Fabry, Johannes (1860–1930), German dermatologist.

FACC *abbr* Fellow of the American College of Cardiology

FACD *abbr* Fellow of the American College of Dentists

face \'fās\ *n, often attrib* : the front part of the head including the chin, mouth, nose, cheeks, eyes, and usu. the forehead

face–bow \'fās-ˌbō\ *n* : a device used in dentistry to determine the positional relationships of the maxillae to the temporomandibular joints of a patient

face fly *n* : a European fly of the genus *Musca* (*M. autumnalis*) that is similar to the house fly, is widely established in No. America, and causes distress in livestock by clustering about the face

face–lift \'fās-ˌlift\ *n* : a plastic surgical operation for removal of facial defects (as wrinkles) typical of aging — called also *rhytidectomy* — **face–lift** *vb*

face–lifting \-ˌlif-tiŋ\ *n* : FACE-LIFT

fac·et \'fa-sət\ *n* : a smooth flat or nearly flat circumscribed anatomical surface (the articular ∼ of a bone) — **fac·et·ed** *or* **fac·et·ted** \'fa-sə-təd\ *adj*

fac·et·ec·to·my \ˌfa-sə-'tek-tə-mē\ *n, pl* **-mies** : excision of a facet esp. of a vertebra

¹fa·cial \'fā-shəl\ *adj* **1** : of, relating to, or affecting the face (∼ neuralgia) **2** : concerned with or used in improving the appearance of the face **3** : relating to or being the buccal and labial surface of a tooth — **fa·cial·ly** \-shə-lē\ *adv*

²facial *n* : a treatment to improve the appearance of the face

facial artery *n* : an artery that arises from the external carotid artery and gives off branches supplying the neck and face — called also *external maxillary artery;* compare MAXILLARY ARTERY

facial bone *n* : any of the 14 bones of the facial region of the human skull that do not take part in forming the braincase

facial canal *n* : a passage in the petrous part of the temporal bone that transmits various branches of the facial nerve

facial colliculus *n* : a medial eminence on the floor of the fourth ventricle of the brain produced by the nucleus of the abducens nerve and the flexure of the facial nerve around it

facial nerve *n* : either of the seventh pair of cranial nerves that supply motor fibers esp. to the muscles of the face and jaw and sensory and parasympathetic fibers to the tongue, palate, and fauces — called also *seventh cranial nerve, seventh nerve*

facial vein *n* : a vein that arises as the angular vein, drains the superficial structures of the face, and empties into the internal jugular vein — called also *anterior facial vein;* see DEEP FACIAL VEIN, POSTERIOR FACIAL VEIN

-fa·cient \\'fā-shənt\ *adj comb form* : making : causing ⟨abortifacient⟩ ⟨rubefacient⟩

fa·cies \\'fā-ıshēz, -shē-ıēz\ *n, pl* **facies** **1** : an appearance and expression of the face characteristic of a particular condition esp. when abnormal ⟨adenoid ∼⟩ **2** : an anatomical surface

fa·cil·i·ta·tion \fə-ısil-ə-'tā-shən\ *n* **1** : the lowering of the threshold for reflex conduction along a particular neural pathway **2** : the increasing of the ease or intensity of a response by repeated stimulation — **fa·cil·i·tate** \\-'sil-ə-ıtāt\ *vb* — **fa·cil·i·ta·to·ry** \\-'sil-lə-tə-ıtōr-ē\ *adj*

fac·ing \\'fā-siŋ\ *n* : a front of porcelain or plastic used in dental crowns and bridgework to face the metal replacement and simulate the natural tooth

facio- *comb form* : facial and ⟨*facio*scapulohumeral⟩

fa·cio·scap·u·lo·hu·mer·al \ıfā-shē-ō-ıska-pyə-lō-'hyü-mə-rəl\ *adj* : relating to or affecting the muscles of the face, scapula, and arm

FACOG *abbr* Fellow of the American College of Obstetricians and Gynecologists

FACP *abbr* Fellow of the American College of Physicians

FACR *abbr* Fellow of the American College of Radiology

FACS *abbr* Fellow of the American College of Surgeons

F–ac·tin \\'ef-ıak-tən\ *n* : a fibrous actin polymerized in the form of a double helix that is produced in the presence of some salts (as divalent calcium) and ATP — compare G-ACTIN

fac·ti·tious \fak-'ti-shəs\ *adj* : not produced by natural means

fac·tor \\'fak-tər\ *n* **1 a** : something that actively contributes to the production of a result **b** : a substance that functions or promotes the function of a particular physiological process or bodily system **2** : GENE — **fac·to·ri·al** \fak-'tōr-ē-əl\ *adj*

factor VIII \\-'āt\ *n* : a glycoprotein of blood plasma that is essential for blood clotting and is absent or inactive in hemophilia — called also *antihemophilic factor, thromboplastinogen*

factor XI \\-i-'le-vən\ *n* : PLASMA THROMBOPLASTIN ANTECEDENT

factor V \\-'fiv\ *n* : a globulin occurring in inactive form in blood plasma that in its active form is one of the factors accelerating the formation of thrombin from prothrombin and is one of the factors of the clotting of blood — called also *accelerator globulin, labile factor, proaccelerin*

factor IX \\-'nīn\ *n* : a clotting factor whose absence is associated with Christmas disease — called also *autoprothrombin II, Christmas factor*

factor VII \\-'se-vən\ *n* : a clotting fac-

tor in normal blood that is formed in the kidney under the influence of vitamin K and may be deficient due to a hereditary disorder or to a vitamin K deficiency — called also *autoprothrombin I, cothromboplastin, proconvertin, stable factor*

factor X \\-'ten\ *n* : a clotting factor that is converted to a proteolytic enzyme which converts prothrombin to thrombin in a reaction dependent on calcium ions and other clotting factors — called also *Stuart-Prower factor*

factor XIII \\-ıthərt-'tēn\ *n* : a substance that aids in clotting blood by causing monomeric fibrin to polymerize and become stable and insoluble — called also *fibrinase;* see TRANSGLUTAMINASE

factor XII \\-'twelv\ *n* : a clotting factor that facilitates blood coagulation in vivo and initiates coagulation on a firm surface (as glass) in vitro but whose deficiency tends not to promote hemorrhage — called also *Hageman factor*

facts of life *n pl* : the fundamental physiological processes and behavior involved in sex and reproduction

fac·ul·ta·tive \\'fa-kəl-ıtā-tiv\ *adj* **1** : taking place under some conditions but not under others ⟨∼ parasitism⟩ **2** : exhibiting an indicated lifestyle under some environmental conditions but not under others ⟨∼ anaerobes⟩ — **fac·ul·ta·tive·ly** *adv*

FAD \ıef-(ı)ā-'dē\ *n* : FLAVIN ADENINE DINUCLEOTIDE

Each boldface word in the list below is a chiefly British variant of the word to its right in small capitals.

faecal	FECAL
faecalith	FECALITH
faecaloid	FECALOID
faeces	FECES

fag·o·py·rism \ıfa-gō-'pī-ıri-zəm\ *n* : a photosensitization esp. of swine and sheep that is due to eating large quantities of buckwheat (esp. *Fagopyrum esculentum* of the family Polygonaceae) and that appears principally on the nonpigmented parts of the skin as an intense redness and swelling with severe itching and the formation of vesicles and later sores and scabs — compare BIGHEAD b, HYPERICISM

Fahr·en·heit \\'far-ən-ıhīt\ *adj* : relating or conforming to a thermometric scale on which under standard atmospheric pressure the boiling point of water is at 212 degrees above the zero of the scale and the freezing point is at 32 degrees above zero — abbr. *F*

Fahrenheit, Daniel Gabriel (1686–1736), German physicist.

fail \\'fāl\ *vb* **1** : to weaken or lose strength **2** : to stop functioning ⟨the patient's heart ∼*ed*⟩

fail·ure \\'fāl-yər\ *n* : a state of inability

to perform a vital function ⟨acute renal ∼⟩ ⟨respiratory ∼⟩ — see HEART FAILURE

¹faint \ˈfānt\ adj : weak, dizzy, and likely to faint — faint·ness \-nəs\ n

²faint vb : to lose consciousness because of a temporary decrease in the blood supply to the brain

³faint n : the physiological action of fainting; also : the resulting condition : SYNCOPE

faith healing n : a method of treating diseases by prayer and exercise of faith in God — faith healer n

falces pl of FALX

falciform ligament n : an anteroposterior fold of peritoneum attached to the under surface of the diaphragm and sheath of the rectus muscle and along a line on the anterior and upper surfaces of the liver extending back from the notch on the anterior margin

fal·cip·a·rum malaria \fal-ˈsi-pə-rəm-, fôl-\ n : severe malaria caused by a parasite of the genus Plasmodium (P. falciparum) and marked by recurrence of paroxysms usu. in less than 48 hours — called also malignant malaria, malignant tertian malaria; compare VIVAX MALARIA

fallen arch n : FLATFOOT

falling sickness n : EPILEPSY

fal·lo·pian tube \fə-ˈlō-pē-ən-\ n, often cap F : either of the pair of tubes that carry the eggs from the ovary to the uterus — called also uterine tube

Fal·lop·pio \fäl-ˈlóp-yō\ or Fal·lop·pia \-ˈlóp-yä\, Gabriele (Latin Gabriel Fal·lo·pi·us \fə-ˈlō-pē-əs\) (1523–1562), Italian anatomist.

Fallot's tetralogy \(ˌ)fa-ˈlōz-\ n : TETRALOGY OF FALLOT

fall·out \ˈfȯ-ˌlau̇t\ n 1 : the often radioactive particles stirred up by or resulting from a nuclear explosion and descending through the atmosphere; also : other polluting particles (as volcanic ash) descending likewise 2 : descent (as of fallout) through the atmosphere

false \ˈfȯls\ adj fals·er; fals·est 1 : not corresponding to truth or reality ⟨a test for syphilis which gave ∼ results⟩ 2 : artificially made ⟨a set of ∼ teeth⟩

false joint n : PSEUDARTHROSIS

false labor n : pains resembling those of normal labor but occurring at irregular intervals and without dilation of the cervix

false membrane n : a fibrinous deposit with enmeshed necrotic cells formed esp. in croup and diphtheria — called also pseudomembrane

false mo·rel \-mȯ-ˈrel\ n : any fungus of the genus Gyromitra

false–negative adj : relating to or being an individual or a test result that is erroneously classified in a negative category (as of diagnosis) because of imperfect testing methods or procedures — compare FALSE-POSITIVE — false negative n

false pelvis n : the upper broader portion of the pelvic cavity — called also false pelvic cavity; compare TRUE PELVIS

false–positive adj : relating to or being an individual or a test result that is erroneously classified in a positive category (as of diagnosis) because of imperfect testing methods or procedures — compare FALSE-NEGATIVE — false positive n

false pregnancy n : PSEUDOCYESIS, PSEUDOPREGNANCY

false rib n : a rib whose cartilages unite indirectly or not at all with the sternum — compare FLOATING RIB

false vocal cords n pl : the upper pair of vocal cords that are not directly concerned with speech production — called also superior vocal cords, ventricular folds, vestibular folds

falx \ˈfalks, ˈfȯlks\ n, pl fal·ces \ˈfal-ˌsēz, ˈfȯl-\ : a sickle-shaped part or structure: as a : FALX CEREBRI b : FALX CEREBELLI

falx cer·e·bel·li \-ˌser-ə-ˈbe-ˌlī\ n : the smaller of the two folds of dura mater separating the hemispheres of the brain that lies between the lateral lobes of the cerebellum

falx cer·e·bri \-ˈser-ə-ˌbrī\ n : the larger of the two folds of dura mater separating the hemispheres of the brain that lies between the cerebral hemispheres and contains the sagittal sinuses

FAMA abbr Fellow of the American Medical Association

fa·mil·ial \fə-ˈmil-yəl\ adj : tending to occur in more members of a family than expected by chance alone ⟨a ∼ disorder⟩ — compare ACQUIRED 2, CONGENITAL 2, HEREDITARY

fam·i·ly \ˈfam-lē, ˈfa-mə-\ n, pl -lies 1 : the basic unit in society having as its nucleus two or more adults living together and cooperating in the care and rearing of their own or adopted children 2 : a group of related plants or animals forming a category ranking above a genus and below an order and usu. comprising several to many genera — family adj

family doctor n 1 : a doctor regularly consulted by a family 2 : a doctor specializing in family practice

family physician n : FAMILY DOCTOR

family planning n : planning intended to determine the number and spacing of one's children through effective methods of birth control

family practice n : a medical practice or specialty which provides continuing general medical care for the individual and family — called also family medicine

family practitioner n : FAMILY DOCTOR

Fan·co·ni's anemia \ˌfän-ˈkō-nēz-, fan-\ n : a rare disease inherited as an autosomal recessive trait that is characterized by progressive hypoplastic pancytopenia, skeletal anomalies (as short stature), and a predisposition to cancer and esp. leukemia

Fanconi, Guido (b 1892), Swiss pediatrician.

Fanconi syndrome n : a disorder of reabsorption in the proximal convoluted tubules of the kidney marked esp. by the presence of glucose, amino acids, and phosphates in the urine

fang \'faŋ\ n 1 : a long sharp tooth: as **a** : one by which an animal's prey is seized and held or torn **b** : one of the long hollow or grooved and often erectile teeth of a venomous snake 2 : the root of a tooth or one of the processes or prongs into which a root divides — **fanged** \'faŋd\ adj

fan-go \'faŋ-(ˌ)gō, 'fäŋ-\ n : mud and esp. a clay mud from hot springs at Battaglio, Italy, that is used in the form of hot external applications in the therapeutic treatment of certain medical conditions (as rheumatism)

fan-ta-size \'fan-tə-ˌsīz\ vb **-sized; -siz-ing** 1 : to indulge in fantasy 2 : to portray in the mind by fantasy

¹fan-ta-sy \'fan-tə-sē, -zē\ n, pl **-sies** : the power or process of creating esp. unrealistic or improbable mental images in response to psychological need; also : a mental image or a series of mental images (as a daydream) so created (sexual fantasies)

²fantasy vb **-sied; -sy-ing** : FANTASIZE

FAPA abbr Fellow of the American Psychological Association

fa-rad-ic \fə-'ra-dik, far-'a-\ also **far-a-da-ic** \far-ə-'dā-ik\ adj : of or relating to an asymmetric alternating current of electricity ⟨∼ muscle stimulation⟩

Far-a-day \'far-ə-ˌdā\, **Michael (1791–1867),** British physicist and chemist.

far-a-dism \'far-ə-ˌdi-zəm\ n : the application of a faradic current of electricity (as for therapeutic purposes)

far-cy \'fär-sē\ n, pl **far-cies** : GLANDERS; esp : cutaneous glanders

farmer's lung n : an acute pulmonary disorder that is characterized by sudden onset, fever, cough, expectoration, and breathlessness and that results from the inhalation of dust from moldy hay or straw

far point n : the point farthest from the eye at which an object is accurately focused on the retina when the accommodation is completely relaxed — compare NEAR POINT

far-sight-ed \'fär-ˌsī-təd\ adj 1 : seeing or able to see to a great distance 2 : affected with hyperopia — **far-sight-ed-ly** adv

far-sight-ed-ness n 1 : the quality or state of being farsighted 2 : HYPEROPIA

FAS abbr fetal alcohol syndrome

fasc abbr fasciculus

fas-cia \'fa-shə, 'fā-, -shē-ə\ n, pl **-ci-ae** \-shē-ˌē\ or **-cias** : a sheet of connective tissue (as an aponeurosis) covering or binding together body structures; also : tissue occurring in such a sheet — see DEEP FASCIA, SUPERFICIAL FASCIA — **fas-cial** \-shəl, -shē-\ adj

fasciae — see TENSOR FASCIAE LATAE

fascia la-ta \-'lä-tə, -'lä-\ n, pl **fasciae la-tae** \-'lä-tē, -'lä-\ : the deep fascia that forms a complete sheath for the thigh

fas-ci-cle \'fa-si-kəl\ n : a small bundle; esp : FASCICULUS

fasciculata — see ZONA FASCICULATA

fas-cic-u-la-tion \fə-ˌsik-yə-'lā-shən, fa-\ n : muscular twitching involving the simultaneous contraction of contiguous groups of muscle fibers

fas-cic-u-lus \fə-'si-kyə-ləs, fa-\ n, pl **-li** \-ˌlī\ : a slender bundle of fibers: **a** : a bundle of skeletal muscle cells bound together by fasciae and forming one of the constituent elements of a muscle **b** : a bundle of nerve fibers that follow the same course but do not necessarily have like functional connections **c** : TRACT 2

fasciculus cu-ne-a-tus \-ˌkyü-nē-'ā-təs\ n : either of a pair of nerve tracts of the posterior funiculus of the spinal cord that are situated on opposite sides of the posterior median septum lateral to the fasciculus gracilis and that carry nerve fibers from the upper part of the body — called also column of Burdach

fasciculus grac-i-lis \-'gra-sə-ləs\ n : either of a pair of nerve tracts of the posterior funiculus of the spinal cord that carry nerve fibers from the lower part of the body — called also gracile fasciculus

fas-ci-ec-to-my \ˌfa-shē-'ek-tə-mē, -sē-\ n, pl **-mies** : surgical excision of strips of fascia

fas-ci-itis \ˌfa-shē-'ī-təs, -sē-\ n : inflammation of a fascia

Fas-ci-o-la \fə-'sī-ə-lə, -'sī-\ n : a genus of digenetic trematode worms (family Fasciolidae) including common liver flukes of various mammals

fa-sci-o-li-a-sis \fə-ˌsē-ə-'lī-ə-səs, -ˌsī-\ n, pl **-a-ses** \-ˌsēz\ : infestation with or disease caused by liver flukes of the genus Fasciola

fas-ci-o-li-cide \fə-'sē-ə-lə-ˌsīd, fa-\ n : an agent that destroys liver flukes of the genus Fasciola

Fas-ci-o-loi-des \fə-ˌsē-ə-'lȯi-(ˌ)dēz, -ˌsī-\ n : a genus of trematode worms (family Fasciolidae) including the giant liver flukes of ruminant mammals

fas-ci-o-lop-si-a-sis \-ˌläp-'sī-ə-səs\ n, pl **-a-ses** \-ˌsēz\ : infestation with or disease caused by a large intestinal fluke of the genus Fasciolopsis (F. buski)

Fas-ci-o-lop-sis \-'läp-səs\ n : a genus of trematode worms (family Fasciolidae) that includes an important intestinal parasite (*F. buski*) of humans, swine, dogs, and rabbits in much of eastern Asia

fas·ci·ot·o·my \fa-shē-'ä-tə-mē\ *n, pl* **-mies** : surgical incision of a fascia

fas·ci·itis \-'shī-təs, -'sī-\ *var of* FASCIITIS

¹**fast** \'fast\ *adj* : resistant to change (as from destructive action) — used chiefly of organisms and in combination with the agent resisted ⟨acid-*fast* bacteria⟩

²**fast** *vb* **1 a** : to abstain from food **b** : to eat sparingly or abstain from some foods **2** : to deny food to ⟨the patient was ~*ed* before treatment⟩

³**fast** *n* **1** : the practice of fasting **2** : a time of fasting

fastigial nucleus \fa-'sti-jē-əl-\ *n* : a nucleus lying near the midline in the roof of the fourth ventricle of the brain

fas·tig·i·um \fa-'sti-jē-əm\ *n* : the period at which the symptoms of a disease (as a febrile disease) are most pronounced

fast–twitch \'fast-ˌtwich\ *adj* : of, relating to, or being muscle fiber that contracts quickly esp. during brief high-intensity physical activity requiring strength — compare SLOW-TWITCH

¹**fat** \'fat\ *adj* **fat·ter; fat·test** : fleshy with superfluous flabby tissue that is not muscle : OBESE — **fat·ness** *n*

²**fat** *n* **1** : animal tissue consisting chiefly of cells distended with greasy or oily matter — compare BROWN FAT **2 a** : oily or greasy matter making up the bulk of adipose tissue **b** : any of numerous compounds of carbon, hydrogen, and oxygen that are glycerides of fatty acids, are the chief constituents of plant and animal fat, are a major class of energy-rich food, and are soluble in organic solvents but not in water **c** : a solid or semisolid fat as distinguished from an oil **3** : the condition of fatness : OBESITY

fa·tal \'fāt-ᵊl\ *adj* : causing death — **fa·tal·ly** *adv*

fa·tal·i·ty \fā-'ta-lə-tē, fə-\ *n, pl* **-ties 1** : the quality or state of causing death or destruction : DEADLINESS **2 a** : death resulting from a disaster **b** : one who suffers such a death

fat cell *n* : a fat-containing cell of adipose tissue — called also *adipocyte*

fat de·pot \-'de-(ˌ)pō, -'dē-\ *n* : ADIPOSE TISSUE

fat farm *n* : a health spa that specializes in weight reduction

father figure *n* : one often of particular power or influence who serves as an emotional substitute for a father

father image *n* : an idealization of one's father often projected onto someone to whom one looks for guidance and protection

fa·ti·ga·bil·i·ty *also* **fa·ti·gua·bil·i·ty** \fə-ˌtē-gə-'bi-lə-tē, ˌfa-ti-\ *n, pl* **-ties** : susceptibility to fatigue

fa·tigue \fə-'tēg\ *n* **1** : weariness or exhaustion from labor, exertion, or stress **2** : the temporary loss of power to respond induced in a sensory receptor or motor end organ by continued stimulation — **fatigue** *vb*

fat pad *n* : a flattened mass of fatty tissue

fat·ty \'fa-tē\ *adj* **fat·ti·er; -est 1 a** : unduly stout **b** : marked by an abnormal deposit of fat ⟨a ~ liver⟩ ⟨~ cirrhosis⟩ **2** : derived from or chemically related to fat — **fat·ti·ness** *n*

fatty acid *n* **1** : any of numerous saturated acids $C_nH_{2n+1}COOH$ containing a single carboxyl group and including many that occur naturally usu. in the form of esters in fats, waxes, and essential oils **2** : any of the saturated or unsaturated acids (as palmitic acid) with a single carboxyl group and usu. an even number of carbon atoms that occur naturally in the form of glycerides in fats and fatty oils

fatty degeneration *n* : a process of tissue degeneration marked by the deposition of fat globules in the cells — called also *steatosis*

fatty infiltration *n* : infiltration of the tissue of an organ with excess amounts of fat

fatty oil *n* : a fat that is liquid at ordinary temperatures — called also *fixed oil;* compare ESSENTIAL OIL, OIL 1

fau·ces \'fȯ-ˌsēz\ *n sing or pl* : the narrow passage from the mouth to the pharynx situated between the soft palate and the base of the tongue — called also *isthmus of the fauces* — **fau·cial** \'fȯ-shəl\ *adj*

fau·na \'fȯn-ə, 'fän-\ *n, pl* **faunas** *also* **fau·nae** \-ˌē, -ˌī\ : animal life; *esp* : the animals characteristic of a region, period, or special environment — compare FLORA — **fau·nal** \-ᵊl\ *adj* — **fau·nal·ly** \-ᵊl-ē\ *adv*

fava bean \'fä-və-\ *n* : BROAD BEAN

fa·vism \'fä-ˌvi-zəm, 'fä-\ *n* : a hereditary allergic condition esp. of males of Mediterranean descent that causes a severe reaction to the broad bean or its pollen which is characterized by hemolytic anemia, fever, and jaundice

fa·vus \'fä-vəs\ *n* : a contagious skin disease of humans and many domestic animals and fowls that is caused by a fungus (as *Trichophyton schoenleinii*) — **fa·vic** \-vik\ *adj*

FDA *abbr* Food and Drug Administration

Fe *symbol* iron

febri- *comb form* : fever ⟨febrifuge⟩

feb·ri·fuge \'fe-brə-ˌfyüj\ *n or adj* : ANTIPYRETIC

fe·brile \'fe-ˌbrīl, 'fē-\ *adj* : FEVERISH

fe·cal \'fē-kəl\ *adj* : of, relating to, or constituting feces — **fe·cal·ly** *adv*

fe·ca·lith \'fē-kə-ˌlith\ *n* : a concretion

of dry compact feces formed in the intestine or vermiform appendix

fe·cal·oid \'fē-kə-ˌlȯid\ *adj* : resembling dung

fe·ces \'fē-(ˌ)sēz\ *n pl* : bodily waste discharged through the anus : EXCREMENT

Fech·ner's law \'fek-nərz-, 'fek-\ *n* : WEBER-FECHNER LAW

fec·u·lent \'fe-kyə-lənt\ *adj* : foul with impurities : FECAL

fe·cund \'fe-kənd, 'fē-\ *adj* 1 : characterized by having produced many offspring 2 : capable of producing : not sterile or barren — **fe·cun·di·ty** \fi-'kən-də-tē, fe-\ *n*

fe·cun·date \'fe-kən-ˌdāt, 'fē-\ *vb* -**dated; -dat·ing** : IMPREGNATE — **fe·cun·da·tion** \ˌfe-kən-'dā-shən, ˌfē-\ *n*

fee·ble-mind·ed \ˌfē-bəl-'mīn-dəd\ *adj* : mentally deficient — **fee·ble-mind·ed·ness** *n*

feed·back \'fēd-ˌbak\ *n* 1 : the partial reversion of the effects of a process to its source or to a preceding stage 2 : the return to a point of origin of evaluative or corrective information about an action or process; *also* : the information so transmitted

feedback inhibition *n* : inhibition of an enzyme controlling an early stage of a series of biochemical reactions by the end product when it reaches a critical concentration

fee-for-service *n* : separate payment to a health-care provider for each medical service rendered to a patient

feel·ing \'fē-liŋ\ *n* 1 : the one of the basic physical senses of which the skin contains the chief end organs and of which the sensations of touch and temperature are characteristic : TOUCH; *also* : a sensation experienced through this sense 2 : an emotional state or reaction (guilt ∼s) 3 : the overall quality of one's awareness esp. as measured along a pleasantness-unpleasantness continuum — compare AFFECT, EMOTION

fee splitting *n* : payment by a medical specialist (as a surgeon) of a part of the specialist's fee to the physician who made the referral — **fee splitter** *n*

feet *pl of* FOOT

Feh·ling's solution \'fā-liŋz-\ *or* **Fehling solution** \-liŋ-\ *n* : a blue solution of Rochelle salt and copper sulfate used as an oxidizing agent in a test for sugars and aldehydes in which the precipitation of a red oxide of copper indicates a positive result

Fehling, Hermann von (1812–1885), German chemist.

fe·line \'fē-ˌlīn\ *adj* : of, relating to, or affecting cats or the cat family (Felidae) — **feline** *n*

feline distemper *n* : PANLEUKOPENIA

feline enteritis *n* : PANLEUKOPENIA

feline infectious anemia *n* : a widespread contagious disease of cats characterized by weakness, lethargy, loss of appetite, and hemolytic anemia and caused by a bacterial parasite of red blood cells belonging to the genus *Haemobartonella* (*H. felis*)

feline infectious peritonitis *n* : an almost invariably fatal infectious disease of cats caused by one or more coronaviruses and characterized by fever, weight and appetite loss, and ascites with a thick yellow fluid

feline leukemia *n* : a disease of cats caused by the feline leukemia virus, characterized by leukemia and lymphoma, and often resulting in death

feline leukemia virus *n* : a retrovirus that is widespread in cat populations, is prob. transmitted by direct contact, and in cats is associated with or causes malignant lymphoma, feline leukemia, anemia, glomerulonephritis, and immunosuppression

feline panleukopenia *n* : PANLEUKOPENIA

feline pneumonitis *n* : an infectious disease of the eyes and upper respiratory tract of cats that is caused by a bacterium of the genus *Chlamydia* (*C. psittaci*) and is characterized esp. by conjunctivitis and rhinitis

fel·late \'fe-ˌlāt, fə-'lāt\ *vb* **fel·lat·ed; fel·lat·ing** : to perform fellatio on someone — **fel·la·tor** \-ˌlā-tər, -'lā-\ *n*

fel·la·tio \fə-'lā-shē-ˌō, fe-, -'lā-tē-\ *also* **fel·la·tion** \-'lā-shən\ *n, pl* -**tios** *also* -**tions** : oral stimulation of the penis

fel·la·tor \'fe-ˌlā-tər, fə-'lā-\ *n* : one and esp. a man who performs fellatio

fel·la·trice \'fe-lə-ˌtrēs\ *n* : FELLATRIX

fel·la·trix \fe-'lā-triks\ *n, pl* -**trix·es** *or* -**tri·ces** \-trə-ˌsēz, ˌfe-lə-'trī-(ˌ)sēz\ : a woman who performs fellatio

fel·on \'fe-lən\ *n* : WHITLOW

Fel·ty's syndrome \'fel-tēz-\ *n* : a condition characterized esp. by rheumatoid arthritis, neutropenia, and splenomegaly

Felty, Augustus Roi (1895–1964), American physician.

FeLV *abbr* feline leukemia virus

fe·male \'fē-ˌmāl\ *n* : an individual that bears young or produces eggs as distinguished from one that produces sperm; *esp* : a woman or girl as distinguished from a man or boy — **female** *adj* — **fe·male·ness** *n*

female hormone *n* : a sex hormone (as an estrogen) primarily produced and functioning in the female

fem·i·nize \'fe-mə-ˌnīz\ *vb* -**nized; -nizing** : to cause (a male or castrate) to take on feminine characters (as by implantation of ovaries or administration of estrogenic substances) — **fem·i·ni·za·tion** \ˌfe-mə-nə-'zā-shən\ *n*

femora *pl of* FEMUR

fem·o·ral \'fe-mə-rəl\ *adj* : of or relating to the femur or thigh

femoral artery *n* : the chief artery of the thigh that lies in the anterior part of the thigh — see DEEP FEMORAL ARTERY

femoral canal *n* : the space that is situated between the femoral vein and the inner wall of the femoral sheath

femoral nerve *n* : the largest branch of the lumbar plexus that supplies extensor muscles of the thigh and skin areas on the front of the thigh and medial surface of the leg and foot and that sends articular branches to the hip and knee joints

femoral ring *n* : the oval upper opening of the femoral canal often the seat of a hernia

femoral sheath *n* : the fascial sheath investing the femoral vessels

femoral triangle *n* : an area in the upper anterior part of the thigh bounded by the inguinal ligament, the sartorius, and the adductor longus — called also *femoral trigone, Scarpa's triangle*

femoral vein *n* : the chief vein of the thigh that is a continuation of the popliteal vein and continues above Poupart's ligament as the external iliac vein

femoris — see BICEPS FEMORIS, PROFUNDA FEMORIS, PROFUNDA FEMORIS ARTERY, QUADRATUS FEMORIS, QUADRICEPS FEMORIS, RECTUS FEMORIS

femoro- *comb form* : femoral and *(femoro*popliteal)

fem•o•ro•pop•li•te•al \,fe-mə-rō-'pä-plə-'tē-əl, -pä-'pli-tē-əl\ *adj* : of, relating to, or connecting the femoral and popliteal arteries (a ~ bypass)

fe•mur \'fē-mər\ *n, pl* **fe•murs** *or* **fem•o•ra** \'fe-mə-rə\ : the proximal bone of the hind or lower limb that is the longest and largest bone in the human body, extends from the hip to the knee, articulates above with the acetabulum, and articulates with the tibia below by a pair of condyles — called also *thighbone*

fe•nes•tra \fə-'nes-trə\ *n, pl* **-trae** \-,trē, -,trī\ **1** : a small anatomical opening (as in a bone): as **a** : OVAL WINDOW **b** : ROUND WINDOW **2 a** : an opening like a window cut in bone **b** : a window cut in a surgical instrument (as an endoscope) — **fe•nes•tral** \-trəl\ *adj*

fenestra coch•le•ae \-'kä-klē-,ē, -'kō-klē-,ī\ *n* : ROUND WINDOW

fenestra oval•is \-ō-'vä-ləs\ *n* : OVAL WINDOW

fenestra ro•tun•da \-,rō-'tən-də\ *n* : ROUND WINDOW

fen•es•trat•ed \'fe-nə-,strā-təd\ *adj* : having one or more openings or pores (~ blood capillaries)

fen•es•tra•tion \,fe-nə-'strā-shən\ *n* **1 a** : a natural or surgically created opening in a surface **b** : the presence of such openings **2** : the operation of cutting an opening in the bony labyrinth between the inner ear and tympanum to replace natural fenestrae that are not functional

fenestra ves•ti•bu•li \-ves-'ti-byə-,lī\ *n* : OVAL WINDOW

fen•flur•amine \fen-'flür-ə-,mēn\ *n* : an amphetamine derivative $C_{12}H_{16}F_3N$ used esp. as the hydrochloride salt to suppress appetite in the treatment of obesity

fen•o•pro•fen \,fe-nə-'prō-fən\ *n* : an anti-inflammatory analgesic $C_{15}H_{14}O_3$ used esp. in the treatment of arthritis

fen•ta•nyl \'fent-ⁿn-,il\ *n* : a narcotic analgesic $C_{22}H_{28}N_2O$ with pharmacological action similar to morphine that is administered esp. as the citrate

fer•ment \'fər-,ment, (,)fər-'\ *n* : ENZYME; *also* : FERMENTATION

fer•men•ta•tion \,fər-mən-'tā-shən, -,men-\ *n* : an enzymatically controlled anaerobic breakdown of an energy-rich compound (as a carbohydrate to carbon dioxide and alcohol); *broadly* : an enzymatically controlled transformation of an organic compound — **fer•ment** \(,)fər-'ment\ *vb* — **fer•men•ta•tive** \(,)fər-'men-tə-tiv\ *adj*

fer•mi•um \'fer-mē-əm, 'fər-\ *n* : a radioactive metallic element artificially produced — symbol *Fm*; see ELEMENT table

fer•ric \'fer-ik\ *adj* **1** : of, relating to, or containing iron **2** : being or containing iron usu. with a valence of three

ferric chloride *n* : a salt $FeCl_3$ that is used in medicine in a water solution or tincture usu. as an astringent or styptic

ferric oxide *n* : the red or black oxide of iron Fe_2O_3

ferric py•ro•phos•phate \-,pī-rō-'fäs-,fāt\ *n* : a green or yellowish green salt, approximately $Fe_4(P_2O_7)_3 \cdot 9H_2O$, used as a source of iron esp. when dietary intake is inadequate

fer•ri•he•mo•glo•bin \fer-,ī-'hē-mə-glō-bən, ,fer-i-\ *n* : METHEMOGLOBIN

fer•ri•tin \'fer-ət-ⁿn\ *n* : a crystalline iron-containing protein that functions in the storage of iron and is found esp. in the liver and spleen

fer•rous \'fer-əs\ *adj* **1** : of, relating to, or containing iron **2** : being or containing iron with a valence of two

ferrous fumarate *n* : a reddish orange to red-brown powder $C_4H_2FeO_4$ used orally in the treatment of iron-deficiency anemia

ferrous gluconate *n* : a yellowish gray or pale greenish yellow powder or granules $C_{12}H_{22}FeO_{14}$ used as a hematinic in the treatment of iron-deficiency anemia

ferrous sulfate *n* : an astringent iron salt obtained usu. in pale green crystalline form $FeSO_4 \cdot 7H_2O$ and used in medicine chiefly for treating iron=deficiency anemia

fer•tile \'fərt-ᵊl, 'fər-,tīl\ *adj* **1** : capable of growing or developing (~ egg) **2** : developing spores or spore-bearing organs **3 a** : capable of breeding or reproducing **b** *of an estrous cycle* : marked by the production of one or more viable eggs

fer·til·i·ty \(ˌ)fər-'ti-lə-tē\ *n, pl* **-ties 1** : the quality or state of being fertile **2** : the birthrate of a population — compare MORTALITY 2b

fer·til·i·za·tion \ˌfərt-ᵊl-ə-'zā-shən\ *n* : an act or process of making fertile; *specif* : the process of union of two gametes whereby the somatic chromosome number is restored and the development of a new individual is initiated — **fer·til·ize** \'fərt-ᵊl-ˌīz\ *vb*

fertilization membrane *n* : a resistant membranous layer in eggs of many animals that forms following fertilization by the thickening and separation of the vitelline membrane from the cell surface and that prevents multiple fertilization

fes·cue foot \'fes-(ˌ)kyü-\ *n* : a disease of the feet of cattle resembling ergotism that is associated with feeding on fescue grass (genus *Festuca* and esp. *F. elatior* var. *arundinacea*)

¹**fes·ter** \'fes-tər\ *n* : a suppurating sore — : PUSTULE

²**fester** *vb* **fes·tered; fes·ter·ing** : to generate pus

fes·ti·nat·ing \'fes-tə-ˌnā-tiŋ\ *adj* : being a walking gait (as in Parkinson's disease) characterized by involuntary acceleration — **fes·ti·na·tion** \ˌfes-tə-'nā-shən\ *n*

fe·tal \'fēt-ᵊl\ *adj* : of, relating to, or being a fetus

fetal alcohol syndrome *n* : a highly variable group of birth defects including mental retardation, deficient growth, and defects of the skull, face, and brain that tend to occur in the infants of women who consume large amounts of alcohol during pregnancy — abbr. FAS

fetal hemoglobin *n* : a hemoglobin variant that predominates in the blood of a newborn and persists in increased proportions in some forms of anemia (as thalassemia) — called also *hemoglobin F*

fe·ta·lis \fi-'ta-ləs\ — see ERYTHROBLASTOSIS FETALIS, HYDROPS FETALIS

fetal position *n* : a position (as of a sleeping person) in which the body lies curled up on one side with the arms and legs drawn up toward the chest and the head bowed forward and which is assumed in some forms of psychic regression

feti- — see FETO-

fe·ti·cide \'fē-tə-ˌsīd\ *n* : the action or process of causing the death of a fetus

fe·tish *also* **fe·tich** \'fe-tish, 'fē-\ *n* : an object or bodily part whose real or fantasized presence is psychologically necessary for sexual gratification and that is an object of fixation to the extent that it may interfere with complete sexual expression

fe·tish·ism *also* **fe·tich·ism** \-ˌti-ˌshi-zəm\ *n* : the pathological displacement of erotic interest and satisfaction to a fetish — **fe·tish·ist** \-shist\ *n* — **fe·tish·is·tic** \ˌfe-ti-ᵊshis-tik *also* ˌfē-\ *adj* — **fe·tish·is·ti·cal·ly** \-ti-k(ə-)lē\ *adv*

fet·lock \'fet-ˌläk\ *n* **1 a** : a projection bearing a tuft of hair on the back of the leg above the hoof of a horse or similar animal **b** : the tuft of hair itself **2** : the joint of the limb at the fetlock

feto- *or* **feti-** *comb form* : fetus (*feticide*) (*fetology*)

fe·tol·o·gist \fē-'tä-lə-jist\ *n* : a specialist in fetology

fe·tol·o·gy \fē-'tä-lə-jē\ *n, pl* **-gies** : a branch of medical science concerned with the study and treatment of the fetus in the uterus

fe·to·pro·tein \ˌfē-tō-'prō-ˌtēn, -tē-ən\ *n* : any of several fetal antigens present in the adult in some abnormal conditions; *esp* : ALPHA-FETOPROTEIN

fe·tor he·pat·i·cus \'fē-tər-hi-'pa-ti-kəs, -ˌtor\ *n* : a characteristically disagreeable odor to the breath that is a sign of liver failure

fe·to·scope \'fē-tə-ˌskōp\ *n* : a fiber-optic tube used to perform fetoscopy

fe·tos·co·py \fē-'täs-kə-pē\ *n, pl* **-pies** : examination of the pregnant uterus by means of a fiber-optic tube

fe·to·tox·ic \ˌfē-tō-'täk-sik\ *adj* : toxic to fetuses — **fe·to·tox·i·ci·ty** \-täk-'si-sə-tē\ *n*

fe·tus \'fē-təs\ *n, pl* **fe·tus·es** : an unborn or unhatched vertebrate esp. after attaining the basic structural plan of its kind; *specif* : a developing human from usu. three months after conception to birth — compare EMBRYO

Feul·gen reaction \'foil-gən\ *n* : the development of a purple color by DNA in a microscopic preparation stained with a modified Schiff's reagent

Feulgen, Robert Joachim (1884–1955), German biochemist.

¹**fe·ver** \'fē-vər\ *n* **1** : a rise of body temperature above the normal **2** : an abnormal bodily state characterized by increased production of heat, accelerated heart action and pulse, and systemic debility with weakness, loss of appetite, and thirst **3** : any of various diseases of which fever is a prominent symptom — see YELLOW FEVER, TYPHOID FEVER — **fe·ver·ish** \-və-rish\ *adj*

²**fever** *vb* **fe·vered; fe·ver·ing** : to affect with or be in a fever

fever blister *n* : COLD SORE

fever therapy *n* : a treatment of disease by fever induced by various artificial means

fever thermometer *n* : CLINICAL THERMOMETER

FFA *abbr* free fatty acids

¹**fi·ber** *or* **fi·bre** \'fī-bər\ *n* **1 a** : a strand of nerve tissue : AXON, DENDRITE **b** : one of the filaments composing most of the intercellular matrix of connec-

tive tissue **c** : one of the elongated contractile cells of muscle tissue **2** : indigestible material in food that stimulates the intestine to peristalsis — called also *bulk, dietary fiber, roughage*

fiber of Mül·ler \-ˈmyü-lər, -ˈmə-\ *n* : any of the neuroglia fibers that extend through the entire thickness of the retina — called also *Müller cell, sustentacular fiber of Müller*

H. Müller — see MÜLLER CELL

fiber optics *n pl* **1** : thin transparent fibers of glass or plastic that transmit light throughout their length by internal reflections; *also* : a bundle of such fibers used in an instrument (as for viewing body cavities) **2** : the technique of the use of fiber optics — used with a sing. verb — **fi·ber-op·tic** *adj*

fi·ber·scope \ˈfī-bər-ˌskōp\ *n* : a flexible instrument utilizing fiber optics for examination of inaccessible areas (as the stomach)

fiber tract *n* : TRACT 2

fibr- *or* **fibro-** *comb form* **1** : fiber : fibrous tissue ⟨*fibro*genesis⟩ **2** : fibrous and ⟨*fibro*elastic⟩

fi·bril \ˈfī-brəl, ˈfib-\ *n* : a small filament or fiber: as **a** : one of the fine threads into which a striated muscle fiber can be longitudinally split **b** : NEUROFIBRIL

fi·bril·la \fī-ˈbril-ə, fi-; ˈfib-ri-lə, ˈfib-\ *n, pl* **fi·bril·lae** \-ˌlē\ : FIBRIL

fi·bril·lar \ˈfib-rə-lər, ˈfib-; fī-ˈbril-, fi-\ *adj* **1** : of or like fibrils or fibers ⟨a ∼ network⟩ **2** : of or exhibiting fibrillation

fi·bril·lary \ˈfib-rə-ˌler-ē, ˈfib-; fī-ˈbril-ə-rē, fi-\ *adj* **1** : of or relating to fibrils or fibers ⟨∼ overgrowth⟩ **2** : of, relating to, or marked by fibrillation ⟨∼ chorea⟩

fi·bril·la·tion \ˌfib-rə-ˈlā-shən, ˌfīb-\ *n* **1** : an act or process of forming fibers or fibrils **2 a** : a muscular twitching involving individual muscle fibers acting without coordination **b** : very rapid irregular contractions of the muscle fibers of the heart resulting in a lack of synchronism between heartbeat and pulse — **fi·bril·late** \ˈfib-rə-ˌlāt, ˈfīb-\ *vb*

fi·bril·lo·gen·e·sis \ˌfib-rə-lō-ˈje-nə-səs, ˌfīb-\ *n, pl* **-e·ses** \-ˌsēz\ : the development of fibrils

fi·brin \ˈfī-brən\ *n* : a white insoluble fibrous protein formed from fibrinogen by the action of thrombin esp. in the clotting of blood

fi·brin·ase \-brə-ˌnās, -ˌnāz\ *n* : FACTOR XIII

fi·brin·o·gen \fī-ˈbri-nə-jən\ *n* : a plasma protein that is produced in the liver and is converted into fibrin during blood clot formation

fi·brin·o·gen·o·pe·nia \(ˌ)fī-ˌbri-nə-ˌje-nə-ˈpē-nē-ə, -nyə\ *n* : a deficiency of

fibrin or fibrinogen or both in the blood

fi·bri·noid \ˈfī-brə-ˌnȯid, ˈfib-\ *n, often attrib* : a homogeneous material that resembles fibrin and is formed in the walls of blood vessels and in connective tissue in some pathological conditions and normally in the placenta

fi·bri·no·ly·sin \ˌfī-brən-ᵊl-ˈīs-ᵊn\ *n* : any of several proteolytic enzymes that promote the dissolution of blood clots; *esp* : PLASMIN

fi·bri·no·ly·sis \-ˈsäs, -brə-ˈnä-lə-səs\ *n, pl* **-ly·ses** \-ˌsēz\ : the usu. enzymatic breakdown of fibrin — **fi·bri·no·lyt·ic** \-brən-ᵊl-ˈi-tik\ *adj*

fi·bri·no·pe·nia \ˌfī-brə-nō-ˈpē-nē-ə, -nyə\ *n* : FIBRINOGENOPENIA

fi·bri·no·pep·tide \-ˈpep-ˌtīd\ *n* : any of the polypeptides that are cleaved from fibrinogen by thrombin during blood clot formation

fi·bri·no·pur·u·lent \-ˈpyur-yə-lənt, -ə-lənt\ *adj* : containing, characterized by, or exuding fibrin and pus (as in certain inflammations)

fi·bri·nous \ˈfī-brə-nəs, ˈfib-\ *adj* : marked by the presence of fibrin

fibro- — see FIBR-

fi·bro·ad·e·no·ma \ˌfī-(ˌ)brō-ˌad-ᵊn-ˈō-mə\ *n, pl* **-mas** *or* **-ma·ta** \-mə-tə\ : adenoma with a large amount of fibrous tissue

fi·bro·blast \ˈfī-brə-ˌblast, ˈfib-\ *n* : a connective-tissue cell of mesenchymal origin that secretes proteins and esp. molecular collagen from which the extracellular fibrillar matrix of connective tissue forms — **fi·bro·blas·tic** \ˌfī-brə-ˈblas-tik, ˌfib-\ *adj*

fi·bro·car·ti·lage \ˌfī-(ˌ)brō-ˈkärt-ᵊl-ij\ *n* : cartilage in which the matrix except immediately about the cells is largely composed of fibers like those of ordinary connective tissue; *also* : a structure or part composed of such cartilage — **fi·bro·car·ti·lag·i·nous** \-ˌkärt-ᵊl-ˈa-jə-nəs\ *adj*

fi·bro·cys·tic \ˌfī-brə-ˈsis-tik, ˌfib-\ *adj* : characterized by the presence or development of fibrous tissue and cysts

fibrocystic disease of the pancreas *n* : CYSTIC FIBROSIS

fi·bro·cyte \ˈfī-brə-ˌsīt, ˈfib-\ *n* : FIBROBLAST; *specif* : a spindle-shaped cell of fibrous tissue

fi·bro·elas·tic \ˌfī-(ˌ)brō-i-ˈlas-tik\ *adj* : consisting of both fibrous and elastic elements ⟨∼ tissue⟩

fi·bro·elas·to·sis \-ˌlas-ˈtō-səs\ *n, pl* **-to·ses** \-ˌsēz\ : a condition of the body or one of its organs characterized by proliferation of fibroelastic tissue — see ENDOCARDIAL FIBROELASTOSIS

fi·bro·gen·e·sis \ˌfī-brə-ˈje-nə-səs, ˌfib-\ *n, pl* **-e·ses** \-ˌsēz\ : the development or proliferation of fibers or fibrous tissue

fi·bro·gen·ic \-ˈje-nik\ *adj* : promoting the development of fibers ⟨a ∼ agent⟩

¹fi·broid \ˈfī-ˌbrȯid, ˈfib-\ *adj* : resembling, forming, or consisting of fibrous tissue

²**fibroid** *n* : a benign tumor that consists of fibrous and muscular tissue and occurs esp. in the uterine wall

fi·bro·ma \fī-'brō-mə\ *n, pl* **-mas** *also* **-ma·ta** \-tə\ : a benign tumor consisting mainly of fibrous tissue — **fi·bro·ma·tous** \-təs\ *adj*

fi·bro·ma·toid \fī-'brō-mə-ˌtòid\ *adj* : resembling a fibroma

fi·bro·ma·to·sis \(ˌ)fī-ˌbrō-mə-'tō-səs\ *n, pl* **-to·ses** \-ˌsēz\ : a condition marked by the presence of or a tendency to develop multiple fibromas

fi·bro·my·al·gia \-ˌmī-'al-jə, -jē-ə\ *n* : any of a group of nonarticular rheumatic disorders characterized by pain, tenderness, and stiffness of muscles and associated connective tissue structures — called also *fibromyositis*

fi·bro·my·o·ma \-ˌmī-'ō-mə\ *n, pl* **-mas** *also* **-ma·ta** \-mə-tə\ : a mixed tumor containing both fibrous and muscle tissue — **fi·bro·my·o·ma·tous** \-mə-təs\ *adj*

fi·bro·my·o·si·tis \-ˌmī-ə-'sī-təs\ *n* : FIBROMYALGIA

fi·bro·myx·o·ma \-mik-'sō-mə\ *n, pl* **-mas** *or* **-ma·ta** \-mə-tə\ : a myxoma containing fibrous tissue

fi·bro·nec·tin \ˌfī-brə-'nek-tən\ *n* : any of a group of glycoproteins of cell surfaces, blood plasma, and connective tissue that promote cellular adhesion and migration

fi·bro·pla·sia \ˌfī-brə-'plā-zhə, -zhē-ə\ *n* : the process of forming fibrous tissue — **fi·bro·plas·tic** \-'plas-tik\ *adj*

fibrosa — see OSTEITIS FIBROSA, OSTEITIS FIBROSA CYSTICA, OSTEITIS FIBROSA CYSTICA GENERALISATA, OSTEODYSTROPHIA FIBROSA

fi·bro·sar·co·ma \-sär-'kō-mə\ *n, pl* **-mas** *or* **-ma·ta** \-mə-tə\ : a sarcoma of relatively low malignancy consisting chiefly of spindle-shaped cells that tend to form collagenous fibrils

fi·brose \'fī-ˌbrōs\ *vb* **-brosed; -brosing** : to form fibrous tissue *⟨a fibrosed wound⟩*

fi·bro·se·rous \ˌfī-brō-'sir-əs\ *adj* : composed of a serous membrane supported by a firm layer of fibrous tissue

fi·bro·sis \fī-'brō-səs\ *n, pl* **-bro·ses** \-ˌsēz\ : a condition marked by increase of interstitial fibrous tissue : fibrous degeneration — **fi·brot·ic** \-'brä-tik\ *adj*

fi·bro·si·tis \ˌfī-brə-'sī-təs\ *n* : a muscular condition that is commonly accompanied by the formation of painful subcutaneous nodules — **fi·bro·sit·ic** \-'si-tik\ *adj*

fibrosus — see ANNULUS FIBROSUS

fi·brous \'fī-brəs\ *adj* **1** : containing, consisting of, or resembling fibers **2** : characterized by fibrosis

fibrous ankylosis *n* : ankylosis due to the growth of fibrous tissue

fib·u·la \'fi-byə-lə\ *n, pl* **-lae** \-lē, -ˌlī\ *or* **-las** : the outer or postaxial and usu. the smaller of the two bones of the hind or lower limb below the knee that is the slenderest bone of the human body in proportion to its length and articulates above with the external tuberosity of the tibia and below with the talus — called also *calf bone* — **fib·u·lar** \-lər\ *adj*

fibular collateral ligament *n* : LATERAL COLLATERAL LIGAMENT

Fick principle \'fik-\ *n* : a generalization in physiology which states that blood flow is proportional to the difference in concentration of a substance (as oxygen) in the blood as it enters and leaves an organ and which is used to determine cardiac output — called also *Fick method*

Fick, Adolf Eugen (1829–1901), German physiologist.

FICS *abbr* Fellow of the International College of Surgeons

field \'fēld\ *n* **1** : a complex of forces that serve as causative agents in human behavior **2** : a region of embryonic tissue potentially capable of a particular type of differentiation **3 a** : an area that is perceived or under observation **b** : the site of a surgical operation

field hospital *n* : a military organization of medical personnel with equipment for establishing a temporary hospital in the field

field of vision *n* : VISUAL FIELD

fièvre bou·ton·neuse \'fyev-rə-ˌbü-tò-'nēz\ *n* : BOUTONNEUSE FEVER

fifth cranial nerve *n* : TRIGEMINAL NERVE

fifth disease *n* : ERYTHEMA INFECTIOSUM

fifth nerve *n* : TRIGEMINAL NERVE

figure–ground \'fi-gyər-'graùnd\ *adj* : relating to or being the relationships between the parts of a perceptual field which is perceived as divided into a part consisting of figures having form and standing out from the part comprising the background and being relatively formless

fil·a·ment \'fi-lə-mənt\ *n* : a single thread or a thin flexible threadlike object, process, or appendage; *esp* : an elongated thin series of cells attached one to another (as of some bacteria) — **fil·a·men·tous** \ˌfi-lə-'men-təs\ *adj*

fi·lar·ia \fə-'lar-ē-ə\ *n, pl* **fi·lar·i·ae** \-ē-ˌē, -ˌī\ : any of numerous slender filamentous nematodes that as adults are parasites in the blood or tissues and as larvae usu. develop in biting insects and that for the most part were once included in one genus (*Filaria*) but are now divided among various genera (as *Wuchereria* and *Onchocerca*) — **fi·lar·i·al** \-ē-əl\ *adj* — **fi·lar·i·id** \-ē-əd\ *adj or n*

fil·a·ri·a·sis \ˌfi-lə-'rī-ə-səs\ *n, pl* **-a-**

ses \-₁sēz\ : infestation with or disease caused by filariae

fi·lar·i·cide \fə-ˈlar-ə-₁sīd\ n : an agent that is destructive to filariae — **fi·lar·i·cid·al** \₁lar-ə-ˈsīd-ᵊl\ adj

fi·lar·i·form \-ə-₁form\ adj, of a larval nematode : resembling a filaria esp. in having a slender elongated form and in possessing a delicate capillary esophagus

fili- or **filo-** comb form : thread (fili-form)

fil·ial generation \ˈfi-lē-əl-, ˈfil-yəl\ n : a generation in a breeding experiment that is successive to a parental generation — symbol F_1 for the first, F_2 for the second, etc.

fi·li·form \ˈfi-lə-₁form, ˈfī-\ n : an extremely slender bougie

filiform papilla n : any of numerous minute pointed papillae on the tongue

fil·i·pin \ˈfi-lə-pin\ n : an antifungal antibiotic $C_{35}H_{58}O_{11}$ produced by a bacterium of the genus *Streptomyces* (*S. filipinensis*)

fill \ˈfil\ vb **1** : to repair the cavities of (teeth) **2** : to supply as directed ⟨~ a prescription⟩

fil·let \ˈfi-lət\ n : a band of anatomical fibers; specif : LEMNISCUS

fill·ing \ˈfi-liŋ\ n **1** : material (as gold or amalgam) used to fill a cavity in a tooth **2** : simple sporadic lymphangitis of the leg of a horse commonly due to overfeeding and insufficient exercise

film \ˈfilm\ n **1 a** : a thin skin or membranous covering **b** : an abnormal growth on or in the eye **2** : an exceedingly thin layer : LAMINA

film badge n : a small pack of sensitive photographic film worn as a badge for indicating exposure to radiation

filo- — see FILI-

fil·ter \ˈfil-tər\ n **1** : a porous article or mass (as of paper) through which a gas or liquid is passed to separate out matter in suspension **2** : an apparatus containing a filter medium — **filter** vb

fil·ter·able \ˈfil-tə-rə-bəl\ also **fil·tra·ble** \-trə-bəl\ adj : capable of being filtered or of passing through a filter — **fil·ter·abil·i·ty** \ˌfil-tə-rə-ˈbi-lə-tē\ n

filterable virus n : any of the infectious agents that pass through a fine filter (as of unglazed porcelain) with the filtrate and remain virulent and that include the viruses as presently understood and various other groups (as the mycoplasmas and rickettsias) which were orig. considered viruses before their cellular nature was established

filter paper n : porous paper used esp. for filtering

fil·trate \ˈfil-₁trāt\ n : fluid that has passed through a filter

fil·tra·tion \fil-ˈtrā-shən\ n **1** : the process of filtering **2** : the process of passing through or as if through a filter; also : DIFFUSION

fi·lum ter·mi·na·le \ˈfī-ləm-₁tər-mə-ˈnā-(₁)lē, ˈfē-ləm-₁ter-mə-ˈnā-₁lā\ n, pl **fi·la ter·mi·na·lia** \ˈfī-lə-tər-mə-ˈnā-lē-ə, ˈfē-lə-₁ter-mə-ˈnā-lē-ə\ : the slender threadlike prolongation of the spinal cord below the origin of the lumbar nerves : the last portion of the pia mater

fim·bria \ˈfim-brē-ə\ n, pl **-bri·ae** \-brē-₁ē, -₁ī\ **1** : a bordering fringe esp. at the entrance of the fallopian tubes **2** : a band of nerve fibers bordering the hippocampus and joining the fornix — **fim·bri·al** \-brē-əl\ adj

fimbriata — see PLICA FIMBRIATA

fim·bri·at·ed \ˈfim-brē-₁ā-tad\ also **fim·bri·ate** \-₁āt\ adj : having the edge or extremity fringed or bordered by slender processes

fi·nas·te·ride \fə-ˈnas-tə-₁rīd\ n : an antineoplastic drug $C_{23}H_{36}N_2O_2$ used esp. to shrink an enlarged prostate gland by inhibiting an enzyme catalyzing conversion of testosterone to dihydrotestosterone — see PROSCAR

fin·ger \ˈfiŋ-gər\ n : any of the five terminating members of the hand : a digit of the forelimb; esp : one other than the thumb — **fin·gered** \ˈfiŋ-gərd\ adj

finger fracture n : valvulotomy of the mitral commissures performed by a finger thrust through the valve

fin·ger·nail \ˈfiŋ-gər-₁nāl\ n : the nail of a finger

fin·ger·print \-₁print\ n **1** : an ink impression of the lines on the fingertip taken for purpose of identification **2** : chromatographic, electrophoretic, or spectrographic evidence of the presence or identity of a substance — compare DNA FINGERPRINTING — **fingerprint** vb — **fin·ger·print·ing** n

fin·ger·stall \-₁stöl\ n : COT

fin·ger·tip \-₁tip\ n : the tip of a finger

fire \ˈfir\ vb **fired; fir·ing** : to transmit or cause to transmit a nerve impulse

fire ant n : any ant of the genus *Solenopsis; esp* : IMPORTED FIRE ANT

fire·damp \-₁damp\ n : a combustible mine gas that consists chiefly of methane; also : the explosive mixture of this gas with air — compare BLACK DAMP

first aid n : emergency care or treatment given to an ill or injured person before regular medical aid can be obtained

first cranial nerve n : OLFACTORY NERVE

first–degree burn n : a mild burn characterized by heat, pain, and reddening of the burned surface but not exhibiting blistering or charring of tissues

first intention n : the healing of an incised wound by the direct union of skin edges without granulations — compare SECOND INTENTION

first polar body n : POLAR BODY a

fish–liv·er oil \ˈfish-₁li-vər-\ n : a fatty oil from the livers of various fishes (as cod, halibut, or sharks) used chiefly as a source of vitamin A — compare COD-LIVER OIL

fish tapeworm *n* : a large tapeworm of the genus *Diphyllobothrium* (*D. latum*) that as an adult infests the human intestine and goes through its intermediate stages in freshwater fishes from which it is transmitted to humans when raw fish is eaten

fis·sion \'fĭ-shən, -zhən\ *n* 1 : a method of reproduction in which a living cell or body divides into two or more parts each of which grows into a whole new individual 2 : the splitting of an atomic nucleus resulting in the release of large amounts of energy — called also *nuclear fission* — **fis·sion·able** \'fĭ-shə-nə-bəl, -zhə-\ *adj*

fis·sure \'fĭ-shər\ *n* 1 : a natural cleft between body parts or in the substance of an organ: as **a** : any of several clefts separating the lobes of the liver **b** : any of various clefts between bones or parts of bones in the skull **c** : any of the deep clefts of the brain; *esp* : one of those located at points of elevation in the walls inside of the ventricles — compare SULCUS **d** : ANTERIOR MEDIAN FISSURE; *also* : POSTERIOR MEDIAN SEPTUM 2 : a break or slit in tissue usu. at the junction of skin and mucous membrane ⟨∼ of the lip⟩ 3 : a linear developmental imperfection in the enamel of a tooth — **fis·sured** \'fĭ-shərd\ *adj*

fissure of Ro·lan·do \-rō-'lan-(₁)dō, -'län-\ *n* : CENTRAL SULCUS
   Rolando, Luigi (1773–1831), Italian anatomist and physiologist.

fissure of Syl·vi·us \-'sil-vē-əs\ *n* : a deep fissure of the lateral aspect of each cerebral hemisphere that divides the temporal from the parietal and frontal lobes — called also *lateral fissure, lateral sulcus, Sylvian fissure*
   Du·bois \dü-'bwä\ *or* **De Le Boë** \də-lä-'bō-ä\, **François** *or* **Franz** (*Latin* **Franciscus Sylvius**) **1614–1672),** Dutch anatomist, physician, and chemist.

fis·tu·la \'fĭs-chə-lə, -tyü-lə\ *n, pl* **-las** *or* **-lae** \-₁lē, -₁lī\ : an abnormal passage leading from an abscess or hollow organ to the body surface or from one hollow organ to another or permitting passage of fluids or secretions — **fis·tu·lat·ed** \-₁lā-təd\ *adj*

fis·tu·lec·to·my \₁fĭs-chə-'lek-tə-mē, -tyü-\ *n, pl* **-mies** : surgical excision of a fistula

fis·tu·li·za·tion \-lə-'zā-shən, -₁lī-\ *n* 1 : the condition of having a fistula 2 : surgical production of an artificial channel

fis·tu·lous \-ləs\ *adj* : of, relating to, or having the form or nature of a fistula

fistulous withers *n sing or pl* : a deep-seated chronic inflammation of the withers of the horse that discharges seropurulent or bloody fluid through

one or more openings and is prob. associated with infection by bacteria of the genus *Brucella* (esp. *B. abortus*)

¹**fit** \'fĭt\ *n* 1 : a sudden violent attack of a disease (as epilepsy) esp. when marked by convulsions or unconsciousness : PAROXYSM 2 : a sudden but transient attack of a physical disturbance

²**fit** *adj* **fit·ter; fit·test** : sound physically and mentally : HEALTHY — **fit·ness** *n*

¹**fix** \'fĭks\ *vb* 1 **a** : to make firm, stable, or stationary **b** (1) : to change into a stable compound or available form ⟨bacteria that ∼ nitrogen⟩ (2) : to kill, harden, and preserve for microscopic study 2 : SPAY, CASTRATE

²**fix** *n* : a shot of a narcotic

fix·at·ed \'fĭk-₁sā-təd\ *adj* : arrested in development or adjustment; *esp* : arrested at a pregenital level of psychosexual development

fix·a·tion \fĭk-'sā-shən\ *n* 1 **a** : the act or an instance of focusing the eyes upon an object **b** (1) : a persistent concentration of libidinal energies upon objects characteristic of psychosexual stages of development preceding the genital stage (2) : an obsessive or unhealthy preoccupation or attachment 2 : the immobilization of the parts of a fractured bone esp. by the use of various metal attachments — **fix·ate** \'fĭk-₁sāt\ *vb*

fixation point *n* : the point in the visual field that is fixated by the two eyes in normal vision and for each eye is the point that directly stimulates the fovea of the retina

fix·a·tive \'fĭk-sə-tĭv\ *n* : a substance used to fix living tissue

fix·a·tor \'fĭk-₁sā-tər\ *n* : a muscle that stabilizes or fixes a part of the body to which a muscle in the process of moving another part is attached

fixed idea *n* : IDÉE FIXE

fixed oil *n* : a nonvolatile oil; *esp* : FATTY OIL — compare ESSENTIAL OIL

fl *abbr* fluid

flac·cid \'fla-səd, 'flak-\ *adj* : not firm or stiff; *also* : lacking normal or youthful firmness ⟨∼ muscles⟩ — **flac·cid·i·ty** \fla-'sĭ-də-tē, flak-\ *n*

flaccid paralysis *n* : paralysis in which muscle tone is lacking in the affected muscles and in which tendon reflexes are decreased or absent

fla·gel·lant \'fla-jə-lənt, flə-'je-lənt\ *n* : a person who responds sexually to being beaten by or to beating another person — **flagellant** *adj* — **fla·gel·lant·ism** \-lən-₁ti-zəm\ *n*

fla·gel·lar \flə-'je-lər, 'fla-jə-\ *adj* : of or relating to a flagellum

¹**fla·gel·late** \'fla-jə-lət, -₁lāt; flə-'je-lət\ *adj* 1 **a** *also* **flag·el·lat·ed** \'fla-jə-₁lā-təd\ : having flagella **b** : shaped like a flagellum 2 : of, relating to, or caused by flagellates

²**flagellate** *n* : a flagellate protozoan or alga

¹**flag·el·la·tion** \ˌfla-jə-ˈlā-shən\ n : the practice of a flagellant

²**flagellation** n : the formation or arrangement of flagella

fla·gel·lum \flə-ˈje-ləm\ n, pl **-la** \-lə\ also **-lums** : a long tapering process that projects singly or in groups from a cell and is the primary organ of motion of many microorganisms

flail \ˈflāl\ adj : exhibiting abnormal mobility and loss of response to normal controls — used of body parts (as joints) damaged by paralysis, accident, or surgery (∼ foot)

flame photometer n : a spectrophotometer in which a spray of metallic salts in solution is vaporized in a very hot flame and subjected to quantitative analysis by measuring the intensities of the spectral lines of the metals present — **flame photometric** adj — **flame photometry** n

flammeus — see NEVUS FLAMMEUS

flank \ˈflaŋk\ n : the fleshy part of the side between the ribs and the hip; broadly : the side of a quadruped

flap \ˈflap\ n : a piece of tissue partly severed from its place of origin for use in surgical grafting

¹**flare** \ˈflar\ vb **flared; flar·ing** : to break out or intensify rapidly : become suddenly worse or more painful — often used with up

²**flare** n 1 : a sudden outburst or worsening of a disease — see FLARE-UP 2 : an area of skin flush resulting from and spreading out from a local center of vascular dilation and hyperemia (urticaria ∼) 3 : the presence of floating particles in the fluid of the anterior chamber of the eye — called also aqueous flare

flare–up \-ˌəp\ n : a sudden increase in the symptoms of a latent or subsiding disease (a ∼ of malaria)

flash \ˈflash\ n : RUSH 2 — see HOT FLASH

flat \ˈflat\ adj **flat·ter; flat·test 1** : being or characterized by a horizontal line or tracing without peaks or depressions **2** : characterized by general impoverishment in the presence of emotion-evoking stimuli — **flat·ness** n

flat bone n : any of various bones (as of the skull, the jaw, the pelvis, or the rib cage) not rounded in cross section

flat·foot \-ˌfut\ n, pl **flat·feet** \-ˌfēt\ **1** : a condition in which the arch of the foot is flattened so that the entire sole rests upon the ground **2** : a foot affected with flatfoot — **flat–foot·ed** \-ˈfu̇-təd\ adj

flat plate n : a radiograph esp. of the abdomen taken with the subject lying flat

flat·u·lence \ˈfla-chə-ləns\ n : the quality or state of being flatulent

flat·u·lent \-lənt\ adj **1** : marked by or affected with gases generated in the intestine or stomach **2** : likely to cause digestive flatulence — **flat·u·lent·ly** adv

fla·tus \ˈflā-təs\ n : gas generated in the stomach or bowels

flat·worm \ˈflat-ˌwərm\ n : PLATYHELMINTH; esp : TURBELLARIAN

fla·vin \ˈflā-vən\ n : any of a class of yellow water-soluble nitrogenous pigments derived from isoalloxazine and occurring in the form of nucleotides as coenzymes of flavoproteins; esp : RIBOFLAVIN

flavin adenine di·nu·cle·o·tide \-ˌdī-ˈnü-klē-ō-ˌtīd, -ˈnyü-\ n : a coenzyme $C_{27}H_{33}N_9O_{15}P_2$ of some flavoproteins — called also FAD

flavin mononucleotide n : FMN

fla·vi·vi·rus \ˈflā-vi-ˌvī-rəs\ n : any of a group of arboviruses that contain a single strand of RNA, are transmitted by ticks and mosquitoes, and include the causative agents of dengue, Japanese B encephalitis, and yellow fever

fla·vo·noid \ˈflā-və-ˌnȯid, ˈfla-\ n : any of a group of compounds that includes many common pigments — **flavonoid** adj

fla·vo·pro·tein \ˌflā-vō-ˈprō-ˌtēn, ˌfla-, -ˈprō-tē-ən\ n : a dehydrogenase that contains a flavin and often a metal and plays a major role in biological oxidations

flavum — see LIGAMENTUM FLAVUM

flax·seed \ˈflaks-ˌsēd\ n : the seed of flax that is used medicinally as a demulcent and emollient

flea \ˈflē\ n : any of an order (Siphonaptera) comprising small wingless bloodsucking insects that have a hard laterally compressed body and legs adapted to leaping and that feed on warm-blooded animals

flea·bite \-ˌbīt\ n : the bite of a flea; also : the red spot caused by such a bite — **flea–bit·ten** \-ˌbit-ᵊn\ adj

flea collar n : a collar for animals that contains insecticide for killing fleas

flea·wort \-ˌwərt, -ˌwȯrt\ n : any of three Old World plantains of the genus Plantago (esp. P. psyllium) that are the source of psyllium seed — called also psyllium

flec·tion var of FLEXION

flesh \ˈflesh\ n : the soft parts of the body; esp : the parts composed chiefly of skeletal muscle as distinguished from visceral structures, bone, and integuments — see GOOSE BUMPS, PROUD FLESH — **fleshed** \ˈflesht\ adj — **fleshy** \ˈfle-shē\ adj

flesh fly n : any of a family (Sarcophagidae) of dipteran flies some of which cause myiasis

flesh wound n : an injury involving penetration of the body musculature without damage to bones or internal organs

Fletch·er·ism \ˈfle-chər-ˌi-zəm\ n : the practice of eating in small amounts and only when hungry and of chewing one's food thoroughly — **fletch·er·ize** \-ˌīz\ *vb*

Fletcher, Horace (1849–1919), American dietitian.

flex \ˈfleks\ *vb* **1** : to bend esp. repeatedly **2 a** : to move muscles so as to cause flexion of (a joint) **b** : to move or tense (a muscle) by contraction

flexibilitas — see CEREA FLEXIBILITAS

flex·i·ble \ˈflek-sə-bəl\ *adj* : capable of being flexed : capable of being turned, bowed, or twisted without breaking — **flex·i·bil·i·ty** \ˌflek-sə-ˈbi-lə-tē\ *n*

flex·ion \ˈflek-shən\ *n* **1** : a bending movement around a joint in a limb (as the knee or elbow) that decreases the angle between the bones of the limb at the joint — compare EXTENSION 2 **2** : a forward raising of the arm or leg by a movement at the shoulder or hip joint

flex·or \ˈflek-sər, -ˌsȯr\ *n* : a muscle serving to bend a body part (as a limb) — called also *flexor muscle*

flexor car·pi ra·di·al·is \-ˈkär-ˌpī-ˌrā-dē-ˈā-ləs, -ˈkär-ˌpē-\ *n* : a superficial muscle of the palmar side of the forearm that flexes the hand and assists in abducting it

flexor carpi ul·nar·is \-ˌəl-ˈnar-əs\ *n* : a superficial muscle of the ulnar side of the forearm that flexes the hand and assists in adducting it

flexor dig·i·ti min·i·mi brev·is \-ˈdi-jə-ˌtī-ˈmi-nə-ˌmī-ˈbre-vəs, -ˈdi-jə-ˌtē-ˈmi-nə-ˌmē-\ *n* **1** : a muscle of the ulnar side of the palm of the hand that flexes the little finger **2** : a muscle of the sole of the foot that flexes the first proximal phalanx of the little toe

flexor dig·i·to·rum brevis \-ˌdi-jə-ˈtȯr-əm-\ *n* : a muscle of the middle part of the sole of the foot that flexes the second phalanx of each of the four small toes

flexor digitorum lon·gus \-ˈlȯŋ-gəs\ *n* : a muscle of the tibial side of the leg that flexes the terminal phalanx of each of the four small toes

flexor digitorum pro·fund·us \-prō-ˈfən-dəs\ *n* : a deep muscle of the ulnar side of the forearm that flexes esp. the terminal phalanges of the four fingers

flexor digitorum su·per·fi·ci·al·is \-ˌsü-pər-ˌfi-shē-ˈā-ləs\ *n* : a superficial muscle of the palmar side of the forearm that flexes esp. the second phalanges of the four fingers

flexor hal·lu·cis brev·is \-ˈha-lü-səs-ˈbre-vəs, -lyü-, -ˈha-lə-kəs-\ *n* : a short muscle of the sole of the foot that flexes the proximal phalanx of the big toe

flexor hallucis longus *n* : a long deep muscle of the fibular side of the leg that flexes esp. the second phalanx of the big toe

flexor muscle *n* : FLEXOR

flexor pol·li·cis brevis \-ˈpä-lə-səs-, -kəs-\ *n* : a short muscle of the palm that flexes and adducts the thumb

flexor pollicis longus *n* : a muscle of the radial side of the forearm that flexes esp. the second phalanx of the thumb

flexor ret·in·ac·u·lum \-ˌret-ən-ˈa-kyə-ləm\ *n* **1** : a fibrous band of fascia on the medial side of the ankle that extends downward from the medial malleolus of the tibia to the calcaneus and that covers over the bony grooves containing the tendons of the flexor muscles, the posterior tibial artery and vein, and the tibial nerve as they pass into the sole of the foot **2** : a fibrous band of fascia on the palm side of the wrist and base of the hand that forms the roof of the carpal tunnel and covers the tendons of the flexor muscles and the median nerve as they pass into the hand — called also *transverse carpal ligament*

flex·ure \ˈflek-shər\ *n* **1** : the quality or state of being flexed : FLEXION **2** : an anatomical turn, bend, or fold; *esp* : one of three sharp bends of the anterior part of the primary axis of the vertebrate embryo that serve to establish the relationship of the parts of the developing brain — see CEPHALIC FLEXURE, HEPATIC FLEXURE, PONTINE FLEXURE; SPLENIC FLEXURE — **flex·ur·al** \-shər-əl\ *adj*

flick·er \ˈfli-kər\ *n* : the wavering or fluttering visual sensation produced by intermittent light when the interval between flashes is not small enough to produce complete fusion of the individual impressions

flicker fusion *n* : FUSION b(2)

flight of ideas *n* : a rapid shifting of ideas that is expressed as a disconnected rambling and occurs esp. in the manic phase of the manic-depressive psychosis

flight surgeon *n* : a medical officer (as in the U.S. Air Force) qualified by additional training for specialization in the psychological and medical problems associated with flying

float·er \ˈflō-tər\ *n* : a bit of optical debris (as a dead cell) in the vitreous humor or lens that may be perceived as a spot before the eye — usu. used in pl. ; compare MUSCAE VOLITANTES

float·ing \ˈflōt-iŋ\ *adj* : located out of the normal position or abnormally movable ⟨a ~ kidney⟩

floating rib *n* : any rib in the last two pairs of ribs that have no attachment to the sternum — compare FALSE RIB

floc·cu·lar \ˈflä-kyə-lər\ *adj* : of or relating to a flocculus

floc·cu·late \ˈflä-kyə-ˌlāt\ *vb* **-lat·ed; -lat·ing** : to aggregate or cause to aggregate into a flocculent mass — **floc·cu·la·tion** \ˌflä-kyə-ˈlā-shən\ *n*

floc·cu·la·tion test \ˌflä-kyə-ˈlā-shən-\ *n* : any of various serological tests (as the Mazzini test for syphilis) in which a positive result depends on the combination of an antigen and antibody to produce a flocculent precipitate

floc·cu·lent \-kyə-lənt\ *adj* : made up of loosely aggregated particles (a ~ precipitate)

floc·cu·lo·nod·u·lar lobe \ˌflä-kyə-(ˌ)lō-ˈnä-jə-lər-\ *n* : the posterior lobe of the cerebellum that consists of the nodulus and paired lateral flocculi and is concerned with equilibrium

floc·cu·lus \-ləs\ *n, pl* **-li** \-ˌlī, -ˌlē\ : a small irregular lobe on the undersurface of each hemisphere of the cerebellum that is linked with the corresponding side of the nodulus by a peduncle

floor \ˈflȯr\ *n* : the lower inside surface of a hollow anatomical structure (the ~ of the pelvis)

flo·ra \ˈflȯr-ə\ *n, pl* **floras** *also* **flo·rae** \ˈflȯr-ˌē, -ˌī\ : plant life; *esp* : the plant life characteristic of a region, period, or special environment (the bacterial ~ of the human intestine) — compare FAUNA a — **flo·ral** \ˈflȯr-əl\ *adj*

flor·id \ˈflȯr-əd, ˈflär-\ *adj* : fully developed : manifesting a complete and typical clinical syndrome (~ schizophrenia) (~ adolescent acne) — **flor·id·ly** *adv*

¹**floss** \ˈfläs, ˈflȯs\ *n* : DENTAL FLOSS

²**floss** *vb* : to use dental floss on (one's teeth)

¹**flow** \ˈflō\ *vb* **1** : to move with a continual change of place among the constituent particles **2** : MENSTRUATE

²**flow** *n* **1** : the quantity that flows in a certain time **2** : MENSTRUATION

flow cy·tom·e·try \-sī-ˈtä-mə-trē\ *n* : a technique for identifying and sorting cells and their components (as DNA) by staining with a fluorescent dye and detecting the fluorescence usu. by laser beam illumination

flowers of zinc *n pl* : zinc oxide esp. as obtained as a light white powder by burning zinc for use in pharmaceutical and cosmetic preparations — called also *pompholyx*

flow·me·ter \ˈflō-ˌmē-tər\ *n* : an instrument for measuring the velocity of flow of a fluid (as blood) in a tube or pipe

fl oz *abbr* fluid ounce

flu \ˈflü\ *n* **1** : INFLUENZA **2** : any of several virus or bacterial diseases marked esp. by respiratory symptoms — see INTESTINAL FLU

fluc·tu·ant \ˈflək-chə-wənt\ *adj* : movable and compressible — used of abnormal body structures (as some abscesses or tumors)

fluc·tu·a·tion \ˌflək-chə-ˈwā-shən\ *n* : the wavelike motion of a fluid collected in a natural or artificial cavity of the body observed by palpation or percussion

flu·cy·to·sine \flü-ˈsī-tə-sēn\ *n* : a white crystalline drug $C_4H_4FN_3O$ used to treat fungal infections esp. by mem-

bers of the genera *Candida* and *Cryptococcus* (esp. *Cryptococcus neoformans*)

flu·dro·cor·ti·sone \ˌflü-drō-ˈkȯr-tə-ˌsōn, -ˌzōn\ *n* : a potent mineralocorticoid drug $C_{21}H_{31}FO_6$ with some glucocorticoid activity that is administered esp. as the acetate

fluid *n* : a substance (as a liquid or gas) tending to flow or conform to the outline of its container; *specif* : one in the body of an animal or plant — see CEREBROSPINAL FLUID, SEMINAL FLUID — **fluid** *adj*

fluid dram *or* **flu·i·dram** \ˈflü-ə-ˈdram\ *n* : either of two units of liquid capacity: **a** : a U.S. unit equal to ⅛ U.S. fluid ounce or 0.226 cubic inch or 3.697 milliliters **b** : a British unit equal to ⅛ British fluid ounce or 0.2167 cubic inch or 3.5516 milliliters

flu·id·ex·tract \ˌflü-əd-ˈek-ˌstrakt\ *n* : an alcohol preparation of a vegetable drug containing the active constituents of one gram of the dry drug in each milliliter

fluid ounce *n* **1** : a U.S. unit of liquid capacity equal to ¹⁄₁₆ pint or 1.805 cubic inches or 29.573 milliliters **2** : a British unit of liquid capacity equal to ¹⁄₂₀ pint or 1.7339 cubic inches or 28.412 milliliters

fluke \ˈflük\ *n* : a flattened digenetic trematode worm; *broadly* : TREMATODE — see LIVER FLUKE

flu·o·cin·o·lone ace·ton·ide \ˌflü-ə-ˈsin-əl-ˌōn-ə-sə-ˈtō-ˌnīd\ *n* : a glucocorticoid steroid $C_{24}H_{30}F_2O_6$ used esp. as an anti-inflammatory agent in the treatment of skin diseases

fluor- *or* **fluoro-** *comb form* **1** : fluorine (fluorosis) **2** *also* **fluori-** : fluorescence (fluoroscope)

flu·o·res·ce·in \ˌflu̇-ə-ˈre-sē-ən, ˌflȯr-\ *n* : a dye $C_{20}H_{12}O_5$ with a bright yellow-green fluorescence in alkaline solution that is used as the sodium salt as an aid in diagnosis (as of brain tumors)

flu·o·res·cence \-ˈes-ᵊns\ *n* : emission of or the property of emitting electromagnetic radiation usu. as visible light resulting from and occurring only during the absorption of radiation from some other source; *also* : the radiation emitted — **flu·o·resce** \-ˈes\ *vb* — **flu·o·res·cent** \-ˈes-ᵊnt\ *adj*

fluorescence microscope *n* : ULTRAVIOLET MICROSCOPE

flu·o·ri·date \ˈflu̇r-ə-ˌdāt, ˈflȯr-\ *vb* **-dat·ed; -dat·ing** : to add a fluoride to (as drinking water) to reduce tooth decay — **flu·o·ri·da·tion** \ˌflu̇r-ə-ˈdā-shən, ˌflȯr-\ *n*

flu·o·ride \ˈflu̇-ər-ˌīd\ *n* **1** : a compound of fluorine usu. with a more electrically positive element or radical **2** : the monovalent anion of fluorine — **fluoride** *adj*

flu·o·rine \ˈflu̇-ər-ˌēn, ˈflȯr-, -ən\ *n* : a nonmetallic halogen element having a chemical valence of one that is normally a pale yellowish flammable irritating toxic gas — symbol *F*; see ELEMENT table

flu·o·rom·e·ter \ˌflü-ə-ˈrä-mə-tər\ *or* **flu·o·rim·e·ter** \-ˈi-mə-tər\ *n* : an instrument for measuring fluorescence and related phenomena (as intensity of radiation) — **flu·o·ro·met·ric** *or* **flu·o·ri·met·ric** \ˌflü-ə-ə-ˈme-trik, ˌflȯr-\ *adj* — **flu·o·rom·e·try** *or* **flu·o·rim·e·try** \-ˈi-mə-trē\ *n*

flu·o·ro·pho·tom·e·ter \ˌflü-ər-ō-fō-ˈtä-mə-tər, ˌflȯr-ō-\ *n* : FLUOROMETER — **flu·o·ro·pho·to·met·ric** \-ˌfō-tə-ˈme-trik\ *adj* — **flu·o·ro·pho·tom·e·try** \-fō-ˈtä-mə-trē\ *n*

flu·o·ro·scope \ˈflu̇r-ə-ˌskōp, ˈflȯr-\ : an instrument used in medical diagnosis for observing the internal structure of the body by means of X rays — **fluoroscope** *vb* — **flu·o·ro·scop·ic** \ˌflu̇r-ə-ˈskä-pik, ˌflȯr-\ *adj* — **flu·o·ro·scop·i·cal·ly** \-i-k(ə-)lē\ *adv* — **flu·o·ros·co·pist** \-ˈäs-kə-pist\ *n* — **flu·o·ros·co·py** \-pē\ *n*

flu·o·ro·sis \ˌflü-ər-ˈō-səs, ˌflȯr-\ *n* : an abnormal condition (as mottled enamel of human teeth) caused by fluorine or its compounds

flu·o·ro·ura·cil \ˌflü-ər-ō-ˈyu̇r-ə-ˌsil, -ˌsəl\ *or* **5–flu·o·ro·ura·cil** \ˈfiv-\ *n* : a fluorine-containing pyrimidine base $C_4H_3FN_2O_2$ used to treat some kinds of cancer

flu·ox·e·tine \ˌflü-ˈäk-sə-ˌtēn\ *n* : an antidepressant drug $C_{17}H_{18}F_3NO$ that enhances serotonin activity

flu·phen·azine \ˌflü-ˈfe-nə-ˌzēn\ *n* : a phenothiazine tranquilizer $C_{22}H_{26}-F_3N_3OS$ used esp. combined as a salt or ester — see PROLIXIN

flur·az·e·pam \ˌflu̇r-ˈa-zə-ˌpam\ *n* : a benzodiazepine closely related structurally to diazepam that is used as a hypnotic in the form of its hydrochloride $C_{21}H_{23}ClFN_3O·2HCl$ — see DALMANE

flur·o·thyl \ˈflu̇r-ə-thil\ *n* : a clear colorless volatile liquid convulsant $C_4H_4-F_6O$ that has been used in place of electroshock therapy in the treatment of mental illness — see INDOKLON

¹**flush** \ˈfləsh\ *n* : a transitory sensation of extreme heat (as in response to some physiological states)

²**flush** *vb* **1** : to blush or become suddenly suffused with color due to vasodilation **2** : to cleanse or wash out with or as if with a rush of liquid

flut·ter \ˈflə-tər\ *n* : an abnormal rapid spasmodic and usu. rhythmic motion or contraction of a body part ⟨a serious ventricular ∼⟩ — **flutter** *vb*

flux \ˈfləks\ *n* **1** : a flowing of fluid from the body; *esp* : an excessive abnormal discharge from the bowels **2** : the matter discharged in a flux

fly \ˈflī\ *n, pl* **flies 1** : any of a large order (Diptera) of usu. winged insects (as the housefly or a mosquito) that have the anterior wings functional and the posterior wings modified to function as sensory flight stabilizers and that have a segmented larva often without a head, eyes, or legs **2** : a large stout-bodied fly (as a horsefly)

fly agar·ic \-ˈa-gə-rik, -ə-ˈgar-ik\ *n* : a poisonous mushroom of the genus *Amanita* (*A. muscaria*) that has a usu. bright red cap and that with the related death cap is responsible for most cases of severe mushroom poisoning — called also *fly amanita, fly mushroom*

¹**fly·blow** \ˈflī-ˌblō\ *vb* **-blew; -blown** : to deposit eggs or young larvae of a flesh fly or blowfly in

²**flyblow** *n* : FLY-STRIKE

fly·blown \-ˌblōn\ *adj* **1** : infested with fly maggots **2** : covered with fly-specks

fly-strike \-ˌstrīk\ *n* : infestation with fly maggots — **fly-struck** \-ˌstrək\ *adj*

Fm *symbol* fermium

FMN \ˌef-(ˌ)em-ˈen\ *n* : a yellow crystalline phosphoric ester $C_{17}H_{21}N_4-O_9P$ of riboflavin that is a coenzyme of several flavoprotein enzymes — called also *flavin mononucleotide, riboflavin phosphate*

foam \ˈfōm\ *n* : a light frothy mass of fine bubbles formed in or on the surface of a liquid ⟨a contraceptive ∼⟩ — **foam** *vb*

foam cell *n* : a swollen vacuolate reticuloendothelial cell filled with lipid inclusions and characteristic of some conditions of disturbed lipid metabolism

focal infection *n* : a persistent bacterial infection of some organ or region; *esp* : one causing symptoms elsewhere in the body

focal length *n* : the distance of a focus from the surface of a lens or concave mirror — symbol *f*

focal point *n* : FOCUS 1

fo·cus \ˈfō-kəs\ *n, pl* **foci** \ˈfō-ˌsī, -ˌkī\ *also* **fo·cus·es 1** : a point at which rays (as of light) converge or from which they diverge or appear to diverge usu. giving rise to an image after reflection by a mirror or refraction by a lens or optical system **2** : a localized area of disease or the chief site of a generalized disease or infection — **focus** *vb*

foe·ti·cide *chiefly Brit var of* FETICIDE

foeto- *or* **foeti-** *chiefly Brit var of* FETO-

foe·tol·o·gy, foe·tus *chiefly Brit var of* FETOLOGY, FETUS

fog \ˈfäg, ˈfȯg\ *vb* **fogged; fog·ging** : to blur (a field of vision) with lenses that prevent a sharp focus in order to relax accommodation before testing vision

foil \ˈfȯil\ *n* : very thin sheet metal (as of gold or platinum) used esp. in filling teeth

fo·la·cin \ˈfō-lə-sən\ *n* : FOLIC ACID

fo·late \ˈfō-ˌlāt\ *n* : FOLIC ACID; *also* : a salt or ester of folic acid

fold \\'fōld\\ *n* : a margin apparently formed by the doubling upon itself of a flat anatomical structure (as a membrane)

Fo·ley catheter \\'fō-lē-\\ *n* : a catheter with an inflatable balloon tip for retention in the bladder

Foley, Frederic Eugene Basil (1891–1966), American urologist.

fo·lic acid \\'fō-lik-\\ *n* : a crystalline vitamin $C_{19}H_{19}N_7O_6$ of the B complex that is used esp. in the treatment of nutritional anemias — called also *folacin, folate, pteroylglutamic acid, vitamin B_c, vitamin M*

folie à deux \\fo-'lē-(¸)ä-'dœ̄, -'dər\\ *n, pl* **folies à deux** *same or* -'lēz-\\ : the presence of the same or similar delusional ideas in two persons closely associated with one another

fo·lin·ic acid \\fō-'li-nik-\\ *n* : CITROVORUM FACTOR

fo·li·um \\'fō-lē-əm\\ *n, pl* **fo·lia** \\-lē-ə\\ : one of the lamellae of the cerebellar cortex

folk medicine *n* : traditional medicine as practiced esp. by people isolated from modern medical services and usu. involving the use of plant=derived remedies on an empirical basis

fol·li·cle \\'fä-li-kəl\\ *n* **1** : a small anatomical cavity or deep narrow=mouthed depression; *esp* : a small simple or slightly branched gland : CRYPT **2** : a small lymph node **3** : a vesicle in the mammalian ovary that contains a developing egg surrounded by a covering of cells : OVARIAN FOLLICLE; *esp* : GRAAFIAN FOLLICLE — **fol·lic·u·lar** \\fə-'li-kyə-lər, fä-\\ *adj*

follicle mite *n* : any of several minute mites of the genus *Demodex* that are parasitic in the hair follicles

follicle–stimulating hormone *n* : a hormone from an anterior lobe of the pituitary gland that stimulates the growth of the ovum-containing follicles in the ovary and that activates sperm-forming cells

follicularis — see KERATOSIS FOLLICULARIS

folliculi — see LIQUOR FOLLICULI, THECA FOLLICULITI

fol·lic·u·lin \\fə-'li-kyə-lən, fä-\\ *n* : ESTROGEN; *esp* : ESTRONE

fol·lic·u·li·tis \\fə-¸li-kyə-'lī-təs\\ *n* : inflammation of one or more follicles esp. of the hair

fol·li·tro·pin \\¸fä-lə-'trō-pən\\ *n* : FOLLICLE-STIMULATING HORMONE

follow–up \\'fä-lō-¸əp\\ *n* : maintenance of contact with or reexamination of a patient at usu. prescribed intervals following diagnosis or treatment; *also* : a patient with whom such contact is maintained — **follow–up** *adj* — **follow up** *vb*

fo·men·ta·tion \\¸fō-mən-'tā-shən, -¸men-\\ *n* **1** : the application of hot moist substances to the body to ease pain **2** : the material applied in fomentation : POULTICE

fomi·tes \\'fä-mə-¸tēz, 'fō-\\ *n pl* : inanimate objects (as clothing, dishes, toys, or books) that may be contaminated with infectious organisms and serve in their transmission

fon·ta·nel *or* **fon·ta·nelle** \\¸fänt-ən-'el\\ *n* : any of the spaces closed by membranous structures between the uncompleted angles of the parietal bones and the neighboring bones of a fetal or young skull

food \\'füd\\ *n, often attrib* **1** : material consisting essentially of protein, carbohydrate, and fat used in the body of an organism to sustain growth, repair, and vital processes and to furnish energy; *also* : such food taken together with supplementary substances (as minerals, vitamins, and condiments) **2** : nutriment in solid form

food poisoning *n* **1** : either of two acute gastrointestinal disorders caused by bacteria or their toxic products: **a** : a rapidly developing intoxication marked by nausea, vomiting, prostration, and often severe diarrhea and caused by the presence in food of toxic products produced by bacteria (as some staphylococci) **b** : a less rapidly developing infection esp. with salmonellas that has generally similar symptoms and that results from multiplication of bacteria ingested with contaminated food **2** : a gastrointestinal disturbance occurring after consumption of food that is contaminated with chemical residues or food (as some fungi) that is inherently unsuitable for human consumption

food·stuff \\'füd-¸stəf\\ *n* : a substance with food value; *esp* : a specific nutrient (as a fat or protein)

foot \\'füt\\ *n, pl* **feet** \\'fēt\\ *also* **foot 1** : the terminal part of the vertebrate leg upon which an individual stands **2** : a unit equal to ⅓ yard and comprising 12 inches or 30.48 centimeters — *pl foot* used between a number and a noun ⟨a 10-*foot* pole⟩; *pl feet* or *foot* used between a number and an adjective ⟨6 *feet* tall⟩

foot–and–mouth disease *n* : an acute contagious febrile disease esp. of cloven-hoofed animals that is caused by a picornavirus related to the rhinoviruses and is marked by ulcerating vesicles in the mouth, about the hoofs, and on the udder and teats — called also *aftosa, aphthous fever, foot-and-mouth, hoof-and-mouth disease;* compare HAND-FOOT-AND=MOUTH DISEASE

foot·bath \\'füt-¸bath\\ *n* : a bath for cleansing, warming, or disinfecting the feet

foot drop *n* : an extended position of the foot caused by paralysis of the flexor muscles of the leg

foot·ed \\'fü-təd\\ *adj* : having a foot or

feet esp. of a specified kind or number — often used in combination ⟨a 4-*footed* animal⟩

foot·plate \'fut-ˌplāt\ n : the flat oval base of the stapes

foot–pound \-'paund\ n, pl **foot–pounds** : a unit of work equal to the work done by a force of one pound acting through a distance of one foot in the direction of the force

foot–pound–second \ˌfut-ˌpaund-'se-kənd\ adj : being or relating to a system of units based upon the foot as the unit of length, the pound as the unit of weight or mass, and the second as the unit of time — abbr. *fps*

foot·print \'fut-ˌprint\ n : an impression of the foot on a surface

foot rot n : a necrobacillosis of tissues of the foot esp. of sheep and cattle that is marked by sloughing, ulceration, suppuration, and sometimes loss of the hoof

fo·ra·men \fə-'rā-mən\ n, pl **fo·ram·i·na** \-'ra-mə-nə\ or **fo·ra·mens** \-'rā-mənz\ : a small opening, perforation, or orifice : FENESTRA 1 — **fo·ram·i·nal** \fə-'ra-mən-ᵊl\ adj

foramen ce·cum \-'sē-kəm\ n : a shallow depression in the posterior dorsal midline of the tongue that is the remnant of the more cranial part of the embryonic duct from which the thyroid gland developed

foramen lac·er·um \-'la-sər-əm\ n : an irregular aperture on the lower surface of the skull bounded by parts of the temporal, sphenoid, and occipital bones that gives passage to the internal carotid artery

foramen mag·num \-'mag-nəm\ n : the opening in the skull through which the spinal cord passes to become the medulla oblongata

foramen of Lusch·ka \-'lush-kə\ n : either of two openings each of which is situated on one side of the fourth ventricle of the brain and communicates with the subarachnoid space

Luschka, Hubert von (1820–1875), German anatomist.

foramen of Ma·gen·die \-mə-ˌzhän-'dē\ n : a passage through the midline of the roof of the fourth ventricle of the brain that gives passage to the cerebrospinal fluid from the ventricles to the subarachnoid space

F. Magendie — see BELL-MAGENDIE LAW

foramen of Mon·ro \-mən-'rō\ n : INTERVENTRICULAR FORAMEN

Monro, Alexander (Secundus) (1733–1817), British anatomist.

foramen of Wins·low \-'winz-ˌlō\ n : EPIPLOIC FORAMEN

Winsløw, Jacob (or Jacques–Bénigne) (1669–1760), Danish anatomist.

foramen ova·le \-ō-'va-(ˌ)lē, -'vā-, -'vä-\ n 1 : an opening in the septum between the two atria of the heart that is normally present only in the fe-

tus 2 : an oval opening in the greater wing of the sphenoid for passage of the mandibular nerve

foramen ro·tun·dum \-rō-'tən-dəm\ n : a circular aperture in the anterior and medial part of the greater wing of the sphenoid that gives passage to the maxillary nerve

foramen spin·o·sum \-spi-'nō-səm\ n : an aperture in the great wing of the sphenoid that gives passage to the middle meningeal artery

foramina pl of FORAMEN

for·ceps \'for-səps, -ˌseps\ n, pl **forceps** : an instrument for grasping, holding firmly, or exerting traction upon objects esp. for delicate operations

For·dyce's disease \'for-ˌdī-səz-\ also **For·dyce disease** \'for-ˌdīs-\ n : a common anomaly of the oral mucosa in which misplaced sebaceous glands form yellowish white nodules on the lips or the lining of the mouth

Fordyce, John Addison (1858–1925), American dermatologist.

fore- comb form 1 : situated at the front : in front ⟨*fore*leg⟩ 2 : front part of (something specified) ⟨*fore*arm⟩

fore·arm \'for-ˌärm\ n : the part of the arm between the elbow and the wrist

fore·brain \-ˌbrān\ n : the anterior of the three primary divisions of the developing vertebrate brain or the corresponding part of the adult brain that includes esp. the cerebral hemispheres, the thalamus, and the hypothalamus and that esp. in higher vertebrates is the main control center for sensory and associative information processing, visceral functions, and voluntary motor functions — called also *prosencephalon*; see DIENCEPHALON, TELENCEPHALON

forebrain bundle — see MEDIAL FOREBRAIN BUNDLE

fore·fin·ger \'for-ˌfin-gər\ n : the finger next to the thumb — called also *index finger*

fore·foot \-ˌfut\ n 1 : one of the anterior feet esp. of a quadruped 2 : the front part of the human foot

fore·gut \-ˌgət\ n : the anterior part of the alimentary canal of a vertebrate embryo that develops into the pharynx, esophagus, stomach, and extreme anterior part of the intestine

fore·head \'for-əd, 'fär-; 'for-ˌhed\ n : the part of the face above the eyes — called also *brow*

for·eign \'for-ən, 'fär-\ adj : occurring in an abnormal situation in the living body and often introduced from outside

fore·leg \'for-ˌleg\ n : a front leg

fore·limb \-ˌlim\ n : a limb (as an arm, wing, fin, or leg) that is situated anteriorly

fo·ren·sic \fə-'ren-sik, -zik\ adj : relating to or dealing with the application of scientific knowledge to legal problems ⟨∼ pathologist⟩ ⟨∼ experts⟩

forensic medicine *n* : a science that deals with the relation and application of medical facts to legal problems — called also *legal medicine*

forensic psychiatry *n* : the application of psychiatry in courts of law (as for the determination of criminal responsibility or liability to commitment for insanity) — **forensic psychiatrist** *n*

fore·play \'fōr-ˌplā\ *n* : erotic stimulation preceding sexual intercourse

fo·re·skin \-ˌskin\ *n* : a fold of skin that covers the glans of the penis — called also *prepuce*

-form \ˌform\ *adj comb form* : in the form or shape of : resembling ⟨chore*iform*⟩ ⟨epilepti*form*⟩

form·al·de·hyde \for-'mal-də-ˌhīd, fər-\ *n* : a colorless pungent irritating gas CH_2O used as a disinfectant and preservative

for·ma·lin \'fōr-mə-lən, -ˌlēn\ *n* : a clear aqueous solution of formaldehyde containing a small amount of methanol

formed element *n* : one of the red blood cells, white blood cells, or blood platelets as contrasted with the fluid portion of the blood

forme fruste \form-'früest, -'früst\ *n*, *pl* **formes frustes** *same or* -'früsts\ : an atypical and usu. abortive manifestation of a disease

for·mic acid \'fōr-mik-\ *n* : a colorless pungent fuming vesicant liquid acid CH_2O_2 found esp. in ants and in many plants

for·mi·ca·tion \ˌfōr-mə-'kā-shən\ *n* : an abnormal sensation resembling that made by insects creeping in or on the skin

for·mu·la \'fōr-myə-lə\ *n*, *pl* **-las** *or* **-lae** \-ˌlē, -ˌlī\ **1 a** : a recipe or prescription giving method and proportions of ingredients for the preparation of some material (as a medicine) **b** : a milk mixture or substitute for feeding an infant typically consisting of prescribed proportions and forms of cow's milk, water, and sugar; *also* : a batch of this made up at one time to meet an infant's future requirements (as during a 24-hour period) **2** : a symbolic expression showing the composition or constitution of a chemical substance and consisting of symbols for the elements present and subscripts to indicate the relative or total number of atoms present in a molecule ⟨the ∼s for water and ethyl alcohol are H_2O and C_2H_5OH respectively⟩

for·mu·lary \'fōr-myə-ˌler-ē\ *n*, *pl* **-ies** : a book containing a list of medicinal subtances and formulas

for·ni·ca·tion \ˌfōr-nə-'kā-shən\ *n* : consensual sexual intercourse between two persons not married to each other — **for·ni·cate** \'fōr-nə-ˌkāt\ *vb* — **for·ni·ca·tor** \-ˌkā-tər\ *n* — **for·ni·ca·trix** \-'kā-triks\ *n*, *pl* **-tri·ces**

\-kə-'trī-ˌsēz\ : a woman who engages in fornication

for·nicis — see CRURA FORNICIS

for·nix \'fōr-niks\ *n*, *pl* **for·ni·ces** \-nə-ˌsēz\ : an anatomical arch or fold: as **a** : the vault of the cranium **b** : the part of the conjunctiva overlying the cornea **c** : a body of nerve fibers lying beneath the corpus callosum and serving to integrate the hippocampus with other parts of the brain **d** : the vaulted upper part of the vagina surrounding the uterine cervix **e** : the fundus of the stomach **f** : the vault of the pharynx

fos·sa \'fä-sə\ *n*, *pl* **fos·sae** \-ˌsē, -ˌsī\ : an anatomical pit, groove, or depression ⟨the temporal ∼ of the skull⟩

fossa na·vic·u·lar·is \-nə-ˌvi-kyə-'lar-əs\ *n* : a depression between the posterior margin of the vaginal opening and the fourchette

fossa oval·is \-ō-'va-ləs, -'vä-, -'vä-\ *n* **1** : a depression in the septum between the right and left atria that marks the position of the foramen ovale in the fetus **2** : SAPHENOUS OPENING

Fos·sar·ia \fä-'sar-ē-ə, fō-\ *n* : a genus of small freshwater snails (family Lymnaeidae) including intermediate hosts of liver flukes — compare GALBA, LYMNAEA

¹foun·der \'faun-dər\ *vb* **foun·dered**; **foun·der·ing 1** : to become disabled; *esp* : to go lame **2** : to disable (an animal) esp. by inducing laminitis through excessive feeding

²founder *n* : LAMINITIS

four·chette *or* **four·chet** \fur-'shet\ *n* : a small fold of membrane connecting the labia minora in the posterior part of the vulva

fourth cranial nerve *n* : TROCHLEAR NERVE

fourth ventricle *n* : a somewhat rhomboidal ventricle of the posterior part of the brain that connects at the front with the third ventricle through the aqueduct of Sylvius and at the back with the central canal of the spinal cord

fo·vea \'fō-vē-ə\ *n*, *pl* **fo·ve·ae** \-vē-ˌē, -ˌī\ **1** : a small fossa **2** : a small area of the retina without rods that affords acute vision — **fo·ve·al** \-əl\ *adj*

fovea cen·tra·lis \-sen-'tra-ləs, -'trä-, -'trä-\ *n* : FOVEA 2

fo·ve·o·la \fō-'vē-ə-lə\ *n*, *pl* **-lae** \-ˌlē, -ˌlī\ *or* **-las** : a small pit; *specif* : one of the pits in the embryonic gastric mucosa from which the gastric glands develop — **fo·ve·o·lar** \-lər\ *adj*

fowl cholera *n* : an acute contagious septicemic disease of birds that is marked by fever, weakness, diarrhea, and petechial hemorrhages in the mucous membranes and is caused by a bacterium of the genus *Pasteurella* (*P. multocida*)

fowl mite *n* : CHICKEN MITE — see NORTHERN FOWL MITE

fowl pest *n* : NEWCASTLE DISEASE

fowl plague *n* : AVIAN INFLUENZA

fowl pox *n* : either of two forms of a virus disease esp. of chickens and turkeys that is characterized by head lesions: **a** : a cutaneous form marked by pustules, warty growths, and scabs esp. on skin that lacks feathers **b** : a more serious form occurring as cheesy lesions of the mucous membranes of the mouth, throat, and eyes

fowl tick *n* : any of several ticks of the genus *Argas* (as *A. persicus*) that attack fowl in the warmer parts of the world causing anemia and transmitting various diseases (as spirochetosis)

fowl typhoid *n* : an infectious disease of poultry characterized by diarrhea, anemia, and prostration and caused by a bacterium of the genus *Salmonella* (*S. gallinarum*)

fox·glove \'fäks-₁gləv\ *n* : any plant of the genus *Digitalis*; *esp* : a common European biennial or perennial (*D. purpurea*) cultivated for its stalks of showy dotted white or purple tubular flowers and as a source of digitalis

fps *abbr* foot-pound-second

Fr *symbol* francium

FR *abbr* flocculation reaction

frac·tion \'frak-shən\ *n* : one of several portions (as of a distillate) separable by fractionation

frac·tion·al \-shə-nəl\ *adj* : of, relating to, or involving a process for fractionating components of a mixture

frac·tion·ate \-shə-₁nāt\ *vb* **-at·ed; -at·ing** : to separate (as a mixture) into different portions (as by distillation or precipitation) — **frac·tion·a·tion** \-₁nā-shən\ *n*

frac·ture \'frak-chər, -shər\ *n* **1** : the act or process of breaking or the state of being broken; *specif* : the breaking of hard tissue (as bone) — see POTT'S FRACTURE **2** : the rupture (as by tearing) of soft tissue (kidney ~) — **fracture** *vb*

fragile X syndrome \-'eks-\ *n* : an inherited disorder that is associated with an abnormal X chromosome, that is characterized esp. by moderate to severe mental retardation, by large ears, chin, and forehead, and by enlarged testes in males, and that often has limited or no effect in heterozygous females

fra·gil·i·tas os·si·um \frə-'ji-lə-təs-'ä-sē-əm\ *n* : OSTEOGENESIS IMPERFECTA

fram·be·sia \fram-'bē-zhə, -zhē-ə\ *n* : YAWS

frame \'frām\ *n* **1** : the physical make-up of an animal and esp. a human body : PHYSIQUE **2 a** : a part of a pair of glasses that holds one of the lenses **b** *pl* : that part of a pair of glasses other than the lenses

frame·shift \-₁shift\ *adj* : relating to, being, or causing a mutation in which a number of nucleotides is not divisible by three is inserted or deleted so that some triplet codons are read incorrectly during genetic translation — **frameshift** *n*

fran·ci·um \'fran-sē-əm\ *n* : a radioactive element discovered as a disintegration product of actinium and obtained artificially by the bombardment of thorium with protons — symbol *Fr*; see ELEMENT table

frank \'fraŋk\ *adj* : clinically evident ⟨~ pus⟩ ⟨~ gout⟩

Frank·fort horizontal plane \'fraŋk-fart-\ *n* : a plane used in craniometry that is determined by the highest point on the upper margin of the opening of each external auditory meatus and the low point on the lower margin of the left orbit and that is used to orient a human skull or head usu. so that the plane is horizontal — called also *Frankfort horizontal, Frankfort plane*

Frank–Star·ling law \'fräŋk-'stär-liŋ-\ *n* : STARLING'S LAW OF THE HEART

Frank, Otto (1865–1944), German physiologist.

Starling, Ernest Henry (1866–1927), British physiologist.

Frank–Starling law of the heart *n* : STARLING'S LAW OF THE HEART

fra·ter·nal \frə-'tərn-əl\ *adj* : derived from two ova : DIZYGOTIC ⟨~ twins⟩

FRCP *abbr* Fellow of the Royal College of Physicians

FRCS *abbr* Fellow of the Royal College of Surgeons

freck·le \'fre-kəl\ *n* : one of the small brownish spots in the skin that are usu. due to precipitation of pigment and that increase in number and intensity on exposure to sunlight — called also *ephelis*; compare LENTIGO — **freckle** *vb* — **freck·led** \-kəld\ *adj*

free \'frē\ *adj* **fre·er; fre·est 1 a** (1) : not united with, attached to, combined with, or mixed with something else (a ~ surface of a bodily part) (2) : having the bare axon exposed in tissue (a ~ nerve ending) **b** : not chemically combined ⟨~ oxygen⟩ **2** : having all living connections severed before removal to another site ⟨a ~ graft⟩

free association *n* **1 a** : the expression (as by speaking or writing) of the content of consciousness without censorship as an aid in gaining access to unconscious processes esp. in psychoanalysis **b** : the reporting of the first thought that comes to mind in response to a given stimulus (as a word) **2** : an idea or image elicited by free association **3** : a method using free association — **free·as·so·ci·ate** \'frē-ə-'sō-shē-₁āt, -sē-\ *vb*

¹free·base \'frē-₁bās\ *vb* **-based; -bas·ing** : to prepare or use (cocaine) as freebase — **free·bas·er** \-₁bā-sər\ *n*

²freebase *n* : cocaine freed from impurities by treatment (as with ether) and heated to produce vapors for inhalation or smoked as crack

free fall *n* : the condition of unrestrained motion in a gravitational field; *also* : such motion

free–float·ing \'frē-'flō-tiŋ\ *adj* : felt as an emotion without apparent cause (∼ anxiety)

free–liv·ing \-'li-viŋ\ *adj* **1** : not fixed to the substrate but capable of motility (a ∼ protozoan) **2** : being metabolically independent : neither parasitic nor symbiotic

free·mar·tin \'frē-₁märt-ᵊn\ *n* : a sexually imperfect usu. sterile female calf born as a twin with a male

free radical *n* an esp. reactive atom or group of atoms that has one or more unpaired electrons

free–swimming *adj* : able to swim about : not attached (a ∼ larva of a trematode)

freeze \'frēz\ *vb* **froze** \'frōz\; **fro·zen** \'frōz-ᵊn\; **freez·ing 1** : to harden or cause to harden into a solid (as ice) by loss of heat **2** : to chill or become chilled with cold **3** : to anesthetize (a part) by cold

freeze–dry \'frēz-'drī\ *vb* **freeze–dried**; **freeze–dry·ing** : to dry and preserve (as food, vaccines, or tissue) in a frozen state under high vacuum — **freeze–dried** *adj*

freeze–etch·ing \-'e-chiŋ\ *n* : preparation of a specimen (as of tissue) for electron microscopic examination by freezing, fracturing along natural structural lines, and preparing a replica (as by simultaneous vapor deposition of carbon and platinum) — **freeze–etch** \-'ech\ *adj* — **freeze–etched** \-₁echt\ *adj*

freeze fracture *also* **freeze–fracturing** *n* : FREEZE-ETCHING — **freeze–fracture** *vb*

freezing point *n* : the temperature at which a liquid solidifies

Frei test \'frī-\ *n* : a serological test for the identification of lymphogranuloma venereum — called also *Frei skin test*

Frei, Wilhelm Siegmund (1885–1943), German dermatologist.

frem·i·tus \'fre-mə-təs\ *n* : a sensation felt by a hand placed on a part of the body (as the chest) that vibrates during speech

fren·ec·to·my \frə-'nek-tə-mē\ *n, pl* **-mies** : excision of a frenulum

fren·u·lum \'fren-yə-ləm\ *n, pl* **-la** \-lə\ : a connecting fold of membrane serving to support or restrain a part (as the tongue)

fre·num \'frē-nəm\ *n, pl* **frenums** *or* **fre·na** \-nə\ : FRENULUM

freq *abbr* frequency

fre·quen·cy \'frē-kwən-sē\ *n, pl* **-cies 1** : the number of individuals in a single class when objects are classified according to variations in a set of one or more specified attributes **2** : the num-

ber of repetitions of a periodic process in a unit of time

Freud·ian \'frȯi-dē-ən\ *adj* : of, relating to, or according with the psychoanalytic theories or practices of Freud — **Freudian** *n* — **Freud·ian·ism** \-ə-₁ni-zəm\ *n*

Freud \'frȯid\, **Sigmund (1856–1939),** Austrian neurologist and psychiatrist.

Freudian slip *n* : a slip of the tongue that is motivated by and reveals some unconscious aspect of the mind

Freund's adjuvant \'frȯindz-\ *n* : any of several oil and water emulsions that contain antigens and are used to stimulate antibody production in experimental animals

Freund \'frȯind\, **Jules Thomas (1890–1960),** American immunologist.

fri·a·ble \'frī-ə-bəl\ *adj* : easily crumbled or pulverized (∼ carcinomatous tissue) — **fri·a·bil·i·ty** \₁frī-ə-'bi-lə-tē\ *n*

friar's balsam *n* : an alcoholic solution containing essentially benzoin, storax, balsam of Tolu, and aloes used chiefly as a local application (as for small fissures) and after addition to hot water as an inhalant (as in laryngitis) — called also *compound benzoin tincture*

Fried·man test \'frēd-mən-\ *also* **Friedman's test** *n* : a modification of the Aschheim-Zondek test for pregnancy using rabbits as test animals

Friedman, Maurice Harold (1903–1991), American physiologist.

Fried·reich's ataxia \'frēd-riks-, 'frēt-rīks-\ *n* : a recessive hereditary degenerative disease affecting the spinal column, cerebellum, and medulla, marked by muscular incoordination and twitching, and usu. becoming manifest in the adult

Friedreich \'frēt-rīk\, **Nikolaus (1825–1882),** German neurologist.

frig·id \'fri-jəd\ *adj* **1** : abnormally averse to sexual intercourse — used esp. of women **2** *of a female* : unable to achieve orgasm during sexual intercourse — **fri·gid·i·ty** \fri-'ji-də-tē\ *n*

fringed tapeworm *n* : a tapeworm of the genus *Thysanosoma* (*T. actinioides*) found in the intestine and bile ducts of ruminants esp. in the western U.S.

frog \'frȯg, 'fräg\ *n* **1** : the triangular elastic horny pad in the middle of the sole of the foot of a horse **2** : a condition in the throat that produces hoarseness (had a ∼ in his throat)

Fröh·lich's syndrome *or* **Froeh·lich's syndrome** \'frā-liks-, 'frœ-liks-\ *n* : *also* **Fröhlich syndrome** *n* : ADIPOSOGENITAL DYSTROPHY

Fröhlich \'frœ-lik\, **Alfred (1871–1953),** Austrian pharmacologist and neurologist.

frondosum — see CHORION FRONDOSUM

fron·tal \'frənt-ᵊl\ *adj* **1** : of, relating to,

or adjacent to the forehead or the frontal bone **2** : of, relating to, or situated at the front or anteriorly **3** : parallel to the main axis of the body and at right angles to the sagittal plane (a ~ plane) — **fron·tal·ly** *adv*

frontal bone *n* : a bone that forms the forehead and roofs over most of the orbits and nasal cavity and that at birth consists of two halves separated by a suture

frontal eminence *n* : the prominence of the human frontal bone above each superciliary ridge

frontal gyrus *n* : any of the convolutions of the outer surface of the frontal lobe of the brain — called also *frontal convolution*

fron·ta·lis \frän-ˈtā-ləs\ *n* : the muscle of the forehead that forms part of the occipitofrontalis — called also *frontalis muscle*

frontal lobe *n* : the anterior division of each cerebral hemisphere having its lower part in the anterior fossa of the skull and bordered behind by the central sulcus

frontal lobotomy *n* : PREFRONTAL LOBOTOMY

frontal nerve *n* : a branch of the ophthalmic nerve supplying the forehead, scalp, and adjoining parts

frontal process *n* **1** : a long plate that is part of the maxillary bone and contributes to the formation of the lateral part of the nose and of the nasal cavity — called also *nasal process* **2** : a process of the zygomatic bone articulating superiorly with the frontal bone, forming part of the orbit anteriorly, and articulating with the sphenoid bone posteriorly

frontal sinus *n* : either of two air spaces lined with mucous membrane each of which lies within the frontal bone above one of the orbits

fronto- *comb form* : frontal bone and ⟨*fronto*parietal⟩

fron·to·oc·cip·i·tal \ˌfrän-tō-äk-ˈsip-ət-ᵊl, ˌfrän-\ *adj* : of or relating to the forehead and occiput

fron·to·pa·ri·e·tal \-pə-ˈrī-ət-ᵊl\ *adj* : of, relating to, or involving both frontal and parietal bones of the skull

frontoparietal suture *n* : CORONAL SUTURE

fron·to·tem·po·ral \-ˈtem-pə-rəl\ *adj* : of or relating to the frontal and the temporal bones

frost·bite \ˈfrost-ˌbīt\ *n* : the freezing or the local effect of a partial freezing of some part of the body — **frostbite** *vb*

frot·tage \fro-ˈtäzh\ *n* : masturbation by rubbing against another person

frot·teur \fro-ˈtər\ *n* : one who engages in frottage

froze *past of* FREEZE

frozen *past part of* FREEZE

frozen shoulder *n* : a shoulder affected by severe pain and stiffening

fruc·to·kin·ase \ˌfrək-tō-ˈkī-ˌnās, -ˈki-

-ˌnāz, ˌfrük-\ *n* : a kinase that catalyzes the transfer of phosphate groups to fructose

fruc·tose \ˈfrak-ˌtōs, ˈfrük-, ˈfrük-, -ˌtōz\ *n* **1** : a sugar $C_6H_{12}O_6$ known in three forms that are optically different with respect to polarized light **2** : the very sweet soluble levorotatory D-form of fructose that occurs esp. in fruit juices and honey — called also *levulose*

fruc·tos·uria \ˌfrək-tə-ˈsur-ē-ə\ *n* : the presence of fructose in the urine

fruit·ar·i·an \frü-ˈter-ē-ən\ *n* : one who lives chiefly on fruit

fruiting body *n* : a plant organ specialized for producing spores; *esp* : SPOROPHORE

fruit sugar *n* : FRUCTOSE 2

fru·se·mide \ˈfrü-sə-ˌmīd\ *n*, *chiefly Brit* : FUROSEMIDE

frus·trat·ed *adj* : filled with a sense of frustration : feeling deep insecurity, discouragement, or dissatisfaction

frus·tra·tion \(ˌ)frəs-ˈtrā-shən\ *n* **1** : a deep chronic sense or state of insecurity and dissatisfaction arising from unresolved problems or unfulfilled needs **2** : something that frustrates — **frus·trate** \ˈfrəs-ˌtrāt\ *vb*

FSH *abbr* follicle-stimulating hormone

ft *abbr* feet; foot

fuch·sin *or* **fuch·sine** \ˈfyük-sən, -ˌsēn\ *n* : a dye that yields a brilliant bluish red and is used in carbolfuchsin paint, in Schiff's reagent, and as a biological stain

fu·cose \ˈfyü-ˌkōs, -ˌkōz\ *n* : an aldose sugar that occurs in bound form in the dextrorotatory D-form in various glycosides and in the levorotatory L-form in some brown algae and in mammalian polysaccharides typical of some blood groups

fu·co·si·dase \ˌfyü-ˈkō-sə-ˌdās, -ˌdāz\ *n* : an enzyme existing in stereoisomeric alpha and beta forms that catalyzes the metabolism of fucose

fu·co·si·do·sis \-ˌkō-sə-ˈdō-səs\ *n*, *pl* **-do·ses** \-ˌsēz\ : a disorder of metabolism inherited as a recessive trait and characterized by progressive neurological degeneration, deficiency of the alpha stereoisomer of fucosidase, and accumulation of fucose-containing carbohydrates

fugax — see AMAUROSIS FUGAX, PROCTALGIA FUGAX

-fuge \ˌfyüj\ *n comb form* : one that drives away ⟨febri*fuge*⟩ ⟨vermi*fuge*⟩

fu·gi·tive \ˈfyü-jə-tiv\ *adj* : tending to be inconstant or transient

fu·gu \ˈfyü-(ˌ)gü, ˈfü-\ *n* : any of various very poisonous puffers that contain tetrodotoxin and that are used as food in Japan after the toxin-containing organs are removed

fugue \ˈfyüg\ *n* : a disturbed state of consciousness in which the one affected seems to perform acts in full awareness but upon recovery cannot recollect them

ful·gu·ra·tion \ˌful-gə-ˈrā-shən, fəl-, -gyə-, -jə-\ n : ELECTRODESICCATION — **ful·gu·rate** \ˈful-gə-ˌrāt, ˈfəl-, -gyə-, -jə-\ vb

full-mouthed \ˈfül-ˈmau̇thd, -ˈmau̇tht\ adj : having a full complement of teeth — used esp. of sheep and cattle

ful·mi·nant \ˈfül-mə-nənt, ˈfəl-\ adj : FULMINATING

ful·mi·nat·ing \-ˌnā-tiŋ\ adj : coming on suddenly with great severity ⟨∼ infection⟩ — **ful·mi·na·tion** \ˌful-mə-ˈnā-shən, ˌfəl-\ n

fu·ma·rate \ˈfyü-mə-ˌrāt\ n : a salt or ester of fumaric acid

fu·mar·ic acid \fyü-ˈmar-ik-\ n : a crystalline acid $C_4H_4O_4$ formed from succinic acid as an intermediate in the Krebs cycle

fu·mi·gant \ˈfyü-mi-gənt\ n : a substance used in fumigating

fu·mi·gate \ˈfyü-mə-ˌgāt\ vb **-gat·ed; -gat·ing** : to apply smoke, vapor, or gas to esp. for the purpose of disinfecting or of destroying pests — **fu·mi·ga·tion** \ˌfyü-mə-ˈgā-shən\ n — **fu·mi·ga·tor** \ˈfyü-mə-ˌgā-tər\ n

func·tion \ˈfəŋk-shən\ n : any of a group of related actions contributing to a larger action; esp : the normal and specific contribution of a bodily part to the economy of a living organism — **function** vb — **func·tion·less** \-ləs\ adj

func·tion·al \ˈfəŋk-shə-nəl\ adj 1 a : of, connected with, or being a function — compare STRUCTURAL 1 b : affecting physiological or psychological functions but not organic structure ⟨∼ heart disease⟩ ⟨a ∼ psychosis⟩ 2 : performing or able to perform a regular function — **func·tion·al·ly** adv

fun·dal \ˈfənd-ᵊl\ adj : FUNDIC

fun·da·ment \ˈfən-də-mənt\ n 1 : BUTTOCKS 2 : ANUS

fun·dic \ˈfən-dik\ adj : of or relating to a fundus

fundic gland n : one of the tubular glands of the fundus of the stomach secreting pepsin and mucus — compare CHIEF CELL 1

fun·do·pli·ca·tion \ˌfən-dō-pli-ˈkā-shən\ n : surgical plication of the fundus of the stomach around the lower end of the esophagus as a treatment for the reflux of stomach contents into the esophagus

fun·dus \ˈfən-dəs\ n, pl **fun·di** \-ˌdī, -ˌdē\ : the bottom of or part opposite the aperture of the internal surface of a hollow organ: as **a** : the greater curvature of the stomach **b** : the lower back part of the bladder **c** : the large upper end of the uterus **d** : the part of the eye opposite the pupil

fun·du·scop·ic also **fun·do·scop·ic** \ˌfən-də-ˈskä-pik\ adj : of, relating to, or by means of ophthalmoscopic examina-

tion of the fundus of the eye — **fun·dus·co·py** \ˌfən-ˈdəs-kə-pē\ also **fun·dos·co·py** \-ˈdäs-\ n

fun·gae·mia Brit var of FUNGEMIA

fun·gal \ˈfəŋ-gəl\ adj 1 : of, relating to, or having the characteristics of fungi 2 : caused by a fungus ⟨∼ infections⟩

fun·gate \ˈfəŋ-ˌgāt\ vb **-gat·ed; -gat·ing** : to assume a fungal form or grow rapidly like a fungus ⟨a fungating lesion⟩ — **fun·ga·tion** \ˌfəŋ-ˈgā-shən\ n

fun·ge·mia \fən-ˈgē-mē-ə\ n : the presence of fungi in the blood

fungi pl of FUNGUS

fungi- comb form : fungus ⟨fungicide⟩

fun·gi·cid·al \ˌfən-jə-ˈsīd-ᵊl, ˌfəŋ-gə-\ adj : destroying fungi; broadly : inhibiting the growth of fungi — **fun·gi·cid·al·ly** adv

fun·gi·cide \ˈfən-jə-ˌsīd, ˈfəŋ-gə-\ n : an agent that destroys fungi or inhibits their growth

fun·gi·form \ˈfən-jə-ˌfȯrm, ˈfəŋ-gə-\ adj : shaped like a mushroom

fungiform papilla n : any of numerous papillae on the upper surface of the tongue that are flat-topped and noticeably red from the richly vascular stroma and usu. contain taste buds

fun·gi·stat \ˈfən-jə-ˌstat, ˈfəŋ-gə-\ n : a fungistatic agent

fun·gi·stat·ic \ˌfən-jə-ˈsta-tik, ˌfəŋ-gə-\ adj : capable of inhibiting the growth and reproduction of fungi without destroying them ⟨a ∼ agent⟩ — **fun·gi·stat·i·cal·ly** \-ti-k(ə-)lē\ adv

Fun·gi·zone \ˈfən-jə-ˌzōn\ trademark — used for a preparation of amphotericin B

fun·goid \ˈfəŋ-ˌgȯid\ adj : resembling, characteristic of, caused by, or being a fungus ⟨a ∼ ulcer⟩ ⟨a ∼ growth⟩

fungoides — see MYCOSIS FUNGOIDES

fun·gous \ˈfəŋ-gəs\ adj : FUNGAL

fun·gus \ˈfəŋ-gəs\ n, pl **fun·gi** \ˈfən-ˌjī, ˈfəŋ-ˌgī\ also **fun·gus·es** \ˈfəŋ-gə-səz\ often attrib 1 : any of a major group (Fungi) of saprophytic and parasitic spore-producing organisms that lack chlorophyll, are usu. classified as plants, and include molds, rusts, mildews, smuts, mushrooms, and yeasts 2 : infection with a fungus

fu·nic·u·li·tis \fyü-ˌni-kyə-ˈlī-təs, fə-\ n : inflammation of the spermatic cord

fu·nic·u·lus \fyü-ˈni-kyə-ləs, fə-\ n, pl **-li** \-ˌlī, -ˌlē\ : any of various bodily structures more or less like a cord in form: as **a** : one of the longitudinal subdivisions of white matter in each lateral half of the spinal cord — see ANTERIOR FUNICULUS, LATERAL FUNICULUS, POSTERIOR FUNICULUS; compare COLUMN a **b** : SPERMATIC CORD

funnel chest n : a depression of the anterior wall of the chest produced by a sinking in of the sternum — called also funnel breast, pectus excavatum

funny bone n : the place at the back of

the elbow where the ulnar nerve rests against a prominence of the humerus — called also *crazy bone*

FUO *abbr* fever of undetermined origin

fur \'fər\ *n* : a coat of epithelial debris on the tongue

fu·ra·zol·i·done \ˌfyùr-ə-'zä-lə-ˌdōn\ *n* : an antimicrobial drug $C_8H_7N_3O_5$ used against bacteria and some protozoa esp. in infections of the gastrointestinal tract

furious rabies *n* : rabies characterized by spasm of the muscles of throat and diaphragm, choking, salivation, extreme excitement, and evidence of fear often manifested by indiscriminate snapping at objects — compare PARALYTIC RABIES

fu·ro·se·mide \fyü-'rō-sə-ˌmīd\ *n* : a powerful diuretic $C_{12}H_{11}ClN_2O_5S$ used esp. to treat edema — called also *frusemide, fursemide*; see LASIX

furred \'fərd\ *adj* : having a coating consisting chiefly of mucus and dead epithelial cells (a ~ tongue)

fur·row \'fər-(ˌ)ō\ *n* 1 : a marked narrow depression or groove 2 : a deep wrinkle

fur·se·mide \'fər-sə-ˌmīd\ *n* : FUROSEMIDE

fu·run·cle \'fyùr-ˌəŋ-kəl\ *n* : BOIL — **fu·run·cu·lar** \fyü-'rəŋ-kyə-lər\ *adj* — **fu·run·cu·lous** \-ləs\ *adj*

fu·run·cu·lo·sis \ˌfyü-ˌrəŋ-kyə-'lō-səs\ *n, pl* **-lo·ses** \-ˌsēz\ 1 : the condition of having or tending to develop multiple furuncles 2 : a highly infectious disease of various salmon and trout

(genera *Salmo* and *Oncorhynchus*) and their relatives that is caused by a bacterium (*Aeromonas salmonicida* of the family Vibrionaceae)

fuse \'fyüz\ *vb* **fused; fus·ing** : to undergo or cause to undergo fusion

fusi- *comb form* : spindle ⟨*fusi*form⟩

fu·si·form \'fyü-zə-ˌfòrm\ *adj* : tapering toward each end ⟨a ~ aneurysm⟩

fu·sion \'fyü-zhən\ *n, often attrib* : a union by or as if by melting together: as **a** : a merging of diverse elements into a unified whole; *specif* : the blending of retinal images in binocular vision **b** (1) : a blend of sensations, perceptions, ideas, or attitudes such that the component elements can seldom be identified by introspective analysis (2) : the perception of light from a source that is intermittent above a critical frequency as if the source were continuous — called also *flicker fusion*; compare FLICKER **c** : the surgical immobilization of a joint — see SPINAL FUSION

fu·so·bac·te·ri·um \ˌfyü-zō-bak-'tir-ē-əm\ *n* 1 *cap* : a genus of gram-negative anaerobic strictly parasitic rod-shaped bacteria (family Bacteroidaceae) that include some pathogens occurring esp. in purulent or gangrenous infections 2 *pl* **-ria** \-ē-ə\ : any bacterium of the genus *Fusobacterium*

fu·so·spi·ro·chet·al \-ˌspī-rə-'kēt-ᵊl\ *adj* : of, relating to, or caused by fusobacteria and spirochetes

G

¹g \'jē\ *n, pl* **g's** *or* **gs** \'jēz\ : a unit of force equal to the force exerted by gravity on a body at rest and used to indicate the force to which a body is subjected when accelerated

²g *abbr* 1 gram 2 gravity; acceleration of gravity

G *abbr* guanine

Ga *symbol* gallium

GABA *abbr* gamma-aminobutyric acid

G–ac·tin \'jē-ˌak-tən\ *n* : a globular monomeric form of actin produced in solutions of low ionic concentration — compare F-ACTIN

gad·fly \'gad-ˌflī\ *n, pl* **-flies** : any of various flies (as a horsefly or botfly) that bite or annoy livestock

gad·o·lin·i·um \ˌgad-ᵊl-'i-nē-əm\ *n* : a magnetic metallic element — symbol *Gd*; see ELEMENT table

gag reflex *n* : reflex contraction of the muscles of the throat caused esp. by stimulation (as by touch) of the pharynx

gal *abbr* gallon

galact- *or* **galacto-** *comb form* 1 : milk ⟨*galacto*rrhea⟩ 2 : galactose ⟨*galacto*kinase⟩

ga·lac·to·cele \gə-'lak-tə-ˌsēl\ *n* : a cystic tumor containing milk or a milky fluid; *esp* : such a tumor of a mammary gland

ga·lac·to·ki·nase \gə-ˌlak-tō-'kī-ˌnās, -'ki-, -ˌnāz\ *n* : a kinase that catalyzes the transfer of phosphate groups to galactose

ga·lac·tor·rhea \gə-ˌlak-tə-'rē-ə\ *n* : a spontaneous flow of milk from the nipple

ga·lac·tor·rhoea *chiefly Brit var of* GALACTORRHEA

ga·lac·tos·ae·mia *chiefly Brit var of* GALACTOSEMIA

ga·lac·tos·amine \gə-ˌlak-'tō-sə-ˌmēn, -zə-\ *n* : an amino derivative $C_6H_{13}O_5N$ of galactose that occurs in cartilage

ga·lac·tose \gə-'lak-ˌtōs, -ˌtōz\ *n* : a sugar $C_6H_{12}O_6$ that is less soluble and less sweet than glucose and is known in dextrorotatory, levorotatory, and racemic forms

ga·lac·tos·emia \gə-ˌlak-tə-'sē-mē-ə\ *n* : an inherited metabolic disorder in which galactose accumulates in the blood due to deficiency of an enzyme catalyzing its conversion to glucose — **ga·lac·tos·emic** \-mik\ *adj*

ga·lac·to·si·dase \gə-ˈlak-ˈtō-sə-ˌdās, -zə-ˌdāz\ *n* : an enzyme (as lactase) that hydrolyzes a galactoside

ga·lac·to·side \gə-ˈlak-tə-ˌsīd\ *n* : a glycoside that yields galactose on hydrolysis

ga·lac·tos·uria \gə-ˌlak-(ˌ)tō-ˈsùr-ē-ə, -ˈsyùr-\ *n* : an excretion of urine containing galactose

Gal·ba \ˈgal-bə, ˈgól-\ *n* : a genus of freshwater snails (family Lymnaeidae) that include hosts of a liver fluke of the genus *Fasciola* (*F. hepatica*) and that are sometimes considered indistinguishable from the genus *Lymnaea* — compare FOSSARIA

ga·lea \ˈgā-lē-ə, ˈga-\ *n* : GALEA APONEUROTICA

galea apo·neu·rot·i·ca \-ˌa-pō-nù-ˈrä-ti-kə, -nyù-\ *n* : the aponeurosis underlying the scalp and linking the frontalis and occipitalis muscles — called also *epicranial aponeurosis*

ga·len·i·cal \gə-ˈle-ni-kəl\ *n* : a standard medicinal preparation (as an extract or tincture) containing usu. one or more active constituents of a plant — **ga·len·ic** \-nik\ *also* **galenical** *adj*

Ga·len \ˈgā-lən\, (*ca* 129–*ca* 199), Greek physician.

Ga·len·ist \ˈgā-lə-nist\ *n* : a follower or disciple of the ancient physician Galen — **Ga·len·ism** \-ˌni-zəm\ *n*

Galen's vein *n* 1 : either of a pair of cerebral veins in the roof of the third ventricle that drain the interior of the brain 2 : GREAT CEREBRAL VEIN

¹**gall** \ˈgól\ *n* : BILE; *esp* : bile obtained from an animal and used in the arts or medicine

²**gall** *n* : a skin sore caused by chronic irritation

³**gall** *vb* : to fret and wear away by friction : CHAFE

gal·la·mine tri·eth·io·dide \ˈga-lə-ˌmēn-ˌtrī-ə-ˈthī-ə-ˌdīd\ *n* : an iodide salt $C_{30}H_{60}I_3N_3O_3$ that is used to produce muscle relaxation esp. during anesthesia — called also *gallamine*

gal·late \ˈga-ˌlāt, ˈgó-\ *n* : a salt or ester of gallic acid — see PROPYL GALLATE

gall·blad·der \ˈgól-ˌbla-dər\ *n* : a membranous muscular sac in which bile from the liver is stored

galli — see CRISTA GALLI

gal·lic acid \ˈga-lik-, ˈgó-\ *n* : a white crystalline acid $C_7H_6O_5$ found widely in plants or combined in tannins

gal·li·um \ˈga-lē-əm\ *n* : a rare bluish white metallic element — symbol *Ga*; see ELEMENT table

gal·lon \ˈga-lən\ *n* 1 : a U.S. unit of liquid capacity equal to four quarts or 231 cubic inches or 3.785 liters 2 : a British unit of liquid and dry capacity equal to four quarts or 277.42 cubic inches or 4.544 liters — called also *imperial gallon*

gal·lop \ˈga-ləp\ *n* : GALLOP RHYTHM

galloping *adj*, *of a disease* : progressing rapidly toward a fatal conclusion

gallop rhythm *n* : an abnormal heart rhythm marked by the occurrence of three distinct sounds in each heartbeat like the sound of a galloping horse — called also *gallop*

gall sickness *n* : ANAPLASMOSIS

gall·stone \ˈgól-ˌstōn\ *n* : a calculus formed in the gallbladder or biliary passages — called also *cholelith*

gal·van·ic \gal-ˈva-nik\ *adj* : of, relating to, involving, or producing galvanism (~ stimulation of flaccid muscles) — **gal·van·i·cal·ly** \-ni-k(ə-)lē\ *adv*

Gal·va·ni \gäl-ˈvä-nē\, **Luigi** (1737–1798), Italian physician and physicist.

galvanic skin response *n* : a change in the electrical resistance of the skin in response to a change in emotional state — abbr. *GSR*

gal·va·nism \ˈgal-və-ˌni-zəm\ *n* : the therapeutic use of direct electric current

gal·va·nom·e·ter \ˌgal-və-ˈnä-mə-tər\ *n* : an instrument for detecting or measuring a small electric current

gamet- *or* **gameto-** *comb form* : gamete (*gametic*) (*gametogenesis*)

gam·ete \ˈga-ˌmēt, gə-ˈmēt\ *n* : a mature male or female germ cell usu. possessing a haploid chromosome set and capable of initiating formation of a new diploid individual by fusion with a gamete of the opposite sex — called also *sex cell* — **ga·met·ic** \gə-ˈme-tik\ *adj* — **ga·met·i·cal·ly** \-ti-k(ə-)lē\ *adv*

ga·me·to·cide \gə-ˈmē-tə-ˌsīd\ *n* : an agent that destroys the gametocytes of a malaria parasite

ga·me·to·cyte \-ˌsīt\ *n* : a cell (as of a protozoan causing malaria) that divides to produce gametes

gam·e·to·gen·e·sis \ˌga-mə-tə-ˈje-nə-səs, gə-ˌmē-tə-\ *n*, *pl* **-e·ses** \-ˌsēz\ : the production of gametes — **gam·e·tog·e·nous** \ˌga-mə-ˈtä-jə-nəs\ *adj*

-gam·ic \ˈgam-ik\ *adj comb form* : -GAMOUS (*monogamic*)

¹**gam·ma** \ˈga-mə\ *n* 1 : the 3d letter of the Greek alphabet — symbol Γ or γ 2 : GAMMA RAY

²**gamma** *or* **γ-** *adj* 1 : of or relating to one of three or more closely related chemical substances (the *gamma* chain of hemoglobin) — used somewhat arbitrarily to specify ordinal relationship or a particular physical form 2 *of streptococci* : producing no hemolysis on blood agar plates

gam·ma–ami·no·bu·tyr·ic acid *also* **γ-ami·no·bu·tyr·ic acid** \ˌga-mə-ə-ˌmē-(ˌ)nō-byü-ˈtir-ik-, ˌga-mə-ˌa-mə-(ˌ)nō-\ *n* : an amino acid $C_4H_9NO_2$ that is a neurotransmitter in the central nervous system — abbr. *GABA*

gamma benzene hexa·chlo·ride \-ˌhek-sə-ˈklór-ˌīd\ *n* : the gamma isomer of benzene hexachloride that comprises the insecticide lindane and is used in medicine esp. as a scabicide and pediculicide in a one-percent cream, lotion, or shampoo — called also *gamma BHC*

gamma camera *n* : a camera that detects the gamma-ray photons produced by radionuclide decay and is used esp. in medical diagnostic scanning to create a visible record of a radioactive substance injected into the body

gamma globulin *n* **1 a** : a protein fraction of blood rich in antibodies **b** : a sterile solution of gamma globulin from pooled human blood administered esp. for passive immunity against measles, German measles, hepatitis A, or poliomyelitis **2** : any of numerous globulins of blood plasma or serum that have less electrophoretic mobility at alkaline pH than serum albumins, alpha globulins, or beta globulins and that include most antibodies

gamma ray *n* **1** : a photon emitted spontaneously by a radioactive substance; *also* : a high-energy photon — usu. used in pl. **2** : a continuous stream of gamma rays — called also *gamma radiation*

gam·mop·a·thy \ga-ˈmä-pə-thē\ *n, pl* **-thies** : a disorder characterized by a disturbance in the body's synthesis of antibodies

-g·a·mous \gə-məs\ *adj comb form* **1** : characterized by having or practicing (such) a marriage or (such or so many) marriages ⟨monoga*mous*⟩ **2** : having (such) gametes or reproductive organs or (such) a mode of fertilization ⟨hetero*gamous*⟩

-g·a·my \gə-mē\ *n comb form* **1** : marriage ⟨monoga*my*⟩ **2** : possession of (such) gametes or reproductive organs or (such) a mode of fertilization ⟨hetero*gamy*⟩

gan·ci·clo·vir \gan-ˈsī-klə-(ˌ)vir\ *n* : an antiviral drug $C_9H_{13}N_5O_4$ related to acyclovir and used esp. in the treatment of cytomegalovirus retinitis in immunocompromised patients — called also *DHPG*

gangli- *or* **ganglio-** *comb form* : ganglion ⟨gangli*oma*⟩ ⟨ganglio*neuroma*⟩

gan·gli·al \ˈgaŋ-glē-əl\ *adj* : of, relating to, or resembling a ganglion

gan·gli·at·ed cord \ˈgaŋ-glē-ˌā-təd-\ *n* : either of the two main trunks of the sympathetic nervous system of which one lies on each side of the spinal column

gan·gli·o·ma \ˌgaŋ-glē-ˈō-mə\ *n, pl* **-mas** *or* **-ma·ta** \-mə-tə\ : a tumor of a ganglion

gan·gli·on \ˈgaŋ-glē-ən\ *n, pl* **-glia** \-glē-ə\ *also* **-gli·ons 1** : a small cystic tumor (as on the back of the wrist) containing viscid fluid and connected either with a joint membrane or tendon sheath **2** : a mass of nerve tissue containing nerve cells: **a** : an aggregation of such cells forming an enlargement upon a nerve or upon two or more nerves at their point of junction or separation **b** : a mass of gray matter within the brain or spinal cord : NUCLEUS 2 — see BASAL GANGLION

gan·gli·on·at·ed \-ə-ˌnā-təd\ *adj* : furnished with ganglia

ganglion cell *n* : a nerve cell having its body outside the central nervous system

gan·gli·on·ec·to·my \ˌgaŋ-glē-ə-ˈnek-tə-mē\ *n, pl* **-mies** : surgical removal of a nerve ganglion

gan·glio·neu·ro·ma \-(ˌ)ō-nu̇-ˈrō-mə, -nyu̇-\ *n, pl* **-mas** *or* **-ro·ma·ta** \-mə-tə\ : a neuroma derived from ganglion cells

gan·gli·on·ic \ˌgaŋ-glē-ˈä-nik\ *adj* : of, relating to, or affecting ganglia or ganglion cells

ganglionic blocking agent *n* : a drug used to produce blockade at a ganglion

gan·gli·on·it·is \ˌgaŋ-glē-ə-ˈnī-təs\ *n* : inflammation of a ganglion

gan·gli·o·side \ˈgaŋ-glē-ə-ˌsīd\ *n* : any of a group of glycolipids that are found esp. in the plasma membrane of cells of the gray matter and have sialic acid, hexoses, and hexosamines in the carbohydrate part and ceramide as the lipid

gan·gli·o·si·do·sis \ˌgaŋ-glē-ˌō-sī-ˈdō-səs\ *n, pl* **-do·ses** \-ˌsēz\ : any of several inherited metabolic diseases (as Tay-Sachs disease) characterized by an enzyme deficiency which causes accumulation of gangliosides in the tissues

gan·go·sa \gaŋ-ˈgō-sə\ *n* : a destructive ulcerative condition believed to be a manifestation of yaws that usu. originates about the soft palate and spreads into the hard palate, nasal structures, and outward to the face — compare GOUNDOU

gan·grene \ˈgaŋ-ˌgrēn, gaŋ-ˈ\ *n* : local death of soft tissues due to loss of blood supply — **gangrene** *vb* — **gan·gre·nous** \ˈgaŋ-grə-nəs\ *adj*

gangrenous stomatitis *n* : CANCRUM ORIS

gan·ja \ˈgän-jə, ˈgan-\ *n* : a potent preparation of marijuana used esp. for smoking; *broadly* : MARIJUANA

Gan·ser syndrome \ˈgän-zər-\ *or* **Gan·ser's syndrome** *n* : a pattern of psychopathological behavior characterized by the giving of approximate answers (as $2 \times 2 = $ about 5)

Ganser, Sigbert Joseph Maria (1853–1931), German psychiatrist.

gapes \ˈgāps\ *n* : a disease of birds and esp. young birds in which gapeworms invade and irritate the trachea

gape·worm \ˈgāp-ˌwərm\ *n* : a nematode worm of the genus *Syngamus* (*S. trachea*) that causes gapes of birds

gap junction *n* : an area of contact between adjacent cells characterized by modification of the cell membranes for intercellular communication or transfer of low molecular-weight substances — **gap-junc·tion·al** \'gap-¦jəŋk-shə-nəl\ *adj*

Gard·ner·el·la \gärd-nə-'re-lə\ *n* : a genus of bacteria of uncertain taxonomic affinities that includes one (*G. vaginalis* syn. *Haemophilus vaginalis*) often present in the flora of the healthy vagina and present in greatly increased numbers in nonspecific vaginitis

Gard·ner, \'gärd-nər\ **Herman L. (fl 1955–80),** American physician.

gar·get \'gär-gət\ *n* : mastitis of domestic animals; *esp* : chronic bovine mastitis

¹**gar·gle** \'gär-gəl\ *vb* **gar·gled; gar·gling** : to hold (a liquid) in the mouth or throat and agitate with air from the lungs; *also* : to cleanse or disinfect (the oral cavity) in this manner

²**gargle** *n* : a liquid used in gargling

gar·goyl·ism \'gar-¦gȯi-¦li-zəm\ *n* : MUCOPOLYSACCHARIDOSIS; *esp* : HURLER'S SYNDROME

Gärt·ner's bacillus \'gert-nərz-\ *n* : a motile bacterium of the genus *Salmonella* (*S. enteritidis*) that causes enteritis

Gärtner, August Anton Hieronymus (1848–1934), German hygienist and bacteriologist.

Gart·ner's duct \'gart-nərz-, 'gert-\ *n* : the remains in the female mammal of a part of the Wolffian duct of the embryo — called also *duct of Gartner*

Gart·ner \'gert-nər\ **Hermann Treschow (1785–1827),** Danish surgeon and anatomist.

gas \'gas\ *n, pl* **gas·es** *also* **gas·ses** 1 : a fluid (as air) that has neither independent shape nor volume but tends to expand indefinitely 2 : a gaseous product of digestion; *also* : discomfort from this 3 : a gas or gaseous mixture used to produce anesthesia 4 : a substance that can be used to produce a poisonous, asphyxiating, or irritant atmosphere

gas chromatograph *n* : an instrument used to separate a sample into components in gas chromatography

gas chromatography *n* : chromatography in which the sample mixture is vaporized and injected into a stream of carrier gas (as helium) moving through a column containing a stationary phase composed of a liquid or a particulate solid and is separated into its component compounds according to the affinity of the compounds for the stationary phase — **gas chromatographic** *adj*

gas·e·ous \'ga-sē-əs, 'ga-shəs\ *adj* : having the form of or being gas; *also* : of or relating to gases

gas gangrene *n* : progressive gangrene marked by impregnation of the dead

and dying tissue with gas and caused by one or more toxin-producing bacteria of the genus *Clostridium*

gash \'gash\ *n* : a deep long cut esp. in flesh — **gash** *vb*

gas–liquid chromatography *n* : gas chromatography in which the stationary phase is a liquid — **gas–liquid chromatographic** *adj*

gas·se·ri·an ganglion \ga-'sir-ē-ən-\ *n, often cap 1st G* : TRIGEMINAL GANGLION

Gas·ser \'gä-sər\ **Johann Laurentius (1723–1765),** Austrian anatomist.

Gas·ter·oph·i·lus \ˌgas-tə-'rä-fə-ləs\ *n* : a genus of botflies including several (esp. *G. intestinalis* in the U.S.) that infest horses and rarely humans

gastr- *or* **gastro-** *also* **gastri-** *comb form* 1 : stomach ⟨*gastr*itis⟩ 2 : gastric and ⟨*gastro*intestinal⟩

gas·tral \'gas-trəl\ *adj* : of or relating to the stomach or digestive tract

gas·tral·gia \ga-'stral-jə\ *n* : pain in the stomach or epigastrium esp. of a neuralgic type — **gas·tral·gic** \-jik\ *adj*

gas·trec·to·my \ga-'strek-tə-mē\ *n, pl* **-mies** : surgical removal of all or part of the stomach

gas·tric \'gas-trik\ *adj* : of or relating to the stomach

gastrica — see ACHYLIA GASTRICA

gastric artery *n* 1 : a branch of the celiac artery that passes to the cardiac end of the stomach and along the lesser curvature — called also *left gastric artery;* see RIGHT GASTRIC ARTERY 2 : any of several branches of the splenic artery distributed to the greater curvature of the stomach

gastric gland *n* : any of various glands in the walls of the stomach that secrete gastric juice

gastric juice *n* : a thin watery acid digestive fluid secreted by the glands in the mucous membrane of the stomach and containing 0.2 to 0.4 percent free hydrochloric acid and several enzymes (as pepsin)

gastric pit *n* : any of the numerous depressions in the mucous membrane lining the stomach into which the gastric glands discharge their secretions

gastric ulcer *n* : a peptic ulcer situated in the stomach

gas·trin \'gas-trən\ *n* : any of various polypeptide hormones that are secreted by the gastric mucosa and induce secretion of gastric juice

gas·tri·no·ma \ˌgas-trə-'nō-mə\ *n, pl* **-mas** *or* **-ma·ta** \-mə-tə\ : a neoplasm that often involves blood vessels, usu. occurs in the pancreas or the wall of the duodenum, and produces excessive amounts of gastrin — see ZOLLINGER-ELLISON SYNDROME

gas·tri·tis \ga-'strī-təs\ *n* : inflammation esp. of the mucous membrane of the stomach

gastro- — see GASTR-

gas·troc·ne·mi·us \ˌgas-(ˌ)träk-'nē-mē-əs, -trək-\ n, pl -mii \-mē-ı1\ : the largest and most superficial muscle of the calf of the leg that arises by two heads from the condyles of the femur and has its tendon of insertion incorporated as part of the Achilles tendon — called also *gastrocnemius muscle*

gas·tro·col·ic \ıgas-trō-'kä-lik, -'kō-\ *adj* : of, relating to, or uniting the stomach and colon ⟨a ~ fistula⟩

gastrocolic reflex *n* : the occurrence of peristalsis following the entrance of food into the empty stomach

Gas·tro·dis·coi·des \ıgas-trō-dis-'kȯi-(ı)dēz\ *n* : a genus of amphistome trematode worms including a common intestinal parasite (*G. hominis*) of humans and swine in southeastern Asia

gas·tro·du·o·de·nal \ıgas-trō-ıdü-ə-'dēn-ə1, -dyü-; -dü-'äd-ᵊn-ə1, -dyü-\ *adj* : of, relating to, or involving both the stomach and the duodenum

gastroduodenal artery *n* : an artery that arises from the hepatic artery and divides to form the right gastroepiploic artery and a branch supplying the duodenum and pancreas

gas·tro·du·o·de·nos·to·my \-ıdü-ə-(ı)dē-'näs-tə-mē, -ıdyü-; -dü-ıäd-ᵊn-'äs-tə-mē, -dyü-\ *n, pl* **-mies** : surgical formation of a passage between the stomach and the duodenum

gas·tro·en·ter·i·tis \-ıen-tə-'rī-təs\ *n, pl* **-en·ter·it·i·des** \-'ri-tə-ıdēz\ : inflammation of the lining membrane of the stomach and the intestines

gas·tro·en·ter·ol·o·gist \-ıen-tə-'rä-lə-jist\ *n* : a specialist in gastroenterology

gas·tro·en·ter·ol·o·gy \-ıen-tə-'rä-lə-jē\ *n, pl* **-gies** : a branch of medicine concerned with the structure, functions, diseases, and pathology of the stomach and intestines — **gas·tro·en·ter·o·log·i·cal** \-rə-'lä-ji-kəl\ *or* **gas·tro·en·ter·o·log·ic** \-'lä-jik\ *adj*

gas·tro·en·ter·op·a·thy \-ıen-tə-'rä-pə-thē\ *n, pl* **-thies** : a disease of the stomach and intestines

gas·tro·en·ter·os·to·my \-'räs-tə-mē\ *n, pl* **-mies** : the surgical formation of a passage between the stomach and small intestine

gas·tro·ep·i·plo·ic artery \-ıe-pə-'plō-ik\ *n* : either of two arteries forming an anastomosis along the greater curvature of the stomach: **a** : one that is larger, arises as one of the two terminal branches of the gastroduodenal artery, and passes from right to left — called also *right gastroepiploic artery* **b** : one that is smaller, arises as a branch of the splenic artery, and passes from left to right — called also *left gastroepiploic artery*

gas·tro·esoph·a·ge·al \ıgas-trō-i-ısä-fə-'jē-əl\ *adj* : of, relating to, or involving the stomach and esophagus ⟨~ reflux⟩

gas·tro·in·tes·ti·nal \-in-'tes-tən-ə1\ *adj*

: of, relating to, or affecting both stomach and intestine

gastrointestinal tract *n* : the stomach and intestine as a functional unit

gas·tro·je·ju·nal \-ji-'jün-ə1\ *adj* : of, relating to, or involving both stomach and jejunum ⟨~ lesions⟩

gas·tro·je·ju·nos·to·my \-ji-(ı)jü-'näs-tə-mē\ *n, pl* **-mies** : the surgical formation of a passage between the stomach and jejunum : GASTROENTEROSTOMY

gas·tro·lith \'ga-strə-ılith\ *n* : a gastric calculus

gas·trop·a·thy \ga-'strä-pə-thē\ *n, pl* **-thies** : a disease of the stomach

gas·tro·pexy \'gas-trə-ıpek-sē\ *n, pl* **-pex·ies** : a surgical operation in which the stomach is sutured to the abdominal wall

gas·tro·pod \'gas-trə-ıpäd\ *n* : any of a large class (Gastropoda) of mollusks (as snails and cones) usu. with a one-piece shell or none and a distinct head bearing sensory organs — **gastropod** *adj*

gas·tros·chi·sis \ga-'sträs-kə-səs\ *n, pl* **-chi·ses** \-ısēz\ : congenital fissure of the ventral abdominal wall

gas·tro·scope \'gas-trə-ıskōp\ *n* : an instrument for viewing the interior of the stomach — **gas·tro·scop·ic** \ıgas-trə-'skä-pik\ *adj* — **gas·tros·co·pist** \ga-'sträs-kə-pist\ *n* — **gas·tros·co·py** \-pē\ *n*

gas·tro·splen·ic ligament \ıgas-trō-'sple-nik-\ *n* : a mesenteric fold passing from the greater curvature of the stomach to the spleen

gas·tros·to·my \ga-'sträs-tə-mē\ *n, pl* **-mies 1** : the surgical formation of an opening through the abdominal wall into the stomach **2** : the opening made by gastrostomy

gas·trot·o·my \ga-'strä-tə-mē\ *n, pl* **-mies** : surgical incision into the stomach

gas·tru·la \'gas-trə-lə\ *n, pl* **-las** *or* **-lae** \-ılē, -ılī\ : an early embryo that develops from the blastula and in mammals is formed by the differentiation of the upper layer of the blastodisc into the ectoderm and the lower layer into the endoderm and by the inward migration of cells through the primitive streak to form the mesoderm — compare BLASTULA, MORULA — **gas·tru·lar** \-lər\ *adj*

gas·tru·la·tion \ıgas-trə-'lä-shən\ *n* : the process of becoming or of forming a gastrula — **gas·tru·late** \'gas-trə-ılāt\ *n*

Gatch bed \'gach-\ *n* : HOSPITAL BED
  Gatch, Willis Dew (1878–1954), American surgeon.

gath·er \'ga-thər\ *vb* **gath·ered; gath·er·ing** : to swell and fill with pus ⟨the boil is ~*ing*⟩

gathering *n* : a suppurating swelling : ABSCESS

Gau·cher's disease \ıgō-'shāz-\ *n* : a

rare hereditary disorder of lipid metabolism that is caused by an enzyme deficiency of glucocerebrosidase, that is characterized by enormous enlargement of the spleen, pigmentation of the skin, and bone lesions, and that is marked by the presence of large amounts of glucocerebroside in the cells of the reticuloendothelial system

Gaucher, Philippe Charles Ernest (1854–1918), French physician.

gaul·the·ria \gol-'thir-ē-ə\ n 1 cap : a genus of evergreen shrubs of the heath family (Ericaceae) that includes the wintergreen (G. procumbens) which is a source of methyl salicylate 2 : a plant of the genus Gaultheria

Gaultier \gō-'tyä\, **Jean François (1708–1756),** Canadian physician and botanist.

gaultheria oil n : OIL OF WINTERGREEN

gauze \'goz\ n : a loosely woven cotton surgical dressing

ga·vage \gə-'väzh, gä-\ n : introduction of material into the stomach by a tube

gave past of GIVE

¹**GB** \jē-'bē\ n : SARIN

²**GB** abbr gallbladder

GC abbr 1 gas chromatograph; gas chromatography 2 gonococcus

G–CSF abbr granulocyte colony-stimulating factor

Gd symbol gadolinium

Ge symbol germanium

GE abbr gastroenterology

Gei·ger counter \'gī-gər-\ n : an instrument for detecting the presence and intensity of radiations (as cosmic rays or particles from a radioactive substance) by means of the ionizing effect on an enclosed gas which results in a pulse that is amplified and fed to a device giving a visible or audible indication

Geiger, Hans (Johannes) Wilhelm (1882–1945), and **Müller** \'mue-ler\, **Walther** (fl 1928), German physicists.

Geiger–Mül·ler counter \-'myü-lər-\ n : GEIGER COUNTER

¹**gel** \'jel\ n : a colloid in a more solid form than a sol

²**gel** vb **gelled; gel·ling** : to change into or take on the form of a gel — **gel·able** \'je-lə-bəl\ adj

gel·ate \'je-,lāt\ vb **gel·at·ed; gel·at·ing** : GEL

gel·a·tin also **gel·a·tine** \'je-lə-tən\ n 1 : glutinous material obtained from animal tissues by boiling; esp : a colloidal protein used as a food and in medicine 2 a : any of various substances (as agar) resembling gelatin b : an edible jelly made with gelatin — **ge·lat·i·nous** \jə-'lat-ᵊn-əs\ adj

gelatinosa — see SUBSTANTIA GELATINOSA

gel·ation \je-'lā-shən\ n : the formation of a gel from a sol

geld \'geld\ vb : CASTRATE; also : SPAY

geld·ing \'gel-diŋ\ n : a castrated animal; specif : a castrated male horse

gel electrophoresis n : electrophoresis in which molecules (as proteins and nucleic acids) migrate through a gel and esp. a polyacrylamide gel and separate into bands according to size

gel filtration n : chromatography in which the material to be fractionated separates primarily according to molecular size as it moves into a column of a gel and is washed with a solvent so that the fractions appear successively at the end of the column — called also gel chromatography

ge·mel·lus \jə-'me-ləs\ n, pl **ge·mel·li** \-,lī\ also **ge·mel·lus·es** : either of two small muscles of the hip that insert into the tendon of the obturator internus: **a** : a superior one originating chiefly from the outer surface of the ischial spine — called also gemellus superior **b** : an inferior one originating chiefly from the ischial tuberosity — called also gemellus inferior

gem·fi·bro·zil \jem-'fi-brə-(,)zil, -'fi-\ n : a drug $C_{15}H_{22}O_3$ that reduces the level of triglycerides in the blood and is used to treat hyperlipoproteinemia

gem·i·na·tion \,je-mə-'nā-shən\ n : a doubling, duplication, or repetition; esp : a formation of two teeth from a single tooth germ

gen- or **geno-** comb form : gene ⟨genome⟩

-gen \jən, ,jen\ also **-gene** \,jēn\ n comb form 1 : producer ⟨allergen⟩ ⟨carcinogen⟩ 2 : one that is (so) produced ⟨phosgene⟩

gen·der \'jen-dər\ n 1 : SEX 1 2 : the behavioral, cultural, or psychological traits typically associated with one sex

gender identity n : the totality of physical and behavioral traits that are designated by a culture as masculine or feminine

gene \'jēn\ n : a specific sequence of nucleotides in DNA or RNA that is located in the germ plasm usu. on a chromosome and that is the functional unit of inheritance controlling the transmission and expression of one or more traits by specifying the structure of a particular polypeptide and esp. a protein or controlling the function of other genetic material — called also determinant, determiner, factor

gene amplification n : replication and esp. massive replication (as in the polymerase chain reaction) of the genetic material in part of a genome

gene complex n : a group of genes of an individual or of a potentially interbreeding group that constitute an interacting functional unit

gene flow n : the passage and establishment of genes typical of one breeding population into the gene pool of another by hybridization and back-crossing

gene frequency n : the ratio of the number of a specified allele in a population to the total of all alleles at its genetic locus

gene mutation n : POINT MUTATION

gene pool n : the collection of genes of all the individuals in an interbreeding population

genera pl of GENUS

gen·er·al \'je-nə-rəl, 'jen-rəl\ adj 1 : not confined by specialization or careful limitation (a ∼ surgeon) 2 : involving or affecting practically the entire organism : not local (∼ nervousness)

general anesthesia n : anesthesia affecting the entire body and accompanied by loss of consciousness

general anesthetic n : an anesthetic used to produce general anesthesia

general hospital n : a hospital in which patients with many different types of ailments are given care

gen·er·al·ist \'jen-rə-list, 'je-nə-rə-\ n : one whose skills or interests extend to several different medical fields; esp : GENERAL PRACTITIONER

generalista — see OSTEITIS FIBROSA CYSTICA GENERALISTA

gen·er·al·i·za·tion \jen-rə-lə-'zā-shən, je-nə-rə-\ n 1 : the action or process of generalizing 2 : the process whereby a response is made to a stimulus similar to but not identical with a reference stimulus

gen·er·al·ize \'jen-rə-līz, 'je-nə-rə-\ vb -ized; -iz·ing : to spread or extend throughout the body

general paresis n : insanity caused by syphilitic alteration of the brain that leads to dementia and paralysis — called also *dementia paralytica*, *general paralysis of the insane*

general practitioner n : a physician or veterinarian whose practice is not limited to a specialty

gen·er·a·tion \je-nə-'rā-shən\ n 1 : a body of living beings constituting a single step in the line of descent from an ancestor 2 : the average span of time between the birth of parents and that of their offspring 3 : the action or process of producing offspring : PROCREATION

gen·er·a·tive \'je-nə-rə-tiv, -ˌrā-\ adj : having the power or function of propagating or reproducing (∼ organs)

gen·er·a·tiv·i·ty \je-nə-rə-'ti-və-tē\ n : a concern for people besides self and family that usu. develops during middle age; esp : a need to nurture and guide younger people and contribute to the next generation — used in the psychology of Erik Erikson

¹**ge·ner·ic** \jə-'ner-ik\ adj 1 : not protected by trademark registration : NONPROPRIETARY 2 : relating to or having the rank of a biological genus — **gen·er·i·cal·ly** \-i-k(ə-)lē\ adv

²**generic** n : a generic drug — usu. used in pl.

gene–splic·ing \'jēn-'splī-siŋ\ n : any of various techniques by which recombinant DNA is produced and made to function in an organism

gene therapy n : the insertion of normal or genetically altered genes into cells usu. to replace defective genes esp. in the treatment of genetic disorders

ge·net·ic \jə-'ne-tik\ also **ge·net·i·cal** \-ti-kəl\ adj 1 : of, relating to, or involving genetics 2 : GENIC — **ge·net·i·cal·ly** \-ti-k(ə-)lē\ adv

-ge·net·ic \jə-'ne-tik\ adj comb form : -GENIC (osteogenetic)

genetic code n : the biochemical basis of heredity consisting of codons in DNA and RNA that determine the specific amino acid sequence in proteins and that appear to be uniform for all known forms of life — **genetic coding** n

genetic counseling n : medical education of affected individuals and the general public concerning inherited disorders that includes discussion of the probability of producing offspring with a disorder, diagnostic tests, and available treatment

genetic drift n : random changes in gene frequency esp. in small populations when leading to preservation or extinction of particular genes

genetic engineering n : the directed alteration of genetic material by intervention in genetic processes; esp : GENE-SPLICING — **genetically engineered** adj — **genetic engineer** n

genetic map n : MAP

genetic marker n : a usu. dominant gene or trait that serves esp. to identify genes or traits linked with it — called also *marker*

ge·net·ics \jə-'ne-tiks\ n 1 a : a branch of biology that deals with the heredity and variation of organisms b : a treatise or textbook on genetics 2 : the genetic makeup and phenomena of an organism, type, group, or condition — **ge·net·i·cist** \jə-'ne-tə-sist\ n

ge·ni·al \ji-'nī-əl\ adj : of or relating to the chin

genial tubercle n : MENTAL TUBERCLE

gen·ic \'jē-nik, 'je-\ adj : of, relating to, or being a gene — **gen·i·cal·ly** \-ni-k(ə-)lē\ adv

-gen·ic \'je-nik, 'jē-\ adj comb form 1 : producing : forming (carcinogenic) 2 : produced by : formed from (nephrogenic)

ge·nic·u·lar artery \jə-'ni-kyə-lər-\ n : any of several branches of the femoral and popliteal arteries that supply the region of the knee — called also *genicular*

ge·nic·u·late \-lət, -ˌlāt\ adj 1 : bent abruptly at an angle like a bent knee 2 : relating to, comprising, or belonging to a geniculate body or geniculate ganglion (∼ cells) (∼ neurons)

geniculate body • genus

geniculate body *n* : either of two prominences of the diencephalon that comprise the metathalamus: **a** : LATERAL GENICULATE BODY **b** : MEDIAL GENICULATE BODY

geniculate ganglion *n* : a small reddish ganglion consisting of sensory and sympathetic nerve cells located at the sharp backward bend of the facial nerve

ge·nic·u·lo·cal·ca·rine \jə-ˌni-kyə-(ˌ)lō-ˈkal-kə-ˌrīn\ *adj* : relating to or comprising the optic radiation from the lateral geniculate body and the pulvinar to the occipital lobe ⟨~ tracts⟩

genio- *comb form* : chin and ⟨*genio*-glossus⟩

ge·nio·glos·sus \ˌjē-nē-ō-ˈglä-səs, -ˈglò-\ *n, pl* **-glos·si** \-ˌsī\ : a fan-shaped muscle that arises from the superior mental spine, inserts on the hyoid bone and into the tongue, and serves to advance and retract and also to depress the tongue

ge·nio·hyo·glos·sus \-ˌhī-ō-ˈglä-səs, -ˈglò-\ *n, pl* **-glos·si** \-ˌsī\ : GENIOGLOSSUS

ge·nio·hy·oid \-ˈhī-ˌòid\ *adj* : of or relating to the chin and hyoid bone

ge·nio·hy·oid·eus \-ˌhī-ˈòi-dē-əs\ *n, pl* **-oid·ei** \-dē-ˌī\ : GENIOHYOID MUSCLE

geniohyoid muscle *n* : a slender muscle that arises from the inferior mental spine, is inserted on the hyoid bone, and acts to raise the hyoid bone and draw it forward and to retract and depress the lower jaw — called also *geniohyoid*

gen·i·tal \ˈje-nə-tᵊl\ *adj* **1** : GENERATIVE **2** : of, relating to, or being a sexual organ **3** : of, relating to, or characterized by the stage of psychosexual development in psychoanalytic theory during which oral and anal impulses are subordinated to adaptive interpersonal mechanisms — compare ANAL 2a, ORAL 2a, PHALLIC 2 — **gen·i·tal·ly** *adv*

genital herpes *n* : HERPES GENITALIS

genital herpes simplex *n* : HERPES GENITALIS

gen·i·ta·lia \ˌje-nə-ˈtāl-yə\ *n pl* : the organs of the reproductive system; *esp* : the external genital organs

genitalis — see HERPES GENITALIS

gen·i·tal·i·ty \ˌta-lə-tē\ *n, pl* **-ties** : possession of full genital sensitivity and capacity to develop orgasmic potency in relation to a sexual partner of the opposite sex

genital ridge *n* : a ridge of embryonic mesoblast developing from the mesonephros and giving rise to the gonad on either side of the body

gen·i·tals \ˈje-nə-tᵊlz\ *n pl* : GENITALIA

genital tubercle *n* : a conical protuberance on the belly wall of an embryo that develops into the penis in the male and the clitoris in the female

genital wart *n* : CONDYLOMA ACUMINATUM

genito- *comb form* : genital and ⟨*genito*urinary⟩

gen·i·to·cru·ral nerve \ˌjə-nə-(ˌ)tō-ˈkrür-əl-\ *n* : GENITOFEMORAL NERVE

gen·i·to·fem·o·ral nerve \-ˈfe-mə-rəl-\ *n* : a nerve that arises from the first and second lumbar nerves and is distributed by way of branches to the skin of the scrotum, labia majora, and the upper anterior aspect of the thigh

gen·i·to·uri·nary \-ˈyür-ə-ˌner-ē\ *adj* : UROGENITAL

genitourinary system *n* : GENITOURINARY TRACT

genitourinary tract *n* : the system of organs comprising those concerned with the production and excretion of urine and those concerned with reproduction — called also *genitourinary system, urogenital system, urogenital tract*

geno- — see GEN-

ge·nome \ˈjē-ˌnōm\ *n* : one haploid set of chromosomes with the genes they contain — **ge·no·mic** \ji-ˈnō-mik, -ˈnä-\ *adj*

ge·no·type \ˈjē-nə-ˌtīp, ˈje-\ *n* : all or part of the genetic constitution of an individual or group — compare PHENOTYPE — **ge·no·typ·ic** \ˌjē-nə-ˈti-pik, ˌje-\ *also* **ge·no·typ·i·cal** \-pi-kəl\ *adj* — **ge·no·typ·i·cal·ly** \-pi-k(ə-)lē\ *adv*

²**genotype** *vb* **-typed; -typ·ing** : to determine the genotype of

-ge·nous \jə-nəs\ *adj comb form* **1** : producing : yielding ⟨erogen*ous*⟩ **2** : produced by : arising or originating in ⟨neurogen*ous*⟩ ⟨endogen*ous*⟩

gen·ta·mi·cin \ˌjen-tə-ˈmis-ᵊn\ *n* : a broad-spectrum antibiotic mixture that is derived from an actinomycete of the genus *Micromonospora* (*M. purpurea* and *M. echinospora*) and is extensively used in the form of the sulfate in treating infections esp. of the urinary tract

gen·tian violet \ˈjen-chən-\ *n, often cap G&V* : a greenish mixture that contains not less than 96% of the derivative of pararosaniline containing six methyl groups in each molecule and is used esp. as a bactericide, fungicide, and anthelmintic

gen·tis·ic acid \jen-ˈti-sik-, -zik\ *n* : a crystalline acid $C_7H_6O_4$ used medicinally as an analgesic and diaphoretic

ge·nu \ˈjē-ˌnü, ˈjen-yü\ *n, pl* **gen·ua** \ˈjen-yə-wə\ : an abrupt flexure; *esp* : the bend in the anterior part of the corpus callosum — compare GENU VALGUM, GENU VARUM

ge·nus \ˈjē-nəs, ˈje-\ *n, pl* **gen·era** \ˈje-nə-rə\ : a category of biological classification ranking between the family and the species, comprising structurally or phylogenetically related species or an isolated species exhibiting unusual differentiation, and being designated by a capitalized singular noun that is Latin or has a Latin form

genu val·gum \-ˈval-gəm\ n : KNOCK-KNEE

genu va·rum \-ˈvar-əm\ n : BOWLEG

-g·e·ny \jə-nē\ n comb form : generation : production ⟨embryogeny⟩ ⟨lysogeny⟩

geo·med·i·cine \ˌjē-ō-ˈme-də-sən\ n : a branch of medicine that deals with geographic factors in disease

ge·o·pha·gia \-ˈfā-jē-ə-, -jə\ n : GEOPHAGY

ge·oph·a·gy \jē-ˈä-fə-jē\ n, pl **-gies** : a practice of eating earthy substances (as clay) among primitive or economically depressed peoples to augment a scanty or mineral-deficient diet — compare PICA

ge·ot·ri·cho·sis \ˌjē-ä-trə-ˈkō-səs\ n : infection of the bronchi or lungs and sometimes the mouth and intestines by a fungus of the genus Geotrichum (G. candidum)

Ge·ot·ri·chum \jē-ˈä-tri-kəm\ n : a genus of fungi (family Moniliaceae) including one (G. candidum) that causes human geotrichosis

ge·ri·at·ric \ˌjer-ē-ˈa-trik, ˌjir-\ n **1** geriatrics \-triks\ : a branch of medicine that deals with the problems and diseases of old age and aging people — used with a sing. verb; compare GERONTOLOGY **2** : an aged person — **geriatric** adj

ger·i·a·tri·cian \ˌjer-ē-ə-ˈtri-shən, ˌjir-\ n : a specialist in geriatrics

ge·ri·a·trist \ˌjer-ē-ˈa-trist, ˌjir-; jə-ˈrī-ə-, n : GERIATRICIAN

germ \ˈjərm\ n **1** : a small mass of living substance capable of developing into an organism or one of its parts **2** : MICROORGANISM; esp : a microorganism causing disease

Ger·man cockroach \ˈjər-mən-\ n : a small active winged cockroach of the genus Blattella (B. germanica) prob. of African origin but now common in many urban buildings in the U.S. — called also Croton bug

ger·ma·nin \jər-ˈmā-nən\ n : SURAMIN

ger·ma·ni·um \(ˌ)jər-ˈmā-nē-əm\ n : a grayish white hard brittle element — symbol Ge; see ELEMENT table

German measles n sing or pl : an acute contagious virus disease that is milder than typical measles but is damaging to the fetus when occurring early in pregnancy — called also rubella

germ cell n : an egg or sperm cell or one of their antecedent cells

germ-free \ˈjərm-ˈfrē\ adj : free of microorganisms : AXENIC

ger·mi·cid·al \ˌjər-mə-ˈsīd-əl\ adj : of or relating to a germicide; also : destroying germs

ger·mi·cide \ˈjər-mə-ˌsīd\ n : an agent that destroys germs

ger·mi·nal \ˈjər-mə-nəl\ adj : of, relating to, or having the characteristics of a germ cell or early embryo

germinal cell n : an embryonic cell of the early vertebrate nervous system that is the source of neuroblasts and neuroglial cells

germinal center n : the lightly staining central proliferative area of a lymphoid follicle

germinal disk n **1** : BLASTODISC **2** : the part of the blastoderm that forms the embryo proper of an amniote vertebrate

germinal epithelium n : the epithelial covering of the genital ridges and of the gonads derived from them

germinal vesicle n : the enlarged nucleus of the egg before completion of meiosis

ger·mi·na·tive layer \ˈjər-mə-ˌnā-tiv-, -nə-\ n : the innermost layer of the epidermis from which new tissue is constantly formed

germinativum — see STRATUM GERMINATIVUM

germ layer n : any of the three primary layers of cells differentiated in most embryos during and immediately following gastrulation

germ plasm n **1** : germ cells and their precursors serving as the bearers of heredity and being fundamentally independent of other cells **2** : the hereditary material of the germ cells : GENES

germ·proof \ˈjərm-ˌprüf\ adj : impervious to the penetration or action of germs

germ theory n : a theory in medicine: infections, contagious diseases, and various other conditions (as suppurative lesions) result from the action of microorganisms

geront- or **geronto-** comb form : aged one : old age ⟨gerontology⟩

ger·on·tol·o·gist \ˌjer-ən-ˈtä-lə-jist\ n : a specialist in gerontology

ger·on·tol·o·gy \-jē\ n, pl **-gies** : the comprehensive study of aging and the problems of the aged — compare GERIATRIC 1 — **ge·ron·to·log·i·cal** \jə-ˌränt-əl-ˈä-ji-kəl\ also **ge·ron·to·log·ic** \-jik\ adj

Gerst·mann's syndrome \ˈgerst-mänz-, ˈgarst-mənz-\ n : cerebral dysfunction characterized esp. by finger agnosia, disorientation with respect to right and left, agraphia, and acalculia and caused by a lesion in the dominant cerebral hemisphere

Gerstmann, Josef (1887–1969), Austrian neurologist and psychiatrist.

Gerst·mann–Sträus·sler–Schein·ker syndrome \ˈgerst-män-ˈshtrois-lər-ˈshiŋ-kər-\ n : GERSTMANN'S SYNDROME — called also Gerstmann-Sträussler-Scheinker disease

ge·stalt \gə-ˈstält, -ˈshtält, -ˈstolt, -ˈshtolt\ n, pl **ge·stalt·en** \-ᵊn\ or **ge·stalts** \-ˈstälts, -ˈshtälts\ : a structure, arrangement, or pattern of physical, biological, or psychological phenomena so integrated as to constitute a functional unit with properties not derivable by summation of its parts

ge·stalt·ist \gə-ˈstäl-tist, -ˈshtäl-, -ˈstol-, -ˈshtol-\ n, often cap : a specialist in Gestalt psychology

Gestalt psychology n : the study of perception and behavior from the standpoint of an individual's response to gestalten with stress on the uniformity of psychological and physiological events and rejection of analysis into discrete events of stimulus, percept, and response — **Gestalt psychologist** n

ges·ta·tion \je-ˈstā-shən\ n 1 : the carrying of young in the uterus from conception to delivery : PREGNANCY 2 : GESTATION PERIOD — **ges·tate** \ˈjes-ˌtāt\ vb — **ges·ta·tion·al** \-shə-nəl\ adj

gestation period n : the length of time during which gestation takes place — called also **gestation**

ges·to·sis \je-ˈstō-səs\ n, pl **-to·ses** \-ˌsēz\ : any disorder of pregnancy; esp : TOXEMIA OF PREGNANCY

-geu·sia \ˈgü-zē-ə, ˈjü-, -sē-ə, -zhə\ n comb form : a (specified) condition of the sense of taste ⟨ageusia⟩ ⟨dysgeusia⟩

GG abbr gamma globulin

GH abbr growth hormone

ghost \ˈgōst\ n : a structure (as a cell or tissue) that does not stain normally because of degenerative changes; specif : a red blood cell that has lost its hemoglobin

GI abbr gastrointestinal

giant cell n : a large multinucleate often phagocytic cell (as those characteristic of tubercular lesions or various sarcomas)

giant cell arteritis n : arterial inflammation that often involves the temporal arteries and may lead to blindness when the ophthalmic artery and its branches are affected, is characterized by the formation of giant cells, and may be accompanied by fever, malaise, fatigue, anorexia, weight loss, and arthralgia — called also **temporal arteritis**

giant–cell tumor n : an osteolytic tumor affecting the metaphyses and epiphyses of long bones that is usually benign but sometimes malignant — called also **osteoclastoma**

gi·gant·ism \ˈjī-ən-ˌti-zəm\ n : GIGANTISM

giant kidney worm n : a blood-red nematode worm of the genus Dioctophyme (D. renale) that sometimes exceeds a yard in length and invades mammalian kidneys esp. of the dog and occas. of humans

giant urticaria n : ANGIOEDEMA

giant water bug n : any of a family (Belostomatidae and esp. genus Lethocerus) of very large predatory bugs capable of inflicting a painful bite

giar·dia \jē-ˈär-dē-ə, ˈjär-\ n 1 cap : a genus of flagellate protozoans inhabiting the intestines of various mammals and including one (G. lamblia)

that is associated with diarrhea in humans 2 : any flagellate of the genus Giardia

Giard \zhē-ˈär\, **Alfred Mathieu** (1846–1908), French biologist.

giar·di·a·sis \(ˌ)jē-ˌär-ˈdī-ə-səs, ˌjē-ər-, (ˌ)jär-\ n, pl **-a·ses** \-ˌsēz\ : infestation with or disease caused by a flagellate protozoan of the genus Giardia (esp. G. lamblia) that is often characterized by diarrhea — called also **lambliasis**

gid \ˈgid\ n : a disease esp. of sheep that is caused by the presence in the brain of the coenurus of a tapeworm of the genus Multiceps (M. multiceps) — called also **sturdy**

Gi·em·sa stain \gē-ˈem-zə-\ also **Giemsa's stain** n : a stain consisting of a mixture of eosin and a blue dye and used chiefly in differential staining of blood films — called also **Giemsa**

Giemsa, Gustav (1867–1948), German chemist and pharmacist.

gi·gan·tism \jī-ˈgan-ˌti-zəm, jə-; ˈjī-gən-\ n : development to abnormally large size from excessive growth of the long bones accompanied by muscular weakness and sexual impotence and usu. caused by hyperpituitarism before normal ossification is complete — called also **macrosomia**; compare ACROMEGALY

Gi·la monster \ˈhē-lə-\ n : a large orange and black venomous lizard of the genus Heloderma (H. suspectum) of the southwestern U.S.; also : the beaded lizard (H. horridum) of Mexico

Gil·bert's disease \zhil-ˈberz-\ n : a metabolic disorder prob. inherited as an autosomal dominant with variable penetrance and characterized by elevated levels of serum bilirubin caused esp. by defective uptake of bilirubin by the liver

Gilbert, Augustin–Nicholas (1858–1927), French physician.

Gil·christ's disease \ˈgil-ˌkrists-\ n : NORTH AMERICAN BLASTOMYCOSIS

Gilchrist, Thomas Caspar (1862–1927), American dermatologist.

¹**gill** \ˈjil\ n : either of two units of capacity: **a** : a British unit equal to ¼ imperial pint or 8.669 cubic inches **b** : a U.S. liquid unit equal to ¼ U.S. liquid pint or 7.218 cubic inches

²**gill** \ˈgil\ n 1 : an organ (as of a fish) for obtaining oxygen from water 2 : one of the radiating plates forming the undersurface of the cap of a mushroom — **gilled** \ˈgild\ adj

gill arch n : one of the bony or cartilaginous arches placed one behind the other on each side of the pharynx and supporting the gills of fishes and amphibians; also : BRANCHIAL ARCH

gill cleft n : GILL SLIT

Gilles de la Tou·rette syndrome \ˈzhēl-də-lä-tü-ˈret\ also **Gilles de la Tourette's syndrome** n : TOURETTE'S SYNDROME

gill slit *n* : one of the openings or clefts between the gill arches in vertebrates that breathe by gills through which water taken in at the mouth passes to the exterior and bathes the gills; *also* : BRANCHIAL CLEFT

gingiv- *or* **gingivo-** *comb form* 1 : gum : gums (*gingivitis*) 2 : gums and (*gingivostomatitis*)

gin·gi·va \'jin-jə-və, jin-'jī-\ *n, pl* **-vae** \-ˌvē, -ˌvī\ *or* : ¹GUM — **gin·gi·val** \'jin-jə-vəl\ *adj*

gingival crevice *n* : a narrow space between the free margin of the gingival epithelium and the adjacent enamel of a tooth — called also *gingival trough*

gingival papilla *n* : INTERDENTAL PAPILLA

gingival trough *n* : GINGIVAL CREVICE

gin·gi·vec·to·my \ˌjin-jə-'vek-tə-mē\ *n, pl* **-mies** : the excision of a portion of the gingiva

gin·gi·vi·tis \ˌjin-jə-'vī-təs\ *n* : inflammation of the gums

gin·gi·vo·plas·ty \'jin-jə-və-ˌplas-tē\ *n, pl* **-ties** : a surgical procedure that involves reshaping the gums for aesthetic or functional purposes

gin·gi·vo·sto·ma·ti·tis \ˌjin-jə-vō-ˌstō-mə-'tī-təs\ *n, pl* **-tit·i·des** \-'ti-tə-ˌdēz\ *or* **-ti·tis·es** : inflammation of the gums and of the mouth

gin·gly·mus \'jiŋ-glə-məs, 'giŋ-\ *n, pl* **gin·gly·mi** \-ˌmī, -ˌmē\ : a hinge joint (as between the humerus and ulna) allowing motion in one plane only

gin·seng \'jin-ˌseŋ, -ˌsiŋ\ *n* : the aromatic root of a Chinese perennial herb (*Panax schinseng* of the family Araliaceae, the ginseng family) valued esp. locally as a medicine; *also* : the plant

gir·dle \'gərd-ᵊl\ *n* : either of two more or less complete bony rings at the anterior and posterior ends of the vertebrate trunk supporting the arms and legs respectively: **a** : PECTORAL GIRDLE **b** : PELVIC GIRDLE

gi·tal·in \'ji-tə-lən; jə-'tā-lən, -'ta-\ *n* 1 : a crystalline glycoside $C_{35}H_{56}O_{12}$ obtained from digitalis 2 : an amorphous water-soluble mixture of glycosides of digitalis used similarly to digitalis

gi·tox·in \jə-'täk-sən\ *n* : a poisonous crystalline steroid glycoside $C_{41}H_{64}O_{14}$ that is obtained from digitalis and from lanatoside B by hydrolysis

give \'giv\ *vb* **gave** \'gāv\; **giv·en** \'gi-vən\; **giv·ing** 1 : to administer as a medicine 2 : to cause a person to catch by contagion, infection, or exposure

giz·zard \'gi-zərd\ *n* : the muscular usu. horny-lined enlargement of the alimentary canal of a bird used for churning and grinding food

gla·bel·la \glə-'be-lə\ *n, pl* **-bel·lae** \-'be-(ˌ)lē, -ˌlī\ : the smooth prominence between the eyebrows — **gla·bel·lar** \-'be-lər\ *adj*

gla·brous \'glā-brəs\ *adj* : having or being a smooth hairless surface (~ skin)

glacial acetic acid *n* : acetic acid containing usu. less than 1 percent of water

glad·i·o·lus \ˌgla-dē-'ō-ləs\ *n, pl* **-li** \-(ˌ)lē, -ˌlī\ : the large middle portion of the sternum lying between the upper manubrium and the lower xiphoid process — called also *mesosternum*

glairy \'glar-ē\ *adj* **glair·i·er; -est** : having a slimy viscid consistency suggestive of an egg white

gland \'gland\ *n* 1 : a cell, group of cells, or organ of endothelial origin that selectively removes materials from the blood, concentrates or alters them, and secretes them for further use in the body or for elimination from the body 2 : any of various animal structures (as a lymph node) suggestive of glands though not secretory in function — **gland·less** *adj*

glan·dered \'glan-dərd\ *adj* : affected with glanders

glan·ders \-dərz\ *n sing or pl* : a contagious and destructive disease esp. of horses caused by a bacterium of the genus *Pseudomonas* (*P. mallei*) and characterized by caseating nodular lesions esp. of the respiratory mucosae and lungs

glandes *pl of* GLANS

gland of Bartholin *n* : BARTHOLIN'S GLAND

gland of Bow·man \-'bō-mən\ *n* : any of the tubular and often branched glands occurring beneath the olfactory epithelium of the nose — called also *Bowman's gland, olfactory gland*

  W. Bowman — see BOWMAN'S CAPSULE

gland of Brunner *n* : BRUNNER'S GLAND

gland of external secretion *n* : EXOCRINE GLAND

gland of internal secretion *n* : ENDOCRINE GLAND

gland of Lit·tré \-lē-'trā\ *n* : any of the urethral glands of the male

  Littré, Alexis (1658–1726), French surgeon and anatomist.

gland of Moll \-'mōl, -'mȯl, -'mäl\ *n* : any of the small glands near the free margin of each eyelid regarded as modified sweat glands

  Moll \'mȯl\, **Jacob Antonius (1832–1914),** Dutch ophthalmologist.

gland of Ty·son \-'tīs-ᵊn\ *n* : any of the small glands at the base of the glans penis that secrete smegma — called also *preputial gland*

  Tyson, Edward (1650–1708), British anatomist.

glan·du·lar \'glan-jə-lər\ *adj* 1 : of, relating to, or involving glands, gland cells, or their products 2 : having the characteristics or function of a gland (~ tissue)

glandular fever *n* : INFECTIOUS MONO-NUCLEOSIS

glan·du·lous \'glan-jə-ləs\ *adj* : GLAN-DULAR

glans \'glanz\ *n, pl* **glan·des** \'glan-ˌdēz\ **1** : a conical vascular body forming the extremity of the penis **2** : a conical vascular body that forms the extremity of the clitoris and is similar to the glans penis

glans cli·tor·i·dis \-klə-'tor-ə-(ˌ)dis\ *n* : GLANS 2

glans penis *n* : GLANS 1

Gla·se·ri·an fissure \glə-'zir-ē-ən-\ *n* : PETROTYMPANIC FISSURE

    Glaser \'glä-zər\, **Johann Heinrich (1629–1675)**, Swiss anatomist and surgeon.

glass·es \'gla-səz\ *n pl* : a device used to correct defects of vision or to protect the eyes that consists typically of a pair of glass or plastic lenses and the frame by which they are held in place — called also *eyeglasses*

glass eye *n* **1** : an artificial eye made of glass **2** : an eye having a pale, whitish, or colorless iris — **glass–eyed** \-'īd\ *adj*

Glau·ber's salt \'glau-bərz-\ *also* **Glauber salt** \-bər-\ *n* : a colorless crystal-line sodium sulfate $Na_2SO_4 \cdot 10H_2O$ used as a cathartic — sometimes used in pl.

    Glauber, Johann Rudolf (1604–1670), German physician and chemist.

glau·co·ma \glau-'kō-mə, glȯ-\ *n* : a disease of the eye marked by increased pressure within the eyeball that can result in damage to the optic disk and gradual loss of vision — **glau·co·ma·tous** \-'kō-mə-təs, -'kä-\ *adj*

GLC *abbr* gas-liquid chromatography

gleet \'glēt\ *n* : a chronic inflammation (as gonorrhea) of a bodily orifice usu. accompanied by an abnormal discharge; *also* : the discharge itself

gle·no·hu·mer·al \ˌgle-(ˌ)nō-'hyü-mə-rəl, ˌglē-\ *adj* : of, relating to, or connecting the glenoid cavity and the humerus

glen·oid \'gle-ˌnȯid, 'glē-\ *adj* **1** : having the form of a smooth shallow depression — used chiefly of skeletal articulatory sockets **2** : of or relating to the glenoid cavity or glenoid fossa

glenoid cavity *n* : the shallow cavity of the upper part of the scapula by which the humerus articulates with the pectoral girdle

glenoid fossa *n* : the depression in each lateral wall of the skull with which the mandible articulates — called also *mandibular fossa*

glenoid labrum *or* **glen·oid·al labrum** \gli-'nȯid-əl-\ *n* : a fibrocartilaginous ligament forming the margin of the glenoid cavity of the shoulder joint that serves to broaden and deepen the cavity and gives attachment to the long head of the biceps brachii — called also *labrum*

gli- *or* **glio-** *comb form* **1** : gliomatous ⟨*glio*blastoma⟩ **2** : neuroglial ⟨*glio*ma⟩

glia \'glē-ə, 'glī-ə\ *n* : NEUROGLIA — **gli·al** \-əl\ *adj*

-glia \glē-ə\ *n comb form* : neuroglia made up of a (specified) kind or size of element ⟨micro*glia*⟩ ⟨oligodendrog*lia*⟩

gli·a·din \'glī-ə-dən\ *n* : PROLAMIN; *esp* : one obtained by alcoholic extraction of gluten from wheat and rye

gliding joint *n* : a diarthrosis in which the articular surfaces glide upon each other without axial motion — called also *arthrodia, plane joint*

glio·blas·to·ma \ˌglī-(ˌ)ō-bla-'stō-mə\ *n, pl* **-mas** *or* **-ma·ta** \-mə-tə\ : a malignant tumor of the central nervous system and usu. of a cerebral hemisphere — called also *spongio-blastoma*

glioblastoma mul·ti·for·me \-ˌməl-tə-'for-mē\ *n* : GLIOBLASTOMA

Glio·cla·di·um \ˌglī-ō-'klä-dē-əm\ *n* : a genus of molds resembling those of the genus *Penicillium* — see GLIOTOX-IN

gli·o·ma \glī-'ō-mə, glē-\ *n, pl* **-mas** *or* **-ma·ta** \-mə-tə\ : a tumor arising from neuroglia — **gli·o·ma·tous** \-mə-təs\ *adj*

gli·o·ma·to·sis \ˌglī-ō-mə-'tō-səs\ *n, pl* **-to·ses** \-ˌsēz\ : a glioma with diffuse proliferation of glial cells or with multiple foci

gli·o·sis \glī-'ō-səs\ *n, pl* **gli·o·ses** \-ˌsēz\ : excessive development of neuroglia esp. interstitially — **gli·ot·ic** \-'ä-tik\ *adj*

glio·tox·in \ˌglī-ō-'täk-sən\ *n* : a toxic antibiotic $C_{13}H_{14}N_2O_4S_2$ that is produced by various fungi esp. of the genus *Gliocladium*

Glis·son's capsule \'glis-ᵊnz-\ *n* : an investment of loose connective tissue entering the liver with the portal vessels and sheathing the larger vessels in their course through the organ

    Glisson, Francis (1597–1677), British physician and anatomist.

globe \'glōb\ *n* : EYEBALL

globe·fish \'glōb-ˌfish\ *n* : PUFFER

glo·bin \'glō-bən\ *n* : a colorless protein obtained by removal of heme from a conjugated protein and esp. hemoglobin

glo·bo·side \'glō-bə-ˌsīd\ *n* : a complex glycolipid that occurs in the red blood cells, serum, liver, and spleen of humans and accumulates in tissues in one of the variants of Tay-Sachs disease

glob·u·lar \'glä-byə-lər\ *adj* **1 a** : having the shape of a globe or globule **b** : having a compact folded molecular structure ⟨~ proteins⟩ **2** : having or consisting of globules — **glob·u·lar·ly** \-lē\ *adv*

glob·ule \'glä-(ˌ)byül\ *n* : a small globular body or mass (as a drop of water, fat, or sweat)

glob·u·lin \'glä-byə-lən\ *n* : any of a class of simple proteins (as myosin) that occur widely in plant and animal tissues — see ALPHA GLOBULIN, BETA GLOBULIN, GAMMA GLOBULIN

glo·bus hys·ter·i·cus \'glō-bəs-his-'ter-i-kəs\ *n* : a choking sensation commonly experienced in hysteria

globus pal·li·dus \-'pa-lə-dəs\ *n* : the median portion of the lentiform nucleus — called also *pallidum*

glom·an·gi·o·ma \glō-man-jē-'ō-ma\ *n, pl* **-mas** *or* **-ma·ta** \-mə-tə\ : GLOMUS TUMOR

glo·mec·to·my \glō-'mek-tə-mē\ *n, pl* **-mies** : excision of a glomus (as the carotid body)

glomerul- *or* **glomerulo-** *comb form* : glomerulus of the kidney (*glomerulo*litis) (*glomerulo*nephritis)

glo·mer·u·lar \glə-'mer-ə-lər, glō-, -ə-lər\ *adj* : of, relating to, or produced by a glomerulus (~ nephritis)

glomerular capsule *n* : BOWMAN'S CAPSULE

glo·mer·u·li·tis \glə-,mer-yə-'lī-təs, glō-, -ə-'lī-\ *n* : inflammation of the glomeruli of the kidney

glo·mer·u·lo·ne·phri·tis \-,mer-yə-lō-ni-'frī-təs, -ə-lō-\ *n, pl* **-phrit·i·des** \-'fri-tə-,dēz\ : nephritis marked by inflammation of the capillaries in the renal glomeruli

glo·mer·u·lo·sa \glə-,mer-yə-'lō-sə, -ə-'lō-, -zə\ *n, pl* **-sae** \-,sē, -,sī, -,zē, -,zī\ : ZONA GLOMERULOSA

glo·mer·u·lo·scle·ro·sis \-,lō-sklə-'rō-səs\ *n, pl* **-ro·ses** \-,sēz\ : nephrosclerosis involving the renal glomeruli

glo·mer·u·lus \glə-'mer-yə-ləs, glō-, -ə-ləs\ *n, pl* **-li** \-,lī, -,lē\ : a small convoluted or intertwined mass: as **a** : a tuft of capillaries at the point of origin of each nephron that passes a protein-free filtrate to the surrounding Bowman's capsule **b** : a dense entanglement of nerve fibers situated in the olfactory bulb and containing the primary synapses of the olfactory pathway

glo·mus \'glō-məs\ *n, pl* **glom·era** \'glä-mə-rə\ *also* **glo·mi** \'glō-,mī, -,mē\ : a small arteriovenous anastomosis together with its supporting structures: as **a** : a vascular tuft that suggests a renal glomerulus and that develops from the embryonic aorta in relation to the pronephros **b** : CAROTID BODY **c** : a tuft of the choroid plexus protruding into each lateral ventricle of the brain

glomus ca·rot·i·cum \-kə-'rä-ti-kəm\ *n* : CAROTID BODY

glomus coc·cy·ge·um \-käk-'si-jē-əm\ *n* : a small mass of vascular tissue situated near the tip of the coccyx — called also *coccygeal body, coccygeal gland*

glomus jug·u·la·re \-,jə-gyə-'lar-ē\ *n* : a mass of chemoreceptors in the adventitia of the dilation in the internal jug-

ular vein where it arises from the transverse sinus in the jugular foramen

glomus tumor *n* : a painful benign tumor that develops by hypertrophy of a glomus — called also *glomangioma*

gloss- *or* **glosso-** *comb form* **1** : tongue (*gloss*itis) (*glosso*pathy) **2** : language (*gloss*olalia)

glos·sal \'glä-səl, 'glò-\ *adj* : of or relating to the tongue

-glos·sia \'glä-sē-ə, 'glò-\ *n comb form* : condition of having (such) a tongue (micro*glossia*)

glos·si·na \glä-'sī-nə, glò-, -'sē-\ *n* **1** *cap* : an African genus of dipteran flies with a long slender sharp proboscis that includes the tsetse flies — compare SLEEPING SICKNESS **2** : any dipteran fly of the genus *Glossina* : TSETSE FLY

glos·si·tis \-'sī-təs\ *n* : inflammation of the tongue

glosso- — see GLOSS-

gloss·odyn·ia \glä-sō-'di-nē-ə, glò-\ *n* : pain localized in the tongue

glos·so·la·lia \glä-sə-'lā-lē-ə, glò-\ *n* : profuse and often emotionally charged speech that mimics coherent speech but is usu. unintelligible to the listener and that is uttered in some states of religious ecstasy and in some schizophrenic states

glos·so·pal·a·tine arch \glä-sō-'pa-lə-,tīn-, glò-\ *n* : PALATOGLOSSAL ARCH

glossopalatine nerve *n* : NERVUS INTER-MEDIUS

glos·so·pal·a·ti·nus \-,pa-lə-'tī-nəs\ *n, pl* **-ni** \-,nī, -,nē\ : PALATOGLOSSUS

glos·sop·a·thy \glä-'sä-pə-thē\ *n, pl* **-thies** : a disease of the tongue

glos·so·pha·ryn·geal \glä-sō-fə-'rin-jē-əl, glò-, -jəl; -,far-ən-'jē-əl\ *adj* **1** : of or relating to both tongue and pharynx **2** : of, relating to, or affecting the glossopharyngeal nerve (~ lesions)

glossopharyngeal nerve *n* : either of the 9th pair of cranial nerves that are mixed nerves and supply chiefly the pharynx, posterior tongue, and parotid gland with motor and sensory fibers — called also *glossopharyngeal, ninth cranial nerve*

glottidis — see RIMA GLOTTIDIS

glot·tis \'glä-təs\ *n, pl* **glot·tis·es** *or* **glot·ti·des** \-tə-,dēz\ : the space between one of the true vocal cords and the arytenoid cartilage on one side of the larynx and those on the other side; *also* : the structures that surround this space — compare EPIGLOTTIS

gluc- *or* **gluco-** *comb form* : glucose (*gluco*kinase) (*gluco*neogenesis)

glu·ca·gon \'glü-kə-,gän\ *n* : a protein hormone that is produced esp. by the pancreatic islets of Langerhans and that promotes an increase in the sugar content of the blood by increasing the rate of breakdown of glycogen in the liver — called also *hyperglycemic factor*

glu·can \'glü-ˌkan, -kən\ *n* : a polysaccharide (as glycogen) that is a polymer of glucose

glu·co·ce·re·bro·si·dase \ˌglü-kō-ˌser-ə-'brō-sə-ˌdās, -ˌdāz\ *n* : an enzyme that catalyzes the hydrolysis of the glucose part of a glucocerebroside and is deficient in patients affected with Gaucher's disease

glu·co·ce·re·bro·side \-'ser-ə-brə-ˌsīd, -sə-'rē\ *n* : a lipid composed of a ceramide and glucose that accumulates in the tissues of patients affected with Gaucher's disease

glu·co·cor·ti·coid \-'kòr-ti-ˌkòid\ *n* : any of a group of corticosteroids (as hydrocortisone or dexamethasone) that are involved in carbohydrate, protein, and fat metabolism, that tend to increase liver glycogen and blood sugar by increasing gluconeogenesis, that are anti-inflammatory and immunosuppressive, and that are used widely in medicine (as in the alleviation of the symptoms of rheumatoid arthritis) — compare MINERALOCORTICOID

glu·co·ki·nase \-'kī-ˌnās, -ˌnāz\ *n* : a hexokinase found esp. in the liver that catalyzes the phosphorylation of glucose

glu·co·nate \'glü-kə-ˌnāt\ *n* : a salt or ester of a crystalline acid $C_6H_{12}O_7$ — see CALCIUM GLUCONATE, FERROUS GLUCONATE

glu·co·neo·gen·e·sis \ˌglü-kə-ˌnē-ə-'jenə-səs\ *n, pl* **-e·ses** \-ˌsēz\ : formation of glucose esp. by the liver and kidney from substances (as fats and proteins) other than carbohydrates — **glu·co·neo·gen·ic** \-'je-nik\ *adj*

glu·cos·amine \glü-'kō-sə-ˌmēn, -zə-\ *n* : an amino derivative $C_6H_{13}NO_5$ of glucose that occurs esp. as a constituent of polysaccharides in animal supporting structures and some plant cell walls

glu·cose \'glü-ˌkōs, -ˌkōz\ *n* : a sugar $C_6H_{12}O_6$ known in dextrorotatory, levorotatory, and racemic forms; *esp* : the sweet soluble dextrorotatory form that occurs widely in nature and is the usual form in which carbohydrate is assimilated by animals

glucose–1–phosphate *n* : an ester C_6-$H_{13}O_9P$ that reacts in the presence of a phosphorylase with aldoses and ketoses to yield disaccharides or with itself in liver and muscle to yield glycogen and phosphoric acid

glucose phosphate *n* : a phosphate ester of glucose: as **a** : GLUCOSE-1-PHOSPHATE **b** : GLUCOSE-6-PHOSPHATE

glucose–6–phosphate *n* : an ester C_6-$H_{13}O_9P$ that is formed from glucose and ATP in the presence of a glucokinase and that is an essential early stage in glucose metabolism

glucose–6–phosphate dehydrogenase *n* : an enzyme found esp. in red blood cells that dehydrogenates glucose-6-phosphate in a glucose degradation pathway alternative to the Krebs cycle

glucose–6–phosphate dehydrogenase deficiency *n* : a hereditary metabolic disorder affecting red blood cells that is controlled by a variable gene on the X chromosome, that is characterized by a deficiency of glucose-6-phosphate dehydrogenase conferring marked susceptibility to hemolytic anemia which may be chronic, episodic, or induced by certain foods (as broad beans) or drugs (as primaquine), and that occurs esp. in individuals of Mediterranean or African descent

glucose tolerance test *n* : a test of the body's powers of metabolizing glucose that involves the administration of a measured dose of glucose to the fasting stomach and the determination of glucose levels in the blood and urine at measured intervals thereafter

glu·cos·uria \ˌglü-kō-'shùr-ē-ə, -'syùr-\ *n* : GLYCOSURIA

glu·cur·on·ic acid \ˌglü-kyə-'rä-nik-\ *n* : a compound $C_6H_{10}O_7$ that occurs esp. as a constituent of glycosaminoglycans and combined as a glucuronide

glu·cur·on·i·dase \-'rä-nə-ˌdās, -ˌdāz\ *n* : an enzyme that hydrolyzes a glucuronide

glu·cur·o·nide \glü-'kyùr-ə-ˌnīd\ *n* : any of various derivatives of glucuronic acid that are formed esp. as combinations with often toxic aromatic hydroxyl compounds (as phenols) and are excreted in the urine

glue–sniffing *n* : the deliberate inhalation of volatile organic solvents from plastic glues that may result in symptoms ranging from mild euphoria to disorientation and coma

glu·ta·mate \'glü-tə-ˌmāt\ *n* : a salt or ester of glutamic acid; *esp* : one that is an excitatory neurotransmitter in the central nervous system : MONOSODIUM GLUTAMATE

glutamate dehydrogenase *n* : an enzyme present esp. in liver mitochondria and cytosol that catalyzes the oxidation of glutamate to ammonia and α-ketoglutaric acid

glu·tam·ic acid \(ˌ)glü-'ta-mik-\ *n* : a crystalline amino acid $C_5H_9NO_4$ widely distributed in plant and animal proteins

glutamic–ox·a·lo·ace·tic transaminase \-ˌäk-sə-lō-ə-'sē-tik-\ *also* **glutamic–ox·al·ace·tic transaminase** \-ˌäk-sə-lə-'sē-tik-\ *n* : an enzyme that promotes transfer of an amino group from glutamic acid to oxaloacetic acid and that when present in abnormally high levels in the blood is a diagnostic indication of myocardial infarction or liver disease

glutamic pyruvic transaminase *n* : an enzyme that promotes transfer of an amino group from glutamic acid to pyruvic acid and that when present in abnormally high levels in the blood is a diagnostic indication of liver disease

glu·ta·mine \\'glü-tə-ˌmēn\ *n* : a crystalline amino acid $C_5H_{10}N_2O_3$ that is found free and in proteins in plants and animals and that yields glutamic acid and ammonia on hydrolysis

glu·tar·al·de·hyde \ˌglü-tə-'ral-də-ˌhīd\ *n* : a compound $C_5H_8O_2$ used esp. as a disinfectant and in fixing biological tissues

glu·tar·ic acid \glü-ˌtar-ik-\ *n* : a crystalline acid $C_5H_8O_4$ used esp. in organic synthesis

glu·ta·thi·one \ˌglü-tə-'thī-ˌōn\ *n* : a peptide $C_{10}H_{17}N_3O_6S$ that contains one amino-acid residue each of glutamic acid, cysteine, and glycine, that occurs widely in plant and animal tissues, and that plays an important role in biological oxidation-reduction processes and as a coenzyme

glute \\'glüt\ *n* : GLUTEUS — usu. used in pl.

glu·te·al \\'glü-tē-əl, glü-'tē-\ *adj* : of or relating to the buttocks or the gluteus muscles

gluteal artery *n* : either of two branches of the internal iliac artery that supply the gluteal region: **a** : the largest branch of the internal iliac artery that sends branches esp. to the gluteal muscles — called also *superior gluteal artery* **b** : a branch that is distributed esp. to the buttocks and the backs of the thighs — called also *inferior gluteal artery*

gluteal nerve *n* : either of two nerves arising from the sacral plexus and supplying the gluteal muscles and adjacent parts: **a** : one arising from the posterior part of the fourth and fifth lumbar nerves and from the first sacral nerve and distributed to the gluteus muscles and to the tensor fasciae latae — called also *superior gluteal nerve* **b** : one arising from the posterior part of the fifth lumbar nerve and from the first and second sacral nerves and distributed to the gluteus maximus — called also *inferior gluteal nerve*

gluteal tuberosity *n* : the lateral ridge of the linea aspera of the femur that gives attachment to the gluteus maximus

glu·ten \\'glüt-ᵊn\ *n* : a gluey protein substance that causes dough to be sticky

glutes *pl of* GLUTE

glu·teth·i·mide \glü-'te-thə-ˌmīd, -məd\ *n* : a sedative-hypnotic drug $C_{13}H_{15}NO_2$ that induces sleep with less depression of respiration than occurs with comparable doses of barbiturates

glu·te·us \\'glü-tē-əs, glü-'tē-\ *n, pl* **glu-**

tei \\'glü-tē-ˌī, -tē-ˌē; glü-'tē-ˌī\ : any of three large muscles of the buttocks: **a** : GLUTEUS MAXIMUS **b** : GLUTEUS MEDIUS **c** : GLUTEUS MINIMUS

gluteus max·i·mus \-'mak-sə-məs\ *n, pl* **glutei max·i·mi** \-sə-ˌmī\ : the outermost of the three muscles in each buttock that acts to extend and laterally rotate the thigh

gluteus me·di·us \-'mē-dē-us\ *n, pl* **glutei me·dii** \-dē-ˌī\ : the middle of the three muscles in each buttock that acts to abduct and medially rotate the thigh

gluteus min·i·mus \-'mi-nə-məs\ *n, pl* **glutei min·i·mi** \-ˌmī\ : the innermost of the three muscles in each buttock that acts similarly to the gluteus medius

glyc- or glyco- *comb form* : carbohydrate and esp. sugar ⟨glycolysis⟩ ⟨glycoprotein⟩

gly·cae·mia *chiefly Brit var of* GLYCEMIA

gly·can \\'glī-ˌkan\ *n* : POLYSACCHARIDE

gly·ce·mia \glī-'sē-mē-ə\ *n* : the presence of glucose in the blood — **gly·ce·mic** \-'sē-mik\ *adj*

glycer- or glycero- *comb form* **1** : glycerol ⟨glyceryl⟩ **2** : related to glycerol or glyceric acid ⟨glyceraldehyde⟩

glyc·er·al·de·hyde \ˌgli-sə-'ral-də-ˌhīd\ *n* : a sweet crystalline compound $C_3H_6O_3$ that is formed as an intermediate in carbohydrate metabolism

gly·cer·ic acid \gli-'ser-ik-\ *n* : a syrupy acid $C_3H_6O_4$ obtainable by oxidation of glycerol or glyceraldehyde

glyc·er·ide \\'gli-sə-ˌrīd\ *n* : an ester of glycerol esp. with fatty acids

glyc·er·in or glyc·er·ine \\'gli-sə-rən\ *n* : GLYCEROL

glycero- — see GLYCER-

glyc·er·ol \\'gli-sə-ˌrȯl, -ˌrōl\ *n* : a sweet syrupy hygroscopic alcohol $C_3H_8O_3$ containing three hydroxy groups per molecule, usu. obtained by the saponification of fats, and used as a moistening agent, emollient, and lubricant, and as an emulsifying agent — called also *glycerin*

glyc·er·yl \\'gli-sə-rəl\ *n* : a radical derived from glycerol by removal of hydroxide; *esp* : a trivalent radical CH_2CHCH_2

glyceryl guai·a·col·ate \-'gwī-ə-kȯ-ˌlāt, -'gī-, -kə-\ *n* : GUAIFENESIN

gly·cine \\'glī-ˌsēn, 'glīs-ᵊn\ *n* : a sweet crystalline amino acid $C_2H_5NO_2$ obtained esp. by hydrolysis of proteins and used esp. as an antacid

gly·cin·uria \ˌglīs-ᵊn-'ùr-ē-ə, -'yùr-\ *n* : a kidney disorder characterized by the presence of excessive amounts of glycine in the urine

glyco- — see GLYC-

gly·co·bi·ar·sol \ˌglī-kō-(ˌ)bī-'är-ˌsȯl, -sȯl\ *n* : an antiprotozoal drug $C_8H_9AsBiNO_6$ used esp. in the treatment of intestinal amebiasis — see MILIBIS

gly·co·chol·ic acid \ˌglī-kō-ˈkä-lik-, -ˈkō-\ n : a crystalline acid $C_{26}H_{43}NO_6$ that occurs in bile

gly·co·con·ju·gate \ˌglī-kō-ˈkän-ji-gət, -ˌgāt\ n : any of a group of compounds (as the glycolipids and glycoproteins) consisting of sugars linked to proteins or lipids

gly·co·gen \ˈglī-kə-jən\ n : a white amorphous tasteless polysaccharide $(C_6H_{10}O_5)x$ that constitutes the principal form in which carbohydrate is stored in animal tissues and esp. in muscle and liver tissue — called also *animal starch*

gly·co·ge·nase \ˈglī-ˈkä-jə-ˌnās, -ˌnāz\ n : an enzyme that catalyzes the hydrolysis of glycogen

gly·co·gen·e·sis \ˌglī-kə-ˈje-nə-səs\ n, pl -e·ses \-ˌsēz\ : the formation and storage of glycogen — compare GLYCOGENOLYSIS

gly·co·gen·ic \-ˈje-nik\ adj : of, relating to, or involving glycogen or glycogenesis

gly·co·gen·ol·y·sis \ˌglī-kə-jə-ˈnä-lə-səs\ n, pl -y·ses \-ˌsēz\ : the breakdown of glycogen esp. to glucose in the body — compare GLYCOGENESIS — **gly·co·gen·o·lyt·ic** \-jən-əl-ˈi-tik, -ˌjen-\ adj

gly·co·ge·no·sis \ˌglī-kə-jə-ˈnō-səs\ n, pl -no·ses \-ˌsēz\ : GLYCOGEN STORAGE DISEASE

glycogen storage disease n : any of several metabolic disorders (as McArdle's disease or Pompe's disease) that are characterized esp. by abnormal deposits of glycogen in tissue, are caused by enzyme deficiencies in glycogen metabolism, and are usu. inherited as an autosomal recessive trait

gly·co·lip·id \ˌglī-kō-ˈli-pəd\ n : a lipid (as a ganglioside or a cerebroside) that contains a carbohydrate radical

gly·col·y·sis \glī-ˈkä-lə-səs\ n, pl -y·ses \-ˌsēz\ : the enzymatic breakdown of a carbohydrate (as glucose) by way of phosphate derivatives with the production of pyruvic or lactic acid and energy stored in high-energy phosphate bonds of ATP — **gly·co·lyt·ic** \ˌglī-kə-ˈli-tik\ adj — **gly·co·lyt·i·cal·ly** adv

gly·co·pep·tide \ˌglī-kō-ˈpep-ˌtīd\ n : GLYCOPROTEIN

gly·co·pro·tein \-ˈprō-ˌtēn, -ˈprō-tē-ən\ n : a conjugated protein in which the nonprotein group is a carbohydrate — compare GLYCOPROTEIN

gly·co·pyr·ro·late \-ˈpī-rə-ˌlāt\ n : a synthetic anticholinergic drug $C_{19}H_{28}BrNO_3$ used in the treatment of gastrointestinal disorders (as peptic ulcer) esp. when associated with hyperacidity, hypermotility, or spasm — see ROBINUL

gly·cos·ami·no·gly·can \ˌglī-kō-sə-ˌmē-nō-ˈglī-ˌkan, -kō-ˌsa-mə-nō-\ n : any of various polysaccharides derived from an amino hexose that are constituents of mucoproteins, glycoproteins, and blood-group substances — called also *mucopolysaccharide*

gly·co·side \ˈglī-kə-ˌsīd\ n : any of numerous sugar derivatives that contain a nonsugar group attached through an oxygen or nitrogen bond and that on hydrolysis yield a sugar (as glucose) — **gly·co·sid·ic** \ˌglī-kə-ˈsi-dik\ adj — **gly·co·sid·i·cal·ly** adv

gly·co·sphin·go·lip·id \ˌglī-kō-ˌsfiŋ-gō-ˈli-pəd\ n : any of various lipids (as a cerebroside or a ganglioside) which are derivatives of ceramides and some of which accumulate in disorders of lipid metabolism (as Tay-Sachs disease)

gly·cos·uria \ˌglī-kō-ˈshùr-ē-ə, -ˈsyùr-\ n : the presence in the urine of abnormal amounts of sugar — called also *glucosuria* — **gly·cos·uric** \-ˈshùr-ik, -ˈsyùr-\ adj

glyc·yr·rhi·za \ˌglī-sə-ˈrī-zə\ n : the dried root of a licorice (*Glycyrrhiza glabra* of the legume family, Leguminosae) that is a source of extracts used to mask unpleasant flavors (as in drugs) or to give a pleasant taste (as to confections) — called also *licorice, licorice root*

gm abbr gram

GM and S abbr General Medicine and Surgery

GM–CSF abbr granulocyte-macrophage colony-stimulating factor

GN abbr graduate nurse

gnat \ˈnat\ n : any of various small usu. biting dipteran flies (as a midge or blackfly)

gna·thi·on \ˈnā-thē-ˌän, ˈna-\ n : the midpoint of the lower border of the human mandible

gna·thos·to·mi·a·sis \nə-ˌthäs-tə-ˈmī-ə-səs\ n, pl -a·ses \-ˌsēz\ : infestation with or disease caused by nematode worms (genus *Gnathostoma*) commonly acquired by eating raw fish

-g·na·thous \g-nə-thəs\ adj comb form : having (such) a jaw (prognathous)

-g·no·sia \g-ˈnō-zhə\ n comb form : -GNOSIS (agnosia) (prosopagnosia)

-g·no·sis \g-ˈnō-səs\ n comb form, pl -g·no·ses \-ˌsēz\ : knowledge : cognition : recognition (stereognosis)

-g·nos·tic \g-ˈnäs-tik\ adj comb form : characterized by or relating to (such) knowledge (pharmacognostic)

-g·no·sy \g-nə-sē\ n comb form, pl -g·no·sies : -GNOSIS (pharmacognosy)

GnRH abbr gonadotropin-releasing hormone

goal–directed adj : aimed toward a goal or toward completion of a task (∼ behavior)

goblet cell n : a mucus-secreting epithelial cell (as of columnar epithelium) that is distended with secretion or its precursors at the free end

goi·ter \ˈgȯi-tər\ n : an enlargement of the thyroid gland that is commonly visible as a swelling of the anterior part of the neck, that often results from insufficient intake of iodine and then is usu. accompanied by hypothyroidism, and that in other cases is associated with hyperthyroidism usu. together with toxic symptoms and exophthalmos — called also *struma* — **goi·trous** \'gȯi-trəs\ *also* **goi·ter·ous** \'gȯi-tə-rəs\ *adj*

goi·tre *chiefly Brit var of* GOITER

goi·tro·gen \'gȯi-trə-jən\ *n* : a substance (as thiourea or thiouracil) that induces goiter formation

goi·tro·gen·ic \ˌgȯi-trə-'je-nik\ *also* **goi·ter·o·gen·ic** \ˌgȯi-tə-rō-'je-nik\ *adj* : producing or tending to produce goiter (a ~ agent) — **goi·tro·ge·nic·i·ty** \ˌgȯi-trə-jə-'ni-sə-tē\ *n*

gold \'gōld\ *n, often attrib* : a malleable ductile yellow metallic element used in the form of its salts (as gold sodium thiomalate) esp. in the treatment of rheumatoid arthritis — symbol *Au;* see ELEMENT table

gold sodium thio·ma·late \-ˌthī-ō-'ma-lāt, -'mä-\ *n* : a gold salt $C_4H_3Au-Na_2O_4S\cdot H_2O$ used in the treatment of rheumatoid arthritis — called also *gold thiomalate;* see MYOCHRYSINE

gold sodium thiosulfate *n* : a soluble gold compound $Na_3Au(S_2O_3)_2\cdot 2H_2O$ administered by intravenous injection in the treatment of rheumatoid arthritis and lupus erythematosus

gold thio·glu·cose \-ˌthī-ō-'glü-ˌkōs\ *n* : an enzyme organic compound of gold $C_6H_{11}AuO_5S$ injected intramuscularly in the treatment of active rheumatoid arthritis and nondisseminated lupus erythematosus — called also *aurothioglucose*

Gol·gi \'gōl-(ˌ)jē\ *adj* : of or relating to the Golgi apparatus, Golgi bodies, or the Golgi method of staining nerve tissue

Golgi, Camillo (1843 *or* 1844–1926), Italian histologist and pathologist.

Golgi apparatus *n* : a cytoplasmic organelle that consists of a stack of smooth membranous saccules and associated vesicles and that is active in the modification and transport of proteins — called also *Golgi complex*

Golgi body *n* : GOLGI APPARATUS; *also* : DICTYOSOME

Golgi cell *n* : a neuron with short dendrites and with either a long axon or an axon that breaks into processes soon after leaving the cell body

Golgi complex *n* : GOLGI APPARATUS

Golgi tendon organ *n* : a spindle-shaped sensory end organ within a tendon that provides information about muscle tension — called also *neurotendinous spindle*

go·mer \'gō-mər\ *n, med slang* : a chronic problem patient who does not respond to treatment — usu. used disparagingly

gom·pho·sis \gäm-'fō-səs\ *n* : an im-

movable articulation in which a hard part is received into a bone cavity (as the teeth into the jaws)

go·nad \'gō-ˌnad\ *n* : a gamete-producing reproductive gland (as an ovary or testis) — **go·nad·al** \gō-'nad-ᵊl\ *adj*

go·nad·o·troph \gō-'na-də-ˌtrōf\ *n* : a cell of the adenohypophysis that secretes a gonadotropic hormone (as luteinizing hormone)

go·nad·o·trop·ic \ˌgō-ˌna-də-'trä-pik\ *also* **go·nad·o·tro·phic** \-'trō-fik, -'trä-\ *adj* : acting on or stimulating the gonads

go·nad·o·tro·pin \-'trō-pən\ *also* **go·nad·o·tro·phin** \-fən\ *n* : a gonadotropic hormone (as follicle-stimulating hormone)

gonadotropin–releasing hormone *n* : a hormone produced by the hypothalamus that stimulates the adenohypophysis to release gonadotropins (as luteinizing hormone and follicle-stimulating hormone) — called also *luteinizing hormone-releasing hormone*

G₁ phase \ˌjē-'wən-\ *n* : the period in the cell cycle from the end of cell division to the beginning of DNA replication — compare G₂ PHASE, M PHASE, S PHASE

goni- *or* **gonio-** *comb form* : corner : angle (*gonio*meter)

gonial angle *n* : the angle formed by the junction of the posterior and lower borders of the human lower jaw — called also *angle of the jaw, angle of the mandible*

go·ni·om·e·ter \ˌgō-nē-'ä-mə-tər\ *n* : an instrument for measuring angles (as of a joint or the skull) — **go·nio·met·ric** \-nē-ə-'me-trik\ *adj* — **go·ni·om·e·try** \-nē-'ä-mə-trē\ *n*

go·nio·punc·ture \'gō-nē-ə-ˌpəŋk-chər\ *n* : a surgical operation for congenital glaucoma that involves making a puncture into the sclera with a knife at the site of discharge of aqueous fluid at the periphery of the anterior chamber of the eye

go·ni·o·scope \-ˌskōp\ *n* : an instrument consisting of a contact lens to be fitted over the cornea and an optical system with which the interior of the eye can be viewed — **go·ni·os·co·py** \ˌgō-nē-'äs-kə-pē\ *n*

go·ni·ot·o·my \ˌgō-nē-'ä-tə-mē\ *n, pl* **-mies** : surgical relief of glaucoma used in some congenital types and achieved by opening the canal of Schlemm

go·ni·tis \gō-'nī-təs\ *n* : inflammation of the knee

gono·coc·cae·mia *chiefly Brit var of* GONOCOCCEMIA

gono·coc·ce·mia \ˌgä-nə-ˌkäk-'sē-mē-ə\ *n* : the presence of gonococci in the blood — **gono·coc·ce·mic** \-'sē-mik\ *adj*

gono·coc·cus \ˌgä-nə-'kä-kəs\ *n, pl* **-coc-**

ci \-ˈkäk-ˌsī, -ˌsē; -ˈkä-ˌkī, -ˌkē\ : a pus-producing bacterium of the genus *Neisseria* (*N. gonorrhoeae*) that causes gonorrhea — **gono·coc·cal** \-ˈkä-kəl\ *adj*

gon·or·rhea \ˌgä-nə-ˈrē-ə\ *n* : a contagious inflammation of the genital mucous membrane caused by the gonococcus — called also *clap* — **gon·or·rhe·al** \-ˈrē-əl\ *adj*

gon·or·rhoea *chiefly Brit var of* GONORRHEA

-g·o·ny \gə-nē\ *n comb form, pl* **-g·o·nies** : manner of generation or reproduction ⟨schizo*gony*⟩

go·ny·au·lax \ˌgō-nē-ˈȯ-ˌlaks\ *n* **1** *cap* : a large genus of phosphorescent marine dinoflagellates that when unusually abundant cause red tide **2** : any dinoflagellate of the genus *Gonyaulax*

Good·pas·ture's syndrome \ˈgu̇d-ˌpas-chərz-\ *also* **Good·pas·ture syndrome** \-chər-\ *n* : a hypersensitivity disorder of unknown cause that is characterized by the presence of circulating antibodies in the blood which react with antigens in the basement membrane of the kidney's glomeruli and with antigens in the lungs producing combined glomerulonephritis and pulmonary hemorrhages

Goodpasture, Ernest William (1886–1960), American pathologist.

goose bumps *n pl* : a roughness of the skin produced by erection of its papillae esp. from cold, fear, or a sudden feeling of excitement — called also *goose pimples*

goose·flesh \-ˌflesh\ *n* : GOOSE BUMPS

gork \ˈgȯrk\ *n, med slang* : a terminal patient whose brain is nonfunctional and the rest of whose body can be kept functioning only by the extensive use of mechanical devices and nutrient solutions — usu. used disparagingly — **gorked** \ˈgȯrkt\ *adj, med slang*

goun·dou \ˈgün-(ˌ)dü\ *n* : a tumorous swelling of the nose often considered a late lesion of yaws — compare GANGOSA

gout \ˈgau̇t\ *n* : a metabolic disease marked by a painful inflammation of the joints, deposits of urates in and around the joints, and usu. an excessive amount of uric acid in the blood — **gouty** \ˈgau̇-tē\ *adj*

GP *abbr* general practitioner

G₁ phase, G₂ phase — see entries alphabetized as G ONE PHASE, G TWO PHASE

G protein \ˈjē-\ *n* : any of a group of proteins in cell membranes that upon activation by a hormone initiate a series of molecular events inside the cell

gr *abbr* **1** grain **2** gram **3** gravity

graaf·ian follicle \ˈgrä-fē-ən-, ˈgra-\ *n, often cap G* : a liquid-filled cavity in a mammalian ovary containing a ma-

ture egg before ovulation — called also *vesicular ovarian follicle*

Graaf \də-ˈgräf\, **Reinier de (1641–1673),** Dutch physician and anatomist.

grac·ile fasciculus \ˈgra-səl-, -ˌsil-\ *n, pl* **gracile fasciculi** : FASCICULUS GRACILIS

grac·i·lis \ˈgra-sə-ləs\ *n* : the most superficial muscle of the inside of the thigh that acts to adduct the thigh and to flex the leg at the knee and assist in rotating it medially

graduate nurse *n* : a person who has completed the regular course of study and practical hospital training in nursing school — called also *trained nurse;* abbr. GN

¹graft \ˈgraft\ *vb* : to implant (living tissue) surgically

²graft *n* **1** : the act of grafting **2** : something grafted; *specif* : living tissue used in grafting

graft–versus–host *adj* : relating to or being the bodily condition that results when cells from a tissue or organ transplant mount an immunological attack against the cells or tissues of the host ⟨~ disease⟩

grain \ˈgrān\ *n* : a unit of avoirdupois, Troy, and apothecaries' weight equal to 0.0648 gram or 0.002286 avoirdupois ounce or 0.002083 Troy ounce — abbr. *gr*

grain alcohol *n* : ETHANOL

grain itch *n* : an itching rash caused by the bite of a mite of the genus *Pyemotes* (*P. ventricosus*) that occurs chiefly on grain, straw, or straw products — compare GROCER'S ITCH

gram \ˈgram\ *n* : a metric unit of mass and weight equal to ¹⁄₁₀₀₀ kilogram and nearly equal to one cubic centimeter of water at its maximum density — abbr. *g*

-gram \ˌgram\ *n comb form* : drawing : writing : record ⟨cardio*gram*⟩

gram calorie *n* : CALORIE 1a

gram·i·ci·din \ˌgra-mə-ˈsīd-ᵊn\ *n* : an antibacterial mixture produced by a soil bacterium of the genus *Bacillus* (*B. brevis*) and used topically against gram-positive bacteria in local infections esp. of the eye

gramme *chiefly Brit var of* GRAM

gram–negative *adj* : not holding the purple dye when stained by Gram's stain — used chiefly of bacteria

gram–positive *adj* : holding the purple dye when stained by Gram's stain — used chiefly of bacteria

Gram's solution \ˈgramz-\ *n* : a watery solution of iodine and the iodide of potassium used in staining bacteria by Gram's stain

Gram \ˈgräm\, **Hans Christian Joachim (1853–1938),** Danish physician.

Gram's stain *or* **Gram stain** \ˈgram-\ *n* **1** : a method for the differential staining of bacteria by treatment with Gram's solution after staining with a triphenylmethane dye — called also *Gram's method* **2** : the chemicals used in Gram's stain

gram–variable *adj* : staining irregularly or inconsistently by Gram's stain

gran·di·ose \'gran-dē-₁ōs, ₁gran-dē-'\ *adj* : characterized by affectation of grandeur or splendor or by absurd exaggeration ⟨∼ delusions⟩ — **gran·di·os·i·ty** \₁gran-dē-'äs-ət-ē\ *n*

grand mal \'grän-₁mäl, 'grän-, 'grand-, -'mäl\ *n* : epilepsy due to an inborn usu. inherited dysrhythmia of the electrical pulsations of the brain as demonstrated by an electroencephalogram and characterized by attacks of violent convulsions, coma, constitutional disturbances, and usu. amnesia — compare PETIT MAL

grand rounds *n* : rounds involving the formal presentation by an expert of a clinical issue sometimes in the presence of selected patients

granul- *or* **granuli-** *or* **granulo-** *comb form* : granule ⟨*granulocyte*⟩

gran·u·lar \'gran-yə-lər\ *adj* **1** : consisting of or appearing to consist of granules : having a grainy texture **2** : having or marked by granulations ⟨∼ tissue⟩ — **gran·u·lar·i·ty** \₁gran-yə-'lar-ə-tē\ *n*

granular conjunctivitis *n* : TRACHOMA

granular leukocyte *n* : a blood granulocyte; *esp* : a polymorphonuclear leukocyte

gran·u·late \'gran-yə-₁lāt\ *vb* **-lat·ed; -lat·ing 1** : to form or crystallize (as sugar) into grains or granules **2** : to form granulations ⟨a *granulating* wound⟩

gran·u·la·tion \₁gran-yə-'lā-shən\ *n* **1** : the act or process of granulating : the condition of being granulated **2 a** : one of the small elevations of a granulated surface: (1) : a minute mass of tissue projecting from the surface of an organ (as on the eyelids in trachoma) (2) : one of the minute red granules made up of loops of newly formed capillaries that form on a raw surface (as of a wound) and that with fibroblasts are the active agents in the process of healing — see GRANULATION TISSUE **b** : the act or process of forming such elevations or granules

granulation tissue *n* : tissue made up of granulations that temporarily replaces lost tissue in a wound

gran·ule \'gran-(₁)yül\ *n* : a little grain or small particle; *esp* : one of a number of particles forming a larger unit

granule cell *n* : one of the small neurons of the cortex of the cerebellum and cerebrum

granuli- — see GRANUL-

granulo- — see GRANUL-

gran·u·lo·cyte \'gran-yə-lō-₁sīt\ *n* : a polymorphonuclear white blood cell with granule-containing cytoplasm — compare AGRANULOCYTE — **gran·u·lo·cyt·ic** \₁gran-yə-lō-'si-tik\ *adj*

granulocytic leukemia *n* : MYELOGENOUS LEUKEMIA

gran·u·lo·cy·to·pe·nia \₁gran-yə-lō-₁sī-tə-'pē-nē-ə\ *n* : deficiency of blood granulocytes; *esp* : AGRANULOCYTOSIS — **gran·u·lo·cy·to·pe·nic** \-'pē-nik\ *adj*

gran·u·lo·cy·to·poi·e·sis \-₁sī-tə-₁pòi-'ē-səs\ *n, pl* **-e·ses** \-₁sēz\ : GRANULOPOIESIS

gran·u·lo·cy·to·sis \₁gran-yə-lō-₁sī-'tō-səs\ *n, pl* **-to·ses** \-₁sēz\ : an increase in the number of blood granulocytes — compare LYMPHOCYTOSIS, MONOCYTOSIS

gran·u·lo·ma \₁gran-yə-'lō-mə\ *n, pl* **-mas** *or* **-ma·ta** \-mə-tə\ : a mass or nodule of chronically inflamed tissue with granulations that is usu. associated with an infective process

granuloma an·nu·la·re \-₁a-nyü-'lar-ē\ *n* : a benign chronic rash of unknown cause characterized by one or more flat spreading ringlike spots with lighter centers esp. on the feet, legs, hands, or fingers

granuloma in·gui·na·le \-₁iŋ-gwə-'na-lē, -'nä-, -'nä-l\ *n* : a sexually transmitted disease characterized by ulceration and formation of granulations on the genitalia and in the groin area and caused by a bacterium of the genus *Calymmatobacterium* (*C. granulomatis* syn. *Donovania granulomatis*) which is usu. recovered from lesions as Donovan bodies

gran·u·lo·ma·to·sis \₁gran-yə-₁lō-mə-'tō-səs\ *n, pl* **-to·ses** \-₁sēz\ : a chronic condition marked by the formation of numerous granulomas

gran·u·lo·ma·tous \-'lō-mə-təs\ *adj* : of, relating to, or characterized by granuloma

gran·u·lo·poi·e·sis \-(₁)lō-₁pòi-'ē-səs\ *n, pl* **-e·ses** \-₁sēz\ : the formation of blood granulocytes typically in the bone marrow — **gran·u·lo·poi·et·ic** \-₁pòi-'e-tik\ *adj*

gran·u·lo·sa cell \₁gran-yə-'lō-sə-, -zə-\ *n* : one of the estrogen-secreting cells of the epithelial lining of a graafian follicle or its follicular precursor

granulosum — see STRATUM GRANULOSUM

grapes \'grāps\ *n sing or pl* **1** : a cluster of raw red nodules of granulation tissue in the hollow of the fetlock of horses that is characteristic of advanced or chronic grease heel **2** : tuberculous disease of the pleura in cattle — called also *grape disease*

grape sugar \'grāp-\ *n* : DEXTROSE

-graph \₁graf\ *n comb form* **1** : something written ⟨mono*graph*⟩ **2** : instrument for making or transmitting records ⟨electrocardio*graph*⟩

-graph·ia \'gra-fē-ə\ *n comb form* : writing characteristic of a (specified) usu. psychological abnormality ⟨dys*graphia*⟩ ⟨dermo*graphia*⟩

grapho- *comb form* : writing ⟨*graphol-ogy*⟩

gra·phol·o·gy \gra-ˈfä-lə-jē\ *n, pl* **-gies** : the study of handwriting esp. for the purpose of character analysis — **graph·o·log·i·cal** \ˌgra-fə-ˈlä-ji-kəl\ *adj* — **gra·phol·o·gist** \gra-ˈfä-lə-jist\ *n*

grapho·ma·nia \ˌgra-fō-ˈmā-nē-ə, -nyə\ *n* : a morbid and compulsive desire for writing — **grapho·ma·ni·ac** \-nē-ˌak\ *n*

grapho·spasm \ˈgra-fə-ˌspa-zəm\ *n* : WRITER'S CRAMP

gras — see TULLE GRAS

GRAS *abbr* generally recognized as safe

grass \ˈgras\ *n* : MARIJUANA

grass sickness *n* : a frequently fatal disease of grazing horses of unknown cause that affects gastrointestinal functioning by causing difficulty in swallowing, interruption of peristalsis, and fecal impaction — called also *grass disease*

grass staggers *n* : GRASS TETANY

grass tetany *n* : a disease of cattle and esp. milk cows marked by tetanic staggering, convulsions, coma, and frequently death and caused by reduction of blood calcium and magnesium when overeating on lush pasture — called also *hypomagnesia*; compare MILK FEVER 2, STAGGERS 1

grav *abbr* gravida

grave \ˈgrāv\ *adj* : very serious : dangerous to life — used of an illness or its prospects ⟨a ∼ prognosis⟩

grav·el \ˈgra-vəl\ *n* **1** : a deposit of small calculous concretions in the kidneys and urinary bladder **2** : the condition that results from the presence of deposits of gravel

Graves' disease \ˈgrāvz-\ *n* : a common form of hyperthyroidism characterized by goiter and often a slight protrusion of the eyeballs — called also *Basedow's disease, exophthalmic goiter*

Graves, Robert James (1796–1853), British physician.

grav·id \ˈgra-vəd\ *adj* : PREGNANT

grav·i·da \ˈgra-və-də\ *n, pl* **-i·das** *or* **-i·dae** \-ˌdē\ : a pregnant woman — often used in combination with a number or figure to indicate the number of pregnancies a woman has had ⟨a 4-*gravida*⟩; compare PARA — **gra·vid·ic** \gra-ˈvi-dik\ *adj*

gra·vid·i·ty \gra-ˈvi-də-tē\ *n, pl* **-ties** : PREGNANCY, PARITY

gravior — see ICHTHYOSIS HYSTRIX GRAVIOR

gravis — see ICTERUS GRAVIS, ICTERUS GRAVIS NEONATORUM, MYASTHENIA GRAVIS

grav·i·ta·tion \ˌgra-və-ˈtā-shən\ *n* : a natural force of attraction that tends to draw bodies together and that occurs because of the mass of the bodies — **grav·i·ta·tion·al** \-shə-nəl\ *adj* — **grav·i·ta·tion·al·ly** *adv*

gravitational field *n* : the space around an object having mass in which the object's gravitational influence can be detected

grav·i·ty \ˈgra-və-tē\ *n, pl* **-ties** : the gravitational attraction of the mass of a celestial object (as earth) for bodies close to it; *also* : GRAVITATION

gray \ˈgrā\ *n* : the mks unit of absorbed dose of ionizing radiation equal to an energy of one joule per kilogram of irradiated material — abbr. *Gy*

Gray, Louis Harold (1905–1965), British radiobiologist.

gray column *n* : any of the longitudinal columns of gray matter in each lateral half of the spinal cord — compare COLUMN a

gray commissure *n* : a transverse band of gray matter in the spinal cord appearing in sections as the transverse bar of the H-shaped mass of gray matter

gray matter *n* : neural tissue esp. of the brain and spinal cord that contains cell bodies as well as nerve fibers, has a brownish gray color, and forms most of the cortex and nuclei of the brain, the columns of the spinal cord, and the bodies of ganglia — called also *gray substance*

gray·out \ˈgrā-ˌau̇t\ *n* : a transient dimming or haziness of vision resulting from temporary impairment of cerebral circulation — compare BLACK-OUT, REDOUT — **gray out** *vb*

gray ramus *n* : RAMUS COMMUNICANS b

gray substance *n* : GRAY MATTER

gray syndrome *n* : a potentially fatal toxic reaction to chloramphenicol esp. in premature infants that is characterized by abdominal distension, cyanosis, vasomotor collapse, and irregular respiration

grease heel *n* : a chronic inflammation of the skin of the fetlocks and pasterns of horses marked by an excess of oily secretion, ulcerations, and in severe cases general swelling of the legs, nodular excrescences, and a foul-smelling discharge and usu. affecting horses with thick coarse legs kept or worked under unsanitary conditions — called also *greasy heel*; see GRAPES 1

great cerebral vein *n* : a broad unpaired vein formed by the junction of Galen's veins and uniting with the inferior sagittal sinus to form the straight sinus

great·er cornu \ˈgrāt-ər-\ *n* : THYROHYAL

greater curvature *n* : the boundary of the stomach that forms a long usu. convex curve on the left from the opening for the esophagus to the opening into the duodenum — compare LESSER CURVATURE

greater multangular *n* : TRAPEZIUM — called also *greater multangular bone*

greater occipital nerve n : OCCIPITAL NERVE a

greater omentum n : a part of the peritoneum attached to the greater curvature of the stomach and to the colon and hanging down over the small intestine — called also *caul*; compare LESSER OMENTUM

greater palatine artery n : PALATINE ARTERY 1b

greater palatine foramen n : a foramen in each posterior side of the palate giving passage to the greater palatine artery and to a palatine nerve

greater petrosal nerve n : a mixed nerve that contains mostly sensory and some parasympathetic fibers, arises in the geniculate ganglion, joins with the deep petrosal nerve at the entrance of the pterygoid canal to form the Vidian nerve, and as part of this nerve sends sensory fibers to the soft palate with some to the eustachian tube and sends parasympathetic fibers forming the motor root of the pterygopalatine ganglion — called also *greater superficial petrosal nerve*

greater sciatic foramen n : SCIATIC FORAMEN a

greater sciatic notch n : SCIATIC NOTCH a

greater splanchnic nerve n : SPLANCHNIC NERVE a

greater superficial petrosal nerve n : GREATER PETROSAL NERVE

greater trochanter *also* **great trochanter** n : TROCHANTER a

greater tubercle n : a prominence on the upper lateral part of the end of the humerus that serves as the insertion for the supraspinatus, infraspinatus, and teres minor — compare LESSER TUBERCLE

greater vestibular gland n : BARTHOLIN'S GLAND

greater wing *also* **great wing** n : a broad curved winglike expanse on each side of the sphenoid bone — called also *alisphenoid*; compare LESSER WING

great ragweed n : RAGWEED b

great saphenous vein n : SAPHENOUS VEIN a

great toe n : BIG TOE

great white shark n : a large shark (*Carcharodon carcharias* of the family Lamnidae) that is bluish when young but becomes whitish with age and is noted for aggressively attacking humans — called also *white shark*

green \'grēn\ *adj* **1** *of a wound* : being recently incurred and unhealed **2** *of hemolytic streptococci* : tending to produce green pigment when cultured on blood media

green monkey n : a long-tailed African monkey (*Cercopithecus aethiops*) with greenish-appearing hair that is often used in medical research

green monkey disease n : a febrile infectious often fatal virus disease characterized esp. by encephalitis, hepatitis, and renal involvement and orig. transmitted to humans from green monkeys — called also *Marburg disease*; see MARBURG VIRUS

green·sick·ness \'grēn-ˌsik-nəs\ n : CHLOROSIS — **green·sick** *adj*

green soap n : a soft soap made from vegetable oils and used esp. in the treatment of skin diseases

green·stick fracture \'grēn-ˌstik-\ n : a bone fracture in a young individual in which the bone is partly broken and partly bent

grew *past of* GROW

grey·out *chiefly Brit var of* GRAYOUT

¹**gripe** \'grīp\ vb **griped**; **grip·ing** : to cause or experience pinching and spasmodic pain in the bowels of

²**gripe** n : a pinching spasmodic intestinal pain — usu. used in pl.

grippe \'grip\ n : an acute febrile contagious virus disease; *esp* : INFLUENZA 1a — **grippy** \'gri-pē\ *adj*

gris·eo·ful·vin \ˌgri-zē-ō-ˈful-vən,-sē-, -ˈfal-\ n : a fungistatic antibiotic $C_{17}H_{17}ClO_6$ used systemically in treating superficial infections by fungi esp. of the genera *Epidermophyton*, *Microsporum*, and *Trichophyton*

grocer's itch n : an itching dermatitis that results from prolonged contact with some mites (esp. family Acaridae), their products, or materials (as feeds) infested with them — called also *baker's itch*; compare GRAIN ITCH

groin \'groin\ n : the fold or depression marking the juncture of the lower abdomen and the inner part of the thigh; *also* : the region of this line

groove \'grüv\ n : a long narrow depression occurring naturally on the surface of an anatomical part

gross \'grōs\ *adj* **1** : glaringly or flagrantly obvious **2** : visible without the aid of a microscope : MACROSCOPIC (~ lesions) — compare OCCULT

gross anatomist n : a specialist in gross anatomy

gross anatomy n : a branch of anatomy that deals with the macroscopic structure of tissues and organs — compare HISTOLOGY

ground itch n : an itching inflammation of the skin marking the point of entrance into the body of larval hookworms

ground substance n : a more or less homogeneous matrix that forms the background in which the specific differentiated elements of a system are suspended: **a** : the intercellular substance of tissues **b** : CYTOSOL

group dynamics n *sing or pl* : the interacting forces within a small human group; *also* : the sociological study of these forces

group practice n : medicine practiced by a group of associated physicians or dentists (as specialists in different fields) working as partners or as partners and employees

group psychotherapy n : GROUP THERAPY

group therapy n : therapy in the presence of a therapist in which several patients discuss and share their personal problems — **group therapist** n

grow \'grō\ vb **grew** \'grü\; **grown** \'grōn\; **grow·ing 1 a :** to spring up and develop to maturity **b :** to be able to grow in some place or situation **c :** to assume some relation through or as if through a process of natural growth ⟨the cut edges of the wound grew together⟩ **2 :** to increase in size by addition of material by assimilation into the living organism or by accretion in a nonbiological process (as crystallization)

growing pains n pl : pains occurring in the legs of growing children having no demonstrable relation to growth

growth \'grōth\ n **1 a** (1) : a stage in the process of growing (2) : full growth **b** : the process of growing **2 a :** something that grows or has grown **b :** an abnormal proliferation of tissue (as a tumor)

growth factor n : a substance (as a vitamin B_{12} or an interleukin) that promotes growth and esp. cellular growth

growth hormone n : a polypeptide hormone that is secreted by the anterior lobe of the pituitary gland and regulates growth — called also somatotropic hormone, somatotropin

growth plate n : the region in a long bone between the epiphysis and diaphysis where growth in length occurs — called also physis

g's or **gs** pl of G

G6PD abbr glucose-6-phosphate dehydrogenase

GSR abbr galvanic skin response

G suit n : a suit designed to counteract the physiological effects of acceleration on an aviator or astronaut

GSW abbr gunshot wound

GTP \ˌjē-(ˌ)tē-ˈpē\ n : an energy-rich nucleotide analogous to ATP that is composed of guanine linked to ribose and three phosphate groups and is necessary for peptide-bond formation during protein synthesis — called also guanosine triphosphate

G₂ phase \ˌjē-ˈtü-\ n : the period in the cell cycle from the completion of DNA replication to the beginning of cell division — compare G₁ PHASE, M PHASE, S PHASE

GU abbr genitourinary

guai·ac \'gwī-ˌak\ n : GUAIACUM

guai·a·col \'gwī-ə-ˌkȯl, -ˌkōl\ n : a liquid or solid $C_7H_8O_2$ with an aromatic odor used chiefly as an expectorant and as a local anesthetic

guaiac test n : a test for blood in urine or feces using a reagent containing guaiacum that yields a blue color when blood is present — see HEMOCCULT

guai·a·cum \'gwī-ə-kəm\ n : a resin with a faint balsamic odor obtained as tears or masses from the trunk of either of two trees (Guaiacum officinale and G. sanctum of the family Zygophyllaceae) and used in various tests (as the guaiac test)

guai·fen·e·sin \gwī-ˈfe-nə-sən\ n : the glyceryl ether of guaiacol $C_{10}H_{14}O_4$ that is used esp. as an expectorant — called also glyceryl guaiacolate

gua·neth·i·dine \gwä-ˈne-thə-ˌdēn\ n : a drug $C_{10}H_{22}N_4$ used esp. as the sulfate in treating severe high blood pressure

gua·ni·dine \'gwä-nə-ˌdēn\ n : a base CH_5N_3 derived from guanine and used as a parasympathetic stimulant in medicine esp. as the hydrochloride salt

gua·nine \'gwä-ˌnēn\ n : a purine base $C_5H_5N_5O$ that codes genetic information in the polynucleotide chain of DNA or RNA — compare ADENINE, CYTOSINE, THYMINE, URACIL

gua·no·sine \'gwä-nə-ˌsēn\ n : a nucleoside $C_{10}H_{13}N_5O_5$ composed of guanine and ribose

guanosine 3', 5'–monophosphate n : CYCLIC GMP

guanosine triphosphate n : GTP

gua·nyl·ate cy·clase \ˈgwän-ᵊl-ˌāt-ˈsī-ˌklās, -ˈklāz\ n : an enzyme that catalyzes the formation of cyclic GMP from GTP

guard·ing \'gär-diŋ\ n : involuntary reaction to protect an area of pain (as by spasm of muscle on palpation of the abdomen over a painful lesion)

gu·ber·nac·u·lum \ˌgü-bər-ˈna-kyü-ləm\ n, pl **-la** \-lə\ : a fibrous cord that connects the fetal testis with the bottom of the scrotum and by failing to elongate in proportion to the rest of the fetus causes the descent of the testis

guide \'gīd\ n : a grooved director for a surgical probe or knife

Guil·lain–Bar·ré syndrome \ˌgē-ˈlan-ˌbä-ˈrā-, ˌgē-ˈyaⁿ-\ n : a polyneuritis of unknown cause characterized esp. by muscle weakness and paralysis — called also Landry's paralysis

Guillain \gē-ˈyaⁿ\, **Georges Charles** (1876–1961), and **Barré** \bä-ˈrā\, **Jean Alexander** (b 1880), French neurologists.

guil·lo·tine \'gi-lə-ˌtēn, ˈgē-ə-\ n : a surgical instrument that consists of a ring and handle with a knife blade which slides down the handle and across the ring and that is used for cutting out a protruding structure (as a tonsil) capable of being placed in the ring

Guil·lo·tin \gē-yō-ˈtaⁿ\, **Joseph–Ignace** (1738–1814), French surgeon.

guillotine amputation n : an emergency surgical amputation (as of a leg) in which the skin is incised around the part being amputated and is allowed to retract, successive layers of muscle are then divided around the part, and finally the bone is divided

guilt \'gilt\ *n* : feelings of culpability esp. for imagined offenses or from a sense of inadequacy : morbid self-reproach often manifest in marked preoccupation with the moral correctness of one's behavior

guin·ea worm \'gi-nē-\ *n* : a slender nematode worm of the genus *Dracunculus* (*D. medinensis*) attaining a length of several feet, being parasitic as an adult in the subcutaneous tissues of mammals including humans in tropical regions, and having a larva that develops in small freshwater crustaceans (as of the genus *Cyclops* of the order Copepoda) and when ingested with drinking water passes through the intestinal wall and tissues to lodge beneath the skin of a mammalian host where it matures — called also *Medina worm*

gul·let \'gə-lət\ *n* : ESOPHAGUS; *broadly* : THROAT

gum \'gəm\ *n* : the tissue that surrounds the necks of teeth and covers the alveolar parts of the jaws; *broadly* : the alveolar portion of a jaw with its enveloping soft tissues

gum ar·a·bic \-'ar-ə-bik\ *n* : a water-soluble gum obtained from several leguminous plants (genus *Acacia* and esp. *A. senegal* and *A. arabica*) and used esp. in pharmacy to suspend insoluble substances in water, to prepare emulsions, and to make pills and lozenges — called also *acacia, gum acacia*

gum·boil \'gəm-ˌbȯil\ *n* : an abscess in the gum

gum karaya *n* : KARAYA GUM

gum·line \'gəm-ˌlīn\ *n* : the line separating the gum from the exposed part of the tooth

gum·ma \'gə-mə\ *n, pl* **gummas** *also* **gum·ma·ta** \-mə-tə\ : a tumor of gummy or rubbery consistency that is characteristic of the tertiary stage of syphilis — **gum·ma·tous** \-mə-təs\ *adj*

gum tragacanth *n* : TRAGACANTH

gur·ney \'gər-nē\ *n, pl* **gurneys** : a wheeled cot or stretcher

gus·ta·tion \ˌgəs-'tā-shən\ *n* : the act or sensation of tasting

gus·ta·to·ry \'gəs-tə-ˌtȯr-ē\ *adj* : relating to, affecting, associated with, or being the sense of taste

gut \'gət\ *n* **1 a** : the alimentary canal or part of it (as the intestine or stomach) **b** : ABDOMEN 1a, BELLY — usu. used in pl.; not often in formal use **2** : CATGUT

Guthrie test \'gə-thrē-\ *n* : a test for phenylketonuria in which the plasma phenylalanine of an affected individual reverses the inhibition of a strain of bacteria of the genus *Bacillus* (*B. subtilis*) needing it for growth

Guthrie, Robert (*b* 1916), American microbiologist.

gut·ta–per·cha \ˌgə-tə-'pər-chə\ *n* : a tough plastic substance from the latex of several Malaysian trees (genera *Payena* and *Palaquium*) of the sapodilla family (Sapotaceae) that is used in dentistry in temporary fillings

gut·tate \'gə-ˌtāt\ *adj* : having small usu. colored spots or drops

gut·ter \'gə-tər\ *n* : a depressed furrow between body parts (as on the surface between a pair of adjacent ribs)

Gut·zeit test \'güt-ˌsīt-\ *n* : a test for arsenic used esp. in toxicology

Gutzeit, Ernst Wilhelm Heinrich (1845–1888), German chemist.

GVH *abbr* graft-versus-host

Gy *abbr* gray

Gym·no·din·i·um \ˌjim-nə-'di-nē-əm\ *n* : a large genus of marine and freshwater dinoflagellates (family Gymnodiniidae) that includes a few forms which cause red tide

gyn *abbr* gynecologic; gynecologist; gynecology

gynaec- *or* **gynaeco-** *chiefly Brit var of* GYNEC-

gy·nae·coid, gy·nae·col·o·gy *chiefly Brit var of* GYNECOID, GYNECOLOGY

gyn·an·dro·blas·to·ma \(ˌ)gī-ˌnan-drə-bla-'stō-mə, ˌ(ˌ)ji-, ˌji-\ *n, pl* **-mas** *or* **-ma·ta** \-mə-tə\ : a rare tumor of the ovary with both masculinizing and feminizing effects — compare ARRHENOBLASTOMA

gynec- *or* **gyneco-** *comb form* : woman (*gyneco*id) (*gyneco*logy)

gy·ne·cog·ra·phy \ˌgī-nə-'kä-grə-fē, ˌji-\ *n, pl* **-phies** : roentgenographic visualization of the female reproductive tract

gy·ne·coid \'gī-ni-ˌkȯid, 'ji-\ *adj, of the pelvis* : having the rounded form typical of the human female — compare ANDROID, ANTHROPOID, PLATYPELLOID

gy·ne·col·o·gist \ˌgī-nə-'kä-lə-jist, ˌji-, ˌji-\ *n* : a specialist in gynecology

gy·ne·col·o·gy \ˌgī-nə-'kä-lə-jē, ˌji-, ˌji-\ *n, pl* **-gies** : a branch of medicine that deals with the diseases and routine physical care of the reproductive system of women — **gy·ne·co·log·ic** \-ni-kə-'lä-jik\ *or* **gy·ne·co·log·i·cal** \-i-kəl\ *adj*

gy·ne·co·mas·tia \ˌgī-nə-kō-'mas-tē-ə, 'ji-, ˌji-\ *n* : excessive development of the breast in the male

gyp·py tummy \'ji-pē-\ *n* : diarrhea contracted esp. by travelers

gy·rase \'ji-ˌrās, -ˌrāz\ *n* : an enzyme that catalyzes the breaking and rejoining of bonds linking adjacent nucleotides in DNA to generate supercoiled DNA helices

gy·rate \'ji-ˌrāt\ *adj* : winding or coiled around : CONVOLUTED

gyrate atrophy *n* : progressive degeneration of the choroid and pigment epithelium of the retina that is inherited as an autosomal recessive trait and is characterized esp. by myopia, constriction of the visual field, night blindness, and cataracts

gy·ra·tion \jī-ˈrā-shən\ *n* : the pattern of convolutions of the brain

Gy·ro·mi·tra \ˌjī-rō-ˈmī-trə, ˌjir-ə-\ *n* : a genus of ascomycetous fungi (family Helvellaceae) that include the false morels and typically contain toxins causing illness or death

gy·rus \ˈjī-rəs\ *n, pl* **gy·ri** \-ˌrī\ : a convoluted ridge between anatomical grooves; *esp* : CONVOLUTION

H

h *abbr* **1** height **2** [Latin *hora*] hour — used in writing prescriptions; see QH

¹H *abbr* heroin

²H *symbol* hydrogen

ha·ben·u·la \hə-ˈben-yə-lə\ *n, pl* **-lae** \-ˌlī, -ˌlē\ **1** : TRIGONUM HABENULAE **2** : either of two nuclei of which one lies on each side of the pineal gland under the corresponding trigonum habenulae, is composed of two groups of nerve cells, and forms a correlation center for olfactory stimuli — called also *habenular nucleus* — **ha·ben·u·lar** \-lər\ *adj*

habenular commissure *n* : a band of nerve fibers situated in front of the pineal gland that connects the habenular nucleus on one side with that on the other

hab·it \ˈha-bət\ *n* **1** : a behavior pattern acquired by frequent repetition or physiological exposure that shows itself in regularity or increased facility of performance **2** : an acquired mode of behavior that has become nearly or completely involuntary **3** : ADDICTION

hab·i·tat \ˈha-bə-ˌtat\ *n* : the place or environment where a plant or animal naturally occurs

habit–forming *adj* : inducing the formation of an addiction

ha·bit·u·al \hə-ˈbi-chə-wəl\ *adj* **1** : having the nature of a habit : being in accordance with habit **2** : doing, practicing, or acting in some manner by force of habit — **ha·bit·u·al·ly** *adv*

habitual abortion *n* : spontaneous abortion occurring in three or more successive pregnancies

ha·bit·u·a·tion \-ˌbi-chə-ˈwā-shən\ *n* **1** : the act or process of making habitual or accustomed **2 a** : tolerance to the effects of a drug acquired through continued use **b** : psychological dependence on a drug after a period of use — compare ADDICTION **3** : a form of nonassociative learning characterized by a decrease in responsiveness upon repeated exposure to a stimulus — compare SENSITIZATION **3** — **ha·bit·u·ate** \-ˈbi-chə-ˌwāt\ *vb*

hab·i·tus \ˈha-bə-təs\ *n, pl* **habitus** \-təs, -ˌtüs\ : HABIT; *specif* : body-build and constitution esp. as related to predisposition to disease (ulcer ∼)

Hab·ro·ne·ma \ˌha-brō-ˈnē-mə\ *n* : a genus of parasitic nematode worms (family Spiruridae) that live as adults in the stomach of the horse or the proventriculus of various birds — see HABRONEMIASIS, SUMMER SORES

hab·ro·ne·mi·a·sis \ˌha-brə-nē-ˈmī-ə-səs\ *n, pl* **-a·ses** \-ˌsēz\ : infestation with or disease caused by roundworms of the genus *Habronema*

hack \ˈhak\ *n* : a short dry cough — **hack** *vb*

haem- *or* **haemo-** *chiefly Brit var of* HEM-

haema- *chiefly Brit var of* HEMA-

hae·ma·cy·tom·e·ter, hae·mal, haem·an·gi·o·ma *chiefly Brit var of* HEMACYTOMETER, HEMAL, HEMANGIOMA

Hae·ma·phy·sa·lis \ˌhē-mə-ˈfī-sə-ləs, ˌhe-\ *n* : a cosmopolitan genus of small ixodid ticks including some that are disease carriers — see KYASANUR FOREST DISEASE

haemat- *or* **haemato-** *chiefly Brit var of* HEMAT-

hae·ma·tem·e·sis, hae·ma·tog·e·nous *chiefly Brit var of* HEMATEMESIS, HEMATOGENOUS

haematobium — see SCHISTOSOMIASIS HAEMATOBIUM

Hae·ma·to·pi·nus \-tə-ˈpī-nəs\ *n* : a genus of sucking lice including the hog louse (*H. suis*) and short-nosed cattle louse (*H. eurysternus*)

-haemia \ˈhē-mē-ə\ — see -EMIA

hae·mo·bar·ton·el·la \ˌhē-mō-ˌbär-tə-ˈne-lə, ˌhe-\ *n* **1** *cap* : a genus of bacteria (family Anaplasmataceae) that are blood parasites in various mammals **2** *pl* **-lae** \-ˌlē, -ˌlī\ : a bacterium of the genus *Haemobartonella*

hae·mo·bar·ton·el·lo·sis \-tə-nə-ˈlō-səs\ *n, pl* **-lo·ses** \-ˌsēz\ : an infection or disease caused by bacteria of the genus *Haemobartonella*

hae·mo·glo·bin *chiefly Brit var of* HEMOGLOBIN

Hae·mon·chus \hē-ˈmäŋ-kəs\ *n* : a genus of nematode worms (family Trichostrongylidae) including a parasite (*H. contortus*) of the abomasum of ruminants (as sheep) and occurring rarely in humans

hae·mo·phil·ia *chiefly Brit var of* HEMOPHILIA

hae·moph·i·lus \hē-ˈmä-fə-ləs\ *n* **1** *cap* : a genus of nonmotile gram-negative facultatively anaerobic rod bacteria (family Pasteurellaceae) that include several important pathogens (as *H. influenzae* associated with human respiratory infections, conjunctivitis, and meningitis and *H. ducreyi* of chancroid) **2** *pl* **-li** \-₁lī, -₁lē\ : any bacterium of the genus *Haemophilus*

Hae·mo·pro·te·us \₁hē-mō-'prō-tē-əs, ₁he-mə-\ *n* : a genus of protozoan parasites (family Haemoproteidae) occurring in the blood of some birds

haem·or·rhage, haem·or·rhoid *chiefly Brit var of* HEMORRHAGE, HEMORRHOID

haf·ni·um \'haf-nē-əm\ *n* : a metallic element that readily absorbs neutrons — symbol *Hf*; see ELEMENT table

Hage·man factor \'ha-gə-mən-, 'häg-mən-\ *n* : FACTOR XII

Hageman (*fl* 1963), hospital patient.

hair \'har\ *n, often attrib* **1** : a slender threadlike outgrowth of the epidermis of an animal; *esp* : one of the usu. pigmented filaments that form the characteristic coat of a mammal **2** : the hairy covering of an animal or a body part; *esp* : the coating of hairs on a human head — **hairlike** *adj*

hair ball *n* : a compact mass of hair formed in the stomach esp. of a shedding animal (as a cat) that cleanses its coat by licking — called also *trichobezoar*

hair bulb *n* : the bulbous expansion at the base of a hair from which the hair shaft develops

hair cell *n* : a cell with hairlike processes; *esp* : one of the sensory cells in the auditory epithelium of the organ of Corti

haired \'hard\ *adj* : having hair esp. of a specified kind — usu. used in combination ⟨red–*haired*⟩

hair follicle *n* : the tubular epithelial sheath that surrounds the lower part of the hair shaft and encloses at the bottom a vascular papilla supplying the growing basal part of the hair with nourishment

hair·line \'har-₁lin\ *n* : the outline of scalp hair esp. on the forehead

hairline fracture *n* : a fracture that appears as a narrow crack along the surface of a bone

hair root *n* : ROOT 2

hair shaft *n* : the part of a hair projecting beyond the skin

hair·worm \'har-₁wərm\ *n* : any nematode worm of the genus *Capillaria*

hairy cell leukemia \'har-ē-\ *n* : a lymphocytic leukemia usu. of B cell origin and characterized by malignant cells with a ciliated appearance that replace bone marrow and infiltrate the spleen causing splenomegaly

hal·a·zone \'ha-lə-₁zōn\ *n* : a white crystalline powdery acid C₇H₅Cl₂NO₄S used as a disinfectant for drinking water

Hal·dol \'hal-₁dȯl, -₁dōl\ *trademark* — used for a preparation of haloperidol

half–life \'haf-₁lif\ *n* **1** : the time required for half of the atoms of a radioactive substance to become disintegrated **2** : the time required for half the amount of a substance (as a

drug or radioactive tracer) in or introduced into a living system or ecosystem to be eliminated or disintegrated by natural processes

half–moon \-₁mün\ *n* : LUNULA a

half–value layer *n* : the thickness of an absorbing substance necessary to reduce by one half the initial intensity of the radiation passing through it

halfway house *n* : a center for formerly institutionalized individuals (as mental patients or drug addicts) that is designed to facilitate their readjustment to private life

halibut–liver oil *n* : a yellowish to brownish fatty oil from the liver of the halibut used chiefly as a source of vitamin A

hal·i·to·sis \₁ha-lə-'tō-səs\ *n, pl* **-to·ses** \-₁sēz\ : a condition of having fetid breath

hal·lu·ci·na·tion \hə-₁lüs-ᵊn-'ā-shən\ *n* **1** : a perception of something (as a visual image or a sound) with no external cause usu. arising from a disorder of the nervous system (as in delirium tremens) or in response to drugs (as LSD) **2** : the object of an hallucinatory perception — compare DELUSION, ILLUSION — **hal·lu·ci·nate** \-'lüs-ᵊn-₁āt\ *vb* — **hal·lu·ci·na·tor** \-'lüs-ᵊn-₁ā-tər\ *n* — **hal·lu·ci·na·to·ry** \-'lüs-ᵊn-ə-₁tōr-ē\ *adj*

hal·lu·ci·no·gen \hə-'lüs-ᵊn-ə-jən\ *n* : a substance and esp. a drug that induces hallucinations

¹hal·lu·ci·no·gen·ic \hə-₁lüs-ᵊn-ə-'je-nik\ *adj* : causing hallucinations — **hal·lu·ci·no·gen·i·cal·ly** \-ni-k(ə-)lē\ *adv*

²hallucinogenic *n* : HALLUCINOGEN

hal·lu·ci·no·sis \hə-₁lüs-ᵊn-'ō-səs\ *n, pl* **-no·ses** \-₁sēz\ : a pathological mental state characterized by hallucinations

hallucis — see ABDUCTOR HALLUCIS, ADDUCTOR HALLUCIS, EXTENSOR HALLUCIS BREVIS, EXTENSOR HALLUCIS LONGUS, FLEXOR HALLUCIS BREVIS, FLEXOR HALLUCIS LONGUS

hal·lux \'ha-ləks\ *n, pl* **hal·lu·ces** \'ha-lə-₁sēz, 'hal-yə-\ : the innermost digit of the foot : BIG TOE

hallux rig·id·us \-'ri-jə-dəs\ *n* : restricted mobility of the big toe due to stiffness of the metatarsophalangeal joint esp. when due to arthritic changes in the joint

hallux val·gus \-'val-gəs\ *n* : an abnormal deviation of the big toe away from the midline of the body or toward the other toes of the foot that is associated esp. with the wearing of ill-fitting shoes — compare BUNION

ha·lo \'hā-(₁)lō\ *n, pl* **halos** *or* **haloes** **1** : a circle of light appearing to surround a luminous body; *esp* : one seen as the result of the presence of glaucoma **2** : a differentiated zone surrounding a central object (the ~ around a boil) **3** : the aura of glory, veneration, or sentiment surrounding an idealized person or thing

halo effect *n* : generalization from the perception of one outstanding personality trait to an overly favorable evaluation of the whole personality

hal·o·gen \'ha-lə-jən\ *n* : any of the five elements fluorine, chlorine, bromine, iodine, and astatine that exist in the free state normally with two atoms per molecule

hal·o·ge·ton \ˌha-lə-'jē-ˌtän\ *n* : a coarse annual herb (*Halogeton glomeratus*) of the goosefoot family (Chenopodiaceae) that in western American ranges is dangerous to sheep and cattle because of its high oxalate content

halo·per·i·dol \ˌha-lō-'per-ə-ˌdȯl, -ˌdōl\ *n* : a depressant $C_{21}H_{23}ClFNO_2$ of the central nervous system used esp. as an antipsychotic drug — see HALDOL

halo·thane \'ha-lə-ˌthān\ *n* : a nonexplosive inhalational anesthetic C_2HBrClF$_3$

Hal·sted radical mastectomy \'halˌsted-\ *n* : RADICAL MASTECTOMY

hal·zoun \'hal-ˌzün, 'hal-zün\ *n* : infestation of the larynx and pharynx esp. by tongue worms (genus *Linguatula* and esp. *L. serrata*) consumed in raw liver

ham \'ham\ *n* 1 : the part of the leg behind the knee : the hollow of the knee : POPLITEAL SPACE 2 : a buttock with its associated thigh or with the posterior part of a thigh — usu. used in pl.

hama·dry·ad \ˌha-mə-'drī-əd, -ˌad\ *n* : KING COBRA

ham·ar·to·ma \ˌha-ˌmar-'tō-mə\ *n*, *pl* **-mas** *or* **-ma·ta** \-mə-tə\ : a mass resembling a tumor that represents anomalous development of tissue natural to a part or organ rather than a true tumor

ha·mate \'hā-ˌmāt, 'ha-mət\ *n* : a bone on the little-finger side of the second row of the carpus — called also *unciform, unciform bone*

ham·mer \'ha-mər\ *n* : MALLEUS

ham·mer·toe \'ha-mər-ˌtō\ *n* : a deformed claw-shaped toe esp. the second that results from permanent angular flexion between one or both phalangeal joints — called also *claw toe*

¹ham·string \'ham-ˌstriŋ\ *n* 1 **a** : either of two groups of tendons bounding the upper part of the popliteal space at the back of the knee and forming the tendons of insertion of some muscles of the back of the thigh **b** : HAMSTRING MUSCLE 2 : a large tendon above and behind the hock of a quadruped

²hamstring *vb* **-strung** \-ˌstrəŋ\; **-string·ing** \-ˌstriŋ-iŋ\ : to cripple by cutting the leg tendons

hamstring muscle *n* : any of three muscles at the back of the thigh that function to flex and rotate the leg and extend the thigh: **a** : SEMIMEMBRANOSUS **b** : SEMITENDINOSUS **c** : BICEPS **b**

ham·u·lus \'ha-myə-ləs\ *n*, *pl* **-u·li** \-ˌlī, -ˌlē\ : a hook or hooked process

hand \'hand\ *n*, *often attrib* : the terminal part of the vertebrate forelimb when modified (as in humans) as a grasping organ

hand·ed \'han-dəd\ *adj* 1 : having a hand or hands esp. of a specified kind or number — usu. used in combination ⟨a large-*handed* man⟩ 2 : using a specified hand or number of hands — used in combination ⟨right-*handed*⟩

hand·ed·ness \-nəs\ *n* : a tendency to use one hand rather than the other

hand–foot–and–mouth disease *n* : a usu. mild contagious disease esp. of young children that is caused by a picornavirus of the coxsackievirus group and is characterized by vesicular lesions in the mouth, on the hands and feet, and sometimes in the diaper-covered area — compare FOOT-AND-MOUTH DISEASE

hand·i·cap \'han-di-ˌkap, -dē-\ *n* : a disadvantage that makes achievement unusually difficult; *esp* : a physical disability

hand·i·capped \-ˌkapt\ *adj* : having a physical or mental disability that substantially limits activity esp. in relation to employment or education

hand·piece \'hand-ˌpēs\ *n* : the hand-held part of an electrically powered dental apparatus that holds the revolving instruments (as a bur)

Hand–Schül·ler–Chris·tian disease \'hand-'shü-lər-'kris-chən-\ *n* : an inflammatory histiocytosis associated with disturbances in cholesterol metabolism that occurs chiefly in young children and is marked by cystic defects of the skull, exophthalmos, and diabetes insipidus — called also *Schüller-Christian disease*

Hand, Alfred (1868–1949), American physician.

Schüller \'shue-ler\, **Artur (1874–1958),** Austrian neurologist.

Christian, Henry Asbury (1876–1951), American physician.

hang·nail \'haŋ-ˌnāl\ *n* : a bit of skin hanging loose at the side or root of a fingernail

hang·over \-ˌō-vər\ *n* 1 : disagreeable physical effects following heavy consumption of alcohol 2 : disagreeable aftereffects from the use of drugs

hang–up \-ˌəp\ *n* : a source of mental or emotional difficulty

Han·sen's bacillus \'han-sənz-\ *n* : a bacterium of the genus *Mycobacterium* (*M. leprae*) that causes leprosy

Han·sen \'hän-sen\, **Gerhard Henrik Armauer (1841–1912),** Norwegian physician.

Hansen's disease *n* : LEPROSY

han·ta·vi·rus \'han-tə-ˌvī-rəs\ *n* : any of a group of closely related arboviruses that cause hemorrhagic fever accompanied by leakage of plasma and red blood cells through the endothelium of blood vessels and by necrosis of the kidney

H antigen \'āch-\ n : any of various antigens associated with the flagella of motile bacteria and used in serological identification of various bacteria — compare O ANTIGEN

hap·a·lo·nych·ia \,ha-pə-lō-'ni-kē-ə\ n : abnormal softness of the fingernails or toenails

hap·loid \'ha-,plȯid\ adj : having the gametic number of chromosomes or half the number characteristic of somatic cells : MONOPLOID — **haploid** n — **hap·loi·dy** \-,plȯi-dē\ n

hap·lo·scope \'ha-plə-,skōp\ n : a simple stereoscope that is used in the study of depth perception

hap·lo·type \-,tīp\ n : a set of genes that determine different antigens but are closely enough linked to be inherited as a unit; also : the antigenic phenotype determined by a haplotype

hapt- or **hapto-** comb form : contact : touch : combination (hapten) (haptic) (haptoglobin)

hap·ten \'hap-,ten\ n : a small separable part of an antigen that reacts specif. with an antibody but is incapable of stimulating antibody production except in combination with an associated protein molecule — **hap·ten·ic** \hap-'te-nik\ adj

hap·tic \'hap-tik\ adj 1 : relating to or based on the sense of touch 2 : characterized by a predilection for the sense of touch

hap·tics \-tiks\ n : a science concerned with the sense of touch

hap·to·glo·bin \'hap-tə-,glō-bən\ n : any of a family of glycoproteins that are serum alpha globulins and can combine with free hemoglobin in the plasma

hard \'härd\ adj 1 : not easily penetrated : not easily yielding to pressure 2 : of or relating to radiation of relatively high penetrating power (∼ X rays) 3 : being at once addictive and gravely detrimental to health (such ∼ drugs as heroin) 4 : resistant to biodegradation (∼ pesticides like DDT) — **hard·ness** n

hard·en·ing \'härd-ᵊn-iŋ\ n : SCLEROSIS 1 (∼ of the arteries)

hard–of–hearing adj : of or relating to a defective but functional sense of hearing

hard pad n : a serious and frequently fatal virus disease of dogs now considered to be a form of distemper — called also **hard pad disease**

hard palate n : the bony anterior part of the palate forming the roof of the mouth

hardware disease n : traumatic damage to the viscera of cattle due to ingestion of a foreign body (as a nail or barbed wire)

Har·dy–Wein·berg law \'här-dē-'wīn-,bərg-\ n : a fundamental principle of population genetics that is approximately true for small populations and holds with increasing exactness for larger and larger populations: population gene frequencies and population genotype frequencies remain constant from generation to generation if mating is random and if mutation, selection, immigration, and emigration do not occur — called also **Hardy-Weinberg principle**

Hardy, Godfrey Harold (1877–1947), British mathematician.

Wein·berg \'vīn-berk\, **Wilhelm (1862–1937),** German physician and geneticist.

hare·lip \'har-,lip\ n : CLEFT LIP — **hare·lipped** \-,lipt\ adj

har·ma·line \'här-mə-,lēn\ n : a hallucinogenic alkaloid $C_{13}H_{14}N_2O$ found in several plants (Peganum harmala of the family Zygophyllaceae and Banisteriopsis spp. of the family Malpighiaceae) and used in medicine as a stimulant of the central nervous system

har·mine \'här-,mēn\ n : a hallucinogenic alkaloid $C_{13}H_{12}N_2O$ similar to harmaline

Hart·nup disease \'härt-,nəp-\ n : an inherited metabolic disease that is caused by abnormalities of the renal tubules and is characterized esp. by aminoaciduria involving only monoamines having a single carboxyl group, a dry red scaly rash, and episodic muscular incoordination due to the effects of the disease on the cerebellum

Hartnup (fl 1950s), British family.

harts·horn \'härts-,hȯrn\ n : a preparation of ammonia used as smelling salts

hash \'hash\ n : HASHISH

Ha·shi·mo·to's disease \,hä-shē-'mō-(,)tōz-\ n : chronic thyroiditis characterized by goiter, thyroid fibrosis, infiltration of thyroid tissue by lymphoid tissue, and the production of autoantibodies that attack the thyroid — called also **Hashimoto's struma, Hashimoto's thyroiditis, struma lymphomatosa**

Hashimoto, Hakaru (1881–1934), Japanese surgeon.

hash·ish \'ha-,shēsh, ha-'shēsh\ n : the concentrated resin from the flowering tops of the female hemp plant (Cannabis sativa) that is smoked, chewed, or drunk for its intoxicating effect — called also **charas**; compare BHANG, MARIJUANA

Has·sall's corpuscle \'ha-səlz-\ n : one of the small bodies of the medulla of the thymus having granular cells at the center surrounded by concentric layers of modified epithelial cells — called also **thymic corpuscle**

Hassall, Arthur Hill (1817–1894), British physician and chemist.

hatch•et \'ha-chət\ *n* : a dental excavator

haus•tra•tion \hȯ-'strā-shən\ *n* **1** : the property or state of having haustra **2** : HAUSTRUM

haus•trum \'hȯ-strəm\ *n, pl* **haus•tra** \-strə\ : one of the pouches or sacculations into which the large intestine is divided — **haus•tral** \-strəl\ *adj*

ha•ver•sian canal \hə-'vər-zhən-\ *n, often cap H* : any of the small canals through which the blood vessels ramify in bone

Ha•vers \'hā-vərz, 'ha-\, **Clopton** (1655?–1702), British osteologist.

haversian system *n, often cap H* : a haversian canal with the laminae of bone that surround it — called also *osteon*

haw \'hȯ\ *n* : NICTITATING MEMBRANE; *esp* : an inflamed nictitating membrane of a domesticated mammal

hawk \'hȯk\ *vb* : to make a harsh coughing sound in or as if in clearing the throat; *also* : to raise by hawking ⟨∼ up phlegm⟩ — **hawk** *n*

hay fever *n* : an acute allergic rhinitis and conjunctivitis that is sometimes accompanied by asthmatic symptoms; *specif* : POLLINOSIS

Hb *abbr* hemoglobin

H band \'äch-\ *n* : a relatively pale band in the middle of the A band of striated muscle

HBsAg *abbr* hepatitis B surface antigen

HBV *abbr* hepatitis B virus

HCG *abbr* human chorionic gonadotropin

HCT *abbr* hematocrit

HDL \ach-(ₐ)dē-'el\ *n* : a lipoprotein of blood plasma that is composed of a high proportion of protein with little triglyceride and cholesterol and that is associated with decreased probability of developing atherosclerosis — called also *alpha-lipoprotein, high≠density lipoprotein*; compare LDL, VLDL

He *symbol* helium

head \'hed\ *n* **1** : the division of the human body that contains the brain, the eyes, the ears, the nose, and the mouth; *also* : the corresponding anterior division of the body of all vertebrates, most arthropods, and many other animals **2** : HEADACHE **3** : a projection or extremity esp. of an anatomical part: as **a** : the rounded proximal end of a long bone (as the humerus) **b** : the end of a muscle nearest the origin **4** : the part of a boil, pimple, or abscess at which it is likely to break — **head** *adj*

head•ache \'he-ₐdāk\ *n* : pain in the head — called also *cephalalgia* — **head•achy** \-dā-kē\ *adj*

head cold *n* : a common cold centered in the nasal passages and adjacent mucous tissues

head louse *n* : one of a variety of louse of the genus *Pediculus* (*P. humanus capitis*) that lives on the human scalp

head nurse *n* : CHARGE NURSE; *esp* : one with overall responsibility for the supervision of the administrative and clinical aspects of nursing care

head•shrink•er \'hed-ₐshriŋ-kər\ *n* : SHRINK

heal \'hēl\ *vb* **1** : to make or become sound or whole esp. in bodily condition **2** : to cure of disease or affliction — **heal•er** \'hē-lər\ *n*

¹heal•ing \'hē-liŋ\ *n* **1** : the act or process of curing or of restoring to health **2** : the process of getting well

²healing *adj* : tending to heal or cure : CURATIVE ⟨a ∼ art⟩

health \'helth\ *n, often attrib* **1** : the condition of an organism or one of its parts in which it performs its vital functions normally or properly : the state of being sound in body or mind; *esp* : freedom from physical disease and pain — compare DISEASE **2** : the condition of an organism with respect to the performance of its vital functions esp. as evaluated subjectively ⟨how is your ∼ today⟩

health care *n* : the maintenance and restoration of health by the treatment and prevention of disease esp. by trained and licensed professionals — **health–care** *adj*

health department *n* : a division of a local or larger government responsible for the oversight and care of matters relating to public health

health•ful \'helth-fəl\ *adj* : beneficial to health of body or mind — **health•ful•ly** *adv* — **health•ful•ness** *n*

health insurance *n* : insurance against loss through illness of the insured; *esp* : insurance providing compensation for medical expenses

health maintenance organization *n* : HMO

health spa *n* : a commercial establishment (as a resort) providing facilities devoted to health and fitness

health visitor *n, Brit* : a trained person who is usu. a qualified nurse and is employed by a local British authority to visit people (as nursing mothers) in their homes and advise them on health matters

healthy \'hel-thē\ *adj* **health•i•er; -est 1** : enjoying health and vigor of body, mind, or spirit **2** : revealing a state of health **3** : conducive to health — **health•i•ly** \-thə-lē\ *adv* — **health•i•ness** \-thē-nəs\ *n*

hear \'hir\ *vb* **heard** \'hərd\; **hear•ing** : to perceive or have the capacity to perceive sound

hearing *n* : one of the senses that is concerned with the perception of sound, is mediated through the organ of Corti, is normally sensitive in humans to sound vibrations between 16 and 27,000 cycles per second but most receptive to those between 2000 and 5000 cycles per second, is conducted centrally by the cochlear branch of the auditory nerve, and is coordinated esp. in the medial geniculate body

hearing aid *n* : an electronic device usu. worn by a person for amplifying sound before it reaches the receptor organs

hearing dog *n* : a dog trained to alert its deaf or hearing-impaired owner to sounds (as of a doorbell, alarm, or telephone) — called also *hearing ear dog*

heart \'härt\ *n* : a hollow muscular organ of vertebrate animals that by its rhythmic contraction acts as a pump maintaining the circulation of the blood and that in the human adult is about five inches (13 centimeters) long and three and one half inches (9 centimeters) broad, is of conical form, is enclosed in a serous pericardium, and consists as in other mammals and in birds of four chambers divided into an upper pair of rather thin-walled atria which receive blood from the veins and a lower pair of thick-walled ventricles into which the blood is forced and which in turn pump it into the arteries

heart attack *n* : an acute episode of heart disease (as myocardial infarction) due to insufficient blood supply to the heart muscle itself esp. when caused by a coronary thrombosis or a coronary occlusion

heart·beat \'härt-ˌbēt\ *n* : one complete pulsation of the heart

heart block *n* : incoordination of the heartbeat in which the atria and ventricles beat independently due to defective transmission through the bundle of His and which is marked by decreased cardiac output often with cerebral ischemia

heart·burn \-ˌbərn\ *n* : a burning discomfort behind the lower part of the sternum usu. related to spasm of the lower end of the esophagus or of the upper part of the stomach — called also *cardialgia, pyrosis;* compare WATER BRASH

heart disease *n* : an abnormal organic condition of the heart or of the heart and circulation

heart failure *n* 1 : a condition in which the heart is unable to pump blood at an adequate rate or in adequate volume — compare ANGINA PECTORIS, CONGESTIVE HEART FAILURE, CORONARY FAILURE 2 : cessation of heartbeat : DEATH

heart–lung machine *n* : a mechanical pump that maintains circulation during heart surgery by shunting blood away from the heart, oxygenating it, and returning it to the body

heart murmur *n* : MURMUR

heart rate *n* : a measure of cardiac ac-

tivity usu. expressed as number of beats per minute

heart·wa·ter \'härt-ˌwȯ-tər, -ˌwä-\ *n* : a serious febrile disease of sheep, goats, and cattle in southern Africa that is caused by a bacterium of the genus *Cowdria* (*C. ruminantium*) transmitted by a bont tick — called also *heartwater disease, heartwater fever*

heart·worm \-ˌwərm\ *n* : a filarial worm of the genus *Dirofilaria* (*D. immitis*) that is a parasite esp. in the right heart of dogs and is transmitted by mosquitoes; *also* : infestation with or disease caused by the heartworm

heat \'hēt\ *n* 1 **a** : a feverish state of the body : pathological excessive bodily temperature (as from inflammation) **b** : a warm flushed condition of the body (as after exercise) 2 : sexual excitement esp. in a female mammal; *specif* : ESTRUS

heat cramps *n pl* : a condition that is marked by sudden development of cramps in skeletal muscles and that results from prolonged work in high temperatures accompanied by profuse perspiration with loss of sodium chloride from the body

heat exchanger *n* : a device (as in an apparatus for extracorporeal blood circulation) for transferring heat from one fluid to another without allowing them to mix

heat exhaustion *n* : a condition marked by weakness, nausea, dizziness, and profuse sweating that results from physical exertion in a hot environment — called also *heat prostration;* compare HEATSTROKE

heat prostration *n* : HEAT EXHAUSTION

heat rash *n* : PRICKLY HEAT

heat·stroke \'hēt-ˌstrōk\ *n* : a condition marked esp. by cessation of sweating, extremely high body temperature, and collapse that results from prolonged exposure to high temperature — compare HEAT EXHAUSTION

heave \'hēv\ *vb* **heaved; heav·ing** : VOMIT, RETCH

heaves \'hēvz\ *n sing or pl* 1 : chronic emphysema of the horse affecting the alveolae of the lungs — called also *broken wind* 2 : a spell of retching or vomiting

heavy chain *n* : either of the two larger of the four polypeptide chains comprising antibodies — compare LIGHT CHAIN

he·be·phre·nia \ˌhē-bə-'frē-nē-ə, -'fre-\ *n* : a disorganized form of schizophrenia characterized by incoherence, delusions which if present lack an underlying theme, and affect that is flat, inappropriate, or silly — **he·be·phre·nic** \-'fre-nik, -'frē-\ *adj or n*

Heb·er·den's node \'he-bər-dənz-\ *n* : any of the bony knots at joint margins (as at the terminal joints of the fingers) commonly associated with osteoarthritis

Heberden, William (1710–1801), British physician.

hec•tic \'hek-tik\ *adj* **1** : of, relating to, or being a fluctuating but persistent fever (as in tuberculosis) **2** : having a hectic fever

heel \'hēl\ *n* **1** : the back of the human foot below the ankle and behind the arch **2** : the part of the palm of the hand nearest the wrist

heel bone *n* : CALCANEUS

heel fly *n* : CATTLE GRUB; *esp* : one in the adult stage

Heer•fordt's syndrome \'hār-ˌförts-\ *n* : UVEOPAROTID FEVER

Heerfordt, Christian Frederik (b 1871), Danish ophthalmologist.

height \'hīt\ *n* : the distance from the bottom to the top of something standing upright; *esp* : the distance from the lowest to the highest point of an animal body esp. of a human being in a natural standing position or from the lowest point to an arbitrarily chosen upper point

Heim•lich maneuver \'hīm-lik-\ *n* : the manual application of sudden upward pressure on the upper abdomen of a choking victim to force a foreign object from the windpipe

Heimlich, Henry Jay (b 1920), American surgeon.

Heinz body \'hīnts-, 'hīnz-\ *n* : a cellular inclusion in a red blood cell that consists of damaged aggregated hemoglobin and is associated with some forms of hemolytic anemia

Heinz \'hīnts\, **Robert (1865–1924),** German physician.

hela cell \'hē-lə-\ *n, often cap H & 1st L* : a cell of a continuously cultured strain isolated from a human uterine cervical carcinoma in 1951 and used in biomedical research esp. to culture viruses

Lacks \'laks\, **Henrietta (fl 1951),** American hospital patient.

heli- *or* **helio-** *comb form* : sun ⟨*helio*therapy⟩

helic- *or* **helico-** *comb form* : helix : spiral ⟨*helical*⟩ ⟨*helico*trema⟩

he•li•cal \'he-li-kəl, 'hē-\ *adj* : of, relating to, or having the form of a helix; *broadly* : SPIRAL 1a — **he•li•cal•ly** *adv*

hel•i•cine artery \'he-lə-ˌsēn-, 'hē-lə-ˌsin-\ *n* : any of various convoluted and dilated arterial vessels that empty directly into the cavernous spaces of erectile tissue and function in its erection

hel•i•co•bac•ter \'he-li-kō-ˌbak-tər\ *n* **1** *cap* : a genus of bacteria formerly placed in the genus *Campylobacter* and including one (*H. pylori*) associated with gastritis and implicated in gastric and duodenal ulcers and gastric cancer **2** : any bacterium of the genus *Helicobacter*

hel•i•co•trema \ˌhe-lə-kō-'trē-mə\ *n*

: the minute opening by which the scala tympani and scala vestibuli communicate at the top of the cochlea of the ear

he•lio•ther•a•py \ˌhē-lē-ō-'ther-ə-pē\ *n, pl* **-pies** : the use of sunlight or of an artificial source of ultraviolet, visible, or infrared radiation for therapeutic purposes

he•li•um \'hē-lē-əm\ *n* : a light nonflammable gaseous element — symbol *He*; see ELEMENT table

he•lix \'hē-liks\ *n, pl* **he•li•ces** \'he-lə-ˌsēz, 'hē-\ *also* **he•lix•es** \'hē-lik-səz\ **1** : the inward curved rim of the external ear **2** : a curve traced on a cylinder by the rotation of a point crossing its right sections at a constant oblique angle; *broadly* : SPIRAL 2 — see ALPHA-HELIX, DOUBLE HELIX

hel•le•bore \'he-lə-ˌbōr\ *n* **1** : any of a genus (*Helleborus*) of poisonous herbs of the buttercup family (Ranunculaceae) that have showy flowers with sepals like petals; *also* : the dried rhizome or an extract or powder of this formerly used in medicine **2 a** : a poisonous herb of the genus *Veratrum* **b** : the dried rhizome of either of two hellebores (*Veratrum viride* of America and *V. album* of Europe) or a powder or extract of this containing alkaloids used as a cardiac and respiratory depressant and as an insecticide — called also *veratrum*

hel•minth \'hel-ˌminth\ *n* : a parasitic worm (as a tapeworm, liver fluke, ascarid, or leech); *esp* : an intestinal worm — **hel•min•thic** \hel-'min-thik\ *adj*

helminth- *or* **helmintho-** *comb form* : helminth ⟨*helminth*iasis⟩ ⟨*helmin-tho*logy⟩

hel•min•thi•a•sis \ˌhel-mən-'thī-ə-səs\ *n, pl* **-a•ses** \-ˌsēz\ : infestation with or disease caused by parasitic worms

hel•min•thol•o•gy \-'thä-lə-jē\ *n, pl* **-gies** : a branch of zoology concerned with helminths; *esp* : the study of parasitic worms — **hel•min•thol•o•gist** \-'thä-lə-jist\ *n*

Helo•der•ma \ˌhē-lō-'dər-mə, ˌhe-\ *n* : a genus of lizards (family Helodermatidae) including the Gila monsters

helper T cell *n* : a T cell that participates in an immune response by recognizing a foreign antigen and secreting lymphokines to activate T cell and B cell proliferation, that usu. carries CD4 molecular markers on its cell surface, and that is reduced to 20 percent or less of normal numbers in AIDS — called also *helper cell, helper lymphocyte, helper T lymphocyte*

hem- *or* **hemo-** *comb form* : blood ⟨*he*mal⟩ ⟨*hem*angioma⟩ ⟨*hemo*philia⟩

hema- *comb form* : HEM- ⟨*hema*cytometer⟩

he•ma•cy•tom•e•ter \ˌhē-mə-sī-'tä-mə-tər\ *n* : an instrument for counting blood cells — called also *hemocytometer*

hem·ad·sorp·tion \hē-(ˌ)mad-'sȯrp-shən, -'zȯrp-\ n : adherence of red blood cells to the surface of something (as a virus or cell) — **hem·ad·sorb·ing** \-'sȯr-biŋ, -'zȯr-\ adj

hem·ag·glu·ti·na·tion \hē-mə-ˌglüt-ᵊn-'ā-shən\ n : agglutination of red blood cells — **hem·ag·glu·ti·nate** \-'glüt-ᵊn-ˌāt\ vb

hem·ag·glu·ti·nin \-'glüt-ᵊn-ən\ n : an agglutinin (as an antibody or viral capsid protein) that causes hemagglutination — compare LEUKOAGGLUTININ

he·mal \'hē-məl\ adj 1 : of or relating to the blood or blood vessels 2 : relating to or situated on the side of the spinal cord where the heart and chief blood vessels are placed — compare NEURAL 2

he·man·gio·en·do·the·li·o·ma \hē-ˌman-jē-ō-ˌen-dō-ˌthē-lē-'ō-mə\ n, pl -mas or -ma·ta \-mə-tə\ : an often malignant tumor originating by proliferation of capillary endothelium

hem·an·gi·o·ma \hē-ˌman-jē-'ō-mə\ n, pl -mas or -ma·ta \-mə-tə\ : a usu. benign tumor made up of blood vessels that typically occurs as a purplish or reddish slightly elevated area of skin

he·man·gio·ma·to·sis \-jē-ō-mə-'tō-səs\ n, pl -to·ses \-ˌsēz\ : a condition in which hemangiomas are present in several parts of the body

hem·an·gio·peri·cy·to·ma \hē-ˌman-jē-ō-ˌper-ə-ˌsī-'tō-mə\ n, pl -mas or -ma·ta \-mə-tə\ : a vascular tumor composed of spindle cells that are held to be derived from pericytes

he·man·gio·sar·co·ma \-jē-ō-sär-'kō-mə\ n, pl -mas or -ma·ta \-mə-tə\ : a malignant hemangioma

he·mar·thro·sis \hē-mär-'thrō-səs, ˌhe-\ n, pl -thro·ses \-ˌsēz\ : hemorrhage into a joint

hemat- or **hemato-** comb form : HEM- ⟨hematemesis⟩ ⟨hematogenous⟩

he·ma·tem·e·sis \hē-mə-'te-mə-səs, ˌhē-mə-tə-'mē-səs\ n, pl -e·ses \-ˌsēz\ : the vomiting of blood

he·ma·tin \'hē-mə-tən\ n 1 : a brownish black or bluish black derivative $C_{34}H_{33}N_4O_5Fe$ of oxidized heme containing iron with a valence of three; also : any of several similar compounds 2 : HEME

he·ma·tin·ic \hē-mə-'ti-nik\ n : an agent that tends to stimulate blood cell formation or to increase the hemoglobin in the blood — **hematinic** adj

he·ma·to·cele \'hē-mə-tə-ˌsēl, hi-'ma-tə-\ n : a blood-filled cavity of the body; also : the effusion of blood into a body cavity (as the scrotum)

he·ma·to·che·zia \hē-mə-tə-'kē-zē-ə, ˌhe-; hi-ˌma-tə-\ n : the passage of blood in the feces — compare MELENA

he·ma·to·col·pos \hē-mə-tō-'käl-pəs, ˌhe-, -ˌpäs; hi-ˌma-tə-\ n : an accumulation of blood within the vagina

he·mat·o·crit \hi-'ma-tə-krət, -ˌkrit\ 1 : an instrument for determining usu. by centrifugation the relative amounts of plasma and corpuscles in blood 2 : the ratio of the volume of packed red blood cells to the volume of whole blood as determined by a hematocrit

he·ma·to·gen·ic \hē-mə-tə-'je-nik\ adj : HEMATOGENOUS 2

he·ma·tog·e·nous \hē-mə-'tä-jə-nəs\ adj 1 : producing blood 2 : involving, spread by, or arising in the blood — **he·ma·tog·e·nous·ly** adv

he·ma·to·log·ic \hē-mət-ᵊl-'ä-jik\ also **he·ma·to·log·i·cal** \-ji-kəl\ adj : of or relating to blood or to hematology

he·ma·tol·o·gy \hē-mə-'tä-lə-jē\ n, pl -gies : a medical science that deals with the blood and blood-forming organs — **he·ma·tol·o·gist** \-jist\ n

he·ma·to·ma \-'tō-mə\ n, pl -mas or -ma·ta \-mə-tə\ : a mass of usu. clotted blood that forms in a tissue, organ, or body space as a result of a broken blood vessel

he·ma·to·me·tra \hē-mə-tə-'mē-trə, ˌhe-\ n : an accumulation of blood or menstrual fluid in the uterus

he·ma·to·my·e·lia \hi-ˌma-tə-ˌmī-'ē-lē-ə, ˌhē-mə-tō-\ n : a hemorrhage into the spinal cord

he·ma·to·pa·thol·o·gy \hi-ˌma-tə-pə-'thä-lə-jē, ˌhē-mə-tō-\ n, pl -gies : the medical science concerned with diseases of the blood and related tissues — **he·ma·to·pa·thol·o·gist** \-jist\ n

he·ma·toph·a·gous \hē-mə-'tä-fə-gəs\ adj : feeding on blood ⟨∼ insects⟩

he·ma·to·poi·e·sis \hi-ˌma-tə-poi-'ē-səs, ˌhē-mə-tō-\ n, pl -e·ses \-ˌsēz\ : the formation of blood or of blood cells in the living body — called also *hemopoiesis* — **he·ma·to·poi·et·ic** \-'e-tik\ adj

he·ma·to·por·phy·rin \hē-mə-tə-'pȯr-fə-rən, ˌhe-\ n : any of several isomeric porphyrins $C_{34}H_{38}O_6N_4$ that are hydrated derivatives of protoporphyrins; esp : the deep red crystalline pigment obtained by treating hematin or heme with acid

he·ma·to·sal·pinx \hē-mə-tə-'sal-(ˌ)piŋks, ˌhe-, hi-ˌma-tə-\ n, pl -sal·pin·ges \-sal-'pin-(ˌ)jēz\ : accumulation of blood in a fallopian tube

he·ma·tox·y·lin \hē-mə-'täk-sə-lən\ n : a crystalline phenolic compound $C_{16}H_{14}O_6$ used chiefly as a biological stain

he·ma·tu·ria \hē-mə-'tur-ē-ə, -'tyur-\ n : the presence of blood or blood cells in the urine

heme \'hēm\ n : the deep red iron-containing prosthetic group $C_{34}H_{32}N_4O_4Fe$ of hemoglobin and myoglobin

hem·er·a·lo·pia \he-mə-rə-'lō-pē-ə\ n 1

: a defect of vision characterized by reduced visual capacity in bright lights **2** : NIGHT BLINDNESS — not considered good medical usage in this sense

hemi- *prefix* : half 〈hemiblock〉 〈hemipelvectomy〉

-hemia \ˈhē-mē-ə\ — see -EMIA

hemi·an·es·the·sia \ˌhe-mē-ˌa-nəs-ˈthē-zhə\ *n* : loss of sensation in either lateral half of the body

hemi·an·op·ia \-ə-ˈnō-pē-ə\ *or* **hemi·an·op·sia** \-ˈnäp-sē-ə\ *n* : blindness in one half of the visual field of one or both eyes — called also *hemiopia* — **hemi·an·op·tic** \-ˈnäp-tik\ *adj*

hemi·at·ro·phy \-ˈa-trə-fē\ *n, pl* **-phies** : atrophy that affects one half of an organ or part or one side of the whole body — compare HEMIHYPERTROPHY

hemi·a·zy·gos vein \-(ˌ)ā-ˈzī-gəs-, -ˈa-zə-gəs-\ *n* : a vein that receives blood from the lower half of the left thoracic wall and the left abdominal wall, ascends along the left side of the spinal column, and empties into the azygos vein near the middle of the thorax

hemi·bal·lis·mus \ˌhe-mi-ba-ˈliz-məs\ *also* **hemi·bal·lism** \-ˈba-li-zəm\ *n* : violent uncontrollable movements of one lateral half of the body usu. due to a lesion in the subthalamic nucleus of the contralateral side of the body

hemi·block \ˈhe-mi-ˌbläk\ *n* : inhibition or failure of conduction of the muscular excitatory impulse in either of the two divisions of the left branch of the bundle of His

he·mic \ˈhē-mik\ *adj* : of, relating to, or produced by the blood or the circulation of the blood

hemi·cho·lin·ium \-ˌkō-ˈli-nē-əm\ *n* : any of several blockers of the parasympathetic nervous system that interfere with the synthesis of acetylcholine

hemi·cho·rea \ˌhe-mi-kə-ˈrē-ə\ *n* : chorea affecting only one lateral half of the body

hemi·col·ec·to·my \-kə-ˈlek-tə-mē, -kō-\ *n, pl* **-mies** : surgical excision of part of the colon

hemi·cra·nia \-ˈkrā-nē-ə\ *n* : pain in one side of the head — **hemi·cra·ni·al** \-nē-əl\ *adj*

hemi·des·mo·some \-ˈdez-mə-ˌsōm\ *n* : a specialization of the plasma membrane of an epithelial cell that serves to connect the basal surface of the cell to the basement membrane

hemi·di·a·phragm \-ˈdī-ə-ˌfram\ *n* : one of the two lateral halves of the diaphragm separating the chest and abdominal cavities

hemi·fa·cial \-ˈfā-shəl\ *adj* : involving or affecting one lateral half of the face

hemi·field \ˈhe-mi-ˌfēld\ *n* : one of two halves of a sensory field (as of vision)

hemi·gas·trec·to·my \ˌhe-mi-ˌga-ˈstrek-tə-mē\ *n, pl* **-mies** : surgical removal of one half of the stomach

hemi·glos·sec·to·my \-ˌglä-ˈsek-tə-mē,

-ˌglö-\ *n, pl* **-mies** : surgical excision of one lateral half of the tongue

hemi·hy·per·tro·phy \-hī-ˈpər-trə-fē\ *n, pl* **-phies** : hypertrophy of one half of an organ or part or of one side of the whole body 〈facial ∼〉 — compare HEMIATROPHY

hemi·lam·i·nec·to·my \-ˌla-mə-ˈnek-tə-mē\ *n, pl* **-mies** : laminectomy involving the removal of vertebral laminae on only one side

hemi·me·lia \-ˈmē-lē-ə\ *n* : a congenital abnormality (as total or partial absence) affecting only the distal half of a limb

he·min \ˈhē-mən\ *n* : a red-brown to blue-black crystalline salt $C_{34}H_{32}N_4O_4FeCl$ that inhibits the biosynthesis of porphyrin and is used to ameliorate the symptoms of some forms of porphyria

hemi·opia \ˌhe-mē-ˈō-pē-ə\ *or* **hemi·op·sia** \-ˈäp-sē-ə\ *n* : HEMIANOPIA

hemi·pa·re·sis \ˌhe-mi-pə-ˈrē-səs, -ˈpar-ə-\ *n, pl* **-re·ses** \-ˌsēz\ : muscular weakness or partial paralysis restricted to one side of the body — **hemi·pa·ret·ic** \-pə-ˈre-tik\ *adj*

hemi·pel·vec·to·my \-pel-ˈvek-tə-mē\ *n, pl* **-mies** : amputation of one leg together with removal of the half of the pelvis on the same side of the body

hemi·ple·gia \ˌhe-mi-ˈplē-jə, -jē-ə\ *n* : total or partial paralysis of one side of the body that results from disease of or injury to the motor centers of the brain

¹hemi·ple·gic \-ˈplē-jik\ *adj* : relating to or marked by hemiplegia

²hemiplegic *n* : a hemiplegic individual

hemi·ret·i·na \ˌhe-mi-ˈret-ᵊn-ə\ *n, pl* **-i·nas** *or* **-i·nae** \-ᵊn-ˌē, -ˌī\ : one half of the retina of one eye

hemi·sect \ˈhe-mi-ˌsekt\ *vb* : to divide along the mesial plane

hemi·sphere \-ˈsfir\ *n* : half of a spherical structure or organ: as **a** : CEREBRAL HEMISPHERE **b** : either of the two lobes of the cerebellum of which one projects laterally and posteriorly from each side of the vermis

hemi·spher·ec·to·my \-ˌsfi-ˈrek-tə-mē\ *n, pl* **-mies** : surgical removal of a cerebral hemisphere

hemi·spher·ic \ˌhe-mi-ˈsfir-ik, -ˈsfer-\ *adj* : of, relating to, or affecting a hemisphere (as a cerebral hemisphere)

hemi·tho·rax \-ˈthor-ˌaks\ *n, pl* **-tho·rax·es** *or* **-tho·ra·ces** \-ˈthor-ə-ˌsēz\ : a lateral half of the thorax

hemi·thy·roid·ec·to·my \-ˌthī-ˌröi-ˈdek-tə-mē\ *n, pl* **-mies** : surgical removal of one lobe of the thyroid gland

hemi·zy·gote \-ˈzī-ˌgōt\ *n* : one that is hemizygous

hemi·zy·gous \-ˈzī-gəs\ *adj* : having or characterized by one or more genes (as in a genetic deficiency or in an X chromosome paired with a Y chromosome) that have no allelic counterparts

hem·lock \'hem-ˌläk\ *n* **1** : any of several poisonous herbs (as a poison hemlock) of the carrot family (Umbelliferae) having finely cut leaves and small white flowers **2** : a drug or lethal drink prepared from the poison hemlock

hemo- — see HEM-

he·mo·ag·glu·ti·nin *var of* HEMAGGLUTININ

he·mo·bar·to·nel·lo·sis *var of* HAEMOBARTONELLOSIS

he·mo·bil·ia \ˌhē-mə-'bi-lē-ə\ *n* : bleeding into the bile ducts and gallbladder

he·mo·blas·to·sis \ˌhē-mə-ˌblas-'tō-səs\ *n*, *pl* **-to·ses** \-ˌsēz\ : abnormal proliferation of the blood-forming tissues

he·mo·cult \'hē-mə-ˌkəlt\ *adj* : relating to or being a modified guaiac test for occult blood

he·mo·cho·ri·al \ˌhē-mə-'kōr-ē-əl\ *adj*, *of a placenta* : having the fetal epithelium bathed in maternal blood

he·mo·chro·ma·to·sis \ˌhē-mə-ˌkrō-mə-'tō-səs\ *n*, *pl* **-to·ses** \-ˌsēz\ : a metabolic disorder esp. of males that is characterized by deposition of iron-containing pigments in the tissues and frequently by diabetes and weakness — compare HEMOSIDEROSIS — **he·mo·chro·ma·tot·ic** \-'tä-tik\ *adj*

he·mo·co·ag·u·la·tion \ˌhē-mō-kō-ˌa-gyə-'lā-shən\ *n* : coagulation of blood

he·mo·con·cen·tra·tion \ˌhē-mō-ˌkän-sən-'trā-shən\ *n* : increased concentration of cells and solids in the blood usu. resulting from loss of fluid to the tissues — compare HEMODILUTION

he·mo·cul·ture \'hē-mə-ˌkəl-chər\ *n* : a culture made from blood to detect the presence of pathogenic microorganisms

he·mo·cy·to·blast \ˌhē-mə-'sī-tə-ˌblast\ *n* : a stem cell for blood-cellular elements; *esp* : one considered competent to produce all types of blood cell — **he·mo·cy·to·blas·tic** \-ˌsī-tə-'blas-tik\ *adj*

he·mo·cy·tom·e·ter \-sī-'tä-mə-tər\ *n* : HEMACYTOMETER

he·mo·di·al·y·sis \ˌhē-mō-dī-'a-lə-səs\ *n*, *pl* **-y·ses** \-ˌsēz\ : the process of removing blood from an artery (as of a kidney patient), purifying it by dialysis, adding vital substances, and returning it to a vein

he·mo·di·a·lyz·er \-'dī-ə-ˌlī-zər\ *n* : ARTIFICIAL KIDNEY

he·mo·di·lu·tion \-dī-'lü-shən, -də-\ *n* : decreased concentration (as after hemorrhage) of cells and solids in the blood resulting from gain of fluid from the tissues — compare HEMOCONCENTRATION — **he·mo·di·lute** \-'lüt\ *vb*

he·mo·dy·nam·ic \-dī-'na-mik, -də-\ *adj* **1** : of, relating to, or involving hemodynamics **2** : relating to or functioning in the mechanics of blood circulation — **he·mo·dy·nam·i·cal·ly** *adv*

he·mo·dy·nam·ics \-miks\ *n sing or pl* **1** : a branch of physiology that deals with the circulation of the blood **2 a** : the forces or mechanisms involved in circulation **b** : hemodynamic effect (as of a drug)

he·mo·glo·bin \'hē-mə-ˌglō-bən\ *n* : an iron-containing respiratory pigment of red blood cells that functions primarily in the transport of oxygen from the lungs to the tissues of the body, that consists of a globin of four subunits each of which is linked to a heme molecule, that combines loosely and reversibly with oxygen in the lungs or gills to form oxyhemoglobin and with carbon dioxide in the tissues to form carbhemoglobin, and that in humans is present normally in blood to the extent of 14 to 16 grams in 100 milliliters — compare CARBOXYHEMOGLOBIN, METHEMOGLOBIN — **he·mo·glo·bin·ic** \ˌhē-mə-glō-'bi-nik\ *adj* — **he·mo·glo·bi·nous** \-'glō-bə-nəs\ *adj*

hemoglobin A *n* : the hemoglobin in the red blood cells of normal human adults

hemoglobin C *n* : an abnormal hemoglobin that differs from hemoglobin A in having a lysine residue substituted for the glutamic-acid residue at position 6 in two of the four polypeptide chains making up the hemoglobin molecule

hemoglobin C disease *n* : an inherited hemolytic anemia that occurs esp. in blacks and is characterized esp. by splenomegaly and the presence of target cells and hemoglobin C in the blood

he·mo·glo·bin·emia \-ˌglō-bə-'nē-mē-ə\ *n* : the presence of free hemoglobin in the blood plasma resulting from the solution of hemoglobin out of the red blood cells or from their disintegration

hemoglobin F *n* : FETAL HEMOGLOBIN

he·mo·glo·bin·om·e·ter \-ˌglō-bə-'nä-mə-tər\ *n* : an instrument for the colorimetric determination of hemoglobin in blood — **he·mo·glo·bin·om·e·try** \-'nä-mə-trē\ *n*

he·mo·glo·bin·op·a·thy \ˌhē-mə-ˌglō-bə-'nä-pə-thē\ *n*, *pl* **-thies** : a blood disorder (as sickle-cell anemia) caused by a genetically determined change in the molecular structure of hemoglobin

hemoglobin S *n* : an abnormal hemoglobin occurring in the red blood cells in sickle-cell anemia and sickle-cell trait and differing from hemoglobin A in having a valine residue substituted for the glutamic-acid residue in position 6 of two of the four polypeptide chains making up the hemoglobin molecule

he·mo·glo·bin·uria \ˌhē-mə-ˌglō-bə-'nür-ē-ə, -'nyür-\ *n* : the presence of free hemoglobin in the urine — **he·mo·glo·bin·uric** \-ˈnu̇r-ik, -ˈnyu̇r-\ *adj*

he·mo·gram \ˈhē-mə-ˌgram\ *n* : a systematic report of the findings from a blood examination

he·mol·y·sate or **he·mol·y·zate** \hi-ˈmäl-ə-ˌzāt, -ˌsät\ *n* : a product of hemolysis

he·mol·y·sin \ˌhē-mə-ˈlīs-ᵊn, hi-ˈmäl-ə-sən\ *n* : a substance that causes the dissolution of red blood cells — called also *hemotoxin*

he·mol·y·sis \hi-ˈmäl-ə-səs, ˌhē-mə-ˈlī-səs\ *n, pl* **-ly·ses** \-ˌsēz\ : lysis of red blood cells with liberation of hemoglobin — see BETA HEMOLYSIS — **he·mo·lyt·ic** \ˌhē-mə-ˈli-tik\ *adj*

hemolytic anemia *n* : anemia caused by excessive destruction (as in infection or sickle-cell anemia) of red blood cells

hemolytic disease of the newborn *n* : ERYTHROBLASTOSIS FETALIS

hemolytic jaundice *n* : a condition characterized by excessive destruction of red blood cells accompanied by jaundice — compare HEREDITARY SPHEROCYTOSIS

he·mo·lyze \ˈhē-mə-ˌlīz\ *vb* **-lyzed; -lyz·ing** : to cause or undergo hemolysis of

he·mo·par·a·site \ˌhē-mō-ˈpar-ə-ˌsīt\ *n* : an animal parasite (as a filarial worm) living in the blood of a vertebrate — **he·mo·par·a·sit·ic** \-ˌpar-ə-ˈsi-tik\ *adj*

he·mop·a·thy \hē-ˈmä-pə-thē\ *n, pl* **-thies** : a pathological state (as anemia or agranulocytosis) of the blood or blood-forming tissues

he·mo·per·fu·sion \ˌhē-mō-pər-ˈfyü-zhən\ *n* : blood cleansing by adsorption on an extracorporeal medium (as activated charcoal) of impurities of larger molecular size than are removed by dialysis

he·mo·peri·car·di·um \-ˌper-ə-ˈkär-dē-əm\ *n, pl* **-dia** \-dē-ə\ : blood in the pericardial cavity

he·mo·peri·to·ne·um \-ˌper-ət-ᵊn-ˈē-əm\ *n* : blood in the peritoneal cavity

he·mo·pex·in \-ˈpek-sən\ *n* : a glycoprotein that binds heme preventing its excretion in urine and that is part of the beta-globulin fraction of human serum

¹**he·mo·phile** \ˈhē-mə-ˌfīl\ *adj* **1** : HEMO-PHILIAC **2** : HEMOPHILIC **2**

²**hemophile** *n* **1** : HEMOPHILIAC **2** : a hemophilic organism (as a bacterium)

he·mo·phil·ia \ˌhē-mə-ˈfi-lē-ə\ *n* : a sex-linked hereditary blood defect that occurs almost exclusively in males and is characterized by delayed clotting of the blood and consequent difficulty in controlling hemorrhage even after minor injuries

hemophilia A *n* : hemophilia caused by the absence of factor VIII from the blood

hemophilia B *n* : CHRISTMAS DISEASE

¹**he·mo·phil·i·ac** \-ˈfi-lē-ˌak\ *adj* : of, resembling, or affected with hemophilia

²**hemophiliac** *n* : one affected with hemophilia — called also *bleeder*

¹**he·mo·phil·ic** \-ˈfi-lik\ *adj* **1** : HEMOPHIL-IAC **2** : tending to thrive in blood ⟨∼ bacteria⟩

²**hemophilic** *n* : HEMOPHILIAC

He·moph·i·lus \hē-ˈmä-fə-ləs\ *n, syn of* HAEMOPHILUS

he·mo·pneu·mo·tho·rax \ˌhē-mə-ˌnü-mə-ˈthȯr-ˌaks, -ˌnyü-\ *n, pl* **-rax·es** or **-ra·ces** \-ˈthȯr-ə-ˌsēz\ : the accumulation of blood and air in the pleural cavity

he·mo·poi·e·sis \ˌhē-mə-pȯi-ˈē-səs, *n, pl* **-e·ses** \-ˌsēz\ : HEMATOPOIESIS — **he·mo·poi·et·ic** \-ˈe-tik\ *adj*

he·mo·pro·tein \-ˈprō-ˌtēn\ *n* : a conjugated protein (as hemoglobin or cytochrome) whose prosthetic group is a porphyrin combined with iron

he·mop·ty·sis \hi-ˈmäp-tə-səs\ *n, pl* **-ty·ses** \-ˌsēz\ : expectoration of blood from some part of the respiratory tract

he·mo·rhe·ol·o·gy \ˌhē-mə-rē-ˈä-lə-jē\ *n, pl* **-gies** : the science of the physical properties of blood flow in the circulatory system

hem·or·rhage \ˈhem-rij, ˈhe-mə-\ *n* : a copious discharge of blood from the blood vessels — **hemorrhage** *vb* — **hem·or·rhag·ic** \ˌhe-mə-ˈra-jik\ *adj*

hemorrhagica — see PURPURA HEMOR-RHAGICA

hemorrhagic diathesis *n* : an abnormal tendency to spontaneous often severe bleeding — compare HEMOPHILIA, PURPURA HEMORRHAGICA

hemorrhagic fever *n* : any of a diverse group of virus diseases (as Korean hemorrhagic fever) usu. transmitted by arthropods or rodents and characterized by a sudden onset, fever, aching, bleeding in the internal organs (as of the gastrointestinal tract), petechiae, and shock — see HANTAVI-RUS

hemorrhagic septicemia *n* : any of several pasteurelloses of domestic animals that are caused by a bacterium of the genus *Pasteurella* (*P. multoci-da*)

hemorrhagic shock *n* : shock resulting from reduction of the volume of blood in the body due to hemorrhage

hemorrhagicum — see CORPUS HEMOR-RHAGICUM

hem·or·rhoid \ˈhem-ˌrȯid, ˈhe-mə-\ *n* : a mass of dilated veins in swollen tissue at the margin of the anus or nearby within the rectum — usu. used in pl.; called also *piles*

¹**hem·or·rhoid·al** \ˌhem-ˈrȯid-ᵊl, ˌhe-mə-\ *adj* **1** : of, relating to, or involving hemorrhoids **2** : RECTAL

²**hemorrhoidal** *n* : a hemorrhoidal part (as an artery or vein)

hemorrhoidal artery *n* : RECTAL ARTERY

hemorrhoidal vein *n* : RECTAL VEIN

hem·or·rhoid·ec·to·my \ˌhe-mə-ˌrȯi-'dek-tə-mē\ *n, pl* **-mies** : surgical removal of a hemorrhoid

he·mo·sid·er·in \ˌhē-mō-'si-də-rən\ *n* : a yellowish brown granular pigment formed by breakdown of hemoglobin, found in phagocytes and in tissues esp. in disturbances of iron metabolism (as in hemochromatosis, hemosiderosis, or some anemias) — compare FERRITIN

he·mo·sid·er·o·sis \-ˌsi-də-'rō-səs\ *n, pl* **-o·ses** \-ˌsēz\ : excessive deposition of hemosiderin in bodily tissues as a result of the breakdown of red blood cells — compare HEMOCHROMATOSIS

he·mo·sta·sis \ˌhē-mə-'stā-səs\ *n, pl* **-sta·ses** \-ˌsēz\ **1** : stoppage or sluggishness of blood flow **2** : the arrest of bleeding (as by a hemostatic agent)

he·mo·stat \'hē-mə-ˌstat\ *n* **1** : HEMOSTATIC **2** : an instrument and esp. forceps for compressing a bleeding vessel

¹he·mo·stat·ic \ˌhē-mə-'sta-tik\ *n* : an agent that checks bleeding; *esp* : one that shortens the clotting time of blood

²hemostatic *adj* **1** : of or caused by hemostasis **2** : serving to check bleeding

he·mo·ther·a·py \-'ther-ə-pē\ *n, pl* **-pies** : treatment involving the administration of fresh blood, a blood fraction, or a blood preparation

he·mo·tho·rax \ˌhē-mə-'thȯr-ˌaks\ *n, pl* **-tho·rax·es** *or* **-tho·ra·ces** \'-thȯr-ə-ˌsēz\ : blood in the pleural cavity

he·mo·tox·ic \-'täk-sik\ *adj* : destructive to red blood corpuscles

he·mo·tox·in \-'täk-sən\ *n* : HEMOLYSIN

he·mo·zo·in \ˌhē-mə-'zō-ən\ *n* : an iron-containing pigment which accumulates as cytoplasmic granules in malaria parasites and is a breakdown product of hemoglobin

hemp \'hemp\ *n* **1** : a tall widely cultivated Asian herb of the genus *Cannabis* (*C. sativa*) with a strong woody fiber used esp. for cordage **2** : the fiber of hemp **3** : a psychoactive drug (as marijuana or hashish) from hemp

hen·bane \'hen-ˌbān\ *n* : a poisonous fetid Old World herb of the genus *Hyoscyamus* (*H. niger*) that contains the alkaloids hyoscyamine and scopolamine and is the source of hyoscyamus — called also *black henbane*

Hen·le's layer \'hen-lēz-\ *n* : a single layer of cuboidal epithelium forming the outer boundary of the inner stratum of a hair follicle — compare HUXLEY'S LAYER

Hen·le \'hen-lə\, **Friedrich Gustav Jacob (1809–1885),** German anatomist and histologist.

Henle's loop *n* : LOOP OF HENLE

Henoch–Schönlein *adj* : SCHÖNLEIN-HENOCH (〜 *purpura*)

He·noch's purpura \'he-nȯks-\ *n* : Schönlein-Henoch purpura that is

characterized esp. by gastrointestinal bleeding and pain — compare SCHÖNLEIN'S DISEASE

E. H. Henoch — see SCHÖNLEIN-HENOCH

hep·a·ran sulfate \'he-pə-ˌran-\ *n* : a sulfated glycosaminoglycan that accumulates in bodily tissues in abnormal amounts in some mucopolysaccharidoses — called also *heparitin sulfate*

hep·a·rin \'he-pə-rən\ *n* : a glycosaminoglycan sulfuric acid ester that occurs esp. in the liver and lungs, that prolongs the clotting time of blood by preventing the formation of fibrin, and that is administered parenterally as the sodium salt in vascular surgery and in the treatment of postoperative thrombosis and embolism — see LIQUAEMIN

hep·a·rin·ize \'he-pə-rə-ˌnīz\ *vb* **-ized; -iz·ing** : to treat with heparin — **hep·a·rin·iza·tion** \-rə-nə-'zā-shən\ *n*

hep·a·rin·oid \-ˌnȯid\ *n* : any of various sulfated polysaccharides that have anticoagulant activity resembling that of heparin — **heparinoid** *adj*

hep·a·ri·tin sulfate \'he-pə-ˌrī-tin-\ *n* : HEPARAN SULFATE

hepat- *or* **hepato-** *comb form* **1** : liver 〈*hepat*itis〉 〈*hepato*toxic〉 **2** : hepatic and 〈*hepato*biliary〉

hep·a·tec·to·my \ˌhe-pə-'tek-tə-mē\ *n, pl* **-mies** : excision of the liver or of part of the liver — **hep·a·tec·to·mized** \-tə-ˌmīzd\ *adj*

he·pat·ic \hi-'pa-tik\ *adj* : of, relating to, affecting, or associated with the liver

hepatic artery *n* : the branch of the celiac artery that supplies the liver with arterial blood

hepatic cell *n* : HEPATOCYTE

hepatic coma *n* : a coma that is induced by severe liver disease

hepatic duct *n* : a duct conveying the bile away from the liver and uniting with the cystic duct to form the common bile duct

hepatic flexure *n* : the right-angle bend in the colon on the right side of the body near the liver that marks the junction of the ascending colon and the transverse colon — called also *right colic flexure*

he·pat·i·cos·to·my \hi-ˌpa-ti-'käs-tə-mē\ *n, pl* **-mies** : an operation to provide an artificial opening into the hepatic duct

he·pat·i·cot·o·my \-'kä-tə-mē\ *n, pl* **-mies** : surgical incision of the hepatic duct

hepatic portal system *n* : a group of veins that carry blood from the capillaries of the stomach, intestines, spleen, and pancreas to the sinusoids of the liver

hepatic portal vein *n* : a portal vein carrying blood from the digestive organs and spleen to the liver

hepaticus — see FETOR HEPATICUS

hepatic vein n : any of the veins that carry the blood received from the hepatic artery and from the hepatic portal vein away from the liver and that in humans are usu. three in number and open into the inferior vena cava

hepatis — see PORTA HEPATIS

hep·a·ti·tis \ˌhe-pə-ˈtī-təs\ n, pl **-tit·i·des** \-ˈti-tə-ˌdēz\ 1 : inflammation of the liver 2 : a disease or condition (as hepatitis A or hepatitis B) marked by inflammation of the liver — **hep·a·tit·ic** \-ˈti-tik\ adj

hepatitis A n : an acute virus hepatitis caused by an RNA-containing virus that does not persist in the blood serum and is transmitted esp. in food and water contaminated with infected fecal matter — called also *infectious hepatitis*

hepatitis B n : a sometimes fatal hepatitis caused by a double-stranded DNA virus that tends to persist in the blood serum and is transmitted esp. by contact with infected blood (as by transfusion) or blood products — called also *serum hepatitis*

hepatitis B surface antigen n : an antigen that resembles a virus and is found in the sera esp. of patients with hepatitis B — called also *Australia antigen*; abbr. *HBsAg*

hepatitis C n : hepatitis that is caused by a single-stranded RNA-containing virus usu. transmitted by parenteral means (as by injection of an illicit drug, blood transfusion, or exposure to blood or blood products) and that accounts for most cases of non-A, non-B hepatitis

hep·a·ti·za·tion \ˌhe-pə-tə-ˈzā-shən\ n : conversion of tissue (as of the lungs in pneumonia) into a substance which resembles liver tissue — **hep·a·tized** \ˈhe-pə-ˌtīzd\ adj

hepato- — see HEPAT-

hep·a·to·bil·i·ary \ˌhe-pə-tō-ˈbi-lē-ˌer-ē, hi-ˌpa-tə-\ adj : of, relating to, situated in or near, produced in, or affecting the liver and bile, bile ducts, and gallbladder ⟨∼ disease⟩

hep·a·to·car·cin·o·gen \-ˈkär-ˈsi-nə-jən, -ˈkärs-ⁿn-ə-ˌjen\ n : a substance or agent causing cancer of the liver — **hep·a·to·car·cin·o·gen·ic** \-ˈje-nik\ adj — **hep·a·to·car·cin·o·gen·ic·i·ty** \-jə-ˈni-sə-tē\ n

hep·a·to·car·cin·o·gen·e·sis \-ˌkärs-ⁿn-ō-ˈje-nə-səs\ n, pl **-e·ses** \-ˌsēz\ : the production of cancer of the liver

hep·a·to·car·ci·no·ma \-ˌkärs-ⁿn-ˈō-mə\ n, pl **-mas** or **-ma·ta** \-mə-tə\ : carcinoma of the liver

hep·a·to·cel·lu·lar \ˌhep-ət-ō-ˈsel-yə-lər, hi-ˌpat-ə-ˈsel-\ adj : of or involving hepatocytes ⟨∼ carcinomas⟩

hep·a·to·cyte \hi-ˈpa-tə-ˌsit, ˈhe-pə-tə-\ n : any of the polygonal epithelial parenchymatous cells of the liver that se-

crete bile — called also *hepatic cell, liver cell*

hep·a·to·gen·ic \ˌhe-pə-tō-ˈje-nik, hi-ˌpa-tə-\ or **hep·a·tog·e·nous** \ˌhe-pə-ˈtä-jə-nəs\ adj : produced or originating in the liver

hep·a·to·len·tic·u·lar degeneration \hi-ˌpa-tə-len-ˌti-kyə-lər-, ˌhe-pə-tō-\ n : WILSON'S DISEASE

hep·a·tol·o·gy \ˌhe-pə-ˈtä-lə-jē\ n, pl **-gies** : a branch of medicine concerned with the liver — **hep·a·tol·o·gist** \-jist\ n

hep·a·to·ma \ˌhe-pə-ˈtō-mə\ n, pl **-mas** or **-ma·ta** \-mə-tə\ : a usu. malignant tumor of the liver — **hep·a·to·ma·tous** \-mə-təs\ adj

hep·a·to·meg·a·ly \ˌhe-pə-tō-ˈme-gə-lē, hi-ˌpa-tə-ˈme-\ n, pl **-lies** : enlargement of the liver — **hep·a·to·meg·a·lic** \-ˈme-gə-lik\ adj

hep·a·to·pan·cre·at·ic \hi-ˌpa-tə-ˌpaŋ-krē-ˈa-tik, ˌhe-pə-tō-, -ˌpan-\ adj : of or relating to the liver and the pancreas

hep·a·top·a·thy \ˌhe-pə-ˈtä-pə-thē\ n, pl **-thies** : an abnormal or diseased state of the liver

hep·a·to·por·tal \ˌhe-pə-tō-ˈpòrt-ᵊl, hi-ˌpa-tə-\ adj : of or relating to the hepatic portal system

hep·a·to·re·nal \-ˈrē-nəl\ adj : of, relating to, or affecting the liver and the kidneys ⟨fatal ∼ dysfunction⟩

hepatorenal syndrome n : functional kidney failure associated with cirrhosis of the liver and characterized typically by jaundice, ascites, hypoalbuminemia, hypoprothrombinemia, and encephalopathy

hep·a·tor·rha·phy \ˌhe-pə-ˈtòr-ə-fē\ n, pl **-phies** : suture of a wound or injury to the liver

hep·a·to·sis \ˌhe-pə-ˈtō-səs\ n, pl **-to·ses** \-ˌsēz\ : any noninflammatory functional disorder of the liver

hep·a·to·splen·ic \ˌhe-pə-tō-ˈsple-nik, hi-ˌpa-tə-\ adj : of or affecting the liver and spleen ⟨∼ schistosomiasis⟩

hep·a·to·spleno·meg·a·ly \-ˌsple-nō-ˈme-gə-lē\ n, pl **-lies** : coincident enlargement of the liver and spleen

hep·a·tot·o·my \ˌhe-pə-ˈtä-tə-mē\ n, pl **-mies** : surgical incision of the liver

hep·a·to·tox·ic \ˌhe-pə-tō-ˈtäk-sik, hi-ˌpa-tə-ˈtäk-\ adj : relating to or causing injury to the liver — **hep·a·to·tox·ic·i·ty** \-ˌtäk-ˈsi-sə-tē\ n

hep·a·to·tox·in \-ˈtäk-sən\ n : a substance toxic to the liver

hep·ta·chlor \ˈhep-tə-ˌklòr\ n : a persistent chlorinated hydrocarbon pesticide $C_{10}H_5Cl_7$ that causes liver disease in animals and is a suspected human carcinogen

herb \ˈərb, ˈhərb\ n, often attrib 1 : a seed plant that lacks woody tissue and dies to the ground at the end of a growing season 2 : a plant or plant part valued for medicinal or savory qualities

¹**herb·al** \'ər-bəl, 'hər-\ n : a book about plants esp. with reference to their medical properties

²**herbal** adj : of, relating to, or made of herbs

herb·al·ist \'ər-bə-list, 'hər-\ n 1 : one who practices healing by the use of herbs 2 : one who collects or grows herbs

herb doctor n : HERBALIST 1

herd immunity n : a reduction in the probability of infection that is held to apply to susceptible members of a population in which a significant proportion of the individuals are immune because the chance of coming in contact with an infected individual is less

he·red·i·tary \hə-'re-də-ˌter-ē\ adj 1 : genetically transmitted or transmittable from parent to offspring — compare ACQUIRED 2, CONGENITAL 2, FAMILIAL 2 : of or relating to inheritance or heredity — **he·red·i·tar·i·ly** \-ˌre-də-'ter-ə-lē\ adv

hereditary hemorrhagic telangiectasia n : a hereditary abnormality that is characterized by multiple telangiectasias and by bleeding into the tissues and mucous membranes because of abnormal fragility of the capillaries — called also *Rendu-Osler-Weber disease*

hereditary spherocytosis n : a disorder of red blood cells that is inherited as a dominant trait and is characterized by anemia, small thick fragile spherocytes which are extremely susceptible to hemolysis, enlargement of the spleen, reticulocytosis, and mild jaundice

he·red·i·ty \hə-'re-də-tē\ n, pl **-ties** 1 : the sum of the qualities and potentialities genetically derived from one's ancestors 2 : the transmission of traits from ancestor to descendant through the molecular mechanism lying primarily in the DNA or RNA of the genes — compare MEIOSIS

heredo- comb form : hereditary ⟨*heredo*familial⟩

her·e·do·fa·mil·ial \ˌher-ə-dō-fə-'mil-yəl\ adj : tending to occur in more than one member of a family and suspected of having a genetic basis ⟨a ~ disease⟩

Her·ing–Breu·er reflex \'her-iŋ-'broi-ər-\ n : any of several reflexes that control inflation and deflation of the lungs; esp : reflex inhibition of inspiration triggered by pulmonary muscle spindles upon expansion of the lungs and mediated by the vagus nerve

Hering, Karl Ewald Konstantin (1834–1918), German physiologist and psychologist.

Breuer, Josef (1842–1925), Austrian physician and physiologist.

her·i·ta·bil·i·ty \ˌher-ə-tə-'bi-lə-tē\ n, pl **-ties** 1 : the quality or state of being heritable 2 : the proportion of observed variation in a particular trait (as intelligence) that can be attributed to inherited genetic factors in contrast to environmental ones

her·i·ta·ble \'her-ə-tə-bəl\ adj : HEREDITARY

her·maph·ro·dite \(ˌ)hər-'ma-frə-ˌdīt\ n 1 : an abnormal individual having both male and female reproductive organs 2 : a plant or animal that normally has both male and female reproductive organs : BISEXUAL — **her·maphrodite** adj — **her·maph·ro·dit·ic** \-ˌma-frə-'di-tik\ adj — **her·maph·ro·dit·ism** \-'ma-frə-ˌdi-ˌti-zəm\ n

her·met·ic \(ˌ)hər-'me-tik\ adj : being airtight or impervious to air — **her·met·i·cal·ly** \-ti-k(ə-)lē\ adv

her·nia \'hər-nē-ə\ n, pl **-ni·as** or **-ni·ae** \-nē-ˌē, -nē-ˌī\ : a protrusion of an organ or part through connective tissue or through a wall of the cavity in which it is normally enclosed — called also *rupture* — **her·ni·al** \-nē-əl\ adj

hernial sac n : a protruding pouch of peritoneum that contains a herniated organ or tissue

her·ni·ate \'hər-nē-ˌāt\ vb **-at·ed; -at·ing** : to protrude through an abnormal body opening : RUPTURE

her·ni·a·tion \ˌhər-nē-'ā-shən\ n 1 : the act or process of herniating 2 : HERNIA

hernio- comb form : hernia ⟨*hernior*rhaphy⟩ ⟨*hernio*tomy⟩

her·nio·plas·ty \'hər-nē-ə-ˌplas-tē\ n, pl **-ties** : HERNIORRHAPHY

her·ni·or·rha·phy \ˌhər-nē-'or-ə-fē\ n, pl **-phies** : an operation for hernia that involves opening the coverings, returning the contents to their normal place, obliterating the hernial sac, and closing the opening with strong sutures

her·ni·ot·o·my \-'ä-tə-mē\ n, pl **-mies** : the operation of cutting through a band of tissue that constricts a strangulated hernia

he·ro·ic \hi-'rō-ik\ adj 1 : of a kind that is likely to be undertaken only to save life ⟨~ surgery⟩ 2 : having a pronounced effect — used chiefly of medicaments or dosage ⟨~ doses⟩ ⟨a ~ drug⟩

her·o·in \'her-ə-wən\ n : a strongly physiologically addictive narcotic $C_{21}H_{23}NO_5$ that is made by acetylation of but is more potent than morphine and that is prohibited for medical use in the U.S. but is used illicitly for its euphoric effects — called also *diacetylmorphine, diamorphine*

her·o·in·ism \-wə-ˌni-zəm\ n : addiction to heroin

her·pan·gi·na \ˌhər-pan-'jī-nə, ˌhər-'pan-jə-nə\ n : a contagious disease of children characterized by fever, headache, and a vesicular eruption in the throat and caused by a coxsack-ievirus

her•pes \'hər-(₁)pēz\ *n* : any of several inflammatory diseases of the skin caused by a herpesvirus and characterized by clusters of vesicles; *esp* : HERPES SIMPLEX

her•pes gen•i•tal•is \-hər-(₁)pēz-₁je-nə-'ta-ləs\ *n* : herpes simplex of the type affecting the genitals — called also *genital herpes, genital herpes simplex*

herpes keratitis *n* : keratitis caused by any of the herpesviruses that produce herpes simplex or shingles

herpes la•bi•al•is \-₁lā-bē-'a-ləs\ *n* : herpes simplex affecting the lips and nose

herpes sim•plex \-'sim-₁pleks\ *n* : either of two diseases caused by a herpesvirus and marked in one case by groups of watery blisters on the skin or mucous membranes (as of the mouth and lips) above the waist and in the other by such blisters on the genitals

her•pes•vi•rus \-'vī-rəs\ *n* : any of a group of DNA-containing viruses (as cytomegalovirus, Epstein-Barr virus, or varicella zoster) that replicate in the nuclei of cells and include the causative agents of a number of diseases (as herpes simplex, chicken pox, and shingles) characterized esp. by blisters or vesicles on the skin and mucous membranes and often by recurrence sometimes after a long period of latency

herpes zos•ter \-'zäs-tər\ *n* : SHINGLES

herpet- *or* **herpeto-** *comb form* : herpes ⟨*herpeti*form⟩

her•pet•ic \(₁)hər-'pe-tik\ *adj* : of, relating to, or resembling herpes

her•pet•i•form \-'pe-tə-₁fŏrm\ *adj* : resembling herpes

herpetiformis — see DERMATITIS HERPETIFORMIS

Herx•heim•er reaction \'hərks-₁hī-mər-\ *n* : JARISCH-HERXHEIMER REACTION

Heschl's gyrus \'he-shəlz-\ *n* : a convolution of the temporal lobe that is the cortical center for hearing and runs obliquely outward and forward from the posterior part of the lateral sulcus

   Heschl, Richard Ladislaus (1824–1881), Austrian anatomist.

het•a•cil•lin \₁he-tə-'si-lən\ *n* : a semisynthetic oral penicillin $C_{19}H_{23}N_3O_4S$ that is converted to ampicillin in the body

heter- *or* **hetero-** *comb form* : other than usual : other : different ⟨*hetero*graft⟩

Het•er•a•kis \-'rā-kəs\ *n* : a genus (family Heterakidae) of nematode worms including one (*H. gallinae*) that infests esp. chickens and turkeys and serves as an intermediate host and transmitter of the protozoan causing blackhead

¹**het•ero** \'he-tə-₁rō\ *n, pl* **-er•os** : HETEROSEXUAL

het•ero•an•ti•body \₁he-tə-rō-'an-ti-₁bä-

dē\ *n, pl* **-dies** : an antibody specific for a heterologous antigen

het•ero•an•ti•gen \-'an-ti-jən, -₁jen\ *n* : an antibody produced by an individual of one species that is capable of stimulating an immune response in an individual of another species

het•ero•chro•ma•tin \-'krō-mə-tən\ *n* : densely staining chromatin that appears as nodules in or along chromosomes and contains relatively few genes — **het•ero•chro•mat•ic** \-krə-'ma-tik\ *adj*

het•ero•chro•mia \₁he-tə-rō-'krō-mē-ə\ *n* : a difference in coloration in two anatomical structures or two parts of the same structure which are normally alike in color ⟨∼ of the iris⟩

heterochromia ir•i•dis \-'ir-i-dəs\ *n* : a difference in color between the irises of the two eyes or between parts of one iris

het•ero•cy•clic \₁he-tə-rō-'sī-klik, -'si-\ *adj* : relating to, characterized by, or being a ring composed of atoms of more than one kind

het•ero•du•plex \₁he-tə-rō-'dü-₁pleks, -'dyü-\ *n* : a nucleic-acid molecule composed of two chains with each derived from a different parent molecule — **heteroduplex** *adj*

het•ero•gam•ete \₁he-tə-rō-'ga-₁mēt, -gə-'mēt\ *n* : either of a pair of gametes that differ in form, size, or behavior and occur typically as large nonmotile female gametes and small motile sperm

het•ero•ga•met•ic \-gə-'me-tik, -'mē-\ *adj* : forming two kinds of gametes of which one determines offspring of one sex and the other determines offspring of the opposite sex — **het•ero•gam•e•ty** \-'ga-mə-tē\ *n*

het•er•og•a•my \₁he-tə-'rä-gə-mē\ *n, pl* **-mies** 1 : sexual reproduction involving fusion of unlike gametes 2 : the condition of reproducing by heterogamy — **het•er•og•a•mous** \-məs\ *adj*

het•ero•ge•neous \₁he-tə-rə-'jē-nē-əs\ *adj* : not uniform in structure or composition — **het•ero•ge•ne•ity** \₁he-tə-rō-jə-'nē-ə-tē\ *n* — **het•ero•ge•neous•ly** *adv*

het•ero•gen•ic \₁he-tər-ə-'je-nik\ *adj* : derived from or involving individuals of a different species ⟨∼ antigens⟩ ⟨∼ transplantation⟩

het•er•og•e•nous \₁he-tə-'rä-jə-nəs\ *adj* 1 : originating in an outside source; *esp* : derived from another species ⟨∼ bone graft⟩ 2 : HETEROGENEOUS

het•ero•graft \'he-tə-rō-₁graft\ *n* : XENOGRAFT

het•er•ol•o•gous \₁he-tə-'rä-lə-gəs\ *adj* 1 : derived from a different species ⟨∼ DNAs⟩ ⟨∼ transplants⟩ — compare AUTOLOGOUS, HOMOLOGOUS 2 2 : characterized by cross-reactivity ⟨a ∼ vaccine⟩ — **het•er•ol•o•gous•ly** *adv*

¹**het•ero•phile** \'he-tə-rə-₁fīl\ *or* **het•er•o•phil** \-₁fil\ *adj* : relating to or being any of a group of antigens in organ-

isms of different species that induce the formation of antibodies which will cross-react with the other antigens of the group; *also* : being or relating to any of the antibodies produced and capable of cross-reacting in this way

²**heterophile** *or* **heterophil** *n* : NEUTRO-PHIL — used esp. in veterinary medicine

het·ero·pho·ria \‚he-tə-rō-'fōr-ē-ə\ *n* : latent strabismus in which one eye tends to deviate either medially or laterally — compare EXOPHORIA

het·ero·plas·tic \‚he-tə-rə-'plas-tik\ *adj* : HETEROLOGOUS — **het·ero·plas·ti·cal·ly** *adv*

het·ero·plas·ty \'he-tə-rə-‚plas-tē\ *n, pl* **-ties** : the operation of making a xenograft

¹**het·ero·sex·u·al** \‚he-tə-rō-'sek-shə-wəl\ *adj* **1 a** : of, relating to, or characterized by a tendency to direct sexual desire toward individuals of the opposite sex — compare HOMO-SEXUAL 1 **b** : of, relating to, or involving sexual intercourse between individuals of the opposite sex — compare HOMOSEXUAL 2 **2** : of or relating to different sexes — **het·ero·sex·u·al·i·ty** \-‚sek-shə-'wa-lə-tē\ *n* — **het·ero·sex·u·al·ly** *adv*

²**heterosexual** *n* : a heterosexual individual

het·ero·top·ic \‚he-tə-rə-'tä-pik\ *adj* **1** : occurring in an abnormal place ⟨∼ bone formation⟩ **2** : grafted or transplanted into an abnormal position ⟨∼ liver transplantation⟩ — **het·ero·to·pia** \-'tō-pē-ə\ *also* **het·er·ot·o·py** \‚he-tə-'rä-tə-pē\ *n* — **het·ero·top·i·cal·ly** *adv*

het·ero·trans·plant \‚he-tə-rō-'trans-‚plant\ *n* : XENOGRAFT — **het·ero·trans·plan·ta·tion** \-‚trans-‚plan-'tā-shən\ *n*

het·ero·tro·pia \-'trō-pē-ə\ *n* : STRABISMUS

het·ero·typ·ic \‚he-tə-rō-'ti-pik\ *adj* : different in kind, arrangement, or form ⟨∼ aggregations of cells⟩

het·ero·zy·go·sis \‚he-tə-rō-(‚)zī-'gō-səs\ *n, pl* **-go·ses** \-‚sēz\ : HETEROZYGOSITY

het·ero·zy·gos·i·ty \-(‚)zī-'gä-sə-tē\ *n, pl* **-ties** : the state of being heterozygous

het·ero·zy·gote \-'zī-‚gōt\ *n* : a heterozygous individual — **het·ero·zy·got·ic** \-(‚)zī-'gä-tik\ *adj*

het·ero·zy·gous \-'zī-gəs\ *adj* : having the two genes at corresponding loci on homologous chromosomes different for one or more loci — compare HOMOZYGOUS

HEW *abbr* Department of Health, Education, and Welfare

hexachloride — see BENZENE HEXA-CHLORIDE, GAMMA BENZENE HEXA-CHLORIDE

hexa·chlo·ro·eth·ane \‚hek-sə-‚klōr-ō-'eth-‚ān\ *or* **hexa·chlor·eth·ane** \-‚klōr-'eth-‚ān\ *n* : a toxic compound C_2Cl_6

used in the control of liver flukes in veterinary medicine

hexa·chlo·ro·phane \-'klōr-ə-‚fān\ *n, Brit* : HEXACHLOROPHENE

hexa·chlo·ro·phene \-'klōr-ə-‚fēn\ *n* : a powdered phenolic bacteria-inhibiting agent $C_{13}Cl_6H_6O_2$

hexa·dac·ty·ly \'dak-tə-lē\ *n, pl* **-lies** : the condition of having six fingers or toes on a hand or foot

hexa·flu·o·re·ni·um \-‚flü-ər-'ē-nē-əm\ *n* : a cholinesterase inhibitor used as the bromide $C_{36}H_{12}Br_2N_2$ in surgery to extend the skeletal-muscle relaxing activity of succinylcholine

hexa·me·tho·ni·um \‚hek-sə-mə-'thō-nē-əm\ *n* : either of two compounds $C_{12}H_{30}Br_2N_2$ or $C_{12}H_{30}Cl_2N_2$ used as ganglionic blocking agents in the treatment of hypertension — see METHIUM

hexa·meth·y·lene·tet·ra·mine \-‚me-thə-‚lēn-'te-trə-‚mēn\ *n* : METHENAMINE

hex·amine \'hek-sə-‚mēn\ *n* : METHENAMINE

hexanitrate — see MANNITOL HEXANITRATE

hex·es·trol \'hek-sə-‚strōl, -‚strōl\ *n* : a synthetic derivative $C_{18}H_{22}O_2$ of diethylstilbestrol

hexo·bar·bi·tal \‚hek-sə-'bär-bə-‚tol\ *n* : a barbiturate $C_{12}H_{16}N_2O_3$ used as a sedative and hypnotic and in the form of its soluble sodium salt as an intravenous anesthetic of short duration

hexo·bar·bi·tone \-'bar-bə-‚tōn\ *n, chiefly Brit* : HEXOBARBITAL

hexo·cy·cli·um meth·yl·sul·fate \‚hek-sə-'sī-klē-əm-‚me-thəl-'səl-‚fāt\ *n* : a white crystalline anticholinergic agent $C_{21}H_{36}N_2O_5S$ that tends to suppress gastric secretion and has been used in the treatment of peptic ulcers — see TRAL

hex·oes·trol \'hek-sē-‚strōl, -‚strōl\ *chiefly Brit var of* HEXESTROL

hexo·ki·nase \‚hek-sə-'kī-‚nās, -‚nāz\ *n* : any of a group of enzymes that accelerate the phosphorylation of hexoses (as in the formation of glucose-6-phosphate from glucose and ATP) in carbohydrate metabolism

hex·os·a·mine \hek-'sä-sə-‚mēn\ *n* : an amine derived from a hexose by replacement of hydroxyl by the amino group

hex·os·a·min·i·dase \‚hek-‚sä-sə-'mi-nə-‚dās, -‚dāz\ *n* : either of two hydrolytic enzymes that catalyze the splitting off of a hexose from a gangli-oside and are deficient in some metabolic diseases: **a** : HEXOSAMINIDASE A **b** : HEXOSAMINIDASE B

hexosaminidase A *n* : the more thermolabile hexosaminidase that is deficient in both typical Tay-Sachs disease and Sandhoff's disease

hexosaminidase B *n* : the more thermostable hexosaminidase that is deficient in Sandoff's disease but present in elevated quantities in typical Tay=Sachs disease

hex·ose \'hek-ısōs, -ısōz\ n : any monosaccharide (as glucose) containing six carbon atoms in the molecule

hex·yl·res·or·cin·ol \ıhek-səl-rə-'zórs-ən-ıòl, -ıōl\ n : a crystalline phenol $C_{12}H_{18}O_2$ used as an antiseptic (as in a throat lozenge) and as an anthelmintic against ascarids (esp. *Ascaris lumbricoides*), hookworms, and whipworms (esp. *Trichuris trichiura*)

Hf *symbol* hafnium

Hg *symbol* [New Latin *hydrargyrum*] mercury

Hgb *abbr* hemoglobin

HGH *abbr* human growth hormone

HHS *abbr* Department of Health and Human Services

HI *abbr* hemagglutination inhibition

hi·a·tal \hī-'āt-əl\ adj : of, relating to, or involving a hiatus

hiatal hernia n : a hernia in which an anatomical part (as the stomach) protrudes through the esophageal hiatus of the diaphragm — called also *hiatus hernia*

hi·a·tus \hī-'ā-təs\ n : a gap or passage through an anatomical part or organ; *esp* : a gap through which another part or organ passes

hiatus semi·lu·nar·is \ı-se-mi-lü-'nar-əs\ n : a curved fissure in the nasal passages into which the frontal and maxillary sinuses open

Hib *abbr* — used to denote a bacterium of the genus *Haemophilus* (*H. influenzae*) belonging to serotype B ⟨∼ vaccine⟩

hi·ber·no·ma \ıhī-bər-'nō-mə\ n, pl -mas or -ma·ta \-mə-tə\ : a rare benign tumor that contains fat cells

hic·cup *also* **hic·cough** \'hi-(ı)kəp\ n 1 : a spasmodic inhalation with closure of the glottis accompanied by a peculiar sound 2 : an attack of hiccuping — usu. used in pl. but with a sing. or pl. verb — **hiccup** vb

hick·ey \'hi-kē\ n, pl **hickeys** : a temporary red mark produced esp. in lovemaking by biting and sucking the skin

hide·bound \'hid-ıbaund\ adj 1 : having a dry skin lacking in pliancy and adhering closely to the underlying flesh — used of domestic animals 2 : having scleroderma — used of human beings

hidr- *or* **hidro-** *comb form* : sweat glands ⟨*hidradenitis*⟩

hi·drad·e·ni·tis \hi-ıdrad-ən-'ī-təs, ıhī-\ n : inflammation of a sweat gland

hidradenitis sup·pur·a·ti·va \-ısə-pyùr-ə-'tī-və\ n : a chronic suppurative inflammatory disease of the apocrine sweat glands

hi·drad·e·no·ma \hī-ıdrad-ən-'ō-mə\ n, pl -mas *or* -ma·ta \-mə-tə\ : any benign tumor derived from epithelial cells of sweat glands

hi·dro·sis \hi-'drō-səs, hī-\ n, pl -dro-ses \-ısēz\ : excretion of sweat : PERSPIRATION

hi·drot·ic \hi-'drät-ik, hī-\ adj : causing perspiration : DIAPHORETIC, SUDORIFIC

¹high \'hī\ adj 1 : having a complex organization : greatly differentiated or developed phylogenetically — usu. used in the comparative degree of advanced types of plants and animals (the ∼er apes) — compare LOW 2 a : exhibiting elation or euphoric excitement ⟨a ∼ patient⟩ b : being intoxicated; *also* : excited or stupefied by or as if by a drug (as marijuana or heroin)

²high n : an excited, euphoric, or stupefied state; *esp* : one produced by or as if by a drug (as heroin)

high blood pressure n : HYPERTENSION

high colonic n : an enema injected deeply into the colon

high–density lipoprotein n : HDL

high forceps n : a rare procedure for delivery of an infant by the use of forceps before engagement has occurred — compare LOW FORCEPS, MIDFORCEPS

high–grade \'hī-'grād\ adj : being near the upper or most favorable extreme of a specified range — compare LOW=GRADE

high–performance liquid chromatography n : a form of chromatography in which the mobile phase is a liquid under pressure and the stationary phase is in the form of small particles so that the rate of flow is increased to shorten the separation time — abbr. *HPLC*

high–power adj : of, relating to, being, or made with a lens that magnifies an image a relatively large number of times and esp. about 40 times

high–strung \'hī-'strəŋ\ adj : having an extremely nervous or sensitive temperament

hi·lar \'hī-lər\ adj : of, relating to, affecting, or located near a hilum

hill·ock \'hi-lək\ n : any small anatomical prominence or elevation

hi·lum \'hī-ləm\ n, pl **hi·la** \-lə\ : a notch in or opening from a bodily part esp. when it is where the blood vessels, nerves, or ducts leave and enter: as a : the indented part of a kidney b : the depression in the medial surface of a lung that forms the opening through which the bronchus, blood vessels, and nerves pass c : a shallow depression in one side of a lymph node through which blood vessels pass and efferent lymphatic vessels emerge

hi·lus \-ləs\ n, pl **hi·li** \-ılī\ : HILUM

hind·brain \'hīnd-ıbrān\ n : the posterior division of the three primary divisions of the developing vertebrate brain or the corresponding part of the adult brain that includes the cerebellum, pons, and medulla oblongata and that controls the autonomic functions and equilibrium — called also *rhombencephalon;* see METENCEPH-ALON, MYELENCEPHALON

hind·foot \-ˌfūt\ *n* **1** *usu* **hind foot** : one of the posterior feet of a quadruped **2** : the posterior part of the embryonic foot that contains the calcaneus, talus, navicular, and cuboid bones

hind·gut \-ˌgət\ *n* : the posterior part of the embryonic alimentary canal

hind leg *n* : the posterior leg of a quadruped

hind limb *n* : a posterior limb esp. of a quadruped

hinge joint \ˈhinj-\ *n* : a joint between bones (as at the elbow or knee) that permits motion in only one plane; *esp* : GINGLYMUS

hip \ˈhip\ *n* **1** : the laterally projecting region of each side of the lower or posterior part of the mammalian trunk formed by the lateral parts of the pelvis and upper part of the femur together with the fleshy parts covering them **2** : HIP JOINT

hip·bone \-ˌbōn\ *n* : the large flaring bone that makes a lateral half of the pelvis in mammals and is composed of the ilium, ischium, and pubis which are consolidated into one bone in the adult — called also *innominate bone, os coxae, pelvic bone*

hip joint *n* : the ball-and-socket joint comprising the articulation between the femur and the hipbone

hipped \ˈhipt\ *adj* : having hips esp. of a specified kind — often used in combination ⟨broad-*hipped*⟩

hip·po·cam·pal \ˌhi-pə-ˈkam-pəl\ *adj* : of or relating to the hippocampus

hippocampal commissure *n* : a triangular band of nerve fibers joining the two crura of the fornix of the rhinencephalon anteriorly before they fuse to form the body of the fornix — called also *psalterium*

hippocampal gyrus *n* : a convolution of the cerebral cortex that borders the hippocampus and contains elements of both archipallium and neopallium — called also *hippocampal convolution*

hippocampal sulcus *n* : a fissure of the mesial surface of each cerebral hemisphere extending from behind the posterior end of the corpus callosum forward and downward to the hippocampal gyrus — called also *hippocampal fissure*

hip·po·cam·pus \ˌhi-pə-ˈkam-pəs\ *n, pl* **-pi** \-ˌpī, -(ˌ)pē\ : a curved elongated ridge that is an important part of the limbic system, extends over the floor of the descending horn of each lateral ventricle of the brain, and consists of gray matter covered on the ventricular surface with white matter

Hip·po·crat·ic \ˌhi-pə-ˈkra-tik\ *adj* : of or relating to Hippocrates or to the school of medicine that took his name

Hip·poc·ra·tes \hi-ˈpä-krə-ˌtēz\ (*ca*

460 BC–*ca* 370 BC), Greek physician.

Hippocratic facies *n* : the face as it appears near death and in some debilitating conditions marked by sunken eyes and temples, pinched nose, and tense hard skin

Hippocratic oath *n* : an oath that embodies a code of medical ethics and is usu. taken by those about to begin medical practice

hip pointer *n* : a deep bruise to the iliac crest or to the attachments of the muscles attached to it that occurs esp. in contact sports (as football)

hip·pu·ran \ˈhi-pyū-ˌran\ *n* : a white crystalline iodine-containing powder $C_9H_7INNaO_3·2H_2O$ used as a radiopaque agent in urography of the kidney — called also *iodohippurate sodium, sodium iodohippurate*

hip·pus \ˈhi-pəs\ *n* : a spasmodic variation in the size of the pupil of the eye caused by a tremor of the iris

Hirsch·sprung's disease \ˈhirsh-ˌprunz-\ *n* : megacolon that is caused by congenital absence of ganglion cells in the muscular wall of the distal part of the colon with resulting loss of peristaltic function in this part and dilatation of the colon proximal to the aganglionic part — called also *congenital megacolon*

Hirschsprung, Harold (1830–1916), Danish pediatrician.

hir·sute \ˈhər-ˌsüt, ˈhir-, ˌhər-ˈ, hir-ˈ\ *adj* : very hairy — **hir·sute·ness** *n*

hir·sut·ism \ˈhər-sə-ˌti-zəm, ˈhir-\ *n* : excessive growth of hair of normal or abnormal distribution : HYPERTRICHOSIS

hi·ru·din \hir-ˈüd-ᵊn, ˈhir-yü-dən\ *n* : an anticoagulant extracted from the buccal glands of a leech

Hi·ru·do \hi-ˈrü-(ˌ)dō\ *n* : a genus of leeches (family Hirudinidae) that includes the common medicinal leech (*H. medicinalis*)

His bundle \ˈhis-\ *n* : BUNDLE OF HIS

hist- *or* **histo-** *comb form* : tissue ⟨*hist*amine⟩ ⟨*histo*compatibility⟩

His·ta·log \ˈhis-tə-ˌläg\ *trademark* — used for a preparation of an isomer of histamine which is a gastric stimulant and is used to test gastric secretion

his·ta·mine \ˈhis-tə-ˌmēn, -mən\ *n* : a compound $C_5H_9N_3$ esp. of mammalian tissues that causes dilatation of capillaries, contraction of smooth muscle, and stimulation of gastric acid secretion, that is released during allergic reactions, and that is formed by decarboxylation of histidine — **his·ta·min·ic** \ˌhis-tə-ˈmi-nik\ *adj*

his·ta·min·er·gic \ˌhis-tə-mə-ˈnər-jik\ *adj* : liberating or activated by histamine ⟨∼ receptors⟩

his·ta·mi·no·lyt·ic \ˌhis-tə-ˌmi-nə-ˈli-tik, hi-ˌsta-mə-nə-\ *adj* : breaking down or tending to break down histamine

hist·i- *or* **histio-** *comb form* : tissue 〈*histiocyte*〉

hist·i·di·nae·mia *chiefly Brit var of* HISTIDINEMIA

his·ti·dine \ˈhis-tə-ˌdēn\ *n* : a crystalline essential amino acid $C_6H_9N_3O_2$ formed by the hydrolysis of most proteins

his·ti·di·ne·mia \ˌhis-tə-də-ˈnē-mē-ə\ *n* : a recessive autosomal metabolic defect that results in an excess amount of histidine in the blood and urine due to an enzyme deficiency and is characterized by speech defects and mild mental retardation

his·ti·din·uria \-ˈnur-ē-ə, -ˈnyur-\ *n* : the presence of an excessive amount of histidine in the urine (as in pregnancy)

his·tio·cyte \ˈhis-tē-ə-ˌsīt\ *n* : MACROPHAGE — **his·tio·cyt·ic** \ˌhis-tē-ə-ˈsit-ik\ *adj*

his·tio·cy·to·ma \ˌhis-tē-ō-sī-ˈtō-mə\ *n, pl* **-mas** *also* **-ma·ta** \-mə-tə\ : a tumor that consists predominantly of macrophages

his·tio·cy·to·sis \-ˈtō-səs\ *n, pl* **-to·ses** \-ˌsēz\ : abnormal multiplication of macrophages; *broadly* : a condition characterized by such multiplication

histo- — see HIST-

his·to·chem·is·try \-ˈke-mə-strē\ *n, pl* **-tries** : a science that combines the techniques of biochemistry and histology in the study of the chemical constitution of cells and tissues — **his·to·chem·i·cal** \-ˈke-mə-kəl\ *adj* — **his·to·chem·i·cal·ly** *adv*

his·to·com·pat·i·bil·i·ty \ˌhis-(ˌ)tō-kəm-ˌpa-tə-ˈbi-lə-tē\ *n, pl* **-ties** *often attrib* : a state of mutual tolerance between tissues that allows them to be grafted effectively — see MAJOR HISTOCOMPATIBILITY COMPLEX — **his·to·com·pat·i·ble** \-kəm-ˈpa-tə-bəl\ *adj*

histocompatibility antigen *n* : any of the antigenic glycoproteins on the surface membranes of cells that enable the body's immune system to recognize a cell as native or foreign and that are determined by the major histocompatibility complex

his·to·flu·o·res·cence \-ˌflor-ˈes-ᵊns, -ˌflur-\ *n* : fluorescence by a tissue upon radiation after introduction of a fluorescent substance into the body and its uptake by the tissue — **his·to·flu·o·res·cent** \-ˈes-ᵊnt\ *adj*

his·to·gen·e·sis \ˌhis-tə-ˈje-nə-səs\ *n, pl* **-e·ses** \-ˌsēz\ : the formation and differentiation of tissues — **his·to·ge·net·ic** \-jə-ˈne-tik\ *adj* — **his·to·ge·net·i·cal·ly** *adv*

his·toid \ˈhis-ˌtȯid\ *adj* **1** : resembling the normal tissues 〈∼ tumors〉 **2** : developed from or consisting of but one tissue

his·to·in·com·pat·i·bil·i·ty \ˌhis-(ˌ)tō-ˌin-kəm-ˌpa-tə-ˈbi-lə-tē\ *n, pl* **-ties** : a state of mutual intolerance between tissues (as of a fetus and its mother or

a graft and its host) that normally leads to reaction against or rejection of one by the other — **his·to·in·com·pat·i·ble** \-kəm-ˈpa-tə-bəl\ *adj*

his·tol·o·gy \hi-ˈstä-lə-jē\ *n, pl* **-gies** **1** : a branch of anatomy that deals with the minute structure of animal and plant tissues as discernible with the microscope **2** : a treatise on histology **3** : tissue structure or organization — **his·to·log·i·cal** \ˌhis-tə-ˈlä-ji-kəl\ *or* **his·to·log·ic** \-ˈlä-jik\ *adj* — **his·to·log·i·cal·ly** *adv* — **his·tol·o·gist** \hi-ˈstä-lə-jist\ *n*

His·to·mo·nas \ˌhis-tə-ˈmō-nəs\ *n* : a genus of flagellate protozoans (family Mastigamoebidae) that are parasites in the liver and intestinal mucosa esp. of poultry and are usu. considered to include a single species (*H. meleagridis*) that causes blackhead

his·to·mo·ni·a·sis \ˌhis-tə-mə-ˈnī-ə-səs\ *n, pl* **-a·ses** \-ˌsēz\ : infection with or disease caused by protozoans of the genus *Histomonas* : BLACKHEAD 2

his·tone \ˈhis-ˌtōn\ *n* : any of various simple water-soluble proteins that are rich in the basic amino acids lysine and arginine and are complexed with DNA in nucleosomes

his·to·patho·gen·e·sis \ˌhis-tə-ˌpa-thə-ˈje-nə-səs\ *n, pl* **-e·ses** \-ˌsēz\ : the origin and development of diseased tissue

his·to·pa·thol·o·gist \ˌhis-tō-pə-ˈthä-lə-jist, -pa-\ *n* : a pathologist who specializes in the detection of the effects of disease on body tissues; *esp* : one who identifies neoplasms by their histological characteristics

his·to·pa·thol·o·gy \ˌhis-tō-pə-ˈthä-lə-jē, -pa-\ *n, pl* **-gies** **1** : a branch of pathology concerned with the tissue changes characteristic of disease **2** : the tissue changes that affect a part or accompany a disease — **his·to·patho·log·ic** \-ˌpa-thə-ˈlä-jik\ *or* **his·to·patho·log·i·cal** \-ji-kəl\ *adj* — **his·to·patho·log·i·cal·ly** *adv*

his·to·plas·ma \ˌhis-tə-ˈplaz-mə\ *n* **1** *cap* : a genus of fungi (family Coccidioidaceae) that includes one (*H. capsulatum*) causing histoplasmosis and another (*H. farciminosum*) causing epizootic lymphangitis **2** : any fungus of the genus *Histoplasma*

his·to·plas·min \-ˈplaz-mən\ *n* : a sterile filtrate of a culture of a fungus of the genus *Histoplasma* (*H. capsulatum*) used in a cutaneous test for histoplasmosis

his·to·plas·mo·sis \-ˌplaz-ˈmō-səs\ *n, pl* **-mo·ses** \-ˌsēz\ : a respiratory disease with symptoms like those of influenza that is endemic in the Mississippi and Ohio river valleys of the U.S., is caused by a fungus of the genus *Histoplasma* (*H. capsulatum*), and is marked by benign involvement of lymph nodes of the trachea and bronchi usu. without symptoms or by severe progressive generalized involvement of the lymph nodes and the reticuloendothelial system with fever, anemia, leukopenia and often with local lesions (as of the skin, mouth, or throat)

his·to·ry \'his-tə-rē\ n, pl **-ries** : an account of a patient's family and personal background and past and present health

his·to·tox·ic \.his-tə-'täk-sik\ adj : toxic to tissues (~ agents)

histotoxic anoxia n : anoxia caused by poisoning of the tissues (as by alcohol) that impairs their ability to utilize oxygen

histotoxic hypoxia n : a deficiency of oxygen reaching the bodily tissues due to impairment of cellular respiration esp. by a toxic agent (as cyanide or alcohol)

HIV \.āch-(.)ī-'vē\ n : any of a group of retroviruses and esp. HIV-1 that infect and destroy helper T cells of the immune system causing the marked reduction in their numbers that is diagnostic of AIDS — called also *AIDS virus, human immunodeficiency virus*

hive \'hīv\ n : an urticarial wheal

hives \'hīvz\ n sing or pl : an allergic disorder marked by raised edematous patches of skin or mucous membrane and usu. by intense itching and caused by contact with a specific precipitating factor (as a food, drug, or inhalant) either externally or internally — called also *urticaria*

HIV-1 \.āch-(.)ī-(.)vē-'wən\ n : a retrovirus that is the most common HIV — called also *HTLV-III, LAV*

HLA also **HL-A** \.āch-(.)el-'ā\ n [*human leukocyte antigen*] 1 : the major histocompatibility complex in humans 2 : a genetic locus, gene, or antigen of the major histocompatibility complex in humans — often used in attribution (*HLA* antigens) (*HLA* typing); often used with one or more letters to designate a locus or with letters and a number to designate an allele at the locus or the antigen corresponding to the locus and allele (*HLA*-B27 antigen)

HMD abbr hyaline membrane disease

HMO \.āch-(.)em-'ō\ n, pl **HMOs** : an organization that provides comprehensive health care to voluntarily enrolled individuals and families in a particular geographic area by member physicians with limited referral to outside specialists and that is financed by fixed periodic payments determined in advance — called also *health maintenance organization*

Ho symbol holmium

hoarse \'hōrs\ adj **hoars·er; hoars·est** 1 : rough or harsh in sound (a ~ voice) 2 : having a hoarse voice — **hoarse·ly** adv — **hoarse·ness** n

hob·nail liver \'häb-.nāl-\ or **hob·nailed**

liver \'häb-.nāld-\ n 1 : the liver as it appears in one form of cirrhosis in which it is shrunken and hard and covered with small projecting nodules 2 : the cirrhosis associated with hobnail liver : LAENNEC'S CIRRHOSIS

hock \'häk\ n : the joint or region of the joint that unites the tarsal bones in the hind limb of a quadruped (as the horse) and that corresponds to the human ankle but is elevated and bends backward

hock disease n : PEROSIS

Hodg·kin's disease \'häj-kənz-\ n : a neoplastic disease that is characterized by progressive enlargement of lymph nodes, spleen, and liver and by progressive anemia

    Hodgkin, Thomas (1798–1866), British physician.

Hodgkin's paragranuloma n : PARAGRANULOMA 2

hog cholera n : a highly infectious often fatal disease of swine caused by a togavirus and characterized by fever, loss of appetite, weakness, erythematous lesions esp. in light-skinned animals, and severe leukopenia — called also *swine fever*

hog louse n : a large sucking louse of the genus *Haematopinus* (*H. suis*) that is parasitic on the hog

hol- or **holo-** comb form 1 : complete : total (*holo*enzyme) 2 : completely : totally (*holo*endemic)

hold·fast \'hōld-.fast\ n : an organ by which a parasitic animal (as a tapeworm) attaches itself to its host

ho·lism \'hō-.li-zəm\ n 1 : a theory that the universe and esp. living nature is correctly seen in terms of interacting wholes (as of living organisms) that are more than the mere sum of elementary particles 2 : a holistic study or method of treatment

ho·lis·tic \hō-'lis-tik\ adj 1 : of or relating to holism 2 : relating to or concerned with wholes or with complete systems rather than with the analysis of, treatment of, or dissection into parts (~ medicine attempts to treat both the mind and the body) — **ho·lis·ti·cal·ly** adv

Hol·land·er test \'hä-lən-dər-\ n : a test for function of the vagus nerve (as after vagotomy for peptic ulcer) in which insulin is administered to induce hypoglycemia and gastric acidity tends to increase if innervation by the vagus nerve remains and decrease if severance is complete

    Hollander, Franklin (1899–1966), American physiologist.

hol·low \'hä-(.)lō\ n : a depressed part of a surface or a concavity (the ~ at the back of the knee)

hollow organ n : a visceral organ that is a hollow tube or pouch (as the stomach or intestine) or that includes a cavity (as of the heart or bladder) which serves a vital function

hol·mi·um \\'hōl-mē-əm\\ *n* : a metallic element that occurs with yttrium and forms highly magnetic compounds — symbol *Ho;* see ELEMENT table

ho·lo·blas·tic \\,hō-lə-'blas-tik, ,hä-\\ *adj* : characterized by cleavage planes that divide the whole egg into distinct and separate though coherent blastomeres ⟨∼ eggs⟩ — compare MERO-BLASTIC

ho·lo·crine \\'hō-lə-krən, 'hä-, -,krīn, -,krēn\\ *adj* : producing or being a secretion resulting from lysis of secretory cells ⟨∼ gland⟩ — compare APOCRINE, ECCRINE, MEROCRINE

ho·lo·en·dem·ic \\,hō-lō-en-'de-mik\\ *adj* : affecting all or characterized by the infection of essentially all the inhabitants of a particular area

ho·lo·en·zyme \\,hō-lō-'en-,zīm\\ *n* : a catalytically active enzyme consisting of an apoenzyme combined with its cofactor

ho·lo·sys·tol·ic \\,hō-lō-sis-'tä-lik\\ *adj* : relating to an entire systole ⟨a ∼ murmur⟩

Hol·ter monitor \\'hōl-tər-\\ *n* : a portable device that makes a continuous record of electrical activity of the heart and that can be worn by an ambulatory patient during the course of daily activities for the purpose of detecting fleeting episodes of abnormal heart rhythms — **Holter monitoring** *n*

hom- — see HOMO-

Ho·mans' sign \\'hō-mənz-\\ *n* : pain in the calf of the leg upon dorsiflexion of the foot with the leg extended that is diagnostic of thrombosis in the deep veins of the area

Homans, John (1877–1954), American surgeon.

hom·at·ro·pine \\hō-'ma-trə-,pēn\\ *n* : a poisonous drug $C_{16}H_{21}NO_3$ used esp. in the form of its hydrobromide for dilating the pupil of the eye — see MESOPIN

home- *or* **homeo-** *also* **homoi-** *or* **homoio-** *comb form* : like : similar ⟨*homeo*stasis⟩ ⟨*homoio*thermy⟩

ho·meo·box \\'hō-mē-ō-,bäks\\ *n* : a short usu. highly conserved DNA sequence in various genes (as many homeotic genes) that codes for a peptide which may be a DNA-binding protein

ho·meo·path \\'hō-mē-ə-,path\\ *n* : a practitioner or adherent of homeopathy

ho·me·op·a·thy \\,hō-mē-'ä-pə-thē, ,hä-\\ *n, pl* **-thies** : a system of medical practice that treats a disease esp. by the administration of minute doses of a remedy that would in healthy persons produce symptoms similar to those of the disease — compare ALLOPATHY 2 — **ho·meo·path·ic** \\,hō-mē-ə-'pa-thik\\ *adj* — **ho·meo·path·i·cal·ly** *adv*

ho·meo·sta·sis \\,hō-mē-ō-'stā-səs\\ *n* : the maintenance of relatively stable internal physiological conditions (as body temperature or the pH of blood)

under fluctuating environmental conditions — **ho·meo·stat·ic** \\-'sta-tik\\ *adj* — **ho·meo·stat·i·cal·ly** *adj*

ho·meo·ther·my \\'hō-mē-ə-,thər-mē\\ *n, pl* **-mies** : the condition of being warm-blooded : WARM-BLOODEDNESS — **ho·meo·therm** \\-,thərm\\ *n* — **ho·meo·ther·mic** \\,hō-mē-ō-'thər-mik\\ *adj*

ho·me·ot·ic \\,hō-mē-'ä-tik\\ *adj* : relating to, caused by, or being a gene producing a usu. major shift in structural development ⟨∼ mutation⟩

home remedy *n* : a simply prepared medication or tonic often of unproven effectiveness administered without prescription or professional supervision — compare FOLK MEDICINE

ho·mi·cid·al \\,hä-mə-'sīd-əl, ,hō-\\ *adj* : of, relating to, or tending toward homicide — **ho·mi·cid·al·ly** *adv*

ho·mi·cide \\'hä-mə-,sīd, 'hō-\\ *n* : a killing of one human being by another

hom·i·nid \\'hä-mə-nəd, -,nid\\ *n* : any of a family (Hominidae) of bipedal primate mammals comprising recent humans together with extinct ancestral and related forms — **hominid** *adj*

ho·mo \\'hō-(,)mō\\ *n* **1** *cap* : a genus of primate mammals (family Hominidae) that includes modern humans (*H. sapiens*) and several extinct related species (as *H. erectus*) **2** *pl* **homos** : any primate mammal of the genus *Homo*

homo- *or* **hom-** *comb form* **1** : one and the same : similar : alike ⟨*homo*zygous⟩ **2** : derived from the same species ⟨*homo*graft⟩ **3** : homosexual ⟨*homo*phobia⟩

ho·mo·cys·te·ine \\,hō-mō-'sis-tə-,ēn, ,hä-\\ *n* : an amino acid $C_4H_9NO_2S$ that is produced in animal metabolism by removal of a methyl group from methionine and forms a complex with serine that breaks up to produce cysteine and homoserine

ho·mo·cys·tine \\-'sis-,tēn\\ *n* : an amino acid $C_8H_{16}N_2O_4S_2$ formed by oxidation of homocysteine and excreted in the urine in homocystinuria

ho·mo·cys·tin·uria \\-,sis-ti-'nur-ē-ə, -'nyur-\\ *n* : a metabolic disorder inherited as a recessive autosomal trait, caused by deficiency of an enzyme important in the metabolism of homocystine with resulting accumulation of homocystine in the body and its excretion in the urine, and characterized typically by mental retardation, dislocation of the crystalline lenses, and cardiovascular and skeletal involvement — **ho·mo·cys·tin·uric** \\-'nur-ik, -'nyur-\\ *n*

ho·mo·cy·to·tro·pic \\-,sī-tə-'trō-pik\\ *adj* : of, relating to, or being any antibody that attaches to cells of the species in which it originates but not to cells of other species

homoe- *or* **homoeo-** *chiefly Brit var of* HOME-

ho·moe·o·path, **ho·moe·op·a·thy**, **ho·moeo·sta·sis**, **ho·moeo·ther·my**, **ho·moe·ot·ic** *chiefly Brit var of* HOMEO-PATH, HOMEOPATHY, HOMEOSTASIS, HO-MEOTHERMY, HOMEOTIC

ho·mo·erot·ic \hō-mō-i-'rä-tik\ *adj* : HOMOSEXUAL — **ho·mo·erot·i·cism** \-i-'rä-tə-ˌsi-zəm\ *also* **ho·mo·erot·ism** \-'er-ə-ˌti-zəm\ *n*

ho·mo·ga·met·ic \-gə-'me-tik, -'mē-\ *adj* : forming gametes which all have the same type of sex chromosome

ho·mo·ge·nate \hō-'mä-jə-ˌnāt, hə-\ *n* : a product of homogenizing

ho·mo·ge·neous \ˌhō-mō-'jē-nē-əs, -nyəs\ *adj* : of uniform structure or composition throughout — **ho·mo·ge·ne·ity** \ˌhō-mə-jə-'nē-ə-tē, -'hä-, -'nā-\ *adj* — **ho·mo·ge·neous·ly** *adv* — **ho·mo·ge·neous·ness** *n*

ho·mog·e·nize \hō-'mä-jə-ˌnīz, hə-\ *vb* **-nized; -niz·ing 1** : to reduce to small particles of uniform size and distribute evenly usu. in a liquid **2** : to reduce the particles of so that they are uniformly small and evenly distributed; *specif* : to break up the fat globules of (milk) into very fine particles — **ho·mog·e·ni·za·tion** \hō-ˌmä-jə-nə-'zā-shən, hə-\ *n* — **ho·mog·e·niz·er** \-'mä-jə-ˌnī-zər\ *n*

ho·mog·e·nous \-nəs\ *adj* **1** : HOMOPLAS-TIC (~ bone grafts) **2** : HOMOGENEOUS

ho·mo·gen·tis·ic acid \ˌhō-mō-ˌjen-'ti-zik, -hä-\ *n* : a crystalline acid $C_8H_8O_4$ formed as an intermediate in the metabolism of phenylalanine and tyrosine and found esp. in the urine of those affected with alkaptonuria

ho·mo·graft \'hō-mə-ˌgraft, -hä-\ *n* : a graft of tissue from a donor of the same species as the recipient — called also *homotransplant*; compare XENOGRAFT — **homograft** *vb*

homoi- *or* **homoio-** — see HOME-

ho·moio·ther·my *var of* HOMEOTHERMY

ho·mo·lat·er·al \ˌhō-mō-'la-tər-əl, -hä-\ *adj* : IPSILATERAL

ho·mo·log *var of* HOMOLOGUE

ho·mol·o·gous \hō-'mä-lə-gəs, hə-\ *adj* **1 a** : having the same relative position, value, or structure **b** : having the same or allelic genes with genetic loci usu. arranged in the same order (~ chromosomes) **2** : derived from or involving organisms of the same species (~ tissue graft) — compare AU-TOLOGOUS, HETEROLOGOUS **1 3** : relating to or being immunity or a serum produced by or containing a specific antibody corresponding to a specific antigen — **ho·mol·o·gous·ly** *adv*

ho·mo·logue \'hō-mə-ˌlòg, -hä-, -ˌläg\ *n* : something (as a chromosome) that is homologous

ho·mol·o·gy \hō-'mä-lə-jē, hə-\ *n, pl* **-gies 1** : likeness in structure between parts of different organisms due to evolutionary differentiation from the same or a corresponding part of a re-

mote ancestor — compare ANALOGY **2** : correspondence in structure between different parts of the same individual **3** : similarity of nucleotide or amino-acid sequence in nucleic acids, peptides, or proteins

hom·on·y·mous \hō-'mä-nə-məs\ *adj* **1** : affecting the same part of the visual field of each eye (right ~ hemianopia) **2** : relating to or being diplopia in which the image that is seen by the right eye is to the right of the image that is seen by the left eye

¹**ho·mo·phile** \'hō-mə-ˌfīl\ *adj* : of, relating to, or concerned with homosexuals or homosexuality (~ lifestyles); *also* : being homosexual

²**homophile** *n* : HOMOSEXUAL

ho·mo·pho·bia \ˌhō-mə-'fō-bē-ə\ *n* : irrational fear of, aversion to, or discrimination against homosexuality or homosexuals — **ho·mo·phobe** \'hō-mə-ˌfōb\ *n* — **ho·mo·pho·bic** \ˌhō-mə-'fō-bik\ *adj*

ho·mo·plas·tic \ˌhō-mə-'plas-tik, -hä-\ *adj* : of, relating to, or derived from another individual of the same species (~ grafts)

ho·mo·sal·ate \ˌhō-mō-'sa-ˌlāt, -hä-\ *n* : a salicylate $C_{16}H_{22}O_3$ that is used in sunscreen lotions to absorb ultraviolet rays and promote tanning

ho·mo·ser·ine \ˌhō-mō-'ser-ˌēn, -hä-, -'sir-\ *n* : an amino acid $C_4H_9NO_3$ that is formed in the conversion of methionine to cysteine — see HOMO-CYSTEINE

¹**ho·mo·sex·u·al** \ˌhō-mə-'sek-shə-wəl\ *adj* **1** : of, relating to, or characterized by a tendency to direct sexual desire toward individuals of one's own sex — compare HETEROSEXUAL 1a **2** : of, relating to, or involving sexual intercourse between individuals of the same sex — compare HETEROSEXUAL 1b — **ho·mo·sex·u·al·ly** *adv*

²**homosexual** *n* : a homosexual individual and esp. a male

ho·mo·sex·u·al·i·ty \ˌhō-mə-ˌsek-shə-'wa-lə-tē\ *n, pl* **-ties 1** : the quality or state of being homosexual **2** : erotic activity with another of the same sex

ho·mo·trans·plant \ˌhō-mō-'trans-ˌplant, -hä-\ *n* : HOMOGRAFT — **ho·motransplant** *vb* — **ho·mo·trans·plan·ta·tion** \-ˌtrans-ˌplan-'tā-shən\ *n*

ho·mo·va·nil·lic acid \-və-ˈni-lik-\ *n* : a dopamine metabolite excreted in human urine

ho·mo·zy·go·sis \-zī-'gō-səs\ *n, pl* **-go·ses** \-ˌsēz\ : HOMOZYGOSITY

ho·mo·zy·gos·i·ty \-zī-'gä-sə-tē\ *n, pl* **-ties** : the state of being homozygous

ho·mo·zy·gote \-'zī-ˌgōt\ *n* : a homozygous individual

ho·mo·zy·gous \-'zī-gəs\ *adj* : having the two genes at corresponding loci on homologous chromosomes identical for one or more loci — compare HET-EROZYGOUS

hon·ey·bee \'hə-nē-ˌbē\ *n* : a honey≠

producing bee (*Apis* and related genera); *esp* : a European bee (*A. mellifera*) introduced worldwide and kept in hives for the honey it produces

hon·ey·comb \'hə-nē-ˌkōm\ *n* : RETICULUM 1

Hong Kong flu \'häŋ-'käŋ-\ *n* : a relatively mild pandemic influenza that first appeared in 1968 and is caused by a variant strain of the influenza virus

hoof \'húf, 'hüf\ *n, pl* **hooves** \'húvz, 'hüvz\ *or* **hoofs** : a horny covering that protects the ends of the toes of numerous plant-eating 4-footed mammals (as horses or cattle); *also* : a hoofed foot — **hoofed** \'húft, 'hüft, 'húvd, 'hüvd\ *or* **hooved** \'húvd, 'hüvd\ *adj*

hoof–and–mouth disease *n* : FOOT-AND-MOUTH DISEASE

hook \'húk\ *n* **1** : an instrument used in surgery to take hold of tissue **2** : an anatomical part that resembles a hook

hook·worm \-ˌwərm\ *n* **1** : any of several parasitic nematode worms (family Ancylostomatidae) that have strong buccal hooks or plates for attaching to the host's intestinal lining and that include serious bloodsucking pests **2** : ANCYLOSTOMIASIS

hookworm disease *n* : ANCYLOSTOMIASIS

hoose \'hüz\ *n* : verminous bronchitis of cattle, sheep, and goats caused by larval strongylid roundworms irritating the bronchial tubes — called also *husk*

hor·de·o·lum \hór-'dē-ə-ləm\ *n, pl* **-o·la** \-lə\ : STY

hore·hound \'hór-ˌhaúnd\ *n* **1** : a European aromatic plant (*Marrubium vulgare*) of the mint family (Labiatae) that is naturalized in the U.S., has a very bitter taste, and is used as a tonic and anthelmintic **2** : an extract or confection made from horehound and used as a remedy for coughs and colds

hor·i·zon·tal \ˌhór-ə-'zänt-ᵊl, ˌhär-\ *adj* **1** : relating to or being a transverse plane or section of the body **2** : relating to or being transmission (as of a disease) by physical contact or proximity in contrast with inheritance — compare VERTICAL — **hor·i·zon·tal·ly** *adv*

horizontal cell *n* : any of the retinal neurons whose axons pass along a course in the plexiform layer following the contour of the retina and whose dendrites synapse with the rods and cones

horizontal fissure *n* : a fissure of the right lung that begins at the oblique fissure and runs horizontally dividing the lung into superior and middle lobes

horizontal plate *n* : a plate of the palatine bone that is situated horizontally,

joins the bone of the opposite side, and forms the back part of the hard palate — compare PERPENDICULAR PLATE 2

hor·mone \'hór-ˌmōn\ *n* **1** : a product of living cells that circulates in body fluids and produces a specific effect on the activity of cells remote from its point of origin; *esp* : one exerting a stimulatory effect on a cellular activity **2** : a synthetic substance that acts like a hormone — **hor·mon·al** \hór-'mōn-ᵊl\ *adj* — **hor·mon·al·ly** *adv* — **hor·mone·like** *adj*

horn \'hórn\ *n* **1** : one of the hard projections of bone or keratin on the head of many hoofed mammals; *also* : the material of which horns are composed or a similar material **2** : CORNU — **horned** \'hórnd\ *adj*

horn cell *n* : a nerve cell lying in one of the gray columns of the spinal cord

horned rattlesnake *n* : SIDEWINDER

Hor·ner's syndrome \'hór-nərz-\ *n* : a syndrome marked by sinking in of the eyeball, contraction of the pupil, drooping of the upper eyelid, and vasodilation and anhidrosis of the face, and caused by injury to the cervical sympathetic nerve fibers on the affected side

Horner, Johann Friedrich (1831–1886), Swiss ophthalmologist.

horn fly *n* : a small black European dipteran fly (*Haematobia irritans* of the family Muscidae) that has been introduced into No. America where it is a bloodsucking pest of cattle

horny \'hór-nē\ *adj* **horn·i·er; -est** **1** : composed of or resembling tough fibrous material consisting chiefly of keratin : KERATINOUS ⟨~ tissue⟩ **2** : being hard or callous

horny layer *n* : STRATUM CORNEUM

hor·rip·i·la·tion \hō-ˌri-pə-'lā-shən, hä-\ *n* : a bristling of the hair of the head or body (as from disease, terror, or chilliness) : GOOSE BUMPS — **hor·rip·i·late** \'ri-pə-ˌlāt\ *vb*

horror au·to·tox·i·cus \-ˌó-tō-'täk-sə-kəs\ *n* : SELF-TOLERANCE

horse \'hórs\ *n, pl* **hors·es** *also* **horse** : a large solid-hoofed herbivorous mammal (*Equus caballus* of the family Equidae) domesticated since a prehistoric period

horse bot *n* : HORSE BOTFLY; *specif* : a larva of a horse botfly

horse botfly *n* : a cosmopolitan botfly of the genus *Gasterophilus* (*G. intestinalis*) whose larvae parasitize the stomach lining of the horse

horse·fly \'hórs-ˌflī\ *n, pl* **-flies** : any of a family (Tabanidae) of usu. large dipteran flies with bloodsucking females

horse·pox \-ˌpäks\ *n* : a virus disease of horses related to cowpox and marked by a vesiculopustular eruption of the skin

horse·shoe kidney \-ˌshü\ *n* : a congenital partial fusion of the kidneys resulting in a horseshoe shape

Hor·ton's syndrome \\ˈhȯr-tənz-\\
: CLUSTER HEADACHE
Horton, Bayard Taylor (1895–1980), American physician.

hosp *abbr* hospital

hos·pice \\ˈhäs-pəs\\ *n* : a facility or program designed to provide a caring environment for supplying the physical and emotional needs of the terminally ill

hos·pi·tal \\ˈhäs-ˌpit-ᵊl\\ *n, often attrib* **1** : a charitable institution for the needy, aged, infirm, or young **2 a** : an institution where the sick or injured are given medical or surgical care — when used in British English following as a preposition, the article is usu. omitted ⟨came and saw me in ∼ — Robert Graves⟩ **b** : a place for the care and treatment of sick and injured animals

hospital bed *n* : a bed with a frame in three movable sections equipped with mechanical spring parts that permit raising the head end, foot end, or middle as required — called also *Gatch bed*

hos·pi·tal·ism \\ˈhäs-(ˌ)pit-ᵊl-ˌi-zəm\\ *n* **1 a** : the factors and influences that adversely affect the health of hospitalized persons **b** : the effect of such factors on mental or physical health **2** : the deleterious physical and mental effects on infants and children resulting from their living in institutions without the benefit of a home environment and parents

hos·pi·tal·iza·tion \\ˌhäs-(ˌ)pit-ᵊl-ə-ˈzā-shən\\ *n* **1** : the act or process of being hospitalized **2** : the period of stay in a hospital

hospitalization insurance *n* : insurance that provides benefits to cover or partly cover hospital expenses

hos·pi·tal·ize \\ˈhäs-(ˌ)pit-ᵊl-ˌīz, häs-ˈpit-ᵊl-ˌīz\\ *vb* **-ized; -iz·ing** : to place in a hospital as a patient

host \\ˈhōst\\ *n* **1** : a living animal or plant on or in which a parasite lives — see DEFINITIVE HOST, INTERMEDIATE HOST **2 a** : an individual into which a tissue or part is transplanted from another **b** : an individual in whom an abnormal growth (as a cancer) is proliferating

hos·til·i·ty \\hä-ˈsti-lə-tē\\ *n, pl* **-ties** : conflict, opposition, or resistance in thought or principle — **hos·tile** \\ˈhäs-tᵊl, -ˌtil\\ *adj*

hot \\ˈhät\\ *adj* **hot·ter; hot·test 1** : having heat in a degree exceeding normal body heat **2** : RADIOACTIVE; *esp* : exhibiting a relatively great amount of radioactivity when subjected to radionuclide scanning

hot flash *n* : a sudden brief flushing and sensation of heat caused by dilation of skin capillaries usu. associated

with menopausal endocrine imbalance — called also *hot flush*

hot line *n* : a telephone service by which usu. unidentified callers can talk confidentially about personal problems to a sympathetic listener

hot pack *n* : absorbent material (as squares of gauze) wrung out in hot water, wrapped around the body or a portion of the body, and covered with dry material to hold in the moist heat — compare COLD PACK

hot–water bottle *n* : a usu. rubber bag that has a stopper and is filled with hot water to provide warmth

hourglass stomach *n* : a stomach divided into two communicating cavities by a circular constriction usu. caused by the scar tissue around an ulcer

house·bro·ken \\ˈhaus-ˌbrō-kən\\ *adj* : trained to excretory habits acceptable in indoor living — used of a household pet — **house·break** \\-ˌbrāk\\ *vb*

house call *n* : a visit (as by a doctor) to a home to provide medical care

house doctor *n* : a physician in residence at an establishment (as a hotel) or on the premises temporarily in the event of a medical emergency

house·fly \\-ˌflī\\ *n, pl* **-flies** : a cosmopolitan dipteran fly of the genus *Musca* (*M. domestica*) that is often found about human habitations and may act as a mechanical vector of diseases (as typhoid fever); *also* : any of various flies of similar appearance or habitat

house·maid's knee \\ˈhaus-ˌmādz-\\ *n* : a swelling over the knee due to an enlargement of the bursa in the front of the patella

house·man \\ˈhaus-mən\\ *n, pl* **-men** \\-mən\\ *chiefly Brit* : INTERN

house mouse *n* : a common nearly cosmopolitan mouse of the genus *Mus* (*M. musculus*) that usu. lives and breeds about buildings, is an important laboratory animal, and is an important pest as a consumer of human food and as a vector of diseases

house officer *n* : an intern or resident employed by a hospital

house physician *n* : a physician and esp. a resident employed by a hospital

house staff *n* : the physicians and esp. the interns and residents sometimes along with other health professionals (as physician's assistants and physical therapists) employed by a hospital

house surgeon *n* : a surgeon fully qualified in a specialty and resident in a hospital

Hous·ton's valve \\ˈhü-stənz-\\ *n* : any of the usu. three but sometimes four or two permanent transverse crescent-shaped folds of the rectum
Houston, John (1802–1845), British surgeon.

How·ard test \\ˈhau-ərd-\\ *n* : a test of renal function that involves the catheterization of each ureter so that the urinary output of each kidney can be determined and analyzed separately

Howard, John Eager (1902–1985), American internist and endocrinologist.

How·ell–Jol·ly body \'haù-əl-zhō-'lē-, -'jä-lē-\ *n* : one of the basophilic granules that are probably nuclear fragments, that sometimes occur in red blood cells, and that indicate by their appearance in circulating blood that red cells are leaving the marrow while incompletely mature (as in certain anemias)

Howell, William Henry (1860–1945), American physiologist.

Jolly \zhò-'lē\, **Justin Marie Jules (1870–1953),** French histologist.

How·ship's lacuna \'haù-ships-\ *n* : a groove or cavity usu. containing osteoclasts that occurs in bone which is undergoing reabsorption

Howship, John (1781–1841), British anatomist.

HPI *abbr* history of present illness

HPLC *abbr* high-performance liquid chromatography

hr *abbr* [Latin *hora*] hour — used in writing prescriptions; see QH

hs *abbr* [Latin *hora somni*] at bedtime — used esp. in writing prescriptions

HS *abbr* house surgeon

HSA *abbr* human serum albumin

HSV *abbr* herpes simplex virus

ht *abbr* height

HTLV \aāch-(a)tē-(a)el-'vē\ *n* : any of several retroviruses (as HIV-1) — often used with a number or Roman numeral to indicate the type and order of discovery ⟨*HTLV*-III⟩; called also *human T-cell leukemia virus, human T-cell lymphotropic virus, human T-lymphotropic virus*

HTLV-III *n* : HIV-1

Hub·bard tank \'hə-bərd-\ *n* : a large tank in which a patient can easily be assisted in exercises while in the water

Hubbard, Leroy Watkins (1857–1938), American orthopedic surgeon.

hue \'hyü\ *n* : the one of the three psychological dimensions of color perception that permits them to be classified as red, yellow, green, blue, or an intermediate between any contiguous pair of these colors and that is correlated with the wavelength or the combination of wavelengths comprising the stimulus — compare BRIGHTNESS, SATURATION 4

Huh·ner test \'hyü-nər-\ *n* : a test used in sterility studies that involves postcoital examination of fluid aspirated from the vagina and cervix to determine the presence or survival of spermatozoa in these areas

Huhner, Max (1873–1947), American surgeon.

¹hu·man \'hyü-mən, 'yü-\ *adj* **1 a** : of, relating to, or characteristic of humans ⟨∼ chorionic gonadotropin⟩ ⟨∼ growth hormone⟩ **b** : primarily or usu. harbored by, affecting, or attacking humans ⟨∼ appendicitis⟩ ⟨the common ∼ flea⟩ **2** : being or consisting of humans ⟨the ∼ race⟩ **3** : consisting of hominids — **hu·man·ness** *n*

²human *n* : a bipedal primate mammal of the genus *Homo* (*H. sapiens*) : MAN; *broadly* : any living or extinct member of the family (Hominidae) to which this primate belongs — **hu·man·like** \-ˌlīk\ *adj*

human being *n* : HUMAN

human botfly *n* : a large fly of the genus *Dermatobia* (*D. hominis*) that is widely distributed in tropical America and undergoes its larval development subcutaneously in some mammals including humans

human ecology *n* : the ecology of human communities and populations esp. as concerned with preservation of environmental quality (as of air or water) through proper application of conservation and civil engineering practices

human engineering *n* : ERGONOMICS

human factors *n* : ERGONOMICS

human factors engineering *n* : ERGONOMICS

human immunodeficiency virus *n* : HIV

human relations *n* **1** : the social and interpersonal relations between human beings **2** : a course, study, or program designed to develop better interpersonal and intergroup adjustments

human T-cell leukemia virus *n* : HTLV

human T-cell leukemia virus type III *n* : HIV-1

human T-cell lym·pho·tro·pic virus \-ˌlim-fə-'trō-pik-\ *n* : HTLV

human T-cell lymphotropic virus type III *n* : HIV-1

human T-lymphotropic virus *n* : HTLV

human T-lymphotropic virus type III *n* : HIV-1

hu·mec·tant \hyü-'mek-tənt\ *n* : a substance (as glycerol or sorbitol) that promotes retention of moisture — **humectant** *adj*

hu·mer·al \'hyü-mə-rəl\ *adj* : of, relating to, or situated in the region of the humerus or shoulder

humeral circumflex artery — see ANTERIOR HUMERAL CIRCUMFLEX ARTERY, POSTERIOR HUMERAL CIRCUMFLEX ARTERY

hu·mer·us \'hyü-mə-rəs\ *n, pl* **hu·meri** \-ˌrī, -ˌrē\ : the longest bone of the upper arm or forelimb extending from the shoulder to the elbow, articulating above by a rounded head with the glenoid fossa, having below a broad articular surface divided by a ridge into a medial pulley-shaped portion and a lateral rounded eminence that articulate with the ulna and radius respectively

hu·mid·i·fi·er \hyü-'mi-də-ˌfī-ər, yü-\ *n* :

: a device for supplying or maintaining humidity

hu·mid·i·fy \-ˌfī\ *vb* **-fied; -fy·ing** : to make humid — **hu·mid·i·fi·ca·tion** \-ˌmi-də-fə-ˈkā-shən\ *n*

hu·mid·i·ty \hyü-ˈmi-də-tē, yü-\ *n, pl* **-ties** : a moderate degree of wetness esp. of the atmosphere — see ABSOLUTE HUMIDITY, RELATIVE HUMIDITY

hu·mor \ˈhyü-mər, ˈyü-\ *n* **1** : a normal functioning bodily semifluid or fluid (as the blood or lymph) **2** : a secretion (as a hormone) that is an excitant of activity

hu·mor·al \ˈhyü-mə-rəl, ˈyü-\ *adj* **1** : of, relating to, proceeding from, or involving a bodily humor (as a hormone) **2** : relating to or being the part of immunity or the immune response that involves antibodies secreted by B cells and circulating in bodily fluids ⟨∼ immunity⟩ — compare CELL-MEDIATED

hu·mour *chiefly Brit var of* HUMOR

hump \ˈhəmp\ *n* : a rounded protuberance; *esp* : HUMPBACK

hump·back \-ˌbak, *for 1 also* -ˈbak\ *n* **1** : a humped or crooked back; *also* : KYPHOSIS **2** : HUNCHBACK **2** — **hump·backed** \-ˌbakt\ *adj*

hunch·back \ˈhənch-ˌbak\ *n* **1** : HUMPBACK **1 2** : a person with a humpback — **hunch·backed** \-ˌbakt\ *adj*

hun·ger \ˈhəŋ-gər\ *n* **1** : a craving, desire, or urgent need for food **2** : an uneasy sensation occasioned normally by the lack of food and resulting directly from stimulation of the sensory nerves of the stomach by the contraction and churning movement of the empty stomach **3** : a weakened disordered condition brought about by prolonged lack of food ⟨die of ∼⟩

hunger pangs *n pl* : pains in the abdominal region which occur in the early stages of hunger or fasting and are correlated with contractions of the empty stomach or intestines

Hun·ner's ulcer \ˈhə-nərz-\ *n* : a painful ulcer affecting all layers of the bladder wall and usu. associated with inflammation of the wall

Hunner, Guy Leroy (1868–1957), American gynecologist.

Hun·ter's canal \ˈhən-tərz-\ *n* : an aponeurotic canal in the middle third of the thigh through which the femoral artery passes

Hunter, John (1728–1793), British anatomist and surgeon.

Hunter's syndrome *or* **Hunter syndrome** \ˈhən-tər-\ *n* : a mucopolysaccharidosis that is similar to Hurler's syndrome but is inherited as a sex-linked recessive trait and has milder symptoms

Hunter, Charles (fl 1917), Canadian physician.

Hun·ting·ton's chorea \ˈhən-tiŋ-tənz-\ *n* : HUNTINGTON'S DISEASE

Huntington, George (1850–1916), American neurologist.

Huntington's disease *n* : a hereditary chorea usu. developing in adult life and progressing to dementia

Hur·ler's syndrome \ˈhər-lərz-, ˈhür-\ *or* **Hur·ler syndrome** \-lər-\ *n* : a mucopolysaccharidosis that is inherited as an autosomal recessive trait and is characterized by deformities of the skeleton and features, hepatosplenomegaly, restricted joint flexibility, clouding of the cornea, mental deficiency, and deafness — called also *Hurler's disease*

Hur·ler \ˈhür-lər\, **Gertrud (fl 1920),** German pediatrician.

husk \ˈhəsk\ *n* : HOOSE

Hutch·in·son's teeth \ˈhə-chən-sənz-\ *n* : peg-shaped teeth having a crescent-shaped notch in the cutting edge and occurring esp. in children with congenital syphilis

Hutchinson, Sir Jonathan (1828–1913), British surgeon and pathologist.

Hutchinson's triad *n* : a triad of symptoms that comprises Hutchinson's teeth, interstitial keratitis, and deafness and occurs in children with congenital syphilis

Hux·ley's layer \ˈhəks-lēz-\ *n* : a layer of the inner stratum of a hair follicle composed of one or two layers of horny, flattened, epithelial cells with nuclei and situated between Henle's layer and the cuticle next to the hair

Huxley, Thomas Henry (1825–1895), British biologist.

hy- *or* **hyo-** *comb form* : of, relating to, or connecting with the hyoid bone ⟨*hyo*glossus⟩

hyal- *or* **hyalo-** *comb form* : glass : glassy : hyaline ⟨*hyal*uronic acid⟩

¹hy·a·line \ˈhī-ə-lən, -ˌlin\ *adj* : transparent or nearly transparent and usu. homogeneous

²hy·a·line \-ə-lən\ *n* : any of several translucent nitrogenous substances that collect around cells and are capable of being stained by eosin

hyaline cartilage *n* : translucent bluish white cartilage consisting of cells embedded in an apparently homogeneous matrix, present in joints and respiratory passages, and forming most of the fetal skeleton

hyaline cast *n* : a renal cast of mucoprotein characterized by homogeneity of structure

hyaline degeneration *n* : tissue degeneration chiefly of connective tissues in which structural elements of affected cells are replaced by homogeneous translucent material that stains intensely with acid stains

hyaline membrane disease *n* : a respiratory disease of unknown cause that occurs in newborn premature infants and is characterized by deficiency of the surfactant coating the inner surface of the lungs, by failure of the lungs to expand and contract properly during breathing with resulting collapse, and by the accumulation of a protein-containing film lining the alveoli and their ducts — abbr. *HMD*; called also *respiratory distress syndrome*

hy·a·lin·i·za·tion \ˌhī-ə-lə-nə-ˈzā-shən\ *n* : the process of becoming hyaline or of undergoing hyaline degeneration; *also* : the resulting state — **hy·a·lin·ized** \ˈhī-ə-lə-ˌnīzd\ *adj*

hy·a·li·no·sis \ˌhī-ə-lə-ˈnō-səs\ *n, pl* **-no·ses** \-ˌsēz\ **1** : HYALINE DEGENERATION **2** : a condition characterized by hyaline degeneration

hy·a·li·tis \ˌhī-ə-ˈlī-təs\ *n* **1** : inflammation of the vitreous humor of the eye **2** : inflammation of the hyaloid membrane of the vitreous humor

hyalo- — see HYAL-

hy·a·loid \ˈhī-ə-ˌloid\ *adj* : being glassy or transparent ⟨a ∼ appearance⟩

hyaloid membrane *n* : a very delicate membrane enclosing the vitreous humor of the eye

hy·a·lo·mere \ˈhī-ˈa-lə-ˌmir\ *n* : the pale portion of a blood platelet that is not refractile — compare CHROMOMERE

Hy·a·lom·ma \ˌhī-ə-ˈlä-mə\ *n* : a genus of Old World ticks that attack wild and domestic mammals and sometimes humans, produce severe lesions by their bites, and often serve as vectors of viral and protozoal diseases (as east coast fever)

hy·a·lo·plasm \ˈhī-ˈa-lə-ˌpla-zəm, ˈhī-ə-lō-\ *n* : CYTOSOL — **hy·a·lo·plas·mic** \ˌhī-ˌa-lə-ˈplaz-mik, ˌhī-ə-lō-\ *adj*

hy·al·uron·ic acid \ˌhī-əl-ˈyu̇-ˈra-nik-, -əl-yu̇-\ *n* : a viscous glycosaminoglycan that occurs esp. in the vitreous humor, the umbilical cord, and synovia and as a cementing substance in the subcutaneous tissue

hy·al·uron·i·dase \-ˈrä-nə-ˌdās, -ˌdāz\ *n* : a mucolytic enzyme that facilitates the spread of fluids through tissues by lowering the viscosity of hyaluronic acid and is used esp. to aid in the dispersion of fluids (as local anesthetics) injected subcutaneously for therapeutic purposes — called also *spreading factor*

H–Y antigen *n* : a male histocompatibility antigen determined by genes on the Y chromosome

hy·brid \ˈhī-brəd\ *n* **1** : an offspring of two animals or plants of different races, breeds, varieties, species, or genera **2** : something heterogeneous in origin or composition ⟨artificial ∼s of DNA and RNA⟩ ⟨somatic cell ∼s of mouse and human cells⟩ — **hybrid** *adj* — **hy·brid·ism** \-brə-ˌdi-zəm\ *n*

hy·brid·ize \ˈhī-brə-ˌdīz\ *vb* **-ized; -iz·ing** : to cause to interbreed or combine so as to produce hybrids — **hy·brid·i·za·tion** \ˌhī-brə-də-ˈzā-shən\ *n*

hy·brid·o·ma \ˌhī-brə-ˈdō-mə\ *n* : a hybrid cell produced by the fusion of an antibody-producing lymphocyte and a tumor cell and used to culture continuously a specific monoclonal antibody

hy·can·thone \hī-ˈkan-ˌthōn\ *n* : a lucanthone analog $C_{20}H_{24}N_2O_2S$ used to treat schistosomiasis

Hy·co·dan \ˈhī-kə-ˌdan\ *trademark* — used for a preparation of dihydrocodeinone

hy·dan·to·in \hī-ˈdan-tə-wən\ *n* **1** : a crystalline weakly acidic compound $C_3H_4N_2O_2$ with a sweetish taste that is found in beet juice **2** : a derivative of hydantoin (as phenytoin)

hy·dan·to·in·ate \-wə-ˌnāt\ *n* : a salt of hydantoin or of one of its derivatives

hy·da·tid \ˈhī-də-təd, -ˌtid\ *n* **1** : the larval cyst of a tapeworm of the genus *Echinococcus* that usu. occurs as a fluid-filled sac containing daughter cysts in which scolices develop but that occas. forms a proliferating spongy mass which actively metastasizes in the host's tissues — called also *hydatid cyst*; see ECHINOCOCCUS **2 a** : an abnormal cyst or cystic structure; *esp* : HYDATIDIFORM MOLE **b** : HYDATID DISEASE

hydatid disease *n* : a form of echinococcosis caused by the development of hydatids of a tapeworm of the genus *Echinococcus* (*E. granulosus*) in the tissues esp. of the liver or lungs of humans and some domestic animals (sheep and dogs)

hy·da·tid·i·form mole \ˌhī-də-ˈti-də-ˌform-\ *n* : a mass in the uterus consisting of enlarged edematous degenerated placental villi growing in clusters resembling grapes and usu. associated with death of the fetus

hy·da·tid·o·sis \ˌhī-də-ˌti-ˈdō-səs\ *n, pl* **-o·ses** \-ˌsēz\ : ECHINOCOCCOSIS; *specif* : HYDATID DISEASE

Hyd·er·gine \ˈhī-dər-ˌjēn\ *trademark* — used for a preparation of ergoloid mesylates

hydr- *or* **hydro-** *comb form* **1** : water ⟨hydrotherapy⟩ **2** : an accumulation of fluid in a (specified) bodily part ⟨hydrocephalus⟩ ⟨hydronephrosis⟩

hy·drae·mia *chiefly Brit var of* HYDREMIA

hy·dra·gogue \ˈhī-drə-ˌgäg\ *n* : a cathartic that causes copious watery discharges from the bowels

hy·dral·azine \hī-ˈdra-lə-ˌzēn\ *n* : an antihypertensive drug $C_8H_8N_4$ used in the form of its hydrochloride and acting to produce peripheral arteriolar dilation by relaxing vascular smooth muscle

hy·dram·ni·os \hī-ˈdram-nē-ˌäs\ *n* : excessive accumulation of the amniotic fluid — called also *polyhydramnios* — **hy·dram·ni·ot·ic** \hī-ˌdram-nē-ˈä-tik\ *adj*

hy·dran·en·ceph·a·ly \ˌhī-ˌdra-nen-ˈse-fə-lē\ *n, pl* **-lies** : a congenital defect of the brain in which fluid-filled cavities take the place of the cerebral hemispheres

hy·drar·gy·rism \hī-ˈdrär-jə-ˌri-zəm\ n : MERCURIALISM

hy·drar·thro·sis \ˌhī-(ˌ)drär-ˈthrō-səs\ n, pl **-thro·ses** \-ˌsēz\ : a watery effusion into a joint cavity

¹hy·drate \ˈhī-ˌdrāt\ n 1 : a compound or complex ion formed by the union of water with some other substance 2 : HYDROXIDE

²hydrate vb **hy·drat·ed; hy·drat·ing 1** : to cause to take up or combine with water or the elements of water 2 : to become a hydrate

hy·dra·tion \hī-ˈdrā-shən\ n 1 : the act or process of combining or treating with water: as **a** : the introduction of additional fluid into the body **b** : a chemical reaction in which water takes part with the formation of only one product 2 : the quality or state of being hydrated; esp : the condition of having adequate fluid in the body tissues

hy·dra·zide \ˈhī-drə-ˌzīd\ n : any of a class of compounds resulting from the replacement by an acid group of hydrogen in hydrazine or in one of its derivatives

hy·dra·zine \ˈhī-drə-ˌzēn\ n : a colorless fuming corrosive strongly reducing liquid base N_2H_4 used in the production of numerous materials (as pharmaceuticals and plastics); also : an organic base derived from this

hy·dra·zone \ˈhī-drə-ˌzōn\ n : any of a class of compounds containing the grouping $>C=NNHR$

hy·dre·mia \hī-ˈdrē-mē-ə\ n : an abnormally watery state of the blood — **hy·dre·mic** \-mik\ adj

hy·dren·ceph·a·ly \ˌhī-dren-ˈse-fə-lē\ n, pl **-lies** : HYDROCEPHALUS

hydro- see HYDR-

hy·droa \hī-ˈdrō-ə\ n : an itching usu. vesicular eruption of the skin; esp : one induced by exposure to light

hy·dro·bro·mide \ˌhī-drō-ˈbrō-ˌmīd\ n : a chemical complex composed of an organic compound in association with hydrogen bromide

hy·dro·car·bon \-ˈkär-bən\ n : an organic compound (as benzene) containing only carbon and hydrogen and often occurring esp. in petroleum, natural gas, and coal

hy·dro·cele \ˈhī-drə-ˌsēl\ n : an accumulation of serous fluid in a sacculated cavity (as the scrotum)

hy·dro·ce·lec·to·my \ˌhī-drə-sē-ˈlek-tə-mē\ n, pl **-mies** : surgical removal of a hydrocele

¹hy·dro·ce·phal·ic \ˌhī-drō-sə-ˈfa-lik\ adj : relating to, characterized by, or affected with hydrocephalus

²hydrocephalic n : an individual affected with hydrocephalus

hy·dro·ceph·a·lus \-ˈse-fə-ləs\ n, pl **-li** \-ˌlī\ : an abnormal increase in the amount of cerebrospinal fluid within the cranial cavity that is accompanied by expansion of the cerebral ventricles and enlargement of the skull

hy·dro·ceph·a·ly \ˌhī-drō-ˈse-fə-lē\ n, pl **-lies** : HYDROCEPHALUS

hy·dro·chlo·ric acid \ˌhī-drə-ˌklor-ik-\ n : an aqueous solution of hydrogen chloride HCl that is a strong corrosive irritating acid and is normally present in dilute form in gastric juice — called also muriatic acid

hy·dro·chlo·ride \-ˈklor-ˌīd\ n : a chemical complex composed of an organic base (as an alkaloid) in association with hydrogen chloride

hy·dro·chlo·ro·thi·a·zide \-ˌklor-ə-ˈthī-ə-ˌzīd\ n : a diuretic and antihypertensive drug $C_7H_8ClN_3O_4S_2$ — see HYDRODIURIL, ORETIC

hy·dro·cho·le·re·sis \-ˌkō-lər-ˈē-səs, -ˌkä-\ n, pl **-re·ses** \-ˌsēz\ : increased production of watery liver bile without necessarily increased secretion of bile solids — compare CHOLERESIS

¹hy·dro·cho·le·ret·ic \-ˈe-tik\ adj : of, relating to, or characterized by hydrocholeresis

²hydrocholeretic n : an agent that produces hydrocholeresis

hy·dro·co·done \ˌhī-drō-ˈkō-ˌdōn\ n : DIHYDROCODEINONE

hy·dro·cor·ti·sone \-ˈkor-tə-ˌsōn, -ˌzōn\ n : a glucocorticoid $C_{21}H_{30}O_5$ of the adrenal cortex that is a derivative of cortisone and is used in the treatment of rheumatoid arthritis — called also cortisol

hy·dro·cy·an·ic acid \ˌhī-drō-sī-ˈa-nik-\ n : an aqueous solution of hydrogen cyanide HCN that is an extremely poisonous weak acid used esp. in fumigating — called also prussic acid

Hy·dro·di·ur·il \-ˈdī-yə-ˌril\ trademark — used for a preparation of hydrochlorothiazide

hy·dro·dy·nam·ics \ˌhī-drō-dī-ˈna-miks\ n : a science that deals with the motion of fluids and the forces acting on moving bodies immersed in fluids — **hy·dro·dy·nam·ic** \-mik\ adj

hy·dro·flu·me·thi·a·zide \-ˌflü-mə-ˈthī-ə-ˌzīd\ n : a diuretic and antihypertensive drug $C_8H_8F_3N_3O_4S_2$ — see SALURON

hy·dro·gel \ˈhī-drə-ˌjel\ n : a gel in which the liquid is water

hy·dro·gen \ˈhī-drə-jən\ n : a nonmetallic element that is the simplest and lightest of the elements and is normally a colorless odorless highly flammable gas, having two atoms in a molecule — symbol H; see ELEMENT table — **hy·drog·e·nous** \hī-ˈdrä-jə-nəs\ adj

hy·dro·ge·nate \hī-ˈdrä-jə-ˌnāt, ˈhī-drə-jə-\ vb **-nat·ed; -nat·ing** : to add hydro-

hy·dras·ti·nine \hī-ˈdras-tə-ˌnēn, -nən\ n : a crystalline base $C_{11}H_{13}NO_3$ useful in controlling uterine hemorrhage

gen to the molecule of (an unsaturated organic compound) — **hy·dro·ge·na·tion** \hī-₁drä-jə-'nā-shən, ₁hī-drə-jə-\ n

hydrogen bond n : a linkage consisting of a hydrogen atom bonded between two negatively charged atoms (as fluorine, oxygen, or nitrogen) with one side of the linkage being a covalent bond and the other being electrostatic in nature; also : the electrostatic bond in this linkage

hydrogen bromide n : a colorless irritating gas HBr that fumes in moist air and yields a strong acid resembling hydrochloric acid when dissolved in water

hydrogen chloride n : a colorless pungent poisonous gas HCl that fumes in moist air and yields hydrochloric acid when dissolved in water

hydrogen cyanide n 1 : a poisonous usu. gaseous compound HCN that has the odor of bitter almonds 2 : HYDROCYANIC ACID

hydrogen peroxide n : an unstable compound H_2O_2 used esp. as an oxidizing and bleaching agent and as an antiseptic

hy·dro·lase \'hī-drə-₁lās, -₁lāz\ n : a hydrolytic enzyme (as an esterase)

hy·drol·o·gy \hī-'drä-lə-jē\ n, pl **-gies** : the body of medical knowledge and practice concerned with the therapeutic use of bathing and water

hy·dro·ly·sate \hī-'drä-lə-₁sāt, ₁hī-drə-'lī-\ or **hy·dro·ly·zate** \-₁zāt\ n : a product of hydrolysis

hy·dro·ly·sis \hī-'drä-lə-səs, ₁hī-drə-'lī-\ n : a chemical process of decomposition involving splitting of a bond and addition of the elements of water — **hy·dro·lyt·ic** \₁hī-drə-'li-tik\ adj — **hy·dro·lyze** \'hī-drə-₁līz\ vb — **hy·dro·lyz·able** \₁hī-drə-'lī-zə-bəl\ adj

hy·dro·me·tro·col·pos \₁hī-drō-₁mē-trō-'käl-₁päs\ n : an accumulation of watery fluid in the uterus and vagina

hy·dro·mor·phone \-'mór-₁fōn\ n : a morphine derivative $C_{17}H_{19}NO_3$ used as an analgesic in the form of its hydrochloride salt

hy·dro·ne·phro·sis \-ni-'frō-səs, n, pl **-phro·ses** \-₁sēz\ : cystic distension of the kidney caused by the accumulation of urine in the renal pelvis as a result of obstruction to outflow and accompanied by atrophy of the kidney structure and cyst formation — **hy·dro·ne·phrot·ic** \-ni-'frä-tik\ adj

hy·drop·a·thy \hī-'drä-pə-thē\ n, pl **-thies** : a method of treating disease by copious and frequent use of water both externally and internally — compare HYDROTHERAPY — **hy·dro·path·ic** \₁hī-drə-'pa-thik\ adj

hy·dro·pe·nia \₁hī-drə-'pē-nē-ə\ n : a condition in which the body is deficient in water — **hy·dro·pe·nic** \-'pē-nik\ adj

hy·dro·peri·car·di·um \₁hī-drō-per-ə-

'kär-dē-əm\ n, pl **-dia** \-dē-ə\ : an excess of watery fluid in the pericardial cavity

hy·dro·phil·ic \-'fi-lik\ adj : of, relating to, or having a strong affinity for water (~ colloids) — compare LIPOPHILIC — **hy·dro·phi·lic·i·ty** \-₁fi-'li-sə-tē\ n

hy·dro·pho·bia \₁hī-drə-'fō-bē-ə\ n 1 : a morbid dread of water 2 : RABIES

hy·dro·pho·bic \-'fō-bik\ adj 1 : of, relating to, or suffering from hydrophobia 2 : resistant to or avoiding wetting (a ~ lens) 3 : of, relating to, or having a lack of affinity for water (~ colloids) — **hy·dro·pho·bic·i·ty** \-₁fō-'bi-sə-tē\ n

hy·droph·thal·mos \₁hī-₁dräf-'thal-məs\ n : general enlargement of the eyeball due to a watery effusion within it

hy·drop·ic \hī-'drä-pik\ adj 1 : exhibiting hydrops; esp : EDEMATOUS 2 : characterized by swelling and taking up of fluid — used of a type of cellular degeneration

hy·dro·pneu·mo·tho·rax \₁hī-drə-₁nü-mə-'thor-₁aks, -nyü-\ n, pl **-tho·rax·es** or **-tho·ra·ces** \-'thor-ə-₁sēz\ : the presence of gas and serous fluid in the pleural cavity

hy·drops \'hī-₁dräps\ n, pl **hy·drop·ses** \-₁dräp-₁sēz\ 1 : EDEMA 2 : distension of a hollow organ with fluid 3 : HYDROPS FETALIS

hydrops fe·tal·is \-fē-'ta-ləs\ n : serious and extensive edema of the fetus (as in erythroblastosis fetalis)

hy·dro·qui·none \₁hī-drō-kwi-'nōn, -'kwi-₁nōn\ n : a bleaching agent $C_6H_6O_2$ used topically to remove pigmentation from hyperpigmented areas of skin (as a lentigo or freckle)

hy·dro·sal·pinx \-'sal-(₁)piŋks\ n, pl **-sal·pin·ges** \-sal-'pin-(₁)jēz\ : abnormal distension of one or both fallopian tubes with fluid usu. due to inflammation

hy·dro·ther·a·py \₁hī-drō-'ther-ə-pē\ n, pl **-pies** : the therapeutic use of water (as in a whirlpool bath) — compare HYDROPATHY — **hy·dro·ther·a·peu·tic** \-₁ther-ə-'pyü-tik\ adj

hy·dro·tho·rax \-'thor-₁aks, n, pl **-tho·rax·es** or **-tho·ra·ces** \-'thor-ə-₁sēz\ : an excess of serous fluid in the pleural cavity; esp : an effusion resulting from failing circulation (as in heart disease)

hy·dro·ure·ter \₁hī-drō-'yur-ə-tər, -yu-'rē-tər\ n : abnormal distension of the ureter with urine

hydrous wool fat \'hī-drəs-\ n : LANOLIN

hy·drox·ide \hī-'dräk-₁sīd\ n 1 : the anion OH⁻ consisting of one atom of hydrogen and one of oxygen — called also hydroxide ion 2 a : an ionic compound of hydroxide with an element or group b : any of various hydrated oxides

hy·droxo·co·bal·amin \hī-₁dräk-(₁)sō-kō-'ba-lə-mən\ n : a member C_{62}-

$H_{89}CoN_{13}O_{15}P$ of the vitamin B_{12} group used in treating and preventing vitamin B_{12} deficiency

hy·droxy \hī-ˈdräk-sē\ *adj* : being or containing hydroxyl; *esp* : containing hydroxyl in place of hydrogen — often used in combination (*hydroxy-butyric acid*)

hy·droxy·am·phet·amine \hī-ˌdräk-sē-am-ˈfe-tə-ˌmēn, -mən\ *n* : a sympathomimetic drug $C_9H_{13}NO$ used esp. as a decongestant and mydriatic

hydroxyanisole — see BUTYLATED HYDROXYANISOLE

hy·droxy·ap·a·tite \hī-ˌdräk-sē-ˈa-pə-ˌtīt\ *n* : a complex phosphate of calcium $Ca_5(PO_4)_3OH$ that is the chief structural element of bone

hy·droxy·ben·zo·ic acid \-ben-ˈzō-ik-\ *n* : SALICYLIC ACID

hy·droxy·bu·ty·rate \-ˈbyü-tə-ˌrāt\ *n* : a salt or ester of hydroxybutyric acid

hy·droxy·bu·tyr·ic acid \-byü-ˈtir-ik-\ *n* : a derivative $C_4H_8O_3$ of butyric acid that is excreted in urine in increased quantities in diabetes — called also *oxybutyric acid*

hy·droxy·chlor·o·quine \-ˈklōr-ə-ˌkwēn, -kwin\ *n* : a drug $C_{18}H_{26}ClN_3O$ derived from quinoline that is administered as the sulfate and is used in the treatment of malaria, rheumatoid arthritis, and lupus erythematosus — see PLAQUENIL

25-hy·droxy·cho·le·cal·cif·er·ol \ˈtwen-tē-ˈfiv-hī-ˌdräk-sē-ˌkō-lə-ˌ(ˌ)kal-ˈsi-fə-ˌrȯl, -rōl\ *n* : a sterol $C_{27}H_{44}O$ that is a metabolite of cholecalciferol formed in the liver and is the circulating form of vitamin D

17-hy·droxy·cor·ti·co·ste·roid \ˌse-vən-ˈtēn-hī-ˌdräk-sē-ˈkȯrt-i-kō-ˈstir-ˌȯid, -ˈster-\ *n* : any of several adrenocorticosteroids (as hydrocortisone) with an —OH group and an $HOCH_2CO^-$ group attached to carbon 17 of the fused ring structure of the steroid

hy·droxy·di·one sodium suc·ci·nate \hī-ˌdräk-sē-ˈdī-ˌōn ... ˈsək-sə-ˌnāt\ *n* : a steroid $C_{25}H_{35}NaO_6$ given intravenously as a general anesthetic

6-hy·droxy·do·pa·mine \ˈsiks-hī-ˌdräk-sē-ˈdō-pə-ˌmēn\ *n* : an isomer of norepinephrine that is taken up by catecholaminergic nerve fibers and causes the degeneration of their terminals

5-hy·droxy·in·dole·ace·tic acid \ˈfiv-hī-ˌdräk-sē-ˌin-(ˌ)dōl-ə-ˈsē-tik-\ *n* : a metabolite $C_{10}H_9NO_3$ of serotonin that is present in cerebrospinal fluid and in urine

hy·drox·yl \hī-ˈdräk-səl\ *n* **1** : the chemical group or ion OH that consists of one atom of hydrogen and one of oxygen and is neutral or positively charged **2** : HYDROXIDE 1

hy·drox·yl·ap·a·tite \hī-ˌdräk-sə-ˈla-pə-ˌtīt\ *var of* HYDROXYAPATITE

hy·drox·y·lase \hī-ˈdräk-sə-ˌlās, -ˌlāz\ *n* : any of a group of enzymes that cat-

alyze oxidation reactions in which one of the two atoms of molecular oxygen is incorporated into the substrate and the other is used to oxidize NADH or NADPH

hy·droxy·ly·sine \hī-ˌdräk-sē-ˈlī-ˌsēn\ *n* : an amino acid $C_6H_{14}N_2O_3$ that is found esp. in collagen

hy·droxy·pro·ges·ter·one \hī-ˌdräk-sē-prō-ˈjes-tə-ˌrōn\ *or* **17α–hydroxyprogesterone** \ˌse-vən-ˈtēn-ˈal-fə-\ *n* : a synthetic derivative $C_{21}H_{30}O_3$ of progesterone used esp. as the caproate in progestational therapy (as for amenorrhea)

hy·droxy·pro·line \-ˈprō-ˌlēn\ *n* : an amino acid $C_5H_9NO_3$ that occurs naturally as a constituent of collagen

8-hy·droxy·quin·o·line \ˈāt-hī-ˌdräk-sē-ˈkwin-ᵊl-ˌēn\ *n* : a derivative C_9H_7NO of quinoline used esp. in the form of its sulfate as a disinfectant, topical antiseptic, antiperspirant, and deodorant — called also *oxyquinoline*

hy·droxy·ste·roid \-ˈstir-ˌȯid, -ˈster-\ *n* : any of several ketosteroids (as androsterone) found esp. in urine

hydroxytoluene — see BUTYLATED HYDROXYTOLUENE

5-hy·droxy·tryp·ta·mine \ˈfiv-hī-ˌdräk-sē-ˈtrip-tə-ˌmēn\ *n* : SEROTONIN

hy·droxy·urea \-yü-ˈrē-ə\ *n* : an antineoplastic drug $CH_4N_2O_2$ used to treat some forms of leukemia

hy·droxy·zine \hī-ˈdräk-sə-ˌzēn\ *n* : a compound $C_{21}H_{27}ClN_2O_2$ that is administered usu. in the form of the hydrochloride or the pamoate and is used as an antihistamine and tranquilizer — see VISTARIL

hy·giene \ˈhī-ˌjēn\ *n* **1** : a science of the establishment and maintenance of health — see MENTAL HYGIENE **2** : conditions or practices (as of cleanliness) conducive to health — **hy·gien·ic** \ˌhī-jē-ˈe-nik, hī-ˈje-, hī-ˈjē-\ *adj* — **hy·gien·i·cal·ly** *adv*

hy·gien·ics \-iks\ *n* : HYGIENE 1

hy·gien·ist \hī-ˈjē-nist, -ˈje-; ˈhī-ˌjē-\ *n* : a specialist in hygiene; *esp* : one skilled in a specified branch of hygiene — see DENTAL HYGIENIST

hy·gro·ma \hī-ˈgrō-mə\ *n*, *pl* **-mas** *or* **-ma·ta** \-mə-tə\ : a cystic tumor of lymphatic origin

hy·grom·e·ter \hī-ˈgrä-mə-tər\ *n* : any of several instruments for measuring the humidity of the atmosphere — **hy·gro·met·ric** \ˌhī-grə-ˈme-trik\ *adj*

hy·gro·my·cin B \ˌhī-grə-ˈmīs-ᵊn-ˈbē\ *n* : an antibiotic $C_{20}H_{37}N_3O_{13}$ obtained from a bacterium of the genus *Streptomyces* (*S. hygroscopicus*) and used as an anthelmintic in swine and chickens

hy·gro·scop·ic \ˌhī-grə-ˈskä-pik\ *adj* : readily taking up and retaining moisture (glycerol is ~)

Hy·gro·ton \ˈhī-grə-ˌtän\ *trademark* — used for a preparation of chlorthalidone

hy·men \'hī-mən\ *n* : a fold of mucous membrane partly or wholly closing the orifice of the vagina — **hy·men·al** \-mən-ᵊl\ *adj*

hymen- *or* **hymeno-** *comb form* : hymen : membrane ⟨hymen*ectomy*⟩ ⟨hymen*otomy*⟩

hy·men·ec·to·my \ˌhī-mə-'nek-tə-mē\ *n, pl* **-mies** : surgical removal of the hymen

Hy·me·nol·e·pis \ˌhī-mə-'nä-lə-pəs\ *n* : a genus of small taenioid tapeworms (family Hymenolepididae) that are parasites of mammals and birds and include one (*H. nana*) that is an intestinal parasite of humans

hy·me·nop·ter·an \ˌhī-mə-'näp-tə-rən\ *n* : any of an order (Hymenoptera) of highly specialized and often colonial insects (as bees, wasps, and ants) that have usu. four thin transparent wings and the abdomen on a slender stalk — **hymenopteran** *adj* — **hy·me·nop·ter·ous** \-tə-rəs\ *adj*

hy·me·nop·ter·ism \-'näp-tə-ˌri-zəm\ *n* : poisoning resulting from the bite or sting of a hymenopteran insect

hy·me·not·o·my \ˌhī-mə-'nä-tə-mē\ *n, pl* **-mies** : surgical incision of the hymen

hyo- — see HY-

hyo·glos·sal \ˌhī-ō-'gläs-əl, -'glós-\ *adj* : of, relating to, or connecting the tongue and hyoid bone

hyo·glos·sus \-'glä-səs, -'gló-\ *n, pl* **-si** \-ˌsī, -ˌsē\ : a flat muscle on each side of the tongue

hy·oid \'hī-ˌoid\ *adj* : of or relating to the hyoid bone

hyoid bone *n* : a bone or complex of bones situated at the base of the tongue and supporting the tongue and its muscles — called also *hyoid*

hyo·man·dib·u·lar \ˌhī-ō-man-'di-byü-lər\ *n* : a bone or cartilage that forms the columella or stapes of the ear of higher vertebrates — **hyomandibular** *adj*

hyo·scine \'hī-ə-ˌsēn\ *n* : SCOPOLAMINE; *esp* : the levorotatory form of scopolamine

hyo·scy·a·mine \ˌhī-ə-'sī-ə-ˌmēn\ *n* : a poisonous crystalline alkaloid $C_{17}H_{23}NO_3$ of which atropine is a racemic mixture; *esp* : its levorotatory form found esp. in the plants belladonna and henbane and used similarly to atropine

hyo·scy·a·mus \-məs\ *n* **1** *cap* : a genus of poisonous Eurasian herbs of the nightshade family (Solanaceae) that includes the henbane (*H. niger*) **2** : the dried leaves of the henbane containing the alkaloids hyoscyamine and scopolamine and used as an antispasmodic and sedative

Hyo·stron·gy·lus \-ˈsträn-jə-ləs\ *n* : a genus of nematode worms (family Trichostrongylidae) that includes the common small red stomach worm (*H. rubidus*) of swine

¹hyp·acu·sic \ˌhī-pə-'kü-sik, -'kyü-\ *adj* : affected with hypoacusis

²hypacusic *n* : one affected with hypoacusis

hyp·acu·sis \-'kü-səs, -'kyü-\ *n* : HYPOACUSIS

hyp·aes·the·sia *Brit var of* HYPESTHESIA

hyp·al·ge·sia \ˌhī-pəl-'jē-zhə, ˌhī-pal-, -zē-ə, -zhē-ə\ *n* : diminished sensitivity to pain — **hyp·al·ge·sic** \-'jē-zik, -sik\ *adj*

Hy·paque \'hī-ˌpāk\ *trademark* — used for a diatrizoate preparation for use in radiographic diagnosis

hyper- *prefix* **1** : excessively ⟨hyper*sensitive*⟩ **2** : excessive ⟨hyper*emia*⟩ ⟨hyper*tension*⟩

hy·per·acid·i·ty \ˌhī-pə-rə-'si-də-tē\ *n, pl* **-ties** : the condition of containing more than the normal amount of acid — **hy·per·acid** \ˌhī-pə-'ra-səd\ *adj*

¹hy·per·ac·tive \ˌhī-pə-'rak-tiv\ *adj* : affected with or exhibiting hyperactivity; *broadly* : more active than is usual or desirable

²hyperactive *n* : one who is hyperactive

hy·per·ac·tiv·i·ty \ˌhī-pə-ˌrak-'ti-və-tē\ *n, pl* **-ties** : a state or condition of being excessively or pathologically active; *esp* : ATTENTION DEFICIT DISORDER

hy·per·acu·sis \ˌhī-pə-rə-'kü-səs, -'kyü-\ *n* : abnormally acute hearing

hy·per·acute \ˌhī-pə-rə-'kyüt\ *adj* : extremely or excessively acute ⟨~ hearing⟩

hy·per·adren·a·lin·ae·mia *chiefly Brit var of* HYPERADRENALINEMIA

hy·per·adren·a·lin·emia \ˌhī-pə-rə-ˌdren-ᵊl-ə-'nē-mē-ə\ *n* : the presence of an excess of adrenal hormones (as epinephrine) in the blood

hy·per·ad·re·no·cor·ti·cism \ˌhī-pə-rə-ˌdrē-nō-'kor-tə-ˌsi-zəm\ *n* : the presence of an excess of adrenocortical products in the body

hy·per·ae·mia, hy·per·aes·the·sia *chiefly Brit var of* HYPEREMIA, HYPERESTHESIA

hy·per·ag·gres·sive \ˌhī-pə-rə-'gre-səv\ *adj* : extremely or excessively aggressive ⟨~ patients⟩

hy·per·al·do·ste·ron·ae·mia *chiefly Brit var of* HYPERALDOSTERONEMIA

hy·per·al·do·ste·ron·emia \ˌhī-pə-ral-ˌdäs-tə-ˌrō-'nē-mē-ə, ˌral-dō-stə-ˌrō-\ *n* : the presence of an excess of aldosterone in the blood

hy·per·al·do·ste·ron·ism \ˌhī-pə-ral-'däs-tə-ˌrō-ˌni-zəm, ˌral-dō-stə-'rō-\ *n* : ALDOSTERONISM

hy·per·al·ge·sia \ˌhī-pə-ral-'jē-zhə, -zē-ə, -zhē-ə\ *n* : increased sensitivity to pain or enhanced intensity of pain sensation — **hy·per·al·ge·sic** \-'jē-zik, -sik\ *adj*

hy·per·al·i·men·ta·tion \ˌhī-pə-ˌra-lə-mən-'tā-shən\ *n* : the administration of nutrients by intravenous feeding

hy·per·ami·no·ac·id·uria \ˌhī-pə-rə-ˌmē-nō-ˌa-sə-'dur-ē-ə, -'dyür-\ *n* : the presence of an excess of amino acids in the urine

hy·per·am·mo·nae·mia *also* **hy·per·am·mon·i·ae·mia** *chiefly Brit var of* HYPERAMMONEMIA

hy·per·am·mo·ne·mia \\hī-pə-ra-mo-ˈnē-mē-ə\ *also* **hy·per·am·mon·i·emia** \\hī-pə-rə-ˌmō-nē-ˈyē-mē-ə\ *n* : the presence of an excess of ammonia in the blood — **hy·per·am·mo·ne·mic** \\hī-pe-ˌrra-mə-ˈnē-mik\ *adj*

hy·per·am·y·las·ae·mia *chiefly Brit var of* HYPERAMYLASEMIA

hy·per·am·y·las·emia \\hī-pə-ˌra-mə-ˌlā-ˈsē-mē-ə\ *n* : the presence of an excess of amylase in the blood

hy·per·arous·al \\hī-pə-rə-ˈrau-zəl\ *n* : excessive arousal

hy·per·bar·ic \\hī-pər-ˈbar-ik\ *adj* **1** : having a specific gravity greater than that of cerebrospinal fluid — used of solutions for spinal anesthesia; compare HYPOBARIC **2** : of, relating to, or utilizing greater than normal pressure esp. of oxygen (a ∼ chamber) (∼ medicine) — **hy·per·bar·i·cal·ly** *adv*

hy·per·be·ta·li·po·pro·tein·emia \-ˌbā-tə-ˌli-pō-ˌprō-ˌtē-ˈnē-mē-ə, -ˌli-, -ˌprō-tē-ə-\ *n* : the presence of excess LDLs in the blood

hy·per·bil·i·ru·bin·emia \-ˌbi-lē-ˌrü-bi-ˈnē-mē-ə\ *n* : the presence of an excess of bilirubin in the blood — called also *bilirubinemia*

hy·per·cal·cae·mia *chiefly Brit var of* HYPERCALCEMIA

hy·per·cal·ce·mia \\hī-pər-kal-ˈsē-mē-ə\ *n* : the presence of an excess of calcium in the blood — **hy·per·cal·ce·mic** \-ˈsē-mik\ *adj*

hy·per·cal·ci·uria \-ˌkal-sē-ˈyùr-ē-ə\ *also* **hy·per·cal·cin·uria** \-ˌkal-sə-ˈnùr-ē-ə\ *n* : the presence of an excess amount of calcium in the urine

hy·per·cap·nia \-ˈkap-nē-ə\ *n* : the presence of an excess of carbon dioxide in the blood — **hy·per·cap·nic** \-nik\ *adj*

hy·per·car·bia \-ˈkär-bē-ə\ *n* : HYPERCAPNIA

hy·per·cel·lu·lar·i·ty \-ˌsel-yə-ˈlar-ə-tē\ *n, pl* **-ties** : the presence of an abnormal excess of cells (as in bone marrow) — **hy·per·cel·lu·lar** \-ˈsel-yə-lər\ *adj*

hy·per·ce·men·to·sis \-ˌsē-men-ˈtō-səs\ *n, pl* **-to·ses** \-ˌsēz\ : excessive formation of cementum at the root of a tooth

hy·per·chlor·ae·mia *chiefly Brit var of* HYPERCHLOREMIA

hy·per·chlor·emia \-ˌklōr-ˈē-mē-ə\ *n* : the presence of excess chloride ions in the blood — **hy·per·chlor·emic** \-ˈē-mik\ *adj*

hy·per·chlor·hy·dria \-ˌklōr-ˈhī-drē-ə\ *n* : the presence of a greater than typical proportion of hydrochloric acid in gastric juice — compare ACHLORHYDRIA, HYPOCHLORHYDRIA

hy·per·cho·les·ter·ol·emia \\hī-pər-kə-

les-tə-rə-ˈlē-mē-ə\ *or* **hy·per·cho·les·ter·emia** \-tə-ˈrē-mē-ə\ *n* : the presence of excess cholesterol in the blood — **hy·per·cho·les·ter·ol·emic** \-tə-rə-ˈlē-mik\ *or* **hy·per·cho·les·ter·emic** \-tə-ˈrē-mik\ *adj*

hy·per·chro·ma·sia \-krō-ˈmā-zhə, -zē-ə, -zhē-ə\ *n* : HYPERCHROMATISM

hy·per·chro·ma·tism \-ˈkrō-mə-ˌti-zəm\ *n* : the development of excess chromatin or of excessive nuclear staining esp. as a part of a pathological process — **hy·per·chro·mat·ic** \-krō-ˈma-tik\ *adj*

hy·per·chro·mia \-ˈkrō-mē-ə\ *n* **1** : excessive pigmentation (as of the skin) **2** : a state of the red blood cells marked by increase in the hemoglobin content — **hy·per·chro·mic** \-ˈkrō-mik\ *adj*

hyperchromic anemia *n* : an anemia with increase of hemoglobin in individual red blood cells and reduction in the number of red blood cells — compare HYPOCHROMIC ANEMIA; see PERNICIOUS ANEMIA

hy·per·chy·lo·mi·cro·ne·mia \\hī-pər-ˌki-lō-ˌmī-krō-ˈnē-mē-ə\ *n* : the presence of excess chylomicrons in the blood

hy·per·co·ag·u·la·bil·i·ty \-kō-ˌa-gyə-lə-ˈbi-lə-tē\ *n, pl* **-ties** : excessive coagulability — **hy·per·co·ag·u·la·ble** \-kō-ˈa-gyə-lə-bəl\ *adj*

hy·per·cor·ti·sol·ism \-ˈkȯr-ti-ˌsȯ-li-zəm, -sō-\ *n* : hyperadrenocorticism produced by excess hydrocortisone in the body

hy·per·cu·prae·mia *chiefly Brit var of* HYPERCUPREMIA

hy·per·cu·pre·mia \-kü-ˈprē-mē-ə, -kyü-\ *n* : the presence of an excess of copper in the blood

hy·per·cy·thae·mia *chiefly Brit var of* HYPERCYTHEMIA

hy·per·cy·the·mia \-sī-ˈthē-mē-ə\ *n* : the presence of an excess of red blood cells in the blood — **hy·per·cy·the·mic** \-ˈthē-mik\ *adj*

hy·per·dip·loid \-ˈdi-ˌplȯid\ *adj* : having slightly more than the diploid number of chromosomes

hy·per·em·e·sis \-ˈe-mə-səs, -i-ˈmē-\ *n, pl* **-eme·ses** \-ˌsēz\ : excessive vomiting

hyperemesis grav·i·dar·um \-ˌgra·və-ˈdar-əm\ *n* : excessive vomiting during pregnancy

hy·per·emia \\hī-pə-ˈrē-mē-ə\ *n* : excess of blood in a body part : CONGESTION — **hy·per·emic** \-mik\ *adj*

hy·per·en·dem·ic \-en-ˈde-mik, -in-\ *adj* **1** : exhibiting a high and continued incidence — used chiefly of human diseases **2** : marked by hyperendemic disease — used of geographic areas — **hy·per·en·de·mic·i·ty** \-ˌen-ˌde-ˈmi-sə-tē\ *n*

hy·per·er·gic \\hī-pər-ˈər-jik\ *adj* : characterized by or exhibiting a greater than normal sensitivity to an allergen — **hy·per·er·gy** \'hī-pər-ˌər-jē\ n

hy·per·es·the·sia \ˌhī-pər-es-'thē-zhə, -zhē-ə\ n : unusual or pathological sensitivity of the skin or of a particular sense to stimulation — **hy·per·es·thet·ic** \-'the-tik\ adj

hy·per·es·trin·ism \-'es-trə-ˌni-zəm\ n : a condition marked by the presence of excess estrins in the blood

hy·per·es·tro·gen·ism \-'es-trə-jə-ˌni-zəm\ n : a condition marked by the presence of excess estrogens in the body

hy·per·ex·cit·abil·i·ty \ˌhī-pər-ik-ˌsī-tə-'bi-lə-tē\ n, pl **-ties** : the state or condition of being unusually or excessively excitable — **hy·per·ex·cited** \-ik-'sī-təd\ adj — **hy·per·ex·cite·ment** n

hy·per·ex·tend \ˌhī-pər-ik-'stend\ vb : to extend so that the angle between bones of a joint is greater than normal ⟨a ∼ed elbow⟩ — **hy·per·ex·ten·sion** \-'sten-chən\ n

hy·per·ex·ten·si·ble \-ik-'sten-sə-bəl\ adj : having the capacity to be hyperextended or stretched to a greater than normal degree ⟨∼ joints⟩ — **hy·per·ex·ten·si·bil·i·ty** \-sten-sə-'bi-lə-tē\ n

hy·per·flex \'hī-pər-ˌfleks\ vb : to flex so that the angle between the bones of a joint is smaller than normal — **hy·per·flex·ion** \-ˌflek-shən\ n

hy·per·func·tion \-ˌfəŋk-shən\ n : excessive or abnormal activity ⟨cardiac ∼⟩ — **hy·per·func·tion·al** \-shə-nəl\ adj — **hy·per·func·tion·ing** n

hy·per·gam·ma·glob·u·lin·ae·mia chiefly Brit var of HYPERGAMMAGLOBULIN-EMIA

hy·per·gam·ma·glob·u·lin·emia \ˌhī-pər-ˌga-mə-ˌglä-byə-lə-'nē-mē-ə\ n : the presence of an excess of gamma globulins in the blood — **hy·per·gam·ma·glob·u·lin·emic** \-'nē-mik\ adj

hy·per·gas·trin·ae·mia chiefly Brit var of HYPERGASTRINEMIA

hy·per·gas·trin·emia \ˌgas-trə-'nē-mē-ə\ n : the presence of an excess of gastrin in the blood — **hy·per·gas·trin·emic** \-'nē-mik\ adj

hy·per·glob·u·lin·ae·mia chiefly Brit var of HYPERGLOBULINEMIA

hy·per·glob·u·lin·emia \-ˌglä-byə-lə-'nē-mē-ə\ n : the presence of excess globulins in the blood — **hy·per·glob·u·lin·emic** \-'nē-mik\ adj

hy·per·glu·ca·gon·ae·mia chiefly Brit var of HYPERGLUCAGONEMIA

hy·per·glu·ca·gon·emia \-ˌglü-kə-gä-'nē-mē-ə\ n : the presence of excess glucagon in the blood

hy·per·gly·ce·mia \ˌhī-pər-glī-'sē-mē-ə\ n : an excess of sugar in the blood — **hy·per·gly·ce·mic** \-mik\ adj

hyperglycemic factor n : GLUCAGON

hy·per·gly·ci·nae·mia chiefly Brit var of HYPERGLYCINEMIA

hy·per·gly·ci·ne·mia \ˌhī-pər-ˌglī-sə-'nē-mē-ə\ n : a hereditary disorder characterized by the presence of excess glycine in the blood

hy·per·go·nad·ism \ˌhī-pər-'gō-ˌna-ˌdi-zəm\ n : excessive hormonal secretion by the gonads

hy·per·hi·dro·sis \-hi-'drō-səs, -hī-\ also **hy·peri·dro·sis** \-i-'drō-\ n, pl **-dro·ses** \-ˌsēz\ : generalized or localized excessive sweating — compare HYPO-HIDROSIS

hy·per·hy·dra·tion \-hī-'drā-shən\ n : an excess of water in the body

hy·per·i·cism \hī-'pər-ə-ˌsi-zəm\ n : a severe dermatitis of domestic animals due to photosensitivity resulting from eating Saint-John's-wort — compare FAGOPYRISM

hy·per·im·mune \ˌhī-pər-i-'myün\ adj : exhibiting an unusual degree of immunization: **a** of a serum : containing exceptional quantities of antibody **b** of an antibody : having the characteristics of a blocking antibody

hy·per·im·mu·nize \-'i-myə-ˌnīz\ vb **-nized; -niz·ing** : to induce a high level of immunity or of circulating antibodies in — **hy·per·im·mu·ni·za·tion** \-ˌi-myə-nə-'zā-shən\ n

hy·per·in·fec·tion \-in-'fek-shən\ n : repeated reinfection with larvae produced by parasitic worms already in the body — compare AUTOINFECTION

hy·per·in·fla·tion \-in-'flā-shən\ n : excessive inflation (as of the lungs)

hy·per·in·su·lin·emia \-ˌin-sə-lə-'nē-mē-ə\ n : the presence of excess insulin in the blood — **hy·per·in·su·lin·emic** \-mik\ adj

hy·per·in·su·lin·ism \-'in-sə-lə-ˌni-zəm\ n : the presence of excess insulin in the body resulting in hypoglycemia

hy·per·ir·ri·ta·bil·i·ty \-ir-ə-tə-'bi-lə-tē\ n, pl **-ties** : abnormally great or uninhibited response to stimuli — **hy·per·ir·ri·ta·ble** \-'ir-ə-tə-bəl\ adj

hy·per·ka·lae·mia chiefly Brit var of HYPERKALEMIA

hy·per·ka·le·mia \-kā-'lē-mē-ə\ n : the presence of an abnormally high concentration of potassium in the blood — called also hyperpotassemia — **hy·per·ka·le·mic** \-'lē-mik\ adj

hy·per·ker·a·ti·ni·za·tion \-ˌker-ə-tə-nə-'zā-shən, -kə-ˌrat-ᵊn-ə-\ n : HYPER-KERATOSIS

hy·per·ker·a·to·sis \-ˌker-ə-'tō-səs\ n, pl **-to·ses** \-'tō-ˌsēz\ **1** : hypertrophy of the stratum corneum of the skin **2** : any of various conditions marked by hyperkeratosis — **hy·per·ker·a·tot·ic** \-'tät-ik\ adj

hy·per·ke·to·ne·mia \-ˌkē-tə-'nē-mē-ə\ n : KETONEMIA 1

hy·per·ki·ne·sia \-kə-'nē-zhə, -kī-, -zhē-ə\ n : HYPERKINESIS

hy·per·ki·ne·sis \-'nē-səs\ n **1** : abnormally increased and sometimes uncontrollable activity or muscular movements **2** : a condition esp. of childhood characterized by hyperactivity

hy·per·ki·net·ic \-kə-'ne-tik, -kī-\ *adj* : of, relating to, or affected with hyperkinesis or hyperactivity

hy·per·lex·ia \-'lek-sē-ə\ *n* : precocious reading ability in a retarded child — **hy·per·lex·ic** \-sik\ *adj*

hy·per·li·pe·mia \-hī-pər-li-'pē-mē-ə\ *n* : the presence of excess fat or lipids in the blood — **hy·per·li·pe·mic** \-mik\ *adj*

hy·per·lip·id·ae·mia *chiefly Brit var of* HYPERLIPIDEMIA

hy·per·lip·id·emia \-li-pə-'dē-mē-ə\ *n* : HYPERLIPEMIA — **hy·per·lip·id·emic** \-mik\ *adj*

hy·per·li·po·pro·tein·ae·mia *chiefly Brit var of* HYPERLIPOPROTEINEMIA

hy·per·li·po·pro·tein·emia \-lī-pə-prō-tē-'nē-mē-ə, -li-\ *n* : the presence of excess lipoprotein in the blood

hy·per·mag·ne·sae·mia *chiefly Brit var of* HYPERMAGNESEMIA

hy·per·mag·ne·se·mia \-mag-ni-'sē-mē-ə\ *n* : the presence of excess magnesium in the blood serum

hy·per·men·or·rhea \-me-nə-'rē-ə\ *n* : abnormally profuse or prolonged menstrual flow — *compare* MENORRHAGIA

hy·per·me·tab·o·lism \-mə-'ta-bə-li-zəm\ *n* : metabolism at an increased or excessive rate — **hy·per·meta·bol·ic** \-me-tə-'bä-lik\ *adj*

hy·per·me·tria \-'mē-trē-ə\ *n* : a condition of cerebellar dysfunction in which voluntary muscular movements tend to result in the movement of bodily parts (as the arm and hand) beyond the intended goal

hy·per·me·tro·pia \-hī-pər-mi-'trō-pē-ə\ *n* : HYPEROPIA — **hy·per·me·tro·pic** \-'trō-pik, -'trä-\ *adj*

hy·per·mne·sia \-hī-(-)pərm-'nē-zhə, -zhē-ə\ *n* : abnormally vivid or complete memory or recall of the past (as at times of extreme danger) — **hy·perm·ne·sic** \-'nē-zik, -sik\ *adj*

hy·per·mo·bil·i·ty \-hī-pər-mō-'bi-lə-tē\ *n, pl* **-ties** : an increase in the range of movement of which a bodily part and esp. a joint is capable — **hy·per·mo·bile** \-'mō-bəl, -bil, -bēl\ *adj*

hy·per·mo·til·i·ty \-hī-pər-mō-'ti-lə-tē\ *n, pl* **-ties** : abnormal or excessive movement; *specif* : excessive motility of all or part of the gastrointestinal tract — *compare* HYPERPERISTALSIS, HYPOMOTILITY — **hy·per·mo·tile** \-'mōt-əl, -'mō-til\ *adj*

hy·per·na·trae·mia *chiefly Brit var of* HYPERNATREMIA

hy·per·na·tre·mia \-nā-'trē-mē-ə\ *n* : the presence of an abnormally high concentration of sodium in the blood — **hy·per·na·tre·mic** \-mik\ *adj*

hy·per·neph·roid \-'ne-froid\ *adj* : resembling the adrenal cortex in histological structure (∼ *tumors*)

hy·per·ne·phro·ma \-ni-'frō-mə\ *n, pl* **-mas** *or* **-ma·ta** \-mə-tə\ : a tumor of the kidney resembling the adrenal cortex in its histological structure

hy·per·oes·trin·ism, hy·per·oes·tro·gen·ism *chiefly Brit var of* HYPERESTRINISM, HYPERESTROGENISM

hy·per·ope \'hī-pər-ōp\ *n* : a person affected with hyperopia

hy·per·opia \-hī-pər-'ō-pē-ə\ *n* : a condition in which visual images come to a focus behind the retina of the eye and vision is better for distant than for near objects — *called also* farsightedness, hypermetropia — **hy·per·opic** \-'ō-pik, -'ä-\ *adj*

hy·per·os·mia \-hī-pər-'äz-mē-ə\ *n* : extreme acuteness of the sense of smell

hy·per·os·mo·lal·i·ty \-äz-mō-'la-lə-tē\ *n, pl* **-ties** : the condition esp. of a bodily fluid of having abnormally high osmolality

hy·per·os·mo·lar·i·ty \-'lar-ə-tē\ *n, pl* **-ties** : the condition esp. of a bodily fluid of having abnormally high osmolarity — **hy·per·os·mo·lar** \-äz-'mō-lər\ *adj*

hy·per·os·mot·ic \-äz-'mä-tik\ *adj* : HYPERTONIC 2

hy·per·os·to·sis \-äs-'tō-səs\ *n, pl* **-to·ses** \-sēz\ : excessive growth or thickening of bone tissue — **hy·per·os·tot·ic** \-'tä-tik\ *adj*

hy·per·ox·al·uria \-ak-sə-'lùr-ē-ə\ *n* : the presence of excess oxalic acid or oxalates in the urine

hy·per·ox·ia \-'äk-sē-ə\ *n* : a bodily condition characterized by a greater oxygen content of the tissues and organs than normally exists at sea level

hy·per·para·thy·roid·ism \-hī-pər-par-ə-'thī-roi-di-zəm\ *n* : the presence of excess parathyroid hormone in the body resulting in disturbance of calcium metabolism

hy·per·path·ia \-'pa-thē-ə\ *n* **1** : disagreeable or painful sensation in response to a normally innocuous stimulus (as touch) **2** : a condition in which the sensations of hyperpathia occur — **hy·per·path·ic** \-thik\ *adj*

hy·per·peri·stal·sis \-per-ə-'stol-səs, -'stäl-, -'stal-\ *n, pl* **-stal·ses** \-sēz\ : excessive or excessively vigorous peristalsis — *compare* HYPERMOTILITY

hy·per·pha·gia \-'fā-jə, -jē-ə\ *n* : abnormally increased appetite for food frequently associated with injury to the hypothalamus — *compare* POLYPHAGIA — **hy·per·phag·ic** \-'fa-jik\ *adj*

hy·per·phe·nyl·al·a·nin·ae·mia *chiefly Brit var of* HYPERPHENYLALANINEMIA

hy·per·phe·nyl·al·a·nin·emia \-fen-əl-a-lə-nə-'nē-mē-ə, -fēn-\ *n* : the presence of excess phenylalanine in the blood (as in phenylketonuria) — **hy-**

per·phe·nyl·al·a·nin·emic \-'nē-mik\ *adj*

hy·per·pho·ria \-'fōr-ē-ə\ *n* : latent strabismus in which one eye deviates upward in relation to the other

hy·per·phos·pha·tae·mia *chiefly Brit var of* HYPERPHOSPHATEMIA

hy·per·phos·pha·te·mia \-ɹfäs-fə-'tē-mē-ə\ *n* : the presence of excess phosphate in the blood

hy·per·phos·pha·tu·ria \-ɹfäs-fə-'tur̄-ē-ə, -'tyūr-\ *n* : the presence of excess phosphate in the urine

hy·per·pi·e·sia \-ɹpī-'ē-zhə, -zhē-ə\ *n* : HYPERTENSION; *esp* : ESSENTIAL HYPERTENSION

hy·per·pig·men·ta·tion \-ɹpig-mən-'tā-shən, -ɹmen-\ *n* : excess pigmentation in a bodily part or tissue (as the skin) — **hy·per·pig·ment·ed** \-'pig-mən-təd, -ɹmen-\ *adj*

hy·per·pi·tu·ita·rism \-pə-'tü-ə-tə-ɹri-zəm, -'tyü-, -ɹtri-zəm\ *n* : excessive production of growth hormones by the pituitary gland — **hy·per·pi·tu·itary** \-pə-'tü-ə-ter-ē, -'tyü-\ *adj*

hy·per·pla·sia \ɹhī-pər-'plā-zhə, -zhē-ə\ *n* : an abnormal or unusual increase in the elements composing a part (as cells composing a tissue) — **hy·per·plas·tic** \-'plas-tik\ *adj*

hy·per·ploid \'hī-pər-ɹplȯid\ *adj* : having a chromosome number slightly greater than an exact multiple of the haploid number — **hy·per·ploi·dy** \-ɹplȯid-ē\ *n*

hy·per·pnea \ɹhī-pərp-'nē-ə, -pər-\ *n* : abnormally rapid or deep breathing — **hy·per·pne·ic** \-'nē-ik\ *adj*

hy·per·pnoea *chiefly Brit var of* HYPERPNEA

hy·per·po·lar·ize \ɹhī-pər-'pō-lə-ɹrīz\ *vb* **-ized; -iz·ing** 1 : to produce an increase in potential difference across (a biological membrane) 2 : to undergo or produce an increase in potential difference across something — **hy·per·po·lar·iza·tion** \-ɹpō-lə-rə-'zā-shən\ *n*

hy·per·po·tas·sae·mia *chiefly Brit var of* HYPERPOTASSEMIA

hy·per·po·tas·se·mia \-pə-ɹta-'sē-mē-ə\ *n* : HYPERKALEMIA — **hy·per·po·tas·se·mic** \-'sē-mik\ *adj*

hy·per·pro·duc·tion \-prə-'dək-shən, -prō-\ *n* : excessive production

hy·per·pro·lac·tin·ae·mia *chiefly Brit var of* HYPERPROLACTINEMIA

hy·per·pro·lac·tin·ae·mia \-prō-ɹlak-tin-'ē-mē-ə\ *n* : the presence of an abnormally high concentration of prolactin in the blood — **hy·per·pro·lac·tin·emic** \-'nē-mik\ *adj*

hy·per·pro·lin·ae·mia *chiefly Brit var of* HYPERPROLINEMIA

hy·per·pro·lin·emia \-prō-lə-'nē-mē-ə\ *n* : a hereditary metabolic disorder characterized by an abnormally high concentration of proline in the blood and often associated with mental retardation

hy·per·py·rex·ia \-pī-'rek-sē-ə\ *n* : exceptionally high fever

hy·per·re·ac·tive \-rē-'ak-tiv\ *adj* : having or showing abnormally high sensitivity to stimuli — **hy·per·re·ac·tiv·i·ty** \-(ɹ)rē-ɹak-'ti-və-tē\ *n*

hy·per·re·flex·ia \-rē-'flek-sē-ə\ *n* : overactivity of physiological reflexes

hy·per·re·nin·ae·mia *chiefly Brit var of* HYPERRENINEMIA

hy·per·re·nin·emia \-ɹrē-nə-'nē-mē-ə, -ɹre-\ *n* : the presence of an abnormally high concentration of renin in the blood

hy·per·re·spon·sive \-ri-'spän-siv\ *adj* : characterized by an abnormal degree of responsiveness (as to a physical stimulus) — **hy·per·re·spon·siv·i·ty** \-ri-ɹspän-'si-və-tē\ *n*

hy·per·sal·i·va·tion \-ɹsa-lə-'vā-shən\ *n* : excessive salivation

hy·per·se·cre·tion \-si-'krē-shən\ *n* : excessive production of a bodily secretion — **hy·per·se·crete** \-si-'krēt\ *vb* — **hy·per·se·cre·to·ry** \-'sē-krə-ɹtor-ē, -si-'krē-tə-rē\ *adj*

hy·per·sen·si·tive \ɹhī-pər-'sen-sə-tiv\ *adj* **1** : excessively or abnormally sensitive **2** : abnormally susceptible physiologically to a specific agent (as a drug) — **hy·per·sen·si·tive·ness** \-nəs\ *n* — **hy·per·sen·si·tiv·i·ty** \-ɹsen-sə-'ti-və-tē\ *n* — **hy·per·sen·si·ti·za·tion** \-sə-tə-'zā-shən\ *n* — **hy·per·sen·si·tize** \-'sen-sə-ɹtiz\ *vb*

hy·per·sex·u·al \-'sek-shə-wəl\ *adj* : exhibiting unusual or excessive concern with or indulgence in sexual activity — **hy·per·sex·u·al·i·ty** \-ɹsek-shə-'wa-lə-tē\ *n*

hy·per·sid·er·ae·mia *chiefly Brit var of* HYPERSIDEREMIA

hy·per·sid·er·emia \-ɹsi-də-'rē-mē-ə\ *n* : the presence of an abnormally high concentration of iron in the blood — **hy·per·sid·er·emic** \-mik\ *adj*

hy·per·som·nia \-'säm-nē-ə\ *n* **1** : sleep of excessive depth or duration **2** : the condition of sleeping for excessive periods at intervals with intervening periods of normal duration of sleeping and waking — compare NARCOLEPSY

hy·per·sple·nism \-'splē-ɹni-zəm, -'sple-\ *n* : a condition marked by excessive destruction of one or more kinds of blood cells in the spleen

hy·per·sthen·ic \ɹhī-pərs-'the-nik\ *adj* : of, relating to, or characterized by excessive muscle tone

hy·per·sus·cep·ti·ble \-sə-'sep-tə-bəl\ *adj* : HYPERSENSITIVE — **hy·per·sus·cep·ti·bil·i·ty** \-ɹsep-tə-'bi-lə-tē\ *n*

hy·per·tel·or·ism \-'te-lə-ɹri-zəm\ *n* : excessive width between two bodily parts or organs (as the eyes)

hy·per·tense \ɹhī-pər-'tens\ *adj* : excessively tense ⟨a ~ emotional state⟩

Hy·per·ten·sin \-'ten-sən\ *trademark* — used for a preparation of the amide of angiotensin

hy·per·ten·sin·ase \-'ten-sə-ˌnās, -ˌnāz\ n : ANGIOTENSINASE

hy·per·ten·sin·o·gen \-ˌten-'si-nə-jən, -ˌjen\ n : ANGIOTENSINOGEN

hy·per·ten·sion \ˌhī-pər-'ten-chən\ n 1 : abnormally high arterial blood pressure: **a** : such blood pressure occurring without apparent or determinable prior organic changes in the tissues possibly because of hereditary tendency, emotional tensions, faulty nutrition, or hormonal influence **b** : such blood pressure with demonstrable organic changes (as in nephritis, diabetes, and hyperthyroidism) 2 : a systemic condition resulting from hypertension that is either symptomless or is accompanied by nervousness, dizziness, or headache

¹**hy·per·ten·sive** \-'ten-siv\ adj : marked by a rise in blood pressure : suffering or caused by hypertension

²**hypertensive** n : a person affected with hypertension

hy·per·ther·mia \-'thər-mē-ə\ n : exceptionally high fever esp. when induced artificially for therapeutic purposes — **hy·per·ther·mic** \-mik\ adj

hy·per·thy·roid \-'thī-ˌroid\ adj : of, relating to, or affected with hyperthyroidism ⟨a ~ state⟩

hy·per·thy·roid·ism \-ˌroi-di-zəm\ n : excessive functional activity of the thyroid gland; also : the resulting condition marked esp. by increased metabolic rate, enlargement of the thyroid gland, rapid heart rate, and high blood pressure — called also *thyrotoxicosis;* see GRAVES' DISEASE

hy·per·to·nia \ˌhī-pər-'tō-nē-ə\ n : HYPERTONICITY

hy·per·ton·ic \-'tä-nik\ adj 1 : exhibiting excessive tone or tension ⟨a ~ bladder⟩ 2 : having a higher osmotic pressure than a surrounding medium or a fluid under comparison — compare HYPOTONIC 2, ISOSMOTIC

hy·per·to·nic·i·ty \-tə-'ni-sə-tē\ n, pl -ties : the quality or state of being hypertonic

hy·per·to·nus \-'tō-nəs\ n : HYPERTONICITY

hy·per·tri·cho·sis \-tri-'kō-səs\ n, pl -cho·ses \-ˌsēz\ : excessive growth of hair

hy·per·tri·glyc·er·i·dae·mia *chiefly Brit var of* HYPERTRIGLYCERIDEMIA

hy·per·tri·glyc·er·i·de·mia \-ˌtrī-ˌgli-sə-ˌrī-'dē-mē-ə\ n : the presence of an excess of triglycerides in the blood — **hy·per·tri·glyc·er·i·de·mic** \-'dē-mik\ adj

hypertrophic arthritis n : OSTEOARTHRITIS

hy·per·tro·phy \hī-'pər-trə-fē\ n, pl -phies : excessive development of an organ or part; *specif* : increase in bulk (as by thickening of muscle fibers) without multiplication of parts — **hy·per·tro·phic** \ˌhī-pər-'trō-fik\ adj — **hypertrophy** vb

hy·per·tro·pia \ˌhī-pər-'trō-pē-ə\ n : elevation of the line of vision of one eye above that of the other : upward strabismus

hy·per·uri·ce·mia \ˌhī-pər-ˌyùr-ə-'sē-mē-ə\ n : excess uric acid in the blood (as in gout) — called also *uricemia* — **hy·per·uri·ce·mic** \-'sē-mik\ adj

hy·per·uri·cos·uria \-ˌyùr-i-kō-'shùr-ē-ə, -'syùr-\ n : the excretion of excessive amounts of uric acid in the urine

hy·per·ven·ti·late \-'vent-əl-ˌāt\ vb -lat·ed; -lat·ing : to breathe rapidly and deeply : undergo hyperventilation

hy·per·ven·ti·la·tion \-ˌvent-əl-'ā-shən\ n : excessive rate and depth of respiration leading to abnormal loss of carbon dioxide from the blood — called also *overventilation*

hy·per·vis·cos·i·ty \-vis-'kä-sə-tē\ n, pl -ties : excessive viscosity (as of the blood)

hy·per·vi·ta·min·osis \-ˌvī-tə-mə-'nō-səs\ n, pl -oses \-ˌsēz\ : an abnormal state resulting from excessive intake of one or more vitamins

hy·per·vol·ae·mia *chiefly Brit var of* HYPERVOLEMIA

hy·per·vol·emia \-vä-'lē-mē-ə\ n : an excessive volume of blood in the body — **hy·per·vol·emic** \-'lē-mik\ adj

hyp·es·the·sia \ˌhī-pes-'thē-zhə, ˌhi-, -zhē-ə\ n : impaired or decreased tactile sensibility — **hyp·es·thet·ic** \-'thē-tik\ adj

hy·phae·ma *chiefly Brit var of* HYPHEMA

hy·phe·ma \hī-'fē-mə\ n : a hemorrhage in the anterior chamber of the eye

hypn- *or* **hypno-** *comb form* 1 : sleep ⟨*hypn*agogic⟩ 2 : hypnotism ⟨*hypno*therapy⟩

hyp·na·go·gic *also* **hyp·no·go·gic** \ˌhip-nə-'gä-jik, -'gō-\ adj : of, relating to, or associated with the drowsiness preceding sleep ⟨~ hallucinations⟩ — compare HYPNOPOMPIC

hyp·no·anal·y·sis \ˌhip-nō-ə-'na-lə-səs\ n, pl -y·ses \-ˌsēz\ : the treatment of mental disease by hypnosis and psychoanalytic methods

hyp·no·pom·pic \ˌhip-nə-'päm-pik\ adj : associated with the semiconsciousness preceding waking ⟨~ illusions⟩ — compare HYPNAGOGIC

hyp·no·sis \hip-'nō-səs\ n, pl -no·ses \-ˌsēz\ 1 : a state that resembles sleep but is induced by a person whose suggestions are readily accepted by the subject 2 : any of various conditions that resemble sleep 3 : HYPNOTISM 1

hyp·no·ther·a·pist \ˌhip-nō-'ther-ə-pist\ n : a specialist in hypnotherapy

hyp·no·ther·a·py \-'ther-ə-pē\ n, pl -pies 1 : the treatment of disease by hypnotism 2 : psychotherapy that facilitates suggestion, reeducation, or analysis by means of hypnosis

¹**hyp·not·ic** \hip-'nä-tik\ adj 1 : tending to produce sleep : SOPORIFIC 2 : of or

relating to hypnosis or hypnotism — **hyp·not·i·cal·ly** *adv*

²**hypnotic** *n* **1** : a sleep-inducing agent : SOPORIFIC **2** : one that is or can be hypnotized

hyp·no·tism \'hip-nə-₁ti-zəm\ *n* **1** : the study or act of inducing hypnosis — compare MESMERISM **2** : HYPNOSIS **1**

hyp·no·tist \-tist\ *n* : an expert in hypnotism : a person who induces hypnosis

hyp·no·tize \-₁tīz\ *vb* **-tized; -tiz·ing** : to induce hypnosis in — **hyp·no·tiz·abil·i·ty** \₁hip-nə-₁tī-zə-'bi-lə-tē\ *n* — **hyp·no·tiz·able** \'hip-nə-'tī-zə-bəl\ *adj*

¹**hy·po** \'hī-(₁)pō\ *n, pl* **hypos** : HYPOCHONDRIA

²**hypo** *n, pl* **hypos** **1** : HYPODERMIC SYRINGE **2** : HYPODERMIC INJECTION

hypo- *or* **hyp-** *prefix* **1** : under : beneath : down ⟨*hypo*blast⟩ ⟨*hypo*dermic⟩ **2** : less than normal or normally ⟨*hypes*thesia⟩ ⟨*hypo*tension⟩

hy·po·acid·i·ty \₁hī-pō-a-'si-də-tē\ *n, pl* **-ties** : abnormally low acidity (gastric ∼)

hy·po·ac·tive \-'ak-tiv\ *adj* : less than normally active ⟨∼ children⟩ ⟨∼ bowel sounds⟩ — **hy·po·ac·tiv·i·ty** \-ak-'ti-və-tē\ *n*

hy·po·acu·sis \-ə-'kü-səs, -'kyü-\ *n* : partial loss of hearing — called also *hypacusis*

hy·po·adren·al·ism \-ə-'dren-ᵊl-₁i-zəm\ *n* : abnormally decreased activity of the adrenal glands; *specif* : HYPOADRENOCORTICISM

hy·po·ad·re·no·cor·ti·cism \-ə-₁drē-nō-'kȯr-tə-₁si-zəm\ *n* : abnormally decreased activity of the adrenal cortex (as in Addison's disease)

hy·po·aes·the·sia \₁hī-pō-es-'thē-zhə, -hi-, -zhē-ə\ *Brit var of* HYPESTHESIA

hy·po·al·bu·min·ae·mia *chiefly Brit var of* HYPOALBUMINEMIA

hy·po·al·bu·min·emia \-al-₁byü-mə-'nē-mē-ə\ *n* : hypoproteinemia marked by reduction in serum albumins — **hy·po·al·bu·min·emic** \-'nē-mik\ *adj*

hy·po·al·ge·sia \-al-'jē-zhə, -zhē-ə, -zē-ə\ *n* : decreased sensitivity to pain

hy·po·al·ler·gen·ic \-₁a-lər-'je-nik\ *adj* : having little likelihood of causing an allergic response ⟨∼ food⟩

hy·po·ami·no·ac·id·emia \-ə-₁mē-nō-₁a-sə-'dē-mē-ə\ *n* : the presence of abnormally low concentrations of amino acids in the blood

hy·po·bar·ic \-'bar-ik\ *adj* : having a specific gravity less than that of cerebrospinal fluid — used of solutions for spinal anesthesia; compare HYPERBARIC **1**

hy·po·bar·ism \-'bar-₁i-zəm\ *n* : a condition which occurs when the ambient pressure is lower than the pressure of gases within the body and which may be marked by the distension of bodily cavities and the release of gas bubbles within bodily tissues

hy·po·blast \'hī-pə-₁blast\ *n* : the endoderm of an embryo — **hy·po·blas·tic** \₁hī-pə-'blas-tik\ *adj*

hy·po·cal·cae·mia *chiefly Brit var of* HYPOCALCEMIA

hy·po·cal·ce·mia \₁hī-pō-₁kal-'sē-mē-ə\ *n* : a deficiency of calcium in the blood — **hy·po·cal·ce·mic** \-mik\ *adj*

hy·po·cal·ci·fi·ca·tion \-₁kal-sə-fə-'kā-shən\ *n* : decreased or deficient calcification (as of tooth enamel)

hy·po·cap·nia \-'kap-nē-ə\ *n* : a deficiency of carbon dioxide in the blood — **hy·po·cap·nic** \-nik\ *adj*

hy·po·chlor·ae·mia *chiefly Brit var of* HYPOCHLOREMIA

hy·po·chlor·emia \₁hī-pō-klȯr-'ē-mē-ə\ *n* : abnormal decrease of chlorides in the blood — **hy·po·chlor·emic** \-klȯr-'ē-mik\ *adj*

hy·po·chlor·hy·dria \-klȯr-'hī-drē-ə\ *n* : deficiency of hydrochloric acid in the gastric juice — compare ACHLORHYDRIA, HYPERCHLORHYDRIA — **hy·po·chlor·hy·dric** \-'hī-drik\ *adj*

hy·po·chlo·rite \₁hī-pə-'klȯr-₁īt\ *n* : a salt or ester of hypochlorous acid

hy·po·chlo·rous acid \-'klȯr-əs-\ *n* : an unstable strongly oxidizing but weak acid HClO obtained in solution along with hydrochloric acid by reaction of chlorine with water and used esp. in the form of salts as an oxidizing agent, bleaching agent, disinfectant, and chlorinating agent

hy·po·cho·les·ter·ol·emia \₁hī-pō-kə-₁les-tə-rə-'lē-mē-ə\ *or* **hy·po·cho·les·ter·emia** \-tə-'rē-mē-ə\ *n* : an abnormal deficiency of cholesterol in the blood — **hy·po·cho·les·ter·ol·emic** \-'lē-mik\ *or* **hy·po·cho·les·ter·emic** \-'rē-mik\ *adj*

hy·po·chon·dria \₁hī-pə-'kän-drē-ə\ *n* : extreme depression of mind or spirits often centered on imaginary physical ailments; *specif* : HYPOCHONDRIASIS

¹**hy·po·chon·dri·ac** \-drē-₁ak\ *adj* **1** : HYPOCHONDRIACAL **2 a** : situated below the costal cartilages **b** : of, relating to, or being the two abdominal regions lying on either side of the epigastric region and above the lumbar regions

²**hypochondriac** *n* : a person affected by hypochondria or hypochondriasis

hy·po·chon·dri·a·cal \-kən-'drī-ə-kəl, -₁kän-\ *adj* : affected with or produced by hypochondria

hy·po·chon·dri·a·sis \-'drī-ə-səs\ *n, pl* **-a·ses** \-₁sēz\ : morbid concern about one's health esp. when accompanied by delusions of physical disease

hy·po·chon·dri·um \-'kän-drē-əm\ *n, pl* **-dria** \-drē-ə\ : either hypochondriac region of the body

hy·po·chro·mia \₁hī-pə-'krō-mē-ə\ *n* **1** : deficiency of color or pigmentation **2** : deficiency of hemoglobin in the red blood cells (as in nutritional anemia) — **hy·po·chro·mic** \-'krō-mik\ *adj*

hypochromic anemia *n* : an anemia marked by deficient hemoglobin and usu. microcytic red blood cells — compare HYPERCHROMIC ANEMIA

hy·po·co·ag·u·la·bil·i·ty \ˌhī-pō-kō-ˌa-gyə-lə-ˈbil-ə-tē\ *n, pl* **-ties** : decreased or deficient coagulability of blood — **hy·po·co·ag·u·la·ble** \-kō-ˈa-gyə-lə-bəl\ *adj*

hy·po·com·ple·men·tae·mia *chiefly Brit var of* HYPOCOMPLEMENTEMIA

hy·po·com·ple·men·te·mia \-ˌkäm-plə-(ˌ)men-ˈtē-mē-ə\ *n* : an abnormal deficiency of complement in the blood — **hy·po·com·ple·men·te·mic** \-ˈtē-mik\ *adj*

hy·po·cu·prae·mia *chiefly Brit var of* HYPOCUPREMIA

hy·po·cu·pre·mia \-kü-ˈprē-mē-ə, -kyü-\ *n* : an abnormal deficiency of copper in the blood

hy·po·cu·pro·sis \-kü-ˈprō-səs, -kyü-\ *n, pl* **-pro·ses** \-ˌsēz\ : HYPOCUPREMIA

hy·po·der·ma \ˌhī-pə-ˈdər-mə\ *n* 1 *cap* : a genus (family Hypodermatidae) of dipteran flies that have parasitic larvae and include the common cattle grub (*H. lineatum*) 2 : any insect or maggot of the genus *Hypoderma*

hy·po·der·ma·to·sis \-ˌdər-mə-ˈtō-səs\ *n* : infestation with maggots of flies of the genus *Hypoderma*

hy·po·der·mi·a·sis \-dər-ˈmī-ə-səs\ *n, pl* **-a·ses** \-ˌsēz\ : HYPODERMATOSIS

¹hy·po·der·mic \ˌhī-pə-ˈdər-mik\ *adj* 1 : of or relating to the parts beneath the skin 2 : adapted for use in or administered by injection beneath the skin — **hy·po·der·mi·cal·ly** *adv*

²hypodermic *n* 1 : HYPODERMIC INJECTION 2 : HYPODERMIC SYRINGE

hypodermic injection *n* : an injection made into the subcutaneous tissues

hypodermic needle *n* 1 : NEEDLE 2 2 : a hypodermic syringe complete with needle

hypodermic syringe *n* : a small syringe used with a hollow needle for injection of material into or beneath the skin

hy·po·der·mis \ˌhī-pə-ˈdər-məs\ *n* : SUPERFICIAL FASCIA

hy·po·der·moc·ly·sis \-dər-ˈmä-klə-səs\ *n, pl* **-ly·ses** \-ˌsēz\ : subcutaneous injection of fluids (as saline solution)

hy·po·dip·loid \ˌhī-pō-ˈdi-ˌplȯid\ *adj* : having slightly fewer than the diploid number of chromosomes — **hy·po·dip·loi·dy** \-ˌplȯi-dē\ *n*

hy·po·don·tia \-ˈdän-chə, -chē-ə\ *n* : an esp. congenital condition marked by a less than normal number of teeth : partial anodontia — **hy·po·don·tic** \-ˈdän-tik\ *adj*

hy·po·dy·nam·ic \-dī-ˈna-mik\ *adj* : marked by or exhibiting a decrease in strength or power ⟨the ∼ heart⟩

hy·po·es·the·sia \ˌhī-pō-es-ˈthē-zhə, -zhē-ə, -zē-ə\ *var of* HYPESTHESIA

hy·po·fer·rae·mia *chiefly Brit var of* HYPOFERREMIA

hy·po·fer·re·mia \ˌhī-pō-fə-ˈrē-mē-ə\ *n* : an abnormal deficiency of iron in the blood — **hy·po·fer·re·mic** \-ˈrē-mik\ *adj*

hy·po·fi·brin·o·gen·ae·mia *chiefly Brit var of* HYPOFIBRINOGENEMIA

hy·po·fi·brin·o·gen·emia \-fī-ˌbri-nə-jə-ˈnē-mē-ə\ *n* : an abnormal deficiency of fibrinogen in the blood

hy·po·func·tion \ˈhī-pō-ˌfəŋk-shən\ *n* : decreased or insufficient function esp. of an endocrine gland

hy·po·gam·ma·glob·u·lin·emia \-ˌga-mə-ˌglä-byə-lə-ˈnē-mē-ə\ *n* : a deficiency of gamma globulins in the blood — **hy·po·gam·ma·glob·u·lin·emic** \-ˈnē-mik\ *adj*

hy·po·gas·tric \ˌhī-pə-ˈgas-trik\ *adj* 1 : of or relating to the lower median abdominal region 2 : relating to or situated along or near the internal iliac arteries or the internal iliac veins

hypogastric artery *n* : ILIAC ARTERY 3

hypogastric nerve *n* : a nerve or several parallel nerve bundles situated dorsal and medial to the common and the internal iliac arteries

hypogastric plexus *n* : the sympathetic nerve plexus that supplies the pelvic viscera

hypogastric vein *n* : ILIAC VEIN c

hy·po·gas·tri·um \ˌhī-pə-ˈgas-trē-əm\ *n, pl* **-tria** \-trē-ə\ : the hypogastric region of the abdomen

hy·po·gen·i·tal·ism \-ˈje-nə-tə-ˌli-zəm\ *n* : subnormal development of genital organs : genital infantilism

hy·po·geu·sia \-ˈgü-sē-ə, -ˈjü-, -zē-ə\ *n* : decreased sensitivity to taste ⟨idiopathic ∼⟩

hy·po·glos·sal \ˌhī-pə-ˈglä-səl\ *adj* : of or relating to the hypoglossal nerves

hypoglossal nerve *n* : either of the 12th and final pair of cranial nerves which are motor nerves arising from the medulla oblongata and supplying muscles of the tongue and hyoid apparatus — called also *hypoglossal*, *twelfth cranial nerve*

hypoglossal nucleus *n* : a nucleus in the floor of the fourth ventricle of the brain that is the origin of the hypoglossal nerve

hy·po·glos·sus \-ˈglä-səs\ *n, pl* **-glos·si** \-ˌsī, -ˌsē\ : HYPOGLOSSAL NERVE

hy·po·gly·ce·mia \ˌhī-pō-glī-ˈsē-mē-ə\ *n* : abnormal decrease of sugar in the blood

¹hy·po·gly·ce·mic \-ˈsē-mik\ *adj* 1 : of, relating to, caused by, or affected with hypoglycemia 2 : producing a decrease in the level of sugar in the blood ⟨∼ drugs⟩

²hypoglycemic *n* 1 : one affected with hypoglycemia 2 : an agent that lowers the level of sugar in the blood

hy·po·go·nad·al \-gō-ˈnad-əl\ *adj* 1 : relating to or affected with hypogonadism 2 : marked by or exhibiting deficient development of secondary sexual characteristics

hy·po·go·nad·ism \-ˈgō-ˌna-ˌdi-zəm\ *n* 1 : functional incompetence of the gonads esp. in the male **2** : a condition (as Klinefelter's syndrome) involving gonadal incompetence

hy·po·go·nad·o·trop·ic \-gō-ˌna-də-ˈträ-pik\ or **hy·po·go·nad·o·tro·phic** \-ˈtrō-fik, -ˈträ-\ adj : characterized by a deficiency of gonadotropins

hy·po·hi·dro·sis \-hi-ˈdrō-səs, -hī-\ n, pl **-dro·ses** \-ˌsēz\ : abnormally diminished sweating — compare HYPER-HIDROSIS

hy·po·his·ti·di·ne·mia \-ˌhis-tə-də-ˈnē-mē-ə\ n : a low concentration of histidine in the blood that is characteristic of rheumatoid arthritis — **hy·po·his·ti·di·ne·mic** \-ˈnē-mik\ adj

hy·po·in·su·lin·emia \-ˌin-sə-lə-ˈnē-mē-ə\ n : an abnormally low concentration of insulin in the blood — **hy·po·in·su·lin·emic** \-ˈnē-mik\ adj

hy·po·ka·lae·mia chiefly Brit var of HY-POKALEMIA

hy·po·ka·le·mia \-kā-ˈlē-mē-ə\ n : a deficiency of potassium in the blood — called also hypopotassemia — **hy·po·ka·le·mic** \-ˈlē-mik\ adj

hy·po·ki·ne·sia \-kə-ˈnē-zhə, -kī-, -zhē-ə\ n : abnormally decreased muscular movement — compare HYPERKINESIS

hy·po·ki·ne·sis \-ˈnē-səs\ n, pl **-ne·ses** \-ˌsēz\ : HYPOKINESIA

hy·po·ki·net·ic \-ˈne-tik\ adj : characterized by, associated with, or caused by decreased motor activity (~ hypoxia)

hy·po·lip·id·ae·mia chiefly Brit var of HYPOLIPIDEMIA

hy·po·lip·id·emia \-ˌli-pə-ˈdē-mē-ə\ n : a deficiency of lipids in the blood — **hy·po·lip·id·emic** \-ˈdē-mik\ adj

hy·po·mag·ne·sae·mia chiefly Brit var of HYPOMAGNESEMIA

hy·po·mag·ne·se·mia \ˌhī-pə-ˌmag-nə-ˈsē-mē-ə\ n : a deficiency of magnesium in the blood — **hy·po·mag·ne·se·mic** \-mik\ adj

hy·po·mag·ne·sia \-mag-ˈnē-shə, -zhə\ n : GRASS TETANY

hy·po·ma·nia \ˌhī-pə-ˈmā-nē-ə, -nyə\ n : a mild mania esp. when part of a manic-depressive cycle

[1]**hy·po·man·ic** \-ˈma-nik\ adj : of, relating to, or affected with hypomania

[2]**hypomanic** n : one affected with hypomania

hy·po·men·or·rhea \-ˌme-nə-ˈrē-ə\ n : decreased menstrual flow

hy·po·me·tab·o·lism \ˌhī-pō-mə-ˈta-bə-ˌli-zəm\ n : a condition (as in myxedema) marked by an abnormally low metabolic rate — **hy·po·meta·bol·ic** \-ˌme-tə-ˈbä-lik\ adj

hy·po·me·tria \-ˈmē-trē-ə\ n : a condition of cerebellar dysfunction in which voluntary muscular movements tend to result in the movement of bodily parts (as the arm and hand) short of the intended goal — compare HYPERMETRIA

hy·po·min·er·al·ized \-ˈmi-nə-rə-ˌlīzd\ adj : relating to or characterized by a deficiency of minerals (~ defects in tooth enamel)

hy·po·mo·til·i·ty \ˌhī-pō-mō-ˈti-lə-tē\ n, pl **-ties** : abnormal deficiency of movement; specif : decreased motility of all or part of the gastrointestinal tract — compare HYPERMOTILITY

hy·po·na·trae·mia chiefly Brit var of HY-PONATREMIA

hy·po·na·tre·mia \-nā-ˈtrē-mē-ə\ n : deficiency of sodium in the blood — **hy·po·na·tre·mic** \-mik\ adj

hy·po·os·mo·lal·i·ty \-ˌäz-mō-ˈla-lə-tē, -ˌäs-\ var of HYPOSMOLALITY

hy·po·os·mot·ic \-ˌäz-ˈmä-tik\ adj : HY-POTONIC 2

hy·po·para·thy·roid·ism \-ˌpar-ə-ˈthī-ˌroi-ˌdi-zəm\ n : deficiency of parathyroid hormone in the body; also : the resultant abnormal state marked by low serum calcium and a tendency to chronic tetany — **hy·po·para·thy·roid** \-ˈthī-ˌroid\ adj

hy·po·per·fu·sion \ˌhī-pō-pər-ˈfyü-zhən\ n : decreased blood flow through an organ (cerebral ~)

hy·po·phar·ynx \-ˈfar-iŋks\ n, pl **-pha·ryn·ges** \-fə-ˈrin-(ˌ)jēz\ also **-phar·ynx·es** : the laryngeal part of the pharynx extending from the hyoid bone to the lower margin of the cricoid cartilage — **hy·po·pha·ryn·geal** \-ˌfar-ən-ˈjē-əl, -fə-ˈrin-jəl, -jē-əl\ adj

hy·po·phos·pha·tae·mia chiefly Brit var of HYPOPHOSPHATEMIA

hy·po·phos·pha·ta·sia \ˌhī-pō-ˌfäs-fə-ˈtā-zhə, -zhē-ə\ n : a congenital metabolic disorder characterized by a deficiency of alkaline phosphatase and usu. resulting in demineralization of bone

hy·po·phos·pha·te·mia \-ˌfäs-fə-ˈtē-mē-ə\ n : deficiency of phosphates in the blood — **hy·po·phos·pha·te·mic** \-ˈtē-mik\ adj

hy·po·phys·e·al also **hy·po·phys·i·al** \(ˌ)hī-ˌpä-fə-ˈsē-əl, ˌhī-pə-fə-, -ˈzē-; ˌhī-pə-ˈfi-zē-əl\ adj : of or relating to the hypophysis

hypophyseal fossa n : the depression in the sphenoid bone that contains the hypophysis

hy·poph·y·sec·to·mize \(ˌ)hī-ˌpä-fə-ˈsek-tə-ˌmīz\ vb **-mized; -miz·ing** : to remove the pituitary gland from

hy·poph·y·sec·to·my \-mē\ n, pl **-mies** : surgical removal of the pituitary gland

hy·po·phys·io·tro·pic \ˌhī-pō-ˌfi-zē-ō-ˈtrō-pik, -ˈträ-\ or **hy·po·phys·io·tro·phic** \-ˈtrō-fik\ adj : acting on or stimulating the hypophysis (~ hormones)

hy·poph·y·sis \hī-ˈpä-fə-səs\ n, pl **-y·ses** \-ˌsēz\ : PITUITARY GLAND

hypophysis ce·re·bri \-sə-ˈrē-ˌbrī, -ˈser-ə-\ n : PITUITARY GLAND

hy·po·pig·men·ta·tion \ˌhī-pō-ˌpig-mən-ˈtā-shən, -ˌmen-\ n : diminished pigmentation in a bodily part or tissue (as the skin) — **hy·po·pig·ment·ed** \-ˈpig-mən-təd, -ˌmen-\ adj

hy·po·pi·tu·i·ta·rism \ˌhī-pō-pə-ˈtü-ə-tə-ˌri-zəm, -ˈtyü-\ *n* : deficient production of growth hormones by the pituitary gland — **hy·po·pi·tu·i·tary** \-ˈtü-ə-ˌter-ē, -ˈtyü-\ *adj*

hy·po·pla·sia \-ˈplā-zhə, -zhē-ə\ *n* : a condition of arrested development in which an organ or part remains below the normal size or in an immature state — **hy·po·plas·tic** \-ˈplas-tik\ *adj*

hypoplastic anemia *n* : APLASTIC ANEMIA

hypoplastic left heart syndrome *n* : a congenital malformation of the heart in which the left side is underdeveloped resulting in insufficient blood flow

hy·po·pnea \ˌhī-pō-ˈnē-ə\ *n* : abnormally slow or esp. shallow respiration

hy·po·pnoea *chiefly Brit var of* HYPOPNEA

hy·po·po·tas·sae·mia *chiefly Brit var of* HYPOPOTASSEMIA

hy·po·po·tas·se·mia \-pə-ˌta-ˈsē-mē-ə\ *n* : HYPOKALEMIA — **hy·po·po·tas·se·mic** \-ˈsē-mik\ *adj*

hy·po·pro·tei·nae·mia *chiefly Brit var of* HYPOPROTEINEMIA

hy·po·pro·tein·emia \-ˌprō-tə-ˈnē-mē-ə, -ˌprō-ˌtē-, -ˌprō-tē-ə-\ *n* : abnormal deficiency of protein in the blood — **hy·po·pro·tein·emic** \-ˈnē-mik\ *adj*

hy·po·pro·throm·bin·ae·mia *chiefly Brit var of* HYPOPROTHROMBINEMIA

hy·po·pro·throm·bin·emia \-prō-ˌthräm-bə-ˈnē-mē-ə\ *n* : deficiency of prothrombin in the blood usu. due to vitamin K deficiency or liver disease and resulting in delayed clotting of blood or spontaneous bleeding (as from the nose) — **hy·po·pro·throm·bin·emic** \-ˈnē-mik\ *adj*

hy·po·py·on \hī-ˈpō-pē-ˌän\ *n* : an accumulation of white blood cells in the anterior chamber of the eye

hy·po·re·ac·tive \ˌhī-pō-rē-ˈak-tiv\ *adj* : having or showing abnormally low sensitivity to stimuli — **hy·po·re·ac·tiv·i·ty** \-(ˌ)rē-ˌak-ˈti-və-tē\ *n*

hy·po·re·flex·ia \-rē-ˈflek-sē-ə\ *n* : underactivity of bodily reflexes

hy·po·re·spon·sive \-ri-ˈspän-siv\ *adj* : characterized by a diminished degree of responsiveness (as to a physical or emotional stimulus) — **hy·po·re·spon·sive·ness** *n*

hypos *pl of* HYPO

hy·po·sal·i·va·tion \-ˌsa-lə-ˈvā-shən\ *n* : diminished salivation

hy·po·se·cre·tion \ˌhī-pō-si-ˈkrē-shən\ *n* : production of a bodily secretion at an abnormally slow rate or in abnormally small quantities

hy·po·sen·si·tive \-ˈsen-sə-tiv\ *adj* : exhibiting or marked by deficient response to stimulation — **hy·po·sen·si·tiv·i·ty** \-ˌsen-sə-ˈti-və-tē\ *n*

hy·po·sen·si·ti·za·tion \-ˌsen-sə-tə-ˈzā-shən\ *n* : the state or process of being reduced in sensitivity esp. to an aller-

gen : DESENSITIZATION — **hy·po·sen·si·tize** \-ˈsen-sə-ˌtīz\ *vb*

hy·pos·mia \hī-ˈpäz-mē-ə, hi-\ *n* : impairment of the sense of smell

hy·pos·mo·lal·i·ty \ˌhī-ˌpäz-mō-ˈla-lə-tē\ *n, pl* **-ties** : the condition esp. of a bodily fluid of having abnormally low osmolality

hy·pos·mo·lar·i·ty \ˌhī-ˌpäz-mō-ˈlar-ə-tē\ *n, pl* **-ties** : the condition esp. of a bodily fluid of having abnormally low osmolarity — **hy·pos·mo·lar** \ˌhi-ˌpäz-ˈmō-lər\ *adj*

hy·pos·mot·ic \-ˌpäz-ˈmä-tik\ *var of* HYPOOSMOTIC

hy·po·spa·di·as \ˌhī-pə-ˈspā-dē-əs\ *n* : an abnormality of the penis in which the urethra opens on the underside

Hy·po·spray \ˈhī-pō-ˌsprā\ *trademark* — used for a device with a spring and plunger for administering a medicated solution by forcing it in extremely fine jets through the unbroken skin

hy·pos·ta·sis \hī-ˈpäs-tə-səs\ *n, pl* **-ta·ses** \-ˌsēz\ : the settling of blood in relatively lower parts of an organ or the body due to impaired or absent circulation — **hy·po·stat·ic** \ˌhī-pə-ˈsta-tik\ *adj*

hypostatic pneumonia *n* : pneumonia that usu. results from the collection of fluid in the dorsal region of the lungs and occurs esp. in those (as the bedridden or elderly) confined to a supine position for extended periods

hy·po·sthe·nia \ˌhī-pəs-ˈthē-nē-ə\ *n* : lack of strength : bodily weakness — **hy·po·sthen·ic** \ˌhī-pəs-ˈthe-nik\ *adj*

hy·pos·the·nu·ria \hī-ˌpäs-thə-ˈnur-ē-ə, -ˈnyur-\ *n* : the secretion of urine of low specific gravity due to inability of the kidney to concentrate the urine normally

hy·po·ten·sion \ˌhī-pō-ˈten-chən\ *n* **1** : abnormally low pressure of the blood — called also *low blood pressure* **2** : abnormally low pressure of the intraocular fluid

¹hy·po·ten·sive \-ˈten-siv\ *adj* **1** : characterized by or due to hypotension (~ shock) **2** : causing low blood pressure or a lowering of blood pressure (~ drugs)

²hypotensive *n* : one with hypotension

hy·po·tha·lam·ic \ˌhī-pō-thə-ˈla-mik\ *adj* : of or relating to the hypothalamus — **hy·po·tha·lam·i·cal·ly** *adv*

hypothalamic releasing factor *n* : any hormone that is secreted by the hypothalamus and stimulates the pituitary gland directly to secrete a hormone — called also *hypothalamic releasing hormone, releasing factor*

hypothalamo- *comb form* : hypothalamus ⟨*hypothalamo*tomy⟩

hy·po·thal·a·mot·o·my \ˌhī-pō-ˌtha-lə-ˈmä-tə-mē\ *n, pl* **-mies** : psychosurgery in which lesions are made in the hypothalamus

hy·po·thal·a·mus \-ˈtha-lə-məs\ *n, pl* **-mi** \-ˌmī\ : a basal part of the diencephalon that lies beneath the thalamus on each side, forms the floor of the third ventricle, and includes vital autonomic regulatory centers

hy·po·the·nar eminence \ˌhī-pō-ˈthē-ˌnär-, -nər-; hī-ˈpä-thə-ˌnär-, -nər-\ *n* : the prominent part of the palm of the hand above the base of the little finger

hypothenar muscle *n* : any of four muscles located in the area of the hypothenar eminence: **a** : ABDUCTOR DIGITI MINIMI **b** : FLEXOR DIGITI MINIMI BREVIS **c** : PALMARIS BREVIS **d** : OPPONENS DIGITI MINIMI

hy·po·ther·mia \-ˈthər-mē-ə\ *n* : subnormal temperature of the body — **hy·po·ther·mic** \-mik\ *adj*

hy·po·thy·re·o·sis \ˌhī-pō-ˌthī-rē-ˈō-səs\ *n* : HYPOTHYROIDISM

hy·po·thy·roid·ism \ˌhī-pō-ˈthī-ˌroi-ˌdi-zəm\ *n* : deficient activity of the thyroid gland; *also* : a resultant bodily condition characterized by lowered metabolic rate and general loss of vigor — **hy·po·thy·roid** \-ˌroid\ *adj*

hy·po·thy·ro·sis \-ˌthī-ˈrō-səs\ *n* : HYPOTHYROIDISM

hy·po·thy·rox·in·ae·mia *chiefly Brit var of* HYPOTHYROXINEMIA

hy·po·thy·rox·in·emia \ˌhī-pō-thī-ˌräk-sə-ˈnē-mē-ə\ *n* : the presence of an abnormally low concentration of thyroxine in the blood — **hy·po·thy·rox·in·emic** \-ˈnē-mik\ *adj*

hy·po·to·nia \ˌhī-pə-ˈtō-nē-ə, -pō-\ *n* 1 : abnormally low pressure of the intraocular fluid 2 : the state of having hypotonic muscle tone

hy·po·ton·ic \ˌhī-pə-ˈtä-nik, -pō-\ *adj* 1 : having deficient tone or tension 2 : having a lower osmotic pressure than a surrounding medium or a fluid under comparison — compare HYPERTONIC 2, ISOSMOTIC

hy·po·to·nic·i·ty \-tə-ˈni-sə-tē\ *n, pl* **-ties** 1 : the state or condition of having hypotonic osmotic pressure 2 : HYPOTONIA 2

hy·pot·o·ny \hī-ˈpä-tə-nē\ *n, pl* **-onies** : HYPOTONIA

hy·po·tri·cho·sis \-tri-ˈkō-səs\ *n, pl* **-cho·ses** \-ˌsēz\ : congenital deficiency of hair

hy·pot·ro·phy \hī-ˈpä-trə-fē\ *n, pl* **-phies** : subnormal growth

hy·po·tym·pa·num \ˌhī-pō-ˈtim-pə-nəm\ *n, pl* **-na** \-nə\ *also* **-nums** : the lower part of the middle ear — compare EPITYMPANUM

hy·po·uri·ce·mia \-ˌyur-ə-ˈsē-mē-ə\ *n* : deficient uric acid in the blood — **hy·po·uri·ce·mic** \-ˈsē-mik\ *adj*

hy·po·ven·ti·la·tion \-ˌvent-ᵊl-ˈā-shən\ *n* : deficient ventilation of the lungs that results in reduction in the oxygen content or increase in the carbon dioxide content of the blood or both — **hy·po·ven·ti·lat·ed** \-ˈvent-ᵊl-ˌā-təd\ *adj*

hy·po·vi·ta·min·osis \-ˌvī-tə-mə-ˈnō-səs\

n : AVITAMINOSIS — **hy·po·vi·ta·min·ot·ic** \-ˈnä-tik\ *adj*

hy·po·vo·lae·mia *chiefly Brit var of* HYPOVOLEMIA

hy·po·vo·le·mia \-vä-ˈlē-mē-ə\ *n* : decrease in the volume of the circulating blood — **hy·po·vo·le·mic** \-ˈlē-mik\ *adj*

hy·pox·ae·mia *chiefly Brit var of* HYPOXEMIA

hy·po·xan·thine \ˌhī-pō-ˈzan-ˌthēn\ *n* : a purine base $C_5H_4N_4O$ of plant and animal tissues that is an intermediate in uric acid synthesis

hypoxanthine–guanine phosphoribosyltransferase *n* : an enzyme that conserves hypoxanthine in the body by limiting its conversion to uric acid and that is lacking in Lesch-Nyhan syndrome — called also *hypoxanthine phosphoribosyltransferase*

hyp·ox·emia \ˌhī-ˌpäk-ˈsē-mē-ə, ˌhī-\ *n* : deficient oxygenation of the blood — **hyp·ox·emic** \-mik\ *adj*

hyp·ox·ia \hī-ˈpäk-sē-ə, hi-\ *n* : a deficiency of oxygen reaching the tissues of the body — **hyp·ox·ic** \-sik\ *adj*

hyps- *or* **hypsi-** *or* **hypso-** *comb form* : high ⟨*hyps*arrhythmia⟩

hyps·ar·rhyth·mia *or* **hyps·arrhyth·mia** \ˌhips-ä-ˈrith-mē-ə\ *n* : an abnormal encephalogram that is characterized by slow waves of high voltage and a disorganized arrangement of spikes, occurs esp. in infants, and is indicative of a condition that leads to severe mental retardation if left untreated

hyster- *or* **hystero-** *comb form* 1 : womb ⟨*hystero*tomy⟩ 2 : hysteria ⟨*hystero*id⟩

hys·ter·ec·to·my \ˌhis-tə-ˈrek-tə-mē\ *n, pl* **-mies** : surgical removal of the uterus — **hys·ter·ec·to·mized** \-tə-ˌmīzd\ *adj*

hys·te·ria \hi-ˈster-ē-ə, -ˈstir-\ *n* 1 : a psychoneurosis marked by emotional excitability and disturbances of the psychic, sensory, vasomotor, and visceral functions without an organic basis 2 : behavior exhibiting overwhelming or unmanageable fear or emotional excess

hys·ter·ic \hi-ˈster-ik\ *n* : one subject to or affected with hysteria

hys·ter·i·cal \-ˈster-i-kəl\ *also* **hys·ter·ic** \-ˈster-ik\ *adj* : of, relating to, or marked by hysteria — **hys·ter·i·cal·ly** *adv*

hysterical personality *n* : a personality characterized by superficiality, egocentricity, vanity, dependence, and manipulativeness, by dramatic, reactive, and intensely expressed emotional behavior, and often by disturbed interpersonal relationships

hys·ter·ics \-iks\ *n sing or pl* : a fit of uncontrollable laughter or crying : HYSTERIA

hystericus — see GLOBUS HYSTERICUS

hys·ter·o·gram \ˈhis-tə-rō-ˌgram\ *n* : a roentgenogram made of the uterus

hys·ter·og·ra·phy \ˌhis-tə-ˈrä-grə-fē\ *n,*

pl **-phies** : examination of the uterus by roentgenography after the injection of an opaque medium

hys·ter·oid \'his-tə-ˌroid\ *adj* : resembling or tending toward hysteria

hys·ter·o·plas·ty \'his-tə-rō-ˌplas-tē\ *n, pl* **-ties** : plastic surgery of the uterus

hys·ter·or·rha·phy \ˌhis-tə-'ror-ə-fē\ *n, pl* **-phies** : a suturing of an incised or ruptured uterus

hys·ter·o·sal·pin·go·gram \ˌhis-tə-rō-ˌsal-'piŋ-gə-ˌgram\ *n* : a roentgenogram made by hysterosalpingography

hys·ter·o·sal·pin·gog·ra·phy \-ˌsal-ˌpin-'gä-gre-fē\ *n, pl* **-phies** : examination of the uterus and fallopian tubes by roentgenography after injection of an opaque medium — called also *uterosalpingography*

hys·ter·o·sal·pin·gos·to·my \-'gäs-tə-mē\

n, pl **-mies** : surgical establishment of an anastomosis between the uterus and an occluded fallopian tube

hys·ter·o·scope \'his-tə-rō-ˌsköp\ *n* : an instrument used in inspection of the uterus — **hys·ter·o·scop·ic** \ˌhis-tə-rō-'skä-pik\ *adj* — **hys·ter·os·co·py** \ˌhis-tə-'räs-kə-pē\ *n*

hys·ter·o·sto·mat·o·my \ˌhis-tə-rō-ˌstō-'ma-tə-mē\ *n, pl* **-mies** : surgical incision of the uterine cervix

hys·ter·ot·o·my \ˌhis-tə-'rä-tə-mē\ *n, pl* **-mies** : surgical incision of the uterus; *esp* : CESAREAN SECTION

hystrix — see ICHTHYOSIS HYSTRIX GRAVIOR

H zone \'äch-ˌzōn\ *n* : a narrow and less dense zone of myosin filaments bisecting the A band in striated muscle — compare M LINE

I

i *abbr* incisor

I *symbol* iodine

-i·a·sis \'i-ə-səs\ *n suffix, pl* **-i·a·ses** \-ˌsēz\ : disease having characteristics of or produced by (something specified) ⟨amebi*asis*⟩ ⟨onchocerci*asis*⟩ ⟨ancylostomi*asis*⟩

-i·at·ric \ē-'a-trik\ *also* **-i·at·ri·cal** \-tri-kəl\ *adj comb form* : of or relating to (such) medical treatment or healing ⟨pediatric⟩

-i·at·rics \ē-'a-triks\ *n pl comb form* : medical treatment ⟨pedi*atrics*⟩

-i·a·trist \'ī-ə-trəst\ *n comb form* : physician : healer ⟨psychi*atrist*⟩ ⟨podi*atrist*⟩

iatro- *comb form* : physician : medicine : healing ⟨*iatro*genic⟩

iat·ro·gen·ic \(ˌ)ī-ˌa-trə-'je-nik\ *adj* : induced inadvertently by a physician or surgeon or by medical treatment or diagnostic procedures ⟨~ rash⟩ — **iat·ro·gen·e·sis** \-'je-nə-səs\ *n* — **iat·ro·gen·i·cal·ly** \-i-k(ə-)lē\ *adv*

-i·a·try \'ī-ə-trē\ *n comb form, pl* **-iatries** : medical treatment : healing ⟨podi*atry*⟩ ⟨psychi*atry*⟩

I band \'ī-\ *n* : a pale band across a striated muscle fiber that consists of actin and is situated between two A bands — called also *isotropic band*

ibo·te·nic acid \ˌī-bō-ˌtē-nik-\ *n* : a neurotoxic compound $C_5H_6N_2O_4$ found esp. in fly agaric

ibu·pro·fen \ˌī-byü-'prō-fən\ *n* : a nonsteroidal anti-inflammatory drug $C_{13}H_{18}O_2$ used in over-the-counter preparations to relieve pain and fever and in prescription strength esp. to relieve the symptoms of rheumatoid arthritis and degenerative arthritis — see MOTRIN

ice bag *n* : a waterproof bag to hold ice for local application of cold to the body

ice pack *n* : crushed ice placed in a container (as an ice bag) or folded in a towel and applied to the body

ich·tham·mol \'ik-thə-ˌmol, -ˌmöl\ *n* : a brownish black viscous tarry liquid prepared from a distillate of some hydrocarbon-containing rocks and used as an antiseptic and emollient — see ICHTHYOL

ichthy- *or* **ichthyo-** *comb form* : fish ⟨*ichthyo*sarcotoxism⟩

Ich·thy·ol \'ik-thē-ˌol, -ˌōl\ *trademark* — used for a preparation of ichthammol

ich·thyo·sar·co·tox·ism \ˌik-thē-ō-ˌsär-kə-'täk-ˌsi-zəm\ *n* : poisoning caused by the ingestion of fish whose flesh contains a toxic substance

ich·thyo·si·form \ˌik-thē-'ō-sə-ˌform\ *adj* : resembling ichthyosis or that of ichthyosis ⟨~ erythroderma⟩

ich·thy·o·sis \ˌik-thē-'ō-səs\ *n, pl* **-o·ses** \-ˌsēz\ : any of several congenital diseases of hereditary origin characterized by rough, thick, and scaly skin — **ich·thy·ot·ic** \-'ä-tik\ *adj*

ichthyosis hys·trix gra·vi·or \-'his-triks-'gra-vē-ˌor, -'grä\ *n* : a rare hereditary abnormality characterized by the formation of brown, verrucose, and often linear lesions of the skin

ichthyosis vul·ga·ris \-ˌvəl-'gar-əs\ *n* : the common hereditary form of ichthyosis

ICN *abbr* International Council of Nurses

-ics \iks\ *n sing or pl suffix* **1** : study : knowledge : skill : practice ⟨opt*ics*⟩ ⟨pediatr*ics*⟩ **2** : characteristic actions or activities ⟨hyster*ics*⟩ **3** : characteristic qualities, operations, or phenomena ⟨acoust*ics*⟩ ⟨phonet*ics*⟩

ICSH *abbr* interstitial-cell stimulating hormone

ICT *abbr* insulin coma therapy

ic·tal \'ik-təl\ *adj* : of, relating to, or caused by ictus

icter- *or* **ictero-** *comb form* : jaundice ⟨*icterogenic*⟩

ic·ter·ic \ik-'ter-ik\ *adj* : of, relating to, or affected with jaundice

icteric index *n* : ICTERUS INDEX

ic·ter·o·gen·ic \ik-tə-rō-'je-nik, ik-₁ter-ə-\ *adj* : causing or tending to cause jaundice ⟨∼drugs⟩

ic·ter·us \'ik-tə-rəs\ *n* : JAUNDICE

icterus gra·vis \-'gra-vəs, -'grä-\ *n* : ICTERUS GRAVIS NEONATORUM

icterus gravis neo·na·tor·um \-₁nē-ō-nā-'tòr-əm\ *n* : severe jaundice in a new-born child due esp. to erythroblastosis fetalis

icterus index *n* : a figure representing the amount of bilirubin in the blood as determined by comparing the color of a sample of test serum with a set of color standards ⟨an *icterus index* of 15 or above indicates active jaundice⟩ — called also *icteric index*

icterus neo·na·tor·um \-₁nē-ō-nā-'tòr-əm\ *n* : jaundice in a newborn

ic·tus \'ik-təs\ *n* **1** : a beat or pulsation esp. of the heart **2** : a sudden attack or seizure esp. of stroke

ICU *abbr* intensive care unit

¹id \'id\ *n* : the one of the three divisions of the psyche in psychoanalytic theory that is completely unconscious and is the source of psychic energy derived from instinctual needs and drives — compare EGO, SUPEREGO

²id *n* : a skin rash that is an allergic reaction to an agent causing an infection ⟨a syphilitic ∼⟩

ID *abbr* intradermal

¹-id \əd, (₁)id\ *also* **-ide** \'id\ *n suffix* : skin rash caused by (something specified) ⟨syphil*id*⟩

²-id *n suffix* : structure, body, or particle of a (specified) kind ⟨chromat*id*⟩

-i·da \ə-də\ *n pl suffix* : animals that are or have the form of — in names of higher taxa (as orders and classes) ⟨Arachn*ida*⟩ — **-i·dan** \ə-dən, əd-ⁿn\ *or adj suffix*

-i·dae \ə-₁dē\ *n pl suffix* : members of the family of — in names of zoological families ⟨Homin*idae*⟩ ⟨Ixod*idae*⟩

IDDM *abbr* insulin-dependent diabetes mellitus

idea \i-'dē-ə\ *n* : something imagined or pictured in the mind

idea of reference *n* : a delusion that the remarks one overhears and people one encounters seem to be concerned with and usu. hostile to oneself — called also *delusion of reference*

ide·ation \i-dē-'ā-shən\ *n* : the capacity for or the act of forming or entertaining ideas ⟨suicidal ∼⟩ — **ide·ation·al** \-shə-nəl\ *adj*

idée fixe \(₁)ē-₁dā-'fēks\ *n, pl* **idées fixes** *same or* -(₁)fēk-səz\ : a usu. delusional idea that dominates the whole mental life during a prolonged period (as in certain mental disorders) — called also *fixed idea*

iden·ti·cal \i-'den-ti-kəl\ *adj* : MONOZYGOTIC

iden·ti·fi·ca·tion \ī-₁den-tə-fə-'kā-shən\ *n* **1** : psychological orientation of the self in regard to something (as a person or group) with a resulting feeling of close emotional association **2** : a largely unconscious process whereby an individual models thoughts, feelings, and actions after those attributed to an object that has been incorporated as a mental image — **iden·ti·fy** \ī-'den-tə-₁fī\ *vb*

iden·ti·ty \ī-'den-tə-tē\ *n, pl* **-ties 1** : the distinguishing character or personality of an individual **2** : the relation established by psychological identification

identity crisis *n* : personal psychosocial conflict esp. in adolescence that involves confusion about one's social role and often a sense of loss of continuity to one's personality

ideo·mo·tor \₁id-ē-ə-'mō-tər, ₁i-\ *adj* **1** : not reflex but motivated by an idea ⟨∼ muscular activity⟩ **2** : of, relating to, or concerned with ideomotor activity

ID₅₀ *symbol* — used for the dose of an infectious organism required to produce infection in 50% of the experimental subjects

idio- *comb form* **1** : one's own : personal : separate : distinct ⟨*idio*type⟩ ⟨*idio*syncrasy⟩ **2** : self-produced : arising within ⟨*idio*pathic⟩ ⟨*idio*ventricular⟩

id·i·o·cy \'i-dē-ə-sē\ *n, pl* **-cies** : extreme mental retardation commonly due to incomplete or abnormal development of the brain

id·io·path·ic \₁i-dē-ə-'pa-thik\ *adj* : arising spontaneously or from an obscure or unknown cause : PRIMARY ⟨∼ epilepsy⟩ ⟨∼ hypertension⟩ ⟨∼ thrombocytopenic purpura⟩ — **id·io·path·i·cal·ly** *adv*

id·io·syn·cra·sy \₁i-dē-ə-'sin-krə-sē\ *n, pl* **-sies 1** : a peculiarity of physical or mental constitution or temperament **2** : individual hypersensitiveness (as to a food) — **id·io·syn·crat·ic** \₁i-dē-ō-sin-'kra-tik\ *adj*

id·i·ot \'i-dē-ət\ *n* : a person affected with idiocy; *esp* : a feebleminded person having a mental age not exceeding three years and requiring complete custodial care — **idiot** *adj*

idiot sa·vant \'ē-₁dyō-sä-'väⁿ\ *n, pl* **id·iots savants** *or* **idiot savants** *same or* -'väⁿz\ : a mentally defective person who exhibits exceptional skill or brilliance in some limited field

id·io·type \'i-dē-ə-₁tīp\ *n* : the molecular structure and conformation in the variable region of an antibody that confers its antigenic specificity — compare ALLOTYPE, ISOTYPE — **id·io·typ·ic** \₁i-dē-ə-'ti-pik\ *adj*

id·io·ven·tric·u·lar \₁i-dē-ə-ven-'tri-kyə-lər, -vən-\ *adj* : of, relating to, associated with, or arising in the ventricles of the heart independently of the atria

idox·uri·dine \ˌi-ˈdäks-ˈyur-ə-ˌdēn\ *n* : a drug $C_9H_{11}N_2O_5$ used to treat keratitis caused by the herpesviruses producing herpes simplex — abbr. *IDU;* called also *iododeoxyuridine, IUDR*

-i·dro·sis \i-ˈdrō-səs\ *n comb form, pl* **-i·dro·ses** \-ˌsēz\ : a specified form of sweating ⟨chrom*idrosis*⟩ ⟨brom*idrosis*⟩

IDU *abbr* idoxuridine

IF *abbr* interferon

IFN *abbr* interferon

Ig *abbr* immunoglobulin

IgA \ˌī-(ˌ)jē-ˈā\ *n* : a class of antibodies found in external bodily secretions (as saliva, tears, and sweat) — called also *immunoglobulin A*

IgD \ˌī-(ˌ)jē-ˈdē\ *n* : a minor class of antibodies of undetermined function — called also *immunoglobulin D*

IgE \ˌī-(ˌ)jē-ˈē\ *n* : a class of antibodies that function esp. in allergic reactions — called also *immunoglobulin E*

IgG \ˌī-(ˌ)jē-ˈjē\ *n* : a class of antibodies including those most commonly circulating in the blood and active esp. against bacteria, viruses, and proteins foreign to the body — called also *immunoglobulin G*

IgM \ˌī-(ˌ)jē-ˈem\ *n* : a class of antibodies of high molecular weight including those appearing early in the immune response to be replaced later by IgG of lower molecular weight — called also *immunoglobulin M*

Il *symbol* illinium

il- — see IN-

ile- *also* **ileo-** *comb form* **1** : ileum ⟨*ile*itis⟩ **2** : ileal and ⟨*ileo*cecal⟩

ilea *pl of* ILEUM

il·e·al \ˈi-lē-əl\ *also* **il·e·ac** \-ˌak\ *adj* : of, relating to, or affecting the ileum

il·e·itis \ˌi-lē-ˈi-təs\ *n, pl* **-it·i·des** \-ˈi-tə-ˌdēz\ : inflammation of the ileum — see REGIONAL ILEITIS

il·eo·ce·cal \ˌi-lē-ō-ˈsē-kəl\ *adj* : of, relating to, or connecting the ileum and cecum

ileocecal valve *n* : the valve formed by two folds of mucous membrane at the opening of the ileum into the large intestine — called also *Bauhin's valve*

il·eo·col·ic \-ˈkä-lik, -ˈkä-\ *adj* : relating to, situated near, or involving the ileum and the colon

ileocolic artery *n* : a branch of the superior mesenteric artery that supplies the terminal part of the ileum and the beginning of the colon

il·eo·co·li·tis \ˌi-lē-ō-kō-ˈlī-təs\ *n* : inflammation of the ileum and colon

il·eo·co·los·to·my \-kə-ˈläs-tə-mē\ *n, pl* **-mies** : a surgical operation producing an artificial opening connecting the ileum and the colon

il·eo·cy·to·plas·ty \-ˈsī-tə-ˌplas-tē\ *n, pl* **-ties** : a surgical operation that in-

volves anastomosing a segment of the ileum to the bladder esp. in order to increase bladder capacity and preserve the function of the kidneys and ureters

il·eo·il·e·al \-ˈi-lē-əl\ *adj* : relating to or involving two different parts of the ileum ⟨an ~ anastomosis⟩

il·eo·proc·tos·to·my \-ˌpräk-ˈtäs-tə-mē\ *n, pl* **-mies** : a surgical operation producing a permanent artificial opening connecting the ileum and rectum

il·e·os·to·my \ˌi-lē-ˈäs-tə-mē\ *n, pl* **-mies** **1** : surgical formation of an artificial anus by connecting the ileum to an opening in the abdominal wall **2** : the artificial opening made by ileostomy

ileostomy bag *n* : a container designed to receive feces discharged through an ileostomy

Iletin \ˈī-lə-tən\ *trademark* — used for a preparation of insulin

il·e·um \ˈi-lē-əm\ *n, pl* **il·ea** \-lē-ə\ : the last division of the small intestine extending between the jejunum and large intestine

il·e·us \ˈi-lē-əs\ *n* : obstruction of the bowel; *specif* : a condition that is commonly marked by a painful distended abdomen, vomiting of dark or fecal matter, toxemia, and dehydration and that results when the intestinal contents back up because peristalsis fails although the lumen is not occluded — compare VOLVULUS

ilia *pl of* ILIUM

il·i·ac \ˈi-lē-ˌak\ *adj* **1** : of, relating to, or located near the ilium ⟨the ~ bone⟩ **2** : of or relating to either of the lowest lateral abdominal regions

iliac artery *n* **1** : either of the large arteries supplying blood to the lower trunk and hind limbs and arising by bifurcation of the aorta to form one vessel for each side of the body — called also *common iliac artery* **2** : the outer branch of the common iliac artery on either side that becomes the femoral artery — called also *external iliac artery* **3** : the inner branch of the common iliac artery on either side of the body that supplies blood chiefly to the pelvic and gluteal areas — called also *hypogastric artery, internal iliac artery*

iliac crest *n* : the thick curved upper border of the ilium

iliac fossa *n* : the inner concavity of the ilium

iliac node *n* : any of the lymph nodes grouped around the iliac arteries and the iliac veins — see EXTERNAL ILIAC NODE, INTERNAL ILIAC NODE

iliac spine *n* : any of four projections on the ilium: **a** : ANTERIOR INFERIOR ILIAC SPINE **b** : ANTERIOR SUPERIOR ILIAC SPINE **c** : POSTERIOR INFERIOR ILIAC SPINE **d** : POSTERIOR SUPERIOR ILIAC SPINE

il·i·a·cus \i-ˈlī-ə-kəs\ *n, pl* **il·i·a·ci** \-ə-ˌsī\ : a muscle of the iliac region of the abdomen that flexes the thigh or bends the pelvis and lumbar region forward

iliac vein *n* : any of several veins on each side of the body corresponding to and accompanying the iliac arteries: **a** : either of two veins of which one is formed on each side of the body by the union of the external and internal iliac veins and which unite to form the inferior vena cava — called also *common iliac vein* **b** : a vein that drains the leg and lower part of the anterior abdominal wall, is an upward continuation of the femoral vein — called also *external iliac vein* **c** : a vein that drains the pelvis and gluteal and perineal regions and that unites with the external iliac vein to form the common iliac vein — called also *hypogastric vein, internal iliac vein*

il·i·al \ˈil-ē-əl\ *var of* ILIAC

ilio- *comb form* : iliac and ⟨*ilio*inguinal⟩

il·io·coc·cy·geus \ˌil-ē-ō-käk-ˈsij-əs, -jē-əs\ *n* : a muscle of the pelvis that is a subdivision of the levator ani and helps support the pelvic viscera — compare PUBOCOCCYGEUS

il·io·cos·ta·lis \-käs-ˈtā-ləs\ *n* : the lateral division of the sacrospinalis muscle that helps to keep the trunk erect and consists of three parts: **a** : ILIOCOSTALIS CERVICIS **b** : ILIOCOSTALIS LUMBORUM **c** : ILIOCOSTALIS THORACIS

iliocostalis cer·vi·cis \-ˈsər-və-səs\ *n* : a muscle that extends from the ribs to the cervical transverse processes and acts to draw the neck to the same side and to elevate the ribs

iliocostalis dor·si \-ˈdȯr-ˌsī\ *n* : ILIOCOSTALIS THORACIS

iliocostalis lum·bor·um \-ˌləm-ˈbȯr-əm\ *n* : a muscle that extends from the ilium to the lower ribs and acts to draw the trunk to the same side or to depress the ribs

iliocostalis tho·ra·cis \-thə-ˈrā-səs\ *n* : a muscle that extends from the lower to the upper ribs and acts to draw the trunk to the same side and to approximate the ribs

il·io·fem·o·ral \ˌil-ē-ō-ˈfe-mə-rəl\ *adj* **1** : of or relating to the ilium and the femur **2** : relating to or involving an iliac vein and a femoral vein ⟨∼ bypass graft⟩

iliofemoral ligament *n* : a ligament that extends from the anterior inferior iliac spine to the intertrochanteric line of the femur and divides below into two branches — called also *Y ligament*

il·io·hy·po·gas·tric nerve \ˌil-ē-ō-ˌhī-pə-ˈgas-trik-\ *n* : a branch of the first lumbar nerve distributed to the skin of the lateral part of the buttocks, the skin of the pubic region, and the muscles of the anterolateral abdominal wall

il·io·in·gui·nal \-ˈiŋ-gwən-ᵊl\ *adj* : of, re-

lating to, or affecting the iliac and inguinal regions

ilioinguinal nerve *n* : a branch of the first lumbar nerve distributed to the muscles of the anterolateral wall of the abdomen, the skin of the proximal and medial part of the thigh, the base of the penis and the scrotum in the male, and the mons veneris and labia majora in the female

il·io·lum·bar artery \ˌil-ē-ō-ˈləm-bər-, -ˌbär-\ *n* : a branch of the internal iliac artery that supplies muscles in the lumbar region and the iliac fossa

iliolumbar ligament *n* : a ligament connecting the transverse process of the last lumbar vertebra with the iliac crest

il·io·pec·tin·e·al eminence \ˌil-ē-ō-pek-ˈti-nē-əl-\ *n* : a ridge on the hipbone marking the junction of the ilium and the pubis

iliopectineal line *n* : a line or ridge on the inner surface of the hipbone marking the border between the true and false pelvis

il·io·pso·as \ˌil-ē-ō-ˈsō-əs, -lē-ˈäp-sō-əs\ *n* : a muscle consisting of the iliacus and psoas major muscles

iliopsoas tendon *n* : the tendon that is common to the iliacus and psoas major

il·io·tib·i·al \ˌil-ē-ō-ˈti-bē-əl\ *adj* : of or relating to the ilium and the tibia

iliotibial band *n* : a fibrous thickening of the fascia lata that extends from the iliac crest down the lateral part of the thigh to the lateral condyle of the tibia — called also *iliotibial tract*

il·i·um \ˈil-ē-əm\ *n, pl* **il·ia** \-ē-ə\ : the dorsal, upper, and largest one of the three bones composing either lateral half of the pelvis that is broad and expanded above and narrower below where it joins with the ischium and pubis to form part of the acetabulum

¹ill \ˈil\ *adj* **worse** \ˈwərs\ *also* **ill·er; worst** \ˈwərst\ **1** : affected with some ailment : not in good health ⟨incurably ∼⟩ ⟨emotionally ∼⟩ **2** : affected with nausea often to the point of vomiting

²ill *n* : AILMENT, SICKNESS

il·lin·i·um \i-ˈli-nē-əm\ *n* : PROMETHIUM

ill·ness \ˈil-nəs\ *n* : an unhealthy condition of body or mind : SICKNESS

il·lu·sion \i-ˈlü-zhən\ *n* **1** : perception of something objectively existing in such a way as to cause misinterpretation of its actual nature; *esp* : OPTICAL ILLUSION **2** : HALLUCINATION **1 3** : a pattern capable of reversible perspective

IL–1 *abbr* interleukin-1

Il·o·sone \ˈi-lə-ˌsōn\ *trademark* — used for a preparation of a salt of erythromycin

Il·o·ty·cin \ˌi-lə-ˈtī-sən\ *trademark* — used for a preparation of erythromycin

IL–2 *abbr* interleukin-2

IM *abbr* intramuscular; intramuscularly

im- — see IN-

¹**im·age** \'i-mij\ *n* : a mental picture or impression of something: as **a** : an idealized conception of a person and esp. a parent that is formed by an infant or child, is retained in the unconscious, and influences behavior in later life — called also *imago* **b** : the memory of a perception in psychology that is modified by subsequent experience; *also* : the representation of the source of a stimulus on a receptor mechanism

²**image** *vb* **im·aged; im·ag·ing 1** : to call up a mental picture of **2** : to create a representation of; *also* : to form an image of

image intensifier *n* : a device used esp. for diagnosis in radiology that provides a more intense image for a given amount of radiation than can be obtained by the usual fluorometric methods — **image intensification** *n*

im·ag·ery \'i-mij-rē, -mi-jə-\ *n, pl* **-eries** : mental images; *esp* : the products of imagination ⟨psychotic ~⟩

im·ag·ing *n* : the action or process of producing an image esp. of a part of the body by radiographic techniques ⟨diagnostic ~⟩ ⟨cardiac ~⟩ — see MAGNETIC RESONANCE IMAGING

ima·go \i-'mā-(ˌ)gō, -'mä-\ *n, pl* **imagoes** *or* **ima·gi·nes** \-'mā-gə-ˌnēz, -'mä-\ : IMAGE a

im·bal·ance \(ˌ)im-'ba-ləns\ *n* : lack of balance : the state of being out of equilibrium or out of proportion: as **a** : loss of parallel relation between the optical axes of the eyes caused by faulty action of the extrinsic muscles and often resulting in diplopia **b** : absence of biological equilibrium ⟨a vitamin ~⟩ — **im·bal·anced** \-lənst\ *adj*

im·be·cile \'im-bə-səl, -ˌsil\ *n* : a mentally retarded person having a mental age of three to seven years and requiring help in routine personal care — **imbecile** *or* **im·be·cil·ic** \ˌim-bə-'si-lik\ *adj* — **im·be·cil·i·ty** \ˌim-bə-'si-lə-tē\ *n*

im·bed \im-'bed\ *var of* EMBED

im·bri·ca·tion \ˌim-brə-'kā-shən\ *n* : an overlapping esp. of successive layers of tissue in the surgical closure of a wound — **im·bri·cate** \'im-brə-ˌkāt\ *vb*

im·id·az·ole \ˌi-mə-'da-ˌzōl\ *n* **1** : a white crystalline heterocyclic base $C_3H_4N_2$ that is an antimetabolite related to histidine **2** : any of a large class of derivatives of imidazole including histidine and histamine

im·id·az·o·line \ˌi-mə-'da-zə-ˌlēn\ *n* : any of three derivatives $C_3H_6N_2$ of imidazole with adrenergic blocking activity

im·i·no·gly·cin·uria \ˌi-mə-ˌnō-ˌgli-sə-'nur-ē-ə, -'nyur-\ *n* : an abnormal inherited condition of the kidney associated esp. with hyperprolinemia and characterized by the presence of proline, hydroxyproline, and glycine in the urine

imip·ra·mine \i-'mi-prə-ˌmēn\ *n* : a tricyclic antidepressant drug $C_{19}H_{24}N_2$ administered esp. in the form of its hydrochloride — see TOFRANIL

im·ma·ture \ˌi-mə-'tur, -'tyur, -'chur\ *adj* : lacking complete growth, differentiation, or development — **im·ma·ture·ly** *adv* — **im·ma·tu·ri·ty** \-'tur-ə-tē, -'tyur-, -'chur-\ *n*

im·me·di·ate \i-'mē-dē-ət\ *adj* **1** : acting or being without the intervention of another object, cause, or agency : being direct ⟨the ~ cause of death⟩ **2** : present to the mind independently of other states or factors ⟨~ awareness⟩

immediate auscultation *n* : auscultation performed without a stethoscope by laying the ear directly against the patient's body

immediate hypersensitivity *n, pl* **-ties** : hypersensitivity in which exposure to an antigen produces an immediate or almost immediate reaction

immersion foot *n* : a painful condition of the feet marked by inflammation and stabbing pain and followed by discoloration, swelling, ulcers, and numbness due to prolonged exposure to moist cold usu. without actual freezing

im·mo·bile \ˌi-'mō-bəl, -ˌbēl, -ˌbīl\ *adj* **1** : incapable of being moved **2** : not moving ⟨keep the patient ~⟩ — **im·mo·bil·i·ty** \ˌi-mō-'bi-lə-tē\ *n*

im·mo·bi·lize \i-'mō-bə-ˌlīz\ *vb* **-ized; -iz·ing** : to make immobile; *esp* : to fix (as a body part) so as to reduce or eliminate motion usu. by means of a cast or splint, by strapping, or by strict bed rest — **im·mo·bi·li·za·tion** \-ˌmō-bə-lə-'zā-shən\ *n*

im·mune \i-'myün\ *adj* **1** : not susceptible or responsive; *esp* : having a high degree of resistance to a disease **2 a** : having or producing antibodies or lymphocytes capable of reacting with a specific antigen ⟨an ~ serum⟩ **b** : produced by, involved in, or concerned with immunity or an immune response ⟨~ agglutinins⟩

immune complex *n* : any of various molecular complexes formed in the blood by combination of an antigen and an antibody that tend to accumulate in bodily tissue and are associated with various pathological conditions (as glomerulonephritis and systemic lupus erythematosus)

immune globulin *n* : globulin from the blood of a person or animal immune to a particular disease — called also *immune serum globulin*

immune response *n* : a bodily response to an antigen that occurs when lymphocytes identify the antigenic molecule as foreign and induce the for-

mation of antibodies and lymphocytes capable of reacting with it and
rendering it harmless — called also
immune reaction

immune serum *n* : ANTISERUM

immune system *n* : the bodily system
that protects the body from foreign
substances, cells, and tissues by producing the immune response and that
includes esp. the thymus, spleen,
lymph nodes, special deposits of lymphoid tissue (as in the gastrointestinal
tract and bone marrow), lymphocytes
including the B cells and T cells, and
antibodies

immune therapy *n* : IMMUNOTHERAPY
im·mu·ni·ty \i-ˈmyü-nə-tē\ *n, pl* **-ties**
: the quality or state of being immune;
esp : a condition of being able to resist a particular disease esp. through
preventing development of a pathogenic microorganism or by counteracting the effects of its products —
see ACQUIRED IMMUNITY, ACTIVE IM-
MUNITY, NATURAL IMMUNITY, PAS-
SIVE IMMUNITY

im·mu·ni·za·tion \i-myə-nə-ˈzā-shən\ *n*
: the creation of immunity usu.
against a particular disease; *esp* : treatment of an organism for the purpose
of making it immune to subsequent
attack by a particular pathogen — **im·
mu·nize** \ˈi-myə-ˌnīz\ *vb*

immuno- *comb form* **1** : physiological
immunity (*immuno*logy) **2** : immunologic (*immuno*chemistry) : immunologically (*immuno*compromised) : immunology and (*immuno*genetics)

im·mu·no·ad·sor·bent \i-myə-nō-ad-
ˈsȯr-bənt, i-ˌmyü-nō-, -ˈzȯr-\ *n* : IM-
MUNOSORBENT — **immunoadsorbent**
adj

im·mu·no·as·say \-ˈas-ˌā, -a-ˈsā\ *n* : the
identification of a substance (as a
protein) based on its capacity to act
as an antigen — **immunoassay** *vb* —
im·mu·no·as·say·able \-a-ˈsā-ə-bəl\ *adj*
im·mu·no·bi·ol·o·gy \-bī-ˈä-lə-jē\ *n, pl*
-gies : a branch of biology concerned
with the physiological reactions characteristic of the immune state — **im·
mu·no·bi·o·log·i·cal** \-ˌbī-ə-ˈlä-ji-kəl\
or **im·mu·no·bi·o·log·ic** \-ˈlä-jik\ *adj* —
im·mu·no·bi·ol·o·gist \-bī-ˈä-lə-jist\ *n*
im·mu·no·blast \i-ˈmyü-nō-ˌblast, ˈi-
myə-nō-\ *n* : a cell formed by transformation of a T cell after antigenic
stimulation and giving rise to a population of T cells with specificity
against the stimulating antigen — **im·
mu·no·blas·tic** \i-myə-nō-ˈblas-tik,
i-ˌmyü-nō-\ *adj*
im·mu·no·blot \-ˌblät\ *n* : a blot in
which a radioactively labeled antibody is used as the molecular probe
— **im·mu·no·blot·ting** *n*
im·mu·no·chem·is·try \-ˈke-mə-strē\ *n,
pl* **-tries** : a branch of chemistry that
deals with the chemical aspects of immunology — **im·mu·no·chem·i·cal**
\-ˈke-mə-kəl\ *adj* — **im·mu·no·chem-**

i·cal·ly *adv* — **im·mu·no·chem·ist**
\-ˈke-mist\ *n*
im·mu·no·che·mo·ther·a·py \-ˌkē-mō-
ˈther-ə-pē\ *n, pl* **-pies** : the combined
use of immunotherapy and chemotherapy in the treatment or control of
disease
im·mu·no·com·pe·tence \-ˈkäm-pə-təns\
n : the capacity for a normal immune
response — **im·mu·no·com·pe·tent**
\-tənt\ *adj*
im·mu·no·com·pro·mised \-ˈkäm-prə-
ˌmīzd\ *adj* : having the immune system impaired or weakened (as by
drugs or illness)
im·mu·no·cyte \i-ˈmyü-nō-ˌsīt, ˈi-myə-
nō-\ *n* : a cell (as a lymphocyte) that
has an immunologic function
im·mu·no·cy·to·chem·is·try \i-myə-nō-
ˌsī-tō-ˈke-mə-strē, i-ˌmyü-nō-\ *n, pl*
-tries : the application of biochemistry to cellular immunology — **im·mu·
no·cy·to·chem·i·cal** \-ˈke-mi-kəl\ *adj*
im·mu·no·de·fi·cien·cy \-di-ˈfi-shən-sē\
n, pl **-cies** : inability to produce a normal complement of antibodies or immunologically sensitized T cells esp.
in response to specific antigens — see
AIDS — **im·mu·no·de·fi·cient** \-shənt\
adj
im·mu·no·de·pres·sion \-di-ˈpre-shən\ *n*
: IMMUNOSUPPRESSION — **im·mu·no·
de·pres·sant** \-di-ˈpres-ənt\ *n*
im·mu·no·di·ag·no·sis \-ˌdī-ig-ˈnō-səs\
n, pl **-no·ses** \-ˌsēz\ : diagnosis (as of
cancer) by immunological methods —
im·mu·no·di·ag·nos·tic \-ˈnäs-tik\ *adj*
im·mu·no·dif·fu·sion \-di-ˈfyü-zhən\ *n*
: any of several techniques for obtaining a precipitate between an antibody
and its specific antigen by suspending
one in a gel and letting the other migrate through it from a well or by letting both antibody and antigen
migrate through the gel from separate
wells to form an area of precipitation
im·mu·no·elec·tro·pho·re·sis \-ə-ˌlek-trə-
fə-ˈrē-səs\ *n, pl* **-re·ses** \-ˌsēz\ : electrophoretic separation of proteins
followed by identification by the formation of precipitates through specific immunologic reactions — **im·mu·
no·elec·tro·pho·ret·ic** \-ˈre-tik\ *adj* —
im·mu·no·elec·tro·pho·ret·i·cal·ly *adv*
im·mu·no·flu·o·res·cence \-ˌflȯ-ˈres-əns,
-flü-\ *n* : the labeling of antibodies or
antigens with fluorescent dyes esp.
for the purpose of demonstrating the
presence of a particular antigen or
antibody in a tissue preparation or
smear — **im·mu·no·flu·o·res·cent** \-ənt\
adj
im·mu·no·gen \i-ˈmyü-nə-jən, ˈi-myə-
nə-, -ˌjen\ *n* : an antigen that pro-
vokes an immune response
im·mu·no·ge·net·ics \-jə-ˈne-tiks\ *n* : a
branch of immunology concerned
with the interrelations of heredity,
disease, and the immune system and
its components (as antibodies) — **im·
mu·no·ge·net·ic** \-tik\ *adj* — **im·mu·no-**

ge·net·i·cal·ly \-∂de\ adv — im·mu·no·ge·net·i·cist \-j∂-'ne-t∂-sist\ n

im·mu·no·gen·ic \₁i-my∂-nō-'jen-ik, i-₁myü-nō-\ adj : relating to or producing an immune response ⟨∼ substances⟩ — im·mu·no·gen·i·cal·ly adv — im·mu·no·ge·nic·i·ty \-j∂-'ni-s∂-tē\ n

im·mu·no·glob·u·lin \-'glä-by∂-l∂n\ n : ANTIBODY — abbr. Ig

immunoglobulin A n : IGA
immunoglobulin D n : IGD
immunoglobulin E n : IGE
immunoglobulin G n : IGG
immunoglobulin M n : IGM

im·mu·no·he·ma·tol·o·gy \-₁hē-m∂-'tä-l∂-jē\ n, pl -gies : a branch of immunology that deals with the immunologic properties of blood — im·mu·no·he·ma·to·log·ic \-₁hē-m∂-t∂-'lä-jik\ or im·mu·no·he·ma·to·log·i·cal \-ji-k∂l\ adj — im·mu·no·he·ma·tol·o·gist \-hē-m∂-'tä-l∂-jist\ n

im·mu·no·his·to·chem·i·cal \-₁his-tō-'ke-mi-k∂l\ adj : of or relating to the application of histochemical and immunologic methods to chemical analysis of living cells and tissues — im·mu·no·his·to·chem·i·cal·ly adv — im·mu·no·his·to·chem·is·try \-'ke-m∂-strē\ n

im·mu·no·his·to·log·i·cal \-₁his-t∂-'lä-ji-k∂l\ also im·mu·no·his·to·log·ic \-'lä-jik\ adj : of or relating to the application of immunologic methods to histology — im·mu·no·his·tol·o·gy \-hi-'stä-l∂-jē\ n

immunological surveillance n : IMMUNOSURVEILLANCE

im·mu·nol·o·gist \₁i-my∂-'nä-l∂-jist\ n : a specialist in immunology

im·mu·nol·o·gy \₁i-my∂-'nä-l∂-jē\ n, pl -gies : a science that deals with the immune system and the cell-mediated and humoral aspects of immunity and immune responses — im·mu·no·log·ic \-n∂-'lä-jik\ or im·mu·no·log·i·cal \-ji-k∂l\ adj — im·mu·no·log·i·cal·ly adv

im·mu·no·mod·u·la·tor \₁i-my∂-nō-'mä-j∂-₁lā-t∂r, i-₁myü-nō-\ n : a substance that affects the functioning of the immune system — im·mu·no·mod·u·la·to·ry \-'mä-j∂-l∂-₁tōr-ē\ adj

im·mu·no·patho·gen·e·sis \-₁pa-th∂-'je-n∂-s∂s\ n, pl -e·ses \-₁sēz\ : the development of disease as affected by the immune system

im·mu·no·pa·thol·o·gist \-p∂-'thä-l∂-jist, -pa-\ n : a specialist in immunopathology

im·mu·no·pa·thol·o·gy \-p∂-'thä-l∂-jē, -pa-\ n, pl -gies : a branch of medicine that deals with immune responses associated with disease — im·mu·no·path·o·log·ic \-₁pa-th∂-'lä-jik\ or im·mu·no·path·o·log·i·cal \-ji-k∂l\ adj

im·mu·no·pre·cip·i·ta·tion \-pri-₁si-p∂-'tā-sh∂n\ n : precipitation of a complex of an antibody and its specific antigen — im·mu·no·pre·cip·i·tate

\-'si-p∂-tāt, -₁tāt\ n — im·mu·no·pre·cip·i·tate \-₁tāt\ vb

im·mu·no·pro·phy·lax·is \-₁prō-f∂-'lak-s∂s, -₁prä-\ n, pl -lax·es \-₁sēz\ : the prevention of disease by the production of active or passive immunity

im·mu·no·ra·dio·met·ric assay \-₁rā-dē-ō-'me-trik-\ n : immunoassay of a substance by combining it with a radioactively labeled antibody

im·mu·no·re·ac·tive \-rē-'ak-tiv\ adj : reacting to particular antigens or haptens ⟨serum ∼ insulin⟩ ⟨lymphocytes⟩ — im·mu·no·re·ac·tion \-'ak-sh∂n\ n — im·mu·no·re·ac·tiv·i·ty \-(₁)rē-₁ak-'ti-v∂-tē\ n

im·mu·no·reg·u·la·to·ry \-'re-gy∂-l∂-₁tōr-ē\ adj : of or relating to the regulation of the immune system ⟨∼ T cells⟩ — im·mu·no·reg·u·la·tion \-₁re-gy∂-'lā-sh∂n\ n

im·mu·no·sor·bent \-'sòr-b∂nt, -'zòr-\ adj : relating to or using a substrate consisting of a specific antibody or antigen chemically combined with an insoluble substance (as cellulose) to selectively remove the corresponding specific antigen or antibody from solution — immunosorbent n

im·mu·no·stim·u·lant \-'sti-my∂-l∂nt\ n : an agent that stimulates an immune response — immunostimulant n — im·mu·no·stim·u·la·tion \-₁sti-my∂-'lā-sh∂n\ n

im·mu·no·sup·pres·sion \-s∂-'pre-sh∂n\ n : suppression (as by drugs) of natural immune responses — im·mu·no·sup·press \-s∂-'pres\ vb — im·mu·no·sup·pres·sant \-'pres-ənt\ n or adj — im·mu·no·sup·pres·sive \-'pre-sòv\ adj

im·mu·no·sur·veil·lance \-s∂r-'vā-l∂ns\ n : a monitoring process of the immune system which detects and destroys neoplastic cells and which tends to break down in immunosuppressed individuals — called also immunological surveillance

im·mu·no·ther·a·py \-'ther-∂-pē\ n, pl -pies : treatment of or prophylaxis against disease by attempting to produce active or passive immunity — called also immune therapy — im·mu·no·ther·a·peu·tic \-ther-∂-'pyü-tik\ adj

IMP \₁i-(₁)em-'pē\ n : INOSINIC ACID

im·pact·ed \im-'pak-t∂d\ adj 1 a : blocked by material (as feces) that is firmly packed or wedged in position ⟨an ∼ colon⟩ b : wedged or lodged in a bodily passage ⟨an ∼ mass of feces⟩ 2 : characterized by broken ends of bone driven together ⟨an ∼ fracture⟩ 3 of a tooth : wedged between the jawbone and another tooth ⟨an ∼ wisdom tooth⟩ — im·pac·tion \im-'pak-sh∂n\ n

impaction fracture n : a fracture that is impacted

im·paired \im-'pard\ adj : being in a less than perfect or whole condition: as a : handicapped or functionally defective — often used in combination ⟨hearing-*impaired*⟩ **b** *chiefly Canad* : intoxicated by alcohol or narcotics ⟨driving while ∼⟩ — **im·pair·ment** \-ᵖar-mənt\ *n*

im·pal·pa·ble \(ˌ)im-ᵖpal-pə-bəl\ *adj* : incapable of being felt by touch

im·ped·ance \im-ᵖpēd-ᵊns\ *n* : opposition to blood flow in the circulatory system

im·ped·i·ment \im-ᵖpe-də-mənt\ *n* : something that impedes; *esp* : an organic obstruction to speech

imperfecta — see AMELOGENESIS IMPERFECTA, OSTEOGENESIS IMPERFECTA, OSTEOGENESIS IMPERFECTA CONGENITA, OSTEOGENESIS IMPERFECTA TARDA

im·per·fect fungus \(ˌ)im-ᵖpər-fikt-\ *n* : any of various fungi (order Fungi Imperfecti syn. Deuteromycetes) of which only the asexual spore-producing stage is known

im·per·fo·rate \(ˌ)im-ᵖpər-fə-rət, -ˌrāt\ *adj* : having no opening or aperture; *specif* : lacking the usual or normal opening ⟨an ∼ hymen⟩ ⟨an ∼ anus⟩

im·pe·ri·al gallon \im-ᵖpir-ē-əl-\ *n* : GALLON 2

im·per·me·able \(ˌ)im-ᵖpər-mē-ə-bəl\ *adj* : not permitting passage (as of a fluid) through its substance — **im·per·me·abil·i·ty** \-mē-ə-ᵇbi-lə-tē\ *n*

im·pe·tig·i·nized \im-pə-ᵗti-jə-ˌnīzd\ *adj* : affected with impetigo on top of an underlying dermatologic condition

im·pe·tig·i·nous \im-pə-ᵗti-jə-nəs\ *adj* : of, relating to, or resembling impetigo ⟨∼ skin lesions⟩

im·pe·ti·go \im-pə-ᵗtē-(ˌ)gō, -ᵗtī-\ *n* : an acute contagious staphylococcal or streptococcal skin disease characterized by vesicles, pustules, and yellowish crusts

impetigo con·ta·gi·o·sa \-kən-ˌtā-jē-ᵗō-sə\ *n* : IMPETIGO

im·plant \ᵗim-ˌplant\ *n* : something (as a graft, a small container of radioactive material for treatment of cancer, or a pellet containing hormones) to be gradually absorbed) that is implanted esp. in tissue — **im·plant** \im-ᵗplant\ *vb* — **im·plant·able** \-ᵗplan-tə-bəl\ *adj*

im·plan·ta·tion \ˌim-ˌplan-ᵗtā-shən\ *n* : the act or process of implanting or the state of being implanted: as **a** : the placement of a natural or artificial tooth in an artificially prepared socket or in the jawbone **b** *in placental mammals* : the process of attachment of the embryo to the maternal uterine wall — called also *nidation* **c** : medical treatment by the insertion of an implant

im·plant·ee \ˌim-ˌplan-ᵗtē\ *n* : the recipient of an implant

im·plan·tol·o·gist \ˌim-ˌplan-ᵗtä-lə-jist\ *n* : a dentist who specializes in implantology

im·plan·tol·o·gy \-ᵗtä-lə-jē\ *n, pl* **-gies** : a branch of dentistry dealing with dental implantation

im·plo·sion therapy \im-ᵖplō-zhən-\ *n* : IMPLOSIVE THERAPY

im·plo·sive therapy \im-ᵖplō-siv-\ *n* : psychotherapy esp. for treating phobias in which the patient is directly confronted with what he or she fears

imported fire ant *n* : either of two mound-building So. American fire ants of the genus *Solenopsis* (*S. invicta* and *S. richteri*) that have been introduced into the southeastern U.S. and can inflict stings requiring medical attention

im·po·tence \ᵗim-pə-təns\ *n* : the quality or state of being impotent; *esp* : an abnormal physical or psychological state of a male characterized by inability to copulate because of failure to have or maintain an erection

im·po·ten·cy \-tən-sē\ *n, pl* **-cies** : IMPOTENCE

im·po·tent \ᵗim-pə-tənt\ *adj* **1** : not potent **2** : unable to engage in sexual intercourse because of inability to have and maintain an erection; *broadly* : STERILE — usu. used of males

im·preg·nate \im-ᵖpreg-ˌnāt, ᵗim-ˌ\ *vb* **-nat·ed; -nat·ing 1 a** : to make pregnant **b** : to introduce sperm cells into : FERTILIZE **2** : to cause to be filled, imbued, permeated, or saturated — **im·preg·na·tion** \(ˌ)im-ˌpreg-ᵗnā-shən\ *n*

im·pres·sion \im-ᵖpre-shən\ *n* : an imprint in plastic material of the surfaces of the teeth and adjacent portions of the jaw from which a likeness may be produced in dentistry

im·print·ing \ᵗim-ˌprint-iŋ, im-ᵗ\ *n* : a rapid learning process that takes place early in the life of a social animal and establishes a behavior pattern (as recognition of and attraction to its own kind or a substitute) — **im·print** *vb*

im·pulse \ᵗim-ˌpəls\ *n* **1** : a wave of excitation transmitted through tissues and esp. nerve fibers and muscles that results in physiological activity or inhibition **2** : a sudden spontaneous inclination or incitement to some usu. unpremeditated action — **im·pul·sive** \im-ᵗpəl-siv\ *adj*

Im·u·ran \ᵗi-myə-ˌran\ *trademark* — used for a preparation of azathioprine

in *abbr* inch

In *symbol* indium

¹in- or **il-** or **im-** or **ir-** *prefix* : not — usu. **il-** before *l* ⟨*illegitimate*⟩ and **im-** before *b, m,* or *p* ⟨*imbalance*⟩ ⟨*immobile*⟩ ⟨*impalpable*⟩ and **ir-** before *r* ⟨*irreducible*⟩ and **in-** before other sounds ⟨*inoperable*⟩

²in- or **il-** or **im-** or **ir-** *prefix* : in : within : into : toward : on ⟨*irradiation*⟩ — usu. **il-** before *l,* **im-** before *b, m,* or *p,* **ir-** before *r,* and **in-** before other sounds

-in \ən,ᵊn, ˌin\ *n suffix* **1 a** : neutral

chemical compound ⟨insul*in*⟩ **b** : enzyme ⟨pancreat*in*⟩ **c** : antibiotic ⟨penicill*in*⟩ **2** : pharmaceutical product ⟨niac*in*⟩

in·ac·ti·vate \(ˌ)i-ˈnak-tə-ˌvāt\ vb **-vat·ed; -vat·ing** : to make inactive: as **a** : to destroy certain biological activities of ⟨~ the complement of normal serum by heat⟩ **b** : to cause (as an infective agent) to lose disease-producing capacity ⟨~ bacteria⟩ — **in·ac·ti·va·tion** \i-ˌnak-tə-ˈvā-shən\ n

in·ac·tive \in-ˈak-tiv\ adj : not active: as **a** : marked by deliberate or enforced absence of activity or effort ⟨forced by illness to lead an ~ life⟩ **b** of a disease : not progressing or fulminating : QUIESCENT **c** : chemically inert ⟨~ charcoal⟩ **d** : biologically inert esp. because of the loss of some quality (as infectivity or antigenicity) — **in·ac·tiv·i·ty** \i-ˌnak-ˈti-və-tē\ n

in·ad·e·quate \i-ˈna-də-kwət\ adj : not adequate; specif : lacking the capacity for psychological maturity or adequate social adjustment

in·a·ni·tion \ˌi-nə-ˈni-shən\ n : the exhausted condition that results from lack of food and water

in·ap·pe·tence \i-ˈna-pə-təns\ n : loss or lack of appetite

in·ap·pro·pri·ate \ˌi-nə-ˈprō-prē-ət\ adj : ABNORMAL 1

in·born \ˈin-ˈbȯrn\ adj : HEREDITARY, INHERITED ⟨~ errors of metabolism⟩

in·breed·ing \ˈin-ˌbrē-diŋ\ n : the interbreeding of closely related individuals — **in·bred** \-ˈbred\ adj — **in·breed** \-ˈbrēd\ vb — compare OUTBREEDING

in·ca·pac·i·tant \ˌin-kə-ˈpa-sə-tənt\ n : a chemical or biological agent (as tear gas) used to temporarily incapacitate people or animals (as in war or a riot)

in·car·cer·at·ed \in-ˈkär-sə-ˌrā-təd\ adj, of a hernia : constricted but not strangulated

in·car·cer·a·tion \in-ˌkär-sə-ˈrā-shən\ n **1** : a confining or state of being confined **2** : abnormal retention or confinement of a body part; specif : a constriction of the neck of a hernial sac so that the hernial contents become irreducible

in·cest \ˈin-ˌsest\ n : sexual intercourse between persons so closely related that they are forbidden by law to marry; also : the statutory crime of such a relationship — **in·ces·tu·ous** \in-ˈses-chə-wəs\ adj

inch \ˈinch\ n : a unit of length equal to ⅟₃₆ yard or 2.54 centimeters

in·ci·dence \ˈin-sə-dəns, -ˌdens\ n : rate of occurrence or influence; esp : the rate of occurrence of new cases of a particular disease in a population being studied — compare PREVALENCE

in·cip·i·ent \in-ˈsi-pē-ənt\ adj : beginning to come into being or to become apparent ⟨the ~ stage of a fever⟩

in·ci·sal \in-ˈsī-zəl\ adj : relating to, bearing, or involving the cutting edge or surface of a tooth (as an incisor)

in·cise \in-ˈsīz, -ˈsīs\ vb **in·cised; in·cis·ing** : to cut into : to make an incision in ⟨incised the swollen tissue⟩

incised adj, of a cut or wound : made with or as if with a sharp knife or scalpel : clean and well-defined

in·ci·sion \in-ˈsi-zhən\ n **1** : a cut or wound of body tissue made esp. in surgery **2** : an act of incising something — **in·ci·sion·al** \-zhə-nəl\ adj

in·ci·sive \in-ˈsī-siv\ adj : INCISAL; also : of, relating to, or situated near the incisors

incisive canal n : a narrow branched passage that extends from the floor of the nasal cavity to the incisive fossa and transmits the nasopalatine nerve and a branch of the greater palatine artery

incisive fossa n : a depression on the front of the maxillary bone above the incisor teeth

in·ci·sor \in-ˈsī-zər\ n : a front tooth adapted for cutting; esp : any of the eight cutting human teeth that are located between the canines with four in the lower and four in the upper jaw

in·ci·su·ra \ˌin-sī-ˈzhur-ə, -sə-\ n, pl **in·ci·su·rae** \-ˌē, -ˌī\ **1** : a notch, cleft, or fissure of a body part or organ **2** : a downward notch in the curve recording aortic blood pressure that occurs between systole and diastole and is caused by backward flow of blood for a short time before the aortic valve closes

incisura an·gu·lar·is \-ˌaŋ-gyə-ˈlar-əs\ n : a notch or bend in the lesser curvature of the stomach near its pyloric end

in·cli·na·tion \ˌin-klə-ˈnā-shən\ n : a deviation from the true vertical or horizontal; esp : the deviation of the long axis of a tooth or of the slope of a cusp from the vertical

in·clu·sion \in-ˈklü-zhən\ n : something that is included; esp : a passive usu. temporary product of cell activity (as a starch grain) within the cytoplasm or nucleus

inclusion blennorrhea n : INCLUSION CONJUNCTIVITIS

inclusion body n : an inclusion, abnormal structure, or foreign cell within a cell; specif : an intracellular body that is characteristic of some virus diseases and that is the site of virus multiplication

inclusion conjunctivitis n : an infectious disease esp. of newborn infants characterized by acute conjunctivitis and the presence of large inclusion bodies and caused by a chlamydia (C. trachomatis)

inclusion disease n : CYTOMEGALIC INCLUSION DISEASE

in·co·her·ent \ˌin-kō-ˈhir-ənt, -ˈher-\ adj : lacking clarity or intelligibility usu. by reason of some emotional stress ⟨∼ speech⟩ — **in·co·her·ence** \-əns\ n — **in·co·her·ent·ly** adv

in·com·pat·i·ble \in-kəm-'pa-tə-bəl\ adj **1** : unsuitable for use together because of chemical interaction or antagonistic physiological effects ⟨∼ drugs⟩ **2** of blood or serum : unsuitable for use in a particular transfusion because of the presence of agglutinins that act against the recipient's red blood cells — **in·com·pat·i·bil·i·ty** \-¡pa-tə-'bi-lə-tē\ n

in·com·pe·tence \in-'käm-pə-təns\ n **1** : lack of legal qualification **2** : inability of an organ or part to perform its function adequately — **in·com·pe·tent** \-tənt\ adj

in·com·pe·ten·cy \-tən-sē\ n, pl **-cies** : INCOMPETENCE

in·com·plete \in-kəm-'plēt\ adj **1** of insect metamorphosis : having no pupal stage between the immature stages and the adult with the young insect usu. resembling the adult — compare COMPLETE 1 **2** of a bone fracture : not broken entirely across — compare COMPLETE 2

incomplete dominance n : the property of being expressed or inherited as a semidominant gene or trait

in·con·stant \in-'kän-stənt\ adj : not always present ⟨an ∼ muscle⟩

in·con·ti·nence \in-'känt-ᵊn-əns\ n **1** : inability or failure to restrain sexual appetite **2** : inability of the body to control the evacuative functions — **in·con·ti·nent** \-ənt\ adj

in·co·or·di·na·tion \¡in-kō-¡ȯrd-ᵊn-'ā-shən\ n : lack of coordination esp. of muscular movements resulting from loss of voluntary control

in·cre·men·tal lines \¡iŋ-krə-'ment-ᵊl-, ¡in-\ n pl : lines seen in a tooth in section showing the periodic depositions of dentin, enamel, and cementum occurring during growth

incremental lines of Ret·zi·us \-'ret-sē-əs\ n pl : incremental lines in the enamel of a tooth

Retzius, Magnus Gustaf (1842–1919), Swedish anatomist and anthropologist.

in·crus·ta·tion \¡in-¡krəs-'tā-shən\ n **1** : the act of encrusting : the state of being encrusted **2** : a crust or hard coating

in·cu·bate \'iŋ-kyə-¡bāt, 'in-\ vb **-bat·ed; -bat·ing 1** : to maintain (as embryos or bacteria) under conditions favorable for hatching or development **2** : to undergo incubation

in·cu·ba·tion \¡iŋ-kyə-'bā-shən, ¡in-\ n **1** : the act or process of incubating **2** : INCUBATION PERIOD

incubation period n : the period between the infection of an individual by a pathogen and the manifestation of the disease it causes

in·cu·ba·tor \'iŋ-kyə-¡bā-tər, 'in-\ n : one that incubates; esp : an apparatus with a chamber used to provide

controlled environmental conditions esp. for the cultivation of microorganisms or the care and protection of premature or sick babies

in·cur·able \in-'kyūr-ə-bəl\ adj : impossible to cure — **in·cur·ably** \-blē\ adv

in·cus \'iŋ-kəs\ n, pl **in·cu·des** \iŋ-'kyū-(¡)dēz, 'iŋ-kyə-¡dēz\ : the middle bone of a chain of three small bones in the ear — called also anvil

IND \¡ī-(¡)en-'dē\ abbr investigational new drug

in·dane·di·one \¡in-dān-'dī-¡ōn\ or **in·dan·di·one** \in-dan-\ n : any of a group of synthetic anticoagulants

indecent assault n : a sexually aggressive act or series of acts exclusive of rape committed against another person without consent

indecent exposure n : intentional exposure of part of one's body (as the genitalia) in a place where such exposure is likely to be an offense against the generally accepted standards of decency in a community

independent assortment n : formation of random combinations of chromosomes in meiosis and of genes on different pairs of homologous chromosomes by the passage at random of one of each diploid pair of homologous chromosomes into each gamete independently of each other pair

In·der·al \'in-də-¡ral\ trademark — used for a preparation of propranolol

in·de·ter·mi·nate \¡in-di-'tər-mə-nət\ adj : relating to, being, or undergoing indeterminate cleavage ⟨an ∼ egg⟩

indeterminate cleavage n : cleavage in which all the early divisions produce cells with the potencies of the entire zygote — compare DETERMINATE CLEAVAGE

in·dex \'in-¡deks\ n, pl **in·dex·es** or **in·di·ces** \-də-¡sēz\ **1** : a ratio or other number derived from a series of observations and used as an indicator or measure (as of a condition, property, or phenomenon) **2** : the ratio of one dimension of a thing (as an anatomical structure) to another dimension — see CEPHALIC INDEX, CRANIAL INDEX

index case n : a case of a disease or condition which is discovered first and which leads to the discovery of others in a family or group; also : the first case of a contagious disease

index finger n : FOREFINGER

index of refraction n : the ratio of the speed of radiation (as light) in one medium to that in another medium — called also refractive index

Indian hemp n : HEMP 1

indica — see CANNABIS INDICA

in·di·can \'in-də-¡kan\ n : an indigo=forming substance $C_8H_7NO_4S$ found as a salt in urine and other animal fluids; also : its potassium salt C_8H_6-KNO_4S

in·di·cate \'in-də-¡kāt\ vb **-cat·ed; -cat·ing 1** : to be a fairly certain symptom of : show the presence or existence of **2** : to call for esp. as treatment for a particular condition ⟨radical surgery is *indicated*⟩

in·di·ca·tion \ˌin-də-ˈkā-shən\ *n* **1** : a symptom or particular circumstance that indicates the advisability or necessity of a specific medical treatment or procedure **2** : something that is indicated as advisable or necessary

in·di·ca·tor \ˈin-də-ˌkā-tər\ *n* : a substance (as a dye) used to show visually usu. by its capacity for color change the condition of a solution with respect to the presence of free acid or alkali or some other substance

indices *pl of* INDEX

indicis — *see* EXTENSOR INDICIS, EXTENSOR INDICIS PROPRIUS

in·dig·e·nous \in-ˈdi-jə-nəs\ *adj* : having originated in and being produced, growing, or living naturally in a particular region or environment ⟨a disease ∼ to the tropics⟩

in·di·gest·ible \ˌin-(ˌ)dī-ˈjes-tə-bəl, -də-\ *adj* : not digestible : not easily digested — **in·di·gest·ibil·i·ty** \-ˌjes-tə-ˈbi-lə-tē\ *n*

in·di·ges·tion \-ˈjes-chən\ *n* **1** : inability to digest or difficulty in digesting food : incomplete or imperfect digestion of food **2** : a case or attack of indigestion

in·di·go car·mine \ˌin-di-ˌgō-ˈkär-mən, -ˌmin\ *n* : a soluble blue dye $C_{16}H_8N_2Na_2O_8S_2$ that is used chiefly as a biological stain and food color and since it is rapidly excreted by the kidneys is used as a dye to mark ureteral structures (as in cystoscopy and catheterization)

in·dis·posed \ˌin-di-ˈspōzd\ *adj* : being usu. temporarily in poor physical health : slightly ill — **in·dis·po·si·tion** \(ˌ)in-ˌdis-pə-ˈzi-shən\ *n*

in·di·um \ˈin-dē-əm\ *n* : a malleable fusible silvery metallic element — *abbr. In;* see ELEMENT table

individual psychology *n* : a modification of psychoanalysis developed by the Austrian psychologist Alfred Adler emphasizing feelings of inferiority and a desire for power as the primary motivating forces in human behavior

in·di·vid·u·a·tion \ˌin-də-ˌvi-jə-ˈwā-shən\ *n* : the process in the analytic psychology of C. G. Jung by which the self is formed by integrating elements of the conscious and unconscious mind — **in·di·vid·u·ate** \-ˈvi-jə-ˌwāt\ *vb*

In·do·cin \ˈin-də-sən\ *trademark* — used for a preparation of indomethacin

in·do·cy·a·nine green \ˌin-dō-ˈsī-ə-ˌnēn-, -nən-\ *n* : a green dye $C_{43}H_{47}N_2NaO_6S_2$ used esp. in testing liver blood flow and cardiac output

In·do·klon \ˈin-də-ˌklän\ *trademark* — used for a preparation of flurothyl

in·dole \ˈin-ˌdōl\ *n* : a crystalline compound C_8H_7N that is found in the intestines and feces as a decomposition product of proteins containing tryptophan; *also* : a derivative of indole

in·dole·ace·tic acid \ˌin-dō-lə-ˌsē-tik-\ *n* : a compound $C_{10}H_9NO_2$ formed from tryptophan in plants and animals that is present in small amounts in normal urine and acts as a growth hormone in plants

in·do·lent \ˈin-də-lənt\ *adj* **1** : causing little or no pain ⟨an ∼ tumor⟩ **2 a** : growing or progressing slowly ⟨an ∼ disease⟩ **b** : slow to heal ⟨an ∼ ulcer⟩ — **in·do·lence** \-ləns\ *n*

in·do·meth·a·cin \ˌin-dō-ˈme-thə-sən\ *n* : a nonsteroidal drug $C_{19}H_{16}ClNO_4$ with anti-inflammatory, analgesic, and antipyretic properties used esp. in treating arthritis — *see* INDOCIN

in·duce \in-ˈdüs, -ˈdyüs\ *vb* **in·duced; in·duc·ing 1** : to cause or bring about: as **a** : to cause to form through embryonic induction **b** : to cause or initiate by artificial means ⟨*induced* labor⟩ **2** : to produce anesthesia in

in·duc·er \-ˈdü-sər, -ˈdyü-\ *n* : one that induces; *specif* : a substance that is capable of activating a structural gene by combining with and inactivating a genetic repressor

in·duc·ible \in-ˈdü-sə-bəl, -ˈdyü-\ *adj* : capable of being induced; *esp* : formed by a cell in response to the presence of its substrate ⟨∼ enzymes⟩ — **in·duc·ibil·i·ty** \in-ˌdü-sə-ˈbi-lə-tē, -ˌdyü-\ *n*

in·duc·tion \in-ˈdək-shən\ *n* **1** : the act of causing or bringing on or about ⟨∼ of labor⟩; *specif* : the establishment of the initial state of anesthesia often with an agent other than that used subsequently to maintain the anesthetic state **2 a** : arousal of a part or area (as of the retina) by stimulation of an adjacent part or area **b** : the sum of the processes by which the fate of embryonic cells is determined and differentiation brought about — **in·duct** \in-ˈdəkt\ *vb* — **in·duc·tive** \-ˈdək-tiv\ *adj* — **in·duc·tive·ly** *adv*

in·duc·tor \in-ˈdək-tər\ *n* : one that inducts; *esp* : ORGANIZER

in·du·rat·ed \ˈin-dü-ˌrā-təd, -dyü-\ *adj* : having become firm or hard esp. by increase of fibrous elements ⟨∼ tissue⟩ ⟨an ulcer with an ∼ border⟩

in·du·ra·tion \ˌin-dü-ˈrā-shən, -dyü-\ *n* **1** : an increase in the fibrous elements in tissue commonly associated with inflammation and marked by loss of elasticity and pliability : SCLEROSIS **2** : a hardened mass or formation — **in·du·ra·tive** \ˈin-du-ˌrā-tiv, -ˌdyü-; in-ˈdur-ə-tiv, -ˈdyür-\ *adj*

in·du·si·um gris·e·um \in-ˈdü-zē-əm-ˈgri-zē-əm, -ˌdyü-, -zhē-\ *n* : a thin layer of gray matter over the dorsal surface of the corpus callosum

industrial disease *n* : OCCUPATIONAL DISEASE

in·dwell·ing \ˈin-ˌdwe-liŋ\ *adj* : left

within a bodily organ or passage to maintain drainage, prevent obstruction, or provide a route for administration of food or drugs — used of an implanted tube (as a catheter)

in·elas·tic \,i-nə-'las-tik\ *adj* : not elastic

in·ert \i-'nərt\ *adj* 1 : lacking the power to move 2 : deficient in active properties; *esp* : lacking a usual or anticipated chemical or biological action ⟨an ∼ drug⟩ — **in·ert·ness** *n*

inert gas *n* : NOBLE GAS

in·er·tia \i-'nər-shə\ *n* : lack of activity or movement — used esp. of the uterus in labor when its contractions are weak or irregular

in ex·tre·mis \,in-ik-'strē-məs, -'strā-\ *adv* : at the point of death

in·fan·cy \'in-fən-sē\ *n, pl* **-cies** 1 : early childhood 2 : the legal status of an infant

in·fant \'in-fənt\ *n* 1 a : a child in the first year of life : BABY b : a child several years of age 2 : a person who is not of full age : MINOR — **infant** *adj*

in·fan·ti·cide \in-'fan-tə-,sīd\ *n* : the killing of an infant — **in·fan·ti·ci·dal** \-,fan-tə-'sīd-ᵊl\ *adj*

in·fan·tile \'in-fən-,tīl, -,tēl, -(,)til\ *adj* 1 : of, relating to, or occurring in infants or infancy ⟨∼ eczema⟩ 2 : suitable to or characteristic of an infant; *esp* : very immature

infantile amaurotic idiocy *n* 1 : TAY-SACHS DISEASE 2 : SANDHOFF'S DISEASE

infantile autism *n* : a severe autism that first occurs before 30 months of age — called also *Kanner's syndrome*

infantile paralysis *n* : POLIOMYELITIS

infantile scurvy *n* : acute scurvy during infancy caused by malnutrition — called also *Barlow's disease*

in·fan·ti·lism \'in-fən-,tī-,li-zəm, -tə-; in-'fant-ᵊl-,i-\ *n* : retention of childish physical, mental, or emotional qualities in adult life; *esp* : failure to attain sexual maturity

infantum — see ROSEOLA INFANTUM

in·farct \'in-,färkt, in-'\ *n* : an area of necrosis in a tissue or organ resulting from obstruction of the local circulation by a thrombus or embolus — **in·farct·ed** \in-'färk-təd\ *adj*

in·farc·tion \in-'färk-shən\ *n* 1 : the process of forming an infarct 2 : INFARCT

in·fect \in-'fekt\ *vb* 1 : to contaminate with a disease-producing substance or agent (as bacteria) 2 a : to communicate a pathogen or a disease to b of *a pathogenic organism* : to invade (an individual or organ) usu. by penetration — compare INFEST

in·fec·tant \in-'fek-tənt\ *n* : an agent of infection (as a bacterium or virus)

in·fec·tion \in-'fek-shən\ *n* 1 : an infective agent or material contaminated with an infective agent 2 a : the state produced by the establishment of an infective agent in or on a suitable host

b : a disease resulting from infection : INFECTIOUS DISEASE 3 : an act or process of infecting; *also* : the establishment of a pathogen in its host after invasion

infectiosum — see ERYTHEMA INFECTIOSUM

in·fec·tious \in-'fek-shəs\ *adj* 1 : capable of causing infection 2 : communicable by invasion of the body of a susceptible organism — compare CONTAGIOUS 1 — **in·fec·tious·ly** *adv* — **in·fec·tious·ness** *n*

infectious abortion *n* : CONTAGIOUS ABORTION

infectious anemia *n* 1 : EQUINE INFECTIOUS ANEMIA 2 : FELINE INFECTIOUS ANEMIA

infectious bovine rhinotracheitis *n* : a disease of cattle caused by a virus serologically related to the virus causing herpes simplex in humans

infectious coryza *n* : an acute infectious respiratory disease of chickens that is caused by a bacterium of the genus *Haemophilus* (*H. paragallinarum* syn. *H. gallinarum*) and is characterized by catarrhal inflammation of the mucous membranes of the nasal passages and sinuses frequently with conjunctivitis and subcutaneous edema of the face and wattles and sometimes with pneumonia

infectious disease *n* : a disease caused by the entrance into the body of organisms (as bacteria) which grow and multiply there — see COMMUNICABLE DISEASE, CONTAGIOUS DISEASE

infectious enterohepatitis *n* : BLACKHEAD 2

infectious hepatitis *n* : HEPATITIS A

infectious jaundice *n* 1 : HEPATITIS A 2 : WEIL'S DISEASE

infectious laryngotracheitis *n* : a severe highly contagious and often fatal disease of chickens and pheasants that affects chiefly adult birds, is caused by a herpesvirus, and is characterized by inflammation of the trachea and larynx often marked by local necrosis and hemorrhage and by the formation of purulent or cheesy exudate interfering with breathing

infectious mononucleosis *n* : an acute infectious disease associated with Epstein-Barr virus and characterized by fever, swelling of lymph nodes, and lymphocytosis — called also *glandular fever, kissing disease, mono*

in·fec·tive \in-'fek-tiv\ *adj* : producing or capable of producing infection : INFECTIOUS

in·fec·tiv·i·ty \,in-,fek-'ti-və-tē\ *n, pl* **-ties** : the quality of being infective : the ability to produce infection; *specif* : a tendency to spread rapidly from host to host — compare VIRULENCE b

in·fec·tor \in-'fek-tər\ *n* : one that infects

in·fe·ri·or \in-ᵊfir-ē-ǝr\ *adj* **1** : situated below and closer to the feet than another and esp. another similar part of an upright body esp. of a human being — compare SUPERIOR 1 **2** : situated in a more posterior or ventral position in the body of a quadruped — compare SUPERIOR 2

inferior alveolar artery *n* : a branch of the maxillary artery that is distributed to the mucous membrane of the mouth and to the teeth of the lower jaw — called also *mandibular artery, inferior dental artery*

inferior alveolar nerve *n* : a branch of the mandibular nerve that is distributed to the teeth of the lower jaw and to the skin of the chin and the skin and mucous membrane of the lower lip — called also *inferior alveolar, inferior dental nerve*

inferior alveolar vein *n* : the vein accompanying the inferior alveolar artery

inferior articular process *n* : ARTICULAR PROCESS b

inferior cerebellar peduncle *n* : CEREBELLAR PEDUNCLE c

inferior colliculus *n* : either member of the posterior and lower pair of corpora quadrigemina that are situated next to the pons and together constitute one of the lower centers for hearing — compare SUPERIOR COLLICULUS

inferior concha *n* : NASAL CONCHA a

inferior constrictor *n* : a muscle of the pharynx that acts to constrict part of the pharynx in swallowing — called also *constrictor pharyngis inferior, inferior pharyngeal constrictor muscle*; compare MIDDLE CONSTRICTOR, SUPERIOR CONSTRICTOR

inferior dental artery *n* : INFERIOR ALVEOLAR ARTERY

inferior dental nerve *n* : INFERIOR ALVEOLAR NERVE

inferior extensor retinaculum *n* : EXTENSOR RETINACULUM 1a

inferior ganglion *n* **1** : the lower and larger of the two sensory ganglia of the glossopharyngeal nerve — called also *petrosal ganglion*; compare SUPERIOR GANGLION 1 **2** : the lower of the two ganglia of the vagus nerve that forms a swelling just beyond the exit of the nerve from the jugular foramen — called also *inferior vagal ganglion, nodose ganglion*; compare SUPERIOR GANGLION 2

inferior gluteal artery *n* : GLUTEAL ARTERY b

inferior gluteal nerve *n* : GLUTEAL NERVE b

inferior hemorrhoidal artery *n* : RECTAL ARTERY a

inferior hemorrhoidal vein *n* : RECTAL VEIN a

inferior horn *n* : the cornu in the lateral ventricle of each cerebral hemisphere that curves downward into the temporal lobe — compare ANTERIOR HORN 2, POSTERIOR HORN 2

in·fe·ri·or·i·ty \(ˌ)in-ˌfir-ē-ᵊȯr-ǝ-tē, -ᵊär-\ *n, pl* **-ties** : a condition or state of being or having a sense of being inferior or inadequate esp. with respect to one's apparent equals or with respect to the world at large

inferiority complex *n* : an acute sense of personal inferiority resulting either in timidity or through overcompensation in exaggerated aggressiveness

inferior laryngeal artery *n* : LARYNGEAL ARTERY a

inferior laryngeal nerve *n* **1** : LARYNGEAL NERVE b — called also *inferior laryngeal* **2** : any of the terminal branches of the inferior laryngeal nerve

inferior longitudinal fasciculus *n* : a band of association fibers in each cerebral hemisphere that connects the occipital and temporal lobes

in·fe·ri·or·ly *adv* : in a lower position

inferior maxillary bone *n* : JAW 1b

inferior maxillary nerve *n* : MANDIBULAR NERVE

inferior meatus *n* : a space extending along the lateral wall of the nasal cavity between the inferior nasal concha and the floor of the nasal cavity — compare MIDDLE MEATUS, SUPERIOR MEATUS

inferior mesenteric artery *n* : MESENTERIC ARTERY a

inferior mesenteric ganglion *n* : MESENTERIC GANGLION a

inferior mesenteric plexus *n* : MESENTERIC PLEXUS a

inferior mesenteric vein *n* : MESENTERIC VEIN a

inferior nasal concha *n* : NASAL CONCHA a

inferior nuchal line *n* : NUCHAL LINE c

inferior oblique *n* : OBLIQUE b(2)

inferior olive *n* : a large gray nucleus that forms the interior of the olive on each side of the medulla oblongata — called also *inferior olivary nucleus*; see ACCESSORY OLIVARY NUCLEUS; compare SUPERIOR OLIVE

inferior ophthalmic vein *n* : OPHTHALMIC VEIN b

inferior orbital fissure *n* : ORBITAL FISSURE b

inferior pancreaticoduodenal artery *n* : PANCREATICODUODENAL ARTERY a

inferior pectoral nerve *n* : PECTORAL NERVE b

inferior peroneal retinaculum *n* : PERONEAL RETINACULUM b

inferior petrosal sinus *n* : PETROSAL SINUS b

inferior pharyngeal constrictor muscle *n* : INFERIOR CONSTRICTOR

inferior phrenic artery *n* : PHRENIC ARTERY b

inferior phrenic vein *n* : PHRENIC VEIN b

inferior radioulnar joint *n* : DISTAL RADIOULNAR JOINT

inferior ramus *n* : RAMUS b(2), c
inferior rectal artery *n* : RECTAL ARTERY a
inferior rectal vein *n* : RECTAL VEIN a
inferior rectus *n* : RECTUS 2d
inferior sagittal sinus *n* : SAGITTAL SINUS b
inferior temporal gyrus *n* : TEMPORAL GYRUS c
inferior thyroarytenoid ligament *n* : VOCAL LIGAMENT
inferior thyroid artery *n* : THYROID ARTERY b
inferior turbinate *n* : NASAL CONCHA a
inferior turbinate bone *also* **inferior turbinated bone** \-'tər-bə-₁nā-təd-\ *n* : NASAL CONCHA a
inferior ulnar collateral artery *n* : a small artery that arises from the brachial artery just above the elbow and branches to anastomose with other arteries in the region of the elbow — compare SUPERIOR ULNAR COLLATERAL ARTERY
inferior vagal ganglion *n* : INFERIOR GANGLION 2
inferior vena cava *n* : a vein that is the largest vein in the human body, is formed by the union of the two common iliac veins at the level of the fifth lumbar vertebra, and returns blood to the right atrium of the heart from bodily parts below the diaphragm
inferior vermis *n* : VERMIS 1b
inferior vesical *n* : VESICAL ARTERY b
inferior vesical artery *n* : VESICAL ARTERY b
inferior vestibular nucleus *n* : the one of the four vestibular nuclei on each side of the medulla oblongata that sends fibers down both sides of the spinal cord to synapse with motoneurons of the ventral roots
inferior vocal cords *n pl* : TRUE VOCAL CORDS
infero- *comb form* : below and ⟨*infero*medial⟩
in·fe·ro·me·di·al \₁in-fə-rō-'mē-dē-əl\ *adj* : situated below and in the middle
in·fer·tile \in-'fərt-ᵊl\ *adj* : not fertile : BARREN — compare STERILE 1 — **in·fer·til·i·ty** \₁in-(₁)fər-'til-ə-tē\ *n*
in·fest \in-'fest\ *vb* : to live in or on as a parasite — compare INFECT — **in·fes·tant** \in-'fes-tənt\ *n* — **in·fes·ta·tion** \₁in-₁fes-'tā-shən\ *n*
in·fib·u·la·tion \(₁)in-₁fi-byə-'lā-shən\ *n* : an act or practice of fastening by ring, clasp, or stitches the labia majora in girls and the prepuce in boys in order to prevent sexual intercourse
in·fil·trate \in-'fil-₁strāt, 'in-(₁)fil-\ *vb* : something that passes or is caused to pass into or through something by permeating or filtering; *esp* : a substance that passes into the bodily tissues and forms an abnormal accumulation ⟨a lung ∼⟩ — **infiltrate** *vb* — **in·fil·tra·tion** \₁in-(₁)fil-'trā-shən\ *n* — **in·fil·tra·tive** \'in-fil-₁trā-tiv, in-'fil-trə-\ *adj*

infiltration anesthesia *n* : anesthesia of an operative site accomplished by local injection of anesthetics
in·firm \in-'fərm\ *adj* : of poor or deteriorated vitality; *esp* : feeble from age
in·fir·ma·ry \in-'fər-mə-rē\ *n, pl* **-ries** : a place where the infirm or sick are lodged for care and treatment
in·fir·mi·ty \in-'fər-mə-tē\ *n, pl* **-ties** : the quality or state of being infirm; *esp* : an unsound, unhealthy, or debilitated state
in·flame \in-'flām\ *vb* **in·flamed; in·flam·ing** 1 : to cause inflammation in (bodily tissue) 2 : to become affected with inflammation
in·flam·ma·tion \₁in-flə-'mā-shən\ *n* : a local response to cellular injury that is marked by capillary dilatation, leukocytic infiltration, redness, heat, pain, swelling, and often loss of function and that serves as a mechanism initiating the elimination of noxious agents and of damaged tissue — **in·flam·ma·to·ry** \in-'fla-mə-₁tōr-ē\ *adj*
inflammatory bowel disease *n* : an inflammatory disease of the bowel: **a** : CROHN'S DISEASE **b** : ULCERATIVE COLITIS
in·flu·en·za \₁in-(₁)flü-'en-zə\ *n* **1 a** : an acute highly contagious virus disease that is caused by various strains of an orthomyxovirus belonging to three major types and that is characterized by sudden onset, fever, prostration, severe aches and pains, and progressive inflammation of the respiratory mucous membrane — often used with the letter *A*, *B*, or *C* to denote disease caused by a strain of virus of one of the three major types **b** : any human respiratory infection of undetermined cause — not used technically **2** : any of numerous febrile usu. virus diseases of domestic animals marked esp. by respiratory symptoms — **in·flu·en·zal** \-zəl\ *adj*
influenza vaccine *n* : a vaccine against influenza; *specif* : a mixture of strains of inactivated influenza virus from chick embryo culture
informed consent *n* : consent to surgery by a patient or to participation in a medical experiment by a subject after achieving an understanding of what is involved
infra- *prefix* **1** : below ⟨*infra*hyoid⟩ **2** : below in a scale or series ⟨*infra*red⟩
in·fra·car·di·ac \₁in-frə-'kär-dē-₁ak\ *adj* : situated below the heart
in·fra·cla·vic·u·lar \₁in-frə-kla-'vi-kyə-lər\ *adj* : situated at or occurring below the clavicle
in·fra·di·a·phrag·mat·ic \₁in-frə-₁dī-ə-frə-'ma-tik, -₁frag-\ *adj* : situated, occurring, or performed below the diaphragm ⟨an ∼ abscess⟩
in·fra·gle·noid tubercle \₁in-frə-'glē-₁nȯid-, -'gle-\ *n* : a tubercle on the scapula for the attachment of the long head of the triceps muscle

in·fra·hy·oid \ˌin-frə-ˈhī-ˌȯid\ *adj* : situated below the hyoid bone

infrahyoid muscle *n* : any of four muscles on each side that are situated next to the larynx and comprise the sternohyoid, sternothyroid, thyrohyoid, and omohyoid muscles

in·fra·mam·ma·ry \ˌin-frə-ˈma-mə-rē\ *adj* : situated or occurring below the mammary gland ⟨∼ pain⟩

in·fra·or·bit·al \ˌin-frə-ˈȯr-bət-ᵊl\ *adj* : situated beneath the orbit

infraorbital artery *n* : a branch or continuation of the maxillary artery that runs along the infraorbital groove with the infraorbital nerve and passes through the infraorbital foramen to give off branches which supply the face just below the eye

infraorbital fissure *n* : ORBITAL FISSURE b

infraorbital foramen *n* : an opening in the maxillary bone just below the lower rim of the orbit that gives passage to the infraorbital artery, nerve, and vein

infraorbital groove *n* : a groove in the middle of the posterior part of the bony floor of the orbit that gives passage to the infraorbital artery, vein, and nerve

infraorbital nerve *n* : a branch of the maxillary nerve that divides into branches distributed to the skin of the upper part of the cheek, the upper lip, and the lower eyelid

infraorbital vein *n* : a vein that drains the inferior structures of the orbit and the adjacent area of the face and that empties into the pterygoid plexus

in·fra·pa·tel·lar \ˌin-frə-pə-ˈte-lər\ *adj* : situated below the patella or its ligament

in·fra·red \ˌin-frə-ˈred\ *adj* **1** : lying outside the visible spectrum at its red end — used of radiation of wavelengths longer than those of visible light **2** : relating to, producing, or employing infrared radiation ⟨∼ therapy⟩ — **infrared** *n*

in·fra·re·nal \ˌin-frə-ˈrēn-ᵊl\ *adj* : situated or occurring below the kidneys

in·fra·spi·na·tus \ˌin-frə-spī-ˈnā-təs\ *n*, *pl* **-na·ti** \-ˈnā-ˌtī\ : a muscle that occupies the chief part of the infraspinous fossa of the scapula and rotates the arm laterally

in·fra·spi·nous \ˌin-frə-ˈspī-nəs\ *adj* : lying below a spine; *esp* : lying below the spine of the scapula

infraspinous fossa *n* : the part of the dorsal surface of the scapula below the spine of the scapula

in·fra·tem·po·ral \ˌin-frə-ˈtem-pə-rəl\ *adj* : situated below the temporal fossa

infratemporal crest *n* : a transverse ridge on the outer surface of the greater wing of the sphenoid bone that divides it into a superior portion that contributes to the formation of

the temporal fossa and an inferior portion that contributes to the formation of the infratemporal fossa

infratemporal fossa *n* : a fossa that is bounded above by the plane of the zygomatic arch, laterally by the ramus of the mandible, and medially by the pterygoid plate, and that contains the masseter and pterygoid muscles and the mandibular nerve

in·fra·ten·to·ri·al \ˌin-frə-ten-ˈtōr-ē-əl\ *adj* : occurring or made below the tentorium cerebelli ⟨∼ burr holes⟩

in·fun·dib·u·lar \ˌin-(ˌ)fən-ˈdi-byə-lər\ *adj* : of, relating to, affecting, situated near, or having an infundibulum

infundibular process *n* : NEURAL LOBE

infundibular recess *n* : a funnel-shaped downward prolongation of the floor of the third ventricle of the brain

in·fun·dib·u·lo·pel·vic ligament \ˌin-fən-ˌdi-byə-lō-ˈpel-vik-\ *n* : SUSPENSORY LIGAMENT OF THE OVARY

in·fun·dib·u·lum \ˌin-(ˌ)fən-ˈdi-byə-ləm\ *n*, *pl* **-la** \-lə\ : any of various conical or dilated organs or parts: as **a** : the hollow conical process of gray matter that constitutes the stalk of the neurohypophysis by which the pituitary gland is continuous with the brain **b** : any of the small spaces having walls beset with air sacs in which the bronchial tubes terminate in the lungs **c** : CONUS ARTERIOSUS **d** : the abdominal opening of a fallopian tube

in·fu·sion \in-ˈfyü-zhən\ *n* **1** : the introducing of a solution (as of salt) into a vein; *also* : the solution so used **2 a** : the steeping or soaking usu. in water of a substance (as a plant drug) in order to extract its soluble constituents or principles — compare DECOCTION 1 **b** : the liquid extract obtained by this process — **in·fuse** \in-ˈfyüz\ *vb*

infusion pump *n* : a device that releases a measured amount of a substance in a specific period of time

in·ges·ta \in-ˈjes-tə\ *n pl* : material taken into the body by way of the digestive tract

in·gest·ible \in-ˈjes-tə-bəl\ *adj* : capable of being ingested ⟨∼ capsules⟩

in·ges·tion \in-ˈjes-chən\ *n* : the taking of material (as food) into the digestive system — **in·gest** \-ˈjest\ *vb* — **in·ges·tive** \in-ˈjes-tiv\ *adj*

in·grow·ing \ˈin-ˌgrō-iŋ\ *adj* : INGROWN

in·grown \ˈin-ˌgrōn\ *adj* : grown in; *specif* : having the normally free tip or edge embedded in the flesh ⟨an ∼ toenail⟩

in·growth \ˈin-ˌgrōth\ *n* **1** : a growing inward (as to fill a void) ⟨∼ of cells⟩ **2** : something that grows in or into a space ⟨lymphoid ∼s⟩

in·gui·nal \ˈiŋ-gwən-ᵊl\ *adj* **1** : of, relating to, or situated in the region of the groin **2** : ILIAC 2

inguinal canal *n* **1** : a passage in the male through which the testis descends into the scrotum and in which the spermatic cord lies **2** : a passage in the female accommodating the round ligament

inguinale — see GRANULOMA INGUINALE, LYMPHOGRANULOMA INGUINALE

inguinal hernia *n* : a hernia into the inguinal canal

inguinal ligament *n* : the thickened lower border of the aponeurosis of the external oblique muscle of the abdomen — called also *Poupart's ligament*

inguinal node *n* : any of the superficial lymph nodes of the groin

inguinal ring *n* : either of two openings in the fasciae of the abdominal muscles on each side of the body that are the inlet and outlet of the inguinal canal, give passage to the spermatic cord in the male and the round ligament in the female, and are a frequent site of hernia formation: **a** : DEEP INGUINAL RING **b** : SUPERFICIAL INGUINAL RING

INH *abbr* isoniazid

¹in·hal·ant \in-ˈhā-lənt\ *n* : something (as an allergen) that is inhaled

²inhalant *adj* : used for inhaling or constituting an inhalant 〈∼ anesthetics〉

in·ha·la·tion \ˌin-hə-ˈlā-shən, ˌin-ᵊl-ˈā-\ *n* **1** : the act or an instance of inhaling; *specif* : the action of drawing air into the lungs by means of a complex of essentially reflex actions **2** : material (as medication) to be taken in by inhaling — **in·ha·la·tion·al** \-shə-nəl\ *adj*

inhalation therapist *n* : a specialist in inhalation therapy

inhalation therapy *n* : the therapeutic use of inhaled gases and esp. oxygen (as in the treatment of respiratory disease)

in·ha·la·tor \ˈin-hə-ˌlā-tər, ˈin-ᵊl-ˌā-\ *n* : a device providing a mixture of oxygen and carbon dioxide for breathing that is used esp. in conjunction with artificial respiration — compare INHALER

in·hale \in-ˈhāl\ *vb* **in·haled; in·hal·ing** : to breathe in

in·hal·ant *var of* INHALANT

in·hal·er \in-ˈhā-lər\ *n* : a device by means of which usu. medicinal material is inhaled — compare INHALATOR

in·her·it \in-ˈher-ət\ *vb* : to receive from a parent or ancestor by genetic transmission — **in·her·it·able** \in-ˈher-ə-tə-bəl\ *adj* — **in·her·it·abil·i·ty** \-ˌher-ə-tə-ˈbi-lə-tē\ *n*

in·her·i·tance \in-ˈher-ə-təns\ *n* **1** : the reception of genetic qualities by transmission from parent to offspring **2** : the sum total of genetic characters or qualities transmitted from parent to offspring — compare PHENOTYPE

in·hib·in \in-ˈhi-bən\ *n* : a hormone that is secreted by Sertoli cells in the male and granulosa cells in the female and

that inhibits the secretion of follicle-stimulating hormone

in·hib·it \in-ˈhi-bət\ *vb* **1 a** : to restrain from free or spontaneous activity esp. through the operation of inner psychological or external social constraints **b** : to check or restrain the force or vitality of 〈∼ aggressive tendencies〉 **2 a** : to reduce or suppress the activity of 〈∼ a nerve〉 **b** : to retard or prevent the formation of **c** : to retard, interfere with, or prevent (a process or reaction) 〈∼ ovulation〉 — **in·hib·i·tor** \in-ˈhi-bə-tər\ *n* — **in·hib·i·to·ry** \in-ˈhi-bə-ˌtōr-ē\ *adj*

in·hib·it·able \-bə-tə-bəl\ *adj* : capable of being inhibited

in·hi·bi·tion \ˌin-hə-ˈbi-shən, ˌi-nə-\ *n* : the act or an instance of inhibiting or the state of being inhibited: as **a** (1) : a restraining of the function of a bodily organ or an agent (as an enzyme) 〈∼ of the heartbeat〉 (2) : interference with or retardation or prevention of a process or activity 〈∼ of bacterial growth〉 **b** (1) : a desirable restraint or check upon the free or spontaneous instincts or impulses of an individual guided or directed by social and cultural forces (2) : a neurotic restraint upon a normal or beneficial impulse or activity caused by psychological inner conflicts or by sociocultural forces

inhibitory postsynaptic potential *n* : increased negativity of the membrane potential of a neuron on the postsynaptic side of a nerve synapse that is caused by a neurotransmitter and that tends to inhibit the neuron — abbr. *IPSP*

in·i·en·ceph·a·lus \ˌi-nē-in-ˈse-fə-ləs\ *n* : a teratological fetus with a fissure in the occiput through which the brain protrudes — **in·i·en·ceph·a·ly** \-lē\ *n*

in·i·on \ˈi-nē-ˌän, -ən\ *n* : OCCIPITAL PROTUBERANCE a

initiation codon *n* : a codon that stimulates the binding of a transfer RNA which starts protein synthesis — called also *initiator codon*; compare TERMINATOR

ini·ti·a·tor \i-ˈni-shē-ˌā-tər\ *n* **1** : a substance that initiates a chemical reaction **2** : a substance that produces an irreversible change in bodily tissue causing it to respond to other substances which promote the growth of tumors

in·ject \in-ˈjekt\ *vb* : to introduce a fluid into (a living body); *also* : to treat (an individual) with injections

¹in·ject·able \-ˈjek-tə-bəl\ *adj* : capable of being injected 〈∼ medications〉

²injectable *n* : an injectable substance (as a drug)

in·jec·tion \in-ˈjek-shən\ *n* **1 a** : the act or an instance of injecting a drug or other substance into the body **b** : a solution (as of a drug) intended for injection (as by catheter or hypodermic syringe) either under or through the skin or into the tissues, a vein, or a body cavity **2** : the state of being injected : CONGESTION — see CIRCUMCORNEAL INJECTION

in·jure \'in-jər\ *vb* **in·jured; in·jur·ing 1** : to inflict bodily hurt on **2** : to impair the soundness of — **in·ju·ri·ous** \in-'jūr-ē-əs\ *adj* — **in·ju·ri·ous·ly** *adv*

in·ju·ry \'in-jə-rē\ *n, pl* **-ries** : hurt, damage, or loss sustained

injury potential *n* : the difference in electrical potential between the injured and uninjured parts of a nerve or muscle

inkblot test *n* : any of several psychological tests (as a Rorschach test) based on the interpretation of irregular figures (as blots of ink)

in·lay \'in-ˌlā\ *n* **1** : a tooth filling shaped to fit a cavity and then cemented into place **2** : a piece of tissue (as bone) laid into the site of missing tissue to cover a defect

in·let \'in-ˌlet, -lət\ *n* : the upper opening of a bodily cavity; *esp* : that of the cavity of the true pelvis bounded by the pelvic brim

in·mate \'in-ˌmāt\ *n* : a person confined (as in a psychiatric hospital) esp. for a long time

in·nards \'i-nərdz\ *n pl* : the internal organs of a human being or animal; *esp* : VISCERA

in·nate \i-'nāt, 'i-ˌ\ *adj* : existing in, belonging to, or determined by factors present in an individual from birth : INBORN ⟨∼ behavior⟩ — **in·nate·ly** *adv* — **in·nate·ness** *n*

inner cell mass *n* : the portion of the blastocyst of an embryo that is destined to become the embryo proper

inner-directed *adj* : directed in thought and action by one's own scale of values as opposed to external norms — **inner-direction** *n*

inner ear *n* : the essential organ of hearing and equilibrium that is located in the temporal bone, is innervated by the auditory nerve, and includes the vestibule, the semicircular canals, and the cochlea — called also *internal ear*

in·ner·vate \i-'nər-ˌvāt, 'i-(ˌ)nər-\ *vb* **-vat·ed; -vat·ing 1** : to supply with nerves **2** : to arouse or stimulate (a nerve or an organ) to activity — **in·ner·va·tion** \ˌi-(ˌ)nər-'vā-shən, i-ˌnər-\ *n*

in·no·cent \'i-nə-sənt\ *adj* : lacking capacity to injure : BENIGN ⟨an ∼ tumor⟩ ⟨∼ heart murmurs⟩

innominata — see SUBSTANTIA INNOMINATA

in·nom·i·nate artery \i-'nä-mə-nət-\ *n* : BRACHIOCEPHALIC ARTERY

innominate bone *n* : HIPBONE

innominate vein *n* : BRACHIOCEPHALIC VEIN

ino- *comb form* : fiber : fibrous ⟨*inotropic*⟩

in·oc·u·lant \i-'nä-kyə-lənt\ *n* : INOCULUM

in·oc·u·late \-ˌlāt\ *vb* **-lat·ed; -lat·ing 1** : to communicate a disease to (an organism) by inserting its causative agent into the body **2** : to introduce (as a microorganism) into a suitable situation for growth **3** : to introduce immunologically active material (as an antibody or antigen) into esp. in order to treat or prevent a disease

in·oc·u·la·tion \i-ˌnä-kyə-'lā-shən\ *n* **1** : the act or process or an instance of inoculating: as **a** : the introduction of a pathogen or antigen into a living organism to stimulate the production of antibodies **b** : the introduction of a vaccine or serum into a living organism to confer immunity **2** : INOCULUM

in·oc·u·lum \i-'nä-kyə-ləm\ *n, pl* **-la** \-lə\ : material used for inoculation

in·op·er·a·ble \i-'nä-pə-rə-bəl\ *adj* : not treatable or remediable by surgery ⟨∼ cancer⟩ — **in·op·er·a·bil·i·ty** \i-ˌnä-pə-rə-'bi-lə-tē\ *n*

in·or·gan·ic \ˌin-ȯr-'ga-nik\ *adj* **1** : being of composed of matter other than plant or animal ⟨an ∼ heart⟩ **2** : of, relating to, or dealt with by a branch of chemistry concerned with substances not usu. classed as organic — **in·or·gan·i·cal·ly** *adv*

in·or·gas·mic \ˌin-ȯr-'gaz-mik\ *adj* : not experiencing or having experienced orgasm

ino·si·nate \i-'nō-si-ˌnāt\ *n* : a salt or ester of inosinic acid

ino·sine \'i-nə-ˌsēn, 'i-, -sən\ *n* : a crystalline nucleoside $C_{10}H_{12}N_4O_5$

ino·sin·ic acid \ˌi-nə-'si-nik-, ˌī-\ *n* : a nucleotide $C_{10}H_{13}N_4O_8P$ that is found in muscle and is formed by deamination of AMP — called also *IMP*

ino·si·tol \i-'nō-sə-ˌtȯl, ī-, -ˌtōl\ *n* : any of several stereoisomeric cyclic alcohols $C_6H_{12}O_6$; *esp* : MYOINOSITOL

ino·tro·pic \ˌē-nə-'trō-pik, ˌi-, -'trä-\ *adj* : relating to or influencing the force of muscular contractions

in·pa·tient \'in-ˌpā-shənt\ *n* : a hospital patient who receives lodging and food as well as treatment — compare OUTPATIENT

in·quest \'in-ˌkwest\ *n* : a judicial or official inquiry esp. before a jury to determine the cause of a violent or unexpected death ⟨a coroner's ∼⟩

in·sane \(ˌ)in-'sān\ *adj* **1** : mentally disordered : exhibiting insanity **2** : used by, typical of, or intended for insane persons — **in·sane·ly** *adv*

in·san·i·tary \(ˌ)in-'sa-nə-ˌter-ē\ *adj* : unclean enough to endanger health

in·san·i·ty \in-'sa-nə-tē\ *n, pl* **-ties 1 a** : a deranged state of the mind usu. occurring as a specific disorder (as schizophrenia) and usu. excluding such states as mental retardation, psychoneurosis, and various character disorders **b** : a mental disorder **2** : such unsoundness of mind or lack of understanding as prevents one from having the mental capacity required by law to enter into a particular relationship, status, or transaction or as removes one from criminal or civil responsibility

in·scrip·tion \in-ˈskrip-shən\ *n* : the part of a medical prescription that contains the names and quantities of the drugs to be compounded

in·sect \ˈin-ˌsekt\ *n* : any of a class (Insecta) of arthropods with well-defined head, thorax, and abdomen, three pairs of legs, and typically one or two pairs of wings — **insect** *adj*

in·sec·ti·cide \in-ˈsek-tə-ˌsīd\ *n* : an agent that destroys insects — **in·sec·ti·cid·al** \(ˌ)in-ˌsek-tə-ˈsīd-əl\ *adj*

in·se·cu·ri·ty \ˌin-si-ˈkyùr-ə-tē\ *n, pl* **-ties** : a feeling of apprehensiveness and uncertainty : lack of assurance or stability — **in·se·cure** \-ˈkyùr\ *adj*

in·sem·i·nate \in-ˈse-mə-ˌnāt\ *vb* **-nat·ed; -nat·ing** : to introduce semen into the genital tract of (a female) — **in·sem·i·na·tion** \-ˌse-mə-ˈnā-shən\ *n*

in·sem·i·na·tor \-ˌnā-tər\ *n* : one that inseminates cattle artificially

in·sen·si·ble \(ˌ)in-ˈsen-sə-bəl\ *adj* **1** : incapable or bereft of feeling or sensation: as **a** : UNCONSCIOUS **b** : lacking sensory perception or ability to react **c** : lacking emotional response — APATHETIC **2** : not perceived by the senses (⟨∼ perspiration⟩) — **in·sen·si·bil·i·ty** \(ˌ)in-ˌsen-sə-ˈbi-lə-tē\ *n*

in·sert \in-ˈsərt\ *vb, of a muscle* : to be in attachment to the part to be moved

inserted *adj* : attached by natural growth (as a muscle or tendon)

in·ser·tion \in-ˈsər-shən\ *n* **1** : the part of a muscle by which it is attached to the part to be moved — compare ORIGIN 2 **2** : the mode or place of attachment of an organ or part **3 a** : a section of genetic material inserted into an existing gene sequence **b** : the mutational process producing a genetic insertion — **in·ser·tion·al** \-shə-nəl\ *adj*

in·sid·i·ous \in-ˈsi-dē-əs\ *adj* : developing so gradually as to be well established before becoming apparent (⟨∼ disease⟩) — **in·sid·i·ous·ly** *adv*

in·sight \ˈin-ˌsīt\ *n* **1** : understanding or awareness of one's mental or emotional condition; *esp* : recognition that one is mentally ill **2** : immediate and clear understanding (as seeing the solution to a problem or the means to reaching a goal) that takes place without recourse to overt trial-and-error behavior — **in·sight·ful** \ˈin-ˌsīt-fəl, in-ˈ\ *adj* — **in·sight·ful·ly** *adv*

insipidus — see DIABETES INSIPIDUS

in si·tu \in-ˈsī-(ˌ)tü, -ˈsi-, -ˈsē-, -(ˌ)tyü, -(ˌ)chü\ *adv or adj* : in the natural or original position

in·som·nia \in-ˈsäm-nē-ə\ *n* : prolonged and usu. abnormal inability to obtain adequate sleep

¹in·som·ni·ac \-nē-ˌak\ *n* : one affected with insomnia

²insomniac *adj* : affected with insomnia

in·spec·tion \in-ˈspek-shən\ *n* : visual observation of the body in the course of a medical examination — compare PALPATION 2 — **in·spect** \in-ˈspekt\ *vb*

in·spi·ra·tion \ˌin-spə-ˈrā-shən\ *n* : the drawing of air into the lungs — **in·spi·ra·to·ry** \in-ˈspī-rə-ˌtȯr-ē, ˈin-spə-rə-\ *adj*

inspiratory capacity *n* : the total amount of air that can be drawn into the lungs after normal expiration

inspiratory reserve volume *n* : the maximal amount of additional air that can be drawn into the lungs by determined effort after normal inspiration — compare EXPIRATORY RESERVE VOLUME

in·spire \in-ˈspīr\ *vb* **in·spired; in·spir·ing** : to draw in by breathing : breathe in : INHALE

in·spis·sat·ed \in-ˈspi-ˌsā-təd, ˈin-spə-ˌsä-\ *adj* : made or having become thickened in consistency

in·sta·bil·i·ty \ˌin-stə-ˈbi-lə-tē\ *n, pl* **-ties** : lack of emotional or mental stability

in·step \ˈin-ˌstep\ *n* : the arched middle portion of the human foot in front of the ankle joint; *esp* : its upper surface

in·still \in-ˈstil\ *vb* **in·stilled; in·still·ing** : to cause to enter esp. drop by drop (⟨∼ medication into the infected eye⟩) — **in·stil·la·tion** \ˌin-stə-ˈlā-shən\ *n*

in·stinct \ˈin-ˌstiŋkt\ *n* **1** : a largely inheritable and unalterable tendency of an organism to make a complex and specific response to environmental stimuli without involving reason **2** : behavior that is mediated by reactions below the conscious level — **in·stinc·tive** \in-ˈstiŋk-tiv\ *adj* — **in·stinc·tive·ly** *adv* — **in·stinc·tu·al** \in-ˈstiŋk-chə-wəl\ *adj*

in·sti·tu·tion·al·ize \ˌin-stə-ˈtü-shə-nə-ˌlīz, -ˈtyü-\ *vb* **1** : to place in or commit to the care of a specialized institution (as for the mentally ill) **2** : to accustom (a person) so firmly to the care and supervised routine of an institution as to make incapable of managing a life outside — **in·sti·tu·tion·al·iza·tion** \-ˌtü-shə-nə-lə-ˈzā-shən, -ˌtyü-\ *n*

in·stru·men·tal \ˌin-strə-ˈmen-təl\ *adj* : OPERANT (⟨∼ conditioning⟩)

in·stru·men·ta·tion \ˌin-strə-mən-ˈtā-shən, -ˌmen-\ *n* : a use of or operation with instruments

in·suf·fi·cien·cy \ˌin-sə-ˈfi-shən-sē\ *n, pl* **-cies** : the quality or state of not being sufficient: as **a** : lack of adequate supply of something **b** : lack of physical power or capacity; *esp* : inability of an organ or bodily part to function normally — compare AORTIC REGURGITATION — **in·suf·fi·cient** \-shənt\ *adj*

in·suf·fla·tion \ˌin-sə-ˈflā-shən\ *n* : the act of blowing something (as a gas) into a body cavity (as the uterus) — **in·suf·flate** \'in-sə-₁flāt, in-'sə-₁flāt\ *vb* — **in·suf·fla·tor** \'in-sə-₁flā-tər, in-'sə-₁flā-tər\ *n*

in·su·la \'in-sü-lə, -syü-, -shü-\ *n, pl* **in·su·lae** \-₁lē, -₁lī\ : the lobe in the center of the cerebral hemisphere that is situated deeply between the lips of the fissure of Sylvius — called also *central lobe, island of Reil*

in·su·lar \-lər\ *adj* : of or relating to an island of cells or tissue (as the islets of Langerhans or the insula)

in·su·lin \'in-sə-lən\ *n* : a protein pancreatic hormone secreted by the islets of Langerhans that is essential esp. for the metabolism of carbohydrates and is used in the treatment and control of diabetes mellitus — see ILETIN

in·su·lin·ae·mia *chiefly Brit var of* INSULINEMIA

in·su·lin·ase \-lə-₁nās, -₁nāz\ *n* : an enzyme found esp. in liver that inactivates insulin

insulin–dependent diabetes mellitus *n* : a form of diabetes mellitus that usu. develops during childhood or adolescence and is characterized by a severe deficiency in insulin secretion resulting from atrophy of the islets of Langerhans and causing hyperglycemia and a marked tendency toward ketoacidosis — abbr. *IDDM;* called also *juvenile diabetes, juvenile-onset diabetes, insulin-dependent diabetes, type I diabetes*

in·su·lin·emia \₁in-sə-lə-'nē-mē-ə\ *n* : the presence of an abnormally high concentration of insulin in the blood

in·su·lin·o·ma \₁in-sə-lə-'nō-mə\ *n, pl* **-mas** *or* **-ma·ta** \-mə-tə\ : a usu. benign insulin-secreting tumor of the islets of Langerhans

in·su·li·no·tro·pic \₁in-sə-₁li-nə-'trō-pik, -'trä-\ *adj* : stimulating or affecting the production and activity of insulin ⟨an ~ hormone⟩

insulin shock *n* : hypoglycemia associated with the presence of excessive insulin in the system and characterized by progressive development of coma

in·su·lo·ma \₁in-sə-'lō-mə\ *n, pl* **-mas** *or* **-ma·ta** \-mə-tə\ : INSULINOMA

in·sult \'in-₁səlt\ *n* 1 : injury to the body or one of its parts 2 : something that causes or has a potential for causing insult to the body — **insult** *vb*

in·tact \in-'takt\ *adj* 1 : physically and functionally complete 2 : mentally unimpaired — **in·tact·ness** *n*

in·te·gra·tion \₁in-tə-'grā-shən\ *n* 1 : coordination of mental processes into a normal effective personality or with the individual's environment 2 : the process by which the different parts of an organism are made a functional and structural whole esp. through the activity of the nervous system and of hormones — **in·te·grate** \'in-tə-₁grāt\ *vb* — **in·te·gra·tive** \'in-tə-₁grā-tiv\ *adj*

in·teg·ri·ty \in-'te-grə-tē\ *n, pl* **-ties** : an unimpaired condition ⟨~ of brain function⟩

in·teg·u·ment \in-'te-gyə-mənt\ *n* : an enveloping layer (as a skin or membrane) of an organism or one of its parts — **in·teg·u·men·ta·ry** \-'men-tə-rē\ *adj*

in·tel·lec·tu·al·ize \₁int-əl-'ek-chə-wə-₁līz\ *vb* **-ized; -iz·ing** : to avoid conscious recognition of the emotional basis of (an act or feeling) by substituting a superficially plausible explanation — **in·tel·lec·tu·al·iza·tion** \-₁ek-chə-wə-lə-'zā-shən\ *n*

in·tel·li·gence \in-'te-lə-jəns\ *n* **1 a** : the ability to learn or understand or to deal with new or trying situations **b** : the ability to apply knowledge to manipulate one's environment or to think abstractly as measured by objective criteria (as tests) **2** : mental acuteness — **in·tel·li·gent** \-jənt\ *adj* — **in·tel·li·gent·ly** *adv*

intelligence quotient *n* : a number used to express the apparent relative intelligence of a person that is the ratio multiplied by 100 of the mental age as reported on a standardized test to the chronological age — called also *IQ*

intelligence test *n* : a test designed to determine the relative mental capacity of a person

intensifying screen *n* : a fluorescent screen placed next to an X-ray photographic film in order to intensify the image initially produced on the film by the action of X rays

in·ten·si·ty \in-'ten-sə-tē\ *n, pl* **-ties** : SATURATION 4

in·ten·sive \in-'ten-siv\ *adj* : of, relating to, or marked by intensity; *esp* : involving the use of large doses or substances having great therapeutic activity — **in·ten·sive·ly** *adv*

intensive care *adj* : having special medical facilities, services, and monitoring devices to meet the needs of gravely ill patients ⟨an *intensive care* unit⟩ — **intensive care** *n*

in·ten·tion \in-'ten-chən\ *n* : a process or manner of healing of incised wounds — see FIRST INTENTION , SECOND INTENTION

intention tremor *n* : a slow tremor of the extremities that increases on attempted voluntary movement and is observed in certain diseases (as multiple sclerosis) of the nervous system

inter- *comb form* : between : among ⟨*inter*cellular⟩ ⟨*inter*costal⟩

in·ter·al·ve·o·lar \₁in-tə-ral-'vē-ə-lər\ *adj* : situated between alveoli esp. of the lungs

in·ter·atri·al septum \₁in-tər-'ā-trē-əl-\ *n* : the wall separating the right and left atria of the heart — called also *atrial septum*

in·ter·au·ral \-'ȯr-əl\ *adj* **1** : situated between or connecting the ears **2** : of or relating to sound reception and perception by each ear considered separately

in·ter·body \'in-tər-ˌbä-dē\ *adj* : performed between the bodies of two contiguous vertebrae (an ~ fusion)

in·ter·breed \ˌin-tər-'brēd\ *vb* **-bred** \-'bred\; **-breed·ing** : to breed together: as **a** : CROSSBREED **b** : to breed within a closed population

in·ter·ca·lat·ed disk \in-'tər-kə-ˌlā-təd-\ *n* : any of the apparent striations across cardiac muscle that are actually membranes separating adjacent cells

intercalated duct *n* : a duct from a tubule or acinus of the pancreas that drains into an intralobular duct

in·ter·cap·il·lary \ˌin-tər-'ka-pə-ˌler-ē\ *adj* : situated between capillaries (~ thrombi)

in·ter·car·pal \-'kär-pəl\ *adj* : situated between, occurring between, or connecting carpal bones

in·ter·cav·ern·ous \-'ka-vər-nəs\ *adj* : situated between and connecting the cavernous sinuses behind and in front of the pituitary gland (~ sinus)

in·ter·cel·lu·lar \-'sel-yə-lər\ *adj* : occurring between cells (~ spaces) — **in·ter·cel·lu·lar·ly** *adv*

in·ter·con·dy·lar \-'kän-də-lər\ *adj* : situated between two condyles

in·ter·con·dy·loid \-'kän-də-ˌloid\ *adj* : INTERCONDYLAR

¹**in·ter·cos·tal** \ˌin-tər-'käs-tᵊl\ *adj* : situated or extending between the ribs (~ spaces) (~ muscles)

²**intercostal** *n* : an intercostal part or structure (as a muscle or nerve)

intercostal artery *n* : any of the arteries supplying or lying in the intercostal spaces: **a** : any of the arteries branching in front directly from the internal thoracic artery — called also *anterior intercostal artery* **b** : any of the arteries that branch from the costocervical trunk of the subclavian artery — called also *posterior intercostal artery*

intercostal muscle *n* : any of the short muscles that extend between the ribs and serve to move the ribs in respiration: **a** : any of 11 muscles on each side between the vertebrae and the junction of the ribs and their cartilages — called also *external intercostal muscle* **b** : any of 11 muscles on each side between the sternum and the line on a rib marking an insertion of the iliocostalis — called also *internal intercostal muscle*

intercostal nerve *n* : any of 11 nerves on each side of which each is an anterior division of a thoracic nerve lying between a pair of adjacent ribs

intercostal vein *n* : any of the veins of the intercostal spaces — see SUPERIOR INTERCOSTAL VEIN

in·ter·cos·to·bra·chi·al nerve \ˌin-tər-ˌkäs-tō-'brā-kē-əl-\ *n* : a branch of the second intercostal nerve that supplies the skin of the inner and back part of the upper half of the arm

in·ter·course \'int-ər-ˌkörs\ *n* : physical sexual contact between individuals that involves the genitalia of at least one person; *esp* : SEXUAL INTERCOURSE 1

in·ter·cris·tal \ˌin-tər-'kris-tᵊl\ *adj* : measured between two crests (as of bone)

in·ter·crit·i·cal \-'kri-ti-kəl\ *adj* : being in the period between attacks (~ gout)

in·ter·cur·rent \-'kər-ənt\ *adj* : occurring during and modifying the course of another disease

in·ter·den·tal \-'dent-ᵊl\ *adj* : situated or intended for use between the teeth — **in·ter·den·tal·ly** \-ᵊl-ē\ *adv*

interdental papilla *n* : the triangular wedge of gingiva between two adjacent teeth — called also *gingival papilla*

in·ter·dig·i·tal \-'di-jə-tᵊl\ *adj* : occurring between digits (~ neuroma)

in·ter·dig·i·tate \-'di-jə-ˌtāt\ *vb* **-tat·ed**; **-tat·ing** : to become interlocked like the fingers of folded hands — **in·ter·dig·i·ta·tion** \-ˌdij-ə-'tā-shən\ *n*

in·ter·fere \ˌin-tər-'fir\ *vb* **-fered**; **-fer·ing** : to be inconsistent with and disturb the performance of previously learned behavior

in·ter·fer·ence \-'fir-əns\ *n* **1** : partial or complete inhibition or sometimes facilitation of other genetic crossovers in the vicinity of a chromosomal locus where a preceding crossover has occurred **2** : the disturbing effect of new learning on the performance of previously learned behavior with which it is inconsistent — compare NEGATIVE TRANSFER **3** : prevention of typical growth and development of a virus in a suitable host by the presence of another virus in the same host individual

in·ter·fer·on \ˌin-tər-'fir-ˌän\ *n* : any of a group of heat-stable soluble basic antiviral glycoproteins of low molecular weight that are produced usu. by cells exposed to the action of a virus, sometimes to the action of another intracellular parasite (as a bacterium), or experimentally to the action of some chemicals, and that include some used medically as antiviral or antineoplastic agents

in·ter·fi·bril·lar \ˌin-tər-'fī-brə-lər, -'fī-\ *or* **in·ter·fi·bril·lary** \-'fī-brə-ˌler-ē, -'fī\ *adj* : situated between fibrils

in·ter·gen·ic \-'jē-nik\ *adj* : occurring between genes : involving more than one gene

in·ter·glob·u·lar \-'glä-byə-lər\ *adj* : resulting from or situated in an area of faulty dentin formation (~ dentin)

in·ter·hemi·spher·ic \-ˌhe-mə-'sfir-ik, -'sfer-\ *also* **in·ter·hemi·spher·al** \-əl\ *adj* : extending or occurring between hemispheres (as of the cerebrum)

in·ter·ic·tal \-'ik-təl\ *adj* : occurring between seizures (as of epilepsy)

in·ter·ki·ne·sis \-kə-'nē-səs, -kī-\ *n, pl* **-ne·ses** \-ˌsēz\ : the period between the first and second meiotic divisions

in·ter·leu·kin \in-tər-'lü-kən\ *n* : any of several compounds of low molecular weight that are produced by lymphocytes, macrophages, and monocytes and that function esp. in regulation of the immune system and esp. cell-mediated immunity

interleukin–1 \-'wən\ *n* : an interleukin produced esp. by monocytes and macrophages that regulates cell-mediated and humoral immune responses by activating lymphocytes and mediates other biological processes (as the onset of fever) usu. associated with infection and inflammation — abbr. *IL-1*

interleukin–2 \-'tü\ *n* : an interleukin produced by antigen-stimulated helper T cells in the presence of interleukin-1 that induces proliferation of immune cells (as T cells and B cells) and is used experimentally esp. in treating certain cancers — abbr. *IL-2*

in·ter·lo·bar \int-ər-'lō-bər, -ˌbär\ *adj* : situated between the lobes of an organ or structure

interlobar artery *n* : any of various secondary branches of the renal arteries that branch to form the arcuate arteries

interlobar vein *n* : any of the veins of the kidney that are formed by convergence of arcuate veins and empty into the renal veins or their branches

in·ter·lob·u·lar \-'lä-byə-lər\ *adj* : lying between, connecting, or transporting the secretions of lobules

interlobular artery *n* : any of the branches of an arcuate artery that pass radially in the cortex of the kidney toward the surface

interlobular vein *n* : any of the veins in the cortex of the kidney that empty into the arcuate veins

in·ter·max·il·lary \-'mak-sə-ˌler-ē\ *adj* **1** : lying between maxillae; *esp* : joining the two maxillary bones (\~ suture) **2** : of or relating to the premaxilla

intermedia — see MASSA INTERMEDIA, PARS INTERMEDIA

intermediary metabolism *n* : the intracellular process by which nutritive material is converted into cellular components

intermediate cuneiform bone *n* : CUNEIFORM BONE 1b — called also INTERMEDIATE CUNEIFORM

intermediate host *n* **1** : a host which is normally used by a parasite in the course of its life cycle and in which it may multiply asexually but not sexually — compare DEFINITIVE HOST 2 **a** : RESERVOIR 2 **b** : VECTOR 1

intermediate metabolism *n* : INTERMEDIARY METABOLISM

intermediate temporal artery *n* : TEMPORAL ARTERY 3b

in·ter·me·din \in-tər-'mēd-ən\ *n* : MELANOCYTE-STIMULATING HORMONE

in·ter·me·dio·lat·er·al \in-tər-ˌmē-dē-ō-'la-tə-rəl\ *adj* : of, relating to, or being the lateral column of gray matter in the spinal cord

intermedium — see STRATUM INTERMEDIUM

intermedius — see NERVUS INTERMEDIUS, VASTUS INTERMEDIUS

in·ter·men·stru·al \-'men-strə-wəl\ *adj* : occurring between menstrual periods (\~ pain)

in·ter·mis·sion \in-tər-'mi-shən\ *n* : the space of time between two paroxysms of a disease — compare REMISSION

in·ter·mit·tent \-'mit-ənt\ *adj* : coming and going at intervals : not continuous (\~ fever) — **in·ter·mit·tence** \-əns\ *n*

intermittent claudication *n* : cramping pain and weakness in the legs and esp. the calves on walking that disappears after rest and is usu. associated with inadequate blood supply to the muscles

intermittent positive pressure breathing *n* : enforced periodic inflation of the lungs by the intermittent application of an increase of pressure to a reservoir of air (as in a bag) supplying the lungs — abbr. *IPPB*

in·ter·mus·cu·lar \-'məs-kyə-lər\ *adj* : lying between and separating muscles (\~ fat)

in·tern \'in-ˌtərn\ *n* : a physician gaining supervised practical experience in a hospital after graduating from medical school — **intern** *vb*

interna — see THECA INTERNA

in·ter·nal \in-'tərn-əl\ *adj* **1 a** : situated near the inside of the body **b** : situated on the side toward the midsagittal plane of the body (the \~ surface of the lung) **2** : present or arising within an organism or one of its parts (\~ stimulus) **3** : applied or intended for application through the stomach by being swallowed (an \~ remedy) — **in·ter·nal·ly** *adv*

internal acoustic meatus *n* : INTERNAL AUDITORY MEATUS

internal anal sphincter *n* : ANAL SPHINCTER b

internal auditory artery *n* : a long slender artery that arises from the basilar artery or one of its branches and is distributed to the inner ear — called also *internal auditory*, *labyrinthine artery*

internal auditory meatus *n* : a short canal in the petrous portion of the temporal bone through which pass the facial and auditory nerves and the nervus intermedius — called also *internal acoustic meatus*, *internal auditory canal*

internal capsule *n* : CAPSULE 1b(1)

internal carotid artery *n* : the inner branch of the carotid artery that supplies the brain, eyes, and other internal structures of the head — called also *internal carotid*

internal ear *n* : INNER EAR

internal iliac artery *n* : ILIAC ARTERY 3

internal iliac node *n* : any of the lymph nodes grouped around the internal iliac artery and the internal iliac vein — compare EXTERNAL ILIAC NODE

internal iliac vein *n* : ILIAC VEIN c

internal inguinal ring *n* : DEEP INGUINAL RING

internal intercostal muscle *n* : INTERCOSTAL MUSCLE b — called also *internal intercostal*

in·ter·nal·ize \in-ˈtərn-əl-ˌīz\ *vb* **-ized; -iz·ing** : to incorporate (as values) within the self as conscious or subconscious guiding principles through learning or socialization — **in·ter·nal·iza·tion** \-ˌtərn-əl-ə-ˈzā-shən\ *n*

internal jugular vein *n* : JUGULAR VEIN a — called also *internal jugular*

internal malleolus *n* : MALLEOLUS b

internal mammary artery *n* : INTERNAL THORACIC ARTERY

internal maxillary artery \ *n* : MAXILLARY ARTERY

internal medicine *n* : a branch of medicine that deals with the diagnosis and treatment of nonsurgical diseases

internal oblique *n* : OBLIQUE a(2)

internal occipital crest *n* : OCCIPITAL CREST b

internal occipital protuberance *n* : OCCIPITAL PROTUBERANCE b

internal os *n* : the opening of the cervix into the body of the uterus

internal pterygoid muscle *n* : PTERYGOID MUSCLE b

internal pudendal artery *n* : a branch of the internal iliac artery that is distributed esp. to the external genitalia and the perineum — compare EXTERNAL PUDENDAL ARTERY

internal pudendal vein *n* : any of several veins that receive blood from the external genitalia and the perineum and unite to form a single vein that empties into the internal iliac vein

internal respiration *n* : the exchange of gases (as oxygen and carbon dioxide) between the cells of the body and the blood — compare EXTERNAL RESPIRATION

internal spermatic artery *n* : TESTICULAR ARTERY

internal thoracic artery *n* : a branch of the subclavian artery of each side that runs down along the anterior wall of the thorax — called also *internal mammary artery*

internal thoracic vein *n* : a vein of the trunk on each side of the body that accompanies the corresponding internal thoracic artery and empties into the brachiocephalic vein

In·ter·na·tion·al System of Units \ˌint-ər-ˈnash-nəl-, -ən-əl-\ *n* : a system of units based on the metric system and developed and refined by international convention esp. for scientific work

international unit *n* : a quantity of a biologic (as a vitamin) that produces a particular biological effect agreed upon as an international standard

in·terne, in·terne·ship *var of* INTERN, INTERNSHIP

in·ter·neu·ron \ˌin-tər-ˈnü-ˌrän, -ˈnyü-\ *n* : INTERNUNCIAL NEURON — **in·ter·neu·ro·nal** \-ˈnür-ən-əl, -ˈnyür-ən-, -nyü-ˈrōn-\ *adj*

in·ter·nist \ˈin-tər-nist\ *n* : a specialist in internal medicine esp. as distinguished from a surgeon

in·tern·ship \ˈin-ˌtərn-ˌship\ *n* **1** : the state or position of being an intern **2 a** : a period of service as an intern **b** : the phase of medical training covered during such service

in·ter·nun·ci·al \ˌint-ər-ˈnən-sē-əl, -ˈnun-\ *adj* : of, relating to, or being internuncial neurons (∼ fibers)

internuncial neuron *n* : a nerve fiber intercalated in the path of a reflex arc in the central nervous system and tending to modify the arc and coordinate it with other bodily activities — called also *interneuron, internuncial*

internus — see MEATUS ACUSTICUS INTERNUS, OBLIQUUS INTERNUS ABDOMINIS, OBTURATOR INTERNUS, SPHINCTER ANI INTERNUS, VASTUS INTERNUS

in·ter·oc·clu·sal \-ə-ˈklü-səl, -zəl\ *adj* : situated or occurring between the occlusal surfaces of opposing teeth (∼ clearance)

in·tero·cep·tive \ˌin-tə-rō-ˈsep-tiv\ *adj* : of, relating to, or being stimuli arising within the body and esp. in the viscera

in·tero·cep·tor \-tər\ *n* : a sensory receptor excited by interoceptive stimuli — compare EXTEROCEPTOR

in·ter·os·se·ous \ˌin-tər-ˈä-sē-əs\ *adj* : situated between bones

interosseous artery — see COMMON INTEROSSEOUS ARTERY

interosseous membrane *n* : either of two thin strong sheets of fibrous tissue: **a** : one extending between and connecting the shafts of the radius and ulna **b** : one extending between and connecting the shafts of the tibia and fibula

interosseous muscle *n* : INTEROSSEUS

in·ter·os·se·us \ˌin-tər-ˈä-sē-əs\ *n, pl* **-sei** \-sē-ˌī\ : any of various small muscles arising from the metacarpals and metatarsals and inserted into the bases of the first phalanges: **a** : DORSAL INTEROSSEUS **b** : PALMAR INTEROSSEUS **c** : PLANTAR INTEROSSEUS

interossei dorsalis *n, pl* **interossei dorsales** : DORSAL INTEROSSEUS

interossei palmaris *n, pl* **interossei palmares** : PALMAR INTEROSSEUS

interosseus plantaris *n, pl* **interossei plantares** : PLANTAR INTEROSSEUS

in·ter·par·ox·ys·mal \-ˌpar-ək-ˈsiz-məl, -pə-ˈräk-\ *adj* : occurring between paroxysms

in·ter·pe·dun·cu·lar nucleus \ˌin-tər-pi-ˈdəŋ-kyə-lər-\ *n* : a mass of nerve cells lying between the cerebral peduncles in the midsagittal plane just dorsal to the pons — called also *interpeduncular ganglion*

in·ter·per·son·al \-ˈpərs-ᵊn-əl\ *adj* : being, relating to, or involving relations between persons ⟨∼ therapy⟩ — **in·ter·per·son·al·ly** *adv*

in·ter·pha·lan·ge·al \ˌin-tər-ˌfā-lən-ˈjē-əl, -ˌfa-; -fə-ˈlan-jē-əl, -fā-\ *adj* : situated or occurring between phalanges; *also* : of or relating to an interphalangeal joint

in·ter·phase \ˈin-tər-ˌfāz\ *n* : the interval between the end of one mitotic or meiotic division and the beginning of another — called also *resting stage*

in·ter·po·lat·ed \in-ˈtər-pə-ˌlā-təd\ *adj* : occurring between normal heartbeats without disturbing the succeeding beat or the basic rhythm of the heart

in·ter·pris·mat·ic \ˌin-tər-priz-ˈma-tik\ *adj* : situated or occurring between prisms esp. of enamel

in·ter·prox·i·mal \-ˈpräk-sə-məl\ *adj* : situated, occurring, or used in the areas between adjoining teeth ⟨∼ space⟩

in·ter·pu·pil·lary \-ˈpyü-pə-ˌler-ē\ *adj* : extending between the pupils of the eyes; *also* : extending between the centers of a pair of spectacle lenses ⟨∼ distance⟩

in·ter·ra·dic·u·lar \-rə-ˈdi-kyə-lər\ *adj* : situated between the roots of a tooth

interruptus — see COITUS INTERRUPTUS

in·ter·scap·u·lar \ˌin-tər-ˈska-pyə-lər\ *adj* : of, relating to, situated in, or occurring between in the region between the scapulae

in·ter·sen·so·ry \-ˈsens-ə-rē\ *adj* : involving two or more sensory systems

in·ter·sep·tal \-ˈsept-ᵊl\ *adj* : situated between septa

in·ter·sex \ˈin-tər-ˌseks\ *n* : an intersexual individual

in·ter·sex·u·al \ˌin-tər-ˈsek-shə-wəl\ *adj* 1 : existing between sexes ⟨∼ hostility⟩ 2 : intermediate in sexual characters between a typical male and a typical female — **in·ter·sex·u·al·i·ty** \-ˌsek-shə-ˈwa-lə-tē\ *n*

in·ter·space \ˈin-tər-ˌspās\ *n* : the space between two related body parts whether void or filled by another kind of structure

in·ter·spi·na·lis \ˌint-ər-ˌspī-ˈna-ləs, -ˈnā-\ *n, pl* **-na·les** \-ˌlēz\ : any of various short muscles that have their origin on the superior surface of the spinous process of one vertebra and their insertion on the inferior surface of the contiguous vertebra above

in·ter·spi·nal ligament \ˌin-tər-ˈspin-ᵊl-\ *n* : any of the thin membranous ligaments that connect the spinous processes of contiguous vertebrae — called also *interspinous ligament*

in·ter·stim·u·lus \-ˈstim-yə-ləs\ *adj* : of, relating to, or being the interval between the presentation of two discrete stimuli

in·ter·sti·tial \-ˈsti-shəl\ *adj* 1 : situated within but not restricted to or characteristic of a particular organ or tissue — used esp. of fibrous tissue 2 : affecting the interstitial tissues of an organ or part ⟨∼ hepatitis⟩ 3 : occuring in the part of a fallopian tube in the wall of the uterus ⟨∼ pregnancy⟩ — **in·ter·sti·tial·ly** *adv*

interstitial cell *n* : a cell situated between the germ cells of the gonads; *esp* : LEYDIG CELL

interstitial cell of Leydig *n* : LEYDIG CELL

interstitial–cell stimulating hormone *n* : LUTEINIZING HORMONE

interstitial cystitis *n* : a chronic idiopathic cystitis characterized by painful inflammation of the subepithelial connective tissue and often accompanied by Hunner's ulcer

interstitial keratitis *n* : a chronic progressive keratitis of the corneal stroma often resulting in blindness and frequently associated with congenital syphilis

interstitial pneumonia *n* : any of several chronic lung diseases of unknown etiology that affect interstitial tissues of the lung

in·ter·sti·tium \ˌin-tər-ˈsti-shē-əm\ *n, pl* **-tia** \-ē-ə\ : interstitial tissue

in·ter·sub·ject \ˈin-tər-ˌsəb-jekt\ *adj* : occurring between subjects in an experiment ⟨∼ variability⟩

in·ter·tar·sal \ˌin-tər-ˈtär-səl\ *adj* : situated, occurring, or performed between tarsal bones ⟨∼ joint⟩ ⟨∼ arthrotomy⟩

in·ter·trans·ver·sar·ii \-ˌtrans-vər-ˈser-ē-ˌī\ *n pl* : a series of small muscles connecting the transverse processes of contiguous vertebrae

in·ter·tri·go \ˈtrī-ˌgō\ *n* : inflammation produced by chafing of adjacent areas of skin — **in·ter·trig·i·nous** \-ˈtri-jə-nəs\ *adj*

in·ter·tro·chan·ter·ic \-ˌtrō-kən-ˈter-ik, -ˌkan-\ *adj* : situated, performed, or occurring between trochanters ⟨∼ fractures⟩

intertrochanteric line *n* : a line on the anterior surface of the femur that runs obliquely from the greater trochanter to the lesser trochanter

in·ter·tu·ber·cu·lar groove \ˌin-tər-tü-ˈbər-kyə-lər-, -tyü-\ *n* : BICIPITAL GROOVE

intertubercular line *n* : an imaginary line passing through the iliac crests of the hipbones that separates the umbilical and lumbar regions of the abdomen from the hypogastric and iliac regions

in·ter·ven·tion \ˌin-tər-ˈven-chən\ *n* : the act or fact of interfering with a condition to modify it or with a process to change its course — **in·ter·ven·tion·al** \-ˈven-chə-nəl\ *adj*

in·ter·ven·tric·u·lar \-ven-ˈtri-kyə-lər\ *adj* : situated between ventricles ⟨∼ septal defect⟩

interventricular foramen *n* : the opening from each lateral ventricle into the third ventricle of the brain — called also *foramen of Monro*

interventricular groove *n* : INTERVENTRICULAR SULCUS

interventricular septum *n* : the curved slanting wall that separates the right and left ventricles of the heart

interventricular sulcus *n* : either of the anterior and posterior grooves on the surface of the heart that lie over the interventricular septum and join at the apex

in·ter·ver·te·bral \ˌin-tər-ˈvər-tə-brəl, -(ˌ)vər-ˈtē-\ *adj* : situated between vertebrae — **in·ter·ver·te·bral·ly** *adv*

intervertebral disk *n* : any of the tough elastic disks that are interposed between the centra of adjoining vertebrae

intervertebral foramen *n* : any of the openings that give passage to the spinal nerves from the vertebral canal

in·tes·ti·nal \in-ˈtes-tən-ᵊl\ *adj* **1 a** : affecting or occurring in the intestine **b** : living in the intestine ⟨the ∼ flora⟩ **2** : of, relating to, or being the intestine ⟨the ∼ canal⟩ — **in·tes·ti·nal·ly** *adv*

intestinal artery *n* : any of 12 to 15 arteries that arise from the superior mesenteric artery and supply the jejunum and ileum

intestinal flu *n* : an acute usu. transitory attack of gastroenteritis that is marked by nausea, vomiting, diarrhea, and abdominal cramping and is typically caused by a virus (as the Norwalk virus) or a bacterium (as *Escherichia coli*) — not usu. used technically

intestinal gland *n* : CRYPT OF LIEBERKÜHN

intestinal juice *n* : a fluid that is secreted in small quantity by the crypts of Lieberkühn of the small intestine — called also *succus entericus*

intestinal lipodystrophy *n* : WHIPPLE'S DISEASE

in·tes·tine \in-ˈtes-tən\ *n* : the tubular portion of the alimentary canal that lies posterior to the stomach from which it is separated by the pyloric sphincter and consists of a slender but long anterior part made up of duodenum, jejunum, and ileum and a broader shorter posterior part made up of cecum, colon, and rectum — often used in pl.; see LARGE INTESTINE, SMALL INTESTINE

in·ti·ma \ˈin-tə-mə\ *n, pl* **-mae** \-ˌmē, -ˌmī\ *or* **-mas** : the innermost coat of an organ (as a blood vessel) consisting usu. of an endothelial layer backed by connective tissue and elastic tissue — called also *tunica intima* — **in·ti·mal** \-məl\ *adj*

in·tol·er·ance \(ˌ)in-ˈtä-lə-rəns\ *n* **1** : lack of an ability to endure ⟨an ∼ to light⟩ **2** : exceptional sensitivity (as to a drug) — **in·tol·er·ant** \-rənt\ *adj*

in·tox·i·cant \in-ˈtäk-si-kənt\ *n* : something that intoxicates; *esp* : an alcoholic drink — **intoxicant** *adj*

in·tox·i·cate \-sə-ˌkāt\ *vb* **-cat·ed; -cat·ing** **1** : POISON **2** : to excite or stupefy by alcohol or a drug esp. to the point where physical and mental control is markedly diminished

in·tox·i·cat·ed \-ˌkā-təd\ *adj* : affected by an intoxicant and esp. by alcohol

in·tox·i·ca·tion \in-ˌtäk-sə-ˈkā-shən\ *n* **1** : an abnormal state that is essentially a poisoning ⟨intestinal ∼⟩ **2** : the condition of being drunk or inebriated

in·tra- \in-trə, (ˌ)trä\ *prefix* **1 a** : within ⟨*intra*cerebellar⟩ **b** : during ⟨*intra*operative⟩ **c** : between layers of ⟨*intra*dermal⟩ **2** : INTRO- ⟨an *intra*muscular injection⟩

in·tra-ab·dom·i·nal \ˌin-trə-ab-ˈdä-mən-ᵊl\ *adj* : situated within, occurring within, or administered by entering the abdomen ⟨an ∼ injection⟩

in·tra-al·ve·o·lar \ˌin-trə-al-ˈvē-ə-lər\ *adj* : situated or occurring within an alveolus

in·tra-am·ni·ot·ic \-ˌam-nē-ˈä-tik\ *adj* : situated within, occurring within, or administered by entering the amnion — **in·tra-am·ni·ot·i·cal·ly** *adv*

in·tra-aor·tic \-ā-ˈor-tik\ *adj* **1** : situated or occurring within the aorta **2** : of, relating to, or used in intra-aortic balloon counterpulsation

intra–aortic balloon counterpulsation *n* : counterpulsation in which cardiocirculatory assistance is provided by a balloon inserted in the thoracic aorta which is inflated during diastole and deflated just before systole

in·tra-ar·te·ri·al \-är-ˈtir-ē-əl\ *adj* : situated or occurring within, administered into, or involving entry by way of an artery ⟨an ∼ catheter⟩ — **in·tra-ar·te·ri·al·ly** *adv*

in·tra-ar·tic·u·lar \-är-ˈti-kyə-lər\ *adj* : situated within, occurring within, or administered by entering a joint — **in·tra-ar·tic·u·lar·ly** *adv*

in·tra-atri·al \-ˈā-trē-əl\ *adj* : situated or occurring within an atrium esp. of the heart ⟨an ∼ block⟩

in·tra·can·a·lic·u·lar \-ˌkan-ᵊl-ˈi-kyə-lər\ *adj* : situated or occurring within a canaliculus ⟨∼ biliary stasis⟩

in·tra·cap·su·lar \-ˈkap-sə-lər\ *adj* **1** : situated or occurring within a capsule **2** *of a cataract operation* : involving removal of the entire lens and its capsule — compare EXTRACAPSULAR 2

in·tra·car·di·ac \-ˈkär-dē-ˌak\ *also* **in-**

in·tra·car·di·al \-ˈdē-əl\ *adj* : situated within, occurring within, introduced into, or involving entry into the heart

in·tra·ca·rot·id \-kə-ˈrä-təd\ *adj* : situated within, occurring within, or administered by entering a carotid artery

in·tra·cav·i·tary \-ˈka-və-ˌter-ē\ *adj* : situated or occurring within a body cavity; *esp* : of, relating to, or being treatment (as of cancer) characterized by the insertion of esp. radioactive substances in a cavity

in·tra·cel·lu·lar \-ˈsel-yə-lər\ *adj* : existing, occurring, or functioning within a cell ⟨∼ parasites⟩ — **in·tra·cel·lu·lar·ly** *adv*

in·tra·cer·e·bel·lar \-ˌser-ə-ˈbe-lər\ *adj* : situated or occurring within the cerebellum

in·tra·ce·re·bral \-sə-ˈrē-brəl, -ˈser-ə-\ *adj* : situated within, occurring within, or administered by entering the cerebrum ⟨∼ injections⟩ ⟨∼ bleeding⟩ — **in·tra·ce·re·bral·ly** *adv*

in·tra·cis·ter·nal \-sis-ˈtər-nəl\ *adj* : situated within, occurring within, or administered by entering a cisterna ⟨an ∼ injection⟩ — **in·tra·cis·ter·nal·ly** *adv*

in·tra·co·ro·nal \-ˈkȯr-ən-əl, -ˈkär-; -ˌkə-ˈrōn-\ *adj* : situated or made within the crown of a tooth

in·tra·cor·o·nary \-ˈkȯr-ə-ˌner-ē, -ˈkär-\ *adj* : situated within, occurring within, or administered by entering the heart

in·tra·cor·ti·cal \-ˈkȯr-ti-kəl\ *adj* : situated or occurring within a cortex and esp. the cerebral cortex ⟨∼ injection⟩

in·tra·cra·ni·al \-ˈkrā-nē-əl\ *adj* : situated or occurring within the cranium ⟨∼ pressure⟩; *also* : affecting or involving intracranial structures — **in·tra·cra·ni·al·ly** *adv*

in·trac·ta·ble \(ˌ)in-ˈtrak-tə-bəl\ *adj* **1** : not easily managed or controlled (as by antibiotics or psychotherapy) **2** : not easily relieved or cured ⟨∼ pain⟩ — **in·trac·ta·bil·i·ty** \(ˌ)in-ˌtrak-tə-ˈbi-lə-tē\ *n*

in·tra·cu·ta·ne·ous \ˌin-trə-kyü-ˈtā-nē-əs, -(ˌ)trā-\ *adj* : INTRADERMAL ⟨∼ lesions⟩ — **in·tra·cu·ta·ne·ous·ly** *adv*

intracutaneous test *n* : INTRADERMAL TEST

in·tra·cy·to·plas·mic \-ˌsī-tə-ˈplaz-mik\ *adj* : lying or occurring in the cytoplasm

in·tra·der·mal \-ˈdər-məl\ *adj* : situated, occurring, or done within or between the layers of the skin; *also* : administered by entering the skin ⟨∼ injections⟩ — **in·tra·der·mal·ly** *adv*

intradermal test *n* : a test for immunity or hypersensitivity made by injecting a minute amount of diluted antigen into the skin — called also *intracutaneous test*; compare PATCH TEST, SCRATCH TEST

in·tra·duc·tal \ˌin-trə-ˈdəkt-əl\ *adj* : situated within, occurring within, or introduced into a duct ⟨∼ carcinoma⟩

in·tra·du·o·de·nal \-ˌdü-ə-ˈdēn-əl, -ˌdyü-, ˈäd-ən-əl\ *adj* : situated in or introduced into the duodenum

in·tra·du·ral \-ˈdur-əl, -ˈdyur-\ *adj* : situated, occurring, or performed within or between the membranes of the dura mater

in·tra·epi·der·mal \-ˌe-pə-ˈdər-məl\ *adj* : located or occurring within the epidermis

in·tra·ep·i·the·li·al \-ˌe-pə-ˈthē-lē-əl\ *adj* : occurring in or situated among the cells of the epithelium

in·tra·eryth·ro·cyt·ic \-i-ˌri-thrə-ˈsi-tik\ *adj* : situated or occurring within the red blood cells

in·tra·fa·mil·ial \-fə-ˈmil-yəl\ *adj* : occurring within a family ⟨∼ conflict⟩

in·tra·fol·lic·u·lar \-fə-ˈli-kyə-lər, -fä-\ *adj* : situated within a follicle

in·tra·fu·sal \-ˈfyü-zəl\ *adj* : situated within a muscle spindle ⟨∼ muscle fibers⟩ — compare EXTRAFUSAL

in·tra·gen·ic \-ˈje-nik\ *adj* : being or occurring within a gene

in·tra·he·pat·ic \-hi-ˈpa-tik\ *adj* : situated or occurring within or originating in the liver ⟨∼ cholestasis⟩

in·tra·le·sion·al \-ˈlē-zhən-əl\ *adj* : introduced into or performed within a lesion ⟨∼ injection⟩ — **in·tra·le·sion·al·ly** *adv*

in·tra·lo·bar \-ˈlō-bər, -ˌbär\ *adj* : situated within a lobe

in·tra·lob·u·lar \-ˈlä-byə-lər\ *adj* : situated or occurring within a lobule (as of the liver or pancreas)

intralobular vein *n* : CENTRAL VEIN

in·tra·lu·mi·nal \-ˈlü-mən-əl\ *adj* : situated within, occurring within, or introduced into the lumen

in·tra·mam·ma·ry \-ˈma-mə-rē\ *adj* : situated or introduced within the mammary tissue ⟨∼ infusion⟩

in·tra·med·ul·lary \-ˈmed-əl-ˌer-ē, -ˈmej-əl-; -mə-ˈdə-lə-rē\ *adj* : situated or occurring within a medulla; *esp* : involving use of the marrow space of a bone for support ⟨∼ pinning of a fracture⟩

in·tra·mem·brane \-ˈmem-ˌbrān\ *adj* : INTRAMEMBRANOUS 2

in·tra·mem·bra·nous \-ˈmem-brə-nəs\ *adj* **1** : relating to, formed by, or being ossification of a membrane ⟨∼ bone development⟩ **2** : situated within a membrane

in·tra·mi·to·chon·dri·al \-ˌmī-tə-ˈkän-drē-əl\ *adj* : situated or occurring within mitochondria ⟨∼ inclusions⟩

in·tra·mu·co·sal \-myü-ˈkō-zəl\ *adj* : situated within, occurring within, or administered by entering a mucous membrane

in·tra·mu·ral \-ˈmyur-əl\ *adj* : situated or occurring within the substance of the walls of an organ ⟨∼ infarction⟩

in·tra·mus·cu·lar \-ˈməs-kyə-lər\ *adj* : situated within, occurring within, or administered by entering a muscle — **in·tra·mus·cu·lar·ly** adv

in·tra·myo·car·di·al \-ˌmī-ə-ˈkär-dē-əl\ adj : situated within, occurring within, or administered by entering the myocardium (an ~ injection)

in·tra·na·sal \-ˈnā-zəl\ adj : lying within or administered by way of the nasal structures — **in·tra·na·sal·ly** adv

in·tra·neu·ral \-ˈnur-əl, -ˈnyur-\ adj : situated within, occurring within, or administered by entering a nerve or nervous tissue — **in·tra·neu·ral·ly** adv

in·tra·neu·ro·nal \-ˈnur-ən-əl, -ˈnyur-; -nu-ˈrōn-əl, -nyu-\ adj : situated or occurring within a neuron (excess ~ sodium)

in·tra·nu·cle·ar \-ˈnü-klē-ər, -ˈnyü-\ adj : situated of occurring within a nucleus (cells with prominent ~ inclusions)

in·tra·oc·u·lar \ˌin-trə-ˈä-kyə-lər\ adj : implanted in, occurring within, or administered by entering the eyeball — **in·tra·oc·u·lar·ly** adv

intraocular pressure n : the pressure within the eyeball that gives it a round firm shape and is caused by the aqueous and vitreous humors — called also *intraocular tension*

in·tra·op·er·a·tive \ˌin-trə-ˈä-pə-rə-tiv\ adj : occurring, carried out, or encountered in the course of surgery (~ irradiation) (~ infarction) — **in·tra·op·er·a·tive·ly** adv

in·tra·oral \-ˈōr-əl, -ˈär-\ adj : situated, occurring, or performed within the mouth (~ treatments)

in·tra·os·se·ous \-ˈä-sē-əs\ adj : situated within, occurring within, or administered by entering a bone (~ vasculature) (~ anesthesia)

in·tra·ovu·lar \-ˈä-vyə-lər, -ˈō-\ adj : situated or occurring within the ovum

in·tra·pan·cre·at·ic \-ˌpaŋ-krē-ˈa-tik, -ˌpan-\ adj : situated or occurring within the pancreas

in·tra·pa·ren·chy·mal \-pə-ˈreŋ-kə-məl, -ˌpar-ən-ˈkī-\ adj : situated or occurring within the parenchyma of an organ

in·tra·par·tum \-ˈpär-təm\ adj : occurring chiefly with reference to a mother during the act of birth (~ complications)

in·tra·pel·vic \-ˈpel-vik\ adj : situated or performed within the pelvis

in·tra·peri·car·di·al \-ˌper-ə-ˈkär-dē-əl\ adj : situated within or administered by entering the pericardium

in·tra·peri·to·ne·al \ˌin-trə-ˌper-ət-ᵊn-ˈē-əl\ adj : situated within or administered by entering the peritoneum — **in·tra·peri·to·ne·al·ly** adv

in·tra·pleu·ral \-ˈplur-əl\ adj : situated within, occurring within, or administered by entering the pleura or pleural cavity — **in·tra·pleu·ral·ly** adv

intrapleural pneumonolysis n : PNEUMONOLYSIS b

in·tra·psy·chic \ˌin-trə-ˈsī-kik\ adj : being or occurring within the psyche, mind, or personality

in·tra·pul·mo·nary \-ˈpul-mə-ˌner-ē, -ˈpəl-\ also **in·tra·pul·mon·ic** \-ˌpul-ˈmä-nik, -pəl-\ adj : situated within, occurring within, or administered by entering the lungs — **in·tra·pul·mo·nar·i·ly** \-ˌpul-mə-ˈner-ə-ˌlē\ adv

in·tra·rec·tal \-ˈrekt-ᵊl\ adj : situated within, occurring within, or administered by entering the rectum

in·tra·re·nal \-ˈrēn-ᵊl\ adj : situated within, occurring within, or administered by entering the kidney — **in·tra·re·nal·ly** adv

in·tra·ret·i·nal \-ˈret-ᵊn-əl\ adj : situated or occurring within the retina

in·tra·scro·tal \-ˈskrōt-ᵊl\ adj : situated or occurring within the scrotum

in·tra·spi·nal \-ˈspin-ᵊl\ adj : situated within, occurring within, or introduced into the spine and esp. the vertebral canal (~ nerve terminals)

in·tra·splen·ic \-ˈsple-nik\ adj : situated within or introduced into the spleen — **in·tra·splen·i·cal·ly** adv

in·tra·the·cal \-ˈthē-kəl\ adj : introduced into or occurring in the space under the arachnoid membrane of the brain or spinal cord — **in·tra·the·cal·ly** adv

in·tra·tho·rac·ic \-thə-ˈra-sik\ adj : situated, occurring, or performed within the thorax (~ pressure)

in·tra·thy·roi·dal \-thī-ˈroid-ᵊl\ adj : situated or occurring within the thyroid

in·tra·tra·che·al \-ˈtrā-kē-əl\ adj : occurring within or introduced into the trachea — **in·tra·tra·che·al·ly** adv

in·tra·uter·ine \-ˈyü-tə-rən, -ˌrīn\ adj : of, situated in, used in, or occurring within the uterus; also : involving or occurring during the part of development that takes place in the uterus

intrauterine contraceptive device n : INTRAUTERINE DEVICE

intrauterine device n : a device inserted and left in the uterus to prevent effective conception — called also *IUCD, IUD*

in·tra·vag·i·nal \-ˈva-jən-ᵊl\ adj : situated within, occurring within, or introduced into the vagina — **in·tra·vag·i·nal·ly** adv

in·tra·vas·cu·lar \ˌin-trə-ˈvas-kyə-lər\ adj : situated in, occurring in, or administered by entry into a blood vessel — **in·tra·vas·cu·lar·ly** adv

in·tra·ve·nous \ˌin-trə-ˈvē-nəs\ adj 1 : situated within, performed within, occurring within, or administered by entering a vein (an ~ feeding) 2 : used in intravenous procedures — **in·tra·ve·nous·ly** adv

intravenous pyelogram n : a pyelogram in which roentgenographic visualization is obtained after intravenous administration of a radiopaque medium which collects in the kidneys

in·tra·ven·tric·u·lar \ˌin-trə-ven-ˈtri-kyə-lər\ adj : situated within, occurring within, or administered into a ventricle — **in·tra·ven·tric·u·lar·ly** *adv*

in·tra·ver·te·bral \-\(ˌ\)vər-ˈtē-brəl, -ˈvər-tə-\ *adj* : situated within a vertebra

in·tra·ves·i·cal \-ˈve-si-kəl\ *adj* : situated or occurring within the bladder

in·tra·vi·tal \-ˈvīt-ᵊl\ *adj* 1 : performed upon or found in a living subject 2 : having or utilizing the property of staining cells without killing them — compare SUPRAVITAL — **in·tra·vi·tal·ly** *adv*

in·tra·vi·tam \-ˈvī-ˌtam, -ˈwē-ˌtäm\ *adj* : INTRAVITAL

in·tra·vit·re·al \-ˈvi-trē-əl\ *adj* : INTRAVITREOUS \(~ injection\)

in·tra·vit·re·ous \-trē-əs\ *adj* : situated within, occurring within, or introduced into the vitreous humor \(~ hemorrhage\)

in·trin·sic \in-ˈtrin-zik, -sik\ *adj* 1 : originating or due to causes or factors within a body, organ, or part \(~ asthma\) 2 : originating and included wholly within an organ or part \(~ muscles\) — compare EXTRINSIC 2

intrinsic factor *n* : a substance produced by the normal gastrointestinal mucosa that facilitates absorption of vitamin B₁₂

intro- *prefix* 1 : in : into \(*introjection*\) 2 : inward : within \(*introvert*\) — compare EXTRO-

in·troi·tus \in-ˈtrō-ə-təs\ *n, pl* **introitus** : the vaginal opening — **in·troi·tal** \in-ˈtrō-ət-ᵊl\ *adj*

in·tro·ject \ˌin-trə-ˈjekt\ *vb* 1 : to incorporate \(attitudes or ideas\) into one's personality unconsciously 2 : to turn toward oneself \(the love felt for another\) or against oneself \(the hostility felt toward another\) — **in·tro·jec·tion** \-ˈjek-shən\ *n*

in·tro·mis·sion \ˌin-trə-ˈmi-shən\ *n* : the insertion or period of insertion of the penis in the vagina in copulation

in·tron \ˈin-ˌträn\ *n* : a polynucleotide sequence in a nucleic acid that does not code information for protein synthesis and is removed before translation of messenger RNA — compare EXON

In·tro·pin \ˈin-trə-ˌpin\ *trademark* — used for a preparation of the hydrochloride of dopamine

in·tro·spec·tion \ˌin-trə-ˈspek-shən\ *n* : an examination of one's own thoughts and feelings — **in·tro·spec·tive** \-tiv\ *adj*

in·tro·ver·sion \ˌin-trə-ˈvər-zhən, -shən\ *n* 1 : the act of directing one's attention toward or getting gratification from one's own interests, thoughts, and feelings 2 : the state or tendency toward being wholly or predominantly concerned with and interested in one's own mental life — compare EXTROVERSION

in·tro·vert \ˈin-trə-ˌvərt\ *n* : one whose personality is characterized by introversion; *broadly* : a reserved or shy person — compare EXTROVERT — **in·tro·vert·ed** \ˈin-trə-ˌvər-təd\ *also* **in·tro·vert** \ˈin-trə-ˌvərt\ *adj*

in·tu·ba·tion \ˌin-tü-ˈbā-shən, -tyü-\ *n* : the introduction of a tube into a hollow organ \(as the trachea or intestine\) to keep it open or restore its patency if obstructed — compare EXTUBATION — **in·tu·bate** \ˈin-tü-ˌbāt, -tyü-\ *vb*

in·tu·mes·cence \ˌin-tü-ˈmes-ᵊns, -tyü-\ *n* 1 a : the action or process of becoming enlarged or swollen **b** : the state of being swollen 2 : something \(as a tumor\) that is swollen or enlarged

in·tus·sus·cep·tion \ˌin-tə-sə-ˈsep-shən\ *n* : INVAGINATION; *esp* : the slipping of a length of intestine into an adjacent portion usu. producing obstruction — **in·tus·sus·cept** \ˌin-tə-sə-ˈsept\ *vb*

in·u·lin \ˈin-yə-lən\ *n* : a tasteless white polysaccharide found esp. dissolved in the sap of the roots and rhizomes of composite plants and used as a source of levulose and as a diagnostic agent in a test for kidney function

in·unc·tion \i-ˈnəŋk-shən\ *n* 1 : the rubbing of an ointment into the skin for therapeutic purposes 2 : OINTMENT, UNGUENT

in utero \in-ˈyü-tə-ˌrō\ *adv or adj* : in the uterus : before birth

in·vade \in-ˈvād\ *vb* **in·vad·ed; in·vad·ing** 1 : to enter and spread within either normally \(as in development\) or abnormally \(as in infection\) often with harmful effects 2 : to affect injuriously and progressively

in·vag·i·na·tion \in-ˌva-jə-ˈnā-shən\ *n* 1 : an act or process of folding in so that an outer surface becomes an inner surface: as **a** : the formation of a gastrula by an infolding of part of the wall of the blastula **b** : intestinal intussusception 2 : an invaginated part — **in·vag·i·nate** \in-ˈva-jə-ˌnāt\ *vb*

¹**in·va·lid** \ˈin-və-ləd\ *adj* 1 : suffering from disease or disability : SICKLY 2 : of, relating to, or suited to one that is sick \(an ~ chair\)

²**invalid** *n* : one that is sickly or disabled

³**in·va·lid** \ˈin-və-ləd, -ˌlid\ *vb* 1 : to remove from active duty by reason of sickness or disability \(was ~ed out of the army\) 2 : to make sickly or disabled

in·va·lid·ism \ˈin-və-lə-ˌdi-zəm\ *n* : a chronic condition of being an invalid

in·va·sion \in-ˈvā-zhən\ *n* : the act of invading: as **a** : the penetration of the body of a host by a microorganism **b** : the spread and multiplication of a pathogenic microorganism or of malignant cells in the body of a host

in·va·sive \-siv, -ziv\ *adj* 1 : tending to spread; *esp* : tending to invade healthy tissue \(~ cancer cells\) 2 : involving entry into the living body \(as by incision or by insertion of an instrument\) \(~ diagnostic techniques\) — **in·va·sive·ness** *n*

in·ven·to·ry \'in-vən-ıtōr-ē\ *n, pl* **-ries 1** : a questionnaire designed to provide an index of individual interests or personality traits **2** : a list of traits, preferences, attitudes, interests, or abilities that is used in evaluating personal characteristics or skills

in·ver·sion \in-'vər-zhən, -shən\ *n* **1** : a reversal of position, order, form, or relationship: as **a** : a dislocation of a bodily structure in which it is turned partially or wholly inside out ⟨~ of the uterus⟩ **b** : the condition (as of the foot) of being turned or rotated inward — compare EVERSION 2 **c** : a breaking off of a chromosome section and its subsequent reattachment in inverted position; *also* : a chromosomal section that has undergone this process **2** : HOMOSEXUALITY — **in·vert** \in-'vərt\ *vb*

inversus — see SITUS INVERSUS

in·ver·tase \in-'vər-ıtās, 'in-vər-, -ıtāz\ *n* : an enzyme found in many microorganisms and plants and in animal intestines that catalyzes the hydrolysis of sucrose — called also *saccharase, sucrase*

¹**in·ver·te·brate** \(ı)in-'vər-tə-brət, -ıbrāt\ *n* : an animal having no backbone or internal skeleton

²**invertebrate** *adj* : lacking a spinal column; *also* : of or relating to invertebrate animals

in·vest \in-'vest\ *vb* : to envelop or cover completely (the pleura ~s the lung)

in·ves·ti·ga·tion·al new drug \in-ıves-ti-'gā-shə-nəl-\ *n* : a drug that has not been approved for general use by the Food and Drug Administration but is under investigation in clinical trials regarding its safety and efficacy first by clinical investigators and then by practicing physicians using subjects who have given informed consent to participate — abbr. *IND*; called also *investigational drug*

in·vest·ment \-mənt\ *n* : an external covering of a cell, part, or organism

in·vi·a·ble \(ı)in-'vī-ə-bəl\ *adj* : incapable of surviving esp. because of a deleterious genetic constitution — **in·vi·a·bil·i·ty** \-ıvī-ə-'bi-lə-tē\ *n*

in vi·tro \in-'vē-(ı)trō, -'vi-\ *adv or adj* : outside the living body and in an artificial environment

in vi·vo \in-'vē-(ı)vō\ *adv or adj* **1** : in the living body of a plant or animal **2** : in a real-life situation

in·vo·lu·crum \ıin-və-'lü-krəm\ *n, pl* **-cra** \-krə\ : a formation of new bone about a sequestrum (as in osteomyelitis)

in·vol·un·tary \(ı)in-'vä-lən-ıter-ē\ *adj* : not subject to control of the will : REFLEX ⟨~ contractions⟩

involuntary muscle *n* : muscle governing reflex functions and not under direct voluntary control; *esp* : SMOOTH MUSCLE

in·vo·lute \in-və-'lüt\ *vb* **-lut·ed; -lut·ing 1** : to return to a former condition **2** : to become cleared up

in·vo·lu·tion \in-və-'lü-shən\ *n* **1 a** : an inward curvature or penetration **b** : the formation of a gastrula by ingrowth of cells formed at the dorsal lip **2** : a shrinking or return to a former size ⟨~ of the uterus after pregnancy⟩ **3** : the regressive alterations of a body or its parts characteristic of the aging process; *specif* : decline marked by a decrease of bodily vigor and in women by menopause

in·vo·lu·tion·al \ıin-və-'lü-shə-nəl\ *adj* **1** : of or relating to involutional melancholia **2** : of or relating to the climacterium and its associated bodily and psychic changes

involutional melancholia *n* : a depression that occurs at the time of menopause or the climacteric and is usu. characterized by somatic and nihilistic delusions — called also *involutional psychosis*

in·volve \in-'välv, -'vȯlv\ *vb* **in·volved; in·volv·ing** : to affect with a disease or condition : include in an area of damage, trauma, or insult ⟨herpes *involved* the trigeminal nerve⟩ — **in·volve·ment** \-mənt\ *n*

lod·amoe·ba \ıī-ō-də-'mē-bə\ *n* : a genus of amebas commensal in the intestine of mammals including humans

io·dide \'ī-ə-ıdīd\ *n* : a compound of iodine usu. with a more electrically positive element or radical

io·dine \'ī-ə-ıdīn, -dən, -ıdēn\ *n* **1** : a nonmetallic halogen element used in medicine (as in antisepsis and in the treatment of goiter and cretinism) **2** : a tincture of iodine used esp. as a topical antiseptic — symbol *I*; see ELEMENT table

iodine–131 *n* : a heavy radioactive isotope of iodine that has the mass number 131 and a half-life of eight days, gives off beta and gamma rays, and is used esp. in the form of its sodium salt in the diagnosis of thyroid disease and the treatment of goiter

iodine–125 *n* : a light radioactive isotope of iodine that has a mass number of 125 and a half-life of 60 days, gives off soft gamma rays, and is used as a tracer in thyroid studies and as therapy in hyperthyroidism

io·dip·amide \ıī-ə-'di-pə-ımīd\ *n* : a radiopaque substance $C_{20}H_{14}I_6N_2O_6$ used as the sodium or meglumine salts esp. in cholecystography

io·dism \'ī-ə-ıdi-zəm\ *n* : an abnormal local and systemic condition resulting from overdosage with, prolonged use of, or sensitivity to iodine or iodine compounds and marked by ptyalism, coryza, frontal headache, emaciation, and skin eruptions

io·dize \'ī-ə-ıdīz\ *vb* **io·dized; io·diz·ing** : to treat with iodine or an iodide ⟨*iodized* salt⟩

io·do·chlor·hy·droxy·quin \ˌī-ō-də-ˌklȯr-hi-'dräk-sē-ˌkwin, ˌī-ā-də-\ *n* : an antimicrobial and mildly irritant drug C_9H_5ClINO formerly used esp. as an antidiarrheal but now used mainly as an antibacterial

io·do·de·oxy·uri·dine \ˌī-ō-də-ˌdē-ˌäk-sē-'yur-ə-ˌdēn\ *or* **5-io·do·de·oxy·uri·dine** \fīv-\ *n* : IDOXURIDINE

io·do·form \ī-'ō-də-ˌfȯrm, -'ä-\ *n* : a yellow crystalline volatile compound CHI_3 that is used as an antiseptic dressing

iodohippurate — see SODIUM IODOHIPPURATE

io·do·hip·pur·ate sodium \ˌī-ˌō-də-'hi-pyə-ˌrāt-, -ˌā-, -hi-'pyur-ˌāt-\ *n* : HIPPURAN

io·do·phor \ī-'ō-də-ˌfȯr, ī-'ä-\ *n* : a complex of iodine and a surface-active agent that releases iodine gradually and serves as a disinfectant

io·dop·sin \ˌī-ə-'däp-sən\ *n* : a photosensitive violet pigment in the retinal cones that is similar to rhodopsin but more labile, is formed from vitamin A, and is important in photopic vision

io·do·pyr·a·cet \ˌī-ˌō-də-'pir-ə-ˌset, ī-ˌä-\ *n* : a salt $C_8H_{19}I_2N_2O_3$ used as a radiopaque medium esp. in urography — see DIODRAST

io·do·quin·ol \ˌī-ˌō-də-'kwi-ˌnȯl, -ä-, -ˌnōl\ *n* : a drug $C_9H_5I_2NO$ used esp. in the treatment of amebic dysentery — called also diiodohydroxyquin, diiodohydroxyquinoline

ion \'ī-ˌän, 'ī-ən\ *n* : an electrically charged particle, atom, or group of atoms — **ion·ic** \ī-'ä-nik\ *adj* — **ion·i·cal·ly** *adv*

ion·ize \'ī-ə-ˌnīz\ *vb* **ion·ized; ion·iz·ing 1** : to convert wholly or partly into ions **2** : to become ionized — **ion·iz·able** \ˌī-ə-'nī-zə-bəl\ *adj* — **ion·iza·tion** \ˌī-ə-nə-'zā-shən\ *n*

ion·o·phore \ī-'ä-nə-ˌfȯr\ *n* : a compound that facilitates transmission of an ion (as of calcium) across a lipid barrier (as in a cell membrane) by combining with the ion or by increasing the permeability of the barrier to it — **ion·oph·o·rous** \ˌī-ə-'nä-fə-rəs\ *adj*

ion·to·pho·re·sis \(ˌ)ī-ˌän-tə-fə-'rē-səs\ *n, pl* **-re·ses** \-ˌsēz\ : the introduction of an ionized substance (as a drug) through intact skin by the application of a direct electric current — **ion·to·pho·ret·ic** \-'re-tik\ *adj* — **ion·to·pho·ret·i·cal·ly** *adv*

io·pa·no·ic acid \ˌī-ə-pə-'nō-ik-\ *n* : a crystalline powder $C_{11}H_{12}I_3NO_2$ used as a radiopaque medium in cholecystography

io·phen·dyl·ate \ˌī-ə-'fen-də-ˌlāt\ *n* : a radiopaque liquid $C_{19}H_{29}IO_2$ used esp. in myelography

io·thal·a·mate \ˌī-ə-'tha-lə-ˌmāt\ *n* : any of several salts of iothalamic acid that are administered by injection as radiopaque media

io·thal·am·ic acid \ˌī-ə-thə-'la-mik-\ *n*

: a white odorless powder $C_{11}H_9$-$I_3N_2O_4$ used as a radiopaque medium

IP *abbr* intraperitoneal; intraperitoneally

ipe·cac \'i-pi-ˌkak\ *or* **ipe·ca·cu·a·nha** \ˌi-pi-ˌka-kü-'a-nə\ *n* **1** : the dried rhizome and roots of either of two tropical American plants (*Cephaelis acuminata* and *C. ipecacuanha*) of the madder family (Rubiaceae) used esp. as a source of emetine **2** : an emetic and expectorant drug that contains emetine and is prepared from ipecac esp. as a syrup for use in treating accidental poisoning

ipo·date \'ī-pə-ˌdāt\ *n* : a compound $C_{12}H_{13}I_3N_2O_2$ that is administered as the sodium or calcium salt for use as a radiopaque medium in cholecystography and cholangiography

IPPB *abbr* intermittent positive pressure breathing

ipro·ni·a·zid \ˌī-prə-'nī-ə-zəd\ *n* : a derivative $C_9H_{13}N_3O$ of isoniazid that is a monoamine oxidase inhibitor used as an antidepressant and formerly used in treating tuberculosis — see MARSILID

ip·si·lat·er·al \ˌip-si-'la-tə-rəl\ *adj* : situated or appearing on or affecting the same side of the body — compare CONTRALATERAL — **ip·si·lat·er·al·ly** *adv*

IPSP *abbr* inhibitory postsynaptic potential

IQ \ˌī-'kyü\ *n* : INTELLIGENCE QUOTIENT

Ir *symbol* iridium

IR *abbr* infrared

ir- — see IN-

irid- *or* **irido-** *comb form* **1** : iris of the eye ⟨*iridectomy*⟩ **2** : iris and ⟨*iridocyclitis*⟩

irid·ec·to·my \ˌir-ə-'dek-tə-mē, ˌīr-\ *n, pl* **-mies** : the surgical removal of part of the iris of the eye

irid·en·clei·sis \ˌir-ə-den-'klī-səs, ˌīr-\ *n, pl* **-clei·ses** \-ˌsēz\ : a surgical procedure esp. for relief of glaucoma in which a small portion of the iris is implanted in a corneal incision to facilitate drainage of aqueous humor

irides *pl of* IRIS

irid·ic \i-'ri-dik, ī-\ *adj* : of or relating to the iris of the eye

iridis — see HETEROCHROMIA IRIDIS, RUBEOSIS IRIDIS

irid·i·um \i-'ri-dē-əm\ *n* : a silver-white brittle metallic element of the platinum group — symbol *Ir*; see ELEMENT table

irido·cy·cli·tis \ˌir-ə-dō-sī-'klī-təs, ˌīr-, -si-\ *n* : inflammation of the iris and the ciliary body

irid·o·di·al·y·sis \ˌir-ə-dō-dī-'a-lə-səs, ˌīr-\ *n, pl* **-y·ses** \-ˌsēz\ : separation of the iris from its attachments to the ciliary body

ir·i·dol·o·gy \ˌī-rə-'dä-lə-jē\ *n, pl* **-gies** : the study of the iris of the eye for indications of bodily health and disease — **ir·i·dol·o·gist** \-jist\ *n*

iri·do·ple·gia \ˌir-ə-dō-ˈplē-jə, ˌir-, -jē-ə\ *n* : paralysis of the sphincter of the iris

iri·dot·o·my \ˌir-ə-ˈdä-tə-mē, ˌir-\ *n, pl* **-mies** : incision of the iris

iris \ˈī-rəs\ *n, pl* **iris·es** *or* **iri·des** \ˈī-rə-ˌdēz, ˈir-ə-\ : the opaque muscular contractile diaphragm that is suspended in the aqueous humor in front of the lens of the eye, is perforated by the pupil and is continuous peripherally with the ciliary body, has a deeply pigmented posterior surface which excludes the entrance of light except through the pupil and a colored anterior surface which determines the color or of the eyes

iris bom·bé \-ˌbäm-ˈbā\ *n* : a condition in which the iris is bowed forward by an accumulation of fluid between the iris and the lens

Irish moss *n* : the dried and bleached plants of a red alga (esp. *Chondrus crispus*) used as an agent for thickening or emulsifying or as a demulcent; *also* : the red alga itself

iri·tis \ī-ˈrī-təs\ *n* : inflammation of the iris of the eye

iron \ˈīrn, ˈī-ərn\ *n* **1** : a heavy malleable ductile magnetic silver-white metallic element vital to biological processes (as in transport of oxygen in the body) — symbol *Fe*; see ELEMENT table **2** : iron chemically combined ⟨∼ in the blood⟩ — **iron** *adj*

iron–deficiency anemia *n* : anemia that is caused by a deficiency of iron and characterized by hypochromic microcytic red blood cells

iron lung *n* : a device for artificial respiration in which rhythmic alternations in the air pressure in a chamber surrounding a patient's chest force air into and out of the lungs esp. when the nerves governing the chest muscles fail to function because of poliomyelitis — called also *Drinker respirator*

ir·ra·di·ate \i-ˈrā-dē-ˌāt\ *vb* **-at·ed; -at·ing** : to affect or treat by radiant energy (as heat); *specif* : to treat by exposure to radiation (as ultraviolet light or gamma rays) — **ir·ra·di·a·tor** \-ā-tər\ *n*

ir·ra·di·a·tion \ir-ˌā-dē-ˈā-shən\ *n* **1** : the radiation of a physiologically active agent from a point of origin within the body; *esp* : the spread of a nervous impulse beyond the usual conduction path **2 a** : exposure to radiation (as ultraviolet light, X rays, or alpha rays) **b** : application of radiation (as X rays or gamma rays) esp. for therapeutic purposes

ir·re·duc·ible \ˌir-i-ˈdü-sə-bəl, -ˈdyü-\ *adj* : impossible to bring into a desired or normal position or state ⟨an ∼ hernia⟩

ir·reg·u·lar \i-ˈre-gyə-lər\ *adj* **1** : lack-

ing perfect symmetry of form : not straight, smooth, even, or regular ⟨∼ teeth⟩ **2 a** : lacking continuity or regularity of occurrence, activity, or function ⟨∼ breathing⟩ **b** *of a physiological function* : failing to occur at regular or normal intervals **c** *of an individual* : failing to defecate at regular or normal intervals — **ir·reg·u·lar·i·ty** \i-ˌre-gyə-ˈlar-ə-tē\ *n* — **ir·reg·u·lar·ly** *adv*

ir·re·me·di·a·ble \ir-i-ˈmē-dē-ə-bəl\ *adj* : impossible to remedy or cure

ir·re·vers·ible \ˌir-i-ˈvər-sə-bəl\ *adj, of a pathological process* : of such severity that recovery is impossible ⟨∼ brain damage⟩ — **ir·re·vers·ibil·i·ty** \-ˌvər-sə-ˈbi-lə-tē\ *n* — **ir·re·vers·ibly** \-ˈvər-sə-blē\ *adv*

ir·ri·gate \ˈir-ə-ˌgāt\ *vb* **-gat·ed; -gat·ing** : to flush (a body part) with a stream of liquid (as in removing a foreign body or medicating) — **ir·ri·ga·tion** \ˌir-ə-ˈgā-shən\ *n* — **ir·ri·ga·tor** \ˈir-ə-ˌgā-tər\ *n*

ir·ri·ta·bil·i·ty \ˌir-ə-tə-ˈbi-lə-tē\ *n, pl* **-ties 1** : the property of protoplasm and of living organisms that permits them to react to stimuli **2 a** : quick excitability to annoyance, impatience, or anger **b** : abnormal or excessive excitability of an organ or part of the body (as the stomach or bladder) — **ir·ri·ta·ble** \ˈir-ə-tə-bəl\ *adj*

irritable bowel syndrome *n* : a functional commonly psychosomatic disorder of the colon characterized by the secretion and passage of large amounts of mucus, by constipation alternating with diarrhea, and by cramping abdominal pain — called also *irritable colon, irritable colon syndrome, mucous colitis, spastic colon*

ir·ri·tant \ˈir-ə-tənt\ *adj* : causing irritation; *specif* : tending to produce inflammation — **irritant** *n*

ir·ri·tate \ˈir-ə-ˌtāt\ *vb* **-tat·ed; -tat·ing 1** : to provoke impatience, anger, or displeasure in **2** : to cause (an organ or tissue) to be irritable : produce irritation in **3** : to produce excitation in (as a nerve) : cause (as a muscle) to contract — **ir·ri·ta·tion** \ˌir-ə-ˈtā-shən\ *n*

ir·ri·ta·tive \ˈir-ə-ˌtā-tiv\ *adj* **1** : serving to excite : IRRITATING ⟨an ∼ agent⟩ **2** : accompanied with or produced by irritation ⟨∼ coughing⟩

is- *or* **iso-** *comb form* **1** : equal : homogeneous : uniform ⟨*isosmotic*⟩ **2** : for or from different individuals of the same species ⟨*isoagglutinin*⟩

isch·ae·mia *chiefly Brit var of* ISCHEMIA

isch·emia \is-ˈkē-mē-ə\ *n* : localized tissue anemia due to obstruction of the inflow of arterial blood (as by the narrowing of arteries by spasm or disease) — **isch·emic** \-mik\ *adj* — **isch·emi·cal·ly** *adv*

ischi- *or* **ischio-** *comb form* **1** : ischium

⟨*ischi*ectomy⟩ **2** : ischial and ⟨*ischio*-rectal⟩

ischia *pl of* ISCHIUM

is·chi·al \\'is-kē-əl\\ *adj* : of, relating to, or situated near the ischium

ischial spine *n* : a thin pointed triangular eminence that projects from the dorsal border of the ischium and gives attachment to the gemellus superior on its external surface and to the coccygeus, levator ani, and pelvic fascia on its internal surface

ischial tuberosity *n* : a bony swelling on the posterior part of the superior ramus of the ischium that gives attachment to various muscles and bears the weight of the body in sitting

is·chi·ec·to·my \\,is-kē-'ek-tə-mē\\ *n, pl* **-mies** : surgical removal of a segment of the hipbone including the ischium

is·chio·cav·er·no·sus \\,is-kē-ō-,ka-vər-'nō-səs\\ *n, pl* **-no·si** \\-,sī\\ : a muscle on each side that arises from the ischium near the crus of the penis or clitoris and is inserted on the crus near the pubic symphysis

is·chio·coc·cy·geus \\-käk-'si-jē-əs\\ *n, pl* **-cy·gei** \\-jē-,ī, -,ē\\ : COCCYGEUS

is·chio·fem·o·ral \\-'fe-mə-rəl\\ *adj* : of, relating to, or being an accessory ligament of the hip joint passing from the ischium below the acetabulum to blend with the articular capsule

is·chio·pu·bic ramus \\,is-kē-ō-'pyü-bik-\\ *n* : the flattened inferior projection of the hipbone below the obturator foramen consisting of the united inferior rami of the pubis and ischium

is·chio·rec·tal \\,is-kē-ō-'rekt-ᵊl\\ *adj* : of, relating to, or adjacent to both ischium and rectum ⟨pelvic ∼ abscess⟩

is·chi·um \\'is-kē-əm\\ *n, pl* **is·chia** \\-ə\\ : the dorsal and posterior of the three principal bones composing either half of the pelvis consisting in humans of a thick portion, a large rough eminence on which the body rests when sitting, and a forwardly directed ramus which joins that of the pubis

Ishi·ha·ra \\,i-shē-'här-ə\\ *adj* : of, relating to, or used in an Ishihara test

Ishihara, Shinobu (1879–1963), Japanese ophthalmologist.

Ishihara test *n* : a widely used test for color blindness that consists of a set of plates covered with colored dots which the test subject views in order to find a number composed of dots of one color which a person with various defects of color vision will confuse with surrounding dots of color

is·land \\'ī-lənd\\ *n* : an isolated anatomical structure, tissue, or group of cells

island of Lang·er·hans \\-'läŋ-ər-,hänz, -,häns\\ *n* : ISLET OF LANGERHANS

island of Reil \\-'rīl\\ *n* : INSULA

Reil, Johann Christian (1759–1813), German anatomist.

is·let \\'ī-lət\\ *n* : ISLET OF LANGERHANS

islet cell *n* : one of the endocrine cells making up an islet of Langerhans

islet of Lang·er·hans \\-'läŋ-ər-,hänz, -,häns\\ *n* : any of the groups of small slightly granular endocrine cells that form anastomosing trabeculae among the tubules and alveoli of the pancreas and secrete insulin and glucagon — called also *islet*

Langerhans, Paul (1847–1888), German pathologist.

-ism \\,i-zəm\\ *n suffix* **1** : act, practice, or process ⟨hypnot*ism*⟩ **2 a** : state, condition, or property ⟨polymorph*ism*⟩ **b** : abnormal state or condition resulting from excess of a (specified) thing or marked by resemblance to a (specified) person or thing ⟨alcohol*ism*⟩ ⟨morphin*ism*⟩ ⟨mongol*ism*⟩

iso- — see IS-

iso·ag·glu·ti·na·tion \\,ī-(,)sō-ə-,glüt-ᵊn-'ā-shən\\ *n* : agglutination of an agglutinogen of one individual by the serum of another of the same species

iso·ag·glu·ti·nin \\-ə-'glüt-ᵊn-ən\\ *n* : an antibody produced by one individual that causes agglutination of cells (as red blood cells) of other individuals of the same species

iso·ag·glu·tin·o·gen \\-ə-glü-'ti-nə-jən\\ *n* : an antigenic substance capable of provoking formation of or reacting with an isoagglutinin

iso·al·lox·a·zine \\-ə-'läk-sə-,zēn\\ *n* : a yellow solid $C_{10}H_6N_4O_2$ that is the precursor of various flavins (as riboflavin)

iso·am·yl nitrite \\,ī-sō-'a-məl-\\ *n* : AMYL NITRITE

iso·an·ti·body \\,ī-(,)sō-'an-ti-,bä-dē\\ *n, pl* **-bod·ies** : ALLOANTIBODY

iso·an·ti·gen \\-'an-ti-jən\\ *n* : ALLOANTIGEN

iso·bor·nyl thio·cyano·ace·tate \\,ī-sō-'bor-nil-,thī-ō-,sī-ə-nō-'a-sə-,tāt, -sī-,a-nō-\\ *n* : a yellow oily liquid $C_{13}H_{19}N_2OS$ used as a pediculicide

iso·bu·tyl nitrite \\,ī-sō-'byüt-ᵊl-\\ *n* : a colorless pungent liquid $C_4H_9NO_2$ inhaled by drug abusers for its stimulating effects which are similar to those of amyl nitrite — called also *butyl nitrite*

iso·car·box·az·id \\-,kär-'bäk-sə-zəd\\ *n* : a hydrazide monoamine oxidase inhibitor $C_{12}H_{13}N_3O_2$ used as an antidepressant — see MARPLAN

iso·chro·mo·some \\-'krō-mə-,sōm, -,zōm\\ *n* : a chromosome produced by transverse splitting of the centromere so that both arms are from the same side of the centromere, are of equal length, and possess identical genes

iso·ci·trate \\,ī-sō-'si-,trāt\\ *n* : any salt or ester of isocitric acid; *also* : ISOCITRIC ACID

isocitrate de·hy·dro·gen·ase \\-dē-(,)hī-'drä-jə-,nās, -'hī-drə-jə-, -,nāz\\ *n* : either of two enzymes which catalyze the oxidation of isocitric acid (as in the Krebs cycle — called also *isocitric dehydrogenase*

iso·cit·ric acid \ˌī-sə-ˈsi-trik-\ *n* : a crystalline isomer of citric acid that occurs esp. as an intermediate stage in the Krebs cycle

isocitric dehydrogenase *n* : ISOCITRATE DEHYDROGENASE

iso·dose \ˈī-sə-ˌdōs\ *adj* : of or relating to points or zones in a medium that receive equal doses of radiation

iso·elec·tric \ˌī-sō-i-ˈlek-trik\ *adj* : being the pH at which the electrolyte will not migrate in an electrical field ⟨the ∼ point of a protein⟩

isoelectric focusing *n* : an electrophoretic technique for separating proteins by causing them to migrate under the influence of an electric field through a medium (as a gel) having a pH gradient to locations with pH values corresponding to their isoelectric points

iso·en·zyme \ˌī-sō-ˈen-ˌzīm\ *n* : any of two or more chemically distinct but functionally similar enzymes — called also *isozyme* — **iso·en·zy·mat·ic** \ˌī-sō-ˌen-zə-ˈma-tik, -zī-\ *adj* — **iso·en·zy·mic** \-en-ˈzī-mik\ *adj*

iso·eth·a·rine \-ˈe-thə-ˌrēn\ *n* : an adrenergic drug $C_{13}H_{21}NO_3$ used as a bronchodilator

iso·fluro·phate \-ˈflür-ə-ˌfāt\ *n* : a volatile irritating liquid ester $C_6H_{14}FO_3P$ that acts as a nerve gas by inhibiting cholinesterases and as a miotic and that is used chiefly in treating glaucoma — called also *DFP, diisopropyl fluorophosphate*

iso·ge·ne·ic \ˌī-sō-jə-ˈnē-ik, -ˈnā-\ *adj* : SYNGENEIC ⟨an ∼ graft⟩

iso·gen·ic \-ˈje-nik\ *adj* : characterized by essentially identical genes

iso·graft \ˈī-sə-ˌgraft\ *n* : a homograft between genetically identical or nearly identical individuals — **isograft** *vb*

iso·hem·ag·glu·ti·nin \-ˌhē-mə-ˈglüt-ᵊn-ən\ *n* : a hemagglutinin causing isoagglutination

iso·hy·dric shift \ˌī-sō-ˈhī-drik-\ *n* : the set of chemical reactions in a red blood cell by which oxygen is released to the tissues and carbon dioxide is taken up while the blood remains at constant pH

iso·im·mu·ni·za·tion \ˌī-sō-ˌi-myə-nə-ˈzā-shən\ *n* : production by an individual of antibodies against constituents of the tissues of another individual of the same species (as when transfused with blood from one belonging to a different blood group)

¹**iso·late** \ˈī-sə-ˌlāt\ *vb* **-lat·ed; -lat·ing** : to set apart from others: as **a** : to separate (one with a contagious disease) from others not similarly infected **b** : to separate (as a chemical compound) from all other substances : obtain pure or in a free state

²**iso·late** \ˈī-sə-lət, -ˌlāt\ *n* **1** : an individual (as a single organism), viable part

of an organism (as a cell), or a strain that has been isolated (as from diseased tissue); *also* : a pure culture produced from such an isolate **2** : a socially withdrawn individual

iso·la·tion \ˌī-sə-ˈlā-shən\ *n* **1** : the action of isolating or condition of being isolated ⟨put the patient in ∼⟩ **2** : a psychological defense mechanism consisting of the separating of ideas or memories from the emotions connected with them

Iso·lette \ˌī-sə-ˈlet\ *trademark* — used for an incubator for premature infants that provides controlled temperature and humidity and an oxygen supply

iso·leu·cine \ˌī-sō-ˈlü-ˌsēn\ *n* : a crystalline essential amino acid $C_6H_{13}NO_2$ isomeric with leucine

isol·o·gous \ī-ˈsä-lə-gəs\ *adj* : SYNGENEIC

iso·mer \ˈī-sə-mər\ *n* : any of two or more compounds, radicals, ions, or nuclides that contain the same number of atoms of the same elements but differ in structural arrangement and properties — **iso·mer·ic** \ˌī-sə-ˈmer-ik\ *adj* — **isom·er·ism** \ī-ˈsä-mə-ˌri-zəm\ *n*

iso·me·thep·tene \ˌī-sō-me-ˈthep-ˌtēn\ *n* : a vasoconstrictive and antispasmodic drug $C_9H_{19}N$ administered as the hydrochloride or mucate

iso·met·ric \ˌī-sə-ˈme-trik\ *adj* : of, relating to, involving, or being muscular contraction (as in isometrics) against resistance, without significant shortening of muscle fibers, and with marked increase in muscle tone — compare ISOTONIC 2 — **iso·met·ri·cal·ly** *adv*

iso·met·rics \ˌī-sə-ˈme-triks\ *n sing or pl* : isometric exercise or an isometric system of exercises

iso·ni·a·zid \ˌī-sō-ˈnī-ə-zəd\ *n* : a crystalline compound $C_6H_7N_3O$ used in treating tuberculosis

isonicotinic acid hydrazide *n* : ISONIAZID

iso·nip·e·caine \ˌī-sō-ˈni-pə-ˌkān\ *n* : MEPERIDINE

Iso·nor·in \ˌī-sə-ˈnor-ən\ *trademark* — used for a preparation of isoproterenol

iso·os·mot·ic \ˌī-sō-äz-ˈmä-tik\ *adj* : ISOSMOTIC

Iso·paque \ˌī-sō-ˈpāk\ *trademark* — used for a preparation of metrizoate sodium

iso·peri·stal·tic \ˌī-sō-ˌper-ə-ˈstol-tik, -ˈstäl-, -ˈstal-\ *adj* : performed or arranged so that the grafted or anastomosed parts exhibit peristalsis in the same direction ⟨∼ gastroenterostomy⟩ — **iso·peri·stal·ti·cal·ly** *adv*

iso·phane \ˈī-sə-ˌfān\ *adj* : of, relating to, or being a ratio of protamine to insulin equal to that in a solution made by mixing equal parts of a solution of the two in which all the protamine precipitates and a solution of the two in which all the insulin precipitates

iso·phane insulin *n* : an isophane mixture of protamine and insulin — called also *isophane*

iso·preg·nen·one \-'preg-ne-₁nōn\ *n* : DYDROGESTERONE

iso·pren·a·line \₁ī-sə-'pren-əl-ən\ *n* : ISOPROTERENOL

iso·pro·pa·mide iodide \₁ī-sō-'prō-pə-₁mēd-\ *n* : an anticholinergic $C_{23}H_{33}IN_2O$ used esp. for its antispasmodic and antisecretory effect on the gastrointestinal tract — called also *isopropamide*

iso·pro·pa·nol \-'prō-pə-₁nȯl, -₁nōl\ *n* : ISOPROPYL ALCOHOL

iso·pro·pyl alcohol \₁ī-sə-'prō-pəl-\ *n* : a volatile flammable alcohol C_3H_8O used as a rubbing alcohol — called also *isopropanol*

iso·pro·pyl·ar·te·re·nol \₁ī-sə-₁prō-pə-₁lär-tə-¹rē-₁nȯl, -₁nōl\ *n* : ISOPROTERENOL

isopropyl my·ris·tate \-mə-'ris-₁tāt\ *n* : an ester $C_{17}H_{34}O_2$ of isopropyl alcohol that is used as an emollient to promote absorption through the skin

iso·pro·ter·e·nol \₁ī-sə-prō-'ter-ə-₁nȯl, -nəl\ *n* : a drug $C_{11}H_{17}NO_3$ used in the treatment of asthma — called also *isoprenaline, isopropylarterenol; see* ISONORIN, ISUPREL

isop·ter \'ī-'säp-tər\ *n* : a contour line in a representation of the visual field around the points representing the macula lutea that passes through the points of equal visual acuity

Isor·dil \'ī-sor-₁dil\ *trademark* — used for a preparation of isosorbide dinitrate

is·os·mot·ic \₁ī-₁säz-'mä-tik, -₁säs-\ *adj* : of, relating to, or exhibiting equal osmotic pressure ($\sim$ solutions) — compare HYPERTONIC 2, HYPOTONIC 2 — **is·os·mot·i·cal·ly** *adv*

iso·sor·bide \₁ī-sō-'sȯr-₁bīd\ *n* 1 : a diuretic $C_6H_{10}O_4$ 2 : ISOSORBIDE DINITRATE

isosorbide di·ni·trate \-dī-'nī-₁trāt\ *n* : a coronary vasodilator $C_6H_8N_2O_8$ used esp. in the treatment of angina pectoris — see ISORDIL

Isos·po·ra \ī-'säs-pə-rə\ *n* : a genus of coccidian protozoans closely related to the genus *Eimeria* and including the only coccidian (*I. hominis*) known to be parasitic in humans

isothiocyanate — see ALLYL ISOTHIOCYANATE

iso·thio·pen·dyl \₁ī-sō-thī-ō-'pen-₁dil\ *n* : an antihistaminic drug $C_{16}H_{19}N_3S$

iso·ton·ic \₁ī-sə-'tä-nik\ *adj* 1 : ISOSMOTIC — used of solutions 2 : of, relating to, or being muscular contraction in the absence of significant resistance, with marked shortening of muscle fibers, and without great increase in muscle tone — compare ISOMETRIC — **iso·ton·i·cal·ly** *adv* — **iso·to·nic·i·ty** \-tō-¹ni-sə-tē\ *n*

iso·tope \'ī-sə-₁tōp\ *n* 1 : any of two or more species of atoms of a chemical element with the same atomic number that differ in the number of neutrons in an atom and have different physical properties 2 : NUCLIDE — **iso·to·pic** \₁ī-sə-'tä-pik, -'tō-\ *adj* — **iso·to·pi·cal·ly** *adv*

iso·trans·plant \₁ī-sō-'trans-₁plant\ *n* : a graft between syngeneic individuals

iso·tret·i·no·in \₁ī-sō-'tre-tə-₁nō-ən\ *n* : a synthetic vitamin A derivative $C_{20}H_{28}O_2$ that inhibits sebaceous gland function and keratinization and that is used in the treatment of acne but is contraindicated in pregnancy because of implication as a cause of birth defects — see ACCUTANE

isotropic band *n* : I BAND

iso·type \'ī-sə-₁tīp\ *n* : any of the categories of antibodies determined by their physicochemical properties (as molecular weight) and antigenic characteristics that occur in all individuals of a species — compare ALLOTYPE, IDIOTYPE — **iso·typ·ic** \₁ī-sə-'ti-pik\ *adj*

iso·va·ler·ic acid \₁ī-sō-və-'lir-ik-, -'ler-\ *n* : a liquid acid $C_5H_{10}O_2$ that has a disagreeable odor

isovaleric ac·i·de·mia \-₁a-sə-'dē-mē-ə\ *n* : a metabolic disorder characterized by the presence of an abnormally high concentration of isovaleric acid in the blood causing acidosis, coma, and an unpleasant body odor

iso·vol·ume \'ī-sə-₁väl-yəm, -(₁)yüm\ *adj* : ISOVOLUMETRIC

iso·vol·u·met·ric \₁ī-sə-₁väl-yù-¹me-trik\ *adj* : of, relating to, or characterized by unchanging volume; *esp* : relating to or being an early phase of ventricular systole in which the cardiac muscle exerts increasing pressure on the contents of the ventricle without significant change in the muscle fiber length and the ventricular volume remains constant

iso·vo·lu·mic \-və-¹lü-mik\ *adj* : ISOVOLUMETRIC

is·ox·az·o·lyl \(₁)ī-₁säk-'sa-zə-₁lil\ *adj* : relating to or being any of a group of semisynthetic penicillins (as oxacillin and cloxacillin) that are resistant to penicillinase, stable in acids, and active against gram-positive bacteria

is·ox·su·prine \ī-'säk-sə-₁prēn\ *n* : a sympathomimetic drug $C_{18}H_{23}NO_3$ used chiefly as a vasodilator

iso·zyme \'ī-sə-₁zīm\ *n* : ISOENZYME — **iso·zy·mic** \₁ī-sə-'zī-mik\ *adj*

is·sue \'i-(₁)shü\ *n* : a discharge (as of blood) from the body that is caused by disease or other physical disorder or that is produced artificially; *also* : an incision made to produce such a discharge

isth·mus \'is-məs\ *n* : a contracted anatomical part or passage connecting two larger structures or cavities: as **a** : an embryonic constriction separating the midbrain from the hindbrain **b** : the lower portion of the uterine corpus — **isth·mic** \'is-mik\ *adj*

isthmus of the fauces *n* : FAUCES

Isu·prel \'ī-sù-ˌprel\ *trademark* — used for a preparation of isoproterenol

itai–itai \i-'tī-i-ˌtī\ *n* : an extremely painful condition caused by poisoning following the ingestion of cadmium and characterized by bone decalcification — called also *itai-itai disease*

itch \'ich\ *n* **1** : an uneasy irritating sensation in the upper surface of the skin usu. held to result from mild stimulation of pain receptors **2** : a skin disorder accompanied by an itch; *esp* : a contagious eruption caused by an itch mite of the genus *Sarcoptes* (*S. scabiei*) that burrows in the skin and causes intense itching — **itch** *vb* — **itch·i·ness** \'i-chē-nəs\ *n* — **itchy** \'i-chē\ *adj*

¹itch·ing *adj* : having, producing, or marked by an uneasy sensation in the skin (an ~ skin eruption)

²itching *n* : ITCH 1

itch mite *n* : any of several minute parasitic mites that burrow into the skin and cause itch; *esp* : a mite of any of several varieties of a species of the genus *Sarcoptes* (*S. scabiei*) that causes the itch

-ite \ˌīt\ *n suffix* **1** : substance produced through some (specified) process (catabol*ite*) **2** : segment or constituent part of a body or of a bodily part (somi*te*) (dendr*ite*)

-it·ic \'i-tik\ *adj suffix* : of, resembling, or marked by — in adjectives formed from nouns usu. ending in -ite (dendr*itic*) and -*itis* (bronch*itic*)

-i·tis \'ī-təs\ *n suffix, pl* **-i·tis·es** *also* **-it·i·des** \'i-tə-ˌdēz\ *or* **-i·tes** \'i-(ˌ)tēz\

: disease usu. inflammatory of a (specified) part or organ : inflammation of (laryng*itis*) (appendic*itis*) (bronch*itis*)

ITP *abbr* idiopathic thrombocytopenic purpura

IU *abbr* : international unit

IUCD \ˌī-(ˌ)yü-(ˌ)sē-'dē\ *n* : INTRA-UTERINE DEVICE

IUD \ˌī-(ˌ)ü-'dē\ *n* : INTRAUTERINE DEVICE

IUDR \ˌī-(ˌ)yü-(ˌ)dē-'är\ *n* : IDOXURI-DINE

¹IV \'ī-'vē\ *n, pl* **IVs** : an apparatus used to administer an intravenous injection or feeding; *also* : such an injection or feeding

²IV *abbr* **1** intravenous; intravenously **2** intraventricular

iver·mec·tin \ˌī-vər-'mek-tən\ *n* : a drug mixture of two structurally similar semisynthetic lactones that is used in veterinary medicine as an anthelmintic, acaricide, and insecticide and in human medicine to treat onchocerciasis

IVF *abbr* in vitro fertilization

IVP *abbr* intravenous pyelogram

Ix·o·des \ik-'sō-(ˌ)dēz\ *n* : a widespread genus of ixodid ticks (as the deer tick) many of which are bloodsucking parasites of humans and animals, and sometimes cause paralysis or other severe reactions

ix·o·di·cide \ik-'sä-di-ˌsid, -'sō-\ *n* : an agent that destroys ticks

ixo·did \ik-'sä-did, -'sō-\ *adj* : of or relating to a family (Ixodidae) of ticks (as the deer tick, American dog tick, and lone star tick) having a hard outer shell and feeding on two or three hosts during the life cycle — **ixodid** *n*

J

jaag·siek·te *also* **jaag·ziek·te** \'yäg-ˌsēk-tə, -ˌzēk-\ *n* : a chronic contagious pneumonitis of sheep and sometimes goats that is caused by a virus

jack·et \'ja-kət\ *n* **1** : a rigid covering that envelops the upper body and provides support, correction, or restraint **2** : JACKET CROWN

jacket crown *n* : an artificial crown that is placed over the remains of a natural tooth

jack·so·ni·an \jak-'sō-nē-ən\ *adj, often cap* : of, relating to, associated with, or resembling Jacksonian epilepsy

Jack·son \'jak-sən\, **John Hughlings (1835–1911)**, British neurologist.

Jacksonian epilepsy *n* : epilepsy that is characterized by progressive spreading of the abnormal movements or sensations from a focus affecting a muscle group on one side of the body to adjacent muscles or by becoming generalized and that corresponds to

the spread of epileptic activity in the motor cortex

Ja·cob·son's nerve \'jä-kəb-sənz-\ *n* : TYMPANIC NERVE

Jacobson \'yä-kóp-sən\, **Ludwig Levin (1783–1843)**, Danish anatomist.

Jacobson's organ *n* : a slender canal in the nasal mucosa that ends in a blind pouch, has an olfactory function, and is rudimentary in adult humans — called also *vomeronasal organ*

jac·ti·ta·tion \ˌjak-tə-'tā-shən\ *n* : a tossing to and fro or jerking and twitching of the body or its parts : excessive restlessness esp. in certain psychiatric disorders — **jac·ti·tate** \'jak-tə-ˌtāt\ *vb*

Jaf·fé reaction \'yä-ˌfā-, zhä-\ *also* **Jaf·fé's reaction** \-'fāz-\ *n* : a reaction between creatinine and picric acid in alkaline solution that results in the formation of a red compound and is used to determine creatinine (as in creatinuria)

Jaffé \yä-'fā\. **Max (1841–1911),** German biochemist.

jag·siek·te *or* **jag·ziek·te** *var of* JAAGSIEKTE

jail fever \'jāl-\ *n* : TYPHUS a

jake leg \'jāk-\ *n* : a paralysis caused by drinking improperly distilled or contaminated liquor

Ja·kob–Creutz·feldt disease \'yä-(₌)kōb-'kroits-₌felt-\ *n* : CREUTZ-FELDT-JAKOB DISEASE

jal·ap \'ja-ləp, 'jä-\ *n* 1 : the dried tuberous root of a Mexican plant (*Ipomoea purga*) of the morning-glory family (Convolvulaceae); *also* : a powdered purgative drug prepared from it that contains resinous glycosides 2 : a plant yielding jalap

JAMA *abbr* Journal of the American Medical Association

ja·mais vu \₌zhä-₌me-'vœ, ₌jä-₌mä-'vü\ *n* : a disorder of memory characterized by the illusion that the familiar is being encountered for the first time — compare AMNESIA, PARAMNESIA b

Jamestown weed \'jāmz-₌taun-\ *n* : JIMSONWEED

jani·ceps \'ja-nə-₌seps, 'jä-\ *n* : a malformed double fetus joined at the thorax and skull and having two equal faces looking in opposite directions

Japanese B encephalitis *n* : an encephalitis that occurs epidemically esp. in Japan in the summer, is caused by an arbovirus, and usu. produces a subclinical infection

japonica — see SCHISTOSOMIASIS JAPONICA

jar·gon \'jär-gən\ *n* : gibberish or babbling speech associated with aphasia, extreme mental retardation, or a severe mental illness

Ja·risch–Herx·hei·mer reaction \'yärish-'herks-₌hi-mər-\ *n* : an increase in the symptoms of a spirochetal disease (as syphilis, Lyme disease, or relapsing fever) occurring in some persons when treatment with spirocheticidal drugs is started — called also *Herxheimer reaction*

    Jarisch, Adolf (1850–1902), Austrian dermatologist.

    Herxheimer, Karl (1861–1944), German dermatologist.

jaun·dice \'jȯn-dəs, 'jän-\ *n* 1 : a yellowish pigmentation of the skin, tissues, and certain body fluids caused by the deposition of bile pigments that follows interference with normal production and discharge of bile (as in certain liver diseases) or excessive breakdown of red blood cells (as after internal hemorrhage or in various hemolytic states) 2 : any disease or abnormal condition (as hepatitis A or leptospirosis) that is characterized by jaundice — **jaun·diced** \-dəst\ *adj*

jaw \'jȯ\ *n* 1 : either of two complex cartilaginous or bony structures in most vertebrates that border the mouth, support the soft parts enclosing it, and usu. bear teeth on their oral margin: **a** : an upper structure more or less firmly fused with the skull — called also *upper jaw, maxilla* **b** : a lower structure that consists of a single bone or of completely fused bones and that is hinged, movable, and articulated by a pair of condyles with the temporal bone of either side — called also *inferior maxillary bone, lower jaw, mandible* 2 : the parts constituting the walls of the mouth and serving to open and close it — usu. used in pl.

jaw·bone \'jȯ-₌bōn\ *n* : JAW 1; *esp* : MANDIBLE

jawed \'jȯd\ *adj* : having jaws — usu. used in combination ⟨square-*jawed*⟩

JCAH *abbr* Joint Commission on Accreditation of Hospitals

J chain \'jā-\ *n* : a relatively short polypeptide chain with a high number of cysteine residues that is found in antibodies of the IgM and IgA classes

jejun- *or* **jejuno-** *comb form* 1 : jejunum ⟨*jejun*itis⟩ 2 : jejunum and ⟨*jejuno*ileitis⟩

je·ju·nal \ji-'jün-ᵊl\ *adj* : of or relating to the jejunum

je·ju·ni·tis \₌je-jü-'nī-təs\ *n* : inflammation of the jejunum

je·ju·no·il·e·al bypass \ji-₌jü-nō-'i-lē-əl-\ *n* : a surgical bypass operation performed esp. to reduce absorption in the small intestine that involves joining the first part of the jejunum with the more distal segment of the ileum

je·ju·no·il·e·itis \ji-₌jü-nō-₌i-lē-'i-təs, ₌je-jü-nō-\ *n* : inflammation of the jejunum and the ileum

je·ju·no·il·e·os·to·my \ji-₌jü-nō-₌i-lē-'äs-tə-mē, ₌je-jü-nō-\ *n, pl* **-mies** : the formation of an anastomosis between the jejunum and the ileum

je·ju·nos·to·my \₌ji-jü-'näs-tə-mē, ₌je-jü-\ *n, pl* **-mies** 1 : the surgical formation of an opening through the abdominal wall into the jejunum 2 : the opening made by jejunostomy

je·ju·num \ji-'jü-nəm\ *n, pl* **je·ju·na** \-nə\ : the section of the small intestine that comprises the first two fifths beyond the duodenum and that is larger, thicker-walled, and more vascular and has more circular folds and fewer Peyer's patches than the ileum

jel·ly \'je-lē\ *n, pl* **jellies** : a semisolid gelatinous substance: as **a** : a medicated preparation usu. intended for local application ⟨ephedrine ∼⟩ **b** : a jellylike preparation used in electrocardiography to obtain better conduction of electricity ⟨electrode ∼⟩

jel·ly·fish \-₌fish\ *n* : a free-swimming marine sexually reproducing coelenterate of either of two classes (Hydrozoa and Scyphozoa) that has a nearly transparent saucer-shaped body and marginal tentacles studded with stinging cells

je·quir·i·ty bean \jə-ˈkwir-ə-tē-\ *n* 1 : the poisonous scarlet and black seed of the rosary pea 2 : ROSARY PEA 1

jerk \ˈjərk\ *n* : an involuntary spasmodic muscular movement due to reflex action; *esp* : one induced by an external stimulus — see KNEE JERK

jet fa·tigue \ˈjet-fə-ˌtēg\ *n* : JET LAG

jet in·jec·tor \-in-ˈjek-tər\ *n* : a device used to inject subcutaneously a fine stream of fluid under high pressure without puncturing the skin — **jet injec·tion** \-ˈjek-shən\ *n*

jet lag \ˈjet-ˌlag\ *n* : a condition that is characterized by various psychological and physiological effects (as fatigue and irritability), occurs following long flight through several time zones, and prob. results from disruption of circadian rhythms in the human body — called also *jet fatigue* — **jet-lagged** *adj*

jig·ger \ˈji-gər\ *n* : CHIGGER

jim·son·weed \ˈjim-sən-ˌwēd\ *n* : a poisonous tall annual weed of the genus *Datura* (*D. stramonium*) with rank-smelling foliage, large white or violet trumpet-shaped flowers, and globe-shaped prickly fruits that is a source of stramonium — called also *Jamestown weed*

jit·ters \ˈji-tərz\ *n pl* : a state of extreme nervousness or nervous shaking — **jit·ter** \-tər\ *vb* — **jit·teri·ness** \-tə-rē-nəs\ *n* — **jit·tery** *adj*

JND *abbr* just noticeable difference

jock itch \ˈjäk-\ *n* : ringworm of the crotch : TINEA CRURIS — called also *jockey itch*

jock·strap \ˈjäk-ˌstrap\ *n* : ATHLETIC SUPPORTER

John's bacillus \ˈyō-nēz-\ *n* : a bacillus of the genus *Mycobacterium* (*M. paratuberculosis*) that causes Johne's disease

Johne \ˈyō-nə\, **Heinrich Albert (1839–1910),** German bacteriologist.

Joh·ne's disease \ˈyō-nəz-\ *n* : a chronic often fatal enteritis esp. of cattle that is caused by Johne's bacillus — called also *paratuberculosis*

john·ny *also* **john·nie** \ˈjä-nē\ *n, pl* **john·nies** : a short-sleeved collarless gown with an opening in the back for wear by persons (as hospital patients) undergoing medical examination or treatment

joint \ˈjoint\ *n* : the point of contact between skeletal elements whether movable or rigidly fixed together with the surrounding and supporting parts (as membranes, tendons, ligaments) — **out of joint** *of a bone* : having the head slipped from its socket

joint capsule *n* : ARTICULAR CAPSULE

joint·ed \ˈjoin-təd\ *adj* : having joints

joint ill *n* : NAVEL ILL

joint mouse \-ˈmaůs\ *n* : a loose fragment (as of cartilage) within a synovial space

joule \ˈjül\ *n* : the absolute mks unit of work or energy equal to 10^7 ergs or approximately 0.7375 foot-pounds

Joule, James Prescott (1818–1889), British physicist.

¹ju·gal \ˈjü-gəl\ *adj* : MALAR

²jugal *n* : ZYGOMATIC BONE — called also *jugal bone*

¹jug·u·lar \ˈjə-gyə-lər, ˈjü-\ *adj* **1** : of or relating to the throat or neck **2** : of or relating to the jugular vein ⟨~ pulsations⟩

²jugular *n* : JUGULAR VEIN

jugulare — see GLOMUS JUGULARE

jugular foramen *n* : a large irregular opening from the posterior cranial fossa that is bounded anteriorly by the petrous part of the temporal bone and posteriorly by the jugular notch of the occipital bone and that transmits the inferior petrosal sinus, the glossopharyngeal, vagus, and accessory nerves, and the internal jugular vein

jugular fossa *n* : a depression on the basilar surface of the petrous portion of the temporal bone or neck that contains a dilation of the internal jugular vein

jugular ganglion *n* : SUPERIOR GANGLION

jugular notch \-ˈnäch\ *n* **1** : SUPRASTERNAL NOTCH **2 a** : a notch in the inferior border of the occipital bone behind the jugular process that forms the posterior part of the jugular foramen **b** : a notch in the petrous portion of the temporal bone that corresponds to the jugular notch of the occipital bone and with it makes up the jugular foramen

jugular process *n* : a quadrilateral or triangular process of the occipital bone on each side that articulates with the temporal bone and is situated lateral to the condyle of the occipital bone on each side articulating with the atlas

jugular trunk *n* : either of two major lymph vessels of which one lies on each side of the body and drains the head and neck

jugular vein *n* : any of several veins of each side of the neck: as **a** : a vein that collects the blood from the interior of the cranium, the superficial part of the face, and the neck, runs down the neck on the outside of the internal and common carotid arteries, and unites with the subclavian vein to form the innominate vein — called also *internal jugular vein* **b** : a smaller and more superficial vein that collects most of the blood from the exterior of the cranium and deep parts of the face and opens into the subclavian vein — called also *external jugular vein* **c** : a vein that commences near the hyoid bone and joins the terminal part of the external jugular vein or the subclavian vein — called also *anterior jugular vein*

juice \'jüs\ *n* : a natural bodily fluid (as blood, lymph, or a secretion) — see GASTRIC JUICE, PANCREATIC JUICE

junc·tion \'jəŋk-shən\ *n* : a place or point of meeting — see NEUROMUSCULAR JUNCTION — **junc·tion·al** \-shə-nəl\ *adj*

junctional nevus *n* : a nevus that develops at the junction of the dermis and epidermis and is potentially cancerous

junctional rhythm *n* : a cardiac rhythm resulting from impulses coming from a locus of tissue in the area of the atrioventricular node

junctional tachycardia *n* : tachycardia associated with the generation of impulses in a locus in the region of the atrioventricular node

Jung·ian \'yuŋ-ē-ən\ *adj* : of, relating to, or characteristic of C. G. Jung or his psychological doctrines which stress the opposition of introversion and extroversion and the concept of mythology and cultural and racial inheritance in the psychology of individuals — **Jungian** *n*

Jung \'yuŋ\, **Carl Gustav** (1875–1961), Swiss psychologist and psychiatrist.

jungle fever *n* : a severe form of malaria or yellow fever — compare JUNGLE YELLOW FEVER

jungle rot *n* : any of various esp. pyogenic skin infections contracted in tropical environments

jungle yellow fever *n* : yellow fever endemic in or near forest or jungle areas in Africa and So. America and transmitted by mosquitoes (esp. genus *Haemagogus*) other than members of the genus *Aedes*

ju·ni·per \'jü-nə-pər\ *n* : an evergreen shrub or tree (genus *Juniperus*) of the cypress family (Cupressaceae)

juniper tar *n* : a dark tarry liquid used locally in treating skin diseases and obtained by distillation from the wood of a Eurasian juniper (*Juniperus oxycedrus*) — called also *cade oil, juniper tar oil*

just noticeable difference *n* : the minimum amount of change in a physical stimulus required for a subject to detect reliably a difference in the level of stimulation

jus·to ma·jor \'jəs-tō-'mā-jər\ *adj*, *of pelvic dimensions* : greater than normal

justo mi·nor \-'mī-nər\ *adj*, *of pelvic dimensions* : smaller than normal

ju·ve·nile \'jü-və-ˌnīl, -nəl\ *adj* **1** : physiologically immature or undeveloped **2** : reflecting psychological or intellectual immaturity — **juvenile** *n*

juvenile amaurotic idiocy *n* : SPIELMEYER-VOGT DISEASE

juvenile delinquency *n* **1** : conduct by a juvenile characterized by antisocial behavior that is beyond parental control and therefore subject to legal action **2** : a violation of the law committed by a juvenile and not punishable by death or life imprisonment — **juvenile delinquent** *n*

juvenile diabetes *n* : INSULIN-DEPENDENT DIABETES MELLITUS

juvenile–onset diabetes *n* : INSULIN-DEPENDENT DIABETES MELLITUS

juxta- *comb form* : situated near (*juxtaglomerular*)

jux·ta–ar·tic·u·lar \ˌjək-stə-är-'ti-kyə-lər\ *adj* : situated near a joint

jux·ta·glo·mer·u·lar \-glō-'mer-yə-lər, -glō-, -ə-lər\ *adj* : situated near a kidney glomerulus

juxtaglomerular apparatus *n* : a functional unit near a kidney glomerulus that controls renin release and is composed of juxtaglomerular cells and a macula densa

juxtaglomerular cell *n* : any of a group of cells that are situated in the wall of each afferent arteriole of a kidney glomerulus near its point of entry adjacent to a macula densa and that produce and secrete renin

jux·ta·med·ul·lary \ˌjək-stə-'med-əl-ˌer-ē, -'mej-əl-; -mə-'də-lə-rē\ *adj* : situated or occurring near the edge of the medulla of the kidney

K

K *symbol* [New Latin *kalium*] potassium

Kahn test \'kän-\ *n* : a serum-precipitation reaction for the diagnosis of syphilis — called also *Kahn, Kahn reaction*

Kahn, Reuben Leon (*b* 1887), American immunologist.

kai·nic acid \'kī-nik-, 'kā-\ *n* : the neurotoxic active principle $C_{10}H_{15}NO_4$ from a dried red alga (*Digenia simplex*) used as an ascaricide

kala–azar \'kä-lə-ə-'zär, 'ka-\ *n* : a severe infectious disease chiefly of Asia marked by fever, progressive anemia, leukopenia, and enlargement of the spleen and liver and caused by a flagellate of the genus *Leishmania* (*L. donovani*) that is transmitted by the bite of sand flies and proliferates in reticuloendothelial cells — called also *dumdum fever*; see LEISHMAN-DONOVAN BODY

ka·li·ure·sis \ˌkä-lē-yü-'rē-səs, ˌka-\ *n*, *pl* **-ure·ses** \-ˌsēz\ : excretion of potassium in the urine esp. in excessive amounts — **ka·li·uret·ic** \-'re-tik\ *adj*

kal·li·din \'ka-lə-din\ *n* : either of two

vasodilator kinins formed from blood plasma globulin by the action of kallikrein

kal·li·kre·in \ˌka-lə-ˈkrē-ən, kə-ˈli-krē-ən\ *n* : a hypotensive proteinase that liberates kinins from blood plasma proteins and is used therapeutically for vasodilation

Kall·mann's syndrome \ˈköl-mənz-\ : a hereditary condition marked by hypogonadism caused by a deficiency of gonadotropins and anosmia caused by failure of the olfactory lobes to develop

Kallmann, Franz Josef (1897–1965), American geneticist and psychiatrist.

kal·ure·sis \ˌkā-lü-ˈrē-səs, ˌka-, -lyü-\ *var of* KALIURESIS

ka·ma·la \ˈkä-mə-lə\ *n* : an orange red cathartic powder derived from the fruit of an East Indian tree (*Mallotus philippinensis*) of the spurge family (Euphorbiaceae) and used as a vermifuge chiefly in veterinary practice

kana·my·cin \ˌka-nə-ˈmīs-ən\ *n* : a broad-spectrum antibiotic from a Japanese soil bacterium of the genus *Streptomyces* (*S. kanamyceticus*)

Kan·ner's syndrome \ˈka-nərz-\ *n* : INFANTILE AUTISM

Kanner, Leo (1894–1981), American psychiatrist.

Kan·trex \ˈkan-ˌtreks\ *trademark* — used for a preparation of kanamycin

ka·olin \ˈkā-ə-lin\ *n* : a fine usu. white clay that is used in medicine esp. as an adsorbent in the treatment of diarrhea (as in food poisoning or dysentery)

Kao·pec·tate \ˌkā-ō-ˈpek-ˌtāt\ *trademark* — used for a preparation of kaolin used as an antidiarrheal

Ka·po·si's sarcoma \ˈka-pə-zēz-, kə-ˈpō-, -sēz-\ *n* : a neoplastic disease affecting esp. the skin and mucous membranes, characterized usu. by the formation of pink to reddish-brown or bluish tumorous plaques, macules, papules, or nodules esp. on the lower extremities, and formerly limited primarily to elderly men in whom it followed a benign course but now being a major and sometimes fatal disease associated with immunodeficient individuals with AIDS — abbr. *KS*

Kaposi \ˈkô-pō-sē\, **Moritz (1837–1902),** Hungarian dermatologist.

kap·pa chain *or* **κ chain** \ˈka-pə-\ *n* : a polypeptide chain of one of the two types of light chain that are found in antibodies and can be distinguished antigenically and by the sequence of amino acids in the chain — compare LAMBDA CHAIN

ka·ra·ya gum \kə-ˈrī-ə-\ *n* : any of several laxative vegetable gums obtained from tropical Asian trees (genera *Sterculia* of the family Sterculiaceae and *Cochlospermum* of the family Bixaceae) — called also *gum karaya, karaya, sterculia gum*

ka·rez·za \kä-ˈret-sə\ *n* : COITUS RESERVATUS

Kar·ta·ge·ner's syndrome \kär-ˈtä-gə-nərz-, ˌkär-tə-ˈgä-nərz-\ *n* : an abnormal condition inherited as an autosomal recessive trait and characterized by situs inversus, abnormalities in the protein structure of cilia, and chronic bronchiectasis and sinusitis

Kartagener, Manes (*b* 1897), Swiss physician.

kary- *or* **karyo-** *also* **cary-** *or* **caryo-** *comb form* : nucleus of a cell ⟨*karyokinesis*⟩ ⟨*caryokinesis*⟩

kary·og·a·my \ˌkar-ē-ˈä-gə-mē\ *n, pl* **-mies** : the fusion of cell nuclei (as in fertilization)

karyo·gram \ˈkar-ē-ō-ˌgram\ *n* : KARYOTYPE; *esp* : a diagrammatic representation of the chromosome complement of an organism

karyo·ki·ne·sis \ˌkar-ē-ō-kə-ˈnē-səs, -kī-\ *n, pl* **-ne·ses** \-ˌsēz\ **1** : the nuclear phenomena characteristic of mitosis **2** : the whole process of mitosis — compare CYTOKINESIS — **karyo·ki·net·ic** \-ˈne-tik\ *adj*

kary·ol·o·gy \ˌkar-ē-ˈä-lə-jē\ *n, pl* **-gies** **1** : the minute cytological characteristics of the cell nucleus esp. with regard to the chromosomes of a single cell or of the cells of an organism or group of organisms **2** : a branch of cytology concerned with the karyology of cell nuclei — **karyo·log·i·cal** \-ē-ə-ˈlä-ji-kəl\ *also* **karyo·log·ic** \-jik\ *adj* — **karyo·log·i·cal·ly** *adv*

karyo·lymph \ˈkar-ē-ō-ˌlimf\ *n* : NUCLEAR SAP

kary·ol·y·sis \ˌkar-ē-ˈä-lə-səs\ *n, pl* **-y·ses** \-ˌsēz\ : dissolution of the cell nucleus with loss of its affinity for basic stains sometimes occurring normally but usu. in necrosis — compare KARYORRHEXIS

karyo·plasm \ˈkar-ē-ō-ˌpla-zəm\ *n* : NUCLEOPLASM

karyo·pyk·no·sis \ˌkar-ē-(ˌ)ō-pik-ˈnō-səs\ *n* : shrinkage of the cell nuclei of epithelial cells (as of the vagina) with breakup of the chromatin into unstructured granules — **karyo·pyk·not·ic** \-ˈnä-tik\ *adj*

karyopyknotic index *n* : an index that is calculated as the percentage of epithelial cells with karyopyknotic nuclei exfoliated from the vagina and is used in the hormonal evaluation of a patient

kary·or·rhex·is \ˌkar-ē-ō-ˈrek-səs\ *n, pl* **-rhex·es** \-ˌsēz\ : a degenerative cellular process involving fragmentation of the nucleus and the breakup of the chromatin into unstructured granules — compare KARYOLYSIS

karyo·some \ˈkar-ē-ə-ˌsōm\ *n* : a mass of chromatin in a cell nucleus that resembles a nucleolus

¹karyo·type \ˈkar-ē-ə-ˌtīp\ *n* : the chromosomal characteristics of a cell; *also* : the chromosomes themselves or a representation of them — **karyo-typ·ic** \,kar-ē-ə-'ti-pik\ *adj* — **karyo-typ·i·cal·ly** *adv*

²**karyotype** *vb* **-typed; -typ·ing** : to determine the karyotype of

karyo-typ·ing \-,tīp-iŋ\ *n* : the action or process of studying karyotypes or of making representations of them

Ka·ta·ya·ma \,kä-tə-'yä-mə\ *n* : a genus of Asian freshwater snails (family Bulimidae) including important intermediate hosts of human trematode worms of the genus *Schistosoma* (as *S. japonicum*)

Ka·wa·sa·ki disease \,kä-wə-'sä-kē-\ *n* : an acute febrile disease affecting young children that is characterized by erythema of the conjunctivae and of the mucous membranes of the upper respiratory tract, erythema and edema of the hands and feet, a rash followed by desquamation, and cervical lymphadenopathy — called also *Kawasaki syndrome, mucocutaneous lymph node disease, mucocutaneous lymph node syndrome*

Kawasaki, Tomisaku (*fl* 1961), Japanese pediatrician.

Kay·ser–Fleis·cher ring \'kī-zər-'flī-shər-\ *n* : a brown or greenish brown ring of copper deposits around the cornea that is characteristic of Wilson's disease

Kayser, Bernhard (1869–1954) and **Fleischer, Bruno Otto (*b* 1874),** German ophthalmologists.

kb *abbr* kilobase

ked \'ked\ *n* : SHEEP KED

Ke·gel exercises \'kā-gəl-, 'kē-\ *n pl* : repetitive contractions by a woman of the muscles that are used to stop the urinary flow in urination in order to increase the tone of the pubococcygeal muscle esp. to control incontinence or to enhance sexual responsiveness during intercourse

Kegel, Arnold Henry (*b* 1894), American physician.

Kell \'kel\ *adj* : of, relating to, or being a group of allelic red-blood-cell antigens of which some are important causes of transfusion reactions and some forms of erythroblastosis fetalis

Kell, medical patient.

Kel·ler \'ke-lər\ *adj* : relating to or being an operation to correct hallux valgus by excision of the proximal part of the proximal phalanx of the big toe with resulting shortening of the toe

Keller, William Lorden (1874–1959), American surgeon.

ke·loid \'kē-,lȯid\ *n* : a thick scar resulting from excessive growth of fibrous tissue and occurring esp. after burns or radiation injury — **keloid** *adj* — **ke·loi·dal** \kē-'lȯid-ᵊl\ *adj*

kelp \'kelp\ *n* : any of various seaweeds that are large brown algae (orders Laminariales and Fucales) and esp. laminarias

kel·vin \'kel-vin\ *n* : a unit of temperature equal to $\frac{1}{273.16}$ of the Kelvin scale temperature of the triple point of water and equal to the Celsius degree

Thom·son \'täm-sən\, **Sir William (1st Baron Kelvin of Largs) (1824–1907),** British physicist.

Kelvin *adj* : relating to, conforming to, or being a temperature scale according to which absolute zero is 0 K, the equivalent of −273.15°C

Ken·a·cort \'ke-nə-,kȯrt\ *trademark* — used for a preparation of triamcinolone

kennel cough *n* : tracheobronchitis of dogs or cats

Ken·ny method \'ke-nē-\ *n* : a method of treating poliomyelitis consisting basically of application of hot fomentations and rehabilitation of muscular activity by passive movement and then guided active coordination — called also *Kenny treatment*

Kenny, Elizabeth (1880–1952), Australian nurse.

ker·a·sin \'ker-ə-sən\ *n* : a cerebroside $C_{48}H_{93}NO_8$ that occurs esp. in Gaucher's disease

keratan sulfate \'ker-ə-,tan-\ *n* : any of several sulfated glycosaminoglycans that have been found esp. in the cornea, cartilage, and bone

ker·a·tec·to·my \,ker-ə-'tek-tə-mē\ *n, pl* **-mies** : surgical excision of part of the cornea

ke·rat·ic precipitates \kə-'ra-tik-\ *n pl* : accumulations on the posterior surface of the cornea esp. of macrophages and epithelial cells that occur in chronic inflammatory conditions — called also *keratitis punctata*

ker·a·tin \'ker-ət-ᵊn\ *n* : any of various sulfur-containing fibrous proteins that form the chemical basis of horny epidermal tissues (as hair and nails)

ke·ra·ti·ni·za·tion \,ker-ə-tə-nə-'zā-shən, kə-,rat-ᵊn-ə-\ *n* : conversion into keratin or keratinous tissue — **ke·ra·ti·nize** \'ker-ə-tə-,nīz, kə-'rat-ᵊn-,īz\ *vb*

ke·ra·ti·no·cyte \kə-'rat-ᵊn-ə-,sīt, ,ker-ə-'ti-nə-\ *n* : an epidermal cell that produces keratin

ke·ra·ti·nous \kə-'rat-ᵊn-əs, ,ker-ə-'tī-nəs\ *adj* : composed of or containing keratin : HORNY

ker·a·ti·tis \,ker-ə-'tī-təs\ *n, pl* **-tit·i·des** \-'ti-tə-,dēz\ : inflammation of the cornea of the eye characterized by burning or smarting, blurring of vision, and sensitiveness to light and caused by infectious or noninfectious agents — compare KERATOCONJUNCTIVITIS

keratitis punc·ta·ta \-pəŋk-'tä-tə, -'tā-\ *n* : KERATIC PRECIPITATES

ker·a·to·ac·an·tho·ma \,ker-ə-tō-,a-,kan-'thō-mə\ *n, pl* **-mas** *or* **-ma·ta**

\-mə-tə\ : a rapidly growing skin tumor that occurs esp. in elderly individuals, resembles a carcinoma of squamous epithelial cells but does not spread, and tends to heal spontaneously with some scarring if left untreated

ker·a·to·con·junc·ti·vi·tis \'ker-ə-(ˌ)tō-kən-ˌjəŋk-tə-'vī-təs\ n : combined inflammation of the cornea and conjunctiva; *esp* : EPIDEMIC KERATOCONJUNCTIVITIS — compare KERATITIS

keratoconjunctivitis sic·ca \-'si-kə\ n : a condition associated with reduction in lacrimal secretion and marked by redness of the conjunctiva, by itching and burning of the eye, and usu. by filaments of desquamated epithelial cells adhering to the cornea

ker·a·to·co·nus \ˌker-ə-tō-'kō-nəs\ n : cone-shaped protrusion of the cornea

ker·a·to·der·ma \-'dər-mə\ n : a horny condition of the skin

keratoderma blen·nor·rhag·i·cum \-ˌble-nō-'ra-ji-kəm\ n : KERATOSIS BLENNORRHAGICA

ker·a·to·der·mia \ˌker-ə-tō-'dər-mē-ə\ n : KERATODERMA

ker·a·to·hy·a·lin \-'hī-ə-lən\ also **ker·a·to·hy·a·line** \-lən, -ˌlēn\ n : a colorless translucent protein that occurs esp. in granules of the stratum granulosum of the epidermis

ker·a·tol·y·sis \ˌker-ə-'tä-lə-səs\ n, pl **-y·ses** \-ˌsēz\ : 1 : the process of breaking down or dissolving keratin 2 : a skin disease marked by peeling of the horny layer of the epidermis

¹ker·a·to·lyt·ic \ˌker-ə-tō-'li-tik\ adj : relating to or causing keratolysis

²keratolytic n : a keratolytic agent

ker·a·to·ma·la·cia \ˌker-ə-tō-mə-'lā-shə, -sē-ə\ n : a softening and ulceration of the cornea of the eye resulting from severe systemic deficiency of vitamin A — compare XEROPHTHALMIA

ker·a·tome \'ker-ə-ˌtōm\ n : a surgical instrument used for making an incision in the cornea in cataract operations

ker·a·tom·e·ter \ˌker-ə-'tä-mə-tər\ n : an instrument for measuring the curvature of the cornea

ker·a·tom·e·try \ˌker-ə-'tä-mə-trē\ n, pl **-tries** : measurement of the form and curvature of the cornea — **ker·a·to·met·ric** \-tō-'me-trik\ adj

ker·a·to·mil·eu·sis \ˌker-ə-tō-mi-'lü-səs, -'lyü-\ n : keratoplasty in which a piece of the cornea is removed, frozen, shaped to correct refractive error, and reinserted

ker·a·top·a·thy \ˌker-ə-'tä-pə-thē\ n, pl **-thies** : any noninflammatory disease of the eye — see BAND KERATOPATHY

ker·a·to·pha·kia \ˌker-ə-tō-'fā-kē-ə\ n : keratoplasty in which corneal tissue from a donor is frozen, shaped, and

inserted into the cornea of a recipient

ker·a·to·plas·ty \'ker-ə-tō-ˌplas-tē\ n, pl **-ties** : plastic surgery on the cornea; *esp* : corneal grafting

ker·a·to·pros·the·sis \ˌker-ə-tō-präs-'thē-səs, -ˌpräs-thə-\ n, pl **-theses** \-ˌsēz\ : a plastic replacement for an opacified inner part of a cornea

ker·a·to·scope \'ker-ə-tō-ˌskōp\ n : an instrument for examining the cornea esp. to detect irregularities of its anterior surface

ker·a·to·sis \ˌker-ə-'tō-səs\ n, pl **-to·ses** \-ˌsēz\ 1 : a disease of the skin marked by overgrowth of horny tissue 2 : an area of the skin affected with keratosis — **ker·a·tot·ic** \-'tä-tik\ adj

keratosis blen·nor·rhag·i·ca \-ˌble-nō-'ra-ji-kə\ n : a disease that is characterized by a scaly rash esp. on the palms and soles and is associated esp. with Reiter's syndrome — called also *keratoderma blennorrhagicum*

keratosis fol·li·cu·lar·is \-ˌfä-lə-kyə-'ler-əs\ n : DARIER'S DISEASE

keratosis pi·la·ris \-pi-'ler-əs\ n : a condition marked by the formation of hard conical elevations in the openings of the sebaceous glands esp. of the thighs and arms that resemble permanent goose bumps

ker·a·tot·o·mist \ˌker-ə-'tä-tə-mist\ n : a surgeon who performs keratotomies

ker·a·tot·o·my \-mē\ n, pl **-mies** : incision of the cornea

ke·ri·on \'kir-ē-ˌän\ n : inflammatory ringworm of the hair follicles of the beard and scalp usu. accompanied by secondary bacterial infection

ker·nic·ter·us \kər-'nik-tə-rəs\ n : a condition marked by the deposit of bile pigments in the nuclei of the brain and spinal cord and by degeneration of nerve cells that occurs usu. in infants as a part of the syndrome of erythroblastosis fetalis — **ker·nic·ter·ic** \-rik\ adj

Ker·nig sign \'ker-nig-\ or **Kernig's sign** \'ker-nigz-\ n : an indication usu. present in meningitis that consists of pain and resistance on attempting to extend the leg at the knee with the thigh flexed at the hip

Kernig, Vladimir Mikhailovich (1840–1917), Russian physician.

ke·ta·mine \'kē-tə-ˌmēn\ n : a general anesthetic that is administered intravenously and intramuscularly in the form of its hydrochloride $C_{13}H_{16}$-ClNO·HCl

ke·thox·al \kē-'thäk-səl\ n : an antiviral agent $C_6H_{12}O_4$

ke·to \'kē-(ˌ)tō\ adj : of or relating to a ketone; *also* : containing a ketone group

keto acid n : a compound that is both a ketone and an acid

ke·to·ac·i·do·sis \ˌkē-tō-ˌa-sə-'dō-səs\ n, pl **-do·ses** \-ˌsēz\ : acidosis accompanied by ketosis ⟨diabetic ∼⟩

ke·to·co·na·zole \ˌkē-tō-ˈkō-nə-ˌzōl\ *n* : a broad-spectrum antifungal agent used to treat chronic internal and cutaneous disorders

ke·to·gen·e·sis \ˌkē-tō-ˈje-nə-səs\ *n, pl* **-e·ses** \-ˌsēz\ : the production of ketone bodies (as in diabetes) — **ke·to·gen·ic** \-ˈjen-ik\ *adj*

ketogenic diet *n* : a diet supplying a large amount of fat and minimal amounts of carbohydrate and protein

ke·to·glu·tar·ic acid \ˌkē-tō-glü-ˈtar-ik-\ *n* : either of two crystalline keto derivatives $C_5H_6O_5$ of glutaric acid; *esp* : ALPHA-KETOGLUTARIC ACID

α–**ketoglutaric acid** *var of* ALPHA–KETOGLUTARIC ACID

ke·to·nae·mia *chiefly Brit var of* KETONEMIA

ke·tone \ˈkē-ˌtōn\ *n* : an organic compound (as acetone) with a CO group attached to two carbon atoms

ketone body *n* : any of the three compounds acetoacetic acid, acetone, and hydroxybutyric acid which are normal intermediates in lipid metabolism and accumulate in the blood and urine in abnormal amounts in conditions of impaired metabolism (as in diabetes mellitus) — called also *acetone body*

ke·to·ne·mia \ˌkē-tə-ˈnē-mē-ə\ *n* **1** : a condition marked by an abnormal increase of ketone bodies in the circulating blood — called also *hyperketonemia* **2** : KETOSIS 2 — **ke·to·ne·mic** \-ˈnē-mik\ *adj*

ke·to·nuria \ˌkē-tə-ˈnür-ē-ə, -ˈnyür-\ *n* : the presence of excess ketone bodies in the urine in conditions (as diabetes mellitus and starvation acidosis) involving reduced or disturbed carbohydrate metabolism — called also *acetonuria*

ke·tose \ˈkē-ˌtōs, -ˌtōz\ *n* : a sugar (as fructose) containing one ketone group per molecule

ke·to·sis \kē-ˈtō-səs\ *n, pl* **-to·ses** \-ˌsēz\ **1** : an abnormal increase of ketone bodies in the body in conditions of reduced or disturbed carbohydrate metabolism (as in uncontrolled diabetes mellitus) — compare ACIDOSIS, ALKALOSIS **2** : a nutritional disease esp. of cattle that is marked by reduction of blood sugar and the presence of ketone bodies in the blood, tissues, milk, and urine — **ke·tot·ic** \-ˈtä-tik\ *adj*

ke·to·ste·roid \ˌkē-tō-ˈstir-ˌoid, -ˈster-\ *n* : a steroid (as cortisone or estrone) containing a ketone group; *esp* : 17–KETOSTEROID

17–ketosteroid *n* : any of the ketosteroids (as androsterone, dehydroepiandrosterone, and estrone) that have the keto group attached to carbon atom 17 of the steroid ring structure, are present in normal human urine, and may be an indication of a tumor of the adrenal cortex or ovary when present in excess

Ke·ty method \ˈkē-tē-\ *n* : a method of determining coronary blood flow by measurement of nitrous oxide levels in the blood of a patient breathing nitrous oxide

Kety, Seymour Solomon (*b* 1915), American physiologist.

kg *abbr* kilogram

khel·lin \ˈke-lən\ *n* : a crystalline compound $C_{14}H_{12}O_5$ obtained from the fruit of a Middle Eastern plant (*Ammi visnaga*) of the carrot family (Umbelliferae) and used esp. as a coronary vasodilator

kid·ney \ˈkid-nē\ *n, pl* **kidneys** : one of a pair of vertebrate organs situated in the body cavity near the spinal column that excrete waste products of metabolism, in humans are bean-shaped organs about 4½ inches (11½ centimeters) long lying behind the peritoneum in a mass of fatty tissue, and consist chiefly of nephrons by which urine is secreted, collected, and discharged into the pelvis of the kidney whence it is conveyed by the ureter to the bladder — compare MESONEPHROS, METANEPHROS, PRONEPHROS

kidney stone *n* : a calculus in the kidney — called also *renal calculus*

kidney worm *n* : any of several nematode worms parasitic in the kidneys: as **a** : GIANT KIDNEY WORM **b** : a common worm of the genus *Stephanurus* (*S. dentatus*) that is related to the gapeworm and is parasitic in the kidneys, lungs, and other viscera of the hog in warm regions

Kien·böck's disease \ˈkēn-ˌbeks-\ *n* : osteochondrosis affecting the lunate bone

Kien·böck, \ˈkēn-ˌbœk\, **Robert** (1871–1953), Austrian roentgenologist.

killer bee *n* : AFRICANIZED BEE

killer cell *n* : a T cell that functions in cell-mediated immunity by destroying a cell (as a tumor cell) having a specific antigenic molecule on its surface by causing lysis of the cell or by releasing a nonspecific toxin — called also *killer T cell*

ki·lo·base \ˈki-lə-ˌbās\ *n* : a unit of measure of the length of a nucleic-acid chain (as of DNA or RNA) that equals one thousand base pairs

ki·lo·cal·o·rie \ˌka-lə-rē\ *n* : CALORIE 1b

ki·lo·gram \ˈki-lə-ˌgram, ˈkē-\ *n* **1** : the basic metric unit of mass and weight that is nearly equal to 1000 cubic centimeters of water at its maximum density **2** : the weight of a kilogram mass under earth's gravity

kilogram calorie *n* : CALORIE 1b

ki·lo·joule \ˈki-lə-ˌjül\ *n* : 1000 joules

ki·lo·me·ter \ˈki-lə-ˌmē-tər, kə-ˈlä-mə-tər\ *n* : 1000 meters

ki·lo·rad \ˈki-lə-ˌrad\ *n* : 1000 rads

ki·lo·volt \-ˌvōlt\ *n* : a unit of potential difference equal to 1000 volts

kin- *or* **kine-** *or* **kino-** *or* **cin-** *or* **cino-** *comb form* : motion : action ⟨kinesthesia⟩

kin·aes·the·sia *chiefly Brit var of* KINESTHESIA

ki·nase \ˈkī-ˌnās, -ˌnāz\ *n* : an enzyme that catalyzes the transfer of phosphate groups from a high-energy phosphate-containing molecule (as ATP or ADP) to a substrate — called also *phosphokinase*

ki·ne·mat·ics \ˌki-nə-ˈma-tiks, ˌkī-\ *n* 1 : a science that deals with aspects of motion apart from considerations of mass and force 2 : the properties and phenomena of an object or system in motion of interest to kinematics ⟨the ∼ of the human ankle joint⟩ — **ki·ne·mat·ic** \-tik\ *or* **ki·ne·mat·i·cal** \-ti-kəl\ *adj*

ki·ne·plas·ty \ˈkī-nə-ˌplas-tē, ˈkī-\ *var of* CINEPLASTY

kinesi- *or* **kinesio-** *comb form* : movement ⟨kinesiology⟩

-ki·ne·sia \kə-ˈnē-zhə, kī-, -zhē-ə\ *comb form* : movement : motion ⟨hyperkinesia⟩

ki·ne·si·ol·o·gy \kə-ˌnē-sē-ˈä-lə-jē, kī-, -zē-\ *n, pl* **-gies** : the study of the principles of mechanics and anatomy in relation to human movement — **ki·ne·si·o·log·ic** \-ō-ˈlä-jik\ *or* **ki·ne·si·o·log·i·cal** \-ji-kəl\ *adj* — **ki·ne·si·ol·o·gist** \kə-ˌnē-sē-ˈä-lə-jist, kī-, -zē-\ *n*

ki·ne·sis \kə-ˈnē-səs, kī-\ *n, pl* **ki·ne·ses** \-ˌsēz\ : a movement that lacks directional orientation and depends upon the intensity of stimulation

-ki·ne·sis \kə-ˈnē-sis, kī-\ *n, pl* **-ki·ne·ses** \-ˌsēz\ 1 : division ⟨karyokinesis⟩ 2 : production of motion ⟨psychokinesis⟩ ⟨telekinesis⟩

kin·es·the·sia \ˌkin-əs-ˈthē-zhə, ˌkī-, -zhē-ə\ *or* **kin·es·the·sis** \-ˈthē-səs\ *n, pl* **-the·sias** *or* **-the·ses** \-ˌsēz\ : a sense mediated by end organs located in muscles, tendons, and joints and stimulated by bodily movements and tensions; *also* : sensory experience derived from this sense — see MUSCLE SENSE — **kin·es·thet·ic** \-ˈthe-tik\ *adj* — **kin·es·thet·i·cal·ly** *adv*

kinet- *or* **kineto-** *comb form* : movement : motion ⟨kinetochore⟩

ki·net·ic \kə-ˈne-tik, kī-\ *adj* : of or relating to the motion of material bodies and the forces and energy associated therewith — **ki·net·i·cal·ly** *adv*

ki·net·ics \kə-ˈne-tiks, kī-\ *n sing or pl* 1 **a** : a science that deals with the effects of forces upon the motions of material bodies or with changes in a physical or chemical system **b** : the rate of change in such a system 2 : the mechanism by which a physical or chemical change is effected

ki·net·o·chore \kə-ˈne-tə-ˌkōr, kī-\ *n* : CENTROMERE

king co·bra \-ˈkō-brə\ *n* : a large cobra (*Ophiophagus hannah*) of southeastern Asia and the Philippines — called also *hamadryad*

king·dom \ˈkiŋ-dəm\ *n* : any of the three primary divisions of lifeless material, plants, and animals into which natural objects are grouped; *also* : a biological category (as Protista) that ranks above the phylum

king's evil *n, often cap K & E* : SCROFULA

ki·nin \ˈkī-nən\ *n* : any of various polypeptide hormones that are formed locally in the tissues and cause dilation of blood vessels and contraction of smooth muscle

ki·nin·ase \ˈkī-nə-ˌnās, -ˌnāz\ *n* : an enzyme in blood that destroys a kinin

ki·nin·o·gen \kī-ˈni-nə-jən\ *n* : an inactive precursor of a kinin — **ki·nin·o·gen·ic** \ˌkī-ˌni-nə-ˈje-nik\ *adj*

kino- — see KIN-

ki·no·cil·i·um \ˌkī-nō-ˈsi-lē-əm\ *n, pl* **-cil·ia** \-lē-ə\ : a motile cilium; *esp* : one that occurs alone at the end of a sensory hair cell of the inner ear among numerous nonmotile stereocilia

Kirsch·ner wire \ˈkərsh-nər-\ *n* : metal wire inserted through bone and used to achieve internal traction or immobilization of bone fractures

   Kirschner, Martin (1879–1942), German surgeon.

kissing bug *n* : CONENOSE

kissing disease *n* : INFECTIOUS MONONUCLEOSIS

kiss of life *n, chiefly Brit* : artificial respiration by the mouth-to-mouth method

kleb·si·el·la \ˌkleb-zē-ˈe-lə\ *n* 1 *cap* : a genus of nonmotile gram-negative rod-shaped and frequently encapsulated bacteria (family Enterobacteriaceae) 2 : any bacterium of the genus *Klebsiella*

   Klebs \ˈkleps\, (Theodor Albrecht) Edwin (1834–1913), German bacteriologist.

Klebs-Löff·ler bacillus \ˈkleps-ˈlef-lər-, ˈklebz-\ *n* : a bacterium of the genus *Corynebacterium* (*C. diphtheriae*) that causes human diphtheria

   Löff·ler \ˈlœf-lər\, Friedrich August Johannes (1852–1915), German bacteriologist.

klee·blatt·schä·del \ˈklä-ˌblät-ˌshäd-əl\ *n* : CLOVERLEAF SKULL

Klein·ian \ˈklī-nē-ən\ *adj* : of, relating to, or according with the psychoanalytic theories or practices of Melanie Klein — **Kleinian** *n*

   Klein \ˈklīn\, Melanie (1882–1960), Austrian psychoanalyst.

klept- *or* **klepto-** *comb form* : stealing : theft ⟨kleptomania⟩

klep·to·lag·nia \ˌklep-tə-ˈlag-nē-ə\ *n* : sexual arousal and gratification produced by committing an act of theft

klep·to·ma·nia \ˌklep-tə-ˈmā-nē-ə, -nyə\ *n* : a persistent neurotic impulse to steal esp. without economic motive

klep·to·ma·ni·ac \-nē-ˌak\ *n* : an individual exhibiting kleptomania

Kline·fel·ter's syndrome \ˈklīn-ˌfel-tərz-\ *also* **Kline·fel·ter syndrome** \-tər-\ *n* : an abnormal condition in a male characterized by two X chromosomes and one Y chromosome, infertility, and smallness of the testicles

Klinefelter, Harry Fitch (*b* 1912), American physician.

Kline reaction \ˈklīn-\ *n* : KLINE TEST

Kline test *n* : a rapid precipitation test for the diagnosis of syphilis

Kline, Benjamin Schoenbrun (*b* 1886), American pathologist.

Klip·pel–Feil syndrome \kli-ˈpel-ˈfīl-\ *n* : congenital fusion of the cervical vertebrae resulting in a short and relatively immobile neck

Klip·pel \klē-ˈpel\, **Maurice (1858–1942)** and **Feil** \ˈfāl\, **André** (*b* 1884), French neurologists.

Klump·ke's paralysis \ˈklŭmp-kēz-\ *n* : atrophic paralysis of the forearm and the hand due to injury to the eighth cervical and first thoracic nerves

Dé·jé·rine–Klump·ke \dā-zhā-ˌrēn-klŭm-ˈkē\, **Augusta (1859–1927)**, French neurologist.

km *abbr* kilometer

knee \ˈnē\ *n* **1** : a joint in the middle part of the leg that is the articulation between the femur, tibia, and patella — called also *knee joint* **2** : the part of the leg that includes this joint — **kneed** \ˈnēd\ *adj*

knee·cap \ˈnē-ˌkap\ *n* : PATELLA

knee jerk *n* : an involuntary forward jerk or kick produced by a light blow or sudden strain upon the patellar ligament of the knee that causes a reflex contraction of the quadriceps muscle — called also *patellar reflex*

knee joint *n* : KNEE 1

Kne·mi·do·kop·tes \ˌnē-mə-dō-ˈkäp-(ˌ)tēz\ *n* : a genus of itch mites (family Sarcoptidae) that attack birds

knife \ˈnīf\ *n, pl* **knives** \ˈnīvz\ **1** : any of various instruments used in surgery primarily to sever tissues: as **a** : a cutting instrument consisting of a sharp blade attached to a handle **b** : an instrument that cuts by means of an electrical current **2** : SURGERY 3 — usu. used in the phrase *under the knife* (went under the ~ this morning)

knit \ˈnit\ *vb* **knit** *or* **knit·ted; knit·ting** : to grow or cause to grow together (a fracture that *knitted* slowly)

knock–knee \ˈnäk-ˌnē\ *n* : a condition in which the legs curve inward at the knees — called also *genu valgum* — **knock–kneed** \-ˌnēd\ *adj*

knot \ˈnät\ *n* **1** : an interlacing of the parts of one or more flexible bodies (as threads or sutures) in a lump to prevent their spontaneous separation — see SURGEON'S KNOT **2** : a usu. firm or hard lump or swelling or protuberance in or on a part of the body or a bone or process — compare SURFER'S KNOT — **knot** *vb*

knuck·le \ˈnə-kəl\ *n* **1 a** : the rounded prominence formed by the ends of the two adjacent bones at a joint — used esp. of those at the joints of the fingers **b** : the joint of a knuckle **2** : a sharply flexed loop of intestines incarcerated in a hernia

Koch·er's forceps \ˈkō-kərz-\ *n* : a strong forceps for controlling bleeding in surgery having serrated blades with interlocking teeth at the tips

Kocher \ˈkō-kər\, **Emil Theodor (1841–1917)**, Swiss surgeon.

Koch's bacillus \ˈkōks-, ˈkä-chəz-\ *or* **Koch bacillus** \ˈkōk-, ˈkäch-\ *n* : a bacillus of the genus *Mycobacterium* (*M. tuberculosis*) that causes human tuberculosis

Koch \ˈkok\, **(Heinrich Hermann) Robert** (1843–1910), German bacteriologist.

Koch's postulates *n pl* : a statement of the steps required to establish a microorganism as the cause of a disease: (1) it must be found in all cases of the disease; (2) it must be isolated from the host and grown in pure culture; (3) it must reproduce the original disease when introduced into a susceptible host; (4) it must be found present in the experimental host so infected — called also *Koch's laws*

Koch–Weeks bacillus \-ˈwēks-\ *n* : a bacterium of the genus *Haemophilus* (*H. aegyptius*) associated with an infectious form of human conjunctivitis

Weeks, John Elmer (1853–1949), American ophthalmologist.

Koch–Weeks conjunctivitis *n* : conjunctivitis caused by the Koch–Weeks bacillus

koil·onych·ia \ˌkȯi-lō-ˈni-kē-ə\ *n* : abnormal thinness and concavity of fingernails occurring esp. in hypochromic anemias — called also *spoon nails*

Kop·lik's spots \ˈkä-pliks-\ *or* **Kop·lik spots** \-plik-\ *n pl* : small bluish white dots surrounded by a reddish zone that appear on the mucous membrane of the cheeks and lips before the appearance of the skin eruption in a case of measles

Koplik, Henry (1858–1927), American pediatrician.

Korean hemorrhagic fever *n* : a hemorrhagic fever that is endemic to Korea, Manchuria, and Siberia, is caused by a hantavirus, and is characterized by acute renal failure in addition to the usual symptoms of the hemorrhagic

Ko·rot·koff sounds *also* **Ko·rot·kow sounds** *or* **Ko·rot·kov sounds** \kō-ˈrȯt-kȯf-\ *n pl* : arterial sounds heard through a stethoscope applied to the brachial artery distal to the cuff of a sphygmomanometer that change with varying cuff pressure and that are used to determine systolic and diastolic blood pressure

Korotkoff, Nikolai Sergieyevich (*b* 1874), Russian physician.

Kor·sa·koff's psychosis \'kȯr-sə-ˌkȯfs-\ *n* : an abnormal mental condition that is usu. a sequel of chronic alcoholism, is often associated with polyneuritis, and is characterized by an impaired ability to acquire new information and by an irregular memory loss for which the patient often attempts to compensate through confabulation

Korsakoff (*or* **Korsakov), Sergei Sergeyevich (1853–1900),** Russian psychiatrist.

Korsakoff's syndrome *or* **Korsakoff syndrome** *n* : KORSAKOFF'S PSYCHOSIS

Kr *symbol* krypton

Krab·be's disease \'kra-bēz-\ *n* : a rapidly progressive demyelinating familial leukoencephalopathy with onset in infancy characterized by irritability followed by tonic convulsions, quadriplegia, blindness, deafness, dementia, and death

Krabbe \'krä-bə\, **Knud H. (1885–1961),** Danish neurologist.

krad \'kā-ˌrad\ *n, pl* **krad** *also* **krads** : KILORAD

krait \'krīt\ *n* : any of a genus (*Bungarus*) of brightly banded extremely venomous nocturnal elapid snakes of Pakistan, India, southeastern Asia, and adjacent islands

krau·ro·sis \krȯ-'rō-səs\ *n, pl* **-ro·ses** \-ˌsēz\ : atrophy and shriveling of the skin or mucous membrane esp. of the vulva where it is often a precancerous lesion — **krau·rot·ic** \-'rä-tik\ *adj*

kraurosis vul·vae \-'vəl-vē\ *n* : kraurosis of the vulva

Krau·se's corpuscle \'kraù-zəz-\ *n* : any of various rounded sensory end organs occurring in mucous membranes (as of the conjunctiva or genitals) — called also *corpuscle of Krause*

Krause, Wilhelm Johann Friedrich (1833–1910), German anatomist.

Krause's end–bulb *n* : KRAUSE'S CORPUSCLE

kre·bi·o·zen \krə-'bī-ə-zən\ *n* : a drug used in the treatment of cancer esp. in the 1950's that was of unproved effectiveness, is not now used in the U.S., and was of undisclosed formulation but was reported to contain creatine

Krebs cycle \'krebz-\ *n* : a sequence of reactions in the living organism in which oxidation of acetic acid or acetyl equivalent provides energy for storage in phosphate bonds (as in ATP) — called also *citric acid cycle, tricarboxylic acid cycle*

Krebs, Sir Hans Adolf (1900–1981), German-British biochemist.

Kru·ken·berg tumor \'krü-kən-ˌbərg-\

n : a metastatic ovarian tumor of mucin-producing epithelial cells usu. derived from a primary gastrointestinal tumor

Kru·ken·berg \-ˌberk\, **Friedrich Ernst (1871–1946),** German pathologist.

kryp·ton \'krip-ˌtän\ *n* : a colorless relatively inert gaseous element — symbol *Kr*; see ELEMENT table

KS *abbr* Kaposi's sarcoma

KUB *abbr* kidney, ureter, and bladder

Kupf·fer cell \'kùp-fər-\ *also* **Kupf·fer's cell** \-fərz-\ *n* : a fixed macrophage of the walls of the liver sinusoids that is stellate with a large oval nucleus and the cytoplasm commonly packed with fragments resulting from phagocytic action

Kupffer, Karl Wilhelm von (1829–1902), German anatomist.

ku·ru \'kü-ˌrü, 'kùr-ü\ *n* : a rare progressive fatal encephalopathy that is caused by a slow virus, resembles Creutzfeldt-Jakob disease, occurs among tribesmen in eastern New Guinea, and is characterized esp. by spongiform changes and proliferation of astrocytes in the brain — called also *laughing death, laughing sickness*

Kuss·maul breathing \'kùs-ˌmaùl-\ *n* : abnormally slow deep respiration characteristic of air hunger and occurring esp. in acidotic states — called also *Kussmaul respiration*

Kussmaul, Adolf (1822–1902), German physician.

Kveim test \'kvām-\ *n* : an intradermal test for sarcoidosis in which an antigen prepared from the lymph nodes or spleen of human sarcoidosis patients is injected intracutaneously and which is positive when an infiltrated area, papule, nodule, or superficial necrosis appears around the site of injection or a skin biopsy yields typical tubercles and giant cell formations upon histological examination

Kveim, Morten Ansgar (*b* 1892), Norwegian physician.

kwa·shi·or·kor \ˌkwä-shē-'ȯr-kȯr, -ȯr-ˈkȯr\ *n* : severe malnutrition in infants and children that is characterized by failure to grow and develop, changes in the pigmentation of the skin and hair, edema, fatty degeneration of the liver, anemia, and apathy and is caused by a diet excessively high in carbohydrate and extremely low in protein — compare PELLAGRA

Kwell \'kwel\ *trademark* — used for a preparation of lindane

Kya·sa·nur For·est disease \ˌkya-sə-ˈnùr-'fȯr-əst-\ *n* : a disease caused by a flavivirus that is characterized by fever, headache, diarrhea, and intestinal bleeding and is transmitted by immature ticks of the genus *Haemaphysalis*

ky·mo·gram \'kī-mə-ˌgram\ *n* : a record made by a kymograph

ky·mo·graph \-ˌgraf\ *n* : a device which graphically records motion or pressure; *esp* : a recording device including an electric motor or clockwork that drives a usu. slowly revolving drum which carries a roll of plain or smoked paper and also having an arrangement for tracing on the paper by means of a stylus a graphic record of motion or pressure (as of the organs of speech, blood pressure, or respiration) often in relation to particular intervals of time — **ky·mo·graph·ic** \ˌkī-mə-ˈgra-fik\ *adj* — **ky·mog·ra·phy** \kī-ˈmä-grə-fē\ *n*

ky·pho·sco·li·o·sis \ˌkī-fō-ˌskō-lē-ˈō-səs\ *n, pl* **-o·ses** \-ˌsēz\ : backward and lateral curvature of the spine

ky·pho·sis \kī-ˈfō-səs\ *n, pl* **-pho·ses** \-ˌsēz\ : exaggerated backward curvature of the thoracic region of the spinal column — compare LORDOSIS, SCOLIOSIS — **ky·phot·ic** \-ˈfä-tik\ *adj*

L

L *abbr* lumbar — used esp. with a number from 1 to 5 to indicate a vertebra or segment of the spinal cord in the lumbar region

l- *prefix* **1** \ˈlē-(ˌ)vō, ˌel, ˈel\ : levorotatory (*l*-tartaric acid) **2** \ˌel, ˈel\ : having a similar configuration at a selected carbon atom to the configuration of levorotatory glyceraldehyde — usu. printed as a small capital (L-fructose)

La *symbol* lanthanum

lab \'lab\ *n* : LABORATORY

¹la·bel \'lā-bəl\ *n* : material used in isotopic labeling

²label *vb* **la·beled** *or* **la·belled**; **la·bel·ing** *or* **la·bel·ling 1** : to distinguish (an element or atom) by using a radioactive isotope or an isotope of unusual mass for tracing through chemical reactions or biological processes **2** : to distinguish (as a compound or cell) by introducing a traceable constituent (as a dye or labeled atom)

la·bet·a·lol \lə-ˈbe-tə-ˌlȯl, -ˌlōl\ *n* : a beta-adrenergic blocking agent used as the hydrochloride $C_{19}H_{24}O_3 \cdot HCl$

labia *pl of* LABIUM

la·bi·al \'lā-bē-əl\ *adj* : of, relating to, or situated near the lips or labia — **la·bi·al·ly** *adv*

labial artery *n* : either of two branches of the facial artery of which one is distributed to the upper and one to the lower lip

labial gland *n* : one of the small tubular mucous and serous glands lying beneath the mucous membrane of the lips

labialis — see HERPES LABIALIS

la·bia ma·jo·ra \'lā-bē-ə-mə-ˈjōr-ə\ *n pl* : the outer fatty folds of the vulva bounding the vestibule

labia mi·no·ra \-mə-ˈnōr-ə\ *n pl* : the inner highly vascular largely connective-tissue folds of the vulva bounding the vestibule — called also *nymphae*

labii — see LEVATOR LABII SUPERIORIS, LEVATOR LABII SUPERIORIS ALAEQUE NASI, QUADRATUS LABII SUPERIORIS

la·bile \'lā-ˌbil, -bəl\ *adj* : readily or frequently changing: as **a** : readily or continually undergoing chemical, physical, or biological change or breakdown **b** : characterized by wide fluctuations (as in blood pressure or glucose tolerance) (~ hypertension) **c** : emotionally unstable — **la·bil·i·ty** \lā-ˈbi-lə-tē\ *n*

labile factor *n* : FACTOR V

labio- *comb form* : labial and (*labio*lingual)

la·bio·buc·cal \ˌlā-bē-ō-ˈbə-kəl\ *adj* : of, relating to, or lying against the inner surface of the lips and cheeks; *also* : administered to labio-buccal tissue

la·bio·glos·so·pha·ryn·geal \ˌlā-bē-ō-ˌglä-sō-ˌfar-ən-ˈjē-əl, -ˌglō-, -fə-ˈrin-jəl, -jē-əl\ *adj* : of, relating to, or affecting the lips, tongue, and pharynx

la·bio·lin·gual \-ˈliŋ-gwəl, -gyə-wəl\ *adj* **1** : of or relating to the lips and the tongue **2** : of or relating to the labial and lingual aspects of a tooth — **la·bio·lin·gual·ly** *adv*

la·bio·scro·tal \-ˈskrōt-əl\ *adj* : relating to or being a swelling or ridge on each side of the embryonic rudiment of the penis or clitoris which develops into one of the scrotal sacs in the male and one of the labia majora in the female

la·bi·um \'lā-bē-əm\ *n, pl* **la·bia** \-ə\ : any of the folds at the margin of the vulva — compare LABIA MAJORA, LABIA MINORA

la·bor \'lā-bər\ *n* : the physical activities involved in parturition consisting essentially of a prolonged series of involuntary contractions of the uterine musculature together with both reflex and voluntary contractions of the abdominal wall; *also* : the period of time during which such labor takes place — **labor** *vb*

lab·o·ra·to·ry \'la-brə-ˌtōr-ē\ *n, pl* **-ries** *often attrib* : a place equipped for experimental study in a science or for testing and analysis

la·bored \'lā-bərd\ *adj* : produced or performed with difficulty or strain (~ breathing)

labor room *n* : a hospital room where a

woman in labor is kept before being taken to the delivery room

la·brum \'lā-brəm\ *n* : a fibrous ring of cartilage attached to the rim of a joint; *esp* : GLENOID LABRUM

lab·y·rinth \'la-bə-ˌrinth\ *n* : a tortuous anatomical structure; *esp* : the internal ear or its bony or membranous part — see BONY LABYRINTH, MEMBRANOUS LABYRINTH

lab·y·rin·thec·to·my \ˌlab-ə-ˌrin-'thek-tə-mē\ *n, pl* **-mies** : surgical removal of the labyrinth of the ear

lab·y·rin·thine \-'rin-thən, -ˌthīn, -ˌthēn\ *adj* : of, relating to, affecting, or originating in the internal ear ⟨human ~ lesions⟩

labyrinthine artery *n* : INTERNAL AUDITORY ARTERY

labyrinthine sense *n* : a complex sense concerned with the perception of bodily position and motion, mediated by end organs in the vestibular apparatus and the semicircular canals, and stimulated by alterations in the pull of gravity and by head movements

lab·y·rin·thi·tis \ˌla-bə-rin-'thī-təs\ *n* : inflammation of the labyrinth of the internal ear

lab·y·rin·thot·o·my \ˌla-bə-rin-'thä-tə-mē\ *n, pl* **-mies** : surgical incision into the labyrinth of the internal ear

lac·er·a·tion \ˌla-sə-'rā-shən\ *n* **1** : the act of making a rough or jagged wound or tear **2** : a torn and ragged wound — **lac·er·ate** \'la-sə-ˌrāt\ *vb*

lacerum — see FORAMEN LACERUM

Each boldface word in the list below is a variant of the word to its right in small capitals.

lachrymal	LACRIMAL
lachrymation	LACRIMATION
lachrymator	LACRIMATOR
lachrymatory	LACRIMATORY

lac operon \'lak-\ *n* : the operon which controls lactose metabolism and has been isolated from one of the colon bacilli of the genus *Escherichia* (*E. coli*)

¹lac·ri·mal \'la-krə-məl\ *adj* **1** : of, relating to, associated with, located near, or constituting the glands that produce tears **2** : of or relating to tears ⟨~ effusions⟩

²lacrimal *n* : a lacrimal anatomical part (as a lacrimal bone)

lacrimal apparatus *n* : the bodily parts which function in the production of tears including the lacrimal glands, lacrimal ducts, lacrimal sacs, nasolacrimal ducts, and lacrimal puncta

lacrimal artery *n* : a large branch of the ophthalmic artery that arises near the optic foramen and supplies the lacrimal gland

lacrimal bone *n* : a small thin bone making up part of the front inner wall of each orbit and providing a groove for the passage of the lacrimal ducts

lacrimal canal *n* : LACRIMAL DUCT 1

lacrimal canaliculus *n* : LACRIMAL DUCT 1

lacrimal caruncle *n* : a small reddish follicular elevation at the medial angle of the eye

lacrimal duct *n* **1** : a short canal leading from a minute orifice on a small elevation at the medial angle of each eyelid to the lacrimal sac — called also *lacrimal canal, lacrimal canaliculus* **2** : any of several small ducts that carry tears from the lacrimal gland to the fornix of the conjunctiva

lacrimal gland *n* : an acinous gland that is about the size and shape of an almond, secretes tears, and is situated laterally and superiorly to the bulb of the eye in a shallow depression on the inner surface of the frontal bone — called also *tear gland*

lacrimal nerve *n* : a small branch of the ophthalmic nerve that enters the lacrimal gland with the lacrimal artery and supplies the lacrimal gland and the adjacent conjunctiva and the skin of the upper eyelid

lacrimal punc·tum \-'pəŋk-təm\ *n* : the opening of either the upper or the lower lacrimal duct at the inner canthus of the eye

lacrimal sac *n* : the dilated oval upper end of the nasolacrimal duct that is situated in a groove formed by the lacrimal bone and the frontal process of the maxilla, is closed at its upper end, and receives the lacrimal ducts

lac·ri·ma·tion \ˌla-krə-'mā-shən\ *n* : the secretion of tears; *specif* : abnormal or excessive secretion of tears due to local or systemic disease

lac·ri·ma·tor \'la-krə-ˌmā-tər\ *n* : a tear-producing substance (as tear gas)

lac·ri·ma·to·ry \'la-kri-mə-ˌtōr-ē\ *adj* : of, relating to, or prompting tears

lact- *or* **lacti-** *or* **lacto-** *comb form* **1** : milk ⟨*lacto*genesis⟩ **2 a** : lactic acid ⟨*lactate*⟩ **b** : lactose ⟨*lactase*⟩

lact·aci·de·mia \ˌlak-ˌta-sə-'dē-mē-ə\ *n* : the presence of excess lactic acid in the blood

lact·al·bu·min \ˌlak-ˌtal-'byü-mən\ *n* : an albumin that is found in milk and is similar to serum albumin; *esp* : a protein fraction from whey

lac·tam \'lak-ˌtam\ *n* : any of a class of amides of amino carboxylic acids that are characterized by the grouping $-CONH-$ in a ring and that include many antibiotics

β–lactam *var of* BETA-LACTAM

β–lactamase *var of* BETA-LACTAMASE

lac·tase \'lak-ˌtās, -ˌtāz\ *n* : an enzyme that hydrolyzes lactose to glucose and galactose and occurs esp. in the intestines of young mammals and in yeasts

¹lac·tate \'lak-ˌtāt\ *n* : a salt or ester of lactic acid

²**lactate** *vb* **lac·tat·ed; lac·tat·ing** : to secrete milk

lactate dehydrogenase *n* : any of a
group of isoenzymes that catalyze reversibly the conversion of pyruvic
acid to lactic acid, are found esp. in
the liver, kidneys, striated muscle,
and the myocardium, and tend to accumulate in the body when these organs or tissues are diseased or injured
— called also *lactic dehydrogenase*

lac·ta·tion \lak-'tā-shən\ *n* **1** : the secretion and yielding of milk by the mam-
mary gland **2** : one complete period of
lactation extending from about the
time of parturition to weaning

lactation tetany *n* : MILK FEVER 1

¹**lac·te·al** \'lak-tē-əl\ *adj* **1** : relating to,
consisting of, producing, or resem-
bling milk (∼ fluid) **2 a** : conveying or
containing a milky fluid (as chyle) (a
∼ channel) **b** : of or relating to the
lacteals (impaired ∼ function)

²**lacteal** *n* : any of the lymphatic vessels
arising from the villi of the small intestine and conveying chyle to the
thoracic duct

lacti- — see LACT-

lac·tic acid \'lak-tik-\ *n* : an organic acid
$C_3H_6O_3$ that is known in three optically isomeric forms: **a** *or* **D–lactic
acid** \'dē-\ : the dextrorotatory form
present normally in blood and muscle
tissue as a product of the metabolism
of glucose and glycogen **b** *or* **L–lactic
acid** \'el-\ : the levorotatory form obtained by biological fermentation of
sucrose **c** *or* **DL–lactic acid** \'dē-'el-\
: the racemic form present in food
products and made usu. by bacterial
fermentation

lactic acidosis *n* : a condition characterized by the accumulation of lactic
acid in bodily tissues

lactic dehydrogenase *n* : LACTATE DEHY-
DROGENASE

lac·tif·er·ous duct \lak-'ti-fə-rəs-\ *n*
: any of the milk-carrying ducts of the
mammary gland that open on the nipple

lactiferous sinus *n* : an expansion in a
lactiferous duct at the base of the nipple in which milk accumulates

lacto- — see LACT-

lac·to·ba·cil·lus \lak-tō-bə-'si-ləs\ *n* **1**
cap : a genus of gram-positive nonmotile lactic-acid-forming bacteria
(family Lactobacillaceae) **2** *pl* **-li** \-ʌi
also -ʌe\ : any bacterium of the genus
Lactobacillus

lac·to·fer·rin \lak-tō-'fer-ən\ *n* : a red
iron-binding protein synthesized by
neutrophils and glandular epithelial
cells, found in many human secretions (as tears and milk), and retard-
ing bacterial and fungal growth

lac·to·fla·vin \lak-tō-'flā-vən\ *n* : RIBO-
FLAVIN

lac·to·gen \'lak-tə-jən, -ˌjen\ *n* : any
hormone (as prolactin) that stimulates the production of milk

lac·to·gen·e·sis \lak-tō-'je-nə-səs\ *n, pl*
-e·ses \-ˌsēz\ : initiation of lactation

lac·to·gen·ic \lak-tō-'je-nik\ *adj* : stimulating lactation

lactogenic hormone *n* : LACTOGEN; *esp*
: PROLACTIN

lac·tone \'lak-ˌtōn\ *n* : any of various
cyclic esters formed from acids containing one or more OH groups

lac·to–ovo–veg·e·tar·i·an \lak-tō-ˌō-vō-
ˌve-jə-'ter-ē-ən\ *n* : a vegetarian
whose diet includes milk, eggs, vegetables, fruits, grains, and nuts —
compare LACTO-VEGETARIAN —
lacto-ovo–vegetarian *adj*

lac·to·per·ox·i·dase \lak-tō-pə-'räk-sə-
ˌdās, -ˌdāz\ *n* : a peroxidase that is
found in milk and saliva and is used to
catalyze the addition of iodine to
tyrosine-containing proteins (as thyroglobulin)

lac·tose \'lak-ˌtōs, -ˌtōz\ *n* : a disaccharide sugar $C_{12}H_{22}O_{11}$ that is present
in milk, yields glucose and galactose
upon hydrolysis, yields esp. lactic
acid upon fermentation, and is used
chiefly in foods, medicines, and culture media (as for the manufacture of
penicillin) — called also *milk sugar*

lac·tos·uria \lak-tō-'shur-ē-ə, -'syur-\
n : the presence of lactose in the urine

lac·to–veg·e·tar·i·an \lak-tō-ˌve-jə-
'ter-ē-ən\ *n* : a vegetarian whose diet
includes milk, vegetables, fruits,
grains, and nuts — compare LACTO-
OVO-VEGETARIAN — **lacto–vegetarian**
adj

lac·tu·lose \'lak-tyù-ˌlōs, -tù-, -ˌlōz\ *n*
: a cathartic disaccharide $C_{12}H_{22}O_{11}$
used to treat chronic constipation and
disturbances of function in the central
nervous system accompanying severe liver disease

la·cu·na \lə-'kü-nə, -'kyü-\ *n, pl* **la-
cu·nae** \-ˌnē, -ˌnī\ : a small cavity, pit,
or discontinuity in an anatomical
structure: as **a** : one of the follicles in
the mucous membrane of the urethra
b : one of the minute cavities in bone
or cartilage occupied by the osteo-
cytes — **la·cu·nar** \-nər\ *adj*

Laen·nec's cirrhosis *or* **Laën·nec's cirrhosis** \'lā-neks-\ *n* : hepatic cirrhosis
in which increased connective tissue
spreads out from the portal spaces
compressing and distorting the lobules, causing impairment of liver
function, and ultimately producing
the typical hobnail liver — called also
portal cirrhosis

    **Laennec, René–Théophile–Hyacinthe
(1781–1826),** French physician.

la·e·trile \'lā-ə-(ˌ)tril\ *n, often cap* : a
drug derived esp. from pits of the
apricot (*Prunus armeniaca* of the
rose family, Rosaceae) that contains
amygdalin and has been used in the
treatment of cancer although of unproved effectiveness

laev- *or* **laevo-** *Brit var of* LEV-

lae·vo·car·dia, lae·vo·do·pa *Brit var of* LEVOCARDIA, LEVODOPA

La·fora body \lä-ᵛför-ə-\ *n* : any of the cytoplasmic inclusion bodies found in neurons of parts of the central nervous system in myoclonic epilepsy and consisting of a complex of glycoprotein and glycosaminoglycan

   Lafora, Gonzalo Rodriguez (*b* 1886), Spanish neurologist.

Lafora's disease *n* : MYOCLONIC EPILEPSY

-lag·nia \ᵛlag-nē-ə\ *comb form* : lust (klepto*lagnia*) (uro*lagnia*)

lag·oph·thal·mos *or* **lag·oph·thal·mus** \la-ᵢgäf-ᵗthal-məs\ *n* : pathological incomplete closure of the eyelids : inability to close the eyelids fully

la grippe \lä-ᵛgrip\ *n* : INFLUENZA

LAK \ᵛlak; ᵢel-(ᵢ)ā-ᵗkā\ *n* : LYMPHOKINE-ACTIVATED KILLER CELL

LAK cell *n* : LYMPHOKINE-ACTIVATED KILLER CELL

lake \ᵛlāk\ *vb* **laked; lak·ing** : to undergo or cause (blood) to undergo a physiological change in which the hemoglobin becomes dissolved in the plasma

-la·lia \ᵛlā-lē-ə\ *n comb form* : speech disorder (of a specified type) (echo*lalia*)

lal·la·tion \la-ᵛlā-shən\ *n* **1** : infantile speech whether in infants or in older speakers (as by mental retardation) **2** : a defective articulation of the letter *l*, the substitution of \l\ for another sound, or the substitution of another sound for \l\ — compare LAMBDACISM

La·maze \lə-ᵛmäz\ *adj* : relating to or being a method of childbirth that involves psychological and physical preparation by the mother in order to suppress pain and facilitate delivery without drugs

   Lamaze, Fernand (1890–1957), French obstetrician.

lamb·da \ᵛlam-də\ *n* **1** : the point of junction of the sagittal and lambdoid sutures of the skull **2** : PHAGE LAMBDA

lambda chain *or* **λ chain** *n* : a polypeptide chain of one of the two types of light chain that are found in antibodies and that can be distinguished antigenically and by the sequence of amino acids in the chain — compare KAPPA CHAIN

lamb·da·cism \ᵛlam-də-ᵢsi-zəm\ *n* : a defective articulation of \l\, the substitution of other sounds for it, or the substitution of \l\ for another sound — compare LALLATION 2

lambda phage *n* : PHAGE LAMBDA

lamb·doid \ᵛlam-ᵢdoid\ *or* **lamb·doi·dal** \lam-ᵛdoid-ᵊl\ *adj* : of, relating to, or being the suture shaped like the Greek letter lambda (λ) that connects the occipital and parietal bones

lam·bli·a·sis \lam-ᵛblī-ə-səs\ *n, pl* **-a·ses** \-ᵢsēz\ : GIARDIASIS

   Lambl \ᵛlämb-ᵊl\, **Wilhelm Dusan** (1824–1895), Austrian physician.

lame \ᵛlām\ *adj* **lam·er; lam·est** : having a body part and esp. a limb so disabled as to impair freedom of movement : physically disabled — **lame·ly** *adv* — **lame·ness** *n*

la·mel·la \lə-ᵛme-lə\ *n, pl* **la·mel·lae** \-ᵢlē, -ᵢlī\ *also* **lamellas 1** : an organ, process, or part resembling a plate: as **a** : one of the bony concentric layers surrounding the Haversian canals in bone **b** (1) : one of the incremental layers of cementum laid down in a tooth (2) : a thin sheetlike organic structure in the enamel of a tooth extending inward from a surface crack **2** : a small medicated disk prepared from gelatin and glycerin for use esp. in the eyes — **la·mel·lar** \lə-ᵛme-lər\ *adj* — **lam·el·lat·ed** \ᵛla-mə-ᵢlā-təd\ *adj*

lamellar ichthyosis *n* : a rare inherited form of ichthyosis characterized by large coarse scales

lamin- *or* **lamini-** *or* **lamino-** *comb form* : lamina (lam*initis*) (lam*inogram*)

lam·i·na \ᵛla-mə-nə\ *n, pl* **-nae** \-ᵢnē, -ᵢnī\ *or* **-nas** : a thin plate or layer esp. of an anatomical part

lamina cri·bro·sa \-ᵢkri-ᵛbrō-sə\ *n, pl* **laminae cri·bro·sae** \-ᵢsē, -ᵢsī\ : any of several anatomical structures having the form of a perforated plate: as **a** : CRIBRIFORM PLATE 1 **b** : the part of the sclera of the eye penetrated by the fibers of the optic nerve **c** : a perforated plate that closes the internal auditory meatus

lamina du·ra \-ᵛdur-ə, -ᵛdyur-\ *n* : the thin hard layer of bone that lines the socket of a tooth and that appears as a dark line in radiography

lam·i·na·gram, lam·i·na·graph *var of* LAMINOGRAM, LAMINOGRAPH

lamina pro·pria \-ᵛprō-prē-ə\ *n, pl* **laminae pro·pri·ae** \-prē-ᵢē, -ᵢī\ : a highly vascular layer of connective tissue under the basement membrane lining a layer of epithelium

lam·i·nar \ᵛla-mə-nər\ *adj* : arranged in, consisting of, or resembling laminae

lam·i·nar·ia \ᵢla-mə-ᵛnar-ē-ə\ *n* : any of a genus (*Laminaria*) of kelps of which some have been used to dilate the cervix in performing an abortion

lamina spi·ral·is \-spə-ᵛra-ləs, -ᵛrä-\ *n* : SPIRAL LAMINA

lam·i·nat·ed \ᵛla-mə-ᵢnā-təd\ *adj* : composed or arranged in layers or laminae (~ membranes)

lamina ter·mi·nal·is \-ᵢtər-mi-ᵛna-ləs, -ᵛnä-\ *n* : a thin layer of gray matter in the telencephalon that extends backward from the corpus callosum above the optic chiasma and forms the median portion of the rostral wall of the third ventricle of the cerebrum

lam·i·na·tion \ᵢla-mə-ᵛnā-shən\ *n* : a laminated structure or arrangement

lam·i·nec·to·my \ᵢla-mə-ᵛnek-tə-mē\ *n,*

pl **-mies** : surgical removal of the posterior arch of a vertebra

lamini- *or* **lamino-** — see LAMIN-

lam·i·nin \ˈla-mə-nən\ *n* : a glycoprotein that is a component of connective tissue basement membrane and that promotes cell adhesion

lam·i·ni·tis \ˌla-mə-ˈnī-təs\ *n* : inflammation of a lamina esp. in the hoof of a horse, cow, or goat that is typically caused by excessive ingestion of a dietary substance (as carbohydrate) — called also *founder*

lam·i·no·gram \ˈla-mə-nə-ˌgram\ *n* : a roentgenogram of a layer of the body made by means of a laminograph; *broadly* : TOMOGRAM

lam·i·no·graph \-ˌgraf\ *n* : an X-ray machine that makes roentgenography of body tissue possible at any desired depth; *broadly* : TOMOGRAPH — **lam·i·no·graph·ic** \ˌla-mə-nə-ˈgra-fik\ *adj* — **lam·i·nog·ra·phy** \ˌla-mə-ˈnä-grə-fē\ *n*

lam·i·not·o·my \ˌla-mə-ˈnä-tə-mē\ *n, pl* **-mies** : surgical division of a vertebral lamina

lamp \ˈlamp\ *n* : any of various devices for producing light or heat — see SLIT LAMP

lam·pas \ˈlam-pəs\ *n* : a congestion of the mucous membrane of the hard palate just posterior to the incisor teeth of the horse due to irritation and bruising from harsh coarse feeds

lam·siek·te \ˈlam-ˌsēk-tə, ˈläm-\ *or* **lam·ziek·te** \-ˌzēk-\ *n* : botulism of phosphorus-deficient cattle esp. in southern Africa due to ingestion of bones and carrion containing clostridial toxins

la·nat·o·side \lə-ˈna-tə-ˌsīd\ *n* : any of three poisonous crystalline cardiac steroid glycosides occurring in the leaves of a foxglove (*Digitalis lanata*): **a** : the glycoside $C_{49}H_{76}O_{19}$ yielding digitoxin, glucose, and acetic acid on hydrolysis — called also *digilanid A, lanatoside A* **b** : the glycoside $C_{49}H_{76}O_{20}$ yielding gitoxin, glucose, and acetic acid on hydrolysis — called also *digilanid B, lanatoside B* **c** : the bitter glycoside $C_{49}H_{76}O_{20}$ yielding digoxin, glucose, and used similarly to digitalis — called also *digilanid C, lanatoside C*

¹**lance** \ˈlans\ *n* : LANCET

²**lance** *vb* **lanced; lanc·ing** : to open with a lancet : make an incision in or into (~ a boil) (~ a vein)

Lance·field group \ˈlans-ˌfēld-\ *also* **Lance·field's group** \-ˌfēldz-\ *n* : one of the serologically distinguishable groups (as group A, group B) into which streptococci can be divided

Lancefield, Rebecca Craighill (1895–1981), American bacteriologist.

lan·cet \ˈlan-sət\ *n* : a sharp-pointed and commonly two-edged surgical instrument used to make small incisions (as in a vein or a boil)

lancet fluke *n* : a small liver fluke of the genus *Dicrocoelium* (*D. dendriticum*) widely distributed in sheep and cattle and rarely infecting humans

lan·ci·nat·ing \ˈlan-sə-ˌnā-tiŋ\ *adj* : characterized by piercing or stabbing sensations (~ pain)

land·mark \ˈland-ˌmärk\ *n* : an anatomical structure used as a point of orientation in locating other structures

Lan·dolt ring \ˈlän-dōlt-\ *n* : one of a series of incomplete rings or circles used in some eye charts to determine visual discrimination or acuity

Landolt, Edmond (1846–1926), French ophthalmologist.

Lan·dry's paralysis \ˈlan-drēz-\ *n* : GUILLAIN-BARRÉ SYNDROME

Landry, Jean–Baptiste–Octave (1826–1865), French physician.

Lang·er·hans cell \ˈläŋ-ər-ˌhäns-\ *n* : a dendritic cell of the interstitial spaces of the epidermis

P. Langerhans — see ISLET OF LANGERHANS

Lang·hans cell \ˈläŋ-häns-\ *n* : any of the cells of cuboidal epithelium that make up the cytotrophoblast

Langhans, Theodor (1839–1915), German pathologist and anatomist.

Langhans giant cell *n* : any of the large cells found in the lesions of some granulomatous conditions (as leprosy) and containing a number of peripheral nuclei arranged in a circle or in the shape of a horseshoe

lan·o·lin \ˈlan-əl-ən\ *n* : wool grease that can be absorbed by the skin, contains from 25% to 30% water, and is used chiefly in ointments and cosmetics — called also *hydrous wool fat*

Lan·ox·in \lə-ˈnäk-sən\ *trademark* — used for a preparation of digoxin

lan·tha·num \ˈlan-thə-nəm\ *n* : a white soft malleable metallic element — symbol *La*; see ELEMENT table

la·nu·go \lə-ˈnü-(ˌ)gō, -ˈnyü-\ *n* : a dense cottony or downy growth; *specif* : the soft downy hair that covers the fetus

lap *abbr* laparotomy

lap·a·ro·scope \ˈla-pə-rə-ˌskōp\ *n* : a fiberoptic instrument that is inserted through an incision in the abdominal wall and is used to examine visually the interior of the peritoneal cavity — called also *peritoneoscope*

lap·a·ros·co·pist \ˌla-pə-ˈräs-kə-pist\ *n* : a physician or surgeon who performs laparoscopies

lap·a·ros·co·py \-pē\ *n, pl* **-pies 1** : visual examination of the abdomen by means of a laparoscope **2** : an operation involving laparoscopy; *esp* : one for sterilization of the female or for removal of ova that involves use of a laparoscope to guide surgical procedures within the abdomen — **lap·a·**

ro·scop·ic \-rə-ˈskä-pik\ *adj* — **lap·a·ro·scop·i·cal·ly** *adv*

lap·a·rot·o·my \ˌla-pə-ˈrä-tə-mē\ *n, pl* **-mies** : surgical section of the abdominal wall

La·place's law \lä-ˈplä-səz-\ *n* : LAW OF LAPLACE

Lar·gac·til \lär-ˈgak-til\ *trademark* — used for a preparation of chlorpromazine

large bowel *n* : LARGE INTESTINE

large calorie *n* : CALORIE 1b

large intestine *n* : the more terminal division of the intestine that is wider and shorter than the small intestine, typically divided into cecum, colon, and rectum, and concerned esp. with the resorption of water and the formation of feces

Lar·gon \ˈlär-ˌgän\ *trademark* — used for a preparation of propiomazine

lark·spur \ˈlärk-ˌspər\ *n* : DELPHINIUM 2

Lar·o·tid \ˈlär-ə-ˌtid\ *trademark* — used for a preparation of amoxicillin

Lar·sen's syndrome \ˈlär-sənz-\ *n* : a syndrome characterized by cleft palate, flattened facies, multiple congenital joint dislocations and deformities of the foot

Larsen, Loren Joseph (*b* 1914), American orthopedic surgeon.

lar·va \ˈlär-və\ *n, pl* **lar·vae** \-(ˌ)vē, -ˌvī\ *also* **larvas** : the immature, wingless, and often wormlike feeding form that hatches from the egg of many insects — **lar·val** \-vəl\ *adj*

lar·va·cide *var of* LARVICIDE

larval mi·grans \-ˈmī-ˌgranz\ *n* : CREEPING ERUPTION

larva migrans *n, pl* **larvae mi·gran·tes** \-ˌmi-ˈgran-ˌtēz\ : CREEPING ERUPTION

lar·vi·cide \ˈlär-və-ˌsīd\ *n* : an agent for killing larvae — **lar·vi·cid·al** \ˌlär-və-ˈsīd-ᵊl\ *adj* — **lar·vi·cid·al·ly** *adv*

laryngo- *or* **laryng-** *comb form* 1 : larynx ⟨*laryng*itis⟩ 2 a : laryngeal ⟨*laryngo*spasm⟩ b : laryngeal and ⟨*laryngo*pharyngeal⟩

¹**la·ryn·ge·al** \lə-ˈrin-jəl, -jē-əl; ˌlar-ən-ˈjē-əl\ *adj* : of, relating to, affecting, or used on the larynx — **la·ryn·geal·ly** *adv*

²**laryngeal** *n* : an anatomical part (as a nerve or artery) that supplies or is associated with the larynx

laryngeal artery *n* : either of two arteries supplying blood to the larynx: a : a branch of the inferior thyroid artery that supplies the muscles and mucous membranes of the dorsal part of the larynx — called also *inferior laryngeal artery* b : a branch of the superior thyroid artery or sometimes of the external carotid artery that supplies the muscles, mucous membranes, and glands of the larynx — called also *superior laryngeal artery*

laryngeal nerve *n* : either of two branches of the vagus nerve supplying the larynx: **a** : one that arises from the ganglion of the vagus situated below the jugular foramen and supplies the cricothyroid muscle — called also *superior laryngeal nerve* **b** : one that arises below the larynx and supplies all the muscles of the thyroid except the cricothyroid — called also *inferior or laryngeal nerve, recurrent laryngeal nerve*; see INFERIOR LARYNGEAL NERVE 2

lar·yn·gec·to·mee \ˌlar-ən-ˌjek-tə-ˈmē\ *n* : a person who has undergone laryngectomy

lar·yn·gec·to·my \-ˈjek-tə-mē\ *n, pl* **-mies** : surgical removal of all or part of the larynx — **lar·yn·gec·to·mized** \-tə-ˌmīzd\ *adj*

lar·yn·gis·mus stri·du·lus \ˌlar-ən-ˈjiz-məs-ˈstri-jə-ləs\ *n, pl* **lar·yn·gis·mi strid·u·li** \-ˌmī-ˈstri-jə-ˌlī\ : a sudden spasm of the larynx that occurs in children esp. in rickets and is marked by difficult breathing with prolonged noisy inspiration — compare LARYNGOSPASM

lar·yn·gi·tis \ˌlar-ən-ˈjī-təs\ *n, pl* **-git·i·des** \-ˈji-tə-ˌdēz\ : inflammation of the larynx

laryngo- — see LARYNG-

la·ryn·go·cele \lə-ˈriŋ-gə-ˌsēl\ *n* : an air-containing evagination of laryngeal mucous membrane having its opening communicating with the ventricle of the larynx

la·ryn·go·fis·sure \lə-ˌriŋ-gō-ˈfi-shər\ *n* : surgical opening of the larynx by an incision through the thyroid cartilage esp. for the removal of a tumor

lar·yn·gog·ra·phy \ˌlar-ən-ˈgä-grə-fē\ *n, pl* **-phies** : X-ray depiction of the larynx after use of a radiopaque material

laryngol *abbr* laryngological

la·ryn·go·log·i·cal \lə-ˌriŋ-gə-ˈlä-ji-kəl\ *also* **la·ryn·go·log·ic** \-ˈlä-jik\ *adj* : of or relating to laryngology or the larynx

lar·yn·gol·o·gist \ˌlar-ən-ˈgä-lə-jist\ *n* : a physician specializing in laryngology

lar·yn·gol·o·gy \ˌlar-ən-ˈgä-lə-jē\ *n, pl* **-gies** : a branch of medicine dealing with diseases of the larynx and nasopharynx

la·ryn·go·pha·ryn·ge·al \lə-ˌriŋ-gō-ˌfar-ən-ˈjē-əl, -fə-ˈrin-jəl, -jē-əl\ *adj* : of or common to both the larynx and the pharynx ⟨∼ cancer⟩

la·ryn·go·phar·yn·gi·tis \-ˌfar-ən-ˈjī-təs\ *n, pl* **-git·i·des** \-ˈji-tə-ˌdēz\ : inflammation of both the larynx and the pharynx

la·ryn·go·phar·ynx \-ˈfar-iŋks\ *n* : the lower part of the pharynx lying behind or adjacent to the larynx — compare NASOPHARYNX

la·ryn·go·plas·ty \lə-ˈriŋ-gə-ˌplas-tē\ *n, pl* **-ties** : plastic surgery to repair laryngeal defects

la·ryn·go·scope \lə-ˈriŋ-gə-ˌskōp, -ˈriŋ-jə-\ *n* : an instrument for examining the interior of the larynx — **la·ryn-**

go·scop·ic \-₁riŋ-gə-'skä-pik, -₁rin-jə-\ *or* **la·ryn·go·scop·i·cal** \-pi-kəl\ *adj*

lar·yn·gos·co·py \₁lar-ən-'gäs-kə-pē\ *n, pl* **-pies** : examination of the interior of the larynx (as with a laryngoscope)

la·ryn·go·spasm \lə-'riŋ-gə-₁spa-zəm\ *n* : spasmodic closure of the larynx — compare LARYNGISMUS STRIDULUS

lar·yn·got·o·my \₁lar-ən-'gä-tə-mē\ *n, pl* **-mies** : surgical incision of the larynx

la·ryn·go·tra·che·al \lə-₁riŋ-gō-'trā-kē-əl\ *adj* : of or common to the larynx and trachea (~ stenosis)

la·ryn·go·tra·che·itis \-₁trā-kē-'ī-təs\ *n* : inflammation of both larynx and trachea — see INFECTIOUS LARYNGOTRACHEITIS

la·ryn·go·tra·cheo·bron·chi·tis \-₁trā-kē-ō-bräŋ-'kī-təs, -brän-\ *n, pl* **-chit·i·des** \-'ki-tə-₁dēz\ : inflammation of the larynx, trachea, and bronchi

lar·ynx \'lar-iŋks\ *n, pl* **la·ryn·ges** \lə-'rin-(₁)jēz\ *or* **lar·ynx·es** : the modified upper part of the respiratory passage that is bounded above by the glottis, is continuous below with the trachea, has a complex cartilaginous or bony skeleton capable of limited motion through the action of associated muscles, and has a set of elastic vocal cords that play a major role in sound production and speech — called also *voice box*

la·ser \'lā-zər\ *n* : a device that utilizes the natural oscillations of atoms or molecules between energy levels for generating coherent electromagnetic radiation in the ultraviolet, visible, or infrared regions of the spectrum

lash \'lash\ *n* : EYELASH

La·six \'lā-ziks, -siks\ *trademark* — used for a preparation of furosemide

L–as·par·a·gi·nase \'el-as-'par-ə-jə-₁nās, -₁nāz\ *n* : an enzyme that breaks down the physiologically commoner form of asparagine, is obtained esp. from bacteria, and is used esp. to treat leukemia

Las·sa fever \'la-sə-\ *n* : a disease esp. of Africa that is caused by an arenavirus and is characterized by a high fever, headaches, mouth ulcers, muscle aches, small hemorrhages under the skin, heart and kidney failure, and a high mortality rate

Lassa virus *n* : an arenavirus that is the causative agent of Lassa fever

las·si·tude \'la-sə-₁tüd, -₁tyüd\ *n* : a condition of weariness, debility, or fatigue

lat \'lat\ *n* : LATISSIMUS DORSI — usu. used in pl.

lata — see FASCIA LATA

latae — see FASCIA LATA, TENSOR FASCIAE LATAE

la·tah \'lä-tə\ *n* : a neurotic condition marked by automatic obedience, echolalia, and echopraxia observed esp. among Malays

la·ten·cy \'lāt-ən-sē\ *n, pl* **-cies** **1** : the quality or state of being latent; *esp*

: the state or period of living or developing in a host without producing symptoms — used of an infective agent or disease **2** : LATENCY PERIOD 1 **3** : the interval between stimulation and response — called also *latent period*

latency period *n* **1** : a stage of personality development that extends from about the age of five to the beginning of puberty and during which sexual urges often appear to lie dormant — called also *latency* **2** : LATENT PERIOD

la·tent \'lāt-ᵊnt\ *adj* : existing in hidden or dormant form: as **a** : present or capable of living or developing in a host without producing visible symptoms of disease (a ~ virus) **b** : not consciously expressed (~ anxiety) **c** : relating to or being the latent content of a dream or thought — **la·tent·ly** *adv*

latent content *n* : the underlying meaning of a dream or thought that is exposed in psychoanalysis by interpretation of its symbols or by free association — compare MANIFEST CONTENT

latent learning *n* : learning that is not demonstrated by behavior at the time it is held to take place but that is inferred to exist based on a greater than expected number of favorable or desired responses at a later time when reinforcement is given

latent period *n* **1** : the period between exposure to a disease-causing agent or process and the appearance of symptoms **2** : LATENCY 3

lat·er·al \'la-tə-rəl, -trəl\ *adj* : of or relating to the side; *esp, of a body part* : lying at or extending toward the right or left side : lying away from the median axis of the body

lateral arcuate ligament *n* : a fascial band that extends from the tip of the transverse process of the first lumbar vertebra to the twelfth rib and provides attachment for part of the diaphragm — compare MEDIAL ARCUATE LIGAMENT, MEDIAN ARCUATE LIGAMENT

lateral brachial cutaneous nerve *n* : a continuation of the posterior branch of the axillary nerve that supplies the skin of the lateral aspect of the upper arm over the distal part of the deltoid muscle and the adjacent head of the triceps brachii

lateral collateral ligament *n* : a ligament that connects the lateral epicondyle of the femur with the lateral side of the head of the fibula and that helps to stabilize the knee by preventing lateral dislocation — called also *fibular collateral ligament*; compare MEDIAL COLLATERAL LIGAMENT

lateral column *n* **1** : a lateral extension of the gray matter in each lateral half of the spinal cord present in the thoracic and upper lumbar regions — called also *lateral horn*; compare

DORSAL HORN, VENTRAL HORN 2 : LATERAL FUNICULUS

lateral condyle *n* : a condyle on the outer side of the lower extremity of the femur; *also* : a corresponding eminence on the upper part of the tibia that articulates with the lateral condyle of the femur — compare MEDIAL CONDYLE

lateral cord *n* : a cord of nerve tissue that is formed by union of the superior and middle trunks of the brachial plexus and that forms one of the two roots of the median nerve — compare MEDIAL CORD, POSTERIOR CORD

lateral corticospinal tract *n* : a band of nerve fibers that descends in the posterolateral part of each side of the spinal cord and consists mostly of fibers arising in the motor cortex of the contralateral side of the brain

lateral cricoarytenoid *n* : CRICOARYTENOID 1

lateral cuneiform bone *n* : CUNEIFORM BONE 1c — called also *lateral cuneiform*

lateral decubitus *n* : a position in which a patient lies on his or her side and which is used esp. in radiography and in making a lumbar puncture

lateral epicondyle *n* : EPICONDYLE a

lateral femoral circumflex artery *n* : an artery that branches from the deep femoral artery or from the femoral artery itself and that supplies the muscles of the lateral part of the thigh and hip joint — compare MEDIAL FEMORAL CIRCUMFLEX ARTERY

lateral femoral circumflex vein *n* : a vein accompanying the lateral femoral circumflex artery and emptying into the femoral vein — compare MEDIAL FEMORAL CIRCUMFLEX VEIN

lateral femoral cutaneous nerve *n* : a nerve that arises from the lumbar plexus and that supplies the anterior and lateral aspects of the thigh down to the knee — compare POSTERIOR FEMORAL CUTANEOUS NERVE

lateral fissure *n* : FISSURE OF SYLVIUS

lateral funiculus *n* : a longitudinal division on each side of the spinal cord comprising white matter between the dorsal and ventral roots — compare ANTERIOR FUNICULUS, POSTERIOR FUNICULUS

lateral gastrocnemius bursa *n* : a bursa of the knee joint that is situated between the lateral head of the gastrocnemius muscle and the joint capsule

lateral geniculate body *n* : a part of the metathalamus that is the terminus of most fibers of the optic tract and receives nerve impulses from the retinas which are relayed to the visual area by way of the geniculocalcarine tracts — compare MEDIAL GENICULATE BODY

lateral geniculate nucleus *n* : a nucleus of the lateral geniculate body

lateral horn *n* : LATERAL COLUMN 1

lateral inhibition *n* : a visual process in which the firing of a retinal cell inhibits the firing of surrounding retinal cells and which is held to enhance the perception of areas of contrast

lateralis — see RECTUS LATERALIS, VASTUS LATERALIS

lat·er·al·i·ty \ˌla-tə-ˈra-lə-tē\ *n, pl* **-ties** : preference in use of homologous parts on one lateral half of the body over those on the other : dominance in function of one of a pair of lateral homologous parts

lat·er·al·i·za·tion \ˌla-tə-rə-lə-ˈzā-shən, ˌla-trə-lə-\ *n* : localization of function or activity (as of verbal processes in the brain) on one side of the body in preference to the other — **lat·er·al·ize** \ˈla-tə-rə-ˌlīz, -trə-\ *vb*

lateral lemniscus *n* : a band of nerve fibers that arises in the cochlear nuclei and terminates in the inferior colliculus and the lateral geniculate body of the opposite side of the brain

lateral ligament *n* : any of various ligaments (as the lateral collateral ligament of the knee) that are in a lateral position or that prevent lateral dislocation of a joint

lateral malleolus *n* : MALLEOLUS a

lateral meniscus *n* : MENISCUS a(1)

lateral nucleus *n* : any of a group of nuclei of the thalamus situated in the dorsolateral region extending from its anterior to posterior ends

lateral pectoral nerve *n* : PECTORAL NERVE a

lateral plantar artery *n* : PLANTAR ARTERY a

lateral plantar nerve *n* : PLANTAR NERVE a

lateral plantar vein *n* : PLANTAR VEIN a

lateral popliteal nerve *n* : COMMON PERONEAL NERVE

lateral pterygoid muscle *n* : PTERYGOID MUSCLE a

lateral pterygoid nerve *n* : PTERYGOID NERVE a

lateral pterygoid plate *n* : PTERYGOID PLATE a

lateral rectus *n* : RECTUS 2b

lateral reticular nucleus *n* : a nucleus of the reticular formation that receives fibers esp. from the dorsal horn of the spinal cord and sends axons to the cerebellum on the same side of the body

lateral sacral artery *n* : either of two arteries on each side which arise from the posterior division of the internal iliac artery and supply muscles and skin in the area

lateral sacral crest *n* : SACRAL CREST b

lateral sacral vein *n* : any of several veins that accompany the corresponding lateral sacral arteries and empty into the internal iliac veins

lateral semilunar cartilage *n* : MENISCUS a(1)

lateral spinothalamic tract *n* : SPINOTHALAMIC TRACT b

lateral sulcus *n* : FISSURE OF SYLVIUS

lateral thoracic artery *n* : THORACIC ARTERY 1b

lateral umbilical ligament *n* : MEDIAL UMBILICAL LIGAMENT

lateral ventricle *n* : an internal cavity in each cerebral hemisphere that consists of a central body and three cornua — see ANTERIOR HORN 2, INFERIOR HORN, POSTERIOR HORN 2

lateral vestibular nucleus *n* : the one of the four vestibular nuclei on each side of the medulla oblongata that sends fibers down the same side of the spinal cord through the vestibulospinal tract — called also *Deiters' nucleus*

latex agglutination test *n* : a test for a specific antibody and esp. rheumatoid factor in which the corresponding antigen is adsorbed on spherical polystyrene latex particles which undergo agglutination upon addition of the specific antibody — called also *latex fixation test, latex test*

lath·y·rism \'la-thə-ˌri-zəm\ *n* : a diseased condition of humans and domestic animals that results from poisoning by a substance found in some legumes (genus *Lathyrus* and esp. *L. sativus*) and is characterized esp. by spastic paralysis of the hind or lower limbs — **lath·y·rit·ic** \ˌla-thə-'ri-tik\ *adj*

lath·y·ro·gen \'la-thə-rə-jən, -ˌjen\ *n* : any of a group of compounds that tend to cause lathyrism and inhibit the formation of links between chains of collagen

la·tis·si·mus dor·si \lə-'ti-sə-məs-'dôr-ˌsī\ *n, pl* **la·tis·si·mi dorsi** \-ˌmī-\ : a broad flat superficial muscle of the lower part of the back that extends, adducts, and rotates the arm medially and draws the shoulder downward and backward

Lat·ro·dec·tus \ˌla-trō-'dek-təs\ *n* : a genus of nearly cosmopolitan spiders (family Theridiidae) that includes most of the well-known venomous spiders (as the black widow, *L. mactans*)

lats \'lats\ *pl of* LAT

LATS *abbr* long-acting thyroid stimulator

laud·able pus \ˌlô-də-bəl-\ *n* : pus discharged freely (as from a wound) and formerly supposed to facilitate the elimination of unhealthy humors from the injured body

lau·da·num \'lôd-nəm, -ᵊn-əm\ *n* 1 : any of various formerly used preparations of opium 2 : a tincture of opium

laughing death *n* : KURU

laughing gas *n* : NITROUS OXIDE

laughing sickness *n* : KURU

Lau·rence–Moon–Biedl syndrome \'lôr-əns-ˌmün-'bēd-ᵊl-, ˌlär-\ *n* : an inherited disorder affecting esp. males and characterized by obesity, mental retardation, the presence of extra fingers or toes, subnormal development of the genital organs, and sometimes by retinitis pigmentosa

Laurence, John Zachariah (1830–1874), British physician.

Moon, Robert Charles (1844–1914), American ophthalmologist.

Biedl, Artur (1869–1933), German physician.

lau·ryl \'lôr-əl, 'lär-\ *n* : the chemical group $C_{12}H_{25}$– having a valence of one — see SODIUM LAURYL SULFATE

LAV \ˌel-(ˌ)ā-'vē\ *n* : HIV-1

la·vage \lə-'väzh, 'la-vij\ *n* : the act or action of washing; *esp* : the therapeutic washing out of an organ — **lavage** *vb*

law of dominance *n* : MENDEL'S LAW 3

law of independent assortment *n* : MENDEL'S LAW 2

law of La·place \-lä-'pläs\ *n* : a law in physics that in medicine is applied in the physiology of blood flow: under equilibrium conditions the pressure tangent to the circumference of a vessel storing or transmitting fluid equals the product of the pressure across the wall and the radius of the vessel for a sphere and half this for a tube — called also *Laplace's law*

Laplace, Pierre–Simon (1749–1827), French astronomer and mathematician.

law of segregation *n* : MENDEL'S LAW 1

law·ren·ci·um \lȯ-'ren-sē-əm\ *n* : a short-lived radioactive element that is produced artificially from californium — symbol Lr; see ELEMENT table

Lawrence, Ernest Orlando (1901–1958), American physicist.

lax \'laks\ *adj* 1 *of the bowels* : LOOSE 3 2 : having loose bowels

lax·a·tion \lak-'sā-shən\ *n* : a bowel movement

¹**lax·a·tive** \'lak-sə-tiv\ *adj* 1 : having a tendency to loosen or relax; *specif* : relieving constipation 2 : LAX 2 — **lax·a·tive·ly** *adv*

²**laxative** *n* : a usu. mild laxative drug

lax·i·ty \'lak-sə-tē\ *n, pl* **-ties** : the quality or state of being loose (a certain ~ of the bowels) (ligamentous ~)

laz·a·ret·to \ˌla-zə-'re-(ˌ)tō\ *or* **laz·a·ret** \-'re, -'rē\ *n, pl* **-rettos** *or* **-rets** 1 *usu* lazaretto : an institution (as a hospital) for those with contagious diseases 2 : a building or a ship used for detention or quarantine

lazy eye *n* : AMBLYOPIA; *also* : an eye affected with amblyopia

lazy–eye blindness *n* : AMBLYOPIA

lb *abbr* pound

LC *abbr* liquid chromatography

L chain *n* : LIGHT CHAIN

LD *abbr* 1 learning disabled; learning disability 2 lethal dose

LD50 *or* **LD₅₀** \ˌel-ˌdē-'fif-tē\ *n* : the amount of a toxic agent (as a poison, virus, or radiation) that is sufficient to kill 50% of a population of animals usu. within a certain time — called also *median lethal dose*

LDH *abbr* lactate dehydrogenase; lactic dehydrogenase

LDL \ˌel-(ˌ)dē-ˈel\ *n* : a lipoprotein of blood plasma that is composed of a moderate proportion of protein with little triglyceride and a high proportion of cholesterol and that is associated with increased probability of developing atherosclerosis — called also *beta-lipoprotein, low-density lipoprotein*; compare HDL, VLDL

L-do·pa \ˌel-ˈdō-pə\ *n* : the levorotatory form of dopa that is obtained esp. from broad beans or prepared synthetically, stimulates the production of dopamine in the brain, and is used in treating Parkinson's disease — called also *levodopa*

LE *abbr* lupus erythematosus

¹**lead** \ˈlēd\ *n* : a flexible or solid insulated conductor connected to or leading out from an electrical device (as an electroencephalograph)

²**lead** \ˈled\ *n, often attrib* : a heavy soft malleable bluish white metallic element found mostly in combination and used esp. in pipes, cable sheaths, batteries, solder, type metal, and shields against radioactivity — symbol *Pb*; see ELEMENT table

lead acetate \ˈled-\ *n* : a poisonous soluble lead salt $PbC_4H_6O_4 \cdot 3H_2O$ used in medicine esp. formerly as an astringent

lead arsenate *n* : an arsenate of lead; *esp* : an acid salt $PbHAsO_4$ or a basic salt $Pb_3(AsO_4)_2$ or a mixture of the two used as an insecticide

lead palsy *n* : localized paralysis caused by lead poisoning esp. of the extensor muscles of the forearm

lead poisoning *n* : chronic intoxication that is produced by the absorption of lead into the system and is characterized by severe colicky pains, a dark line along the gums, and local muscular paralysis — called also *plumbism, saturnism*

leaf·let \ˈlē-flət\ *n* : a leaflike organ, structure, or part; *esp* : any of the flaps of the biscuspid valve or the tricuspid valve

learn·ing \ˈlər-niŋ\ *n* : the process of acquiring a modification in a behavioral tendency by experience (as exposure to conditioning); *also* : the modified behavioral tendency itself — **learn** \ˈlərn\ *vb*

learning disabled *adj* : having difficulty in learning a basic scholastic skill and esp. reading, writing, or arithmetic because of a psychological or organic disorder (as dyslexia or attention deficit disorder) that interferes with the learning process — **learning disability** *n*

least splanchnic nerve \ˈlēst-\ *n* : SPLANCHNIC NERVE c

Le·boy·er \lə-bȯi-ˈā\ *adj* : of or relating to a method of childbirth designed to reduce trauma for the newborn esp. by avoiding use of forceps and bright lights in the delivery room and by giving the newborn a warm bath

　Leboyer, Frédérick (*b* 1918), French obstetrician.

LE cell \ˌel-ˈē-ˌsel\ *n* : a polymorphonuclear leukocyte that is found esp. in patients with lupus erythematosus — called also *lupus erythematosus cell*

lecith- *or* **lecitho-** *comb form* : yolk of an egg (*lecith*al) (*ovolecith*in)

lec·i·thal \ˈle-sə-thəl\ *adj* : having a yolk — often used in combination

lec·i·thin \ˈle-sə-thən\ *n* : any of several waxy hygroscopic phospholipids that are widely distributed in animals and plants, form colloidal solutions in water, and have emulsifying, wetting, and antioxidant properties; *also* : a mixture of or a substance rich in lecithins — called also *phosphatidylcholine*

lec·i·thin·ase \-thə-ˌnās, -ˌnāz\ *n* : PHOSPHOLIPASE

lec·tin \ˈlek-tin\ *n* : any of a group of proteins rich of plants that are not antibodies and do not originate in an immune system but bind specifically to carbohydrate-containing receptors on cell surfaces (as of red blood cells)

leech \ˈlēch\ *n* : any of numerous carnivorous or bloodsucking usu. freshwater annelid worms (class Hirudinea) that have typically a flattened segmented lance-shaped body with a sucker at each end — see MEDICINAL LEECH

LE factor \ˌel-ˈē-\ *n* : an antibody found in the serum esp. of patients with systemic lupus erythematosus

left *adj* : of, relating to, or being the side of the body in which the heart is mostly located; *also* : located nearer to this side than to the right

left atrioventricular valve *n* : BICUSPID VALVE

left colic flexure *n* : SPLENIC FLEXURE

left gastric artery *n* : GASTRIC ARTERY 1

left gastroepiploic artery *n* : GASTROEPIPLOIC ARTERY b

left-hand \ˈleft-ˈhand\ *adj* **1** : situated on the left **2** : LEFT-HANDED

left hand *n* **1** : the hand on a person's left side **2** : the left side

left–hand·ed \ˈleft-ˈhan-dəd\ *adj* **1** : using the left hand habitually or more easily than the right **2** : relating to, designed for, or done with the left hand **3** : having a direction contrary to that of movement of the hands of a watch viewed from in front **4** : LEVOROTATORY — **left–handed** *adv* — **left–hand·ed·ness** *n*

left heart *n* : the left atrium and ventricle : the half of the heart that receives oxygenated blood from the pulmonary circulation and passes it to the aorta

left lymphatic duct *n* : THORACIC DUCT

left pulmonary artery *n* : PULMONARY ARTERY c

left subcostal vein *n* : SUBCOSTAL VEIN b

leg \'leg\ *n* : a limb of an animal used esp. for supporting the body and for walking: as **a** : either of the two lower human limbs that extend from the top of the thigh to the foot and esp. the part between the knee and the ankle **b** : any of the rather generalized appendages of an arthropod used in walking and crawling — **leg·ged** \'leg·əd, 'legd\ *adj*

legal age *n* : the age at which a person enters into full adult legal rights and responsibilities (as of making contracts or wills)

legal blindness *n* : blindness as recognized by law which in most states of the U.S. means that the better eye using the best possible methods of correction has visual acuity of 20/200 or worse or that the visual field is restricted to 20 degrees or less — **legal·ly blind** *adj*

legal medicine *n* : FORENSIC MEDICINE

Legg-Cal·vé-Per·thes disease \'leg-,kal-'vā-'pər,tēz\ *n* : osteochondritis affecting the bony knob at the upper end of the femur — called also *Perthes disease*

> **Legg, Arthur Thornton (1874–1939),** American orthopedic surgeon.
>
> **Calvé, Jacques (1875–1954),** French surgeon.
>
> **Perthes, Georg Clemens (1869–1927),** German surgeon.

Legg-Perthes disease *n* : LEGG-CALVÉ-PERTHES DISEASE

Le·gion·el·la \,lē-jə-'ne-lə\ *n* : a genus of gram-negative rod-shaped bacteria (family Legionellaceae) that includes the causative agent (*L. pneumophila*) of Legionnaires' disease

le·gion·el·lo·sis \,lē-jə-,ne-'lō-səs\ *n* : LEGIONNAIRES' DISEASE

Le·gion·naires' bacillus \,lē-jə-'narz-\ *n* : a bacterium of the genus *Legionella* (*L. pneumophila*) that causes Legionnaires' disease

Legionnaires' disease *also* **Legionnaire's disease** *n* : a lobar pneumonia caused by a bacterium of the genus *Legionella* (*L. pneumophila*)

le·gume \'le-,gyüm, li-'gyüm\ *n* : any of a large family (Leguminosae) of plants having fruits that are dry pods and split when ripe and including important food and forage plants (as beans and clover); *also* : the part (as seeds or pods) of a legume used as food — **le·gu·mi·nous** \li-'gyü-mə-nəs, le-\ *adj*

leio- *or* **lio-** *comb form* : smooth ⟨*leiomyoma*⟩

leio·myo·blas·to·ma \,lī-ō-,mī-ō-blas-'tō-mə\ *n*, *pl* **-mas** *or* **-ma·ta** \-mə-tə\ : LEIOMYOMA; *esp* : one resembling epithelium

leio·my·o·ma \,lī-ō-mī-'ō-mə\ *n*, *pl* **-mas** *or* **-ma·ta** \-mə-tə\ : a tumor consisting of smooth muscle fibers — **leio·my·o·ma·tous** \-mə-təs\ *adj*

leio·myo·sar·co·ma \,lī-ō-,mī-ō-sär-'kō-mə\ *n*, *pl* **-mas** *or* **-ma·ta** \-mə-tə\ : a sarcoma composed in part of smooth muscle cells

Leish·man-Don·o·van body \'lēsh-mən-'dä-nə-vən-\ *n* : a protozoan of the genus *Leishmania* (esp. *L. donovani*) in its nonmotile stage that is found esp. in cells of the skin, spleen, and liver of individuals affected with leishmaniasis and esp. kala-azar — compare DONOVAN BODY

> **Leishman, Sir William Boog (1865–1926),** British bacteriologist.
>
> **Donovan, Charles (1863–1951),** British surgeon.

leish·man·ia \lēsh-'ma-nē-ə, -'mä-\ *n* **1** *cap* : a genus of flagellate protozoans (family Trypanosomatidae) that are parasitic in the tissues of vertebrates and include one (*L. donovani*) causing kala-azar and another (*L. tropica*) causing oriental sore **2** : any protozoan of the genus *Leishmania*; *broadly* : a protozoan resembling the leishmanias that is included in the family (Trypanosomatidae) to which they belong — **leish·man·ial** \-nē-əl\ *adj*

leish·man·i·a·sis \,lēsh-mə-'nī-ə-səs\ *n*, *pl* **-a·ses** \-,sēz\ : infection with or disease (as kala-azar or oriental sore) caused by leishmanias

lem·nis·cus \lem-'nis-kəs\ *n*, *pl* **-nis·ci** \-'nis-,kī, -,kē; -'ni-,sī\ : a band of fibers and esp. nerve fibers — called also *fillet*; see LATERAL LEMNISCUS, MEDIAL LEMNISCUS — **lem·nis·cal** \-'nis-kəl\ *adj*

len·i·tive \'le-nə-tiv\ *adj* : alleviating pain or harshness — **lenitive** *n*

lens *also* **lense** \'lenz\ *n* **1** : a curved piece of glass or plastic used singly or combined in eyeglasses or an optical instrument (as a microscope) for forming an image; *also* : a device for focusing radiation other than light **2** : a highly transparent biconvex lens-shaped or nearly spherical body in the eye that focuses light rays entering the eye typically onto the retina and that lies immediately behind the pupil — **lensed** *adj* — **lens·less** *adj*

lens·om·e·ter \len-'zä-mə-tər\ *n* : an instrument used to determine the optical properties (as the focal length and axis) of ophthalmic lenses

Len·te insulin \'len-tā-\ *n* : a suspension of insulin for injection in a buffered solution containing zinc chloride in which forms of insulin which are relatively slowly and rapidly absorbed are in the approximate ratio of 3:7

len·ti·co·nus \,len-tə-'kō-nəs\ *n* : a rare abnormal and usu. congenital condition of the lens of the eye in which the surface is conical esp. on the posterior side

len·tic·u·lar \len-ˈti-kyə-lər\ *adj* **1 :** having the shape of a double-convex lens **2 :** of or relating to a lens esp. of the eye **3 :** relating to or being the lentiform nucleus of the brain

lenticular nucleus *n* : LENTIFORM NUCLEUS

lenticular process *n* : the tip of the long process of the incus which articulates with the stapes

lentiform nucleus *n* : the one of the four basal ganglia in each cerebral hemisphere that comprises the larger and external nucleus of the corpus striatum — called also *lenticular nucleus*

len·ti·go \len-ˈtī-(ˌ)gō, -ˈtē-\ *n, pl* **len·tig·i·nes** \len-ˈtij-ə-ˌnēz\ **1 :** a small melanotic spot in the skin in which the formation of pigment is unrelated to exposure to sunlight and which is potentially malignant; *esp* : NEVUS — compare FRECKLE 2 : FRECKLE

lentigo ma·lig·na \-mə-ˈlig-nə\ *n* : a precancerous lesion on the skin esp. in areas exposed to the sun (as the face) that is flat, mottled, and brownish with an irregular outline and grows slowly over a period of years

lentigo se·nil·is \-sə-ˈni-ləs\ *n* : flat spots evenly colored with darker pigment that occur on the exposed skin esp. of persons aged 50 and over — see LIVER SPOTS

len·ti·vi·rus \ˈlen-tə-ˌvī-rəs\ *n* : any of a group of retroviruses that cause slowly progressive often fatal diseases (as AIDS)

le·on·ti·a·sis os·sea \ˌlē-ən-ˈtī-ə-səs-ˈä-sē-ə\ *n* : an overgrowth of the bones of the head producing enlargement and distortion of the face

lep·er \ˈle-pər\ *n* : an individual affected with leprosy

LE phenomenon \ˌel-ˈē-\ *n* : the process which a leukocyte undergoes in becoming a lupus erythematosus cell

lep·ra \ˈle-prə\ *n* : LEPROSY

lep·re·chaun·ism \ˈle-prə-ˌkä-ˌni-zəm, -ˌkȯ-\ *n* : a rare genetically-determined disorder characterized by mental and physical retardation, by endocrine disorders, by hirsutism, and esp. by a facies marked by large wide-set eyes and large low-set ears

lep·rol·o·gist \le-ˈprä-lə-jist\ *n* : a specialist in the study of leprosy and its treatment — **lep·rol·o·gy** \-jē\ *n*

lep·ro·ma \le-ˈprō-mə\ *n, pl* **-mas** *or* **-ma·ta** \-mə-tə\ : a nodular lesion of leprosy

lep·ro·ma·tous \lə-ˈprä-mə-təs, -ˈprō-\ *adj* : of, relating to, characterized by, or affected with lepromas or lepromatous (~ patients)

lepromatous leprosy *n* : the one of the two major forms of leprosy that is characterized by the formation of lep-

romas, the presence of numerous Hansen's bacilli in the lesions, and a negative skin reaction to lepromin and that remains infectious to others until treated — compare TUBERCULOID LEPROSY

lep·ro·min \le-ˈprō-mən\ *n* : an extract of human leprous tissue used in a skin test for leprosy infection

lep·ro·sar·i·um \ˌle-prə-ˈser-ē-əm\ *n, pl* **-iums** *or* **-ia** \-ē-ə\ : a hospital for leprosy patients

lep·ro·ser·ie *also* **lep·ro·sery** \ˈle-prə-ˌser-ē\ *n, pl* **-series** : LEPROSARIUM

lep·ro·stat·ic \ˌle-prə-ˈsta-tic\ *n* : an agent that inhibits the growth of Hansen's bacillus

lep·ro·sy \ˈle-prə-sē\ *n, pl* **-sies** : a chronic disease caused by infection with an acid-fast bacillus of the genus *Mycobacterium* (*M. leprae*) and characterized by the formation of nodules on the surface of the body and esp. on the face or by the appearance of tuberculoid macules on the skin that enlarge and spread and are accompanied by loss of sensation followed sooner or later in both types if not treated by involvement of nerves with eventual paralysis, wasting of muscle, and production of deformities and mutilations — called also *Hansen's disease, lepra*; see LEPROMATOUS LEPROSY, TUBERCULOID LEPROSY

lep·rot·ic \le-ˈprä-tik\ *adj* : of, caused by, or infected with leprosy

lep·rous \ˈle-prəs\ *adj* **1 :** infected with leprosy **2 :** of, relating to, or associated with leprosy or a leper

-lep·sy \ˌlep-sē\ *n comb form, pl* **-lep·sies** : taking : seizure (narco*lepsy*)

lept- *or* **lepto-** *comb form* : small : weak : thin : fine (*lepto*meninges) (*lepto*tene)

lep·ta·zol \ˈlep-tə-ˌzȯl, -ˌzōl\ *n, chiefly Brit* : PENTYLENETETRAZOL

lep·to \ˈlep-ˌtō\ *n* : LEPTOSPIROSIS

lep·to·me·nin·ges \ˌlep-tō-mə-ˈnin-(ˌ)jēz\ *n pl* : the pia mater and the arachnoid considered together as investing the brain and spinal cord — called also *pia-arachnoid* — **lep·to·men·in·ge·al** \-me-nən-ˈgē-əl\ *adj*

lep·to·men·in·gi·tis \-ˌme-nən-ˈjī-təs\ *n, pl* **-git·i·des** \-ˈji-tə-ˌdēz\ : inflammation of the pia mater and the arachnoid membrane

lep·to·ne·ma \ˌlep-tə-ˈnē-mə\ *n* : a chromatin thread or chromosome at the leptotene stage of meiotic prophase

lep·to·phos \ˈlep-tō-ˌfäs\ *n* : an organophosphorus pesticide $C_{13}H_{10}BrCl_2$-O_2PS that has been associated with the occurrence of neurological damage in individuals exposed to it esp. in the early and mid 1970s

lep·to·spi·ra \ˈlep-tō-ˌspī-rə\ *n* **1** *cap* : a genus of extremely slender aerobic spirochetes (family Treponemataceae) that are free-living or parasitic in mammals and include a number of important pathogens (as *L. ictero-haemorrhagiae* of Weil's disease or *L. canicola* of canicola fever) 2 *pl* **-ra** *or* **-ras** *or* **-rae** \-ˌrē\ : LEPTOSPIRE

lep·to·spire \ˈlep-tə-ˌspīr\ *n* : any spirochete of the genus *Leptospira* — called also *leptospira* — **lep·to·spi·ral** \ˌlep-tə-ˈspī-rəl\ *adj*

lep·to·spi·ro·sis \ˌlep-tə-spī-ˈrō-səs\ *n*, *pl* **-ro·ses** \-ˌsēz\ : any of several diseases of humans and domestic animals that are caused by infection with spirochetes of the genus *Leptospira* — called also *lepto;* see WEIL'S DISEASE

lep·to·tene \ˈlep-tə-ˌtēn\ *n* : a stage of meiotic prophase immediately preceding synapsis in which the chromosomes appear as fine discrete threads — **leptotene** *adj*

Le·riche's syndrome \lə-ˈrē-shəz-\ *n* : occlusion of the descending continuation of the aorta in the abdomen typically resulting in impotence, the absence of a pulse in the femoral arteries, and weakness and numbness in the lower back, buttocks, hips, thighs, and calves

Leriche, René (1879–1955), French surgeon.

¹**les·bi·an** \ˈlez-bē-ən\ *adj, often cap* : of or relating to homosexuality between females

²**lesbian** *n, often cap* : a female homosexual — called also *sapphic, sapphist*

les·bi·an·ism \ˈlez-bē-ə-ˌni-zəm\ *n* : female homosexuality — called also *sapphism*

Lesch–Ny·han syndrome \ˈlesh-ˈnī-ən-\ *n* : a rare and usu. fatal genetic disorder of male children that is transmitted as a recessive trait linked to the X chromosome and that is characterized by hyperuricemia, mental retardation, spasticity, compulsive biting of the lips and fingers, and a deficiency of hypoxanthine-guanine phosphoribosyltransferase — called also *Lesch-Nyhan disease*

Lesch, Michael (b 1939) and **Nyhan, William Leo (b 1926),** American pediatricians.

¹**le·sion** \ˈlē-zhən\ *n* : an abnormal change in structure of an organ or part due to injury or disease; *esp* : one that is circumscribed and well defined — **le·sioned** \-zhənd\ *adj*

²**lesion** *vb* : to produce lesions in

les·ser cornu \ˈles-ər-\ *n* : CERATOHYAL

lesser curvature *n* : the boundary of the stomach that in humans forms a relatively short concave curve on the right from the opening for the esophagus to the opening into the duodenum — compare GREATER CURVATURE

lesser multangular *n* : TRAPEZOID — called also *lesser multangular bone*

lesser occipital nerve *n* : OCCIPITAL NERVE b

lesser omentum *n* : a part of the peritoneum attached to the liver and to the lesser curvature of the stomach and supporting the hepatic vessels — compare GREATER OMENTUM

lesser petrosal nerve *n* : the continuation of the tympanic nerve beyond the inferior ganglion of the glossopharyngeal nerve that terminates in the otic ganglion which it supplies with preganglionic parasympathetic fibers

lesser sciatic foramen *n* : SCIATIC FORAMEN b

lesser sciatic notch *n* : SCIATIC NOTCH b

lesser splanchnic nerve *n* : SPLANCHNIC NERVE b

lesser trochanter *n* : TROCHANTER b

lesser tubercle *n* : a prominence on the upper anterior part of the end of the humerus that serves as the insertion for the subscapularis — compare GREATER TUBERCLE

lesser wing *n* : an anterior triangular process on each side of the sphenoid bone in front of and much smaller than the corresponding greater wing — compare GREATER WING

¹**le·thal** \ˈlē-thəl\ *adj* : of, relating to, or causing death ⟨a ~ injury⟩; *also* : capable of causing death ⟨~ chemicals⟩ ⟨a ~ dose⟩ — **le·thal·i·ty** \lē-ˈtha-lə-tē\ *n* — **le·thal·ly** *adv*

²**lethal** *n* **1** : an abnormality of genetic origin causing the death of the organism possessing it usu. before maturity **2** : LETHAL GENE

lethal gene *n* : a gene that in some (as homozygous) conditions may prevent development or cause the death of an organism or its germ cells — called also *lethal factor, lethal mutant, lethal mutation*

lethargica — see ENCEPHALITIS LETHARGICA

leth·ar·gy \ˈle-thər-jē\ *n, pl* **-gies 1** : abnormal drowsiness **2** : the quality or state of being lazy, sluggish, or indifferent — **lethargic** *adj*

Let·ter·er–Si·we disease \ˈle-tər-ər-ˈsē-və-\ *n* : an acute disease of children characterized by fever, hemorrhages, and other evidences of a disturbance in the reticuloendothelial system and by severe bone lesions esp. of the skull

Letterer, Erich (b 1895), German physician.

Siwe, Sture August (b 1897), Swedish pediatrician.

Leu *abbr* leucine

leuc- *or* **leuco-** *chiefly Brit var of* LEUK-

leu·cine \ˈlü-ˌsēn\ *n* : a white crystalline essential amino acid $C_6H_{13}NO_2$ obtained by the hydrolysis of most dietary proteins

leucine aminopeptidase *n* : an aminopeptidase that is found in all bodily tissues and is increased in the serum in some conditions or diseases (as pancreatic carcinoma)

leu·cine—en·keph·a·lin \-en-ˈke-fə-lən\ *n* : a pentapeptide having a terminal leucine residue that is one of the two enkephalins occurring naturally in the brain — called also *Leu-enkephalin*

leu·ci·no·sis \ˌlü-sə-ˈnō-səs\ *n, pl* **-no·ses** \-ˌsēz\ *or* **-no·sis·es** : a condition characterized by an abnormally high concentration of leucine in bodily tissues and the presence of leucine in the urine

leucocyt- *or* **leucocyto-** *chiefly Brit var of* LEUKOCYT-

leu·co·cy·to·zo·on \ˌlü-kō-ˌsī-tə-ˈzō-ˌän, -ən\ *n* **1** *cap* : a genus of sporozoans parasitic in birds **2** *pl* **-zoa** \-ˈzō-ə\ : any sporozoan of the genus *Leucocytozoon*

leu·co·cy·to·zoo·no·sis \-ˌzō-ə-ˈnō-səs\ *n, pl* **-no·ses** \-ˌsēz\ : infection by or a disease caused by infection with sporozoans of the genus *Leucocytozoon*

leu·co·vor·in \ˌlü-ˈkä-və-rin\ *n* : CITROVORUM FACTOR

Leu—en·keph·a·lin \ˌlü-en-ˈke-fə-lin\ *n* : LEUCINE-ENKEPHALIN

leuk- *or* **leuko-** *comb form* **1** : white : colorless : weakly colored ⟨*leuko*cyte⟩ ⟨*leuk*orrhea⟩ **2** : leukocyte ⟨*leuk*emia⟩ **3** : white matter of the brain ⟨*leuko*encephalopathy⟩

leu·kae·mia, leu·kae·mic *chiefly Brit var of* LEUKEMIA, LEUKEMIC

leu·ka·phe·re·sis \ˌlü-kə-fə-ˈrē-səs\ *n, pl* **-phe·re·ses** \-ˌsēz\ : a procedure by which the leukocytes are removed from a donor's blood which is then transfused back into the donor — called also *leukopheresis*

leu·ke·mia \lü-ˈkē-mē-ə\ *n* : an acute or chronic disease characterized by an abnormal increase in the number of white blood cells in bodily tissues with or without a corresponding increase of those in the circulating blood — see MONOCYTIC LEUKEMIA, MYELOGENOUS LEUKEMIA

¹leu·ke·mic \lü-ˈkē-mik\ *adj* **1** : of, relating to, or affected by leukemia **2** : characterized by an increase in white blood cells ⟨∼ blood⟩

²leukemic *n* : a person affected with leukemia

leu·ke·mo·gen·e·sis \ˌlü-ˌkē-mə-ˈje-nə-səs\ *n, pl* **-e·ses** \-ˌsēz\ : induction or production of leukemia — **leu·ke·mo·gen·ic** \-ˈjen-ik\ *adj*

leu·ke·moid \lü-ˈkē-mȯid\ *adj* : resembling leukemia

leuko- — see LEUK-

leu·ko·ag·glu·ti·nin \ˌlü-kō-ə-ˈglüt-ᵊn-ən\ *n* : an antibody that agglutinates leukocytes — compare HEMAGGLUTININ

leukocyt- *or* **leukocyto-** *comb form* : leukocyte ⟨*leukocyto*sis⟩

leu·ko·cyte \ˈlü-kə-ˌsīt\ *n* **1** : WHITE BLOOD CELL **2** : a cell (as a macro-

phage) of the tissues comparable to or derived from a leukocyte

leu·ko·cyt·ic \ˌlü-kə-ˈsi-tik\ *adj* **1** : of, relating to, or involving leukocytes **2** : characterized by an excess of leukocytes

leu·ko·cy·to·sis \ˌlü-kə-sī-ˈtō-səs, -kə-sə-\ *n, pl* **-to·ses** \-ˌsēz\ : an increase in the number of leukocytes in the circulating blood that occurs normally (as after meals) or abnormally (as in some infections) — **leu·ko·cy·tot·ic** \-ˈtä-tik\ *adj*

leu·ko·der·ma \ˌlü-kə-ˈdər-mə\ *n* : a skin abnormality that is characterized by a usu. congenital lack of pigment in spots or bands and produces a patchy whiteness — compare VITILIGO

leu·ko·dys·tro·phy \ˌlü-kō-ˈdis-trə-fē\ *n, pl* **-phies** : any of several genetically determined diseases characterized by degeneration of the white matter of the brain

leu·ko·en·ceph·a·lop·a·thy \-in-ˌse-fə-ˈlä-pə-thē\ *n, pl* **-thies** : any of various diseases (as leukodystrophy) affecting the brain's white matter

leuk·onych·ia \ˌlü-kō-ˈni-kē-ə\ *n* : a white spotting, streaking, or discoloration of the fingernails caused by injury or ill health

leu·ko·pe·nia \ˌlü-kō-ˈpē-nē-ə\ *n* : a condition in which the number of leukocytes circulating in the blood is abnormally low and which is most commonly due to a decreased production of new cells in conjunction with various infectious diseases, as a reaction to various drugs or other chemicals, or in response to irradiation — **leu·ko·pe·nic** \-ˈpē-nik\ *adj*

leu·ko·phe·re·sis \-fə-ˈrē-səs\ *n, pl* **-re·ses** \-ˌsēz\ : LEUKAPHERESIS

leu·ko·pla·kia \ˌlü-kō-ˈplā-kē-ə\ *n* : a condition commonly considered precancerous in which thickened white patches of epithelium occur on the mucous membranes esp. of the mouth, vulva, and renal pelvis; *also* : a lesion or lesioned area of leukoplakia — **leu·ko·pla·kic** \-ˈplā-kik\ *adj*

leu·ko·poi·e·sis \-pȯi-ˈē-səs\ *n, pl* **-e·ses** \-ˌsēz\ : the formation of white blood cells — **leu·ko·poi·et·ic** \-ˈe-tik\ *adj*

leu·kor·rhea \ˌlü-kə-ˈrē-ə\ *n* : a white, yellowish, or greenish white viscid discharge from the vagina resulting from inflammation or congestion of the uterine or vaginal mucous membrane — **leu·kor·rhe·al** \-ˈrē-əl\ *adj*

leu·ko·sar·co·ma \ˌlü-kō-sär-ˈkō-mə\ *n, pl* **-mas** *or* **-ma·ta** \-mə-tə\ : lymphosarcoma accompanied by leukemia — **leu·ko·sar·co·ma·to·sis** \-sär-ˌkō-mə-ˈtō-səs\ *n*

leu·ko·sis \lü-ˈkō-səs\ *n, pl* **-ko·ses** \-ˌsēz\ : LEUKEMIA; *esp* : any of various leukemic diseases of poultry — **leu·kot·ic** \-ˈkä-tik\ *adj*

leu·ko·tac·tic \,lü-kō-'tak-tik\ *adj* : tending to attract leukocytes

leu·ko·tome \'lü-kə-,tōm\ *n* : a cannula through which a wire is inserted and used to cut the white matter in the brain in lobotomy

leu·kot·o·my \lü-'kä-tə-mē\ *n, pl* **-mies** : LOBOTOMY

leu·ko·tox·in \,lü-kō-'täk-sən\ *n* : a substance specif. destructive to leukocytes

leu·ko·tri·ene \,lü-kə-'trī-,ēn\ *n* : any of a group of eicosanoids that are generated in basophils, mast cells, macrophages, and human lung tissue by lipoxygenase-catalyzed oxygenation esp. of arachidonic acid and that participate in allergic responses (as bronchoconstriction in asthma) — see SLOW-REACTING SUBSTANCE OF ANAPHYLAXIS

leu·ro·cris·tine \,lur-ō-'kris-,tēn\ *n* : VINCRISTINE

lev- *or* **levo-** *comb form* : left : on the left side *or* : to the left ⟨*levo*cardia⟩

lev·al·lor·phan \,le-və-'lȯr-,fan, -fən\ *n* : a drug $C_{19}H_{25}NO$ related to morphine that is used to counteract morphine poisoning

le·vam·i·sole \lə-'va-mə-,sōl\ *n* : an anthelmintic drug $C_{11}H_{12}N_2S$ administered in the form of its hydrochloride that also possesses immunostimulant properties and is used esp. in the treatment of colon cancer

Le·vant storax \lə-'vant-\ *n* : STORAX 1

lev·ar·ter·e·nol \le-vär-'tir-ə-,nȯl, -'ter-, -,nōl\ *n* : levorotatory norepinephrine

le·va·tor \li-'vā-tər\ *n, pl* **lev·a·to·res** \,le-və-'tȯr-(,)ēz\ *or* **le·va·tors** \li-'vā-tərz\ : a muscle that serves to raise a body part — compare DEPRESSOR a

levator an·gu·li oris \-'aŋ-gyə-,lī-'ȯr-əs\ *n* : a facial muscle that arises from the maxilla, inclines downward to be inserted into the corner of the mouth, and draws the lips up and back — called also *caninus*

levator ani \-'ā-,nī\ *n* : a broad thin muscle that is attached in a sheet to each side of the inner surface of the pelvis and descends to form the floor of the pelvic cavity where it supports the viscera and surrounds structures which pass through it and inserts into the sides of the apex of the coccyx, the margins of the anus, the side of the rectum, and the central tendinous point of the perineum — see ILIOCOCCYGEUS, PUBOCOCCYGEUS

le·va·to·res cos·tar·um \-,käs-'tär-əm, -'tär-\ *n pl* : a series of 12 muscles on each side that arise from the transverse processes of the seventh cervical and upper 11 thoracic vertebrae, that insert into the ribs, and that raise the ribs increasing the volume of the thoracic cavity and extend, bend, and rotate the spinal column

levator la·bii su·pe·ri·or·is \-'lā-bē-,ī-sù-,pir-ē-'ȯr-əs\ *n* : a facial muscle arising from the lower margin of the orbit and inserting into the muscular substance of the upper lip which it elevates — called also *quadratus labii superioris*

levator labii superioris alae·que na·si \-ā-'lē-kwē-'nā-,zī\ *n* : a muscle that arises from the nasal process of the maxilla, that passes downward and laterally, that divides into a part inserting into the alar cartilage and one inserting into the upper lip, and that dilates the nostril and raises the upper lip

levator pal·pe·brae su·pe·ri·or·is \-'pal-'pē-,brē-su-,pir-ē-'ȯr-əs\ *n* : a thin flat extrinsic muscle of the eye arising from the lesser wing of the sphenoid bone and inserting into the tarsal plate of the skin of the upper eyelid which it raises

levator pros·ta·tae \-'präs-tə-,tē\ *n* : a part of the pubococcygeus comprising the more medial and ventral fasciculi that insert into the tissue in front of the anus and serve to support and elevate the prostate gland

levator scap·u·lae \-'ska-pyə-,lē\ *n* : a back muscle that arises in the transverse processes of the first four cervical vertebrae and descends to insert into the vertebral border of the scapula which it elevates

levator ve·li pal·a·ti·ni \-'vē-,lī-,pa-lə-'tī-,nī\ *n* : a muscle arising from the temporal bone and the cartilage of the eustachian tube and descending to insert into the midline of the soft palate which it elevates esp. to close the nasopharynx while swallowing is taking place

Le·Veen shunt \lə-'vēn-'shənt\ *n* : a plastic tube that passes from the jugular vein to the peritoneal cavity where a valve permits absorption of ascitic fluid which is carried back to venous circulation by way of the superior vena cava

LeVeen, Harry Henry (b 1916), American surgeon.

Le·vin tube \lə-'vēn-, lə-'vin-\ *n* : a tube designed to be passed into the stomach or duodenum through the nose

Levin, Abraham Louis (1880–1940), American physician.

le·vo \'lē-(,)vō\ *adj* : LEVOROTATORY

levo- — see LEV-

le·vo·car·dia \,lē-və-'kär-dē-ə\ *n* : normal position of the heart when associated with situs inversus of other abdominal viscera and usu. with structural defects of the heart itself

le·vo·di·hy·droxy·phe·nyl·al·a·nine \,lē-vō-,dī-hī-,dräk-sē-,fen-əl-'a-lə-,nēn, -,fēn-\ *n* : L-DOPA

le·vo·do·pa \'lē-və-,dō-pə, ,lē-və-'dō-pə\ *n* : L-DOPA

Le·vo-Dro·mo·ran \,lē-vō-'drō-mə-

ˌran\ *trademark* — used for a preparation of levorphanol

le·vo·nor·ges·trel \ˌlē-və-nȯr-ˈjes-trəl\ *n* : the levorotatory form of norgestrel used in oral contraceptives and contraceptive implants — see NORPLANT

Levo·phed \ˈle-və-ˌfed\ *trademark* — used for a preparation of norepinephrine

Levo·prome \ˈlē-və-ˌprōm\ *trademark* — used for a preparation of methotrimeprazine

le·vo·pro·poxy·phene \ˌlē-və-ˌprō-ˈpäk-si-ˌfēn\ *n* : a drug $C_{22}H_{29}NO_2$ used esp. in the form of the napsylate as an antitussive

le·vo·ro·ta·to·ry \-ˈrō-tə-ˌtōr-ē\ *or* **le·vo·ro·ta·ry** \-ˈrō-tə-rē\ *adj* : turning toward the left or counterclockwise; *esp* : rotating the plane of polarization of light to the left — compare DEXTROROTATORY

lev·or·pha·nol \le-ˈvȯr-fə-ˌnȯl\ *n* : an addictive drug $C_{17}H_{23}NO$ used esp. in the form of the tartrate as a potent analgesic with properties similar to morphine — see LEVO-DROMORAN

le·vo·thy·rox·ine \ˌlē-vō-thī-ˈräk-ˌsēn, -sən\ *n* : the levorotatory isomer of thyroxine that is administered in the form of the sodium salt for treatment of hypothyroidism

lev·u·lose \ˈle-vyə-ˌlōs, -ˌlōz\ *n* : FRUCTOSE 2

lev·u·los·uria \ˌle-vyə-lō-ˈsyur-ē-ə, -ˈshur-\ *n* : the presence of fructose in the urine

Lew·is blood group \ˈlü-əs-\ *n* : any of a system of blood groups controlled by a pair of dominant-recessive alleles and characterized by antigens which are adsorbed onto the surface of red blood cells and tend to interreact with the antigens produced by secretors although they are genetically independent of them

Lewis, H. D. G., British hospital patient.

lew·is·ite \ˈlü-ə-ˌsīt\ *n* : a colorless or brown vesicant liquid $C_2H_2AsCl_3$ developed as a poison gas for war use

Lewis, Winford Lee (1878–1943), American chemist.

-lex·ia \ˈlek-sē-ə\ *n comb form* : reading of (such) a kind or with (such) an impairment ⟨dys*lexia*⟩

Ley·dig cell \ˈlī-dig-\ *also* **Ley·dig's cell** \-digz-\ *n* : an interstitial cell of the testis usu. considered the chief source of testicular androgens and perhaps other hormones — called also *cell of Leydig, interstitial cell of Leydig*

Leydig, Franz von (1821–1908), German anatomist.

L-form \ˈel-ˌfȯrm\ *n* : a variant form of some bacteria that usu. lacks a cell wall — called also *L-phase*

LH *abbr* luteinizing hormone

LHRH *abbr* luteinizing hormone-releasing hormone

Li *symbol* lithium

lib — see AD LIB

li·bi·do \lə-ˈbē-(ˌ)dō, -ˈbī-, ˈli-bə-ˌdō\ *n, pl* **-dos 1** : emotional or psychic energy that in psychoanalytic theory is derived from primitive biological urges and that is usu. goal-directed **2** : sexual drive — **li·bid·i·nal** \lə-ˈbid-ᵊn-əl\ *adj*

libitum — see AD LIBITUM

Lib·man–Sacks endocarditis \ˈlib-mən-ˈsaks-\ *n* : a noninfectious form of verrucous endocarditis associated with systemic lupus erythematosus — called also *Libman-Sacks disease, Libman-Sacks syndrome*

Libman, Emanuel (1872–1946) and **Sacks, Benjamin (b 1896),** American physicians.

li·brary \ˈlī-ˌbrer-ē\ *n* : a collection of sequences of DNA and esp. recombinant DNA that are maintained in a suitable cellular environment and that represent the genetic material of a particular organism or tissue

Lib·ri·um \ˈli-brē-əm\ *trademark* — used for a preparation of chlordiazepoxide

lice *pl of* LOUSE

licensed practical nurse *n* : a person who has undergone training and obtained a license (as from a state) to provide routine care for the sick — called also *LPN*

licensed vocational nurse *n* : a licensed practical nurse authorized by license to practice in the states of California or Texas — called also *LVN*

li·chen \ˈlī-kən\ *n* **1** : any of several skin diseases characterized by the eruption of flat papules; *esp* : LICHEN PLANUS **2** : any of numerous complex plants (group Lichenes) made up of an alga and a fungus growing in symbiotic association on a solid surface (as a rock)

li·chen·i·fi·ca·tion \ˌlī-ˌke-nə-fə-ˈkā-shən, ˌli-kə-\ *n* : the process by which skin becomes hardened and leathery or lichenoid usu. as a result of chronic irritation; *also* : a patch of skin so modified — **li·chen·i·fied** \ˈlī-ˈke-nə-ˌfīd, ˈli-kə-\ *adj*

li·chen·oid \ˈlī-kə-ˌnȯid\ *adj* : resembling lichen ⟨a ~ eruption⟩

lichenoides — see PITYRIASIS LICHENOIDES ET VARIOLIFORMIS ACUTA

lichen pla·nus \-ˈplā-nəs\ *n* : a skin disease characterized by an eruption of wide flat papules covered by a horny glazed film, marked by intense itching, and often accompanied by lesions on the oral mucosa

lichen scle·ro·sus et atro·phi·cus \-ˌsklə-ˈrō-səs-et-ˌā-ˈtrō-fi-kəs\ *n* : a chronic skin disease that is characterized by the eruption of flat white hardened papules with central hair follicles often having black keratotic plugs

lichen sim·plex chron·i·cus \-ˈsim-ˌpleks-ˈkrä-ni-kəs\ *n* : dermatitis marked by one or more clearly defined patches produced by chronic rubbing of the skin

lic·o·rice \'li-kə-rish, -ris\ *n* : GLYCYRRHIZA

licorice root *n* : GLYCYRRHIZA

lid \'lid\ *n* : EYELID

li·do·caine \'lī-də-ˌkān\ *n* : a crystalline compound $C_{14}H_{22}N_2O$ that is used in the form of its hydrochloride as a local anesthetic — called also *ligno·caine*; see XYLOCAINE

Lie·ber·mann–Bur·chard reaction \'lē-bər-mən-'bur-ˌkärt-\ *n* : a test for unsaturated steroids (as cholesterol) and for terpenes having the formula $C_{30}H_{48}$ — called also *Liebermann= Burchard test*

Liebermann, Carl Theodore (1842–1914), German chemist. H. Burchard may have been one of his many student-research assistants.

lie detector \'lī-di-ˌtek-tər\ *n* : an instrument for detecting physiological evidence (as changes in pulse or blood pressure) of the tension that accompanies lying

li·en \'lī-ən, 'lī-ˌen\ *n* : SPLEEN — **li·en·al** \-ᵊl\ *adj*

lienal vein *n* : SPLENIC VEIN

life \'līf\ *n, pl* **lives** \'līvz\ **1 a** : the quality that distinguishes a vital and functional plant or animal from a dead body **b** : a state of living characterized by capacity for metabolism, growth, reaction to stimuli, and reproduction **2 a** : the sequence of physical and mental experiences that make up the existence of an individual **b** : a specific part or aspect of the process of living ⟨sex ~⟩ ⟨adult ~⟩ — **life·less** \'līf-ləs\ *adj*

life cycle *n* : the series of stages in form and functional activity through which an organism passes between successive recurrences of a specified primary stage

life expectancy *n* : an expected number of years of life based on statistical probability

¹life·sav·ing \'līf-ˌsā-viŋ\ *adj* : designed for or used in saving lives ⟨~ drugs⟩

²lifesaving *n* : the skill or practice of saving or protecting the lives esp. of drowning persons

life science *n* : a branch of science (as biology, medicine, anthropology, or sociology) that deals with living organisms and life processes — usu. used in pl. — **life scientist** *n*

life space *n* : the physical and psychological environment of an individual or group

life span \'līf-ˌspan\ *n* **1** : the duration of existence of an individual **2** : the average length of life of a kind of organism or of a material object

life–sup·port \'līf-sə-ˌpōrt\ *adj* : providing support necessary to sustain life; *esp* : of, relating to, or being a life-support system ⟨~ equipment⟩

life support *n* : medical life-support equipment ⟨the patient was placed on *life support*⟩

life–support system *n* : a system that provides all or some of the items (as oxygen, food, water, and disposition of carbon dioxide and body wastes) necessary for maintaining life or health

lift \'lift\ *n* : FACE-LIFT — **lift** *vb*

lig·a·ment \'li-gə-mənt\ *n* **1** : a tough band of tissue that serves to connect the articular extremities of bones or to support or retain an organ in place and is usu. composed of coarse bundles of dense white fibrous tissue parallel or closely interlaced, pliant, and flexible, but not extensible **2** : any of various folds or bands of pleura, peritoneum, or mesentery connecting parts or organs

ligament of the ovary *n* : a rounded cord of fibrous and muscular tissue extending from each superior angle of the uterus to the inner extremity of the ovary of the same side — called also *ovarian ligament*; see SUSPENSORY LIGAMENT OF THE OVARY

ligament of Treitz \-'trīts\ *n* : a band of smooth muscle extending from the junction of the duodenum and jejunum to the left crus of the diaphragm and functioning as a suspensory ligament

Treitz, Wenzel (1819–1872), Austrian physician.

ligament of Zinn \-'zin, -'tsin\ *n* : the common tendon of the inferior rectus and the internal rectus muscles of the eye — called also *tendon of Zinn*

Zinn \'tsin\, **Johann Gottfried (1727–1759),** German anatomist and botanist.

lig·a·men·tous \ˌli-gə-'men-təs\ *adj* **1** : of or relating to a ligament **2** : forming or formed of a ligament

lig·a·men·tum \ˌli-gə-'men-təm\ *n, pl* **-ta** \-tə\ : LIGAMENT

ligamentum ar·te·ri·o·sum \-är-ˌtir-ē-'ō-səm\ *n* : a cord of tissue that connects the pulmonary trunk and the aorta and that is the vestige of the ductus arteriosus

ligamentum fla·vum \-'flā-vəm\ *n, pl* **ligamenta fla·va** \-və\ : any of a series of ligaments of yellow elastic tissue connecting the laminae of adjacent vertebrae from the axis to the sacrum

ligamentum nu·chae \-'nü-ˌkē, -'nyü-, -ˌkī\ *n, pl* **ligamenta nuchae** : a medium ligament of the back of the neck that is rudimentary in humans but highly developed and composed of yellow elastic tissue in many quadrupeds where it assists in supporting the head

ligamentum te·res \-'tē-ˌrēz\ *n* : ROUND LIGAMENT; *esp* : ROUND LIGAMENT 1

ligamentum ve·no·sum \-vē-'nō-səm\ *n* : a cord of tissue connected to the liver that is the vestige of the ductus venosus

li·gase \'lī-₁gās, -₁gāz\ *n* : SYNTHETASE
li·ga·tion \lī-'gā-shən\ *n* **1 a** : the surgical process of tying up an anatomical channel (as a blood vessel) **b** : the process of joining together chemical chains (as of DNA or protein) **2** : something that binds : LIGATURE — **li·gate** \'lī-₁gāt, lī-'\ *vb*
lig·a·ture \'li-gə-₁chúr, -chər, -₁tyúr\ *n* **1** : something that is used to bind; *specif* : a filament (as a thread) used in surgery (as for tying blood vessels) **2** : the action or result of binding or tying — **ligature** *vb*
light \'līt\ *n* **1 a** : the sensation aroused by stimulation of the visual receptors **b** : an electromagnetic radiation in the wavelength range including infrared, visible, ultraviolet, and X rays and traveling in a vacuum with a speed of about 186,281 miles (300,000 kilometers) per second; *specif* : the part of this range that is visible to the human eye **2** : a source of light
light adaptation *n* : the adjustments including narrowing of the pupillary opening and decrease in rhodopsin by which the retina of the eye is made efficient as a visual receptor under conditions of strong illumination — compare DARK ADAPTATION — **light–adapt·ed** \'līt-ə-₁dap-təd\ *adj*
light chain *n* : either of the two smaller of the four polypeptide chains that are subunits of antibodies — called also L chain; compare HEAVY CHAIN
light·en·ing \'līt-ᵊn-iŋ\ *n* : a sense of decreased weight and abdominal tension felt by a pregnant woman on descent of the fetus into the pelvic cavity prior to labor
light–head·ed \'līt-'he-dəd\ *adj* : mentally disordered : DIZZY — **light–head·ed·ness** *n*
light microscope *n* : an ordinary microscope that uses light as distinguished from an electron microscope — **light microscopy** *n*
light·ning pains \'līt-niŋ-\ *n pl* : intense shooting or lancinating pains occurring in tabes dorsalis
lig·no·caine \'lig-na-₁kān\ *n, Brit* : LIDOCAINE
limb \'lim\ *n* **1** : one of the projecting paired appendages of an animal body concerned esp. with movement and grasping; *esp* : a human leg or arm **2** : a branch or arm of something (as an anatomical part)
lim·bal \'lim-bəl\ *adj* : of or relating to the limbus ⟨a ~ incision⟩
limb bud *n* : a proliferation of embryonic tissue shaped like a mound from which a limb develops
lim·ber·neck \'lim-bər-₁nek\ *n* : a botulism of birds (esp. poultry) characterized by paralysis of the neck muscles and pharynx
lim·bic \'lim-bik\ *adj* : of, relating to, or

being the limbic system of the brain
limbic lobe *n* : the marginal medial portion of the cortex of a cerebral hemisphere
limbic system *n* : a group of subcortical structures (as the hypothalamus, the hippocampus, and the amygdala) of the brain that are concerned esp. with emotion and motivation
lim·bus \'lim-bəs\ *n* : a border distinguished by color or structure; *esp* : the marginal region of the cornea of the eye by which it is continuous with the sclera
lime \'līm\ *n* : a caustic powdery white solid that consists of the oxide of calcium often together with magnesia
li·men \'lī-mən\ *n* : THRESHOLD
lim·i·nal \'li-mə-nəl\ *adj* **1** : of or relating to a sensory threshold **2** : barely perceptible
limp \'limp\ *vb* **1** : to walk lamely; *esp* : to walk favoring one leg **2** : to go unsteadily — **limp** *n*
Lin·co·cin \liŋ-'kō-sən\ *trademark* — used for a preparation of lincomycin
lin·co·my·cin \₁liŋ-kə-'mīs-ᵊn\ *n* : an antibiotic obtained from an actinomycete of the genus *Streptomyces* (*S. lincolnensis*) and effective esp. against gram-positive bacteria
linc·tus \'liŋk-təs\ *n, pl* **linc·tus·es** : a syrupy or sticky preparation containing medicaments exerting a local action on the mucous membrane of the throat
lin·dane \'lin-₁dān\ *n* : an insecticide consisting of not less than 99 percent gamma benzene hexachloride that is biodegraded very slowly
Lin·dau's disease \'lin-₁daúz-\ *n* : VON HIPPEL-LINDAU DISEASE
line \'līn\ *n* : a strain produced and maintained esp. by selective breeding or biological culture
lin·ea al·ba \₁li-nē-ə-'al-bə\ *n, pl* **lin·e·ae al·bae** \₁li-nē-₁ē-'al-₁bē\ : a median vertical tendinous line on the abdomen formed of fibers from the aponeuroses of the two rectus abdominis muscles and extending from the xiphoid process to the pubic symphysis
linea as·pe·ra \-'as-pə-rə\ *n, pl* **lineae as·pe·rae** \-₁rē\ : a longitudinal ridge on the posterior surface of the middle third of the femur
lineae al·bi·can·tes \-₁al-bə-'kan-₁tēz\ *n pl* : whitish marks in the skin esp. of the abdomen and breasts that often follow pregnancy
linea semi·lu·nar·is \-₁se-mi-lü-'nar-əs\ *n, pl* **lineae semi·lu·nar·es** \-'nar-₁ēz\ : a curved line on the ventral abdominal wall parallel to the midline and halfway between it and the side of the body that marks the lateral border of the rectus abdominis muscle — called also *semilunar line*
line of sight *n* : a line from an observer's eye to a distant point

line of vision n : a straight line joining the fovea of the eye with the fixation point

linguae — see LONGITUDINALIS LINGUAE

lin·gual \'liŋ-gwəl, -gyə-wəl\ adj 1 : of, relating to, or resembling the tongue 2 : lying near or next to the tongue; esp : relating to or being the surface of tooth next to the tongue

lingual artery n : an artery arising from the external carotid artery between the superior thyroid and facial arteries and supplying the tongue

lingual gland n : any of the mucous, serous, or mixed glands that empty their secretions onto the surface of the tongue

lin·gual·ly \'liŋ-gwə-lē\ adv : toward the tongue ⟨a tooth displaced ∼⟩

lingual nerve n : a branch of the mandibular division of the trigeminal nerve supplying the anterior two thirds of the tongue and responding to stimuli of pressure, touch, and temperature

lingual tonsil n : a variable mass or group of small nodules of lymphoid tissue lying at the base of the tongue just anterior to the epiglottis

lin·gu·la \'liŋ-gyə-lə\ n, pl **lin·gu·lae** \-ˌlē\ : a tongue-shaped process or part: as a : a ridge of bone in the angle between the body and the greater wing of the sphenoid b : an elongated prominence of the superior vermis of the cerebellum c : a dependent projection of the upper lobe of the left lung — **lin·gu·lar** \-lər\ adj

lin·i·ment \'li-nə-mənt\ n : a liquid or semifluid preparation that is applied to the skin as an anodyne or a counterirritant — called also *embrocation*

li·ni·tis plas·ti·ca \lə-ˈnī-təs-ˈplas-ti-kə\ n : carcinoma of the stomach characterized by thickening and diffuse infiltration of the wall rather than localization of the tumor in a discrete lump

link·age \'liŋ-kij\ n : the relationship between genes on the same chromosome that causes them to be inherited together — compare MENDEL'S LAW 2

linkage group n : a set of linked genes at different loci on the same chromosome

linked \'liŋkt\ adj : marked by linkage ⟨∼ genes⟩

Li·nog·na·thus \li-ˈnäg-nə-thəs\ n : a genus of sucking lice including parasites of several domestic mammals

lio- — see LEIO-

li·o·thy·ro·nine \ˌlī-ō-ˈthī-rə-ˌnēn\ n : TRIIODOTHYRONINE

lip \'lip\ n 1 : either of the two fleshy folds that surround the mouth and organs of speech essential to certain articulations; *also* : the pink or reddish margin of the human lip composed of nonglandular mucous membrane 2 : an edge of a wound 3 : either of a pair of fleshy folds surrounding an orifice 4 : an anatomical part or structure (as a labium) resembling a lip — **lip·like** \'lip-ˌlīk\ adj

lip- or **lipo-** comb form : fat : fatty tissue : fatty ⟨lipoid⟩ ⟨lipoprotein⟩

li·pae·mia chiefly Brit var of LIPEMIA

li·pase \'lī-ˌpās, 'lī-, -ˌpāz\ n : an enzyme that hydrolyzes glycerides

li·pec·to·my \lī-ˈpek-tə-mē, li-\ n, pl **-mies** : the excision of subcutaneous fatty tissue esp. as a cosmetic surgical procedure

li·pe·mia \li-ˈpē-mē-ə\ n : the presence of an excess of fats or lipids in the blood; *specif* : HYPERCHOLESTEROLEMIA — **li·pe·mic** \-mik\ adj

lip·id \'li-pəd\ *also* **lip·ide** \-ˌpīd\ n : any of various substances that are soluble in nonpolar organic solvents, that with proteins and carbohydrates constitute the principal structural components of living cells, and that include fats, waxes, phospholipids, cerebrosides, and related and derived compounds — **li·pid·ic** \li-ˈpi-dik\ adj

lip·i·do·sis \ˌli-pə-ˈdō-səs\ n, pl **-do·ses** \-ˌsēz\ : a disorder of fat metabolism esp. involving the deposition of fat in an organ (as the liver or spleen) — called also *lipoidosis*; compare LIPODYSTROPHY

li·po·at·ro·phy \ˌli-pō-ˈa-trə-fē\ n, pl **-phies** : an allergic reaction to insulin medication that is manifested as a loss of subcutaneous fat — **li·po·atro·phic** \-(ˌ)ä-ˈtrō-fik\ adj

li·po·chon·dro·dys·tro·phy \-ˌkän-drə-ˈdis-trə-fē\ n, pl **-phies** : MUCOPOLYSACCHARIDOSIS; *esp* : HURLER'S SYNDROME

li·po·chrome \'li-pə-ˌkrōm, 'lī-\ n : any of the naturally occurring pigments soluble in fats or in solvents for fats; *esp* : CAROTENOID

li·po·dys·tro·phy \ˌli-pō-ˈdis-trə-fē, ˌlī-\ n, pl **-phies** : a disorder of fat metabolism esp. involving loss of fat from or deposition of fat in tissue — compare LIPIDOSIS

li·po·fi·bro·ma \ˌli-pō-fī-ˈbrō-mə, ˌlī-\ n, pl **-mas** *also* **-ma·ta** \-mə-tə\ : a lipoma containing fibrous tissue

li·po·fus·cin \ˌli-pə-ˈfəs-ᵊn, ˌli-, -ˈfyü-sᵊn\ n : a dark brown lipochrome found esp. in the tissue (as of the heart) of the aged

li·po·fus·cin·o·sis \-ˌfə-sə-ˈnō-səs, -ˌfyü-\ n : any condition characterized by disordered storage of lipofuscins

li·po·gen·e·sis \-ˈje-nə-səs\ n, pl **-e·ses** \-ˌsēz\ 1 : formation of fat in the living body esp. when excessive or abnormal 2 : the formation of fatty acids from acetyl coenzyme A in the living body

li·po·ic acid \li-ˈpō-ik-, lī-\ n : any of several microbial growth factors; *esp* : a crystalline compound $C_8H_{14}O_2S_2$

that is essential for the oxidation of alpha-keto acids (as pyruvic acid) in metabolism

¹li•poid \'li-ˌpȯid, 'lī-\ *or* **li•poi•dal** \li-'pȯid-ᵊl\ *adj* : resembling fat

²lipoid *n* : LIPID

lipoidica — see NECROBIOSIS LIPOIDI-CA, NECROBIOSIS LIPOIDICA DIABETI-CORUM

li•poid•o•sis \ˌli-ˌpȯi-'dō-səs, ˌlī-\ *n, pl* **-o•ses** \-ˌsēz\ : LIPIDOSIS

li•pol•y•sis \li-'päl-ə-səs, lī-\ *n, pl* **-y•ses** \-ˌsēz\ : the hydrolysis of fat — **li•po•lyt•ic** \ˌli-pə-'lit-ik, ˌlī-\ *adj*

li•po•ma \li-'pō-mə, lī-\ *n, pl* **-mas** *or* **-ma•ta** \-mə-tə\ : a tumor of fatty tissue — **li•po•ma•tous** \-mə-təs\ *adj*

li•po•ma•to•sis \ˌli-ˌpō-mə-'tō-səs, ˌlī-\ *n, pl* **-to•ses** \-ˌsēz\ : any of several abnormal conditions marked by local or generalized deposits of fat or replacement of other tissue by fat; *specif* : the presence of multiple lipomas

li•po•phil•ic \ˌli-pə-'fil-ik, ˌlī-\ *adj* : having an affinity for lipids (as fats) ⟨a ∼ metabolite⟩ — compare HYDROPHILIC — **li•po•phi•lic•i•ty** \-ˌfi-'li-sə-tē\ *n*

li•po•poly•sac•cha•ride \ˌli-pō-ˌpä-li-'sa-kə-ˌrīd, ˌlī-\ *n* : a large molecule consisting of lipids and sugars joined by chemical bonds

li•po•pro•tein \-'prō-ˌtēn\ *n* : any of a large class of conjugated proteins composed of a complex of protein and lipid and separable on the basis of solubility and mobility properties — see HDL, LDL, VLDL

li•po•sar•co•ma \-sär-'kō-mə\ *n, pl* **-mas** *or* **-ma•ta** \-mə-tə\ : a sarcoma arising from immature fat cells of the bone marrow

li•po•some \'li-pə-ˌsōm, 'lī-\ *n* **1** : one of the fatty droplets in the cytoplasm of a cell **2** : a vesicle composed of one or more concentric phospholipid bilayers and used medically esp. to deliver a drug into the body — **li•po•so•mal** \ˌli-pə-'sō-məl, ˌlī-\ *adj*

li•po•suc•tion \-ˌsək-shən\ *n* : surgical removal of local fat deposits (as in the thighs) esp. for cosmetic purposes by applying suction through a small tube inserted into the body

li•po•tro•pin \ˌli-pə-'trō-pən, ˌlī-\ *n* : either of two protein hormones of the anterior part of the pituitary gland that function in the mobilization of fat reserves; *esp* : BETA-LIPOTROPIN

li•pox•y•gen•ase \li-'päk-sə-jə-ˌnäs, lī-, -ˌnāz\ *n* : a crystallizable enzyme that catalyzes the oxidation primarily of unsaturated fatty acids or unsaturated fats by oxygen

Lippes loop \'li-pēz-\ *n* : an S-shaped plastic intrauterine device

Lippes, Jack (*b* 1924), American obstetrician and gynecologist.

Li•quae•min \'li-kwə-ˌmin\ *trademark* — used for a preparation of heparin

liq•ue•fac•tion \ˌli-kwə-'fak-shən\ *n* **1** : the process of making or becoming

liquid **2** : the state of being liquid

liq•uid \'lik-wəd\ *adj* **1** : flowing freely like water **2** : neither solid nor gaseous : characterized by free movement of the constituent molecules among themselves but without the tendency to separate ⟨∼ mercury⟩

²liquid *n* : a liquid substance

liq•uid•am•bar \ˌli-kwə-'dam-bər\ *n* **1** *cap* : a genus of trees of the witch hazel family (Hamamelidaceae) **2** : STORAX 2

liquid chromatography *n* : chromatography in which the mobile phase is a liquid

liquid protein diet *n* : a reducing diet consisting of high-protein liquids

Li•qui•prin \'li-kwə-ˌprin\ *trademark* — used for a preparation of acetaminophen

li•quor \'li-kər\ *n* : a liquid substance (as a medicinal solution) — compare TINCTURE

liquor am•nii \'lī-ˌkwȯr-'am-nē-ˌī, 'lī-\ *n* : AMNIOTIC FLUID

liquor fol•li•cu•li \-'fä-'li-kyə-ˌlī\ *n* : the fluid surrounding the ovum in the ovarian follicle

li•quo•rice *chiefly Brit var of* LICORICE

li•sin•o•pril \li-'si-nə-ˌpril, lī-\ *n* : an antihypertensive drug $C_{21}H_{31}N_3O_5 \cdot 2H_2O$ that is an ACE inhibitor — see PRINIVIL, ZESTRIL

lisp \'lisp\ *vb* **1** : to pronounce the sibilants \s\ and \z\ imperfectly esp. by giving them the sounds \th\ and \th\ **2** : to speak with a lisp — **lisp** *n* — **lisp•er** \'lis-pər\ *n*

liss- *or* **lisso-** *comb form* : smooth ⟨*liss*encephaly⟩

lis•sen•ceph•a•ly \ˌli-sen-'se-fə-lē\ *n, pl* **-lies** : the condition of having a smooth cerebrum without convolutions — **lis•sen•ce•phal•ic** \-sə-'fa-lik\ *adj*

lis•te•ria \li-'stir-ē-ə\ *n* **1** *cap* : a genus of small gram-positive flagellated rod-shaped bacteria (family Corynebacteriaceae) including one (*L. monocytogenes*) that causes infectious mononucleosis **2** : any bacterium of the genus *Listeria* — **lis•te•ri•al** \li-'stir-ē-əl\ *adj* — **lis•te•ric** \-ik\ *adj*

Lis•ter \'lis-tər\, **Joseph (1827–1912),** British surgeon and medical scientist.

lis•te•ri•o•sis \(ˌ)li-ˌstir-ē-'ō-səs\ *n, pl* **-ri•o•ses** \-ˌsēz\ : a serious commonly fatal disease of a great variety of mammals and birds and occas. humans caused by a bacterium of the genus *Listeria* (*L. monocytogenes*) and taking the form of a severe encephalitis accompanied by disordered movements usu. ending in paralysis, fever, and monocytosis — see CIRCLING DISEASE

li•ter \'lē-tər\ *n* : a metric unit of capacity equal to the volume of one kilogram of water at 4°C (39°F) and at standard atmospheric pressure of 760 millimeters of mercury

lith- *or* **litho-** *comb form* : calculus ⟨*li-thiasis*⟩ ⟨*litho*tripsy⟩

-lith \ˌlith\ *n comb form* : calculus ⟨uro*lith*⟩

li·thi·a·sis \li-ˈthī-ə-səs\ *n, pl* **-a·ses** \-ˌsēz\ : the formation of stony concretions in the body (as in the urinary tract or gallbladder) — often used in combination ⟨chole*lithiasis*⟩

lith·i·um \ˈli-thē-əm\ *n* **1** : a soft silver-white element that is the lightest metal known — symbol *Li*; see ELEMENT table **2** : a lithium salt and esp. lithium carbonate used in psychiatric medicine

lithium carbonate *n* : a crystalline salt Li_2CO_3 used in medicine in the treatment of mania and hypomania in manic-depressive psychosis

lith·o·gen·ic \ˌli-thə-ˈje-nik\ *adj* : of, promoting, or undergoing the formation of calculi ⟨a ∼ diet⟩ — **lith·o·gen·e·sis** \-ˈje-nə-ə-səs\ *n*

lith·ol·a·paxy \li-ˈthä-lə-ˌpak-sē, ˈli-thə-lə-\ *n, pl* **-pax·ies** : LITHOTRIPSY

lith·o·pe·di·on \ˌli-thə-ˈpē-dē-ˌän\ *n* : a fetus calcified in the body of the mother

li·thot·o·my \li-ˈthä-tə-mē\ *n, pl* **-mies** : surgical incision of the urinary bladder for removal of a stone

lith·o·trip·sy \ˈli-thə-ˌtrip-sē\ *n, pl* **-sies** : the breaking (as by shock waves or crushing with a surgical instrument) of a stone in the urinary system into pieces small enough to be voided or washed out — called also *litholapaxy*

lith·o·trip·ter *also* **lith·o·trip·tor** \ˈli-thə-ˌtrip-tər\ *n* : a device for performing lithotripsy; *esp* : a noninvasive device that pulverizes stones by focusing shock waves on a patient immersed in a water bath

lit·mus \ˈlit-məs\ *n* : a coloring matter from lichens that turns red in acid solutions and blue in alkaline solutions and is used as an acid-base indicator

litmus paper *n* : paper colored with litmus and used as an acid-base indicator

li·tre \ˈlē-tər\ *chiefly Brit var of* LITER

¹lit·ter \ˈli-tər\ *n* **1** : a device (as a stretcher) for carrying a sick or injured person **2** : the offspring at one birth of a multiparous animal

²litter *vb* : to give birth to young

little finger *n* : the fourth and smallest finger of the hand counting the forefinger as the first

Little League elbow *n* : inflammation of the medial epicondyle and adjacent tissues of the elbow esp. in preteen and teenage baseball players who make too strenuous use of the muscles of the forearm — called also *Little Leaguer's elbow*

little toe *n* : the outermost and smallest digit of the foot

live birth \ˈlīv-\ *n* : birth in such a state

that acts of life are manifested after the extrusion of the whole body — compare STILLBIRTH

live–born \ˈlīv-ˈbȯrn\ *adj* : born alive — compare STILLBORN

li·ve·do re·tic·u·lar·is \li-ˈvē-dō-ri-ˌti-kyə-ˈlar-əs\ *n* : a condition of the peripheral blood vessels characterized by reddish blue mottling of the skin esp. of the extremities usu. upon exposure to cold

liv·er \ˈli-vər\ *n* : a large very vascular glandular organ of vertebrates that secretes bile and causes important changes in many of the substances contained in the blood which passes through it (as by converting sugars into glycogen which it stores up until required and by forming urea) and that in humans is the largest gland in the body, weighs from 40 to 60 ounces (1100 to 1700 grams), is a dark red color, and occupies the upper right portion of the abdominal cavity immediately below the diaphragm

liver cell *n* : HEPATOCYTE

liver fluke *n* : any of various trematode worms that invade the mammalian liver; *esp* : one of the genus *Fasciola* (*F. hepatica*) that is a major parasite of the liver, bile ducts, and gallbladder of cattle and sheep, causes fascioliasis in humans, and uses snails of the genus *Lymnaea* as an intermediate host — see CHINESE LIVER FLUKE

liver rot *n* : a disease caused by liver flukes esp. in sheep and cattle and marked by great local damage to the liver — see DISTOMATOSIS; compare BLACK DISEASE

liver spots *n pl* : spots of darker pigmentation (as lentigo senilis or those of chloasma and tinea versicolor) on the skin

lives *pl of* LIFE

liv·id \ˈli-vəd\ *adj* : discolored by bruising : BLACK-AND-BLUE — **li·vid·i·ty** \li-ˈvi-də-tē\ *n*

living will *n* : a document in which the signer requests to be allowed to die rather than be kept alive by artificial means in the event of becoming disabled beyond a reasonable expectation of recovery

LLQ *abbr* left lower quadrant (abdomen)

Loa \ˈlō-ə\ *n* : a genus of African filarial worms (family Dipetalonematidae) that infect the subcutaneous tissues and blood, include the eye worm (*L. loa*) causing Calabar swellings, are transmitted by the bite of flies of the genus *Chrysops*, and are associated with some allergic manifestations (as hives)

load \ˈlōd\ *n* **1** : BURDEN ⟨the worm ∼ in rats⟩ **2** : the decrease in capacity for survival of the average individual in a population due to the presence of deleterious genes in the gene pool

load·ing \ˈlō-diŋ\ *n* **1** : administration of

a factor or substance to the body or a bodily system in sufficient quantity to test capacity to deal with it **2** : the relative contribution of each component factor in a psychological test or in an experimental, clinical, or social situation

lo·a·i·a·sis \ˌlō-ə-ˈī-ə-səs, -sēz\ *n, pl* **-a·ses** \-ˌsēz\ : infestation with or disease caused by an eye worm of the genus *Loa* (L. *loa*) that migrates through the subcutaneous tissue and across the cornea of the eye — compare CALABAR SWELLING

loa loa \ˈlō-ə-ˈlō-ə\ *n* : LOAIASIS

lob- *or* **lobi-** *or* **lobo-** *comb form* : lobe ⟨*lobectomy*⟩ ⟨*lobotomy*⟩

lo·bar \ˈlō-bər, -ˌbär\ *adj* : of or relating to a lobe

lobar pneumonia *n* : acute pneumonia involving one or more lobes of the lung characterized by sudden onset, chill, fever, difficulty in breathing, cough, and blood-stained sputum, marked by consolidation, and normally followed by resolution and return to normal of the lung tissue

lobe \ˈlōb\ *n* : a curved or rounded projection or division: as **a** : a more or less rounded projection of a body organ or part (∼ of the ear) **b** : a division of a body organ marked off by a fissure on the surface (as of the brain, lungs, or liver) — **lobed** \ˈlōbd\ *adj*

lo·bec·to·my \lō-ˈbek-tə-mē\ *n, pl* **-mies** : surgical removal of a lobe of an organ (as a lung) or gland (as the thyroid); *specif* : excision of a lobe of the lung — compare LOBOTOMY

lo·be·line \ˈlō-bə-ˌlēn\ *n* : an alkaloid $C_{22}H_{27}NO_2$ that is obtained from an American herb (*Lobelia inflata* of the family Lobeliaceae) and is used esp. in nonprescription drugs as a smoking deterrent

lobi-, lobo- — see LOB-

lo·bot·o·my \lō-ˈbä-tə-mē\ *n, pl* **-mies** : surgical severance of nerve fibers connecting the frontal lobes to the thalamus for the relief of some mental disorders — called also *leukotomy*; compare LOBECTOMY — **lo·bot·o·mize** \-ˌmīz\ *vb*

lobster claw \ˈläb-stər-ˌklȯ\ *n* : an incompletely dominant genetic anomaly marked by variable reduction of the skeleton of the extremities and cleaving of the hands and feet into two segments

lob·u·lar \ˈlä-byə-lər\ *adj* : of, relating to, affecting, or resembling a lobule

lob·u·lat·ed \ˈlä-byə-ˌlā-təd\ *adj* : made up of, provided with, or divided into lobules ⟨a ∼ tumor⟩ — **lob·u·la·tion** \ˌlä-byə-ˈlā-shən\ *n*

lob·ule \ˈlä-ˌbyül\ *n* **1** : a small lobe (the ∼ of the ear) **2** : a subdivision of a lobe; *specif* : one of the small masses of tissue of which various organs (as the liver) are made up

lob·u·lus \ˈlä-byə-ləs\ *n, pl* **lob·u·li** \-ˌlī\ **1** : LOBE **2** : LOBULE

¹lo·cal \ˈlō-kəl\ *adj* : involving or affecting only a restricted part of the organism : TOPICAL — compare SYSTEMIC a — **lo·cal·ly** *adv*

²local *n* : LOCAL ANESTHETIC; *also* : LOCAL ANESTHESIA

local anesthesia *n* : loss of sensation in a limited and usu. superficial area esp. from the effect of a local anesthetic

local anesthetic *n* : an anesthetic for topical and usu. superficial application

lo·cal·ize \ˈlō-kə-ˌlīz\ *vb* **-ized; -iz·ing 1** : to make local; *esp* : to fix in or confine to a definite place or part **2** : to accumulate in or be restricted to a specific or limited area — **lo·cal·iza·tion** \ˌlō-kə-lə-ˈzā-shən\ *n*

lo·chia \ˈlō-kē-ə, ˈlä-\ *n, pl* **lochia** : a discharge from the uterus and vagina following delivery — **lo·chi·al** \-əl\ *adj*

loci *pl of* LOCUS

locked \ˈläkt\ *adj, of the knee joint* : having a restricted mobility and incapable of complete extension

lock·jaw \ˈläk-ˌjȯ\ *n* : an early symptom of tetanus characterized by spasm of the jaw muscles and inability to open the jaws; *also* : TETANUS 1a

lo·co·ism \ˈlō-kō-ˌi-zəm\ *n* **1** : a disease of horses, cattle, and sheep caused by chronic poisoning with locoweeds and characterized by motor and sensory nerve damage resulting in peculiarities of gait, impairment of vision, lassitude or extreme excitement, emaciation, and ultimately paralysis and death if not controlled **2** : any of several intoxications of domestic animals (as selenosis) that are sometimes confused with locoweed poisoning

lo·co·mo·tion \ˌlō-kə-ˈmō-shən\ *n* : an act or the power of moving from place to place : progressive movement (as of an animal body) — **lo·co·mo·tor** \ˌlō-kə-ˈmō-tər\ *adj* — **lo·co·mo·to·ry** \ˌlō-kə-ˈmō-tə-rē\ *adj*

locomotor ataxia *n* : TABES DORSALIS

lo·co·weed \ˈlō-(ˌ)kō-ˌwēd\ *n* : any of several leguminous plants (genera *Astragalus* and *Oxytropis*) of western No. America that cause locoism

loc·u·lus \ˈlä-kyə-ləs\ *n, pl* **-li** \-ˌlī, -ˌlē\ : a small chamber or cavity esp. in a plant or animal body — **loc·u·lat·ed** \ˈlä-kyə-ˌlā-təd\ *adj* — **loc·u·la·tion** \ˌlä-kyə-ˈlā-shən\ *n*

lo·cum te·nens \ˌlō-kəm-ˈtē-ˌnenz, -nənz\ *n, pl* **locum te·nen·tes** \-ˌti-ˈnen-ˌtēz\ : a medical practitioner who temporarily takes the place of another

lo·cus \ˈlō-kəs\ *n, pl* **lo·ci** \ˈlō-ˌsī, -ˌkī, -ˌkē\ **1** : a place or site of an event, activity, or thing **2** : the position in a chromosome of a particular gene or allele

lo·cus coe·ru·le·us also **lo·cus ce·ru·le·us** \lō-kəs-si-'rü-lē-əs\ n, pl **loci coe·ru·lei** also **loci ce·ru·lei** \-lē-ī\ : a blue area of the brain stem with many norepinephrine-containing neurons

Loef·fler's syndrome \'le-flərz-\ n : a mild pneumonitis marked by transitory pulmonary infiltration and eosinophilia and usu. considered to be basically an allergic reaction — called also *Loeffler's pneumonia*

Löf·fler \'lœ-flər\, **Wilhelm** (b 1887), Swiss physician.

log- or **logo-** comb form : word : thought : speech : discourse ⟨*logorrhea*⟩

log·o·pe·dics \ˌlȯ-gə-'pē-diks, ˌlä-\ n sing or pl : the scientific study and treatment of speech defects

log·or·rhea \ˌlȯ-gə-'rē-ə, ˌlä-\ n : pathologically excessive and often incoherent talkativeness or wordiness

log·or·rhoea chiefly Brit var of LOGORRHEA

log·o·ther·a·py \ˌlȯ-gə-'ther-ə-pē, ˌlä-\ n : a highly directive existential psychotherapy that emphasizes the importance of meaning in the patient's life esp. as gained through spiritual values

-l·o·gy \l-ə-jē\ n comb form, pl **-logies** : doctrine : theory : science ⟨*physiology*⟩

lo·i·a·sis \ˌlō-ī-ə-səs\ var of LOAIASIS

loin \'lȯin\ n **1** : the part of the body on each side of the spinal column between the hipbone and the false ribs **2** pl **a** : the upper and lower abdominal regions and the region about the hips **b** (1) : the pubic region (2) : the generative organs — not usu. used technically in senses 2a, b

loin disease n : aphosphorosis of cattle often complicated by botulism

Lo·mo·til \'lō-mə-ˌtil, lō-'mät-ᵊl\ trademark — used for a preparation of diphenoxylate

lo·mus·tine \lō-'məs-ˌtēn\ n : an antineoplastic drug $C_9H_{16}ClN_3O_2$ used esp. in the treatment of brain tumors and Hodgkin's disease

lone star tick n : a No. American ixodid tick of the genus *Amblyomma* (*A. americanum*) that is a vector of Rocky Mountain spotted fever

long–acting thyroid stimulator n : a protein that often occurs in the plasma of patients with Graves' disease and may be an IgG immunoglobulin — abbr. *LATS*

long bone n : any of the elongated bones supporting a limb and consisting of an essentially cylindrical shaft that contains marrow and ends in enlarged heads for articulation with other bones

long ciliary nerve n : any of two or three nerves that are given off by the nasociliary nerve and are distributed to the iris and cornea — compare SHORT CILIARY NERVE

long head n : the longest of the three heads of the triceps muscle that arises from the infraglenoid tubercle of the scapula

longi pl of LONGUS

lon·gis·si·mus \län-'ji-si-məs\ n, pl **lon·gis·si·mi** \-ˌmī\ : the intermediate division of the sacrospinalis muscle that consists of the longissimus capitis, longissimus cervicis, and longissimus thoracis; also : any of these three muscles

longissimus cap·i·tis \-'ka-pi-təs\ n : a muscle that arises by tendons from the upper thoracic and lower cervical vertebrae, is inserted into the posterior margin of the mastoid process, and extends the head and bends it and rotates it to one side — called also *trachelomastoid muscle*

longissimus cer·vi·cis \-'sər-vi-səs\ n : a muscle medial to the longissimus thoracis that arises by long thin tendons from the transverse processes of the upper four or five thoracic vertebrae, is inserted by similar tendons into the transverse processes of the second to sixth cervical vertebrae, and extends the spinal column and bends it to one side

longissimus dor·si \-'dȯr-ˌsī\ n : LONGISSIMUS THORACIS

longissimus thor·a·cis \-'thȯr-ə-səs, -thō-'rā-səs\ n : a muscle that arises as the middle and largest division of the sacrospinalis muscle, that is attached by some of its fibers to the lumbar vertebrae, that is inserted into all the thoracic vertebrae and the lower 9 or 10 ribs and that depresses the ribs and with the longissimus cervicis extends the spinal column and bends it to one side

lon·gi·tu·di·nal \ˌlän-jə-'tüd-ᵊn-əl, -'tyüd-\ adj **1** : of, relating to, or occurring in the lengthwise dimension ⟨a ∼ bone fracture⟩ **2** : extending along or relating to the anteroposterior axis of a body or part **3** : involving the repeated observation or examination of a set of subjects over time with respect to one or more study variables — **lon·gi·tu·di·nal·ly** adv

longitudinal fissure n : the deep groove that divides the cerebrum into right and left hemispheres

lon·gi·tu·di·na·lis linguae \ˌlän-jə-ˌtü-də-'nā-ləs-, -ˌtyü-\ n : either of two bands of muscle comprising the intrinsic musculature of the tongue — called also *longitudinalis*

long–nosed cattle louse n : a sucking louse of the genus *Linognathus* (*L. vituli*) that feeds on cattle

long posterior ciliary artery n : either of usu. two arteries of which one arises from the ophthalmic artery on each side of the optic nerve, passes forward along the optic nerve, enters the sclera, and at the junction of the ciliary process and the iris divides into upper and lower branches which form a ring of arteries around the iris — compare SHORT POSTERIOR CILIARY ARTERY

long saphenous vein *n* : SAPHENOUS VEIN a

long·sight·ed \'loṅ-ˈsī-təd\ *adj* : FAR-SIGHTED — **long·sight·ed·ness** *n*

long–term memory *n* : memory that involves the storage and recall of information over a long period of time (as days, weeks, or years)

lon·gus \'loṅ-gəs\ *n, pl* **lon·gi** \-ˌgī\ : a long structure (as a muscle) in the body — see ABDUCTOR POLLICIS LONGUS, ADDUCTOR LONGUS, EXTENSOR CARPI RADIALIS LONGUS, EXTENSOR DIGITORUM LONGUS, EXTENSOR HALLUCIS LONGUS, EXTENSOR POLLICIS LONGUS, FLEXOR DIGITORUM LONGUS, FLEXOR HALLUCIS LONGUS, FLEXOR POLLICIS LONGUS, PALMARIS LONGUS, PERONEUS LONGUS

longus cap·i·tis \-ˈka-pi-təs\ *n* : a muscle of either side of the front and upper portion of the neck that arises from the third to sixth cervical vertebrae, is inserted into the basilar portion of the occipital bone, and bends the neck forward

Lon·i·ten \'lä-ni-tən\ *trademark* — used for a preparation of minoxidil

loop — see LIPPES LOOP

loop of Hen·le \-ˈhen-lē\ *n* : the U= shaped part of a nephron that lies between and is continuous with the proximal and distal convoluted tubules, that leaves the cortex of the kidney descending into the medullary tissue and then bending back and reentering the cortex, and that functions in water resorption — called also *Henle's loop*

F. G. J. Henle — see HENLE'S LAYER

loose \'lüs\ *adj* **loos·er; loos·est** **1 a** (1) : having worked partly free from attachments ⟨a ~ tooth⟩ (2) : having relative freedom of movement **b** : produced freely and accompanied by raising of mucus ⟨a ~ cough⟩ **2** : not dense, close, or compact in structure or arrangement ⟨~ connective tissue⟩ **3** : lacking in restraint or power of restraint ⟨~ bowels⟩ **4** : not tightly drawn or stretched — **loose·ly** *adv* — **loose·ness** *n*

lor·az·e·pam \lȯr-ˈa-zə-ˌpam\ *n* : an anxiolytic benzodiazepine $C_{15}H_{10}Cl_2N_2O_2$ — see ATIVAN

lor·do·sis \lȯr-ˈdō-səs\ *n* : exaggerated forward curvature of the lumbar and cervical regions of the spinal column — compare KYPHOSIS, SCOLIOSIS — **lor·dot·ic** \-ˈdä-tik\ *adj*

lo·tion \'lō-shən\ *n* **1** : a liquid usu. aqueous medicinal preparation containing one or more insoluble substances and applied externally for skin disorders **2** : a liquid cosmetic preparation usu. containing alcohol and a cleansing, softening, or astringent agent and applied to the skin

Lo·tri·min \'lō-trə-min\ *trademark* — used for a preparation of clotrimazole

Lou Geh·rig's disease \'lü-ˈger-igz-\ *n* : AMYOTROPHIC LATERAL SCLEROSIS

Gehrig, Lou (1903–1941), American baseball player.

loupe \'lüp\ *n* : a magnifying lens worn esp. by surgeons performing microsurgery; *also* : two such lenses mounted on a single frame

loup·ing ill \'laü-piṅ-, 'lō-\ *n* : a tick-borne disease of sheep and other domestic animals that is caused by a flavivirus and is related to or identical with the Russian spring-summer encephalitis of humans

louse \'laüs\ *n, pl* **lice** \'līs\ : any of the small wingless usu. flattened insects that are parasitic on warm-blooded animals and constitute two orders (Anoplura and Mallophaga)

louse–borne typhus *n* : TYPHUS a

lousy \'laü-zē\ *adj* **lous·i·er; -est** : infested with lice — **lous·i·ness** \'laü-zē-nəs\ *n*

lov·a·stat·in \'lō-və-ˌsta-tən, 'lə-\ *n* : a drug $C_{24}H_{36}O_5$ that decreases the level of cholesterol in the blood stream by inhibiting the liver enzyme that controls cholesterol synthesis and is used in the treatment of hypercholesterolemia

love object *n* : a person on whom affection is centered or on whom one is dependent for affection or needed help

low \'lō\ *adj* : having a relatively less complex organization : not greatly differentiated or developed phylogenetically — usu. used in the comparative degree of less advanced types of plants and animals ⟨the ~*er* vertebrates⟩; compare HIGH 1

low–back \'lō-ˈbak\ *adj* : of, relating to, suffering, or being pain in the lowest portion of the back ⟨~ pain⟩

low blood pressure *n* : HYPOTENSION 1

low–density lipoprotein *n* : LDL

low·er \'lō-ər\ *n* : the lower member of a pair; *esp* : a lower denture

lower jaw *n* : JAW 1b

lower respiratory *adj* : of, relating to, or affecting the lower respiratory tract ⟨*lower respiratory* infections⟩

lower respiratory tract *n* : the part of the respiratory system including the larynx, trachea, bronchi, and lungs — compare UPPER RESPIRATORY TRACT

lowest splanchnic nerve *n* : SPLANCHNIC NERVE c

low forceps *n* : a procedure for delivery of an infant by the use of forceps when the head is visible at the outlet of the birth canal — called also *outlet forceps*; compare HIGH FORCEPS, MID-FORCEPS

low–grade \'lō-ˈgrād\ *adj* : being near that extreme of a specified range which is lowest, least intense, or least competent ⟨a ~ fever⟩ ⟨a ~ infection⟩ — compare HIGH-GRADE

low–power *adj* : of, relating to, or being a lens that magnifies an image a relatively small number of times and esp. 10 times — compare HIGH≠ POWER

low–salt diet n : LOW-SODIUM DIET

low–sodium diet n : a diet restricted to foods naturally low in sodium content and prepared without added salt that is used esp. in the management of certain circulatory or kidney disorders

low vision n : impaired vision in which there is a significant reduction in visual function that cannot be corrected by conventional glasses but which may be improved with special aids or devices

Lox·os·ce·les \läk-ˈsä-sə-ˌlēz\ n : a genus of spiders (family Loxoscelidae) native to So. America that includes the brown recluse spider (*L. reclusa*)

lox·os·ce·lism \läk-ˈsä-sə-ˌli-zəm\ n : a painful condition resulting from the bite of a spider of the genus *Loxosceles* and esp. the brown recluse spider (*L. reclusa*) that is characterized esp. by local necrosis of tissue

loz·enge \ˈläz-ᵊnj\ n : a small usu. sweetened solid piece of medicated material that is designed to be held in the mouth for slow dissolution and often contains a demulcent — called also *pastille, troche*

L–PAM \ˈel-ˌpam\ n : MELPHALAN

L–phase \ˈel-ˌfāz\ n : L-FORM

LPN \ˌel-(ˌ)pē-ˈen\ n : LICENSED PRACTICAL NURSE

Lr *symbol* lawrencium

LSD \ˌel-(ˌ)es-ˈdē\ n : an organic compound $C_{20}H_{25}N_3O$ that induces psychotic symptoms similar to those of schizophrenia — called also *acid, lysergic acid diethylamide, lysergide*

LSD–25 n : LSD

LTH *abbr* luteotropic hormone

Lu *symbol* lutetium

lubb–dupp *also* **lub–dup** *or* **lub–dub** \ˈləb-ˈdəp, -ˈdəb\ n : the characteristic sounds of a normal heartbeat as heard in auscultation

lu·can·thone \lü-ˈkan-ˌthōn\ n : an antischistosomal drug $C_{20}H_{24}N_2OS$ administered in the form of its hydrochloride — called also *miracil D*

lu·cid \ˈlü-səd\ *adj* : having, showing, or characterized by an ability to think clearly and rationally — **lu·cid·i·ty** \lü-ˈsi-də-tē\ n

lucid interval n : a temporary period of rationality between periods of insanity or delirium

lucidum — see STRATUM LUCIDUM

Lu·cil·ia \lü-ˈsi-lē-ə\ n : a genus of blowflies whose larvae are sometimes the cause of intestinal myiasis and infest open wounds

lüc·ken·schä·del \ˈlᵫe-kən-ˌshäd-ᵊl\ n : a

condition characterized by incomplete ossification of the bones of the skull

Lud·wig's angina \ˈlüd-(ˌ)vigz-\ n : an acute streptococcal or sometimes staphylococcal infection of the deep tissues of the floor of the mouth and adjoining parts of the neck and lower jaw marked by severe rapid swelling that may close the respiratory passage and accompanied by chills and fever

Ludwig, **Wilhelm Friedrich von** (1790–1865), German surgeon.

Lu·er syringe \ˈlü-ər-\ n : a glass syringe with a glass piston that has the apposing surfaces ground and that is used esp. for hypodermic injection

Luer (d 1883), German instrument maker.

lu·es \ˈlü-(ˌ)ēz\ n, pl lues : SYPHILIS

lu·et·ic \lü-ˈe-tik\ *adj* : SYPHILITIC

Lu·gol's solution \lü-ˈgolz-\ n : any of several deep brown solutions of iodine and potassium iodide in water or alcohol — called also *Lugol's iodine, Lugol's iodine solution*

Lugol, **Jean Guillaume Auguste** (1786–1851), French physician.

lumb- *or* **lumbo-** *comb form* : lumbar and ⟨*lumbo*sacral⟩

lum·ba·go \ˌləm-ˈbā-(ˌ)gō\ n : usu. painful rheumatism involving muscular and fibrous tissue of the lower back region

lum·bar \ˈləm-bər, -ˌbär\ *adj* **1** : of, relating to, or constituting the loins or the vertebrae between the thoracic vertebrae and sacrum **2** : of, relating to, or being the abdominal region lying on either side of the umbilical region and above the corresponding iliac region

lumbar artery n : any artery of the usu. four pairs that arise from the back of the aorta opposite the lumbar vertebrae and supply the muscles of the loins, the skin of the sides of the abdomen, and the spinal cord

lumbar nerve n : any nerve of the five pairs of spinal nerves of the lumbar region of which one on each side passes out below each lumbar vertebra and the upper four unite by connecting branches into a lumbar plexus

lumbar plexus n : a plexus embedded in the psoas major and formed by the anterior or ventral divisions of the four upper lumbar nerves of which the first is usu. supplemented by a communication from the twelfth thoracic nerve

lumbar puncture n : puncture of the subarachnoid space in the lumbar region of the spinal cord to withdraw cerebrospinal fluid or inject anesthetic drugs — called also *spinal tap*

lumbar vein n : any vein of the four pairs collecting blood from the muscles and integument of the loins, the walls of the abdomen, and adjacent parts and emptying into the dorsal part of the inferior vena cava — see ASCENDING LUMBAR VEIN

lumbar vertebra *n* : any of the five vertebrae situated between the thoracic vertebrae above and the sacrum below

lumbo- — see LUMB-

lum·bo·dor·sal fascia \ˌləm-bō-ˈdȯr-səl-\ *n* : a large fascial band on each side of the back extending from the iliac crest and the sacrum to the ribs and the intermuscular septa of the muscles of the neck

lumborum — see ILIOCOSTALIS LUMBORUM, QUADRATUS LUMBORUM

lum·bo·sa·cral \ˌləm-bō-ˈsa-krəl, -ˈsā-\ *adj* : of, relating to, or being the lumbar and sacral regions or parts

lumbosacral joint *n* : the joint between the fifth lumbar vertebra and the sacrum

lumbosacral plexus *n* : a network of nerves comprising the lumbar plexus and the sacral plexus

lumbosacral trunk *n* : a nerve trunk that is formed by the fifth lumbar nerve and a smaller branch of the fourth lumbar nerve and that connects the lumbar plexus to the sacral plexus

lum·bri·ca·lis \ˌləm-brə-ˈkā-ləs\ *n, pl* **-les** \-ˌlēz\ **1** : any of the four small muscles of the palm of the hand that arise from tendons of the flexor digitorum profundus, are inserted at the base of the digit to which the tendon passes, and flex the proximal phalanx and extend the two distal phalanges of each finger **2** : any of four small muscles of the foot homologous to the lumbricales of the hand that arise from tendons of the flexor digitorum longus and are inserted into the first phalanges of the four small toes of which they flex the proximal phalanges and extend the two distal phalanges — **lum·bri·cal** \ˈləm-bri-kəl\ *adj*

lu·men \ˈlü-mən\ *n, pl* **lu·mi·na** \-mə-nə\ or **lumens 1** : the cavity of a tubular organ ⟨the ∼ of a blood vessel⟩ **2** : the bore of a tube (as of a catheter) — **lu·mi·nal** *also* **lu·me·nal** \ˈlü-mən-ᵊl\ *adj*

Lu·mi·nal \ˈlü-mə-ˌnal, -ˌnȯl\ *trademark* — used for a preparation of phenobarbital

lump \ˈləmp\ *n* **1** : a piece or mass of indefinite size and shape **2** : an abnormal swelling

lump·ec·to·my \ˌləm-ˈpek-tə-mē\ *n, pl* **-mies** : excision of a breast tumor with a limited amount of associated tissue — called also *tylectomy*

lumpy jaw \ˈləm-pē-\ *also* **lump jaw** *n* : ACTINOMYCOSIS; *esp* : actinomycosis of the head in cattle

lu·na·cy \ˈlü-nə-sē\ *n, pl* **-cies** : any of various forms of insanity

lu·nar caustic \ˈlü-nər-, -ˌnär-\ *n* : silver nitrate esp. when fused and molded into sticks or small cones for use as a caustic

lu·nate bone \ˈlü-ˌnāt-\ *n* : a crescent-shaped bone that is the middle bone in the proximal row of the carpus between the scaphoid bone and the triquetral bone and that has a deep concavity on the distal surface articulating with the capitate — called also *lunate, semilunar bone*

lunate sulcus *n* : a sulcus of the cerebrum on the lateral part of the occipital lobe that marks the front boundary of the visual area

¹**lu·na·tic** \ˈlü-nə-ˌtik\ *adj* : INSANE; *also* : used for the care of insane individuals

²**lunatic** *n* : an insane individual

lung \ˈləŋ\ *n* **1** : one of the usu. two compound saccular organs that constitute the basic respiratory organ of air-breathing vertebrates, that normally occupy the entire lateral parts of the thorax and consist essentially of an inverted tree of intricately branched bronchioles communicating with thin-walled terminal alveoli swathed in a network of delicate capillaries where the actual gaseous exchange of respiration takes place, and that in humans are somewhat flattened with a broad base resting against the diaphragm and have the right lung divided into three lobes and the left into two lobes **2** : a mechanical device for regularly introducing fresh air into and withdrawing stale air from the lungs : RESPIRATOR — see IRON LUNG — **lunged** *adj*

lung·er \ˈləŋ-ər\ *n* : one affected with a chronic disease of the lungs; *esp* : one who is tubercular

lung fluke *n* : a fluke invading the lungs; *esp* : either of two Old World forms of the genus *Paragonimus* (*P. westermanii* and *P. kellicotti*) that produce lesions in humans which are comparable to those of tuberculosis and that are acquired by eating inadequately cooked freshwater crustaceans which act as intermediate hosts

lung·worm \ˈləŋ-ˌwərm\ *n* : any of various nematodes (esp. genera *Dictyocaulus* and *Metastrongylus* of the family Metastrongylidae) that infest the lungs and air passages of mammals

lu·nu·la \ˈlü-nyə-lə\ *n, pl* **-lae** \-ˌlē *also* -ˌlī\ : a crescent-shaped body part: as **a** : the whitish mark at the base of a fingernail — called also *half-moon* **b** : the crescentic unattached border of a semilunar valve

lu·nule \ˈlü-ˌnyül\ *n* : LUNULA

lu·pine *also* **lu·pin** \ˈlü-pən\ *n* : any of a genus (*Lupinus*) of leguminous herbs some of which cause lupinosis

lu·pi·no·sis \ˌlü-pə-ˈnō-səs\ *n, pl* **-no·ses** \-ˌsēz\ : acute liver atrophy of domestic animals (as sheep) due to poisoning by ingestion of various lupines

lu·poid hepatitis \'lü-ˌpȯid-\ n : chronic active hepatitis associated with lupus erythematosus

lu·pus \'lü-pəs\ n : any of several diseases (as lupus vulgaris or systemic lupus erythematosus) characterized by skin lesions

lupus band test n : a test to determine the presence of antibodies and complement deposits at the junction of the dermal and epidermal skin layers of patients with systemic lupus erythematosus

lupus er·y·the·ma·to·sus \-ˌer-ə-ˌthē-mə-'tō-səs\ n : a disorder characterized by skin inflammation; esp : SYSTEMIC LUPUS ERYTHEMATOSUS

lupus erythematosus cell n : LE CELL

lupus ne·phri·tis \-ni-'frī-təs\ n : glomerulonephritis associated with systemic lupus erythematosus that is typically characterized by proteinuria and hematuria and that often leads to renal failure

lupus vul·gar·is \-ˌvəl-'gar-əs\ n : a tuberculous disease of the skin marked by formation of soft brownish nodules with ulceration and scarring

LUQ abbr left upper quadrant (abdomen)

Lur·ide \'lur-ˌīd\ trademark — used for a preparation of sodium fluoride

lute- or **luteo-** comb form : corpus luteum ⟨luteal⟩ ⟨luteolysis⟩

lutea — see MACULA LUTEA

lu·te·al \'lü-tē-əl\ adj : of, relating to, characterized by, or involving the corpus luteum ⟨~ activity⟩

lu·te·cium var of LUTETIUM

lu·tein \'lü-tē-ən, 'lü-ˌtēn\ n : an orange xanthophyll $C_{40}H_{56}O_2$ occurring in plants usu. with carotenes and chlorophylls and in animal fat, egg yolk, and the corpus luteum

lu·tein·iza·tion \ˌlü-tē-ə-nə-'zā-shən, ˌlü-ˌtē-\ n : the process of forming corpora lutea — **lu·tein·ize** \'lü-tē-ə-ˌnīz, 'lü-ˌtē-ˌnīz\ vb

luteinizing hormone n : a hormone of the adenohypophysis of the pituitary gland that in the female stimulates the development of the corpora lutea and together with follicle-stimulating hormone the secretion of progesterone and in the male the development of interstitial tissue in the testis and the secretion of testosterone — abbr LH; called also interstitial-cell stimulating hormone, lutropin

luteinizing hormone–releasing factor n : GONADOTROPIN-RELEASING HORMONE

luteinizing hormone–releasing hormone n : GONADOTROPIN-RELEASING HORMONE

lu·te·ol·y·sis \ˌlü-tē-'ä-lə-səs\ n, pl **-ses** \-ˌsēz\ : regression of the corpus luteum — **lu·teo·lyt·ic** \ˌlü-tē-ə-'li-tik\ adj

lu·te·oma \ˌlü-tē-'ō-mə\ n, pl **-mas** or **-ma·ta** \-mə-tə\ : an ovarian tumor derived from a corpus luteum — **lu·te·o·ma·tous** \-mə-təs\ adj

lu·teo·tro·pic \ˌlü-tē-ə-'trō-pik, -'trä-\ or **lu·teo·tro·phic** \-'trō-fik, -'trä-\ adj : acting on the corpora lutea

luteotropic hormone n : PROLACTIN

lu·teo·tro·pin \ˌlü-tē-ə-'trō-pən\ or **lu·teo·tro·phin** \-fən\ n : PROLACTIN

lu·te·tium \lü-'tē-shē-əm, -shəm\ n : a metallic element — symbol Lu; see ELEMENT table

luteum — see CORPUS LUTEUM

lu·tro·pin \lü-'trō-pən\ n : LUTEINIZING HORMONE

lux·a·tion \ˌlək-'sā-shən\ n : dislocation of an anatomical part — **lux·ate** \'lək-ˌsät\ vb

LVN \ˌel-(ˌ)vē-'en\ n : LICENSED VOCATIONAL NURSE

ly·can·thro·py \lī-'kan-thrə-pē\ n, pl **-pies** : a delusion that one has become or has assumed the characteristics of a wolf

Ly·ell's syndrome \'lī-əlz-\ n : TOXIC EPIDERMAL NECROLYSIS

Lyell, Alan (fl 1950–1972), British dermatologist.

ly·ing–in \ˌlī-iŋ-'in\ n, pl **lyings–in** or **lying–ins** : the state attending and consequent to childbirth : CONFINEMENT

Lyme disease \'līm-\ n : an acute inflammatory disease that is usu. characterized initially by the skin lesion erythema chronicum migrans and by fatigue, fever, and chills and if left untreated may later manifest itself in cardiac and neurological disorders, joint pain, and arthritis and that is caused by a spirochete of the genus Borrelia (B. burgdorferi) transmitted by the bite of a tick esp. of the genus Ixodes (I. scapularis in the eastern and midwestern U.S., I. pacificus in the Pacific northwestern U.S., and I. ricinus in Europe) — called also Lyme arthritis

Lym·naea \lim-'nē-ə, 'lim-nē-ə\ n : a genus of snails (family Lymnaeidae) including some medically important intermediate hosts of flukes — compare FOSSARIA, GALBA

lymph \'limf\ n : a pale coagulable fluid that bathes the tissues, passes into lymphatic channels and ducts, is discharged into the blood by way of the thoracic duct, and consists of a liquid portion resembling blood plasma and containing white blood cells but normally no red blood cells — see CHYLE

lymph- or **lympho-** comb form : lymph : lymphatic tissue ⟨lymphedema⟩ ⟨lymphogranuloma⟩

lymph·ad·e·nec·to·my \ˌlim-ˌfad-ᵊn-'ek-tə-mē\ n, pl **-mies** : surgical removal of a lymph node

lymph·ad·e·ni·tis \ˌlim-ˌfad-ᵊn-'ī-təs\ n : inflammation of lymph nodes — **lymph·ad·e·nit·ic** \-'i-tik\ adj

lymph·ad·e·nop·a·thy \ˌlim-ˌfad-ᵊn-'ä-pə-thē\ n, pl **-thies** : abnormal enlargement of the lymph nodes — **lymph-ad·e·no·path·ic** \ₗlim-ₗfad-ᵊn-ō-ᵗpa-thik\ *adj*

lymphadenopathy–associated virus *n* : HIV-1

lymph·ad·e·no·sis \ₗlim-ₗfad-ᵊn-ᵗō-səs\ *n, pl* **-no·ses** \-ₗsēz\ : any of certain abnormalities or diseases affecting the lymphatic system: as **a** : leukosis involving lymphatic tissues **b** : LYMPHOCYTIC LEUKEMIA

lymphangi- *or* **lymphangio-** *comb form* : lymphatic vessels ⟨*lymphangiography*⟩

lymph·an·gi·ec·ta·sia \ₗlim-ₗfan-jē-ek-ᵗtā-zhə, -zhē-ə\ *or* **lymph·an·gi·ec·ta·sis** \-ᵗek-tə-səs\ *n, pl* **-ta·sias** *or* **-ta·ses** \-ₗsēz\ : dilatation of the lymphatic vessels

lymph·an·gio·gram \(ₗ)lim-ᵗfan-jē-ə-ₗgram\ *n* : an X-ray picture made by lymphangiography

lymph·an·gi·og·ra·phy \ₗlim-ₗfan-jē-ᵗä-grə-fē\ *n, pl* **-phies** : X-ray depiction of lymphatic vessels and lymph nodes after use of a radiopaque material — called also *lymphography* — **lymph·an·gio·graph·ic** \ₗlim-ₗfan-jē-ə-ᵗgra-fik\ *adj*

lymph·an·gi·o·ma \ₗlim-ₗfan-jē-ᵗō-mə\ *n, pl* **-mas** *or* **-ma·ta** \-mə-tə\ : a tumor formed of dilated lymphatic vessels

lymph·an·gio·sar·co·ma \ₗlim-ₗfan-jē-ō-(ₗ)sär-ᵗkō-mə\ *n, pl* **-mas** *or* **-ma·ta** \-mə-tə\ : a sarcoma arising from the endothelial cells of lymphatic vessels

lymph·an·gi·ot·o·my \ₗlim-ₗfan-ᵗä-tə-mē\ *n, pl* **-mies** : incision of a lymphatic vessel

lym·phan·gi·tis \ₗlim-ₗfan-ᵗjī-təs\ *n, pl* **-git·i·des** \-ᵗji-tə-ₗdēz\ : inflammation of the lymphatic vessels

¹**lym·phat·ic** \lim-ᵗfa-tik\ *adj* **1** : of, relating to, or produced by lymph, lymphoid tissue, or lymphocytes **2** : conveying lymph — **lym·phat·i·cal·ly** *adv*

²**lymphatic** *n* : a vessel that contains or conveys lymph, that originates as an interfibrillar or intercellular cleft or space in a tissue or organ, and that if small has no distinct walls or walls composed only of endothelial cells and if large resembles a vein in structure — called also *lymphatic vessel, lymph vessel*; see THORACIC DUCT

lymphatic capillary *n* : any of the smallest lymphatic vessels that are blind at one end and collect lymph in organs and tissues — called also *lymph capillary*

lymphatic duct *n* : any of the lymphatic vessels that are part of the system collecting lymph from the lymphatic capillaries and pouring it into the subclavian veins by way of the right lymphatic duct and the thoracic duct — called also *lymph duct*

lymphatic leukemia *n* : LYMPHOCYTIC LEUKEMIA

lym·phat·i·co·ve·nous \ₗlim-ₗfa-ti-kō-ᵗvē-nəs\ *adj* : of, relating to, or connecting the veins and lymphatic vessels

lymphatic vessel *n* : LYMPHATIC

lymph capillary *n* : LYMPHATIC CAPILLARY

lymph duct *n* : LYMPHATIC DUCT

lymph·ede·ma \ₗlim-fi-ᵗdē-mə\ *n* : edema due to faulty lymphatic drainage — **lymph·edem·a·tous** \ₗlim-fi-ᵗde-mə-təs\ *adj*

lymph follicle *n* : LYMPH NODE; *esp* : LYMPH NODULE

lymph gland *n* : LYMPH NODE

lymph node *n* : any of the rounded masses of lymphoid tissue that are surrounded by a capsule of connective tissue, are distributed along the lymphatic vessels, and contain numerous lymphocytes which filter the flow of lymph passing through the node — called also *lymph gland*

lymph nodule *n* : a small simple lymph node

lympho- — see LYMPH-

lym·pho·blast \ᵗlim-fə-ₗblast\ *n* : a lymphocyte that has enlarged following stimulation by an antigen, has the capacity to recognize the stimulating antigen, and is undergoing proliferation and differentiation either to an effector state in which it functions to eliminate the antigen or to a memory state in which it functions to recognize the future reappearance of the antigen — **lym·pho·blas·tic** \ₗlim-fə-ᵗblas-tik\ *adj*

lymphoblastic leukemia *n* : lymphocytic leukemia characterized by an abnormal increase in the number of lymphoblasts

lym·pho·blas·toid \ₗlim-fə-ᵗblas-ₗtöid\ *adj* : resembling a lymphoblast

lym·pho·blas·to·ma \ₗlim-fə-blas-ᵗtō-mə\ *n, pl* **-mas** *or* **-ma·ta** \-mə-tə\ : any of several diseases of lymph nodes marked by the formation of tumorous masses composed of mature or immature lymphocytes

lym·pho·blas·to·sis \-ₗblas-ᵗtō-səs\ *n, pl* **-to·ses** \-ₗsēz\ : the presence of lymphoblasts in the peripheral blood

lym·pho·cele \ᵗlim-fə-ₗsēl\ *n* : a cyst containing lymph

lym·pho·cyte \ᵗlim-fə-ₗsīt\ *n* : any of the colorless weakly motile cells originating from stem cells and differentiating in lymphoid tissue (as of the thymus or bone marrow) that are the typical cellular elements of lymph, include the cellular mediators of immunity, and constitute 20 to 30 percent of the leukocytes of normal human blood — see B CELL, T CELL — **lym·pho·cyt·ic** \ₗlim-fə-ᵗsi-tik\ *adj*

lymphocyte transformation *n* : a transformation caused in lymphocytes by a mitosis-inducing agent (as phytohemagglutinin) or by a second exposure to an antigen and characterized by an increase in size and in the amount of cytoplasm, by visibility of nucleoli in the nucleus, and after about 72 hours by a marked resemblance to blast cells

lym·pho·cyt·ic cho·rio·men·in·gi·tis \-ˌkōr-ē-ō-i-me-nən-ˈjī-təs\ n : an acute disease caused by an arenavirus, characterized by fever, nausea and vomiting, headache, stiff neck, and slow pulse, and transmitted esp. by rodents

lymphocytic leukemia n : leukemia marked by proliferation of lymphoid tissue, abnormal increase of leukocytes in the circulating blood, and enlarged lymph nodes — called also *lymphatic leukemia, lymphoid leukemia*; see LYMPHOBLASTIC LEUKEMIA

lym·pho·cy·to·pe·nia \ˌlim-fō-ˌsī-tə-ˈpē-nē-ə\ n : a decrease in the normal number of lymphocytes in the circulating blood

lym·pho·cy·to·poi·e·sis \-ˌpoi-ˈē-səs\ n, pl **-e·ses** \-ˌsēz\ : formation of lymphocytes usu. in the lymph nodes

lym·pho·cy·to·sis \ˌlim-fə-ˌsī-ˈtō-səs, -fə-sə-\ n, pl **-to·ses** \-ˌsēz\ : an increase in the number of lymphocytes in the blood usu. associated with chronic infections or inflammations — compare GRANULOCYTOSIS, MONOCYTOSIS

lym·pho·cy·to·tox·ic \ˌlim-fə-ˌsī-tə-ˈtäk-sik\ adj 1 : being or relating to toxic effects on lymphocytes 2 : being toxic to lymphocytes — **lym·pho·cy·to·tox·ic·i·ty** \-ˌtäk-ˈsi-sə-tē\ n

lym·phog·e·nous \lim-ˈfä-jə-nəs\ also **lym·pho·gen·ic** \ˌlim-fə-ˈje-nik\ adj 1 : producing lymph or lymphocytes 2 : arising, resulting from, or spread by way of lymphocytes or lymphatic vessels

lym·pho·gran·u·lo·ma \ˌlim-fō-ˌgran-yə-ˈlō-mə\ n, pl **-mas** or **-ma·ta** \-mə-tə\ 1 : a nodular swelling of a lymph node 2 : LYMPHOGRANULOMA VENEREUM — **lym·pho·gran·u·lo·mat·ous** \-ˈlō-mə-təs\ adj

lymphogranuloma in·gui·na·le \-ˌiŋ-gwə-ˈnä-lē, -ˈna-, -ˈnal-ē\ n : LYMPHOGRANULOMA VENEREUM

lym·pho·gran·u·lo·ma·to·sis \-ˌlō-mə-ˈtō-səs\ n, pl **-to·ses** \-ˌsēz\ : the development of benign or malignant lymphogranulomas in various parts of the body; also : a condition characterized by lymphogranulomas

lymphogranuloma ve·ne·re·um \-və-ˈnir-ē-əm\ n : a contagious venereal disease that is caused by various strains of a bacterium of the genus *Chlamydia* (*C. trachomatis*) and is marked by swelling and ulceration of lymphatic tissue in the iliac and inguinal regions — called also *lymphogranuloma inguinale, lymphopathia venereum*

lym·phog·ra·phy \lim-ˈfä-grə-fē\ n, pl **-phies** : LYMPHANGIOGRAPHY — **lym·pho·graph·ic** \ˌlim-fə-ˈgra-fik\ adj

lym·phoid \ˈlim-ˌfoid\ adj 1 : of, relating to, or being tissue (as the lymph nodes or thymus) containing lymphocytes 2 : of, relating to, or resembling lymph

lymphoid cell n : any of the cells responsible for the production of immunity mediated by cells or antibodies and including lymphocytes, lymphoblasts, and plasma cells

lymphoid leukemia n : LYMPHOCYTIC LEUKEMIA

lym·pho·kine \ˈlim-fə-ˌkīn\ n : any of various substances (as interleukin-2) of low molecular weight that are not antibodies, are secreted by T cells in response to stimulation by antigens, and have a role (as the activation of macrophages or the enhancement or inhibition of antibody production) in cell-mediated immunity

lym·pho·kine–activated killer cell n : a lymphocyte that has been turned into a cancer-killing cell by being cultured with interleukin-2 — called also *LAK*

lym·pho·ma \lim-ˈfō-mə\ n, pl **-mas** or **-ma·ta** \-mə-tə\ : a usu. malignant tumor of lymphoid tissue — **lym·pho·ma·tous** \-mə-təs\ adj

lym·pho·ma·toid \lim-ˈfō-mə-ˌtoid\ adj : characterized by or resembling lymphomas (a ~ tumor)

lymphomatosa — see STRUMA LYMPHOMATOSA

lym·pho·ma·to·sis \(ˌ)lim-ˌfō-mə-ˈtō-səs\ n, pl **-to·ses** \-ˌsēz\ : the presence of multiple lymphomas in the body

lym·pho·path·ia ve·ne·re·um \ˌlim-fə-ˌpa-thē-ə-və-ˈnir-ē-əm\ n : LYMPHOGRANULOMA VENEREUM

lym·pho·pe·nia \ˌlim-fə-ˈpē-nē-ə\ n : reduction in the number of lymphocytes circulating in the blood — **lym·pho·pe·nic** \-ˈpē-nik\ adj

lym·pho·poi·e·sis \ˌlim-fə-poi-ˈē-səs\ n, pl **-e·ses** \-ˌsēz\ : the formation of lymphocytes or lymphatic tissue — **lym·pho·poi·et·ic** \-poi-ˈe-tik\ adj

lym·pho·pro·lif·er·a·tive \ˌlim-fō-prə-ˈli-fə-ˌrā-tiv, -rə-tiv\ adj : of or relating to the proliferation of lymphoid tissue (~ syndrome)

lym·pho·re·tic·u·lar \ˌlim-fō-ri-ˈti-kyə-lər\ adj : RETICULOENDOTHELIAL

lymphoreticular system n : RETICULOENDOTHELIAL SYSTEM

lym·pho·sar·co·ma \ˌlim-fō-sär-ˈkō-mə\ n, pl **-mas** or **-ma·ta** \-mə-tə\ : a malignant lymphoma that tends to metastasize freely

lym·pho·tox·in \ˌlim-fō-ˈtäk-sən\ n : a lymphokine that lyses various cells and esp. tumor cells — **lym·pho·tox·ic** \-ˈtäk-sik\ adj

lymph vessel n : LYMPHATIC

Ly·on hypothesis \ˈlī-ən-\ n : a hypothesis explaining why the phenotypic effect of the X chromosome is the same in the mammalian female which has two X chromosomes as it is in the male which has only one X chromosome: one of each two somatic X chromosomes in mammalian females is selected at random and inactivated early in embryonic development

Lyon, Mary Frances (b 1925), British geneticist.

ly·oph·i·lize \lī-ˈä-fə-ˌlīz\ vb **-lized; -lizing** : FREEZE-DRY — **ly·oph·i·li·za·tion** n

ly·pres·sin \lī-ˈpres-ᵊn\ n : a lysine-containing vasopressin $C_{46}H_{65}N_{13}O_{12}S_2$ used esp. as a nasal spray in the control of diabetes insipidus

lys- or **lysi-** or **lyso-** comb form : lysis ⟨lysin⟩ ⟨lysolecithin⟩

lyse \ˈlīs, ˈlīz\ vb **lysed; lys·ing** : to cause to undergo lysis : produce lysis in

ly·ser·gic acid \lə-ˈsər-jik-, (ˌ)lī-\ n : a crystalline acid $C_{16}H_{16}N_2O_2$ from ergot alkaloids; also : LSD

lysergic acid di·eth·yl·am·ide \-ˌdī-e-thə-ˈla-ˌmīd\ n : LSD

ly·ser·gide \lə-ˈsər-ˌjid, lī-\ n : LSD

lysi- — see LYS-

ly·sin \ˈlīs-ᵊn\ n : a substance (as an antibody) capable of causing lysis

ly·sine \ˈlī-ˌsēn\ n : a crystalline essential amino acid $C_6H_{14}N_2O_2$ obtained from the hydrolysis of various proteins

ly·sis \ˈlī-səs\ n, pl **ly·ses** \-ˌsēz\ **1** : the gradual decline of a disease process (as fever) — compare CRISIS 1 **2** : a process of disintegration or dissolution (as of cells)

-ly·sis \l-ə-səs, ˈl-ə-ˌsis\ n comb form, pl **-ly·ses** \l-ə-ˌsēz\ **1** : decomposition ⟨hydrolysis⟩ **2** : disintegration : breaking down ⟨autolysis⟩ **3 a** : relief or reduction ⟨neurolysis⟩ **b** : detachment ⟨epidermolysis⟩

lyso- — see LYS-

ly·so·gen \ˈlī-sə-jən\ n : a lysogenic bacterium or bacterial strain

ly·so·gen·ic \ˌlī-sə-ˈje-nik\ adj **1** : harboring a prophage as hereditary material ⟨∼ bacteria⟩ **2** : TEMPERATE — **ly·sog·e·ny** \lī-ˈsä-jə-nē\ n

Ly·sol \ˈlī-ˌsȯl, -ˌsōl\ trademark — used for a disinfectant consisting of a brown emulsified solution containing cresols

ly·so·lec·i·thin \ˌlī-sə-ˈle-sə-thən\ n : LYSOPHOSPHATIDYLCHOLINE

ly·so·phos·pha·ti·dyl·cho·line \ˌlī-sō-ˌfäs-fə-ˌtid-ᵊl-ˈkō-ˌlēn, -(ˌ)fäs-ˌfa-təd-ᵊl-\ n : a hemolytic substance produced by the removal of a fatty acid group (as by the action of cobra venom) from a lecithin

ly·so·some \ˈlī-sə-ˌsōm\ n : a saclike cellular organelle that contains various hydrolytic enzymes — **ly·so·som·al** \ˌlī-sə-ˈsō-məl\ adj — **ly·so·so·mal·ly** adv

ly·so·zyme \ˈlī-sə-ˌzīm\ n : a basic bacteriolytic protein that hydrolyzes peptidoglycon and is present in egg white and in saliva and tears — called also muramidase

-lyte \ˌlīt\ n comb form : substance capable of undergoing (such) decomposition ⟨electrolyte⟩

lyt·ic \ˈli-tik\ adj : of or relating to lysis or a lysin; also : productive of or effecting lysis (as of cells) ⟨∼ viruses⟩ — **lyt·i·cal·ly** adv

-lyt·ic \ˈli-tik\ adj suffix : of, relating to, or effecting (such) decomposition ⟨hydrolytic⟩

M

m abbr **1** meter **2** molar **3** molarity **4** mole **5** muscle

M abbr [Latin misce] mix — used in writing prescriptions

MA mental age

McArdle's disease, McBurney's point — see entries alphabetized as MC-

Mace \ˈmās\ trademark — used for a temporarily disabling liquid that when sprayed in the face of a person causes tears, dizziness, immobilization, and sometimes nausea

¹mac·er·ate \ˈma-sə-ˌrāt\ vb **-at·ed; -at·ing** : to soften (as tissue) by steeping or soaking so as to separate into constituent elements — **mac·er·at·ed** \-ˌrā-təd\ adj — **mac·er·a·tion** \ˌma-sə-ˈrā-shən\ n

²mac·er·ate \-rət\ n : a product of macerating : something prepared by maceration — compare HOMOGENATE

Ma·chu·po virus \mä-ˈchü-pō-\ n : an arenavirus associated with hemorrhagic fever in Bolivia

mackerel shark n : any of a family (Lamnidae) of large aggressive sharks that include the great white shark

Mac·leod's syndrome \mə-ˈklaüdz-\ n : abnormally increased translucence of one lung usu. accompanied by reduction in ventilation and perfusion with blood

Macleod, William Mathieson (1911–1977), British physician.

macr- or **macro-** comb form : large ⟨macromolecule⟩ ⟨macrocyte⟩

Mac·ra·can·tho·rhyn·chus \ˌma-krə-ˌkan-thə-ˈriŋ-kəs\ n : a genus of intestinal worms (phylum Acanthocephala) that include the common acanthocephalan (M. hirudinaceus) of swine

Mac·rob·del·la \ˌma-ˌkräb-ˈde-lə\ n : a genus of large blood-sucking leeches including one (M. decora) that has been used medicinally

mac·ro·bi·ot·ic \ˌma-krō-bī-ˈä-tik, -bē-\

adj : of, relating to, or being an extremely restricted diet (as one containing chiefly whole grains)

mac·ro·bi·ot·ics \-tiks\ *n* : a macrobiotic dietary system

mac·ro·ceph·a·lous \,ma-krō-'se-fə-ləs\ *or* **mac·ro·ce·phal·ic** \-sə-'fa-lik\ *adj* : having or being an exceptionally large head or cranium — **mac·ro·ceph·a·ly** \-'se-fə-lē\ *n*

mac·ro·cy·clic \,ma-krō-'si-klik, -'sī-\ *adj* : containing or being a chemical ring that consists usu. of 15 or more atoms (a ~ antibiotic) — **macrocyclic** *n*

mac·ro·cyte \'ma-krə-,sīt\ *n* : an exceptionally large red blood cell occurring chiefly in anemias (as pernicious anemia) — called also *megalocyte*

mac·ro·cyt·ic \,ma-krə-'si-tik\ *adj* : of, or relating to macrocytes; *specif* : of an anemia : characterized by macrocytes in the blood

mac·ro·cy·to·sis \,ma-krə-sī-'tō-səs\, *pl* **-to·ses** \-,sēz\ : the occurrence of macrocytes in the blood

mac·ro·ga·mete \,ma-krō-gə-'mēt, -'ga-,mēt\ *n* : the larger and usu. the female gamete of a heterogamous organism — compare MICROGAMETE

mac·ro·ga·me·to·cyte \-gə-'mē-tə-,sīt\ *n* : a gametocyte producing macrogametes

mac·ro·gen·i·to·so·mia \,ma-krō-,je-ni-tə-'sō-mē-ə\ *n* : premature excessive development of the external genitalia

mac·ro·glia \ma-'krä-glē-ə, ,ma-krō-'glī-ə\ *n* : neuroglia made up of astrocytes — **mac·ro·gli·al** \-əl\ *adj*

mac·ro·glob·u·lin \,ma-krō-'glä-byə-lən\ *n* : a highly polymerized globulin (as IgM) of high molecular weight

mac·ro·glob·u·lin·ae·mia *chiefly Brit var of* MACROGLOBULINEMIA

mac·ro·glob·u·lin·emia \-,glä-byə-lə-'nē-mē-ə\ *n* : a disorder characterized by increased blood serum viscosity and the presence of macroglobulins in the serum — **mac·ro·glob·u·lin·emic** \-mik\ *adj*

mac·ro·glos·sia \,ma-krō-'glä-sē-ə, -'glō-\ *n* : pathological and commonly congenital enlargement of the tongue

mac·ro·lide \'ma-krə-,līd\ *n* : any of several antibiotics that are produced by actinomycetes of the genus *Streptomyces*

mac·ro·mol·e·cule \,ma-krō-'mä-li-,kyül\ *n* : a large molecule (as of a protein) built up from smaller chemical structures — compare MICROMOLECULE — **mac·ro·mo·lec·u·lar** \-mə-'le-kyə-lər\ *adj*

mac·ro·nu·tri·ent \-'nü-trē-ənt, 'nyü-\ *n* : a chemical element or substance (as protein, carbohydrate, or fat) required in relatively large quantities in nutrition

mac·ro·phage \'ma-krə-,fāj, -,fäzh\ *n* : a phagocytic tissue cell of the reticuloendothelial system that may be

fixed or freely motile, is derived from a monocyte, and functions in the protection of the body against infection and noxious substances — called also *histiocyte* — **mac·ro·phag·ic** \,ma-krə-'fa-jik\ *adj*

mac·ro·scop·ic \,ma-krə-'skä-pik\ *adj* : large enough to be observed by the naked eye — compare MICROSCOPIC 2, SUBMICROSCOPIC, ULTRAMICROSCOPIC 1 — **mac·ro·scop·i·cal·ly** *adv*

mac·ro·so·mia \,ma-krə-'sō-mē-ə\ *n* : GIGANTISM — **mac·ro·so·mic** \-'sō-mik\ *adj*

mac·ro·struc·ture \'ma-krō-,strək-chər\ *n* : the structure (as of a body part) revealed by visual examination with little or no magnification — **mac·ro·struc·tur·al** \,ma-krō-'strək-chə-rəl, -shə-rəl\ *adj*

macul- *or* **maculo-** *comb form* : macule : macular and ⟨*maculo*papular⟩

mac·u·la \'ma-kyə-lə\ *n, pl* **-lae** \-,lē, -,lī\ *also* **-las** 1 : any spot or blotch; *esp* : MACULE 2 2 : an anatomical structure having the form of a spot differentiated from surrounding tissues: as **a** : MACULA ACUSTICA **b** : MACULA LUTEA

macula acus·ti·ca \-ə-'küs-ti-kə\ *n, pl* **maculae acus·ti·cae** \-ti-,sē\ : either of two small areas of sensory hair cells in the ear that are covered with gelatinous material on which are located crystals or concretions of calcium carbonate and that are associated with the perception of equilibrium: **a** : one located in the saccule **b** : one located in the utricle

macula den·sa \-'den-sa\ *n* : a group of modified epithelial cells in the distal convoluted tubule of the kidney that control renin release by relaying information about the sodium concentration in the fluid passing through the convoluted tubule to the renin-producing juxtaglomerular cells of the afferent arteriole

macula lu·tea \-'lü-tē-ə\ *n, pl* **maculae lu·te·ae** \-tē-,ē, -tē-,ī\ : a small yellowish area lying slightly lateral to the center of the retina that constitutes the region of maximum visual acuity and is made up almost wholly of retinal cones

mac·u·lar \'ma-kyə-lər\ *adj* 1 : of, relating to, or characterized by a spot or spots ⟨a ~ skin rash⟩ 2 : of, relating to, affecting, or mediated by the macula lutea ⟨~ vision⟩

macular degeneration *n* : a loss of central vision in both eyes produced by pathological changes in the macula lutea and characterized by spots of pigmentation or other abnormalities

mac·ule \'ma-(,)kyül\ *n* 1 : MACULE 2 2 : a patch of skin that is altered in color or but usu. not elevated and that is a characteristic feature of various diseases (as smallpox)

maculo- — see MACUL-

mac·u·lo·pap·u·lar \ˌma-kyə-(ˌ)lō-ˈpa-pyə-lər\ *adj* : combining the characteristics of macules and papules ⟨a ∼ rash⟩ ⟨a ∼ lesion⟩

mac·u·lo·pap·ule \-ˈpa-(ˌ)pyül\ *n* : a maculopapular elevation of the skin

mad \ˈmad\ *adj* **mad·der; mad·dest 1** : arising from, indicative of, or marked by mental disorder **2** : affected with rabies : RABID

mad itch *n* : PSEUDORABIES

mad·ness \ˈmad-nəs\ *n* **1** : INSANITY **2** : one of several ailments of animals marked by frenzied behavior; *specif* : RABIES

Ma·du·ra foot \ˈma-dyûr-ə-, -dûr-; mə-ˈ\ *n* : maduromycosis of the foot

mad·u·ro·my·co·sis \ˌma-dyü-rō-mī-ˈkō-səs, -dü-\ *n, pl* **-co·ses** \-ˌsēz\ : a destructive chronic disease usu. restricted to the feet, marked by swelling and deformity resulting from the formation of granulomatous nodules and caused esp. by an aerobic form of actinomycetes and sometimes by fungi — compare NOCARDIOSIS — **mad·u·ro·my·cot·ic** \-ˈkä-tik\ *adj*

maf·e·nide \ˈma-fə-ˌnīd\ *n* : a sulfonamide $C_7H_{10}N_2O_2S$ applied topically as an antibacterial ointment esp. in the treatment of burns — see SULFAMYLON

mag·got \ˈma-gət\ *n* : a soft-bodied legless grub that is the larva of a dipteran fly (as the housefly) and develops usu. in decaying organic matter or as a parasite in plants or animals

magic bullet *n* : a substance or therapy capable of destroying pathogenic agents (as bacteria or cancer cells) without deleterious side effects

magic mushroom *n* : any fungus containing hallucinogenic alkaloids (as psilocybin)

mag·ma \ˈmag-mə\ *n* : a suspension of a large amount of precipitated material (as in milk of magnesia or milk of bismuth) in a small volume of a watery vehicle

magna — see CISTERNA MAGNA

Mag·na·my·cin \ˌmag-nə-ˈmis-ᵊn\ *trademark* — used for a preparation of carbomycin

mag·ne·sia \mag-ˈnē-shə, -ˈnē-zhə\ *n* : MAGNESIUM OXIDE

magnesia magma *n* : MILK OF MAGNESIA

mag·ne·sium \mag-ˈnē-zē-əm, -zhəm\ *n* : a silver-white light malleable ductile metallic element that occurs abundantly in nature (as in bones) — symbol *Mg*; see ELEMENT table

magnesium carbonate *n* : a carbonate of magnesium; *esp* : the very white crystalline salt $MgCO_3$ used as an antacid and laxative

magnesium chloride *n* : a bitter crystalline salt $MgCl_2$ used esp. to replenish body electrolytes

magnesium citrate *n* : a crystalline salt used in the form of a lemony acidulous effervescent solution as a saline laxative

magnesium hydroxide *n* : a slightly alkaline crystalline compound $Mg(OH)_2$ used as an antacid and laxative — see MILK OF MAGNESIA

magnesium oxide *n* : a white compound MgO used as an antacid and mild laxative

magnesium sil·i·cate \-ˈsi-lə-ˌkāt, -kət\ *n* : a silicate that is approximately $Mg_3Si_2O_8 \cdot nH_2O$ and that is used chiefly in medicine as a gastric antacid adsorbent and coating (as in the treatment of ulcers)

magnesium sulfate *n* : a sulfate of magnesium $MgSO_4$ that occurs in nature and serves as the basis of Epsom salts

magnetic field *n* : the portion of space near a magnetic body or a current-carrying body in which the magnetic forces due to the body or current can be detected

magnetic resonance *n* : the absorption of energy exhibited by particles (as atomic nuclei or electrons) in a static magnetic field when the particles are exposed to electromagnetic radiation of certain frequencies — see NUCLEAR MAGNETIC RESONANCE

magnetic resonance imaging *n* : a noninvasive diagnostic technique that produces computerized images of internal body tissues and is based on nuclear magnetic resonance of atoms within the body induced by the application of radio waves — abbr. *MRI*

mag·ne·to·en·ceph·a·log·ra·phy \mag-ˌnē-tō-in-ˌse-fə-ˈlä-grə-fē\ *n, pl* **-phies** : the process of detecting and recording the magnetic field of the brain

mag·ni·fi·ca·tion \ˌmag-nə-fə-ˈkā-shən\ *n* : the apparent enlargement of an object by an optical instrument that is the ratio of the dimensions of an image formed by the instrument to the corresponding dimensions of the object — called also *power* — **mag·ni·fy** \ˈmag-nə-ˌfī\ *vb*

mag·no·cel·lu·lar \ˌmag-nō-ˈsel-yə-lər\ *adj* : having or consisting of large cells (∼ hypothalamic nuclei)

magnum — see FORAMEN MAGNUM

magnus — see ADDUCTOR MAGNUS

maid·en·head \ˈmād-ᵊn-ˌhed\ *n* : HYMEN

maim \ˈmām\ *vb* **1** : to commit the felony of mayhem upon **2** : to wound seriously : MUTILATE, DISABLE

main·line \ˈmān-ˌlīn\ *vb* **-lined; -lining** *slang* : to inject a narcotic drug (as heroin) into a vein

main·stream \-ˌstrēm\ *adj* : relating to or being tobacco smoke that is drawn (as from a cigarette) directly into the mouth of the smoker and is usu. inhaled into the lungs — compare SIDESTREAM

main·te·nance \ˈmānt-ᵊn-əns\ *adj* : designed or adequate to maintain a patient in a stable condition : serving to maintain a gradual process of healing or to prevent a relapse ⟨a ∼ dose⟩ ⟨∼ chemotherapy⟩

ma·jor \'mā-jər\ *adj* : involving grave risk : SERIOUS ⟨a ∼ illness⟩ ⟨a ∼ operative procedure⟩ — compare MINOR

majora — see LABIA MAJORA

major histocompatibility complex *n* : a group of genes that function esp. in determining the histocompatibility antigens found on cell surfaces and that in humans comprise the alleles occurring at four loci on the short arm of chromosome 6 — abbr. *MHC*

major labia *n pl* : LABIA MAJORA

major–medical *adj* : of, relating to, or being a form of insurance designed to pay all or part of the medical bills of major illnesses usu. after deduction of a fixed initial sum

major surgery *n* : surgery involving a risk to the life of the patient; *specif* : an operation upon an organ within the cranium, chest, abdomen, or pelvic cavity — compare MINOR SURGERY

mal \'mäl, 'mal\ *n* : DISEASE, SICKNESS

mal- *comb form* **1** : bad ⟨*mal*practice⟩ **2 a** : abnormal ⟨*mal*formation⟩ **b** : abnormally ⟨*mal*formed⟩ **3 a** : inadequate ⟨*mal*adjustment⟩ **b** : inadequately ⟨*mal*nourished⟩

mal·ab·sorp·tion \,ma-ləb-'sórp-shən, -'zórp-\ *n* : faulty absorption of nutrient materials from the alimentary canal — **mal·ab·sorp·tive** \-tiv\ *adj*

malabsorption syndrome *n* : a syndrome resulting from malabsorption that is typically characterized by weakness, diarrhea, muscle cramps, edema, and loss of weight

malac- *or* **malaco-** *comb form* : soft ⟨*malaco*plakia⟩

ma·la·cia \mə-'lā-shə, -shē-ə\ *n* : abnormal softening of a tissue — often used in combination ⟨osteo*malacia*⟩ — **ma·lac·ic** \-sik\ *adj*

mal·a·co·pla·kia \,ma-lə-kō-'plā-kē-ə\ *n* : inflammation of the mucous membrane of a hollow organ (as the urinary bladder) characterized by the formation of soft granulomatous lesions

mal·ad·ap·ta·tion \,mal-,a-,dap-'tā-shən\ *n* : poor or inadequate adaptation ⟨psychological ∼⟩ — **mal·adap·tive** \,ma-lə-'dap-tiv\ *adj* — **mal·adap·tive·ly** *adv*

mal·a·die de Ro·ger \,ma-lə-'dē-də-rō-'zhā\ *n* : a small usu. asymptomatic ventricular septal defect

Roger, Henri–Louis (1809–1891), French physician.

mal·ad·just·ment \,ma-lə-'jəst-mənt\ *n* : poor, faulty, or inadequate adjustment — **mal·ad·just·ed** \-'jəs-təd\ *adj*

mal·ad·min·is·tra·tion \,ma-ləd-,mi-nə-'strā-shən\ *n* : incorrect administration (as of a drug)

mal·a·dy \'ma-lə-dē\ *n, pl* **-dies** : DISEASE, SICKNESS ⟨a fatal ∼⟩

mal·aise \mə-'lāz, ma-, -'lez\ *n* : an indefinite feeling of debility or lack of health often indicative of or accompanying the onset of an illness

mal·a·ko·pla·kia *var of* MALACOPLAKIA

mal·align·ment \,ma-lə-'līn-mənt\ *n* : incorrect or imperfect alignment (as of teeth) — **mal·aligned** \-'līnd\ *adj*

ma·lar \'mā-lər, -,lär\ *adj* : of or relating to the cheek, the side of the head, or the zygomatic bone

malar bone *n* : ZYGOMATIC BONE — called also *malar*

malari- *or* **malario-** *comb form* : malaria ⟨*malario*logy⟩

ma·lar·ia \mə-'ler-ē-ə\ *n* **1** : an acute or chronic disease caused by the presence of sporozoan parasites of the genus *Plasmodium* in the red blood cells, transmitted from an infected to an uninfected individual by the bite of anopheline mosquitoes, and characterized by periodic attacks of chills and fever that coincide with mass destruction of blood cells and the release of toxic substances by the parasite at the end of each reproductive cycle — see FALCIPARUM MALARIA, VIVAX MALARIA **2** : any of various diseases of birds and mammals that are more or less similar to malaria of human beings and are caused by blood protozoans — **ma·lar·i·al** \-əl\ *adj*

ma·lar·i·ae malaria \mə-'ler-ē-,ē-\ *n* : malaria caused by a malaria parasite (*Plasmodium malariae*) and marked by recurrence of paroxysms at 72-hour intervals — called also *quartan malaria*

malarial mosquito *or* **malaria mosquito** *n* : a mosquito of the genus *Anopheles* (esp. *A. quadrimaculatus*) that transmits the malaria parasite

malaria parasite *n* : a protozoan of the sporozoan genus *Plasmodium* that is transmitted to humans or to certain other mammals or birds by the bite of a mosquito in which its sexual reproduction takes place, that multiplies asexually in the vertebrate host by schizogony in the red blood cells or in certain tissue cells, and that causes destruction of red blood cells and the febrile disease malaria — see MEROZOITE, PHANEROZITE, SCHIZONT, SPOROZOITE

ma·lar·i·ol·o·gy \mə-,ler-ē-'ä-lə-jē\ *n, pl* **-gies** : the scientific study of malaria — **ma·lar·i·ol·o·gist** \-jist\ *n*

ma·lar·i·ous \mə-'ler-ē-əs\ *adj* : characterized by the presence of or infected with malaria ⟨∼ regions⟩

ma·late \'ma-,lāt, 'mā-\ *n* : a salt or ester of malic acid

mal·a·thi·on \,ma-lə-'thī-ən, -,än\ *n* : an insecticide $C_{10}H_{19}O_6PS_2$ with a lower mammalian toxicity than parathion

mal de mer \ˌmal-də-ˈmer\ *n* : SEASICK-NESS

mal·des·cent \ˌmal-di-ˈsent\ *n* : an improper or incomplete descent of a testis into the scrotum — **mal·des·cend·ed** \-ˈsen-dəd\ *adj*

mal·de·vel·op·ment \ˌmal-di-ˈve-ləp-mənt\ *n* : abnormal growth or development : DYSPLASIA

¹**male** \ˈmāl\ *n* : an individual that produces small usu. motile gametes (as sperm or spermatozoa) which fertilize the eggs of a female

²**male** *adj* : of, relating to, or being the sex that produces gametes which fertilize the eggs of a female

ma·le·ate \ˈmā-lē-ˌāt, -lē-ət\ *n* : a salt or ester of maleic acid

male bonding *n* : bonding between males through shared activities excluding females

male climacteric *n* : CLIMACTERIC 2

ma·le·ic acid \mə-ˈlē-ik-, -ˈlā-\ *n* : an isomer of fumaric acid

male menopause *n* : CLIMACTERIC 2

male–pattern baldness *n* : typical hereditary baldness in the male characterized by loss of hair on the crown and temples

mal·for·ma·tion \ˌmal-fȯr-ˈmā-shən\ *n* : irregular, anomalous, abnormal, or faulty formation or structure — **malformed** \(ˌ)mal-ˈfȯrmd\ *adj*

mal·func·tion \(ˌ)mal-ˈfəŋk-shən\ *vb* : to function imperfectly or badly : fail to operate in the normal or usual manner — **malfunction** *n*

ma·lic acid \ˈma-lik, ˈmā-\ *n* : any of three optical isomers of an acid $C_4H_6O_5$; *esp* : the one formed as an intermediate in the Krebs cycle

maligna — see LENTIGO MALIGNA

ma·lig·nan·cy \mə-ˈlig-nən-sē\ *n*, *pl* **-cies 1** : the quality or state of being malignant **2 a** : exhibition (as by a tumor) of malignant qualities : VIRULENCE **b** : a malignant tumor

ma·lig·nant \-nənt\ *adj* **1** : tending to produce death or deterioration; *esp* : tending to infiltrate, metastasize, and terminate fatally (∼ tumor) — compare BENIGN 1 **2** : of unfavorable prognosis : not responding favorably to treatment

malignant catarrhal fever *n* : an acute infectious often fatal disease esp. of cattle and deer that is caused by one or more herpesviruses and is characterized by fever, depression, enlarged lymph nodes, discharge from the eyes and nose, and lesions affecting most organ systems — called also *catarrhal fever, malignant catarrh*

malignant edema *n* : an acute often fatal toxemia of wild and domestic animals that follows wound infection by an anaerobic toxin-producing bacterium of the genus *Clostridium (C. septicum)* and is characterized by anorexia, intoxication, fever, and soft fluid-filled swellings — compare BLACK DISEASE, BRAXY

malignant hypertension *n* : essential hypertension characterized by acute onset, severe symptoms, rapidly progressive course, and poor prognosis

malignant hyperthermia *n* : a rare inherited condition characterized by a rapid, extreme, and often fatal rise in body temperature following the administration of general anesthesia

malignant malaria *n* : FALCIPARUM MALARIA

malignant malnutrition *n* : KWASHIORKOR

malignant pustule *n* : localized anthrax of the skin taking the form of a pimple surrounded by a zone of edema and hyperemia and tending to become necrotic and ulcerated

malignant tertian malaria *n* : FALCIPARUM MALARIA

malignant transformation *n* : the transformation that a cell undergoes to become a rapidly dividing tumor-producing cell

ma·lig·ni·za·tion \mə-ˌlig-nə-ˈzā-shən\ *n* : a process or instance of becoming malignant (∼ of a tumor)

ma·lin·ger \mə-ˈliŋ-gər\ *vb* **-gered; -gering** : to pretend or exaggerate incapacity or illness so as to avoid duty or work — **ma·lin·ger·er** \-ər-\ *n*

mal·le·o·lar \mə-ˈlē-ə-lər\ *adj* : of or relating to a malleolus esp. of the ankle

mal·le·o·lus \mə-ˈlē-ə-ləs\ *n*, *pl* **-li** \-ˌlī\ : an expanded projection or process at the distal extremity of each bone of the leg: **a** : the expanded lower extremity of the fibula situated on the lateral side of the leg at the ankle — called also *external malleolus, lateral malleolus* **b** : a strong pyramid-shaped process of the tibia that projects distally on the medial side of its lower extremity at the ankle — called also *internal malleolus, medial malleolus*

mal·let finger \ˈma-lət-\ *n* : involuntary flexion of the distal phalanx of a finger caused by avulsion of the extensor tendon

mal·le·us \ˈma-lē-əs\ *n*, *pl* **mal·lei** \-lē-ˌī, -lē-ˌē\ : the outermost of the three auditory ossicles of the middle ear consisting of a head, neck, short process, long process, and handle with the short process and handle being fastened to the tympanic membrane and the head articulating with the head of the incus — called also *hammer*

mal·nour·ished \(ˌ)mal-ˈnər-isht\ *adj* : UNDERNOURISHED

mal·nour·ish·ment \-ˈnər-ish-mənt\ *n* : MALNUTRITION

mal·nu·tri·tion \ˌmal-nu̇-ˈtri-shən, -nyu̇-\ *n* : faulty nutrition due to inadequate or unbalanced intake of nutrients or their impaired assimilation or utilization — **mal·nu·tri·tion·al** \-ˈl\ *adj*

mal·oc·clu·sion \ˌma-lə-ˈklü-zhən\ *n*

: improper occlusion; *esp* : abnormality in the coming together of teeth — **mal·oc·clu·ded** \-'klü-dəd\ *adj*

Mal·pi·ghi·an body \mal-'pi-gē-ən-, -'pē-\ *n* : RENAL CORPUSCLE; *also* : MALPIGHIAN CORPUSCLE 2

Malpighi \mäl-'pē-gē\, **Marcello** (1628–1694), Italian anatomist.

Malpighian corpuscle *n* 1 : RENAL CORPUSCLE 2 : any of the small masses of adenoid tissue formed around the branches of the splenic artery in the spleen

Malpighian layer *n* : the deeper part of the epidermis consisting of cells whose protoplasm has not yet changed into horny material — called also *stratum germinativum*

Malpighian pyramid *n* : RENAL PYRAMID

mal·posed \mal-'pōzd\ *adj* : characterized by malposition (~ teeth)

mal·po·si·tion \mal-pə-'zi-shən\ *n* : wrong or faulty position

mal·prac·tice \(ˌ)mal-'prak-təs\ *n* : a dereliction of professional duty or a failure to exercise an accepted degree of professional skill or learning by a physician rendering professional services which results in injury, loss, or damage — **malpractice** *vb*

mal·pre·sen·ta·tion \mal-ˌprē-zen-'tā-shən, -ˌpre-\ *n* : abnormal presentation of the fetus at birth

mal·ro·ta·tion \mal-rō-'tā-shən\ *n* : improper rotation of a bodily part and esp. of the intestines — **mal·ro·tat·ed** \-'rō-ˌtāt-əd\ *adj*

Mal·ta fever \ˈmȯl-tə-\ *n* : BRUCELLOSIS a

malt·ase \'mȯl-ˌtās, -ˌtāz\ *n* : an enzyme that catalyzes the hydrolysis of maltose to glucose

malt·ose \'mȯl-ˌtōs, -ˌtōz\ *n* : a crystalline dextrorotatory sugar $C_{12}H_{22}O_{11}$ formed esp. from starch by amylase (as in saliva)

mal·union \mal-'yün-yən\ *n* : incomplete or faulty union (as of the fragments of a fractured bone)

mam·ba \'mäm-bə, 'mam-\ *n* : any of several venomous elapid snakes (genus *Dendroaspis*) of sub-Saharan Africa

mam·il·la·ry, mam·il·lat·ed, ma·mil·lo·tha·lam·ic tract *var of* MAMMILLARY, MAMMILLATED, MAMMILLOTHALAMIC TRACT

mamm- *or* **mamma-** *or* **mammi-** *or* **mammo-** *comb form* : breast (*mammogram*)

mam·ma \'ma-mə\ *n*, *pl* **mam·mae** \'ma-ˌmē, -ˌmī\ : a mammary gland and its accessory parts

mam·mal \'ma-məl\ *n* : any of a class (Mammalia) of warm-blooded higher vertebrates (as dogs, cats, and humans) that nourish their young with milk secreted by mammary glands and have the skin more or less covered by hair — **mam·ma·li·an** \mə-'mā-lē-ən, ma-\ *adj* or *n*

mam·ma·plas·ty \'ma-mə-ˌplas-tē\ *n*, *pl* **-ties** : plastic surgery of the breast

¹**mam·ma·ry** \'ma-mə-rē\ *adj* : of, relating to, lying near, or affecting the mammae

²**mammary** *n*, *pl* **-aries** : MAMMARY GLAND

mammary artery — see INTERNAL THORACIC ARTERY

mammary gland *n* : any of the large compound sebaceous glands that in female mammals are modified to secrete milk, are situated ventrally in pairs, and usu. terminate in a nipple

mam·mil·la·ry \'ma-mə-ˌler-ē, ma-'mil-lə-rē\ *adj* 1 : of, relating to, or resembling the breasts 2 : studded with breast-shaped protuberances

mammillary body *n* : either of two small rounded eminences on the underside of the brain behind the tuber cinereum

mam·mil·lat·ed \'ma-mə-ˌlā-təd\ *adj* 1 : having nipples or small protuberances 2 : having the form of a bluntly rounded protuberance

mam·mil·lo·tha·lam·ic tract \mə-ˌmi-lō-thə-'la-mik-\ *n* : a bundle of nerve fibers that runs from the mammillary body to the anterior nucleus of the thalamus — called also *mammillothalamic fasciculus*

mammo- — see MAMM-

mam·mo·gram \'ma-mə-ˌgram\ *n* : a photograph of the breasts made by X rays

mam·mo·graph \-ˌgraf\ *n* : MAMMOGRAM

mam·mog·ra·phy \ma-'mä-grə-fē\ *n*, *pl* **-phies** : X-ray examination of the breasts (as for early detection of cancer) — **mam·mo·graph·ic** \ˌma-mə-'gra-fik\ *adj*

mam·mo·plas·ty \'ma-mə-ˌplas-tē\ *n*, *pl* **-ties** : plastic surgery of the breast

mam·mo·tro·pin \ˌma-mə-'trōp-ᵊn\ *n* : PROLACTIN

man \'man\ *n*, *pl* **men** \'men\ : a bipedal primate mammal of the genus *Homo* (*H. sapiens*) that is anatomically related to the family (Pongidae) of larger more advanced apes but is distinguished esp. by notable development of the brain with a resultant capacity for articulate speech and abstract reasoning, is usu. considered to form a variable number of freely interbreeding races, and is the sole representative of a natural family (Hominidae); *broadly* : any living or extinct member of this family

managed care *n* : a system of providing health care through managed programs (as HMOs or PPOs) that is designed esp. to control costs

man·age·ment \'ma-nij-mənt\ *n* : the whole system of care and treatment of a disease or a sick individual — **man·age** \'ma-nij\ *vb*

Man·del·amine \man-'de-lə-mēn\ *trade-mark* — used for a preparation of the mandelate of methenamine

man·del·ate \'man-də-ˌlāt\ *n* : a salt or ester of mandelic acid

man·del·ic acid \man-'de-lik-\ *n* : an acid $C_8H_8O_3$ that is used chiefly in the form of its salts as a bacteriostatic agent for genitourinary tract infections

man·di·ble \'man-də-bəl\ *n* **1** : JAW 1; *esp* : JAW 1b **2** : the lower jaw with its investing soft parts — **man·dib·u·lar** \man-'di-byə-lər\ *adj*

mandibul- *or* **mandibuli-** *or* **mandibulo-** *comb form* : mandibular and ⟨*mandibulo*facial dysostosis⟩

mandibular arch *n* : the first branchial arch of the vertebrate embryo from which in humans are developed the lower lip, the mandible, the masticatory muscles, and the anterior part of the tongue

mandibular artery *n* : INFERIOR ALVEOLAR ARTERY

mandibular canal *n* : a bony canal within the mandible that gives passage to blood vessels and nerves supplying the lower teeth

mandibular foramen *n* : the opening on the medial surface of the ramus of the mandible that leads into the mandibular canal and transmits blood vessels and nerves supplying the lower teeth

mandibular fossa *n* : GLENOID FOSSA

mandibular nerve *n* : the one of the three major branches or divisions of the trigeminal nerve that supplies sensory fibers to the lower jaw, the floor of the mouth, the anterior two-thirds of the tongue, and the lower teeth and motor fibers to the muscles of mastication — called also *inferior maxillary nerve*; compare MAXILLARY NERVE, OPHTHALMIC NERVE

mandibuli-, mandibulo- — see MANDIBUL-

man·di·bu·lo·fa·cial dysostosis \man-ˌdi-byə-lō-'fā-shəl-\ *n* : a dysostosis of the face and lower jaw inherited as an autosomal dominant trait and characterized by bilateral malformations, deformities of the outer and middle ear, and a usu. smaller lower jaw — called also *Treacher Collins syndrome*

man-eat·er \'man-ˌē-tər\ *n* : one (as a great white shark) having an appetite for human flesh — **man-eat·ing** *adj*

man-eater shark *n* : MACKEREL SHARK; *esp* : GREAT WHITE SHARK

man-eating shark *n* : MAN-EATER SHARK

ma·neu·ver \mə-'nü-vər, -'nyü-\ *n* **1** : a movement, procedure, or method performed to achieve a desired result and esp. to restore a normal physiological state or to promote normal function — see HEIMLICH MANEUVER, VALSALVA MANEUVER **2** : a manipula-

tion to accomplish a change of position; *specif* : a rotation or other movement applied to a fetus within the uterus to alter its position and facilitate delivery — see SCANZONI MANEUVER

man·ga·nese \'maŋ-gə-ˌnēz, -ˌnēs\ *n* : a grayish white usu. hard and brittle metallic element — symbol *Mn*; see ELEMENT table

mange \'mānj\ *n* : any of various more or less severe, persistent, and contagious skin diseases that are marked esp. by eczematous inflammation and loss of hair and that affect domestic animals or sometimes humans; *esp* : a skin disease caused by a minute parasitic mite of *Sarcoptes*, *Psoroptes*, *Chorioptes*, or related genera that burrows in or lives on the skin or by one of the genus *Demodex* that lives in the hair follicles or sebaceous glands — see CHORIOPTIC MANGE, DEMODECTIC MANGE, SARCOPTIC MANGE, SCABIES

mange mite *n* : any of the small parasitic mites that infest the skin of animals and cause mange

man·go fly \'maŋ-gō-\ *n* : any of various horseflies of the genus *Chrysops* that are vectors of filarial worms

man·gy \'mān-jē\ *adj* **man·gi·er; -est 1** : infected with mange ⟨a ~ dog⟩ **2** : relating to, characteristic of, or resulting from mange ⟨a ~ itch⟩

ma·nia \'mā-nē-ə, -nyə\ *n* : excitement of psychotic proportions manifested by mental and physical hyperactivity, disorganization of behavior, and elevation of mood; *specif* : the manic phase of manic-depressive psychosis

ma·ni·ac \'mā-nē-ˌak\ *n* : an individual affected with or exhibiting madness — **ma·ni·a·cal** \mə-'nī-ə-kəl\ *also* **ma·ni·ac** \'mā-nē-ak\ *adj*

¹man·ic \'ma-nik\ *adj* : affected with, relating to, or resembling mania — **man·i·cal·ly** *adv*

²manic *n* : an individual affected with mania

manic–depression *n* : MANIC-DEPRESSIVE PSYCHOSIS

¹manic–depressive *adj* : characterized by mania, by psychotic depression, or by alternating mania and depression

²manic–depressive *n* : a manic-depressive person

manic–depressive psychosis *n* : a major mental disorder characterized by manic-depressive episodes — called also *manic-depressive reaction*

man·i·fes·ta·tion \ˌma-nə-fə-'stā-shən, -fe-\ *n* : a perceptible, outward, or visible expression (as of a disease or abnormal condition)

manifest content *n* : the content of a dream as it is recalled by the dreamer in psychoanalysis — compare LATENT CONTENT

ma·nip·u·late \mə-'ni-pyə-ˌlāt\ *vb* -lat-ed; -lat·ing 1 : to treat or operate with the hands or by mechanical means esp. in a skillful manner (~ the fragments of a broken bone into correct position) 2 : to control or play upon by artful, unfair, or insidious means esp. to one's own advantage — **ma·nip·u·la·tive** \mə-ˈni-pyə-ˌlā-tiv, -lə-\ *adj* — **ma·nip·u·la·tive·ness** *n*

ma·nip·u·la·tion \mə-ˌni-pyə-ˈlā-shən\ *n* 1 : the act, process, or an instance of manipulating esp. a body part by manual examination and treatment; *esp* : adjustment of faulty structural relationships by manual means (as in the reduction of fractures or dislocations) 2 : the condition of being manipulated

man·ner·ism \ˈma-nə-ˌri-zəm\ *n* : a characteristic and often unconscious mode or peculiarity of action, bearing, or treatment; *esp* : any pointless and compulsive activity performed repeatedly

man·ni·tol \ˈma-nə-ˌtȯl, -ˌtōl\ *n* : a slightly sweet crystalline alcohol $C_6H_14O_6$ found in many plants and used esp. as a diuretic and in testing kidney function

mannitol hexa·ni·trate \-ˌhek-sə-ˈnī-ˌtrāt\ *n* : an explosive crystalline ester $C_6H_8(NO_3)_6$ made from mannitol and used mixed with a carbohydrate (as lactose) in the treatment of angina pectoris and vascular hypertension

man·nose \ˈma-ˌnōs, -ˌnōz\ *n* : an aldose $C_6H_{12}O_6$ found esp. in plants

man·nos·i·do·sis \ˌma-ˌnō-sə-ˈdō-səs\ *n, pl* **-do·ses** \-ˌsēz\ : a rare inherited metabolic disease characterized by deficiency of an enzyme catalyzing the metabolism of mannose with resulting accumulation of mannose in the body and marked esp. by facial and skeletal deformities and by mental retardation

ma·noeu·vre *chiefly Brit var of* MANEUVER

ma·nom·e·ter \mə-ˈnä-mə-tər\ *n* 1 : an instrument for measuring the pressure of gases and vapors 2 : SPHYGMOMANOMETER — **mano·met·ric** \ˌma-nə-ˈme-trik\ *adj* — **mano·met·ri·cal·ly** *adv* — **ma·nom·e·try** \mə-ˈnä-mə-trē\ *n*

Man·son·el·la \ˌman-sə-ˈne-lə\ *n* : a genus of filarial worms (family Dipetalonematidae) including one (*M. ozzardi*) that is common and apparently nonpathogenic in human visceral fat and mesenteries in So. and Central America

Man·son \ˈman-sən\, **Sir Patrick (1844–1922),** British parasitologist.

mansoni — *see* SCHISTOSOMIASIS MANSONI

Man·son's disease \ˈman-sənz-\ *n* : SCHISTOSOMIASIS MANSONI

man·tle \ˈmant-ᵊl\ *n* 1 : something that covers, enfolds, or envelops 2 : CEREBRAL CORTEX

Man·toux test \man-ˈtü-, ˌmäⁿ-\ *n* : an intradermal test for hypersensitivity to tuberculin that indicates past or present infection with tubercle bacilli — *compare* TUBERCULIN TEST

Mantoux, Charles (1877–1947), French physician.

ma·nu·bri·um \mə-ˈnü-brē-əm, -ˈnyü-\ *n, pl* **-bria** \-brē-ə\ *also* **-bri·ums** : an anatomical process or part shaped like a handle: as **a** : the cephalic segment of the sternum that is a somewhat triangular flattened bone with anterolateral borders which articulate with the clavicles **b** : the process of the malleus of the ear

ma·nus \ˈmā-nəs, ˈmä-\ *n, pl* **ma·nus** \-nəs, -ˌnüs\ : the distal segment of the vertebrate forelimb from the carpus to the end of the limb

many·plies \ˈme-nē-ˌplīz\ *n* : OMASUM

MAO *abbr* monoamine oxidase

MAOI *abbr* monoamine oxidase inhibitor

Mao·late \ˈmā-ō-ˌlāt\ *trademark* — used for a preparation of chlorphenesin carbamate

¹**map** \ˈmap\ *n* : the arrangement of genes on a chromosome — called also *genetic map*

²**map** *vb* **mapped; map·ping** 1 : to locate (a gene) on a chromosome 2 *of a gene* : to be located (a repressor ~s near the corresponding structural gene)

maple syrup urine disease *n* : a hereditary aminoaciduria caused by a deficiency of decarboxylase leading to high concentrations of valine, leucine, isoleucine, and alloisoleucine in the blood, urine, and cerebrospinal fluid and characterized by an odor of maple syrup to the urine, vomiting, hypertonicity, severe mental retardation, seizures, and eventually death unless the condition is treated with dietary measures

ma·pro·ti·line \mə-ˈprō-tə-ˌlēn\ *n* : an antidepressant drug used in the form of its hydrochloride $C_{20}H_{23}N·HCl$ to relieve major depression (as in manic depressive psychosis) and anxiety associated with depression

ma·ras·mus \mə-ˈraz-məs\ *n* : a condition of chronic undernourishment occurring esp. in children and usu. caused by a diet deficient in calories and proteins but sometimes by disease (as congenital syphilis) or parasitic infection — **ma·ras·mic** \-mik\ *adj*

marble bone disease *n* : OSTEOPETROSIS

Mar·bor·an \ˈmär-bə-ˌran\ *trademark* — used for a preparation of methisazone

Mar·burg disease \ˈmär-bərg-\ *n* : GREEN MONKEY DISEASE

Marburg virus *n* : an African RNA arbovirus that causes green monkey disease

march \ˈmärch\ *n* : the progression of epileptic activity through the motor centers of the cerebral cortex that is manifested in localized convulsions in first one and then an adjacent part of the body

Mar·ek's disease \'mar-iks-\ n : a highly contagious viral disease of poultry that is characterized esp. by proliferation of lymphoid cells and is caused by a herpesvirus

Marek, Jozsef (1867–1952), Hungarian veterinarian.

Ma·rey's law \mə-'rāz-\ n : a statement in physiology: heart rate is related inversely to arterial blood pressure

Marey, Étienne–Jules (1830–1904), French physiologist.

Mar·e·zine \'mar-ə-₁zēn\ trademark — used for a preparation of the hydrochloride of cyclizine

Mar·fan's syndrome \'mär-₁fanz-\ or **Mar·fan syndrome** \-₁fan-\ n : a disorder of connective tissue inherited as a simple dominant and characterized by abnormal elongation of the long bones and often by ocular and circulatory defects

Marfan \mär-'fäⁿ\, **Antonin Bernard Jean (1858–1942),** French pediatrician.

mar·gin \'mär-jən\ n 1 : the outside limit or edge of something (as a bodily part or a wound) 2 : the part of consciousness at a particular moment that is felt only vaguely and dimly — **mar·gin·al** \'mär-jə-nəl\ adj

mar·gin·a·tion \₁mär-jə-'nā-shən\ n 1 : the act or process of forming a margin; specif : the adhesion of white blood cells to the walls of damaged blood vessels 2 : the action of finishing a dental restoration or a filling for a cavity (~ of an amalgam with a bur)

Ma·rie–Strüm·pell disease also **Ma·rie–Strüm·pell's disease** \mä-'rē-'strüm-pəl(z)-\ n : ANKYLOSING SPONDYLITIS

Marie, Pierre (1853–1940), French neurologist.

Strümpell \'shtruem-pəl\, **Ernst Adolf Gustav Gottfried von (1853–1925),** German neurologist.

mar·i·jua·na also **mar·i·hua·na** \₁mar-ə-'wä-nə, -'hwä-\ n 1 : HEMP 1 2 : the dried leaves and flowering tops of the pistillate hemp plant that yield THC and are sometimes smoked in cigarettes for their intoxicating effect — compare BHANG, CANNABIS, HASHISH

mark \'märk\ n : an impression or trace made or occurring on something — see BIRTHMARK, STRAWBERRY MARK

mark·er \'mär-kər\ n 1 : something that serves to characterize or distinguish (a surface ~ on a cell that acts as an antigen) 2 : GENETIC MARKER — called also marker gene

Mar·o·teaux–La·my syndrome \mär-ō-'tō-lä-'mē-\ n : a mucopolysaccharidosis that is inherited as an autosomal recessive trait and that is similar to Hurler's syndrome except that

intellectual development is not retarded

Maroteaux, Pierre (b 1926), French physician.

Lamy, Maurice Emile Joseph (b 1895), French physician.

Mar·plan \'mär-₁plan\ trademark — used for a preparation of isocarboxazid

mar·row \'mar-(₁)ō\ n 1 : a soft highly vascular modified connective tissue that occupies the cavities and cancellous part of most bones and occurs in two forms: **a** : a whitish or yellowish marrow consisting chiefly of fat cells and predominating in the cavities of the long bones — called also yellow marrow **b** : a reddish marrow containing little fat, being the chief seat of red blood cell and blood granulocyte production, and occurring in the normal adult only in cancellous tissue esp. in certain flat bones — called also red marrow 2 : the substance of the spinal cord

Mar·seilles fever \mär-'sā-\ n : BOUTONNEUSE FEVER

Mar·si·lid \'mär-sə-lid\ trademark — used for a preparation of iproniazid

mar·su·pi·al·ize \mär-'sü-pē-ə-₁līz\ vb **-ized; -iz·ing** : to open (as the bladder or a cyst) and sew by the edges to the abdominal wound to permit further treatment (as of an enclosed tumor) or to discharge pathological matter (as from a hydatid cyst) — **mar·su·pi·al·i·za·tion** \-₁sü-pē-ə-li-'zā-shən\ n

mas·cu·line \'mas-kyə-lən\ adj 1 : MALE 2 : having the qualities distinctive of or appropriate to a male 3 : having a mannish bearing or quality — **mas·cu·lin·i·ty** \₁mas-kyə-'li-nə-tē\ n

mas·cu·lin·ize \'mas-kyə-lə-₁nīz\ vb **-ized; -iz·ing** : to give a preponderantly masculine character to; esp : to cause (a female) to take on male characteristics — **mas·cu·lin·i·za·tion** \₁mas-kyə-lə-nə-'zā-shən\ n

MASH abbr mobile army surgical hospital

¹mask \'mask\ n 1 : a protective covering for the face 2 **a** : a device covering the mouth and nose to facilitate inhalation **b** : a comparable device to prevent exhalation of infective material **c** : a cosmetic preparation for the skin of the face that produces a tightening effect as it dries

²mask vb 1 : to modify or reduce the effect or activity of (as a process or a reaction) 2 : to raise the audibility threshold of (a sound) by the simultaneous presentation of another sound

masked adj : failing to present or produce the usual symptoms : not obvious : LATENT (a ~ fever)

mas·och·ism \'ma-sə-₁ki-zəm, 'ma-zə-, 'mä-sə-\ n : a sexual perversion characterized by pleasure in being subjected to pain or humiliation esp. by a love object — compare ALGO-

LAGNIA, SADISM — **mas·och·is·tic** \ˌma-sə-ˈkis-tik, ˌma-zə-, ˌmä-sə-\ *adj* — **mas·och·is·ti·cal·ly** *adv*

Sa·cher–Ma·soch \ˈzä-kər-ˈmä-zók\, **Leopold von** (1836–1895), Austrian novelist.

mas·och·ist \-kist\ *n* : an individual who is given to masochism

mass \ˈmas\ *n* **1** : the property of a body that is a measure of its inertia, that is commonly taken as a measure of the amount of material it contains and causes it to have weight in a gravitational field **2** : a homogeneous pasty mixture compounded for making pills, lozenges, and plasters

mas·sage \mə-ˈsäzh, -ˈsäj\ *n* : manipulation of tissues (as by rubbing, stroking, kneading, or tapping) with the hand or an instrument for therapeutic purposes — **massage** *vb*

mas·sa in·ter·me·dia \ˈma-sə-ˌin-tər-ˈmē-dē-ə\ *n* : an apparently functionless mass of gray matter in the midline of the third ventricle that is found in many but not all human brains and is formed when the surfaces of the thalami protruding inward from opposite sides of the third ventricle make contact and fuse

mas·se·ter \mə-ˈsē-tər, ma-\ *n* : a large muscle that raises the lower jaw and assists in mastication, arises from the zygomatic arch and the zygomatic process of the temporal bone, and is inserted into the mandibular ramus and gonial angle — **mas·se·ter·ic** \ˌma-sə-ˈter-ik\ *adj*

mas·seur \ma-ˈsər, mə-\ *n* : a man who practices massage

mas·seuse \-ˈsərz, -ˈsüz\ *n* : a woman who practices massage

mas·sive \ˈma-siv\ *adj* **1** : large in comparison to what is typical — used esp. of medical dosage or of an infective agent ⟨a ∼ dose of penicillin⟩ **2** : being extensive and severe — used of a pathologic condition ⟨a ∼ hemorrhage⟩

mass number *n* : an integer that approximates the mass of an isotope and designates the total number of protons and neutrons in the nucleus ⟨the symbol for carbon of *mass number* 14 is ^{14}C or C^{14}⟩

mas·so·ther·a·py \ˌma-sō-ˈther-ə-pē\ *n*, *pl* **-pies** : the practice of massage for remedial or hygienic purposes

mass spectrometry *n* : an instrumental method for identifying the chemical constitution of a substance by means of the separation of gaseous ions according to their differing mass and charge — **mass spectrometer** *n* — **mass spectrometric** *adj*

mass spectroscopy *n* : MASS SPECTROMETRY — **mass spectroscope** *n* — **mass spectroscopic** *adj*

mast- *or* **masto-** *comb form* : breast : nipple : mammary gland ⟨*mastitis*⟩

mas·tal·gia \mas-ˈtal-jə\ *n* : MASTODYNIA

mast cell \ˈmast-\ *n* : a large cell that occurs esp. in connective tissue and has basophilic granules containing substances (as histamine and heparin) which mediate allergic reactions

mas·tec·to·mee \ma-ˌstek-tə-ˈmē\ *n* : a person who has had a mastectomy

mas·tec·to·my \ma-ˈstek-tə-mē\ *n*, *pl* **-mies** : excision or amputation of a mammary gland and usu. associated tissue

master gland *n* : PITUITARY GLAND

-mas·tia \ˈmas-tē-ə\ *n comb form* : condition of having (such or so many) breasts or mammary glands ⟨gynecomastia⟩

mas·ti·cate \ˈmas-tə-ˌkāt\ *vb* **-cat·ed; -cat·ing 1** : to grind, crush, and chew (food) with or as if with the teeth in preparation for swallowing **2** : to soften or reduce to pulp by crushing or kneading — **mas·ti·ca·tion** \ˌmas-tə-ˈkā-shən\ *n* — **mas·ti·ca·to·ry** \ˈmas-tə-kə-ˌtōr-ē\ *adj*

mas·ti·tis \ma-ˈstī-təs\ *n*, *pl* **-tit·i·des** \-ˈti-tə-ˌdēz\ : inflammation of the mammary gland or udder usu. caused by infection — see BLUE BAG, BOVINE MASTITIS, GARGET — **mas·tit·ic** \ma-ˈsti-tik\ *adj*

masto- — see MAST-

mas·to·cy·to·ma \ˌmas-tə-ˌsī-ˈtō-mə\ *n*, *pl* **-mas** *or* **-ma·ta** \-mə-tə\ : a tumorous mass produced by proliferation of mast cells

mas·to·cy·to·sis \-ˈtō-səs\ *n*, *pl* **-to·ses** \-ˌsēz\ : excessive proliferation of mast cells in the tissue

mas·to·dyn·ia \ˌmas-tə-ˈdī-nē-ə\ *n* : pain in the breast — called also *mastalgia*

¹mas·toid \ˈmas-ˌtóid\ *adj* : of, relating to, or being the mastoid process; *also* : occurring in the region of the mastoid process

²mastoid *n* : a mastoid bone or process

mastoid air cell *n* : MASTOID CELL

mastoid antrum *n* : TYMPANIC ANTRUM

mastoid cell *n* : one of the small cavities in the mastoid process that develop after birth and are filled with air — called also *mastoid air cell*

mas·toid·ec·to·my \ˌmas-ˌtói-ˈdek-tə-mē\ *n*, *pl* **-mies** : surgical removal of the mastoid cells or of the mastoid process of the temporal bone

mas·toid·itis \ˌmas-ˌtói-ˈdī-təs\ *n*, *pl* **-it·i·des** \-ˈdi-tə-ˌdēz\ : inflammation of the mastoid and esp. of the mastoid cells

mas·toid·ot·o·my \ˌmas-ˌtói-ˈdä-tə-mē\ *n*, *pl* **-mies** : incision of the mastoid

mastoid process *n* : the process of the temporal bone behind the ear that is well developed and of somewhat conical form in adults but inconspicuous in children

mas·top·a·thy \ma-ˈstä-pə-thē\ *n*, *pl*

-thies : a disorder of the breast; *esp* : a painful disorder of the breast

mas·tot·o·my \ma-'stä-tə-mē\ *n, pl* **-mies** : incision of the breast

mas·tur·ba·tion \₁mas-tər-'bā-shən\ *n* : erotic stimulation esp. of one's own genital organs commonly resulting in orgasm and achieved by manual or other bodily contact exclusive of sexual intercourse, by instrumental manipulation, occasionally by sexual fantasies, or by various combinations of these agencies — called also *onanism, self-abuse* — **mas·tur·bate** \'mas-tər-₁bāt\ *vb* — **mas·tur·ba·tor** \-₁bā-tər\ *n*

mas·tur·ba·tory \'mas-tər-bə-₁tōr-ē\ *adj* : of, relating to, or associated with masturbation ⟨∼ fantasies⟩

mate *vb* **mated; mat·ing 1** : to pair or join for breeding **2** : COPULATE

ma·te·ria al·ba \mə-'tir-ē-ə-'al-bə\ *n pl* : a soft whitish deposit of epithelial cells, white blood cells, and microorganisms esp. at the gumline

materia med·i·ca \-'me-di-kə\ *n* **1** : substances used in the composition of medical remedies : DRUGS, MEDICINE **2 a** : a branch of medical science that deals with the sources, nature, properties, and preparation of drugs **b** : a treatise on materia medica

ma·ter·nal \mə-'tərn-əl\ *adj* **1** : of, relating to, belonging to, or characteristic of a mother ⟨∼ instinct⟩ **2 a** : related through a mother **b** : inherited or derived from the female parent ⟨∼ genes⟩ — **ma·ter·nal·ly** *adv*

maternal inheritance *n* : inheritance of characters transmitted through the cytoplasm of the egg

maternal rubella *n* : German measles in a pregnant woman that may cause developmental anomalies in the fetus when occurring during the first trimester

¹**ma·ter·ni·ty** \mə-'tər-nə-tē\ *n, pl* **-ties** : a hospital facility designed for the care of women before and during childbirth and for the care of newborn babies

²**maternity** *adj* : of or relating to pregnancy or the period close to and including childbirth

ma·ter·no·fe·tal \me-₁tər-nō-'fēt-əl\ *adj* : involving a fetus and its mother ⟨the human ∼ interface⟩

ma·tri·cide \'ma-trə-₁sīd, 'mā-\ *n* : murder of a mother by her son or daughter

ma·trix \'mā-triks\ *n, pl* **ma·tri·ces** \'mā-trə-₁sēz, 'ma-\ *or* **matrixes 1 a** : the intercellular substance in which tissue cells (as of connective tissue) are embedded **b** : the thickened epithelium at the base of a fingernail or toenail from which new nail substance develops — called also *nail bed, nail matrix* **2** : a mass by which something is enclosed or in which something is embedded **3 a** : a strip or band placed so as to serve as a retaining outer wall of a tooth in filling a cavity **b** : a metal or porcelain pattern in which an inlay is cast or fused

mat·ter \'ma-tər\ *n* **1** : material (as feces or urine) discharged for or discharge from the living body **2** : material discharged by suppuration : PUS

mattress suture *n* : a surgical stitch in which the suture is passed back and forth through both edges of a wound so that the needle is reinserted each time on the side of exit and passes through to the side of insertion

mat·u·rate \'ma-chə-₁rāt\ *vb* **-rat·ed; -rat·ing** : MATURE

mat·u·ra·tion \₁ma-chə-'rā-shən\ *n* **1 a** : the process of becoming mature **b** : the emergence of personal and behavioral characteristics through growth processes **c** : the final stages of differentiation of cells, tissues, or organs **d** : the achievement of intellectual or emotional maturity **2 a** : the entire process by which diploid gamete-producing cells are transformed into haploid gametes that includes both meiosis and physiological and structural changes fitting the gamete for its future role **b** : SPERMIOGENESIS **2** — **mat·u·ra·tion·al** \₁ma-chə-'rā-shə-nəl\ *adj*

ma·ture \mə-'túr, -'túr, -chúr\ *adj* **ma·tur·er; -est 1** : having completed natural growth and development **2** : having undergone maturation — **mature** *vb*

ma·tu·ri·ty \mə-'túr-ə-tē, -'tyúr-, -'chúr-\ *n, pl* **-ties** : the quality or state of being mature; *esp* : full development

maturity-onset diabetes *n* : NON-INSULIN-DEPENDENT DIABETES MELLITUS

max *abbr* maximum

Max·ib·o·lin \mak-'si-bə-lin, ₁mak-si-'bō-lin\ *trademark* — used for a preparation of ethylestrenol

maxill- *or* **maxilli-** *or* **maxillo-** *comb form* **1** : maxilla ⟨*maxillectomy*⟩ **2** : maxillary and ⟨*maxillofacial*⟩

max·il·la \mak-'si-lə\ *n, pl* **max·il·lae** \-'si-(₁)lē, -₁lī\ *or* **maxillas 1** : JAW 1a **2 a** : an upper jaw esp. of humans or other mammals in which the bony elements are closely fused **b** : either of two membrane bone elements of the upper jaw that lie lateral to the premaxillae and bear most of the teeth

¹**max·il·lary** \'mak-sə-₁ler-ē\ *adj* : of, relating to, being, or associated with a maxilla ⟨∼ blood vessels⟩

²**maxillary** *n, pl* **-lar·ies 1** : MAXILLA 2b **2** : a maxillary part (as a nerve or blood vessel)

maxillary air sinus *n* : MAXILLARY SINUS

maxillary artery *n* : an artery supplying the deep structures of the face (as the nasal cavities, palate, tonsils, and pharynx) and sending a branch to the meninges of the brain — called also *internal maxillary artery;* compare FACIAL ARTERY

maxillary bone *n* : MAXILLA 2b

maxillary nerve *n* : the one of the three major branches or divisions of the trigeminal nerve that supplies sensory fibers to the skin areas of the middle part of the face, the upper jaw and its teeth, and the mucous membranes of the palate, nasal cavities, and nasopharynx — called also *maxillary division;* compare MANDIBULAR NERVE, OPHTHALMIC NERVE

maxillary process *n* : a triangular embryonic process that grows out from the dorsal end of the mandibular arch on each side and forms the lateral part of the upper lip, the cheek, and the upper jaw except the premaxilla

maxillary sinus *n* : an air cavity in the body of the maxilla that communicates with the middle meatus of the nose — called also *antrum of Highmore*

maxillary vein *n* : a short venous trunk of the face that is formed by the union of veins from the pterygoid plexus and that joins with the superficial temporal vein to form a vein which contributes to the formation of the external jugular vein

max·il·lec·to·my \₁mak-sə-'lek-tə-mē\ *n, pl* **-mies** : surgical removal of the maxilla

maxilli-, maxillo- — see MAXILL-

max·il·lo·fa·cial \mak-₁si-(₁)lō-'fā-shəl, ₁mak-sə-(₁)lō-\ *adj* : of, relating to, treating, or affecting the maxilla and the face ⟨∼ lesions⟩

max·i·mal \'mak-sə-məl\ *adj* **1** : most complete or effective ⟨∼ vasodilation⟩ **2** : being an upper limit — **max·i·mal·ly** *adv*

max·i·mum \'mak-sə-məm\ *n, pl* **max·i·ma** \-sə-mə\ *or* **maximums 1 a** : the greatest quantity or value attainable or attained **b** : the period of highest, greatest, or utmost development **2** : an upper limit allowed (as by a legal authority) or allowable (as by the circumstances of a particular case) — **maximum** *adj*

maximum permissible concentration *n* : the maximum concentration of radioactive material in body tissue that is regarded as acceptable and not producing significant deleterious effects on the human organism — abbr. *MPC*

maximum permissible dose *n* : the amount of ionizing radiation a person may be exposed to supposedly without being harmed

Max·i·pen \'mak-si-₁pen\ *trademark* — used for a preparation of the potassium salt of phenethicillin

may·ap·ple \'mā-₁ap-əl\ *n, often cap* : a No. American herb of the genus *Podophyllum* (*P. peltatum*) having a poisonous rootstock and rootlets that are a source of the drug podophyllum

Ma·ya·ro virus \mä-'yä-rō-\ *n* : a So. American togavirus that is the causative agent of a febrile disease

may·hem \'mā-₁hem, 'mā-əm\ *n* **1** : willful and permanent deprivation of a bodily member resulting in impairment of a person's fighting ability and constituting a grave felony under English common law **2** : willful and permanent crippling, mutilation, or disfiguring of any part of the body constituting a grave felony under modern statutes and in some jurisdictions requiring a specific intent as distinguished from general malice

may·tan·sine \'mā-₁tan-₁sēn\ *n* : an antineoplastic agent $C_{34}H_{46}ClN_3O_{10}$ isolated from several members of a genus (*Maytenus* of the family Celastraceae) of tropical American shrubs and trees

maz- *or* **mazo-** *comb form* : breast ⟨*mazoplasia*⟩

ma·zin·dol \'mā-zin-₁dȯl\ *n* : an adrenergic drug $C_{16}H_{13}ClN_2O$ used as an appetite suppressant

ma·zo·pla·sia \₁mā-zə-'plā-zhə, -zhē-ə\ *n* : a degenerative condition of breast tissue

Maz·zi·ni test \mə-'zē-nē-\ *n* : a flocculation test for the diagnosis of syphilis

Mazzini, Louis Yolando (1894–1973), American serologist.

MB *abbr* [New Latin *medicinae baccalaureus*] bachelor of medicine

M band \'em-₁band\ *n* : M LINE

MBD *abbr* minimal brain dysfunction

mc *abbr* millicurie

MC *abbr* **1** medical corps **2** [New Latin *magister chirurgiae*] master of surgery

Mc·Ar·dle's disease \mə-'kärd-əlz-\ *n* : glycogenosis that is due to a deficiency of muscle phosphorylase and affects skeletal muscle — called also *McArdle's syndrome*

McArdle, Brian (fl 1936–1972), British physician.

MCAT *abbr* Medical College Admissions Test

Mc·Bur·ney's point \mək-'bər-nēz-\ *n* : a point on the abdominal wall that lies between the navel and the right anterior superior iliac spine and that is the point where most pain is elicited by pressure in acute appendicitis

McBurney, Charles (1845–1913), American surgeon.

mcg *abbr* microgram

MCh *abbr* [New Latin *magister chirurgiae*] master of surgery

MCH *abbr* **1** maternal and child health **2** mean corpuscular hemoglobin (concentration)

MCHC *abbr* mean corpuscular hemoglobin concentration

mCi *abbr* millicurie

MCV *abbr* mean corpuscular volume

Md *symbol* mendelevium

¹MD \₁em-'dē\ *n* **1** [Latin *medicinae*

doctor] : an earned academic degree conferring the rank and title of doctor of medicine **2** : a person who has a doctor of medicine

²**MD** *abbr* muscular dystrophy

MDMA \ₑem-(ₑ)dē-(ₑ)em-ˈā\ *n* : ECSTASY 2

MDR *abbr* minimum daily requirement

MDS *abbr* master of dental surgery

ME *abbr* medical examiner

meadow mushroom *n* : a common edible brown-spored mushroom (*Agaricus campestris*) that occurs naturally in moist open organically rich soil and is often cultivated

mean corpuscular hemoglobin concentration *n* : the number of grams of hemoglobin per unit volume and usu. 100 ml of packed red blood cells that is found by multiplying the number of grams of hemoglobin per unit volume of the original blood sample of whole blood by 100 and dividing by the hematocrit — abbr. *MCHC*

mean corpuscular volume *n* : the volume of the average red blood cell in a given blood sample that is found by multiplying the hematocrit by 10 and dividing by the estimated number of red blood cells — abbr. *MCV*

mea·sle \ˈmē-zəl\ *n* : CYSTICERCUS; *specif* : one found in the muscles of a domesticated mammal — compare TAENIA 1

mea·sles \ˈmē-zəlz\ *n sing or pl* **1 a** : an acute contagious disease caused by a paramyxovirus, commencing with catarrhal symptoms, conjunctivitis, cough, and Koplik's spots on the oral mucous membrane, and marked by the appearance on the third or fourth day of an eruption of distinct red circular spots which coalesce in a crescentic form, are slightly raised, and after the fourth day of the eruption gradually decline — called also *rubeola* **b** : any of various eruptive diseases (as German measles) **2** : infestation with or disease caused by larval tapeworms in the muscles and tissues; *specif* : infestation of cattle and swine with cysticerci of tapeworms that as adults parasitize humans — see MEASLE

mea·sly \ˈmē-zə-lē, ˈmēz-lē\ *adj* **mea·sli·er; -est 1** : infected with measles **2 a** : containing larval tapeworms **b** : infected with trichinae

meat- or **meato-** *comb form* : meatus ⟨*meato*plasty⟩

me·a·tal \mē-ˈāt-ᵊl\ *adj* : of, relating to, or forming a meatus

me·a·to·plas·ty \mē-ˈa-tə-ₑplast-ē\ *n, pl* **-ties** : plastic surgery of a meatus ⟨urethral ∼⟩

me·a·tot·o·my \ₑmē-ə-ˈtä-tə-mē\ *n, pl* **-mies** : incision of the urethral meatus esp. to enlarge it

me·atus \mē-ˈā-təs\ *n, pl* **me·atus·es** \-tə-səz\ *or* **me·atus** \-ˈā-təs, -ₑtüs\ : a natural body passage : CANAL, DUCT

meatus acus·ti·cus ex·ter·nus \-ə-ˈküs-ti-kəs-ek-ˈstər-nəs\ *n* : EXTERNAL AUDITORY MEATUS

meatus acusticus in·ter·nus \-in-ˈtər-nəs\ *n* : INTERNAL AUDITORY MEATUS

me·ban·a·zine \me-ˈba-nə-ₑzēn\ *n* : a monoamine oxidase inhibitor $C_8H_{12}N_2$ used as an antidepressant

Meb·a·ral \ˈme-bə-ₑral\ *trademark* — used for a preparation of mephobarbital

me·ben·da·zole \me-ˈben-də-ₑzōl\ *n* : a broad-spectrum anthelmintic agent $C_{16}H_{13}N_3O_3$

me·bu·ta·mate \me-ˈbyü-tə-ₑmāt\ *n* : a central nervous system depressant $C_{10}H_{20}N_2O_4$ used to treat mild hypertension

mec·a·myl·a·mine \ₑme-kə-ˈmi-lə-ₑmēn\ *n* : a drug that is used orally in the form of its hydrochloride $C_{11}H_{21}N·HCl$ as a ganglionic blocking agent to effect a rapid lowering of severely elevated blood pressure

me·chan·i·cal \mi-ˈka-ni-kəl\ *adj* : caused by, resulting from, or relating to physical as opposed to biological or chemical processes or change ⟨∼ injury⟩ ⟨∼ asphyxiation⟩ — **me·chan·i·cal·ly** *adv*

mechanical heart *n* : a mechanism designed to maintain the flow of blood to the tissues of the body esp. during a surgical operation on the heart

mech·a·nism \ˈme-kə-ₑni-zəm\ *n* **1** : a piece of machinery **2 a** : a bodily process or function ⟨the ∼ of healing⟩ **b** : the combination of mental processes by which a result is obtained ⟨psychological ∼s⟩ **3** : the fundamental physical or chemical processes involved in or responsible for an action, reaction, or other natural phenomenon — **mech·a·nis·tic** \ₑme-kə-ˈnis-tik\ *adj*

mech·a·no·chem·is·try \ₑme-kə-nō-ˈke-mə-strē\ *n, pl* **-tries** : chemistry that deals with the conversion of chemical energy into mechanical work (as in the contraction of a muscle) — **mech·a·no·chem·i·cal** \-ˈke-mi-kəl\ *adj*

mech·a·no·re·cep·tor \-ri-ˈsep-tər\ *n* : a neural end organ (as a tactile receptor) that responds to a mechanical stimulus (as a change in pressure) — **mech·a·no·re·cep·tion** \-ˈsep-shən\ *n* — **mech·a·no·re·cep·tive** \-ˈsep-tiv\ *adj*

mech·a·no·sen·so·ry \-ˈsen-sə-rē\ *adj* : of or relating to the sensing of mechanical stimuli ⟨∼ terminals⟩

mech·lor·eth·amine \ₑme-ₑklór-ˈe-thə-ₑmēn\ *n* : a nitrogen mustard $C_5H_{11}Cl_2N$ used in the form of its hydrochloride in palliative treatment of some neoplastic diseases

Mech·o·lyl \ˈme-kə-ₑlil\ *trademark* — used for a preparation of methacholine

Me·cis·to·cir·rus \mə-ₑsis-tō-ˈsir-əs\ *n* : a genus of nematode worms (family Trichostrongylidae) including a common parasite (*M. digitatus*) of the abomasum of domesticated ruminants and the stomach of swine

Meck·el–Gru·ber syndrome \'me-kəl-ˌgrü-bər-\ n : a syndrome inherited as an autosomal recessive trait and typically characterized by occipital encephalocele, microcephaly, cleft palate, polydactyly, and polycystic kidneys — called also *Meckel's syndrome*

Meckel, Johann Friedrich, the Younger (1781–1833), German anatomist.

Gruber, Georg Benno Otto (b 1884), German pathologist.

Meck·el's cartilage \'me-kəlz-\ n : the cartilaginous bar of the embryonic mandibular arch of which the distal end ossifies to form the malleus

J. F. Meckel the Younger — see MECKEL–GRUBER SYNDROME

Meckel's diverticulum n : the proximal part of the omphalomesenteric duct when persistent as a blind fibrous tube connected with the lower ileum

J. F. Meckel the Younger — see MECKEL–GRUBER SYNDROME

Meckel's ganglion n : PTERYGOPALATINE GANGLION

Meckel, Johann Friedrich, the Elder (1724–1774), German anatomist.

mec·li·zine \'me-klə-ˌzēn\ n : a drug $C_{25}H_{27}ClN_2$ used usu. in the form of its hydrochloride to treat nausea and vertigo — see ANTIVERT

mec·lo·fen·a·mate sodium \ˌme-klō-'fe-nə-ˌmāt-\ n : a mild analgesic and anti-inflammatory drug $C_{14}H_{10}Cl_2N-NaO_2 \cdot H_2O$ used orally to treat rheumatoid arthritis and osteoarthritis — called also *meclofenamate*

mec·lo·zine \'me-klō-ˌzēn\ Brit var of MECLIZINE

me·co·ni·um \mi-'kō-nē-əm\ n : a dark greenish mass of desquamated cells, mucus, and bile that accumulates in the bowel of a fetus and is discharged shortly after birth

meconium ileus n : congenital intestinal obstruction by inspissated meconium that is often associated with cystic fibrosis of newborn infants

med \'med\ adj : MEDICAL ⟨∼ school⟩

me·daz·e·pam \me-'da-zə-ˌpam\ n : a drug $C_{16}H_{15}ClN_2$ used in the form of its hydrochloride as a tranquilizer

med·e·vac \'me-də-ˌvak\ n 1 : emergency evacuation of the sick or wounded (as from a combat area) 2 : a helicopter used for medevac — **medevac** vb

medi- or **medio-** comb form : middle ⟨*medio*lateral⟩

¹**media** pl of MEDIUM

²**me·dia** \'mē-dē-ə\ n, pl **me·di·ae** \-dē-ˌē\ : the middle coat of the wall of a blood or lymph vessel consisting chiefly of circular muscle fibers — called also *tunica media*

media — see AERO-OTITIS MEDIA, OTITIS MEDIA, SCALA MEDIA, SEROUS OTITIS MEDIA

me·di·ad \'mē-dē-ˌad\ adv : toward the median line or plane of a body or part

me·di·al \'mē-dē-əl\ adj 1 : lying or extending in the middle; esp, of a body part : lying or extending toward the median axis of the body ⟨the ∼ surface of the tibia⟩ 2 : of or relating to the media of a blood vessel — **me·di·al·ly** adv

medial arcuate ligament n : an arched band of fascia that covers the upper part of the psoas major muscle, extends from the body of the first or second lumbar vertebra to the transverse process of the first and sometimes also the second lumbar vertebra, and provides attachment for part of the lumbar portion of the diaphragm — compare LATERAL ARCUATE LIGAMENT

medial collateral ligament n : a ligament that connects the medial epicondyle of the femur with the medial surface of the tibia and medial condyle and that helps to stabilize the knee by preventing lateral dislocation — called also *tibial collateral ligament*; compare LATERAL COLLATERAL LIGAMENT

medial condyle n : a condyle on the inner side of the lower extremity of the femur; also : a corresponding eminence on the upper part of the tibia that articulates with the medial condyle of the femur — compare LATERAL CONDYLE

medial cord n : a cord of nerve tissue that is continuous with the anterior division of the inferior trunk of the brachial plexus and that is one of the two roots forming the median nerve — compare LATERAL CORD, POSTERIOR CORD

medial cuneiform bone n : CUNEIFORM BONE 1a — called also *medial cuneiform*

medial epicondyle n : EPICONDYLE b

medial femoral circumflex artery n : an artery that branches from the deep femoral artery or from the femoral artery itself and that supplies the muscles of the medial part of the thigh and hip joint — compare LATERAL FEMORAL CIRCUMFLEX ARTERY

medial femoral circumflex vein n : a vein accompanying the medial femoral circumflex artery and emptying into the femoral vein or sometimes into one of its tributaries corresponding to the deep femoral artery — compare LATERAL FEMORAL CIRCUMFLEX VEIN

medial forebrain bundle n : a prominent tract of nerve fibers that connects the subcallosal area of the cerebral cortex with the lateral areas of the hypothalamus and that has fibers passing to the tuber cinereum, the brain stem, and the mammillary bodies

medial geniculate body n : a part of the

metathalamus consisting of a small oval tubercle situated between the pulvinar, colliculi, and cerebral peduncle that receives nerve impulses from the inferior colliculus and relays them to the auditory area — compare LATERAL GENICULATE BODY

medialis — see RECTUS MEDIALIS, VASTUS MEDIALIS

medial lemniscus *n* : a band of nerve fibers that transmits proprioceptive impulses from the spinal cord to the thalamus

medial longitudinal fasciculus *n* : any of four longitudinal bundles of white matter of which there are two on each side that extend from the midbrain to the upper parts of the spinal cord where they are located close to the midline ventral to the gray commissure and that are composed of fibers esp. from the vestibular nuclei

medial malleolus *n* : MALLEOLUS b

medial meniscus *n* : MENISCUS a(2)

medial pectoral nerve *n* : PECTORAL NERVE b

medial plantar artery *n* : PLANTAR ARTERY b

medial plantar nerve *n* : PLANTAR NERVE b

medial plantar vein *n* : PLANTAR VEIN b

medial popliteal nerve *n* : TIBIAL NERVE

medial pterygoid muscle *n* : PTERYGOID MUSCLE b

medial pterygoid nerve *n* : PTERYGOID NERVE b

medial pterygoid plate *n* : PTERYGOID PLATE b

medial rectus *n* : RECTUS 2c

medial semilunar cartilage *n* : MENISCUS a(2)

medial umbilical ligament *n* : a fibrous cord sheathed in peritoneum and extending from the pelvis to the umbilicus that is a remnant of part of the umbilical artery in the fetus — called also *lateral umbilical ligament*

medial vestibular nucleus *n* : the one of the four vestibular nuclei on each side of the medulla oblongata that sends ascending fibers to the oculomotor and trochlear nuclei in the cerebrum on the opposite side of the brain and sends descending fibers down both sides of the spinal cord to synapse with motoneurons of the ventral roots

¹**me·di·an** \'mē-dē-ən\ *n* : a medial part (as a vein or nerve)

²**median** *adj* : situated in the middle; *specif* : lying in a plane dividing a bilateral animal into right and left halves

median an·te·bra·chi·al vein \-ˌan-ti-ˈbrā-kē-əl-\ *n* : a vein usu. present in the forearm that drains the plexus of veins in the palm of the hand and that runs up the little finger side of the forearm

median arcuate ligament *n* : a tendinous arch that lies in front of the aorta and that connects the attachments

of the lumbar portion of the diaphragm to the lumbar vertebrae on each side — compare LATERAL ARCUATE LIGAMENT

median cubital vein *n* : a continuation of the cephalic vein of the forearm that passes obliquely toward the inner side of the arm in the bend of the elbow to join with the ulnar veins in forming the basilic vein and is often selected for venipuncture

median eminence *n* : a raised area in the floor of the third ventricle of the brain produced by the infundibulum of the hypothalamus

median lethal dose *n* : LD50

median nerve *n* : a nerve that arises by two roots from the brachial plexus and passes down the middle of the front of the arm

median nuchal line *n* : OCCIPITAL CREST a

median plane *n* : MIDSAGITTAL PLANE

median sacral crest *n* : SACRAL CREST a

median sacral vein *n* : an unpaired vein that accompanies the middle sacral artery and usu. empties into the left common iliac vein

median umbilical ligament *n* : a fibrous cord extending from the urinary bladder to the umbilicus that is the remnant of the fetal urachus

me·di·as·ti·nal \ˌmē-dē-ə-ˈstī-nəl\ *adj* : of or relating to a mediastinum

me·di·as·ti·ni·tis \ˌmē-dē-ˌas-tə-ˈnī-təs\ *n*, *pl* **-nit·i·des** \-ˈni-tə-ˌdēz\ : inflammation of the tissues of the mediastinum

me·di·as·tin·o·scope \ˌmē-dē-a-ˈsti-nə-ˌskōp\ *n* : an optical instrument used in mediastinoscopy

me·di·as·ti·nos·co·py \ˌmē-dē-ˌas-tə-ˈnäs-kə-pē\ *n*, *pl* **-pies** : examination of the mediastinum through an incision above the sternum

me·di·as·ti·not·o·my \-ˈnä-tə-mē\ *n*, *pl* **-mies** : surgical incision into the mediastinum

me·di·as·ti·num \ˌmē-dē-ə-ˈstī-nəm\ *n*, *pl* **-na** \-nə\ **1** : the space in the chest between the pleural sacs of the lungs that contains all the viscera of the chest except the lungs and pleurae; *also* : this space with its contents **2** : MEDIASTINUM TESTIS

mediastinum testis *n* : a mass of connective tissue at the back of the testis that is continuous externally with the tunica albuginea and internally with the interlobular septa and encloses the rete testis

¹**me·di·ate** \'mē-dē-ət\ *adj* **1** : occupying a middle position **2** : acting through an intervening agency : exhibiting indirect causation, connection, or relation

²**me·di·ate** \'mē-dē-ˌāt\ *vb* **-at·ed; -at·ing** : to transmit or carry (as a physical process or effect) as intermediate mechanism or agency — **me·di·a·tion** \ˌmē-dē-ˈā-shən\ *n*

me·di·a·tor \'mē-dē-ˌā-tər\ *n* : one that mediates; *esp* : a mediating agent (as an enzyme or hormone) in a chemical or biological process

med·ic \'me-dik\ *n* : one engaged in medical work; *esp* : CORPSMAN

medica — see MATERIA MEDICA

med·i·ca·ble \'me-di-kə-bəl\ *adj* : CURABLE, REMEDIABLE

med·ic·aid \'me-di-ˌkād\ *n, often cap* : a program of medical aid designed for those unable to afford regular medical service and financed jointly by the state and federal governments

¹**med·i·cal** \'me-di-kəl\ *adj* 1 : of, relating to, or concerned with physicians or the practice of medicine often as distinguished from surgery 2 : requiring or devoted to medical treatment — **med·i·cal·ly** *adv*

²**medical** *n* : a medical examination

medical examiner *n* 1 : a usu. appointed public officer who must be a person trained in medicine and whose functions are to make postmortem examinations of the bodies of persons dead by violence or suicide or under circumstances suggesting crime, to investigate the cause of their deaths, to conduct autopsies, and sometimes to initiate inquests 2 : a physician employed to make medical examinations (as of applicants for military service or of claimants of workers' compensation) 3 : a physician appointed to examine and license candidates for the practice of medicine in a political jurisdiction (as a state)

medical jurisprudence *n* : FORENSIC MEDICINE

medical psychology *n* : theories of personality and behavior not necessarily derived from academic psychology that provide a basis for psychotherapy in psychiatry and in general medicine

medical record *n* : a record of a person's illnesses and their treatment

medical tran·scrip·tion·ist \-tran-ˈskrip-shə-nist\ *n* : a typist who transcribes dictated medical reports

me·di·ca·ment \mi-ˈdi-kə-mənt, ˈme-di-kə-\ *n* : a substance used in therapy — **med·i·ca·men·tous** \ˌmi-ˌdi-kə-ˈmen-təs, ˌme-di-kə-\ *adj*

med·i·cant \'me-di-kənt\ *n* : a medicinal substance

med·i·care \'me-di-ˌkar\ *n, often cap* : a government program of medical care esp. for the elderly

med·i·cate \'me-də-ˌkāt\ *vb* **-cat·ed; -cat·ing** 1 : to treat medicinally 2 : to impregnate with a medicinal substance (*medicated* soap)

med·i·ca·tion \ˌme-də-ˈkā-shən\ *n* 1 : the act or process of medicating 2 : a medicinal substance : MEDICAMENT

¹**me·dic·i·nal** \mə-ˈdis-ʰn-əl\ *adj* : of, relating to, or being medicine : tending or used to cure disease or relieve pain — **me·dic·i·nal·ly** *adv*

²**medicinal** *n* : a medicinal substance : MEDICINE

medicinal leech *n* : a large European freshwater leech of the genus *Hirudo* (*H. medicinalis*) that is a source of hirudin, is now sometimes used to drain blood (as from a hematoma), and was formerly used to bleed patients thought to have excess blood

med·i·cine \'me-də-sən\ *n* 1 : a substance or preparation used in treating disease 2 **a** : the science and art dealing with the maintenance of health and the prevention, alleviation, or cure of disease **b** : the branch of medicine concerned with the nonsurgical treatment of disease

medicine cabinet *n* : CHEST 1

medicine chest *n* : CHEST 1

medicine dropper *n* : DROPPER

med·i·co \'me-di-ˌkō\ *n, pl* **-cos** : a medical practitioner : PHYSICIAN; *also* : a medical student

medico- *comb form* : medical : medical and (*medico*legal)

med·i·co·le·gal \ˌme-di-kō-ˈlē-gəl\ *adj* : of or relating to both medicine and law

Med·i·nal \'me-di-ˌnal\ *trademark* — used for a preparation of the sodium salt of barbital

Me·di·na worm \mə-ˈdē-nə-\ *n* : GUINEA WORM

medio- — see MEDI-

me·dio·car·pal \ˌmē-dē-ō-ˈkär-pəl\ *adj* : located between the two rows of the bones of the carpus (the ∼ joint)

me·dio·lat·er·al \-ˈla-tə-rəl\ *adj* : relating to, extending along, or being a direction or axis from side to side or from median to lateral — **me·dio·lat·er·al·ly** *adv*

Med·i·ter·ra·nean anemia \ˌme-də-tə-ˈrā-nē-ən-\ *n* : THALASSEMIA

Mediterranean fever *n* : any of several febrile conditions often endemic in parts of the Mediterranean region; *specif* : BRUCELLOSIS a

me·di·um \'mē-dē-əm\ *n, pl* **mediums** or **me·dia** \-dē-ə\ 1 : a means of effecting or conveying something 2 *pl* **media** : a nutrient system for the artificial cultivation of cells or organisms and esp. bacteria

medius — see CONSTRICTOR PHARYNGIS MEDIUS, GLUTEUS MEDIUS, PEDUNCULUS CEREBELLARIS MEDIUS, SCALENUS MEDIUS

med·i·vac *var of* MEDEVAC

MED·LARS \'med-ˌlärz\ *n* : a computer system for the storage and retrieval of bibliographical information concerning medical literature

MED·LINE \'med-ˌlīn\ *n* : a system providing rapid access to MEDLARS through a direct telephone linkage

med·ro·ges·tone \ˌme-drō-ˈjes-ˌtōn\ *n* : a synthetic progestin $C_{23}H_{32}O_2$ that has been used in the treatment of fibroid uterine tumors

Med·rol \'me-ˌdrol\ *trademark* — used

for a preparation of methylprednisolone

me·droxy·pro·ges·ter·one acetate \me-ˌdräk-sē-prō-ˈjes-tə-ˌrōn-\ *n* : a synthetic steroid progestational hormone $C_{24}H_{34}O_4$ that is used orally to treat secondary amenorrhea and abnormal uterine bleeding due to hormonal imbalance and parenterally in the palliative treatment of endometrial and renal carcinoma — called also *medroxyprogesterone;* see DEPO-PROVERA

me·dul·la \mə-ˈdə-lə, -ˈdu̇-\ *n, pl* **-las** *or* **-lae** \-(ˌ)lē, -ˌlī\ **1** *pl* **medullae a** : MARROW **1 b** : MEDULLA OBLONGATA **2 a** : the inner or deep part of an organ or structure **b** : MYELIN SHEATH

medulla ob·lon·ga·ta \-ˌä-blȯŋ-ˈgä-tə\ *n, pl* **medulla oblongatas** *or* **medullae ob·lon·ga·tae** \-ˈgä-tē, -ˌtī\ : the somewhat pyramidal last part of the vertebrate brain developed from the posterior portion of the hindbrain and continuous posteriorly with the spinal cord, enclosing the fourth ventricle, and containing nuclei associated with most of the cranial nerves, major fiber tracts and decussations that link spinal with higher centers, and various centers mediating the control of involuntary vital functions (as respiration)

medullaris — see CONUS MEDULLARIS

med·ul·lary \ˈmed-ᵊl-ˌer-ē, ˈme-jə-ˌler-ē; mə-ˈdə-lə-rē\ *adj* **1 a** : of or relating to the medulla of any body part or organ **b** : containing, consisting of, or resembling marrow **c** : of or relating to the medulla oblongata or the spinal cord **d** : of, relating to, or formed of the dorsally located embryonic ectoderm destined to sink below the surface and become neural tissue **2** : resembling marrow in consistency — used of cancers

medullary canal *n* : the marrow cavity of a bone

medullary cavity *n* : MEDULLARY CANAL

medullary cystic disease *n* : a progressive familial kidney disease that is characterized by renal medullary cysts and that manifests itself in anemia and uremia

medullary fold *n* : NEURAL FOLD

medullary groove *n* : NEURAL GROOVE

medullary plate *n* : the longitudinal dorsal zone of epiblast in the early vertebrate embryo that constitutes the primordium of the neural tissue

medulla spi·na·lis \-ˌspī-ˈnä-ləs\ *n* : SPINAL CORD

med·ul·lat·ed \ˈmed-ᵊl-ˌā-təd, ˈme-jə-ˌlā-\ *adj* **1** : MYELINATED **2** : having a medulla — used of fibers other than nerve fibers

med·ul·lec·to·my \ˌmed-ᵊl-ˈek-tə-mē, ˌme-jə-ˈlek-\ *n, pl* **-mies** : surgical excision of a medulla (as of the adrenal glands)

me·dul·lin \me-ˈdə-lən, ˈmed-ᵊl-ən, ˈme-jə-lin\ *n* : a renal prostaglandin effective in reducing blood pressure

me·dul·lo·blas·to·ma \mə-ˌdə-lō-ˌblas-ˈtō-mə\ *n, pl* **-to·mas** *also* **-to·ma·ta** \-ˈtō-mə-tə\ : a malignant tumor of the central nervous system arising in the cerebellum in children

mef·e·nam·ic acid \ˌme-fə-ˈna-mik-\ *n* : a drug $C_{15}H_{15}NO_2$ used as an antiinflammatory

mega- *or* **meg-** *comb form* **1** : great : large ⟨*mega*colon⟩ ⟨*mega*dose⟩ **2** : million : multiplied by one million ⟨*mega*curie⟩

mega·co·lon \ˈme-gə-ˌkō-lən\ *n* : great often congenital dilation of the colon — see HIRSCHSPRUNG'S DISEASE

mega·cu·rie \ˈme-gə-ˌkyu̇r-ē, -kyu̇-ˈrē\ *n* : one million curies

mega·dose \-ˌdōs\ *n* : a large dose (as of a vitamin) — **mega·dos·ing** \-ˌdō-siŋ\ *n*

mega·esoph·a·gus \ˌme-gə-i-ˈsä-fə-gəs\ *n, pl* **-gi** \-ˌgī, -ˌjī\ : enlargement and hypertrophy of the lower portion of the esophagus

mega·kary·o·blast \ˌme-gə-ˈkar-ē-ō-ˌblast\ *n* : a large cell with large reticulate nucleus that gives rise to megakaryocytes

mega·kary·o·cyte \ˌme-gə-ˈkar-ē-ō-ˌsīt\ *n* : a large cell that has a lobulated nucleus, is found esp. in the bone marrow, and is considered to be the source of blood platelets — **mega·kary·o·cyt·ic** \-ˌkar-ē-ō-ˈsi-tik\ *adj*

megal- *or* **megalo-** *comb form* **1** : large ⟨*megalo*cyte⟩ : abnormally large ⟨*megalo*cephaly⟩ **2** : grandiose ⟨*megalo*mania⟩

meg·a·lo·blast \ˈme-gə-lō-ˌblast\ *n* : a large erythroblast that appears in the blood esp. in pernicious anemia — **meg·a·lo·blas·tic** \ˌme-gə-lō-ˈblas-tik\ *adj*

megaloblastic anemia *n* : an anemia (as pernicious anemia) characterized by the presence of megaloblasts in the circulating blood

meg·a·lo·ceph·a·ly \ˌme-gə-lō-ˈse-fə-lē\ *n, pl* **-lies** : largeness and esp. abnormal largeness of the head

meg·a·lo·cyte \ˈme-gə-lə-ˌsīt\ *n* : MACROCYTE — **meg·a·lo·cyt·ic** \ˌme-gə-lə-ˈsi-tik\ *adj*

meg·a·lo·ma·nia \ˌme-gə-lō-ˈmā-nē-ə, -nyə\ *n* : a delusional mental disorder that is marked by infantile feelings of personal omnipotence and grandeur — **meg·a·lo·ma·ni·a·cal** \-mō-ˈnī-ə-kəl\ *or* **megalomaniac** *also* **meg·a·lo·man·ic** \-ˈma-nik\ *adj* — **meg·a·lo·ma·ni·a·cal·ly** *adv*

meg·a·lo·ma·ni·ac \-ˈmā-nē-ˌak\ *n* : an individual affected with or exhibiting megalomania

-megaly \ˈme-gə-lē\ *n comb form, pl* **-lies** : abnormal enlargement (of a specified part) ⟨hepato*megaly*⟩ ⟨spleno*megaly*⟩

mega·rad \'me-gə-ˌrad\ n : one million rads

mega·vi·ta·min \ˌme-gə-'vī-tə-mən\ adj : relating to or consisting of very large doses of vitamins

mega·vi·ta·mins \-mənz\ n pl : a large quantity of vitamins

me·ges·trol acetate \me-'jes-ˌtrȯl-\ n : a synthetic progestational hormone $C_{24}H_{32}O_4$ used in palliative treatment of advanced carcinoma of the breast and in endometriosis

Meg·i·mide \'me-gə-ˌmīd\ trademark — used for a preparation of bemegride

meg·lu·mine \'me-glü-ˌmēn, me-'glü-\ n : a crystalline base $C_7H_{17}NO_5$ used to prepare salts used in radiopaque and therapeutic substances — see IODIPAMIDE

me·grim \'mē-grəm\ n 1 a : MIGRAINE b : VERTIGO 2 : any of numerous diseases of animals marked by disturbance of equilibrium and abnormal gait and behavior — usu. used in pl.

mei·bo·mian gland \mī-'bō-mē-ən-\ n, often cap M : one of the long sebaceous glands of the eyelids that discharge a fatty secretion which lubricates the eyelids — called also tarsal gland; see CHALAZION
Meibom \'mī-ˌbōm\, **Heinrich (1638–1700)**, German physician.

mei·o·sis \mī-'ō-səs\ n, pl **mei·o·ses** \-ˌsēz\ : the cellular process that results in the number of chromosomes in gamete-producing cells being reduced to one half and that involves a reduction division in which one of each pair of homologous chromosomes passes to each daughter cell and a mitotic division — compare MITOSIS 1 — **mei·ot·ic** \mī-'ä-tik\ adj — **mei·ot·i·cal·ly** adv

Meiss·ner's corpuscle \'mīs-nərz-\ n : any of the small elliptical tactile end organs in hairless skin containing numerous transversely placed tactile cells and fine flattened nerve endings
Meissner, Georg (1829–1905), German anatomist and physiologist.

Meissner's plexus n : a plexus of ganglionated nerve fibers lying between the muscular and mucous coats of the intestine — compare MYENTERIC PLEXUS

mel \'mel\ n : a subjective unit of tone pitch equal to $\frac{1}{1000}$ of the pitch of a tone having a frequency of 1000 cycles — used esp. in audiology

me·lae·na chiefly Brit var of MELENA

melan- or **melano-** comb form 1 : black : dark ⟨melanin⟩ ⟨melanoma⟩ 2 : melanin ⟨melanogenesis⟩

mel·an·cho·lia \ˌme-lən-'kō-lē-ə\ n : a mental condition characterized by extreme depression, bodily complaints, and often hallucinations and delusions; esp : MANIC-DEPRESSIVE PSYCHOSIS

mel·an·cho·li·ac \-lē-ˌak\ n : an individual affected with melancholia

[^1]**mel·an·chol·ic** \ˌme-lən-'kä-lik\ adj 1 : of, relating to, or subject to melancholy : DEPRESSED 2 : of or relating to melancholia

[^2]**melancholic** n 1 : a melancholy person 2 : MELANCHOLIAC

mel·an·choly \'me-lən-ˌkä-lē\ n, pl **-chol·ies** 1 : MELANCHOLIA 2 : depression or dejection of spirits — **melancholy** adj

mel·a·nin \'me-lə-nən\ n 1 : any of various dark brown or black pigments of animal or plant structures (as skin or hair) 2 : any of various pigments that are similar to the natural melanins and are obtained esp. by enzymatic oxidation of tyrosine or dopa

mel·a·nism \'me-lə-ˌni-zəm\ n 1 : an increased amount of black or nearly black pigmentation (as of skin, feathers, or hair) of an individual or kind of organism 2 : intense human pigmentation in skin, eyes, and hair — **mel·a·nis·tic** \ˌme-lə-'nis-tik\ adj

mel·a·nize \'me-lə-ˌnīz\ vb **-nized; -niz·ing** : to convert into or infiltrate with melanin ⟨melanized cell granules⟩ — **mel·a·ni·za·tion** \ˌme-lə-nə-'zā-shən\ n

melano- — see MELAN-

me·la·no·blast \mə-'la-nə-ˌblast, 'me-lə-nō-\ n : a cell that is a precursor of a melanocyte

me·la·no·blas·to·ma \mə-ˌla-nə-blas-'tō-mə, ˌme-lə-nō-\ n, pl **-mas** or **-ma·ta** \-mə-tə\ : a malignant tumor derived from melanoblasts

mel·a·no·car·ci·no·ma \-ˌkärs-ᵊn-'ō-mə\ n, pl **-mas** or **-ma·ta** \-mə-tə\ : a melanoma believed to be of epithelial origin

me·la·no·cyte \mə-'la-nə-ˌsīt, 'me-lə-nō-\ n : an epidermal cell that produces melanin

melanocyte–stimulating hormone n : either of two vertebrate hormones of the pituitary gland that darken the skin by stimulating melanin dispersion in pigment-containing cells — abbr. MSH; called also intermedin, melanophore-stimulating hormone, melanotropin

me·la·no·cyt·ic \mə-ˌla-nə-'si-tik, ˌme-lə-nō-\ adj : similar to or characterized by the presence of melanocytes

me·la·no·cy·to·ma \-sī-'tō-mə\ n, pl **-mas** or **-ma·ta** \-mə-tə\ : a benign tumor composed of melanocytes

mel·a·no·der·ma \ˌme-lə-nō-'dər-mə, mə-ˌla-\ n : abnormally intense pigmentation of the skin

me·la·no·gen·e·sis \ˌme-lə-ˌla-nə-'je-nə-səs, ˌme-lə-nō-\ n, pl **-e·ses** \-ˌsēz\ : the formation of melanin

me·la·no·gen·ic \-'je-nik\ adj 1 : of, relating to, or characteristic of melanogenesis 2 : producing melanin

mel·a·no·ma \ˌme-lə-'nō-mə\ n, pl **-mas** also **-ma·ta** \-mə-tə\ 1 : a benign or malignant skin tumor containing dark pigment 2 : a tumor of high malignancy that starts in melanocytes of normal skin or moles and metastasizes rapidly and widely — called also *melanosarcoma*

me·la·no·phage \mə-'la-nə-ˌfāj, 'me-lə-nə-\ *n* : a melanin-containing cell which obtains the pigment by phagocytosis

me·la·no·phore–stimulating hormone \mə-'la-nō-ˌfōr-, 'me-lə-nə-\ *n* : MELANOCYTE-STIMULATING HORMONE

me·la·no·sar·co·ma \-ˌsär-'kō-mə\ *n, pl* **-mas** *or* **-ma·ta** \-mə-tə\ : MELANOMA 2

mel·a·no·sis \ˌme-lə-'nō-səs\ *n, pl* **-no·ses** \-'nō-ˌsēz\ : a condition characterized by abnormal deposition of melanins or sometimes other pigments in the tissues of the body

melanosis co·li \-'kō-ˌlī\ *n* : dark brownish black pigmentation of the mucous membrane of the colon due to the deposition of pigment in macrophages

me·la·no·some \mə-'la-nə-ˌsōm, 'me-lə-nō-\ *n* : a melanin-producing granule in a melanocyte — **me·la·no·som·al** \mə-ˌla-nə-'sō-məl, ˌme-lə-nō-\ *adj*

mel·a·not·ic \ˌme-lə-'nä-tik\ *adj* : having or characterized by black pigmentation ⟨a ～ sarcoma⟩

me·la·no·tro·pin \mə-ˌla-nə-'trō-pən, ˌme-lə-nō-\ *n* : MELANOCYTE-STIMULATING HORMONE

me·lar·so·prol \mə-'lar-sə-ˌpról\ *n* : a drug $C_{12}H_{15}AsN_6OS_2$ used in the treatment of trypanosomiasis esp. in advanced stages

me·las·ma \mə-'laz-mə\ *n* : a dark pigmentation of the skin (as in Addison's disease) — **me·las·mic** \-mik\ *adj*

mel·a·to·nin \ˌme-lə-'tō-nən\ *n* : a vertebrate hormone $C_{13}H_{16}N_2O_2$ that is derived from serotonin, is secreted by the pineal gland especially in response to darkness, and has been linked to the regulation of circadian rhythms

me·le·na \mə-'lē-nə\ *n* : the passage of dark tarry stools containing decomposing blood that is usu. an indication of bleeding in the upper part of the alimentary canal — compare HEMATOCHEZIA

mel·en·ges·trol acetate \ˌme-lən-'jes-ˌtról-, -ˌtról-\ *n* : a progestational and antineoplastic agent $C_{25}H_{32}O_4$ that has been used as a growth-stimulating feed additive for beef cattle

-me·lia \'mē-lē-ə\ *n comb form* : condition of the limbs ⟨micro*melia*⟩ ⟨hemi*melia*⟩

mel·i·oi·do·sis \ˌme-lē-ˌoi-'dō-səs\ *n, pl* **-do·ses** \-ˌsēz\ : a highly fatal bacterial disease closely related to glanders that occurs naturally in rodents of southeastern Asia but is readily transmitted to other mammals and humans by the rat flea or under certain conditions by dissemination in air of the causative bacterium of the

genus *Pseudomonas* (*P. pseudomallei*)

me·lit·tin \mə-'lit-ᵊn\ *n* : a toxic protein in bee venom that causes localized pain and inflammation

Mel·la·ril \'me-lə-ˌril\ *trademark* — used for a preparation of thioridazine

mellitus — see DIABETES MELLITUS, INSULIN-DEPENDENT DIABETES MELLITUS, NON-INSULIN-DEPENDENT DIABETES MELLITUS

Me·loph·a·gus \mə-'lä-fə-gəs\ *n* : a genus of wingless flies (family Hippoboscidae) that includes the sheep ked (*M. ovinus*)

melo·rhe·os·to·sis \ˌme-lə-ˌrē-ä-'stō-səs\ *n, pl* **-to·ses** \-ˌsēz\ *or* **-tosises** : an extremely rare form of osteosclerosis characterized by asymmetrical or local enlargement and sclerotic changes in the long bones of one extremity

Mel·ox·ine \mə-'läk-ˌsēn\ *trademark* — used for a preparation of methoxsalen

mel·pha·lan \'mel-fə-ˌlan\ *n* : an antineoplastic drug $C_{13}H_{18}Cl_2N_2O_2$ that is a derivative of nitrogen mustard and is used esp. in the treatment of multiple myeloma — called also *L-PAM, phenylalanine mustard, sarcolysin*

melting point *n* : the temperature at which a solid melts

-melus \mə-ləs\ *n comb form* : one having a (specified) abnormality of the limbs ⟨phoco*melus*⟩

mem·ber \'mem-bər\ *n* : a body part or organ: as **a** : LIMB **b** : PENIS

membran- *or* **membrani-** *or* **membrano-** *comb form* : membrane ⟨*membrano*proliferative glomerulonephritis⟩

mem·bra·na \mem-'brä-nə, -'brä-\ *n, pl* **mem·bra·nae** \-ˌnē, -ˌnī\ : MEMBRANE

membrana nic·ti·tans \-'nik-tə-ˌtanz\ *n* : NICTITATING MEMBRANE

mem·brane \'mem-ˌbrān\ *n* **1** : a thin soft pliable sheet or layer esp. of animal or plant origin **2** : a limiting protoplasmic surface or interface — see NUCLEAR MEMBRANE, PLASMA MEMBRANE — **mem·braned** \'mem-ˌbränd\ *adj*

membrane bone *n* : a bone that ossifies directly in connective tissue without previous existence as cartilage

membrane of Descemet *n* : DESCEMET'S MEMBRANE

membrane potential *n* : the difference in electrical potential between the interior of a cell and the interstitial fluid beyond the membrane

mem·bra·no·pro·lif·er·a·tive glomerulo·nephritis \ˌmem-ˌbrä-nō-prə-'li-fə-rə-tiv-\ *n* : a slowly progressive chronic glomerulonephritis characterized by proliferation of mesangial cells and irregular thickening of glomerular capillary walls and narrowing of the capillary lumina

mem·bra·nous \'mem-brə-nəs\ *adj* **1** : of, relating to, or resembling membranes **2** : characterized or accompanied by the formation of a usu. abnormal membrane or membranous layer (~ gastritis) — **mem·bra·nous·ly** adv

membranous glomerulonephritis n : a form of glomerulonephritis characterized by thickening of glomerular capillary basement membranes and nephrotic syndrome

membranous labyrinth n : the sensory structures of the inner ear including the receptors of the labyrinthine sense and the cochlea — see BONY LABYRINTH

membranous urethra n : the part of the male urethra that is situated between the layers of the urogenital diaphragm and that connects the parts of the urethra passing through the prostate gland and the penis

mem·o·ry \'mem-rē, 'me-mə-\ n, pl **-ries 1** : the power or process of reproducing or recalling what has been learned and retained esp. through associative mechanisms **2** : the store of things learned and retained from an organism's activity or experience as indicated by modification of structure or behavior or by recall and recognition

memory trace n : ENGRAM

men pl of MAN

men- or **meno-** comb form : menstruation ⟨menopause⟩ ⟨menorrhagia⟩

men·a·di·one \me-nə-'dī-ōn, -dī-'\ n : a yellow crystalline compound $C_{11}H_8O_2$ with the biological activity of natural vitamin K — called also vitamin K_3

me·naph·thone \mə-'naf-thōn\ n, Brit : MENADIONE

men·a·quin·one \me-nə-'kwi-nōn\ n : VITAMIN K 1b; also : a synthetic derivative of vitamin K_2

men·ar·che \'me-när-kē\ n : the beginning of the menstrual function; esp : the first menstrual period of an individual — **men·ar·che·al** \me-'när-kē-əl\ or **men·ar·chal** \-kəl\ adj

¹**mend** \'mend\ vb **1** : to restore to health : CURE **2** : to improve in health; also : HEAL

²**mend** n : an act of mending or repair — **on the mend** : getting better or improving esp. in health

men·de·le·vi·um \men-də-'lē-vē-əm, -'lā-\ n : a radioactive element that is artificially produced — symbol Md or Mv; see ELEMENT table

Men·de·lian \men-'dē-lē-ən, -'dēl-yən\ adj : of, relating to, or according with Mendel's laws or Mendelism — **Mendelian** n

Men·del \'mend-əl\, **Gregor Johann (1822–1884),** Austrian botanist and geneticist.

Mendelian factor n : GENE

Mendelian inheritance n : PARTICULATE INHERITANCE

Men·del·ism \'mend-əl-i-zəm\ n : the principles or the operations of Men-

del's laws; also : PARTICULATE INHERITANCE

Men·del's law \'men-dəlz-\ n **1** : a principle in genetics: hereditary units occur in pairs that separate during gamete formation so that every gamete receives but one member of a pair — called also law of segregation **2** : a principle in genetics limited and modified by the subsequent discovery of the phenomenon of linkage: the different pairs of hereditary units are distributed to the gametes independently of each other, the gametes combine at random, and the various combinations of hereditary pairs occur in the zygotes according to the laws of chance — called also law of independent assortment **3** : a principle in genetics proved subsequently to be subject to many limitations: because one of each pair of hereditary units dominates the other in expression, characters are inherited as alternatives on an all or nothing basis — called also law of dominance

men·go·vi·rus \'men-gō-vī-rəs\ n : an enterovirus that causes encephalomyocarditis and has been found esp. in rodents and primates

Mé·nière's disease \mən-'yerz-, 'men-yərz-\ n : a disorder of the membranous labyrinth of the inner ear that is marked by recurrent attacks of dizziness, tinnitus, and deafness — called also Ménière's syndrome

Ménière, Prosper (1799–1862), French physician.

mening- or **meningo-** also **meningi-** comb form **1** : meninges ⟨meningococcus⟩ **2** : meninges and ⟨meningoencephalitis⟩

men·in·ge·al \me-nən-'jē-əl\ adj : of, relating to, or affecting the meninges

meningeal artery n : any of several arteries supplying the meninges of the brain and neighboring structures; esp : MIDDLE MENINGEAL ARTERY

meningeal vein n : any of several veins draining the meninges of the brain and neighboring structures

meninges pl of MENINX

me·nin·gi·o·ma \mə-nin-jē-'ō-mə\ n, pl **-o·mas** or **-o·ma·ta** \-'ō-mə-tə\ : a slow-growing encapsulated tumor arising from the meninges and often causing damage by pressing upon the brain and adjacent parts

men·in·gism \'me-nən-ji-zəm, mə-'nin-\ n : MENINGISMUS

men·in·gis·mus \me-nən-'jiz-məs\ n, pl **-gis·mi** \-mī\ : a state of meningeal irritation with symptoms suggesting meningitis that often occurs at the onset of acute febrile diseases esp. in children

men·in·gi·tis \me-nən-'jī-təs\ n, pl **-git·i·des** \-'ji-tə-dēz\ **1** : inflammation of the meninges and esp. of the pia mater and the arachnoid **2** : a usu. bacterial disease in which inflammation of the meninges occurs — **men·in·git·ic** \-'ji-tik\ *adj*

me·nin·go·cele \me-'niŋ-gə-,sēl, mə-'nin-jə-\ *n* : a protrusion of meninges through a defect in the skull or spinal column forming a cyst filled with cerebrospinal fluid

me·nin·go·coc·cae·mia *chiefly Brit var of* MENINGOCOCCEMIA

me·nin·go·coc·ce·mia \mə-,niŋ-gō-käk-'sē-mē-ə, -,nin-jə-\ *n* : an abnormal condition characterized by the presence of meningococci in the blood

me·nin·go·coc·cus \mə-,niŋ-gə-'kä-kəs, -,nin-jə-\ *n, pl* **-coc·ci** \-'kä-kī, -,kē; -'käk-,sī, -,sē\ : a bacterium of the genus *Neisseria* (*N. meningitidis*) that causes cerebrospinal meningitis — **me·nin·go·coc·cal** \-'kä-kəl\ *also* **me·nin·go·coc·cic** \-'kä-kik, -'käk-sik\ *adj*

me·nin·go·coele *var of* MENINGOCELE

me·nin·go·en·ceph·a·li·tis \-in-,se-fə-'lī-təs\ *n, pl* **-lit·i·des** \-'li-tə-,dēz\ : inflammation of the brain and meninges — **me·nin·go·en·ceph·a·lit·ic** \mə-,niŋ-(,)gō-ən-,se-fə-'li-tik, -,nin-(,)jō-\ *adj*

me·nin·go·en·ceph·a·lo·cele \-in-'se-fə-lō-,sēl\ *n* : a protrusion of meninges and brain through a defect in the skull

me·nin·go·en·ceph·a·lo·my·eli·tis \-in-,se-fə-lō-,mī-ə-'lī-təs\ *n, pl* **-elit·i·des** \-ə-'li-tə-,dēz\ : inflammation of the meninges, brain, and spinal cord

me·nin·go·my·elo·cele \-'mī-ə-lō-,sēl\ *n* : a protrusion of meninges and spinal cord through a defect in the spinal column

me·nin·go·vas·cu·lar \-'vas-kyə-lər\ *adj* : of, relating to, or affecting the meninges and the cerebral blood vessels

me·ninx \'mē-niŋks, 'me-\ *n, pl* **me·nin·ges** \mə-'nin-(,)jēz\ : any of the three membranes that envelop the brain and spinal cord and include the arachnoid, dura mater, and pia mater

me·nis·cal \mə-'nis-kəl\ *adj* : of or relating to a meniscus ⟨a ∼ tear⟩

men·is·cec·to·my \,me-ni-'sek-tə-mē\ *n, pl* **-mies** : surgical excision of a meniscus of the knee or temporomandibular joint

me·nis·cus \mə-'nis-kəs\ *n, pl* **me·nis·ci** \-'ni-,kī, -,kē; -'ni-,sī\ *also* **me·nis·cus·es** : a fibrous cartilage within a joint: **a** : either of two crescent-shaped lamellae of fibrocartilage that border and partly cover the articulating surfaces of the tibia and femur at the knee : SEMILUNAR CARTILAGE: (1) : one mostly between the lateral condyles of the tibia and femur — called also *lateral meniscus, lateral semilunar cartilage* (2) : one mostly between the medial condyles of the tibia and femur — called also *medial meniscus, medial semilunar cartilage* **b** : a thin oval ligament of the temporomandibular joint that is situated between the condyle of the mandible

and the mandibular fossa and separates the joint into two cavities

meno·met·ror·rha·gia \,me-nō-,me-trə-'rā-jə, -'rä-, -jē-ə, -zhə\ *n* : a combination of menorrhagia and metrorrhagia

meno·pause \'me-nə-,pȯz, 'mē-\ *n* **1** : the period of natural cessation of menstruation occurring usu. between the ages of 45 and 50 **2** : CLIMACTERIC — **meno·paus·al** \,me-nə-'pȯ-zəl, ,mē-\ *adj*

Men·o·pon \'me-nə-,pän\ *n* : a genus of biting lice that includes the shaft louse (*M. gallinae*) of poultry

men·or·rha·gia \,me-nə-'rä-jə, -'rä-, -jē-ə, -zhə\ *n* : abnormally profuse menstrual flow — compare HYPERMENORRHEA, METRORRHAGIA — **men·or·rhag·ic** \-'ra-jik\ *adj*

men·or·rhea \,me-nə-'rē-ə\ *n* : normal menstrual flow

men·or·rhoea *chiefly Brit var of* MENORRHEA

men·ses \'men-,sēz\ *n sing or pl* : the menstrual flow

men·stru·al \'men-strə-wəl\ *adj* : of or relating to menstruation — **men·stru·al·ly** *adv*

menstrual cycle *n* : the whole cycle of physiologic changes from the beginning of one menstrual period to the beginning of the next

menstrual extraction *n* : a procedure for shortening the menstrual period or for early termination of pregnancy by withdrawing the uterine lining and a fertilized egg if present by means of suction

men·stru·a·tion \,men-strə-'wā-shən\ *n* : a discharging of blood, secretions, and tissue debris from the uterus that recurs in nonpregnant human and other primate females of breeding age at approximately monthly intervals and that is considered to represent a readjustment of the uterus to the nonpregnant state following proliferative changes accompanying the preceding ovulation; *also* : PERIOD 1b — **men·stru·ate** \'men-strə-,wāt\ *vb* — **men·stru·ous** \'men-strə-wəs\ *adj*

men·stru·um \'men-strə-wəm\ *n, pl* **-stru·ums** *or* **-strua** \-strə-wə\ : a substance that dissolves a solid or holds it in suspension : SOLVENT

menta *pl of* MENTUM

¹men·tal \'ment-ᵊl\ *adj* **1 a** : of or relating to the mind; *specif* : of or relating to the total emotional and intellectual response of an individual to external reality **b** : of or relating to intellectual as contrasted with emotional activity **2 a** : of, relating to, or affected by a psychiatric disorder **b** : intended for the care or treatment of persons affected by psychiatric disorders ⟨∼ hospitals⟩ — **men·tal·ly** *adv*

²mental *adj* : of or relating to the chin : GENIAL

mental age *n* : a measure used in psychological testing that expresses an individual's mental attainment in terms of the number of years it takes an average child to reach the same level

mental artery n : a branch of the inferior alveolar artery on each side that emerges from the mental foramen and supplies blood to the chin — called also *mental branch*

mental capacity n 1 : sufficient understanding and memory to comprehend in a general way the situation in which one finds oneself and the nature, purpose, and consequence of any act or transaction into which one proposes to enter 2 : the degree of understanding and memory the law requires to uphold the validity of or to charge one with responsibility for a particular act or transaction

mental competence n : MENTAL CAPACITY

mental deficiency n : MENTAL RETARDATION

mental disorder n : MENTAL ILLNESS

mental foramen n : a foramen for the passage of blood vessels and a nerve on the outside of the lower jaw on each side near the chin

mental health n : the condition of being sound mentally and emotionally that is characterized by the absence of mental illness (as neurosis or psychosis) and by adequate adjustment esp. as reflected in feeling comfortable about oneself, positive feelings about others, and ability to meet the demands of life; *also* : the field of mental health : MENTAL HYGIENE

mental hygiene n : the science of maintaining mental health and preventing the development of mental illness

mental illness n : a mental or bodily condition marked primarily by sufficient disorganization of personality, mind, and emotions to seriously impair the normal psychological functioning of the individual — called also *mental disorder*

mental incapacity n 1 : an absence of mental capacity 2 : an inability through mental illness or mental retardation to carry on the everyday affairs of life or to care for one's person or property with reasonable discretion

mental incompetence n : MENTAL INCAPACITY

men·ta·lis \men-ˈtā-lis\ n, pl **men·ta·les** \-ˌlēz\ : a muscle that originates in the incisive fossa of the mandible, inserts in the skin of the chin, and raises the chin and pushes up the lower lip

men·tal·i·ty \men-ˈta-lə-tē\ n, pl **-ties 1** : mental power or capacity **2** : mode or way of thought

mental nerve n : a branch of the inferior alveolar nerve that emerges from the bone of the mandible near the mental

protuberance and divides into branches which are distributed to the skin of the chin and to the skin and mucous membranes of the lower lip

mental protuberance n : the bony protuberance at the front of the lower jaw forming the chin

mental retardation n : subaverage intellectual ability that is equivalent to or less than an IQ of 70, is present from birth or infancy, and is manifested esp. by abnormal development, by learning difficulties, and by problems in social adjustment — **mentally retarded** adj

mental spine n : either of two small elevations on the inner surface of each side of the symphysis of the lower jaw of which the superior one on each side provides attachment for the genioglossus and the inferior for the geniohyoid muscle

mental test n : any of various standardized procedures applied to an individual in order to ascertain ability or evaluate behavior

mental tubercle n : a prominence on each side of the mental protuberance of the mandible — called also *genial tubercle*

men·ta·tion \men-ˈtā-shən\ n : mental activity ⟨unconscious ∼⟩

men·thol \ˈmen-ˌthȯl, -ˌthōl\ n : a crystalline alcohol $C_{10}H_{20}O$ that occurs esp. in mint oils, has the odor and cooling properties of peppermint, and is used in flavoring and in medicine (as locally to relieve pain, itching, and nasal congestion)

men·tho·lat·ed \ˈmen-thə-ˌlā-təd\ adj : containing or impregnated with menthol ⟨a ∼ salve⟩

mentis see COMPOS MENTIS, NON COMPOS MENTIS

men·tum \ˈmen-təm\ n, pl **men·ta** \-tə\ : CHIN

Meo·nine \ˈmē-ə-ˌnīn\ trademark — used for a preparation of methionine

mep·a·crine \ˈme-pə-ˌkrēn, -krən\ n, chiefly Brit : QUINACRINE

mep·a·zine \ˈme-pə-ˌzēn\ n : a phenothiazine tranquilizer $C_{19}H_{22}N_2S$ administered in the form of the acetate or hydrochloride

me·pen·zo·late bromide \mə-ˈpen-zə-ˌlāt-\ n : an anticholinergic drug $C_{21}H_{26}BrNO_3$

me·per·i·dine \mə-ˈper-ə-ˌdēn\ n : a synthetic narcotic drug $C_{15}H_{21}NO_2$ used in the form of its hydrochloride as an analgesic, sedative, and antispasmodic — called also *isonipecaine, pethidine*

me·phen·e·sin \mə-ˈfe-nə-sin\ n : a crystalline compound $C_{10}H_{14}O_3$ used chiefly in the treatment of neuromuscular conditions — called also *myanesin*

meph·en·ox·a·lone \ˌme-fə-ˈnäk-sə-ˌlōn\ n : a tranquilizing drug $C_{11}H_{13}NO_4$

me·phen·ter·mine \mə-ˈfen-tər-ˌmēn\ n : an adrenergic drug $C_{11}H_{17}N$ administered often in the form of the sulfate as a vasopressor and nasal decongestant

me·phen·y·to·in \mə-ˈfe-ni-ˌtō-in\ n : an anticonvulsant drug $C_{12}H_{14}N_2O_2$ — see MESANTOIN

mepho·bar·bi·tal \ˌme-fō-ˈbär-bə-ˌtäl\ n : a crystalline barbiturate $C_{13}H_{14}$-N_2O_3 used as a sedative and in the treatment of epilepsy

Meph·y·ton \ˈme-fə-ˌtän\ trademark — used for a preparation of vitamin K_1

me·piv·a·caine \me-ˈpi-və-ˌkān\ n : a drug $C_{15}H_{22}N_2O$ used esp. in the form of the hydrochloride as a local anesthetic

Me·prane \ˈmē-ˌprān\ trademark — used for a preparation of promethestrol

mep·ro·bam·ate \ˌme-prō-ˈba-ˌmāt, mə-ˈprō-bə-ˌmāt\ n : a bitter carbamate $C_9H_{18}N_2O_4$ used as a tranquilizer — see MEPROSPAN, MILTOWN

Mep·ro·span \ˈme-prō-ˌspan\ trademark — used for a preparation of meprobamate

¹**mer-** or **mero-** comb form : thigh ⟨meralgia⟩

²**mer-** or **mero-** comb form : part : partial ⟨meroblastic⟩

me·ral·gia \mə-ˈral-jə, -jē-ə\ n : pain esp. of a neuralgic kind in the thigh

meralgia par·aes·thet·i·ca Brit var of MERALGIA PARESTHETICA

meralgia par·es·thet·i·ca \-ˌpar-əs-ˈthe-ti-kə\ n : an abnormal condition characterized by pain and paresthesia in the outer surface of the thigh

mer·al·lu·ride \mə-ˈral-yə-ˌrīd, -ˌrid\ n : a diuretic consisting of a chemical combination of an organic mercurial compound $C_9H_{16}HgN_2O_6$ and theophylline and administered chiefly by injection as an aqueous solution of its sodium salt — see MERCUHYDRIN

mer·bro·min \ˌmər-ˈbrō-mən\ n : a green crystalline mercurial compound $C_{20}H_8Br_2HgNa_2O_6$ used as a topical antiseptic and germicide in the form of its red solution — see MERCUROCHROME

mer·cap·tom·er·in \(ˌ)mər-ˌkap-ˈtä-mə-rən\ n : a mercurial diuretic related chemically to mercurophylline and administered by injection of an aqueous solution of its sodium salt $C_{16}H_{25}HgNNa_2O_6S$

mer·cap·to·pu·rine \(ˌ)mər-ˌkap-tə-ˈpyúr-ˌēn\ n : an antimetabolite $C_5H_4N_4S$ that interferes esp. with the metabolism of purine bases and the biosynthesis of nucleic acids and that is sometimes useful in the treatment of acute leukemia

Mer·cu·hy·drin \ˌmər-kyù-ˈhī-drən\ trademark — used for a preparation of meralluride

mer·cu·mat·i·lin \ˌmər-kyù-ˈmat-əl-ən, mər-ˌkyü-mə-ˈti-lən\ n : a mercurial

diuretic consisting of a mercury-containing acid $C_{14}H_{14}HgO_6$ and theophylline that is often administered in the form of the sodium salt

¹**mer·cu·ri·al** \(ˌ)mər-ˈkyúr-ē-əl\ adj : of, relating to, containing, or caused by mercury ⟨∼ salves⟩

²**mercurial** n : a pharmaceutical or chemical containing mercury

mer·cu·ri·al·ism \(ˌ)mər-ˈkyúr-ē-ə-ˌli-zəm\ n : chronic poisoning with mercury (as from industrial contacts with the metal or its fumes) — called also hydrargyrism

mer·cu·ric chloride \(ˌ)mər-ˈkyúr-ik-\ n : a heavy crystalline poisonous compound $HgCl_2$ used as a disinfectant and fungicide — called also bichloride of mercury, corrosive sublimate, mercury bichloride

mercuric cyanide n : the mercury cyanide $Hg(CN)_2$ which has been used as an antiseptic

mercuric iodide n : a red crystalline poisonous salt HgI_2 which has been used as a topical antiseptic

mercuric oxide n : either of two forms of a slightly water-soluble crystalline poisonous compound HgO which has been used in antiseptic ointments

Mer·cu·ro·chrome \(ˌ)mər-ˈkyúr-ə-ˌkrōm\ trademark — used for a preparation of merbromin

mer·cu·ro·phyl·line \ˌmər-kyə-rō-ˈfi-ˌlēn, -lən\ n : a diuretic consisting of a chemical combination of an organic mercurial compound or its sodium salt $C_{14}H_{24}HgNNaO_5$ and theophylline — see MERCUZANTHIN

mer·cu·rous chloride \ˌmər-ˈkyúr-əs-, ˈmər-kyə-rəs-\ n : CALOMEL

mer·cu·ry \ˈmər-kyə-rē\ n, pl **-ries 1** : a heavy silver-white poisonous metallic element that is liquid at ordinary temperatures — symbol Hg; called also quicksilver; see ELEMENT table **2** : a pharmaceutical preparation containing mercury or a compound of it

mercury bi·chlo·ride \-ˌbī-ˈklōr-ˌīd\ n : MERCURIC CHLORIDE

mercury chloride n : a chloride of mercury: as **a** : CALOMEL **b** : MERCURIC CHLORIDE

mercury–vapor lamp n : an electric lamp in which the discharge takes place through mercury vapor and which has been used therapeutically as a source of ultraviolet radiation

Mer·cu·zan·thin \ˌmər-kyü-ˈzan-thən\ trademark — used for a preparation of mercurophylline

mercy killing n : EUTHANASIA

-mere \ˌmir\ n comb form : part : segment ⟨blastomere⟩ ⟨centromere⟩

mer·eth·ox·yl·line procaine \ˌmər-e-ˈthäk-sə-ˌlēn-\ n : a mercurial diuretic $C_{15}H_{19}HgNO_6 \cdot C_{13}H_{20}N_2O_2$

me·rid·i·an \mə-ˈri-dē-ən\ n **1** : an imaginary circle or closed curve on the surface of a sphere or globe-shaped body (as the eyeball) that lies in a plane passing through the poles **2** : any of the pathways along which the body's vital energy flows according to the theory of acupuncture — **meridian** *adj* — **me·rid·i·o·nal** \mə-ˈri-dē-ən-ᵊl\ *adj*

Mer·kel–Ran·vier corpuscle \ˈmer-kəl-ˌrän̄-ˈvyā-\ *n* : MERKEL'S DISK
  Merkel, Friedrich Siegmund (1845–1919), German anatomist.
  Ranvier, Louis–Antoine (1835–1922), French histologist.

Mer·kel's disk \ˈmer-kəlz-\ *n* : a touch receptor of the deep layers of the skin consisting of a flattened or cupped body associated peripherally with a large modified epithelial cell and centrally with an efferent nerve fiber — called also *Merkel's cell, Merkel's corpuscle*

mero- — see MER-

mero·blas·tic \ˌmer-ə-ˈblas-tik\ *adj* : characterized by or being incomplete cleavage as a result of the presence of an impeding mass of yolk material (as in the eggs of birds, class Aves) — compare HOLOBLASTIC — **mero·blas·ti·cal·ly** *adv*

mero·crine \ˈmer-ə-krən, -ˌkrīn, -ˌkrēn\ *adj* : producing a secretion that is discharged without major damage to the secreting cells (~ glands); *also* : of or produced by a merocrine gland (a ~ secretion) — compare APOCRINE, ECCRINE, HOLOCRINE

mero·my·o·sin \ˌmer-ə-ˈmī-ə-sən\ *n* : either of two structural subunits of myosin that are obtained esp. by tryptic digestion

mero·zo·ite \ˌmer-ə-ˈzō-ˌīt\ *n* : a small ameboid sporozoan trophozoite (as of a malaria parasite) produced by schizogony that is capable of initiating a new sexual or asexual cycle of development

mer·sal·yl \(ˌ)mər-ˈsa-lil\ *n* : an organic mercurial $C_{13}H_{16}HgNNaO_6$ administered by injection in combination with theophylline as a diuretic

Mer·thi·o·late \(ˌ)mər-ˈthī-ə-ˌlāt, -lət\ *trademark* — used for a preparation of thimerosal

mes- *or* **meso-** *comb form* **1 a** : mid : in the middle ⟨*meso*derm⟩ **b** : mesentery or membrane supporting a (specified) part ⟨*meso*appendix⟩ ⟨*meso*colon⟩ **2** : intermediate (as in size or type) ⟨*meso*morph⟩

mes·an·gi·um \me-ˈsan-jē-əm, ˌmē-\ *n, pl* **-gia** \-jē-ə\ : a thin membrane that gives support to the capillaries surrounding the tubule of a nephron — **mes·an·gi·al** \-jē-əl\ *adj*

Mes·an·to·in \me-ˈsan-tō-in\ *trademark* — used for a preparation of mephenytoin

mes·aor·ti·tis \ˌme-ˌsā-ȯr-ˈtī-təs, ˌmē-\ *n, pl* **-tit·i·des** \-ˈti-tə-ˌdēz\ : inflammation of the middle layer of the aorta

mes·ar·ter·i·tis \-ˌsär-tə-ˈrī-təs\ *n, pl* **-it-**

i·des \-ˈri-tə-ˌdēz\ : inflammation of the middle layer of an artery

mes·cal \me-ˈskal, mə-\ *n* **1** : a small cactus (*Lophophora williamsii*) with rounded stems covered with jointed tubercles that are used as a stimulant and antispasmodic esp. among the Mexican Indians **2** : a usu. colorless Mexican liquor distilled esp. from the central leaves of any of various fleshy-leaved agaves (genus *Agave* of the family Agavaceae); *also* : a plant from which mescal is produced

mescal button *n* : one of the dried discoid tops of the mescal

mes·ca·line \ˈmes-kə-lən, -ˌlēn\ *n* : a hallucinatory crystalline alkaloid $C_{11}H_{17}NO_3$ that is the chief active principle in mescal buttons

mes·en·ceph·a·lon \ˌme-zən-ˈse-fə-ˌlän, ˌmē-, -sən-, -lən\ *n* : MIDBRAIN — **mes·en·ce·phal·ic** \-zen-sə-ˈfa-lik, -sen-\ *adj*

mes·en·chyme \ˈme-zən-ˌkīm, ˈmē-, -sən-\ *n* : loosely organized undifferentiated mesodermal cells that give rise to such structures as connective tissues, blood, lymphatics, bone, and cartilage — **mes·en·chy·mal** \me-zən-ˈkī-məl, mē-, -sən-\ *adj* — **mes·en·chy·ma·tous** \-mə-təs\ *adj*

mes·en·chy·mo·ma \ˌme-zən-kī-ˈmō-mə, ˌmē-, -sən-\ *n, pl* **-mas** *or* **-ma·ta** \-mə-tə\ : a benign or malignant tumor consisting of a mixture of at least two types of embryonic connective tissue

¹**mes·en·ter·ic** \ˌme-zən-ˈter-ik, -sən-\ *adj* : of, relating to, or located in or near a mesentery

²**mesenteric** *n* : a mesenteric part; *esp* : MESENTERIC ARTERY

mesenteric artery *n* : either of two arteries arising from the aorta and passing between the two layers of the mesentery to the intestine: **a** : one that arises just above the bifurcation of the abdominal aorta into the common iliac arteries and supplies the left half of the transverse colon, the descending colon, the sigmoid colon, and most of the rectum — called also *inferior mesenteric artery* **b** : a large artery that arises from the aorta just below the celiac artery at the level of the first lumbar vertebra and supplies the greater part of the small intestine, the cecum, the ascending colon, and the right half of the transverse colon — called also *superior mesenteric artery*

mesenteric ganglion *n* : either of two ganglionic masses of the sympathetic nervous system associated with the corresponding mesenteric plexus: **a** : a variable amount of massed ganglionic tissue of the inferior mesenteric plexus near the origin of the inferior mesenteric artery — called also *inferior mesenteric ganglion* **b** : a usu. discrete ganglionic mass of the superior mesenteric plexus near the origin of the superior mesenteric artery — called also *superior mesenteric ganglion*

mesenteric node *n* : any of the lymphatic glands of the mesentery — called also *mesenteric gland, mesenteric lymph node*

mesenteric plexus *n* : either of two plexuses of the sympathetic nervous system lying mostly in the mesentery in close proximity to and distributed to the same structures as the corresponding mesenteric arteries: **a** : one associated with the inferior mesenteric artery — called also *inferior mesenteric plexus* **b** : a subdivision of the celiac plexus that is associated with the superior mesenteric artery — called also *superior mesenteric plexus*

mesenteric vein *n* : either of two veins draining the intestine, passing between the two layers of the mesentery, and associated with the corresponding mesenteric arteries: **a** : one that is a continuation of the superior rectal vein, that returns blood from the rectum, the sigmoid colon, and the descending colon, that accompanies the inferior mesenteric artery, and that usu. empties into the splenic vein — called also *inferior mesenteric vein* **b** : one that drains blood from the small intestine, the cecum, the ascending colon, and the transverse colon, that accompanies the superior mesenteric artery, and that joins with the splenic vein to form the portal vein — called also *superior mesenteric vein*

mes·en·tery \'me-zən-ˌter-ē, -sən-\ *n, pl* **-ter·ies 1** : one or more vertebrate membranes that consist of a double fold of the peritoneum and invest the intestines and their appendages and connect them with the dorsal wall of the abdominal cavity; *specif* : such membranes connected with the jejunum and ileum in humans **2** : a fold of membrane comparable to a mesentery and supporting a viscus (as the heart) that is not a part of the digestive tract

mesh \'mesh\ *n* : a flexible netting of fine wire used in surgery esp. in the repair of large hernias and other body defects

me·si·al \'mē-zē-əl, -sē-\ *adj* **1** : being or located in the middle or a median part ⟨the ~ aspect of the metacarpal head⟩ **2** : situated in or near or directed toward the median plane of the body ⟨the heart is ~ to the lungs⟩ — compare DISTAL 1b **3** : of, relating to, or being the surface of a tooth that is next to the tooth in front of it or that is closest to the middle of the front of the jaw — compare DISTAL 1c, PROXIMAL 1b — **me·si·al·ly** *adv*

mesio- *comb form* : mesial and ⟨*mesiodistal*⟩ ⟨*mesiobuccal*⟩

me·sio·buc·cal \ˌmē-zē-ō-ˈbək-əl, -sē-\ *adj* : of or relating to the mesial and buccal surfaces of a tooth — **me·sio·buc·cal·ly** *adv*

me·sio·clu·sion *also* **me·si·oc·clu·sion** \ˌmē-zē-ə-ˈklü-zhən, -sē-\ *n* : malocclusion characterized by mesial displacement of one or more of the lower teeth

me·sio·dis·tal \ˌmē-zē-ō-ˈdist-əl\ *adj* : of or relating to the mesial and distal surfaces of a tooth; *esp* : relating to, lying along, containing, or being a diameter joining the mesial and distal surfaces — **me·sio·dis·tal·ly** *adv*

me·sio·lin·gual \-ˈliŋ-gwəl\ *adj* : of or relating to the mesial and lingual surfaces of a tooth — **me·sio·lin·gual·ly** *adv*

mes·mer·ism \'mez-mə-ˌri-zəm, 'mes-\ *n* : hypnotic induction by the practices of F. A. Mesmer; *broadly* : HYPNOTISM — **mes·mer·ist** \-rist\ *n* — **mes·mer·ize** \-ˌrīz\ *vb*

    Mes·mer \'mes-mər\, **Franz** *or* **Friedrich Anton (1734–1815),** German physician.

meso- — see MES-

me·so·ap·pen·dix \ˌme-zō-ə-ˈpen-diks, ˌmē-, -sō-\ *n, pl* **-dix·es** *or* **-di·ces** \-də-ˌsēz\ : the mesentery of the vermiform appendix — **me·so·ap·pen·di·ce·al** \-ˌpen-də-ˈsē-əl\ *adj*

me·so·blast \'me-zə-ˌblast, 'mē-, -sə-\ *n* : the embryonic cells that give rise to mesoderm; *broadly* : MESODERM — **me·so·blas·tic** \ˌme-zō-ˈblas-tik, ˌmē-, -sō-\ *adj*

me·so·car·di·um \ˌme-zō-ˈkär-dē-əm, ˌmē-, -sō-\ *n* **1** : the transitory mesentery of the embryonic heart **2** : either of two tubular prolongations of the epicardium that enclose the aorta and pulmonary trunk and the venae cavae and pulmonary veins

Me·so·ces·toi·des \-ˌses-ˈtȯi-(ˌ)dēz\ *n* : a genus (family Mesocestoididae) of tapeworms having the adults parasitic in mammals and birds and a slender threadlike contractile larva free in cavities or encysted in tissues of mammals, birds, and sometimes reptiles

me·so·co·lon \ˌme-zə-ˈkō-lən, ˌme-sə-\ *n* : a mesentery joining the colon to the dorsal abdominal wall

me·so·derm \'me-zə-ˌdərm, 'mē-, -sə-\ *n* : the middle of the three primary germ layers of an embryo that is the source esp. of bone, muscle, connective tissue, and dermis; *broadly* : tissue derived from this germ layer — **me·so·der·mal** \ˌme-zə-ˈdər-məl, ˌmē-, -sə-\ *or* **me·so·der·mal·ly** *adv*

me·so·duo·de·num \ˌme-zə-ˌdü-ə-ˈdē-nəm, ˌmē-, -sə-, -ˌdyü-; -dü-ˈäd-ᵊn-əm, -dyü-\ *n, pl* **-de·na** \-ə-ˈdē-nə, -ˈäd-ᵊn-ə\ *or* **-de·nums** : the mesentery of the duodenum usu. not persisting in adult life in humans and other mammals in which the developing intestine undergoes a counterclockwise rotation

me·so·gas·tri·um \-ˈgas-trē-əm\ n, pl **-tria** \-trē-ə\ **1** : a ventral mesentery of the embryonic stomach that persists as the falciform ligament and the lesser omentum — called also *ventral mesogastrium* **2** : a dorsal mesentery of the embryonic stomach that gives rise to ligaments between the stomach and spleen and the spleen and kidney — called also *dorsal mesogastrium*

me·so·ino·si·tol \ˌme-zō-i-ˈnō-sə-ˌtȯl, ˌmē-, -ˈnō-, -ˌtōl\ n : MYOINOSITOL

me·so·morph \ˈme-zə-ˌmȯrf, ˈmē-, -sə-\ n : a mesomorphic body or person

me·so·mor·phic \ˌme-zə-ˈmȯr-fik, ˌmē-, -sə-\ adj **1** : of or relating to the component in W. H. Sheldon's classification of body types that measures esp. the degree of muscularity and bone development **2** : having a husky muscular body build — compare ECTOMORPHIC 1, ENDOMORPHIC 1 — **me·so·mor·phy** \ˈme-zə-ˌmȯr-fē, ˈmē-, -sə-\ n

me·so·neph·ric \ˌme-zə-ˈne-frik, ˌmē-, -sə-\ adj : of or relating to the mesonephros

mesonephric duct n : WOLFFIAN DUCT

me·so·neph·ro·ma \-ni-ˈfrō-mə\ n, pl **-mas** or **-ma·ta** \-mə-tə\ : a benign or malignant tumor esp. of the female genital tract held to be derived from the mesonephros

me·so·neph·ros \ˌme-zə-ˈne-frəs, ˌmē-, -sə-, -ˌfräs\ n, pl **-neph·roi** \-ˈne-ˌfrȯi\ : either member of the second and midmost of the three paired vertebrate renal organs that functions in adult fishes and amphibians but functions only in the embryo of reptiles, birds, and mammals in which it is replaced by a metanephros in the adult — called also *Wolffian body*; compare PRONEPHROS

Mes·o·pin \ˈme-sə-pin\ trademark — used for a preparation of a semisynthetic quaternary antimuscarinic bromide $C_{17}H_{24}BrNO_3$ of homatropine

me·so·rec·tum \ˌme-zə-ˈrek-təm, ˌmē-, -sə-\ n, pl **-tums** or **-ta** \-tə\ : the mesentery that supports the rectum

mes·orid·a·zine \ˌme-zō-ˈri-də-ˌzēn, ˌmē-, -sō-\ n : a phenothiazine tranquilizer $C_{21}H_{26}N_2OS_2$ used in the treatment of schizophrenia, organic brain disorders, alcoholism, and psychoneuroses

me·so·sal·pinx \ˌme-zō-ˈsal-(ˌ)piŋks, ˌmē-, -sō-\ n, pl **-sal·pin·ges** \-sal-ˈpin-(ˌ)jēz\ : a fold of the broad ligament

investing and supporting the fallopian tube

me·so·sig·moid \-ˈsig-ˌmȯid\ n : the mesentery of the sigmoid part of the descending colon

me·so·ster·num \ˌme-zə-ˈstər-nəm, ˌmē-, -sə-\ n, pl **-ster·na** \-nə\ : GLADIOLUS

me·so·ten·don \-ˈten-dən\ n : a fold of synovial membrane connecting a tendon to its synovial sheath

me·so·the·li·o·ma \ˌme-zə-ˌthē-lē-ˈō-mə, ˌmē-, -sə-\ n, pl **-mas** or **-ma·ta** \-mə-tə\ : a tumor derived from mesothelial tissue (as that lining the peritoneum or pleura)

me·so·the·li·um \-ˈthē-lē-əm\ n, pl **-lia** \-lē-ə\ : epithelium derived from mesoderm that lines the body cavity of a vertebrate embryo and gives rise to epithelia (as of the peritoneum, pericardium, and pleurae), striated muscle, heart muscle, and several minor structures — **me·so·the·li·al** \-lē-əl\ adj

mes·ovar·i·um \ˌme-zə-ˈvar-ē-əm, ˌmē-, -sə-\ n, pl **-ovar·ia** \-ē-ə\ : the mesentery uniting the ovary with the body wall

mes·ox·a·ly·lurea \ˌmes-ˌäk-sə-li-ˈlu̇r-ē-ə, ˌlil-ˈyu̇r-\ n : ALLOXAN

mes·sen·ger \ˈmes-ən-jər\ n **1** : a substance (as a hormone) that mediates a biological effect — see SECOND MESSENGER **2** : MESSENGER RNA

messenger RNA n : an RNA produced by transcription that carries the code for a particular protein from the nuclear DNA to a ribosome in the cytoplasm and acts as a template for the formation of that protein — called also *mRNA*; compare TRANSFER RNA

mes·ter·o·lone \me-ˈster-ə-ˌlōn\ n : an androgen $C_{20}H_{32}O_2$ used in the treatment of male infertility

Mes·ti·non \ˈmes-tə-ˌnän\ trademark — used for a preparation of pyridostigmine

mes·tra·nol \ˈmes-trə-ˌnȯl, -ˌnōl\ n : a synthetic estrogen $C_{21}H_{26}O_2$ used in oral contraceptives — see ENOVID

mes·y·late \ˈme-si-ˌlāt\ n : any of the salts or esters of an acid CH_4SO_3 including some in which it is combined with a drug — see ERGOLOID MESYLATES

Met abbr methionine

meta- or **met-** prefix **1** : situated behind or beyond ⟨*met*encephalon⟩ **2** : change in : transformation of ⟨*meta*plasia⟩

met·a·bol·ic \ˌme-tə-ˈbä-lik\ adj **1** : of, relating to, or based on metabolism **2** : VEGETATIVE 1a(2) — used esp. of a cell nucleus that is not dividing — **met·a·bol·i·cal·ly** adv

metabolic acidosis n : acidosis resulting from excess acid due to abnormal metabolism, excessive acid intake, or renal retention or from excessive loss of bicarbonate (as in diabetes)

metabolic alkalosis n : alkalosis resulting from excessive alkali intake or excessive acid loss (as from vomiting)

metabolic pathway *n* : PATHWAY 2

metabolic rate *n* : metabolism per unit time esp. as estimated by food consumption, energy released as heat, or oxygen used in metabolic processes — see BASAL METABOLIC RATE

me·tab·o·lism \mə-'ta-bə-ˌli-zəm\ *n* **1** : the sum of the processes in the buildup and destruction of protoplasm; *specif* : the chemical changes in living cells by which energy is provided for vital processes and activities and new material is assimilated — see ANABOLISM, CATABOLISM **2** : the sum of the processes by which a particular substance is handled (as by assimilation and incorporation or by detoxification and excretion) in the living body

me·tab·o·lite \-ˌlīt\ *n* **1** : a product of metabolism: **a** : a metabolic waste usu. more or less toxic to the organism producing it : EXCRETION **b** : a product of one metabolic process that is essential to another such process in the same organism **c** : a metabolic waste of one organism that is markedly toxic to another : ANTIBIOTIC **2** : a substance essential to the metabolism of a particular organism or to a particular metabolic process

me·tab·o·lize \-ˌlīz\ *vb* **-lized; -liz·ing** : to subject to metabolism — **me·tab·o·liz·able** \mə-ˌta-bə-'lī-zə-bəl\ *adj*

¹meta·car·pal \ˌme-tə-'kär-pəl\ *adj* : of, relating to, or being the metacarpus or a metacarpal

²metacarpal *n* : any bone of the metacarpus of the human hand or the front foot in quadrupeds

meta·car·po·pha·lan·ge·al \ˌme-tə-ˌkär-pō-ˌfā-lən-'jē-əl, -ˌfa-, -fə-'lan-jē-\ *adj* : of, relating to, or involving both the metacarpus and the phalanges

meta·car·pus \-'kär-pəs\ *n* : the part of the human hand or the front foot in quadrupeds between the carpus and the phalanges that contains five more or less elongated bones when all the digits are present (as in humans) but is modified in many animals by the loss or reduction of some bones or the fusing of adjacent bones

meta·cen·tric \ˌme-tə-'sen-trik\ *adj* : having the centromere medially situated so that the two chromosomal arms are of roughly equal length — compare ACROCENTRIC, TELOCENTRIC — **metacentric** *n*

meta·cer·car·ia \ˌme-tə-(ˌ)sər-'kar-ē-ə\ *n, pl* **-iae** \-ē-ˌē\ : a tailless encysted late larva of a digenetic trematode that is usu. the form which is infective for the definitive host — **meta·cer·car·i·al** \-ē-əl\ *adj*

meta·ces·tode \-'ses-ˌtōd\ *n* : a stage of a tapeworm occurring in an intermediate host : a larval tapeworm

metachromatic leukodystrophy *n* : a hereditary neurological disorder of lipid metabolism characterized by the accumulation of cerebroside sulfates, loss of myelin in the central nervous system, and progressive deterioration of mental and motor activity

me·tach·ro·nous \mə-'ta-krə-nəs\ *adj* : occurring or starting at different times (~ cancers)

meta·cre·sol \ˌme-tə-'krē-ˌsòl, -ˌsōl\ *n* : an isomer of cresol that has antiseptic properties

meta·cryp·to·zo·ite \-ˌkrip-tō-'zō-ˌīt\ *n* : a member of a second or subsequent generation of tissue-dwelling forms of a malaria parasite derived from the sporozoite without intervening generations of blood parasites — compare CRYPTOZOITE

Meta·gon·i·mus \-'gä-nə-məs\ *n* : a genus of small intestinal flukes (family Heterophyidae) that includes one (*M. yokogawai*) common in humans, dogs, and cats in parts of eastern Asia as a result of the eating of raw fish containing the larva

Meta·hy·drin \-'hī-drin\ *trademark* — used for a preparation of trichlormethiazide

metall- *or* **metallo-** *comb form* : containing a metal or ion in the molecule ⟨*metallo*porphyrin⟩

me·tal·lo·en·zyme \mə-ˌta-lō-'en-ˌzīm\ *n* : an enzyme consisting of a protein linked with a specific metal

met·al·loid \'met-əl-ˌoid\ *n* : an element (as boron, silicon, or arsenic) intermediate in properties between the typical metals and nonmetals

me·tal·lo·por·phy·rin \-'pòr-fə-rən\ *n* : a compound (as heme) formed from a porphyrin and a metal ion

me·tal·lo·pro·tein \-'prō-ˌtēn, -'prōt-ē-ən\ *n* : a conjugated protein in which the prosthetic group is a metal

me·tal·lo·thi·o·ne·in \-ˌthī-ə-'nē-ən\ *n* : a metal-binding protein involved in the storage of copper in the liver

meta·mere \'me-tə-ˌmir\ *n* : any of a linear series of primitively similar segments into which the body of a higher invertebrate or vertebrate is divisible and which are usu. clearly distinguishable in the embryo, identifiable in somewhat modified form in various invertebrates (as annelid worms), and detectable in the adult higher vertebrate only in specialized segmentally arranged structures (as cranial and spinal nerves or vertebrae) : SOMITE — **meta·mer·ic** \ˌme-tə-'mer-ik\ *adj*

Met·a·mine \'me-tə-ˌmēn\ *trademark* — used for a preparation of the phosphate of trolnitrate

meta·mor·phic \ˌme-tə-'mòr-fik\ *adj* : of or relating to metamorphosis

meta·mor·pho·sis \ˌme-tə-'mòr-fə-səs\ *n, pl* **-pho·ses** \-ˌsēz\ **1** : change of physical form, structure, or substance **2** : a marked and more or less abrupt developmental change in the form or structure of an animal (as a butterfly or a frog) occurring subsequent to birth or hatching — **meta·mor·phose** \-₁fōz, -₁fōs\ vb

Met·a·mu·cil \₁me-tə-'myüs-əl\ trademark — used for a laxative preparation of a hydrophilic mucilloid from the husk of psyllium seed

meta·my·elo·cyte \₁me-tə-'mī-ə-lə-₁sīt\ n : any of the most immature granulocytes present in normal blood that are distinguished by typical cytoplasmic granulation in combination with a simple kidney-shaped nucleus

Me·tan·dren \me-'tan-drən\ trademark — used for a preparation of methyltestosterone

meta·neph·ric \₁me-tə-'ne-frik\ adj : of or relating to the metanephros

meta·neph·rine \-'ne-₁frēn\ n : a catabolite of epinephrine that is found in the urine and some tissues

meta·neph·ro·gen·ic \-₁ne-frə-'je-nik\ adj : giving rise to the metanephroi

meta·neph·ros \-'ne-frəs, -₁fräs\ n, pl **-neph·roi** \-'ne-₁froi\ : either member of the final and most caudal pair of the three successive pairs of vertebrate renal organs that functions as a permanent adult kidney in reptiles, birds, and mammals but is not present at all in lower forms — compare MESONEPHROS, PRONEPHROS

meta·phase \'me-tə-₁fāz\ n : the stage of mitosis and meiosis in which the chromosomes become arranged in the equatorial plane of the spindle

metaphase plate n : a section in the equatorial plane of the metaphase spindle having the chromosomes oriented upon it

Met·a·phen \'me-tə-fən\ trademark — used for a preparation of nitromersol

me·taph·y·se·al also **me·taph·y·si·al** \₁mə-₁ta-fə-'sē-əl, -'zē-, ₁me-tə-'fi-zē-əl\ adj : of or relating to a metaphysis

me·taph·y·sis \mə-'ta-fə-səs\ n, pl **-y·ses** \-₁sēz\ : the transitional zone at which the diaphysis and epiphysis of a bone come together

meta·pla·sia \₁me-tə-'plā-zhə, -zhē-ə\ n **1** : transformation of one tissue into another (∼ of cartilage into bone) **2** : abnormal replacement of cells of one type by cells of another — **meta·plas·tic** \-'plas-tik\ adj

meta·pro·ter·e·nol \-prō-'ter-ə-₁nol, -₁nōl\ n : a beta-adrenergic bronchodilator $C_{11}H_{17}NO_3$ that is used in the treatment of bronchial asthma and reversible bronchospasm associated with bronchitis and emphysema and that is administered as the sulfate — see ALUPENT

meta·ram·i·nol \₁me-tə-'ra-mə-₁nol, -₁nōl\ n : a sympathomimetic drug $C_9H_{13}NO_2$ used esp. as a vasoconstrictor

met·ar·te·ri·ole \₁met-₁är-'tir-ē-₁ōl\ n : any of the delicate blood vessels that branch from the smallest arteri-

oles and connect with the capillary bed — called also precapillary

me·tas·ta·sis \mə-'tas-tə-səs\ n, pl **-ta·ses** \-₁sēz\ : change of position, state, or form: as **a** : transfer of a disease-producing agency (as cancer cells or bacteria) from an original site of disease to another part of the body with development of a similar lesion in the new location **b** : a secondary metastatic growth of a malignant tumor — **me·tas·ta·size** \mə-'tas-tə-₁sīz\ vb — **met·a·stat·ic** \₁me-tə-'sta-tik\ adj

Meta·stron·gy·lus \₁me-tə-'strän-jə-ləs\ n : a genus of nematode worms (family Metastrongylidae) parasitizing as adults the lungs and sometimes other organs of mammals

¹meta·tar·sal \₁me-tə-'tär-səl\ adj : of, relating to, or being the part of the human foot or of the hind foot in quadrupeds between the tarsus and the phalanges

²metatarsal n : a metatarsal bone

meta·tar·sal·gia \-₁tär-'sal-jə, -jē-ə\ n : a cramping burning pain below and between the metatarsal bones where they join the toe bones — see MORTON'S TOE

meta·tar·sec·to·my \-₁tär-'sek-tə-mē\ n, pl **-mies** : surgical removal of the metatarsus or a metatarsal bone

meta·tar·so·pha·lan·ge·al joint \-₁tär-sō-₁fā-lən-'jē-əl-, ₁fa-, -fə-'lan-jē-\ n : any of the joints between the metatarsals and the phalanges

meta·tar·sus \₁me-tə-'tär-səs\ n : the part of the human foot or of the hind foot in quadrupeds that is between the tarsus and phalanges, contains when all the digits are present (as in humans) five more or less elongated bones but is modified in many animals with loss or reduction of some bones or fusing of others, and in humans forms the instep

meta·thal·a·mus \-'tha-lə-məs\ n, pl **-mi** \-₁mī\ : the part of the diencephalon on each side that comprises the lateral and medial geniculate bodies

met·ax·a·lone \mə-'tak-sə-₁lōn\ n : a drug $C_{12}H_{15}NO_3$ used as a skeletal muscle relaxant

meta·zo·an \₁me-tə-'zō-ən\ n : any of a group (Metazoa) that comprises all animals having the body composed of cells differentiated into tissues and organs and usu. a digestive cavity lined with specialized cells — **metazoan** adj

met·en·ceph·a·lon \₁met-₁en-'se-fə-₁län, -lən\ n : the anterior segment of the developing vertebrate hindbrain or the corresponding part of the adult brain composed of the cerebellum and pons — **met·en·ce·phal·ic** \-₁en-sə-'fa-lik\ adj

Met–en·keph·a·lin \₁me-ten-'ke-fə-lin\ n : METHIONINE-ENKEPHALIN

me·te·or·ism \'mē-tē-ə-₁ri-zəm\ n : gaseous distension of the stomach or intestine : TYMPANITES

me·ter \'mē-tər\ *n* : the basic metric unit of length that is equal to 39.37 inches

-meter *n comb form* : instrument or means for measuring ⟨calori*meter*⟩

meter–kilogram–second *adj* : MKS

meth \'meth\ *n* : METHAMPHETAMINE

meth- *or* **metho-** *comb form* : methyl ⟨*meth*amphetamine⟩

metha·cho·line \·me-thə-'kō-·lēn\ *n* : a parasympathomimetic drug C_8H_{19}-NO_3 administered in the form of its crystalline chloride or bromide — see MECHOLYL

metha·cy·cline \·me-thə-'sī-·klēn\ *n* : a semisynthetic tetracycline $C_{22}H_{22}$-N_2O_8 with longer duration of action than most other tetracyclines and used in the treatment of gonorrhea esp. in penicillin-sensitive subjects

meth·a·done \'me-thə-·dōn\ *also* **meth·a·don** \-·dän\ *n* : a synthetic addictive narcotic drug $C_{21}H_{27}NO$ used esp. in the form of its hydrochloride for the relief of pain and as a substitute narcotic in the treatment of heroin addiction — called also *amidone*

met·hae·mo·glo·bi·nae·mia *chiefly Brit var of* METHEMOGLOBINEMIA

meth·am·phet·amine \·me-tham-'fe-tə-·mēn, -thəm-, -mən\ *n* : an amine $C_{10}H_{15}N$ used medically in the form of its crystalline hydrochloride esp. in the treatment of obesity and often used illicitly as a stimulant — called also *methedrine*

meth·an·dro·sten·o·lone \·me-·than-drō-'ste-nə-·lōn\ *n* : an anabolic steroid $C_{20}H_{28}O_2$

meth·a·nol \'me-thə-·nȯl, -·nōl\ *n* : a light volatile pungent flammable poisonous liquid alcohol CH_3OH used esp. as a solvent, antifreeze, or denaturant for ethyl alcohol and in the synthesis of other chemicals — called also *methyl alcohol*, *wood alcohol*

meth·an·the·line \·me-'than-thə-·lēn, -lən\ *n* : an anticholinergic drug usu. administered in the form of its crystalline bromide $C_{21}H_{26}BrNO_3$ in the treatment of peptic ulcers — see BANTHINE

meth·a·phen·i·lene \·me-thə-'fen-əl-·ēn\ *n* : an antihistamine drug $C_{15}H_{20}N_2S$ usu. administered in the form of its hydrochloride

meth·a·pyr·i·lene \-'pir-ə-·lēn\ *n* : an antihistamine drug $C_{14}H_{19}N_3S$ widely used in the form of its fumarate or hydrochloride as a mild sedative in proprietary sleep-inducing drugs

meth·aqua·lone \·me-'tha-kwə-·lōn\ *n* : a sedative and hypnotic nonbarbiturate drug $C_{16}H_{14}N_2O$ that is habit-forming — see QUAALUDE

meth·ar·bi·tal \·me-'thär-bə-·tȯl, -·täl\ *n* : an anticonvulsant barbiturate $C_9H_{14}N_2O_3$

meth·a·zol·amide \·me-thə-'zō-lə-·mīd\ *n* : a sulfonamide $C_5H_8N_4O_3S_2$ that inhibits the production of carbonic anhydrase, reduces intraocular pressure, and is used in the treatment of glaucoma — see NEPTAZANE

meth·dil·a·zine \meth-'di-lə-·zēn, -'dī-lə-·zin\ *n* : a phenothiazine antihistamine $C_{18}H_{20}N_2S$ used in the form of its hydrochloride as an antipruritic

meth·e·drine \'me-thə-drən, -·drēn\ *n* : METHAMPHETAMINE

met·hem·al·bu·min \·met-·hē-mal-'byü-mən\ *n* : an albumin complex with hematin found in plasma during diseases (as blackwater fever) that are associated with extensive hemolysis

met·he·mo·glo·bin \(·)met-'hē-mə-·glō-bin\ *n* : a soluble brown crystalline basic blood pigment that is found in normal blood in much smaller amounts than hemoglobin, that is formed from blood, hemoglobin, and oxyhemoglobin by oxidation, and that differs from hemoglobin in containing ferric iron and in being unable to combine reversibly with molecular oxygen — called also *ferrihemoglobin*

met·he·mo·glo·bi·ne·mia \·met-·hē-mə-·glō-bə-'nē-mē-ə\ *n* : the presence of methemoglobin in the blood due to conversion of part of the hemoglobin to this inactive form

me·the·na·mine \mə-'thē-nə-·mēn, -mən\ *n* : a crystalline compound $C_6H_{12}N_4$ used in medicine as a urinary antiseptic esp. in cystitis and pyelitis — called also *hexamethylenetetramine*, *hexamine*; see MANDELAMINE, UROTROPIN

me·the·no·lone \mə-'thē-nə-·lōn, me-'the-\ *n* : a hormone $C_{20}H_{30}O_2$ that is an anabolic steroid

Meth·er·gine \'me-thər-jən\ *trademark* — used for a preparation of methylergonovine

meth·i·cil·lin \·me-thə-'si-lən\ *n* : a semisynthetic penicillin $C_{17}H_{19}N_2$-O_6NaS that is esp. effective against penicillinase-producing staphylococci

me·thi·ma·zole \me-'thī-mə-·zōl, mə-\ *n* : a drug $C_4H_6N_2S$ used to inhibit activity of the thyroid gland

meth·io·dal sodium \mə-'thī-ə-·dal-\ *n* : a crystalline salt CH_2ISO_3Na used as a radiopaque contrast medium in intravenous urography

me·thi·o·nine \mə-'thī-ə-·nēn\ *n* : a crystalline sulfur-containing essential amino acid $C_5H_{11}NO_2S$ that occurs in the L-form as a constituent of many proteins (as casein and egg albumin) and that is used as a dietary supplement and in the treatment of fatty infiltration of the liver — see MEONINE

methionine–en·keph·a·lin \-en-'kə-fə-lin\ *n* : a pentapeptide having a terminal methionine residue that is one of the two enkephalins occurring naturally in the brain — called also *Met≠ enkephalin*

meth·is·a·zone \me-ʹthi-sə-ˌzōn\ *n* : an antiviral drug $C_{10}H_{10}N_4OS$ that has been used in the preventive treatment of smallpox — see MARBORAN

Meth·ium \ʹme-thē-əm\ *trademark* — used for a preparation of hexamethonium in its chloride form $C_{12}H_{30}$-Cl_2N_2

me·thix·ene \me-ʹthik-ˌsēn\ *n* : an anticholinergic drug $C_{20}H_{23}NS$ used as an antispasmodic in the treatment of functional bowel hypermotility and spasm — see TREST

metho- — see METH-

meth·o·car·ba·mol \ˌme-thə-ʹkär-bə-ˌmȯl\ *n* : a skeletal muscle relaxant drug $C_{11}H_{15}NO_5$

meth·o·hex·i·tal \ˌme-thə-ʹhek-sə-ˌtȯl, -ˌtal\ *n* : a barbiturate with a short period of action usu. used in the form of its sodium salt $C_{14}H_{17}N_3NaO_3$ as an intravenous general anesthetic

meth·o·trex·ate \-ʹtrek-ˌsāt\ *n* : a toxic anticancer drug $C_{20}H_{22}N_8O_5$ that is an analog of folic acid and an antimetabolite — called also *amethopterin*

meth·o·tri·mep·ra·zine \-ˌtrī-ʹmep-prə-ˌzēn\ *n* : a nonnarcotic analgesic and tranquilizer $C_{19}H_{24}N_2OS$ — see LEVOPROME

me·thox·amine \me-ʹthäk-sə-ˌmēn, -mən\ *n* : a sympathomimetic amine $C_{11}H_{17}NO_3$ used in the form of its hydrochloride esp. to raise or maintain blood pressure (as during surgery) by its vasoconstrictor effects — see VASOXYL

me·thox·sa·len \me-ʹthäk-sə-lən\ *n* : a drug $C_{12}H_8O_4$ used to increase the production of melanin in the skin upon exposure to ultraviolet light and in the treatment of vitiligo — called also *xanthotoxin;* see MELOXINE

me·thoxy·flu·rane \me-ˌthäk-sē-ʹflu̇r-ˌān\ *n* : a potent nonexplosive inhalational general anesthetic $C_3H_4Cl_2$-F_2O

8–meth·oxy·psor·a·len \ˌāt-ˌme-ˌthäk-sē-ʹsȯr-ə-lən\ *n* : METHOXSALEN

meth·sco·pol·amine \ˌmeth-skō-ʹpä-lə-ˌmēn, -mən\ *n* : an anticholinergic derivative of scopolamine that is usu. used in the form of its bromide C_{18}-$H_{24}BrNO_4$ for its inhibitory effect on gastric secretion and gastrointestinal motility esp. in the treatment of peptic ulcer and gastric disorders — see PAMINE

meth·sux·i·mide \-ʹsək-si-ˌmīd\ *n* : an anticonvulsant drug $C_{12}H_{13}NO_2$ used esp. in the control of petit mal seizures

meth·y·clo·thi·azide \ˌme-thē-ˌklō-ʹthī-ə-ˌzīd\ *n* : a thiazide drug $C_9H_{11}Cl_2$-$N_3O_4S_2$ used as a diuretic and antihypertensive agent

meth·yl \ʹme-thəl, *Brit also* ʹmē-ˌthīl\ *n* : an alkyl group CH_3 that occurs esp. in combination in many compounds

meth·yl·al \ʹme-thə-ˌlal\ *n* : a volatile flammable liquid $C_3H_8O_2$ used as a hypnotic and anesthetic

methyl alcohol *n* : METHANOL

meth·yl·am·phet·amine \ˌme-thəl-am-ʹfe-tə-ˌmēn\ *n* : METHAMPHETAMINE

meth·yl·ate \ʹme-thə-ˌlāt\ *vb* **-at·ed; -at·ing 1** : to impregnate or mix with methanol **2** : to introduce the methyl group into — **meth·yl·ation** \ˌme-thə-ʹlā-shən\ *n*

methylated spirit *n* : ethyl alcohol denatured with methanol — often used in pl. with a sing. verb

meth·yl·ben·ze·tho·ni·um chloride \ˌme-thəl-ˌben-zə-ˌthō-nē-əm-\ *n* : a quaternary ammonium salt $C_{28}H_{44}ClNO_2$ used as a bactericide and antiseptic esp. in the treatment of diaper rash — called also *methylbenzethonium*

meth·yl·cel·lu·lose \ˌme-thəl-ʹsel-yə-ˌlōs, -ˌlōz\ *n* : any of various gummy products of cellulose methylation that swell in water and are used as bulk laxatives

meth·yl·cho·lan·threne \-kə-ʹlan-ˌthrēn\ *n* : a potent carcinogenic hydrocarbon $C_{21}H_{16}$ obtained from certain bile acids and cholesterol as well as synthetically

meth·yl·do·pa \-ʹdō-pə\ *n* : a drug $C_{10}H_{13}NO_4$ used to lower blood pressure

meth·y·lene blue \ʹme-thə-ˌlēn-, -lən-\ *n* : a basic thiazine dye $C_{16}H_{18}ClN_3S$-$3H_2O$ used in the treatment of methemoglobinemia and as an antidote in cyanide poisoning

meth·yl·er·go·no·vine \ˌme-thəl-ˌər-gə-ʹnō-ˌvēn\ *n* : an oxytocic drug C_{20}-$H_{25}N_3O_2$ used similarly to ergonovine usu. in the form of its maleate salt — see METHERGINE

meth·yl·glu·ca·mine \-ʹglü-kə-ˌmēn\ *n* : MEGLUMINE

meth·yl·hex·ane·amine \ˌme-thəl-ˌhek-sā-ʹna-mēn\ *n* : an amine base C_7-$H_{17}N$ used as a local vasoconstrictor of nasal mucosa in the treatment of nasal congestion

meth·yl·iso·cy·a·nate \-ˌī-sō-ʹsī-ə-ˌnāt\ *n* : an extremely toxic chemical CH_3NCO that is used esp. in the manufacture of pesticides and was the cause of numerous deaths and injuries in a leak at a chemical plant in Bhopal, India, in 1984 — abbr. *MIC*

meth·yl·ma·lon·ic acid \ˌme-thəl-mə-ʹlä-nik-\ *n* : a structural isomer of succinic acid present in minute amounts in healthy human urine but excreted in large quantities in the urine of individuals with a vitamin B_{12} deficiency

methylmalonic aciduria *n* : a metabolic defect which is controlled by an autosomal recessive gene and in which methylmalonic acid is not converted to succinic acid with chronic metabolic acidosis resulting

meth·yl mer·cap·tan \'me-thəl-'kap-,tan\ *n* : a pungent gas CH₄S produced in the intestine by the decomposition of certain proteins and responsible for the characteristic odor of fetor hepaticus

meth·yl·mer·cu·ry \,me-thəl-'mər-kyə-rē\ *n*, *pl* **-ries** : any of various toxic compounds of mercury containing the complex CH₃Hg− that often occur as pollutants formed as industrial by-products or pesticide residues, tend to accumulate in living organisms (as fish) esp. in higher levels of a food chain, are rapidly and easily absorbed through the human intestinal wall, and cause neurological dysfunction in humans — see MINAMATA DISEASE

meth·yl·mor·phine \,me-thəl-'mòr-,fēn\ *n* : CODEINE

meth·yl·para·ben \,me-thəl-'par-ə-,ben\ *n* : a crystalline compound C₈H₈O₃ used as an antifungal preservative (as in pharmaceutical ointments and cosmetic creams)

meth·yl·para·fy·nol \-'par-ə-'fī-,nòl\ *n* : a sedative and hypnotic drug C₆H₁₀O

methyl parathion *n* : a potent synthetic organophosphate insecticide C₈H₁₀NO₅PS that is more toxic than parathion

meth·yl·phe·ni·date \,me-thəl-'fe-nə-,dāt, -'fē-\ *n* : a mild stimulant C₁₄H₁₉NO₂ of the central nervous system used in the form of its hydrochloride to treat narcolepsy and hyperkinetic behavior disorders in children — see RITALIN

meth·yl·pred·nis·o·lone \-pred-'ni-sə-,lōn\ *n* : a glucocorticoid C₂₂H₃₀O₅ that is a derivative of prednisolone and is used as an anti-inflammatory agent; *also* : any of several of its salts (as an acetate) used similarly — see MEDROL

methyl salicylate *n* : a liquid ester C₈H₈O₃ that is obtained from the leaves of a wintergreen (*Gaultheria procumbens*) or the bark of a birch (*Betula lenta*), but is usu. made synthetically, and that is used as a flavoring and a counterirritant — see OIL OF WINTERGREEN

methylsulfate — see PENTAPIPERIDE METHYLSULFATE

meth·yl·tes·tos·ter·one \-te-'stäs-tə-,rōn\ *n* : a synthetically prepared crystalline compound C₂₀H₃₀O₂ administered orally in cases of male sex hormone deficiency — see METANDREN

meth·yl·thio·ura·cil \-,thī-ō-'yùr-ə-,sil\ *n* : a crystalline compound C₅H₆N₂OS used in the suppression of hyperactivity of the thyroid

α-meth·yl·ty·ro·sine \,al-fə-,me-thəl-'tī-rə-,sēn\ *n* : a compound C₁₀H₁₃NO₃ that inhibits the synthesis of catecholamines but not of serotonin

meth·yl·xan·thine \,me-thəl-'zan-,thēn\ *n* : a methylated xanthine derivative (as caffeine, theobromine, or theophylline)

meth·y·pry·lon \,me-thə-'prī-,län\ *n* : a sedative and hypnotic drug C₁₀H₁₇NO₂

meth·y·ser·gide \,me-thə-'sər-,jīd\ *n* : a serotonin antagonist C₂₁H₂₇N₃O₂ used in the form of its maleate esp. in the treatment and prevention of migraine headaches

Met·i·cor·te·lone \,me-ti-'kòr-tə-,lōn\ *trademark* — used for a preparation of prednisolone

met·o·clo·pra·mide \,me-tə-'klō-prə-,mīd\ *n* : an antiemetic drug C₁₄H₂₂ClN₃O₂ administered as the hydrochloride

met·o·cur·ine iodide \,me-tə-'kyùr-,ēn-\ *n* : a crystalline iodine-containing powder C₄₀H₄₈I₂N₂O₆ that is derived from the dextrorotatory form of tubocurarine and is a potent skeletal muscle relaxant — called also *metocurine*; see METUBINE

me·to·la·zone \me-'tō-lə-,zōn\ *n* : a diuretic and antihypertensive drug C₁₆H₁₆ClN₃O₃S

me·top·ic \me-'tä-pik\ *adj* : of or relating to the forehead : FRONTAL; *esp* : of, relating to, or being a suture uniting the frontal bones in the fetus and sometimes persistent after birth

met·o·pim·a·zine \,me-tə-'pi-mə-,zēn\ *n* : an antiemetic drug C₂₂H₂₇N₃O₃S₂

Met·o·pir·one \,me-tə-'pir-,ōn\ *trademark* — used for a preparation of metyrapone

Me·to·pi·um \mə-'tō-pē-əm\ *n* : a genus of trees and shrubs of the cashew family (Anacardiaceae) that includes the poisonwood (*M. toxiferum*)

met·o·pon \'me-tə-,pän\ *n* : a narcotic drug C₁₈H₂₁NO₃ that is derived from morphine and is used in the form of the hydrochloride to relieve pain

met·o·pro·lol \me-'tō-prə-,lòl, -,lōl\ *n* : a beta-blocker C₁₅H₂₅NO₃ used in the treatment of hypertension

metr- *or* **metro-** *comb form* : uterus ⟨*metr*itis⟩

-me·tra \'mē-trə\ *n comb form* : a (specified) condition of the uterus ⟨hemato*metra*⟩

Met·ra·zol \'me-trə-,zòl, -,zōl\ *trademark* — used for pentylenetetrazol

me·tre *chiefly Brit var of* METER

met·ric \'me-trik\ *adj* : of, relating to, or using the metric system — **met·ri·cal·ly** *adv*

-met·ric \me-trik\ *or* **-met·ri·cal** \'me-tri-kəl\ *adj comb form* **1** : of, employing, or obtained by (such) a meter ⟨calori*metric*⟩ **2** : of or relating to (such) an art, process, or science of measuring ⟨psycho*metric*⟩

metric system *n* : a decimal system of weights and measures based on the meter and on the kilogram — compare CGS, MKS

me·tri·tis \mə-'trī-təs\ *n* : inflammation of the uterus

-me·tri·um \'mē-trē-əm\ *n comb form* : part or layer of the uterus (endo*metrium*)

me·triz·a·mide \me-'tri-za-₁mīd\ *n* : a radiopaque medium $C_{18}H_{22}I_3N_3O_8$

met·ri·zo·ate sodium \₁me-tri-'zō-āt-\ *n* : a radiopaque medium $C_{12}H_{10}I_3$-N_2NaO_4 — see ISOPAQUE

met·ro·ni·da·zole \₁me-trə-'nī-də-₁zōl\ *n* : a drug $C_6H_9N_3O_3$ used esp. in treating vaginal trichomoniasis

me·tror·rha·gia \mē-trə-'rā-jə, -jē-ə, -zhə; -'rā-\ *n* : profuse uterine bleeding esp. between menstrual periods — compare MENORRHAGIA — **me·tror·rhag·ic** \-'ra-jik\ *adj*

-me·try \mə-trē\ *n comb form* : art, process, or science of measuring (something specified) ⟨audio*metry*⟩

Me·tu·bine \me-'tü-₁bēn, -'tyü-\ *trademark* — used for a preparation of metocurine iodide

me·tu·re·depa \mə-₁tür-ə-'de-pə, ₁me-tyə-rə-\ *n* : an antineoplastic drug $C_{11}H_{22}N_3O_3P$

Met·y·caine \'me-tə-₁kān\ *trademark* — used for a preparation of the hydrochloride of piperocaine

me·tyr·a·pone \mə-'tir-ə-₁pōn, -'tīr-\ *n* : a metabolic hormone $C_{14}H_{14}N_2O$ that inhibits biosynthesis of cortisol and corticosterone and is used to test for normal functioning of the pituitary gland — see METOPIRONE

me·ze·re·um \mə-'zir-ē-əm\ *n* : the dried bark of various European shrubs (genus *Daphne* and esp. *D. mezereum* of the family Thymelaeaceae) used externally as a vesicant and irritant

mg *abbr* milligram

Mg *symbol* magnesium

MHC *abbr* major histocompatibility complex

MI *abbr* **1** mitral incompetence; mitral insufficiency **2** myocardial infarction

mi·an·ser·in \mī-'an-sər-in\ *n* : a drug $C_{18}H_{20}N_2$ administered in the form of its hydrochloride as a serotonin inhibitor and antihistamine

MIC *abbr* **1** methylisocyanate **2** minimal inhibitory concentration; minimum inhibitory concentration

mice *pl of* MOUSE

mi·con·a·zole \mī-'kä-nə-₁zōl\ *n* : an antifungal agent administered esp. in the form of its nitrate $C_{18}H_{14}Cl_4$-$N_2O \cdot HNO_3$

micr- *or* **micro-** *comb form* **1 a** : minute ⟨*micro*aneurysm⟩ **b** : used for or involving minute quantities or variations ⟨*micro*analysis⟩ **2 a** : using microscopy ⟨*micro*dissection⟩ **b** : revealed by or having its structure discernible only by microscopical examination ⟨*micro*organism⟩ **3** : abnormally small ⟨*micro*cyte⟩

micra *pl of* MICRON

mi·cren·ceph·a·ly \₁mī-₁kren-'se-fə-lē\ *n, pl* **-lies** : the condition of having an abnormally small brain

mi·cro·ab·scess \'mī-krō-₁ab-ses\ *n* : a very small abscess

mi·cro·ad·e·no·ma \₁mī-krō-₁ad-ᵊn-'ō-mə\ *n, pl* **-mas** *or* **-ma·ta** \-mə-tə\ : a very small adenoma

mi·cro·ag·gre·gate \-'a-gri-gət\ *n* : an aggregate of microscopic particles (as of fibrin) formed esp. in stored blood

mi·cro·anal·y·sis \₁mī-krō-ə-'na-lə-səs\ *n, pl* **-y·ses** \-₁sēz\ : chemical analysis on a small or minute scale that usu. requires special, very sensitive, or small-scale apparatus — **mi·cro·an·a·lyt·ic** \-₁an-ᵊl-'i-tik\ *or* **mi·cro·an·a·lyt·i·cal** \-'i-ti-kəl\ *adj*

mi·cro·anat·o·my \-ə-'na-tə-mē\ *n, pl* **-mies** : HISTOLOGY — **mi·cro·ana·tom·i·cal** \-₁a-nə-'tä-mi-kəl\ *adj*

mi·cro·an·eu·rysm *also* **mi·cro·an·eu·rism** \-'a-nyə-₁ri-zəm\ *n* : a saccular enlargement of the venous end of a retinal capillary associated esp. with diabetic retinopathy — **mi·cro·an·eu·rys·mal** \-₁a-nyə-'riz-məl\ *adj*

mi·cro·an·gio·g·ra·phy \-₁an-jē-'ä-grə-fē\ *n, pl* **-phies** : minutely detailed angiography — **mi·cro·an·gio·graph·ic** \-₁an-jē-ə-'gra-fik\ *adj*

mi·cro·an·gi·op·a·thy \-'ä-pə-thē\ *n, pl* **-thies** : a disease of very fine blood vessels ⟨thrombotic ∼⟩ — **mi·cro·an·gio·path·ic** \-₁an-jē-ə-'pa-thik\ *adj*

mi·cro·ar·te·ri·og·ra·phy \-är-₁tir-ē-'ä-grə-fē\ *n, pl* **-phies** : minutely detailed arteriography

mi·crobe \'mī-₁krōb\ *n* : MICROORGANISM, GERM — used esp. of pathogenic bacteria

mi·cro·bi·al \mī-'krō-bē-əl\ *adj* : of, relating to, caused by, or being microbes ⟨∼ infection⟩ ⟨∼ agents⟩

mi·cro·bic \mī-'krō-bik\ *adj* : MICROBIAL

mi·cro·bi·cide \mī-'krō-bə-₁sīd\ *n* : an agent that destroys microbes — **mi·cro·bi·ci·dal** \mī-₁krō-bə-'sīd-ᵊl\ *adj*

mi·cro·bi·ol·o·gy \₁mī-krō-bī-'ä-lə-jē\ *n, pl* **-gies** : a branch of biology dealing esp. with microscopic forms of life (as bacteria, protozoa, viruses, and fungi) — **mi·cro·bi·o·log·i·cal** \'mī-krō-₁bī-ə-'lä-ji-kəl\ *also* **mi·cro·bi·o·log·ic** \-'lä-jik\ *adj* — **mi·cro·bi·o·log·i·cal·ly** *adv* — **mi·cro·bi·ol·o·gist** \-jist\ *n*

mi·cro·body \'mī-krō-₁bä-dē\ *n, pl* **-bod·ies** : PEROXISOME

mi·cro·cap·sule \'mī-krō-₁kap-səl, -(₁)sül\ *n* : a tiny capsule containing material (as a medicine) that is released when the capsule is broken, melted, or dissolved

¹mi·cro·ce·phal·ic \₁mī-krō-sə-'fa-lik\ *adj* : having a small head; *specif* : having an abnormally small head

²microcephalic *n* : an individual with an abnormally small head

mi·cro·ceph·a·lus \-'se-fa-ləs\ *n, pl* **-li** \-₁lī\ : MICROCEPHALY

mi·cro·ceph·a·ly \-'se-fə-lē\ *n, pl* **-lies** : a condition of abnormal smallness of the head usu. associated with mental defects

mi·cro·cir·cu·la·tion \-₁sər-kyə-'lā-shən\ *n* : blood circulation in the microvascular system; *also* : the microvascular system itself — **mi·cro·cir·cu·la·to·ry** \-'sər-kyə-lə-₁tōr-ē\ *adj*

mi·cro·coc·cus \₁mī-krō-'kä-kəs\ *n* **1** *cap* : a genus of nonmotile gram=positive spherical bacteria (family Micrococcaceae) that occur in tetrads or irregular clusters and include nonpathogenic forms found on human and animal skin **2** *pl* **-coc·ci** \-'kä-₁kī, -'käk-₁sī\ : a small spherical bacterium; *esp* : any bacterium of the genus *Micrococcus* — **mi·cro·coc·cal** \₁mī-krō-'kä-kəl\ *adj*

mi·cro·cul·ture \'mī-krō-₁kəl-chər\ *n* : a microscopic culture of cells or organisms (a ∼ of lymphocytes) — **mi·cro·cul·tur·al** \₁mī-krō-'kəlch-(ə-)rəl\ *adj*

mi·cro·cu·rie \'mī-krō-₁kyur-ē, ₁mī-krō-kyu-'rē\ *n* : a unit of quantity of or of radioactivity equal to one millionth of a curie

mi·cro·cyte \'mī-krə-₁sīt\ *n* : an abnormally small red blood cell present esp. in some anemias

mi·cro·cyt·ic \₁mī-krə-'si-tik\ *adj* : of, relating to, being, or characterized by the presence of microcytes

microcytic anemia *n* : an anemia characterized by the presence of microcytes in the blood

mi·cro·cy·to·sis \-sī-'tō-səs\ *n, pl* **-to·ses** \-₁sēz\ : decrease in the size of red blood cells

mi·cro·cy·to·tox·ic·i·ty test \-₁sīt-ō-₁täk-'si-sə-tē\ *n* : a procedure using microscopic quantities of materials (as complement and lymphocytes in cell=mediated immunity) to determine cytotoxicity (as to cancer cells or cells of transplanted tissue) — called also *microcytotoxicity assay*

mi·cro·dis·sec·tion \₁mī-krō-di-'sek-shən, -dī-\ *n* : dissection under the microscope; *specif* : dissection of cells and tissues by means of fine needles that are precisely manipulated by levers — **mi·cro·dis·sect·ed** \-'sek-təd\ *adj*

mi·cro·dose \'mī-krō-₁dōs\ *n* : an extremely small dose

mi·cro·do·sim·e·try \₁mī-krō-dō-'si-mə-trē\ *n, pl* **-tries** : dosimetry involving microdoses of radiation or minute amounts of radioactive material

mi·cro·drop \'mī-krō-₁dräp\ *n* : a very small drop or minute droplet (as 0.1 to 0.01 of a drop)

mi·cro·drop·let \-₁drä-plət\ *n* : MICRODROP

mi·cro·elec·trode \₁mī-krō-i-'lek-₁trōd\ *n* : a minute electrode; *esp* : one that is inserted in a living biological cell or tissue in studying its electrical characteristics

mi·cro·elec·tro·pho·re·sis \-i-₁lek-trə-fə-'rē-səs\ *n, pl* **-re·ses** \-₁sēz\ : electrophoresis in which the movement of single particles is observed in a microscope — **mi·cro·elec·tro·pho·ret·ic** \-'re-tik\ *adj* — **mi·cro·elec·tro·pho·ret·i·cal·ly** *adv*

mi·cro·el·e·ment \₁mī-krō-'e-lə-mənt\ *n* : TRACE ELEMENT

mi·cro·em·bo·lus \-'em-bə-ləs\ *n, pl* **-li** \-₁lī\ : an extremely small embolus

mi·cro·en·cap·su·late \-in-'kap-sə-₁lāt\ *vb* **-lat·ed; -lat·ing** : to enclose in a microcapsule — **mi·cro·en·cap·su·la·tion** \-in-₁kap-sə-'lā-shən\ *n*

mi·cro·en·vi·ron·ment \-in-'vī-rən-mənt, -'vī-ərn-\ *n* : a small usu. distinctly specialized and effectively isolated habitat — called also *microhabitat* — **mi·cro·en·vi·ron·men·tal** \-₁vī-rən-'ment-ᵊl\ *adj*

mi·cro·fi·bril \-'fī-brəl, -'fi-\ *n* : an extremely fine fibril — **mi·cro·fi·bril·lar** \-brə-lər\ *adj*

mi·cro·fil·a·ment \₁mī-krō-'fi-lə-mənt\ *n* : any of the minute actin-containing protein filaments that are widely distributed in the cytoplasm of eukaryotic cells, help maintain their structural framework, and play a role in the movement of cell components — **mi·cro·fil·a·men·tous** \-₁fi-lə-'men-təs\ *adj*

mi·cro·fil·a·rae·mia *chiefly Brit var of* MICROFILAREMIA

mi·cro·fil·a·re·mia \-₁fi-lə-'rē-mē-ə\ *n* : the presence of microfilariae in the blood of one affected with some forms of filariasis

mi·cro·fi·lar·ia \₁mī-krō-fə-'lar-ē-ə\ *n, pl* **-iae** \-ē-₁ē\ : a minute larval filaria — **mi·cro·fi·lar·i·al** \-ē-əl\ *adj*

mi·cro·flo·ra \₁mī-krə-'flōr-ə\ *n* : a small or strictly localized flora (intestinal ∼) — **mi·cro·flo·ral** \-əl\ *adj*

mi·cro·fluo·rom·e·try \-₁flü-'rä-mə-trē\ *n, pl* **-tries** : the detection and measurement of the fluorescence produced by minute quantities of materials (as in cells) — **mi·cro·fluo·rom·e·ter** \-'rä-mə-tər\ *n* — **mi·cro·fluo·ro·met·ric** \-rə-'me-trik\ *adj*

mi·cro·ga·mete \-'ga-₁mēt, -gə-'mēt\ *n* : the smaller and usu. male gamete of an organism producing two types of gametes — compare MACROGAMETE

mi·cro·ga·me·to·cyte \-gə-'mē-tə-₁sīt\ *n* : a gametocyte producing microgametes

mi·crog·lia \mī-'krä-glē-ə\ *n* : neuroglia consisting of small cells with few processes that are scattered throughout the central nervous system, have a phagocytic function as part of the reticuloendothelial system, and are now usu. considered to be of mesodermal origin — **mi·crog·li·al** \-glē-əl\ *adj*

β₂-mi·cro·glob·u·lin \₁bā-tə-₁tü-₁mī-krō-'glä-byə-lən\ *n* : a beta globulin of low molecular weight that is present at a low level in plasma, is normally excreted in the urine, is homologous in structure to part of an antibody, and forms a subunit of histocompatibility antigens

mi·cro·glos·sia \ˌmī-krō-ˈglä-sē-ə, -ˈglȯ-\ *n* : abnormal smallness of the tongue

mi·cro·gna·thia \ˌmī-krō-ˈnā-thē-ə, -ˈna-, ˌmī-ˌkräg-\ *n* : abnormal smallness of one or both jaws

mi·cro·gram \ˈmī-krə-ˌgram\ *n* : one millionth of a gram

mi·cro·graph \-ˌgraf\ *n* : a graphic reproduction (as a photograph) of the image of an object formed by a microscope — **micrograph** *vb*

mi·cro·hab·i·tat \ˌmī-krō-ˈha-bə-ˌtat\ *n* : MICROENVIRONMENT

mi·cro·he·mat·o·crit \-hi-ˈma-tə-ˌkrit\ *n* **1** : a procedure for determining the ratio of the volume of packed red blood cells to the volume of whole blood by centrifuging a minute quantity of blood in a capillary tube coated with heparin **2** : a hematocrit value obtained by microhematocrit (a ∼ of 37%)

mi·cro·in·farct \-in-ˈfärkt\ *n* : a very small infarct

mi·cro·in·jec·tion \ˌmī-krō-in-ˈjek-shən\ *n* : injection under the microscope; *specif* : injection into cells or tissues by means of a fine mechanically controlled capillary tube — **mi·cro·in·ject** \-in-ˈjekt\ *vb*

mi·cro·in·va·sive \-in-ˈvā-siv\ *adj* : of, relating to, or characterized by very slight invasion into adjacent tissues by malignant cells of a carcinoma in situ — **mi·cro·in·va·sion** \-ˈvā-zhən\ *n*

mi·cro·ion·to·pho·re·sis \-ˌ(ˌ)ī-ˌän-tə-fə-ˈrē-səs\ *n, pl* **-re·ses** \-ˌsēz\ : a process for observing or recording the effect of an ionized substance on nerve cells that involves inserting a double micropipette into the brain close to a nerve cell, injecting an ionized fluid through one barrel of the pipette, and using a concentrated saline solution in the other tube as an electrical conductor to pick up and transmit back to an oscilloscope any change in neural activity — **mi·cro·ion·to·pho·ret·ic** \-ˈre-tik\ *adj* — **mi·cro·ion·to·pho·ret·i·cal·ly** *adv*

mi·cro·li·ter \ˈmī-krō-ˈlē-tər\ *n* : a unit of capacity equal to one millionth of a liter

mi·cro·lith \ˈmī-krō-ˌlith\ *n* : a microscopic calculus or concretion — compare GRAVEL 1

mi·cro·li·thi·a·sis \ˌmī-krō-li-ˈthī-ə-səs\ *n, pl* **-a·ses** \-ˌsēz\ : the formation or presence of microliths or gravel

mi·cro·ma·nip·u·la·tion \ˌmī-krō-mə-ˌni-pyə-ˈlā-shən\ *n* : the technique or practice of microdissection and microinjection — **mi·cro·ma·nip·u·late** \-ˈni-pyə-ˌlāt\ *vb* — **mi·cro·ma·nip·u·la·tor** \-ˈni-pyə-ˌlā-tər\ *n*

mi·cro·mas·tia \-ˈmas-tē-ə\ *n* : postpu-bertal immaturity and abnormal smallness of the breasts

mi·cro·me·lia \-ˈmē-lē-ə\ *n* : a condition characterized by abnormally small and imperfectly developed extremities — **mi·cro·me·lic** \-ˈmē-lik\ *adj*

mi·cro·me·tas·ta·sis \ˌmī-krō-mə-ˈtas-tə-səs\ *n, pl* **-ta·ses** \-ˌsēz\ : the spread of cancer cells from a primary site and the formation of microscopic tumors at secondary sites — **mi·cro·met·a·stat·ic** \-ˌme-tə-ˈsta-tik\ *adj*

mi·cro·me·ter \ˈmī-krō-ˌmē-tər\ *n* : a unit of length equal to one millionth of a meter — called also *micron, mu*

mi·cro·meth·od \ˈmī-krō-ˌme-thəd\ *n* : a method (as of microanalysis) that requires only very small quantities of material or that involves the use of the microscope

mi·cro·mi·cro·cu·rie \ˌmī-krō-ˈmī-krō-ˌkyür-ē\ *n* : one millionth of a microcurie

mi·cro·mol·e·cule \-ˈmä-lə-ˌkyül\ *n* : a molecule (as of an amino acid or a fatty acid) of relatively low molecular weight — compare MACROMOLECULE — **mi·cro·mo·lec·u·lar** \-mə-ˈle-kyə-lər\ *adj*

mi·cro·mono·spo·ra \-ˌmä-nə-ˈspȯr-ə\ *n* **1** *cap* : a genus of actinomycetes that includes several antibiotic-producing forms (as *M. purpurea,* the source of gentamicin) **2** *pl* **-rae** \-ˌrē\ : any bacterium of the genus *Micromonospora*

mi·cron \ˈmī-ˌkrän\ *n, pl* **microns** *also* **mi·cra** \-krə\ : MICROMETER

mi·cro·nee·dle \ˈmī-krō-ˌnēd-əl\ *n* : a needle for micromanipulation

mi·cro·nod·u·lar \ˌmī-krō-ˈnä-jə-lər\ *adj* : characterized by the presence of extremely small nodules

mi·cro·nu·tri·ent \-ˈnü-trē-ənt, -ˈnyü-\ *n* : a mineral or organic compound (as a vitamin) essential in minute amounts to the growth and health of an animal — compare TRACE ELEMENT

mi·cro·or·gan·ism \-ˈȯr-gə-ˌni-zəm\ *n* : an organism of microscopic or ultramicroscopic size — **mi·cro·or·gan·is·mal** \-ˌȯr-gə-ˈniz-məl\ *adj*

mi·cro·par·a·site \ˌmī-krō-ˈpar-ə-ˌsīt\ *n* : a parasitic microorganism — **mi·cro·par·a·sit·ic** \-ˌpar-ə-ˈsi-tik\ *adj*

mi·cro·pe·nis \-ˈpē-nəs\ *n, pl* **-pe·nes** \-ˌnēz\ *or* **-pe·nis·es** : MICROPHALLUS

mi·cro·per·fu·sion \-pər-ˈfyü-zhən\ *n* : an act or instance of forcing a fluid through a small organ or tissue by way of a tubule or blood vessel — **mi·cro·per·fused** \-ˈfyüzd\ *adj*

mi·cro·phage \ˈmī-krə-ˌfāj\ *n* : a small phagocyte

mi·cro·pha·kia \ˌmī-krō-ˈfā-kē-ə\ *n* : abnormal smallness of the lens of the eye

mi·cro·phal·lus \-ˈfa-ləs\ *n* : smallness of the penis esp. to an abnormal degree — called also *micropenis*

mi·cro·phon·ic \ˌmī-krō-ˈfä-nik\ *n* : an electrical potential arising in the cochlea when the mechanical energy of a sound stimulus is transformed to electrical energy as the action potential of the transmitting nerve — **mi·crophonic** *adj*

mi·cro·pho·to·graph \-'fō-tə-ɪgraf\ : PHOTOMICROGRAPH — **mi·cro·pho·tog·ra·phy** \-ɪfə-'tä-grə-fē\ *n*

mi·croph·thal·mia \ɪmī-ɪkräf-'thal-mē-ə\ *n* : abnormal smallness of the eye usu. occurring as a congenital anomaly

mi·croph·thal·mic \-'thal-mik\ *adj* : exhibiting microphthalmia : having small eyes

mi·croph·thal·mos \-məs, -ɪmäs\ *or* **mi·croph·thal·mus** \-'thal-məs\ *n, pl* **-moi** \-ɪmȯi\ *or* **-mi** \-ɪmī, -ɪmē\ : MICROPHTHALMIA

mi·cro·pi·pette *or* **mi·cro·pi·pet** \-pī-'pet\ *n* **1** : a pipette for the measurement of minute volumes **2** : a small and extremely fine-pointed pipette used in making microinjections — **mi·cropipette** *vb*

mi·cro·probe \'mī-krō-ɪprōb\ *n* : a device for microanalysis that operates by exciting radiation in a minute area or volume of material so that the composition may be determined from the emission spectrum

mi·crop·sia \mī-'kräp-sē-ə\ *also* **mi·crop·sy** \'mī-ɪkräp-sē\ *n, pl* **-sias** *also* **-sies** : a pathological condition in which objects appear to be smaller than they are in reality

mi·cro·punc·ture \ɪmī-krō-'pəŋk-chər\ *n* : an extremely small puncture (as of a nephron); *also* : an act of making a micropuncture

mi·cro·pyle \'mī-krə-ɪpil\ *n* : a differentiated area of surface in an egg through which a sperm enters — **mi·cro·py·lar** \ɪmī-krə-'pī-lər\ *adj*

mi·cro·ra·dio·gram \ɪmī-krō-'rā-dē-ə-ɪgram\ *n* : MICRORADIOGRAPH

mi·cro·ra·dio·graph \-ɪgraf\ *n* : an X-ray photograph prepared by microradiography

mi·cro·ra·di·og·ra·phy \-ɪrā-dē-'ä-grə-fē\ *n, pl* **-phies** : radiography in which an X-ray photograph is prepared showing minute internal structure — **mi·cro·ra·dio·graph·ic** \-ɪrā-dē-ə-'gra-fik\ *adj*

mi·cro·scis·sors \'mī-krō-ɪsi-zərz\ *n sing or pl* : extremely small scissors for use in microsurgery

mi·cro·scope \'mī-krə-ɪskōp\ *n* : an instrument for making enlarged images of minute objects usu. using light; *esp* : COMPOUND MICROSCOPE — see ELECTRON MICROSCOPE, LIGHT MICROSCOPE, PHASE-CONTRAST MICROSCOPE, POLARIZING MICROSCOPE, ULTRAVIOLET MICROSCOPE

mi·cro·scop·ic \ɪmī-krə-'skä-pik\ *also* **mi·cro·scop·i·cal** \-pi-kəl\ *adj* **1** : of, relating to, or conducted with the microscope or microscopy **2** : so small or fine as to be invisible or indistin-

guishable without the use of a microscope — compare MACROSCOPIC, SUBMICROSCOPIC, ULTRAMICROSCOPIC 1 — **mi·cro·scop·i·cal·ly** *adv*

microscopic anatomy *n* : HISTOLOGY

mi·cros·co·py \mī-'kräs-kə-pē\ *n, pl* **-pies** : the use of or investigation with the microscope — **mi·cros·co·pist** \-pist\ *n*

mi·cro·sec·ond \'mī-krō-ɪse-kənd, -kənt\ *n* : one millionth of a second

mi·cro·sec·tion \-ɪsek-shən\ *n* : a thin section (as of tissue) prepared for microscopic examination — **microsection** *vb*

mi·cro·slide \'mī-krō-ɪslīd\ *n* : a slip of glass on which a preparation is mounted for microscopic examination

mi·cro·some \'mī-krə-ɪsōm\ *n* **1** : any of various minute cellular structures (as a ribosome) **2** : a particle in a particulate fraction that is obtained by heavy centrifugation of broken cells and consists of various amounts of ribosomes, fragmented endoplasmic reticulum, and mitochondrial cristae — **mi·cro·som·al** \ɪmī-krə-'sō-məl\ *adj*

mi·cro·so·mia \ɪmī-krə-'sō-mē-ə\ *n* : abnormal smallness of the body

mi·cro·sphe·ro·cy·to·sis \-ɪsfir-ō-sī-'tō-səs, -ɪsfer-\ *n, pl* **-to·ses** \-'tō-ɪsēz\ : spherocytosis esp. when marked by very small spherocytes

mi·cros·po·rum \mī-'kräs-pə-rəm\ *n* **1** *cap* : a genus of fungi (family Moniliaceae) producing both small, nearly oval single-celled spores and large spindle-shaped multicellular spores with a usu. rough outer wall and including several that cause ringworm, tinea capitis, and tinea corporis **2** *pl* **-ra** : any fungus of the genus *Microsporum*

mi·cro·struc·ture \'mī-krō-ɪstrək-chər\ *n* : microscopic structure (as of a cell) — **mi·cro·struc·tur·al** \ɪmī-krō-'strək-chə-rəl, -'strək-shrəl\ *adj*

mi·cro·sur·gery \ɪmī-krō-'sər-jə-rē\ *n, pl* **-ger·ies** : minute dissection or manipulation (as by a micromanipulator or laser beam) of living structures or tissue — **mi·cro·sur·geon** \'mī-krō-ɪsər-jən\ *n* — **mi·cro·sur·gi·cal** \ɪmī-krō-'sər-ji-kəl\ *adj* — **mi·cro·sur·gi·cal·ly** *adv*

mi·cro·sy·ringe \-sə-'rinj\ *n* : a hypodermic syringe equipped for the precise measurement and injection of minute quantities of fluid

mi·cro·tech·nique \ɪmī-krō-tek-'nēk\ *also* **mi·cro·tech·nic** \'mī-krō-ɪtek-nik, ɪmī-krō-tek-'nēk\ *n* : any of various methods of handling and preparing material for microscopic observation and study

mi·cro·throm·bus \-'thräm-bəs\ *n, pl* **-bi** \-ɪbī\ : a very small thrombus

mi·cro·tia \mī-'krō-shə, -shē-ə\ *n* : abnormal smallness of the external ear

mi·cro·tome \'mī-krə-ɪtōm\ *n* : an instrument for cutting sections (as of organic tissues) for microscopic examination — **microtome** *vb*

mi·cro·trau·ma \'mī-krō-,traú-mə, -,trō-\ *n* : a very slight injury or lesion

mi·cro·tu·bule \,mī-krō-'tü-,byül, -'tyü-\ *n* : any of the minute tubules in eukaryotic cytoplasm that are composed of the protein tubulin and form an important component of the cytoskeleton, mitotic spindle, cilia, and flagella — **mi·cro·tu·bu·lar** \-byə-lər\ *adj*

mi·cro·unit \'mī-krō-,yü-nət\ *n* : one millionth of a standard unit and esp. an international unit ($\sim$s of insulin)

mi·cro·vas·cu·lar \-'vas-kyə-lər\ *adj* : of, relating to, or constituting the part of the circulatory system made up of minute vessels (as venules or capillaries) that average less than 0.3 millimeters in diameter — **mi·cro·vas·cu·la·ture** \-lə-,chur, -,tyùr\ *n*

mi·cro·ves·i·cle \-'ve-si-kəl\ *n* : a very small vesicle

mi·cro·ves·sel \'\-'ve-səl\ *n* : a blood vessel (as a capillary, arteriole, or venule) of the microcirculatory system

mi·cro·vil·lus \-'vi-ləs\ *n, pl* -**vil·li** \-'lī\ : a microscopic projection of a tissue, cell, or cell organelle; *esp* : any of the fingerlike outward projections of some cell surfaces — **mi·cro·vil·lar** \-'vi-lər\ *adj* — **mi·cro·vil·lous** \-'vi-ləs\ *adj*

mi·cro·wave \'mī-krō-,wāv\ *n, often attrib* : a comparatively short electromagnetic wave; *esp* : one between about 1 millimeter and 1 meter in wavelength

microwave sickness *n* : a condition of impaired health reported esp. in the Russian medical literature that is characterized by headaches, anxiety, sleep disturbances, fatigue, and difficulty in concentrating and by changes in the cardiovascular and central nervous systems and that is held to be caused by prolonged exposure to low-intensity microwave radiation

Mi·cru·rus \mī-'krúr-əs\ *n* : a genus of small venomous elapid snakes comprising the American coral snakes

mic·tu·ri·tion \,mik-chə-'ri-shən, ,mik-tyü-\ *n* : URINATION — **mic·tu·rate** \'mik-chə-,rāt, -,tyü-\ *vb*

MID *abbr* minimal infective dose

mid·ax·il·lary line \,mid-'ak-sə-,ler-ē-\ *n* : an imaginary line through the axilla parallel to the long axis of the body and midway between its ventral and dorsal surfaces

mid·brain \'mid-,brān\ *n* : the middle of the three primary divisions of the developing vertebrate brain or the corresponding part of the adult brain that includes a ventral part containing the cerebral peduncles and a dorsal tectum containing the corpora quadrigemina and that surrounds the aqueduct of Sylvius connecting the

third and fourth ventricles — called also *mesencephalon*

mid·cla·vic·u·lar line \-kla-'vi-kyə-lər-, -klə-\ *n* : an imaginary line parallel to the long axis of the body and passing through the midpoint of the clavicle on the ventral surface of the body

middle age *n* : the period of life from about 40 to about 60 — **mid·dle-aged** \,mid-əl-'ājd\ *adj* — **mid·dle-ag·er** \-'ā-jər\ *n*

middle cerebellar peduncle *n* : CEREBELLAR PEDUNCLE b

middle cerebral artery *n* : CEREBRAL ARTERY b

middle concha *n* : NASAL CONCHA b

middle constrictor *n* : a fan-shaped muscle of the pharynx that arises from the ceratohyal and thyrohyal of the hyoid bone and from the stylohyoid ligament, inserts into the median line at the back of the pharynx, and acts to constrict part of the pharynx in swallowing — called also *constrictor pharyngis medius, middle pharyngeal constrictor muscle;* compare INFERIOR CONSTRICTOR, SUPERIOR CONSTRICTOR

middle ear *n* : the intermediate portion of the ear of higher vertebrates consisting typically of a small air-filled membrane-lined chamber in the temporal bone continuous with the nasopharynx through the eustachian tube, separated from the external ear by the tympanic membrane and from the inner ear by fenestrae, and containing a chain of three ossicles that extends from the tympanic membrane to the oval window and transmits vibrations to the inner ear — called also *tympanic cavity;* compare INCUS, MALLEUS, STAPES

middle finger *n* : the midmost of the five digits of the hand

middle hemorrhoidal artery *n* : RECTAL ARTERY b

middle hemorrhoidal vein *n* : RECTAL VEIN b

middle meatus *n* : a curved anteroposterior passage in each nasal cavity that is situated below the middle nasal concha and extends along the entire superior border of the inferior nasal concha — compare INFERIOR MEATUS, SUPERIOR MEATUS

middle meningeal artery *n* : a branch of the first portion of the maxillary artery that is the largest artery supplying the dura mater, enters the cranium through the foramen spinosum, and divides into anterior and posterior branches in a groove in the greater wing of the sphenoid bone

middle nasal concha *n* : NASAL CONCHA b

middle peduncle *n* : CEREBELLAR PEDUNCLE b

middle pharyngeal constrictor muscle *n* : MIDDLE CONSTRICTOR

middle rectal artery *n* : RECTAL ARTERY b

middle rectal vein *n* : RECTAL VEIN b

middle sacral artery *n* : a small artery that arises from the back of the abdominal part of the aorta just before it forks into the two common iliac arteries and that descends near the midline in front of the fourth and fifth lumbar vertebrae, the sacrum, and the coccyx to the glomus coccygeum

middle temporal artery *n* : TEMPORAL ARTERY 2b

middle temporal gyrus *n* : TEMPORAL GYRUS b

middle temporal vein *n* : TEMPORAL VEIN a(2)

middle turbinate *n* : NASAL CONCHA b

middle turbinate bone *also* **middle turbinated bone** *n* : NASAL CONCHA b

mid·dor·sal \(ˌ)mid-ˈdȯr-səl\ *adj* : of, relating to, or situated in the middle part or median line of the back

mid·epi·gas·tric \-ˌe-pi-ˈgas-trik\ *adj* : of, relating to, or located in the middle of the epigastric region of the abdomen ⟨~ tenderness⟩

mid·for·ceps \-ˈfȯr-səps, -ˌseps\ *n* : a procedure for delivery of an infant by the use of forceps after engagement has occurred but before the head has reached the lower part of the birth canal — compare HIGH FORCEPS, LOW FORCEPS

midge \ˈmij\ *n* : any of numerous tiny dipteran flies (esp. families Ceratopogonidae, Cecidomyiidae, and Chironomidae) many of which are capable of giving painful bites and some of which are vectors or intermediate hosts of parasites of humans and various other vertebrates — see BITING MIDGE

midg·et \ˈmi-jət\ *n* : a very small person; *specif* : a person of unusually small size who is physically well-proportioned

midg·et·ism \ˈmi-jə-ˌti-zəm\ *n* : the state of being a midget

mid·gut \ˈmid-ˌgət\ *n* : the middle part of the alimentary canal of a vertebrate embryo that in humans gives rise to the more distal part of the duodenum and to the jejunum, ileum, cecum and appendix, ascending colon, and much of the transverse colon

mid–life \(ˌ)mid-ˈlīf\ *n* : MIDDLE AGE

mid–life crisis *n* : a period of emotional turmoil in middle age caused by the realization that one is no longer young and characterized esp. by a strong desire for change

mid·line \ˈmid-ˌlin, ˌmid-ˈlīn\ *n* : a median line; *esp* : the median line or median plane of the body or some part of the body

mid·preg·nan·cy \(ˌ)mid-ˈpreg-nən-sē\ *n, pl* **-cies** : the middle period of a term of pregnancy

mid·riff \ˈmi-ˌdrif\ *n* **1** : DIAPHRAGM 1 **2** : the mid-region of the human torso

mid·sag·it·tal \(ˌ)mid-ˈsa-jət-əl\ *adj* : median and sagittal

midsagittal plane *n* : the median vertical longitudinal plane that divides a bilaterally symmetrical animal into right and left halves — called also *median plane*

mid·sec·tion \ˈmid-ˌsek-shən\ *n* : a section midway between the extremes; *esp* : MIDRIFF 2

mid·stream \ˌmid-ˈstrēm\ *adj* : of, relating to, or being urine passed during the middle of an act of urination and not at the beginning or end ⟨a ~ specimen⟩

mid·tar·sal \-ˈtär-səl\ *adj* : of, relating to, or being the articulation between the two rows of tarsal bones

midtarsal amputation *n* : amputation of the forepart of the foot through the midtarsal joint

mid·tri·mes·ter \-(ˌ)trī-ˈmes-tər\ *adj* : of, performed during, or occurring during the fourth through sixth months of human pregnancy

mid·ven·tral \-ˈven-trəl\ *adj* : of, relating to, or being the middle of the ventral surface — **mid·ven·tral·ly** *adv*

mid·wife \ˈmid-ˌwif\ *n* : one who assists women in childbirth — see NURSE-MIDWIFE

mid·wife·ry \ˌmid-ˈwi-fə-rē, -ˈwī-; ˈmid-ˌwī-\ *n, pl* **-ries** : the art or act of assisting at childbirth; *also* : OBSTETRICS

mi·fep·ris·tone \mi-ˈfe-pri-ˌstōn\ *n* : RU 486

mi·graine \ˈmī-ˌgrān\ *n* **1** : a condition that is marked by recurrent usu. unilateral severe headache often accompanied by nausea and vomiting and followed by sleep, that tends to occur in more than one member of a family, and that is of uncertain origin though attacks appear to be precipitated by dilatation of intracranial blood vessels **2** : an episode or attack of migraine ⟨suffers from ~s⟩ — called also *sick headache* — **mi·grain·ous** \-ˌgrā-nəs\ *adj*

mi·grain·eur \ˌmē-gre-ˈnər\ *n* : a person who experiences migraines

mi·grain·oid \ˈmī-ˌgrā-ˌnȯid, mī-ˈgrā-\ *adj* : resembling migraine

migrans — see ERYTHEMA CHRONICUM MIGRANS, LARVAL MIGRANS, LARVA MIGRANS

migrantes — see LARVA MIGRANS

mi·grate \ˈmī-ˌgrāt, mī-ˈ\ *vb* **mi·grat·ed; mi·grat·ing** : to move from one place to another: as **a** : to move from one site to another in a host organism esp. as part of a life cycle **b** *of an atom or group* : to shift position within a molecule — **mi·gra·tion** \mī-ˈgrā-shən\ *n* — **mi·gra·to·ry** \ˈmī-grə-ˌtōr-ē\ *adj*

migration inhibitory factor *n* : a lymphokine which inhibits the migration of macrophages away from the site of interaction between lymphocytes and antigens

mi·ka·my·cin \ˌmī-kə-ˈmī-sən\ n : an antibiotic complex isolated from a bacterium of the genus *Streptomyces* (*S. mitakaensis*)

Mi·ku·licz resection \ˈme-kü-ˌlich-\ n : an operation for removal of part of the intestine and esp. the colon in stages that involves bringing the diseased portion out of the body, closing the wound around the two parts of the loop which have been sutured together, and cutting off the diseased part leaving a double opening which is later joined by crushing the common wall and closed from the exterior

  Mikulicz–Ra·dec·ki \-ra-ˈdet-skē\, **Johann von (1850–1905),** Polish surgeon.

Mi·ku·licz's disease \-ˌli-chəz-\ n : abnormal enlargement of the lacrimal and salivary glands

Mikulicz's syndrome n : Mikulicz's disease esp. when occurring as a complication of another disease (as leukemia or sarcoidosis)

mild \ˈmīld\ *adj* 1 : moderate in action or effect ⟨a ~ drug⟩ 2 : not severe

mil·dew \ˈmil-ˌdü, -ˌdyü\ n 1 : a superficial usu. whitish growth produced esp. on organic matter or living plants by fungi (as of the families Erysiphaceae and Peronosporaceae) 2 : a fungus producing mildew

mild silver protein n : SILVER PROTEIN a

mil·i·ar·ia \ˌmi-lē-ˈar-ē-ə\ n : an inflammatory disorder of the skin characterized by redness, eruption, burning or itching, and the release of sweat in abnormal ways (as by the eruption of vesicles) due to blockage of the ducts of the sweat glands; *esp* : PRICKLY HEAT — **mil·i·ar·i·al** \-əl\ *adj*

miliaria crys·tal·li·na \-ˌkris-tə-ˈlē-nə\ n : SUDAMINA

mil·i·ary \ˈmi-lē-ˌer-ē\ *adj* 1 : resembling or suggesting a small seed or many small seeds ⟨a ~ aneurysm⟩ ⟨~ tubercles⟩ 2 : characterized by the formation of numerous small lesions ⟨~ pneumonia⟩

miliary tuberculosis n : acute tuberculosis in which minute tubercles are formed in one or more organs of the body by tubercle bacilli usu. spread by way of the blood

Mil·i·bis \ˈmi-li-bis\ *trademark* — used for a preparation of glycobiarsol

mi·lieu \mēl-ˈyə(r), -ˈyü; ˈmēl-ˌyü, mē-ˈlyœ̄\ n, pl **milieus** or **mi·lieux** \same or -ˈyə(r)z, -ˈyüz; -ˌyüz, -ˈlyœ̄z\ : ENVIRONMENT

milieu therapy n : manipulation of the environment of a mental patient for therapeutic purposes

mil·i·um \ˈmi-lē-əm\ n, pl **mil·ia** \-lē-ə\ : a small pearly firm noninflammatory elevation of the skin (as of the face) due to retention of keratin in an oil gland duct blocked by a thin layer

of epithelium — called also *whitehead;* compare BLACKHEAD 1

¹**milk** \ˈmilk\ n : a fluid secreted by the mammary glands of females for the nourishment of their young; *esp* : cow's milk used as a food by humans

²**milk** *vb* : to draw off the milk of

milk·er's nodules \ˈmil-kərz-\ n : a mild virus infection characterized by reddish blue nodules on the hands, arms, face, or neck acquired by direct contact with the udders of cows infected with a virus similar to that causing cowpox — called also *paravaccinia, pseudocowpox*

milk fever n 1 : a febrile disorder following parturition 2 : a disease of newly lactating cows, sheep, or goats that is caused by excessive drain on the body mineral reserves during the establishment of the milk flow — called also *parturient paresis;* compare GRASS TETANY

milk leg n : postpartum thrombophlebitis of a femoral vein — called also *phlegmasia alba dolens*

Milk·man's syndrome \ˈmilk-mənz-\ n : an abnormal condition marked by porosity of bone and tendency to spontaneous often symmetrical fractures

  Milkman, Louis Arthur (1895–1951), American roentgenologist.

milk of bismuth n : a thick white suspension in water of the hydroxide of bismuth and bismuth subcarbonate that is used esp. in the treatment of diarrhea

milk of magnesia n : a milk-white suspension of magnesium hydroxide in water used as an antacid and laxative — called also *magnesia magma*

milk sickness n : an acute disease characterized by weakness, vomiting, and constipation and caused by eating dairy products or meat from cattle affected with trembles

milk sugar n : LACTOSE

milk tooth n : a temporary tooth of a young mammal; *esp* : one of the human dentition including four incisors, two canines, and four molars in each jaw which fall out during childhood and are replaced by the permanent teeth — called also *baby tooth, deciduous tooth, primary tooth*

Mil·ler–Ab·bott tube \ˈmi-lər-ˈa-bət-\ n : a double-lumen balloon-tipped rubber tube used for the purpose of decompression in treating intestinal obstruction

  Miller, Thomas Grier (b 1886) and **Abbott, William Osler (1902–1943),** American physicians.

milli- *comb form* : thousandth — used esp. in terms belonging to the metric system ⟨*millirad*⟩

mil·li·bar \ˈmi-lə-ˌbär\ n : a unit of atmospheric pressure equal to ¹⁄₁₀₀₀ bar or 1000 dynes per square centimeter

mil·li·cu·rie \ˌmi-lə-ˈkyu̇r-(ˌ)ē, -kyu̇-ˈrē\ *n* : one thousandth of a curie

mil·li·gram \ˈmi-lə-ˌgram\ *n* : one thousandth of a gram

mil·li·li·ter \-ˌlē-tər\ *n* : one thousandth of a liter

mil·li·me·ter \-ˌmē-tər\ *n* : one thousandth of a meter

mil·li·mi·cron \ˌmi-lə-ˈmī-ˌkrän\ *n* : NANOMETER

mil·li·os·mol *or* **mil·li·os·mole** \ˌmi-lē-ˈäz-ˌmōl, -ˈäs-\ *n* : one thousandth of an osmol

mil·li·pede \ˈmi-lə-ˌpēd\ *n* : any of a class (Diplopoda) of arthropods having usu. a cylindrical segmented body, two pairs of legs on most segments, and including some forms that secrete toxic substances causing skin irritation but that unlike centipedes possess no poison fangs

mil·li·rad \-ˌrad\ *n* : one thousandth of a rad

mil·li·rem \-ˌrem\ *n* : one thousandth of a rem

mil·li·roent·gen \ˌmi-lə-ˈrent-gən, -ˈrənt-, -jən; -ˈren-chən, -ˈrən-\ *n* : one thousandth of a roentgen

mil·li·unit \ˈmi-lə-ˌyü-nət\ *n* : one thousandth of a standard unit and esp. of an international unit

Mi·lon·tin \mi-ˈlän-tin\ *trademark* — used for a preparation of phensuximide

Mil·roy's disease \ˈmil-ˌrȯiz-\ *n* : a hereditary lymphedema esp. of the legs
    Milroy, William Forsyth (1855–1942), American physician.

Mil·town \ˈmil-ˌtau̇n\ *trademark* — used for a preparation of meprobamate

Mil·wau·kee brace \mil-ˈwȯ-kē-, -ˈwä-\ *n* : an orthopedic brace that extends from the pelvis to the neck and is used esp. in the treatment of scoliosis

mi·met·ic \mə-ˈme-tik, mī-\ *adj* : simulating the action or effect of — usu. used in combination ⟨sympatho*mimetic* drugs⟩

mim·ic \ˈmi-mik\ *vb* **mim·icked** \-mikt\ ; **mim·ick·ing** : to imitate or resemble closely: as **a** : to imitate the symptoms of **b** : to produce an effect and esp. a physiological effect similar to — **mimic** *n* — **mim·ic·ry** \ˈmi-mi-krē\ *n*

min *abbr* minim

Min·a·mata disease \ˌmi-nə-ˈmä-tə-\ *n* : a toxic neuropathy caused by the ingestion of methylmercury compounds (as in contaminated seafood) and characterized by impairment of cerebral functions, constriction of the visual field, and progressive weakening of muscles

mind \ˈmīnd\ *n* **1** : the element or complex of elements in an individual that feels, perceives, thinks, wills, and esp. reasons **2** : the conscious mental events and capabilities in an organism **3** : the organized conscious and unconscious adaptive mental activity of an organism

mind–set \ˈmīnd-ˌset\ *n* : a mental inclination, tendency, or habit

min·er·al \ˈmi-nə-rəl\ *n* : a solid homogeneous crystalline chemical element or compound that results from the inorganic processes of nature

²mineral *adj* **1** : of or relating to minerals; *also* : INORGANIC **2** : impregnated with mineral substances

min·er·al·ize \ˈmi-nə-rə-ˌlīz\ *vb* **-ized; -iz·ing** : to impregnate or supply with minerals or an inorganic compound — **min·er·al·i·za·tion** \ˌmi-nə-rə-lə-ˈzā-shən\ *n*

min·er·al·o·cor·ti·coid \ˌmi-nə-rə-lō-ˈkȯr-tə-ˌkȯid\ *n* : a corticosteroid (as aldosterone) that affects chiefly the electrolyte and fluid balance in the body — compare GLUCOCORTICOID

mineral oil *n* : a transparent oily liquid obtained usu. by distilling petroleum and used in medicine esp. for treating constipation

min·er's asthma \ˈmī-nərz-\ *n* : PNEUMOCONIOSIS

miner's elbow *n* : bursitis of the elbow that tends to occur in miners who work in small tunnels and rest their weight on their elbows

miner's phthisis *n* : an occupational respiratory disease (as pneumoconiosis or anthracosilicosis) of miners

mini·lap·a·rot·o·my \ˌmi-nē-ˌla-pə-ˈrätə-mē\ *n, pl* **-mies** : a ligation of the Fallopian tubes performed through a small incision in the abdominal wall

min·im \ˈmi-nəm\ *n* : either of two units of capacity equal to ¹⁄₆₀ fluid dram: **a** : a U.S. unit of liquid capacity equivalent to 0.003760 cubic inch or 0.061610 milliliter **b** : a British unit of liquid capacity and dry measure equivalent to 0.003612 cubic inch or 0.059194 milliliter

minimae — see VENAE CORDIS MINIMAE

min·i·mal \ˈmi-nə-məl\ *adj* : relating to or being a minimum : constituting the least possible with respect to size, number, degree, or certain stated conditions

minimal brain damage *n* : ATTENTION DEFICIT DISORDER

minimal brain dysfunction *n* : ATTENTION DEFICIT DISORDER — abbr. *MBD*

minimal infective dose *n* : the smallest quantity of infective material that regularly produces infection — abbr. *MID*

minimal inhibitory concentration *n* : the smallest concentration of an antibiotic that regularly inhibits growth of a bacterium in vitro — abbr. *MIC*

minimi — see ABDUCTOR DIGITI MINIMI, EXTENSOR DIGITI MINIMI, FLEXOR DIGITI MINIMI BREVIS, GLUTEUS MINIMUS, OPPONENS DIGITI MINIMI

min·i·mum \ˈmi-nə-məm\ *n, pl* **-i·ma** \-mə\ *or* **-i·mums** **1** : the least quantity

assignable, admissible. or possible 2 : the lowest degree or amount of variation (as of temperature) reached or recorded — **minimum** *adj*

minimum dose *n* : the smallest dose of a medicine or drug that will produce an effect

minimum inhibitory concentration *n* : MINIMAL INHIBITORY CONCENTRATION

minimum lethal dose *n* : the smallest dose experimentally found to kill any one animal of a test group

minimus — see GLUTEUS MINIMUS

mini·pill \'mi-nē-₁pil\ *n* : a contraceptive pill that is intended to minimize side effects, contains a very low dose of a progestogen and esp. norethindrone but no estrogen, and is taken daily

Mini·press \-₁pres\ *trademark* — used for a preparation of prazosin

Min·ne·so·ta Mul·ti·pha·sic Personality Inventory \₁mi-nə-'sō-tə-₁məl-ti-'fā-zik-, -₁məl-₁tī-\ *n* : a test of personal and social adjustment based on a complex scaling of the answers to an elaborate true or false test

Mi·no·cin \mi-'nō-sin\ *trademark* — used for a preparation of minocycline

min·o·cy·cline \₁mi-nō-'sī-klēn\ *n* : a broad-spectrum tetracycline antibiotic $C_{23}H_{27}N_3O_7$

¹**mi·nor** \'mi-nər\ *adj* : not serious or involving risk to life (~ illness) (a ~ operation) — compare MAJOR

²**minor** *n* : a person of either sex under the age of legal qualification for adult rights and responsibilities that has traditionally been 21 in the U.S. but is now 18 in many states or sometimes less under certain circumstances (as marriage or pregnancy)

minora — see LABIA MINORA

minor surgery *n* : surgery involving little risk to the life of the patient; *specif* : an operation on the superficial structures of the body or a manipulative procedure that does not involve a serious risk — compare MAJOR SURGERY

min·ox·i·dil \mi-'näk-sə-₁dil\ *n* : a peripheral vasodilator $C_9H_{15}N_5O$ used orally to treat hypertension and topically in a propylene glycol solution to promote hair regrowth in male≈pattern baldness — see ROGAINE

minute volume *n* : CARDIAC OUTPUT

mi·o·sis \mi-'ō-səs, mē-\ *n, pl* **mi·o·ses** \-₁sēz\ : excessive smallness or contraction of the pupil of the eye

¹**mi·ot·ic** \-'ä-tik\ *n* : an agent that causes miosis

²**miotic** *adj* : relating to or characterized by miosis

mi·ra·cid·i·um \₁mir-ə-'si-dē-əm, ₁mī-rə-\ *n, pl* **-cid·ia** \-dē-ə\ : the free≈swimming ciliated first larva of a digenetic trematode that seeks out and penetrates a suitable snail intermediate host in which it develops into a

sporocyst — **mi·ra·cid·i·al** \-dē-əl\ *adj*

mir·a·cil D \'mir-ə-₁sil-'dē\ *n* : LUCANTHONE

mir·a·cle drug \'mir-ə-kəl-\ *n* : a drug usu. newly discovered that elicits a dramatic response in a patient's condition — called also *wonder drug*

mi·rage \mə-'räzh\ *n* : an optical effect that is sometimes seen at sea, in the desert, or over a hot pavement, that may have the appearance of a pool of water or a mirror in which distant objects are seen inverted, and that is caused by the bending or reflection of rays of light by a layer of heated air of varying density

mi·rex \'mī-₁reks\ *n* : an organochlorine insecticide $C_{10}Cl_{12}$ formerly used esp. against ants that is a suspected carcinogen

mirror writing *n* : backward writing resembling in slant and order of letters the reflection of ordinary writing in a mirror

mis- *prefix* : badly : wrongly (*mis*diagnose)

mis·car·riage \mis-'kar-ij\ *n* : spontaneous expulsion of a human fetus before it is viable and esp. between the 12th and 28th weeks of gestation — compare ABORTION 1a — **mis·car·ry** \(₁)mis-'kar-ē\ *vb*

mis·di·ag·nose \(₁)mis-'dī-ig-₁nōs, -₁nōz\ *vb* **-nosed; -nos·ing** : to diagnose incorrectly — **mis·di·ag·no·sis** \(₁)mis-₁dī-ig-'nō-səs\ *n*

mi·sog·y·nist \mə-'sä-jə-nist\ *n* : one who hates women — **misogynist** *adj* — **mi·sog·y·ny** \mə-'sä-jə-nē\ *n*

mi·so·pros·tol \₁mi-sō-'präs-₁tōl, -₁tȯl\ *n* : a prostaglandin analog $C_{22}H_{38}O_5$ used to prevent stomach ulcers occurring esp. as a side effect of drugs used to treat arthritis

missed abortion \'mist-\ *n* : an intra-uterine death of a fetus that is not followed by its immediate expulsion

missed labor *n* : a retention of a fetus in the uterus beyond the normal period of pregnancy

¹**mis·sense** \'mis-₁sens\ *adj* : relating to or being a genetic mutation involving alteration of one or more codons so that different amino acids are determined — compare ANTISENSE, NONSENSE

²**missense** *n* : missense genetic mutation

missionary position *n* : a coital position in which the female lies on her back with the male on top and with his face opposite hers

mit- *or* **mito-** *comb form* **1** : thread (*mito*chondrion) **2** : mitosis (*mito*genesis)

mite \'mit\ *n* : any of numerous small to very minute acarid arachnids that include parasites of insects and vertebrates some of which are important disease vectors, parasites of plants, pests of various stored products, and free-living aquatic and terrestrial forms — see ITCH MITE

mith·ra·my·cin \ˌmi-thrə-ˈmīs-ᵊn\ n : PLICAMYCIN

mith·ri·da·tism \ˈmi-thrə-ˌdā-ˌti-zəm\ n : tolerance to a poison acquired by taking gradually increased doses of it — **Mith·ra·da·tes VI Eu·pa·tor** \ˌmi-thrə-ˈdā-tēz-ˈsiks-ˈyü-pə-ˌtor\, (*d* 63 BC), king of Pontus.

mi·ti·cide \ˈmī-tə-ˌsīd\ n : an agent used to kill mites — **mi·ti·cid·al** \ˌmī-tə-ˈsīd-ᵊl\ *adj*

mi·to·chon·dri·on \ˌmī-tə-ˈkän-drē-ən\ n, pl **-dria** \-drē-ə\ : any of various round or long cellular organelles of most eukaryotes that are found outside the nucleus, produce energy for the cell through cellular respiration, and are rich in fats, proteins, and enzymes — **mi·to·chon·dri·al** \-drē-əl\ *adj* — **mi·to·chon·dri·al·ly** *adv*

mi·to·gen \ˈmī-tə-jən\ n : a substance that induces mitosis

mi·to·gen·e·sis \ˌmī-tə-ˈje-nə-səs\ n, *pl* **-e·ses** \-ˌsēz\ : the production of cell mitosis

mi·to·gen·ic \-ˈje-nik\ *adj* : of, producing, or stimulating mitosis

mi·to·my·cin \ˌmī-tə-ˈmīs-ᵊn\ n : a complex of antibiotic substances which is produced by a Japanese bacterium of the genus *Streptomyces* (*S. caespitosus*) and one form of which inhibits DNA synthesis and is used as an antineoplastic agent

mi·to·sis \mī-ˈtō-səs\ n, *pl* **-to·ses** \-ˌsēz\ 1 : a process that takes place in the nucleus of a dividing cell, involves typically a series of steps consisting of prophase, metaphase, anaphase, and telophase, and results in the formation of two new nuclei each having the same number of chromosomes as the parent nucleus — compare MEIOSIS 2 : cell division in which mitosis occurs — **mi·tot·ic** \-ˈtä-tik\ *adj* — **mi·tot·i·cal·ly** *adv*

mitotic index n : the number of cells per thousand cells actively dividing at a particular time

mi·tral \ˈmī-trəl\ *adj* : of, relating to, being, or adjoining a mitral valve or orifice

mitral cell n : any of the pyramidal cells of the olfactory bulb about which terminate numerous fibers from the olfactory cells of the nasal mucosa

mitral insufficiency n : inability of the mitral valve to close perfectly permitting blood to flow back into the atrium and leading to varying degrees of heart failure — called also *mitral incompetence*

mitral orifice n : the left atrioventricular orifice

mitral regurgitation n : backward flow of blood into the atrium due to mitral insufficiency

mitral stenosis n : a condition usu. the result of disease in which the mitral valve is abnormally narrow

mitral valve n : BICUSPID VALVE

mit·tel·schmerz \ˈmi-tᵊl-ˌshmertz\ n : abdominal pain occurring between the menstrual periods and usu. considered to be associated with ovulation

mixed \ˈmikst\ *adj* 1 : combining features or exhibiting symptoms of more than one condition or disease (a ∼ tumor) 2 : producing more than one kind of secretion (∼ salivary glands)

mixed connective tissue disease n : a syndrome characterized by symptoms of various rheumatic diseases (as systemic lupus erythematosus, scleroderma, and polymyositis) and by high concentrations of antibodies to extractable nuclear antigens

mixed glioma n : a glioma consisting of more than one cell type

mixed nerve n : a nerve containing both sensory and motor fibers

mix·ture \ˈmiks-chər\ n : a product of mixing: as **a** : a portion of matter consisting of two or more components in varying proportions that retain their own properties **b** : an aqueous liquid medicine; *specif* : a preparation in which insoluble substances are suspended in watery fluids by the addition of a viscid material (as gum, sugar, or glycerol)

mks \ˌem-ˌkā-ˈes\ *adj, often cap M&K&S* : of, relating to, or being a system of units based on the meter, the kilogram, and the second (∼ system) (∼ units)

ml *abbr* milliliter

MLD *abbr* 1 median lethal dose 2 minimum lethal dose

M line \ˈem-ˌlin\ n : a thin dark line across the center of the H zone of a striated muscle fiber — called also *M band*

MLT *abbr* medical laboratory technician

mm *abbr* millimeter

M–mode \ˈem-ˌmōd\ *adj* : of, relating to, or being an ultrasonographic technique that is used for studying the movement of internal body structures

MMPI *abbr* Minnesota Multiphasic Personality Inventory

MMR *abbr* measles-mumps-rubella (vaccine)

Mn *symbol* manganese

MN *abbr* master of nursing

-m·ne·sia \m-ˈnē-zhə\ n *comb form* : a (specified) type or condition of memory (paramnesia)

Mo *symbol* molybdenum

MO *abbr* medical officer

mo·bile \ˈmō-bəl, -ˌbil\ *adj* : capable of moving or being moved about readily; *specif* : characterized by an extreme degree of fluidity — **mo·bil·i·ty** \mō-ˈbi-lə-tē\ n

mo·bi·lize \ˈmō-bə-ˌlīz\ *vb* **-lized; -lizing** 1 : to put into movement or circulation : make mobile; *specif* : to release (something stored in the body) for body use 2 : to assemble (as resources) and make ready for use 3 : to separate (an organ or part) from associated structures so as to make more accessible for operative procedures 4 : to develop to a state of acute activity — **mo·bi·li·za·tion** \ˌmō-bə-lə-'zā-shən\ n

Mö·bius syndrome \'mü-bē-əs-, 'mœ-\ n : congenital bilateral paralysis of the facial muscles associated with other neurological disorders

Möbius, Paul Julius (1853–1907), German neurologist.

moc·ca·sin \'mä-kə-sən\ n 1 : WATER MOCCASIN 2 : a snake (as of the genus *Natrix*) resembling a water moccasin

mo·dal·i·ty \mō-'da-lə-tē\ n, pl -ties 1 : one of the main avenues of sensation (as vision) 2 a : a usu. physical therapeutic agency b : an apparatus for applying a modality

¹mod·el \'mäd-əl\ n 1 a : a pattern of something to be made b : a cast of a tooth or oral cavity 2 : something (as a similar object or a construct) used to help visualize or explore something else (as the living human body) that cannot be directly observed or experimented on — see ANIMAL MODEL

²model vb mod·eled or mod·elled; mod·el·ing or mod·el·ling : to produce (as by computer) a representation or simulation of

mod·er·ate \'mä-də-rət\ adj : not severe in effect : not serious or permanently disabling or incapacitating

Mod·er·il \'mä-də-ˌril\ trademark — used for a preparation of rescinnamine

modified radical mastectomy n : a mastectomy that is similar to the radical mastectomy but does not include removal of the pectoral muscles

mod·i·fi·er \'mä-də-ˌfī-ər\ n 1 : one that modifies 2 : a gene that modifies the effect of another

mod·i·fy \'mä-də-ˌfī\ vb -fied; -fy·ing : to make a change in (~ behavior by the use of drugs) — **mod·i·fi·ca·tion** \ˌmä-də-fə-'kā-shən\ n

mo·di·o·lar \mə-'dī-ə-lər\ adj : of or relating to the modiolus of the ear

mo·di·o·lus \mə-'dī-ə-ləs\ n, pl -li \-ˌlī\ : a central bony column in the cochlea of the ear

mod·u·late \'mä-jə-ˌlāt\ vb -lat·ed; -lat·ing : to adjust to or keep in proper measure or proportion (~ an immune response) (~ cell activity) — **mod·u·la·tion** \ˌmä-jə-'lā-shən\ n — **mod·u·la·tor** \'mä-jə-ˌlā-tər\ n — **mod·u·la·to·ry** \-lə-ˌtōr-ē\ adj

Moe·bius syndrome var of MÖBIUS SYNDROME

Mohs' technique \'mōz-\ n : a chemosurgical technique for the removal of skin malignancies in which excision is made to a depth at which the tissue is microscopically free of cancer — called also *Mohs' chemosurgery*

Mohs, Frederic Edward (b 1910), American surgeon.

moist \'moist\ adj 1 : slightly or moderately wet 2 a : marked by a discharge or exudation of liquid (~ eczema) b : suggestive of the presence of liquid — used of sounds heard in auscultation (~ rales)

moist gangrene n : gangrene that develops in the presence of combined arterial and venous obstruction, is usu. accompanied by an infection, and is characterized by a watery discharge usu. of foul odor

mol var of ³MOLE

mol·al \'mō-ləl\ adj : of, relating to, or containing a mole of solute per 1000 grams of solvent (a ~ solution) — **mo·lal·i·ty** \mō-'la-lə-tē\ n

¹mo·lar \'mō-lər\ n : a tooth with a rounded or flattened surface adapted for grinding; specif : one of the mammalian teeth behind the incisors and canines sometimes including the premolars but more exactly restricted to the three posterior pairs in each adult human jaw on each side which are not preceded by milk teeth

²molar adj 1 a : pulverizing by friction (~ teeth) b : of, relating to, or located near the molar teeth (~ gland) 2 : of, relating to, possessing the qualities of, or characterized by a uterine mole (~ pregnancy)

³molar adj 1 : of or relating to a mole of a substance (the ~ volume of a gas) 2 : containing one mole of solute in one liter of solution — **mo·lar·i·ty** \mō-'lar-ə-tē\ n

¹mold \'mōld\ n : a cavity in which a fluid or malleable substance is shaped

²mold vb : to give shape to esp. in a mold

³mold vb : to become moldy

⁴mold n 1 : a superficial often woolly growth produced esp. on damp or decaying organic matter or on living organisms 2 : a fungus (as of the order Mucorales) that produces mold

mold·ing \'mōl-diŋ\ n : the shaping of the fetal head to allow it to pass through the birth canal during parturition

moldy \'mōl-dē\ adj mold·i·er; -est : covered with a mold-producing fungus (~ bread)

¹mole \'mōl\ n : a pigmented spot, mark, or small permanent protuberance on the human body; esp : NEVUS

²mole n : an abnormal mass in the uterus: a : a blood clot containing a degenerated fetus and its membranes b : HYDATIDIFORM MOLE

³mole \'mōl\ n : the base unit in the International System of Units for the amount of pure substance that contains the same number of elementary entities as there are atoms in exactly 12 grams of the isotope carbon 12

mo·lec·u·lar \mə-'le-kyə-lər\ adj : of,

relating to, or produced by molecules — **mo·lec·u·lar·ly** *adv*

molecular biology *n* : a branch of biology dealing with the ultimate physicochemical organization of living matter and esp. with the molecular basis of inheritance and protein synthesis — **molecular biologist** *n*

molecular formula *n* : a chemical formula (as $C_6H_{12}O_6$ for glucose) that is based on both analysis and molecular weight and gives the total number of atoms of each element in a molecule — see STRUCTURAL FORMULA

molecular genetics *n pl* : a branch of genetics dealing with the structure and activity of genetic material at the molecular level

molecular weight *n* : the mass of a molecule that may be calculated as the sum of the atomic weights of its constituent atoms

mol·e·cule \'mä-li-ˌkyül\ *n* : the smallest particle of a substance that retains all the properties of the substance and is composed of one or more atoms

mol·in·done \mō-'lin-ˌdōn\ *n* : a drug $C_{16}H_{24}N_2O_2$ used in the form of the hydrochloride as an antipsychotic agent

mol·lus·ci·cide \mə-'ləs-kə-ˌsīd, -'lə-si-ˌsīd\ *n* : an agent for destroying mollusks (as snails) — **mol·lus·ci·cid·al** \-ˌləs-kə-'sīd-əl, -ˌlə-si-'sīd-\ *adj*

mol·lus·cum \mə-'ləs-kəm\ *n, pl* -**ca** \-kə\ : any of several skin diseases marked by soft pulpy nodules; *esp* : MOLLUSCUM CONTAGIOSUM

molluscum body *n* : any of the rounded cytoplasmic bodies found in the central opening of the nodules characteristic of molluscum contagiosum

molluscum con·ta·gi·o·sum \-kən-ˌtä-jē-'ō-səm\ *n, pl* **mollusca con·ta·gi·o·sa** \-sə\ : a mild chronic disease of the skin caused by a poxvirus and characterized by the formation of small nodules with a central opening and contents resembling curd

mol·lusk *or* **mol·lusc** \'mä-ləsk\ *n* : any of a large phylum (Mollusca) of invertebrate animals (as snails) that have a soft unsegmented body lacking segmented appendages and commonly protected by a calcareous shell — **mol·lus·can** *also* **mol·lus·kan** \mə-'les-kən, mä-\ *adj*

molt \'mōlt\ *vb* : to shed hair, feathers, shell, horns, or an outer layer periodically — **molt** *n*

mo·lyb·de·num \mə-'lib-də-nəm\ *n* : a metallic element that is a trace element in plant and animal metabolism — symbol *Mo*; see ELEMENT table

mom·ism \'mä-ˌmi-zəm\ *n* : an excessive popular adoration and sentimentalizing of mothers that is held to be oedipal in nature

mon- *or* **mono-** *comb form* **1** : one : single (*mono*filament) **2** : affecting a single part (*mono*plegia)

mon·ar·tic·u·lar \ˌmä-när-'ti-kyə-lər\ *var of* MONOARTICULAR

mon·au·ral \(ˌ)mä-'nor-əl\ *adj* : of, relating to, affecting, or designed for use with one ear (~ hearing aid systems) — **mon·au·ral·ly** *adv*

Mönckeberg's sclerosis \'mün-kə-ˌbargz-, 'meŋ-\ *n* : arteriosclerosis characterized by the formation of calcium deposits in the mediae of esp. the peripheral arteries

   Mönckeberg \'mœn-kə-ˌberk\, **Johann Georg (1877–1925),** German pathologist.

Monday morning disease *n* : azoturia of horses caused by heavy feeding during a period of inactivity — called also *Monday disease*

mo·nen·sin \mō-'nen-sən\ *n* : an antibiotic $C_{36}H_{62}O_{11}$ obtained from a bacterium of the genus *Streptomyces* (*S. cinnamonensis*) and used as an antiprotozoal, antibacterial, and antifungal agent and as an additive to cattle feed

mo·ner·an \mə-'nir-ən\ *n* : PROKARYOTE — **moneran** *adj*

mon·es·trous \(ˌ)mä-'nes-trəs\ *adj* : experiencing estrus once each year or breeding season

Mon·gol \'mäŋ-gəl, 'mäŋ-ˌgōl, 'mäŋ-\ *n, often not cap* : one affected with Down's syndrome

Mon·go·lian \mäŋ-'gōl-yən, mäŋ-, -'gō-lē-ən\ *adj* : MONGOLOID

Mongolian spot *n* : a bluish pigmented area near the base of the spine that is present at birth esp. in Asian, southern European, American Indian, and black infants and that usu. disappears during childhood

mon·gol·ism \'mäŋ-gə-ˌli-zəm\ *n* : DOWN'S SYNDROME

Mon·gol·oid \'mäŋ-gə-ˌloid\ *adj, often not cap* : of, relating to, or affected with Down's syndrome — **Mongoloid** *n, often not cap*

mo·nie·zia \ˌmä-nē-'e-zē-ə\ *n* **1** *cap* : a genus of tapeworms (family Anoplocephalidae) parasitizing the intestine of various ruminants **2** : any tapeworm of the genus *Moniezia*

   Moniez \mon-'yä\, **Romain–Louis (1852–1936),** French parasitologist.

mo·nil·e·thrix \mə-'ni-lə-ˌthriks\ *n, pl* **mon·i·let·ri·ches** \ˌmä-nə-'le-trə-ˌkēz\ : a disease of the hair in which each hair appears as if strung with small beads or nodes

mo·nil·ia \mə-'ni-lē-ə\ *n, pl* **monilias** *or* **monilia** *also* **mo·nil·i·ae** \-lē-ˌē\ **1** : any fungus of the genus *Candida* **2** *pl* **mo·nil·ias** : CANDIDIASIS

Mo·nil·ia \mə-'ni-lē-ə\ *n, syn of* CANDIDA

mo·nil·i·al \mə-'ni-lē-əl\ *adj* : of, relating to, or caused by a fungus of the genus *Candida* (~ vaginitis)

mo·nil·i·a·sis \ˌmō-nə-ˈlī-ə-səs, ˌmä-\ *n*, *pl* **-a·ses** \-ˌsēz\ : CANDIDIASIS

mo·nil·i·id \mə-ˈni-lē-əd\ *n* : a secondary commonly generalized dermatitis resulting from hypersensitivity developed in response to a primary focus of infection with a fungus of the genus *Candida*

¹**mon·i·tor** \ˈmä-nə-tər\ *n* : one that monitors; *esp* : a device for observing or measuring a biologically important condition or function (a heart ∼)

²**monitor** *vb* **1** : to watch, observe, or check closely or continuously (∼ a patient's vital signs) **2** : to test for intensity of radiations esp. if due to radioactivity

mon·key \ˈmən-kē\ *n* : a nonhuman primate mammal with the exception of the smaller more primitive primates (as the lemurs, family Lemuridae)

mono \ˈmä-(ˌ)nō\ *n* : INFECTIOUS MONONUCLEOSIS

mono- — see MON-

monoacetate — see RESORCINOL MONOACETATE

mono·am·ine \ˌmä-nō-ə-ˈmēn, -ˈa-ˌmēn\ *n* : an amine RNH₂ that has one organic substituent attached to the nitrogen atom; *esp* : one (as serotonin) that is functionally important in neural transmission

monoamine oxidase *n* : an enzyme that deaminates monoamines oxidatively and that functions in the nervous system by breaking down monoamine neurotransmitters oxidatively

monoamine oxidase inhibitor *n* : any of various antidepressant drugs which increase the concentration of monoamines in the brain by inhibiting the action of monoamine oxidase

mono·am·in·er·gic \ˌmä-nō-ˌa-mə-ˈnər-jik\ *adj* : liberating or involving monoamines (as serotonin or norepinephrine) in neural transmission (∼ neurons) (∼ mechanisms)

mono·ar·tic·u·lar \ˌmä-nō-är-ˈti-kyə-lər\ *adj* : affecting only one joint of the body (∼ arthritis)

mono·ben·zone \ˌmä-nō-ˈben-ˌzōn\ *n* : a drug C₁₃H₁₂O₂ applied topically as a melanin inhibitor in the treatment of hyperpigmentation

mono·blast \ˈmä-nō-ˌblast\ *n* : a motile cell of the spleen and bone marrow that gives rise to the monocyte of the circulating blood

mono·cho·ri·on·ic \ˌmä-nō-ˌkōr-ē-ˈä-nik\ *also* **mono·cho·ri·al** \-ˈkō-rē-əl\ *adj*, *of twins* : sharing or developed with a common chorion

mono·chro·ma·cy \-ˈkrō-mə-sē\ *n*, *pl* **-cies** : MONOCHROMATISM

mono·chro·mat \ˈmä-nō-krō-ˌmat, ˌmä-ˈ\ *n* : a person who is completely color-blind

mono·chro·mat·ic \ˌmä-nō-krō-ˈma-tik\ *adj* **1** : having or consisting of one color or hue **2** : consisting of radiation of a single wavelength or of a very small range of wavelengths **3** : of, relating to, or exhibiting monochromatism

mono·chro·ma·tism \-ˈkrō-mə-ˌti-zəm\ *n* : complete color blindness in which all colors appear as shades of gray — called also *monochromacy*

mon·o·cle \ˈmä-ni-kəl\ *n* : an eyeglass for one eye

¹**mono·clo·nal** \ˌmä-nō-ˈklōn-əl\ *adj* : produced by, being, or composed of cells derived from a single cell (a ∼ tumor); *esp* : relating to or being an antibody derived from a single cell in large quantities for use against a specific antigen (as a cancer cell)

²**monoclonal** *n* : a monoclonal antibody

mono·crot·ic \-ˈkrä-tik\ *adj*, *of the pulse* : having a simple beat and forming a smooth single-crested curve on a sphygmogram — compare DICROTIC 1

mon·oc·u·lar \mä-ˈnä-kyə-lər, mə-\ *adj* **1** : of, involving, or affecting a single eye (∼ vision) (a ∼ cataract) **2** : suitable for use with only one eye (a ∼ microscope) — **mon·oc·u·lar·ly** *adv*

mono·cyte \ˈmä-nə-ˌsīt\ *n* : a large leukocyte with finely granulated chromatin dispersed throughout the nucleus that is formed in the bone marrow, enters the blood, and migrates into the connective tissue where it differentiates into a macrophage — **mono·cyt·ic** \ˌmä-nə-ˈsi-tik\ *adj*

monocytic leukemia *n* : leukemia characterized by the presence of large numbers of monocytes in the circulating blood

mono·cy·to·sis \ˌmä-nō-sī-ˈtō-səs\ *n*, *pl* **-to·ses** \-ˌsēz\ : an abnormal increase in the number of monocytes in the circulating blood — compare GRANULOCYTOSIS, LYMPHOCYTOSIS

mono·fac·to·ri·al \-fak-ˈtōr-ē-əl\ *adj* : MONOGENIC

mono·fil·a·ment \-ˈfi-lə-mənt\ *n* : a single untwisted synthetic filament (as of nylon) used to make surgical sutures

mo·nog·a·mist \mə-ˈnä-gə-mist\ *n* : one who practices or upholds monogamy

mo·nog·a·my \-mē\ *n*, *pl* **-mies** : the state or custom of being married to one person at a time or of having only one mate at a time — **mo·nog·a·mous** \mə-ˈnä-gə-məs\ *also* **mono·gam·ic** \ˌmä-nə-ˈga-mik\ *adj*

mono·gas·tric \ˌmä-nō-ˈgas-trik\ *adj* : having a stomach with only a single compartment (as in humans)

mono·gen·ic \-ˈje-nik, -ˈjē-\ *adj* : of, relating to, or controlled by a single gene and esp. by either of an allelic pair — **mono·gen·i·cal·ly** *adv*

mono·graph \ˈmä-nə-ˌgraf\ *n* **1** : a learned detailed thoroughly documented treatise covering exhaustively a small area of a field of learning **2** : a description (as in a pharmacopoeia or formulary) of the name, chemical formula, and uniform method for determining the strength and purity of a drug — **monograph** *vb*

mono·iodo·ty·ro·sine \ˌmä-nō-ˌī-ˌō-də-ˈtī-rə-ˌsēn, -ˌī-ə-\ *n* : an iodine-containing tyrosine $C_9H_{10}INO_3$ that is produced in the thyroid gland and that combines with diiodotyrosine to form triiodothyronine

mono·lay·er \ˈmä-nō-ˌlā-ər\ *n* : a single continuous layer or film that is one cell or molecule in thickness

mono·ma·nia \ˌmä-nō-ˈmā-nē-ə, -nyə\ *n* : mental illness esp. when limited in expression to one idea or area of thought — **mono·ma·ni·a·cal** \-mə-ˈnī-ə-kəl\ *adj*

mono·ma·ni·ac \-nē-ˌak\ *n* : an individual affected by monomania

mono·me·lic \-ˈme-lik\ *adj* : relating to or affecting only one limb

mono·mer \ˈmä-nə-mər\ *n* : a chemical compound that can undergo polymerization — **mono·mer·ic** \ˌmä-nə-ˈmer-ik, ˌmō-\ *adj*

mono·neu·ri·tis \ˌmä-nō-nu̇-ˈrī-təs, -nyu̇-\ *n*, *pl* **-rit·i·des** \-ˈri-tə-ˌdēz\ *or* **-ri·tis·es** : neuritis of a single nerve

mononeuritis multiplex \-ˈməl-ti-ˌpleks\ *n* : neuritis that affects several separate nerves — called also *mononeuropathy multiplex*

mono·neu·rop·a·thy \-nu̇-ˈrä-pə-thē, -nyu̇-\ *n*, *pl* **-thies** : a nerve disease affecting only a single nerve

¹**mono·nu·cle·ar** \ˌmä-nō-ˈnü-klē-ər, -ˈnyü-\ *adj* : having only one nucleus

²**mononuclear** *n* : a mononuclear cell; *esp* : MONOCYTE

mono·nu·cle·at·ed \-ˈnü-klē-ˌā-təd, -ˈnyü-\ *also* **mono·nu·cle·ate** \-klē-ət, -ˌāt\ *adj* : MONONUCLEAR

mono·nu·cle·o·sis \-ˌnü-klē-ˈō-səs, -ˌnyü-\ *n* : an abnormal increase of mononuclear leukocytes in the blood; *specif* : INFECTIOUS MONONUCLEOSIS

mono·nu·cle·o·tide \-ˈnü-klē-ə-ˌtīd, -ˈnyü-\ *n* : a nucleotide that is derived from one molecule each of a nitrogenous base, a sugar, and a phosphoric acid

mono·pha·sic \-ˈfā-zik\ *adj* 1 : having a single phase; *specif* : relating to or being a record of a nerve impulse that is negative or positive but not both ⟨a ∼ action potential⟩ — compare DIPHASIC b, POLYPHASIC 1 2 : having a single period of activity followed by a period of rest in each 24 hour period

mono·phos·phate \-ˈfäs-ˌfāt\ *n* : a phosphate containing a single phosphate group

mono·ple·gia \-ˈplē-jə, -jē-ə\ *n* : paralysis affecting a single limb, body part, or group of muscles — **mono·ple·gic** \-jik\ *adj*

mono·ploid \ˈmä-nō-ˌploid\ *adj* : HAPLOID

mono·po·lar \ˌmä-nō-ˈpō-lər\ *adj* : UNIPOLAR

mon·or·chid \mä-ˈnȯr-kəd\ *n* : an individual who has only one testis or only

one descended into the scrotum — compare CRYPTORCHID — **monorchid** *adj*

mon·or·chid·ism \-kə-ˌdi-zəm\ *also* **mon·or·chism** \ˈmä-ˌnȯr-ˌki-zəm\ *n* : the quality or state of being monorchid — compare CRYPTORCHIDISM

mono·sac·cha·ride \ˌmä-nō-ˈsa-kə-ˌrīd\ *n* : a sugar not decomposable to simpler sugars by hydrolysis — called also *simple sugar*

mono·so·di·um glu·ta·mate \ˌmä-nō-ˈsō-dē-əm-ˈglü-tə-ˌmāt\ *n* : a crystalline salt $C_5H_8O_4NaN$ used to enhance the flavor of food and medicinally to reduce ammonia levels in blood and tissues in ammoniacal azotemia (as in hepatic insufficiency) — abbr. *MSG*; called also *sodium glutamate*; see CHINESE RESTAURANT SYNDROME

monosodium urate *n* : a salt of uric acid that precipitates out in cartilage as tophi in gout

mono·some \ˈmä-nō-ˌsōm\ *n* 1 : a chromosome lacking a synaptic mate; *esp* : an unpaired X chromosome 2 : a single ribosome

mono·so·mic \ˌmä-nō-ˈsō-mik\ *adj* : having one less than the diploid number of chromosomes — **mono·so·my** \ˈmä-nə-ˌsō-mē\ *n*

mono·spe·cif·ic \ˌmä-nō-spə-ˈsi-fik\ *adj* : specific for a single antigen or receptor site on an antigen — **mono·spec·i·fic·i·ty** \-ˌspe-sə-ˈfi-sə-tē\ *n*

mono·sper·mic \-ˈspər-mik\ *adj* : involving or resulting from a single sperm cell ⟨∼ fertilization⟩

mono·sper·my \ˈmä-nō-ˌspər-mē\ *n*, *pl* **-mies** : the entry of a single fertilizing sperm into an egg — compare POLYSPERMY

mon·os·tot·ic \ˌmä-ˌnäs-ˈtä-tik\ *adj* : relating to or affecting a single bone

mono·symp·tom·at·ic \ˌmä-nō-ˌsimp-tə-ˈma-tik\ *adj* : exhibiting or manifested by a single principal symptom

mono·syn·ap·tic \-sə-ˈnap-tik\ *adj* : having or involving a single neural synapse — **mono·syn·ap·ti·cal·ly** *adv*

mono·un·sat·u·rate \-ˌən-ˈsa-chə-rət\ *n* : a monounsaturated oil or fatty acid

mono·un·sat·u·rat·ed \-ˌən-ˈsa-chə-ˌrā-təd\ *adj, of an oil or fatty acid* : containing one double or triple bond per molecule — compare POLYUNSATURATED

mono·va·lent \ˌmä-nə-ˈvā-lənt\ *adj* 1 : having a chemical valence of one 2 : containing antibodies specific for or antigens of a single strain of a microorganism ⟨a ∼ vaccine⟩

mon·ovu·lar \(ˌ)mä-ˈnä-vyə-lər, -ˈnō-\ *adj* : MONOZYGOTIC ⟨∼ twins⟩

mon·ox·ide \mə-ˈnäk-ˌsīd\ *n* : an oxide containing one atom of oxygen per molecule — see CARBON MONOXIDE

mono·zy·got·ic \ˌmä-nō-zī-ˈgä-tik\ *adj* : derived from a single egg ⟨∼ twins⟩ — **mono·zy·gos·i·ty** \-ˈgä-sə-tē\ *n* — **mono·zy·gote** \-ˈzī-ˌgōt\ *n*

mono·zy·gous \ˌmä-nō-ˈzī-gəs, (ˌ)mä-ˈnä-zə-gəs\ *adj* : MONOZYGOTIC

mons \ˈmänz\ *n, pl* **mon·tes** \ˈmän-ˌtēz\ : a body part or area raised above or demarcated from surrounding structures (as the papilla of mucosa through which the ureter enters the bladder)

mons pubis *n, pl* **montes pubis** : a rounded eminence of fatty tissue upon the pubic symphysis esp. of the human female

mon·ster \ˈmän-stər\ *n* : an animal or plant of abnormal form or structure; *esp* : a fetus or offspring with a major developmental abnormality

mon·stros·i·ty \män-ˈsträ-sə-tē\ *n, pl* **-ties 1 a** : a malformation of a plant or animal **b** : MONSTER **2** : the quality or state of deviating greatly from the natural form or character — **monstrous** \ˈmän-strəs\ *adj*

mons ve·ne·ris \-ˈve-nə-rəs\ *n, pl* **montes veneris** : the mons pubis of a female

Mon·teg·gia fracture \män-ˈte-jə-\ *or* **Mon·teg·gia's fracture** \-ˈte-jəz-\ *n* : a fracture in the proximal part of the ulna with dislocation of the head of the radius

   Monteggia, Giovanni Battista (1762–1815), Italian surgeon.

Mon·te·zu·ma's revenge \ˌmän-tə-ˈzü-məz-\ *n* : diarrhea contracted in Mexico esp. by tourists

   Montezuma II (1466–1520), Mexican emperor.

Mont·gom·ery's gland \(ˌ)mənt-ˈgəm-rēz-, mänt-ˈgäm-\ *n* : an apocrine gland in the areola of the mammary gland

   Montgomery, William Fetherston (1797–1859), British obstetrician.

month·lies \ˈmənth-lēz\ *n pl* : a menstrual period

mon·tic·u·lus \män-ˈtik-yə-ləs\ *n* : the median dorsal ridge of the cerebellum formed by the vermis

mood \ˈmüd\ *n* : a conscious state of mind or predominant emotion : affective state : FEELING 3 〈∼ disorders such as mania and depression〉

moon \ˈmün\ *n* : LUNULA a

moon blindness *n* : a recurrent inflammation of the eye of the horse — called also *periodic ophthalmia*

moon face *n* : the full rounded facies characteristic of hyperadrenocorticism — called also *moon facies*

Moon's molar *or* **Moon molar** *n* : a first molar tooth which has become dome-shaped due to malformation by congenital syphilis; *also* : MULBERRY MOLAR

   Moon, Henry (1845–1892), British surgeon.

MOPP \ˈem-(ˌ)ō-(ˌ)pē-ˈpē\ *n* : a combination of four drugs including mechlorethamine, vincristine, procarbazine, and prednisone that is used in the treatment of some forms of cancer (as Hodgkin's disease)

Mor·ax–Ax·en·feld bacillus \ˈmȯr-äks-ˈäk-sən-ˌfeld-\ *n* : a rod-shaped bacterium of the genus *Moraxella* (*M. lacunata*) that causes Morax-Axenfeld conjunctivitis

   Morax, Victor (1866–1935), French ophthalmologist.

   Axenfeld, Karl Theodor Paul Polykarpos (1867–1930), German ophthalmologist.

Morax–Axenfeld conjunctivitis *n* : a chronic conjunctivitis caused by a rod-shaped bacterium of the genus *Moraxella* (*M. lacunata*) and now occurring rarely but formerly more prevalent in persons living under poor hygienic conditions

Mor·ax·el·la \ˌmȯr-ak-ˈse-lə\ *n* : a genus of short rod-shaped gram-negative bacteria (family Neisseriaceae) that includes the causative agent (*M. lacunata*) of Morax-Axenfeld conjunctivitis

mor·bid \ˈmȯr-bəd\ *adj* **1 a** : of, relating to, or characteristic of disease **b** : affected with or induced by disease 〈a ∼ condition〉 **c** : productive of disease 〈∼ substances〉 **2** : abnormally susceptible to or characterized by gloomy or unwholesome feelings

mor·bid·i·ty \mȯr-ˈbi-də-tē\ *n, pl* **-ties 1** : a diseased state or symptom **2** : the incidence of disease : the rate of sickness (as in a specified community or group) — compare MORTALITY 2

mor·bil·li \mȯr-ˈbi-ˌlī\ *n pl* : MEASLES 1

mor·bil·li·form \mȯr-ˈbi-lə-ˌfȯrm\ *adj* : resembling the eruption of measles 〈a ∼ pruritic rash〉

mor·bus \ˈmȯr-bəs\ *n, pl* **mor·bi** \-ˌbī\ : DISEASE — see CHOLERA MORBUS

mor·cel·la·tion \mȯr-sə-ˈlā-shən\ *n* : division and removal in small pieces (as of a tumor)

mor·gan \ˈmȯr-gən\ *n* : a unit of inferred distance between genes on a chromosome that is used in constructing genetic maps and is equal to the distance for which the frequency of crossing-over between specific pairs of genes is 100 percent

   Morgan, Thomas Hunt (1866–1945), American geneticist.

morgue \ˈmȯrg\ *n* : a place where the bodies of persons found dead are kept until identified and claimed by relatives or are released for burial

mor·i·bund \ˈmȯr-ə-(ˌ)bənd, ˈmär-\ *adj* : being in the state of dying : approaching death

morning–after pill *n* : an oral drug usu. containing high doses of estrogen that interferes with pregnancy by blocking implantation of a fertilized egg in the human uterus

morning sickness *n* : nausea and vomiting that occurs on rising in the morning esp. during the earlier months of pregnancy

mo·ron \'mōr-ˌän\ *n* : a mentally retarded person who has a potential mental age of between 8 and 12 years and is capable of doing routine work under supervision

Moro reflex \'mȯr-ō-\ *n* : a reflex reaction of infants upon being startled (as by a loud noise or a bright light) that is characterized by extension of the arms and legs away from the body and to the side and then by drawing them together as if in an embrace

Moro, Ernst (1874–1951), German pediatrician.

Moro test *n* : a diagnostic skin test formerly used to detect infection or past infection by the tubercle bacillus and involving the rubbing of an ointment containing tuberculin directly on the skin with the appearance of reddish papules after one or two days indicating a positive result

morph- *or* **morpho-** *comb form* : form : shape : structure : type ⟨*morpho*logy⟩

-morph \ˌmȯrf\ *n comb form* : one having (such) a form ⟨ecto*morph*⟩

mor·phea \mȯr-'fē-ə\ *n, pl* **mor·phe·ae** \-'fē-ˌē\ : localized scleroderma

mor·phia \'mȯr-fē-ə\ *n* : MORPHINE

-mor·phic \'mȯr-fik\ *adj comb form* : having (such) a form ⟨endo*morphic*⟩

mor·phine \'mȯr-ˌfēn\ *n* : a bitter crystalline addictive narcotic base $C_{17}H_{19}NO_3$ that is the principal alkaloid of opium and is used in the form of a soluble salt (as a hydrochloride or a sulfate) as an analgesic and sedative

mor·phin·ism \'mȯr-ˌfē-ˌni-zəm, -fə-\ *n* : a disordered condition of health produced by habitual use of morphine

mor·phi·no·mi·met·ic \ˌmȯr-fē-nə-mə-'me-tik, -fə-, -ˌmī-\ *adj* : resembling opiates in their affinity for opiate receptors in the brain ⟨the enkephalins are ∼ pentapeptides⟩

-mor·phism \'mȯr-ˌfi-zəm\ *n comb form* : quality or state of having (such) a form ⟨poly*morphism*⟩

mor·pho·dif·fer·en·ti·a·tion \ˌmȯr-fō-ˌdi-fə-ˌren-chē-'ā-shən\ *n* : structure or organ differentiation (as in tooth development)

mor·phoea *Brit var of* MORPHEA

mor·pho·gen \'mȯr-fə-jən, -ˌjen\ *n* : a diffusible chemical substance that exerts control over morphogenesis esp. by forming a gradient in concentration

mor·pho·gen·e·sis \ˌmȯr-fə-'je-nə-səs\ *n, pl* **-e·ses** \-ˌsēz\ : the formation and differentiation of tissues and organs — compare ORGANOGENESIS

mor·pho·ge·net·ic \-jə-'ne-tik\ *adj* : relating to or concerned with the development of normal organic form — **mor·pho·ge·net·i·cal·ly** *adv*

mor·pho·gen·ic \-'je-nik\ *adj* : MORPHOGENETIC

mor·pho·log·i·cal \ˌmȯr-fə-'lä-ji-kəl\ *also* **mor·pho·log·ic** \-'lä-jik\ *adj* : of, relating to, or concerned with form or structure — **mor·pho·log·i·cal·ly** *adv*

mor·phol·o·gy \mȯr-'fä-lə-jē\ *n, pl* **-gies** 1 : a branch of biology that deals with the form and structure of animals and plants esp. with respect to the forms, relations, metamorphoses, and phylogenetic development of organs apart from their functions — see ANATOMY 1; compare PHYSIOLOGY 1 2 : the form and structure of an organism or any of its parts — **mor·phol·o·gist** \-jist\ *n*

-mor·phous \'mȯr-fəs\ *adj comb form* : having (such) a form ⟨poly*morphous*⟩

-mor·phy \ˌmȯr-fē\ *n comb form, pl* **-phies** : quality or state of having (such) a form ⟨meso*morphy*⟩

Mor·quio's disease \'mȯr-kē-ˌōz-\ *n* : an autosomal recessive mucopolysaccharidosis characterized by excretion of keratan sulfate in the urine, dwarfism, a short neck, protruding sternum, kyphosis, a flat nose, prominent upper jaw, and a waddling gait

Morquio, Luis (1867–1935), Uruguayan physician.

mor·tal \'mȯrt-³l\ *adj* 1 : having caused or being about to cause death : FATAL ⟨a ∼ injury⟩ 2 : of, relating to, or connected with death ⟨∼ agony⟩

mor·tal·i·ty \mȯr-'ta-lə-tē\ *n, pl* **-ties** 1 : the quality or state of being mortal 2 a : the number of deaths in a given time or place b : the proportion of deaths to population : DEATH RATE — called also *mortality rate*; compare FERTILITY 2, MORBIDITY 2

mor·tar \'mȯr-tər\ *n* : a strong vessel in which material is pounded or rubbed with a pestle

mor·ti·cian \mȯr-'ti-shən\ *n* : UNDERTAKER

mor·ti·fi·ca·tion \ˌmȯr-tə-fə-'kā-shən\ *n* : local death of tissue in the animal body : NECROSIS, GANGRENE

mortis — see ALGOR MORTIS, RIGOR MORTIS

Mor·ton's toe \'mȯrt-³nz-\ *n* : metatarsalgia that is caused by compression of a branch of the plantar nerve between the heads of the metatarsal bones and tends to occur when the second toe is longer than the big toe — called also *Morton's disease, Morton's foot*

Morton, Thomas George (1835–1903), American surgeon.

mor·tu·ary \'mȯr-chə-ˌwer-ē\ *n, pl* **-ar·ies** : a place in which dead bodies are kept and prepared for burial or cremation

mor·u·la \'mȯr-yù-lə, 'mär-\ *n, pl* **-lae** \-ˌlē, -ˌlī\ : a globular solid mass of blastomeres formed by cleavage of a zygote that typically precedes the blastula — compare GASTRULA —

mor·u·la·tion \ˌmȯr-yu̇-ˈlā-shən, ˌmär-\ n

¹**mo·sa·ic** \mō-ˈzā-ik\ n : an organism or one of its parts composed of cells of more than one genotype : CHIMERA

²**mosaic** adj 1 : exhibiting mosaicism 2 : DETERMINATE — **mo·sa·i·cal·ly** adv

mo·sa·i·cism \mō-ˈzā-ə-ˌsi-zəm\ n : the condition of possessing cells of two or more different genetic constitutions

mos·qui·to \mə-ˈskē-tō\ n, pl **-toes** also **-tos** : any of numerous dipteran flies (family Culicidae) that have a rather narrow abdomen and usu. a long slender rigid proboscis, that have in the male broad feathery antennae and in the female slender antennae and a set of needlelike organs in the proboscis with which they puncture the skin of animals to suck the blood, and that in some species are the only vectors of certain diseases — see AEDES, ANOPHELES, CULEX

mosquito forceps n : a very small surgical forceps — called also mosquito clamp

mossy fiber n : any of the complexly ramifying nerve fibers that surround some nerve cells of the cerebellar cortex

moth·er \ˈmə-thər\ n : a female parent

mother cell n : a cell that gives rise to other cells usu. of a different sort

mo·tile \ˈmōt-ᵊl, ˈmō-ˌtil\ adj : exhibiting or capable of movement

mo·til·i·ty \mō-ˈti-lə-tē\ n, pl **-ties** : the quality or state of being motile : CONTRACTILITY (gastrointestinal ∼)

mo·tion \ˈmō-shən\ n 1 : an act, process, or instance of changing place : MOVEMENT 2 a : an evacuation of the bowels b : the matter evacuated — often used in pl. (blood in the ∼s)

motion sickness n : sickness induced by motion (as in travel by air, car, or ship) and characterized by nausea

mo·ti·vate \ˈmō-tə-ˌvāt\ vb **-vat·ed; -vat·ing** : to provide with a motive or serve as a motive for — **mo·ti·va·tion** \ˌmō-tə-ˈvā-shən\ n — **mo·ti·va·tion·al** \-shnəl, -shən-ᵊl\ adj — **mo·ti·va·tion·al·ly** adv

mo·tive \ˈmō-tiv\ n : something (as a need or desire) that causes a person to act

moto- comb form : motion : motor (motoneuron)

mo·to·neu·ron \ˌmō-tō-ˈnü-ˌrän, -ˈnyü-\ n : a neuron that passes from the central nervous system or a ganglion toward or to a muscle and conducts an impulse that causes movement — called also motor neuron; compare ASSOCIATIVE NEURON, SENSORY NEURON — **mo·to·neu·ro·nal** \-ˈnür-ən-ᵊl, -ˈnyür-; -nü-ˈrōn-, -nyü-\ adj

mo·tor \ˈmō-tər\ adj 1 : causing or imparting motion 2 : of, relating to, or being a motoneuron or a nerve containing motoneurons (∼ fibers) 3 : of, relating to, concerned with, or involving muscular movement

motor aphasia n : the inability to speak or to organize the muscular movements of speech — called also Broca's aphasia

motor area n : any of various areas of cerebral cortex believed to be associated with the initiation, coordination, and transmission of motor impulses to lower centers; specif : a region immediately anterior to the central sulcus having an unusually thick zone of cortical gray matter and communicating with lower centers chiefly through the corticospinal tracts — see PRECENTRAL GYRUS

motor center n : a nervous center that controls or modifies (as by inhibiting or reinforcing) a motor impulse

motor cortex n : the cortex of a motor area; also : the motor areas as a functional whole

motor end plate n : the terminal arborization of a motor axon on a muscle fiber

mo·tor·ic \mō-ˈtȯr-ik, -ˈtär-\ adj : MOTOR (∼ and verbal behavior) — **mo·tor·i·cal·ly** adv

motor neuron n : MOTONEURON

motor paralysis n : paralysis of the voluntary muscles

motor root n : a nerve root containing only motor fibers; specif : the ventral root of a spinal nerve

motor unit n : a motor neuron together with the muscle fibers on which it acts

Mo·trin \ˈmō-trən\ trademark — used for a preparation of ibuprofen

mottled enamel n : spotted tooth enamel caused by drinking water containing excessive fluorides during the time the teeth are calcifying

mou·lage \mü-ˈläzh\ n : a mold of a lesion or defect used as a guide in applying medical treatment (as in radiotherapy) or in performing reconstructive surgery esp. on the face

mould, moulding, mouldy chiefly Brit var of MOLD, MOLDING, MOLDY

moult chiefly Brit var of MOLT

¹**mount** \ˈmau̇nt\ n 1 : a glass slide with its accessories on which objects are placed for examination with a microscope 2 : a specimen mounted on a slide for microscopic examination — **mount** vb

mountain fever n : any of various febrile diseases occurring in mountainous regions

mountain sickness n : altitude sickness experienced esp. above 10,000 feet (about 3000 meters) and caused by insufficient oxygen in the air

mouse \ˈmau̇s\ n, pl **mice** \ˈmīs\ 1 : any of numerous small rodents (as of the genus Mus) with pointed snout, rather small ears, elongated body, and slender hairless or sparsely haired tail **2** : a dark-colored swelling caused by a blow; *specif* : BLACK EYE

mouse·pox \\'maus-ˌpäks\\ *n* : a highly contagious disease of mice that is caused by a poxvirus — called also *ectromelia*

mouth \\'mauth\\ *n, pl* **mouths** \\'mauthz\\ : the natural opening through which food passes into the animal body and which in vertebrates is typically bounded externally by the lips and internally by the pharynx and encloses the tongue, gums, and teeth

mouth breather *n* : a person who habitually inhales and exhales through the mouth rather than through the nose

mouth–to–mouth *adj* : of, relating to, or being a method of artificial respiration in which the rescuer's mouth is placed tightly over the victim's mouth in order to force air into the victim's lungs by blowing forcefully enough every few seconds to inflate them 〈~ resuscitation〉

mouth·wash \\'mauth-ˌwosh, -ˌwäsh\\ *n* : a liquid preparation (as an antiseptic solution) for cleansing the mouth and teeth — called also *collutorium*

move \\'müv\\ *vb* **moved; mov·ing 1** : to go or pass from one place to another **2** *of the bowels* : to eject fecal matter : EVACUATE

move·ment \\'müv-mənt\\ *n* **1** : the act or process of moving **2 a** : an act of voiding the bowels **b** : matter expelled from the bowels at one passage : STOOL

moxa \\'mäk-sə\\ *n* : a soft woolly mass prepared from the young leaves of various wormwoods of eastern Asia and used esp. in Japanese popular medicine as a cautery by being ignited on the skin

mox·i·bus·tion \\ˌmäk-si-'bəs-chən\\ *n* : the use of a moxa as a cautery by igniting it on the skin

MPC *abbr* maximum permissible concentration

MPH *abbr* master of public health

M phase \\'em-ˌfāz\\ *n* : the period in the cell cycle during which cell division takes place — compare G₁ PHASE, G₂ PHASE, S PHASE

MRI *abbr* magnetic resonance imaging

mRNA \\ˌem-(ˌ)är-(ˌ)en-'ā\\ *n* : MESSENGER RNA

MS *abbr* multiple sclerosis

MSG *abbr* monosodium glutamate

MSH *abbr* melanocyte-stimulating hormone

MSN *abbr* master of science in nursing

M substance \\'em-ˌ\\ *n* : a protein that is an antigen tending to occur on the surface of beta-hemolytic bacteria belonging to the genus *Streptococcus* and placed in a particular group (Lancefield group A) and that is closely associated with high virulence (as for scarlet fever)

MSW *abbr* master of social work

MT *abbr* medical technologist

mu \\'myü, 'mü\\ *n, pl* **mu** : MICROMETER

muc- or **muci-** or **muco-** *comb form* **1** : mucus 〈*muc*in〉 〈*muco*protein〉 **2** : mucous and 〈*muco*purulent〉

mu·cate \\'myü-ˌkāt\\ *n* : a salt or ester of a crystalline acid $C_6H_{10}O_8$

mu·ci·lage \\'myü-sə-lij\\ *n* **1** : a gelatinous substance of various plants (as legumes or seaweeds) that contains protein and polysaccharides and is similar to plant gums **2** : an aqueous usu. viscid solution (as of a gum) used in pharmacy as an excipient and in medicine as a demulcent — **mu·ci·lag·i·nous** \\ˌmyü-sə-'la-jə-nəs\\ *adj*

mu·cil·loid \\'myü-sə-ˌloid\\ *n* : a mucilaginous substance

mu·cin \\'myüs-ᵊn\\ *n* : any of a group of mucoproteins that are found in various human and animal secretions and tissues (as in saliva, the lining of the stomach, and the skin) and that are white or yellowish powders when dry and viscid when moist 〈gastric ~〉

mu·cin·o·gen \\myü-'si-nə-jən, -ˌjen\\ *n* : any of various substances which undergo conversion into mucins

mu·ci·nous \\'myüs-ᵊn-əs\\ *adj* : of, relating to, resembling, or containing mucin 〈~ fluid〉 〈~ carcinoma〉

muco- — see MUC-

mu·co·buc·cal fold \\ˌmyü-kō-'bə-kəl-\\ *n* : the fold formed by the oral mucosa where it passes from the mandible or maxilla to the cheek

mu·co·cele \\'myü-kō-ˌsēl\\ *n* : a swelling like a sac that is due to distension of a hollow organ or cavity with mucus 〈a ~ of the appendix〉; *specif* : a dilated lacrimal sac

mu·co·cil·i·ary \\ˌmyü-kō-'si-lē-ˌer-ē\\ *adj* : of, relating to, or involving cilia of the mucous membranes of the respiratory system

mu·co·cu·ta·ne·ous \\ˌmyü-kō-kyu-'tā-nē-əs\\ *adj* : made up of or involving both typical skin and mucous membrane 〈~ candidiasis〉

mucocutaneous lymph node disease *n* : KAWASAKI DISEASE

mucocutaneous lymph node syndrome *n* : KAWASAKI DISEASE

mu·co·epi·der·moid \\ˌmyü-kō-ˌe-pə-'dər-ˌmoid\\ *adj* : of, relating to, or consisting of both mucous and squamous epithelial cells; *esp* : being a tumor of the salivary glands made up of mucous and epithelial elements 〈~ carcinoma〉

mu·co·gin·gi·val \\-'jin-jə-vəl\\ *adj* : of, relating to, or being the junction between the oral mucosa and the gingiva 〈the ~ line〉

¹mu·coid \\'myü-ˌkoid\\ *adj* : resembling mucus

²mucoid *n* : MUCOPROTEIN

mu·co·lyt·ic \\ˌmyü-kə-'li-tik\\ *adj* : hydrolyzing mucopolysaccharides : tending to break down or lower the viscosity of mucin-containing body secretions or components

Mu·co·myst \'myü-kə-ˌmist\ *trademark* — used for a preparation of acetylcysteine

mu·co·pep·tide \ˌmyü-kō-'pep-ˌtīd\ *n* : PEPTIDOGLYCAN

mu·co·peri·os·te·um \-ˌper-ē-'äs-tē-əm\ *n* : a periosteum backed with mucous membrane (as that of the palatine surface of the mouth) — **mu·co·peri·os·te·al** \-'äs-tē-əl\ *adj*

mu·co·poly·sac·cha·ride \ˌmyü-kō-ˌpä-li-'sa-kə-ˌrīd\ *n* : GLYCOSAMINOGLYCAN

mu·co·poly·sac·cha·ri·do·sis \-ˌsa-kə-rī-'dō-səs\ *n, pl* **-do·ses** \-ˌsēz\ : any of a group of genetically determined disorders (as Hunter's syndrome and Hurler's syndrome) of glycosaminoglycan metabolism that are characterized by the accumulation of glycosaminoglycans in the tissues and their excretion in the urine — called also *gargoylism, lipochondrodystrophy*

mu·co·pro·tein \ˌmyü-kə-'prō-ˌtēn\ *n* : any of a group of various complex conjugated proteins (as mucins) that contain glycosaminoglycans (as chondroitin sulfate) combined with amino acid units or polypeptides and that occur in body fluids and tissues — called also *mucoid*; compare GLYCOPROTEIN

mu·co·pu·ru·lent \-'pyür-yə-lənt\ *adj* : containing both mucus and pus 〈∼ discharge〉

mu·co·pus \'myü-kō-ˌpəs\ *n* : mucus mixed with pus

mu·cor \'myü-ˌkȯr\ *n* 1 *cap* : a genus (family Mucoraceae) of molds including several (as *M. corymbifer*) causing infections in humans and animals 2 : any mold of the genus *Mucor*

mu·cor·my·co·sis \ˌmyü-kər-mi-'kō-səs\ *n, pl* **-co·ses** \-ˌsēz\ : mycosis caused by fungi of the genus *Mucor* usu. primarily involving the lungs and invading other tissues by means of metastatic lesions — **mu·cor·my·cot·ic** \-'kä-tik\ *adj*

mu·co·sa \myü-'kō-zə\ *n, pl* **-sae** \-(ˌ)zē, -ˌzī\ *or* **-sas** : MUCOUS MEMBRANE — **mu·co·sal** \-zəl\ *adj*

mucosae — see MUSCULARIS MUCOSAE

mucosal disease *n* : a virus disease of cattle characterized by fever, diarrhea, loss of appetite, dehydration, and excessive salivation

mu·co·si·tis \ˌmyü-kō-'sī-təs\ *n* : inflammation of a mucous membrane

mu·co·stat·ic \ˌmyü-kə-'sta-tik\ *adj* 1 : of, relating to, or representing the mucosal tissues of the jaws as they are in a state of rest 2 : stopping the secretion of mucus

mu·cous \'myü-kəs\ *adj* 1 : covered with or as if with mucus 〈a ∼ surface〉 2 : of, relating to, or resembling mucus 〈a ∼ secretion〉 3 : secreting or containing mucus 〈∼ glands〉

mucous cell *n* : a cell that secretes mucus

mucous colitis *n* : IRRITABLE BOWEL SYNDROME; *esp* : irritable bowel syndrome characterized by the passage of unusually large amounts of mucus

mucous membrane *n* : a membrane rich in mucous glands; *specif* : one that lines body passages and cavities which communicate directly or indirectly with the exterior (as the alimentary, respiratory, and genitourinary tracts), that functions in protection, support, nutrient absorption, and secretion of mucus, enzymes, and salts, and that consists of a deep vascular connective-tissue stroma and a superficial epithelium — compare SEROUS MEMBRANE

mu·co·vis·ci·do·sis \ˌmyü-kō-ˌvi-sə-'dō-səs\ *n, pl* **-do·ses** \-ˌsēz\ : CYSTIC FIBROSIS

mu·cus \'myü-kəs\ *n* : a viscid slippery secretion that is usu. rich in mucins and is produced by mucous membranes which it moistens and protects

mud bath *n* : an immersion of the body or a part of it in mud (as for the alleviation of rheumatism or gout)

mud fever *n* 1 : a chapped inflamed condition of the skin of the legs and belly of a horse due to irritation from mud or drying resulting from washing off mud spatters and closely related or identical in nature to grease heel 2 : a mild leptospirosis that occurs chiefly in European agricultural and other workers in wet soil, is caused by infection with a spirochete of the genus *Leptospira* (*L. grippotyphosa*) present in native field mice, and is marked by fever and headache without accompanying jaundice

Muel·le·ri·an duct *var of* MÜLLERIAN DUCT

Muel·le·ri·us \myü-'lir-ē-əs\ *n* : a genus of lungworms (family Metastrongylidae) that include forms (as *M. capillaris* syn. *M. minutissimus*) infecting the lungs of sheep and goats and having larval stages in various snails and slugs

Mül·ler \'mœ-ler\, **Fritz (Johann Friedrich Theodor) (1822–1897)**, German zoologist.

mulberry molar *n* : a first molar tooth whose occlusal surface is pitted due to congenital syphilis with nodules replacing the cusps — see MOON'S MOLAR

mules·ing \'myül-ziŋ\ *n* : the use of Mules operation to reduce the occurrence of blowfly strike

Mules operation \'myülz-\ *n* : removal of excess loose skin from either side of the crutch of a sheep to reduce the incidence of blowfly strike

Mules, J. H. W., Australian sheep rancher.

Mül·ler cell \'myü-lər-, 'mi-, 'mə-\ *also*
  Mül·ler's cell \-lərz-\ *n* : FIBER OF
  MÜLLER
Mül·ler \'mᵫ-lər, 'myü-\, **Heinrich
  (1820–1864),** German anatomist.
Mül·le·ri·an duct \myü-'lir-ē-ən-, mi-,
  mə-\ *n* : either of a pair of ducts parallel to the Wolffian ducts and giving
  rise in the female to the oviducts —
  called also *paramesonephric duct*
    Mül·ler \'mᵫ-lər, 'myü-\, **Johannes
    Peter (1801–1858),** German physiolo-
    gist and anatomist.
Müllerian tubercle *n* : an elevation on
  the wall of the embryonic urogenital
  sinus where the Müllerian ducts enter
¹**mult·an·gu·lar** \məl-'taŋ-gyə-lər\ *adj*
  : having many angles (a ~ bone)
²**multangular** *n* : a multangular bone —
  see TRAPEZIUM, TRAPEZOID
multi- *comb form* **1 a** : many : multiple
  : much ⟨*multi*neuronal⟩ **b** : consisting
  of, containing, or having more than
  two ⟨*multi*nucleate⟩ **c** : more than one
  ⟨*multi*parous⟩ **2** : affecting many parts
  ⟨*multi*glandular⟩
mul·ti·an·gu·lar \məl-tē-'aŋ-gyə-lər,
  ˌməl-ˌtī-\ *adj* : MULTANGULAR
mul·ti·cel·lu·lar \-'sel-yə-lər\ *adj* : having or consisting of many cells — **mul-
  ti·cel·lu·lar·i·ty** \-ˌsel-yə-'lar-ə-tē\ *n*
mul·ti·cen·ter \-'sen-tər\ *adj* : involving
  more than one medical or research institution ⟨a ~ clinical study⟩
mul·ti·cen·tric \-'sen-trik\ *adj* : having
  multiple centers of origin ⟨a ~ tumor⟩
mul·ti·ceps \'məl-tə-ˌseps\ *n* **1** *cap* : a
  genus of taeniid tapeworms that have
  a coenurus larva parasitic in ruminants, rodents, and rarely humans
  and that include the parasite of gid
  (*M. multiceps*) and other worms typically parasitic on carnivores **2** : COE-
  NURUS
mul·ti·clo·nal \ˌməl-tē-'klō-nəl, -ˌtī-\
  adj : POLYCLONAL
mul·ti·cus·pid \-'kəs-pəd\ *adj* : having
  several cusps ⟨a ~ tooth⟩
mul·ti·cys·tic \-'sis-tik\ *adj* : POLYCYS-
  TIC
mul·ti·dose \'məl-tē-ˌdōs, -ˌtī-\ *adj*
  : utilizing or containing more than
  one dose
mul·ti·drug \-ˌdrəg\ *adj* : utilizing or relating to more than one drug ⟨~ ther-
  apy⟩
mul·ti·en·zyme \ˌməl-tē-'en-ˌzīm, -ˌtī-\
  adj : composed of or involving two or
  more enzymes that function in a biosynthetic pathway ⟨~ complex⟩
mul·ti·fac·to·ri·al \-fak-'tōr-ē-əl\ *adj* **1**
  : having characters or a mode of inheritance dependent on a number of
  genes at different loci **2** *or* **mul·ti·fac-
  tor** \-'fak-tər\ : having, involving, or
  produced by a variety of elements or
  causes ⟨a ~ study⟩ ⟨a disease with a
  ~ etiology⟩ — **mul·ti·fac·to·ri·al·ly**
  adv
mul·tif·i·dus \ˌməl-'ti-fə-dəs\ *n, pl* **-di**
  \-ˌdī\ : a muscle of the fifth and deep-

est layer of the back filling up the
groove on each side of the spinous
processes of the vertebrae from the
sacrum to the skull and consisting of
many fasciculi that pass upward and
inward to the spinous processes and
help to erect and rotate the spine
mul·ti·fo·cal \ˌməl-tē-'fō-kəl\ *adj* **1**
  : having more than one focal length
  ⟨~ lenses⟩ **2** : arising from or occurring in more than one focus or location ⟨~ convulsions⟩
multifocal leukoencephalopathy — see
  PROGRESSIVE MULTIFOCAL LEUKOEN-
  CEPHALOPATHY
¹**mul·ti·form** \'məl-ti-ˌförm\ *adj* : having
  or occurring in many forms
²**multiforme** — see ERYTHEMA MULTI-
  FORME, GLIOBLASTOMA MULTIFORME
mul·ti·gene \ˌməl-tē-'jēn, -ˌtī-\ *adj* : relating to or determined by a group of
  genes which were originally copies of
  the same gene but evolved by mutation to become different from each
  other
mul·ti·gen·ic \-'je-nik, -'jē-\ *adj* : MUL-
  TIFACTORIAL 1
mul·ti·glan·du·lar \-'glan-jə-lər\ *adj*
  : POLYGLANDULAR
mul·ti·grav·i·da \-'gra-vi-də\ *n* : a woman who has been pregnant more than
  once — compare MULTIPARA
mul·ti·han·di·capped \ˌməl-tē-'han-di-
  ˌkapt, -ˌtī-\ *adj* : affected by more
  than one handicap ⟨~ children⟩
mul·ti·hos·pi·tal \-'häs-ˌpit-ᵊl\ *adj* : involving or affiliated with more than
  one hospital
mul·ti·lobed \-'lōbd\ *adj* : having two or
  more lobes
mul·ti·loc·u·lar \-'lä-kyə-lər\ *adj* : having or divided into many small chambers or vesicles ⟨a ~ cyst⟩
mul·ti·mam·mate mouse \-'ma-ˌmāt-\ *n*
  : any of several common African rodents of the genus *Rattus* that have 12
  rather than the usual five or six mammae on each side, are vectors of disease, and are used in medical
  research — called also *multimam-
  mate rat*
mul·ti·mo·dal \-'mōd-ᵊl\ *adj* : relating
  to, having, or utilizing more than one
  mode or modality (as of stimulation
  or treatment)
mul·ti·neu·ro·nal \-'nür-ən-ᵊl, -'nyür-;
  -nu-'rōn-, -nyu-\ *adj* : made up of or
  involving more than one neuron ⟨~
  circuits⟩
mul·ti·nod·u·lar \-'nä-jə-lər\ *adj* : having many nodules ⟨~ goiter⟩
mul·ti·nu·cle·ate \-'nü-klē-ət, -'nyü-\ *or*
  mul·ti·nu·cle·at·ed \-klē-ˌā-təd\ *adj*
  : having more than two nuclei
mul·ti·or·gas·mic \-ˌor-'gaz-mik\ *adj*
  : experiencing one orgasm after another with little or no recovery period
  between them
mul·tip·a·ra \ˌməl-'ti-pə-rə\ *n* : a woman who has borne more than one child
  — compare MULTIGRAVIDA

multiparity • Musca 438

mul·ti·par·i·ty \ˌməl-ti-ˈpar-ə-tē\ *n, pl* **-ties 1** : the production of two or more young at a birth **2** : the condition of having borne a number of children

mul·tip·a·rous \ˌmal-ˈti-pər-əs\ *adj* **1** : producing many or more than one at a birth **2** : having experienced one or more previous parturitions — compare PRIMIPAROUS

mul·ti·ple \ˈmal-tə-pəl\ *adj* **1** : consisting of, including, or involving more than one ⟨∼ births⟩ **2** : affecting many parts of the body at once

multiple allele *n* : an allele of a genetic locus having more than two allelic forms within a population

multiple factor *n* : POLYGENE

multiple myeloma *n* : a disease of bone marrow that is characterized by the presence of numerous myelomas in various bones of the body — called also *myelomatosis*

multiple personality *n* : an hysterical neurosis in which the personality becomes dissociated into two or more distinct but complex and socially and behaviorally integrated parts each of which becomes dominant and controls behavior from time to time to the exclusion of the others — called also *alternating personality*; compare SPLIT PERSONALITY

multiple sclerosis *n* : a demyelinating disease marked by patches of hardened tissue in the brain or the spinal cord and associated esp. with partial or complete paralysis and jerking muscle tremor

multiplex — see ARTHROGRYPOSIS MULTIPLEX CONGENITA, MONONEURITIS MULTIPLEX, PARAMYOCLONUS MULTIPLEX

mul·ti·po·lar \ˌmal-tē-ˈpō-lər, -ˌtī-\ *adj* **1** : having several poles ⟨∼ mitoses⟩ **2** : having several dendrites ⟨∼ nerve cells⟩ — **mul·ti·po·lar·i·ty** \-ˌpō-ˈlar-ə-tē\ *n*

mul·tip·o·tent \ˌmal-ˈti-pə-tənt\ *adj* : having power to do many things

mul·ti·po·ten·tial \ˌmal-tē-pə-ˈten-chəl, -ˌtī-\ *adj* : having the potential of becoming any of several mature cell types ⟨∼ stem cell⟩

mul·ti·re·sis·tant \-ri-ˈzis-tənt\ *adj* : biologically resistant to several toxic agents

mul·ti·spe·cial·ty \-ˈspe-shəl-tē\ *adj* : providing service in or staffed by members of several medical specialties ⟨∼ health center⟩

mul·ti·syn·ap·tic \-sə-ˈnap-tik\ *adj* : relating to or consisting of more than one synapse ⟨∼ pathways⟩

mul·ti·sys·tem \-ˈsis-təm\ *also* **mul·ti·sys·te·mic** \-sis-ˈtē-mik\ *adj* : relating to, consisting of, or involving more than one bodily system

¹**mul·ti·va·lent** \-ˈvā-lənt\ *adj* **1** : represented more than twice in the somatic chromosome number ⟨∼ chromosomes⟩ **2** : POLYVALENT

²**multivalent** *n* : a multivalent group of chromosomes

¹**mul·ti·vi·ta·min** \-ˈvī-tə-mən, -ˈvi-\ *adj* : containing several vitamins and esp. all known to be essential to health ⟨a ∼ formula⟩

²**multivitamin** *n* : a multivitamin preparation

mum·mi·fy \ˈmə-mi-ˌfī\ *vb* **-fied; -fy·ing** : to dry up and shrivel like a mummy ⟨a *mummified* fetus⟩ — **mum·mi·fi·ca·tion** \ˌmə-mi-fə-ˈkā-shən\ *n*

mumps \ˈməmps\ *n sing or pl* : an acute contagious disease caused by a paramyxovirus and marked by fever and by swelling esp. of the parotid gland — called also *epidemic parotitis*

Mun·chau·sen syndrome \ˈmən-ˌchaù-zən-\ *or* **Mun·chau·sen's syndrome** \-zənz-\ *n* : a condition characterized by the feigning of the symptoms of a disease or injury in order to undergo diagnostic tests, hospitalization, or medical or surgical treatment

Münch·hau·sen \ˈmŭnk-ˌhaù-zən\, **Karl Friedrich Hieronymus, Freiherr von (1720–1797),** German soldier.

mu·ral \ˈmyur-əl\ *adj* : attached to and limited to a wall or a cavity ⟨∼ thrombus⟩ ⟨∼ abscess⟩

mu·ram·i·dase \myù-ˈra-mə-ˌdās, -ˌdāz\ *n* : LYSOZYME

mu·rein \ˈmyur-ē-ən, ˈmyur-ˌēn\ *n* : PEPTIDOGLYCAN

mu·ri·at·ic acid \ˌmyür-ē-ˈa-tik-\ *n* : HYDROCHLORIC ACID

mu·rid \ˈmyur-id\ *n* : any of a large family (Muridae) of relatively small rodents including various Old World forms (as the house mouse and the common rats) — **murid** *adj*

¹**mu·rine** \ˈmyur-ˌīn\ *adj* **1 a** : of or relating to the genus *Mus* or its subfamily (Murinae) that includes most of the rats and mice which habitually live in intimate association with humans ⟨∼ rodents⟩ **b** : of, relating to, or produced by the house mouse ⟨a ∼ odor⟩ **2** : affecting or transmitted by rats or mice ⟨∼ rickettsial diseases⟩

²**murine** *n* : a murine animal

murine typhus *n* : a mild febrile disease that is marked by headache and rash, is caused by a rickettsial bacterium of the genus *Rickettsia* (*R. typhi*), is widespread in nature in rodents, and is transmitted to humans by a flea — called also *endemic typhus*

mur·mur \ˈmər-mər\ *n* : an atypical sound of the heart indicating a functional or structural abnormality — called also *heart murmur*

Mus \ˈməs\ *n* : a genus of rodents (family Muridae) that includes the house mouse (*M. musculus*) and a few related small forms

Mus·ca \ˈməs-kə\ *n* : a genus of flies (family Muscidae) that is now restricted to the common housefly (*M. domestica*) and closely related flies

mus·cae vo·li·tan·tes \ˈməs-ˌkē-ˌvä-lə-ˈtan-ˌtēz, ˈmə-ˌsē-\ *n pl* : spots before the eyes due to cells and cell fragments in the vitreous humor and lens — compare FLOATER

mus·ca·rine \ˈməs-kə-ˌrēn\ *n* : a toxic ammonium base [$C_9H_{20}NO_2$]$^+$ that is biochemically related to acetylcholine, is found esp. in fly agaric, acts directly on smooth muscle, and when ingested produces profuse salivation and sweating, abdominal colic with evacuation of bowels and bladder, contracted pupils and blurring of vision, excessive bronchial secretion, bradycardia, and respiratory depression

mus·ca·rin·ic \ˌməs-kə-ˈri-nik\ *adj* : relating to, resembling, producing, or mediating the parasympathetic effects (as a slowed heart rate and increased activity of smooth muscle) produced by muscarine (∼ receptors) — compare NICOTINIC

mus·cle \ˈmə-səl\ *n, often attrib* **1** : a body tissue consisting of long cells that contract when stimulated and produce motion — see CARDIAC MUSCLE, SMOOTH MUSCLE, STRIATED MUSCLE **2** : an organ that is essentially a mass of muscle tissue attached at either end to a fixed point and that by contracting moves or checks the movement of a body part — see AGONIST 1, ANTAGONIST a, SYNERGIST 2

mus·cle–bound \ˈmə-səl-ˌbaùnd\ *adj* : having some of the muscles tense and enlarged and of impaired elasticity sometimes as a result of excessive exercise

muscle fiber *n* : any of the elongated cells characteristic of muscle

muscle sense *n* : the part of kinesthesia mediated by end organs located in muscles

muscle spasm *n* : persistent involuntary hypertonicity of one or more muscles usu. of central origin and commonly associated with pain and excessive irritability

muscle spindle *n* : a sensory end organ in a muscle that is sensitive to stretch in the muscle, consists of small striated muscle fibers richly supplied with nerve fibers, and is enclosed in a connective tissue sheath — called also *stretch receptor*

muscle tone *n* : TONUS 2

muscul- *or* **musculo-** *comb form* **1** : muscle ⟨*muscul*ar⟩ **2** : muscular and ⟨*musculo*skeletal⟩

mus·cu·lar \ˈməs-kyə-lər\ *adj* **1 a** : of, relating to, or constituting muscle **b** : of, relating to, or performed by the muscles **2** : having well-developed musculature — **mus·cu·lar·ly** *adv*

muscular coat *n* : an outer layer of smooth muscle surrounding a hollow or tubular organ (as the bladder, esophagus, large intestine, small intestine, stomach, ureter, uterus, and vagina) that often consists of an inner layer of circular fibers serving to narrow the lumen of the organ and an outer layer of longitudinal fibers serving to shorten its length — called also *muscularis externa, tunica muscularis*

muscular dystrophy *n* : any of a group of hereditary diseases characterized by progressive wasting of muscles

mus·cu·la·ris \ˌməs-kyə-ˈlar-is\ *n* **1** : the smooth muscular layer of the wall of various more or less contractile organs (as the bladder) **2** : the thin layer of smooth muscle that forms part of a mucous membrane (as in the esophagus)

muscularis ex·ter·na \-eks-ˈtər-nə\ *n* : MUSCULAR COAT

muscularis mu·co·sae \-myü-ˈkō-sē\ *also* **muscularis mu·co·sa** \-sə\ *n* : MUSCULARIS 2

mus·cu·lar·i·ty \ˌməs-kyə-ˈlar-ə-tē\ *n, pl* **-ties** : the quality or state of being muscular

mus·cu·la·ture \ˈməs-kyə-lə-ˌchùr, -chər, -ˌtyùr\ *n* : the muscles of all or a part of the body

mus·cu·li pec·ti·na·ti \ˈməs-kyə-ˌlī-ˌpek-ti-ˈnā-ˌtī\ *n pl* : small muscular ridges on the inner wall of the auricular appendage of the left and right atria of the heart

musculo- — see MUSCUL-

mus·cu·lo·cu·ta·ne·ous \ˌməs-kyə-lō-kyü-ˈtā-nē-əs\ *adj* : of, relating to, supplying, or consisting of both muscle and skin

musculocutaneous nerve *n* **1** : a large branch of the brachial plexus supplying various parts of the upper arm (as flexor muscles) and forearm (as the skin) **2** : SUPERFICIAL PERONEAL NERVE

mus·cu·lo·fas·cial \-ˈfa-shəl, -shē-əl\ *adj* : relating to or consisting of both muscular and fascial tissue

mus·cu·lo·fi·brous \-ˈfī-brəs\ *adj* : relating to or consisting of both muscular and fibrous connective tissue

mus·cu·lo·mem·bra·nous \-ˈmem-brə-nəs\ *adj* : relating to or consisting of both muscle and membrane

mus·cu·lo·phren·ic artery \-ˈfre-nik-\ *n* : a branch of the internal thoracic artery that gives off branches to the seventh, eighth, and ninth intercostal spaces as anterior intercostal arteries, to the pericardium, to the diaphragm, and to the abdominal muscles — called also *musculophrenic, musculophrenic branch*

musculorum — see DYSTONIA MUSCULORUM DEFORMANS

mus·cu·lo·skel·e·tal \ˌməs-kyə-lō-ˈske-lət-əl\ *adj* : of, relating to, or involving both musculature and skeleton

mus·cu·lo·ten·di·nous \-ˈten-də-nəs\ *adj* : of, relating to, or affecting muscular and tendinous tissue (∼ injuries)

mus·cu·lo·ten·di·nous cuff *n* : ROTATOR CUFF

mus·cu·lus \'məs-kyə-ləs\ *n, pl* **-li** \-ˌlī\ : MUSCLE

mush·room \'məsh-ˌrüm, -ˌrüm\ *n* **1** : an enlarged complex fleshy fruiting body of a fungus (as most members of the class Basidiomycetes) that arises from an underground mycelium and consists typically of a stem bearing a spore-bearing structure; *esp* : one that is edible — compare TOADSTOOL 2 : FUNGUS 1

mu·si·co·gen·ic \ˌmyü-zi-kō-'je-nik\ *adj* : of, relating to, or being epileptic seizures precipitated by music

music therapy *n* : the treatment of disease (as mental illness) by means of music — **music therapist** *n*

mussel poisoning *n* : a toxic reaction following the eating of mussels; *esp* : a severe often fatal intoxication following the consumption of mussels that have fed on red tide flagellates and esp. gonyaulax and stored up a dangerous alkaloid in their tissues

mus·tard \'məs-tərd\ *n* **1** : a pungent yellow condiment consisting of the pulverized seeds of either of two herbs (*Brassica nigra* and *B. hirta* of the family Cruciferae, the mustard family) either dry or made into a paste and serving as a stimulant and diuretic or in large doses as an emetic and as a counterirritant when applied to the skin as a poultice **2 a** : MUSTARD GAS **b** : NITROGEN MUSTARD

mustard gas *n* : an irritant oily liquid $C_4H_8Cl_2S$ that is a war gas, causes blistering, attacks the eyes and lungs, and is a systemic poison

mustard oil *n* **1** : a colorless to pale yellow pungent irritating essential oil that is obtained by distillation from mustard seeds, that consists largely of allyl isothiocyanate, and that is used esp. in liniments and medicinal plasters **2** : ALLYL ISOTHIOCYANATE

mustard plaster *n* : a counterirritant and rubefacient plaster containing powdered mustard — called also *mustard paper*

mu·ta·gen \'myü-tə-jən\ *n* : a substance (as mustard gas or various radiations) that tends to increase the frequency or extent of mutation

mu·ta·gen·e·sis \ˌmyü-tə-'je-nə-səs\ *n, pl* **-e·ses** \-ˌsēz\ : the occurrence or induction of mutation — **mu·ta·gen·ic** \-'je-nik\ *adj* — **mu·ta·ge·nic·i·ty** \-jə-'ni-sə-tē\ *n*

mu·ta·gen·ize \'myü-tə-jə-ˌnīz\ *vb* **-ized; -iz·ing** : MUTATE

¹**mu·tant** \'myüt-ᵊnt\ *adj* : of, relating to, or produced by mutation

²**mutant** *n* : a mutant individual

mu·ta·tion \myü-'tā-shən\ *n* **1** : a relatively permanent change in hereditary material involving either a physical change in chromosome relations or a biochemical change in the codons that make up genes; *also* : the process of producing a mutation **2** : an individual, strain, or trait resulting from mutation — whether from **mu·tate** \'myü-ˌtāt, myü-'\ *vb* — **mu·ta·tion·al** \-shə-nəl\ *adj* — **mu·ta·tion·al·ly** *adv*

¹**mute** \'myüt\ *adj* **mut·er; mut·est** : unable to speak : DUMB — **mute·ness** *n*

²**mute** *n* : a person who cannot or does not speak

mu·ti·late \'myüt-ᵊl-ˌāt\ *vb* **-lat·ed; -lat·ing** : to cut off or permanently destroy a limb or essential part of; *also* : CASTRATE — **mu·ti·la·tion** \ˌmyüt-ᵊl-'ā-shən\ *n*

mut·ism \'myü-ˌti-zəm\ *n* : the condition of being mute whether from physical, functional, or psychological cause

¹**muz·zle** \'mə-zəl\ *n* **1** : the projecting jaws and nose of an animal **2** : a fastening or covering for the mouth of an animal used to prevent eating or biting

²**muzzle** *vb* **muz·zled; muz·zling** : to fit with a muzzle

Mv *symbol* mendelevium

my- *or* **myo-** *comb form* **1 a** : muscle ⟨*my*asthenia⟩ ⟨*myo*globin⟩ **b** : muscular and ⟨*myo*neural⟩ **2** : myoma and ⟨*myo*edema⟩

my·al·gia \mī-'al-jē, -jē-ə\ *n* : pain in one or more muscles — **my·al·gic** \-jik\ *adj*

My·am·bu·tol \mī-'am-byü-ˌtȯl, -ˌtōl\ *trademark* — used for a preparation of ethambutol

my·an·e·sin \mī-'a-nə-sən\ *n* : MEPHENESIN

my·as·the·nia \ˌmī-əs-'thē-nē-ə\ *n* : muscular debility — **my·as·then·ic** \-'the-nik\ *adj*

myasthenia gra·vis \-'gra-vis, -'grä-\ *n* : a disease characterized by progressive weakness of voluntary muscles without atrophy or sensory disturbance and caused by an autoimmune attack on acetylcholine receptors at neuromuscular junctions

my·a·to·nia \ˌmī-ə-'tō-nē-ə\ *n* : lack of muscle tone : muscular flabbiness

myc- *or* **myco-** *comb form* : fungus ⟨*my*celium⟩ ⟨*myco*logy⟩ ⟨*myco*sis⟩

my·ce·li·um \mī-'sē-lē-əm\ *n, pl* **-lia** \-lē-ə\ : the mass of interwoven filaments that forms esp. the vegetative body of a fungus and is often submerged in another body (as of soil or organic matter or the tissues of a host); *also* : a similar mass of filaments formed by some bacteria (as of the genus *Streptomyces*) — **my·ce·li·al** \-lē-əl\ *adj*

-my·ces \'mī-ˌsēz\ *n comb form* : fungus ⟨Strepto*myces*⟩

mycet- *or* **myceto-** *comb form* : fungus ⟨*myceto*ma⟩

-my·cete \'mī-ˌsēt, ˌmī-'sēt\ *n comb form* : fungus ⟨actino*mycete*⟩

my·ce·tis·mus \ˌmī-sə-'tiz-məs\ *n, pl* **-mi** \-ˌmī\ : mushroom poisoning

my·ce·to·ma \ˌmī-sə-ˈtō-mə\ *n, pl* **-mas** or **-ma·ta** \-mə-tə\ **1** : a condition marked by invasion of the deep subcutaneous tissues with fungi or actinomycetes: **a** : MADUROMYCOSIS **b** : NOCARDIOSIS **2** : a tumorous mass occurring in mycetoma — **my·ce·to·ma·tous** \-mə-təs\ *adj*

-my·cin \ˈmīs-ᵊn\ *n comb form* : substance obtained from a fungus (erythro*mycin*)

my·co·bac·te·ri·o·sis \ˌmī-kō-bak-ˌtir-ē-ˈō-səs\ *n, pl* **-o·ses** \-ˌsēz\ : a disease caused by bacteria of the genus *Mycobacterium*

my·co·bac·te·ri·um \-bak-ˈtir-ē-əm\ *n cap* : a genus of nonmotile acid-fast aerobic bacteria (family Mycobacteriaceae) that include the causative agents of tuberculosis (*M. tuberculosis*) and leprosy (*M. leprae*) as well as numerous purely saprophytic forms **2** *pl* **-ria** : any bacterium of the genus *Mycobacterium* or a closely related genus — **my·co·bac·te·ri·al** \-ē-əl\ *adj*

my·col·o·gy \mī-ˈkä-lə-jē\ *n, pl* **-gies** : a branch of biology dealing with fungi **2** : fungal life — **my·co·log·i·cal** \ˌmī-kə-ˈläj-i-kəl\ *adj* — **my·col·o·gist** \mī-ˈkä-lə-jist\ *n*

my·co·my·cin \ˌmī-kə-ˈmīs-ᵊn\ *n* : an antibiotic acid $C_{13}H_{10}O_2$ obtained from an actinomycete of the genus *Nocardia* (*N. acidophilus*)

my·co·phe·no·lic acid \ˌmī-kō-fi-ˈnō-lik-, -ˈnä-\ *n* : a crystalline antibiotic $C_{17}H_{20}O_6$ obtained from fungi of the genus *Penicillium*

my·co·plas·ma \ˌmī-kō-ˈplaz-mə\ *n 1 cap* : a genus of minute pleomorphic gram-negative chiefly nonmotile prokaryotic microorganisms (family Mycoplasmataceae) without cell walls that are intermediate in some respects between viruses and bacteria and are mostly parasitic usu. in mammals — see PLEUROPNEUMONIA 2 *2 pl* **-mas** *or* **-ma·ta** \-mə-tə\ : any microorganism of the genus *Mycoplasma* or of the family (Mycoplasmataceae) to which it belongs — called also *pleuropneumonia-like organism, PPLO* — **my·co·plas·mal** \-məl\ *adj*

my·co·sis \mī-ˈkō-səs\ *n, pl* **my·co·ses** \-ˌsēz\ : infection with or disease caused by a fungus — **my·cot·ic** \-ˈkä-tik\ *adj*

mycosis fun·goi·des \-fəŋ-ˈgȯi-ˌdēz\ *n* : a form of lymphoma characterized by a chronic, patchy, red, scaly, irregular and often eczematous dermatitis that progresses over a period of years to form elevated plaques and then tumors

my·co·stat \ˈmī-kə-ˌstat\ *n* : an agent that inhibits the growth of molds — **my·co·stat·ic** \ˌmī-kə-ˈsta-tik\ *adj*

My·co·stat·in \ˈmī-kə-ˈsta-tən\ *trademark* — used for a preparation of nystatin

my·cot·ic \mī-ˈkä-tik\ *adj* : of, relating to, or characterized by mycosis

my·co·tox·ic \ˌmī-kō-ˈtäk-sik\ *adj* : of, relating to, or caused by a mycotoxin — **my·co·tox·ic·i·ty** \-ˌtäk-ˈsi-sə-tē\ *n*

my·co·tox·i·co·sis \ˌmī-kō-ˌtäk-sə-ˈkō-səs\ *n, pl* **-co·ses** \-ˈkō-ˌsēz\ : poisoning caused by a mycotoxin

my·co·tox·in \-ˈtäk-sən\ *n* : a poisonous substance produced by a fungus and esp. a mold — see AFLATOXIN

My·dri·a·cyl \mə-ˈdrī-ə-ˌsil\ *trademark* — used for a preparation of tropicamide

myd·ri·a·sis \mə-ˈdrī-ə-səs\ *n, pl* **-a·ses** \-ˌsēz\ : a long-continued or excessive dilatation of the pupil of the eye

¹**myd·ri·at·ic** \ˌmī-drē-ˈa-tik\ *adj* : causing or involving dilatation of the pupil of the eye

²**mydriatic** *n* : a drug that produces dilatation of the pupil of the eye

my·ec·to·my \mī-ˈek-tə-mē\ *n, pl* **-mies** : surgical excision of part of a muscle

myel- *or* **myelo-** *comb form* : marrow: as **a** : bone marrow (*myelo*cyte) **b** : spinal cord (*myelo*dysplasia)

my·el·en·ceph·a·lon \ˌmī-ə-len-ˈse·fə-ˌlän, -lən\ *n* : the posterior part of the developing vertebrate hindbrain or the corresponding part of the adult brain composed of the medulla oblongata — **my·el·en·ce·phal·ic** \-ˌlen-sə-ˈfa-lik\ *adj*

-my·e·lia \mī-ˈē-lē-ə\ *n comb form* : a (specified) condition of the spinal cord (hemato*myelia*) (syringo*myelia*)

my·e·lin \ˈmī-ə-lən\ *n* : a soft white somewhat fatty material that forms a thick myelin sheath about the protoplasmic core of a myelinated nerve fiber — **my·e·lin·ic** \ˌmī-ə-ˈli-nik\ *adj*

my·e·lin·at·ed \ˈmī-ə-lə-ˌnā-təd\ *adj* : having a myelin sheath

my·e·li·na·tion \ˌmī-ə-lə-ˈnā-shən\ *n 1* : the process of acquiring a myelin sheath **2** : the condition of being myelinated

my·e·lin·i·za·tion \ˌmī-ə-ˌli-nə-ˈzā-shən\ *n* : MYELINATION

my·e·li·nol·y·sis \ˌmī-ə-lə-ˈnä-lə-səs\ — see CENTRAL PONTINE MYELINOLYSIS

myelin sheath *n* : a layer of myelin surrounding some nerve fibers

my·e·li·tis \ˌmī-ə-ˈlī-təs\ *n, pl* **my·elit·i·des** \-ˈli-tə-ˌdēz\ : inflammation of the spinal cord or of the bone marrow — **my·e·lit·ic** \-ˈli-tik\ *adj*

my·e·lo·blast \ˈmī-ə-lə-ˌblast\ *n* : a large mononuclear nongranular bone-marrow cell; *esp* : one that is a precursor of a myelocyte — **my·e·lo·blas·tic** \ˌmī-ə-lə-ˈblas-tik\ *adj*

myeloblastic leukemia *n* : MYELOGENOUS LEUKEMIA

my·e·lo·blas·to·sis \ˌmī-ə-lō-blas-ˈtō-səs\ *n, pl* **-to·ses** \-ˌsēz\ : the presence of an abnormally large number of myeloblasts in the tissues, organs, or circulating blood

my·e·lo·cele \ˈmī-ə-lə-ˌsēl\ *n* : spina bifida in which the neural tissue of the spinal cord is exposed — compare MYELOMENINGOCELE

my·e·lo·cyte \'mī-ə-lə-ˌsīt\ n : a bone=marrow cell; esp : a motile white cell with cytoplasmic granules that gives rise to the blood granulocytes and occurs abnormally in the circulating blood (as in myelogenous leukemia) — **my·e·lo·cyt·ic** \ˌmī-ə-lə-'si-tik\ adj

myelocytic leukemia n : MYELOGENOUS LEUKEMIA

my·e·lo·cy·to·ma \-sī-'tō-mə\ n, pl -mas or -ma·ta \-mə-tə\ : a tumor esp. of fowl in which the typical cellular element is a myelocyte or a cell of similar differentiation

my·e·lo·cy·to·sis \-sī-'tō-səs\ n, pl -to·ses \-ˌsēz\ : the presence of excess numbers of myelocytes esp. in the blood or bone marrow

my·e·lo·dys·pla·sia \-dis-'plā-zhə, -zhē-ə\ n : a developmental anomaly of the spinal cord — **my·e·lo·dys·plas·tic** \-'plas-tik\ adj

my·e·lo·fi·bro·sis \ˌmī-ə-lō-fī-'brō-səs\ n, pl -bro·ses \-ˌsēz\ : an anemic condition in which bone marrow becomes fibrotic and the liver and spleen usu. exhibit a development of blood cell precursors — **my·e·lo·fi·brot·ic** \-'brä-tik\ adj

my·e·log·e·nous \ˌmī-ə-'lä-jə-nəs\ also **my·e·lo·gen·ic** \ˌmī-ə-lə-'je-nik\ adj : of, relating to, originating in, or produced by the bone marrow

myelogenous leukemia n : leukemia characterized by proliferation of myeloid tissue (as of the bone marrow and spleen) and an abnormal increase in the number of granulocytes, myelocytes, and myeloblasts in the circulating blood — called also granulocytic leukemia, myeloblastic leukemia, myelocytic leukemia, myeloid leukemia

my·e·lo·gram \'mī-ə-lə-ˌgram\ n 1 : a differential study of the cellular elements present in bone marrow usu. made on material obtained by sternal biopsy 2 : a roentgenogram of the spinal cord made by myelography

my·e·lo·graph·ic \ˌmī-ə-lə-'gra-fik\ adj : of, relating to, or by means of a myelogram or myelography — **my·e·lo·graph·i·cal·ly** \-i-k(ə-)lē\ adv

my·e·log·ra·phy \ˌmī-ə-'lä-grə-fē\ n, pl -phies : roentgenographic visualization of the spinal cord after injection of a contrast medium into the spinal subarachnoid space

my·e·loid \'mī-ə-ˌloid\ adj 1 : of or relating to the spinal cord 2 : of, relating to, or resembling bone marrow

myeloid leukemia n : MYELOGENOUS LEUKEMIA

my·e·lo·li·po·ma \ˌmī-ə-lō-li-'pō-mə, -li-\ n, pl -mas or -ma·ta \-mə-tə\ : a benign tumor esp. of the adrenal glands that consists of fat and hematopoietic tissue

my·e·lo·ma \ˌmī-ə-'lō-mə\ n, pl -mas or -ma·ta \-mə-tə\ : a primary tumor of the bone marrow formed of any one of the bone marrow cells (as myelocytes or plasma cells) and usu. involving several different bones at the same time — see MULTIPLE MYELOMA

my·e·lo·ma·to·sis \ˌmī-ə-lō-mə-'tō-səs\ n, pl -to·ses \-ˌsēz\ : MULTIPLE MYELOMA

my·e·lo·me·nin·go·cele \ˌmī-ə-lō-mə-'nin-gə-ˌsēl, -mə-ˌnin-jə-\ n : spina bifida in which neural tissue and the investing meninges protrude from the spinal column forming a sac under the skin — compare MYELOCELE

my·e·lo·mono·cyt·ic \-ˌmä-nə-'si-tik\ adj : relating to or being a blood cell that has the characteristics of both monocytes and granulocytes

myelomonocytic leukemia n : a kind of monocytic leukemia in which the cells resemble granulocytes

my·e·lop·a·thy \ˌmī-ə-'lä-pə-thē\ n, pl -thies : any disease or disorder of the spinal cord or bone marrow — **my·e·lo·path·ic** \ˌmī-ə-lō-'pa-thik\ adj

my·e·lo·phthis·ic anemia \ˌmī-ə-lō-'ti-zik-, -'tī-sik-\ n : anemia in which the blood-forming elements of the bone marrow are unable to reproduce normal blood cells and which is commonly caused by specific toxins or by overgrowth of tumor cells

my·e·lo·poi·e·sis \ˌmī-ə-lō-(ˌ)poi-'ē-səs\ n, pl -poi·e·ses \-'ē-ˌsēz\ 1 : production of marrow or marrow cells 2 : production of blood cells in the bone marrow; esp : formation of blood granulocytes — **my·e·lo·poi·et·ic** \-(ˌ)poi-'e-tik\ adj

my·e·lo·pro·lif·er·a·tive \ˌmī-ə-lō-prə-'li-fə-ˌrā-tiv, -rə-\ adj : of, relating to, or being a disorder (as leukemia) marked by excessive proliferation of bone marrow elements and esp. blood cell precursors

my·e·lo·sis \ˌmī-ə-'lō-səs\ n, pl -elo·ses \-ˌsēz\ 1 : the proliferation of marrow tissue to produce the changes in cell distribution typical of myelogenous leukemia 2 : MYELOGENOUS LEUKEMIA

my·e·lo·sup·pres·sion \ˌmī-ə-lō-sə-'pre-shən\ n : suppression of the bone marrow's production of blood cells and platelets — **my·e·lo·sup·pres·sive** \-sə-'pre-siv\ adj

my·e·lot·o·my \ˌmī-ə-'lä-tə-mē\ n, pl -mies : surgical incision of the spinal cord; esp : section of crossing nerve fibers at the midline of the spinal cord and esp. of sensory fibers for the relief of intractable pain

my·e·lo·tox·ic \ˌmī-ə-lō-'täk-sik\ adj : destructive to bone marrow or any of its elements (a ~ agent) — **my·e·lo·tox·ic·i·ty** \-täk-'si-sə-tē\ n

my·en·ter·ic \ˌmī-ən-'ter-ik\ adj : of or relating to the muscular coat of the intestinal wall

myenteric plexus n : a network of nerve

fibers and ganglia between the longitudinal and circular muscle layers of the intestine — called also *Auerbach's plexus;* compare MEISSNER'S PLEXUS

myenteric plexus of Auerbach *n* : MYENTERIC PLEXUS

myenteric reflex *n* : a reflex that is responsible for the wave of peristalsis moving along the intestine and that involves contraction of the digestive tube above and relaxation below the place where it is stimulated by an accumulated mass of food

my·ia·sis \mī-ˈī-ə-səs, mē-\ *n, pl* **my·ia·ses** \-ˌsēz\ : infestation with fly maggots

myl- *or* **mylo-** *comb form* : molar ⟨*mylohyoid*⟩

My·lan·ta \mī-ˈlan-tə\ *trademark* — used for an antacid and antiflatulent preparation

Myl·e·ran \ˈmi-lə-ˌran\ *trademark* — used for a preparation of busulfan

My·li·con \ˈmī-lə-ˌkän\ *trademark* — used for a preparation of simethicone

my·lo·hy·oid \ˌmī-lō-ˈhī-ˌoid\ *adj* : of, indicating, or adjoining the mylohyoid muscle

my·lo·hy·oi·de·us \-hī-ˈoi-dē-əs\ *n, pl* **-dei** \-dē-ˌī\ : MYLOHYOID MUSCLE

mylohyoid line *n* : a ridge on the inner side of the bone of the lower jaw giving attachment to the mylohyoid muscle and to the superior constrictor of the pharynx — called also *mylohyoid ridge*

mylohyoid muscle *n* : a flat triangular muscle on each side of the mouth that is located above the anterior belly of the digastric muscle, extends from the inner surface of the mandible to the hyoid bone, and with its mate on the opposite side forms the floor of the mouth — called also *mylohyoid, mylohyoideus*

myo- — see MY-

myo·blast \ˈmī-ə-ˌblast\ *n* : an undifferentiated cell capable of giving rise to muscle cells

myo·blas·to·ma \ˌmī-ə-(ˌ)blas-ˈtō-mə\ *n, pl* **-mas** *or* **-ma·ta** \-mə-tə\ : a tumor that is composed of cells resembling primitive myoblasts and is associated with striated muscle

myo·car·di·al \ˌmī-ə-ˈkär-dē-əl\ *adj* : of, relating to, or involving the myocardium — **myo·car·di·al·ly** *adv*

myocardial infarction *n* : infarction of the myocardium that results typically from coronary occlusion — compare ANGINA PECTORIS, CORONARY INSUFFICIENCY, HEART FAILURE 1

myocardial insufficiency *n* : inability of the myocardium to perform its function : HEART FAILURE

myo·car·di·op·a·thy \-ˌkär-dē-ˈä-pə-thē\ *n, pl* **-thies** : disease of the myocardium

myo·car·di·tis \ˌmī-ə-(ˌ)kär-ˈdī-təs\ *n* : inflammation of the myocardium

myo·car·di·um \ˌmī-ə-ˈkär-dē-əm\ *n, pl* **-dia** \-dē-ə\ : the middle muscular layer of the heart wall

Myo·chry·sine \ˌmī-ō-ˈkrī-ˌsēn, -ˈsən\ *trademark* — used for a preparation of gold sodium thiomalate

myo·clo·nia \ˌmī-ə-ˈklō-nē-ə\ *n* : MYOCLONUS

myo·clon·ic \-ˈklä-nik\ *adj* : of, relating to, characterized by, or being myoclonus ⟨~ seizures⟩

myoclonic epilepsy *n* : an inherited form of epilepsy characterized by myoclonic seizures, progressive mental deterioration, and the presence of Lafora bodies in parts of the central nervous system — called also *Lafora's disease, myoclonus epilepsy*

myo·clo·nus \mī-ˈä-klə-nəs\ *n* : irregular involuntary contraction of a muscle usu. resulting from functional disorder of controlling motoneurons; *also* : a condition characterized by myoclonus

myo·cyte \ˈmī-ə-ˌsīt\ *n* : a contractile cell; *specif* : a muscle cell

myo·ede·ma \ˌmī-ō-i-ˈdē-mə\ *n, pl* **-mas** *or* **-ma·ta** \-mə-tə\ : the formation of a lump in a muscle when struck a slight blow that occurs in states of exhaustion or in certain diseases

myo·elec·tric \ˌmī-ō-i-ˈlek-trik\ *also* **myo·elec·tri·cal** \-tri-kəl\ *adj* : of, relating to, or utilizing electricity generated by muscle

myo·epi·the·li·al \-ˌe-pə-ˈthē-lē-əl\ *adj* : of, relating to, or being large contractile cells of epithelial origin which are located at the base of the secretory cells of various glands (as the salivary and mammary glands)

myo·epi·the·li·o·ma \-ˌe-pə-ˌthē-lē-ˈō-mə\ *n, pl* **-mas** *or* **-ma·ta** \-mə-tə\ : a tumor arising from myoepithelial cells esp. of the sweat glands

myo·epi·the·li·um \-ˌe-pə-ˈthē-lē-əm\ *n, pl* **-lia** : tissue made up of myoepithelial cells

myo·fas·cial \-ˈfa-shəl, -shē-əl\ *adj* : of or relating to the fasciae of muscles

myo·fi·bril \ˌmī-ō-ˈfī-brəl, -ˈfi-\ *n* : one of the longitudinal parallel contractile elements of a muscle cell that are composed of myosin and actin — **myo·fi·bril·lar** \-brə-lər\ *adj*

myo·fi·bro·blast \-ˈfī-brə-ˌblast, -ˈfi-\ *n* : a fibroblast that has developed some of the functional and structural characteristics (as the presence of myofilaments) of smooth muscle cells

myo·fil·a·ment \-ˈfi-lə-mənt\ *n* : one of the individual filaments of actin or myosin that make up a myofibril

myo·func·tion·al \-ˈfəŋk-shə-nəl\ *adj* : of, relating to, or concerned with muscle function esp. in the treatment of orthodontic problems

myo·gen·e·sis \ˌmī-ə-ˈje-nə-səs\ *n, pl* **-e·ses** \-ˌsēz\ : the development of muscle tissue

myo·gen·ic \ˌmī-ə-ˈje-nik\ *also* **my·og·**

e·nous \mī-'ä-jə-nəs\ *adj* **1** : originating in muscle ⟨∼ pain⟩ **2** : taking place or functioning in ordered rhythmic fashion because of inherent properties of cardiac muscle rather than by reason of specific neural stimuli ⟨a ∼ heartbeat⟩ — compare NEUROGENIC 2b — **myo·ge·nic·i·ty** \-jə-'ni-sə-tē\ *n*

myo·glo·bin \'mī-ə-ˌglō-bən, 'mī-ə-ˌ\ *n* : a red iron-containing protein pigment in muscles that is similar to hemoglobin

myo·glo·bin·uria \-ˌglō-bi-'nür-ē-ə, -'nyur-\ *n* : the presence of myoglobin in the urine

myo·gram \'mī-ə-ˌgram\ *n* : a graphic representation of the phenomena (as intensity) of muscular contractions

myo·graph \-ˌgraf\ *n* : an apparatus for producing myograms

my·oid \'mī-ˌoid\ *adj* : resembling muscle

myo·ino·si·tol \ˌmī-ō-i-'nō-sə-ˌtōl, -ˌtōl\ *n* : a biologically active inositol that is a component of the vitamin B complex — called also *mesoinositol*

myom- *or* **myomo-** *comb form* : myoma ⟨*myome*ctomy⟩

my·o·ma \mī-'ō-mə\ *n, pl* **-mas** *or* **-ma·ta** \-mə-tə\ : a tumor consisting of muscle tissue

myo·mec·to·my \ˌmī-ə-'mek-tə-mē\ *n, pl* **-mies** : surgical excision of a myoma

myo·me·tri·tis \-mə-'trī-təs\ *n* : inflammation of the uterine myometrium

myo·me·tri·um \ˌmī-ə-'mē-trē-əm\ *n* : the muscular layer of the wall of the uterus — **myo·me·tri·al** \-'mē-trē-əl\ *adj*

myo·ne·cro·sis \-nə-'krō-səs, -ne-\ *n, pl* **-cro·ses** \-ˌsēz\ : necrosis of muscle

myo·neu·ral \ˌmī-ō-'nur-əl, -'nyur-\ *adj* : of, relating to, or connecting muscles and nerves ⟨∼ effects⟩

myoneural junction *n* : NEUROMUSCULAR JUNCTION

myo·path·ic \ˌmī-ə-'pa-thik\ *adj* **1** : involving abnormality of the muscles ⟨∼ syndrome⟩ **2** : of or relating to myopathy ⟨∼ dystrophy⟩

my·op·a·thy \mī-'ä-pə-thē\ *n, pl* **-thies** : a disorder of muscle tissue or muscles

my·ope \'mī-ˌōp\ *n* : a myopic person — called also *myopic*

myo·peri·car·di·tis \ˌmī-ō-ˌper-ə-ˌkär-'dī-təs\ *n, pl* **-dit·i·des** \-'di-tə-ˌdēz\ : inflammation of both the myocardium and pericardium

myo·pia \mī-'ō-pē-ə\ *n* : a condition in which the visual images come to a focus in front of the retina of the eye because of defects in the refractive media of the eye or of abnormal length of the eyeball resulting esp. in defective vision of distant objects — called also *nearsightedness*; compare ASTIGMATISM 2, EMMETROPIA

¹my·o·pic \-'ō-pik, -'ä-\ *adj* : affected by

myopia : of, relating to, or exhibiting myopia — **my·o·pi·cal·ly** *adv*

²myopic *n* : MYOPE

myo·plasm \'mī-ə-ˌpla-zəm\ *n* : the contractile portion of muscle tissue — compare SARCOPLASM — **myo·plas·mic** \ˌmī-ə-'plaz-mik\ *adj*

¹myo·re·lax·ant \ˌmī-ō-ri-'lak-sənt\ *n* : a drug that causes relaxation of muscle

²myorelaxant *adj* : relating to or causing relaxation of muscle ⟨∼ effects⟩ — **myo·re·lax·ation** \-ˌrē-lak-'sā-shən, -ri-ˌlak-\ *n*

myo·sar·co·ma \ˌmī-ə-ˌsär-'kō-mə\ *n, pl* **-mas** *or* **-ma·ta** \-mə-tə\ : a sarcomatous myoma

my·o·sin \'mī-ə-sən\ *n* : a fibrous globulin of muscle that can split ATP and that reacts with actin to form actomyosin

myo·sis *var of* MIOSIS

myo·si·tis \ˌmī-ə-'sī-təs\ *n* : muscular discomfort or pain

myositis os·sif·i·cans \-ä-'si-fə-ˌkanz\ *n* : myositis accompanied by ossification of muscle tissue or bony deposits in the muscles

myo·tat·ic reflex \ˌmī-ə-'ta-tik-\ *n* : STRETCH REFLEX

my·ot·ic *var of* MIOTIC

myo·tome \'mī-ə-ˌtōm\ *n* **1** : the portion of an embryonic somite from which skeletal musculature is produced **2** : an instrument for myotomy — **myo·to·mal** \ˌmī-ə-'tō-məl\ *adj*

my·ot·o·my \mī-'ä-tə-mē\ *n, pl* **-mies** : incision or division of a muscle

myo·to·nia \ˌmī-ə-'tō-nē-ə\ *n* : tonic spasm of one or more muscles; *also* : a condition characterized by such spasms — **myo·ton·ic** \-'tä-nik\ *adj*

myotonia con·gen·i·ta \-kän-'je-nə-tə\ *n* : an inherited condition that is characterized by delay in the ability to relax muscles after forceful contractions but not by wasting of muscle — called also *Thomsen's disease*

myotonia dys·tro·phi·ca \-dis-'trä-fi-kə, -'trō-\ *n* : MYOTONIC DYSTROPHY

myotonic dystrophy *n* : an inherited condition characterized by delay in the ability to relax muscles after forceful contraction, wasting of muscles, the formation of cataracts, premature baldness, atrophy of the gonads, and often mental deficiency

my·ot·o·nus \mī-'ä-tə-nəs\ *n* : sustained spasm of a muscle or muscle group

myo·trop·ic \ˌmī-ə-'trä-pik, -'trō-\ *adj* : affecting or tending to invade muscles ⟨a ∼ infection⟩

myo·tube \'mī-ə-ˌtüb, -ˌtyüb\ *n* : a developmental stage of a muscle fiber

myring- *or* **myringo-** *comb form* : tympanic membrane ⟨*myring*otomy⟩

myr·in·go·plas·ty \mə-'riŋ-gə-ˌplas-tē\ *n, pl* **-ties** : a plastic operation for the repair of perforations in the tympanic membrane

myr·in·got·o·my \ˌmir-ən-'gä-tə-mē\ *n, pl* **-mies** : incision of the tympanic membrane — called also *tympanotomy*

my·ris·tate \mi-ˈris-ˌtāt\ — see ISOPROPYL MYRISTATE

myx- *or* **myxo-** *comb form* **1** : mucus ⟨*myxoma*⟩ **2** : myxoma ⟨*myxosarcoma*⟩

myx·ede·ma \ˌmik-sə-ˈdē-mə\ *n* : severe hypothyroidism characterized by firm inelastic edema, dry skin and hair, and loss of mental and physical vigor — **myx·ede·ma·tous** \-ˈde-mə-təs, -ˈdē-\ *adj*

myx·oid \ˈmik-ˌsöid\ *adj* : resembling mucus

myx·o·ma \mik-ˈsō-mə\ *n, pl* **-mas** *or* **-ma·ta** \-mə-tə\ : a soft tumor made up of gelatinous connective tissue resembling that found in the umbilical cord — **myx·o·ma·tous** \-mə-təs\ *adj*

myx·o·ma·to·sis \mik-ˌsō-mə-ˈtō-səs\ *n, pl* **-to·ses** \-ˌsēz\ : a condition characterized by the presence of myxomas in the body; *specif* : a severe disease of rabbits that is caused by a poxvirus, is transmitted by mosquitos, biting flies, and direct contact, and has been used in the biological control of wild rabbit populations

myxo·sar·co·ma \-sär-ˈkō-mə\ *n, pl* **-mas** *or* **-ma·ta** \-mə-tə\ : a sarcoma with myxomatous elements

myxo·vi·rus \ˈmik-sə-ˌvī-rəs\ *n* : any of a group of rather large RNA-containing viruses that includes the orthomyxoviruses and the paramyxoviruses — **myxo·vi·ral** \ˌmik-sə-ˈvī-rəl\ *adj*

N

n \ˈen\ *n, pl* **n's** *or* **ns** \ˈenz\ : the haploid or gametic number of chromosomes — compare X

N *symbol* nitrogen — usu. italicized when used as a prefix ⟨*N*-allylnormorphine⟩

Na *symbol* sodium

NA *abbr* **1** Nomina Anatomica **2** nurse's aide

na·bo·thi·an cyst \nə-ˈbō-thē-ən-\ *n* : a mucous gland of the uterine cervix esp. when occluded and dilated — called also *nabothian follicle*
    Na·both \ˈnä-ˌbot\, **Martin (1675–1721),** German anatomist and physician.

NAD \ˌen-(ˌ)ā-ˈdē\ *n* : a coenzyme $C_{21}H_{27}N_7O_{14}P_2$ of numerous dehydrogenases that occurs in most cells and plays an important role in all phases of intermediary metabolism as an oxidizing agent or when in the reduced form as a reducing agent for various metabolites — called also *nicotinamide adenine dinucleotide, diphosphopyridine nucleotide*

NADH \ˌen-(ˌ)ā-(ˌ)dē-ˈāch\ *n* : the reduced form of NAD

na·do·lol \nā-ˈdō-ˌlòl, -ˌlōl\ *n* : a beta-blocker $C_{17}H_{27}NO_4$ used in the treatment of hypertension and angina pectoris

NADP \ˌen-(ˌ)ā-(ˌ)dē-ˈpē\ *n* : a coenzyme $C_{21}H_{28}N_7O_{17}P_3$ of numerous dehydrogenases (as that acting on glucose-6-phosphate) that occurs esp. in red blood cells and plays a role in intermediary metabolism similar to NAD but acting often on different metabolites — called also *nicotinamide adenine dinucleotide phosphate, TPN, triphosphopyridine nucleotide*

NADPH \ˌen-(ˌ)ā-(ˌ)dē-(ˌ)pē-ˈāch\ *n* : the reduced form of NADP

nae·paine \ˈnē-ˌpān\ *n* : a drug $C_{14}H_{22}N_2O_2$ used in the form of its

hydrochloride as a local anesthetic

nae·void, nae·vus *chiefly Brit var of* NEVOID, NEVUS

naf·cil·lin \naf-ˈsi-lən\ *n* : a semisynthetic penicillin $C_{21}H_{22}N_2O_5S$ that is resistant to penicillinase and is used esp. in the form of its sodium salt as an antibiotic

naf·ox·i·dine \na-ˈfäk-sə-ˌdēn\ *n* : an antiestrogen administered in the form of its hydrochloride $C_{29}H_{31}NO_2$·HCl

na·ga·na \nə-ˈgä-nə\ *n* : a highly fatal disease of domestic animals in tropical Africa caused by a flagellated protozoan of the genus *Trypanosoma* and transmitted by tsetse and possibly other biting flies; *broadly* : trypanosomiasis of domestic animals

nail \ˈnāl\ *n* **1** : a horny sheath of thickened and condensed epithelial stratum lucidum that grows out from a vascular matrix of cutis and protects the upper surface of the end of each finger and toe — called also *nail plate* **2** : a rod (as of metal) used to fix the parts of a broken bone in normal relation ⟨medullary ∼⟩

nail bed *n* : MATRIX 1b

nail–biting *n* : habitual biting at the fingernails usu. being symptomatic of emotional tensions and frustrations

nail fold *n* : the fold of the cutis at the margin of a fingernail or toenail

nail·ing \ˈnā-liŋ\ *n* : the act or process of fixing the parts of a broken bone by means of a nail ⟨intramedullary ∼⟩

nail matrix *n* : MATRIX 1b

nail plate *n* : NAIL 1

na·ive *or* **na·ïve** \nä-ˈēv\ *adj* **na·iv·er; -est** : not previously subjected to experimentation or a particular experimental situation ⟨made the test with ∼ rats⟩; *also* : not having previously used a particular drug (as marijuana)

Na·ja \ˈnä-jə\ *n* : a genus of elapid snakes comprising the true cobras

na·ked \ˈnä-kəd\ *adj* : lacking some

natural external covering (as of hair or myelin) — used of the animal body or one of its parts (∼ nerve endings)

na·li·dix·ic acid \ˌnā-lə-ˈdik-sik-\ : an antibacterial agent $C_{12}H_{12}N_2O_3$ that is used esp. in the treatment of genitourinary infections — see NEGGRAM

Nal·line \ˈna-ˌlēn\ *trademark* — used for a preparation of nalorphine

na·lor·phine \na-ˈlȯr-ˌfēn\ *n* : a white crystalline compound $C_{19}H_{21}NO_3$ that is derived from morphine and is used in the form of its hydrochloride as a respiratory stimulant to counteract poisoning by morphine and similar narcotic drugs — called also *N-allylnormorphine*; see NALLINE

nal·ox·one \na-ˈläk-ˌsōn, ˈna-lək-ˌsōn\ *n* : a potent antagonist $C_{19}H_{21}NO_4$ of narcotic drugs and esp. morphine that is administered esp. in the form of its hydrochloride — see NARCAN

nal·trex·one \nal-ˈtrek-ˌsōn\ *n* : a synthetic opiate antagonist $C_{20}H_{23}NO_4$ used esp. to maintain detoxified opiate addicts in a drug-free state

nan- *or* **nano-** *comb form* : dwarf ⟨*nano*cephalic⟩

nan·dro·lone \ˈnan-drə-ˌlōn\ *n* : a synthetic androgen $C_{18}H_{26}O_2$ used as an anabolic steroid

na·nism \ˈna-ˌni-zəm, ˈnā-\ *n* : the condition of being abnormally or exceptionally small in stature : DWARFISM

nano- *comb form* : one billionth (10^{-9}) part of ⟨*nano*second⟩

nano·ce·phal·ic \ˌna-nō-si-ˈfa-lik\ *adj* : having an abnormally small head

nano·cu·rie \ˈna-nō-ˌkyür-ē, -kyü-ˈrē\ *n* : one billionth of a curie

nano·gram \-ˌgram\ *n* : one billionth of a gram

nano·me·ter \-ˌmē-tər\ *n* : one billionth of a meter — abbr. *nm*

nano·sec·ond \-ˌse-kənd, -kənt\ *n* : one billionth of a second — abbr. *ns*, *nsec*

nape \ˈnāp, ˈnap\ *n* : the back of the neck

na·phaz·o·line \nə-ˈfa-zə-ˌlēn\ *n* : a base $C_{14}H_{14}N_2$ used locally in the form of its bitter crystalline hydrochloride esp. to relieve nasal congestion

naph·tha·lene \ˈnaf-thə-ˌlēn\ *n* : a crystalline aromatic hydrocarbon $C_{10}H_8$

naphthoate — see PAMAQUINE NAPHTHOATE

naph·thol \ˈnaf-ˌthȯl, -ˌthōl\ *n* : either of two isomeric derivatives $C_{10}H_8O$ of naphthalene

naph·tho·qui·none *also* **naph·tha·qui·none** \ˌnaf-thə-kwi-ˈnōn, -ˈkwi-ˌnōn\ *n* : any of three isomeric yellow to red crystalline compounds $C_{10}H_6O_2$; *esp* : one that occurs naturally in the form of derivatives (as vitamin K)

naph·thyl·amine \naf-ˈthi-lə-ˌmēn\ *n* : either of two isomeric crystalline bases $C_{10}H_9N$ that are used esp. in synthesizing dyes; *esp* : one (β–**naphthylamine**) with the amino group

in the beta position that has been demonstrated to cause bladder cancer in individuals exposed to it while working in the dye industry

Naph·ur·ide \ˈna-fyü-ˌrīd\ *trademark* — used for a preparation of suramin

nap·kin \ˈnap-kən\ *n* : SANITARY NAPKIN

na·prap·a·thy \nə-ˈpra-pə-thē\ *n, pl* **-thies** : a system of treatment by manipulation of connective tissue and adjoining structures (as ligaments, joints, and muscles) and by dietary measures that is held to facilitate the recuperative and regenerative processes of the body

Na·pro·syn \nə-ˈprōs-ᵊn\ *trademark* — used for a preparation of naproxen

na·prox·en \nə-ˈpräk-sᵊn\ *n* : an antiinflammatory analgesic antipyretic drug $C_{14}H_{14}O_3$ used esp. to treat arthritis — see NAPROSYN

nap·syl·ate \ˈnap-sə-ˌlāt\ *n* : a salt or ester of either of two crystalline acids $C_{10}H_7SO_3H$

Naqua \ˈna-kwə\ *trademark* — used for a preparation of trichlormethiazide

narc- *or* **narco-** *comb form* 1 : numbness : stupor ⟨*narc*osis⟩ 2 : deep sleep ⟨*narco*lepsy⟩

Nar·can \ˈnär-ˌkan\ *trademark* — used for a preparation of naloxone

nar·cis·sism \ˈnär-sə-ˌsi-zəm\ *n* 1 : love of or sexual desire for one's own body 2 : the state or stage of development in which there is considerable erotic interest in one's own body and ego and which in abnormal forms persists through fixation or reappears through regression — **nar·cis·sist** \-sist\ *n* — **nar·cis·sis·tic** \ˌnär-sə-ˈsis-tik\ *adj*

nar·co·anal·y·sis \ˌnär-kō-ə-ˈna-lə-səs\ *n, pl* **-y·ses** \-ˌsēz\ : psychotherapy that is performed under sedation for the recovery of repressed memories together with the emotion accompanying the experience and that is designed to facilitate an acceptable integration of the experience in the patient's personality

nar·co·lep·sy \ˈnär-kə-ˌlep-sē\ *n, pl* **-sies** : a condition characterized by brief attacks of deep sleep — compare HYPERSOMNIA 2

¹nar·co·lep·tic \ˌnär-kə-ˈlep-tik\ *adj* : of, relating to, or affected with narcolepsy

²narcoleptic *n* : an individual who is subject to attacks of narcolepsy

nar·co·sis \när-ˈkō-səs\ *n, pl* **-co·ses** \-ˌsēz\ : a state of stupor, unconsciousness, or arrested activity produced by the influence of narcotics or other chemicals

nar·co·syn·the·sis \ˌnär-kō-ˈsin-thə-səs\ *n, pl* **-the·ses** \-ˌsēz\ : narcoanalysis which has as its goal a reintegration of the patient's personality

¹nar·cot·ic \när-ˈkä-tik\ *n* 1 : a drug (as opium) that in moderate doses dulls the senses, relieves pain, and induces profound sleep but in excessive doses causes stupor, coma, or convulsions **2** : a drug (as marijuana or LSD) subject to restriction similar to that of addictive narcotics whether physiologically addictive and narcotic or not

²**narcotic** *adj* **1** : having the properties of or yielding a narcotic **2** : of, induced by, or concerned with narcotics **3** : of, involving, or intended for narcotic addicts

nar·co·ti·za·tion \ˌnär-kə-tə-ˈzā-shən\ *n* : the act or process of inducing narcosis

nar·co·tize \ˈnär-kə-ˌtīz\ *vb* **-tized; -tizing 1** : to treat with or subject to a narcotic **2** : to put into a state of narcosis

Nar·dil \ˈnär-ˌdil\ *trademark* — used for a preparation of phenelzine

na·res \ˈnar-ˌēz\ *n pl* : the pair of openings of the nose

narrow–angle glaucoma *n* : CLOSED-ANGLE GLAUCOMA

narrow–spectrum *adj* : effective against only a limited range of organisms — compare BROAD-SPECTRUM

nas- *or* **naso-** *also* **nasi-** *comb form* **1** : nose : nasal (*naso*pharyngoscope) **2** : nasal and ⟨*naso*tracheal⟩

¹**na·sal** \ˈnā-zəl\ *n* : a nasal part (as a bone)

²**nasal** *adj* : of or relating to the nose — **na·sal·ly** *adv*

nasal bone *n* : either of two bones of the skull of vertebrates above the fishes that lie in front of the frontal bones and in humans are oblong in shape forming by their junction the bridge of the nose and partly covering the nasal cavity

nasal cavity *n* : the vaulted chamber that lies between the floor of the cranium and the roof of the mouth of higher vertebrates extending from the external nares to the pharynx, being enclosed by bone or cartilage and usu. incompletely divided into lateral halves by the septum of the nose, and having its walls lined with mucous membrane that is rich in venous plexuses and ciliated in the lower part which forms the beginning of the respiratory passage and warms and filters the inhaled air and that is modified as sensory epithelium in the upper olfactory part

nasal concha *n* : any of three thin bony plates on the lateral wall of the nasal fossa on each side with or without their covering of mucous membrane: **a** : a separate curved bony plate that is the largest of the three and separates the inferior and middle meatuses of the nose — called also *inferior concha, inferior nasal concha, inferior turbinate, inferior turbinate bone* **b** : the lower of two thin bony processes of the ethmoid bone on the lateral wall of each nasal fossa that sepa-

rates the superior and middle meatuses of the nose — called also *middle concha, middle nasal concha, middle turbinate, middle turbinate bone* **c** : the upper of two thin bony processes of the ethmoid bone on the lateral wall of each nasal fossa that forms the upper boundary of the superior meatus of the nose — called also *superior concha, superior nasal concha, superior turbinate, superior turbinate bone*

nasal fossa *n* : either lateral half of the nasal cavity

na·sa·lis \nā-ˈzā-ləs, -ˈsā-\ *n* : a small muscle on each side of the nose that constricts the nasal aperture

nasal nerve *n* : NASOCILIARY NERVE

nasal notch *n* : the rough surface on the anterior lower border of the frontal bone between the orbits which articulates with the nasal bones and the maxillae

nasal process *n* : FRONTAL PROCESS 1

nasal septum *n* : the bony and cartilaginous partition between the nasal passages

nasal spine *n* : any of several median bony processes adjacent to the nasal passages: as **a** : ANTERIOR NASAL SPINE **b** : POSTERIOR NASAL SPINE

nasi — see ALA NASI, LEVATOR LABII SUPERIORIS ALAEQUE NASI

nasi- — see NAS-

na·si·on \ˈnā-zē-ˌän\ *n* : the middle point of the nasofrontal suture

Na·smyth's membrane \ˈnā-smiths-\ *n* : the thin cuticular remains of the enamel organ which surrounds the enamel of a tooth during its fetal development and for a brief period after birth

  Nasmyth, Alexander (*d* 1848), British anatomist and dentist.

naso- — see NAS-

na·so·cil·i·ary \ˌnā-zō-ˈsi-lē-ˌer-ē\ *adj* : nasal and ciliary

nasociliary nerve *n* : a branch of the ophthalmic nerve distributed in part to the ciliary ganglion and in part to the mucous membrane and skin of the nose — called also *nasal nerve*

na·so·fron·tal \-ˈfrənt-əl\ *adj* : of or relating to the nasal and frontal bones

nasofrontal suture *n* : the cranial suture between the nasal and frontal bones

na·so·gas·tric \-ˈgas-trik\ *adj* : of, relating to, being, or performed by intubation of the stomach by way of the nasal passages (insertion of a ∼ tube)

na·so·la·bi·al \-ˈlā-bē-əl\ *adj* : of, relating to, located between, or occurring between the nose and the lips

na·so·lac·ri·mal *also* **na·so·lach·ry·mal** \-ˈla-krə-məl\ *adj* : of or relating to the lacrimal apparatus and nose

nasolacrimal duct *n* : a duct that transmits tears from the lacrimal sac to the inferior meatus of the nose

na·so·max·il·lary \-ˈmak-sə-ˌler-ē\ *adj* : of, relating to, or located between the nasal bone and the maxilla 〈~ fracture〉

na·so·pal·a·tine \-'pa-lə-ˌtīn\ *adj* : of, relating to, or connecting the nose and the palate

nasopalatine nerve *n* : a parasympathetic and sensory nerve that arises in the sphenopalatine ganglion, passes through the sphenopalatine foramen, across the roof of the nasal cavity to the nasal septum, and obliquely downward to and through the incisive canal, and innervates esp. the glands and mucosa of the nasal septum and the anterior part of the hard palate

na·so·pha·ryn·geal \ˌnā-zō-fə-'rin-jəl, -jē-əl; -ˌfar-ən-'jē-əl\ *adj* : of, relating to, or affecting the nose and pharynx or the nasopharynx

nasopharyngeal tonsil *n* : PHARYNGEAL TONSIL

na·so·pha·ryn·go·scope \-fə-'riŋ-gə-ˌskōp\ *n* : an instrument equipped with an optical system and used in examining the nasal passages and pharynx — **na·so·pha·ryn·go·scop·ic** \-fə-ˌriŋ-gə-'skä-pik\ *adj* — **na·so·phar·yn·gos·co·py** \-ˌfar-ən-'gäs-kə-pē\ *n*

na·so·phar·ynx \-'far-iŋks\ *n, pl* **-pha·ryn·ges** \-fə-'rin-(ˌ)jēz\ *also* **-phar·ynx·es** : the upper part of the pharynx continuous with the nasal passages — compare LARYNGOPHARYNX

na·so·tra·che·al \-'trā-kē-əl\ *adj* : of, relating to, being, or performed by means of intubation of the trachea by way of the nasal passage

na·tal \'nāt-ᵊl\ *adj* : of or relating to birth 〈the ~ death rate〉

na·tal·i·ty \nā-'ta-lə-tē, nə-\ *n, pl* **-ties** : BIRTHRATE

na·tes \'nā-ˌtēz\ *n pl* : BUTTOCKS

National Formulary *n* : a periodically revised book of officially established and recognized drug names and standards — abbr. *NF*

na·tri·ure·sis \ˌnā-trē-yù-'rē-səs\ *n* : excessive loss of cations and esp. sodium in the urine — **na·tri·uret·ic** \-'re-tik\ *adj or n*

natural childbirth *n* : a system of managing childbirth in which the mother receives preparatory education in order to remain conscious during and assist in delivery with minimal or no use of drugs or anesthetics

natural family planning *n* : a method of birth control that involves abstention from sexual intercourse during the period of ovulation which is determined through observation and measurement of bodily symptoms (as cervical mucus and body temperature)

natural food *n* : food that has undergone minimal processing and contains no preservatives or artificial additives (as synthetic flavorings)

natural history *n* : the natural development of something (as an organism or disease) over a period of time

natural immunity *n* : immunity that is possessed by a group (as a race, strain, or species) and occurs in an individual as part of its natural biologic makeup and that is sometimes considered to include that acquired passively in utero or from mother's milk or actively by exposure to infection — compare ACQUIRED IMMUNITY, ACTIVE IMMUNITY, PASSIVE IMMUNITY

natural killer cell *n* : a large granular lymphocyte capable of killing a tumor or microbial cell without prior exposure to the target cell and without having it presented with or marked by a histocompatibility antigen

na·tu·ro·path \'nā-chə-rə-ˌpath, nə-'tyùr-ə-\ *n* : a practitioner of naturopathy

na·tu·rop·a·thy \ˌnā-chə-'rä-pə-thē\ *n, pl* **-thies** : a system of treatment of disease that avoids drugs and surgery and emphasizes the use of natural agents (as air, water, and sunshine) and physical means (as manipulation and electrical treatment) — **na·tu·ro·path·ic** \ˌnā-chə-rə-'pa-thik, nə-ˌtyùr-ə-\ *adj*

nau·sea \'nȯ-zē-ə, -sē-ə; 'nȯ-zhə, -shə\ *n* : a stomach distress with distaste for food and an urge to vomit

nau·se·ant \'nȯ-zhənt, -zhē-ənt, -shənt, -shē-ənt\ *adj* : inducing nausea : NAUSEATING

nau·se·ate \'nȯ-zē-ˌāt, -zhē-, -sē-, -shē-\ *vb* **-at·ed; -at·ing** : to affect or become affected with nausea

nau·seous \'nȯ-shəs, 'nȯ-zē-əs\ *adj* **1** : causing nausea **2** : affected with nausea

Nav·ane \'na-ˌvān\ *trademark* — used for a preparation of thiothixene

na·vel \'nā-vəl\ *n* : a depression in the middle of the abdomen that marks the point of former attachment of the umbilical cord to the embryo — called also *umbilicus*

navel ill *n* : a serious septicemia of newborn animals caused by pus-producing bacteria entering the body through the umbilical cord or opening — called also *joint ill*

¹**na·vic·u·lar** \nə-'vi-kyə-lər\ *n* : a navicular bone: **a** : the one of the seven tarsal bones of the human foot that is situated on the big-toe side between the talus and the cuneiform bones — called also *scaphoid* **b** : SCAPHOID 2

²**navicular** *adj* **1** : resembling or having the shape of a boat 〈a ~ bone〉 **2** : of, relating to, or involving a navicular bone 〈~ fractures〉

navicular disease *n* : inflammation of the navicular bone and forefoot of the horse

navicular fossa *n* : the dilated terminal portion of the urethra in the glans penis

navicularis — see FOSSA NAVICULARIS

Nb *symbol* niobium

NBRT *abbr* National Board for Respiratory Therapy

NCI *abbr* National Cancer Institute

Nd *symbol* neodymium

NDT *abbr* neurodevelopmental treatment

Ne *symbol* neon

ne- *or* **neo-** *comb form* **1** : new : recent ⟨*neo*natal⟩ **2** : an abnormal new formation ⟨*neo*plasm⟩ **3** : new chemical compound isomeric with or otherwise related to (such) a compound ⟨*neo*stigmine⟩

near point *n* : the point nearest the eye at which an object is accurately focused on the retina when the maximum degree of accommodation is employed — compare FAR POINT

near·sight·ed \'nir-'sī-təd\ *adj* : able to see near things more clearly than distant ones : MYOPIC — **near·sight·ed·ly** *adv*

near·sight·ed·ness *n* : MYOPIA

neb·u·li·za·tion \ ,ne-byə-lə-'zā-shən\ *n* **1** : reduction of a medicinal solution to a fine spray **2** : treatment (as of respiratory diseases) by means of a fine spray — **neb·u·lize** \'ne-byə-,līz\ *vb*

neb·u·liz·er \-lī-zər\ *n* : ATOMIZER; *specif* : an atomizer equipped to produce an extremely fine spray for deep penetration of the lungs

Ne·ca·tor \nə-'kā-tər\ *n* : a genus of common hookworms that include internal parasites of humans and various other mammals, and that are prob. of African origin though first identified in No. America — compare ANCYLOSTOMA

neck \'nek\ *n* **1 a** : the usu. narrowed part of an animal that connects the head with the body; *specif* : the cervical region of a vertebrate **b** : the part of a tapeworm immediately behind the scolex from which new proglottids are produced **2** : a relatively narrow part suggestive of a neck: as **a** : a narrow part of a bone ⟨the ∼ of the femur⟩ **b** : CERVIX 2 **c** : the part of a tooth between the crown and the root

necr- *or* **necro-** *comb form* **1 a** : those that are dead : the dead : corpses ⟨*necro*philia⟩ **b** : one that is dead : corpse ⟨*necro*psy⟩ **2** : death : conversion to dead tissue : atrophy ⟨*necro*sis⟩

nec·ro \'ne-(,)krō\ *n* : NECROTIC ENTERITIS

nec·ro·bac·il·lo·sis \ ,ne-krō-,ba-sə-'lō-səs\ *n, pl* **-lo·ses** \-,sēz\ : any of several infections or diseases (as bullnose or calf diphtheria) that are either localized (as in foot rot) or disseminated through the body of the infected animal and that are characterized by inflammation and ulcerative or necrotic lesions from which a bacterium of the genus *Fusobacterium* (*F. necrophorum* syn. *Sphaerophorus necrophorus*) has been isolated — see QUITTOR

nec·ro·bi·o·sis \-bī-'ō-səs\ *n, pl* **-o·ses** \-,sēz\ : death of a cell or group of

cells within a tissue whether normal (as in various epithelial tissues) or part of a pathologic process — compare NECROSIS

necrobiosis li·poid·i·ca \-li-'pȯi-di-kə\ *n* : a disease of the skin that is characterized by the formation of multiple necrobiotic lesions esp. on the legs and that is often associated with diabetes mellitus

necrobiosis lipoidica dia·bet·i·co·rum \-,dī-ə-,be-ti-'kȯr-əm\ *n* : NECROBIOSIS LIPOIDICA

nec·ro·bi·ot·ic \ ,ne-krə-bī-'ä-tik\ *adj* : of, relating to, or being in a state of necrobiosis

nec·ro·phile \'ne-krə-,fīl\ *n* : one that is affected with necrophilia

nec·ro·phil·ia \ ,ne-krə-'fi-lē-ə\ *n* : obsession with and usu. erotic interest in or stimulation by corpses

¹**nec·ro·phil·i·ac** \-'fi-lē-,ak\ *adj* : of, relating to, or affected with necrophilia

²**necrophiliac** *n* : NECROPHILE

nec·ro·phil·ic \-'fi-lik\ *adj* : NECROPHILIAC

¹**nec·rop·sy** \'ne-,kräp-sē\ *n, pl* **-sies** : AUTOPSY

²**necropsy** *vb* **-sied; -sy·ing** : AUTOPSY

nec·rose \'ne-,krōs, -,krōz, ne-'krōz\ *vb* **nec·rosed; nec·ros·ing** : to undergo or cause to undergo necrosis

ne·cro·sis \nə-'krō-sis, ne-\ *n, pl* **ne·cro·ses** \-,sēz\ : death of living tissue; *specif* : death of a portion of tissue differentially affected by local injury (as loss of blood supply, corrosion, burning, or the local lesion of a disease) — compare *necrobiosis*

nec·ro·sper·mia \ ,ne-krə-'spər-mē-ə\ *n* : a condition in which the spermatozoa in seminal fluid are dead or motionless

ne·crot·ic \nə-'krä-tik, ne-\ *adj* : affected with, characterized by, or producing necrosis ⟨a ∼ gall bladder⟩

necrotic enteritis *n* : a serious infectious disease of young swine caused by a bacterium of the genus *Salmonella* (*S. cholerae-suis*) — called also *necro*; see PARATYPHOID

necrotic rhinitis *n* : BULLNOSE

nec·ro·tiz·ing \'ne-krə-,tī-ziŋ\ *adj* : causing, associated with, or undergoing necrosis ⟨∼ infections⟩ ⟨∼ tissue⟩

necrotizing angiitis *n* : an inflammatory condition of the blood vessels characterized by necrosis of vascular tissue

necrotizing papillitis *n* : necrosis of the papillae of the kidney — called also *necrotizing renal papillitis*

¹**nee·dle** \'nēd-ᵊl\ *n* **1** : a small slender usu. steel instrument designed to carry suture when sewing tissues in surgery **2** : a slender hollow instrument for introducing material into or removing material from the body parenterally

²**needle** *vb* **nee·dled; nee·dling** : to punc-

ture, operate on, or inject with a needle

needle aspiration biopsy *n* : a needle biopsy in which tissue is removed by aspiration into a syringe

needle biopsy *n* : a biopsy esp. of deep tissues done with a hollow needle

nee·dle·stick \'nēd-ᵊl-ˌstik\ *n* : an accidental puncture of the skin with an unsterile instrument (as a syringe) — called also *needlestick injury*

neg·a·tive \'ne-gə-tiv\ *adj* **1** : marked by denial, prohibition, or refusal **2** : marked by features (as hostility or withdrawal) opposing constructive treatment or development **3** : being, relating to, or charged with electricity of which the electron is the elementary unit **4** : not affirming the presence of the organism or condition in question (a ~ TB test) — **neg·a·tive·ly** *adv* — **neg·a·tiv·i·ty** \ˌne-gə-'ti-və-tē\ *n*

negative feedback *n* : feedback that tends to stabilize a process by reducing its rate or output when its effects are too great

negative pressure *n* : pressure that is less than existing atmospheric pressure

negative reinforcement *n* : psychological reinforcement by removal of an unpleasant stimulus when a desired response occurs

negative transfer *n* : the impeding of learning or performance in a situation by the carry-over of learned responses from another situation — compare INTERFERENCE 2

neg·a·tiv·ism \'ne-gə-ti-ˌvi-zəm\ *n* **1** : an attitude of mind marked by skepticism about nearly everything affirmed by others **2** : a tendency to refuse to do, to do the opposite of, or to do something at variance with what is asked — **neg·a·tiv·is·tic** \ˌne-gə-ti-'vis-tik\ *adj*

Neg-Gram \'neg-ˌgram\ *trademark* — used for a preparation of nalidixic acid

Ne·gri body \'nā-grē-\ *n* : an inclusion body found in the nerve cells in rabies
Negri, Adelchi (1876–1912), Italian physician and pathologist.

Neis·se·ria \nī-'sir-ē-ə\ *n* : a genus (family Neisseriaceae) of parasitic bacteria that grow in pairs and occas. tetrads and include the gonococcus (*N. gonorrhoeae*) and meningococcus (*N. meningitidis*)
Neis·ser \'nī-sər\, **Albert Ludwig Sigesmund (1855–1916),** German dermatologist.

neis·se·ri·an \nī-'sir-ē-ən\ *or* **neis·se·ri·al** \-ē-əl\ *adj* : of, relating to, or caused by bacteria of the genus *Neisseria* (~ culture) (~ infection)

nemat- *or* **nemato-** *comb form* **1** : thread (*nematocyst*) **2** : nematode (*nematology*)

ne·ma·to·cide *or* **ne·ma·ti·cide** \'ne-mə-tə-ˌsīd, ni-'ma-tə-\ *n* : a substance or preparation used to destroy nematodes — **ne·ma·to·cid·al** *also* **ne·ma·ti·cid·al** \ˌne-mə-tə-'sīd-ᵊl, ni-ˌma-tə-\ *adj*

ne·ma·to·cyst \'ne-mə-tə-ˌsist, ni-'ma-tə-\ *n* : one of the minute stinging organelles of various coelenterates

nem·a·tode \'ne-mə-ˌtōd\ *n* : any of a phylum (Nematoda) of elongated cylindrical worms parasitic in animals or plants or free-living in soil or water

Nem·a·to·di·rus \ˌne-mə-tə-'dī-rəs\ *n* : a genus of reddish strongylid nematode worms parasitic in the small intestine of ruminants and sometimes other mammals

nem·a·tol·o·gy \ˌne-mə-'tä-lə-jē\ *n, pl* **-gies** : a branch of zoology that deals with nematodes — **nem·a·tol·o·gist** \-jist\ *n*

Nem·bu·tal \'nem-byə-ˌtȯl\ *trademark* — used for the sodium salt of pentobarbital

neo- — see NE-

Neo–Ant·er·gan \ˌnē-ō-'an-'tər-gən\ *trademark* — used for a preparation of pyrilamine

neo·ars·phen·a·mine \ˌnē-ō-ärs-'fe-nə-ˌmēn\ *n* : a yellow powder $C_{13}H_{13}As_2N_2NaO_4S$ similar to arsphenamine in structure and use — called also *neosalvarsan*

neo·cer·e·bel·lum \ˌnē-ō-ˌser-ə-'be-ləm\ *n, pl* **-bellums** *or* **-bel·la** : the part of the cerebellum associated with the cerebral cortex in the integration of voluntary limb movements and comprising most of the cerebellar hemispheres and the superior vermis — compare PALEOCEREBELLUM — **neo·cer·e·bel·lar** \ˌnē-ō-ˌser-ə-'be-lər\ *adj*

neo·cin·cho·phen \ˌnē-ō-'siŋ-kə-ˌfen\ *n* : a white crystalline compound $C_{19}H_{17}NO_2$ used as an analgesic and in the treatment of gout

neo·cor·tex \ˌnē-ō-'kȯr-ˌteks\ *n, pl* **-cor·ti·ces** \-'kȯr-tə-ˌsēz\ *or* **-cortexes** : the dorsal region of the cerebral cortex that is unique to mammals — **neo·cor·ti·cal** \-'kȯr-ti-kəl\ *adj*

neo·dym·i·um \ˌnē-ō-'di-mē-əm\ *n* : a yellow metallic element — symbol *Nd*; see ELEMENT table

¹neo–Freud·ian \-'frȯi-dē-ən\ *adj, often cap N* : of or relating to a school of psychoanalysis that differs from Freudian orthodoxy in emphasizing the importance of social and cultural factors in the development of an individual's personality

²neo–Freudian *n, often cap N* : a member of or advocate of a neo-Freudian school of psychoanalysis
S. Freud — see FREUDIAN

Neo·het·ra·mine \ˌnē-ō-'he-trə-ˌmēn\ *trademark* — used for a preparation of thonzylamine

ne·ol·o·gism \nē-'ä-lə-ˌji-zəm\ *n* **1** : a new word, usage, or expression **2** : a word coined by a psychotic that is meaningless except to the coiner

neo·my·cin \ˌnē-ə-ˈmīs-ᵊn\ *n* : a broad-spectrum highly toxic antibiotic or mixture of antibiotics produced by a bacterium of the genus *Streptomyces* (*S. fradiae*) and used to treat local infections

ne·on \ˈnē-ˌän\ *n* : a colorless odorless primarily inert gaseous element — symbol *Ne*; see ELEMENT table

neo·na·tal \ˌnē-ō-ˈnāt-ᵊl\ *adj* : of, relating to, or affecting the newborn and esp. the human infant during the first month after birth — compare PRENATAL, POSTNATAL — **neo·na·tal·ly** *adv*

ne·o·nate \ˈnē-ə-ˌnāt\ *n* : a newborn child; *esp* : a child less than a month old

neo·na·tol·o·gist \ˌnē-ə-nā-ˈtä-lə-jist\ *n* : a specialist in neonatology

neo·na·tol·o·gy \-jē\ *n, pl* **-gies** : a branch of medicine concerned with the care, development, and diseases of newborn infants

neonatorum — see ICTERUS GRAVIS NEONATORUM, ICTERUS NEONATORUM, OPHTHALMIA NEONATORUM, SCLEREMA NEONATORUM

neo·pal·li·um \ˌnē-ō-ˈpa-lē-əm\ *n, pl* **-lia** \-lē-ə\ : the part of the cerebral cortex that develops from the area between the piriform lobe and the hippocampus, comprises the nonolfactory region of the cortex, and attains its maximum development in humans where it makes up the greater part of the cerebral hemisphere on each side — compare ARCHIPALLIUM

neo·pho·bia \ˌnē-ə-ˈfō-bē-ə\ *n* : dread of or aversion to novelty

neo·pla·sia \ˌnē-ə-ˈplā-zhə, -zhē-ə\ *n* **1** : the process of tumor formation **2** : a tumorous condition of the body

neo·plasm \ˈnē-ə-ˌpla-zəm\ *n* : a new growth of tissue serving no physiological function : TUMOR — compare CANCER 1

neo·plas·tic \ˌnē-ə-ˈplas-tik\ *adj* : of, relating to, or constituting a neoplasm or neoplasia — **neo·plas·ti·cal·ly** *adv*

neo·sal·var·san \ˌnē-ō-ˈsal-vər-ˌsan\ *n* : NEOARSPHENAMINE

neo·stig·mine \ˌnē-ə-ˈstig-ˌmēn\ *n* : a cholinergic drug used in the form of its bromide $C_{12}H_{19}BrN_2O_2$ or a sulfate derivative $C_{13}H_{22}N_2O_6S$ esp. in the treatment of some ophthalmic conditions and in the diagnosis and treatment of myasthenia gravis — see PROSTIGMIN

neo·stri·a·tum \ˌnē-ō-(ˌ)strī-ˈā-təm\ *n, pl* **-tums** *or* **-ta** \-tə\ : the evolutionarily older part of the corpus striatum consisting of the caudate nucleus and putamen — **neo·stri·a·tal** \-ˈāt-ᵊl\ *adj*

Neo-Sy·neph·rine \ˌnē-ō-si-ˈne-frən, -ˌfren\ *trademark* — used for a preparation of phenylephrine

Neo·thyl·line \ˌnē-ō-ˈthi-lən\ *trademark* — used for a preparation of dyphylline

neo·vas·cu·lar·i·za·tion \-ˌvas-kyə-lə-rə-

ˈzā-shən\ *n* : vascularization esp. in abnormal quantity (as in some conditions of the retina) or in abnormal tissue (as a tumor) — **neo·vas·cu·lar** \ˌnē-ō-ˈvas-kyə-lər\ *adj* — **neo·vas·cu·lar·i·ty** \-ˌvas-kyə-ˈlar-ə-tē\ *n*

neph·e·lom·e·ter \ˌne-fə-ˈlä-mə-tər\ *n* : an instrument for measuring turbidity (as to determine the number of bacteria suspended in a fluid) — **neph·e·lo·met·ric** \ˌne-fə-lō-ˈme-trik\ *adj* — **neph·e·lom·e·try** \-ˈläm-ə-trē\ *n*

nephr- *or* **nephro-** *comb form* : kidney ⟨*nephrectomy*⟩ ⟨*nephrology*⟩

ne·phrec·to·my \ni-ˈfrek-tə-mē\ *n, pl* **-mies** : the surgical removal of a kidney — **ne·phrec·to·mize** \-ˌmīz\ *vb*

neph·ric \ˈne-frik\ *adj* : RENAL

ne·phrit·ic \ni-ˈfri-tik\ *adj* **1** : RENAL **2** : of, relating to, or affected with nephritis

ne·phri·tis \ni-ˈfrī-təs\ *n, pl* **ne·phrit·i·des** \-ˈfri-tə-ˌdēz\ : acute or chronic inflammation of the kidney affecting the structure (as of the glomerulus or parenchyma) and caused by infection, degenerative process, or vascular disease — compare NEPHROSCLEROSIS, NEPHROSIS

neph·ri·to·gen·ic \ˌne-frə-tə-ˈje-nik, ni-ˌfri-tə-\ *adj* : causing nephritis

neph·ro·blas·to·ma \ˌne-frō-blas-ˈtō-mə\ *n, pl* **-mas** *or* **-ma·ta** \-mə-tə\ : WILMS' TUMOR

neph·ro·cal·ci·no·sis \ˌne-frō-ˌkal-si-ˈnō-səs\ *n, pl* **-no·ses** \-ˌsēz\ : a condition marked by calcification of the tubules of the kidney

neph·ro·gen·ic \ˌne-frə-ˈje-nik\ *adj* **1** : originating in the kidney : caused by factors originating in the kidney ⟨∼ hypertension⟩ **2** : developing into or producing kidney tissue

neph·ro·gram \ˈne-frə-ˌgram\ *n* : an X ray of the kidney

ne·phrog·ra·phy \ni-ˈfrä-grə-fē\ *n, pl* **-phies** : roentgenography of the kidney

-nephroi *pl of* -NEPHROS

neph·ro·li·thi·a·sis \ˌne-frō-li-ˈthī-ə-səs\ *n, pl* **-a·ses** \-ˌsēz\ : a condition marked by the presence of renal calculi

neph·ro·li·thot·o·my \-li-ˈthä-tə-mē\ *n, pl* **-mies** : the surgical operation of removing a calculus from the kidney

ne·phrol·o·gist \ni-ˈfrä-lə-jist\ *n* : a specialist in nephrology

ne·phrol·o·gy \ni-ˈfrä-lə-jē\ *n, pl* **-gies** : a medical specialty concerned with the kidneys and esp. with their structure, functions, or diseases

ne·phro·ma \ni-ˈfrō-mə\ *n, pl* **-mas** *also* **-ma·ta** \-mə-tə\ : a malignant tumor of the renal cortex

neph·ron \ˈne-ˌfrän\ *n* : a single excretory unit of the vertebrate kidney typically consisting of a Malpighian corpuscle, proximal convoluted tubule, loop of Henle, distal convoluted tubule, collecting tubule, and vascular and supporting tissues and discharging by way of a renal papilla into the renal pelvis

ne·phrop·a·thy \ni-ˈfrä-pə-thē\ *n, pl* **-thies** : an abnormal state of the kidney; *esp* : one associated with or secondary to some other pathological process — **neph·ro·path·ic** \ˌne-frə-ˈpa-thik\ *adj*

neph·ro·pexy \ˈne-frə-ˌpek-sē\ *n, pl* **-pex·ies** : surgical fixation of a floating kidney

neph·rop·to·sis \ˌne-ˌfräp-ˈtō-səs\ *n, pl* **-to·ses** \-ˌsēz\ : abnormal mobility of the kidney : floating kidney

ne·phror·rha·phy \ne-ˈfror-ə-fē\ *n, pl* **-phies** **1** : the fixation of a floating kidney by suturing it to the posterior abdominal wall **2** : the suturing of a kidney wound

-neph·ros \ˈne-frəs, -ˌfräs\ *n comb form, pl* **-neph·roi** \ˈne-ˌfroi\ : kidney ⟨pro*nephros*⟩

neph·ro·scle·ro·sis \ˌne-frō-sklə-ˈrō-səs\ *n, pl* **-ro·ses** \-ˌsēz\ : hardening of the kidney; *specif* : a condition that is characterized by sclerosis of the renal arterioles with reduced blood flow and contraction of the kidney, that is associated usu. with hypertension, and that terminates in renal failure and uremia — compare NEPHRITIS — **neph·ro·scle·rot·ic** \-ˈrä-tik\ *adj*

ne·phro·sis \ni-ˈfrō-səs\ *n, pl* **ne·phro·ses** \-ˌsēz\ *n* : a noninflammatory disease of the kidneys chiefly affecting function of the nephrons; *esp* : NEPHROTIC SYNDROME — compare NEPHRITIS

neph·ros·to·gram \ni-ˈfräs-tə-ˌgram\ *n* : a roentgenogram of the renal pelvis after injection of a radiopaque substance through an opening formed by nephrostomy

ne·phros·to·my \ni-ˈfräs-tə-mē\ *n, pl* **-mies** : the surgical formation of an opening between a renal pelvis and the outside of the body

ne·phrot·ic \ni-ˈfrä-tik\ *adj* : of, relating to, affected by, or associated with nephrosis ⟨∼ edema⟩ ⟨a ∼ patient⟩

nephrotic syndrome *n* : an abnormal condition that is marked by deficiency of albumin in the blood and its excretion in the urine due to altered permeability of the glomerular basement membranes (as by a toxic chemical agent)

neph·ro·to·mo·gram \ˌne-frō-ˈtō-mə-ˌgram\ *n* : a roentgenogram made by nephrotomography

neph·ro·to·mog·ra·phy \-tō-ˈmä-grə-fē\ *n, pl* **-phies** : tomographic visualization of the kidney usu. combined with intravenous nephrography — **neph·ro·to·mo·graph·ic** \-ˌtō-mə-ˈgra-fik\ *adj*

ne·phrot·o·my \ni-ˈfrä-tə-mē\ *n, pl* **-mies** : surgical incision of a kidney (as for the extraction of a stone)

neph·ro·tox·ic \ˌne-frə-ˈtäk-sik\ *adj* : poisonous to the kidney ⟨∼ drugs⟩; *also* : resulting from or marked by poisoning of the kidney ⟨∼ effects⟩ — **neph·ro·tox·ic·i·ty** \-täk-ˈsi-sə-tē\ *n*

neph·ro·tox·in \-ˈtäk-sən\ *n* : a cytotoxin that is destructive to kidney cells

Nep·ta·zane \ˈnep-tə-ˌzän\ *trademark* — used for a preparation of methazolamide

nep·tu·ni·um \nep-ˈtü-nē-əm, -ˈtyü-\ *n* : a radioactive metallic element — symbol *Np*; see ELEMENT table

nerve \ˈnərv\ *n* **1** : any of the filamentous bands of nervous tissue that connect parts of the nervous system with the other organs, conduct nervous impulses, and are made up of axons and dendrites together with protective and supportive structures and that for the larger nerves have the fibers gathered into funiculi surrounded by a perineurium and the funiculi enclosed in a common epineurium **2** *pl* : a state or condition of nervous agitation or irritability **3** : the sensitive pulp of a tooth

nerve block *n* **1** : an interruption of the passage of impulses through a nerve (as with pressure or narcotization) — called also *nerve blocking* **2** : BLOCK ANESTHESIA

nerve cell *n* : NEURON; *also* : CELL BODY

nerve center *n* : CENTER

nerve cord *n* : the dorsal tubular cord of nervous tissue above the notochord that in vertebrates includes or develops an anterior enlargement comprising the brain and a more posterior part comprising the spinal cord with the two together making up the central nervous system

nerve deafness *n* : hearing loss or impairment resulting from injury to or loss of function of the organ of Corti or the auditory nerve — called also *perceptive deafness*; compare CENTRAL DEAFNESS, CONDUCTION DEAFNESS

nerve ending *n* : the structure in which the distal end of the axon of a nerve fiber terminates

nerve fiber *n* : any of the processes (as axons or dendrites) of a neuron

nerve gas *n* : an organophosphate chemical weapon that interferes with normal nerve transmission and induces intense bronchial spasm with resulting inhibition of respiration

nerve growth factor *n* : a protein that promotes development of the sensory and sympathetic nervous systems and is required for maintenance of sympathetic neurons — abbr. *NGF*

nerve impulse *n* : the progressive physicochemical change in the membrane of a nerve fiber that follows stimulation and serves to transmit a record of sensation from a receptor or an instruction to act to an effector — called also *nervous impulse*

nerve of Her·ing \-ˈher-iŋ\ *n* : a nerve

that arises from the main trunk of the glossopharyngeal nerve and runs along the internal carotid artery to supply afferent fibers esp. to the baroreceptors of the carotid sinus

Hering, Heinrich Ewald (1866–1948), German physiologist.

nerve sheath *n* : NEURILEMMA

nerve trunk *n* : a bundle of nerve fibers enclosed in a connective tissue sheath

nervi *pl of* NERVUS

nerv·ing \'nər-vin\ *n* : the removal of part of a nerve trunk in chronic inflammation in order to cure lameness (as of a horse) by destroying sensation in the parts supplied

nervosa — see ANOREXIA NERVOSA, PARS NERVOSA

ner·vous \'nər-vəs\ *adj* **1** : of, relating to, or composed of neurons ⟨the ~ layer of the eye⟩ **2 a** : of or relating to the nerves; *also* : originating in or affected by the nerves ⟨~ energy⟩ **b** : easily excited or irritated — **ner·vous·ly** *adv* — **ner·vous·ness** *n*

nervous breakdown *n* : an attack of mental or emotional disorder esp. when of sufficient severity to require hospitalization

nervous impulse *n* : NERVE IMPULSE

nervous system *n* : the bodily system that in vertebrates is made up of the brain and spinal cord, nerves, ganglia, and parts of the receptor organs and that receives and interprets stimuli and transmits impulses to the effector organs — see CENTRAL NERVOUS SYSTEM; AUTONOMIC NERVOUS SYSTEM, PERIPHERAL NERVOUS SYSTEM

ner·vus \'nər-vəs, 'ner-\ *n, pl* **ner·vi** \'nər-ˌvī, 'ner-ˌvē\ : NERVE 1

nervus er·i·gens \-'er-i-ˌjenz\ *n, pl* **nervi er·i·gen·tes** \-ˌer-i-'jen-(ˌ)tēz\ : PELVIC SPLANCHNIC NERVE

nervus in·ter·me·di·us \-ˌin-tər-'mē-dē-əs\ *n* : the branch of the facial nerve that contains sensory and parasympathetic fibers and that supplies the anterior tongue and parts of the palate and fauces — called also *glossopalatine nerve*

nervus ra·di·a·lis \-ˌrā-dē-'ā-ləs\ *n, pl* **nervi ra·di·a·les** \-(ˌ)lēz\ : RADIAL NERVE

nervus ter·mi·na·lis \-ˌtər-mə-'nā-ləs\ *n, pl* **nervi ter·mi·na·les** \-(ˌ)lēz\ : a group of ganglionated nerve fibers that arise in the cerebral hemisphere near where the nerve tract leading from the olfactory bulb joins the temporal lobe and that pass anteriorly along this tract and the olfactory bulb through the cribriform plate to the nasal mucosa — called also *terminal nerve*

Nes·a·caine \'ne-sə-ˌkān\ *trademark* — used for a preparation of chloroprocaine

neth·a·lide \'ne-thə-ˌlīd\ *n* : PRONETHALOL

net·tle \'net-ᵊl\ *n* **1** : any plant of the genus *Urtica* **2** : any of various prickly or stinging plants other than one of the genus *Urtica*

nettle rash *n* : an eruption on the skin caused by or resembling the condition produced by stinging with nettles : URTICARIA

neur- *or* **neuro-** *comb form* **1** : nerve ⟨neural⟩ ⟨neurology⟩ **2** : neural : neural and ⟨neuromuscular⟩

neu·ral \'nur-əl, -'nyur-\ *adj* **1** : of, relating to, or affecting a nerve or the nervous system **2** : situated in the region of or on the same side of the body as the brain and spinal cord : DORSAL — compare HEMAL 2 — **neu·ral·ly** *adv*

neural arch *n* : the cartilaginous or bony arch enclosing the spinal cord on the dorsal side of a vertebra — called also *vertebral arch*

neural canal *n* **1** : VERTEBRAL CANAL **2** : the cavity or system of cavities in a vertebrate embryo that form the central canal of the spinal cord and the ventricles of the brain

neural crest *n* : the ridge of one of the folds forming the neural tube that gives rise to the spinal ganglia and various structures of the autonomic nervous system — called also *neural ridge;* compare NEURAL PLATE

neural fold *n* : the lateral longitudinal fold on each side of the neural plate that by folding over and fusing with the opposite fold gives rise to the neural tube

neu·ral·gia \nu-'ral-jə, nyu-\ *n* : acute paroxysmal pain radiating along the course of one or more nerves usu. without demonstrable changes in the nerve structure — compare NEURITIS — **neu·ral·gic** \-jik\ *adj*

neural groove *n* : the median dorsal longitudinal groove formed in the vertebrate embryo by the neural plate after the appearance of the neural folds — called also *medullary groove*

neural lobe *n* : the expanded distal portion of the neurohypophysis — called also *infundibular process, pars nervosa*

neural plate *n* : a thickened plate of ectoderm along the dorsal midline of the early embryo that gives rise to the neural tube and crests

neural ridge *n* : NEURAL CREST

neural tube *n* : the hollow longitudinal dorsal tube that is formed by infolding and subsequent fusion of the opposite ectodermal folds in the vertebrate embryo and gives rise to the brain and spinal cord

neur·amin·ic acid \ˌnur-ə-'mi-nik-, ˌnyur-\ *n* : an amino acid $C_9H_{17}NO_8$ of carbohydrate character occurring in the form of acyl derivatives

neur·amin·i·dase \ˌnur-ə-'mi-nə-ˌdās,

ₙnyür-, -ₙdāz\ n : a hydrolytic enzyme that is produced by some bacteria and viruses, splits mucoproteins by breaking a glucoside bond, and occurs as a cell-surface antigen of the influenza virus

neur·aprax·ia \ₙnür-ə-ʹprak-sē-ə, ₙnyür-, -(ₙ)ä-ʺ\ n : an injury to a nerve that interrupts conduction causing temporary paralysis but not degeneration and that is followed by a complete and rapid recovery

neur·as·the·nia \ₙnür-əs-ʹthē-nē-ə, ₙnyür-\ n : an emotional and psychic disorder that is characterized esp. by easy fatigability and often by lack of motivation, feelings of inadequacy, and psychosomatic symptoms

¹**neur·as·then·ic** \-ʹthe-nik\ adj : of, relating to, or having neurasthenia

²**neurasthenic** n : a person affected with neurasthenia

neur·ax·is \nür-ʹak-səs, nyür-\ n, pl **neur·ax·es** \-ₙsēz\ : CENTRAL NERVOUS SYSTEM

neu·rec·to·my \nü-ʹrek-tə-mē, nyü-\ n, pl **-mies** : the surgical excision of part of a nerve

neu·ri·lem·ma \ₙnür-ə-ʹle-mə, ₙnyür-\ n : the plasma membrane surrounding a Schwann cell of a myelinated nerve fiber and separating layers of myelin — **neu·ri·lem·mal** \-ʹle-məl\ adj

neu·ri·lem·mo·ma or **neu·ri·le·mo·ma** \-lə-ʹmō-mə\ n, pl **-mas** or **-ma·ta** \-mə-tə\ : a tumor of the myelinated sheaths of nerve fibers that consist of Schwann cells in a matrix — called also *neurinoma, schwannoma*

neu·ri·no·ma \ₙnür-ə-ʹnō-mə, ₙnyür-\ n, pl **-mas** or **-ma·ta** \-mə-tə\ : NEURILEMMOMA

neu·rite \ʹn(y)ü-ₙrīt\ n : AXON; also : DENDRITE

neu·ri·tis \nü-ʹrī-təs, nyü-\ n, pl **-rit·i·des** \-ʹri-tə-ₙdēz\ or **-ri·tis·es** : an inflammatory or degenerative lesion of a nerve marked esp. by pain, sensory disturbances, and impaired or lost reflexes — compare NEURALGIA — **neu·rit·ic** \-ʹri-tik\ adj

neu·ro \ʹnü-ₙrō, ʹnyü-\ adj : NEUROLOGICAL

neuro- — see NEUR-

neu·ro·ac·tive \ₙnür-ō-ʹak-tiv, ₙnyür-\ adj : stimulating neural tissue

neu·ro·anat·o·my \-ə-ʹna-tə-mē\ n, pl **-mies** : the anatomy of nervous tissue and the nervous system — **neu·ro·ana·tom·i·cal** \-ₙa-nə-ʹtä-mi-kəl\ also **neu·ro·ana·tom·ic** \-mik\ adj — **neu·ro·anat·o·mist** \-mist\ n

neu·ro·ar·throp·a·thy \-är-ʹthrä-pə-thē\ n, pl **-thies** : a joint disease (as Charcot's joint) that is associated with a disorder of the nervous system

neu·ro·be·hav·ior·al \-bi-ʹhā-vyə-rəl\ adj : of or relating to the relationship between the action of the nervous system and behavior

neu·ro·bi·ol·o·gy \-bī-ʹä-lə-jē\ n, pl **-gies** : a branch of biology that deals with the anatomy, physiology, and pathology of the nervous system — **neu·ro·bi·o·log·i·cal** \-ₙbī-ə-ʹlä-ji-kəl\ adj — **neu·ro·bi·ol·o·gist** \-bī-ʹä-lə-jist\ n

neu·ro·blast \ʹnür-ə-ₙblast, ʹnyür-\ n : a cellular precursor of a nerve cell; esp : an undifferentiated embryonic nerve cell — **neu·ro·blas·tic** \ₙnür-ə-ʹblas-tik, ₙnyür-\ adj

neu·ro·blas·to·ma \ₙnür-ō-blas-ʹtō-mə, ₙnyür-\ n, pl **-mas** or **-ma·ta** \-mə-tə\ : a malignant tumor formed of embryonic ganglion cells

neu·ro·cen·trum \-ʹsen-trəm\ n, pl **-trums** or **-tra** \-trə\ : either of the two dorsal elements of a vertebra that unite to form a neural arch from which the vertebral spine is developed — **neu·ro·cen·tral** \-ʹsen-trəl\ adj

neu·ro·chem·is·try \-ʹke-mə-strē\ n, pl **-tries 1** : the study of the chemical makeup and activities of nervous tissue **2** : chemical processes and phenomena related to the nervous system — **neu·ro·chem·i·cal** \-ʹke-mi-kəl\ adj or n — **neu·ro·chem·ist** \-mist\ n

neu·ro·cir·cu·la·to·ry \-ʹsər-kyə-lə-ₙtōr-ē\ adj : of or relating to the nervous and circulatory systems

neurocirculatory asthenia n : a condition marked by shortness of breath, fatigue, rapid pulse, and heart palpitation sometimes with extra beats that occurs chiefly with exertion and is not due to physical disease of the heart — called also *cardiac neurosis, effort syndrome, soldier's heart*

neu·ro·cra·ni·um \-ʹkrā-nē-əm\ n, pl **-ni·ums** or **-nia** \-nē-ə\ : the portion of the skull that encloses and protects the brain — **neu·ro·cra·ni·al** \-nē-əl\ adj

neu·ro·cu·ta·ne·ous \-kyü-ʹtā-nē-əs\ adj : of, relating to, or affecting the skin and nerves

neu·ro·cy·to·ma \-sī-ʹtō-mə\ n, pl **-mas** or **-ma·ta** \-mə-tə\ : any of various tumors of nerve tissue arising in the central or sympathetic nervous system

neu·ro·de·gen·er·a·tive \-di-ʹje-nə-rə-tiv, -ₙrā-\ adj : relating to or characterized by degeneration of nervous tissue — **neu·ro·de·gen·er·a·tion** \-ₙje-nə-ʹrā-shən\ n

neu·ro·der·ma·ti·tis \-ₙdər-mə-ʹtī-təs\ n, pl **-ti·tis·es** or **-tit·i·des** \-ʹti-tə-ₙdēz\ : a chronic allergic disorder of the skin characterized by patches of an itching lichenoid eruption and occurring esp. in persons of nervous and emotional instability

neu·ro·de·vel·op·ment \-di-ʹve-ləp-mənt\ n : the development of the nervous system — **neu·ro·de·vel·op·men·tal** \-ₙve-ləp-ʹment-ᵊl\ adj

neu·ro·di·ag·nos·tic \-ₙdī-ig-ʹnäs-tik\ adj : of or relating to the diagnosis of diseases of the nervous system

neu·ro·dy·nam·ic \-dī-ʹna-mik\ adj : of,

relating to, or involving communication between different parts of the nervous system — **neu·ro·dy·nam·ics** \-miks\ n

neu·ro·ec·to·derm \-'ek-tə-₁dərm\ n : embryonic ectoderm that gives rise to nervous tissue — **neu·ro·ec·to·der·mal** \-₁ek-tə-'dər-məl\ adj

neu·ro·ef·fec·tor \-i-'fek-tər, -₁tȯr\ adj : of, relating to, or involving both neural and effector components

neu·ro·elec·tric \-i-'lek-trik\ also **neu·ro·elec·tri·cal** \-tri-kəl\ adj : of or relating to the electrical phenomena (as potentials or signals) generated by the nervous system

neu·ro·en·do·crine \-'en-də-krən, -₁krīn, -₁krēn\ adj **1** : of, relating to, or being a hormonal substance that influences the activity of nerves **2** : of, relating to, or functioning in neurosecretion

neu·ro·en·do·cri·nol·o·gy \-₁en-də-kri-'nä-lə-jē, -(₁)krī-\ n, pl -gies : a branch of biology dealing with neurosecretion and the physiological interaction between the central nervous system and the endocrine system — **neu·ro·en·do·cri·no·log·i·cal** \-₁kri-nəl-'äj-i-kəl, -₁krī-, -₁krē-\ also **neu·ro·en·do·cri·no·log·ic** \-nə-'lä-jik\ adj — **neu·ro·en·do·cri·nol·o·gist** \-'nä-lə-jist\ n

neu·ro·ep·i·the·li·al \₁nūr-ō-₁e-pə-'thē-lē-əl, ₁nyūr-\ adj **1** : of or relating to neuroepithelium **2** : having qualities of both neural and epithelial cells

neu·ro·epi·the·li·o·ma \-₁thē-lē-'ō-mə\ n, pl -mas or -ma·ta \-mə-tə\ : a neurocytoma or glioma esp. of the retina

neu·ro·epi·the·li·um \-'thē-lē-əm\ n, pl -lia \-lē-ə\ **1** : the part of the embryonic ectoderm that gives rise to the nervous system **2** : the modified epithelium of an organ of special sense

neu·ro·fi·bril \₁nūr-ō-'fī-brəl, ₁nyūr-, -'fī-\ n : a fine proteinaceous fibril that is found in cytoplasm (as of a neuron) and is capable of conducting excitation — **neu·ro·fi·bril·lary** \-brə-₁ler-ē\ also **neu·ro·fi·bril·lar** \-brə-lər\ adj

neurofibrillary tangle n : an abnormality of the cytoplasm of the pyramidal cells of the hippocampus and neurons of the cerebral cortex that occurs esp. in Alzheimer's disease and appears under the light microscope after impregnation and staining with silver as arrays of parallel thick coarse argentophil fibers

neu·ro·fi·bro·ma \-fī-'brō-mə\ n, pl -mas also -ma·ta \-mə-tə\ : a fibroma composed of nervous and connective tissue and produced by proliferation of Schwann cells

neu·ro·fi·bro·ma·to·sis \-fī-₁brō-mə-'tō-səs\ n, pl -to·ses \-₁sēz\ : a disorder inherited as an autosomal dominant and characterized by brown spots on the skin, neurofibromas of peripheral nerves, and deformities of subcutaneous tissues and bone — abbr. *NF;* called also *Recklinghausen's disease, von Recklinghausen's disease*

neu·ro·fi·bro·sar·co·ma \-₁fī-brō-sär-'kō-mə\ n, pl -mas or -ma·ta \-mə-tə\ : a malignant neurofibroma

neu·ro·fil·a·ment \-'fi-lə-mənt\ n : a microscopic filament of protein that is found in the cytoplasm of neurons and that with neurotubules makes up the structure of neurofibrils — **neu·ro·fil·a·men·tous** \-₁fi-lə-'men-təs\ adj

neu·ro·gen·e·sis \₁nūr-ə-'je-nə-səs, ₁nyūr-\ n, pl -e·ses \-₁sēz\ : development of nerves, nervous tissue, or the nervous system

neu·ro·ge·net·ics \-jə-'ne-tiks\ n : a branch of genetics dealing with the nervous system and esp. with its development

neu·ro·gen·ic \₁nūr-ō-'je-nik, ₁nyūr-\ also **neu·rog·e·nous** \nū-'rä-jə-nəs, nyū-\ adj **1 a** : originating in nervous tissue ⟨a ~ tumor⟩ **b** : induced, controlled, or modified by nervous factors; esp : disordered because of abnormally altered neural relations ⟨the ~ kidney⟩ **2 a** : constituting the neural component of a bodily process ⟨~ factors in disease⟩ **b** : taking place or viewed as taking place in ordered rhythmic fashion under the control of a network of nerve cells scattered in the cardiac muscle ⟨a ~ heartbeat⟩ — compare MYOGENIC 2 — **neu·ro·gen·i·cal·ly** adv

neu·ro·glia \nū-'rō-glē-ə, nyū-, -'rä-; ₁nūr-ə-'glē-ə, ₁nyūr-, -₁gli-\ n : supporting tissue that is intermingled with the essential elements of nervous tissue esp. in the brain, spinal cord, and ganglia, is of ectodermal origin, and is composed of a network of fine fibrils and of flattened stellate cells with numerous radiating fibrillar processes — see MICROGLIA — **neu·ro·gli·al** \-əl\ adj

neu·ro·his·tol·o·gy \₁nūr-ō-hi-'stä-lə-jē, ₁nyūr-\ n, pl -gies : a branch of histology concerned with the nervous system — **neu·ro·his·to·log·i·cal** \-₁his-tə-'lä-ji-kəl\ also **neu·ro·his·to·log·ic** \-'lä-jik\ adj — **neu·ro·his·tol·o·gist** \-hi-'stä-lə-jist\ n

neu·ro·hor·mon·al \-hȯr-'mōn-əl\ adj **1** : involving both neural and hormonal mechanisms **2** : of, relating to, or being a neurohormone

neu·ro·hor·mone \-'hȯr-₁mōn\ n : a hormone (as acetylcholine or norepinephrine) produced by or acting on nervous tissue

neu·ro·hu·mor \-'hyü-mər, -'yü-\ n : NEUROHORMONE; esp : NEUROTRANSMITTER — **neu·ro·hu·mor·al** \-mə-rəl\ adj

neu·ro·hy·po·phy·se·al or **neu·ro·hy·po·phys·i·al** \-(₁)hī-₁pä-fə-'sē-əl, -hi-₁pä-fə-, -'zē-; -₁hī-pə-'fi-zē-əl\ adj : of, relating to, or secreted by the neurohypophysis ⟨~ hormones⟩

neu·ro·hy·poph·y·sis \-hī-'pä-fə-səs\ *n* : the portion of the pituitary gland that is derived from the embryonic brain, is composed of the infundibulum and neural lobe, and is concerned with the secretion of various hormones — called also *posterior pituitary gland*

neu·ro·im·mu·nol·o·gy \-i-myə-'nä-lə-jē\ *n, pl* **-gies** : a branch of immunology that deals esp. with the interrelationships of the nervous system and immune responses and autoimmune disorders

neu·ro·lem·mo·ma *var of* NEURILEMMOMA

neu·ro·lept·an·al·ge·sia \-₁lep-₁tan-ᵊl-'jē-zhə, -zhē-ə, -zē-ə\ *also* **neu·ro·lep·to·an·al·ge·sia** \-₁lep-tō-₁an-ᵊl-\ *n* : joint administration of a tranquilizing drug and an analgesic esp. for relief of surgical pain — **neu·ro·lept·an·al·ge·sic** \-'jē-zik, -sik\ *adj*

neu·ro·lep·tic \-'lep-tik\ *n* : any of the powerful tranquilizers (as the phenothiazines or butyrophenones) used esp. to treat psychosis and believed to act by blocking dopamine nervous receptors — called also *antipsychotic* — **neuroleptic** *adj*

neu·ro·lin·guis·tics \-liŋ-'gwis-tiks\ *n* : the study of the relationships between the human nervous system and language esp. with respect to the correspondence between disorders of language and the nervous system — **neu·ro·lin·guis·tic** \-tik\ *adj*

neu·rol·o·gist \nu̇-'rä-lə-jist, nyu̇-\ *n* : one specializing in neurology; *esp* : a physician skilled in the diagnosis and treatment of disease of the nervous system

neu·rol·o·gy \-jē\ *n, pl* **-gies** : the scientific study of the nervous system esp. in respect to its structure, functions, and abnormalities — **neu·ro·log·i·cal** \₁nu̇r-ə-'lä-ji-kəl, ₁nyu̇r-\ *or* **neu·ro·log·ic** \-jik\ *adj* — **neu·ro·log·i·cal·ly** *adv*

neu·rol·y·sis \nu̇-'rä-lə-səs, nyu̇-\ *n, pl* **-y·ses** \-₁sēz\ **1** : the breaking down of nerve substance (as from disease or exhaustion) **2** : the operation of freeing a nerve from adhesions — **neu·ro·lyt·ic** \₁nu̇r-ə-'li-tik, ₁nyu̇r-\ *adj*

neu·ro·ma \nu̇-'rō-mə, nyu̇-\ *n, pl* **-mas** *or* **-ma·ta** \-mə-tə\ **1** : a tumor or mass growing from a nerve and usu. consisting of nerve fibers **2** : a mass of nerve tissue in an amputation stump resulting from abnormal regrowth of the stumps of severed nerves — called also *amputation neuroma*

neu·ro·mod·u·la·tor \₁nu̇r-ō-'mä-jə-₁lā-tər, ₁nyu̇r-\ *n* : something (as a polypeptide) that potentiates or inhibits the transmission of a nerve impulse but is not the actual means of transmission itself — **neu·ro·mod·u·la·to·ry** \-lə-₁tȯr-ē\ *adj*

neu·ro·mo·tor \-'mō-tər\ *adj* : relating to efferent nervous impulses

neu·ro·mus·cu·lar \-'məs-kyə-lər\ *adj* : of or relating to nerves and muscles; *esp* : jointly involving nervous and muscular elements

neuromuscular junction *n* : the junction of an efferent nerve fiber and the muscle fiber plasma membrane — called also *myoneural junction*

neuromuscular spindle *n* : MUSCLE SPINDLE

neu·ro·my·eli·tis \₁nu̇r-ō-₁mī-ə-'lī-təs, ₁nyu̇r-\ *n* **1** : inflammation of the medullary substance of the nerves **2** : inflammation of both spinal cord and nerves

neu·ro·my·op·a·thy \-₁mī-'ä-pə-thē\ *n, pl* **-thies** : a disease of nerves and associated muscle tissue

neu·ron \'nü-₁rän, 'nyü-\ *also* **neu·rone** \-₁rōn\ *n* : one of the cells that constitute nervous tissue, that have the property of transmitting and receiving nervous impulses, and that possess cytoplasmic processes which are highly differentiated frequently as multiple dendrites or usu. as solitary axons and which conduct impulses toward and away from the nerve cell body — **neu·ro·nal** \'nü-rən-ᵊl, 'nyü-; nü-'rōn-ᵊl, nyü-\ *also* **neu·ron·ic** \nü-'rä-nik, nyü-\ *adj*

neu·ro·neu·ro·nal \₁nu̇r-ō-'nü-rən-ᵊl, ₁nyu̇r-ō-'nyu̇-; ₁nu̇r-ō-nü-'rōn-ᵊl, ₁nyu̇r-ō-nyu̇-\ *adj* : between nerve cells or nerve fibers

neu·ron·itis \₁nu̇r-ō-'nī-təs, ₁nyu̇r-\ *n* : inflammation of neurons; *esp* : neuritis involving nerve roots and nerve cells within the spinal cord

neu·ro·no·tro·pic \-'trō-pik, -'trä-\ *adj* : having an affinity for neurons : NEUROTROPIC

neu·ro·oph·thal·mol·o·gy \-₁äf-thəl-'mä-lə-jē, -₁äp-\ *n, pl* **-gies** : the neurological study of the eye — **neu·ro·oph·thal·mo·log·ic** \-mə-'lä-jik\ *or* **neu·ro·oph·thal·mo·log·i·cal** \-'lä-ji-kəl\ *adj*

neu·ro·otol·o·gy \-ō-'tä-lə-jē\ *n, pl* **-gies** : the neurological study of the ear — **neu·ro·oto·log·ic** \-ō-tə-'lä-jik\ *or* **neu·ro·oto·log·i·cal** \-'lä-ji-kəl\ *adj*

neu·ro·par·a·lyt·ic \-₁par-ə-'li-tik\ *adj* : of, relating to, causing, or characterized by paralysis or loss of sensation due to a lesion in a nerve

neu·ro·path·ic \₁nu̇r-ə-'pa-thik, ₁nyu̇r-\ *adj* : of, relating to, characterized by, or being a neuropathy — **neu·ro·path·i·cal·ly** *adv*

neu·ro·patho·gen·e·sis \-₁pa-thə-'je-nə-səs\ *n, pl* **-e·ses** \-₁sēz\ : the pathogenesis of a nervous disease

neu·ro·patho·gen·ic \-'je-nik\ *adj* : causing or capable of causing disease of nervous tissue (∼ viruses)

neu·ro·pa·thol·o·gist \₁nu̇r-ō-pə-'thä-lə-jist, ₁nyu̇r-\ *n* : a specialist in neuropathology

neu·ro·pa·thol·o·gy \-pə-ˈthä-lə-jē, -pa-\ *n, pl* **-gies** : pathology of the nervous system — **neu·ro·path·o·log·ic** \-pə-thə-ˈlä-jik\ *or* **neu·ro·path·o·log·i·cal** \-ji-kəl\ *adj*

neu·rop·a·thy \nu̇-ˈra-pə-thē, nyu̇-\ *n, pl* **-thies** : an abnormal and usu. degenerative state of the nervous system or nerves; *also* : a systemic condition (as muscular atrophy) that stems from a neuropathy

neu·ro·pep·tide \ˌnu̇r-ō-ˈpep-ˌtīd, ˌnyu̇r-\ *n* : an endogenous peptide (as an endorphin or an enkephalin) that influences neural activity or functioning

neu·ro·phar·ma·col·o·gist \-ˌfär-mə-ˈkä-lə-jist\ *n* : a specialist in neuropharmacology

neu·ro·phar·ma·col·o·gy \-ˌfär-mə-ˈkä-lə-jē\ *n, pl* **-gies 1** : a branch of medical science dealing with the action of drugs on and in the nervous system **2** : the properties and reactions of a drug on and in the nervous system — **neu·ro·phar·ma·co·log·i·cal** \-kə-ˈlä-ji-kəl\ *also* **neu·ro·phar·ma·co·log·ic** \-jik\ *adj*

neu·ro·phy·sin \-ˈfī-sᵊn\ *n* : any of several brain hormones that bind with and carry either oxytocin or vasopressin

neu·ro·phys·i·ol·o·gist \-ˌfi-zē-ˈä-lə-jist\ *n* : a specialist in neurophysiology

neu·ro·phys·i·ol·o·gy \-ˌfi-zē-ˈä-lə-jē\ *n, pl* **-gies** : physiology of the nervous system — **neu·ro·phys·i·o·log·i·cal** \-zē-ə-ˈlä-ji-kəl\ *also* **neu·ro·phys·i·o·log·ic** \-jik\ *adj* — **neu·ro·phys·i·o·log·i·cal·ly** *adv*

neu·ro·pil \ˈnu̇r-ō-ˌpil, ˈnyu̇r-\ *also* **neu·ro·pile** \-ˌpīl\ *n* : a fibrous network of delicate unmyelinated nerve fibers found in concentrations of nervous tissue esp. in parts of the brain where it is highly developed — **neu·ro·pi·lar** \ˌnu̇r-ō-ˈpī-lər, ˌnyu̇r-\ *adj*

neu·ro·psy·chi·a·trist \ˌnu̇r-ō-sə-ˈkī-ə-trist, ˌnyu̇r-, -sī-\ *n* : a specialist in neuropsychiatry

neu·ro·psy·chi·a·try \-sə-ˈkī-ə-trē, -sī-\ *n, pl* **-tries** : a branch of medicine concerned with both neurology and psychiatry — **neu·ro·psy·chi·at·ric** \-ˌsī-kē-ˈa-trik\ *adj* — **neu·ro·psy·chi·at·ri·cal·ly** *adv*

neu·ro·psy·chol·o·gist \-sī-ˈkä-lə-jist\ *n* : a specialist in neuropsychology

neu·ro·psy·chol·o·gy \-jē\ *n, pl* **-gies** : a science concerned with the integration of psychological observations on behavior and the mind with neurological observations on the brain and nervous system — **neu·ro·psy·cho·log·i·cal** \-ˌsī-kə-ˈlä-ji-kəl\ *adj* — **neu·ro·psy·cho·log·i·cal·ly** *adv*

neu·ro·psy·cho·phar·ma·col·o·gy \-ˌsī-kō-ˌfär-mə-ˈkä-lə-jē\ *n, pl* **-gies** : a branch of medical science combining neuropharmacology and psychopharmacology

neu·ro·ra·di·ol·o·gist \-ˌrā-dē-ˈä-lə-jist\ *n* : a specialist in neuroradiology

neu·ro·ra·di·ol·o·gy \-ˌrā-dē-ˈä-lə-jē\ *n, pl* **-gies** : radiology of the nervous system — **neu·ro·ra·dio·log·i·cal** \-dē-ə-ˈlä-ji-kəl\ *also* **neu·ro·ra·dio·log·ic** \-jik\ *adj*

neu·ro·ret·i·ni·tis \-ˌret-ᵊn-ˈī-təs\ *n, pl* **-nit·i·des** \-ˈni-tə-ˌdēz\ : inflammation of the optic nerve and the retina

neu·ror·rha·phy \nu̇-ˈrȯr-ə-fē, nyu̇-\ *n, pl* **-phies** : the surgical suturing of a divided nerve

neu·ro·sci·ence \ˈnu̇r-ō-ˈsī-əns, ˈnyu̇r-\ *n* : a branch (as neurophysiology) of biology that deals with the anatomy, physiology, biochemistry, or molecular biology of nerves and nervous tissue and esp. their relation to behavior and learning — **neu·ro·sci·en·tif·ic** \-ˌsī-ən-ˈti-fik\ *adj* — **neu·ro·sci·en·tist** \-ˈsī-ən-tist\ *n*

neu·ro·se·cre·tion \-si-ˈkrē-shən\ *n* **1** : the process of producing a secretion by nerve cells **2** : a secretion produced by neurosecretion — **neu·ro·se·cre·to·ry** \-ˈsē-krə-ˌtȯr-ē\ *adj*

neu·ro·sen·so·ry \-ˈsen-sə-rē\ *adj* : of or relating to afferent nerves

neu·ro·sis \nu̇-ˈrō-səs, nyu̇-\ *n, pl* **-ro·ses** \-ˌsēz\ : a mental and emotional disorder that affects only part of the personality, is accompanied by a less distorted perception of reality than in a psychosis, does not result in disturbance of the use of language, and is accompanied by various physical, physiological, and mental disturbances (as visceral symptoms or phobias)

neu·ro·stim·u·la·tor \ˌnu̇r-ō-ˈsti-myə-ˌlā-tər, ˌnyu̇r-\ *n* : a device that provides electrical stimulation to nerves

neu·ro·sur·geon \-ˈsər-jən\ *n* : a surgeon specializing in neurosurgery

neu·ro·sur·gery \-ˈsər-jə-rē\ *n, pl* **-gies** : surgery of nervous structures (as nerves, the brain, or the spinal cord) — **neu·ro·sur·gi·cal** \-ˈsər-ji-kəl\ *adj* — **neu·ro·sur·gi·cal·ly** *adv*

neu·ro·syph·i·lis \-ˈsi-fə-ləs\ *n* : syphilis of the central nervous system — **neu·ro·syph·i·lit·ic** \-ˌsi-fə-ˈli-tik\ *adj*

neu·ro·ten·di·nous spindle \-ˈten-di-nəs-\ *n* : GOLGI TENDON ORGAN

neu·ro·ten·sin \-ˈten-sən\ *n* : a protein composed of 13 amino acid residues that causes hypertension and vasodilation and is present in the brain

¹neu·rot·ic \nu̇-ˈrä-tik, nyu̇-\ *adj* **1 a** : of, relating to, or involving the nerves (a ~ disorder) **b** : being a neurosis : NERVOUS **2** : affected with, relating to, or characterized by neurosis — **neu·rot·i·cal·ly** *adv*

²neurotic *n* **1** : one affected with a neurosis **2** : an emotionally unstable individual

neu·rot·i·cism \-ˈrä-tə-ˌsi-zəm\ *n* : a neurotic character, condition, or trait

neu·ro·tol·o·gy \ˌnu̇r-ō-ˈtä-lə-jē, ˌnyu̇r-\ *var of* NEURO-OTOLOGY

neu·rot·o·my \-'rä-tə-mē\ *n, pl* **-mies 1** : the dissection or cutting of nerves **2** : the division of a nerve (as to relieve neuralgia)

neu·ro·tox·ic \ˌnùr-ō-'täk-sik, ˌnyùr-\ *adj* : toxic to the nerves or nervous tissue — **neu·ro·tox·ic·i·ty** \-ˌtäk-'si-sə-tē\ *n*

neu·ro·tox·i·col·o·gist \-ˌtäk-sə-'kä-lə-jist\ *n* : a specialist in the study of neurotoxins and their effects

neu·ro·tox·i·col·o·gy \-jē\ *n, pl* **-gies** : the study of neurotoxins and their effects — **neu·ro·tox·i·co·log·i·cal** \-kə-'lä-jə-kəl\ *adj*

neu·ro·tox·in \-'täk-sən\ *n* : a poisonous protein complex that acts on the nervous system

neu·ro·trans·mis·sion \-trans-'mi-shən, -tranz-\ *n* : the transmission of nerve impulses across a synapse

neu·ro·trans·mit·ter \-trans-'mi-tər, -tranz-; -'trans-ˌmi-, -'tranz-\ *n* : a substance (as norepinephrine or acetylcholine) that transmits nerve impulses across a synapse

neu·ro·troph·ic \-'trä-fik, -'trō-\ *adj* **1** : relating to or dependent on the influence of nerves on the nutrition of tissue **2** : NEUROTROPIC

neu·ro·trop·ic \-'trä-pik\ *adj* : having an affinity for or localizing selectively in nerve tissue ⟨~ viruses⟩ — compare PANTROPIC — **neu·rot·ro·pism** \nù-'rä-trə-ˌpi-zəm, nyù-\ *n*

neu·ro·tu·bule \ˌnùr-ō-'tü-byül, ˌnyùr-ō-'tyü-\ *n* : one of the tubular elements sometimes considered to be a fundamental part of the nerve-cell axon

neu·ro·vas·cu·lar \-'vas-kyə-lər\ *adj* : of, relating to, or involving both nerves and blood vessels

neu·ro·vir·u·lence \-'vir-yə-ləns, -'vir-ə-\ *n* : the tendency or capacity of a microorganism to attack the nervous system — **neu·ro·vir·u·lent** \-lənt\ *adj*

neu·ru·la \ˌnùr-yù-lə, ˌnyùr-, -ù-lə\ *n, pl* **-lae** \-ˌlē\ *or* **-las** : an early vertebrate embryo which follows the gastrula and in which nervous tissue begins to differentiate — **neu·ru·la·tion** \ˌnùr-yù-'lā-shən, ˌnyùr-, -ù-'lā-\ *n*

¹**neu·ter** \'nü-tər, 'nyü-\ *n* : a spayed or castrated animal (as a cat)

²**neuter** *vb* : CASTRATE, ALTER

neu·tral \'nü-trəl, 'nyü-\ *adj* **1** : not decided or pronounced as to characteristics **2** : neither acid nor basic : neither acid nor alkaline; *specif* : having a pH value of 7.0 **3** : not electrically charged

neutral fat *n* : TRIGLYCERIDE

neu·tral·ize \'nü-trə-ˌliz, 'nyü-\ *vb* **-ized; -iz·ing 1** : to make chemically neutral **2** : to counteract the activity or effect of : make ineffective **3** : to make electrically inert by combining equal positive and negative quantities

— **neu·tral·i·za·tion** \ˌnü-trə-lə-'zā-shən, ˌnyü-\ *n*

neutro- *comb form* **1** : neutral ⟨*neutro*phil⟩ **2** : neutrophil ⟨*neutro*penia⟩

neu·tron \'nü-ˌträn, 'nyü-\ *n* : an uncharged atomic particle that is nearly equal in mass to the proton

neu·tro·pe·nia \ˌnü-trə-'pē-nē-ə, ˌnyü-\ *n* : leukopenia in which the decrease in white blood cells is chiefly in neutrophils — **neu·tro·pe·nic** \-'pē-nik\ *adj*

¹**neu·tro·phil** \'nü-trə-ˌfil, 'nyü-\ *or* **neu·tro·phil·ic** \ˌnü-trə-'fi-lik, ˌnyü-\ *adj* : staining to the same degree with acid or basic dyes ⟨~ granulocytes⟩

²**neutrophil** *n* : a granulocyte that is the chief phagocytic white blood cell of the blood

neu·tro·phil·ia \ˌnü-trə-'fi-lē-ə, ˌnyü-\ *n* : leukocytosis in which the increase in white blood cells is chiefly in neutrophils

ne·void \'nē-ˌvóid\ *adj* : resembling a nevus ⟨a ~ tumor⟩; *also* : accompanied by nevi or similar superficial lesions

ne·vus \'nē-vəs\ *n, pl* **ne·vi** \-ˌvī\ : a congenital pigmented area on the skin : BIRTHMARK, MOLE; *esp* : a tumor made up chiefly of blood vessels — see BLUE NEVUS

nevus flam·me·us \-'fla-mē-əs\ *n* : PORT≠WINE STAIN

¹**new·born** \'nü-'bórn, 'nyü-\ *adj* **1** : recently born **2** : affecting or relating to the newborn

²**newborn** \-ˌbórn\ *n, pl* **newborn** *or* **newborns** : a newborn individual : NEONATE

New·cas·tle disease \'nü-ˌka-səl-, 'nyü-; nü-'ka-səl-, nyü-\ *n* : a disease of domestic fowl and other birds caused by a paramyxovirus and resembling bronchitis or coryza

new drug *n* : a drug that has not been declared safe and effective by qualified experts under the conditions prescribed, recommended, or suggested in the label and that may be a new chemical formula or an established drug prescribed for use in a new way

New Latin *n* : Latin as used since the end of the medieval period esp. in scientific description and classification

new·ton \'nü-tən, 'nyü-\ *n* : the unit of force in the metric system equal to the force required to impart an acceleration of one meter per second per second to a mass of one kilogram

NF *abbr* **1** National Formulary **2** neurofibromatosis

ng *abbr* nanogram

NG *abbr* nasogastric

n'ga·na \nə-'gä-nə\ *var of* NAGANA

NGF *abbr* nerve growth factor

NGU *abbr* nongonococcal urethritis

NHS *abbr* National Health Service

Ni *symbol* nickel

ni·a·cin \'nī-ə-sən\ *n* : a crystalline acid $C_6H_5NO_2$ that is a member of the vitamin B complex occurring usu. in the form of a complex of niacinamide in various animal and plant parts (as blood, liver, yeast, bran, and legumes) and is effective in preventing and treating human pellagra and blacktongue of dogs — called also *nicotinic acid*

ni·a·cin·amide \ˌnī-ə-ˈsi-nə-ˌmīd\ *n* : a bitter crystalline basic amide $C_6H_6N_2O$ that is a member of the vitamin B complex and is formed from and converted to niacin in the living organism, that occurs naturally usu. as a constituent of coenzymes, and that is used similarly to niacin — called also *nicotinamide*

ni·al·amide \nī-ˈa-lə-ˌmīd\ *n* : a synthetic antidepressant drug $C_{16}H_{18}N_4O_2$ that is an inhibitor of monoamine oxidase

nick \ˈnik\ *n* : a break in one strand of two-stranded DNA caused by a missing phosphodiester bond — **nick** *vb*

nick·el \ˈni-kəl\ *n* : a silver-white hard malleable ductile metallic element — symbol *Ni;* see ELEMENT table

nick·ing \ˈni-kiŋ\ *n* : localized constriction of a retinal vein by the pressure from an artery crossing it seen esp. in arterial hypertension

nicotin- *or* **nicotino-** *comb form* **1** : nicotine (*nicotini*c) **2** : nicotinic acid (*nicotin*amide)

nic·o·tin·amide \ˌni-kə-ˈtē-nə-ˌmīd, -ˈti-\ *n* : NIACINAMIDE

nicotinamide adenine dinucleotide *n* : NAD

nicotinamide adenine dinucleotide phosphate *n* : NADP

nic·o·tine \ˈni-kə-ˌtēn\ *n* : a poisonous alkaloid $C_{10}H_{14}N_2$ that is the chief active principle of tobacco

Ni·cot \nē-ˈkō\, **Jean** (1530?–1600), French diplomat.

nic·o·tin·ic \ˌni-kə-ˈtē-nik, -ˈti-\ *adj* : relating to, resembling, producing, or mediating the effects that are produced by acetylcholine liberated by nerve fibers at autonomic ganglia and at the neuromuscular junctions of voluntary muscle and that are mimicked by nicotine which increases activity in small doses and inhibits it in larger doses (∼ receptors) — compare MUSCARINIC

nicotinic acid *n* : NIACIN

nictitans — see MEMBRANA NICTITANS

nic·ti·tat·ing membrane \ˈnik-tə-ˌtā-tiŋ-\ *n* : a thin membrane found in many vertebrate animals at the inner angle or beneath the lower lid of the eye and capable of extending across the eyeball — called also *membrana nictitans, third eyelid*

ni·da·tion \nī-ˈdā-shən\ *n* **1** : the development of the epithelial membrane lining the inner surface of the uterus following menstruation **2** : IMPLANTATION b

NIDDM *abbr* non-insulin-dependent diabetes mellitus

ni·dus \ˈnī-dəs\ *n, pl* **ni·di** \-ˌdī\ *or* **ni·dus·es 1** : a place or substance in tissue where the germs of a disease or other organisms lodge and multiply **2** : a place where something originates or is fostered or develops

Nie·mann–Pick disease \ˈnē-ˌmän-ˈpik-\ *n* : an error in lipid metabolism that is inherited as an autosomal recessive trait, is characterized by accumulation of phospholipid in macrophages of the liver, spleen, lymph glands, and bone marrow, and leads to gastrointestinal disturbances, malnutrition, enlargement of the spleen, liver, and lymph nodes, and abnormalities of the blood-forming organs

Niemann, Albert (1880–1921) and **Pick, Ludwig (1868–1944),** German physicians.

ni·fed·i·pine \nī-ˈfe-də-ˌpēn\ *n* : a calcium channel blocker $C_{17}H_{18}N_2O_6$ that is a coronary vasodilator used esp. in the treatment of angina pectoris — see PROCARDIA

night blindness *n* : reduced visual capacity in faint light (as at night) — called also *nyctalopia* — **night–blind** \ˈnit-ˌblīnd\ *adj*

night·mare \ˈnīt-ˌmar\ *n* : a frightening dream accompanied by a sense of oppression or suffocation that usu. awakens the sleeper

night·shade \ˈnīt-ˌshād\ *n* **1** : any plant of the genus *Solanum* (family Solanaceae, the nightshade family) which includes some poisonous weeds, various ornamental garden plants, and important crop plants (as the potato and eggplant) **2** : BELLADONNA 1

night sweat *n* : profuse sweating during sleep that is sometimes a symptom of febrile disease

night terrors *n pl* : a sudden awakening in dazed terror occurring in children and often preceded by a sudden shrill cry uttered in sleep — called also *pavor nocturnus*

night vision *n* : ability to see in dim light (as provided by moon and stars)

ni·gra \ˈnī-grə\ *n* : SUBSTANTIA NIGRA — **ni·gral** \-grəl\ *adj*

nigricans — see ACANTHOSIS NIGRICANS

ni·gro·stri·a·tal \ˌnī-grō-strī-ˈāt-əl\ *adj* : of, relating to, or joining the corpus striatum and the substantia nigra

NIH *abbr* National Institutes of Health

ni·hi·lism \ˈnī-ə-ˌli-zəm, ˈnē-, -hə-\ *n* **1** : NIHILISTIC DELUSION **2** : skepticism as to the value of a drug or method of treatment (therapeutic ∼) — **ni·hi·lis·tic** \ˌnī-ə-ˈlis-tik, ˌnē-, -hə-\ *adj*

nihilistic delusion *n* : the belief that oneself, a part of one's body, or the real world does not exist or has been destroyed

nik·eth·amide \ni-ˈke-thə-ˌmīd\ *n* : a

bitter viscous liquid or crystalline compound $C_{10}H_{14}N_2O$ used chiefly in aqueous solution as a respiratory stimulant

NIMH *abbr* National Institute of Mental Health

ni·mo·di·pine \ni-'mō-də-ˌpēn\ *n* : a calcium channel blocker $C_{21}H_{26}N_2O_7$ used as a cerebral vasodilator

ninth cranial nerve *n* : GLOSSOPHARYNGEAL NERVE

ni·o·bi·um \nī-'ō-bē-əm\ *n* : a lustrous ductile metallic element — symbol *Nb*; see ELEMENT table

NIOSH *abbr* National Institute of Occupational Safety and Health

nip·per \'ni-pər\ *n* : an incisor of a horse; *esp* : one of the middle four incisors — compare DIVIDER

nip·ple \'ni-pəl\ *n* **1** : the protuberance of a mammary gland upon which in the female the lactiferous ducts open and from which milk is drawn **2** : an artificial teat through which a bottle-fed infant nurses

Ni·pride \'nī-ˌprīd\ *trademark* — used for a preparation of sodium nitroprusside

ni·sin \'nī-sən\ *n* : a polypeptide antibiotic that is produced by a bacterium of the genus *Streptococcus* (*S. lactis*) and is used as a food preservative esp. for cheese and canned fruits and vegetables

Nissl bodies \'ni-səl-\ *n pl* : discrete granular bodies of variable size that occur in the perikaryon and dendrites but not the axon of neurons and are composed of RNA and polyribosomes — called also *Nissl granules, tigroid substance*

    Nissl, Franz (1860–1919), German neurologist.

Nissl substance *n* : the nucleoprotein material of Nissl bodies — called also *chromidial substance*

nit \'nit\ *n* : the egg of a louse or other parasitic insect; *also* : the insect itself when young

ni·trate \'nī-ˌtrāt, -trət\ *n* : a salt or ester of nitric acid

nitric acid \'nī-trik-\ *n* : a corrosive liquid inorganic acid HNO_3

ni·trite \'nī-ˌtrīt\ *n* : a salt or ester of nitrous acid

ni·tri·toid \'nī-trə-ˌtȯid\ *adj* : resembling a nitrite or a reaction characterized esp. by flushing and faintness that is caused by a nitrite (a severe ~ crisis may follow arsphenamine injection)

ni·tro·ben·zene \ˌnī-trō-'ben-ˌzēn, -ben-'\ *n* : a poisonous yellow insoluble oil $C_6H_5NO_2$

ni·tro·fu·ran \ˌnī-trō-'fyùr-ˌan, -fyù-'ran\ *n* : any of several compounds containing a nitro group that are used as bacteria-inhibiting agents

ni·tro·fu·ran·to·in \-fyù-'ran-tō-in\ *n* : a nitrofuran derivative $C_8H_6N_4O_5$ that is a broad-spectrum antimicrobial

agent used esp. in treating urinary tract infections

ni·tro·fu·ra·zone \-'fyùr-ə-ˌzōn\ *n* : a pale yellow crystalline compound $C_6H_6N_4O_4$ used chiefly externally as a bacteriostatic or bactericidal dressing (as for wounds and infections)

ni·tro·gen \'nī-trə-jən\ *n* : a common nonmetallic element that in the free form is normally a colorless odorless tasteless insoluble inert gas containing two atoms per molecule and comprising 78 percent of the atmosphere by volume and that in the combined form is a constituent of biologically important compounds (as proteins, nucleic acids, alkaloids) — symbol *N*; see ELEMENT table

nitrogen balance *n* : the difference between nitrogen intake and nitrogen excretion in the animal body such that a greater intake results in a positive balance and an increased excretion causes a negative balance

nitrogen base *or* **nitrogenous base** *n* : a nitrogen-containing molecule with basic properties; *esp* : one that is a purine or pyrimidine

nitrogen dioxide *n* : a poisonous strongly oxidizing reddish brown gas NO_2

nitrogen mustard *n* : any of various toxic blistering compounds analogous to mustard gas but containing nitrogen instead of sulfur; *esp* : an amine $C_5H_{11}Cl_2N$ used in the form of its hydrochloride in treating neoplastic diseases (as Hodgkin's disease and leukemia)

nitrogen narcosis *n* : a state of euphoria and exhilaration that occurs when nitrogen in normal air enters the bloodstream at approximately seven times atmospheric pressure (as in deep-water diving) — called also *rapture of the deep*

ni·trog·e·nous \nī-'trä-jə-nəs\ *adj* : of, relating to, or containing nitrogen in combined form (as in proteins)

ni·tro·glyc·er·in *or* **ni·tro·glyc·er·ine** \ˌnī-trə-'gli-sə-rən\ *n* : a heavy oily explosive poisonous liquid $C_3H_5N_3O_9$ used in medicine as a vasodilator (as in angina pectoris)

ni·tro·mer·sol \ˌnī-trō-'mər-ˌsȯl, -ˌsōl\ *n* : a brownish yellow to yellow solid organic mercurial $C_7H_5HgNO_3$ used chiefly in the form of a solution of its sodium salt as an antiseptic and disinfectant — see METAPHEN

nitroprusside — see SODIUM NITROPRUSSIDE

ni·tro·sa·mine \nī-'trō-sə-ˌmēn\ *n* : any of various neutral compounds which are characterized by the grouping NNO and some of which are powerful carcinogens

ni·tro·so·di·meth·yl·amine \ˌnī-ˌtrō-sō-ˌdī-me-thə-'la-ˌmēn, -ə-'mēn\ *n* : DI-METHYLNITROSAMINE

ni·tro·so·urea \-yu̇-'rē-ə\ *n* : any of a group of lipid-soluble drugs that function as alkylating agents, have the ability to enter the central nervous system, and are effective in the treatment of some brain tumors and meningeal leukemias

ni·trous oxide \\'nī-trəs-\ *n* : a colorless gas N_2O that when inhaled produces loss of sensibility to pain preceded by exhilaration and sometimes laughter and is used esp. as an anesthetic in dentistry — called also *laughing gas*

NK cell \\'en-'kā-\ *n* : NATURAL KILLER CELL

nm *abbr* nanometer

NMR *abbr* nuclear magnetic resonance

No *symbol* nobelium

no·bel·i·um \nō-'be-lē-əm\ *n* : a radioactive element produced artificially — symbol *No*; see ELEMENT table

No·bel \nō-'bel\, **Alfred Bernhard (1833–1896),** Swedish inventor and philanthropist.

no·ble gas \\'nō-bəl-\ *n* : any of a group of rare gases that include helium, neon, argon, krypton, xenon, and sometimes radon and that exhibit great stability and extremely low reaction rates — called also *inert gas*

no·car·dia \nō-'kär-dē-ə\ *n* 1 *cap* : a genus of aerobic actinomycetes (family Actinomycetaceae) that include various pathogens as well as some soil-dwelling saprophytes 2 : any actinomycete of the genus *Nocardia* — **no·car·di·al** \-əl\ *adj*

No·card \nō-'kär\, **Edmond–Isidore–Etienne (1850–1903),** French veterinarian and biologist.

no·car·di·o·sis \nō-,kär-dē-'ō-səs\ *n, pl* **-o·ses** \-,sēz\ : actinomycosis caused by actinomycetes of the genus *Nocardia* and characterized by production of spreading granulomatous lesions — compare MADUROMYCOSIS

noci- *comb form* : pain ⟨*nociceptor*⟩

no·ci·cep·tive \,nō-si-'sep-tiv\ *adj* 1 *of a stimulus* : causing pain or injury 2 : of, induced by, or responding to a nociceptive stimulus — used esp. of receptors or protective reflexes

no·ci·cep·tor \-'sep-tər\ *n* : a receptor for injurious or painful stimuli : a pain sense organ

noc·tu·ria \näk-'tur-ē-ə, -'tyur-\ *n* : urination at night esp. when excessive

noc·tur·nal \näk-'tərn-əl\ *adj* 1 : of, relating to, or occurring at night ⟨~ myoclonus⟩ 2 : characterized by nocturnal activity

nocturnal emission *n* : an involuntary discharge of semen during sleep often accompanied by an erotic dream — see WET DREAM

nocturnus — see PAVOR NOCTURNUS

noc·u·ous \\'nä-kyə-wəs\ *adj* : likely to cause injury ⟨a ~ stimulus⟩

nod·al \\'nōd-əl\ *adj* : being, relating to, or located at or near a node — **nod·al·ly** *adv*

node \\'nōd\ *n* 1 : a pathological swelling or enlargement (as of a rheumatic joint) 2 : a body part resembling a knot; *esp* : a discrete mass of one kind of tissue enclosed in tissue of a different kind — see ATRIOVENTRICULAR NODE, LYMPH NODE

node of Ran·vier \-,rän'-vē-'ā\ *n* : a constriction in the myelin sheath of a myelinated nerve fiber

L.–R. Ranvier — see MERKEL–RANVIER CORPUSCLE

no·do·sa — see PERIARTERITIS NODOSA, POLYARTERITIS NODOSA

no·dose ganglion \\'nō-,dōs-\ *n* : INFERIOR GANGLION 2

no·do·sum — see ERYTHEMA NODOSUM

nod·u·lar \\'nä-jə-lər\ *adj* : of, relating to, characterized by, or occurring in the form of nodules ⟨~ lesions⟩ — **nod·u·lar·i·ty** \,nä-jə-'lar-ə-tē\ *n*

nodular disease *n* : infestation with or disease caused by nodular worms of the genus *Oesophagostomum* — called also *nodule worm disease*

nodular worm *n* : any of several nematode worms of the genus *Oesophagostomum* that are parasitic in the large intestine of ruminants and swine — called also *nodule worm*

nod·ule \\'nä-(,)jül\ *n* : a small mass of rounded or irregular shape: as **a** : a small abnormal knobby bodily protuberance (as a tumorous growth or a calcification near an arthritic joint) **b** : the nodulus of the cerebellum

nod·u·lus \\'nä-jə-ləs\ *n, pl* **nod·u·li** \-,lī\ : NODULE; *esp* : a prominence on the inferior surface of the cerebellum forming the anterior end of the vermis

noire — see TACHE NOIRE

noise pollution *n* : environmental pollution consisting of annoying or harmful noise (as of automobiles or jet airplanes) — called also *sound pollution*

no·ma \\'nō-mə\ *n* : a spreading invasive gangrene chiefly of the lining of the cheek and lips that is usu. fatal and occurs most often in persons severely debilitated by disease or profound nutritional deficiency — see CANCRUM ORIS

no·men·cla·ture \\'nō-mən-,klā-chər\ *n* : a system of terms used in a particular science; *esp* : an international system of standardized New Latin names used in biology for kinds and groups of kinds of animals and plants — see BINOMIAL NOMENCLATURE — **no·men·cla·tur·al** \,nō-mən-'klā-chə-rəl\ *adj*

No·mi·na An·a·tom·i·ca \'nä-mi-nə-,a-nə-'tä-mi-kə, 'nō-\ *n* : the Latin anatomical nomenclature that was prepared by revising the Basle Nomina Anatomica, adopted in 1955 at the Sixth International Congress of Anatomists, and modified at subsequent Congresses — abbr. *NA*

no·mo·top·ic \,nä-mə-'tō-pik, ,nō-,

-tä- *adj* : occurring in the normal place

-n•o•my \n-ə-mē\ *n comb form, pl* **-nomies** : system of laws or sum of knowledge regarding a (specified) field ⟨taxo*nomy*⟩

non- *prefix* : not : reverse of : absence of ⟨*non*allergic⟩

non•ab•sorb•able \ˌnän-əb-ˈsȯr-bə-bəl, -ˈzȯr-\ *adj* : not capable of being absorbed ⟨∼ silk sutures⟩

non•ac•id \ˈa-səd\ *adj* : not acid : being without acid properties

non•adap•tive \ˌnän-ə-ˈdap-tiv\ *adj* : not serving to adapt the individual to the environment ⟨∼ traits⟩

non•ad•dict \ˈa-dikt\ *n* : a person who is not addicted to a drug

non•ad•dict•ing \-ə-ˈdik-tiŋ\ *adj* : not causing addiction

non•ad•dic•tive \-ə-ˈdik-tiv\ *adj* : NON-ADDICTING

non•al•le•lic \ˌnän-ə-ˈlē-lik, -ˈle-\ *adj* : not behaving as alleles toward one another ⟨∼ genes⟩

non•al•ler•gen•ic \ˌa-lər-ˈje-nik\ *adj* : not causing an allergic reaction

non•al•ler•gic \-ə-ˈlər-jik\ *adj* : not allergic ⟨∼ individuals⟩ ⟨a ∼ reaction⟩

non•am•bu•la•to•ry \ˈam-byə-lə-ˌtȯr-ē\ *adj* : not able to walk about ⟨∼ patients⟩

non–A, non–B hepatitis \ˌnän-ˈā-ˌnän-ˈbē-\ *n* : hepatitis clinically and immunologically similar to hepatitis A and hepatitis B but caused by different viruses

non•an•ti•bi•ot•ic \-ˌan-tē-bī-ˈä-tik, -ˌan-ˌtī-\ *adj* : not antibiotic

non•an•ti•gen•ic \-ˌan-ti-ˈje-nik\ *adj* : not antigenic ⟨∼ materials⟩

non•ar•tic•u•lar \ˌnän-är-ˈti-kyə-lər\ *adj* : affecting or involving soft tissues (as muscles and connective tissues) rather than joints ⟨∼ rheumatic disorders⟩

non•as•so•cia•tive \-ə-ˈsō-shē-ˌā-tiv, -sē-ˌā-tiv, -shə/tiv\ *adj* : relating to or being learning (as habituation and sensitization) that is not associative learning

non•bac•te•ri•al \-bak-ˈtir-ē-əl\ *adj* : not of, relating to, caused by, or being bacteria ⟨∼ pneumonia⟩

non•bar•bi•tu•rate \-bär-ˈbi-chə-rət, -ˌrāt\ *adj* : not derived from barbituric acid

non•bio•log•i•cal \-ˌbī-ə-ˈlä-ji-kəl\ *adj* : not biological

non•can•cer•ous \-ˈkan-sə-rəs\ *adj* : not affected with or being cancer

non•car•ci•no•gen•ic \-ˌkär-ˌsi-nə-ˈje-nik, -ˌkärs-ᵊn-ə-\ *adj* : not causing cancer — **non•car•cin•o•gen** \-kär-ˈsi-nə-jən, -ˈkärs-ᵊn-ə-ˌjen\ *n*

non•car•di•ac \-kär-dē-ˌak\ *adj* : not cardiac: as **a** : not affected with heart disease **b** : not relating to the heart or heart disease ⟨∼ disorders⟩

non•cel•lu•lar \-ˈsel-yə-lər\ *adj* : not made up of or divided into cells

non•chro•mo•som•al \-ˌkrō-mə-ˈsō-məl\ *adj* **1** : not situated on a chromosome ⟨∼ DNA⟩ **2** : not involving chromosomes ⟨∼ mutations⟩

non•cod•ing \-ˈkō-diŋ\ *adj* : not specifying the genetic code ⟨∼ DNA⟩

non•co•ital \-ˈkō-ət-ᵊl, -kō-ˈēt-ᵊl\ *adj* : not involving heterosexual copulation

non•com•mu•ni•ca•ble \-kə-ˈmyü-ni-kə-bəl\ *adj* : not capable of being communicated; *specif* : not transmissible by direct contact ⟨a ∼ disease⟩

non•com•pli•ance \-kəm-ˈplī-əns\ *n* : failure or refusal to comply (as in the taking of prescribed medication) — **non•com•pli•ant** \-ənt\ *adj*

non com•pos men•tis \ˌnän-ˈkäm-pəs-ˈmen-təs, ˌnōn-\ *adj* : not of sound mind

non•con•scious \-ˈkän-chəs\ *adj* : not conscious

non•con•ta•gious \ˌnän-kən-ˈtā-jəs\ *adj* : not contagious

non•con•trac•tile \-kən-ˈtrakt-ᵊl, -ˌīl\ *adj* : not contractile ⟨∼ fibers⟩

non•con•vul•sive \-kən-ˈvəl-siv\ *adj* : not convulsive ⟨∼ seizures⟩

non•cor•o•nary \-ˈkȯr-ə-ˌner-ē, -ˈkär-\ *adj* : not affecting, affected with disease of, or involving the coronary vessels of the heart

non•de•form•ing \-di-ˈfȯr-miŋ\ *adj* : not causing deformation

¹**non•di•a•bet•ic** \-ˌdī-ə-ˈbe-tik\ *adj* : not affected with diabetes

²**nondiabetic** *n* : an individual not affected with diabetes

non•di•a•lyz•able \-ˌdī-ə-ˈlī-zə-bəl\ *adj* : not dialyzable

non•di•rec•tive \ˌnän-də-ˈrek-tiv, -(ˌ)dī-\ *adj* : of, relating to, or being psychotherapy, counseling, or interviewing in which the counselor refrains from interpretation or explanation but encourages the client (as by repeating phrases) to talk freely

non•dis•junc•tion \-dis-ˈjəŋk-shən\ *n* : failure of homologous chromosomes or sister chromatids to separate subsequent to metaphase in meiosis or mitosis so that one daughter cell has both and the other neither of the chromosomes

non•dis•sem•i•nat•ed \-di-ˈse-mə-ˌnā-təd\ *adj* : not disseminated ⟨∼ lupus erythematosus⟩

non•di•vid•ing \-də-ˈvī-diŋ\ *adj* : not undergoing cell division

non•drug \ˌnän-ˈdrəg\ *adj* : not relating to, being, or employing drugs

non•elas•tic \-i-ˈlas-tik\ *adj* : not elastic ⟨∼ fibrous tissue⟩

non•emer•gen•cy \-i-ˈmər-jən-sē\ *adj* : not being or requiring emergency care ⟨∼ surgery⟩ ⟨∼ patients⟩

non•en•zy•mat•ic \-i-ˈma-tik\ *or* **non•en•zy•mic** \-en-ˈzī-mik\ *also* **non•en•zyme** \-ˈen-ˌzīm\ *adj* : not involving the action of enzymes

non•es•sen•tial \-i-ˈsen-chəl\ *adj* : being a nonessential amino acid

nonessential amino acid *n* : any of various amino acids which are required for normal health and growth, whose carbon chains can be synthesized within the body or which can be derived in the body from essential amino acids, and which include alanine, asparagine, aspartic acid, cystine, glutamic acid, glutamine, glycine, proline, serine, and tyrosine

non·fat \ˈnän-ˈfat\ *adj* : lacking fat solids : having fat solids removed ⟨∼ milk⟩

non·fa·tal \-ˈfāt-ᵊl\ *adj* : not fatal

non·fe·brile \-ˈfe-ˌbril, -ˈfē-\ *adj* : not febrile ⟨∼ illnesses⟩

non·flag·el·lat·ed \-ˈfla-jə-ˌlā-təd\ *adj* : not having flagella

non·func·tion·al \-ˈfeŋk-shə-nəl\ *adj* : not performing or able to perform a regular function ⟨a ∼ muscle⟩

non·ge·net·ic \-jə-ˈne-tik\ *adj* : not genetic ⟨∼ diseases⟩

non·glan·du·lar \-ˈglan-jə-lər\ *adj* : not glandular ⟨the ∼ mucosa⟩

non·gono·coc·cal \-ˌgä-nə-ˈkä-kəl\ *adj* : not caused by a gonococcus ⟨∼ urethritis⟩

non·gran·u·lar \-ˈgra-nyə-lər\ *adj* : not granular; *esp* : characterized by or being cytoplasm which does not contain granules ⟨∼ white blood cells⟩

non·grav·id \-ˈgra-vid\ *adj* : not pregnant

non·heme \-ˈhēm\ *adj* : not containing or being iron that is bound in a porphyrin ring like that of heme

non·he·mo·lyt·ic \-ˌhē-mə-ˈli-tik\ *adj* : not causing or characterized by hemolysis ⟨a ∼ streptococcus⟩

non·hem·or·rhag·ic \-he-mə-ˈra-jik\ *adj* : not causing or associated with hemorrhage ⟨∼ shock⟩

non·he·red·i·tary \-hə-ˈre-də-ˌter-ē\ *adj* : not hereditary

non·her·i·ta·ble \-ˈher-ə-tə-bəl\ *adj* : not heritable ⟨∼ diseases⟩

non·his·tone \-ˈhis-ˌtōn\ *adj* : relating to or being any of the eukaryotic proteins (as DNA polymerase) that form complexes with DNA but are not considered histones

non–Hodgkin's lymphoma \-ˈhäj-kinz-\ *n* : any of the numerous malignant lymphomas (as Burkitt's lymphoma) that are not classified as Hodgkin's disease and that usu. have malignant cells derived from B cells or T cells

non·ho·mol·o·gous \-hō-ˈmä-lə-gəs, -hə-\ *adj* : being of unlike genic constitution — used of chromosomes of one set containing nonallelic genes

non·hor·mon·al \-hȯr-ˈmōn-ᵊl\ *adj* : not hormonal

non·hos·pi·tal \-ˈhäs-ˌpit-ᵊl\ *adj* : not relating to, associated with, or occurring within a hospital ⟨∼ clinics⟩

non·hos·pi·tal·ized \-ˈhäs-ˌpit-ᵊl-ˌīzd\ *adj* : not hospitalized ⟨∼ patients⟩

non·iden·ti·cal \-(ˌ)ī-ˈden-ti-kəl\ *adj* : not identical; *esp* : FRATERNAL

non·im·mune \-i-ˈmyün\ *adj* : not immune

non·in·fect·ed \-in-ˈfek-təd\ *adj* : not having been subjected to infection

non·in·fec·tious \-in-ˈfek-shəs\ *adj* : not infectious ⟨∼ endocarditis⟩

non·in·fec·tive \-tiv\ *adj* : not infective ⟨∼ leukemia⟩

non·in·flam·ma·to·ry \-in-ˈfla-mə-ˌtōr-ē\ *adj* : not inflammatory

non·in·sti·tu·tion·al·ized \-ˌin-stə-ˈtü-shə-nə-ˌlizd, -ˈtyü-\ *adj* : not institutionalized

non–insulin–dependent diabetes mellitus *n* : a common form of diabetes mellitus that develops esp. in adults and most often in obese individuals and that is characterized by hyperglycemia resulting from impaired insulin utilization coupled with the body's inability to compensate with increased insulin production — abbr. *NIDDM;* called also *adult-onset diabetes, maturity-onset diabetes, non-insulin= dependent diabetes, type II diabetes*

non·in·va·sive \-in-ˈvā-siv, -ziv\ *adj* **1** : not tending to spread; *specif* : not tending to infiltrate and destroy healthy tissue ⟨∼ cancer of the bladder⟩ **2** : not involving penetration (as by surgery) of the skin of the intact organism ⟨∼ diagnostic techniques⟩ — **non·in·va·sive·ly** *adv* — **non·in·va·sive·ness** *n*

non·ir·ra·di·at·ed \-i-ˈrā-dē-ˌā-təd\ *adj* : not having been exposed to radiation

non·ke·tot·ic \-kē-ˈtä-tik\ *adj* : not associated with ketosis ⟨∼ diabetes⟩

non·liv·ing \-ˈli-viŋ\ *adj* : not having or characterized by life

non·lym·pho·cyt·ic \-ˌlim-fə-ˈsi-tik\ *adj* : not lymphocytic; *esp* : being or relating to a form of leukemia other than lymphocytic leukemia

non·ma·lig·nant \-mə-ˈlig-nənt\ *adj* : not malignant ⟨a ∼ tumor⟩

non·med·ul·lat·ed \-ˈmed-ᵊl-ˌā-təd, -ˈme-jə-ˌlā-\ *adj* : UNMYELINATED

non·met·al \-ˈmet-ᵊl\ *n* : a chemical element (as carbon) that lacks the characteristics of a metal — **non·me·tal·lic** \-mə-ˈta-lik\ *adj*

non·mi·cro·bi·al \-mī-ˈkrō-bē-əl\ *adj* : not microbial ⟨∼ diseases⟩

non·mo·tile \-ˈmōt-ᵊl, -ˈmō-ˌtīl\ *adj* : not motile ⟨∼ gametes⟩

non·my·elin·at·ed \-ˈmī-ə-lə-ˌnā-təd\ *adj* : UNMYELINATED

non·nar·cot·ic \-när-ˈkä-tik\ *adj* : not narcotic ⟨∼ analgesics⟩

non·neo·plas·tic \-ˌnē-ə-ˈplas-tik\ *adj* : not being or not caused by neoplasms ⟨∼ diseases⟩

non·ner·vous \-ˈnər-vəs\ *adj* : not nervous ⟨∼ tissue⟩

non·nu·cle·at·ed \-ˈnü-klē-ˌā-təd, -ˈnyü-\ *adj* : not nucleated ⟨∼ bacterial cells⟩

non·nu·tri·tive \-ˈnü-trə-tiv, -ˈnyü-\ *adj* : not relating to or providing nutrition

non·obese \-ō-'bēs\ *adj* : not obese

non·ob·struc·tive \-əb-'strək-tiv\ *adj* : not causing or characterized by obstruction (as of a bodily passage)

non·oc·clu·sive \-ə-'klü-siv\ *adj* : not causing or characterized by occlusion

non·of·fi·cial \-ə-'fi-shəl\ *adj* : not described in the current *U.S. Pharmacopeia* and *National Formulary* and never having been described therein — compare OFFICIAL

non·ol·fac·to·ry \-äl-'fak-tə-rē, -ōl-\ *adj* : not olfactory

non·or·gas·mic \-ȯr-'gaz-mik\ *adj* : not capable of experiencing orgasm

no·nox·y·nol·9 \nä-'näk-sə-ˌnȯl-'nīn, -ˌnȯl-\ *n* : a spermicide used in contraceptive products that consists of a mixture of compounds having the general formula $C_{15}H_{23}(OCH_2CH_2)_n$-OH with an average of nine ethylene oxide groups per molecule

non·par·a·sit·ic \-ˌpar-ə-'sit-ik\ *adj* : not parasitic; *esp* : not caused by parasites ⟨∼ diseases⟩

non·patho·gen·ic \-ˌpa-thə-'je-nik\ *adj* : not capable of inducing disease — compare AVIRULENT

non·per·sis·tent \-pər-'sis-tənt\ *adj* : not persistent; *esp* : decomposed rapidly by environmental action ⟨∼ insecticides⟩

non·phy·si·cian \-fə-'zi-shən\ *n* : a person who is not a legally qualified physician

non·pig·ment·ed \-'pig-mən-təd\ *adj* : not pigmented

non·poi·son·ous \-'pȯi-zə-nəs\ *adj* : not poisonous

non·po·lar \-'pō-lər\ *adj* : not polar; *esp* : not having or requiring the presence of electrical poles ⟨∼ molecules⟩

non·preg·nant \-'preg-nənt\ *adj* : not pregnant

non·pre·scrip·tion \-pri-'skrip-shən\ *adj* : available for purchase without a doctor's prescription ⟨∼ drugs⟩

non·pro·duc·tive \-prə-'dək-tiv\ *adj, of a cough* : not effective in raising mucus or exudate from the respiratory tract : DRY 2

non·pro·pri·etary \-prə-'prī-ə-ˌter-ē\ *adj* : not proprietary ⟨a drug's ∼ name⟩

non·pro·tein \-'prō-ˌtēn\ *adj* : not being or derived from protein ⟨the ∼ part of an enzyme⟩

non·psy·chi·at·ric \-ˌsī-kē-'a-trik\ *adj* : not psychiatric

non·psy·chi·a·trist \-sə-'kī-ə-trist, -sī-\ *adj* : not specializing in psychiatry ⟨∼ physicians⟩ — **nonpsychiatrist** *n*

non·psy·chot·ic \-sī-'kä-tik\ *adj* : not psychotic ⟨∼ emotional disorders⟩

non·ra·dio·ac·tive \-ˌrā-dē-ō-'ak-tiv\ *adj* : not radioactive

non·re·ac·tive \-rē-'ak-tiv\ *adj* : not reactive; *esp* : not exhibiting a positive reaction in a particular laboratory test ⟨40% of the serums were ∼⟩

non·re·nal \-'rēn-əl\ *adj* : not renal; *esp*

: not resulting from dysfunction of the kidneys ⟨∼ alkalosis⟩

non·rheu·ma·toid \-'rü-mə-ˌtȯid\ *adj* : not relating to, affected with, or being rheumatoid arthritis

non·rhyth·mic \-'rith-mik\ *adj* : not rhythmic ⟨∼ contractions⟩

¹non·schizo·phren·ic \-ˌskit-sə-'fren-ik\ *adj* : not relating to, affected with, or being schizophrenia ⟨∼ patients⟩

²nonschizophrenic *n* : a nonschizophrenic individual

non·se·cre·tor \-si-'krē-tər\ *n* : an individual of blood group A, B, or AB who does not secrete the antigens characteristic of these blood groups in bodily fluids (as saliva)

non·se·cre·to·ry \-'sē-krə-ˌtȯr-ē\ *adj* : not secretory ⟨∼ cells⟩

non·se·lec·tive \-sə-'lek-tiv\ *adj* : not selective; *esp* : not limited (as to a single body part or organism) in action or effect ⟨∼ anti-infective agents⟩

non·self \ˌnän-'self\ *n* : material that is foreign to the body of an organism — **nonself** *adj*

¹non·sense \'nän-ˌsens, -səns\ *n* : genetic information consisting of one or more codons that do not code for any amino acid and usu. cause termination of the molecular chain in protein synthesis — compare ANTISENSE, MISSENSE

²nonsense *adj* : consisting of one or more codons that are genetic nonsense

non·sen·si·tive \-'sen-sə-tiv\ *adj* : not sensitive

non·sex·u·al \-'sek-shə-wəl\ *adj* : not sexual ⟨∼ reproduction⟩

non·spe·cif·ic \-spi-'si-fik\ *adj* : not specific: as **a** : not caused by a specific agent ⟨∼ enteritis⟩ **b** : having a general purpose or effect — **non·spe·cif·i·cal·ly** *adv*

non·ste·roi·dal \-stə-'rȯid-əl\ *also* **non·ste·roid** \-'stir-ˌȯid, -'ster-\ *adj* : of, relating to, or being a compound and esp. a drug that is not a steroid — see NSAID — **nonsteroid** *n*

nonstriated muscle *n* : SMOOTH MUSCLE

non·sug·ar \-'shu-gər\ *n* : a substance that is not a sugar; *esp* : AGLYCONE

non·sur·gi·cal \-'sər-ji-kəl\ *adj* : not surgical ⟨∼ hospital care⟩ — **non·sur·gi·cal·ly** *adv*

non·sys·tem·ic \-sis-'te-mik\ *adj* : not systemic

non·tast·er \-'tā-stər\ *n* : a person unable to taste the chemical phenylthiocarbamide

non·ther·a·peu·tic \-ˌther-ə-'pyü-tik\ *adj* : not relating to or being therapy

non·throm·bo·cy·to·pe·nic \-ˌthräm-bə-ˌsī-tə-'pē-nik\ *adj* : not relating to, affected with, or associated with thrombocytopenia ⟨∼ purpura⟩

non·tox·ic \-'täk-sik\ *adj* **1** : not toxic **2** *of goiter* : not associated with hyperthyroidism

non·trop·i·cal sprue \-'trä-pi-kəl-\ *n* : CELIAC DISEASE

non·union \-'yün-yən\ *n* : failure of the fragments of a broken bone to knit together

non·vas·cu·lar \-'vas-kyə-lər\ *adj* : lacking blood vessels or a vascular system ⟨a ~ layer of the skin⟩

non·ven·om·ous \-'ve-nə-məs\ *adj* : not venomous

non·vi·a·ble \-'vī-ə-bəl\ *adj* : not capable of living, growing, or developing and functioning successfully

NOPHN *abbr* National Organization for Public Health Nursing

nor·adren·a·line *also* **nor·adren·a·lin** \nȯr-ə-'dren-ᵊl-ən\ *n* : NOREPINEPHRINE

nor·ad·ren·er·gic \nȯr-ˌa-drə-'nər-jik\ *adj* : liberating, activated by, or involving norepinephrine in the transmission of nerve impulses — compare ADRENERGIC 1, CHOLINERGIC 1

nor·epi·neph·rine \nȯr-ˌe-pə-'ne-frən, -ˌfrēn\ *n* : a catecholamine $C_8H_{11}NO_3$ that is the chemical means of transmission across synapses in postganglionic neurons of the sympathetic nervous system and in some parts of the central nervous system, is a vasopressor hormone of the adrenal medulla, and is a precursor of epinephrine in its major biosynthetic pathway — called also *noradrenaline; see* LEVOPHED

nor·eth·in·drone \nȯ-'re-thən-ˌdrōn\ *n* : a synthetic progestational hormone $C_{20}H_{26}O_2$ used in oral contraceptives often in the form of its acetate

nor·ethis·ter·one \nȯr-ə-'this-tə-ˌrōn\ *n, chiefly Brit* : NORETHINDRONE

nor·ethyn·o·drel \nȯr-ə-'thi-nə-ˌdrəl\ *n* : a progesterone derivative $C_{20}H_{26}O_2$ used in oral contraceptives and clinically in the treatment of abnormal uterine bleeding and the control of menstruation — see ENOVID

nor·ges·trel \nȯr-'jes-trel\ *n* : a synthetic progestogen $C_{21}H_{28}O_2$ having two optically active forms of which the biologically active levorotatory form is used in oral contraceptives — see LEVONORGESTREL

norm \'nȯrm\ *n* : an established standard or average: as **a** : a set standard of development or achievement usu. derived from the average or median achievement of a large group **b** : a pattern or trait taken to be typical in the behavior of a social group

norm- *or* **normo-** *comb form* : normal ⟨*normo*blast⟩ ⟨*normo*tensive⟩

¹**nor·mal** \'nȯr-məl\ *adj* **1 a** : according with, constituting, or not deviating from a norm, rule, or principle **b** : conforming to a type, standard, or regular pattern **2** : occurring naturally and not because of disease, inoculation, or any experimental treatment ⟨~ immunity⟩ **3 a** : of, relating to, or characterized by average intelligence

or development **b** : free from mental disorder : SANE **c** : characterized by the balanced well-integrated functioning of the organism as a whole — **nor·mal·ize** \'nȯr-mə-ˌlīz\ *vb* — **nor·mal·ly** \'nȯr-mə-lē\ *adv*

²**normal** *n* : a subject who is normal

nor·meta·neph·rine \ˌnȯr-ˌme-tə-'ne-frən, -ˌfrēn\ *n* : a metabolite of norepinephrine $C_9H_{13}NO_3$ found esp. in the urine

nor·mo·ac·tive \ˌnȯr-mō-'ak-tiv\ *adj* : normally active

nor·mo·blast \'nȯr-mə-ˌblast\ *n* : an immature red blood cell containing hemoglobin and a pyknotic nucleus and normally present in bone marrow but appearing in the blood in many anemias — compare ERYTHROBLAST — **nor·mo·blas·tic** \ˌnȯr-mə-'blas-tik\ *adj*

nor·mo·cal·cae·mia *chiefly Brit var of* NORMOCALCEMIA

nor·mo·cal·ce·mia \ˌnȯr-mō-kal-'sē-mē-ə\ *n* : the presence of a normal concentration of calcium in the blood — **nor·mo·cal·ce·mic** \-mik\ *adj*

nor·mo·chro·mia \ˌnȯr-mə-'krō-mē-ə\ *n* : the color of red blood cells that contain a normal amount of hemoglobin — **nor·mo·chro·mic** \-'krō-mik\ *adj*

normochromic anemia *n* : an anemia marked by reduced numbers of normochromic red blood cells in the circulating blood

nor·mo·cyte \'nȯr-mə-ˌsīt\ *n* : a red blood cell that is normal in size and in hemoglobin content

nor·mo·cyt·ic \ˌnȯr-mə-'si-tik\ *adj* : characterized by red blood cells that are normal in size and usu. also in hemoglobin content ⟨~ blood⟩

normocytic anemia *n* : an anemia marked by reduced numbers of normal red blood cells in the circulating blood

nor·mo·gly·ce·mia \ˌnȯr-mō-glī-'sē-mē-ə\ *n* : the presence of a normal concentration of glucose in the blood — **nor·mo·gly·ce·mic** \-mik\ *adj*

nor·mo·ka·le·mic \ˌnȯr-mō-kā-'lē-mik\ *adj* : having or characterized by a normal concentration of potassium in the blood

nor·mo·ten·sive \ˌnȯr-mō-'ten-siv\ *adj* : having blood pressure typical of the group to which one belongs

nor·mo·ther·mia \-'thər-mē-ə\ *n* : normal body temperature — **nor·mo·ther·mic** \-mik\ *adj*

nor·mo·vo·lae·mia *chiefly Brit var of* NORMOVOLEMIA

nor·mo·vol·emia \ˌnȯr-mō-ˌvä-'lē-mē-ə\ *n* : a normal volume of blood in the body — **nor·mo·vol·emic** \-mik\ *adj*

Nor·plant \'nȯr-ˌplant\ *trademark* — used for contraceptive implants of encapsulated levonorgestrel

North American blastomycosis *n* : blastomycosis that involves esp. the skin, lymph nodes, and lungs and that is caused by infection with a fungus of the genus *Blastomyces* (*B. dermatitidis*) — called also *Gilchrist's disease*

Northern blot *n* : a blot consisting of a sheet of a cellulose derivative that contains spots of RNA for identification by a suitable molecular probe — compare SOUTHERN BLOT, WESTERN BLOT — **Northern blotting** *n*

northern cattle grub *n* : an immature form or adult of a warble fly of the genus *Hypoderma* (*H. bovis*) — called also *cattle grub*

northern fowl mite *n* : a parasitic mite (*Ornithonyssus sylviarum*) that is a pest of birds and esp. poultry and pigeons

northern rat flea *n* : a common and widely distributed flea of the genus *Nosopsyllus* (*N. fasciatus*) that is parasitic on rats and transmits murine typhus and possibly plague

nor·trip·ty·line \nŏr-'trip-tə-ˌlēn\ *n* : a tricyclic antidepressant $C_{19}H_{21}N$ used in the form of its hydrochloride — see AVENTYL

Nor·walk virus \'nŏr-ˌwȯk-\ *n* : a parvovirus that causes an infectious human gastroenteritis — called also *Norwalk agent*

Nor·way rat \'nŏr-wā-\ *n* : BROWN RAT

nos- *or* **noso-** *comb form* : disease (*nosology*)

nose \'nōz\ *n* **1 a** : the part of the face that bears the nostrils and covers the anterior part of the nasal cavity; *broadly* : this part together with the nasal cavity **b** : the anterior part of the head above or projecting beyond the muzzle **2** : the sense of smell — OLFACTION **3** : OLFACTORY ORGAN

nose·bleed \-ˌblēd\ *n* : an attack of bleeding from the nose — called also *epistaxis*

nose botfly *n* : a botfly of the genus *Gasterophilus* (*G. haemorrhoidalis*) that is parasitic in the larval stage esp. on horses and mules — called also *nose fly*

nose job *n* : RHINOPLASTY

nose·piece \'nōz-ˌpēs\ *n* : the bridge of a pair of eyeglasses

nos·o·co·mi·al \ˌnä-sə-'kō-mē-əl\ *adj* : originating or taking place in a hospital (~ infection)

no·sol·o·gy \nō-'sä-lə-jē, -'zä-\ *n*, *pl* **-gies 1** : a classification or list of diseases **2** : a branch of medical science that deals with classification of diseases — **no·so·log·i·cal** \ˌnō-sə-'lä-ji-kəl\ *or* **no·so·log·ic** \-jik\ *adj* — **no·so·log·i·cal·ly** *adv* — **no·sol·o·gist** \nō-'sä-lə-jist\ *n*

Nos·o·psyl·lus \ˌnä-sə-'si-ləs\ *n* : a genus of fleas that includes the northern rat flea (*N. fasciatus*)

nos·tril \'näs-trəl\ *n* **1** : either of the external nares; *broadly* : either of the nares with the adjoining passage on the same side of the nasal septum **2** : either fleshy lateral wall of the nose

nos·trum \'näs-trəm\ *n* : a medicine of secret composition recommended by its preparer but usu. without scientific proof of its effectiveness

not- *or* **noto-** *comb form* : back : back part (*notochord*)

notch \'näch\ *n* : a V-shaped indentation (as on a bone) — see ACETABULAR NOTCH, SCIATIC NOTCH, VERTEBRAL NOTCH — **notched** \'nächt\ *adj*

no·ti·fi·able \ˌnō-tə-'fī-ə-bəl\ *adj* : required by law to be reported to official health authorities (a ~ disease)

no·ti·fy \'nō-tə-ˌfī\ *vb* **-fied; -fy·ing** : to report the occurrence of (a communicable disease or an individual suffering from such disease) in a community to public-health or other authority — **no·ti·fi·ca·tion** \ˌnō-tə-fə-'kā-shən\ *n*

no·to·chord \'nō-tə-ˌkȯrd\ *n* : a longitudinal flexible rod of cells that in all vertebrates and some more primitive forms provides the supporting axis of the body, that is almost obliterated in the adult of higher vertebrates as the body develops, and that arises as an outgrowth from dorsal lip of the blastopore extending forward between epiblast and hypoblast in the middorsal line — **no·to·chord·al** \ˌnō-tə-'kȯrd-əl\ *adj*

No·to·ed·res \ˌnō-tō-'e-ˌdrēz\ *n* : a genus of mites (family Sarcoptidae) containing mange mites that attack various mammals including occas. but rarely seriously humans usu. through contact with cats

nour·ish \'nər-ish\ *vb* : to furnish or sustain with nutriment

nour·ish·ing *adj* : giving nourishment : NUTRITIOUS

nour·ish·ment \'nər-ish-mənt\ *n* **1** : FOOD 1, NUTRIMENT **2** : the act of nourishing or the state of being nourished

no·vo·bi·o·cin \ˌnō-və-'bī-ə-sən\ *n* : a highly toxic antibiotic $C_{31}H_{36}N_2O_{11}$ used in some serious cases of staphylococcal and urinary tract infection

No·vo·cain \'nō-və-ˌkān\ *trademark* — used for a preparation containing the hydrochloride of procaine

no·vo·caine \-ˌkān\ *n* : PROCAINE; *also* : its hydrochloride

noxa \'näk-sə\ *n*, *pl* **nox·ae** \-ˌsē, -ˌsī\ : something that exerts a harmful effect on the body

nox·ious \'näk-shəs\ *adj* : physically harmful or destructive to living beings

Np *symbol* neptunium

NP *abbr* neuropsychiatric; neuropsychiatry

NPN *abbr* nonprotein nitrogen

NR *abbr* no refill

NREM sleep \'en-ˌrem-\ *n* : SLOW-WAVE SLEEP

ns *abbr* nanosecond

NSAID \'en-₁sed, -₁säd\ *n* : a nonsteroidal anti-inflammatory drug (as ibuprofen)

nsec *abbr* nanosecond

NSU *abbr* nonspecific urethritis

nu·chae \'nü-kē, 'nyü-\ — see LIGAMENTUM NUCHAE

nu·chal \'nü-kəl, 'nyü-\ *adj* : of, relating to, or lying in the region of the nape

nuchal line *n* : any of several ridges on the outside of the skull: as **a** : one on each side that extends laterally in a curve from the external occipital protuberance to the mastoid process of the temporal bone — called also *superior nuchal line* **b** : OCCIPITAL CREST **a c** : one on each side that extends laterally from the middle of the external occipital crest below and roughly parallel to the superior nuchal line — called also *inferior nuchal line*

nucle- *or* **nucleo-** *comb form* **1** : nucleus ⟨*nucle*on⟩ ⟨*nucle*oplasm⟩ **2** : nucleic acid ⟨*nucleo*protein⟩

nu·cle·ar \'nü-klē-ər, 'nyü-\ *adj* **1** : of, relating to, or constituting a nucleus **2** : of, relating to, or utilizing the atomic nucleus, atomic energy, the atomic bomb, or atomic power

nuclear family *n* : a family group that consists only of father, mother, and children — see EXTENDED FAMILY

nuclear fission *n* : FISSION 2

nuclear magnetic resonance *n* **1** : the magnetic resonance of an atomic nucleus **2** : chemical analysis that uses nuclear magnetic resonance esp. to study molecular structure — abbr. *NMR;* see MAGNETIC RESONANCE IMAGING

nuclear medicine *n* : a branch of medicine dealing with the use of radioactive materials in the diagnosis and treatment of disease

nuclear membrane *n* : a double membrane enclosing a cell nucleus and having its outer part continuous with the endoplasmic reticulum

nuclear sap *n* : the clear homogeneous ground substance of a cell nucleus — called also *karyolymph*

nu·cle·ase \'nü-klē-₁ās, 'nyü-, -₁āz\ *n* : any of various enzymes that promote hydrolysis of nucleic acids

nu·cle·at·ed \-₁ā-təd\ *or* **nu·cle·ate** \-klē-ət\ *adj* : having a nucleus or nuclei ⟨~ cells⟩

nu·cle·ic acid \nü-'klē-ik-, nyü-, -'klā-\ *n* : any of various acids (as an RNA or a DNA) composed of nucleotide chains

nu·cle·in \'nü-klē-in, 'nyü-\ *n* **1** : NUCLEOPROTEIN **2** : NUCLEIC ACID

nucleo- — see NUCLE-

nu·cleo·cap·sid \₁nü-klē-ō-'kap-səd, ₁nyü-\ *n* : the nucleic acid and surrounding protein coat of a virus

nu·cleo·cy·to·plas·mic \-₁sī-tə-'plaz-mik\ *adj* : of or relating to the nucleus and cytoplasm

nu·cleo·his·tone \-'his-₁tōn\ *n* : a nucleoprotein in which the protein is a histone

nu·cle·oid \'nü-klē-₁oid, 'nyü-\ *n* : the DNA-containing area of a prokaryotic cell (as a bacterium)

nucleol- *or* **nucleolo-** *comb form* : nucleolus ⟨*nucleolar*⟩

nu·cle·o·lar \nü-'klē-ə-lər, nyü-, ₁nü-klē-'ō-lər, ₁nyü-\ *adj* : of, relating to, or constituting a nucleolus ⟨~ proteins⟩

nucleolar organizer *n* : NUCLEOLUS ORGANIZER

nu·cle·o·lus \nü-'klē-ə-ləs, nyü-\, *pl* **-li** \-₁lī\ : a spherical body of the nucleus of most eukaryotes that becomes enlarged during protein synthesis, is associated with a nucleolus organizer, and contains the DNA templates for ribosomal RNA

nucleolus organizer *n* : the specific part of a chromosome with which a nucleolus is associated esp. during its reorganization after nuclear division — called also *nucleolar organizer*

nu·cle·on \'nü-klē-₁än, 'nyü-\ *n* : a proton or neutron esp. in the atomic nucleus

nu·cleo·phil·ic \₁nü-klē-ə-'fil-ik, ₁nyü-\ *adj* : having an affinity for atomic nuclei : electron-donating

nu·cleo·plasm \'nü-klē-ə-₁pla-zəm, 'nyü-\ *n* : the protoplasm of a nucleus; *esp* : NUCLEAR SAP

nu·cleo·pro·tein \₁nü-klē-ō-'prō-₁tēn, ₁nyü-\ *n* : a compound that consists of a protein (as a histone) conjugated with a nucleic acid (as a DNA) and that is the principal constituent of the hereditary material in chromosomes

nu·cleo·side \'nü-klē-ə-₁sīd, 'nyü-\ *n* : a compound (as guanosine or adenosine) that consists of a purine or pyrimidine base combined with deoxyribose or ribose and is found esp. in DNA or RNA — compare NUCLEOTIDE

nu·cleo·some \-₁sōm\ *n* : any of the repeating globular subunits of chromatin that consist of a complex of DNA and histone — called also *nucleosomal* \₁nü-klē-ə-'sō-məl, ₁nyü-\ *adj*

nu·cleo·tide \'nü-klē-ə-₁tīd, 'nyü-\ *n* : any of several compounds that consist of a ribose or deoxyribose sugar joined to a purine or pyrimidine base and to a phosphate group and that are the basic structural units of RNA and DNA — compare NUCLEOSIDE

nu·cle·us \'nü-klē-əs, 'nyü-\ *n, pl* **nu·clei** \-klē-₁ī\ *also* **nu·cle·us·es 1** : a cellular organelle of eukaryotes that is essential to cell functions (as reproduction and protein synthesis), is composed of nuclear sap and a nucleoprotein-rich network from which chromosomes and nucleoli arise, and is enclosed in a definite membrane **2** : a mass of gray matter or group of nerve cells in the central nervous system **3** : the positively charged central portion of an atom that comprises nearly all of the atomic mass and that consists of protons and neutrons except in hydrogen which consists of one proton only

nucleus ac·cum·bens \-ə-'kəm-bənz\ n : a nucleus forming the floor of the caudal part of the anterior prolongation of the lateral ventricle of the brain

nucleus am·big·u·us \-am-'bi-gyə-wəs\ n : an elongated nucleus in the medulla oblongata that is a continuation of a group of cells in the ventral horn of the spinal cord and gives rise to the motor fibers of the glossopharyngeal, vagus, and accessory nerves supplying striated muscle of the larynx and pharynx

nucleus cu·ne·a·tus \-ˌkyü-nē-'ā-təs\ n : the nucleus in the medulla oblongata in which the fibers of the fasciculus cuneatus terminate and synapse with a component of the medial lemniscus — called also *cuneate nucleus*

nucleus grac·i·lis \-'gra-sə-ləs\ n : a nucleus in the posterior part of the medulla oblongata in which the fibers of the fasciculus gracilis terminate

nucleus pul·po·sus \-ˌpəl-'pō-səs\ n, pl **nuclei pul·po·si** \-ˌsī\ : an elastic pulpy mass lying in the center of each intervertebral fibrocartilage

nu·clide \'nü-ˌklīd, 'nyü-\ n : a species of atom characterized by the constitution of its nucleus and hence by the number of protons, the number of neutrons, and the energy content

null cell \'nəl-\ n : a lymphocyte in the blood that does not have on its surface the receptors typical of either mature B cells or T cells

nul·li·grav·i·da \ˌnə-li-'gra-və-də\ n : a woman who has never been pregnant

nul·lip·a·ra \ˌnə-'li-pə-rə\ n, pl **-ras** also **-rae** \-ˌrē\ : a woman who has never borne a child

nul·lip·a·rous \ˌnə-'li-pə-rəs\ adj : of, relating to, or being a female that has not borne offspring — **nul·li·par·i·ty** \ˌnə-lə-'par-ə-tē\ n

numb \'nəm\ adj : devoid of sensation esp. as a result of cold or anesthesia — **numb·ness** n

num·mu·lar \'nə-myə-lər\ adj **1** : circular or oval in shape (∼ lesions) **2** : characterized by circular or oval lesions or drops (∼ dermatitis)

Nu·per·caine \'nü-pər-ˌkān, 'nyü-\ trademark — used for a preparation of dibucaine

¹**nurse** \'nərs\ n **1** : a woman who suckles an infant not her own : WET NURSE **2** : a person who is skilled or trained in caring for the sick or infirm esp. under the supervision of a physician

²**nurse** vb **nursed; nurs·ing a** : to nourish at the breast : SUCKLE **b** : to take

nourishment from the breast : SUCK **a** : to care for and wait on (as an injured or infirm person) **b** : to attempt a cure of (as an ailment) by care and treatment

nurse–anes·the·tist \-ə-'nes-thə-tist\ n : a registered nurse who has completed two years of additional training in anesthesia and is qualified to serve as an anesthetist under the supervision of a physician

nurse clinician n : NURSE-PRACTITIONER

nurse–midwife n, pl **nurse–midwives** : a registered nurse who has received additional training as a midwife, delivers infants, and provides antepartum and postpartum care — **nurse–midwifery** n

nurse–practitioner n : a registered nurse who through advanced training is qualified to assume some of the duties and responsibilities formerly assumed only by a physician — called also *nurse clinician*

nurs·ery \'nər-sə-rē\ n, pl **-er·ies** : the department of a hospital where newborn infants are cared for

nurse's aide n : a worker who assists trained nurses in a hospital by performing general services

nurs·ing \'nər-siŋ\ n **1** : the profession of a nurse (schools of ∼) **2** : the duties of a nurse

nursing bottle n : a bottle with a rubber nipple used in supplying food to infants

nursing home n : a privately operated establishment where maintenance and personal or nursing care are provided for persons (as the aged or the chronically ill) who are unable to care for themselves properly — compare REST HOME

nur·tur·ance \'nər-chə-rəns\ n : affectionate care and attention — **nur·tur·ant** \-rənt\ adj

Nu·tra·Sweet \'nü-trə-ˌswēt, 'nyü-\ trademark — used for a preparation of aspartame

¹**nu·tri·ent** \'nü-trē-ənt, 'nyü-\ adj : furnishing nourishment

²**nutrient** n : a nutritive substance or ingredient

nu·tri·ment \'nü-trə-mənt, 'nyü-\ n : something that nourishes or promotes growth and repairs the natural wastage of organic life

nu·tri·tion \nü-'tri-shən, nyü-\ n : the act or process of nourishing or being nourished; specif : the sum of the processes by which an animal or plant takes in and utilizes food substances — **nu·tri·tion·al** \-'tri-shə-nəl\ adj — **nu·tri·tion·al·ly** adv

nutritional anemia n : anemia (as hypochromic anemia) that results from inadequate intake or assimilation of materials essential for the production of red blood cells and hemoglobin — called also *deficiency anemia*

nu·tri·tion·ist \-ˈtri-shə-nist\ n : a specialist in the study of nutrition

nu·tri·tious \nü-ˈtri-shəs, nyü-\ adj : providing nourishment

nu·tri·tive \ˈnü-trə-tiv, ˈnyü-\ adj 1 : of or relating to nutrition 2 : NOURISHING

nu·tri·ture \ˈnü-trə-ˌchur, ˈnyü-, -chər\ n : bodily condition with respect to nutrition and esp. with respect to a given nutrient (as zinc)

nux vom·i·ca \ˈnəks-ˈvä-mi-kə\ n, pl **nux vomica** 1 : the poisonous seed of an Asian tree of the genus *Strychnos* (*S. nux-vomica*) that contains the alkaloids strychnine and brucine 2 : a drug containing nux vomica

nyc·ta·lo·pia \ˌnik-tə-ˈlō-pē-ə\ n : NIGHT BLINDNESS

ny·li·drin \ˈnī-li-drən\ n : a synthetic adrenergic drug $C_{19}H_{25}NO_2$ that acts as a peripheral vasodilator and is usually administered in the form of its hydrochloride

nymph \ˈnimf\ n 1 : any of various insects in an immature stage and esp. a late larva (as of a true bug) in which rudiments of the wings and genitalia are present; *broadly* : any insect larva that differs chiefly in size and degree of differentiation from the adult 2 : a

mite or tick in the first eight-legged form that immediately follows the last larval molt — **nymph·al** \ˈnim-fəl\ adj

nymph- or **nympho-** also **nymphi-** comb form : nymph : nymphae (*nymphomania*)

nym·phae \ˈnim-(ˌ)fē\ n pl : LABIA MINORA

nym·pho \ˈnim-(ˌ)fō\ n, pl **nymphos** : NYMPHOMANIAC

nym·pho·ma·nia \ˌnim-fə-ˈmā-nē-ə, -nyə\ n : excessive sexual desire by a female — compare SATYRIASIS

¹nym·pho·ma·ni·ac \-nē-ˌak\ n : one affected with nymphomania

²nymphomaniac or **nym·pho·ma·ni·a·cal** \-mə-ˈnī-ə-kəl\ adj : of, affected with, or characterized by nymphomania

nys·tag·mus \ni-ˈstag-məs\ n : a rapid involuntary oscillation of the eyeballs occurring normally with dizziness during and after bodily rotation or abnormally after injuries

nys·ta·tin \ˈnis-tət-ən\ n : an antibiotic that is derived from a soil actinomycete of the genus *Streptomyces* (*S. noursei*) and is used esp. in the treatment of candidiasis

O

¹O abbr [Latin *octarius*] pint — used in writing prescriptions

²O symbol oxygen

o- or **oo-** comb form : egg : ovum ⟨*oocyte*⟩

O antigen \ˈō-\ n : an antigen that occurs in the body of a gram-negative bacterial cell — compare H ANTIGEN

oat–cell \ˈōt-ˌsel\ adj : of, relating to, or being a highly malignant form of cancer esp. of the lungs that is characterized by rapid proliferation of small anaplastic cells ⟨~ carcinomas⟩

oath — see HIPPOCRATIC OATH

OB abbr 1 obstetric 2 obstetrician 3 obstetrics

obese \ō-ˈbēs\ adj : excessively fat

obe·si·ty \ō-ˈbē-sə-tē\ n, pl **-ties** : a condition characterized by excessive bodily fat

obex \ˈō-ˌbeks\ n : a thin triangular lamina of gray matter in the roof of the fourth ventricle of the brain

ob–gyn \ˌō-(ˌ)bē-ˈjin, -(ˌ)jē-(ˌ)wi-ˈen\ n, pl **ob–gyns** : a physician who specializes in obstetrics and gynecology

OB–GYN abbr obstetrics-gynecology

ob·jec·tive \əb-ˈjek-tiv, äb-\ adj 1 : of, relating to, or being an object, phenomenon, or condition in the realm of sensible experience independent of individual thought and perceptible by all observers ⟨~ reality⟩ 2 : perceptible to persons other than the affected individual ⟨an ~ symptom of disease⟩

— compare SUBJECTIVE 2b — **ob·jec·tive·ly** adv

ob·li·gate \ˈä-bli-gət, -ˌgät\ adj 1 : restricted to one particularly characteristic mode of life or way of functioning 2 : biologically essential for survival — **ob·li·gate·ly** adv

oblig·a·to·ry \ə-ˈbli-gə-ˌtōr-ē, ä-\ adj : OBLIGATE 1

¹oblique \ō-ˈblēk, ə-, -ˈblīk\ adj 1 : neither perpendicular nor parallel : being on an incline 2 : situated obliquely and having one end not inserted on bone ⟨~ muscles⟩ — **oblique·ly** adv

²oblique n : any of several oblique muscles: as **a** : either of two flat muscles on each side that form the middle and outer layers of the lateral walls of the abdomen and that act to compress the abdominal contents and to assist in expelling the contents of various visceral organs (as in urination and expiration): (1) : one that forms the outer layer of the lateral abdominal wall — called also *external oblique, obliquus externus abdominis* (2) : one situated under the external oblique in the lateral and ventral part of the abdominal wall — called also *internal oblique, obliquus internus abdominis* **b** (1) : a long thin muscle that arises just above the margin of the optic foramen, is inserted on the upper part of the eyeball, and moves the eye downward and laterally — called also *superior oblique, obliquus superior* *oculi* (2) : a short muscle that arises from the orbital surface of the maxilla, is inserted slightly in front of and below the superior oblique, and moves the eye upward and laterally — called also *inferior oblique, obliquus inferior oculi* c (1) : a muscle that arises from the superior surface of the transverse process of the atlas, passes medially upward to insert into the occipital bone, and functions to extend the head and bend it to the side — called also *obliquus capitis superior* (2) : a muscle that arises from the apex of the spinous process of the axis, inserts into the transverse process of the atlas, and rotates the atlas turning the face in the same direction — called also *obliquus capitis inferior*

oblique fissure *n* : either of two fissures of the lungs of which the one on the left side of the body separates the superior lobe of the left lung from the inferior lobe and the one on the right separates the superior and middle lobes of the right lung from the inferior lobe

oblique popliteal ligament *n* : a strong broad flat fibrous ligament that passes obliquely across and strengthens the posterior part of the knee — compare ARCUATE POPLITEAL LIGAMENT

oblique vein of Mar·shall \-ˈmär-shəl\ *n* : OBLIQUE VEIN OF THE LEFT ATRIUM
Marshall, John (1818–1891), British anatomist and surgeon.

oblique vein of the left atrium *n* : a small vein that passes obliquely down the posterior surface of the left atrium and empties into the coronary sinus — called also *oblique vein, oblique vein of left atrium*

ob·li·quus \ō-ˈbli-kwəs\ *n, pl* **ob·li·qui** \-ˌkwī\ : OBLIQUE

obliquus cap·i·tis inferior \-ˈka-pə-təs-\ *n* : OBLIQUE c(2)

obliquus capitis superior *n* : OBLIQUE c(1)

obliquus externus ab·dom·i·nis \-ab-ˈdä-mə-nəs\ *n* : OBLIQUE a(1)

obliquus inferior *n* : OBLIQUE b(2)

obliquus inferior oc·u·li \-ˈä-kyü-ˌlī, -ˌlē\ *n* : OBLIQUE b(2)

obliquus internus ab·dom·i·nis \-ab-ˈdä-mə-nəs\ *n* : OBLIQUE a(2)

obliquus superior *n* : OBLIQUE b(1)

obliquus superior oc·u·li \-ˈä-kyü-ˌlī, -ˌlē\ *n* : OBLIQUE b(1)

oblit·er·ate \ə-ˈbli-tə-ˌrāt, ō-\ *vb* **-at·ed; -at·ing** : to cause to disappear (as a bodily part) or collapse (as a duct conveying body fluid) — **oblit·er·a·tion** \-ˌbli-tə-ˈrā-shən\ *n* — **oblit·er·a·tive** \ə-ˈbli-tə-ˌrā-tiv, ō-, -rə-\ *adj*

obliterating endarteritis *n* : ENDARTERITIS OBLITERANS

ob·lon·ga·ta \ˌä-ˌbloṅ-ˈgä-tə\ *n, pl* **-tas** *or* **-tae** \-ˌtē\ : MEDULLA OBLONGATA

OBS *abbr* **1** obstetrician **2** obstetrics

ob·ser·va·tion \ˌäb-sər-ˈvā-shən, -zər-\ *n* **1** : the noting of a fact or occurrence (as in nature) often involving the measurement of some magnitude with suitable instruments; *also* : a record so obtained **2** : close watch or examination (as to monitor or diagnose a condition) ⟨postoperative ∼⟩

ob·sess \əb-ˈses, äb-\ *vb* **1** : to preoccupy intensely or abnormally ⟨∼ed with success⟩ **2** : to engage in obsessive thinking ⟨solve problems rather than ∼ about them — Carol Tavris⟩

ob·ses·sion \äb-ˈse-shən, əb-\ *n* : a persistent disturbing preoccupation with an often unreasonable idea or feeling; *also* : something that causes such preoccupation — compare COMPULSION, PHOBIA — **ob·ses·sion·al** \-ˈse-shə-nəl\ *adj*

obsessional neurosis *n* : an obsessive‑compulsive neurosis in which obsessive thinking predominates with little need to perform compulsive acts

¹**ob·ses·sive** \äb-ˈse-siv, əb-\ *adj* : of, relating to, causing, or characterized by obsession : deriving from obsession ⟨∼ behavior⟩ — **ob·ses·sive·ly** *adv* — **ob·ses·sive·ness** *n*

²**obsessive** *n* : an obsessive individual

¹**obsessive–compulsive** *adj* : relating to or characterized by recurring obsessions and compulsions esp. as symptoms of an obsessive-compulsive disorder

²**obsessive–compulsive** *n* : a person affected with an obsessive-compulsive disorder

obsessive–compulsive disorder *n* : a psychoneurotic disorder in which the patient is beset with obsessions or compulsions or both and suffers extreme anxiety or depression through failure to think the obsessive thoughts or perform the compelling acts — called also *obsessive-compulsive neurosis, obsessive-compulsive reaction*

ob·stet·ric \əb-ˈste-trik, äb-\ *or* **ob·stet·ri·cal** \-tri-kəl\ *adj* : of, relating to, or associated with childbirth or obstetrics — **ob·stet·ri·cal·ly** *adv*

obstetric forceps *n* : a forceps for grasping the fetal head or other part to facilitate delivery in difficult labor

ob·ste·tri·cian \ˌäb-stə-ˈtri-shən\ *n* : a physician or veterinarian specializing in obstetrics

ob·stet·rics \əb-ˈste-triks, äb-\ *n sing or pl* : a branch of medical science that deals with birth and with its antecedents and sequels

ob·sti·pa·tion \ˌäb-stə-ˈpā-shən\ *n* : severe and intractable constipation

ob·struct \əb-ˈstrəkt, äb-\ *vb* : to block or close up by an obstacle

ob·struc·tion \əb-ˈstrək-shən, äb-\ *n* **1 a** : an act of obstructing **b** : a condition of being clogged or blocked ⟨intesti-

nal $\sim$) **2** : something that obstructs —
ob·struc·tive \-tiv\ *adj*
obstructive jaundice *n* : jaundice due to obstruction of the biliary passages (as by gallstones or tumor)
ob·tund \äb-'tənd\ *vb* : to reduce the intensity or sensitivity of : make dull ($\sim$ed reflexes) (agents that $\sim$ pain) — **ob·tun·da·tion** \ₐäb-(ₐ)tən-'dā-shən\ *n*
ob·tu·ra·tor \'äb-tyə-ₐrā-tər, -tə-\ *n* **1 a** : either of two muscles arising from the obturator membrane and adjacent bony surfaces: (1) : OBTURATOR EXTERNUS (2) : OBTURATOR INTERNUS **b** : OBTURATOR NERVE **2 a** : a prosthetic device that closes or blocks up an opening (as a fissure in the palate) **b** : a device that blocks the opening of an instrument (as a sigmoidoscope) that is being introduced into the body
obturator artery *n* : an artery that arises from the internal iliac artery or one of its branches, passes out through the obturator canal, and divides into two branches which are distributed to the muscles and fasciae of the hip and thigh
obturator canal *n* : the small patent opening of the obturator foramen through which nerves and vessels pass
obturator ex·ter·nus \-ek-'stər-nəs\ *n* : a flat triangular muscle that arises esp. from the medial side of the obturator foramen and from the medial part of the obturator membrane, that inserts by a tendon into the trochanteric fossa of the femur, and that acts to rotate the thigh laterally
obturator foramen *n* : an opening that is the largest foramen in the human body and is situated between the ischium and pubis of the hipbone
obturator in·ter·nus \-in-'tər-nəs\ *n* : a muscle that arises from the margin of the obturator foramen and from the obturator membrane, that inserts into the greater trochanter of the femur, and that acts to rotate the thigh laterally when it is extended and to abduct it in the flexed position
obturator membrane *n* : a firm fibrous membrane covering most of the obturator foramen except for the obturator canal
obturator nerve *n* : a branch of the lumbar plexus that arises from the second, third, and fourth lumbar nerves and that supplies the hip and knee joints, the adductor muscles of the thigh, and the skin
obturator vein *n* : a tributary of the internal iliac vein that accompanies the obturator artery
occipit- or **occipito-** *comb form* : occipital and (*occipito*temporal)
occipita *pl of* OCCIPUT
¹oc·cip·i·tal \äk-'si-pət-ᵊl\ *adj* : of, relating to, or located within or near the occiput or the occipital bone

²occipital *n* : OCCIPITAL BONE
occipital artery *n* : an artery that arises from the external carotid artery, ascends within the superficial fascia of the scalp, and supplies or gives off branches supplying structures and esp. muscles of the back of the neck and head
occipital bone *n* : a compound bone that forms the posterior part of the skull and surrounds the foramen magnum, bears the condyles for articulation with the atlas, is composed of four united elements, is much curved and roughly trapezoidal in outline, and ends in front of the foramen magnum in the basilar process
occipital condyle *n* : an articular surface on the occipital bone by which the skull articulates with the atlas
occipital crest *n* : either of the two ridges on the occipital bone: **a** : a median ridge on the outer surface of the occipital bone that with the external occipital protuberance gives attachment to the ligamentum nuchae — called also *external occipital crest, median nuchal line* **b** : a median ridge similarly situated on the inner surface of the occipital bone that bifurcates near the foramen magnum to give attachment to the falx cerebelli — called also *internal occipital crest*
occipital fontanel *n* : a triangular fontanel at the meeting of the sutures between the parietal and occipital bones
oc·cip·i·ta·lis \äk-ₐsi-pə-'tā-ləs\ *n* : the posterior belly of the occipitofrontalis that arises from the lateral two-thirds of the superior nuchal lines and from the mastoid part of the temporal bone, inserts into the galea aponeurotica, and acts to move the scalp
occipital lobe *n* : the posterior lobe of each cerebral hemisphere that bears the visual areas and has the form of a 3-sided pyramid
occipital nerve *n* : either of two nerves that arise mostly from the second cervical nerve: **a** : one that innervates the scalp at the top of the head — called also *greater occipital nerve* **b** : one that innervates the scalp esp. in the lateral area of the head behind the ear — called also *lesser occipital nerve*
occipital protuberance *n* : either of two prominences on the occipital bone: **a** : a prominence on the outer surface of the occipital bone midway between the upper border and the foramen magnum — called also *external occipital protuberance, inion* **b** : a prominence similarly situated on the inner surface of the occipital bone — called also *internal occipital protuberance*
occipital sinus *n* : a single or paired venous sinus that arises near the margin of the foramen magnum by the union of several small veins and empties

into the confluence of sinuses or sometimes into one of the transverse sinuses

occipito- — see OCCIPIT-

oc·cip·i·to·fron·ta·lis \ˌäk-ˌsi-pə-tō-frən-ˈtā-ləs\ *n* : a fibrous and muscular sheet on each side of the vertex of the skull that extends from the eyebrow to the occiput, that is composed of the frontalis muscle in front and the occipitalis muscle in back with the galea aponeurotica in between, and that acts to draw back the scalp to raise the eyebrow and wrinkle the forehead — called also *epicranius*

oc·cip·i·to·pa·ri·etal \-pə-ˈrī-ət-ᵊl\ *adj* : of or relating to the occipital and parietal bones of the skull

oc·cip·i·to·tem·po·ral \-ˈtem-pə-rəl\ *adj* : of, relating to, or distributed to the occipital and temporal lobes of a cerebral hemisphere (the ∼ cortex)

oc·ci·put \ˈäk-sə-(ˌ)pət\ *n, pl* **occiputs** *or* **oc·cip·i·ta** \äk-ˈsi-pə-tə\ : the back part of the head or skull

oc·clude \ə-ˈklüd, ä-\ *vb* **oc·clud·ed; oc·clud·ing 1** : to close up or block off : OBSTRUCT **2** : to bring (upper and lower teeth) into occlusion **3** : SORB

occlus- *or* **occluso-** : occlusion ⟨*occlusal*⟩

oc·clu·sal \ə-ˈklü-səl, ä-, -zəl\ *adj* : of, relating to, or being the grinding or biting surface of a tooth; *also* : of or relating to occlusion of the teeth (∼ abnormalities) — **oc·clu·sal·ly** *adv*

occlusal disharmony *n* : a condition in which incorrect positioning of one or more teeth causes an abnormal increase in or change of direction of the force applied to one or more teeth when the upper and lower teeth are occluded

occlusal plane *n* : an imaginary plane formed by the occlusal surfaces of the teeth when the jaw is closed

oc·clu·sion \ə-ˈklü-zhən\ *n* **1** : the act of occluding or the state of being occluded : a shutting off or obstruction of something ⟨a coronary ∼⟩; *esp* : a blocking of the central passage of one reflex by the passage of another **2 a** : the bringing of the opposing surfaces of the teeth of the two jaws into contact; *also* : the relation between the surfaces when in contact **b** : the transient approximation of the edges of a natural opening ⟨∼ of the eyelids⟩ — **oc·clu·sive** \-siv\ *adj*

occlusive dressing *n* : a dressing that seals a wound to protect against infection

oc·cult \ə-ˈkəlt, ˈä-ˌkəlt\ *adj* : not manifest or detectable by clinical methods alone ⟨∼ carcinoma⟩; *also* : not present in macroscopic amounts ⟨∼ blood in a stool specimen⟩ — compare GROSS 2

occulta — see SPINA BIFIDA OCCULTA

oc·cu·pa·tion·al \ˌä-kyə-ˈpā-shə-nəl\ *adj* : relating to or being an occupational disease ⟨∼ deafness⟩ — **oc·cu·pa·tion·al·ly** *adv*

occupational disease *n* : an illness caused by factors arising from one's occupation — called also *industrial disease*

occupational medicine *n* : a branch of medicine concerned with the prevention and treatment of occupational diseases

occupational therapist *n* : a person trained in or engaged in the practice of occupational therapy

occupational therapy *n* : therapy by means of activity; *esp* : creative activity prescribed for its effect in promoting recovery or rehabilitation — compare RECREATIONAL THERAPY

och·ra·tox·in \ˌō-krə-ˈtäk-sən\ *n* : a mycotoxin produced by a fungus of the genus *Aspergillus* (*A. ochraceus*)

och·ro·no·sis \ˌō-krə-ˈnō-səs\ *n, pl* **-no·ses** \-ˌsēz\ : a condition often associated with alkaptonuria and marked by pigment deposits in cartilages, ligaments, and tendons — **och·ro·not·ic** \-ˈnä-tik\ *adj*

oc·ta·pep·tide \ˌäk-tə-ˈpep-ˌtīd\ *n* : a protein fragment or molecule (as oxytocin) that consists of eight amino acids linked in a polypeptide chain

ocul- *or* **oculo-** *comb form* **1** : eye ⟨*oculomotor*⟩ **2** : ocular and ⟨*oculocutaneous*⟩

oc·u·lar \ˈä-kyə-lər\ *adj* : of or relating to the eye ⟨∼ muscles⟩ ⟨∼ diseases⟩

oc·u·lar·ist \ˈä-kyə-lə-rist\ *n* : a person who makes and fits artificial eyes

oculi — see OBLIQUUS INFERIOR OCULI, OBLIQUUS SUPERIOR OCULI, ORBICULARIS OCULI, RECTUS OCULI

oc·u·list \ˈä-kyə-list\ *n* **1** : OPHTHALMOLOGIST **2** : OPTOMETRIST

oc·u·lo·cu·ta·ne·ous \ˌä-kyə-(ˌ)lō-kyü-ˈtā-nē-əs\ *adj* : relating to or affecting both the eyes and the skin

oc·u·lo·gy·ric crisis \ˌä-kyə-lō-ˈjī-rik-\ *n* : a spasmodic attack that occurs in some nervous diseases and is marked by fixation of the eyeballs in one position usu. upward — called also *oculogyric spasm*

oc·u·lo·mo·tor \ˌä-kyə-lə-ˈmō-tər\ *adj* **1** : moving or tending to move the eyeball **2** : of or relating to the oculomotor nerve

oculomotor nerve *n* : either nerve of the third pair of cranial nerves that are motor nerves with some associated autonomic fibers, arise from the midbrain, and supply most muscles of the eye with motor fibers and the ciliary body and iris with autonomic fibers by way of the ciliary ganglion — called also *third cranial nerve*

oculomotor nucleus *n* : a nucleus that is situated under the aqueduct of Sylvius rostral to the trochlear nucleus and is the source of the motor fibers of the oculomotor nerve

oc·u·lo·plas·tic \ˌä-kyə-lō-ˈplas-tik\ *adj*

: of, relating to, or being plastic surgery of the eye and associated structures

od *abbr* [Latin *omnes dies*] every day — used in writing prescriptions

¹**OD** \(ₐ)ō-'dē\ *n* **1** : an overdose of a narcotic **2** : one who has taken an OD

²**OD** *vb* **OD'd** *or* **ODed; OD'ing; OD's** : to become ill or die of an OD

³**OD** *abbr* **1** doctor of optometry **2** [Latin *oculus dexter*] right eye — used in writing prescriptions

Oddi — see SPHINCTER OF ODDI

odont- *or* **odonto-** *comb form* : tooth ⟨*odontitis*⟩ ⟨*odonto*blast⟩

odon·tal·gia \ₐō-ₐdän-'tal-jə, -jē-ə\ *n* : TOOTHACHE — **odon·tal·gic** \-jik\ *adj*

-odon·tia \ə-'dän-chə, -chē-ə\ *n comb form* : form, condition, or mode of treatment of the teeth ⟨orth*odontia*⟩

odon·ti·tis \-'tī-təs\ *n, pl* **odon·tit·i·des** \-'ti-tə-ₐdēz\ : inflammation of a tooth

odon·to·blast \ō-'dän-tə-ₐblast\ *n* : one of the elongated radially arranged outer cells of the dental pulp that secrete dentin — **odon·to·blas·tic** \-ₐdän-tə-'blas-tik\ *adj*

odon·to·gen·e·sis \ō-ₐdän-tə-'je-nə-səs\ *n, pl* **-e·ses** \-ₐsēz\ : the formation and development of teeth

odon·to·gen·ic \ō-ₐdän-tə-'je-nik\ *adj* **1** : forming or capable of forming teeth ⟨~ tissues⟩ **2** : containing or arising from odontogenic tissues ⟨~ tumors⟩

odon·toid process \ō-'dän-ₐtòid-\ *n* : a toothlike process that projects from the anterior end of the centrum of the axis in the spinal column and serves as a pivot on which the atlas rotates — called also **dens**

odon·tol·o·gist \(ₐ)ō-ₐdän-'tä-lə-jist\ *n* : a specialist in odontology

odon·tol·o·gy \(ₐ)ō-ₐdän-'tä-lə-jē\ *n, pl* **-gies** : a science dealing with the teeth, their structure and development, and their diseases — **odon·to·log·i·cal** \-ₐdänt-ᵊl-'ä-ji-kəl\ *adj*

odon·to·ma \(ₐ)ō-ₐdän-'tō-mə\ *n, pl* **-mas** *also* **-ma·ta** \-mə-tə\ : a tumor originating from a tooth and containing dental tissue (as enamel, dentin, or cementum)

odon·tome \ō-'dän-ₐtōm\ *n* : ODONTOMA

odor \'ō-dər\ *n* **1** : a quality of something that affects the sense of smell **2** : a sensation resulting from adequate chemical stimulation of the receptors for the sense of smell — **odored** *adj* — **odor·less** *adj*

odour *chiefly Brit var of* ODOR

-o·dyn·ia \ə-'di-nē-ə\ *n comb form* : pain ⟨pleur*odynia*⟩

odyno·pha·gia \ō-ₐdi-nə-'fā-jə, -jē-ə\ *n* : pain produced by swallowing

oe·de·ma *chiefly Brit var of* EDEMA

oe·di·pal \'e-də-pəl, 'ē-\ *adj, often cap* : of, relating to, or resulting from the Oedipus complex — **oe·di·pal·ly** *adv, often cap*

¹**Oe·di·pus** \-pəs\ *adj* : OEDIPAL

---

²**Oedipus** *n* : OEDIPUS COMPLEX

Oedipus complex *n* : the positive libidinal feelings of a child toward the parent of the opposite sex and hostile or jealous feelings toward the parent of the same sex that may be a source of adult personality disorder when unresolved — used esp. of the male child; see ELECTRA COMPLEX

oesophag- *or* **oesophago-** *chiefly Brit var of* ESOPHAG-

oe·soph·a·ge·al, oe·soph·a·gec·to·my, oe·soph·a·go·gas·trec·to·my, oe·soph·a·go·plas·ty, oe·soph·a·gus *chiefly Brit var of* ESOPHAGEAL, ESOPHAGECTOMY, ESOPHAGOGASTRECTOMY, ESOPHAGOPLASTY, ESOPHAGUS

oe·soph·a·go·sto·mi·a·sis \i-ₐsä-fə-(ₐ)gō-stə-'mī-ə-səs\ *n, pl* **-a·ses** \-ₐsēz\ : infestation with or disease caused by nematode worms of the genus *Oesophagostomum* : NODULAR DISEASE

Oe·soph·a·gos·to·mum \i-ₐsä-fə-'gäs-tə-məm\ *n* : a genus of strongylid nematode worms comprising the nodular worms of ruminants and swine and other worms affecting primates including humans esp. in Africa

oestr- *or* **oestro-** *chiefly Brit var of* ESTR-

oes·tra·di·ol, oes·tro·gen, oes·trus *chiefly Brit var of* ESTRADIOL, ESTROGEN, ESTRUS

Oes·trus \'es-trəs, 'ēs-\ *n* : a genus (family *Oestridae*) of dipteran flies including the sheep botfly (*O. ovis*)

of·fi·cial \ə-'fi-shəl\ *adj* : prescribed or recognized as authorized; *specif* : described by the *U.S. Pharmacopeia* or the *National Formulary* — compare NONOFFICIAL, UNOFFICIAL — **of·fi·cial·ly** *adv*

of·fic·i·nal \ə-'fis-ᵊn-əl, ō-; ä-; ₐö-fə-'sin-ᵊl, ₐä-\ *adj* **1 a** : available without special preparation or compounding ⟨~ medicine⟩ **b** : OFFICIAL **2** : of a plant : MEDICINAL ⟨~ rhubarb⟩

officinal *n* : an officinal drug, medicine, or plant

off·spring \'òf-ₐspriŋ\ *n, pl* **offspring** *also* **offsprings** : the progeny of an animal or plant

ohm \'ōm\ *n* : a unit of electrical resistance equal to the resistance of a circuit in which a potential difference of one volt produces a current of one ampere

oid·ium \ō-'i-dē-əm\ *n* **1** *cap* : a genus (family Moniliaceae) of imperfect fungi including many which are now considered to be asexual spore-producing stages of various powdery mildews ⟨*O. ovis*⟩ **2** \-dē-ə\ : any fungus of the genus *Oidium*

oil \'òil\ *n* **1** : any of numerous fatty or greasy liquid substances obtained from plants, animals, or minerals and used for fuel, food, medicines, and manufacturing **2** : a substance (as a cosmetic preparation) of oily consistency — **oil** *adj*

oil gland *n* : a gland (as of the skin) that produces an oily secretion; *specif* : SEBACEOUS GLAND

oil of wintergreen *n* : a preparation of methyl salicylate obtained by distilling the leaves of wintergreen (*Gaultheria procumbens*) — called also *wintergreen oil*

oily \'oi-lē\ *adj* **oil·i·er; -est 1** : of, relating to, or consisting of oil **2** : excessively high in naturally secreted oils ⟨∼ hair⟩ ⟨∼ skin⟩

oint·ment \'oint-mənt\ *n* : a salve or unguent for application to the skin; *specif* : a semisolid medicinal preparation usu. having a base of fatty or greasy material

-ol \ˌol, ˌōl\ *n suffix* : chemical compound (as an alcohol or phenol) containing hydroxyl ⟨glycer*ol*⟩

OL *abbr* [Latin *oculus laevus*] left eye — used in writing prescriptions

ole- *or* **oleo-** *also* **olei-** *comb form* : oil ⟨*olei*n⟩

olea *pl of* OLEUM

ole·an·der \'ō-lē-ˌan-dər, ˌō-lē-'\ *n* : a poisonous evergreen shrub (*Nerium oleander*) of the dogbane family (Apocynaceae) with fragrant white to red flowers that contains the cardiac glycoside oleandrin

ole·an·do·my·cin \ˌō-lē-ˌan-də-'mīs-ᵊn\ *n* : an antibiotic $C_{35}H_{61}NO_{12}$ produced by a bacterium of the genus *Streptomyces* (*S. antibioticus*)

ole·an·drin \ˌō-lē-'an-drən\ *n* : a poisonous crystalline glycoside $C_{32}H_{48}O_9$ found in oleander leaves and resembling digitalis in its action

ole·ate \'ō-lē-ˌāt\ *n* **1** : a salt or ester of oleic acid **2** : a liquid or semisolid preparation of a medicinal dissolved in an excess of oleic acid

olec·ra·non \ō-'le-krə-ˌnän\ *n* : the large process of the ulna that projects behind the elbow joint, forms the bony prominence of the elbow, and receives the insertion of the triceps muscle

olecranon fossa *n* : the fossa at the distal end of the humerus into which the olecranon fits when the arm is in full extension — compare CORONOID FOSSA

ole·ic acid \ō-'lē-ik-, -'lā-\ *n* : a monounsaturated fatty acid $C_{18}H_{34}O_2$ found in natural fats and oils

ole·in \'ō-lē-ən\ *n* : an ester of glycerol and oleic acid

oleo- — see OLE-

oleo·res·in \ˌō-lē-ō-'rez-ᵊn\ *n* **1** : a natural plant product (as turpentine) containing chiefly essential oil and resin **2** : a preparation consisting essentially of oil holding resin in solution — **oleo·res·in·ous** \-'rez-ᵊn-əs\ *adj*

oleo·tho·rax \'ō-lē-ō-ˌthōr-ˌaks, -ˌak-\ *n, pl* **-tho·rax·es** *or* **-tho·ra·ces** \-'thōr-ə-ˌsēz\ : a state in which oil is present in the pleural cavity usu. as a result of

injection — compare PNEUMOTHORAX 1

ole·um \'ō-lē-əm\ *n, pl* **olea** \-lē-ə\ : OIL 1

ol·fac·tion \äl-'fak-shən, ōl-\ *n* **1** : the sense of smell **2** : the act or process of smelling

ol·fac·to·ry \äl-'fak-tə-rē, ōl-\ *adj* : of, relating to, or connected with the sense of smell

olfactory area *n* **1** : the sensory area for olfaction lying in the hippocampal gyrus **2** : the area of nasal mucosa in which the olfactory organ is situated

olfactory bulb *n* : a bulbous anterior projection of the olfactory lobe that is the place of termination of the olfactory nerves

olfactory cell *n* : a sensory cell specialized for the reception of sensory stimuli caused by odors; *specif* : one of the spindle-shaped neurons buried in the nasal mucous membrane of vertebrates — see OLFACTORY ORGAN

olfactory epithelium *n* : the nasal mucosa containing olfactory cells

olfactory gland *n* : GLAND OF BOWMAN

olfactory gyrus *n* : either a lateral or a medial gyrus on each side of the brain by which the olfactory tract on the corresponding side communicates with the olfactory area

olfactory lobe *n* : a lobe of the brain that rests on the lower surface of a temporal lobe and projects forward from the anterior lower part of each cerebral hemisphere and that consists of an olfactory bulb, an olfactory tract, and an olfactory trigone

olfactory nerve *n* : either of the pair of nerves that are the first cranial nerves, that serve to conduct sensory stimuli from the olfactory organ to the brain, and that arise from the olfactory cells and terminate in the olfactory bulb — called also *first cranial nerve*

olfactory organ *n* : an organ of chemical sense that receives stimuli interpreted as odors, that lies in the walls of the upper part of the nasal cavity, and that forms a mucous membrane continuous with the rest of the lining of the nasal cavity

olfactory pit *n* : a depression on the head of an embryo that becomes converted into a nasal passage

olfactory tract *n* : a tract of nerve fibers in the olfactory lobe on the inferior surface of the frontal lobe of the brain that passes from the olfactory bulb to the olfactory trigone

olfactory trigone *n* : a triangular area of gray matter on each side of the brain forming the junction of an olfactory tract with a cerebral hemisphere near the optic chiasma

olig- *or* **oligo-** *comb form* **1** : few ⟨*oligo*peptide⟩ **2** : deficiency : insufficiency ⟨*olig*uria⟩

ol·i·gae·mia *chiefly Brit var of* OLI-GEMIA

ol·i·ge·mia \ˌä-lə-ˈgē-mē-ə, -ˈjē-\ *n* : a condition in which the total volume of the blood is reduced — **ol·i·ge·mic** \-mik\ *adj*

oli·go·dac·tyl·ism \ˌä-li-gō-ˈdak-tə-ˌli-zəm, ə-ˌli-gō-\ *also* **oli·go·dac·tyly** \-lē\ *n, pl* **-tyl·isms** *also* **-tylies** : the presence of fewer than five digits on a hand or foot

oli·go·den·dro·cyte \-ˈden-drə-ˌsīt\ *n* : a neuroglial cell resembling an astrocyte but smaller with few and slender processes having few branches

oli·go·den·drog·lia \ˌä-li-gō-den-ˈdrä-glē-ə, ˌō-li-, -ˈdrō-\ *n* : neuroglia made up of oligodendrocytes that is held to function in myelin formation in the central nervous system — **oli·go·den·drog·li·al** \-lē-əl\ *adj*

oli·go·den·dro·gli·o·ma \-ˌden-drō-glī-ˈō-mə\ *n, pl* **-mas** *or* **-ma·ta** \-mə-tə\ : a tumor of the nervous system composed of oligodendroglia

oli·go·hy·dram·ni·os \-ˌhī-ˈdram-nē-ˌäs\ *n* : deficiency of amniotic fluid sometimes resulting in an embryonic defect through adherence between embryo and amnion

oli·go·men·or·rhea \-ˌme-nə-ˈrē-ə\ *n* : abnormally infrequent or scanty menstrual flow

oli·go·men·or·rhoea *chiefly Brit var of* OLIGOMENORRHEA

oli·go·nu·cle·o·tide \-ˈnü-klē-ə-ˌtīd, -ˈnyü-\ *n* : a chain of up to 25 nucleotides

oli·go·pep·tide \ˌä-li-gō-ˈpep-ˌtīd, ō-li-\ *n* : a protein fragment or molecule that usu. consists of less than 25 amino acid residues linked in a polypeptide chain

oli·go·phre·nia \-ˈfrē-nē-ə\ *n* : MENTAL RETARDATION

oli·go·sper·mia \-ˈspər-mē-ə\ *n* : deficiency of sperm in the semen — **oli·go·sper·mic** \-mik\ *adj*

ol·i·gu·ria \ˌä-lə-ˈgür-ē-ə, -ˈgyür-\ *n* : reduced excretion of urine — **ol·i·gur·ic** \-ik\ *adj*

ol·i·vary \ˈä-lə-ˌver-ē\ *adj* 1 : shaped like an olive 2 : of, relating to, situated near, or comprising one or more of the olives, inferior olives, or superior olives ⟨the ∼ complex⟩ ⟨∼ fibers⟩

olivary nucleus *n* 1 : INFERIOR OLIVE 2 : SUPERIOR OLIVE

ol·ive \ˈä-liv\ *n* : an oval eminence on each ventrolateral aspect of the medulla oblongata that contains the inferior olive of the same side — called also *olivary body*

olive oil *n* : a pale yellow to yellowish green oil obtained from the pulp of olives (from the olive tree, *Olea europaea* of the family Oleaceae) usu. by expressing and used chiefly as a salad oil and in cooking, in toilet soaps, and as an emollient

ol·i·vo·cer·e·bel·lar tract \ˌä-li-vō-ˌser-ə-ˈbe-lər-\ *n* : a tract of fibers that arises in the olive on one side, crosses to the olive on the other, and enters the cerebellum by way of the inferior cerebellar peduncle

ol·i·vo·pon·to·cer·e·bel·lar atrophy \-ˌpän-tō-ˌser-ə-ˈbe-lər-\ *n* : an inherited disease esp. of mid to late life that is characterized by ataxia, hypotonia, dysarthria, and degeneration of the cerebellar cortex, middle cerebellar peduncles, and inferior olives — called also *olivopontocerebellar degeneration*

ol·i·vo·spi·nal tract \-ˈspīn-əl-\ *n* : a tract of fibers on the peripheral aspect of the ventral side of the cervical part of the spinal cord that communicates with the inferior olive

-o·ma \ˈō-mə\ *n suffix, pl* **-o·mas** \-məz\ *or* **-o·ma·ta** \-mə-tə\ : tumor ⟨adenoma⟩ ⟨fibroma⟩

oma·sum \ō-ˈmä-səm\ *n, pl* **oma·sa** \-sə\ : the third chamber of the ruminant stomach that is situated between the reticulum and the abomasum — called also *manyplies, psalterium* — **oma·sal** \-səl\ *adj*

ome·ga-3 \ō-ˈme-gə-ˈthrē, -ˈmä-\ *adj* : being or composed of polyunsaturated fatty acids that have the final double bond in the hydrocarbon chain between the third and fourth carbon atoms from the end of the molecule opposite that of the carboxylic acid group and that are found esp. in fish, fish oils, vegetable oils, and green leafy vegetables — **omega-3** *n*

oment- *or* **omento-** *comb form* : omentum ⟨omentectomy⟩ ⟨omentopexy⟩

omen·tec·to·my \ˌō-men-ˈtek-tə-mē\ *n, pl* **-mies** : excision or resection of all or part of an omentum — called also *epiploectomy*

omen·to·pexy \ō-ˈmen-tə-ˌpek-sē\ *n, pl* **-pex·ies** : the operation of suturing the omentum esp. to another organ

omen·to·plas·ty \-ˌplas-tē\ *n, pl* **-ties** : the use of a piece or flap of tissue from an omentum as a graft

omen·tor·rha·phy \ˌō-men-ˈtor-ə-fē\ *n, pl* **-phies** : surgical repair of an omentum by suturing

omen·tum \ō-ˈmen-təm\ *n, pl* **-ta** \-tə\ *or* **-tums** : a fold of peritoneum connecting or supporting abdominal structures (as the viscera) — see GREATER OMENTUM, LESSER OMENTUM — **omen·tal** \-ˈment-əl\ *adj*

om·ni·fo·cal \ˌäm-ni-ˈfō-kəl\ *adj* : of, relating to, or being a bifocal eyeglass that is so ground as to permit smooth transition from one correction to the other

omo·hy·oi·de·us \ˌhī-ˈoi-dē-əs\ *n, pl* **-dei** \-dē-ˌī\ : OMOHYOID MUSCLE

omo·hy·oid muscle \ˌō-mō-ˈhī-ˌoid-\ *n* : a muscle that arises from the upper border of the scapula, is inserted in the body of the hyoid bone, and acts to draw the hyoid bone in a caudal direction — called also *omohyoid*

omphal- *or* **omphalo-** *comb form* **1** : umbilicus ⟨*omphalitis*⟩ **2** : umbilical and ⟨*omphalo*mesenteric duct⟩

om·pha·lec·to·my \ˌäm-fə-ˈlek-tə-mē\ *n, pl* **-mies** : surgical excision of the umbilicus — called also *umbilectomy*

om·phal·ic \(ˌ)äm-ˈfa-lik\ *adj* : of or relating to the umbilicus

om·pha·li·tis \ˌäm-fə-ˈlī-təs\ *n, pl* **-lit·i·des** \-ˈli-tə-ˌdēz\ : inflammation of the umbilicus

om·pha·lo·cele \äm-ˈfa-lə-ˌsēl, ˈäm-fə-lə-\ *n* : protrusion of abdominal contents through an opening at the umbilicus occurring esp. as a congenital defect

om·pha·lo·mes·en·ter·ic duct \ˌäm-fə-lō-ˌmez-ᵊn-ˈter-ik-, -ˌmes-\ *n* : the duct by which the yolk sac or umbilical vesicle remains connected with the alimentary tract of the vertebrate embryo — called also *vitelline duct, yolk stalk*

om·pha·lo·phle·bi·tis \-fli-ˈbī-təs\ *n, pl* **-bit·i·des** \-ˈbī-tə-ˌdēz\ : a condition (as navel ill) characterized by or resulting from inflammation and infection of the umbilical vein

onan·ism \ˈō-nə-ˌni-zəm\ *n* **1** : MASTURBATION **2** : COITUS INTERRUPTUS — **onan·is·tic** \ˌō-nə-ˈnis-tik\ *adj*

onan·ist \ˈō-nə-nist\ *n* : one that practices onanism

On·cho·cer·ca \ˌäŋ-kə-ˈsər-kə\ *n* : a genus of long slender filarial worms (family Dipetalonematidae) that are parasites of mammalian subcutaneous and connective tissues

on·cho·cer·ci·a·sis \ˌäŋ-kō-(ˌ)sər-ˈkī-ə-səs, -(ˌ)sē-\ *n, pl* **-a·ses** \-ˌsēz\ : infestation with or disease caused by filarial worms of the genus *Onchocerca; esp* : a human disease caused by a worm (*O. volvulus*) that is native to Africa but now present in parts of tropical America and is transmitted by several blackflies — called also *river blindness*

on·cho·sphere *var of* ONCOSPHERE

onco- *or* **oncho-** *comb form* **1** : tumor ⟨*oncology*⟩ **2** : bulk : mass ⟨*onco*sphere⟩

on·co·cyte \ˈäŋ-kō-ˌsīt\ *n* : an acidophilic granular cell esp. of the parotid gland

on·co·cy·to·ma \ˌäŋ-kō-sī-ˈtō-mə\ *n, pl* **-mas** *or* **-ma·ta** \-mə-tə\ : a tumor (as of the parotid gland) consisting chiefly or entirely of oncocytes

on·co·fe·tal \-ˈfēt-ᵊl\ *adj* : of, relating to, or occurring in both tumorous and fetal tissues

on·co·gene \ˈäŋ-kō-ˌjēn\ *n* : a gene having the potential to cause a normal cell to become cancerous

on·co·gen·e·sis \ˌäŋ-kō-ˈje-nə-səs\ *n, pl* **-e·ses** \-ˌsēz\ : the induction or formation of tumors

on·co·gen·ic \-ˈje-nik\ *adj* **1** : relating to tumor formation **2** : tending to cause tumors — **on·co·gen·i·cal·ly** *adv* — **on·co·ge·nic·i·ty** \-jə-ˈni-sə-tē\ *n*

on·col·o·gist \än-ˈkä-lə-jəst, äŋ-\ *n* : a specialist in oncology

on·col·o·gy \än-ˈkä-lə-jē, äŋ-\ *n, pl* **-gies** : the study of tumors — **on·co·log·i·cal** \ˌäŋ-kə-ˈlä-ji-kəl\ *also* **on·co·log·ic** \-jik\ *adj*

on·col·y·sis \-ˈkä-lə-səs, -ˌsēz\ *n, pl* **-y·ses** \-ˌsēz\ : the destruction of tumor cells — **on·co·lyt·ic** \ˌäŋ-kə-ˈli-tik\ *adj* — **on·co·lyt·i·cal·ly** *adv*

on·cor·na·vi·rus \äŋ-ˌkȯr-nə-ˈvī-rəs\ *n* : any of a group of RNA-containing viruses that produce tumors

on·co·sphere \ˈäŋ-kō-ˌsfir\ *n* : an embryo of a tapeworm (order Cyclophyllidea) that has six hooks and is in the earliest differentiated stage

on·cot·ic pressure \(ˌ)äŋ-ˈkä-tik-, (ˌ)än-\ *n* : the pressure exerted by plasma proteins on the capillary wall

On·co·vin \ˈäŋ-kō-ˌvin\ *trademark* — used for a preparation of vincristine

one–egg *adj* : MONOZYGOTIC ⟨∼ twins⟩

on·lay \ˈȯn-ˌlā, ˈän-\ *n* **1** : a metal covering attached to a tooth to restore one or more of its surfaces **2** : a graft applied to the surface of a tissue (as bone)

on·set \ˈȯn-ˌset, ˈän-\ *n* : the initial existence or symptoms of a disease

ont- *or* **onto-** *comb form* : organism ⟨*ont*ogeny⟩

-ont \ˌänt\ *n comb form* : cell : organism ⟨schiz*ont*⟩

on·to·gen·e·sis \ˌän-tə-ˈje-nə-səs\ *n, pl* **-gen·e·ses** \-ˌsēz\ : ONTOGENY

on·to·ge·net·ic \-jə-ˈne-tik\ *adj* : of, relating to, or appearing in the course of ontogeny ⟨∼ variation⟩ — **on·to·ge·net·i·cal·ly** *adv*

on·tog·e·ny \än-ˈtä-jə-nē\ *n, pl* **-nies** : the development or course of development of an individual organism — called also *ontogenesis; compare* PHYLOGENY 2

onych- *or* **onycho-** *comb form* : nail of the finger or toe ⟨*onycho*lysis⟩

on·ych·ec·to·my \ˌä-ni-ˈkek-tə-mē\ *n, pl* **-mies** : surgical excision of a fingernail or toenail

onych·ia \ō-ˈni-kē-ə\ *n* : inflammation of the matrix of a nail often leading to suppuration and loss of the nail

-onych·ia \ə-ˈni-kē-ə\ *n comb form* : condition of the nails of the fingers or toes ⟨leuk*onychia*⟩

-onych·i·um \ə-ˈni-kē-əm\ *n comb form* : fingernail : toenail : region of the fingernail or toenail ⟨ep*onychium*⟩

on·y·cho·gry·po·sis \ˌä-ni-kō-gri-ˈpō-səs\ *n, pl* **-po·ses** \-ˌsēz\ : an abnormal condition of the nails characterized by marked hypertrophy and increased curvature

on·y·chol·y·sis \ˌä-ni-ˈkä-lə-səs\ *n, pl* **-y·ses** \-ˌsēz\ : a loosening of a nail from the nail bed beginning at the free edge and proceeding to the root

on·y·cho·ma·de·sis \ä-ni-kō-mə-ˈdē-səs\ *n, pl* **-de·ses** \-ˌsēz\ : loosening and shedding of the nails

on·y·cho·my·co·sis \-mi-ˈkō-səs\ *n, pl* **-co·ses** \-ˌsēz\ : a fungal disease of the nails

oo- — see O-

oo·cy·e·sis \ˌō-ə-sī-ˈē-səs\ *n, pl* **-e·ses** \-ˌsēz\ : extrauterine pregnancy in an ovary

oo·cyst \ˈō-ə-ˌsist\ *n* : ZYGOTE; *specif* : a sporozoan zygote undergoing sporogenous development

oo·cyte \ˈō-ə-ˌsit\ *n* : an egg before maturation : a female gametocyte

oo·gen·e·sis \ˌō-ə-ˈje-nə-səs\ *n, pl* **-e·ses** \-ˌsēz\ : formation and maturation of the egg — called also *ovogenesis*

oogon- *or* **oophoro-** *comb form* : ovary ⟨*oophoro*ectomy⟩

oo·go·ni·um \ˌō-ə-ˈgō-nē-əm\ *n* : a descendant of a primordial germ cell that gives rise to oocytes — **oo·go·ni·al** \-nē-əl\ *adj*

oophor- *or* **oophoro-** *comb form* : ovary ⟨*oophoro*ectomy⟩

oo·pho·rec·to·my \ˌō-ə-fə-ˈrek-tə-mē\ *n, pl* **-mies** : OVARIECTOMY — **oo·pho·rec·to·mize** \-ˌmiz\ *vb*

oo·pho·ri·tis \ˌō-ə-fə-ˈri-təs\ *n* : inflammation of one or both ovaries

oophorus — see CUMULUS OOPHORUS

oo·plasm \ˈō-ə-ˌpla-zəm\ *n* : the cytoplasm of an egg — **oo·plas·mic** \-ˈplaz-mik\ *adj*

oo·tid \ˈō-ə-ˌtid\ *n* : an egg cell after meiosis — compare SPERMATID

opac·i·fi·ca·tion \ō-ˌpa-sə-fə-ˈkā-shən\ *n* : an act or the process of becoming or rendering opaque ⟨∼ of the cornea⟩ — **opac·i·fy** \ō-ˈpa-sə-ˌfi\ *vb*

opac·i·ty \ō-ˈpa-sə-tē\ *n, pl* **-ties 1** : the quality or state of a body that makes it impervious to the rays of light; *broadly* : the relative capacity of matter to obstruct by absorption or reflection the transmission of radiant energy **2** : an opaque spot in a normally transparent structure (as the lens of the eye)

opaque \ō-ˈpāk\ *adj* : exhibiting opacity : not allowing passage of radiant energy

OPD *abbr* outpatient department

¹open \ˈō-pən\ *adj* **1 a** : not covered, enclosed, or scabbed over **b** : not involving or encouraging a covering (as by bandages or overgrowth of tissue) or enclosure ⟨∼ treatment of burns⟩ **c** : shedding the infective agent to the exterior ⟨∼ tuberculosis⟩ — compare CLOSED 2 **d** : relating to or being a compound fracture **2 a** : unobstructed by congestion ⟨∼ sinuses⟩ **b** : not constipated ⟨∼ bowels⟩ **3** : using a minimum of physical restrictions and custodial restraints on the freedom of movement of the patients or inmates

²open *vb* **opened; open·ing 1** : to make available for entry or passage by removing (as a cover) or clearing away (as an obstruction); *specif* : to free (a body passage) of an occluding agent **2** : to make one or more openings in ⟨∼ed the boil⟩

open–angle glaucoma *n* : a progressive form of glaucoma in which the drainage channel for the aqueous humor composed of the attachment at the edge of the iris and the junction of the sclera and cornea remains open and in which serious reduction in vision occurs only in the advanced stages of the disease due to tissue changes along the drainage channel — compare CLOSED-ANGLE GLAUCOMA

open chain *n* : an arrangement of atoms represented in a structural formula by a chain whose ends are not joined so as to form a ring

open–heart *adj* : of, relating to, or performed on a heart temporarily relieved of circulatory function and surgically opened for inspection and treatment ⟨∼ surgery⟩

open reduction *n* : realignment of a fractured bone after incision into the fracture site

op·er·a·ble \ˈä-pə-rə-bəl\ *adj* **1** : fit, possible, or desirable to use **2** : likely to result in a favorable outcome upon surgical treatment — **op·er·a·bil·i·ty** \ˌä-pə-rə-ˈbi-lə-tē\ *n*

¹op·er·ant \ˈä-pə-rənt\ *adj* : of, relating to, or being an operant or operant conditioning ⟨∼ behavior⟩ — compare RESPONDENT — **op·er·ant·ly** *adv*

²operant *n* : behavior that operates on the environment to produce rewarding and reinforcing effects

operant conditioning *n* : conditioning in which the desired behavior or increasingly closer approximations to it are followed by a rewarding or reinforcing stimulus — compare CLASSICAL CONDITIONING

op·er·ate \ˈä-pə-ˌrāt\ *vb* **·at·ed; -at·ing** : to perform surgery

op·er·at·ing *adj* : of, relating to, or used for operations

op·er·a·tion \ˌä-pə-ˈrā-shən\ *n* : a procedure carried out on a living body usu. with instruments esp. for the repair of damage or the restoration of health

op·er·a·tive \ˈä-pə-rə-tiv, -ˌrā-\ *adj* : of, relating to, involving, or resulting from an operation

op·er·a·tor \ˈä-pə-ˌrā-tər\ *n* **1** : one (as a dentist or surgeon) who performs surgical operations **2** : a binding site in a DNA chain at which a genetic repressor binds to inhibit the initiation of transcription of messenger RNA by one or more nearby structural genes — called also *operator gene;* compare OPERON

op·er·a·to·ry \ˈä-pə-rə-ˌtōr-ē\ *n, pl* **-ries** : a working space (as of a dentist or surgeon) : SURGERY

oper·cu·lum \ō-ˈpər-kyə-ləm\ *n, pl* **-la** \-lə\ *also* **-lums** : any of several parts of the cerebrum bordering the fissure of Sylvius and concealing the insula

op·er·on \\'ä-pə-ˌrän\\ n : a group of closely linked genes that produces a single messenger RNA molecule in transcription and that consists of structural genes and regulating elements (as an operator and promoter)

ophthalm- or **ophthalmo-** comb form : eye ⟨ophthalmology⟩ : eyeball ⟨ophthalmodynamometry⟩

oph·thal·mia \\äf-'thal-mē-ə, äp-\\ n : inflammation of the conjunctiva or the eyeball

-oph·thal·mia \\äf-'thal-mē-ə, ˌäp-\\ comb form : condition of having (such) eyes ⟨microphthalmia⟩

ophthalmia neo·na·to·rum \\-ˌnē-ə-nə-'tōr-əm\\ n : acute inflammation of the eyes of a newborn from infection during passage through the birth canal

oph·thal·mic \\äf-'thal-mik, äp-\\ adj 1 : of, relating to, or situated near the eye 2 : supplying or draining the eye or structures in the region of the eye

ophthalmic artery n : a branch of the internal carotid artery following the optic nerve through the optic foramen into the orbit and supplying the eye and adjacent structures

ophthalmic nerve n : the one of the three major branches or divisions of the trigeminal nerve that supply sensory fibers to the lacrimal gland, eyelids, ciliary muscle, nose, forehead, and adjoining parts — called also ophthalmic, ophthalmic division; compare MANDIBULAR NERVE, MAXILLARY NERVE

ophthalmic vein n : either of two veins that pass from the orbit: **a** : one that begins at the inner angle of the orbit and empties into the cavernous sinus — called also superior ophthalmic vein **b** : one that drains a venous network in the floor and medial wall of the orbit and divides into two parts of which one joins the pterygoid plexus of veins and the other empties into the cavernous sinus — called also inferior ophthalmic vein

ophthalmo- — see OPHTHALM-

oph·thal·mo·dy·na·mom·e·try \\äf-ˌthal-mō-ˌdī-nə-'mä-mə-trē, äp-\\ n, pl -tries : measurement of the arterial blood pressure in the retina

oph·thal·mol·o·gist \\ˌäf-thəl-'mä-lə-jist, ˌäp-, -thal-\\ n : a physician who specializes in ophthalmology — compare OPTICIAN 2, OPTOMETRIST

oph·thal·mol·o·gy \\-jē\\ n, pl -gies : a branch of medical science dealing with the structure, functions, and diseases of the eye — **oph·thal·mo·log·ic** \\-mə-'lä-jik\\ or **oph·thal·mo·log·i·cal** \\-ji-kəl\\ adj — **oph·thal·mo·log·i·cal·ly** adv

oph·thal·mom·e·ter \\-'mä-mə-tər\\ n : an instrument for measuring the eye; specif : KERATOMETER

oph·thal·mo·ple·gia \\-'plē-jə, -jē-ə\\ n : paralysis of some or all of the muscles of the eye — **oph·thal·mo·ple·gic** \\-jik\\ adj

oph·thal·mo·scope \\äf-'thal-mə-ˌskōp\\ n : an instrument for viewing the interior of the eye consisting of a concave mirror with a hole in the center through which the observer examines the eye, a source of light that is reflected into the eye by the mirror, and lenses in the mirror which can be rotated into the opening in the mirror — **oph·thal·mo·scop·ic** \\äf-ˌthal-mə-'skäpik\\ adj

oph·thal·mos·co·py \\ˌäf-thal-'mäs-kə-pē\\ n, pl -pies : examination of the eye with an ophthalmoscope

-opia \\'ō-pē-ə\\ n comb form 1 : condition of having (such) vision ⟨diplopia⟩ 2 : condition of having (such) a visual defect ⟨hyperopia⟩

¹**opi·ate** \\'ō-pē-ət, -ˌāt\\ n 1 : a preparation (as morphine, heroin, and codeine) containing or derived from opium and tending to induce sleep and to alleviate pain 2 : a synthetic drug capable of producing or sustaining addiction similar to that characteristic of morphine and cocaine : a narcotic or opioid peptide — used esp. in modern law

²**opiate** adj 1 : of, relating to, or being opium or an opium derivative 2 : of, relating to, binding, or being an opiate ⟨∼ receptors⟩

opin·ion \\ə-'pin-yən\\ n : a formal expression of judgment or advice by an expert ⟨wanted a second ∼⟩

opi·oid \\'ō-pē-ˌȯid\\ adj 1 : possessing some properties characteristic of opiate narcotics but not derived from opium 2 : of, involving, or induced by an opioid substance or an opioid peptide

opioid peptide n : any of a group of endogenous neural polypeptides (as an endorphin or enkephalin) that bind esp. to opiate receptors and mimic some of the pharmacological properties of opiates — called also opioid

opisth- or **opistho-** comb form : dorsal : posterior ⟨opisthotonos⟩

opis·thor·chi·a·sis \\ə-ˌpis-ˌthȯr-'kī-ə-səs\\ n : infestation with or disease caused by liver flukes of the genus Opisthorchis

Op·is·thor·chis \\ˌä-pəs-'thȯr-kəs\\ n : a genus of digenetic trematode worms (family Opisthorchiidae) including several that are casual or incidental parasites of the human liver

op·is·thot·o·nos \\ˌä-pəs-'thät-ᵊn-əs\\ n : a condition of spasm of the muscles of the back, causing the head and lower limbs to bend backward and the trunk to arch forward

opi·um \\'ō-pē-əm\\ n : a highly addictive drug that consists of the dried milky juice from the seed capsules of the opium poppy, that is a stimulant narcotic causing coma or death if the dose is excessive, that was formerly used in medicine to soothe pain, and that is smoked as an intoxicant

opium poppy *n* : a Eurasian poppy (*Papaver somniferum*) that is the source of opium

op·po·nens \ə-ˈpō-ˌnenz\ *n, pl* **-nentes** \ˌä-pə-ˈnen-(ˌ)tēz\ *or* **-nens** : any of several muscles of the hand or foot that tend to draw one of the lateral digits across the palm or sole toward the others

opponens dig·i·ti min·i·mi \-ˈdi-jə-ˌtī-ˈmi-nə-ˌmī\ *n* : a triangular muscle of the hand that arises from the hamate and adjacent flexor retinaculum, is inserted along the ulnar side of the metacarpal of the little finger, and functions to abduct, flex, and rotate the fifth metacarpal in opposing the little finger and thumb

opponens pol·li·cis \-ˈpä-lə-səs\ *n* : a small triangular muscle of the hand that is located below the abductor pollicis brevis, arises from the trapezium and the flexor retinaculum of the hand, is inserted along the radial side of the metacarpal of the thumb, and functions to abduct, flex, and rotate the metacarpal of the thumb in opposing the thumb and fingers

op·po·nent \ə-ˈpō-nənt\ *n* : a muscle that opposes or counteracts and limits the action of another

op·por·tun·ist \ˌä-pər-ˈtü-nist, -ˈtyü-\ *n* : an opportunistic microorganism

op·por·tu·nist·ic \-tü-ˈnis-tik, -tyü-\ *adj* **1** : of, relating to, or being a microorganism that is usu. harmless but can become pathogenic when the host's resistance to disease is impaired **2** : of, relating to, or being a disease caused by an opportunistic organism

op·pos·able \ə-ˈpō-zə-bəl\ *adj* : capable of being placed against one or more of the remaining digits of a hand or foot ⟨an ∼ thumb⟩

-op·sia \ˈäp-sē-ə\ *n comb form, pl* **-opsias** : vision of a (specified) kind or condition ⟨hemian*opsia*⟩

op·sin \ˈäp-sən\ *n* : any of various colorless proteins that in combination with retinal or a related prosthetic group form a visual pigment (as rhodopsin) in a reaction which is reversed by light

op·so·nin \ˈäp-sə-nən\ *n* : an antibody of blood serum that makes foreign cells more susceptible to the action of the phagocytes — **op·son·ic** \äp-ˈsä-nik\ *adj*

op·son·iza·tion \ˌäp-sə-nə-ˈzā-shən, -ˌnī-ˈzā-\ *n* : the process of modifying (as a bacterium) by the action of opsonins — **op·son·ize** \ˈäp-sə-ˌnīz\ *vb*

-op·sy \ˌäp-sē, əp-\ *n comb form, pl* **-opsies** : examination ⟨bi*opsy*⟩ ⟨necr*opsy*⟩

opt *abbr* optician

¹op·tic \ˈäp-tik\ *adj* **1** : of or relating to vision ⟨∼ phenomena⟩ **2 a** : of or relating to the eye : OCULAR **b** : affecting the eye or an optic structure

²optic *n* : any of the lenses, prisms, or mirrors of an optical instrument

op·ti·cal \ˈäp-ti-kəl\ *adj* **1** : of or relating to the science of optics **2 a** : of or relating to vision : VISUAL **b** : designed to aid vision **3** : of, relating to, or utilizing light ⟨∼ microscopy⟩ — **op·ti·cal·ly** *adv*

optical activity *n* : ability to rotate the plane of vibration of polarized light to the right or left

optical axis *n* : a straight line perpendicular to the front of the cornea of the eye and extending through the center of the pupil — called also *optic axis*

optical illusion *n* : visual perception of a real object in such a way as to misinterpret its actual nature

optically active *adj* : capable of rotating the plane of vibration of polarized light to the right or left : either dextrorotatory or levorotatory — used of compounds, molecules, or atoms

optic atrophy *n* : degeneration of the optic nerve

optic axis *n* : OPTICAL AXIS

optic canal *n* : OPTIC FORAMEN

optic chiasma *n* : the X-shaped partial decussation on the undersurface of the hypothalamus through which the optic nerves are continuous with the brain — called also *optic chiasm*

optic cup *n* : the optic vesicle after invaginating to form a 2-layered cup from which the retina and pigmented layer of the eye will develop — called also *eyecup*

optic disk *n* : BLIND SPOT

optic foramen *n* : the passage through the orbit of the eye in the lesser wing of the sphenoid bone that is traversed by the optic nerve and ophthalmic artery — called also *optic canal*; see CHIASMATIC GROOVE

op·ti·cian \äp-ˈti-shən\ *n* **1** : a maker of or dealer in optical items and instruments **2** : a person who reads prescriptions for visual correction, orders lenses, and dispenses eyeglasses and contact lenses — compare OPHTHALMOLOGIST, OPTOMETRIST

op·ti·cian·ry \-rē\ *n, pl* **-ries** : the profession or practice of an optician

optic lobe *n* : SUPERIOR COLLICULUS

optic nerve *n* : either of the pair of sensory nerves that comprise the second pair of cranial nerves, arise from the ventral part of the diencephalon, form an optic chiasma before passing to the eye and spreading over the anterior surface of the retina, and conduct visual stimuli to the brain — called also *second cranial nerve*

op·tics \ˈäp-tiks\ *n sing or pl* **1** : a science that deals with the nature and properties of light **2** : optical properties

optic stalk *n* : the constricted part of the optic vesicle by which it remains continuous with the embryonic fore-brain

optic tectum *n* : SUPERIOR COLLICULUS

optic tract *n* : the portion of each optic nerve between the optic chiasma and the diencephalon proper

optic vesicle *n* : an evagination of each lateral wall of the embryonic vertebrate forebrain from which the nervous structures of the eye develop

opto- *comb form* **1** : vision ⟨*opto*metry⟩ **2** : optic and ⟨*opto*kinetic⟩

op·to·ki·net·ic \ˌäp-tō-kə-ˈne-tik, -kī-\ *adj* : of, relating to, or involving movements of the eyes ⟨∼ nystagmus⟩

op·tom·e·trist \äp-ˈtä-mə-trist\ *n* : a specialist licensed to practice optometry — compare OPHTHALMOLOGIST, OPTICIAN 2

op·tom·e·try \-trē\ *n*, *pl* **-tries** : the art or profession of examining the eye for defects and faults of refraction and prescribing corrective lenses or exercises but not drugs or surgery — **op·to·met·ric** \ˌäp-tə-ˈme-trik\ *adj*

OPV *abbr* oral polio vaccine

OR *abbr* operating room

ora *pl of* ²OS

orad \ˈȯr-ˌad\ *adv* : toward the mouth or oral region

orae serratae *pl of* ORA SERRATA

oral \ˈȯr-əl, ˈär-\ *adj* **1 a** : of, relating to, or involving the mouth : BUCCAL ⟨the ∼ mucous membrane⟩ **b** : given or taken through or by way of the mouth ⟨∼ contraceptives⟩ **c** : acting on the mouth **2 a** : of, relating to, or characterized by the first stage of psychosexual development in psychoanalytic theory during which libidinal gratification is derived from intake (as of food), by sucking, and later by biting **b** : of, relating to, or characterized by personality traits of passive dependence and aggressiveness — compare ANAL 2, GENITAL 3, PHALLIC 2 — **oral·ly** *adv*

oral cavity *n* : the cavity of the mouth; *esp* : the part of the mouth behind the gums and teeth that is bounded above by the hard and soft palates and below by the tongue and by the mucous membrane connecting it with the inner part of the mandible

oral sex *n* : oral stimulation of the genitals : CUNNILINGUS : FELLATIO

oral surgeon *n* : a specialist in oral surgery

oral surgery *n* **1** : a branch of dentistry that deals with the diagnosis and treatment of oral conditions requiring surgical intervention **2** : a branch of surgery that deals with conditions of the jaws and mouth structures requiring surgery

ora ser·ra·ta \ˌȯr-ə-sə-ˈrä-tə, -ˈrä-\ *n*, *pl* **orae ser·ra·tae** \ˌȯr-ē-sə-ˈrä-tē\ : the dentate border of the retina

or·bic·u·lar·is oculi \ˌȯr-ˌbi-kyə-ˈlar-əs-ˈä-kyü-ˌlī, -ˌlē\ *n*, *pl* **or·bic·u·lar·es**

oculi \-ˈlar-(ˌ)ēz-\ : the muscle encircling the opening of the orbit and functioning to close the eyelids

orbicularis oris \-ˈȯr-əs\ *n*, *pl* **orbiculares oris** : a muscle made up of several layers of fibers passing in different directions that encircles the mouth and controls most movements of the lips

orbiculus cil·i·ar·is \-ˌsi-lē-ˈer-əs\ *n* : a circular tract in the eye that extends from the ora serrata forward to the posterior part of the ciliary processes — called also *ciliary ring, pars plana*

or·bit \ˈȯr-bət\ *n* : the bony cavity perforated for the passage of nerves and blood vessels that occupies the lateral front of the skull immediately beneath the frontal bone on each side and encloses and protects the eye and its appendages — called also *eye socket, orbital cavity* — **or·bit·al** \-ᵊl\ *adj*

orbital fissure *n* : either of two openings transmitting nerves and blood vessels to or from the orbit: **a** : one situated superiorly between the greater wing and the lesser wing of the sphenoid bone — called also *superior orbital fissure, supraorbital fissure* **b** : one situated inferiorly between the greater wing of the sphenoid bone and the maxilla — called also *inferior orbital fissure, infraorbital fissure, sphenomaxillary fissure*

orbital plate *n* **1** : the part of the frontal bone forming most of the top of the orbit **2** : a thin plate of bone forming the lateral wall enclosing the ethmoidal air cells and forming part of the side of the orbit next to the nose

or·bi·tot·o·my \ˌȯr-bə-ˈtä-tə-mē\ *n*, *pl* **-mies** : incision of the orbit

or·bi·vi·rus \ˈȯr-bi-ˌvī-rəs\ *n* : any of a group of reoviruses that include the causative agents of Colorado tick fever and bluetongue of sheep

or·chi·dec·to·my \ˌȯr-kə-ˈdek-tə-mē\ *n*, *pl* **-mies** : ORCHIECTOMY

-or·chi·dism \ˈȯr-kə-ˌdi-zəm\ *also* **-or·chism** \ˈȯr-ˌki-zəm\ *n comb form* : a (specified) form or condition of the testes ⟨crypt*orchidism*⟩

or·chi·do·pexy \ˈȯr-kə-dō-ˌpek-sē\ *n*, *pl* **-pex·ies** : surgical fixation of a testis — called also *orchiopexy*

or·chi·ec·to·my \ˌȯr-kē-ˈek-tə-mē\ *n*, *pl* **-mies** : surgical excision of a testis or of both testes — called also *orchidectomy*

or·chi·o·pexy \ˈȯr-kē-ō-ˌpek-sē\ *n*, *pl* **-pex·ies** : ORCHIDOPEXY

or·chi·tis \ȯr-ˈkī-təs\ *n* : inflammation of a testis — **or·chit·ic** \ȯr-ˈki-tik\ *adj*

¹**or·der** \ˈȯr-dər\ *vb* **or·dered; or·der·ing** : to give a prescription for : PRESCRIBE

²**order** *n* : a category of taxonomic classification ranking above the family and below the class

or·der·ly \-lē\ *n*, *pl* **-lies** : a hospital attendant who does routine or heavy work (as cleaning, carrying supplies, or moving patients)

Oret·ic \ȯr-ˈe-tik\ *trademark* — used for a preparation of hydrochlorothiazide

-orex·ia \ə-ˈrek-sē-ə, ə-ˈrek-shə\ *n comb form* : appetite ⟨an*orexia*⟩

or·gan \ˈȯr-gən\ *n* : a differentiated structure (as a heart or kidney) consisting of cells and tissues and performing some specific function in an organism

organ- *or* **organo-** *comb form* **1** : organ ⟨*organ*elle⟩ ⟨*organo*genesis⟩ **2** : organic ⟨*organo*phosphorus⟩

or·gan·elle \ˌȯr-gə-ˈnel\ *n* : a specialized cellular part (as a mitochondrion, lysosome, or ribosome) that is analogous to an organ

or·gan·ic \ȯr-ˈga-nik\ *adj* **1 a** : of, relating to, or arising in a bodily organ **b** : affecting the structure of the organism ⟨an ∼ disease⟩ — compare FUNCTIONAL 1b **2 a** : of, relating to, or derived from living organisms **b** (1) : of, relating to, or containing carbon compounds (2) : relating to, being, or dealt with by a branch of chemistry concerned with the carbon compounds of living beings and most other carbon compounds — **or·gan·i·cal·ly** *adv*

organic brain syndrome *n* : any mental disorder (as senile dementia) resulting from or associated with organic changes in brain tissue — called also *organic brain disorder, organic mental syndrome*

or·gan·ism \ˈȯr-gə-ˌni-zəm\ *n* : an individual constituted to carry on the activities of life by means of organs separate in function but mutually dependent : a living being — **or·gan·is·mic** \ˌȯr-gə-ˈniz-mik\ *also* **or·gan·is·mal** \-məl\ *adj* — **or·gan·is·mi·cal·ly** *adv*

or·ga·ni·za·tion \ˌȯr-gə-nə-ˈzā-shən\ *n* : the formation of fibrous tissue from a clot or exudate by invasion of connective tissue cells and capillaries from adjoining tissues — **or·ga·nize** \ˈȯr-gə-ˌnīz\ *vb*

or·ga·niz·er \ˈȯr-gə-ˌnī-zər\ *n* : a region of a developing embryo (as part of the dorsal lip of the blastopore) or a substance produced by such a region that is capable of inducing a specific type of development in undifferentiated tissue — called also *inductor*

organo- — see ORGAN-

or·gano·chlo·rine \ˌȯr-ˌga-nə-ˈklȯr-ˌēn, -ən\ *adj* : of, relating to, or belonging to the chlorinated hydrocarbon pesticides (as aldrin, DDT, or dieldrin) — **organochlorine** *n*

organ of Cor·ti \-ˈkȯr-tē\ *n* : a complex epithelial structure in the cochlea that in mammals is the chief part of the ear by which sound is directly perceived

Cor·ti, Alfonso Giacomo Gaspare (1822–1876), Italian anatomist.

organ of Ro·sen·mül·ler \-ˈrō-zən-ˌmyü-lər\ *n* : EPOOPHORON

Rosenmüller, Johann Christian (1771–1820), German anatomist.

or·gan·o·gen·e·sis \ˌȯr-gə-nō-ˈje-nə-səs, ȯr-ˌga-nə-\ *n, pl* **-gen·e·ses** \-ˌsēz\ : the origin and development of bodily organs — compare MORPHOGENESIS — **or·gan·o·ge·net·ic** \-jə-ˈne-tik\ *adj*

or·gan·oid \ˈȯr-gə-ˌnȯid\ *adj* : resembling an organ in structural appearance or qualities — used esp. of abnormal masses (as tumors)

or·gan·o·lep·tic \ˌȯr-gə-nō-ˈlep-tik, ȯr-ˌga-nə-\ *adj* : being, affecting, or relating to qualities (as taste, color, and odor) of a substance (as a food) that stimulate the sense organs **2** : involving use of the sense organs

or·gan·ol·o·gy \ˌȯr-gə-ˈnä-lə-jē\ *n, pl* **-gies** : the study of the organs of plants and animals

or·gano·mer·cu·ri·al \ȯr-ˌga-nō-(ˌ)mər-ˈkyur-ē-əl\ *n* : an organic compound or a pharmaceutical preparation containing mercury — **organomercurial** *adj*

or·gano·phos·phate \ȯr-gə-nə-ˈfäs-ˌfāt\ *n* : an organophosphorus pesticide — **organophosphate** *adj*

or·gano·phos·pho·rus \-ˈfäs-fə-rəs\ *also* **or·gano·phos·pho·rous** \-fäs-ˈfȯr-əs\ *adj* : of, relating to, or being a phosphorus-containing organic pesticide (as malathion) that acts by inhibiting cholinesterase — **organophosphorus** *n*

or·gasm \ˈȯr-ˌga-zəm\ *n* : the climax of sexual excitement that is usu. accompanied in the male by ejaculation — **or·gas·mic** \ȯr-ˈgaz-mik\ *also* **or·gas·tic** \-ˈgas-tik\ *adj*

ori- *comb form* : mouth ⟨*ori*fice⟩

ori·ent \ˈȯr-ē-ˌent\ *vb* : to acquaint with or adjust according to the existing situation or environment

oriental rat flea *n* : a flea of the genus *Xenopsylla* (*X. cheopis*) that is widely distributed on rodents and is a vector of plague

oriental sore *n* : a skin disease caused by a protozoan of the genus *Leishmania* (*L. tropica*) that is marked by persistent granulomatous and ulcerating lesions and occurs widely in Asia and in tropical regions

ori·en·ta·tion \ˌȯr-ē-ən-ˈtā-shən, -ˌen-\ *n* **1 a** : the act or process of orienting or of being oriented **b** : the state of being oriented **2** : change of position by organs, organelles, or organisms in response to external stimulus **3** : awareness of the existing situation with reference to time, place, and identity of persons — **ori·en·ta·tion·al** \-shə-nəl\ *adj*

oriented *adj* : having psychological orientation ⟨the patient was alert and ∼⟩

or·i·fice \ˈȯr-ə-fəs, ˈär-\ *n* : an opening

through which something may pass
— **or·i·fi·cial** \ˌȯr-ə-ˈfi-shəl, ˌär-\ *adj*

or·i·gin \ˈȯr-ə-jən, ˈär-\ *n* **1** : the point
at which something begins or rises or
from which it derives **2** : the more
fixed, central, or larger attachment of
a muscle — compare INSERTION 1

oris — see CANCRUM ORIS, LEVATOR ANG-
ULI ORIS, ORBICULARIS ORIS

Or·mond's disease \ˈȯr-ˌmändz-\ *n*
: RETROPERITONEAL FIBROSIS
  Ormond, John Kelso (*b* 1886), Amer-
  ican urologist.

or·ni·thine \ˈȯr-nə-ˌthēn\ *n* : a crystalline amino acid $C_5H_{12}N_2O_2$ that functions esp. in urea production

Or·ni·thod·o·ros \ˌȯr-nə-ˈthä-də-rəs\ *n*
: a genus of ticks (family Argasidae)
containing forms that act as carriers
of relapsing fever as well as Q fever

or·ni·tho·sis \ˌȯr-nə-ˈthō-səs\ *n, pl* **-tho-
ses** \-ˌsēz\ : PSITTACOSIS; *esp* : a form
of the disease occurring in or originating in birds (as the turkeys and pigeons) that do not belong to the
family (Psittacidae) containing the
parrots

oro- *comb form* **1** : mouth (*oro*pharynx) **2** : oral and (*oro*facial) (*oro*nasal)

oro·an·tral \ˌȯr-ō-ˈan-trəl\ *adj* : of, relating to, or connecting the mouth
and the maxillary sinus

oro·fa·cial \-ˈfā-shəl\ *adj* : of or relating
to the mouth and face

oro·na·sal \-ˈnā-zəl\ *adj* : of or relating
to the mouth and nose; *esp* : connecting the mouth and the nasal cavity

oro·pha·ryn·geal \ˌȯr-ō-fə-ˈrän-jē-əl, -fə-
ˈrin-jəl, -jē-əl\ *adj* **1** : of or relating to
the oropharynx **2** : of or relating to
the mouth and pharynx

oropharyngeal airway *n* : a tube used to
provide free passage of air between
the mouth and pharynx of an unconscious person

oro·phar·ynx \-ˈfar-iŋks\ *n, pl* **-pha-
ryn·ges** \-fə-ˈrin-(ˌ)jēz\ *also* **-phar-
ynx·es** : the part of the pharynx that is
below the soft palate and above the
epiglottis and is continuous with the
mouth

oro·so·mu·coid \ˌȯr-ə-sō-ˈmyü-ˌkȯid\ *n*
: a plasma glycoprotein believed to be
associated with inflammation

oro·tra·che·al \ˌȯr-ō-ˈtrā-kē-əl\ *adj* : relating to or being intubation of the trachea by way of the mouth

Oroya fever \ȯr-ˈȯi-ə-\ *n* : the acute
first stage of bartonellosis characterized by high fever and severe anemia

orphan drug *n* : a drug that is not developed or marketed because its extremely limited use (as in the treatment of a rare disease) makes it un-
profitable

or·phen·a·drine \ȯr-ˈfe-nə-drən, -ˌdrēn\
n : a drug $C_{18}H_{23}NO$ used in the form
of the citrate and the hydrochloride
as a muscle relaxant and antispasmodic

orth- *or* **ortho-** *comb form* : correct
: corrective (*ortho*dontia)

or·tho·caine \ˈȯr-thə-ˌkān\ *n* : a white
crystalline powder $C_8H_9NO_3$ used as
a local anesthetic

or·tho·chro·mat·ic \ˌȯr-thə-krō-ˈma-tik\
adj : staining in the normal way (∼
tissue) (∼ erythroblast)

orth·odon·tia \ˌȯr-thə-ˈdän-chə, -chē-ə\
n : ORTHODONTICS

orth·odon·tics \-ˈdän-tiks\ *n* : a branch
of dentistry dealing with irregularities
of the teeth and their correction (as
by means of braces) — **orth·odon·tic**
\-tik\ *adj* — **orth·odon·ti·cal·ly** *adv*

or·tho·don·tist \ˌȯr-thə-ˈdän-tist\ *n* : a
specialist in orthodontics

orthodox sleep *n* : SLOW-WAVE SLEEP

or·tho·drom·ic \ˌȯr-thə-ˈdrä-mik\ *adj*
: of, relating to, or inducing nerve impulses along an axon in the normal direction

or·thog·nath·ic \ˌȯr-thag-ˈna-thik,
-ˌthäg-\ *adj* : correcting deformities of
the jaw and the associated malocclusion (∼ surgery)

or·tho·my·xo·vi·rus \ˌȯr-thō-ˈmik-sə-
ˌvī-rəs\ *n* : any of a group of RNA=
containing viruses that cause influenza and are smaller than the related
paramyxoviruses

**or·tho·pae·dic, or·tho·pae·dics, or·tho-
pae·dist** *chiefly Brit var of* ORTHOPE-
DIC, ORTHOPEDICS, ORTHOPEDIST

or·tho·pe·dic \ˌȯr-thə-ˈpē-dik\ *adj* **1**
: of, relating to, or employed in orthopedics **2** : marked by deformities or
crippling — **or·tho·pe·di·cal·ly** *adv*

or·tho·pe·dics \-ˈpē-diks\ *n sing or pl* : a
branch of medicine concerned with
the correction or prevention of skeletal deformities

or·tho·pe·dist \-ˈpē-dist\ *n* : one who
practices orthopedics

or·tho·phos·pho·ric acid \ˌȯr-thə-ˌfäs-
ˈfȯr-ik-, -ˈfär-; -ˌfäs-fə-rik-\ *n* : PHOS-
PHORIC ACID 1

or·thop·nea \ȯr-ˈthäp-nē-ə, ˌȯr-ˌthäp-
ˈnē-ə\ *n* : inability to breathe except
in an upright position (as in congestive heart failure) — **or·thop·ne·ic** \-ik\
adj

or·thop·noea *chiefly Brit var of* ORTHOP-
NEA

or·tho·psy·chi·a·trist \ˌȯr-thə-sə-ˈkī-ə-
trəst, -(ˌ)sī-\ *n* : a specialist in ortho-
psychiatry

or·tho·psy·chi·a·try \-sə-ˈkī-ə-trē,
-(ˌ)sī-\ *n, pl* **-tries** : prophylactic psychiatry concerned esp. with incipient
mental and behavioral disorders in
youth — **or·tho·psy·chi·at·ric** \-ˌsī-kē-
ˈa-trik\ *adj*

or·thop·tics \ȯr-ˈthäp-tiks\ *n sing or pl*
: the treatment or the art of treating
defective visual habits, defects of binocular vision, and muscle imbalance
(as strabismus) by reeducation of visual habits, exercise, and visual training — **or·thop·tic** \-tik\ *adj*

or·thop·tist \-tist\ *n* : a person who is

trained in or practices orthoptics
or·tho·sis \òr-'thō-səs\ *n, pl* **or·tho·ses** \-₁sēz\ : ORTHOTIC
or·tho·stat·ic \₁òr-thə-'sta-tik\ *adj* : of, relating to, or caused by erect posture ⟨~ hypotension⟩
orthostatic albuminuria *n* : albuminuria that occurs only when a person is in an upright position
¹or·thot·ic \òr-'thä-tik\ *adj* **1** : of or relating to orthotics **2** : designed for the support of weak or ineffective joints or muscles ⟨~ devices⟩
²orthotic *n* : a support or brace for weak or ineffective joints or muscles — called also *orthosis*
or·thot·ics \-tiks\ *n* : a branch of mechanical and medical science that deals with the support and bracing of weak or ineffective joints or muscles
or·tho·tist \-tist\ *n* : a person who practices orthotics
or·tho·top·ic \₁òr-thə-'tä-pik\ *adj* : of or relating to the grafting of tissue in a natural position ⟨~ transplant⟩ — **or·tho·top·i·cal·ly** *adv*
or·tho·volt·age \'òr-thō-₁vōl-tij\ *n* : X-ray voltage of about 150 to 500 kilovolts
¹os \'äs\ *n, pl* **os·sa** \'ä-sə\ : BONE
²os \'ōs\ *n, pl* **ora** \'òr-ə\ : ORIFICE
Os *symbol* osmium
OS *abbr* [Latin *oculus sinister*] left eye — used in writing prescriptions
os cal·cis \-'kal-səs\ *n, pl* **ossa calcis** : CALCANEUS
os·cil·late \'ä-sə-₁lāt\ *vb* **-lat·ed; -lat·ing 1** : to swing backward and forward like a pendulum **2** : to move or travel back and forth between two points — **os·cil·la·tion** \₁ä-sə-'lā-shən\ *n* — **os·cil·la·tor** \'ä-sə-₁lā-tər\ *n* — **os·cil·la·to·ry** \'ä-sə-lə-₁tōr-ē\ *adj*
os·cil·lo·scope \ä-'si-lə-₁skōp, ə-\ *n* : an instrument in which the variations in a fluctuating electrical quantity appear temporarily as a visible waveform on the fluorescent screen of a cathode-ray tube — called also *cathode-ray oscilloscope* — **os·cil·lo·scop·ic** \ä-₁si-lə-'skä-pik, ₁ä-sə-lə-\ *adj*
os cox·ae \-'käk-₁sē\ *n, pl* **ossa coxae** : HIPBONE
-ose \₁ōs\ *n suffix* : carbohydrate; *esp* : sugar ⟨fruct*ose*⟩ ⟨pent*ose*⟩
Os·good–Schlat·ter's disease \'äz-₁gùd-'shlä-tərz-\ *n* : an osteochondritis of the tuberosity of the tibia that occurs esp. among adolescent males
 Osgood, Robert Bayley (1873–1956), American orthopedic surgeon.
 Schlatter, Carl (1864–1934), Swiss surgeon.
-o·side \ə-₁sīd\ *n suffix* : glycoside or similar compound ⟨ganglio*side*⟩
-o·sis \'ō-səs\ *n suffix, pl* **-o·ses** \'ō-₁sēz\ *or* **-o·sis·es 1 a** : action : process : condition ⟨hypn*osis*⟩ **b** : abnormal or diseased condition ⟨leuk*osis*⟩ **2** : increase : formation ⟨leukocyt*osis*⟩

os·mic acid \'äz-mik-\ *n* : OSMIUM TETROXIDE
os·mi·um \'äz-mē-əm\ *n* : a hard brittle blue-gray or blue-black polyvalent metallic element — symbol *Os;* see ELEMENT table
osmium tetroxide *n* : a crystalline compound OsO_4 that is an oxide of osmium used as a biological fixative and stain (as for fatty substances in cytology)
osmo- *comb form* : osmosis : osmotic ⟨*osmo*regulation⟩
os·mol *or* **os·mole** \'äz-₁mōl, 'äs-\ *n* : a standard unit of osmotic pressure based on a one molal concentration of an ion in a solution
os·mo·lal·i·ty \₁äz-mō-'la-lə-tē, ₁äs-\ *n, pl* **-ties** : the concentration of an osmotic solution esp. when measured in osmols or milliosmols per 1000 grams of solvent — **os·mo·lal** \äz-'mō-ləl, äs-\ *adj*
os·mo·lar·i·ty \₁äz-mō-'lar-ə-tē, ₁äs-\ *n, pl* **-ties** : the concentration of an osmotic solution esp. when measured in osmols or milliosmols per liter of solution — **os·mo·lar** \äz-'mō-lər, äs-\ *adj*
os·mo·re·cep·tor \'äz-mō-ri-'sep-tər\ *n* : any of a group of cells sensitive to plasma osmolality that are held to exist in the brain and to regulate water balance in the body by controlling thirst and the release of vasopressin
os·mo·reg·u·la·to·ry \-'re-gyə-lə-₁tōr-ē\ *adj* : of, relating to, or concerned with the maintenance of constant osmotic pressure — **os·mo·reg·u·la·tion** \₁äz-mō-₁re-gyə-'lā-shən, ₁äs-\ *n*
os·mo·ses \-₁sēz\ : movement of a solvent through a semipermeable membrane (as of a living cell) into a solution of higher solute concentration that tends to equalize the concentrations of solute on the two sides of the membrane — **os·mot·ic** \-'mä-tik\ *adj* — **os·mot·i·cal·ly** *adv*
osmotic pressure *n* : the pressure produced by or associated with osmosis and dependent on molar concentration and absolute temperature: as **a** : the maximum pressure that develops in a solution separated from a solvent by a membrane permeable only to the solvent **b** : the pressure that must be applied to a solution to just prevent osmosis
ossa *pl of* **¹OS**
os·se·ous \'ä-sē-əs\ *adj* : of, relating to, or composed of bone — **os·se·ous·ly** *adv*
osseous labyrinth *n* : BONY LABYRINTH
ossi- *comb form* : bone ⟨*ossi*fy⟩
os·si·cle \'ä-si-kəl\ *n* : a small bone or bony structure; *esp* : any of three small bones of the middle ear including the malleus, incus, and stapes — **os·sic·u·lar** \ä-'si-kyə-lər\ *adj*
ossificans — see MYOSITIS OSSIFICANS

os·si·fi·ca·tion \ˌä-sə-fə-ˈkā-shən\ *n* **1 a** : the process of bone formation usu. beginning at particular centers in each prospective bone and involving the activities of special osteoblasts that segregate and deposit inorganic bone substance about themselves — compare CALCIFICATION **b** : an instance of this process **2 a** : the condition of being altered into a hard bony substance (∼ of the muscular tissue) **b** : a mass or particle of ossified tissue : a calcareous deposit in the tissues (∼s in the aortic wall) — **os·si·fy** \ˈä-sə-ˌfī\ *vb*

ossium — see FRAGILITAS OSSIUM

oste- *or* **osteo-** *comb form* : bone (*oste*al) (*osteo*myelitis)

os·te·al \ˈäs-tē-əl\ *adj* : of, relating to, or resembling bone; *also* : affecting or involving bone or the skeleton

os·tec·to·my \äs-ˈtek-tə-mē\ *n, pl* **-mies** : surgical removal of all or part of a bone

os·te·itis \ˌäs-tē-ˈī-təs\ *n, pl* **-it·i·des** \-ˈi-tə-ˌdēz\ : inflammation of bone — called also *ostitis* — **os·te·it·ic** \-ˈi-tik\ *adj*

osteitis de·for·mans \-di-ˈfȯr-ˌmanz\ *n* : PAGET'S DISEASE 2

osteitis fi·bro·sa \-fī-ˈbrō-sə\ *n* : a disease of bone that is characterized by fibrous degeneration of the bone and the formation of cystic cavities and that results in deformities of the affected bones and sometimes in fracture — called also *osteodystrophia fibrosa*

osteitis fibrosa cys·ti·ca \-ˈsis-tə-kə\ *n* : OSTEITIS FIBROSA

osteitis fibrosa cystica gen·er·al·is·ta \-ˌje-nə-rə-ˈlis-tə\ *n* : OSTEITIS FIBROSA

os·teo·ar·thri·tis \ˌäs-tē-ō-är-ˈthrī-təs\ *n, pl* **-thrit·i·des** \-ˈthri-tə-ˌdēz\ : arthritis of middle age characterized by degenerative and sometimes hypertrophic changes in the bone and cartilage of one or more joints and a progressive wearing down of apposing joint surfaces with consequent distortion of joint position usu. without bony stiffening — called also *degenerative arthritis, degenerative joint disease, hypertrophic arthritis*; compare RHEUMATOID ARTHRITIS — **os·teo·ar·thrit·ic** \-ˈthri-tik\ *adj*

os·teo·ar·throp·a·thy \-är-ˈthrä-pə-thē\ *n, pl* **-thies** : a disease of joints or bones; *specif* : a condition marked by enlargement of the terminal phalanges, thickening of the joint surfaces, and curving of the nails and sometimes associated with chronic disease of the lungs — called also *acropachy*

os·teo·ar·thro·sis \-är-ˈthrō-sis\ *n* : OSTEOARTHRITIS — **os·teo·ar·throt·ic** \-ˈthrä-tik\ *adj*

os·teo·ar·tic·u·lar \-är-ˈti-kyə-lər\ *adj* : relating to, involving, or affecting bones and joints (∼ diseases)

os·teo·blast \ˈäs-tē-ə-ˌblast\ *n* : a bone-forming cell

os·teo·blas·tic \ˌäs-tē-ə-ˈblas-tik\ *adj* **1** : relating to or involving the formation of bone **2** : composed of or being osteoblasts

os·teo·blas·to·ma \-ˌbla-ˈstō-mə\ *n, pl* **-mas** *or* **-ma·ta** \-mə-tə\ : a benign tumor of bone

os·teo·car·ti·lag·i·nous \-ˌkärt-əl-ˈa-jə-nəs\ *adj* : relating to or composed of bone and cartilage (an ∼ nodule)

osteochondr- *or* **osteochondro-** *comb form* : bone and cartilage (*osteochondr*itis)

os·teo·chon·dral \-ˈkän-drəl\ *adj* : relating to or composed of bone and cartilage

os·teo·chon·dri·tis \-ˌkän-ˈdrī-təs\ *n* : inflammation of bone and cartilage

osteochondritis dis·se·cans \-ˈdi-sə-ˌkanz\ *n* : partial or complete detachment of a fragment of bone and cartilage at a joint

os·teo·chon·dro·dys·pla·sia \-ˌkän-drō-ˌdis-ˈplā-zhə, -zhē-ə\ *n* : abnormal growth or development of cartilage and bone

os·teo·chon·dro·ma \-ˌkän-ˈdrō-mə\ *n, pl* **-mas** *or* **-ma·ta** \-mə-tə\ : a benign tumor containing both bone and cartilage and occurring near the end of a long bone

os·teo·chon·dro·sis \-ˌkän-ˈdrō-səs\ *n, pl* **-dro·ses** \-ˌsēz\ : a disease esp. of children and young animals in which an ossification center esp. in the epiphyses of long bones undergoes degeneration followed by calcification — **os·teo·chon·drot·ic** \-ˈdrä-tik\ *adj*

os·teo·clast \ˈäs-tē-ə-ˌklast\ *n* : any of the large multinucleate cells closely associated with areas of bone resorption (as in a fracture that is healing) — compare CHONDROCLAST — **os·teo·clas·tic** \ˌäs-tē-ə-ˈklas-tik\ *adj*

os·teo·clas·to·ma \ˌäs-tē-ō-kla-ˈstō-mə\ *n, pl* **-mas** *or* **-ma·ta** \-mə-tə\ : GIANT-CELL TUMOR

os·teo·cyte \ˈäs-tē-ə-ˌsīt\ *n* : a cell that is characteristic of adult bone and is isolated in a lacuna of the bone substance

os·teo·dys·tro·phia fi·bro·sa \ˌäs-tē-ō-di-ˈstrō-fē-ə-fī-ˈbrō-sə\ *n* : OSTEITIS FIBROSA

os·teo·dys·tro·phy \-ˈdis-trə-fē\ *n, pl* **-phies** : defective ossification of bone usu. associated with disturbed calcium and phosphorus metabolism

os·teo·gen·e·sis \ˌäs-tē-ə-ˈje-nə-səs\ *n, pl* **-e·ses** \-ˌsēz\ : development and formation of bone

osteogenesis im·per·fec·ta \-ˌim-pər-ˈfek-tə\ *n* : a hereditary disease marked by extreme brittleness of the long bones and a bluish color of the whites of the eyes — called also *fragilitas ossium, osteopsathyrosis*

osteogenesis imperfecta con·gen·i·ta

\-kən-ˈje-nə-tə\ *n* : a severe and often fatal form of osteogenesis imperfecta characterized by usu. multiple fractures in utero

os·te·o·gen·e·sis imperfecta tar·da \-ˈtär-də\ *n* : a less severe form of osteogenesis imperfecta which is not apparent at birth

os·te·o·gen·ic \ˌäs-tē-ə-ˈje-nik\ *also* **os·te·o·ge·net·ic** \-jə-ˈne-tik\ *adj* **1** : of, relating to, or functioning in osteogenesis; *esp* : producing bone **2** : originating in bone

osteogenic sarcoma *n* : OSTEOSARCOMA

¹os·te·oid \ˈäs-tē-ˌoid\ *adj* : resembling bone (∼ tissue)

²osteoid *n* : uncalcified bone matrix

osteoid osteoma *n* : a small benign painful tumor of bony tissue occurring esp. in the extremities of children and young adults

os·te·ol·o·gy \ˌäs-tē-ˈä-lə-jē\ *n, pl* **-gies 1** : a branch of anatomy dealing with the bones **2** : the bony structure of an organism — **os·te·o·log·i·cal** \ˌäs-tē-ə-ˈlä-ji-kəl\ *adj* — **os·te·ol·o·gist** \ˌäs-tē-ˈä-lə-jist\ *n*

os·te·ol·y·sis \ˌäs-tē-ˈä-lə-səs\ *n, pl* **-y·ses** \-ˌsēz\ : dissolution of bone esp. when associated with resorption — **os·te·o·lyt·ic** \ˌäs-tē-ə-ˈli-tik\ *adj*

os·te·o·ma \ˌäs-tē-ˈō-mə\ *n, pl* **-mas** *or* **-ma·ta** \-mə-tə\ : a benign tumor composed of bone tissue

os·te·o·ma·la·cia \ˌäs-tē-ō-mə-ˈlā-shə, -shē-ə\ *n* : a disease of adults that is characterized by softening of the bones and is analogous to rickets in the immature — **os·te·o·ma·la·cic** \-ˈlā-sik\ *adj*

os·te·o·my·eli·tis \-ˌmī-ə-ˈlī-təs\ *n, pl* **-elit·i·des** \-ə-ˈli-tə-ˌdēz\ : an infectious inflammatory disease of bone often of bacterial origin that is marked by local death and separation of tissue — **os·te·o·my·elit·ic** \-ˈli-tik\ *adj*

os·te·on \ˈäs-tē-ˌän\ *n* : HAVERSIAN SYSTEM — **os·te·on·al** \ˌäs-tē-ˈän-əl, -ˈōn-\ *adj*

os·te·o·ne·cro·sis \ˌäs-tē-ō-nə-ˈkrō-səs\ *n, pl* **-cro·ses** \-ˌsēz\ : necrosis of bone

os·te·o·path \ˈäs-tē-ə-ˌpath\ *n* : a practitioner of osteopathy

os·te·op·a·thy \ˌäs-tē-ˈä-pə-thē\ *n, pl* **-thies 1** : a disease of bone **2** : a system of medical practice based on a theory that diseases are due chiefly to loss of structural integrity which can be restored by manipulation of the parts supplemented by therapeutic measures (as use of medicine or surgery) — **os·te·o·path·ic** \ˌäs-tē-ə-ˈpa-thik\ *adj* — **os·te·o·path·i·cal·ly** *adv*

os·te·o·pe·nia \ˌäs-tē-ō-ˈpē-nē-ə\ *n* : reduction in bone volume to below normal levels esp. due to inadequate replacement of bone lost to normal lysis — **os·te·o·pe·nic** \-nik\ *adj*

os·te·o·pe·tro·sis \-pə-ˈtrō-səs\ *n, pl* **-tro·ses** \-ˌsēz\ : a rare hereditary disease

characterized by extreme density and hardness and abnormal fragility of the bones with partial or complete obliteration of the marrow cavities — called also *Albers-Schönberg disease* — **os·te·o·pe·trot·ic** \-pə-ˈträ-tik\ *adj*

os·te·o·phyte \ˈäs-tē-ə-ˌfīt\ *n* : a pathological bony outgrowth — **os·te·o·phyt·ic** \ˌäs-tē-ə-ˈfi-tik\ *adj*

os·te·o·plas·tic \ˌäs-tē-ə-ˈplas-tik\ *adj* : of, relating to, or being osteoplasty

osteoplastic flap *n* : a surgically excised portion of the skull folded back on a hinge of skin to expose the underlying tissues (as in a craniotomy)

os·te·o·plas·ty \ˈäs-tē-ə-ˌplas-tē\ *n, pl* **-ties** : plastic surgery on bone; *esp* : replacement of lost bone tissue or reconstruction of defective bony parts

os·te·o·poi·ki·lo·sis \ˌäs-tē-ō-ˌpȯi-kə-ˈlō-səs\ *n* : an asymptomatic hereditary bone disorder characterized by numerous sclerotic foci giving the bones a mottled or spotted appearance

os·te·o·po·ro·sis \ˌäs-tē-ō-pə-ˈrō-səs\ *n, pl* **-ro·ses** \-ˌsēz\ : a condition that affects esp. older women and is characterized by decrease in bone mass with decreased density and enlargement of bone spaces producing porosity and fragility — **os·te·o·po·rot·ic** \-ˈrä-tik\ *adj*

os·te·op·sath·y·ro·sis \ˌäs-tē-äp-ˌsa-thə-ˈrō-səs\ *n, pl* **-ro·ses** \-ˌsēz\ : OSTEOGENESIS IMPERFECTA

os·te·o·ra·dio·ne·cro·sis \ˌäs-tē-ō-ˌrā-dē-ō-nə-ˈkrō-səs\ *n, pl* **-cro·ses** \-ˌsēz\ : necrosis of bone following irradiation

os·te·o·sar·co·ma \-sär-ˈkō-mə\ *n, pl* **-mas** *or* **-ma·ta** \-mə-tə\ : a sarcoma derived from bone or containing bone tissue — called also *osteogenic sarcoma*

os·te·o·scle·ro·sis \-sklə-ˈrō-səs\ *n, pl* **-ro·ses** \-ˌsēz\ : abnormal hardening of bone or of bone marrow — **os·te·o·scle·rot·ic** \-ˈrä-tik\ *adj*

os·te·o·syn·the·sis \-ˈsin-thə-səs\ *n, pl* **-the·ses** \-ˌsēz\ : the operation of uniting the ends of a fractured bone by mechanical means (as a wire)

os·te·o·tome \ˈäs-tē-ə-ˌtōm\ *n* : a chisel without a bevel that is used for cutting bone

os·te·ot·o·my \ˌäs-tē-ˈä-tə-mē\ *n, pl* **-mies** : a surgical operation in which a bone is divided or a piece of bone is excised (as to correct a deformity)

Os·ter·tag·ia \ˌäs-tər-ˈtä-jə, -jē-ə\ *n* : a genus of nematode worms (family Trichostrongylidae) parasitic in the abomasum of ruminants

os·ti·tis \äs-ˈtī-təs\ *n* : OSTEITIS

os·ti·um \ˈäs-tē-əm\ *n, pl* **os·tia** \-tē-ə\ : a mouthlike opening in a bodily part (as a fallopian tube or a blood vessel) — **os·tial** \ˈäs-tē-əl\ *adj*

os·to·mate \ˈäs-tə-ˌmāt\ *n* : a person who has undergone an ostomy

os·to·my \'äs-tə-mē\ n, pl **-mies** : an operation (as a colostomy, ileostomy, or urostomy) to create an artificial passage for bodily elimination

-os·to·sis \äs-'tō-səs\ n comb form, pl **-os·to·ses** \-ˌsēz\ or **-os·to·sis·es** : ossification of a (specified) part or to a (specified) degree ⟨hyper*ostosis*⟩

OT abbr **1** occupational therapist **2** occupational therapy

ot- or **oto-** comb form **1** : ear ⟨*otitis*⟩ **2** : ear and ⟨*otolaryngology*⟩

otal·gia \ō-'tal-jə, -jē-ə\ n : EARACHE

other–directed adj : directed in thought and action primarily by external norms rather than by one's own scale of values — compare INNER-DIRECTED

otic \'ō-tik\ adj : of, relating to, or located in the region of the ear

¹-ot·ic \'ät-ik\ adj suffix **1 a** : of, relating to, or characterized by a (specified) action, process, or condition ⟨symbi*otic*⟩ **b** : having an abnormal or diseased condition of a (specified) kind ⟨epizo*otic*⟩ **2** : showing an increase or a formation of ⟨leukocyt*otic*⟩

²-otic \'ō-tik\ adj comb form : having (such) a relationship to the ear ⟨dich*otic*⟩

otic ganglion n : a small parasympathetic ganglion that is associated with the mandibular nerve and sends postganglionic fibers to the parotid gland by way of the auriculotemporal nerve

otitis \ō-'tī-təs\ n, pl **otit·i·des** \-'ti-ə-ˌdēz\ : inflammation of the ear — **otit·ic** \-'ti-tik\ adj

otitis ex·ter·na \-ek-'stər-nə\ n : inflammation of the external ear

otitis in·ter·na \-in-'tər-nə\ n : inflammation of the inner ear

otitis me·dia \-'mē-dē-ə\ n : inflammation of the middle ear marked by pain, fever, dizziness, and abnormalities of hearing — see SEROUS OTITIS MEDIA

oto- — see OT-

Oto·bi·us \ō-'tō-bē-əs\ n : a genus of ticks (family Argasidae) that includes the spinose ear tick (*O. megnini*) of southwestern U.S. and Mexico

oto·co·nia \ˌō-tə-'kō-nē-ə\ n pl : small crystals of calcium carbonate in the saccule and utricle of the ear that under the influence of acceleration in a straight line cause stimulation of the hair cells by their movement relative to the gelatinous supporting substrate containing the embedded cilia of the hair cells — called also *statoconia*

Oto·dec·tes \ˌō-tə-'dek-ˌtēz\ n : a genus of mites that includes one (*O. cynotis*) causing otodectic mange — **oto·dec·tic** \-'dek-tik\ adj

otodectic mange n : ear mange caused by a mite (*O. cynotis*) of the genus *Otodectes*

oto·lar·yn·gol·o·gist \ˌō-tō-ˌlar-ən-'gä-lə-jist\ n : a specialist in otorhino-

laryngology — called also *otorhino-laryngologist*

oto·lar·yn·gol·o·gy \-jē\ n, pl **-gies** : a medical specialty concerned esp. with the ear, nose, and throat — called also *otorhinolaryngology* — **oto·lar·yn·go·log·i·cal** \-ˌlar-ən-gə-'lä-ji-kəl\ adj

oto·lith \'ōt-ᵊl-ˌith\ n : a calcareous concretion in the internal ear composed of masses of otoconia — called also *statolith* — **oto·lith·ic** \ˌōt-ᵊl-'i-thik\ adj

otol·o·gist \ō-'tä-lə-jist\ n : a specialist in otology

otol·o·gy \-jē\ n, pl **-gies** : a science that deals with the ear and its diseases — **oto·log·ic** \ˌō-tə-'lä-jik\ also **oto·log·i·cal** \-'lä-ji-kəl\ adj — **oto·log·i·cal·ly** adv

oto·my·co·sis \ˌō-tō-mī-'kō-səs\ n, pl **-co·ses** \-ˌsēz\ : disease of the ear produced by the growth of fungi in the external auditory meatus

oto·plas·ty \'ō-tə-ˌplas-tē\ n, pl **-ties** : plastic surgery of the external ear

oto·rhi·no·lar·yn·gol·o·gist \ˌō-tō-ˌrī-nō-ˌlar-ən-'gä-lə-jist\ n : OTOLARYNGOLOGIST

oto·rhi·no·lar·yn·gol·o·gy \-jē\ n, pl **-gies** : OTOLARYNGOLOGY — **oto·rhi·no·lar·yn·go·log·i·cal** \-gə-'lä-ji-kəl\ adj

otor·rhea \ˌō-tə-'rē-ə\ n : a discharge from the external ear

otor·rhoea chiefly Brit var of OTORRHEA

oto·scle·ro·sis \ˌō-tō-sklə-'rō-səs\ n, pl **-ro·ses** \-ˌsēz\ : growth of spongy bone in the inner ear where it gradually obstructs the oval window or round window or both and causes progressively increasing deafness — **oto·scle·rot·ic** \-sklə-'rä-tik\ adj

oto·scope \'ō-tə-ˌskōp\ n : an instrument fitted with lighting and magnifying lens systems and used to facilitate visual examination of the auditory canal and ear drum — **oto·scop·ic** \ˌō-tə-'skä-pik\ adj — **otos·co·py** \ō-'täs-kə-pē\ n

oto·tox·ic \ˌō-tə-'täk-sik\ adj : producing, involving, or being adverse effects on organs or nerves involved in hearing or balance — **oto·tox·ic·i·ty** \-täk-'si-sə-tē\ n

OTR abbr registered occupational therapist

oua·bain \wä-'bā-ən, 'wä-ˌbān\ n : a poisonous glycoside $C_{29}H_{44}O_{12}$ used medically like digitalis

ounce \'auns\ n **1 a** : a unit of troy weight equal to ¹⁄₁₂ troy pound or 31.103 grams **b** : a unit of avoirdupois weight equal to ¹⁄₁₆ avoirdupois pound or 28.350 grams **2** : FLUID OUNCE

out·breed·ing \'aut-ˌbrē-diŋ\ n : breeding between individuals or stocks that are relatively unrelated — compare INBREEDING — **out·bred** \-ˌbred\ adj — **out·breed** \-ˌbrēd\ vb

out·cross \'aut-ˌkrös\ n **1** : a cross between relatively unrelated individuals **2** : the progeny of an outcross — **out·cross** vb

outer ear n : the outer visible portion of the ear that collects and directs sound waves toward the tympanic membrane by way of a canal which extends inward through the temporal bone

out·growth \'aut-ˌgrōth\ n **1** : the process of growing out **2** : something that grows directly out of something else ⟨an ∼ of hair⟩ ⟨a deformed ∼⟩

out·let \'aut-ˌlet, -lət\ n **1** : an opening or a place through which something is let out ⟨the pelvic ∼⟩ **2** : a means of release or satisfaction for an emotion or impulse

outlet forceps n : LOW FORCEPS

out–of–body adj : relating to or involving the feeling of separation from one's body and of being able to view oneself and others from an external perspective ⟨an ∼ experience⟩

out·pa·tient \'aut-ˌpā-shənt\ n : a patient who is not hospitalized overnight but who visits a hospital, clinic, or associated facility for diagnosis or treatment — compare INPATIENT

out·pock·et·ing \'aut-ˌpä-kə-tiŋ\ n : EVAGINATION 2

out·pouch·ing \-ˌpau̇-chiŋ\ n : EVAGINATION 2

out·put \'aut-ˌpu̇t\ n : the amount of energy or matter discharged usu. within a specified time by a bodily system or organ ⟨renal ∼⟩ ⟨urinary ∼⟩ — see CARDIAC OUTPUT

ov- or **ovi-** or **ovo-** comb form : egg ⟨ovicide⟩ : ovum ⟨oviduct⟩ ⟨ovogenesis⟩

ova pl of OVUM

ovale — see FORAMEN OVALE

ova·le malaria \ō-ˈvä-lē-\ n : a relatively mild form of malaria caused by a protozoan of the genus Plasmodium (P. ovale) that is characterized by tertian chills and febrile paroxysms and that usu. ends spontaneously

ovalis — see FENESTRA OVALIS, FOSSA OVALIS

oval window n : an oval opening between the middle ear and the vestibule having the base of the stapes or columella attached to its membrane — called also fenestra ovalis, fenestra vestibuli

ovari- or **ovario-** also **ovar-** comb form **1** : ovary ⟨ovariectomy⟩ ⟨ovariotomy⟩ **2** : ovarian and ⟨ovariohysterectomy⟩

ovar·i·an \ō-ˈvar-ē-ən\ also **ovar·i·al** \-ē-əl\ adj : of, relating to, affecting, or involving an ovary

ovarian artery n : either of two arteries in the female that arise from the aorta below the renal arteries with one on each side, and are distributed to the ovaries with branches supplying the ureters, the fallopian tubes, the labia majora, and the groin

ovarian follicle n : FOLLICLE 3

ovarian ligament n : LIGAMENT OF THE OVARY

ovarian vein n : either of two veins in the female with one on each side that drain a venous plexus in the broad ligament of the same side and empty on the right into the inferior vena cava and on the left into the left renal vein

ovar·i·ec·to·my \ˌō-ˌvar-ē-ˈek-tə-mē\ n, pl **-mies** : the surgical removal of an ovary — called also oophorectomy — **ovari·ec·to·mize** \ō-ˌvar-ē-ˈek-tə-ˌmīz\ vb

ovar·io·hys·ter·ec·to·my \ō-ˌvar-ē-ō-ˌhis-tə-ˈrek-tə-mē\ n, pl **-mies** : surgical removal of the ovaries and the uterus

ovar·i·ot·o·my \ō-ˌvar-ē-ˈä-tə-mē\ n, pl **-mies 1** : surgical incision of an ovary **2** : OVARIECTOMY

ova·ry \'ō-və-rē\ n, pl **-ries** : one of the typically paired essential female reproductive organs that produce eggs and female sex hormones, that occur in the adult human as oval flattened bodies about one and a half inches (four centimeters) long suspended from the dorsal surface of the broad ligament of either side, that arise from the mesonephros, and that consist of a vascular fibrous stroma enclosing developing egg cells

over·achiev·er \ˌō-vər-ə-ˈchē-vər\ n : one who achieves success over and above the standard or expected level esp. at an early age — **overachieve** vb

over·ac·tive \-ˈak-tiv\ adj : excessively or abnormally active ⟨∼ glands⟩ — **over·ac·tiv·i·ty** \-ˌak-ˈti-və-tē\ n

over·bite \'ō-vər-ˌbīt\ n : the projection of the upper anterior teeth over the lower when the jaws are in the position they occupy in occlusion — compare OVERJET

over·breathe \ˌō-vər-ˈbrēth\ vb **-breathed; -breath·ing** : HYPERVENTILATE

over·com·pen·sa·tion \-ˌkäm-pən-ˈsā-shən, -ˌpen-\ n : excessive compensation; specif : excessive reaction to a feeling of inferiority, guilt, or inadequacy leading to an exaggerated attempt to overcome the feeling — **over·com·pen·sate** \-ˈkäm-pən-ˌsāt\ vb

over·dis·ten·sion or **over·dis·ten·tion** \-dis-ˈten-chən\ n : excessive distension ⟨gastric ∼⟩ ⟨∼ of the alveoli⟩ — **over·dis·tend·ed** \-dis-ˈten-dəd\ adj

over·dose \'ō-vər-ˌdōs\ n : too great a dose (as of a therapeutic agent); also : a lethal or toxic amount (as of a drug) — **over·dos·age** \ˌō-vər-ˈdō-sij\ n — **over·dose** \ˌō-vər-ˈdōs\ vb

over·eat \ˌō-vər-ˈēt\ vb **over·ate** \-ˈāt\; **over·eat·en** \-ˈēt-ən\; **over·eat·ing** n : to eat to excess — **over·eat·er** n

overeating disease n : ENTEROTOXEMIA

over·ex·ert \-ig-ˈzərt\ vb : to exert (oneself) too much — **over·ex·er·tion** \-ˈzər-shən\ n

over·ex·pose \ˌō-vər-ik-ˈspōz\ vb **-posed; -pos·ing** : to expose excessively 〈skin *overexposed* to sunlight〉 — **over·ex·po·sure** \-ˈspō-zhər\ n

over·ex·tend \ik-ˈstend\ vb : to extend too far 〈∼ the back〉 — **over·ex·ten·sion** \-ik-ˈsten-chən\ n

over·fa·tigue \-fə-ˈtēg\ n : excessive fatigue esp. when carried beyond the recuperative contour of the individual

over·feed \-ˈfēd\ vb **-fed** \-ˈfed\; **-feed·ing** : to feed or eat to excess

over·growth \ˈō-vər-ˌgrōth\ n **1 a** : excessive growth or increase in numbers **b** : HYPERTROPHY, HYPERPLASIA **2** : something (as cells or tissue) grown over something else

over·hang \ˈō-vər-ˌhaŋ\ n : a portion of a filling that extends beyond the normal contour of a tooth

over·hy·dra·tion \ˌō-vər-hī-ˈdrā-shən\ n : a condition in which the body contains an excessive amount of fluids

over·jet \ˈō-vər-ˌjet\ n : displacement of the mandibular teeth sideways when the jaws are held in the position they occupy in occlusion — compare OVERBITE

over·med·i·cate \-ˈme-di-ˌkāt\ vb **-cat·ed; -cat·ing** : to administer too much medication to : to prescribe too much medication for — **over·med·i·ca·tion** \-ˌme-di-ˈkā-shən\ n

over·nu·tri·tion \ˌō-vər-nü-ˈtri-shən, -nyü-\ n : excessive food intake esp. when viewed as a factor in pathology

over·pre·scribe \-pri-ˈskrīb\ vb **-scribed; -scrib·ing** : to prescribe excessive or unnecessary medication — **over·pre·scrip·tion** \-pri-ˈskrip-shən\ n

over·reach \-ˈrēch\ vb, of a horse : to strike the toe of the hind foot against the heel or quarter of the forefoot

over·se·da·tion \-si-ˈdā-shən\ n : excessive sedation

over·shot \ˈō-vər-ˌshät\ adj **1** : having the upper jaw extending beyond the lower **2** : projecting beyond the lower jaw

over·stim·u·la·tion \ˌō-vər-ˌsti-myə-ˈlā-shən\ n : excessive stimulation 〈∼ of the pancreas〉 — **over·stim·u·late** \-ˈsti-myə-ˌlāt\ vb

overt \ō-ˈvərt, ˈō-ˌvərt\ adj : open to view : readily perceived

over-the-coun·ter adj : sold lawfully without prescription 〈∼ drugs〉

over·ven·ti·la·tion \ˌō-vər-ˌvent-ᵊl-ˈā-shən\ n : HYPERVENTILATION

over·weight \-ˈwāt\ n **1** : bodily weight in excess of the normal for one's age, height, and build **2** : an individual of more than normal weight — **overweight** adj

over·work \-ˈwərk\ vb : to cause to work too hard, too long, or to exhaustion

ovi- — see OV-

ovi·cide \ˈō-və-ˌsīd\ n : an agent that kills eggs; esp : an insecticide effective against the egg stage — **ovi·cid·al** \ˌō-və-ˈsīd-ᵊl\ adj

ovi·du·cal \ˌō-və-ˈdü-kəl, -ˈdyü-\ adj : OVIDUCTAL

ovi·duct \ˈō-və-ˌdəkt\ n : a tube that serves exclusively or esp. for the passage of eggs from an ovary

ovi·duc·tal \ˌō-və-ˈdəkt-ᵊl\ adj : of, relating to, or affecting an oviduct 〈∼ surgery〉

ovine \ˈō-ˌvīn\ adj : of, relating to, or resembling sheep 〈∼ growth hormone〉

ovip·a·rous \ō-ˈvi-pə-rəs\ adj : producing eggs that develop and hatch outside the maternal body — compare OVOVIVIPAROUS, VIVIPAROUS — **ovi·par·i·ty** \ˌō-və-ˈpar-ə-tē\ n

ovi·pos·it \ˈō-və-ˌpä-zət, ˌō-və-ˈ\ vb : to lay eggs — used esp. of insects — **ovi·po·si·tion** \ˌō-və-pə-ˈzi-shən\ n — **ovi·po·si·tion·al** \-ˈzi-shə-nəl\ adj

ovi·pos·i·tor \ˈō-və-ˌpä-zə-tər, ˌō-və-ˈ\ n : a specialized organ (as of an insect) for depositing eggs

ovo- — see OV-

ovo·gen·e·sis \ˌō-və-ˈje-nə-səs\ n, pl **-e·ses** \-ˌsēz\ : OOGENESIS

ovoid \ˈō-ˌvȯid\ adj : shaped like an egg

ovo·lec·i·thin \ˌō-vō-ˈle-sə-thən\ n : lecithin obtained from egg yolk

ovo·mu·coid \-ˈmyü-ˌkȯid\ n : a mucoprotein present in egg white

ovo·plasm \ˈō-və-ˌpla-zəm\ n : the cytoplasm of an unfertilized egg

ovo·tes·tis \ˌō-vō-ˈtes-təs\ n, pl **-tes·tes** \-ˌtēz\ : a hermaphrodite gonad

ovo·vi·tel·lin \ˌō-vō-ˈte-lən\ n : VITELLIN

ovo·vi·vip·a·rous \ˌō-vō-vī-ˈvi-pə-rəs\ adj : producing eggs that develop within the maternal body — compare OVIPAROUS, VIVIPAROUS — **ovo·vi·vi·par·i·ty** \-ˌvī-və-ˈpar-ə-tē, -ˌvi-\ n

ovu·lar \ˈä-vyə-lər, ˈō-\ adj : of or relating to an ovule or ovum

ovu·la·tion \ˌä-vyə-ˈlā-shən, ˌō-\ n : the discharge of a mature ovum from the ovary — **ovu·late** \ˈä-vyə-ˌlāt\ vb — **ovu·la·to·ry** \ˈä-vyə-lə-ˌtȯr-ē, ˈō-\ adj

ovule \ˈä-ˌvyül, ˈō-\ n **1** : an outgrowth of the ovary of a seed plant that after fertilization develops into a seed **2** : a small egg; esp : one in an early stage of growth

ovum \ˈō-vəm\ n, pl **ova** \-və\ : a female gamete : MACROGAMETE; esp : a mature egg that has undergone reduction, is ready for fertilization, and takes the form of a relatively large inactive gamete providing a comparatively great amount of reserve material and contributing most of the cytoplasm of the zygote

ox \ˈäks\ n, pl **ox·en** \ˈäk-sən\ also **ox** : a domestic bovine mammal (*Bos taurus* of the subfamily Bovinae); also : an adult male castrated domestic ox

ox·a·cil·lin \ˌäk-sə-ˈsi-lən\ n : a semisynthetic penicillin that is esp. effective in the control of infections caused by penicillin-resistant staphylococci

¹**ox·a·late** \ˈäk-sə-ˌlāt\ n : a salt or ester of oxalic acid

²**oxalate** vb **-lat·ed; -lat·ing** : to add an oxalate to (blood or plasma) to prevent coagulation

ox·al·ic acid \(ˌ)äk-ˈsa-lik-\ n : a poisonous strong acid (COOH)₂ or $H_2C_2O_4$ that occurs in various plants as oxalates

ox·a·lo·ace·tic acid \ˌäk-sə-lō-ə-ˈsē-tik-\ also **ox·al·ace·tic acid** \ˌäk-sə-lə-ˈsē-tik-\ n : a crystalline acid $C_4H_4O_5$ that is formed by reversible oxidation of malic acid (as in carbohydrate metabolism via the Krebs cycle) and in reversible transamination reactions (as from aspartic acid)

ox·a·lo·sis \ˌäk-sə-ˈlō-səs\ n : an abnormal condition characterized by hyperoxaluria and the formation of calcium oxalate deposits in tissues throughout the body

ox·an·a·mide \äk-ˈsa-nə-ˌmīd\ n : a tranquilizing drug $C_8H_{15}NO_2$

ox·an·dro·lone \äk-ˈsan-drə-ˌlōn\ n : an anabolic agent $C_{19}H_{30}O_3$

ox·a·pro·zin \ˌäk-sə-ˈprō-zən\ n : an anti-inflammatory drug $C_{18}H_{15}NO_3$

ox·az·e·pam \äk-ˈsa-zə-ˌpam\ n : a benzodiazepine tranquilizer $C_{15}H_{11}ClN_2O_2$

ox·a·zol·i·dine \ˌäk-sə-ˈzō-lə-ˌdēn, -ˈzä-\ n : the heterocyclic compound C_3H_7NO; also : an anticonvulsant derivative (as trimethadione) of this compound

ox·i·dase \ˈäk-sə-ˌdās, -ˌdāz\ n : any of various enzymes that catalyze oxidations; esp : one able to react directly with molecular oxygen

ox·i·da·tion \ˌäk-sə-ˈdā-shən\ n **1** : the act or process of oxidizing **2** : the state or result of being oxidized — **ox·i·da·tive** \ˈäk-sə-ˌdā-tiv\ adj — **ox·i·da·tive·ly** adv

oxidation–reduction n : a chemical reaction in which one or more electrons are transferred from one atom or molecule to another — called also redox

oxidative phosphorylation n : the synthesis of ATP by phosphorylation of ADP for which energy is obtained by electron transport and which takes place in the mitochondria during aerobic respiration

ox·ide \ˈäk-ˌsīd\ n : a binary compound of oxygen with an element or chemical group

ox·i·dize \ˈäk-sə-ˌdīz\ vb **-dized; -diz·ing 1** : to combine with oxygen **2** : to dehydrogenate **3** : to change (a compound) by increasing the proportion of the part tending to attract electrons or change (an element or ion) from a lower to a higher positive valence : remove one or more electrons from (an atom, ion, or molecule) — **ox·i·diz·able** \ˌäk-sə-ˈdī-zə-bəl\ adj

oxidized cellulose n : an acid degradation product of cellulose that is usu. obtained by oxidizing cotton or gauze with nitrogen dioxide, is a useful hemostatic (as in surgery), and is absorbed by body fluids (as when used to pack wounds)

oxidizing agent n : a substance that oxidizes something esp. chemically (as by accepting electrons) — compare REDUCING AGENT

oxi·do·re·duc·tase \ˌäk-sə-dō-ri-ˈdək-ˌtās, -ˌtāz\ n : an enzyme that catalyzes an oxidation-reduction reaction

ox·im·e·ter \äk-ˈsi-mə-tər\ n : an instrument for measuring continuously the degree of oxygen saturation of the circulating blood — **ox·i·met·ric** \ˌäk-sə-ˈme-trik\ adj — **ox·im·e·try** \äk-ˈsi-mə-trē\ n

oxo·phen·ar·sine \ˌäk-sə-fe-ˈnär-ˌsēn, -sən\ n : an arsenical used in the form of its white powdery hydrochloride $C_6H_6AsNO_2·HCl$ esp. in the treatment of syphilis

oxo·trem·o·rine \ˌäk-sō-ˈtre-mə-ˌrēn, -rən\ n : a cholinergic agent $C_{12}H_{18}N_2O$ that induces tremors

ox·pren·o·lol \ˌäks-ˈpre-nə-ˌlol\ n : a beta-adrenergic blocking agent $C_{15}H_{23}NO_3$ used in the form of the hydrochloride as a coronary vasodilator

ox·tri·phyl·line \ˌäks-tri-ˈfi-ˌlēn, -tri-fə-lēn\ n : the choline salt $C_{12}H_{21}N_5O_3$ of theophylline used chiefly as a bronchodilator

ox warble n : the maggot of either the common cattle grub or the northern cattle grub

oxy \ˈäk-sē\ adj : containing oxygen or additional oxygen — often used in combination ⟨oxyhemoglobin⟩

oxy- comb form **1** : sharp : pointed : acute ⟨oxycephaly⟩ **2** : quick ⟨oxytocic⟩ **3** : acid ⟨oxyntic⟩

oxy·ben·zone \ˌäk-sē-ˈben-ˌzōn\ n : a sunscreening agent $C_{14}H_{12}O_3$

oxy·bu·tyr·ic acid \-byü-ˈtir-ik-\ n : HYDROXYBUTYRIC ACID

oxy·ceph·a·ly \-ˈse-fə-lē\ n, pl **-lies** : congenital deformity of the skull due to early synostosis of the parietal and occipital bones with compensating growth in the region of the anterior fontanel resulting in a pointed or pyramidal skull — called also acrocephaly, turricephaly — **oxy·ce·phal·ic** \-si-ˈfa-lik\ adj

oxy·chlo·ro·sene \-ˈklōr-ə-ˌsēn\ n : a topical antiseptic $C_{20}H_{34}O_3S·HOCl$

oxy·co·done \-ˈkō-ˌdōn\ n : a narcotic analgesic $C_{18}H_{21}NO_4$ used esp. in the form of the hydrochloride

oxy·gen \ˈäk-si-jən\ n : an element that is found free as a colorless tasteless odorless gas in the atmosphere of which it forms about 21 percent or combined in water, is active in physiological processes, and is involved esp. in combustion processes — symbol O; see ELEMENT table

oxy·gen·ate \ˈäk-si-jə-ˌnāt, äk-ˈsi-jə-\

vb **-at·ed; -at·ing** : to impregnate, combine, or supply with oxygen ⟨*oxygenated* blood⟩ — **ox·y·gen·ation** \ˌäk-si-jə-ˈnā-shən, ˌäk-ˌsi-jə-\ *n*

ox·y·gen·ator \ˈäk-si-jə-ˌnā-tər, ˌäk-ˈsi-jə-\ *n* : one that oxygenates; *specif* : an apparatus that oxygenates the blood extracorporeally (as during open-heart surgery)

oxygen capacity *n* : the amount of oxygen which a quantity of blood is able to absorb

oxygen debt *n* : a cumulative deficit of oxygen available for oxidative metabolism that develops during periods of intense bodily activity and must be made good when the body returns to rest

oxygen mask *n* : a device worn over the nose and mouth through which oxygen is supplied from a storage tank

oxygen tent *n* : a canopy which can be placed over a bedridden person and within which a flow of oxygen can be maintained

oxy·he·mo·glo·bin \ˌäk-si-ˈhē-mə-ˌglō-bən\ *n* : hemoglobin loosely combined with oxygen that it releases to the tissues

oxy·mor·phone \-ˈmȯr-ˌfōn\ *n* : a semi-synthetic narcotic analgesic drug used in the form of its hydrochloride $C_{17}H_{19}NO_4 \cdot HCl$ and having uses, activity, and side effects like those of morphine

oxy·myo·glo·bin \ˌäk-si-ˈmī-ə-ˌglō-bən\ *n* : a pigment formed by the combination of myoglobin with oxygen

ox·yn·tic \äk-ˈsin-tik\ *adj* : secreting acid — used esp. of the parietal cells of the gastric glands

oxy·phen·bu·ta·zone \ˌäk-sē-ˈfen-ˈbyü-tə-ˌzōn\ *n* : a phenylbutazone derivative $C_{19}H_{20}N_2O_3$ used for its antiinflammatory, analgesic, and antipyretic effects

oxy·phen·cy·cli·mine \-ˈsī-klə-ˌmēn\ *n* : an anticholinergic drug $C_{20}H_{28}N_2O_3$ with actions similar to atropine usu. used in the form of its hydrochloride as an antispasmodic esp. in the treatment of peptic ulcer

oxy·quin·o·line \-ˈkwin-ᵊl-ˌēn\ *n* : 8-HY-DROXYQUINOLINE

Oxy·spi·ru·ra \ˌäk-si-ˌspī-ˈru̇r-ə\ *n* : a genus of nematode worms (family Thelaziidae) comprising the eye worms of birds and esp. domestic poultry

oxy·tet·ra·cy·cline \-ˌte-trə-ˈsī-ˌklēn\ *n* : a yellow crystalline broad-spectrum antibiotic $C_{22}H_{24}N_2O_9$ produced by a soil actinomycete of the genus *Streptomyces* (*S. rimosus*) — see TERRA-MYCIN

¹**oxy·to·cic** \ˌäk-si-ˈtō-sik\ *adj* : hastening parturition; *also* : inducing contraction of uterine smooth muscle

²**oxytocic** *n* : a substance that stimulates contraction of uterine smooth muscle or hastens childbirth

oxy·to·cin \-ˈtōs-ᵊn\ *n* : a postpituitary octapeptide hormone $C_{43}H_{66}N_{12}O_{12}S_2$ that stimulates esp. the contraction of uterine muscle and the secretion of milk — see PITOCIN

oxy·uri·a·sis \ˌäk-si-yü-ˈrī-ə-səs\ *n, pl* **-a·ses** \-ˌsēz\ : infestation with or disease caused by pinworms (as of the genera *Enterobius* and *Oxyuris*)

oxy·urid \ˌäk-sē-ˈyür-əd\ *n* : any of a family (Oxyuridae) of nematode worms that are chiefly parasites of the vertebrate intestinal tract — see PINWORM — **oxyurid** *adj*

oxy·uris \-ˈyür-əs\ *n* **1** *cap* : a genus of parasitic nematodes (family Oxyuridae) **2** : any nematode worm of the genus *Oxyuris* or a related genus (as *Enterobius*) : PINWORM

oz *abbr* ounce; ounces

oze·na \ō-ˈzē-nə\ *n* : a chronic disease of the nose accompanied by a fetid discharge and marked by atrophic changes in the nasal structures

ozone \ˈō-ˌzōn\ *n* : a very reactive form of oxygen containing three atoms per molecule that is a bluish irritating gas of pungent odor, that is formed naturally in the atmosphere by a photochemical reaction and is a major air pollutant in the lower atmosphere but a beneficial component of the upper atmosphere, and that is used for oxidizing, bleaching, disinfecting, and deodorizing

P

¹**P** *abbr* **1** parental **2** pressure **3** pulse

²**P** *symbol* phosphorus

p- *abbr* para- ⟨*p*-dichlorobenzene⟩

Pa *symbol* protactinium

PA *n* : PHYSICIAN'S ASSISTANT

PA *abbr* pernicious anemia

PABA \ˈpä-bə, ˌpē-ˌā-ˈbē-ˌä\ *n* : PARA-AMINOBENZOIC ACID

pab·u·lum \ˈpa-byə-ləm\ *n* : FOOD; *esp* : a suspension or solution of nutrients in a state suitable for absorption

PAC *abbr* physician's assistant, certified

pac·chi·o·ni·an body \ˌpa-kē-ˈō-nē-ən-\ *n* : ARACHNOID GRANULATION

Pac·chi·o·ni \ˌpä-kē-ˈō-nē\ **Antonio** (1665–1726), Italian anatomist.

pace·mak·er \ˈpās-ˌmā-kər\ *n* **1** : a body part (as the sinoatrial node of the heart) that serves to establish and maintain a rhythmic activity **2** : an electrical device for stimulating or steadying the heartbeat or reestablishing the rhythm of an arrested heart — called also *pacer*

pace·mak·ing \-ımā-kiŋ\ n : the act or process of serving as a pacemaker

pac·er \'pā-sər\ n : PACEMAKER 2

pachy- *comb form* : thick ⟨pachytene⟩

pachy·men·in·gi·tis \ıpa-kē-ıme-nən-'ji-təs\ n, pl **-git·i·des** \-'ji-tə-ıdēz\ : inflammation of the dura mater

pachy·men·inx \-'mē-ıniŋks, -'me-\ n, pl **-men·in·ges** \-mə-'nin-(ı)jēz\ : DURA MATER

pachy·o·nych·ia \ıpa-kē-ō-'ni-kē-ə\ n : extreme usu. congenital thickness of the nails

pachy·tene \'pa-ki-ıtēn\ n : the stage of meiotic prophase which immediately follows the zygotene and in which the paired chromosomes are thickened and visibly divided into chromatids — **pachytene** adj

paci·fi·er \'pa-sə-ıfī-ər\ n 1 : a usu. nipple-shaped device for babies to suck or bite on 2 : TRANQUILIZER

pac·ing \'pā-siŋ\ n : the act or process of regulating or changing the timing or intensity of cardiac contractions (as by an artificial pacemaker)

Pa·cin·i·an corpuscle \pə-'si-nē-ən-\ *also* **Pa·ci·ni's corpuscle** \pə-'chē-nēz-\ n : an oval capsule that terminates some sensory nerve fibers esp. in the skin of the hands and feet

Pacini, Filippo (1812–1883), Italian anatomist.

¹**pack** \'pak\ n 1 : a container shielded with lead or mercury for holding radium in large quantities esp. for therapeutic application 2 **a** : absorbent material saturated with water or other liquid for therapeutic application to the body or a body part **b** : a folded square or compress of gauze or other absorbent material used esp. to maintain a clear field in surgery, to stop cavities, to check bleeding by compression, or to apply medication

²**pack** vb : to cover or surround with a pack; *specif* : to envelop (a patient) in a wet or dry sheet or blanket

packed cell volume n : the percentage of the total volume of a blood sample that is represented by the centrifuged red blood cells in it — abbr. PCV

pack·ing \'pa-kiŋ\ n 1 : the therapeutic application of a pack 2 : the material used in packing

¹**pad** \'pad\ n 1 : a usu. square or rectangular piece of often folded typically absorbent material (as gauze) fixed in place over some part of the body as a dressing or other protective covering 2 : a part of the body or of an appendage that resembles or is suggestive of a cushion : a thick fleshy resilient part: as **a** : the sole of the foot or underside of the toes of an animal (as a dog) that is typically thickened so as to form a cushion **b** : the underside of the extremities of the

fingers; *esp* : the ball of the thumb

²**pad** \'pad\ vb

pad·i·mate A \'pa-di-ımāt-'ā\ n : a sunscreen $C_{14}H_{21}NO_2$

paed- *or* **paedo-** *chiefly Brit var of* PED-

pae·di·a·trics, pae·do·don·tics, pae·do·phil·ia *chiefly Brit var of* PEDIATRICS, PEDODONTICS, PEDOPHILIA

PAF *abbr* platelet-activating factor

Pag·et's disease \'pa-jəts-\ n 1 : an eczematous inflammatory condition esp. of the nipple and areola that is the epidermal manifestation of an underlying carcinoma 2 : a chronic disease of bones characterized by their great enlargement and rarefaction with bowing of the long bones and deformation of the flat bones — called also *osteitis deformans*

Pag·et \'pa-jət\ **Sir James (1814–1899),** British surgeon.

pa·go·pha·gia \ıpā-gə-'fā-jə, -jē-ə\ n : the compulsive eating of ice that is a common symptom of a lack of iron

-pa·gus \pə-gəs\ *n comb form, pl* **-pa·gi** \pə-ıji, -ıgi\ : congenitally united twins with a (specified) type of fixation ⟨cranio*pagus*⟩

¹**PAH** \ıpē-(ı)ā-'āch\ n : POLYCYCLIC AROMATIC HYDROCARBON

²**PAH** *abbr* **1** para-aminohippurate; para-aminohippuric acid **2** polynuclear aromatic hydrocarbon

¹**pain** \'pān\ n **1 a** : a usu. localized physical suffering associated with bodily disorder (as a disease or an injury); *also* : a basic bodily sensation that is induced by a noxious stimulus, is received by naked nerve endings, is characterized by physical discomfort (as pricking, throbbing, or aching), and typically leads to evasive action **b** : acute mental or emotional suffering or distress **2 pains** pl : the protracted series of involuntary contractions of the uterine musculature that constitute the major factor in parturient labor and that are often accompanied by considerable pain — **pain·ful** \-fəl\ adj — **pain·ful·ly** adv — **pain·less** \-ləs\ adj — **pain·less·ly** adv

²**pain** vb : to cause or experience pain

pain·kill·er \-ıki-lər\ n : something (as a drug) that relieves pain — **pain·kill·ing** adj

pain spot n : one of many small localized areas of the skin that respond to stimulation (as by pricking or burning) by giving a sensation of pain

paint·er's colic \'pān-tərz-\ n : intestinal colic associated with obstinate constipation due to chronic lead poisoning

pair–bond n : a monogamous relationship — **pair–bond·ing** n

paired–associate learning n : the learning of items (as syllables, digits, or words) in pairs so that one member of the pair evokes recall of the other — compare ASSOCIATIVE LEARNING

palae- *or* **palaeo-** *chiefly Brit var of* PALE-

pal·aeo·cer·e·bel·lum, **pal·aeo·pa·thol·ogy** *chiefly Brit var of* PALEOCEREBELLUM, PALEOPATHOLOGY

pal·a·tal \'pa-lət-ᵊl\ *adj* : of, relating to, forming, or affecting the palate — **pal·a·tal·ly** *adv*

palatal bar *n* : a connector extending across the roof of the mouth to join the parts of a maxillary partial denture

palatal process *n* : PALATINE PROCESS

pal·ate \'pa-lət\ *n* : the roof of the mouth separating the mouth from the nasal cavity — see HARD PALATE, SOFT PALATE

palati — see TENSOR PALATI

¹**pal·a·tine** \'pa-lə-ˌtīn\ *adj* : of, relating to, or lying near the palate

²**palatine** *n* : PALATINE BONE

palatine aponeurosis *n* : a thin fibrous lamella attached to the posterior part of the hard palate that supports the soft palate, includes the tendon of the tensor veli palatini, and supports the other muscles of the palate

palatine artery *n* 1 : either of two arteries of each side of the face: **a** : an inferior artery that arises from the facial artery and divides into two branches of which one supplies the soft palate and the palatine glands and the other supplies esp. the tonsils and the eustachian tube — called also *ascending palatine artery* **b** : a superior artery that arises from the maxillary artery and sends branches to the soft palate, the palatine glands, the mucous membrane of the hard palate, and the gums — called also *greater palatine artery* 2 : any of the branches of the palatine arteries

palatine bone *n* : a bone of extremely irregular form on each side of the skull that is situated in the posterior part of the nasal cavity between the maxilla and the pterygoid process of the sphenoid bone and that consists of a horizontal plate which joins the bone of the opposite side and forms the back part of the hard palate and a vertical plate which is extended into three processes and helps to form the floor of the orbit, the outer wall of the nasal cavity, and several adjoining parts — called also *palatine*

palatine foramen *n* : any of several foramina in the palatine bone giving passage to the palatine vessels and nerves — see GREATER PALATINE FORAMEN

palatine gland *n* : any of numerous small mucous glands in the palate opening into the mouth

palatine nerve *n* : any of several nerves arising from the pterygopalatine ganglion and supplying the roof of the mouth, parts of the nose, and adjoining parts

palatine process *n* : a process of the maxilla that projects medially, articulates posteriorly with the palatine

bone, and forms with the corresponding process on the other side the anterior three-fourths of the hard palate — called also *palatal process*

palatine suture *n* : either of two sutures in the hard palate: **a** : a transverse suture lying between the horizontal plates of the palatine bones and the maxillae **b** : a median suture lying between the maxillae in front and continued posteriorly between the palatine bones

palatine tonsil *n* : TONSIL 1a

palatini — see LEVATOR VELI PALATINI, TENSOR VELI PALATINI

palato- *comb form* 1 : palate : of the palate (*palato*plasty) 2 : palatal and (*palato*glossal arch)

pal·a·to·glos·sal arch \ˌpa-lə-tō-ˈglä-səl-, -ˈglō-\ *n* : the more anterior of the two ridges of soft tissue at the back of the mouth on each side that curves downward from the uvula to the side of the base of the tongue forming a recess for the palatine tonsil as it diverges from the palatopharyngeal arch and is composed of part of the palatoglossus with its covering of mucous membrane — called also *anterior pillar of the fauces, glossopalatine arch*

pal·a·to·glos·sus \-ˈglä-səs, -ˈglō-\ *n, pl* **-glos·si** \-(ˌ)sī\ : a thin muscle that arises from the soft palate on each side, contributes to the structure of the palatoglossal arch, and is inserted into the side and dorsum of the tongue — called also *glossopalatinus*

pal·a·to·pha·ryn·geal arch \-ˌfar-ən-ˈjē-əl-, -fə-ˈrin-jəl-, -jē-əl-\ *n* : the more posterior of the two ridges of soft tissue at the back of the mouth on each side that curves downward from the uvula to the side of the pharynx forming a recess for the palatine tonsil as it diverges from the palatoglossal arch and is composed of part of the palatopharyngeus with its covering of mucous membrane — called also *posterior pillar of the fauces, pharyngopalatine arch*

pal·a·to·pha·ryn·ge·us \-ˌfar-ən-ˈjē-əs; -fə-ˈrin-jəs, -jē-əs\ *n* : a longitudinal muscle of the pharynx that arises from the soft palate, contributes to the structure of the palatopharyngeal arch, and is inserted into the thyroid cartilage and the wall of the pharynx

pal·a·to·plas·ty \'pa-lə-tə-ˌplas-tē\ *n, pl* **-ties** : a plastic operation for repair of the palate (as in cleft palate)

pale \'pāl\ *adj* **pal·er; pal·est** : deficient in color or intensity of color (a ∼ face) — **pale·ness** \-nəs\ *n*

pale- *or* **paleo-** *comb form* : early : old (*paleo*pathology)

pa·leo·cer·e·bel·lum \ˌpā-lē-ō-ˌser-ə-ˈbe-ləm\ *n, pl* **-bel·lums** *or* **-bel·la** \-ˈbe-lə\ : an evolutionarily old part of the cerebellum concerned with maintenance of normal postural relationships and made up chiefly of the anterior lobe of the vermis and of the pyramid — compare NEOCEREBELLUM

pa·leo·pa·thol·o·gy \pā-lē-ō-pǝ-ʹthä-lǝ-jē\ *n, pl* **-gies** : a branch of pathology concerned with diseases of former times as determined esp. from fossil or other remains — **pa·leo·pa·thol·o·gist** \-jist\ *n*

pali- *comb form* : pathological state characterized by repetition of a (specified) act ⟨*pali*lalia⟩

pali·la·lia \pa-lǝ-ʹlā-lē-ǝ\ *n* : a speech defect marked by abnormal repetition of syllables, words, or phrases

pal·in·drome \ʹpa-lǝn-ˌdrōm\ *n* : a palindromic sequence of DNA

pal·in·drom·ic \pa-lǝn-ʹdrō-mik\ *adj* 1 : RECURRENT ⟨∼ rheumatism⟩ 2 : of, relating to, or consisting of a double-stranded sequence of DNA in which the order of the nucleotides is the same on each side but running in opposite directions

pal·isade worm \pa-lǝ-ʹsād-\ *n* : BLOODWORM

pal·la·di·um \pǝ-ʹlā-dē-ǝm\ *n* : a silverwhite ductile malleable metallic element — symbol *Pd;* see ELEMENT table

pal·li·ate \ʹpa-lē-ˌāt\ *vb* **-at·ed; -at·ing** : to reduce the violence of (a disease) : ease without curing — **pal·li·a·tion** \pa-lē-ʹā-shǝn\ *n*

¹pal·lia·tive \ʹpa-lē-ˌā-tiv, ʹpal-yǝ-\ *adj* : serving to palliate ⟨∼ surgery⟩

²palliative *n* : something that palliates

pal·li·dal \ʹpa-lǝd-ǝl\ *adj* : of, relating to, or involving the globus pallidus

pal·li·dum \ʹpa-lǝ-dǝm\ *n* : GLOBUS PALLIDUS

pallidus — see GLOBUS PALLIDUS

pal·li·um \ʹpa-lē-ǝm\ *n, pl* **-lia** \-lē-ǝ\ *or* **-li·ums** : CEREBRAL CORTEX

pal·lor \ʹpa-lǝr\ *n* : deficiency of color esp. of the face : PALENESS

palm \ʹpälm, ʹpäm\ *n* : the somewhat concave part of the hand between the bases of the fingers and the wrist — **pal·mar** \ʹpal-mǝr, ʹpäl-, ʹpä-\ *adj*

palmar aponeurosis *n* : an aponeurosis of the palm of the hand that consists of a superficial longitudinal layer continuous with the tendon of the palmaris longus and of a deeper transverse layer — called also *palmar fascia*

palmar arch *n* : either of two loops of blood vessels in the palm of the hand: **a** : a deeply situated transverse artery that is composed of the terminal part of the radial artery joined to a branch of the ulnar artery and that supplies principally the deep muscles of the hand, thumb, and index finger — called also *deep palmar arch* **b** : a superficial arch that is the continuation of the ulnar artery which anastomoses with a branch derived from the radial artery and that sends branches

mostly to the fingers — called also *superficial palmar arch*

palmar fascia *n* : PALMAR APONEUROSIS

palmar interosseus *n* : any of three small muscles of the palmar surface of the hand each of which arises from, extends along, and inserts on the side of the second, fourth, or fifth finger facing the middle finger and which acts to adduct its finger toward the middle finger, flex its metacarpophalangeal joint, and extend its distal two phalanges — called also *interosseus palmaris, palmar interosseous muscle*

pal·mar·is \pal-ʹmar-ǝs\ *n, pl* **pal·mar·es** \-ˌēz\ : either of two muscles of the palm of the hand: **a** : PALMARIS BREVIS **b** : PALMARIS LONGUS — see PALMAR INTEROSSEUS

palmaris brev·is \-ʹbrev-ǝs\ *n* : a short transverse superficial muscle of the ulnar side of the palm of the hand that arises from the flexor retinaculum and palmar aponeurosis, inserts into the skin on the ulnar edge of the palm, and functions to tense and stabilize the palm (as in making a fist or catching a ball)

palmaris lon·gus \-ʹloŋ-gǝs\ *n* : a superficial muscle of the forearm lying on the medial side of the flexor carpi radialis that arises esp. from the medial epicondyle of the humerus, inserts esp. into the palmar aponeurosis, and acts to flex the hand

pal·mi·tate \ʹpal-mǝ-ˌtāt, ʹpäl-, ʹpä-\ *n* : a salt or ester of palmitic acid

pal·mit·ic acid \(ˌ)pal-ʹmi-tik-, (ˌ)päl-, (ˌ)pä-\ *n* : a waxy crystalline saturated fatty acid $C_{16}H_{32}O_2$ occurring free or in the form of esters (as glycerides) in most fats and fatty oils and in several essential oils and waxes

pal·mi·tin \ʹpal-mǝ-tǝn, ʹpäl-, ʹpä-\ *n* : the triglyceride $C_{51}H_{98}O_6$ of palmitic acid that occurs as a solid with stearin and olein in animal fats — called also *tripalmitin*

pal·mo·plan·tar \pal-mō-ʹplan-tǝr, ˌpäl-, ˌpä-\ *adj* : of, relating to, or affecting both the palms of the hands and the soles of the feet ⟨∼ psoriasis⟩

pal·pa·ble \ʹpal-pǝ-bǝl\ *adj* : capable of being touched or felt; *esp* : capable of being examined by palpation

pal·pa·tion \pal-ʹpā-shǝn\ *n* **1** : an act of touching or feeling **2** : physical examination in medical diagnosis by pressure of the hand or fingers to the surface of the body esp. to determine the condition (as of size or consistency) of an underlying part or organ ⟨∼ of the liver⟩ — compare INSPECTION — **pal·pate** \ʹpal-ˌpāt\ *vb* — **pal·pa·to·ry** \ʹpal-pǝ-ˌtōr-ē\ *adj*

pal·pe·bra \ʹpal-pǝ-brǝ, pal-ʹpē-brǝ\ *n, pl* **pal·pe·brae** \-ˌbrē\ : EYELID — **pal·pe·bral** \pal-ʹpē-brǝl\ *adj*

palpebrae — see LEVATOR PALPEBRAE SUPERIORIS

palpebral fissure *n* : the space between the margins of the eyelids — called also *rima palpebrarum*

palpebrarum — see RIMA PALPEBRARUM, XANTHELASMA PALPEBRARUM

pal·pi·tate \'pal-pə-ˌtāt\ *vb* **-tat·ed; -tat·ing** : to beat rapidly and strongly — used esp. of the heart when its pulsation is abnormally rapid

pal·pi·ta·tion \ˌpal-pə-'tā-shən\ *n* : a rapid pulsation; *esp* : an abnormally rapid beating of the heart when excited by violent exertion, strong emotion, or disease

pal·sied \'pȯl-zēd\ *adj* : affected with palsy ⟨hands weak and ∼⟩

pal·sy \'pȯl-zē\ *n, pl* **pal·sies** 1 : PARALYSIS — used chiefly in combination ⟨oculomotor ∼⟩ — see BELL'S PALSY, CEREBRAL PALSY 2 : a condition that is characterized by uncontrollable tremor or quivering of the body or one or more of its parts — not used technically

Pal·u·drine \'pa-lə-drən\ *trademark* — used for derivatives of biguanide used as antimalarials

L-PAM \'el-ˌpam\ *n* : MELPHALAN

2-PAM \ˌtü-ˌpē-ˌā-'em\ *n* : PRALIDOXIME

pam·a·quine \'pa-mə-ˌkwin, -ˌkwēn\ *n* : a toxic antimalarial drug $C_{19}H_{29}N_3O$; *also* : PAMAQUINE NAPHTHOATE — see PLASMOCHIN

pamaquine naph·tho·ate \-'naf-thə-ˌwāt\ *n* : an insoluble salt $C_{42}H_{45}N_3O_7$ of pamaquine

Pam·ine \'pa-ˌmēn\ *trademark* — used for a preparation of the bromide salt of methscopolamine

pam·o·ate \'pa-mə-ˌwāt\ *n* : any of various salts or esters of an acid $C_{23}H_{16}O_6$ — see HYDROXYZINE

pam·pin·i·form plexus \pam-'pi-nə-ˌform-\ *n* : a venous plexus that is associated with each testicular vein in the male and each ovarian vein in the female — called also *pampiniform venous plexus*

pan- *comb form* : whole : general ⟨pancarditis⟩ ⟨panleukopenia⟩

pan·car·di·tis \ˌpan-kär-'dī-təs\ *n* : general inflammation of the heart

Pan·coast's syndrome \'pan-ˌkȯsts-\ *n* : a complex of symptoms associated with Pancoast's tumor which includes Horner's syndrome and neuralgia of the arm resulting from pressure on the brachial plexus

Pancoast, Henry Khunrath (1875–1939), American radiologist.

Pancoast's tumor *or* **Pancoast tumor** *n* : a malignant tumor formed at the upper extremity of the lung

pan·cre·as \'paŋ-krē-əs, 'pan-\ *n, pl* **-cre·as·es** *also* **-cre·ata** \pan-'krē-ə-tə\ : a large lobulated gland that in humans lies in front of the upper lumbar vertebrae and behind the stomach and is somewhat hammer-shaped and firmly attached anteriorly to the

curve of the duodenum with which it communicates through one or more pancreatic ducts and that consists of (1) tubular acini secreting digestive enzymes which pass to the intestine and function in the breakdown of proteins, fats, and carbohydrates; (2) modified acinar cells that form islets of Langerhans between the tubules and secrete the hormones insulin and glucagon; and (3) a firm connective-tissue capsule that extends supportive strands into the organ

pancreat- *or* **pancreato-** *comb form* 1 : pancreas : pancreatic ⟨pancreatectomy⟩ ⟨pancreatin⟩ 2 : pancreas and ⟨pancreatoduodenectomy⟩

pan·cre·atec·to·my \ˌpaŋ-krē-ə-'tek-tə-mē, ˌpan-\ *n, pl* **-mies** : surgical excision of all or part of the pancreas — **pan·cre·atec·to·mized** \ˌpaŋ-krē-ə-'tek-tə-ˌmīzd, ˌpan-\ *adj*

pan·cre·at·ic \ˌpaŋ-krē-'a-tik, ˌpan-\ *adj* : of, relating to, or produced in the pancreas ⟨∼ amylase⟩

pancreatic cholera *n* : VERNER-MORRISON SYNDROME

pancreatic duct *n* : a duct connecting the pancreas with the intestine: **a** : the chief duct of the pancreas that runs from left to right through the body of the gland, passes out its neck, and empties into the duodenum either through an opening shared with the common bile duct or through one close to it — called also *duct of Wirsung, Wirsung's duct* **b** : ACCESSORY PANCREATIC DUCT

pancreatic juice *n* : a clear alkaline secretion of pancreatic enzymes (as trypsin and lipase) that flows into the duodenum and acts on food already acted on by the gastric juice and saliva

pancreatico- *comb form* : pancreatic : pancreatic and ⟨pancreaticoduodenal⟩

pan·cre·at·i·co·du·o·de·nal \ˌpaŋ-krē-ˌa-ti-(ˌ)kō-ˌdü-ə-'dē-nəl, ˌpan-, -ˌdyü-; dü-'äd-ᵊn-əl, -dyü-\ *adj* : of or relating to the pancreas and the duodenum

pancreaticoduodenal artery *n* : either of two arteries that supply the pancreas and duodenum forming an anastomosis giving off numerous branches to these parts: **a** : one arising from the superior mesenteric artery — called also *inferior pancreaticoduodenal artery* **b** : one arising from the gastroduodenal artery — called also *superior pancreaticoduodenal artery*

pancreaticoduodenal vein *n* : any of several veins that drain the pancreas and duodenum accompanying the inferior and superior pancreaticoduodenal arteries

pan·cre·at·i·co·du·o·de·nec·to·my \-ˌdü-ə-ˌdē-'nek-tə-mē, -ˌdyü-; -dü-ˌä-də-'nek-tə-mē, -dyü-\ *n, pl* **-mies** : partial or complete excision of the pancreas and the duodenum — called also *pancreatoduodenectomy*

pan·cre·at·i·co·du·o·de·nos·to·my \-ˈnäs-tə-mē\ *n, pl* **-mies** : surgical formation of an artificial opening connecting the pancreas to the duodenum

pan·cre·at·i·co·je·ju·nos·to·my \-ji-ˌjü-ˈnäs-tə-mē, -ˌje-jü-\ *n, pl* **-mies** : surgical formation of an artificial passage connecting the pancreas to the jejunum

pan·cre·atin \pan-ˈkrē-ə-tən; ˈpaŋ-krē-, ˈpan-\ *n* : a mixture of enzymes from the pancreatic juice; *also* : a preparation containing such a mixture obtained from the pancreas of the domestic swine or ox and used as a digestant

pan·cre·ati·tis \ˌpaŋ-krē-ə-ˈtī-təs, ˌpan-\ *n, pl* **-atit·i·des** \-ˈti-tə-ˌdēz\ : inflammation of the pancreas

pancreato- — see PANCREAT-

pan·cre·a·to·du·o·de·nec·to·my \ˈpan-krē-ə-tō-ˌdü-ə-də-ˈnek-tə-mē, -ˌdyü-; -ˌdü-ˌäd-ə-ˈnek-tə-mē, -dyü-\ *n, pl* **-mies** : PANCREATICODUODENECTOMY

pan·cre·o·zy·min \ˌpan-krē-ō-ˈzī-mən\ *n* : CHOLECYSTOKININ

pan·cu·ro·ni·um bromide \ˌpan-kyə-ˈrō-nē-əm-\ *n* : a neuromuscular blocking agent $C_{35}H_{60}Br_2N_2O_4$ used as a skeletal muscle relaxant — called also *pancuronium*

pan·cy·to·pe·nia \ˌpan-ˌsī-tə-ˈpē-nē-ə\ *n* : an abnormal reduction in the number of red blood cells, white blood cells, and blood platelets in the blood; *also* : a disorder (as aplastic anemia) characterized by such a reduction — **pan·cy·to·pe·nic** \-ˈpē-nik\ *adj*

¹**pan·dem·ic** \pan-ˈde-mik\ *adj* : occurring over a wide geographic area and affecting an exceptionally high proportion of the population (∼ malaria)

²**pandemic** *n* : a pandemic outbreak of a disease

pan·en·ceph·a·li·tis \ˌpan-in-ˌse-fə-ˈlī-təs\ *n, pl* **-lit·i·des** \-ˈli-tə-ˌdēz\ : inflammation of the brain affecting both white and gray matter — see SUBACUTE SCLEROSING PANENCEPHALITIS

pan·en·do·scope \-ˈen-də-ˌskōp\ *n* : a cystoscope fitted with an obliquely forward telescopic system that permits wide-angle viewing of the interior of the urinary bladder — **pan·en·do·scop·ic** \-ˌen-də-ˈskä-pik\ *adj* — **pan·en·dos·co·py** \-en-ˈdäs-kə-pē\ *n*

Pa·neth cell \ˈpä-net\ *n* : any of the granular epithelial cells with large acidophilic nuclei occurring at the base of the crypts of Lieberkühn in the small intestine and appendix

   Paneth, Josef (1857–1890), Austrian physiologist.

pang \ˈpaŋ\ *n* : a brief piercing spasm of pain — see BIRTH PANG, HUNGER PANGS

pan·hy·po·pi·tu·ita·rism \ˌpan-ˌhī-pō-pə-ˈtü-ə-tə-ˌri-zəm, -ˈtyü-\ *n* : gener-

alized secretory deficiency of the anterior lobe of the pituitary gland; *also* : a disorder (as Simmond's disease) characterized by such deficiency — **pan·hy·po·pi·tu·itary** \-ˈtü-ə-ˌter-ē, -ˈtyü-\ *adj*

pan·hys·ter·ec·to·my \ˌ(ˌ)pan-ˌhis-tə-ˈrek-tə-mē\ *n, pl* **-mies** : surgical excision of the uterus and uterine cervix

pan·ic \ˈpa-nik\ *n* : a sudden overpowering fright; *esp* : a sudden unreasoning terror often accompanied by mass flight — **panic** *vb*

panic disorder *n* : ANXIETY NEUROSIS

pan·leu·ko·pe·nia \ˌpan-ˌlü-kə-ˈpē-nē-ə\ *n* : an acute usu. fatal viral epizootic disease esp. of cats that is caused by a parvovirus and is characterized by fever, diarrhea and dehydration, and extensive destruction of white blood cells — called also *cat distemper, cat fever, feline distemper, feline enteritis, feline panleukopenia*

pan·nic·u·li·tis \pə-ˌni-kyə-ˈlī-təs\ *n* **1** : inflammation of the subcutaneous layer of fat **2** : a syndrome characterized by recurring fever and usu. painful inflammatory and necrotic nodules in the subcutaneous tissues esp. of the thighs, abdomen, or buttocks — called also *relapsing febrile nodular nonsuppurative panniculitis, Weber-Christian disease*

pan·nic·u·lus \pə-ˈni-kyə-ləs\ *n, pl* **-u·li** \-ˌlī\ : a sheet or layer of tissue; *esp* : PANNICULUS ADIPOSUS

panniculus ad·i·po·sus \-ˌa-də-ˈpō-səs\ *n* : any superficial fascia bearing deposits of fat

pan·nus \ˈpa-nəs\ *n, pl* **pan·ni** \-ˌnī\ **1** : a vascular tissue causing a superficial opacity of the cornea and occurring esp. in trachoma **2** : a sheet of inflammatory granulation tissue that spreads from the synovial membrane and invades the joint in rheumatoid arthritis ultimately leading to fibrous ankylosis

pan·oph·thal·mi·tis \ˌ(ˌ)pan-ˌäf-thəl-ˈmī-təs, -ˌäp-\ *n* : inflammation involving all the tissues of the eyeball

pan·sys·tol·ic \ˌ(ˌ)pan-sis-ˈtä-lik\ *adj* : persisting throughout systole (a ∼ heart murmur)

pant \ˈpant\ *vb* : to breathe quickly, spasmodically, or in a labored manner

pan·to·caine \ˈpan-tə-ˌkān\ *n* : TETRACAINE

pan·to·the·nate \ˌpan-tə-ˈthe-ˌnāt, pan-ˈtä-thə-ˌnāt\ *n* : a salt or ester of pantothenic acid — see CALCIUM PANTOTHENATE

pan·to·then·ic acid \ˌpan-tə-ˈthe-nik-\ *n* : a viscous oily acid $C_9H_{17}NO_5$ that belongs to the vitamin B complex, occurs usu. combined (as in coenzyme A) in all living tissues

pan·trop·ic \ˌ(ˌ)pan-ˈträ-pik\ *adj* : affecting various tissues without showing special affinity for one of them ⟨a ~ virus⟩ — compare NEUROTROPIC

pa·pa·in \pə-'pā-ən, -'pī-\ n : a crystallizable proteinase in the juice of the green fruit of the papaya (*Carica papaya* of the family Caricaceae) obtained usu. as a brownish powder and used chiefly as a tenderizer for meat and in medicine as a digestant

Pa·pa·ni·co·laou smear \ˌpä-pə-'nē-kə-ˌlaü-, ˌpa-pə-'ni-kə-\ n : PAP SMEAR

Papanicolaou, George Nicholas (1883–1962), American anatomist and cytologist.

Papanicolaou test n : PAP SMEAR

Pa·pa·ver \pə-'pā-vər, -'pä-\ n : a genus (family Papaveraceae) of chiefly bristly hairy herbs that contains the opium poppy (*P. somniferum*)

pa·pav·er·ine \pə-'pa-və-ˌrēn, -rən\ n : a crystalline alkaloid $C_{20}H_{21}NO_4$ that is used in the form of its hydrochloride chiefly as an antispasmodic (as in spasm of blood vessels due to a blood clot)

paper chromatography n : chromatography that uses paper strips or sheets as the adsorbent stationary phase through which a solution flows and is used esp. to separate amino acids — compare COLUMN CHROMATOGRAPHY, THIN-LAYER CHROMATOGRAPHY

papill- or **papillo-** comb form 1 : papilla ⟨*papill*itis⟩ 2 : papillary ⟨*papill*edema⟩ ⟨*papill*oma⟩

pa·pil·la \pə-'pi-lə\ n, pl **pa·pil·lae** \-'(ˌ)lē, -ˌlī\ : a small projecting body part similar to a nipple in form: as **a** : a vascular process of connective tissue extending into and nourishing the root of a hair or developing tooth **b** : any of the vascular protuberances of the dermal layer of the skin extending into the epidermal layer and often containing tactile corpuscles **c** : RENAL PAPILLA **d** : any of the small protuberances on the upper surface of the tongue — see CIRCUMVALLATE PAPILLA, FILIFORM PAPILLA, FUNGIFORM PAPILLA, INTERDENTAL PAPILLA

papilla of Vater n : AMPULLA OF VATER

pap·il·lary \'pa-pə-ˌler-ē\ adj : of, relating to, or resembling a papilla : PAPILLOSE

papillary carcinoma n : a carcinoma characterized by a papillary structure

papillary layer n : the superficial layer of the dermis raised into papillae that fit into corresponding depressions on the inner surface of the epidermis

papillary muscle n : one of the small muscular columns attached at one end to the chordae tendineae and at the other to the wall of the ventricle and that maintain tension on the chordae tendineae as the ventricle contracts

pap·il·late \'pa-pə-ˌlāt, pə-'pi-lət\ adj : covered with or bearing papillae

pap·il·lec·to·my \ˌpa-pə-'lek-tə-mē\ n,

pl **-mies** : the surgical removal of a papilla

pap·il·le·de·ma \ˌpa-pə-lə-'dē-mə\ n : swelling and protrusion of the blind spot of the eye caused by edema — called also choked disk

pap·il·li·tis \ˌpa-pə-'lī-təs\ n : inflammation of a papilla; esp : inflammation of the optic disk — see NECROTIZING PAPILLITIS

pap·il·lo·ma \ˌpa-pə-'lō-mə\ n, pl **-mas** or **-ma·ta** \-mə-tə\ **1** : a benign tumor (as a wart or condyloma) resulting from an overgrowth of epithelial tissue on papillae of vascularized connective tissue (as of the skin) **2** : an epithelial tumor caused by a virus

pap·il·lo·ma·to·sis \-ˌlō-mə-'tō-səs\ n, pl **-to·ses** \-ˌsēz\ : a condition marked by the presence of numerous papillomas

pap·il·lo·ma·tous \-'lō-mə-təs\ adj **1** : resembling or being a papilloma **2** : marked or characterized by papillomas

pap·il·lo·ma·vi·rus \ˌpa-pə-'lō-mə-ˌvī-rəs\ n : any of a group of papovaviruses that cause papillomas

pap·il·lose \'pa-pə-ˌlōs\ adj : covered with, resembling, or bearing papillae

pa·po·va·vi·rus \pə-'pō-və-ˌvī-rəs\ n : any of a group of viruses that have a capsid composed of 72 capsomers and that are associated with or responsible for various neoplasms (as some warts)

pap·pa·ta·ci fever also **pa·pa·ta·ci fever** \ˌpa-pə-'tä-chē-\ or **pa·pa·ta·si fever** \-'tä-sē-\ n : SANDFLY FEVER

Pap smear \'pap-\ n : a method or a test based on it for the early detection of cancer esp. of the uterine cervix that involves staining exfoliated cells by a special technique which differentiates diseased tissue — called also *Papanicolaou smear, Papanicolaou test, Pap test*

G. N. Papanicolaou — see PAPANICOLAOU SMEAR

pap·u·la \'pa-pyə-lə\ n, pl **pap·u·lae** \-ˌlē\ **1** : PAPULE **2** : a small papilla

pap·u·lar \'pa-pyə-lər\ adj : consisting of or characterized by papules ⟨a ~ rash⟩ ⟨~ lesions⟩

pap·u·la·tion \ˌpa-pyə-'lā-shən\ n **1** : a stage in some eruptive conditions marked by the formation of papules **2** : the formation of papules

pap·ule \'pa-(ˌ)pyül\ n : a small solid usu. conical elevation of the skin caused by inflammation, accumulated secretion, or hypertrophy of tissue elements

papulo- comb form **1** : papula ⟨*papulo*pustular⟩ **2** : papulous and ⟨*papulo*vesicular⟩

pap·u·lo·pus·tu·lar \ˌpa-pyə-lō-'pəs-chə-lar, -'pəs-tyü-\ adj : consisting of both papules and pustules ⟨~ lesions⟩

pap·u·lo·sis \ˌpa-pyə-'lō-səs\ n : the condition of having papular lesions

pap·u·lo·ve·sic·u·lar \ˌpa-pyə-lō-və-'si-kya-lər\ *adj* : marked by the presence of both papules and vesicles

pap·y·ra·ceous \₁pa-pə-ˈrā-shəs\ *adj* : of, relating to, or being one of twin fetuses which has died in the uterus and been compressed to a thinness like paper by the growth of the other

para \ˈpar-ə\ *n, pl* **par·as** *or* **par·ae** \ˈpar-ˌē\ : a woman delivered of a specified number of children — used in combination with a term or figure to indicate the number (multi*para*) (a 36-year-old *para* 5); compare GRAVIDA

para- \ˌpar-ə, ˈpar-ə\ *or* **par-** *prefix* **1** : beside : alongside of : beyond : aside from ⟨*para*thyroid⟩ ⟨*par*enteral⟩ **2 a** : closely related to ⟨*para*ldehyde⟩ **b** : involving substitution at or characterized by two opposite positions that are separated by two carbon atoms in the flat symmetrical ring of six carbon atoms characteristic of benzene ⟨*para*dichlorobenzene⟩ — abbr. *p-* **3 a** : faulty : abnormal ⟨*par*esthesia⟩ **b** : associated in a subsidiary or accessory capacity ⟨*para*medical⟩ **c** : closely resembling : almost ⟨*para*typhoid⟩

para–ami·no·ben·zo·ic acid \ˈpar-ə-ə-ˌmē-ˌno-ˌben-ˈzō-ik-, ˈpar-ə-ˌa-mə-(ˌ)nō-\ *n* : a colorless para-substituted aminobenzoic acid that is a growth factor of the vitamin B complex — called also *PABA*

para–ami·no·hip·pu·rate \ˌhi-pyə-ˌrāt\ *n* : a salt of para-aminohippuric acid

para–ami·no·hip·pu·ric acid \-hi-ˈpyur-ik-\ *n* : a crystalline acid $C_{19}H_{10}N_2O_3$ used chiefly in the form of its sodium salt in testing kidney function

para–ami·no·sal·i·cyl·ic acid \-ˌsal-ə-ˈsi-lik-\ *n* : the white crystalline para-substituted isomer of aminosalicylic acid that is made synthetically and is used in the treatment of tuberculosis

para–aor·tic \ˌpar-ə-ā-ˈor-tik\ *adj* : close to the aorta ⟨~ lymph nodes⟩

para–api·cal \-ˈā-pi-kəl, -ˈa-\ *adj* : close to the apex of the heart

para·ben \ˈpar-ə-ben\ *n* : either of two antifungal agents used as preservatives in foods and pharmaceuticals: **a** : METHYLPARABEN **b** : PROPYLPARABEN

para·bi·o·sis \ˌpar-ə-(ˌ)bī-ˈō-səs, -bē-\ *n, pl* **-o·ses** \-ˌsēz\ : the anatomical and physiological union of two organisms either natural or artificially produced — **para·bi·ot·ic** \-ˈä-tik\ *adj* — **para·bi·ot·i·cal·ly** *adv*

para·cen·te·sis \ˌpar-ə-(ˌ)sen-ˈtē-səs, *pl* **-te·ses** \-ˌsēz\ : a surgical puncture of a cavity of the body with a trocar, aspirator, or other instrument usu. to draw off any abnormal effusion

para·cen·tral \ˌpar-ə-ˈsen-trəl\ *adj* : lying near a center or central part

para·cen·tric \-ˈsen-trik\ *adj* : being an inversion that occurs in a single arm of one chromosome and does not in-

volve the chromomere — compare PERICENTRIC

para·cer·vi·cal \-ˈsər-və-kəl\ *adj* : located or administered next to the uterine cervix ⟨~ injection⟩

para·cet·a·mol \ˌpar-ə-ˈsē-tə-ˌmól\ *n, Brit* : ACETAMINOPHEN

para·chlo·ro·phe·nol \-ˌklór-ə-ˈfē-ˌnól, -ˌnól, -fi-ˈnól\ *n* : a chlorinated phenol C_6H_5ClO used as a germicide

para·chol·era \-ˈkä-lə-rə\ *n* : a disease clinically resembling Asiatic cholera but caused by a different vibrio

Para·coc·cid·i·oi·des \ˌpar-ə-(ˌ)käk-ˌsi-dē-ˈói-ˌdēz\ *n* : a genus of imperfect fungi that includes the causative agent (*P. brasiliensis*) of South American blastomycosis

para·coc·cid·i·oi·do·my·co·sis \-(ˌ)käk-ˌsi-dē-ˌói-dō-(ˌ)mī-ˈkō-sis\ *n, pl* **-co·ses** \-ˌsēz\ : SOUTH AMERICAN BLASTOMYCOSIS

para·co·lic \-ˈkō-lik, -ˈkä-\ *adj* : adjacent to the colon ⟨~ lymph nodes⟩

para·cone \ˈpar-ə-ˌkōn\ *n* : the anterior of the three cusps of a primitive upper molar that in higher forms is the principal anterior and external cusp

par·acu·sis \ˌpar-ə-ˈkyü-səs, -ˈkü-\ *n, pl* **-acu·ses** \-ˌsēz\ : a disorder in the sense of hearing

para·den·tal \-ˈdent-əl\ *adj* : adjacent to a tooth ⟨~ infections⟩

para·di·chlo·ro·ben·zene \ˌpar-ə-ˌdī-ˌklór-ə-ˈben-ˌzēn, -ˌben-\ *n* : a white crystalline compound $C_6H_4Cl_2$ made by chlorinating benzene and used chiefly as a fumigant against clothes moths — called also *PDB*

para·did·y·mis \-ˈdi-də-məs\ *n, pl* **-y·mi·des** \-mə-ˌdēz\ : a group of coiled tubules situated in front of the lower end of the spermatic cord above the enlarged upper extremity of the epididymis and is considered to be a remnant of tubes of the mesonephros

par·a·dox·i·cal \ˌpar-ə-ˈdäk-si-kəl\ *also* **par·a·dox·ic** \-sik\ *adj* : not being the normal or usual kind ⟨~ pulse⟩

paradoxical sleep *n* : REM SLEEP

paradoxus — see PULSUS PARADOXUS

para·esoph·a·ge·al \-i-ˌsä-fə-ˈjē-əl\ *adj* : adjacent to the esophagus; *esp* : relating to or being a hiatal hernia in which the connection between the esophagus and the stomach remains in its normal location but part or all of the stomach herniates through the hiatus into the thorax

par·aes·the·sia *chiefly Brit var of* PARESTHESIA

par·af·fin \ˈpar-ə-fən\ *n* **1** : a waxy crystalline flammable substance obtained esp. from distillates of wood, coal, or petroleum that is a complex mixture of hydrocarbons and is used in pharmaceuticals and cosmetics **2** : ALKANE — **par·af·fin·ic** \ˌpar-ə-ˈfi-nik\ *adj*

para·fol·lic·u·lar \ˌpar-ə-fə-ˈli-kyə-lər\ *adj* : located in the vicinity of or surrounding a follicle ⟨∼ cells of the thyroid⟩

para·for·mal·de·hyde \-fȯr-'mal-də-ˌhīd, -far-\ *n* : a white powder $(CH_2O)_x$ that consists of a polymer of formaldehyde and is used esp. as a fungicide

para·fo·vea \-'fō-vē-ə\ *n, pl* **-fo·ve·ae** \-'fō-vē-ˌē, -vē-ˌī\ : the area surrounding the fovea — **para·fo·ve·al** \-'fō-vē-əl\ *adj*

para·gan·gli·o·ma \-ˌgaŋ-glē-'ō-mə\ *n, pl* **-mas** *or* **-ma·ta** \-mə-tə\ : a ganglioma derived from chromaffin cells — compare PHEOCHROMOCYTOMA

para·gan·gli·on \-'gaŋ-glē-ən\ *n, pl* **-glia** \-glē-ə\ : one of numerous collections of chromaffin cells associated with ganglia and plexuses of the sympathetic nervous system and similar in structure to the medulla of the adrenal glands — **para·gan·gli·on·ic** \-ˌgaŋ-glē-'ä-nik\ *adj*

par·a·gon·i·mi·a·sis \ˌpar-ə-ˌgä-nə-'mī-ə-səs\ *n, pl* **-a·ses** \-ˌsēz\ : infestation with or disease caused by a lung fluke of the genus *Paragonimus* (*P. westermanii*) that invades the lung

Par·a·gon·i·mus \ˌpar-ə-'gä-nə-məs\ *n* : a genus of digenetic trematodes (family Troglotrematidae) comprising forms normally parasitic in the lungs of mammals including humans

para·gran·u·lo·ma \-ˌgra-nyə-'lō-mə\ *n, pl* **-mas** *or* **-ma·ta** \-mə-tə\ **1** : a granuloma esp. of the lymph glands that is characterized by inflammation and replacement of the normal cell structure by an infiltrate **2** : a benign form of Hodgkin's disease in which paragranulomas of the lymph glands are a symptom — called also *Hodgkin's paragranuloma*

para·in·flu·en·za virus \ˌpar-ə-ˌin-flü-'en-zə-\ *n* : any of several paramyxoviruses that are associated with or responsible for some respiratory infections esp. in children — called also *parainfluenza*

para·ker·a·to·sis \ˌpar-ə-ˌker-ə-'tō-səs\ *n, pl* **-to·ses** \-ˌsēz\ : an abnormality of the horny layer of the skin resulting in a disturbance in the process of keratinization

par·al·de·hyde \pa-'ral-də-ˌhīd, pə-\ *n* : a colorless liquid polymeric modification $C_6H_{12}O_3$ of acetaldehyde used as a hypnotic esp. for controlling insomnia, excitement, delirium, and convulsions (as in delirium tremens and withdrawal from alcohol abuse)

pa·ral·y·sis \pə-'ra-lə-səs\ *n, pl* **-y·ses** \-ˌsēz\ : complete or partial loss of function esp. when involving the power of motion or of sensation in any part of the body — see HEMIPLEGIA, PARAPLEGIA, PARESIS 1

paralysis agi·tans \-'a-jə-ˌtanz\ *n* : PARKINSON'S DISEASE

¹par·a·lyt·ic \ˌpar-ə-'li-tik\ *adj* **1** : affected with or characterized by paralysis

2 : of, relating to, or resembling paralysis

²paralytic *n* : one affected with paralysis

paralytica — see DEMENTIA PARALYTICA

paralytic dementia *n* : GENERAL PARESIS

paralytic ileus *n* : ileus resulting from failure of peristalsis

paralytic rabies *n* : rabies marked by sluggishness and by early paralysis esp. of the muscles of jaw and throat — called also *dumb rabies*; compare FURIOUS RABIES

paralytic shellfish poisoning *n* : food poisoning that results from consumption of shellfish and esp. 2-shelled mollusks (as clams, mussels, or scallops) contaminated with dinoflagellates causing red tide and that is characterized by paresthesia, nausea, vomiting, abdominal cramping, muscle weakness, and sometimes paralysis which may lead to respiratory failure

par·a·lyze \'par-ə-ˌlīz\ *vb* **-lyzed; -lyz·ing** : to affect with paralysis — **par·a·ly·za·tion** \ˌpar-ə-lə-'zā-shən\ *n*

para·me·di·an \ˌpar-ə-'mē-dē-ən\ *adj* : situated adjacent to the midline

para·med·ic \ˌpar-ə-'me-dik\ *also* **para·med·i·cal** \-di-kəl\ *n* **1** : a person who works in a health field in an auxiliary capacity to a physician (as by giving injections and taking X rays) **2** : a specially trained medical technician licensed to provide a wide range of emergency medical services (as defibrillation and the intravenous administration of drugs) before or during transportation to the hospital — compare EMT

para·med·i·cal \ˌpar-ə-'me-di-kəl\ *also* **para·med·ic** \-dik\ *adj* : concerned with supplementing the work of highly trained medical professionals

para·me·so·neph·ric duct \-ˌme-zə-'ne-frik-, -ˌmē-, -sə-\ *n* : MÜLLERIAN DUCT

para·metha·di·one \-ˌme-thə-'dī-ˌōn\ *n* : a liquid compound $C_7H_{11}NO_3$ that is a derivative of trimethadione and is used in the treatment of petit mal epilepsy

para·meth·a·sone \-'me-thə-ˌzōn\ *n* : a glucocorticoid with few mineralocorticoid side effects that is used for its anti-inflammatory and antiallergic actions esp. as the acetate $C_{24}H_{31}FO_6$

para·me·tri·tis \-mə-'trī-təs\ *n* : inflammation of the parametrium

para·me·tri·um \-'mē-trē-əm\ *n, pl* **-tria** \-trē-ə\ : the connective tissue and fat adjacent to the uterus

par·am·ne·sia \ˌpar-ˌam-'nē-zhə, -əm-\ *n* : a disorder of memory: as **a** : a condition in which the proper meaning of words cannot be remembered **b** : the illusion of remembering scenes and events when experienced for the first time — called also *déjà vu*; compare JAMAIS VU

para·mo·lar \,par-ə-'mō-lər\ *adj* : of, relating to, or being a supernumerary tooth esp. on the buccal side of a permanent molar or a cusp or tubercle located esp. on the buccal aspect of a molar and representing such a tooth

par·am·y·loid·o·sis \,par-,a-mə-,lȯi-'dō-səs\ *n, pl* **-oses** \-,sēz\ : amyloidosis characterized by the accumulation of an atypical form of amyloid in the tissues

para·myo·clo·nus mul·ti·plex \,par-ə-,mī-'ä-klə-nəs-'məl-tə-,pleks\ *n* : a nervous disease characterized by clonic spasms with tremor in corresponding muscles on the two sides

para·myo·to·nia \,par-ə-,mī-ə-'tō-nē-ə\ *n* : an abnormal state characterized by tonic muscle spasm

para·myxo·vi·rus \,par-ə-'mik-sə-,vī-rəs\ *n* : any of a group of RNA-containing viruses (as the mumps, measles, and parainfluenza viruses) that are larger than the related orthomyxoviruses

para·na·sal \-'nā-zəl\ *adj* : adjacent to the nasal cavities; *esp* : of, relating to, or affecting the paranasal sinuses

paranasal sinus *n* : any of various sinuses (as the maxillary sinus and frontal sinus) in the bones of the face and head that are lined with mucous membrane derived from and continuous with the lining of the nasal cavity

para·neo·plas·tic \,par-ə-,nē-ə-'plas-tik\ *adj* : caused by or resulting from the presence of cancer in the body but not the physical presence of cancerous tissue in the part or organ affected

para·noia \,par-ə-'nȯi-ə\ *n* **1** : a psychosis characterized by systematized delusions of persecution or grandeur usu. without hallucinations **2** : a tendency on the part of an individual or group toward excessive or irrational suspiciousness and distrustfulness of others

¹para·noi·ac \-'nȯi-,ak, -'nȯi-ik\ *also* **para·no·ic** \-'nō-ik\ *adj* : of, relating to, affected with, or characteristic of paranoia or paranoid schizophrenia

²paranoiac *also* **paranoic** *n* : PARANOID

¹para·noid \'par-ə-,nȯid\ *also* **para·noi·dal** \,par-ə-'nȯid-əl\ *adj* **1** : characterized by or resembling paranoia or paranoid schizophrenia **2** : characterized by suspiciousness, persecutory trends, or megalomania

²paranoid *n* : one affected with paranoia or paranoid schizophrenia — called also *paranoiac*

paranoid schizophrenia *n* : schizophrenia characterized esp. by persecutory or grandiose delusions or hallucinations or by delusional jealousy

paranoid schizophrenic *n* : an individual affected with paranoid schizophrenia

para·nor·mal \,par-ə-'nȯr-məl\ *adj* : not understandable in terms of known scientific laws and phenomena — **para·nor·mal·ly** *adv*

para·ol·fac·to·ry \,par-ə-äl-'fak-tə-rē, -ȯl-\ *n* : a small area of the cerebral cortex situated on the medial side of the frontal lobe below the corpus callosum and considered part of the limbic system

para·ox·on \-'äk-,sän\ *n* : a phosphate ester $C_{10}H_{14}NO_6P$ that is formed from parathion in the body and that is a potent anticholinesterase

para·pa·re·sis \,par-ə-pə-'rē-səs, ,par-ə-'par-ə-səs\ *n, pl* **-re·ses** \-,sēz\ : partial paralysis affecting the lower limbs — **para·pa·ret·ic** \-pə-'re-tik\ *adj*

para·per·tus·sis \-(,)pər-'tə-sis\ *n* : a human respiratory disease closely resembling whooping cough but milder and less often fatal and caused by a different bacterium of the genus *Bordetella* (*B. parapertussis*)

para·pha·ryn·ge·al space \-,far-ən-'jē-əl-, -fə-'rin-jəl-, -jē-əl-\ *n* : a space bounded medially by the superior constrictor of the pharynx, laterally by the medial pterygoid muscle, posteriorly by the cervical vertebrae, and below by the muscles arising from the styloid process

par·a·pha·sia \-'fā-zhə, -zhē-ə\ *n* : aphasia in which the patient uses wrong words or uses words or sounds in senseless combinations — **par·a·pha·sic** \-'fā-zik\ *adj*

para·phen·yl·ene·di·amine \-,fen-əl-,ēn-'dī-ə-,mēn\ *n* : a benzene derivative C_6H_8N used esp. in dyeing hair and sometimes causing an allergic reaction

para·phil·ia \-'fil-ē-ə\ *n* : perverted sexual behavior

¹para·phil·iac \-'fil-ē-,ak\ *adj* : of, relating to, or characterized by paraphilia

²paraphiliac *n* : a person who engages in paraphilia

para·phi·mo·sis \-fī-'mō-səs, -fi-\ *n, pl* **-mo·ses** \-,sēz\ : a condition in which the foreskin is retracted behind the glans penis and cannot be replaced

para·phre·nia \-'frē-nē-ə\ *n* **1** : the group of paranoid disorders **2** : any of the paranoid disorders; *also* : SCHIZOPHRENIA — **para·phren·ic** \-'fre-nik\ *adj*

para·ple·gia \,par-ə-'plē-jə, -jē-ə\ *n* : paralysis of the lower half of the body with involvement of both legs usu. due to disease of or injury to the spinal cord

¹para·ple·gic \-'plē-jik\ *adj* : of, relating to, or affected with paraplegia

²paraplegic *n* : an individual affected with paraplegia

para·prax·is \-'prak-səs\ *n, pl* **-praxes** \-'prak-,sēz\ : a faulty act (as a

Freudian slip) of purposeful behavior

para·pro·tein \-'prō-ˌtēn\ *n* : any of various abnormal serum globulins with unique physical and electrophoretic characteristics

para·pro·tein·emia \-ˌprō-tē-'nē-mē-ə, -ˌprō-tē-ə-'nē-\ *n* : the presence of a paraprotein in the blood

para·pso·ri·a·sis \-sə-'rī-ə-səs\ *n, pl* **-a·ses** \-ˌsēz\ : a rare skin disease characterized by red scaly patches similar to those of psoriasis but causing no sensations of pain or itch

para·psy·chol·o·gy \ˌpar-ə-(ˌ)sī-'kä-lə-jē\ *n, pl* **-gies** : a field of study concerned with the investigation of evidence for paranormal psychological phenomena (as telepathy, clairvoyance, and psychokinesis) — **para·psych·o·log·i·cal** \-ˌsī-kə-'lä-ji-kəl\ *adj* — **para·psy·chol·o·gist** \-sī-'kä-lə-jist, -sə-\ *n*

para·quat \'par-ə-ˌkwät\ *n* : an herbicide containing a salt of a cation $C_{12}H_{14}N_2$ that is extremely toxic to the liver, kidneys, and lungs if ingested

para·re·nal \ˌpar-ə-'rēn-ᵊl\ *adj* : adjacent to the kidney

para·ros·an·i·line \ˌpar-ə-'rō-'zan-ᵊl-ən\ *n* : a white crystalline base $C_{19}H_{19}N_3O$ that is the parent compound of many dyes; *also* : its red chloride used esp. as a biological stain

para·sag·it·tal \-'sa-jət-ᵊl\ *adj* : situated alongside of or adjacent to a sagittal location or a sagittal plane

Par·as·ca·ris \(ˌ)par-'as-kə-rəs\ *n* : a genus of nematode worms (family Ascaridae) including the large roundworm (*P. equorum*) of the horse

parasit- *or* **parasito-** *also* **parasiti-** *comb form* : parasite (*parasit*emia) ⟨*parasiti*cide⟩

para·sit·ae·mia *chiefly Brit var of* PARASITEMIA

par·a·site \'par-ə-ˌsīt\ *n* : an organism living in, with, or on another organism in parasitism

par·a·sit·emia \ˌpar-ə-ˌsī-'tē-mē-ə\ *n* : a condition in which parasites are present in the blood — used esp. to indicate the presence of parasites without clinical symptoms (an afebrile ∼ of malaria)

par·a·sit·ic \ˌpar-ə-'sit-ik\ *also* **par·a·sit·i·cal** \-ti-kəl\ *adj* **1** : relating to or having the habit of a parasite : living on another organism **2** : caused by or resulting from the effects of parasites — **par·a·sit·i·cal·ly** *adv*

par·a·sit·i·cide \-'si-tə-ˌsīd\ *n* : an agent that is destructive to parasites — **par·a·sit·i·cid·al** \-ˌsi-tə-'sīd-ᵊl\ *adj*

par·a·sit·ism \'par-ə-sə-ˌti-zəm, -ˌsī-\ *n* **1** : an intimate association between organisms of two or more kinds : *esp* : one in which a parasite obtains benefits from a host which it usu. injures **2** : PARASITOSIS

par·a·sit·ize \-sə-ˌtīz, -ˌsī-\ *vb* **-ized; -iz·ing** : to infest or live on or with as a parasite — **par·a·sit·iza·tion** \ˌpar-ə-sə-tə-'zā-shən, -ˌsī-\ *n*

parasito- — see PARASIT-

par·a·si·tol·o·gist \-'tä-lə-jist\ *n* : a specialist in parasitology; *esp* : one who deals with the worm parasites of animals

par·a·si·tol·o·gy \ˌpar-ə-sə-'tä-lə-jē, -ˌsī-\ *n, pl* **-gies** : a branch of biology dealing with parasites and parasitism esp. among animals — **par·a·si·to·log·i·cal** \-ˌsit-ᵊl-'ä-ji-kəl, -ˌsit-\ *also* **par·a·si·to·log·ic** \-jik\ *adj* — **par·a·si·to·log·i·cal·ly** *adv*

par·a·si·to·sis \-sə-'tō-səs, -ˌsī-\ *n, pl* **-o·ses** \-ˌsēz\ : infestation with or disease caused by parasites

para·spe·cif·ic \-spi-'si-fik\ *adj* : having or being curative actions or properties in addition to the specific one considered medically useful

para·spi·nal \-'spīn-ᵊl\ *adj* : adjacent to the spinal column (∼ muscles)

para·ster·nal \-'stər-nəl\ *adj* : adjacent to the sternum — **para·ster·nal·ly** *adv*

¹para·sym·pa·thet·ic \ˌpar-ə-ˌsim-pə-'the-tik\ *adj* : of, relating to, being, or acting on the parasympathetic nervous system (∼ drugs)

²parasympathetic *n* **1** : a parasympathetic nerve **2** : PARASYMPATHETIC NERVOUS SYSTEM

parasympathetic nervous system *n* : the part of the autonomic nervous system that contains chiefly cholinergic fibers, that tends to induce secretion, to increase the tone and contractility of smooth muscle, and to slow the heart rate, and that consists of a cranial part and a sacral part — called also *parasympathetic system*; compare SYMPATHETIC NERVOUS SYSTEM

¹para·sym·pa·tho·lyt·ic \ˌpar-ə-ˌsim-pə-thō-'li-tik\ *adj* : tending to oppose the physiological results of parasympathetic nervous activity or of parasympathomimetic drugs — compare SYMPATHOLYTIC

²parasympatholytic *n* : a parasympatholytic substance

¹para·sym·pa·tho·mi·met·ic \ˌpar-ə-ˌsim-pə-(ˌ)thō-mi-'me-tik, -mə-\ *adj* : simulating parasympathetic nervous action in physiological effect — compare SYMPATHOMIMETIC

²parasympathomimetic *n* : a parasympathomimetic agent (as a drug)

para·sys·to·le \-'sis-tə-(ˌ)lē\ *n* : an irregularity in cardiac rhythm caused by an ectopic pacemaker in addition to the normal one

para·tax·ic \ˌpar-ə-'tak-sik\ *adj* : relating to or being thinking in which a cause and effect relationship is attributed to events occurring at about the same time but having no logical relationship

para·ten·on \ˌpar-ə-'te-nən, -(ˌ)nän\ *n*

: the areolar tissue filling the space between a tendon and its sheath

para·thi·on \par-ə-ˈthī-ən, -ˌän\ n : an extremely toxic sulfur-containing insecticide $C_{10}H_{14}NO_5PS$

par·a·thor·mone \ˌpar-ə-ˈthor-ˌmōn\ n : PARATHYROID HORMONE

¹para·thy·roid \-ˈthī-ˌroid\ n : PARATHYROID GLAND

²parathyroid adj **1** : adjacent to a thyroid gland **2** : of, relating to, or produced by the parathyroid glands

para·thy·roid·ec·to·my \-ˌthī-ˌroi-ˈdek-tə-mē\ n, pl **-mies** : partial or complete excision of the parathyroid glands — **para·thy·roid·ec·to·mized** \-ˌmizd\ adj

parathyroid gland n : any of usu. four small endocrine glands that are adjacent to or embedded in the thyroid gland, are composed of irregularly arranged secretory epithelial cells lying in a stroma rich in capillaries, and produce parathyroid hormone

parathyroid hormone n : a hormone of the parathyroid gland that regulates the metabolism of calcium and phosphorus in the body — abbr. PTH; called also *parathormone*

para·thy·ro·tro·pic \ˌpar-ə-ˌthī-rō-ˈträ-pik\ adj : acting on or stimulating the parathyroid glands (a ~ hormone)

para·tra·che·al \-ˈtrā-kē-əl\ adj : adjacent to the trachea

para·tu·ber·cu·lo·sis \-tù-ˌbər-kyə-ˈlō-səs, -tyù-\ n, pl **-lo·ses** \-ˌsēz\ : JOHNE'S DISEASE

¹para·ty·phoid \ˌpar-ə-ˈtī-ˌfoid, -(ˌ)tī-\ adj **1** : resembling typhoid fever **2** : of or relating to paratyphoid or its causative organisms (~ infection)

²paratyphoid n : any of numerous salmonelloses (as necrotic enteritis) that resemble typhoid fever and are commonly contracted by eating contaminated food — called also *paratyphoid fever*

para·um·bil·i·cal \-ˌəm-ˈbi-li-kəl\ adj : adjacent to the navel (~ pain)

para·ure·thral \-yù-ˈrē-thrəl\ adj : adjacent to the urethra

paraurethral gland n : any of several small glands that open into the female urethra near its opening and are homologous to glandular tissue in the prostate gland in the male — called also *Skene's gland*

para·vac·cin·ia \-vak-ˈsi-nē-ə\ n : MILKER'S NODULES

para·ven·tric·u·lar nucleus \-ven-ˈtrik-yə-lər-, -vən-\ n : a nucleus in the hypothalamus that produces vasopressin and esp. oxytocin and that innervates the neurohypophysis

para·ver·te·bral \-(ˌ)vər-ˈtē-brəl, -ˈvər-tə-\ adj : situated, occurring, or performed beside or adjacent to the spinal column (~ sympathectomy)

par·e·gor·ic \ˌpar-ə-ˈgor-ik, -ˈgär-\ n : camphorated tincture of opium used esp. to relieve pain

par·en·chy·ma \pə-ˈreŋ-kə-mə\ n : the essential and distinctive tissue of an organ or an abnormal growth as distinguished from its supportive framework

par·en·chy·mal \pə-ˈreŋ-kə-məl, ˌpar-ən-ˈkī-məl\ adj : PARENCHYMATOUS

par·en·chy·ma·tous \ˌpar-ən-ˈkī-mə-təs, -ˈki-\ adj : of, relating to, made up of, or affecting parenchyma

par·ent \ˈpar-ənt\ n **1** : one that begets or brings forth offspring **2** : the material or source from which something is derived — **parent** adj

pa·ren·tal generation \pə-ˈrent-ᵊl-\ n : a generation of individuals of distinctively different genotypes that are crossed to produce hybrids — see FILIAL GENERATION

¹par·en·ter·al \pə-ˈren-tə-rəl\ adj : situated or occurring outside the intestine; esp : introduced otherwise than by way of the intestines — **par·en·ter·al·ly** adv

²parenteral n : an agent (as a drug or solution) intended for parenteral administration

par·ent·ing \ˈpar-ənt-iŋ\ n : the raising of a child by his or her parents

pa·re·sis \pə-ˈrē-səs, ˈpar-ə-səs\ n, pl **pa·re·ses** \-ˌsēz\ **1** : slight or partial paralysis **2** : GENERAL PARESIS

par·es·the·sia \ˌpar-es-ˈthē-zhə, -zhē-ə\ n : a sensation of pricking, tingling, or creeping on the skin having no objective cause and usu. associated with injury or irritation of a sensory nerve or nerve root — **par·es·thet·ic** \-ˈthe-tik\ adj

paresthetica — see MERALGIA PARESTHETICA

¹pa·ret·ic \pə-ˈre-tik\ adj : of, relating to, or affected with paresis

²paretic n : a person affected with paresis

par·gy·line \ˈpär-jə-ˌlēn\ n : a monoamine oxidase inhibitor $C_{11}H_{13}N$ that is used in the form of its hydrochloride esp. as an antihypertensive agent

par·i·es \ˈpar-ē-ˌēz\ n, pl **pa·ri·e·tes** \pə-ˈrī-ə-ˌtēz\ : the wall of a cavity or hollow organ — usu. used in pl.

¹pa·ri·etal \pə-ˈrī-ət-ᵊl\ adj **1** : of or relating to the walls of a part or cavity — compare VISCERAL **2** : of, relating to, or located in the upper posterior part of the head; specif : relating to the parietal bones

²parietal n : a parietal part (as a bone)

parietal bone n : either of a pair of membrane bones of the roof of the skull between the frontal and occipital bones that are large and quadrilateral in outline, meet in the sagittal suture, and form much of the top and sides of the cranium

parietal cell n : any of the large oval cells of the gastric mucous membrane that secrete hydrochloric acid and lie between the chief cells and the basement membrane

parietal emissary vein *n* : a vein that passes from the superior sagittal sinus inside the skull through a foramen in the parietal bone to connect with veins of the scalp

parietalis *see* DECIDUA PARIETALIS

parietal lobe *n* : the middle division of each cerebral hemisphere that is situated behind the central sulcus, above the fissure of Sylvius, and in front of the parieto-occipital sulcus and that contains an area concerned with bodily sensations

parietal pericardium *n* : the tough thickened membranous outer layer of the pericardium that is attached to the central part of the diaphragm and the posterior part of the sternum — compare EPICARDIUM

parietal peritoneum *n* : the part of the peritoneum that lines the abdominal wall — compare VISCERAL PERITONEUM

parieto- *comb form* : parietal and (*parieto*temporal)

pa·ri·e·to-oc·cip·i·tal \pə-ˌrī-ə-tō-äk-ˈsi-pət-ᵊl\ *adj* : of, relating to, or situated between the parietal and occipital bones or lobes

parieto–occipital sulcus *n* : a fissure near the posterior end of each cerebral hemisphere separating the parietal and occipital lobes — called also *parieto-occipital fissure*

pa·ri·e·to·tem·po·ral \-ˈtem-pə-rəl\ *n* : of or relating to the parietal and temporal bones or lobes

Par·i·naud's oc·u·lo·glan·du·lar syndrome \ˌpar-i-ˈnōz-ä-kyə-lō-ˈglan-jə-lər-\ *n* : conjunctivitis that is often unilateral, is usu. characterized by dense local infiltration by lymphoid tissue with tenderness and swelling of the preauricular lymph nodes, and is usu. associated with a bacterial infection (as in cat scratch disease and tularemia) — called also *Parinaud's conjunctivitis*

Parinaud, Henri (1844–1905), French ophthalmologist.

Parinaud's syndrome *n* : paralysis of the upward movements of the two eyes that is associated esp. with a lesion or compression of the superior colliculi of the midbrain

Paris green \ˈpar-əs-\ *n* : a very poisonous copper-based bright green powder $Cu(C_2H_3O_2)_2\cdot3Cu(AsO_2)_2$ that is used as an insecticide and pigment

par·i·ty \ˈpar-ə-tē\ *n, pl* **-ties** : the state or fact of having borne offspring; *also* : the number of children previously borne

¹**par·kin·so·nian** \ˌpär-kən-ˈsō-nē-ən, -nyən\ *adj* 1 : of or similar to that of parkinsonism 2 : affected with parkinsonism and esp. Parkinson's disease

Parkinson \ˈpär-kən-sən\, **James (1755–1824),** British surgeon.

²**parkinsonian** *n* : an individual affected with parkinsonism and esp. Parkinson's disease

par·kin·son·ism \ˈpär-kən-sə-ˌni-zəm\ *n* 1 : PARKINSON'S DISEASE 2 : a nervous disorder that resembles Parkinson's disease

Par·kin·son's disease \ˈpär-kən-sənz-\ *n* : a chronic progressive nervous disease chiefly of later life that is linked to decreased dopamine production in the substantia nigra and is marked by tremor and weakness of resting muscles and by a shuffling gait — called also *paralysis agitans, parkinsonism, Parkinson's, Parkinson's syndrome*

par·odon·tal \ˌpar-ə-ˈdänt-ᵊl\ *adj* : PERIODONTAL 2 — **par·odon·tal·ly** *adv*

par·o·mo·my·cin \ˌpar-ə-mō-ˈmīs-ᵊn\ *n* : a broad-spectrum antibiotic $C_{23}H_{45}N_5O_{14}$ that is obtained from a bacterium of the genus *Streptomyces* (*S. rimosus paromomycinus*) and is used against intestinal amebiasis esp. in the form of its sulfate

par·o·nych·ia \ˌpar-ə-ˈni-kē-ə\ *n* : inflammation of the tissues adjacent to the nail of a finger or toe usu. accompanied by infection and pus formation — compare WHITLOW

par·ooph·o·ron \ˌpar-ō-ˈä-fə-ˌrän\ *n* : a group of rudimentary tubules in the broad ligament between the epoophoron and the uterus that constitutes a remnant of the lower part of the mesonephros in the female

par·os·mia \ˌpar-ˈäz-mē-ə\ *n* : a distortion of the sense of smell (as when affected with a cold)

¹**pa·rot·id** \pə-ˈrä-təd\ *adj* : of, relating to, being, produced by, or located near the parotid gland

²**parotid** *n* : PAROTID GLAND

parotid duct *n* : the duct of the parotid gland opening on the inner surface of the cheek opposite the second upper molar tooth — called also *Stensen's duct*

parotid gland *n* : a salivary gland that is situated on each side of the face below and in front of the ear, in humans is the largest of the salivary glands, is of pure serous type, and communicates with the mouth by the parotid duct

par·o·ti·tis \ˌpar-ə-ˈtī-təs\ *n* 1 : inflammation and swelling of one or both parotid glands or other salivary glands (as in mumps) 2 : MUMPS

par·ous \ˈpar-əs\ *adj* 1 : having produced offspring 2 : of or characteristic of the parous female

-p·a·rous \p-ə-rəs\ *adj comb form* : giving birth to : producing (multi*parous*)

par·o·var·i·um \ˌpar-ō-ˈvar-ē-əm\ *n* : EPOOPHORON — **par·o·var·i·an** \-ē-ən\ *adj*

par·ox·ysm \ˈpar-ək-ˌsi-zəm, pə-ˈräk-\ *n* 1 : a sudden attack or spasm (as of a disease) 2 : a sudden recurrence of symptoms or an intensification of existing symptoms — **par·ox·ys·mal** \par-ək-'siz-məl, pə-ˌräk-\ *adj*

paroxysmal dyspnea *n* : CARDIAC ASTHMA

paroxysmal nocturnal hemoglobinuria *n* : a form of hemolytic anemia that is characterized by an abnormally strong response to the action of complement, by acute episodes of hemolysis esp. at night with hemoglobinuria noted upon urination after awakening, venous occlusion, and often leukopenia and thrombocytopenia

paroxysmal tachycardia *n* : tachycardia that begins and ends abruptly and that is initiated by a premature supraventricular beat originating in the atrium or in the atrioventricular node or bundle of His or by a premature ventricular beat

par·rot fever \'par-ət-\ *n* : PSITTACOSIS

pars \'pärs\ *n, pl* **par·tes** \'pär-(ˌ)tēz\ : an anatomical part

pars com·pac·ta \-käm-'pak-tə\ *n* : the large dorsal part of gray matter of the substantia nigra that is next to the tegmentum

pars dis·ta·lis \-di-'stä-ləs\ *n* : the anterior part of the adenohypophysis that is the major secretory part of the gland

pars in·ter·me·dia \-ˌin-tər-'mē-dē-ə\ *n* : a thin slip of tissue fused with the neurohypophysis and representing the remains of the posterior wall of Rathke's pouch

pars ner·vo·sa \-nər-'vō-sə\ *n* : NEURAL LOBE

pars pla·na \-'plā-nə\ *n* : ORBICULUS CILIARIS

pars tu·ber·a·lis \-ˌtü-bə-'rä-ləs, -ˌtyü-\ *n* : a thin plate of cells that is an extension of the adenohypophysis on the ventral or anterior aspect of the infundibulum

partes *pl of* PARS

parthen- *or* **partheno-** *comb form* : virgin : without fertilization ⟨*partheno*genesis⟩

par·the·no·gen·e·sis \ˌpär-thə-nō-'je-nə-səs\ *n, pl* **-e·ses** \-ˌsēz\ : reproduction by development of an unfertilized usu. female gamete that occurs esp. among lower plants and invertebrate animals — **par·the·no·ge·net·ic** \-jə-'ne-tik\ *also* **par·the·no·gen·ic** \-'je-nik\ *adj*

par·tial denture \'pär-shəl-\ *n* : a usu. removable artificial replacement of one or more teeth

partial pressure *n* : the pressure exerted by a (specified) component in a mixture of gases

par·tic·u·late \pär-'ti-kyə-lət\ *adj* : of, relating to, or existing in the form of minute separate particles

par·tic·u·late *n* : a particulate substance

particulate inheritance *n* : inheritance of characters specif. transmitted by genes in accord with Mendel's laws — called also *Mendelian inheritance*;

compare QUANTITATIVE INHERITANCE

par·tu·ri·ent \pär-'tür-ē-ənt, -'tyür-\ *adj* **1** : bringing forth or about to bring forth young **2** : of or relating to parturition ⟨~ pangs⟩ **3** : typical of parturition ⟨the ~ uterus⟩

par·tu·ri·ent *n* : a parturient individual

parturient paresis *n* : MILK FEVER 2

par·tu·ri·tion \ˌpär-tə-'ri-shən, ˌpär-chə-, ˌpär-tyü-\ *n* : the action or process of giving birth to offspring — **par·tu·ri·tion·al** \-shə-nəl\ *adj*

pa·ru·lis \pə-'rü-ləs\ *n, pl* **-li·des** \-lə-ˌdēz\ : an abscess in the gum : GUMBOIL

par·um·bil·i·cal vein \ˌpar-ˌəm-'bi-li-kəl-\ *n* : any of several small veins that connect the veins of the anterior abdominal wall with the portal vein and the internal and common iliac veins

parv- *or* **parvi-** *also* **parvo-** *comb form* : small ⟨*parvo*virus⟩

par·vo \'pär-ˌvō\ *n* : PARVOVIRUS 2

par·vo·cel·lu·lar *also* **par·vi·cel·lu·lar** \ˌpar-və-'sel-yə-lər\ *adj* : of, relating to, or being small cells

par·vo·vi·rus \'pär-vō-ˌvī-rəs\ *n* **1** : any of a group of small single-stranded DNA viruses that include the causative agent of erythema infectiosum **2** : a highly contagious febrile disease of dogs that is caused by a parvovirus, that is spread esp. by contact with infected feces, and that is marked by loss of appetite, lethargy, often bloody diarrhea and vomiting, and sometimes death — called also *parvo*

PAS \ˌpē-(ˌ)ā-'es\ *adj* : PERIODIC ACID=SCHIFF

PAS *abbr* para-aminosalicylic acid

PASA *abbr* para-aminosalicylic acid

pass \'pas\ *vb* : to emit or discharge from a bodily part and esp. from the bowels : EVACUATE 2, VOID

pas·sage \'pa-sij\ *n* **1** : the action or process of passing from one place, condition, or stage to another **2** : an anatomical channel ⟨the nasal ~s⟩ **3** : a movement or an evacuation of the bowels **4 a** : an act or action of passing something or undergoing a passing ⟨~ of a catheter through the urethra⟩ **b** : incubation of a pathogen (as a virus) in a tissue culture, a developing egg, or a living organism to increase the amount of pathogen or to alter its characteristics

pas·sage *vb* **pas·saged; pas·sag·ing** : to subject to passage

pas·sive \'pa-siv\ *adj* **1 a** (1) : lethargic or lacking in energy or will (2) : tending not to take an active or dominant part **b** : induced by an outside agency ⟨~ exercise of a paralyzed leg⟩ **2 a** : of, relating to, or characterized by a state of chemical inactivity **b** : not involving expenditure of chemical energy ⟨~ transport across a cell membrane) — **pas·sive·ly** *adv* — **pas·sive·ness** *n*

passive congestion *n* : congestion caused by obstruction to the return flow of venous blood — called also *passive hyperemia*

passive immunity *n* : immunity acquired by transfer of antibodies (as by injection of serum from an individual with active immunity) — compare ACQUIRED IMMUNITY, NATURAL IMMUNITY — **passive immunization** *n*

passive smoking *n* : the involuntary inhalation of tobacco smoke (as from another's cigarette) esp. by a nonsmoker

passive transfer *n* : a local transfer of skin sensitivity from an allergic to a normal individual by injection of the allergic individual's serum that is used esp. for identifying specific allergens when a high degree of sensitivity is suspected — called also *Prausnitz-Küstner reaction*

pas·siv·i·ty \pa-'si-və-tē\ *n, pl* **-ties** : the quality or state of being passive or submissive

pass out *vb* : to lose consciousness

paste \'pāst\ *n* : a soft plastic mixture or composition; *esp* : an external medicament that has a stiffer consistency than an ointment but is less greasy because of its higher percentage of powdered ingredients

pas·tern \'pas-tərn\ *n* : a part of the foot of an equine extending from the fetlock to the top of the hoof

pas·teu·rel·la \,pas-tə-'re-lə\ *n* **1** *cap* : a genus of gram-negative facultatively anaerobic rod bacteria (family Pasteurellaceae) that include several important pathogens esp. of domestic animals — see HEMORRHAGIC SEPTICEMIA; YERSINIA **2** *pl* **-las** *or* **-lae** \-,lī\ : any bacterium of the genus *Pasteurella*

Pas·teur \pa-'stər, -'stœr\, **Louis (1822–1895),** French chemist and bacteriologist.

pas·teu·rel·lo·sis \,pas-tə-rə-'lō-səs\ *n, pl* **-lo·ses** \-,sēz\ : infection with or disease caused by bacteria of the genus *Pasteurella*

pas·teur·iza·tion \,pas-chə-rə-'zā-shən, ,pas-tə-\ *n* **1** : partial sterilization of a substance and esp. a liquid (as milk) at a temperature and for a period of exposure that destroys objectionable organisms **2** : partial sterilization of perishable food products (as fruit or fish) with radiation (as gamma rays) — **pas·teur·ize** \'pas-chə-,rīz, 'pas-tə-\ *vb*

Pasteur treatment *n* : a method of aborting rabies by stimulating production of antibodies through successive inoculations with attenuated virus of gradually increasing strength

pas·tille \pas-'tēl\ *also* **pas·til** \'past-ᵊl\ *n* : LOZENGE

past–pointing test \'past-'pȯin-tiŋ-\ *n*

: a test for defective functioning of the vestibular nerve in which a subject is asked to point at an object with eyes open and then closed first after rotation in a chair to the right and then to the left and which indicates an abnormality if the subject does not point to the side of the object in the direction of rotation

PAT *abbr* paroxysmal atrial tachycardia

patch \'pach\ *n* **1 a** : a piece of material (as an adhesive plaster) used medically usu. to cover a wound, repair a defect, or supply medication through the skin — see PATCH GRAFT **b** : a shield worn over the socket of an injured or missing eye **2** : a circumscribed region of tissue (as on the skin or in a section from an organ) that differs from the normal color or composition — **patch** *vb* — **patchy** \'pa-chē\ *adj*

patch graft *n* : a graft of living or synthetic material used to repair a defect in a blood vessel

patch test *n* : a test for determining allergic sensitivity that is made by applying to the unbroken skin small pads soaked with the allergen to be tested and that indicates sensitivity when irritation develops at the point of application — compare INTRADERMAL TEST, SCRATCH TEST

pa·tel·la \pə-'te-lə\ *n, pl* **-lae** \-'te-(,)lē, -,lī\ *or* **-las** : a thick flat triangular movable bone that forms the anterior point of the knee, protects the front of the knee joint, and increases the leverage of the quadriceps — called also *kneecap* — **pa·tel·lar** \-lər\ *adj*

patellar ligament *n* : the part of the tendon of the quadriceps that extends from the patella to the tibia — called also *patellar tendon*

patellar reflex *n* : KNEE JERK

patellar tendon *n* : PATELLAR LIGAMENT

pat·el·lec·to·my \,pa-tə-'lek-tə-mē\ *n, pl* **-mies** : surgical excision of the patella

pa·tel·lo·fem·o·ral \pə-,te-lō-'fe-mə-rəl\ *adj* : of or relating to the patella and femur (the ~ articulation)

pa·ten·cy \'pat-ᵊn-sē, 'pāt-\ *n, pl* **-cies** : the quality or state of being patent or unobstructed

pa·tent \'pat-ᵊnt\ *n* **1** : protected by a trademark or a trade name so as to establish proprietary rights analogous to those conveyed by a patent : PROPRIETARY (~ drugs) **2** \'pāt-\ : affording free passage : being open and unobstructed

pa·tent ductus arteriosus \'pāt-ᵊnt-\ *n* : an abnormal condition in which the ductus arteriosus fails to close after birth

pat·ent medicine \'pat-ᵊnt-\ *n* : a packaged nonprescription drug which is protected by a trademark and whose contents are incompletely disclosed; *also* : any drug that is a proprietary

pa·ter·ni·ty test \pə-'tər-nə-tē-\ n : a test esp. of DNA or genetic traits to determine whether a given man could be the biological father of a given child — **paternity testing** n

¹path \'path\ n, pl **paths** \'pathz, 'paths\ : PATHWAY 2

²path abbr pathological; pathology

path- or **patho-** comb form **1** : pathological ⟨pathobiology⟩ **2** : pathological state : disease ⟨pathogen⟩

-path \¸path\ n comb form **1** : practitioner of a (specified) system of medicine that emphasizes one aspect of disease or its treatment ⟨naturopath⟩ **2** : one affected with a disorder (of such a part or system) ⟨psychopath⟩

-path·ia \'pa-thē-ə\ n comb form : -PATHY 2 ⟨hyperpathia⟩

-path·ic \'pa-thik\ adj comb form **1** : feeling or affected in a (specified) way ⟨telepathic⟩ **2** : affected by disease of a (specified) part or kind ⟨myopathic⟩ **3** : relating to therapy based on a (specified) unitary theory of disease or its treatment ⟨homeopathic⟩

Path·i·lon \'pa-thə-¸län\ trademark — used for a preparation of tridihexethyl chloride

patho·bi·ol·o·gy \¸pa-thō-bī-'ä-lə-jē\ n, pl **-gies** : PATHOLOGY 1, 2

patho·gen \'pa-thə-jən\ n : a specific causative agent (as a bacterium or virus) of disease

patho·gen·e·sis \¸pa-thə-'je-nə-səs\ n, pl **-e·ses** \-¸sēz\ : the origination and development of a disease

patho·ge·net·ic \-jə-'ne-tik\ adj **1** : of or relating to pathogenesis **2** : PATHOGENIC 2

patho·gen·ic \-'je-nik\ adj **1** : PATHOGENETIC 1 2 **2** : causing or capable of causing disease ⟨∼ microorganisms⟩ — **patho·gen·i·cal·ly** adv

patho·ge·nic·i·ty \-jə-'ni-sə-tē\ n, pl **-ties** : the quality or state of being pathogenic : degree of pathogenic capacity

patho·gno·mon·ic \¸pa-thəg-'nä-mik, -thə-\ adj : PATHOGNOMONIC

pa·tho·gno·mon·ic \¸pa-thəg-nō-'mä-nik, -thə-\ adj : distinctively characteristic of a particular disease or condition

pathol abbr pathological; pathologist; pathology

patho·log·i·cal \¸pa-thə-'lä-ji-kəl\ also **patho·log·ic** \-jik\ adj **1** : of or relating to pathology ⟨a ∼ laboratory⟩ **2** : altered or caused by disease ⟨∼ tissue⟩ — **patho·log·i·cal·ly** adv

pathological fracture n : a fracture of a bone weakened by disease

pathological liar n : an individual who habitually tells lies so exaggerated or bizarre that they are suggestive of mental disorder

pa·thol·o·gist \pə-'thä-lə-jist, pa-\ n : a specialist in pathology; specif : a physician who interprets and diagnoses the changes caused by disease in tissues and body fluids

pa·thol·o·gy \-jē\ n, pl **-gies** **1** : the study of the essential nature of diseases and esp. of the structural and functional changes produced by them **2** : the anatomic and physiologic deviations from the normal that constitute disease or characterize a particular disease **3** : a treatise on or compilation of abnormalities

patho·mor·phol·o·gy \¸pa-thō-mȯr-'fä-lə-jē\ n, pl **-gies** : morphology of abnormal conditions — **patho·mor·pho·log·i·cal** \-mȯr-fə-'lä-ji-kəl\ or **patho·mor·pho·log·ic** \-jik\ adj

patho·phys·i·ol·o·gy \-¸fi-zē-'ä-lə-jē\ n, pl **-gies** : the physiology of abnormal states; specif : the functional changes that accompany a particular syndrome or disease — **patho·phys·i·o·log·i·cal** \-¸fi-zē-ə-'lä-ji-kəl\ also **patho·phys·i·o·log·ic** \-jik\ adj

path·way \'path-¸wā\ n **1** : a line of communication over connected neurons extending from one organ or center to another **2** : the sequence of enzyme catalyzed reactions by which an energy-yielding substance is utilized by protoplasm

-pa·thy \pə-thē\ n comb form, pl **-pathies** **1** : feeling ⟨apathy⟩ ⟨telepathy⟩ **2** : disease of a (specified) part or kind ⟨myopathy⟩ **3** : therapy or system of therapy based on a (specified) unitary theory of disease or its treatment ⟨homeopathy⟩

pa·tient \'pā-shənt\ n **1** : a sick individual esp. when awaiting or under the care and treatment of a physician or surgeon **2** : a client for medical service (as of a physician or dentist)

pat·ri·cide \'pa-trə-¸sīd\ n : murder of a father by his son or daughter

pat·tern \'pa-tərn\ n **1** : a model for making a mold used to form a casting **2** : a reliable sample of traits, acts, tendencies, or other observable characteristics of a person, group, or institution ⟨∼s of behavior⟩ **3** : an established mode of behavior or cluster of mental attitudes, beliefs, and values that are held in common by members of a group

pat·tern·ing n : physical therapy intended to improve malfunctioning nervous control by means of feedback from muscular activity imposed by an outside source or induced by other muscles

pat·u·lin \'pa-chə-lən\ n : a colorless crystalline very toxic antibiotic $C_7H_6O_4$ produced by several molds (as Aspergillus clavatus and Penicillium patulum)

pat·u·lous \'pa-chə-ləs\ adj : spread widely apart : wide open or distended

Paul–Bun·nell test \'pȯl-'bə-nəl-\ n : a test for heterophile antibodies used in the diagnosis of infectious mononucleosis — called also *Paul-Bunnell reaction*

Paul, John Rodman (1893–1971), and **Bunnell, Walls Willard** (1902–1965), American physicians.

paunch \'pónch, 'pänch\ *n* : RUMEN

pa·vil·ion \pə-'vil-yən\ *n* : a more or less detached part of a hospital devoted to a special use

Pav·lov·ian \pav-'lò-vē-ən, -'lò-; -'lò-fē-\ *adj* : of or relating to Ivan Pavlov or to his work and theories

Pavlov, Ivan Petrovich (1849–1936), Russian physiologist.

pav·or noc·tur·nus \'pa-₁vor-näk-'tər-nəs\ *n* : NIGHT TERRORS

pay–bed \'pā-₁bed\ *n*, *Brit* : hospital accommodations and services for which the patient is charged

Pb *symbol* lead

PBB \₁pē-(₁)bē-'bē\ *n* : POLYBROMINATED BIPHENYL

PC *abbr* 1 [Latin *post cibos*] after meals — used in writing prescriptions 2 professional corporation

PCB \₁pē-(₁)sē-'bē\ *n* : POLYCHLORINATED BIPHENYL

PCP \₁pē-(₁)sē-'pē\ *n* : PHENCYCLIDINE

PCP *abbr* Pneumocystis carinii pneumonia

PCR *abbr* polymerase chain reaction

PCV *abbr* packed cell volume

PCWP *abbr* pulmonary capillary wedge pressure

Pd *symbol* palladium

PDB \₁pē-(₁)dē-'bē\ *n* : PARADICHLOROBENZENE

PDGF *abbr* platelet-derived growth factor

PDR *abbr* *Physicians' Desk Reference*

PE *abbr* physical examination

pearl \'pərl\ *n* 1 : PERLE 2 : one of the rounded concentric masses of squamous epithelial cells characteristic of certain tumors 3 : a miliary leproma of the iris 4 : a rounded abnormal mass of enamel on a tooth

pec \'pek\ *n* : PECTORALIS — usu. used in pl.

pecking order *also* **peck order** *n* : the basic pattern of social organization within a flock of poultry in which each bird pecks another lower in the scale without fear of retaliation and submits to pecking by one of higher rank

pec·tin \'pek-tən\ *n* 1 : any of various water-soluble substances that bind adjacent cell walls in plant tissues and yield a gel which is the basis of fruit jellies 2 : a product containing mostly pectin obtained as a powder or syrup and used chiefly in making jelly and other foods, in pharmaceutical products esp. for the control of diarrhea, and in cosmetics

pectinati — see MUSCULI PECTINATI

pec·tin·e·al line \pek-'ti-nē-əl-\ *n* : a ridge on the posterior surface of the femur that runs downward from the

lesser trochanter and gives attachment to the pectineus

pec·tin·e·us \pek-'ti-nē-əs\ *n*, *pl* **-tin·ei** \-nē-₁ī, -nē-ē\ : a flat quadrangular muscle of the upper front and inner aspect of the thigh that arises mostly from the iliopectineal line of the pubis and is inserted along the pectineal line of the femur

¹pec·to·ral \'pek-tə-rəl\ *n* 1 : a pectoral part or organ; *esp* : PECTORALIS 2 : a medicinal substance for treating diseases of the respiratory tract

²pectoral *adj* 1 : of, relating to, or occurring in or on the chest (~ arch) 2 : relating to or good for diseases of the respiratory tract (a ~ syrup)

pectoral girdle *n* : the bony or cartilaginous arch supporting the forelimbs of a vertebrate that corresponds to the pelvic girdle of the hind limbs — called also *shoulder girdle*

pec·to·ra·lis \pek-tə-'rä-ləs\ *n*, *pl* **-ra·les** \-₁lēz\ : either of the muscles that connect the ventral walls of the chest with the bones of the upper arm and shoulder of which in humans there are two on each side: **a** : a larger one that arises from the clavicle, the sternum, the cartilages of most or all of the ribs, and the aponeurosis of the external oblique muscle and is inserted by a strong flat tendon into the posterior bicipital ridge of the humerus — called also *pectoralis major* **b** : a smaller one that lies beneath the larger, arises from the third, fourth, and fifth ribs, and is inserted by a flat tendon into the coracoid process of the scapula — called also *pectoralis minor*

pectoralis major *n* : PECTORALIS a

pectoralis minor *n* : PECTORALIS b

pectoralis muscle *n* : PECTORALIS

pectoral muscle *n* : PECTORALIS

pectoral nerve *n* : either of two nerves that arise from the brachial plexus on each side or from the nerve trunks forming it and that supply the pectoral muscles: **a** : one lateral to the axillary artery — called also *lateral pectoral nerve, superior pectoral nerve* **b** : one medial to the axillary artery — called also *inferior pectoral nerve, medial pectoral nerve*

pec·to·ril·o·quy \₁pek-tə-'ri-lə-kwē\ *n*, *pl* **-quies** : the sound of words heard through the chest wall and usu. indicating a cavity or consolidation of lung tissue — compare BRONCHOPHONY

pectoris — see ANGINA PECTORIS

pec·tus ex·ca·va·tum \'pek-təs-₁ek-skə-'vä-təm\ *n* : FUNNEL CHEST

ped- *or* **pedo-** *comb form* : child : children (*pediatrics*)

ped·al \'ped-əl, 'pēd-\ *adj* : of or relating to the foot

ped·er·ast \'pe-də-₁rast\ *n* : one that practices anal intercourse esp. with a boy as a passive partner — **ped·er-**

as·tic \ˌpe-də-ˈras-tik\ *adj* — **ped·er·as·ty** \ˈped-ə-ˌras-tē\ *n*

pe·di·at·ric \ˌpē-dē-ˈa-trik\ *adj* : of or relating to pediatrics

pe·di·a·tri·cian \ˌpē-dē-ə-ˈtri-shən\ *n* : a specialist in pediatrics

pe·di·at·rics \ˌpē-dē-ˈa-triks\ *n* : a branch of medicine dealing with the development, care, and diseases of children

ped·i·cle \ˈpe-di-kəl\ *n* : a basal attachment: as **a** : the basal part of each side of the neural arch of a vertebra connecting the laminae with the centrum **b** : the narrow basal part by which various organs (as kidney or spleen) are continuous with other body structures **c** : the narrow base of a tumor **d** : the part of a pedicle flap left attached to the original site — **ped·i·cled** \-kəld\ *adj*

pedicle flap *n* : a flap which is left attached to the original site by a narrow base of tissue to provide a blood supply during grafting — called also *pedicle graft*

pe·dic·u·li·cide \pi-ˈdi-kyə-lə-ˌsīd\ *n* : an agent for destroying lice

pe·dic·u·lo·sis \pi-ˌdi-kyə-ˈlō-səs\ *n*, *pl* **-lo·ses** \-ˌsēz\ : infestation with lice

pediculosis cap·i·tis \-ˈka-pi-təs\ *n* : infestation of the scalp by head lice

pediculosis cor·po·ris \-ˈkȯr-pə-rəs\ *n* : infestation by body lice

pediculosis pubis *n* : infestation by crab lice

pe·dic·u·lus \pi-ˈdi-kyə-ləs\ *n* **1** *cap* : a genus of lice (family Pediculidae) that includes the body louse (*P. humanus corporis*) and head louse (*P. humanus capitis*) infesting humans **2** *pl* **pe·dic·u·li** \-ˌlī\ *or* **pediculus** : any louse of the genus *Pediculus*

ped·i·gree \ˈpe-də-ˌgrē\ *n* : a record of the ancestry of an individual

pedis — see DORSALIS PEDIS, TINEA PEDIS

pedo- — see PED-

pe·do·don·tics \ˌpē-də-ˈdän-tiks\ *n* : a branch of dentistry that is concerned with the dental care of children — **pe·do·don·tic** *adj*

pe·do·don·tist \ˌpē-də-ˈdän-tist\ *n* : a specialist in pedodontics

pe·do·phile \ˈpē-də-ˌfīl\ *n* : an individual affected with pedophilia

pe·do·phil·ia \ˌpē-də-ˈfi-lē-ə\ *n* : sexual perversion in which children are the preferred sexual object — **pe·do·phil·i·ac** \-ˌak\ *or* **pe·do·phil·ic** \-ˈfi-lik\ *adj*

pe·dun·cle \ˈpē-ˌdəŋ-kəl, pi-ˈ\ *n* **1** : a band of white matter joining different parts of the brain — see CEREBELLAR PEDUNCLE, CEREBRAL PEDUNCLE **2** : a narrow stalk by which a tumor or polyp is attached — **pe·dun·cu·lar** \pi-ˈdəŋ-kyə-lər\ *adj*

pe·dun·cu·lat·ed \pi-ˈdəŋ-kyə-ˌlā-təd\ *also* **pe·dun·cu·late** \-lət\ *adj* : having,

growing on, or being attached by a peduncle ⟨a ∼ tumor⟩

pe·dun·cu·lot·o·my \pi-ˌdəŋ-kyə-ˈlä-tə-mē\ *n*, *pl* **-mies** : surgical incision of a cerebral peduncle for relief of involuntary movements

pe·dun·cu·lus ce·re·bel·la·ris inferior \pi-ˌdəŋ-kyə-ləs-ˌser-ə-be-ˈler-əs-\ *n* : CEREBELLAR PEDUNCLE c

pedunculus cerebellaris me·di·us \-ˈmē-dē-əs\ *n* : CEREBELLAR PEDUNCLE b

pedunculus cerebellaris superior *n* : CEREBELLAR PEDUNCLE a

peel *n* : the surgical removal of skin blemishes by the application of a caustic chemical and esp. an acid to the skin — called also *chemical peel*

peep·er \ˈpē-pər\ *n* : VOYEUR

Peep·ing Tom \ˌpē-piŋ-ˈtäm\ *n* : VOYEUR — **Peeping Tom·ism** \-ˈtä-ˌmi-zəm\ *n*

Peg·a·none \ˈpe-gə-ˌnōn\ *trademark* — used for a preparation of ethotoin

pe·li·o·sis hepatitis \ˌpe-lē-ˈō-səs-, ˌpē-\ *n* : an abnormal condition characterized by the occurrence of numerous small blood-filled cystic lesions throughout the liver

pel·la·gra \pə-ˈla-grə, -ˈlā-, -ˈlä-\ *n* : a disease marked by dermatitis, gastrointestinal disorders, and nervous symptoms and associated with a diet deficient in niacin and protein — compare KWASHIORKOR — **pel·la·grous** \-grəs\ *adj*

pellagra–preventive factor *n* : NIACIN

pel·la·grin \-grən\ *n* : one that is affected with pellagra

pel·let \ˈpe-lət\ *n* : a usu. small rounded or spherical body; *specif* : a small cylindrical or ovoid compressed mass (as of a hormone) that is implanted subcutaneously for slow absorption into bodily tissues

pel·li·cle \ˈpe-li-kəl\ *n* : a thin skin or film: as **a** : an outer membrane of some protozoans **b** : a thin layer of salivary glycoproteins coating the surface of the teeth

pellucida — see SEPTUM PELLUCIDUM, ZONA PELLUCIDA

pel·oid \ˈpe-ˌlȯid\ *n* : mud prepared and used for therapeutic purposes

pel·ta·tin \pel-ˈtā-tən\ *n* : either of two lactones that occur as glycosides in the rootstock of the mayapple (*Podophyllum peltatum*) and have some antineoplastic activity

pelv- *or* **pelvi-** *or* **pelvo-** *comb form* : pelvis ⟨*pelvic*⟩ ⟨*pelvimetry*⟩

pelves *pl of* PELVIS

¹pel·vic \ˈpel-vik\ *adj* : of, relating to, or located in or near the pelvis

²pelvic *n* : a pelvic part

pelvic bone *n* : HIPBONE

pelvic brim *n* : the bony ridge in the cavity of the pelvis that marks the boundary between the false pelvis and the true pelvis

pelvic cavity *n* : the cavity of the pelvis comprising in humans a broad upper and a more contracted lower part — compare FALSE PELVIS, TRUE PELVIS

pelvic colon *n* : SIGMOID FLEXURE

pelvic diaphragm *n* : the muscular floor of the pelvis

pelvic fascia *n* : the fascia lining the pelvic cavity

pelvic girdle *n* : the bony or cartilaginous arch that supports the hind limbs of a vertebrate and that in humans is represented by paired hipbones articulating solidly with the sacrum dorsally and with one another at the pubic symphysis

pelvic inflammatory disease *n* : inflammation of the female reproductive tract and esp. the fallopian tubes that is caused esp. by sexually transmitted disease, occurs more often in women using intrauterine devices, and is a leading cause of female sterility — abbr. *PID*

pelvic outlet *n* : the irregular bony opening bounded by the lower border of the pelvis and closed by muscle and other soft tissues through which the terminal parts of the excretory, reproductive, and digestive systems pass to communicate with the surface of the body

pelvic plexus *n* : a plexus of the autonomic nervous system that is formed by the hypogastric plexus, by branches from the sacral part of the sympathetic chain, and by the visceral branches of the second, third, and fourth sacral nerves and that is distributed to the viscera of the pelvic region

pelvic splanchnic nerve *n* : any of the groups of parasympathetic fibers that originate with cells in the second, third, and fourth sacral segments of the spinal cord, pass through the inferior portion of the hypogastric plexus, and supply the descending colon, rectum, anus, bladder, prostate gland, and external genitalia — called also *nervus erigens*

pel·vim·e·ter \pel-ˈvi-mə-tər\ *n* : an instrument for measuring the dimensions of the pelvis

pel·vim·e·try \ˈpel-ˈvi-mə-trē\ *n, pl* **-tries** : measurement of the pelvis (as by X-ray examination)

pel·vis \ˈpel-vəs\ *n, pl* **pel·vis·es** \-və-səz\ *or* **pel·ves** \-ˌvēz\ **1** : a basin-shaped structure in the skeleton of many vertebrates that in humans is composed of the two hipbones bounding it on each side and in front while the sacrum and coccyx complete it behind **2** : PELVIC CAVITY **3** : RENAL PELVIS

pelvo- — see PELV-

pem·o·line \ˈpem-ə-ˌlēn\ *n* : a synthetic drug $C_9H_8N_2O_2$ that is a mild stimulant of the central nervous system

¹pem·phi·goid \ˈpem-fə-ˌgòid\ *adj* : resembling pemphigus

²pemphigoid *n* : any of several diseases

that resemble pemphigus; *esp* : BULLOUS PEMPHIGOID

pem·phi·gus \ˈpem-fi-gəs, pem-ˈfī-gəs\ *n, pl* **-gus·es** *or* **-gi** \-ˌjī\ : any of several diseases characterized by the formation of successive eruptions of large blisters on apparently normal skin and mucous membranes often in association with sensations of itching or burning and with constitutional symptoms

pemphigus er·y·the·ma·to·sus \-ˌer-i-ˌthē-mə-ˈtō-səs\ *n* : a relatively benign form of chronic pemphigus that is characterized by the eruption esp. on the face and trunk of lesions resembling those which occur in systemic lupus erythematosus

pemphigus vul·gar·is \-ˌvəl-ˈgar-əs\ *n* : a severe and often fatal form of chronic pemphigus

Pen·brit·in \ˈpen-ˈbri-tən\ *trademark* — used for a preparation of ampicillin

pen·cil \ˈpen-səl\ *n* : a small medicated or cosmetic roll or stick for local applications ⟨a menthol ∼⟩

pe·nec·to·my \pē-ˈnek-tə-mē\ *n, pl* **-mies** : surgical removal of the penis

penes *pl of* PENIS

pen·e·trance \ˈpe-nə-trəns\ *n* : the proportion of individuals of a particular genotype that express its phenotypic effect in a given environment — compare EXPRESSIVITY

pen·e·trate \ˈpe-nə-ˌtrāt\ *vb* **-trat·ed; -trat·ing 1** : to pass, extend, pierce, or diffuse into or through something **2** : to insert the penis into the vagina of in copulation — **pen·e·tra·tion** \ˌpe-nə-ˈtrā-shən\ *n*

pen·flur·i·dol \ˌpen-ˈflür-i-ˌdòl\ *n* : a tranquilizing drug $C_{28}H_{27}ClF_5NO$

-penia \ˈpē-nē-ə\ *n comb form* : deficiency of ⟨eosino*penia*⟩

pen·i·cil·la·mine \ˌpe-nə-ˈsi-lə-ˌmēn\ *n* : an amino acid $C_5H_{11}NO_2S$ that is obtained from penicillins and is used esp. to treat cystinuria and metal poisoning (as by copper or lead)

pen·i·cil·lic acid \ˌpe-nə-ˈsi-lik-\ *n* : a crystalline antibiotic $C_8H_{10}O_4$ produced by several molds of the genera *Penicillium* and *Aspergillus*

pen·i·cil·lin \ˌpe-nə-ˈsi-lən\ *n* **1** : a mixture of antibiotic relatively nontoxic acids produced esp. by molds of the genus *Penicillium* (as *P. notatum* or *P. chrysogenum*) and having a powerful bacteriostatic effect against various bacteria (as staphylococci, gonococci, pneumococci, hemolytic streptococci, or some meningococci) **2** : any of numerous often hygroscopic and unstable acids (as penicillin G, penicillin O, and penicillin V) that are components of the penicillin mixture or are produced biosynthetically by the use of different strains of molds or different media or are synthesized chemically **3** : a salt or ester of a penicillin acid or a mixture of such salts or esters

pen·i·cil·lin·ase \-ˈsi-lə-ˌnās, -ˌnāz\ *n* : an enzyme found esp. in staphylococcal bacteria that inactivates the penicillins by hydrolyzing them — called also *beta-lactamase*

penicillin F \-ˈef\ *n* : a penicillin $C_{14}H_{20}N_2O_4S$ that was the first of the penicillins isolated in Great Britain

penicillin G \-ˈjē\ *n* : the penicillin $C_{16}H_{18}N_2O_4S$ that constitutes the principal or sole component of most commercial preparations and is used chiefly in the form of stable salts (as the crystalline sodium salt or the crystalline procaine salt) — called also *benzylpenicillin;* see PROCAINE PENICILLIN G

penicillin O \-ˈō\ *n* : a penicillin $C_{13}H_{18}N_2O_4S_2$ that is similar to penicillin G in antibiotic activity

penicillin V \-ˈvē\ *n* : a crystalline acid $C_{16}H_{18}N_2O_5S$ that is similar to penicillin G in antibacterial action and is more resistant to inactivation by gastric acids — called also *phenoxymethyl penicillin*

pen·i·cil·lio·sis \ˌpe-nə-ˌsi-lē-ˈō-səs\ *n, pl* **-oses** \-ˌsēz\ : infection with or disease caused by molds of the genus *Penicillium*

pen·i·cil·li·um \ˌpe-nə-ˈsi-lē-əm\ *n* **1** *cap* : a genus of fungi (family Moniliaceae) comprising the blue molds found chiefly on moist nonliving organic matter (as decaying fruit) and including molds useful in economic fermentation and the production of antibiotics **2** *pl* **-lia** \-lē-ə\ : any mold of the genus *Penicillium*

pen·i·cil·lo·yl–poly·ly·sine \ˌpe-nə-ˈsi-lō-ˌil-ˌpä-li-ˈlī-ˌsēn\ *n* : a preparation of a penicillic acid and polylysine which is used in a skin test to determine hypersensitivity to penicillin

pen·i·cil·lus \ˌpe-nə-ˈsi-ləs\ *n, pl* **-li** \-ˌlī\ : one of the small straight arteries of the red pulp of the spleen

pe·nile \ˈpē-ˌnīl\ *adj* : of, relating to, or affecting the penis ⟨a ~ prosthesis⟩ ⟨~ lesions⟩

pe·nis \ˈpē-nəs\ *n, pl* **pe·nes** \ˈpē-(ˌ)nēz\ *or* **pe·nis·es** : a male copulatory organ that in mammals including humans usu. functions as the channel by which urine leaves the body and is typically a cylindrical organ that is suspended from the pubic arch, contains a pair of large lateral corpora cavernosa and a smaller ventromedial corpus cavernosum containing the urethra, and has a terminal glans enclosing the ends of the corpora cavernosa, covered by mucous membrane, and sheathed by a foreskin continuous with the skin covering the body of the organ

penis envy *n* : the supposed coveting of the penis by a young human female which is held in psychoanalytic theo-

ry to lead to feelings of inferiority and defensive or compensatory behavior

pen·nate \ˈpe-ˌnāt\ *adj* : having a structure like that of a feather; *esp* : being a muscle in which fibers extend obliquely from either side of a central tendon

pen·ni·form \ˈpe-ni-ˌfòrm\ *adj* : PENNATE

pe·no·scro·tal \ˌpē-nō-ˈskrōt-ᵊl\ *adj* : of or relating to the penis and scrotum

penoscrotal raphe *n* : the ridge on the surface of the scrotum that divides it into two lateral halves and is continued forward on the underside of the penis and backward along the midline of the perineum to the anus

Pen·rose drain \ˈpen-ˌrōz-\ *n* : CIGARETTE DRAIN

Penrose, Charles Bingham (1862–1925), American gynecologist.

pen·ta·chlo·ro·phe·nol \ˌpen-tə-ˌklòr-ə-ˈfē-ˌnòl, -fi-ˈ\ *n* : a crystalline compound C_6Cl_5OH used esp. as a wood preservative, insecticide, and herbicide

pen·ta·eryth·ri·tol tet·ra·ni·trate \-i-ˈri-thrə-ˌtòl-ˌte-trə-ˈnī-ˌtrāt, -ˌtòl-\ *n* : a crystalline ester $C_5H_8N_4O_{12}$ used in the treatment of angina pectoris

pen·ta·gas·trin \ˌpen-tə-ˈgas-trən\ *n* : a pentapeptide $C_{37}H_{49}N_7O_9S$ that stimulates gastric acid secretion

pen·ta·me·tho·ni·um \ˌpen-tə-me-ˈthō-nē-əm\ *n* : an organic ion $[C_{11}H_{28}N_2]^{2+}$ used in the form of its salts (as the bromide and iodide) for its ganglionic blocking activity in the treatment of hypertension

pent·am·i·dine \pen-ˈta-mə-ˌdēn, -dən\ *n* : an antiprotozoal drug used chiefly in the form of its salt $C_{23}H_{36}N_4O_{10}S_2$ to treat protozoal infections (as leishmaniasis) and to prevent Pneumocystis carinii pneumonia in HIV-infected individuals

pen·ta·pep·tide \ˌpen-tə-ˈpep-ˌtīd\ *n* : a polypeptide that contains five amino acid residues

pen·ta·pip·er·ide meth·yl·sul·fate \ˌpen-tə-ˈpi-pər-ˌid-ˌme-thəl-ˈsəl-ˌfāt\ *n* : a synthetic anticholinergic and antisecretory agent $C_{18}H_{27}NO_2\cdot C_2H_6O_4S$ used esp. in the treatment of peptic ulcer — see QUILENE

pen·ta·quine \ˈpen-tə-ˌkwēn\ *n* : an antimalarial drug $C_{18}H_{27}N_3O$ used esp. in the form of its pale yellow crystalline phosphate

pen·taz·o·cine \pen-ˈta-zə-ˌsēn\ *n* : an analgesic drug $C_{19}H_{27}NO$ that is less addictive than morphine — see TALWIN

pen·to·bar·bi·tal \ˌpen-tə-ˈbär-bə-ˌtòl\ *n* : a granular barbiturate $C_{11}H_{18}N_2O_3$ used esp. in the form of its sodium or calcium salt as a sedative, hypnotic, and antispasmodic

pen·to·bar·bi·tone \-ˌtōn\ *n, Brit* : PENTOBARBITAL

pen·to·lin·i·um tartrate \ˌpen-tə-ˈli-nē-əm-\ *n* : a ganglionic blocking agent $C_{23}H_{42}N_2O_{12}$ used as an antihypertensive drug

pen·tose \'pen-₁tōs, -₁tōz\ *n* : any monosaccharide $C_5H_{10}O_5$ (as ribose) that contains five carbon atoms in a molecule

pen·tos·uria \₁pen-tō-'sùr-ē-ə, -'syùr-\ *n* : the excretion of pentoses in the urine; *specif* : a rare hereditary anomaly characterized by regular excretion of pentoses

Pen·to·thal \'pen-tə-₁thòl\ *trademark* — used for a preparation of thiopental

pent·ox·i·fyl·line \₁pen-₁täk-'si-fə-₁lēn\ *n* : a methylxanthine derivative $C_{13}H_{18}N_4O_3$ that reduces blood viscosity, increases microcirculatory blood flow, and is used to treat intermittent claudication resulting from occlusive arterial disease — see TRENTAL

pen·tyl·ene·tet·ra·zol \₁pen-ti-₁lēn-'te-trə-₁zòl, -₁zōl\ *n* : a white crystalline drug $C_6H_{10}N_4$ used as a respiratory and circulatory stimulant and for producing a state of convulsion in treating certain mental disorders — called also *leptazol*; see METRAZOL

pep pill *n* : any of various stimulant drugs (as amphetamine) in pill or tablet form

-pep·sia \'pep-shə, 'pep-sē-ə\ *n comb form* : digestion ⟨dys*pepsia*⟩

pep·sin \'pep-sən\ *n* **1** : a crystallizable protease that in an acid medium digests most proteins to polypeptides, that is secreted by glands in the mucous membrane of the stomach, and that in combination with dilute hydrochloric acid is the chief active principle of gastric juice **2** : a preparation containing pepsin obtained as a powder or scales from the stomach esp. of the hog and used esp. as a digestant

pep·sin·o·gen \pep-'si-nə-jən\ *n* : a granular zymogen of the gastric glands that is readily converted into pepsin in a slightly acid medium

pept- *or* **pepto-** *comb form* : protein fragment or derivative ⟨*pept*ide⟩

pep·tic \'pep-tik\ *adj* **1** : relating to or promoting digestion : DIGESTIVE **2** : of, relating to, producing, or caused by pepsin ⟨~ digestion⟩

peptic ulcer *n* : an ulcer in the wall of the stomach or duodenum resulting from the digestive action of the gastric juice on the mucous membrane when the latter is rendered susceptible to its action (as by psychosomatic or local factors)

pep·ti·dase \'pep-tə-₁dās, -₁dāz\ *n* : an enzyme that hydrolyzes simple peptides or their derivatives

pep·tide \'pep-₁tīd\ *n* : any of various amides that are derived from two or more amino acids by combination of the amino group of one acid with the carboxyl group of another and are usu. obtained by partial hydrolysis of

proteins — **pep·tid·ic** \pep-'ti-dik\ *adj*

peptide bond *n* : the chemical bond between carbon and nitrogen in a peptide linkage

peptide linkage *n* : the group CONH having a chemical valence of two that unites the amino acid residues in a peptide

pep·tid·er·gic \₁pep-tī-'dər-jik\ *adj* : being, relating to, releasing, or activated by neurotransmitters that are short peptide chains ⟨~ neurons⟩

pep·ti·do·gly·can \₁pep-tə-dō-'gli-₁kan\ *n* : a polymer that is composed of polysaccharide and peptide chains and is found esp. in bacterial cell walls — called also *mucopeptide*, *murein*

pep·tone \'pep-₁tōn\ *n* **1** : any of various protein derivatives that are formed by the partial hydrolysis of proteins (as by enzymes of the gastric and pancreatic juices or by acids or alkalies) **2** : a complex water-soluble product containing peptones and other protein derivatives that is obtained by digesting protein (as meat) with an enzyme (as pepsin or trypsin) and is used chiefly in nutrient media in bacteriology

per \'pər\ *prep* : by the means or agency of : by way of : through ⟨blood ~ rectum⟩ — see PER OS

per·acute \₁pər-ə-'kyüt\ *adj* : very acute and violent

per·ceive \pər-'sēv\ *vb* **per·ceived; per·ceiv·ing** : to become aware of through the senses — **per·ceiv·able** \-'sē-və-bəl\ *adj*

per·cept \'pər-₁sept\ *n* : an impression of an object obtained by use of the senses : SENSE-DATUM

per·cep·ti·ble \pər-'sep-tə-bəl\ *adj* : capable of being perceived esp. by the senses — **per·cep·ti·bly** \-blē\ *adv*

per·cep·tion \pər-'sep-shən\ *n* : awareness of the elements of environment through physical sensation ⟨color ~⟩ — compare SENSATION 1a

per·cep·tive \pər-'sep-tiv\ *adj* : responsive to sensory stimulus ⟨a ~ eye⟩ — **per·cep·tive·ly** *adv*

perceptive deafness *n* : NERVE DEAFNESS

per·cep·tu·al \(₁)pər-'sep-chə-wəl, -shə-\ *adj* : of, relating to, or involving perception esp. in relation to immediate sensory experience ⟨auditory ~ deficits⟩ — **per·cep·tu·al·ly** *adv*

per·co·late \'pər-kə-₁lāt, -lət\ *n* : a product of percolation

per·co·la·tion \₁pər-kə-'lā-shən\ *n* **1** : the slow passage of a liquid through a filtering medium **2** : a method of extraction or purification by means of filtration **3** : the process of extracting the soluble constituents of a powdered drug by passage of a liquid through it — **per·co·late** \'pər-kə-₁lāt\ *vb* — **per·co·la·tor** \-₁lā-tər\ *n*

per·cus·sion \pər-'kə-shən\ *n* **1** : the act

or technique of tapping the surface of a body part to learn the condition of the parts beneath by the resulting sound **2** : massage consisting of the striking of a body part with light rapid blows — called also *tapotement* — **per·cuss** \pər-ˈkəs\ *vb*

per·cu·ta·ne·ous \ˌpər-kyü-ˈtā-nē-əs\ *adj* : effected or performed through the skin 〈∼ absorption〉 — **per·cu·ta·ne·ous·ly** *adv*

percutaneous transluminal angioplasty *n* : a surgical procedure used to enlarge the lumen of a partly occluded blood vessel (as one with atherosclerotic plaques on the walls) by passing a balloon catheter through the skin, into the vessel, and through the vessel to the site of the lesion where the tip of the catheter is inflated to expand the lumen of the vessel

percutaneous transluminal coronary angioplasty *n* : percutaneous transluminal angioplasty of a coronary artery — called also *PTCA*

per·fo·rate \ˈpər-fə-ˌrāt\ *vb* **-rat·ed; -rat·ing** : to enter, penetrate, or make a hole through 〈an ulcer ∼s the duodenal wall〉

per·fo·rat·ed \-ˌrā-təd\ *adj* : characterized by perforation 〈a ∼ ulcer〉

per·fo·ra·tion \ˌpər-fə-ˈrā-shən\ *n* **1** : the act or process of perforating; *specif* : the penetration of a body part through accident or disease **2 a** : a rupture in a body part caused esp. by accident or disease **b** : a natural opening in an organ or body part

per·fo·ra·tor \ˈpər-fə-ˌrā-tər\ *n* : one that perforates: as **a** : an instrument used to perforate tissue (as bone) **b** : a nerve or blood vessel forming a connection between a deep system and a superficial one

per·fus·ate \(ˌ)pər-ˈfyü-ˌzāt, -zət\ *n* : a fluid (as a solution pumped through the heart) that is perfused

per·fuse \(ˌ)pər-ˈfyüzd\ *vb* **-fused; -fus·ing 1** : SUFFUSE **2 a** : to cause to flow or spread : DIFFUSE **b** : to force a fluid through (an organ or tissue) esp. by way of the blood vessels

per·fu·sion \-ˈfyü-zhən\ *n* : an act or instance of perfusing; *specif* : the pumping of a fluid through an organ or tissue

per·fu·sion·ist \pər-ˈfyü-zhə-nist\ *n* : a certified medical technician responsible for extracorporeal oxygenation of the blood during open-heart surgery and for the operation and maintenance of equipment (as a heart-lung machine) controlling it

per·hex·i·line \pər-ˈhek-sə-ˌlēn\ *n* : a drug $C_{19}H_{35}N$ used as a coronary vasodilator

peri- *prefix* **1** : near : around 〈*peri*menopausal〉 **2** : enclosing : surrounding 〈*peri*neurium〉

peri·anal \ˌper-ē-ˈān-ᵊl\ *adj* : of, relating to, occurring in, or being the tissues surrounding the anus 〈a ∼ abscess〉

peri·aor·tic \-ā-ˈȯr-tik\ *adj* : of, relating to, occurring in, or being the tissues surrounding the aorta

peri·api·cal \-ˈā-pi-kəl, -ˈa-\ *adj* : of, relating to, occurring in, affecting, or being the tissues surrounding the apex of the root of a tooth

peri·aq·ue·duc·tal \-ˌā-kwə-ˈdəkt-ᵊl\ *adj* : of, relating to, or being the gray matter which surrounds the aqueduct of Sylvius

peri·ar·te·ri·al \-är-ˈtir-ē-əl\ *adj* : of, relating to, occurring in, or being the tissues surrounding an artery

peri·ar·te·ri·o·lar \-är-ˌtir-ē-ˈō-lər\ *adj* : of, relating to, occurring in, or being the tissues surrounding an arteriole

peri·ar·ter·i·tis no·do·sa \ˌper-ē-ˌär-tə-ˈrī-təs-nō-ˈdō-sə\ *n* : POLYARTERITIS NODOSA

peri·ar·thri·tis \-är-ˈthrī-təs\ *n, pl* **-thrit·i·des** \-ˈthri-tə-ˌdēz\ : inflammation of the structures (as the muscles, tendons, and bursa of the shoulder) around a joint

peri·ar·tic·u·lar \-är-ˈti-kyə-lər\ *adj* : of, relating to, occurring in, or being the tissues surrounding a joint

peri·bron·chi·al \per-ə-ˈbräŋ-kē-əl\ *adj* : of, relating to, occurring in, affecting, or being the tissues surrounding a bronchus 〈a ∼ growth〉

peri·cap·il·lary \-ˈka-pə-ˌler-ē\ *adj* : of, relating to, occurring in, or being the tissues surrounding a capillary 〈∼ infiltration〉

pericardi- *or* **pericardio-** *or* **pericardo- comb form* **1** : pericardium 〈*pericardi*ectomy〉 **2** : pericardial and 〈*pericardio*phrenic artery〉

peri·car·di·al \per-ə-ˈkär-dē-əl\ *adj* : of, relating to, or affecting the pericardium; *also* : situated around the heart

pericardial cavity *n* : the fluid-filled space between the two layers of the pericardium

pericardial fluid *n* : the serous fluid that fills the pericardial cavity and protects the heart from friction

peri·car·di·ec·to·my \ˌper-ə-ˌkär-dē-ˈek-tə-mē\ *n, pl* **-mies** : surgical excision of the pericardium

peri·car·dio·cen·te·sis \ˌper-ə-ˌkär-dē-ō-(ˌ)sen-ˈtē-səs\ *n, pl* **-te·ses** \-ˌsēz\ : surgical puncture of the pericardium esp. to aspirate pericardial fluid

peri·car·dio·phren·ic artery \ˌper-ə-ˌkär-dē-ə-ˈfre-nik\ *n* : a branch of the internal thoracic artery that descends through the thorax accompanying the phrenic nerve between the pleura and the pericardium to the diaphragm

peri·car·di·os·to·my \ˌper-ə-ˌkär-dē-ˈäs-tə-mē\ *n, pl* **-mies** : surgical formation of an opening into the pericardium

peri·car·di·ot·o·my \-ˈä-tə-mē\ *n, pl*

-mies : surgical incision of the pericardium

peri·car·di·tis \-ə-ˈkär-ˈdī-təs\ *n, pl* **-dit·i·des** \-ˈdī-tə-ˌdēz\ : inflammation of the pericardium — see ADHESIVE PERICARDITIS

peri·car·di·um \ˌper-ə-ˈkär-dē-əm\ *n, pl* **-dia** \-dē-ə\ : the conical sac of serous membrane that encloses the heart and the roots of the great blood vessels of vertebrates and consists of an outer fibrous coat that loosely invests the heart and is prolonged on the outer surface of the great vessels except the inferior vena cava and a double inner serous coat of which one layer is closely adherent to the heart while the other lines the inner surface of the outer coat with the intervening space being filled with pericardial fluid

pericardo- — see PERICARDI-

peri·cel·lu·lar \-ˈsel-yə-lər\ *adj* : of, relating to, occurring in, or being the tissues surrounding a cell

peri·ce·men·ti·tis \-sē-ˌmen-ˈtī-təs\ *n* : PERIODONTITIS

peri·ce·men·tum \-si-ˈmen-təm\ *n* : PERIODONTAL MEMBRANE

peri·cen·tric \-ˈsen-trik\ *adj* : of, relating to, or involving the centromere of a chromosome (∼ inversion) — compare PARACENTRIC

peri·chol·an·gi·tis \-ˌkō-ˌlan-ˈjī-təs, -ˌkä-\ *n* : inflammation of the tissues surrounding the bile ducts

peri·chon·dri·tis \-ˌkän-ˈdrī-təs\ *n* : inflammation of a perichondrium

peri·chon·dri·um \ˌper-ə-ˈkän-drē-əm\ *n, pl* **-dria** \-drē-ə\ : the membrane of fibrous connective tissue that invests cartilage except at joints — **peri·chon·dri·al** \-drē-əl\ *adj*

peri·co·ro·nal \ˌper-ə-ˈkȯr-ən-ᵊl, -ˈkär-; -kə-ˈrōn-ᵊl\ *adj* : occurring about or surrounding the crown of a tooth

peri·cor·o·ni·tis \-ˌkȯr-ə-ˈnī-təs, -ˌkär-\ *n, pl* **-nit·i·des** \-ˈni-tə-ˌdēz\ : inflammation of the gum about the crown of a partially erupted tooth

peri·cyte \ˈper-ə-ˌsīt\ *n* : a cell of the connective tissue about capillaries or other small blood vessels

peri·du·ral \ˌper-i-ˈdür-əl, -ˈdyür-\ *adj* : occurring or applied about the dura mater

peridural anesthesia *n* : EPIDURAL ANESTHESIA

peri·fo·cal \ˌper-ə-ˈfō-kəl\ *adj* : of, relating to, occurring in, or being the tissues surrounding a focus (as of infection) — **peri·fo·cal·ly** *adv*

peri·fol·lic·u·lar \ˌper-ə-fə-ˈli-kyə-lər, -fä-\ *adj* : of, relating to, occurring in, or being the tissues surrounding a follicle

peri·hep·a·ti·tis \-ˌhe-pə-ˈtī-təs, *n, pl* **-tit·i·des** \-ˈti-tə-ˌdēz\ : inflammation of the peritoneal capsule of the liver

peri·kary·on \-ˈkar-ē-ˌän, -ən\ *n, pl* **-karya** \-ē-ə\ : CELL BODY — **peri·kary·al** \-ē-əl\ *adj*

peri·lymph \ˈper-ə-ˌlimf\ *n* : the fluid between the membranous and bony labyrinths of the ear

peri·lym·phat·ic \ˌper-ə-lim-ˈfa-tik\ *adj* : relating to or containing perilymph

peri·men·o·pau·sal \ˌper-ē-me-nə-ˈpȯ-zəl, -ˌmē-\ *adj* : relating to, being in, or occurring in the period around the onset of menopause (∼ women) (∼ bleeding)

pe·rim·e·ter \pə-ˈri-mə-tər\ *n* : an instrument for examining the discriminative powers of different parts of the retina

peri·me·tri·um \ˌper-ə-ˈmē-trē-əm\ *n, pl* **-tria** \-trē-ə\ : the peritoneum covering the fundus and ventral and dorsal aspects of the uterus

pe·rim·e·try \pə-ˈri-mə-trē\ *n, pl* **-tries** : examination of the eye by means of a perimeter — **peri·met·ric** \ˌper-ə-ˈme-trik\ *adj*

peri·my·si·um \ˌper-ə-ˈmizh-əm, -zē-\ *n, pl* **-sia** \-zhē-ə, -zē-ə\ : the connective-tissue sheath that surrounds a muscle and forms sheaths for the bundles of muscle fibers

peri·na·tal \-ˈnāt-ᵊl\ *adj* : occurring in, concerned with, or being in the period around the time of birth (∼ mortality) — **peri·na·tal·ly** *adv*

peri·na·tol·o·gist \ˌper-ə-nā-ˈtä-lə-jist\ *n* : a specialist in perinatology

peri·na·tol·o·gy \-nā-ˈtä-lə-jē\ *n, pl* **-gies** : a branch of medicine concerned with perinatal care

per·i·ne·al \ˌper-ə-ˈnē-əl\ *adj* : of or relating to the perineum

perineal artery *n* : a branch of the internal pudendal artery that supplies the skin of the external genitalia and the superficial parts of the perineum

perineal body *n* : a mass of muscle and fascia that separates the lower end of the vagina and the rectum in the female and the urethra and the rectum in the male

perinei superficialis — see TRANSVERSUS PERINEI SUPERFICIALIS

perineo- *comb form* : perineum (*perineotomy*)

per·i·ne·o·plas·ty \ˌper-i-ˈnē-ō-ˌplas-tē\ *n, pl* **-ties** : plastic surgery of the perineum

per·i·ne·or·rha·phy \ˌper-ə-nē-ˈȯr-ə-fē\ *n, pl* **-phies** : suture of the perineum usu. to repair a laceration occurring during labor

per·i·ne·ot·o·my \ˌper-ə-nē-ˈä-tə-mē\ *n, pl* **-mies** : surgical incision of the perineum

peri·neph·ric \ˌper-ə-ˈne-frik\ *adj* : PERIRENAL (a ∼ abscess)

per·i·ne·um \ˌper-ə-ˈnē-əm\ *n, pl* **-nea** \-ˈnē-ə\ : an area of tissue that marks externally the approximate boundary of the pelvic outlet and gives passage to the urinogenital ducts and rectum; *also* : the area between the anus and the posterior part of the external genitalia esp. in the female

peri·neu·ral \per-ə-ˈnu̇r-əl, -ˈnyu̇r-\ adj : occurring about or surrounding nervous tissue or a nerve

peri·neu·ri·al \-ˈnu̇r-ē-əl, -ˈnyu̇r-\ adj 1 : of or relating to perineurium 2 : PERINEURAL

peri·neu·ri·um \per-ə-ˈnu̇r-ē-əm, -ˈnyu̇r-\ n, pl -ria \-ē-ə\ : the connective-tissue sheath that surrounds a bundle of nerve fibers

peri·nu·cle·ar \-ˈnü-klē-ər, -ˈnyü-\ adj : situated around or surrounding the nucleus of a cell ⟨∼ structures⟩

peri·oc·u·lar \per-ē-ˈä-kyə-lər\ adj : surrounding the eyeball but within the orbit ⟨∼ space⟩

pe·ri·od \ˈpir-ē-əd\ n 1 a : a portion of time determined by some recurring phenomenon b : a single cyclic occurrence of menstruation 2 : a chronological division

pe·ri·od·ic \pir-ē-ˈä-dik\ adj : occurring or recurring at regular intervals

per·iod·ic acid \pər-(ˌ)ī-ˈä-dik-\ n : any of the strongly oxidizing iodine-containing acids (as H_5IO_6 or HIO_4)

periodic acid–Schiff \-ˈshif\ adj : relating to, being, or involving a reaction testing for polysaccharides and related substances in which tissue sections are treated with periodic acid and then Schiff's reagent with a reddish violet color indicating a positive test

periodic breathing n : abnormal breathing characterized by an irregular respiratory rhythm; esp : CHEYNE–STOKES RESPIRATION

periodic ophthalmia n : MOON BLINDNESS

periodic table n : an arrangement of chemical elements based on their atomic numbers

peri·odon·tal \per-ē-ō-ˈdänt-əl\ adj 1 : investing or surrounding a tooth 2 : of or affecting the periodontium ⟨∼ infection⟩ — **peri·odon·tal·ly** adv

periodontal disease n : any disease affecting the periodontium

periodontal membrane n : the fibrous connective-tissue layer covering the cementum of a tooth and holding it in place in the jawbone — called also pericementum, periodontal ligament

peri·odon·tics \per-ə-ˈdän-tiks\ n : a branch of dentistry that deals with diseases of the supporting and investing structures of the teeth including the gums, cementum, periodontal membranes, and alveolar bone — called also periodontology

peri·odon·tist \-ˈdän-tist\ n : a specialist in periodontics — called also periodontologist

peri·odon·ti·tis \per-ē-(ˌ)ō-ˌdän-ˈtī-təs\ n : inflammation of the periodontium and esp. the periodontal membrane — called also pericementitis

periodontitis sim·plex \-ˈsim-ˌpleks\ n : the common form of chronic peri-

odontitis usu. resulting from local infection and characterized by destruction of the periodontal membrane, formation of pockets around the teeth, and resorption of alveolar bone in a horizontal direction

peri·odon·tium \per-ē-ō-ˈdän-chē-əm, -chəm\ n, pl -tia \-chē-ə, -chə\ : the supporting structures of the teeth including the cementum, the periodontal membrane, the bone of the alveolar process, and the gums

peri·odon·to·cla·sia \-ō-ˌdän-tə-ˈklā-zhə, -zhē-ə\ n : any periodontal disease characterized by destruction of the periodontium

peri·odon·tol·o·gist \per-ē-ō-dän-ˈtä-lə-jist\ n : PERIODONTIST

peri·odon·tol·o·gy \-ˌdän-ˈtä-lə-jē\ n, pl -gies : PERIODONTICS

peri·odon·to·sis \per-ē-ō-ˌdän-ˈtō-səs\ n, pl -to·ses \-ˌsēz\ : a severe degenerative disease of the periodontium which in the early stages of its pure form is characterized by a lack of clinical evidence of inflammation

peri·op·er·a·tive \per-ē-ˈä-pə-rə-tiv, -ˌrā-\ adj : relating to, occurring in, or being the period around the time of a surgical operation ⟨∼ morbidity⟩

peri·oral \-ˈȯr-əl, -ˈär-\ adj : of, relating to, occurring in, or being the tissues around the mouth

peri·or·bit·al \-ˈȯr-bət-əl\ adj : of, relating to, occurring in, or being the tissues surrounding or lining the orbit of the eye ⟨∼ edema⟩

periost- or **perioste-** or **periosteo-** comb form : periosteum ⟨periostitis⟩

peri·os·te·al \per-ē-ˈäs-tē-əl\ adj 1 : situated around or produced internal to bone 2 : of, relating to, or involving the periosteum ⟨a ∼ sarcoma⟩

periosteal elevator n : a surgical instrument used to separate the periosteum from bone

peri·os·te·um \per-ē-ˈäs-tē-əm\ n, pl -tea \-tē-ə\ : the membrane of connective tissue that closely invests all bones except at the articular surfaces

peri·os·ti·tis \-ˌäs-ˈtī-təs\ n : inflammation of the periosteum

peri·pan·cre·at·ic \per-ə-ˌpaŋ-krē-ˈa-tik, -ˌpan-\ adj : of, relating to, occurring in, or being the tissue surrounding the pancreas

pe·riph·er·al \pə-ˈri-fə-rəl\ adj 1 : of, relating to, involving, forming, or located near a periphery or surface part (as of the body) 2 : of, relating to, affecting, or being part of the peripheral nervous system ⟨∼ nerves⟩ ⟨∼ neuropathy⟩ 3 : of, relating to, or being the outer part of the field of vision 4 : of, relating to, or being blood in the systemic circulation ⟨∼ blood⟩ — **pe·riph·er·al·ly** adv

peripheral nervous system n : the part of the nervous system that is outside the central nervous system and comprises the cranial nerves excepting the optic nerve, the spinal nerves, and the autonomic nervous system

peripheral vascular disease *n* : vascular disease (as Raynaud's disease and thromboangiitis obliterans) affecting blood vessels esp. of the extremities

Peri·pla·ne·ta \,per-ē-plə-'nē-tə\ *n* : a genus of large cockroaches that includes the American cockroach (*P. americana*)

peri·plas·mic \,per-ə-'plaz-mik\ *adj* : of, relating to, occurring in, or being the space between the cell wall and the cell membrane

peri·por·tal \,per-ə-'pōrt-³l\ *adj* : of, relating to, occurring in, or being the tissues surrounding a portal vein

peri·rec·tal \-'rek-t³l\ *adj* : of, relating to, occurring in, or being the tissues surrounding the rectum ⟨a ∼ abscess⟩

peri·re·nal \-'rēn-³l\ *adj* : of, relating to, occurring in, or being the tissues surrounding the kidney ⟨a ∼ abscess⟩

peri·stal·sis \,per-ə-'stōl-səs, -'stäl-, -'stal-\ *n, pl* **-stal·ses** \-,sēz\ : successive waves of involuntary contraction passing along the walls of a hollow muscular structure (as the esophagus or intestine) and forcing the contents onward — compare SEGMENTATION 2 — **peri·stal·tic** \-tik\ *adj*

peri·ten·di·ni·tis \,per-ə-,ten-də-'nī-təs\ *n* : inflammation of the tissues around a tendon

periton- *or* **peritone-** *or* **peritoneo-** *comb form* 1 : peritoneum ⟨*peritonitis*⟩ 2 : peritoneal and ⟨*peritoneovenous shunt*⟩

peri·to·nae·um *chiefly Brit var of* PERITONEUM

peri·to·ne·al \,per-ə-tə-'nē-əl\ *adj* : of, relating to, or affecting the peritoneum — **peri·to·ne·al·ly** *adv*

peritoneal cavity *n* : a space formed when the parietal and visceral layers of the peritoneum spread apart

peri·to·neo·scope \,per-ə-tə-'nē-ə-,skōp\ *n* : LAPAROSCOPE — **peri·to·neo·scop·ic** \-,nē-ə-'skä-pik\ *adj*

peri·to·neos·co·py \,per-ə-,tō-nē-'äs-kə-pē\ *n, pl* **-pies** : the study of the abdominal and pelvic cavities by means of the peritoneoscope

peri·to·neo·ve·nous shunt \,per-ə-tə-,nē-ō-'vē-nəs-\ *n* : a shunt between the peritoneum and the jugular vein for relief of peritoneal ascites

peri·to·ne·um \,per-ə-tə-'nē-əm\ *n, pl* **-ne·ums** *or* **-nea** \-'nē-ə\ : the smooth transparent serous membrane that lines the cavity of the abdomen, is folded inward over the abdominal and pelvic viscera, and consists of an outer layer closely adherent to the walls of the abdomen and an inner layer that folds to invest the viscera — see PARIETAL PERITONEUM, VISCERAL PERITONEUM; compare MESENTERY 1

peri·to·ni·tis \,per-ə-tə-'nī-təs\ *n* : inflammation of the peritoneum

peri·ton·sil·lar abscess \,per-ə-'tän-sə-lər-\ *n* : QUINSY

peri·tu·bu·lar \,per-ə-'tü-byə-lər, -'tyü-\ *adj* : being adjacent to or surrounding a tubule

peritubular capillary *n* : any of a network of capillaries surrounding the renal tubules

peri·um·bi·li·cal \,per-ē-,əm-'bi-li-kəl\ *adj* : situated or occurring adjacent to the navel ⟨∼ pain⟩

peri·un·gual \-'əŋ-gwəl, -'ən-\ *adj* : situated or occurring around a fingernail or toenail

peri·ure·thral \-yü-'rē-thrəl\ *adj* : of, relating to, occurring in, or being the tissues surrounding the urethra

peri·vas·cu·lar \,per-ə-'vas-kyə-lər\ *adj* : of, relating to, occurring in, or being the tissues surrounding a blood vessel

peri·vas·cu·li·tis \-,vas-kyə-'lī-təs\ *n* : inflammation of a perivascular sheath ⟨∼ in the retina⟩

peri·ve·nous \,per-ə-'vē-nəs\ *adj* : of, relating to, occurring in, or being the tissues surrounding a vein

peri·ven·tric·u·lar \-ven-'tri-kyə-lər\ *adj* : situated or occurring around a ventricle esp. of the brain

peri·vi·tel·line space \,per-ə-vī-'te-lən-, -,lēn-, -,lin-\ *n* : the fluid-filled space between the fertilization membrane and the ovum after the entry of a sperm into the egg

per·i·win·kle \'per-i-,wiŋ-kəl\ *n* : a commonly cultivated shrub (*Catharanthus roseus* syn. *Vinca rosea*) of the dogbane family (Apocynaceae) that is native to the Old World tropics and is the source of several antineoplastic drugs — see VINBLASTINE, VINCRISTINE

perle \'pərl\ *n* 1 : a soft gelatin capsule for enclosing volatile or unpleasant tasting liquids intended to be swallowed 2 : a fragile glass vial that contains a liquid (as amyl nitrite) and that is intended to be crushed and the vapor inhaled

per·lèche \per-'lesh\ *n* : a superficial inflammatory condition of the angles of the mouth often with fissure formation that is caused esp. by infection or avitaminosis

per·ma·nent \'pər-mə-nənt\ *adj* : of, relating to, or being a permanent tooth ⟨∼ dentition⟩

permanent tooth *n* : one of the second set of teeth of a mammal that follow the milk teeth, typically persist into old age, and in humans are 32 in number including 4 incisors, 2 canines, and 10 premolars and molars in each jaw

per·me·able \'pər-mē-ə-bəl\ *adj* : capable of being permeated; *esp* : having pores or openings that permit liquids or gases to pass through — **per·me·abil·i·ty** \,pər-mē-ə-'bi-lə-tē\ *n*

per·me·ate \'pər-mē-,āt\ *vb* **-at·ed; -at·ing** : to diffuse through or penetrate something — **per·me·ation** \ˌpər-mē-'ā-shən\ *n*

per·mis·sive \pər-'mi-siv\ *adj* : supporting genetic replication (as of a virus)

per·ni·cious \pər-'ni-shəs\ *adj* : highly injurious or destructive : tending to a fatal issue : DEADLY ⟨∼ disease⟩

pernicious anemia *n* : a severe hyperchromic anemia marked by a progressive decrease in number and increase in size and hemoglobin content of the red blood cells and by pallor, weakness, and gastrointestinal and nervous disturbances and associated with reduced ability to absorb vitamin B_{12} due to the absence of intrinsic factor — called also *addisonian anemia*

per·nio \'pər-nē-ˌō\ *n, pl* **per·ni·o·nes** \ˌpər-nē-'ō-(ˌ)nēz\ : CHILBLAIN

pe·ro·me·lia \ˌpē-rə-'mē-lē-ə\ *n* : congenital malformation of the limbs

pe·ro·ne·al \ˌper-ō-'nē-əl, pə-'rō-nē-\ *adj* **1** : of, relating to, or located near the fibula **2** : relating to or involving a peroneal part

peroneal artery *n* : a deeply seated artery running along the back part of the fibular side of the leg to the heel, arising from the posterior tibial artery, and ending in branches near the ankle

peroneal muscle *n* : PERONEUS

peroneal muscular atrophy *n* : a chronic inherited progressive muscular atrophy that affects the parts of the legs and feet innervated by the peroneal nerves and first and later progresses to the hands and arms — called also *Charcot-Marie-Tooth disease, peroneal atrophy*

peroneal nerve *n* : COMMON PERONEAL NERVE — see DEEP PERONEAL NERVE, SUPERFICIAL PERONEAL NERVE

peroneal retinaculum *n* : either of two bands of fascia that support and bind in place the tendons of the peroneus longus and peroneus brevis muscles as they pass along the lateral aspect of the ankle: **a** : one that is situated more superiorly — called also *superior peroneal retinaculum* **b** : one that is situated more inferiorly — called also *inferior peroneal retinaculum*

peroneal vein *n* : any of several veins that drain the muscles in the lateral and posterior parts of the leg, accompany the peroneal artery, and empty into the posterior tibial veins about two-thirds of the way up the leg

pe·ro·ne·us \ˌper-ə-'nē-əs\ *n, pl* **-nei** \-'nē-ˌī\ : any of three muscles of the lower leg: **a** : PERONEUS BREVIS **b** : PERONEUS LONGUS **c** : PERONEUS TERTIUS

peroneus brev·is \-'bre-vis\ *n* : a peroneus muscle that arises esp. from the side of the lower part of the fibula, ends in a tendon that inserts on the tuberosity at the base of the fifth metatarsal bone, and assists in everting and pronating the foot

peroneus lon·gus \-'lȯŋ-gəs\ *n* : a peroneus muscle that arises esp. from the head and side of the fibula, ends in a long tendon that inserts on the side of the first metatarsal bone and the cuneiform bone on the medial side, and aids in everting and pronating the foot

peroneus ter·ti·us \-'tər-shē-əs\ *n* : a branch of the extensor digitorum longus muscle that arises esp. from the lower portion of the fibula, inserts on the dorsal surface of the base of the fifth metatarsal bone, and flexes the foot dorsally and assists in everting it

per·oral \(ˌ)pər-'ȯr-əl, per-, -'är-\ *adj* : done, occurring, or obtained through or by way of the mouth ⟨∼ administration of a drug⟩ ⟨∼ infection⟩ — **per·oral·ly** *adv*

per os \ˌpər-'ōs\ *adv* : by way of the mouth ⟨infection *per os*⟩

pe·ro·sis \pə-'rō-səs\ *n, pl* **pe·ro·ses** \-ˌsēz\ : a disorder of poultry that is characterized by leg deformity and can be prevented by additions of choline to the diet — called also *hock disease, slipped tendon*

per·ox·i·dase \pə-'räk-sə-ˌdās, -ˌdāz\ *n* : an enzyme that catalyzes the oxidation of various substances by peroxides

per·ox·ide \pə-'räk-ˌsīd\ *n* : an oxide containing a high proportion of oxygen; *esp* : a compound (as hydrogen peroxide) in which oxygen is visualized as joined to oxygen

per·ox·i·some \pə-'räk-sə-ˌsōm\ *n* : a cytoplasmic cell organelle containing enzymes (as catalase) which act esp. in the production and decomposition of hydrogen peroxide — called also *microbody* — **per·ox·i·som·al** \-ˌräk-sə-'sō-məl\ *adj*

per·pen·dic·u·lar plate \ˌpər-pən-'di-kyə-lər-\ *n* **1** : a flattened bony lamina of the ethmoid bone that is the largest bony part assisting in forming the nasal septum **2** : a long thin vertical bony plate forming part of the palatine bone — compare HORIZONTAL PLATE

per·phen·a·zine \(ˌ)pər-'fe-nə-ˌzēn\ *n* : a phenothiazine tranquilizer $C_{21}H_{26}ClN_3OS$ that is used to control tension, anxiety, and agitation esp. in psychotic conditions

per·rec·tal \ˌpər-'rekt-əl\ *adj* : done or occurring through or by way of the rectum ⟨∼ administration⟩ — **per·rec·tal·ly** *adv*

per rectum *adv* : by way of the rectum ⟨a solution injected *per rectum*⟩

Per·san·tine \pər-'san-ˌtēn\ *trademark* — used for a preparation of dipyridamole

persecution complex *n* : the feeling of being persecuted esp. without basis in reality

per·se·cu·to·ry \'pər-sə-kyü-ıtōr-ē, pər-'se-kyə-\ *adj* : of, relating to, or being feelings of persecution : PARANOID

per·sev·er·a·tion \pər-ıse-və-'rā-shən\ *n* : continual involuntary repetition of a mental act usu. exhibited by speech or by some other form of overt behavior — **per·sev·er·ate** \pər-'se-və-ırāt\ *vb* — **per·sev·er·a·tive** \pər-'se-və-ırā-tiv\ *adj*

per·sis·tent \pər-'sis-tənt\ *adj* 1 : existing or continuing for a long time: as a : effective in the open for an appreciable time usu. through slow formation of a vapor ⟨mustard gas is ∼⟩ b : degraded only slowly by the environment ⟨∼ pesticides⟩ c : remaining infective for a relatively long time in a vector after an initial period of incubation ⟨∼ viruses⟩ 2 : continuing to exist despite interference or treatment ⟨a ∼ cough⟩

per·so·na \pər-'sō-nə, -ınä\ *n, pl* **perso·nas** : an individual's social facade or front that esp. in the analytic psychology of C.G. Jung reflects the role in life the individual is playing — compare ANIMA

per·son·al·i·ty \ıpər-sə-'na-lə-tē\ *n, pl* **-ties** 1 : the complex of characteristics that distinguishes an individual esp. in relationships with others 2 a : the totality of an individual's behavioral and emotional tendencies b : the organization of the individual's distinguishing character traits, attitudes, and habits

personality disorder *n* : a psychopathological condition or group of conditions in which an individual's entire life pattern is considered deviant or nonadaptive although the individual shows neither neurotic symptoms nor psychotic disorganization

personality inventory *n* : any of several tests that attempt to characterize the personality of an individual by objective scoring of replies to a large number of questions concerning the individual's behavior and attitudes — see MINNESOTA MULTIPHASIC PERSONALITY INVENTORY

personality test *n* : any of several tests that consist of standardized tasks designed to determine various aspects of the personality or the emotional status of the individual examined

per·spi·ra·tion \ıpər-spə-'rā-shən\ *n* 1 : the act or process of perspiring 2 : a saline fluid that is secreted by the sweat glands, that consists chiefly of water containing sodium chloride and other salts, nitrogenous substances (as urea), carbon dioxide, and other solutes, and that serves both as a means of excretion and as a regulator of body temperature through the cooling effect of its evaporation — **per·spire** \pər-'spīr\ *vb*

per·spi·ra·to·ry \'pər-'spī-rə-ıtōr-ē,

'pər-spə-rə-\ *adj* : of, relating to, secreting, or inducing perspiration

per·sua·sion \pər-'swā-zhən\ *n* : a method of treating neuroses consisting essentially in rational conversation and reeducation

Per·thes disease \'pər-ıtēz-\ *n* : LEGG-CALVÉ-PERTHES DISEASE

Per·to·frane \'pər-tə-ıfrān\ *trademark* — used for a preparation of desipramine

per·tus·sis \pər-'tə-səs\ *n* : WHOOPING COUGH

peruana — see VERRUGA PERUANA

Peru balsam *n* : BALSAM OF PERU

Peruvian balsam *n* : BALSAM OF PERU

per·ver·sion \pər-'vər-zhən, -shən\ *n* 1 : the action of perverting or the condition of being perverted 2 : a perverted form : *esp* : an aberrant sexual practice esp. when habitual and preferred to normal coitus — **per·verse** \pər-'vərs\ *adj*

¹**per·vert** \pər-'vərt\ *vb* : to cause to engage in perversion or to become perverted

²**per·vert** \'pər-ıvərt\ *n* : one that has been perverted; *specif* : one given to some form of sexual perversion

perverted *adj* : marked by abnormality or perversion ⟨∼ pancreatic function⟩

pes an·se·ri·nus \'pez-ıan-sə-'rī-nəs\ *n* : the combined tendinous insertion on the medial aspect of the tuberosity of the tibia of the sartorius, gracilis, and semitendinosus muscles

pes ca·vus \-'kā-vəs\ *n* : a foot deformity characterized by an abnormally high arch

pes·sa·ry \'pe-sə-rē\ *n, pl* **-ries** 1 : a vaginal suppository 2 : a device worn in the vagina to support the uterus, remedy a malposition, or prevent conception

pest \'pest\ *n* 1 : an epidemic disease associated with high mortality; *specif* : PLAGUE 2 2 : something resembling a pest in destructiveness; *esp* : a plant or animal detrimental to humans or human concerns

pes·ti·cide \'pes-tə-ısīd\ *n* : an agent used to destroy pests — **pes·ti·ci·dal** \ıpes-tə-'sīd-ᵊl\ *adj*

pes·tif·er·ous \pes-'ti-fə-rəs\ *adj* 1 : carrying or propagating infection : PESTILENTIAL ⟨a ∼ insect⟩ 2 : infected with a pestilential disease

pes·ti·lence \'pes-tə-ləns\ *n* : a contagious or infectious epidemic disease that is virulent and devastating; *specif* : BUBONIC PLAGUE — **pes·ti·len·tial** \ıpes-tə-'len-chəl\ *adj*

pes·tis \'pes-təs\ *n* : PLAGUE 2

pes·tle \'pe-səl, 'pes-tᵊl\ *n* : a usu. club-shaped implement for pounding or grinding substances in a mortar

PET *abbr* positron-emission tomography

pe·te·chia \pə-'tē-kē-ə\ *n, pl* **-chi·ae** \-kē-ıī\ : a minute reddish or purplish spot containing blood that appears in skin or mucous membrane esp. in some infectious diseases (as typhoid fever) — compare ECCHYMOSIS — **pe·te·chi·al** \-kē-əl\ *adj* — **pe·te·chi·a·tion** \pə-ˌtē-kē-ˈā-shən\ *n*

peth·i·dine \ˈpe-thə-ˌdēn, -dən\ *n, chiefly Brit* : MEPERIDINE

pe·tit mal \ˈpe-tē-ˌmal, -ˌmäl\ *n* : epilepsy caused by a usu. inherited dysrhythmia of the electrical pulsations of the brain and characterized by attacks of mild convulsive seizures with transient clouding of consciousness without amnesia and with or without slight movements of the head, eyes, or extremities — compare GRAND MAL

pe·tri dish \ˈpē-trē-\ *n* : a small shallow dish of thin glass or plastic with a loose cover used esp. for cultures in bacteriology

Pe·tri \ˈpā-trē\, **Julius Richard (1852–1921),** German bacteriologist.

pe·tris·sage \pā-tri-ˈsäzh\ *n* : massage in which the muscles are kneaded

pet·ro·la·tum \ˌpe-trə-ˈlā-təm, -ˈlä-\ *n* : PETROLEUM JELLY

pe·tro·leum jelly \pə-ˈtrō-lē-əm-ˈje-lē\ *n* : a neutral unctuous odorless tasteless substance obtained from petroleum and used esp. in ointments and dressings

pe·tro·sal \pə-ˈtrō-səl\ *n* : PETROSAL BONE

petrosal bone *n* : the petrous portion of the human temporal bone

petrosal ganglion *n* : INFERIOR GANGLION 1

petrosal nerve *n* : any of several small nerves passing through foramina in the petrous portion of the temporal bone: as **a** : DEEP PETROSAL NERVE **b** : GREATER PETROSAL NERVE **c** : LESSER PETROSAL NERVE

petrosal sinus *n* : either of two venous sinuses on each side of the base of the brain: **a** : a small superior sinus that connects the cavernous and transverse sinuses of the same side — called also *superior petrosal sinus* **b** : a larger inferior sinus that extends from the posterior inferior end of the cavernous sinus through the jugular foramen to join the internal jugular vein of the same side — called also *inferior petrosal sinus*

pe·tro·tym·pan·ic fissure \ˌpe-trō-tim-ˈpa-nik-, ˌpē-trō-\ *n* : a narrow transverse slit dividing the glenoid fossa of the temporal bone — called also *Glaserian fissure*

pe·trous \ˈpe-trəs, ˈpē-\ *adj* : of, relating to, or constituting the exceptionally hard and dense portion of the human temporal bone that contains the internal auditory organs and is a pyramidal process wedged in at the base of the skull between the sphenoid and occipital bones

PET scan \ˈpet-\ *n* : a sectional view of the body constructed by positron-emission tomography — **PET scanning** *n*

PET scanner *n* : a medical instrument consisting of integrated X-ray and computing equipment and used for positron-emission tomography

Peutz–Je·ghers syndrome \ˈpœts-ˈjā-gərz-\ *n* : a familial polyposis inherited as an autosomal dominant trait and characterized by numerous polyps in the stomach, small intestine, and colon and by melanin-containing spots on the skin and mucous membranes esp. of the lips and gums

Peutz, J.L.A. (fl 1921), Dutch physician.

Jeghers, Harold (b 1904), American physician.

-pexy \ˌpek-sē\ *n comb form, pl* **-pexies** : fixation : making fast ⟨gastropexy⟩

Pey·er's patch \ˈpī-ərz-\ *n* : any of numerous large oval patches of closely aggregated nodules of lymphoid tissue in the walls of the small intestines esp. in the ileum that partially or entirely disappear in advanced life and in typhoid fever become the seat of ulcers which may perforate the intestines — called also *Peyer's gland*

Peyer, Johann Conrad (1653–1712), Swiss physician and anatomist.

pey·o·te \pā-ˈō-tē\ *also* **pey·otl** \-ˈōt-ᵊl\ *n* **1** : any of several American cacti (genus *Lophophora*); *esp* : MESCAL **2** : a stimulant drug derived from mescal buttons

Pey·ro·nie's disease \ˌpā-rə-ˈnēz-, pā-ˈrō-nēz-\ *n* : the formation of fibrous plaques in one or both corpora cavernosa of the penis resulting in distortion or deflection of the erect organ

La Peyronie \lä-pā-rō-ˈnē\, **François Gigot de (1678–1747),** French surgeon.

pg *abbr* picogram

PG *abbr* prostaglandin

PGA *abbr* pteroylglutamic acid

PGR *abbr* psychogalvanic reaction; psychogalvanic reflex; psychogalvanic response

PGY *abbr* postgraduate year

pH \ˌpē-ˈāch\ *n* : a measure of acidity and alkalinity of a solution that is a number on a scale whose values run from 0 to 14 with 7 representing neutrality, numbers less than 7 increasing acidity, and numbers greater than 7 increasing alkalinity

PHA *abbr* phytohemagglutinin

phac- *or* **phaco-** *comb form* : lens ⟨*phaco*emulsification⟩

phaco·emul·si·fi·ca·tion \ˌfa-kō-i-ˌməl-sə-fə-ˈkā-shən\ *n* : a cataract operation in which the diseased lens is reduced to a liquid by ultrasonic vibrations and drained out of the eye — **phaco·emul·si·fi·er** \-ˈməl-sə-ˌfī-ər\ *n*

phaco·ma·to·sis \ˌfa-kō-mə-ˈtō-səs\ *n, pl* **-to·ses** \-ˌsēz\ : any of a group of hereditary or congenital diseases (as neurofibromatosis) affecting the central nervous system and characterized by the development of hamartomas

phaeo·chro·mo·cy·to·ma *Brit var of* PHEOCHROMOCYTOMA

phag- *or* **phago-** *comb form* : eating : feeding ⟨*phage*dena⟩

phage \ˈfāj, ˈfäzh\ *n* : BACTERIOPHAGE

-phage \ˌfāj, ˌfäzh\ *n comb form* : one that eats ⟨bacterio*phage*⟩

phag·e·de·na \ˌfa-jə-ˈdē-nə\ *n* : rapidly spreading destructive ulceration of soft tissue — **phag·e·den·ic** \-ˈde-nik, -ˈdē-\ *adj*

phage lambda *n* : a coliphage that can be integrated as a prophage into the DNA of some lysogenic strains of a bacterium of the genus *Escherichia* (*E. coli*) — called also *bacteriophage lambda, lambda, lambda phage*

phage type *n* : a set of strains of a bacterium susceptible to the same bacteriophages

phage-typing *n* : determination of the phage type of a bacterium

-pha·gia \ˈfā-jə, -jē-ə\ *n comb form* : -PHAGY ⟨dys*phagia*⟩

phago·cyte \ˈfa-gə-ˌsīt\ *n* : a cell (as a white blood cell) that engulfs and consumes foreign material (as microorganisms) and debris — **phago·cyt·ic** \ˌfa-gə-ˈsi-tik\ *adj*

phago·cy·tize \ˈfa-gō-ˌsī-ˌtiz, -sə-\ *vb* **-tized; -tiz·ing** : PHAGOCYTOSE

phago·cy·tose \ˈfa-gō-ˈsī-ˌtōs, -ˌtōz\ *vb* **-tosed; -tos·ing** : to consume by phagocytosis — **phago·cy·tos·able** \ˌfa-gə-sī-ˈtō-zə-bəl, -sə-...-ˈtōs-\ *adj*

phago·cy·to·sis \ˌfa-gə-sī-ˈtō-səs, -sə-\ *n, pl* **-to·ses** \-ˌsēz\ : the engulfing and usu. the destruction of particulate matter by phagocytes that serves as an important bodily defense mechanism against infection by microorganisms and against occlusion of mucous surfaces or tissues by foreign particles and tissue debris — **phago·cy·tot·ic** \-ˈtä-tik\ *adj*

phago·some \ˈfa-gə-ˌsōm\ *n* : a membrane-bound vesicle that encloses particulate matter taken into the cell by phagocytosis

-pha·gous \fə-gəs\ *adj comb form* : feeding esp. on a (specified) kind of food ⟨hemato*phagous*⟩

-ph·agy \f-ə-jē\ *n comb form, pl* **-phagies** : eating : eating of a (specified) type or substance ⟨geo*phagy*⟩

phak- *or* **phako-** — see PHAC-

pha·lan·ge·al \ˌfā-lən-ˈjē-əl, ˌfa-; fə-ˈlan-jē-, fā-\ *adj* : of or relating to a phalanx or the phalanges

pha·lan·gec·to·my \ˌfā-lən-ˈjek-tə-mē, ˌfa-\ *n, pl* **-mies** : surgical excision of a phalanx of a finger or toe

pha·lanx \ˈfā-ˌlaŋks\ *n, pl* **pha·lan·ges** \fə-ˈlan-(ˌ)jēz, fā-, ˈfā-\ : any of the digital bones of the hand or foot distal to the metacarpus or metatarsus that in humans are three to each finger and toe with the exception of the thumb and big toe which have only two each

phall- *or* **phallo-** *comb form* : penis ⟨*phallo*plasty⟩

phal·lic \ˈfa-lik\ *adj* **1** : of, relating to, or resembling a penis **2** : of, relating to, or characterized by the stage of psychosexual development in psychoanalytic theory during which a child becomes interested in his or her own sexual organs — compare ANAL 2a, GENITAL 3, ORAL 2a

phal·loi·din \fa-ˈlòid-ᵊn\ *also* **phal·loi·dine** \fa-ˈlòid-ᵊn, ˈfa-lòi-ˌdēn\ *n* : a very toxic crystalline peptide $C_{35}H_{46}N_8O_{10}S \cdot H_2O$ obtained from the death cap mushroom

phal·lo·plas·ty \ˈfa-lō-ˌplas-tē\ *n, pl* **-ties** : plastic surgery of the penis or scrotum

phal·lus \ˈfa-ləs\ *n, pl* **phal·li** \ˈfa-ˌlī, -ˌlē\ *or* **phal·lus·es 1** : PENIS **2** : the first embryonic rudiment of the penis or clitoris

phan·ero·zo·ite \ˌfa-nə-rō-ˈzō-ˌīt\ *n* : an exoerythrocytic malaria parasite found late in the course of an infection — **phan·ero·zo·it·ic** \-zō-ˈi-tik\ *adj*

phan·tasm \ˈfan-ˌta-zəm\ *n* **1** : a figment of the imagination or disordered mind **2** : an apparition of a living or dead person

phan·ta·sy *var of* FANTASY

¹phan·tom \ˈfan-təm\ *n* **1** : a model of the body or one of its parts **2** : a body of material resembling a body or bodily part in mass, composition, and dimensions and used to measure absorption of radiations

²phantom *adj* : not caused by an anatomical lesion ⟨~ respiratory disorders⟩

phantom limb *n* : an often painful sensation of the presence of a limb that has been amputated — called also *phantom pain, phantom sensations*

phantom tumor *n* : a swelling (as of the abdomen) suggesting a tumor

Phar. D. *abbr* doctor of pharmacy

pharm *abbr* pharmaceutical; pharmacist; pharmacy

¹phar·ma·ceu·ti·cal \ˌfär-mə-ˈsü-ti-kəl\ *also* **phar·ma·ceu·tic** \-tik\ *adj* : of, relating to, or engaged in pharmacy or the manufacture and sale of pharmaceuticals ⟨a ~ company⟩ — **phar·ma·ceu·ti·cal·ly** *adv*

²pharmaceutical *also* **pharmaceutic** *n* : a medicinal drug

phar·ma·ceu·tics \-tiks\ *n* : the science of preparing, using, or dispensing medicines : PHARMACY

phar·ma·cist \ˈfär-mə-sist\ *n* : a person licensed to engage in pharmacy

pharmaco- *comb form* : medicine : drug ⟨*pharmaco*logy⟩ ⟨*pharmaco*therapy⟩

phar·ma·co·dy·nam·ics \ˌfär-mə-kō-dī-ˈna-miks, -də-\ *n* : a branch of pharmacology dealing with the reactions between drugs and living systems — **phar·ma·co·dy·nam·ic** \-mik\ *adj* — **phar·ma·co·dy·nam·i·cal·ly** *adv*

phar·ma·co·ge·net·ics \-jə-'ne-tiks\ *n* : the study of the interrelation of hereditary constitution and response to drugs — **phar·ma·co·ge·net·ic** \-tik\ *adj*

phar·ma·cog·no·sist \ˌfär-mə-'käg-nə-sist\ *n* : a specialist in pharmacognosy

phar·ma·cog·no·sy \ˌfär-mə-'käg-nə-sē\ *n, pl* **-sies** : a science dealing with the composition, production, use, and history of crude drugs and simples — **phar·ma·cog·nos·tic** \-ˌkäg-'näs-tik\ *or* **phar·ma·cog·nos·ti·cal** \-ti-kəl\ *adj*

phar·ma·co·ki·net·ics \-kō-kə-'ne-tiks, -kō-kī-\ *n* 1 : the study of the bodily absorption, distribution, metabolism, and excretion of drugs 2 : the characteristic interactions of a drug and the body in terms of its absorption, distribution, metabolism, and excretion — **phar·ma·co·ki·net·ic** \-tik\ *adj*

phar·ma·col·o·gist \ˌfär-mə-'kä-lə-jist\ *n* : a specialist in pharmacology

phar·ma·col·o·gy \ˌfär-mə-'kä-lə-jē\ *n, pl* **-gies** 1 : the science of drugs including materia medica, toxicology, and therapeutics 2 : the properties and reactions of drugs esp. with relation to their therapeutic value — **phar·ma·co·log·i·cal** \-kə-'lä-ji-kəl\ *also* **phar·ma·co·log·ic** \-jik\ *adj* — **phar·ma·co·log·i·cal·ly** *adv*

phar·ma·co·poe·ia *or* **phar·ma·co·pe·ia** \ˌfär-mə-kə-'pē-ə\ *n* 1 : a book describing drugs, chemicals, and medicinal preparations; *esp* : one issued by an officially recognized authority and serving as a standard 2 : a collection or stock of drugs — **phar·ma·co·poe·ial** *or* **phar·ma·co·pe·ial** \-əl\ *adj*

phar·ma·co·ther·a·peu·tic \-ˌther-ə-'pyü-tik\ *adj* : of or relating to pharmacotherapeutics or pharmacotherapy

phar·ma·co·ther·a·peu·tics \-tiks\ *n sing or pl* : the study of the therapeutic uses and effects of drugs

phar·ma·co·ther·a·py \ˌfär-mə-kō-'ther-ə-pē\ *n, pl* **-pies** : the treatment of disease and esp. mental illness with drugs

phar·ma·cy \'fär-mə-sē\ *n, pl* **-cies** 1 : the art, practice, or profession of preparing, preserving, compounding, and dispensing medical drugs 2 a : a place where medicines are compounded or dispensed ⟨a hospital ∼⟩ b : DRUGSTORE 3 : PHARMACOPOEIA 1

Pharm. D. *abbr* doctor of pharmacy

pharyng- *or* **pharyngo-** *comb form* 1 : pharynx ⟨*pharyng*itis⟩ 2 : pharyngeal and ⟨*pharyngo*esophageal⟩

pha·ryn·geal \ˌfar-ən-'jē-əl; fə-'rin-jəl, -jē-əl\ *adj* 1 : relating to or located in the region of the pharynx 2 a : innervating the pharynx esp. by contributing to the formation of the pharyngeal plexus ⟨the ∼ branch of the vagus nerve⟩ b : supplying or draining the

pharynx ⟨the ∼ branch of the maxillary artery⟩

pharyngeal aponeurosis *n* : the middle or fibrous coat of the walls of the pharynx

pharyngeal arch *n* : BRANCHIAL ARCH

pharyngeal cavity *n* : the cavity of the pharynx that consists of a part continuous anteriorly with the nasal cavity by way of the nasopharynx, a part opening into the oral cavity by way of the fauces, and a part continuous posteriorly with the esophagus and opening into the larynx by way of the epiglottis

pharyngeal cleft *n* : BRANCHIAL CLEFT

pharyngeal plexus *n* : a plexus formed by branches of the glossopharyngeal, vagus, and sympathetic nerves supplying the muscles and mucous membrane of the pharynx and adjoining parts

pharyngeal pouch *n* : any of a series of evaginations of ectoderm on either side of the pharynx that meet the corresponding external furrows and give rise to the branchial clefts of the vertebrate embryo

pharyngeal tonsil *n* : a mass of lymphoid tissue at the back of the pharynx between the eustachian tubes that is usu. best developed in young children, is commonly atrophied in the adult, and is markedly subject to hypertrophy and adenoid formation esp. in children — called also *nasopharyngeal tonsil*

phar·yn·gec·to·my \ˌfar-ən-'jek-tə-mē\ *n, pl* **-mies** : surgical removal of a part of the pharynx

pharyngis — see CONSTRICTOR PHARYNGIS INFERIOR, CONSTRICTOR PHARYNGIS MEDIUS, CONSTRICTOR PHARYNGIS SUPERIOR

phar·yn·gi·tis \ˌfar-ən-'jī-təs\ *n, pl* **-git·i·des** \-'ji-tə-ˌdēz\ : inflammation of the pharynx

pharyngo- — see PHARYNG-

pha·ryn·go·epi·glot·tic fold \fə-ˌriŋ-gō-ˌe-pə-'glä-tik-\ *n* : either of two folds of mucous membrane extending from the base of the tongue to the epiglottis with one on each side of the midline

pha·ryn·go·esoph·a·ge·al \-i-ˌsä-fə-'jē-əl\ *adj* : of or relating to the pharynx and the esophagus

pharyngoesophageal diverticulum *n* : ZENKER'S DIVERTICULUM

pha·ryn·go·lar·yn·gec·to·my \fə-ˌriŋ-gō-ˌlar-ən-'jek-tə-mē\ *n, pl* **-mies** : surgical excision of the hypopharynx and larynx

pha·ryn·go·pal·a·tine arch \-'pa-lə-ˌtīn-\ *n* : PALATOPHARYNGEAL ARCH

pha·ryn·go·plas·ty \fə-'riŋ-gō-ˌplas-tē\ *n, pl* **-ties** : plastic surgery performed on the pharynx

pha·ryn·gos·to·my \ˌfar-iŋ-'gäs-tə-mē\ *n, pl* **-mies** : surgical formation of an artificial opening into the pharynx

phar·yn·got·o·my \ˌfar-iŋ-'gä-tə-mē\ *n,*

pl **-mies** : surgical incision into the pharynx

pha·ryn·go·ton·sil·li·tis \fə-ˌriŋ-gō-ˌtän-sə-ˈlī-təs\ *n* : inflammation of the pharynx and the tonsils

pha·ryn·go·tym·pan·ic tube \-tim-ˈpa-nik-\ *n* : EUSTACHIAN TUBE

phar·ynx \ˈfar-iŋks\ *n, pl* **pha·ryn·ges** \fə-ˈrin-(ˌ)jēz\ *also* **phar·ynx·es** : the part of the alimentary canal situated between the cavity of the mouth and the esophagus and having a conical musculomembranous tube about four and a half inches long that is continuous above with the mouth and nasal passages, communicates through the eustachian tubes with the ears, and extends downward past the opening into the larynx to the lower border of the cricoid cartilage where it is continuous with the esophagus

phase \ˈfāz\ *n* **1** : a particular appearance or state in a regularly recurring cycle of changes **2** : a distinguishable part in a course, development, or cycle ⟨the early ∼s of a disease⟩ **3** : a point or stage in the period of a periodic motion or process (as a light wave or a vibration) in relation to an arbitrary reference or starting point in the period **4** : a homogeneous, physically distinct, and mechanically separable portion of matter present in a nonhomogeneous physicochemical system; *esp* : one of the fundamental states of matter usu. considered to include the solid, liquid, and gaseous forms

phase–contrast microscope *n* : a microscope that translates differences in phase of the light transmitted through or reflected by the object into differences of intensity in the image — **phase–contrast microscopy** *n*

-pha·sia \ˈfā-zhə, -zhē-ə\ *also* **-pha·sy** \fə-sē \ *n comb form, pl* **-phasias** *also* **-phasies** : speech disorder (of a specified type) ⟨dys*phasia*⟩

PhD \ˌpē-(ˌ)āch-ˈdē\ *abbr* **1** an earned academic degree conferring the rank and title of doctor of philosophy **2** a person who has a doctor of philosophy

phe·na·caine \ˈfē-nə-ˌkān, ˈfe-\ *n* : a crystalline base $C_{18}H_{22}N_2O_2$ or its hydrochloride used as a local anesthetic

phen·ac·e·tin \fi-ˈnas-ə-tən\ *n* : a compound $C_{10}H_{13}NO_2$ formerly used to ease pain or fever but now withdrawn from use because of its link to high blood pressure, heart attacks, cancer, and kidney disease — called also *acetophenetidin*

phe·naz·o·cine \fi-ˈna-zə-ˌsēn\ *n* : a drug $C_{22}H_{27}NO$ related to morphine that has greater pain-relieving and slighter narcotic effect

phen·a·zone \ˈfe-nə-ˌzōn\ *n* : ANTIPYRINE

phen·cy·cli·dine \ˌfen-ˈsi-klə-ˌdēn,

-ˈsī-, -dən\ *n* : a piperidine derivative $C_{17}N_{25}N$ used esp. as a veterinary anesthetic and sometimes illicitly as a psychedelic drug to induce vivid mental imagery — called also *angel dust*, *PCP*

phen·el·zine \ˈfen-əl-ˌzēn\ *n* : a monoamine oxidase inhibitor $C_8H_{12}N_2$ that suppresses REM sleep and is used esp. as an antidepressant drug — see NARDIL

Phen·er·gan \fe-ˈnər-ˌgan\ *trademark* — used for a preparation of promethazine

phe·neth·i·cil·lin \fi-ˌne-thə-ˈsi-lən\ *n* : a semisynthetic penicillin $C_{17}H_{20}$-N_2O_5S administered orally in the form of its potassium salt and used esp. in the treatment of less severe infections caused by bacteria that do not produce penicillinase — see MAXIPEN

phen·eth·yl alcohol \fe-ˈne-thəl-\ *n* : PHENYLETHYL ALCOHOL

phen·for·min \fen-ˈfȯr-mən\ *n* : a toxic drug $C_{10}H_{15}N_5$ formerly used to treat diabetes but now banned because of its life-threatening side effects

phen·in·di·one \ˌfen-in-ˈdī-ˌōn\ *n* : an anticoagulant drug $C_{15}H_{10}O_2$

phen·ip·ra·zine \fe-ˈni-prə-ˌzēn\ *n* : a monoamine oxidase inhibitor C_9-$H_{14}N_2$

phen·ir·amine \fe-ˈnir-ə-ˌmēn, -mən\ *n* : a drug $C_{16}H_{20}N_2$ used in the form of its maleate as an antihistamine

phen·met·ra·zine \fen-ˈme-trə-ˌzēn\ *n* : a sympathomimetic stimulant C_{11}-$H_{15}NO$ used in the form of its hydrochloride as an appetite suppressant — see PRELUDIN

phe·no·barb \ˈfē-nō-ˌbärb\ *n* : PHENOBARBITAL; *also* : a pill containing phenobarbital

phe·no·bar·bi·tal \ˌfē-nō-ˈbär-bə-ˌtȯl\ *n* : a crystalline barbiturate $C_{12}H_{12}$-N_2O_3 used as a hypnotic and sedative — see LUMINAL

phe·no·bar·bi·tone \-ˈbär-bə-ˌtōn\ *n, chiefly Brit* : PHENOBARBITAL

phe·no·copy \ˈfē-nə-ˌkä-pē\ *n, pl* **-copies** : a phenotypic variation that is caused by unusual environmental conditions and resembles the normal expression of a genotype other than its own

phe·nol \ˈfē-ˌnōl, -ˌnȯl, fi-ˈ\ *n* **1** : a caustic poisonous crystalline acidic compound C_6H_5OH present in coal tar that is used in the manufacture of some pharmaceuticals and as a topical anesthetic in dilute solution — called also *carbolic*, *carbolic acid* **2** : any of various acidic compounds analogous to phenol — **phe·no·lic** \fi-ˈnō-lik, -ˈnä-\ *adj*

phe·nol·phtha·lein \ˌfēn-əl-ˈtha-lē-ən, -ˈtha-ˌlēn, -ˈthā-\ *n* : a white or yellowish white crystalline compound $C_{20}H_{14}O_4$ used in analysis as an indicator because its solution is brilliant red in alkalies and is decolorized by acids and in medicine as a laxative

phenol red *n* : PHENOLSULFONPHTHALEIN

phe·nol·sul·fon·phtha·lein \ˌfēn-ᵊl-ˌsəl-fän-ˈtha-lē-ən, -ˈtha-ˌlēn, -ˈthā-\ *n* : a red crystalline compound $C_{19}H_{14}O_5$ used chiefly as a test of kidney function and as an acid-base indicator

phenolsulfonphthalein test *n* : a test in which phenolsulfonphthalein is administered by injection and urine samples are subsequently taken at regular intervals to measure the rate at which it is excreted by the kidneys

phe·nom·e·non \fi-ˈnä-mə-ˌnän, -nən\ *n, pl* **-na** \-nə, -ˌnä\ **1** : an observable fact or event **2 a** : an object or aspect known through the senses rather than by thought or intuition **b** : a fact or event of scientific interest susceptible of scientific description and explanation

phe·no·thi·azine \ˌfē-nō-ˈthī-ə-ˌzēn\ *n* **1** : a greenish yellow crystalline compound $C_{12}H_9NS$ used as an anthelmintic and insecticide esp. in veterinary practice **2** : any of various phenothiazine derivatives (as chlorpromazine) that are used as tranquilizing agents esp. in the treatment of schizophrenia

phe·no·type \ˈfē-nə-ˌtīp\ *n* : the visible properties of an organism that are produced by the interaction of the genotype and the environment — compare GENOTYPE — **phe·no·typ·ic** \ˌfē-nə-ˈti-pik\ *also* **phe·no·typ·i·cal** \-pi-kəl\ *adj* — **phe·no·typ·i·cal·ly** *adv*

phe·noxy·ben·za·mine \fi-ˌnäk-sē-ˈben-zə-ˌmēn\ *n* : a drug $C_{18}H_{22}ClNO$ that blocks the activity of alpha-receptors and is used in the form of its hydrochloride esp. to produce peripheral vasodilation

phe·noxy·meth·yl penicillin \-ˈmeth-ᵊl-\ *n* : PENICILLIN V

phen·pro·cou·mon \ˌfen-prō-ˈkü-ˌmän\ *n* : an anticoagulant drug $C_{18}H_{16}O_3$

phen·sux·i·mide \ˌfen-ˈsək-si-ˌmid\ *n* : an anticonvulsant drug $C_{11}H_{11}NO_2$ used esp. in the control of petit mal epilepsy — see MILONTIN

phen·ter·mine \ˈfen-tər-ˌmēn\ *n* : a drug $C_{10}H_{15}N$ used often in the form of its hydrochloride as an appetite suppressant

phen·tol·amine \fen-ˈtä-lə-ˌmēn, -mən\ *n* : an adrenergic blocking agent $C_{17}H_{19}N_3O$ that is used esp. in the diagnosis and treatment of hypertension due to pheochromocytoma — see REGITINE

phe·nyl \ˈfen-ᵊl, ˈfēn-\ *n* : a chemical group C_6H_5 that has a valence of one and is derived from benzene by removal of one hydrogen atom — often used in combination

phe·nyl·al·a·nine \ˌfen-ᵊl-ˈa-lə-ˌnēn, ˌfēn-\ *n* : an essential amino acid $C_9H_{11}NO_2$ that is obtained in its levorotatory L form by the hydrolysis of proteins (as lactalbumin), that is essential in human nutrition, and that is converted in the normal body to tyrosine — see PHENYLKETONURIA, PHENYLPYRUVIC ACID

phenylalanine mustard *or* **L-phenylalanine mustard** \ˈel-\ *n* : MELPHALAN

phen·yl·bu·ta·zone \ˌfen-ᵊl-ˈbyü-tə-ˌzōn\ *n* : a drug $C_{19}H_{20}N_2O_2$ that is used for its analgesic and anti-inflammatory properties esp. in the treatment of arthritis, gout, and bursitis — see BUTAZOLIDIN

phen·yl·eph·rine \ˌfen-ᵊl-ˈe-ˌfrēn, -frən\ *n* : a sympathomimetic agent $C_9H_{13}NO_2$ that is used in the form of the hydrochloride as a vasoconstrictor, a mydriatic, and by injection to raise the blood pressure — see NEO-SYNEPHRINE

phe·nyl·eth·yl alcohol \ˌfen-ᵊl-ˈeth-ᵊl-, ˌfēn-\ *n* : a fragrant liquid alcohol $C_8H_{10}O$ that is used as an antibacterial agent in ophthalmic solutions with limited effectiveness

phe·nyl·eth·yl·amine \ˌfen-ᵊl-ˌeth-ᵊl-ˈa-ˌmēn, ˌfēn-\ *n* : a neurotransmitter $C_8H_{11}N$ that is an amine resembling amphetamine in structure and physiological and pharmacological properties; *also* : any of its derivatives

phe·nyl·ke·ton·uria \ˌfen-ᵊl-ˌkē-tə-ˈnúr-ē-ə, ˌfēn-, -ˈnyúr-\ *n* : an inherited metabolic disease that is characterized by inability to oxidize a metabolic product of phenylalanine and by severe mental retardation — abbr. *PKU*; called *also* *phenylpyruvic amentia, phenylpyruvic oligophrenia*

¹phe·nyl·ke·ton·uric \-ˈnúr-ik, -ˈnyúr-\ *n* : one affected with phenylketonuria

²phenylketonuric *adj* : of, relating to, or affected with phenylketonuria

phen·yl·mer·cu·ric \ˌfen-ᵊl-mər-ˈkyúr-ik\ *adj* : of, relating to, or being the positively charged ion $C_6H_5Hg^+$

phenylmercuric acetate *n* : a crystalline salt $C_8H_8HgO_2$ used chiefly as a fungicide and herbicide

phenylmercuric nitrate *n* : a crystalline basic salt that is a mixture of $C_6H_5HgNO_3$ and C_6H_5HgOH used chiefly as a fungicide and antiseptic

phe·nyl·pro·pa·nol·amine \ˌfen-ᵊl-ˌprō-pə-ˈnó-lə-ˌmēn, -ˈnō-; -nō-ˈla-ˌmēn\ *n* : a sympathomimetic drug $C_9H_{13}NO$ used in the form of its hydrochloride esp. as a nasal and bronchial decongestant and as an appetite suppressant — abbr. *PPA*; see PROPADRINE

phe·nyl·py·ru·vic acid \ˌfen-ᵊl-pī-ˈrü-vik-, ˌfēn-\ *n* : a crystalline keto acid $C_9H_8O_3$ found in the urine as a metabolic product of phenylalanine esp. in phenylketonuria

phenylpyruvic amentia *n* : PHENYLKETONURIA

phenylpyruvic oligophrenia *n* : PHENYL-KETONURIA

phenyl salicylate *n* : a crystalline ester $C_{13}H_{10}O_3$ used as an ingredient of suntan preparations because of its ability to absorb ultraviolet light and also as an analgesic and antipyretic — called also *salol*

phen·yl·thio·car·ba·mide \,fen-ºl-,thī-ō-'kär-bə-,mīd\ *n* : a compound $C_7H_8N_2S$ that is extremely bitter or tasteless depending on the presence or absence of a single dominant gene in the taster — called also *PTC*

phen·yl·thio·urea \-,thī-ō-yu̇-'rē-ə\ *n* : PHENYLTHIOCARBAMIDE

phen·y·to·in \fə-'ni-tə-wən\ *n* : a crystalline anticonvulsant compound $C_{15}H_{12}N_2O_2$ used in the form of its sodium salt in the treatment of epilepsy — called also *diphenylhydantoin*; see DILANTIN

pheo·chro·mo·cy·to·ma \,fē-ə-,krō-mə-sə-'tō-mə, -sī-\ *n, pl* **-mas** *or* **-ma·ta** \-mə-tə\ : a tumor that is derived from chromaffin cells and is usu. associated with paroxysmal or sustained hypertension

phe·re·sis \fə-'rē-səs\ *n, pl* **phe·re·ses** \-,sēz\ : removal of blood from a donor's body, separation of a blood component (as plasma or white blood cells), and transfusion of the remaining blood components back into the donor — called also *apheresis*; see PLASMAPHERESIS, PLATELETPHERESIS

pher·o·mone \'fer-ə-,mōn\ *n* : a chemical substance that is produced by an animal and serves esp. as a stimulus to other individuals of the same species for one or more behavioral responses — **pher·o·mon·al** \,fer-ə-'mōn-ºl\ *adj*

PhG *abbr* graduate in pharmacy

phi·al \'fīl\ *n* : VIAL

Phi·a·loph·o·ra \,fī-ə-'lä-fə-rə\ *n* : a genus (family Dematiaceae) of imperfect fungi of which some forms are important in human mycotic infections (as chromoblastomycosis)

¹-phil \,fil\ *or* **-phile** \,fīl\ *n comb form* : lover : one having an affinity for or a strong attraction to (acido*phil*)

²-phil *or* **-phile** *adj comb form* : loving : having a fondness or affinity for (hemo*phile*)

Philadelphia chromosome *n* : an abnormally short chromosome 22 that is found in the hematopoietic cells of persons suffering from chronic myelogenous leukemia and lacks the major part of its long arm which has usu. undergone translocation to chromosome 9

-phil·ia \'fi-lē-ə\ *n comb form* **1** : tendency toward (hemo*philia*) **2** : abnormal appetite or liking for (necro*philia*)

-phil·iac \'fi-lē-,ak\ *n comb form* **1** : one having a tendency toward (hemo*philiac*) **2** : one having an abnor-mal appetite or liking for (copro*philiac*)

-phil·ic \'fi-lik\ *adj comb form* : having an affinity for : loving (acido*philic*)

phil·trum \'fil-trəm\ *n, pl* **phil·tra** \-trə\ : the vertical groove on the median line of the upper lip

phi·mo·sis \fī-'mō-səs, fi-\ *n, pl* **phi·mo·ses** \-,sēz\ : tightness or constriction of the orifice of the prepuce arising either congenitally or from inflammation, congestion, or other postnatal causes and making it impossible to bare the glans

phi phenomenon \'fī-\ *n* : the appearance of motion resulting from an orderly sequence of stimuli (as lights flashed in rapid succession a short distance apart on a sign) without any actual motion being presented to the eye

phleb- *or* **phlebo-** *comb form* : vein (*phleb*itis)

phle·bi·tis \fli-'bī-təs\ *n, pl* **phle·bit·i·des** \-'bi-tə-,dēz\ : inflammation of a vein

phle·bo·gram \'flē-bə-,gram\ *n* **1** : a tracing made with a sphygmograph that records the pulse in a vein **2** : a roentgenogram of a vein after injection of a radiopaque medium

phle·bo·graph \-,graf\ *n* : a sphygmograph adapted for recording the venous pulse

phle·bog·ra·phy \fli-'bä-grə-fē\ *n, pl* **-phies** : the process of making phlebograms — **phle·bo·graph·ic** \,flē-bə-'gra-fik\ *adj*

phle·bo·lith \'flē-bə-,lith\ *n* : a calculus in a vein usu. resulting from the calcification of an old thrombus

phle·bol·o·gist \fli-'bä-lə-jist\ *n* : a specialist in phlebology

phle·bol·o·gy \fli-'bä-lə-jē\ *n, pl* **-gies** : a branch of medicine concerned with the veins

phle·bo·throm·bo·sis \,flē-bō-thräm-'bō-səs\ *n, pl* **-bo·ses** \-,sēz\ : venous thrombosis accompanied by little or no inflammation — compare THROMBOPHLEBITIS

phle·bot·o·mist \fli-'bä-tə-mist\ *n* : one who practices phlebotomy

phle·bot·o·mize \fli-'bä-tə-,mīz\ *vb* **-mized; -miz·ing** : to draw blood from : BLEED

phle·bot·o·mus \fli-'bä-tə-məs\ *n* **1** *cap* : a genus of small bloodsucking sand flies (family Psychodidae) including one (*P. papatasii*) that is the carrier of sandfly fever and others suspected of carrying other human disease **2** *pl* **-mi** \-,mī\ *also* **-mus·es** : any sand fly of the genus *Phlebotomus*

phlebotomus fever *n* : SANDFLY FEVER

phle·bot·o·my \fli-'bä-tə-mē\ *n, pl* **-mies** : the letting of blood for transfusion, pheresis, diagnostic testing, or experimental procedures and esp. formerly for the treatment of disease — called also *venesection, venotomy*

phlegm \\'flem\\ n : viscid mucus secreted in abnormal quantity in the respiratory passages

phleg·ma·sia \\fleg-'mā-zhə, -zhē-ə\\ n, pl **-siae** \\-zhē, -zhē-ē\\ : INFLAMMATION

phlegmasia al·ba do·lens \\-'al-bə-'dō-lenz\\ n : MILK LEG

phlegmasia ce·ru·lea dolens \\-sə-'rü-lē-ə-\\ n : severe thrombophlebitis with extreme pain, edema, cyanosis, and possible ischemic necrosis

phleg·mon \\'fleg-män\\ n : purulent inflammation and infiltration of connective tissue — compare ABSCESS — **phleg·mon·ous** \\'fleg-mə-nəs\\ adj

phlor·e·tin \\'flōr-ət-ən, flə-'rēt-ən\\ n : a crystalline phenolic ketone $C_{15}H_{14}O_5$ that is a potent inhibitor of transport systems for sugars and anions

phlo·ri·zin or **phlo·rhi·zin** \\'flōr-ə-zən, flə-'riz-ən\\ or **phlo·rid·zin** \\'flōr-əd-zən, flə-'rid-zən\\ n : a bitter crystalline glucoside $C_{21}H_{24}O_{10}$ used chiefly in producing experimental diabetes in animals

phlyc·ten·u·lar \\flik-'ten-yə-lər\\ adj : marked by or associated with phlyctenules (~ conjunctivitis)

phlyc·te·nule \\flik-'ten-(,)yül; 'flik-tə-,nül, -,nyül\\ n : a small vesicle or pustule; esp : one on the conjunctiva or cornea of the eye

PHN abbr public health nurse

-phobe \\,fōb\\ n comb form : one fearing or averse to (something specified) (chromophobe)

pho·bia \\'fō-bē-ə\\ n : an exaggerated and often disabling fear usu. inexplicable to the subject and having sometimes a logical but usu. an illogical or symbolic object, class of objects, or situation — compare COMPULSION, OBSESSION

-pho·bia \\'fō-bē-ə\\ n comb form 1 : abnormal fear of (acrophobia) 2 : intolerance or aversion for (photophobia)

pho·bi·ac \\'fō-bē-,ak\\ n : PHOBIC

¹pho·bic \\'fō-bik\\ adj : of, relating to, affected with, or constituting phobia

²phobic n : one who exhibits a phobia

-pho·bic \\'fō-bik\\ or **-pho·bous** \\-fə-bəs\\ adj comb form 1 : having an aversion for or fear of (agoraphobic) 2 : lacking affinity for (hydrophobic)

phobic reaction n : a psychoneurosis in which the principal symptom is a phobia

pho·co·me·lia \\,fō-kə-'mē-lē-ə\\ n : a congenital deformity in which the limbs are extremely shortened so that the feet and hands arise close to the trunk — **pho·co·me·lic** \\-'mē-lik\\ adj

pho·co·mel·us \\fō-'kä-mə-ləs\\ n, pl **-li** \\-,lī\\ : an individual exhibiting phocomelia

phon \\'fän\\ n : the unit of loudness on a scale beginning at zero for the faintest audible sound and corresponding to the decibel scale of sound intensity with the number of phons of a given sound being equal to the decibels of a pure 1000-cycle tone judged by the average listener to be equal in loudness to the given sound

phon- or **phono-** comb form : sound : voice : speech : tone (phonation)

pho·na·tion \\fō-'nā-shən\\ n : the production of vocal sounds and esp. speech — **pho·nate** \\'fō-,nāt\\ vb

-pho·nia \\'fō-nē-ə, 'fōn-yə\\ or **-pho·ny** \\fə-nē\\ n comb form, pl **-phonias** or **-phonies** : speech disorder (of a specified type esp. relating to phonation) (dysphonia)

pho·no·car·dio·gram \\,fō-nə-'kär-dē-ə-,gram\\ n : a record of heart sounds made by means of a phonocardiograph

pho·no·car·dio·graph \\-,graf\\ n : an instrument used for producing a graphic record of heart sounds

pho·no·car·di·og·ra·phy \\-,kär-dē-'ä-grə-fē\\ n, pl **-phies** : the recording of heart sounds by means of a phonocardiograph — **pho·no·car·dio·graph·ic** \\-,kär-dē-ə-'gra-fik\\ adj

phor·bol \\'fōr-,bōl, -,bōl\\ n : an alcohol $C_{20}H_{28}O_6$ that is the parent compound of tumor-promoting esters occurring in croton oil

-pho·re·sis \\fə-'rē-səs\\ n comb form : transmission (electrophoresis)

pho·ria \\'fō-rē-ə\\ n : any of various tendencies of the lines of vision to deviate from the normal when binocular fusion of the retinal images is prevented

-pho·ria \\'fōr-ē-ə\\ n comb form : bearing : state : tendency (euphoria) (heterophoria)

-phor·ic \\'fōr-ik\\ adj comb form : having (such) a bearing or tendency (thanatophoric)

Phor·mia \\'fōr-mē-ə\\ n : a genus of dipteran flies (family Calliphoridae) including one (C. regina) causing myiasis in sheep

phos- comb form : light (phosphene)

phos·gene \\'fäz-,jēn\\ n : a colorless gas $COCl_2$ of unpleasant odor that is a severe respiratory irritant and has been used in chemical warfare

phosph- or **phospho-** comb form : phosphoric acid : phosphate (phospholipid)

phos·pha·gen \\'fäs-fə-jən, -,jen\\ n : any of several phosphate compounds (as phosphocreatine) occurring esp. in muscle and releasing energy on hydrolysis of the phosphate

phos·pha·tase \\'fäs-fə-,tās, -,tāz\\ n : an enzyme that accelerates the hydrolysis and synthesis of organic esters of phosphoric acid and the transfer of phosphate groups to other compounds: **a** : ALKALINE PHOSPHATASE **b** : ACID PHOSPHATASE

phos·phate \\'fäs-,fāt\\ n 1 **a** : a salt or ester of a phosphoric acid **b** : the negatively charged ion PO_4^{3-} having a chemical valence of three and derived from phosphoric acid H_3PO_4 2 : an organic compound of phosphoric acid in which the acid group is bound to nitrogen or a carboxyl group in a way that permits useful energy to be released (as in metabolism)

phos·pha·tide \'fäs-fə-₁tīd\ *n* : PHOSPHOLIPID

phos·pha·tid·ic acid \₁fäs-fə-'ti-dik-\ *n* : any of several acids (RCOO)₂C₃H₅OPO₃H₂ that are formed from phosphatides and yield on hydrolysis two fatty-acid molecules RCOOH and one molecule each of glycerol and phosphoric acid

phos·pha·ti·dyl·cho·line \₁fäs-fə-₁tīd-ºl-'kō-₁lēn, (₁)fäs-fa-təd-ºl-\ *n* : LECITHIN

phos·pha·ti·dyl·eth·a·nol·amine \-₁e-thə-'nä-lə-₁mēn, -'nō-\ *n* : any of a group of phospholipids that occur esp. in blood plasma and in the white matter of the central nervous system — called also *cephalin*

phos·pha·ti·dyl·ser·ine \-'ser-₁ēn\ *n* : a phospholipid found in mammalian cells

phos·pha·tu·ria \₁fäs-fə-'tùr-ē-ə, -'tyùr-\ *n* : the excessive discharge of phosphates in the urine

phos·phene \'fäs-₁fēn\ *n* : a luminous impression that occurs when the retina undergoes stimulation (as by pressure on the eyeball when the lid is closed)

phospho- — see PHOSPH-

phos·pho·cre·atine \₁fäs-(₁)fō-'krē-ə-₁tēn\ *n* : a compound $C_4H_{10}N_3O_5P$ of creatine and phosphoric acid that is found esp. in vertebrate muscle where it is an energy source for muscle contraction — called also *creatine phosphate*

phos·pho·di·es·ter·ase \-dī-'es-tə-₁rās, -₁rāz\ *n* : a phosphatase (as from snake venom) that acts on compounds (as some nucleotides) having two ester groups to hydrolyze only one of the groups

phos·pho·di·es·ter bond \-dī-'es-tər-\ *n* : a covalent bond in RNA or DNA that holds a polynucleotide chain together by joining a phosphate group at position 5 in the pentose sugar of one nucleotide to the hydroxyl group at position 3 in the pentose sugar of the next nucleotide — called also *phosphodiester linkage*

phos·pho·enol·pyr·uvate \'fäs-₁fō-ə-₁nōl-pī-'rü-₁vāt, -nōl-, -₁pīr-'yü-\ *n* : a salt or ester of phosphoenolpyruvic acid

phos·pho·enol·pyr·uvic acid \-pī-'rü-vik-, -₁pīr-'yü-vik-\ *n* : a phosphate $H_2C=C(OPO_3H_2)COOH$ formed as an intermediate in carbohydrate metabolism

phos·pho·fruc·to·ki·nase \₁fäs-(₁)fō-₁frək-tō-'kī-₁nās, -₁frük-, -₁frük-, -₁nāz\ *n* : an enzyme that functions in carbohydrate metabolism and esp. in

glycolysis by catalyzing the transfer of a second phosphate (as from ATP) to fructose

phos·pho·glu·co·mu·tase \-₁glü-kō-'myü-₁tās, -₁tāz\ *n* : an enzyme that catalyzes the reversible isomerization of glucose-1-phosphate to glucose-6-phosphate

phos·pho·glu·co·nate \-'glü-kə-₁nāt\ *n* : a compound formed by dehydrogenation of glucose-6-phosphate as the first step in a glucose degradation pathway alternative to the Krebs cycle

phosphogluconate dehydrogenase *n* : an enzyme that catalyzes the oxidative decarboxylation of phosphogluconate with the generation of NADPH

phos·pho·glyc·er·al·de·hyde \-₁gli-sə-'ral-də-₁hīd\ *n* : a phosphate of glyceraldehyde $C_3H_5O_3(H_2PO_3)$ that is formed esp. in anaerobic metabolism of carbohydrates by the splitting of a diphosphate of fructose

phos·pho·ino·si·tide \-i-'nō-sə-₁tīd\ *n* : any of a group of inositol-containing derivatives of phosphatidic acid that do not contain nitrogen and are found in the brain

phos·pho·ki·nase \₁fäs-fō-'kī-₁nās, -₁nāz\ *n* : KINASE

phos·pho·li·pase \-'lī-₁pās, -₁pāz\ *n* : any of several enzymes that hydrolyze lecithins or phosphatidylethanolamines — called also *lecithinase*

phos·pho·lip·id \-'li-pəd\ *n* : any of numerous lipids (as lecithins and sphingomyelin) in which phosphoric acid as well as a fatty acid is esterified to glycerol and which are found in all living cells and in the bilayers of plasma membranes — called also *phosphatide*

phos·pho·lip·in \-'li-pən\ *n* : PHOSPHOLIPID

phos·pho·mono·es·ter·ase \-₁mä-nō-'es-tə-₁rās, -₁rāz\ *n* : a phosphatase that acts on esters containing only a single ester group

phos·pho·pro·tein \₁fäs-fō-'prō-₁tēn\ *n* : any of various proteins (as casein) that contain combined phosphoric acid

phosphor- *or* **phosphoro-** *comb form* : phosphoric acid ⟨*phosphoro*lysis⟩

phos·pho·ri·bo·syl·py·ro·phos·phate \₁fäs-fō-₁rī-bə-₁sil-₁pī-rō-'fäs-₁fāt\ *n* : a substance that is formed enzymatically from ATP and the phosphate of ribose and that plays a fundamental role in nucleotide synthesis

phosphoribosyltransferase — see HYPOXANTHINE-GUANINE PHOSPHORIBOSYLTRANSFERASE

phos·phor·ic \fäs-'fȯr-ik, -'fär-; 'fäs-fə-rik\ *adj* : of, relating to, or containing phosphorus esp. with a valence higher than in phosphorous compounds

phosphoric acid *n* 1 : a syrupy or deliquescent acid H_3PO_4 having three replaceable hydrogen atoms — called also *orthophosphoric acid* **2** : a compound consisting of phosphate groups linked directly to each other by oxygen

phos·pho·rol·y·sis \ˌfäs-fə-ˈrä-lə-səs\ *n, pl* **-y·ses** \-ˌsēz\ : a reversible reaction analogous to hydrolysis in which phosphoric acid functions in a manner similar to that of water with the formation of a phosphate (as glucose-1-phosphate in the breakdown of liver glycogen) — **phos·pho·ro·lyt·ic** \-rō-ˈli-tik\ *adj*

phos·pho·rous \ˈfäs-fə-rəs, fäs-ˈfōr-əs\ *adj* : of, relating to, or containing phosphorus esp. with a valence lower than in phosphoric compounds

phos·pho·rus \ˈfäs-fə-rəs\ *n, often attrib* : a nonmetallic element that occurs widely in combined form esp. as inorganic phosphates in minerals, soils, natural waters, bones, and teeth and as organic phosphates in all living cells — symbol *P*; see ELEMENT table

phosphorus 32 *n* : a heavy radioactive isotope of phosphorus having a mass number of 32 and a half-life of 14.3 days that is produced in nuclear reactors and used chiefly in tracer studies (as in biology and in chemical analysis) and in medical diagnosis (as in location of tumors) and therapy (as of polycythemia vera) — symbol P^{32} or ^{32}P

phos·phor·y·lase \ˈfäs-ˈfōr-ə-ˌlāz\ *n* : any of a group of enzymes that catalyze phosphorolysis with the formation of organic phosphates (as glucose-1-phosphate in the breakdown and synthesis of glycogen)

phos·phor·y·la·tion \ˌfäs-ˌfōr-ə-ˈlā-shən\ *n* : the process by which a chemical compound takes up or combines with phosphoric acid or a phosphorus-containing group; *esp* : the enzymatic conversion of carbohydrates into their phosphoric esters in metabolic processes — **phos·phor·y·late** \ˈfäs-ˈfōr-ə-ˌlāt\ *vb* — **phos·phor·y·la·tive** \ˌfäs-ˌfōr-ə-ˈlā-tiv\ *adj*

phos·phor·yl·cho·line \ˌfäs-fə-ˌril-ˈkō-ˌlēn\ *n* : a hapten used medicinally in the form of its chloride $C_5H_{15}ClNO_4P$ to treat hepatobiliary dysfunction

phos·pho·trans·fer·ase \ˌfäs-fō-ˈtrans-(ˌ)fər-ˌās, -ˌāz\ *n* : any of several enzymes that catalyze the transfer of phosphorus-containing groups from one compound to another

phos·sy jaw \ˈfä-sē-\ *n* : a jawbone destroyed by chronic phosphorus poisoning

phot- *or* **photo-** *comb form* : light : radiant energy ⟨*photo*dermatitis⟩

pho·tic \ˈfō-tik\ *adj* : of, relating to, or involving light esp. in relation to organisms ⟨∼ stimulation⟩ — **pho·ti·cal·ly** *adv*

pho·to·ac·ti·va·tion \ˌfō-tō-ˌak-tə-ˈvā-shən\ *n* : the process of activating a

substance by means of radiant energy and esp. light — **pho·to·ac·ti·vate** \-ˈak-tə-ˌvāt\ *vb* — **pho·to·ac·tive** \-ˈak-tiv\ *adj* — **pho·to·ac·tiv·i·ty** \-ˌak-ˈti-və-tē\ *n*

pho·to·ag·ing \ˌfō-tō-ˈā-jiŋ\ *n* : the long-term negative effects on skin (as increased susceptibility to wrinkles and cancer) of exposure to sunlight — **pho·to·aged** \-ˈājd\ *adj*

pho·to·al·ler·gic \ˌfō-tō-ə-ˈlər-jik\ *adj* : of, relating to, caused by, or affected with a photoallergy ⟨∼ dermatitis⟩

pho·to·al·ler·gy \-ˈa-lər-jē\ *n, pl* **-gies** : an allergic sensitivity to light

pho·to·bi·ol·o·gy \-(ˌ)bī-ˈä-lə-jē\ *n, pl* **-gies** : a branch of biology that deals with the effects of radiant energy (as light) on living things — **pho·to·bi·ol·o·gist** \ˌfō-tō-(ˌ)bī-ˈä-lə-jist\ *n*

pho·to·chem·i·cal \ˌfō-tō-ˈke-mi-kəl\ *adj* : of, relating to, or resulting from the chemical action of radiant energy and esp. light ⟨∼ smog⟩

pho·to·che·mo·ther·a·py \-ˌkē-mō-ˈther-ə-pē\ *n, pl* **-pies** : treatment esp. for psoriasis in which administration of a photosensitizing drug (as methoxsalen) is followed by exposure to ultraviolet radiation or sunlight

¹pho·to·chro·mic \ˌfō-tə-ˈkrō-mik\ *adj* **1** : capable of changing color on exposure to radiant energy (as light) ⟨eyeglasses with ∼ lenses⟩ **2** : of, relating to, or utilizing the change of color shown by a photochromic substance ⟨a ∼ process⟩ — **pho·to·chro·mism** \-ˌmi-zəm\ *n*

²photochromic *n* : a photochromic substance — usu. used in pl.

pho·to·co·ag·u·la·tion \-kō-ˌa-gyə-ˈlā-shən\ *n* : a surgical process of coagulating tissue by means of a precisely oriented high-energy light source (as a laser beam) — **pho·to·co·ag·u·la·tor** \-kō-ˈa-gyə-ˌlā-tər\ *n*

pho·to·con·vul·sive \ˌfō-tō-kən-ˈvəl-siv\ *adj* : of or relating to an abnormal electroencephalogram produced in response to a flickering light

pho·to·der·ma·ti·tis \ˌdər-mə-ˈtī-təs\ *n, pl* **-ti·tis·es** *or* **-tit·i·des** \-ˈti-tə-ˌdēz\ : any dermatitis caused or precipitated by exposure to light

pho·to·der·ma·to·sis \-ˌdər-mə-ˈtō-səs\ *n, pl* **-to·ses** \-ˌsēz\ : any dermatosis produced by exposure to light

pho·to·dy·nam·ic \-dī-ˈna-mik\ *adj* : of, relating to, or having the property of intensifying or inducing a toxic reaction to light (as the destruction of cancer cells stained with a light-sensitive dye) in a living system

pho·to·flu·o·rog·ra·phy \-(ˌ)flü-ə-ˈrä-grə-fē\ *n, pl* **-phies** : the photography of the image produced on a fluorescent screen by X rays — **pho·to·flu·o·ro·graph·ic** \-ˈflür-ə-ˈgra-fik\ *adj*

pho·to·gen·ic \ˌfō-tə-ˈje-nik\ *adj* **1** : produced or precipitated by light ⟨∼ epilepsy) ⟨~ dermatitis⟩ 2 : producing or generating light ⟨~ bacteria⟩

pho·tom·e·ter \fō-'tä-mə-tər\ n : an instrument for measuring the intensity of light

pho·to·mi·cro·graph \ˌfō-tə-'mī-krə-ˌgraf\ n : a photograph of a magnified image of a small object — called also *microphotograph* — **pho·to·mi·cro·graph·ic** \-ˌmī-krə-'gra-fik\ adj — **pho·to·mi·cro·graph·i·cal·ly** adv — **pho·to·mi·crog·ra·phy** \-mī-'krä-grə-fē\ n

pho·ton \'fō-ˌtän\ n 1 : a unit of intensity of light at the retina equal to the illumination received per square millimeter of a pupillary area from a surface having a brightness of one candle per square meter — called also *troland* 2 : a quantum of electromagnetic radiation — **pho·ton·ic** \fō-'tä-nik\ adj

pho·to·patch test \'fō-tō-ˌpach-\ n : a test of the capability of a particular substance to photosensitize a particular human skin in which the substance is applied to the skin under a patch and the area is irradiated with ultraviolet light

pho·to·pho·bia \ˌfō-tə-'fō-bē-ə\ n 1 : intolerance to light; *esp* : painful sensitiveness to strong light 2 : an abnormal fear of light — **pho·to·pho·bic** \-'fō-bik\ adj

phot·oph·thal·mia \ˌfōt-ˌäf-'thal-mē-ə, -ˌäp-\ n : inflammation of the eye and esp. of the cornea and conjunctiva caused by exposure to light of short wavelength (as ultraviolet light)

phot·opic \fōt-'ō-pik, -'ä-\ adj : relating to or being vision in bright light with light-adapted eyes that is mediated by the cones of the retina

pho·to·pig·ment \'fō-tō-ˌpig-mənt\ n : a pigment (as a compound in the retina) that undergoes a physical or chemical change under the action of light

pho·top·sia \fō-'täp-sē-ə\ n : the perception of light (as luminous rays or flashes) that is purely subjective and accompanies a pathological condition esp. of the retina or brain

pho·to·re·cep·tor \ˌfō-tō-ri-'sep-tər\ n : a receptor for light stimuli

pho·to·scan \'fō-tō-ˌskan\ n : a photographic representation of variation in tissue state (as of the kidney) determined by gamma-ray emission from an injected radioactive substance — **photoscan** vb

pho·to·sen·si·tive \ˌfō-tō-'sen-sə-tiv\ adj : sensitive or sensitized to the action of radiant energy — **pho·to·sen·si·tiv·i·ty** \-ˌsen-sə-'ti-və-tē\ n

pho·to·sen·si·tize \-'sen-sə-ˌtīz\ vb -tized; -tiz·ing : to make sensitive to the influence of radiant energy and esp. light — **pho·to·sen·si·ti·za·tion** \-ˌsen-sə-tə-'zā-shən\ n — **pho·to·sen·si·tiz·er** n

pho·to·syn·the·sis \-'sin-thə-səs\ n, pl -the·ses \-ˌsēz\ : the formation of carbohydrates from carbon dioxide and a source of hydrogen (as water) in chlorophyll-containing cells (as of green plants) exposed to light involving a photochemical release of oxygen through the decomposition of water followed by various enzymatic synthetic reactions that usu. do not require the presence of light — **pho·to·syn·the·size** \-ˌsīz\ vb — **pho·to·syn·thet·ic** \-sin-'the-tik\ adj — **pho·to·syn·thet·i·cal·ly** adv

pho·to·ther·a·py \-'ther-ə-pē\ n, pl -pies : the application of light for therapeutic purposes

pho·to·tox·ic \ˌfō-tō-'täk-sik\ adj 1 *of a substance ingested or brought into contact with skin* : rendering the skin susceptible to damage (as sunburn or blisters) upon exposure to light and esp. ultraviolet light 2 : induced by a phototoxic substance (a ~ response) — **pho·to·tox·ic·i·ty** \-täk-'si-sə-tē\ n

phren- or **phreno-** comb form 1 : mind ⟨*phreno*logy⟩ 2 : diaphragm ⟨*phreni*cotomy⟩

phren·em·phrax·is \ˌfren-em-'frak-səs\ n, pl -**phrax·es** \-ˌsēz\ : crushing of the phrenic nerve for therapeutic reasons

phreni- comb form : phrenic nerve ⟨*phreni*cotomy⟩

-phre·nia \'frē-nē-ə, 'fre-\ n comb form : disordered condition of mental functions ⟨hebe*phrenia*⟩

¹**phren·ic** \'fre-nik\ adj : of or relating to the diaphragm

²**phrenic** n : PHRENIC NERVE

phrenic artery n : any of the several arteries supplying the diaphragm: **a** : either of two arising from the thoracic aorta and distributed over the upper surface of the diaphragm — called also *superior phrenic artery* **b** : either of two that arise from the abdominal aorta and that supply the underside of the diaphragm and the adrenal glands — called also *inferior phrenic artery*

phren·i·cec·to·my \ˌfre-nə-'sek-tə-mē\ n, pl -**mies** : surgical removal of part of a phrenic nerve to secure collapse of a diseased lung — compare PHRENICOTOMY

phrenic nerve n : a general motor and sensory nerve on each side of the body that arises chiefly from the fourth cervical nerve, passes down through the thorax to the diaphragm, and supplies or gives off branches supplying esp. the pericardium, pleura, and diaphragm — called also *phrenic*

phren·i·cot·o·my \ˌfre-ni-'kä-tə-mē\ n, pl -**mies** : surgical division of a phrenic nerve to secure collapse of a diseased lung — compare PHRENICECTOMY

phrenic vein n : any of the veins that drain the diaphragm and accompany the phrenic arteries: **a** : one that accompanies the pericardiophrenic artery and usu. empties into the internal thoracic vein — called also *superior phrenic vein* **b** : any of two or three veins which follow the course of the inferior phrenic arteries and of which the one on the right empties into the inferior vena cava and the one or two on the left empty into the left renal or suprarenal vein or the inferior vena cava — called also *inferior phrenic vein*

phreno- — see PHREN-

phre·nol·o·gy \fri-ʹnä-lə-jē\ *n, pl* **-gies** : the study of the conformation of the skull based on the belief that it is indicative of mental faculties and character — **phre·no·log·i·cal** \fri-ʹnä-lə-jist\ *n*

phry·no·der·ma \ˌfrī-nə-ʹdər-mə\ *n* : a rough dry skin eruption marked by keratosis and usu. associated with vitamin A deficiency

PHS *abbr* Public Health Service

phthal·yl·sul·fa·thi·a·zole \ˌtha-ˌlil-ˌsəl-fə-ʹthī-ə-ˌzōl\ *n* : a sulfonamide $C_{17}H_{13}N_3O_5S_2$ used in the treatment of intestinal infections

phthi·ri·a·sis \thə-ʹrī-ə-səs, thī-\ *n, pl* **-a·ses** \-ˌsēz\ : PEDICULOSIS; *esp* : infestation with crab lice

Phthir·i·us \ʹthir-ē-əs\ *n* : a genus of lice (family Phthiriidae) containing the crab louse (*P. pubis*)

Phthi·rus \ʹthī-rəs\ *n, syn of* PHTHIRIUS

phthi·sic \ʹti-zik, ʹti-sik\ *n* : PHTHISIS — **phthisic** *or* **phthis·i·cal** \ʹti-zi-kəl, ʹti-si-\ *adj*

phthisio- *comb form* : phthisis ⟨*phthisiology*⟩

phthis·i·ol·o·gy \ˌti-zē-ʹä-lə-jē, ˌthi-\ *n, pl* **-gies** : the care, treatment, and study of tuberculosis — **phthis·i·ol·o·gist** \-jist\ *n*

phthi·sis \ʹtī-səs, ʹthī-, ʹti-, ʹthi-\ *n, pl* **phthi·ses** \-ˌsēz\ : a progressively wasting or consumptive condition; *esp* : pulmonary tuberculosis

phthisis bul·bi \-ʹbəl-ˌbī\ *n* : wasting and shrinkage of the eyeball following destructive diseases of the eye (as panophthalmitis)

phy·co·my·cete \ˌfī-kō-ʹmī-ˌsēt, -ˌmī-ʹsēt\ *n* : any of a group of lower fungi that are in many respects similar to algae and are often grouped in a class (Phycomycetes) or separated into two major taxonomic groups (Mastigomycotina and Zygomycotina)

phy·co·my·co·sis \-ˌmī-ʹkō-səs\, *n, pl* **-co·ses** \-ˌkō-ˌsēz\ : any mycosis caused by a phycomycete (as of the genera *Rhizopus and Mucor*)

phyl- *or* **phylo-** *comb form* : tribe : race : phylum ⟨*phylogeny*⟩

phyl·lode \ʹfi-ˌlōd\ *adj* : having a cross section that resembles a leaf ⟨~ tumors of the breast⟩

phyl·lo·qui·none   \ˌfi-lō-kwi-ʹnōn, -ʹkwi-ˌnōn\ *n* : VITAMIN K 1a

phy·log·e·ny \fī-ʹlä-jə-nē\ *n, pl* **-nies** 1 : the evolutionary history of a kind of organism 2 : the evolution of a genetically related group of organisms as distinguished from the development of the individual organism — compare ONTOGENY — **phy·lo·ge·net·ic** \ˌfī-lō-jə-ʹne-tik\ *adj* — **phy·lo·ge·net·i·cal·ly** *adv*

phy·lum \ʹfī-ləm\ *n, pl* **phy·la** \-lə\ : a major group of animals or in some classifications plants sharing one or more fundamental characteristics that set them apart from all other animals and plants

phys *abbr* **1** physical **2** physician **3** physiological

phy·sa·lia \fī-ʹsā-lē-ə\ *n* **1** *cap* : a genus of large oceanic siphonophores (family Physaliidae) including the Portuguese man-of-wars **2** : any siphonophore of the genus *Physalia*

Phy·sa·lop·tera \ˌfī-sə-ʹläp-tə-rə, ˌfi-\ *n* : a large genus of nematode worms (family Physalopteridae) parasitic in the digestive tract of various vertebrates including humans

physes *pl of* PHYSIS

physi- *or* **physio-** *comb form* **1** : physical ⟨*physio*therapy⟩ **2** : physiological and ⟨*physio*pathologic⟩

phys·i·at·rics \ˌfi-zē-ʹa-triks\ *n* : PHYSICAL MEDICINE

phys·i·at·rist \ˌfi-zē-ʹa-trist\ *n* : a physician who specializes in physical medicine

¹**phys·ic** \ʹfi-zik\ *n* **1 a** : the art or practice of healing disease **b** : the practice or profession of medicine **2** : a medicinal agent or preparation; *esp* : PURGATIVE

²**physic** *vb* **phys·icked; phys·ick·ing** : to treat with or administer medicine to; *esp* : PURGE

¹**phys·i·cal** \ʹfi-zi-kəl\ *adj* **1** : having material existence : perceptible esp. through the senses and subject to the laws of nature **2** : of or relating to the body — **phys·i·cal·ly** *adv*

²**physical** *n* : PHYSICAL EXAMINATION

physical examination *n* : an examination of the bodily functions and condition of an individual

physical medicine *n* : a branch of medicine concerned with the diagnosis and treatment of disease and disability by physical means (as radiation, heat, and electricity)

physical sign *n* : an indication of bodily condition that can be directly perceived

physical therapist *n* : a specialist in physical therapy — called also *physiotherapist*

physical therapy *n* : the treatment of disease by physical and mechanical means (as massage, regulated exercise, water, light, heat, and electricity) — called also *physiotherapy*

phy·si·cian \fə-ʹzi-shən\ *n* : a person skilled in the art of healing; *specif* : a doctor of medicine

physician's assistant *or* **physician assistant** *n* : a person who is certified to provide basic medical services (as the diagnosis and treatment of common ailments) usu. under the supervision of a licensed physician — called also *PA*

phys·i·co·chem·i·cal \ˌfi-zi-kō-ˈke-mi-kəl\ *adj* : being physical and chemical — **phys·i·co·chem·i·cal·ly** *adv*

physio- — see PHYSI-

phys·i·o·log·i·cal \ˌfi-zē-ə-ˈlä-ji-kəl\ *or* **phys·i·o·log·ic** \-jik\ *adj* **1** : of or relating to physiology **2** : characteristic of or appropriate to an organism's healthy or normal functioning **3** : differing in, involving, or affecting physiological factors ⟨a ~ strain of bacteria⟩ — **phys·i·o·log·i·cal·ly** *adv*

physiological chemistry *n* : a branch of science dealing with the chemical aspects of physiological and biological systems : BIOCHEMISTRY

physiological dead space *n* : the total dead space in the entire respiratory system including the alveoli — compare ANATOMICAL DEAD SPACE

physiological psychology *n* : PSYCHOPHYSIOLOGY

physiological saline *n* : a solution of a salt or salts that is essentially isotonic with tissue fluids or blood; *esp* : an approximately 0.9 percent solution of sodium chloride — called also *physiological saline solution, physiological salt solution*

phys·i·ol·o·gy \ˌfi-zē-ˈä-lə-jē\ *n, pl* **-gies 1** : a branch of biology that deals with the functions and activities of life or of living matter (as organs, tissues, or cells) and of the physical and chemical phenomena involved — compare ANATOMY 1, MORPHOLOGY 1 **2** : the organic processes and phenomena of an organism or any of its parts or of a particular bodily process ⟨~ of the thyroid gland⟩ **3** : a treatise on physiology — **phys·i·ol·o·gist** \-jist\ *n*

phys·i·o·pa·thol·o·gy \ˌfi-zē-ō-pə-ˈthä-lə-jē, -pa-\ *n, pl* **-gies** : a branch of biology or medicine that combines physiology and pathology esp. in the study of altered bodily function in disease — **phys·i·o·path·o·log·ic** \-ˌpa-thə-ˈlä-jik\ *or* **phys·i·o·path·o·log·i·cal** \-ji-kəl\ *adj*

phys·i·o·ther·a·peu·tic \ˌfi-zē-ō-ˌther-ə-ˈpyü-tik\ *adj* : of or relating to physical therapy

phys·i·o·ther·a·pist \-ˈther-ə-pist\ *n* : PHYSICAL THERAPIST

phys·i·o·ther·a·py \ˌfi-zē-ō-ˈther-ə-pē\ *n, pl* **-pies** : PHYSICAL THERAPY

phy·sique \fi-ˈzēk\ *n* : the form or structure of a person's body : bodily makeup ⟨a muscular ~⟩

phy·sis \ˈfī-səs\ *n, pl* **phy·ses** \-ˌsēz\ : GROWTH PLATE

Phy·so·ceph·a·lus \ˌfī-sə-ˈse-fə-ləs\ *n* : a genus of nematode worms (family Thelaziidae) including a common parasite (*P. sexalatus*) of the stomach and small intestine of swine

phy·so·stig·mine \ˌfi-sə-ˈstig-ˌmēn\ *n* : a crystalline tasteless alkaloid $C_{15}H_{21}N_3O_2$ from an African vine (*Physostigma venenosum*) of the legume family (Leguminosae) that is used esp. in the form of its salicylate for its anticholinesterase activity — called also *eserine*

phyt- *or* **phyto-** *comb form* : plant ⟨*phyto*toxin⟩

phy·tan·ic acid \fī-ˈta-nik-\ *n* : a fatty acid that accumulates in the blood and tissues of patients affected with Refsum's disease

-phyte \ˌfīt\ *n comb form* **1** : plant having a (specified) characteristic or habitat (*sapro*phyte) **2** : pathological growth (osteo*phyte*)

phy·tic acid \ˈfī-tik-\ *n* : an acid $C_6H_{18}P_6O_{24}$ that occurs in cereal grains and that when ingested interferes with the intestinal absorption of various minerals (as calcium and magnesium)

phy·to·be·zoar \ˌfī-tō-ˈbē-ˌzōr\ *n* : a concretion formed in the stomach or intestine and composed chiefly of undigested compacted vegetable fiber

phy·to·hem·ag·glu·ti·nin \ˌfī-tō-ˌhē-mə-ˈglüt-ᵊn-ən\ *n* : a proteinaceous hemagglutinin of plant origin used esp. to induce mitosis (as in lymphocytes) — abbr. *PHA*

phy·to·na·di·one \ˌfī-tō-nə-ˈdī-ˌon\ *n* : VITAMIN K 1a

phy·to·pho·to·der·ma·ti·tis \ˌfī-tō-ˌfō-tō-ˌdər-mə-ˈtī-təs\ *n, pl* **-ti·tis·es** *or* **-tit·i·des** \-ˈti-tə-ˌdēz\ : a bullous eruption occurring on skin that has been exposed to sunlight after being made hypersensitive by contact with any of various plants

phy·to·ther·a·py \ˌfī-tō-ˈther-ə-pē\ *n, pl* **-pies** : the use of vegetable drugs in medicine

phy·to·tox·in \-ˈtäk-sən\ *n* : a toxin (as ricin) produced by a plant

pia \ˈpī-ə, ˈpē-ə\ *n* : PIA MATER

pia–arach·noid \ˌpī-ə-ə-ˈrak-ˌnoid, ˌpē-\ *n* : LEPTOMENINGES

Pia·get·ian \ˌpē-ə-ˈje-tē-ən\ *adj* : of, relating to, or dealing with Jean Piaget or his writings, theories, or methods esp. with respect to child development

Pia·get \pē-ä-ˈzhä\, **Jean (1896–1980)**, Swiss psychologist.

pi·al \ˈpī-əl, ˈpē-\ *adj* : of or relating to the pia mater ⟨a ~ artery⟩

pia ma·ter \-ˈmä-tər\ *n* : the delicate and highly vascular membrane of connective tissue investing the brain and spinal cord, lying internal to the arachnoid and dura mater, dipping down between the convolutions of the brain, and sending an ingrowth into the anterior fissure of the spinal cord — called also *pia*

pi·an \pē-ˈan, ˈpyän\ *n* : YAWS

pi·blok·to \pi-'bläk-(ˌ)tō\ n : a hysteria among Eskimos characterized by excitement and sometimes by mania, usu. followed by depression, and occurring chiefly in winter and usu. to women

pi·ca \'pī-kə\ n : an abnormal craving for and eating of substances (as chalk, ashes, or bones) not normally eaten that occurs in nutritional deficiency states (as aphosphorosis) in humans or animals or in some forms of mental illness — compare GEOPHAGY

¹Pick's disease \'piks-\ n : a dementia marked by progressive impairment of intellect and judgment and transitory aphasia, caused by progressive atrophic changes of the cerebral cortex, and usu. commencing in late middle age

　　Pick \'pik\, **Arnold (1851–1924)**, Czechoslovakian psychiatrist and neurologist.

²Pick's disease n : pericarditis with adherent pericardium resulting in circulatory disturbances with edema and ascites

　　Pick, Friedel (1867–1926), Czechoslovakian physician.

Pick·wick·ian syndrome \pik-'wi-kē-ən-\ n : obesity accompanied by somnolence and lethargy, hypoventilation, hypoxia, and secondary polycythemia

　　Pick·wick \'pik-ˌwik\, **Samuel**, literary character.

pico- comb form **1** : one trillionth (10^{-12}) part of ⟨picogram⟩ **2** : very small ⟨picornavirus⟩

pi·co·cu·rie \ˌpē-kō-'kyủr-ē, -kyủ-'rē\ n : one trillionth of a curie

pi·co·gram \'pē-kō-ˌgram\ n : one trillionth of a gram — abbr. pg

pi·cor·na·vi·rus \ˌpē-ˌkȯr-nə-'vī-rəs\ n : any of a group of small single-stranded RNA-containing viruses that include the enteroviruses and rhinoviruses

pic·ric acid \'pi-krik-\ n : a bitter toxic explosive yellow crystalline acid $C_6H_3N_3O_7$ — called also trinitrophenol

pic·ro·tox·in \ˌpi-krō-'täk-sən\ n : a poisonous bitter crystalline principle $C_{30}H_{34}O_{13}$ that is found esp. in the berry of an East Indian vine (Anamirta cocculus of the family Menispermaceae) and is a stimulant and convulsant drug administered intravenously as an antidote for poisoning by overdoses of barbiturates

PID abbr pelvic inflammatory disease

pie·dra \pē-'ā-drə\ n : a fungus disease of the hair marked by the formation of small stony nodules along the hair shafts

Pierre Ro·bin syndrome \ˌpyer-rò-'ben-\ n : a congenital defect of the face characterized by micrognathia, abnormal smallness of the tongue, cleft palate, absence of the gag reflex, and sometimes accompanied by bilateral eye defects, glaucoma, or retinal detachment

　　Robin, Pierre (1867–1950), French pediatrician.

pi·geon breast \'pi-jən-\ n : a rachitic deformity of the chest marked by sharp projection of the sternum — **pi·geon–breast·ed** \-'bres-təd\ adj

pigeon chest n : PIGEON BREAST

pigeon–toed \-'tōd\ adj : having the toes turned in

pig·ment \'pig-mənt\ n : a coloring matter in animals and plants esp. in a cell or tissue; also : any of various related colorless substances — **pig·men·tary** \'pig-mən-ˌter-ē\ adj

pigmentary retinopathy n : RETINITIS PIGMENTOSA

pig·men·ta·tion \ˌpig-mən-'tā-shən, -ˌmen-\ n : coloration with or deposition of pigment; esp : an excessive deposition of bodily pigment

pigment cell n : a cell containing a deposition of coloring matter

pig·ment·ed \'pig-ˌmen-təd\ adj : colored by a deposit of pigment

pigmentosa — see RETINITIS PIGMENTOSA

pigmentosum — see XERODERMA PIGMENTOSUM

pig·weed \'pig-ˌwēd\ n : any of several plants of the genus Amaranthus (as A. retroflexus and A. hybridus) producing pollen that is an important hay fever allergen

pil abbr [Latin pilula] pill — used in writing prescriptions

pil- or **pili-** or **pilo-** comb form : hair ⟨pilomotor⟩

pilaris — see KERATOSIS PILARIS, PITYRIASIS RUBRA PILARIS

pile \'pīl\ n **1** : a single hemorrhoid **2** pl : HEMORRHOIDS; also : the condition of one affected with hemorrhoids

pili pl of PILUS

pili — see ARRECTOR PILI MUSCLE

pill \'pil\ n **1** : medicine in a small rounded mass to be swallowed whole **2** often cap : an oral contraceptive — usu. used with the

pil·lar \'pi-lər\ n : a body part likened to a pillar or column (as the margin of the external inguinal ring); specif : PILLAR OF THE FAUCES

pillar of the fauces n : either of two curved folds on each side that bound the fauces and enclose the tonsil — see PALATOGLOSSAL ARCH, PALATOPHARYNGEAL ARCH

pi·lo·car·pine \ˌpī-lə-'kär-ˌpēn\ n : a miotic alkaloid $C_{11}H_{16}N_2O_2$ that is obtained from the dried crushed leaves of two So. American shrubs (Pilocarpus jaborandi and P. microphyllus) of the rue family (Rutaceae) and is used esp. in the treatment of glaucoma

pi·lo·erec·tion \ˌpī-lō-i-'rek-shən\ n : involuntary erection or bristling of

hairs due to a sympathetic reflex usu. triggered by cold, shock, or fright or due to a sympathomimetic agent

pi·lo·mo·tor \\ˌpī-lə-ˈmō-tər\\ *adj* : moving or tending to cause movement of the hairs of the skin (∼ nerves) (∼ erection)

pi·lo·ni·dal \\ˌpī-lə-ˈnīd-ᵊl\\ *adj* **1** : containing hair nested in a cyst — used of congenitally anomalous cysts in the sacrococcygeal area that often become infected and discharge through a channel near the anus **2** : of, relating to, involving, or for use on pilonidal cysts, tracts, or sinuses

pi·lo·se·ba·ceous \\ˌpī-lō-si-ˈbā-shəs\\ *adj* : of or relating to hair and the sebaceous glands

pi·lus \\ˈpī-ləs\\ *n, pl* **pi·li** \\-ˌlī\\ : a hair or a structure (as of a bacterium) resembling a hair

pi·mar·i·cin \\pi-ˈmar-ə-sən\\ *n* : an antifungal antibiotic $C_{34}H_{49}NO_{14}$ derived from a bacterium of the genus *Streptomyces* and effective esp. against aspergillus, candida, and mucor infections

pim·o·zide \\ˈpi-mə-ˌzīd\\ *n* : a tranquilizer $C_{28}H_{29}F_2N_3O$

pim·ple \\ˈpim-pəl\\ *n* **1** : a small inflamed elevation of the skin : PAPULE; *esp* : PUSTULE **2** : a swelling or protuberance like a pimple — **pim·pled** \\-pəld\\ *adj* — **pim·ply** *adj*

pin \\ˈpin\\ *n* **1** : a metal rod driven into or through a fractured bone to immobilize it **2** : a metal rod driven into the root of a reconstructed tooth to provide support for a crown or into the jaw to provide support for an artificial tooth — **pin** *vb*

pin·do·lol \\ˈpin-də-ˌlȯl, -ˌlōl\\ *n* : a beta-blocker $C_{14}H_{20}N_2O_2$ used in the treatment of hypertension

pi·ne·al \\ˈpī-nē-əl, ˈpī-, pī-ˈ\\ *adj* : of, relating to, or being the pineal gland

pi·ne·al·ec·to·my \\ˌpī-nē-ə-ˈlek-tə-mē, ˌpī-nē-, ˌpī-ˌ\\ *n, pl* **-mies** : surgical removal of the pineal gland — **pi·ne·a·lec·to·mize** \\ˌpī-nē-ə-ˈlek-tə-ˌmiz\\ *vb*

pineal gland *n* : a small body that arises from the roof of the third ventricle and is enclosed by the pia mater and that functions primarily as an endocrine organ — called also *pineal, pineal body, pineal organ*

pin·e·a·lo·cyte \\ˈpī-nē-ə-lō-ˌsīt\\ *n* : the parenchymatous epithelioid cell of the pineal gland that has prominent nucleoli and long processes ending in bulbous expansions

pin·e·a·lo·ma \\ˌpī-nē-ə-ˈlō-mə\\ *n, pl* **-mas** *or* **-ma·ta** \\-mə-tə\\ : a tumor of the pineal gland

pineal organ *n* : PINEAL GLAND

pine–needle oil *n* : a colorless or yellowish bitter essential oil obtained from the needles of various pines (esp. *Pinus mugo*) and used in medicine chiefly as an inhalant in treating bronchitis

pine tar *n* : tar obtained from the wood of pine trees (genus *Pinus* and esp. *P. palustris* of the family Pinaceae) and used in soaps and in the treatment of skin diseases

pink disease \\ˈpiŋk-\\ *n* : ACRODYNIA

pink·eye \\ˈpiŋ-ˌkī\\ *n* : an acute highly contagious conjunctivitis of humans and various domestic animals

pink spot *n* : the appearance of pulp through the attenuated hard tissue of the crown of a tooth affected with resorption of dentin

pin·na \\ˈpi-nə\\ *n, pl* **pin·nae** \\ˈpi-ˌnē, -ˌnī\\ *or* **pinnas** : the largely cartilaginous projecting portion of the external ear — **pin·nal** \\ˈpi-nᵊl\\ *adj*

pi·no·cy·to·sis \\ˌpī-nə-sə-ˈtō-səs, ˌpi-, -ˌsī-\\ *n, pl* **-to·ses** \\-ˌsēz\\ : the uptake of fluid by a cell by invagination and pinching off of the plasma membrane — **pi·no·cy·tot·ic** \\-ˈtä-tik\\ *or* **pi·no·cyt·ic** \\-ˈsi-tik\\ *adj*

pins and needles *n pl* : a pricking tingling sensation in a limb growing numb or recovering from numbness

pint \\ˈpint\\ *n* : any of various measures of liquid capacity equal to one-half quart: as **a** : a U.S. measure equal to 16 fluid ounces, 473.176 milliliters, or 28.875 cubic inches **b** : a British measure equal to 20 fluid ounces, 568.26 milliliters, or 34.678 cubic inches

pin·ta \\ˈpin-tə, -ˌtä\\ *n* : a chronic skin disease that is endemic in tropical America, that occurs successively as an initial papule, a generalized eruption, and a patchy loss of pigment, and that is caused by a spirochete of the genus *Treponema* (*T. careteum*) morphologically indistinguishable from the causative agent of syphilis — called also *pinto*

pin·tid \\ˈpin-təd\\ *n* : one of many initially reddish, then brown, slate blue, or black patches on the skin characteristic of the second stage of pinta

pin·worm \\ˈpin-ˌwərm\\ *n* : any of numerous small oxyurid nematode worms that have the tail of the female prolonged into a sharp point and infest the intestines and esp. the cecum of various vertebrates; *esp* : a worm of the genus *Enterobius* (*E. vermicularis*) that is parasitic in humans

pi·per·a·zine \\pī-ˈper-ə-ˌzēn\\ *n* : a crystalline heterocyclic base $C_4H_{10}N_2$ or $C_4H_{10}N_2 \cdot 6H_2O$ used esp. as an anthelmintic

pi·per·i·dine \\pī-ˈper-ə-ˌdēn\\ *n* : a liquid heterocyclic base $C_5H_{11}N$ that has a peppery ammoniacal odor

pi·per·o·caine \\pī-ˈper-ə-ˌkān\\ *n* : a local anesthetic $C_{16}H_{23}NO_2$ derived from piperidine and benzoic acid and used in the form of its crystalline hydrochloride — see METYCAINE

pi·per·o·nyl bu·tox·ide \\pī-ˈper-ə-ˌnil-byü-ˈtäk-ˌsīd, -nəl-\\ *n* : an insecticide $C_{19}H_{30}O_5$ that has the capacity to alter the pharmacological action of some drugs; *also* : an oily liquid containing this compound that is used chiefly as a synergist (as for pyrethrum insecticides)

pip·er·ox·an \,pi-pə-'räk-,san\ *n* : an adrenolytic drug $C_{14}H_{19}NO_2$ that has been used in the form of its crystalline hydrochloride to detect pheochromocytoma by the transient fall in blood pressure it produces

pi·pette *or* **pi·pet** \pī-'pet\ *n* : a small piece of apparatus which typically consists of a narrow tube into which fluid is drawn by suction (as for dispensing or measurement) and retained by closing the upper end — **pipette** *or* **pipet** *vb*

pir·i·form \'pir-ə-,form\ *adj* 1 : having the form of a pear 2 : of or relating to the piriform lobe (the ~ cortex)

piriform aperture *n* : the anterior opening of the nasal cavities in the skull

piriform area *n* : PIRIFORM LOBE

piriform fossa *n* : PIRIFORM RECESS

pir·i·for·mis \,pir-ə-'for-mis\ *n* : a muscle that arises from the front of the sacrum, passes out of the pelvis through the greater sciatic foramen, is inserted into the upper border of the greater trochanter of the femur, and rotates the thigh laterally

piriform lobe *n* : the lateral olfactory gyrus and the hippocampal gyrus taken together

piriform recess *n* : a small cavity or pocket between the lateral walls of the pharynx on each side and the upper part of the larynx — called also *piriform fossa, piriform sinus*

Pi·ro·goff's amputation \,pir-ə-'gofs-\ *or* **Pi·ro·goff amputation** \-'gof-\ *n* : amputation of the foot through the articulation of the ankle with retention of part of the calcaneus — compare SYME'S AMPUTATION

    Pirogoff, Nikolai Ivanovich (1810–1881), Russian surgeon.

piro·plasm \'pir-ə-,pla-zəm\ *or* **piro·plas·ma** \,pir-ə-'plaz-mə\ *n, pl* **piro·plasms** *or* **piro·plas·ma·ta** \,pir-ə-'plaz-mə-tə\ : BABESIA 2

Piro·plas·ma \,pir-ə-'plaz-mə\ *n, syn of* BABESIA

piro·plas·mo·sis \,pir-ə-,plaz-'mō-səs\ *n, pl* **-mo·ses** \-,sēz\ : infection with or disease that is caused by protozoans of a family (Babesiidae) and esp. of the genus *Babesia* and that includes Texas fever and east coast fever of cattle and babesiosis of sheep

pi·rox·i·cam \pi-'räk-sə-,kam\ *n* : a nonsteroidal anti-inflammatory drug $C_{15}H_{13}N_3O_4S$ used in the treatment of rheumatic diseases (as osteoarthritis)

Pir·quet test \pir-'kā-\ *n* : a tuberculin test made by applying a drop of tuberculin to a scarified spot on the skin — called also *Pirquet reaction*

    Pir·quet von Ce·se·na·ti·co \pir-'kā-

fōn-,chä-se-'nä-ti-kō\, **Clemens Peter** (1874–1929), Austrian physician.

pi·si·form \'pi-sə-,form\ *n* : a bone on the little-finger side of the carpus that articulates with the triquetral bone — called also *pisiform bone*

pit \'pit\ *n* : a hollow or indentation esp. in a surface of an organism: as **a** : a natural hollow in the surface of the body **b** : one of the indented scars left in the skin by a pustular disease : POCKMARK **c** : a usu. developmental imperfection in the enamel of a tooth that takes the form of a small pointed depression — **pit** *vb*

pitch \'pich\ *n* : the property of a sound and esp. a musical tone that is determined by the frequency of the waves producing it : highness or lowness of sound

pitch·blende \'pich-,blend\ : a brown to black mineral that has a distinctive luster and contains radium

Pi·to·cin \pi-'tō-sən\ *trademark* — used for a preparation of oxytocin

pi·tot tube \pē-'tō-\ *n, often cap P* : a device that consists of a tube that is used with a manometer to measure the velocity of fluid flow (as in a blood vessel)

    Pitot, Henri (1695–1771), French hydraulic engineer.

Pi·tres·sin \pi-'tres-ən\ *trademark* — used for a preparation of vasopressin

pitting *n* 1 : the action or process of forming pits (as in acned skin, a tooth, or a dental restoration) 2 : the formation of a depression or indentation in living tissue that is produced by pressure with a finger or blunt instrument and disappears only slowly following release of the pressure in some forms of edema

pitting edema *n* : edema in which pitting results in a depression in the edematous tissue which disappears only slowly

pi·tu·i·cyte \pə-'tü-ə-,sīt, -'tyü-\ *n* : one of the pigmented more or less fusiform cells of the stalk and posterior lobe of the pituitary gland that are usu. considered to be derived from neuroglial cells

¹**pi·tu·i·tary** \pə-'tü-ə-,ter-ē, -'tyü-\ *adj* 1 : of or relating to the pituitary gland 2 : caused or characterized by secretory disturbances of the pituitary gland (a ~ dwarf)

²**pituitary** *n, pl* **-tar·ies** 1 : PITUITARY GLAND 2 : the cleaned, dried, and powdered posterior lobe of the pituitary gland of cattle that is used in the treatment of uterine atony and hemorrhage, shock, and intestinal paresis

pituitary ba·soph·i·lism \-bā-'sä-fə-,li-zəm\ *n* : CUSHING'S DISEASE

pituitary gland *n* : a small oval endocrine organ that is attached to the infundibulum of the brain and occupies the sella turcica, that consists essentially of an epithelial anterior lobe derived from a diverticulum of the oral cavity and joined to a posterior lobe of nervous origin by a pars intermedia, and that has the several parts associated with various hormones which directly or indirectly affect most basic bodily functions and include substances exerting a controlling and regulating influence on other endocrine organs, controlling growth and development, or modifying the contraction of smooth muscle, renal function, and reproduction — called also *hypophysis, pituitary body;* see NEUROHYPOPHYSIS

pituitary portal system *n* : a portal system supplying blood to the anterior lobe of the pituitary gland through veins connecting the capillaries of the median eminence of the hypothalamus with those of the anterior lobe

Pi·tu·i·trin \pə-ˈtü-ə-trin, -ˈtyü-\ *trademark* — used for an aqueous extract of the fresh pituitary gland of cattle

pit viper *n* : any of various mostly New World venomous snakes (as the rattlesnake, copperhead, and water moccasin) that belong to a subfamily (Crotalinae of the family Viperidae) and have a small depression on each side of the head and hollow perforated fangs

pit·y·ri·a·sis \ˌpi-tə-ˈrī-ə-səs\ *n, pl* **pit·y·ri·a·ses** \-ˌsēz\ **1** : any of several skin diseases marked by the formation and desquamation of fine scales **2** : a disease of domestic animals marked by dry epithelial scales or scurf

pityriasis li·che·noi·des et var·i·o·li·for·mis acu·ta \-ˌlī-kə-ˈnoi-ˌdēz-et-ˌvar-ē-ō-lə-ˈfor-mis-ə-ˈkyü-tə, -ˈkü-\ *n* : a disease of unknown cause that is characterized by the sudden appearance of polymorphous lesions (as papules, purpuric vesicles, crusts, or ulcerations) resembling chicken pox but tending to persist from a month to as long as years, occurs esp. between the ages of 30 and 50, and is more common in men

pityriasis ro·sea \-ˈrō-zē-ə\ *n* : an acute benign and self-limited skin eruption of unknown cause that consists of dry, scaly, oval, pinkish or fawn-colored papules, usu. lasts six to eight weeks, and affects esp. the trunk, arms, and thighs

pityriasis ru·bra pi·lar·is \-ˈrü-brə-pi-ˈlar-əs\ *n* : a chronic dermatitis characterized by the formation of papular horny plugs in the hair follicles and pinkish macules which tend to spread and become scaly plaques

pityriasis versicolor *n* : TINEA VERSICOLOR

piv·ot \ˈpi-vət\ *n* : a usu. metallic pin holding an artificial crown to the root of a tooth

pivot joint *n* : an anatomical articulation that consists of a bony pivot in a ring of bone and ligament (as that of

the odontoid process and atlas) that permits rotatory movement only — called also *trochoid*

pivot tooth *n* : an artificial crown attached to the root of a tooth by a usu. metallic pin — called also *pivot crown*

PK \ˌpē-ˈkā\ *n* : PSYCHOKINESIS

PKU *abbr* phenylketonuria

pla·ce·bo \plə-ˈsē-(ˌ)bō\ *n, pl* **-bos 1** : a medication prescribed more for the mental relief of the patient than for its actual effect on a disorder **2** : an inert or innocuous substance used esp. in controlled experiments testing the efficacy of another substance (as a drug)

placebo effect *n* : improvement in the condition of a sick person that occurs in response to treatment but cannot be considered due to the specific treatment used

pla·cen·ta \plə-ˈsen-tə\ *n, pl* **-centas** *or* **-cen·tae** \-ˈsen-(ˌ)tē\ : the vascular organ that unites the fetus to the maternal uterus and mediates its metabolic exchanges through a more or less intimate association of uterine mucosal with chorionic and usu. allantoic tissues permitting exchange of material by diffusion between the maternal and fetal vascular systems but without direct contact between maternal and fetal blood and typically involving the interlocking of fingerlike vascular chorionic villi with corresponding modified areas of the uterine mucosa — see ABLATIO PLACENTAE, ABRUPTIO PLACENTAE — **pla·cen·tal** \-təl\ *adj*

placental barrier *n* : a semipermeable membrane made up of placental tissues and limiting the kind and amount of material exchanged between mother and fetus

placentalis — see DECIDUA PLACENTALIS

placenta pre·via \-ˈprē-vē-ə\ *n, pl* **placentae previae** \-vē-ˌē\ : an abnormal implantation of the placenta at or near the internal opening of the uterine cervix so that it tends to precede the child at birth usu. causing severe maternal hemorrhage

plac·en·ti·tis \ˌplas-ᵊn-ˈtī-təs\ *n, pl* **-tit·i·des** \-ˈti-tə-ˌdēz\ : inflammation of the placenta

plac·en·tog·ra·phy \ˌplas-ᵊn-ˈtä-grə-fē\ *n, pl* **-phies** : roentgenographic visualization of the placenta after injection of a radiopaque medium

Plac·i·dyl \ˈpla-sə-ˌdil\ *trademark* — used for a preparation of ethchlorvynol

pla·gio·ceph·a·ly \ˌplā-jē-ō-ˈse-fə-lē\ *n, pl* **-lies** : a malformation of the head marked by an oblique slant to the main axis of the skull and usu. caused by closure of half of the coronal suture

plague \ˈplāg\ *n* **1** : an epidemic disease

causing a high rate of mortality : PESTILENCE (a ∼ of cholera) **2** : a virulent contagious febrile disease that is caused by a bacterium of the genus *Yersinia* (*Y. pestis* syn. *Pasteurella pestis*), that occurs in bubonic, pneumonic, and septicemic forms, and that is usu. transmitted from rats to humans by the bite of infected fleas (as in bubonic plague) or directly from person to person (as in pneumonic plague) — called also *black death*

plana — see PARS PLANA

plane \'plān\ *n* **1 a** : a surface that contains at least three points not all in a straight line and is such that a line drawn through any two points in it lies wholly in the surface **b** : an imaginary plane used to identify parts of the body or a part of the skull — see FRANKFORT HORIZONTAL PLANE, MIDSAGGITAL PLANE **2** : a stage in surgical anesthesia (maintained a light ∼ of anesthesia with cyclopropane)

plane joint *n* : GLIDING JOINT

plane of polarization *n* : the plane in which electromagnetic radiation vibrates when it is polarized so as to vibrate in a single plane

pla·ni·gram \'plā-nə-ˌgram, 'plā-\ *n* : TOMOGRAM

pla·nig·ra·phy \plə-'ni-grə-fē\ *n, pl* **-phies** : TOMOGRAPHY

Planned Par·ent·hood \'pland-'par-əntˌhüd\ *service mark* — used for research and dissemination of information on contraception

Pla·nor·bis \plə-'nor-bis\ *n* : a widely distributed genus of snails (family Planorbidae) that includes several intermediate hosts for schistosomes infecting humans

plantae — see QUADRATUS PLANTAE

plan·ta·go \plan-'tā-(ˌ)gō\ *n* **1** *cap* : a large genus of weeds (family Plantaginaceae) including several (*P. psyllium*, *P. indica*, and *P. ovata*) that have indigestible and mucilaginous seeds used as a mild cathartic — see PSYLLIUM SEED **2** : PLANTAIN

plantago seed *n* : PSYLLIUM SEED

plan·tain \'plant-ᵊn\ *n* : any plant of the genus *Plantago*

plan·tar \'plan-tər, -ˌtär\ *adj* : of, relating to, or typical of the sole of the foot (the ∼ aspect of the foot)

plantar arch *n* : an arterial arch in the sole of the foot formed by the lateral plantar artery and a branch of the dorsalis pedis

plantar artery *n* : either of the two terminal branches into which the posterior tibial artery divides: **a** : one that is larger and passes laterally and then medially to join with a branch of the dorsalis pedis to form the plantar arch — called also *lateral plantar artery* **b** : one that is smaller and follows a more medial course as it passes distally supplying or giving off branches

which supply the plantar part of the foot and the toes — called also *medial plantar artery*

plantar cal·ca·neo·na·vic·u·lar ligament \-(ˌ)kal-ˌkā-nē-ō-nə-'vi-kyə-lər-\ *n* : an elastic ligament of the sole of the foot that connects the calcaneus and navicular bone and supports the head of the talus — called also *spring ligament*

plantar fascia *n* : a very strong dense fibrous membrane of the sole of the foot that lies beneath the skin and superficial layer of fat and binds together the deeper structures

plantar fasciitis *n* : inflammation involving the plantar fascia esp. in the area of its attachment to the calcaneus and causing pain under the heel in walking and running

plantar flexion *n* : movement of the foot that flexes the foot or toes downward toward the sole — compare DORSIFLEXION

plantar interosseus *n* : any of three small muscles of the plantar aspect of the foot each of which lies along the plantar side of one of the third, fourth, and fifth toes facing the second toe and acts to flex the proximal phalanx and extend the distal phalanges of its toe and to adduct its toe toward the second toe — called also *interosseus plantaris*, *plantar interosseous muscle*

plan·tar·is \plan-'tar-əs\ *n, pl* **plan·tar·es** \-'tar-ˌēz\ : a small muscle of the calf of the leg that arises from the lower end of the femur and the posterior ligament of the knee joint, is inserted with the Achilles tendon by a very long slender tendon into the calcaneus, and weakly flexes the leg at the knee and the foot at the ankle — see INTEROSSEUS PLANTARIS, VERRUCA PLANTARIS

plantar nerve *n* : either of two nerves of the foot that are the two terminal branches into which the tibial nerve divides: **a** : a smaller one that supplies most of the deeper muscles of the foot and the skin on the lateral part of the sole and on the fifth toe as well as on the lateral part of the fourth toe — called also *lateral plantar nerve* **b** : a larger one that accompanies the medial plantar artery and supplies a number of muscles of the medial part of the foot, the skin on the medial two-thirds of the sole, and the skin on the first to fourth toes — called also *medial plantar nerve*

plantar reflex *n* : a reflex movement of flexing the foot and toes that after the first year is the normal response to tickling of the sole — compare BABINSKI REFLEX

plantar vein *n* : either of two veins that accompany the plantar arteries: **a** : one accompanying the lateral plantar artery — called also *lateral plan* *tar vein* **b** : one accompanying the medial plantar artery — called also *medial plantar vein*

plantar wart *n* : a wart on the sole of the foot — called also *planter's wart*, *verruca plantaris*

plan·ti·grade \'plan-tə-₁grād\ *adj* : walking on the sole with the heel touching the ground (bears and humans are ∼ animals) — **plantigrade** *n*

pla·num \'plā-nəm\ *n*, *pl* **pla·na** \-nə\ : a flat surface of bone esp. of the skull

planus — see LICHEN PLANUS

plaque \'plak\ *n* **1 a** : a localized abnormal patch on a body part or surface and esp. on the skin (psoriatic ∼) **b** : a film of mucus that harbors bacteria on a tooth **c** : an atherosclerotic lesion **d** : a histopathologic lesion of brain tissue that is characteristic of Alzheimer's disease and consists of a cluster of degenerating nerve endings and dendrites around a core of amyloid **2** : a visibly distinct and esp. a clear or opaque area in a bacterial culture produced by damage to or destruction of cells by a virus

Plaque·nil \'pla-kə-₁nil\ *trademark* — used for a preparation of hydroxychloroquine

-pla·sia \'plā-zhə, -zhē-ə\ *or* **-pla·sy** \₁plā-sē, -plə-sē\ *n comb form*, *pl* **-plasias** *or* **-plasies** : development : formation (dys*plasia*)

plasm- *or* **plasmo-** *comb form* : plasma (*plasm*apheresis)

-plasm \₁pla-zəm\ *n comb form* : formative or formed material (as of a cell or tissue) (cyto*plasm*) (endo*plasm*)

plas·ma \'plaz-mə\ *n* : the fluid part of blood and lymph that is distinguished from suspended material and that in blood differs from serum essentially in containing the precursor substance of fibrin in addition to the constituents of serum

plasma cell *n* : a lymphocyte that is a mature antibody-secreting B cell

plas·ma·cy·to·ma \₁plaz-mə-sī-'tō-mə\ *n*, *pl* **-mas** *or* **-ma·ta** \-mə-tə\ : a myeloma composed of plasma cells

plas·ma·cy·to·sis \₁plaz-mə-sī-'tō-səs\ *n*, *pl* **-to·ses** \-₁sēz\ : the presence of abnormal numbers of plasma cells in the blood

plas·ma·lem·ma \₁plaz-mə-'le-mə\ *n* : PLASMA MEMBRANE

plas·mal·o·gen \plaz-'ma-lə-jən, -₁jen\ *n* : any of a group of phospholipids in which a fatty acid group is replaced by a fatty aldehyde and which include lecithins and phosphatidylethanolamines

plasma membrane *n* : a semipermeable limiting layer of cell protoplasm consisting of three molecular layers of which the inner and outer are composed of protein while the middle layer is composed of a double layer of fat molecules — called also *cell membrane*, *plasmalemma*

plas·ma·pher·e·sis \₁plaz-mə-fə-'rē-səs, -'fer-ə-səs\ *n*, *pl* **-e·ses** \-₁sēz\ : a process for obtaining blood plasma without depleting the donor or patient of other blood constituents (as red blood cells) by separating out the plasma from the whole blood and returning the rest to the donor's or patient's circulatory system

plasma thromboplastin an·te·ced·ent \-₁an-tə-'sēd-ənt\ *n* : a clotting factor whose absence is associated with a form of hemophilia — abbr. *PTA*; called also *factor XI*

plasma thromboplastin component *n* : FACTOR IX

plas·mat·ic \plaz-'ma-tik\ *adj* : of, relating to, or occurring in plasma esp. of blood (∼ fibrils)

plas·mid \'plaz-mid\ *n* : an extrachromosomal ring of DNA that replicates independently and is found esp. in bacteria — compare EPISOME

plas·min \-min\ *n* : a proteolytic enzyme that dissolves the fibrin of blood clots

plas·min·o·gen \plaz-'mi-nə-jən\ *n* : the precursor of plasmin that is found in blood plasma and serum — called also *profibrinolysin*

plasmo- — see PLASM-

Plas·mo·chin \'plaz-mə-kin\ *trademark* — used for a preparation of pamaquine

plas·mo·cy·to·ma *var of* PLASMACYTOMA

plas·mo·di·al \plaz-'mō-dē-əl\ *adj* : of, relating to, or resembling a plasmodium

plas·mo·di·um \plaz-'mō-dē-əm\ *n* **1** *cap* : a genus of sporozoans (family Plasmodiidae) that includes all the malaria parasites affecting humans **2** *pl* **-dia** : any individual malaria parasite

-plast \₁plast\ *n comb form* : organized particle or granule : cell (chloro*plast*)

plas·ter \'plas-tər\ *n* : a medicated or protective dressing that consists of a film (as of cloth or plastic) spread with a usu. medicated substance

plaster cast *n* : a rigid dressing of gauze impregnated with plaster of paris

plaster of par·is \-'par-is\ *n* : a white powdery slightly hydrated calcium sulfate $CaSO_4 \cdot \frac{1}{2}H_2O$ or $2CaSO_4 \cdot H_2O$ that forms a quick-setting paste with water and is used in medicine chiefly in casts and for surgical bandages

plas·tic \'plas-tik\ *adj* **1** : capable of being deformed continuously and permanently in any direction without breaking or tearing **2** : capable of growth, repair, or differentiation (a ∼ tissue) **3** : of, relating to, or involving plastic surgery (∼ repair)

-plas·tic \'plas-tik\ *adj comb form* **1** : developing : forming (thrombo*plastic*) **2** : of or relating to (something designated by a term ending in

-plasia, -plasm, or -plasty\ (neoplas-tic)

plas·tic·i·ty \pla-'sti-sə-tē\ n, pl **-ties 1** : the quality or state of being plastic; esp : capacity for being molded or altered **2** : the ability to retain a shape attained by pressure deformation **3** : the capacity of organisms with the same genotype to vary in developmental pattern, in phenotype, or in behavior according to varying environmental conditions

plastic surgeon n : a specialist in plastic surgery

plastic surgery n : a branch of surgery concerned with the repair, restoration, or improvement of lost, injured, defective, or misshapen parts of the body chiefly by transfer of tissue

plas·ty \'plas-tē\ n, pl **plas·ties** : a surgical procedure for the repair, restoration, or replacement (as by a prosthesis) of a part of the body ⟨quadriceps ∼⟩ ⟨total knee ∼⟩

-plas·ty \plas-tē\ n comb form, pl **-plas·ties** : plastic surgery ⟨osteoplas-ty⟩

-plasy — see -PLASIA

plat- — see PLATY-

¹**plate** \'plāt\ n 1 : a flat thin piece or lamina (as of bone) that is part of the body **2 a** : a flat glass dish used chiefly for culturing microorganisms; esp : PETRI DISH **b** : a culture or culture medium contained in such a dish **3** : a supporting or reinforcing element: as **a** : the part of a denture that fits in the mouth; broadly : DENTURE **b** : a thin flat narrow piece of metal (as stainless steel) that is used to repair a bone defect or fracture

²**plate** vb **plat·ed; plat·ing 1** : to inoculate and culture (microorganisms or cells) on a plate; also : to distribute (an inoculum) on a plate or plates for cultivation **2** : to repair (as a fractured bone) with metal plates

plate·let \'plāt-lət\ n : BLOOD PLATELET

platelet–activating factor n : phospholipid that is produced esp. by mast cells and basophils, causes the aggregation of blood platelets and the release of blood-platelet substances (as histamine or serotonin), and is a mediator of inflammation (as in asthma) — abbr. PAF

platelet–derived growth factor n : a mitogenic growth factor that is found esp. in platelets, consists of two polypeptide chains linked by bonds containing two sulfur atoms each, stimulates cell proliferation (as in connective tissue, smooth muscle, and neuroglia), and plays a role in wound healing — abbr. PDGF

plate·let·phe·re·sis \'plāt-lət-¹fer-ə-səs, -fə-¹rē-səs\ n, pl **-re·ses** \-¹sēz\ : pheresis used to collect blood platelets

plat·ing \'plāt-iŋ\ n 1 : the spreading of a sample of cells or microorganisms on a nutrient medium in a petri dish **2**

: the immobilization of a fractured bone by securing a metal plate to it

Plat·i·nol \'pla-tə-ˌnȯl, -ˌnōl\ trademark — used for a preparation of cis-platin

plat·i·num \'plat-ᵊn-əm\ n : a grayish white ductile malleable metallic element used esp. as a catalyst and in alloys (as in dentistry) — symbol Pt; see ELEMENT table

platy- also **plat-** comb form : flat : broad ⟨platypelloid⟩

platy·ba·sia \ˌpla-ti-¹bā-sē-ə\ n : a developmental deformity of the base of the skull in which the lower occiput is pushed by the upper cervical spine into the cranial fossa

platy·hel·minth \ˌpla-ti-¹hel-ˌminth\ n : any of a phylum (Platyhelminthes) of soft-bodied usu. much flattened worms (as the flukes and tapeworms) — called also flatworm — **platy·hel·min·thic** \-hel-¹min-thik, -tik\ adj

platy·pel·loid \-¹pe-ˌlȯid\ adj, of the pelvis : broad and flat — compare ANDROID, ANTHROPOID, GYNECOID

platys·ma \plə-¹tiz-mə\ n, pl **-ma·ta** \-mə-tə\ also **-mas** : a broad thin layer of muscle that is situated on each side of the neck immediately under the superficial fascia belonging to the group of facial muscles, that is innervated by the facial nerve, and that draws the lower lip and the corner of the mouth to the side and down and when moved forcefully expands the neck and draws its skin upward

play therapy n : psychotherapy in which a child is encouraged to reveal feelings and conflicts in play rather than by verbalization

pleasure principle n : a tendency for individual behavior to be directed toward immediate satisfaction of instinctual drives and immediate relief from pain or discomfort — compare REALITY PRINCIPLE

pledg·et \'ple-jət\ n : a compress or small flat mass usu. of gauze or absorbent cotton that is laid over a wound or into a cavity to apply medication, exclude air, retain dressings, or absorb the matter discharged

-ple·gia \'plē-jə, -jē-ə\ n comb form : paralysis ⟨diplegia⟩

pleio·tro·pic \ˌplī-ə-¹trō-pik, -¹trä-\ adj : producing more than one genic effect; specif : having multiple phenotypic expressions ⟨a ∼ gene⟩ — **plei·ot·ro·py** \plī-¹ä-trə-pē\ n

pleo·cy·to·sis \ˌplē-ō-ˌsī-¹tō-səs\ n, pl **-to·ses** \-ˌsēz\ : an abnormal increase in the number of cells (as lymphocytes) in the cerebrospinal fluid

pleo·mor·phic \ˌplē-ə-¹mȯr-fik\ also **pleio·mor·phic** \ˌplī-ə-\ adj : able to assume different forms : POLYMORPHIC ⟨∼ bacteria⟩ ⟨a ∼ sarcoma⟩ — **pleo·mor·phism** \ˌplē-ə-¹mȯr-ˌfi-zəm\ n

ple·op·tics \plē-¹äp-tiks\ n : a system of treating amblyopia by retraining visual habits using guided exercises — **ple·op·tic** \-'tik\ *adj*

pleth·o·ra \'ple-thə-rə\ *n* : a bodily condition characterized by an excess of blood and marked by turgescence and a florid complexion — **ple·thor·ic** \plə-'thòr-ik, ple-, -'thär-; 'ple-thə-rik\ *adj*

ple·thys·mo·gram \ple-'thiz-mə-ˌgram, plə-\ *n* : a tracing made by a plethysmograph

ple·thys·mo·graph \-ˌgraf\ *n* : an instrument for determining and registering variations in the size of an organ or limb resulting from changes in the amount of blood present or passing through it — **ple·thys·mo·graph·ic** \-ˌthiz-mə-'gra-fik\ *adj* — **ple·thys·mo·graph·i·cal·ly** *adv* — **pleth·ys·mog·ra·phy** \ˌple-thiz-'mä-grə-fē\ *n*

pleur- or **pleuro-** *comb form* 1 : pleura ⟨*pleuro*pneumonia⟩ 2 : pleura and ⟨*pleuro*peritoneal⟩

pleu·ra \'plur-ə\ *n, pl* **pleu·rae** \'plur-ē\ or **pleuras** : either of a pair of two-walled sacs of serous membrane each lining one lateral half of the thorax, having an inner layer closely adherent to the corresponding lung, reflected at the root of the lung to form a parietal layer that adheres to the walls of the thorax, the pericardium, upper surface of the diaphragm, and adjacent parts, and containing a small amount of serous fluid that minimizes the friction of respiratory movements

pleu·ral \'plur-əl\ *adj* : of or relating to the pleura or the sides of the thorax

pleural cavity *n* : the space that is formed when the two layers of the pleura spread apart — called also *pleural space*

pleural effusion *n* 1 : an exudation of fluid from the blood or lymph into a pleural cavity 2 : an exudate in a pleural cavity

pleural space *n* : PLEURAL CAVITY

pleu·rec·to·my \plu-'rek-tə-mē\ *n, pl* **-mies** : surgical excision of part of the pleura

pleu·ri·sy \'plur-ə-sē\ *n, pl* **-sies** : inflammation of the pleura usu. with fever, painful and difficult respiration, cough, and exudation of fluid or fibrinous material into the pleural cavity — **pleu·rit·ic** \plü-'ri-tik\ *adj*

pleu·ri·tis \plü-'rī-təs\ *n, pl* **pleu·rit·i·des** \-'ri-tə-ˌdēz\ : PLEURISY

pleu·ro·dyn·ia \ˌplur-ə-'di-nē-ə\ *n* 1 : a sharp pain in the side usu. located in the intercostal muscles and believed to arise from inflammation of fibrous tissue 2 : EPIDEMIC PLEURODYNIA

pleu·ro·peri·car·di·tis \ˌplur-ō-ˌper-ə-ˌkär-'dī-təs\ *n, pl* **-dit·i·des** \-'di-tə-ˌdēz\ : inflammation of the pleura and the pericardium

pleu·ro·peri·to·ne·al \-ˌper-ə-tə-'nē-əl\ *adj* : of or relating to the pleura and the peritoneum

pleu·ro·pneu·mo·nia \ˌplur-ō-nu̇-'mō-

nyə, -nyu̇-\ *n* 1 : pleurisy accompanied by pneumonia 2 : a highly contagious pneumonia usu. associated with pleurisy of cattle, goats, and sheep that is caused by a microorganism of the genus *Mycoplasma* (esp. *M. mycoides*) 3 : a contagious often fatal respiratory disease esp. of young pigs that is caused by a bacterium of the genus *Haemophilus* (*H. pleuropneumoniae*) 4 : pleurisy of horses that is often accompanied by pneumonia and is caused by various microorganisms

pleuropneumonia–like organism *n* : MYCOPLASMA 2

pleu·ro·pul·mo·nary \ˌplur-ō-'pul-mə-ˌner-ē, -'pəl-\ *adj* : of or relating to the pleura and the lungs

plex·ec·to·my \plek-'sek-tə-mē\ *n, pl* **-mies** : surgical removal of a plexus

plexi·form \'plek-sə-ˌform\ *adj* : of, relating to, or having the form or characteristics of a plexus ⟨~ networks⟩

plexiform layer *n* : either of two reticular layers of the retina consisting of nerve cell processes and situated between layers of ganglion cells and cell bodies

plex·im·e·ter \plek-'si-mə-tər\ *n* : a small hard flat plate (as of ivory) placed in contact with the body to receive the blow in percussion

plex·op·a·thy \plek-'sä-pə-thē\ *n, pl* **-thies** : a disease of a plexus

plex·or \'plek-sər\ *n* : a small hammer with a rubber head used in medical percussion

plex·us \'plek-səs\ *n, pl* **plex·us·es** : a network of anastomosing or interlacing blood vessels or nerves

pli·ca \'plī-kə\ *n, pl* **pli·cae** \-ˌkē, -ˌsē\ : a fold or folded part; *esp* : a groove or fold of skin

plicae cir·cu·la·res \-ˌsər-kyə-'lar-(ˌ)ēz\ *n pl* : the numerous permanent crescentic folds of mucous membrane found in the small intestine esp. in the lower part of the duodenum and the jejunum — called also *valvulae conniventes*

plica fim·bri·a·ta \-ˌfim-brē-'ā-tə\ *n, pl* **plicae fim·bri·a·tae** \-'ā-tē\ : a fold resembling a fringe on the under surface of the tongue on either side of the frenulum

pli·ca·my·cin \ˌplī-kə-'mīs-ᵊn\ *n* : an antineoplastic agent $C_{52}H_{76}O_{24}$ produced by three bacteria of the genus *Streptomyces* (*S. argillaceus, S. tanashiensis,* and *S. plicatus*) and administered intravenously esp. in the treatment of malignant tumors of the testes or in the treatment of hypercalcemia and hypercalciuria associated with advanced neoplastic disease — called also *mithramycin*

plica semi·lu·na·ris \-ˌse-mi-ˌlü-'nar-əs\ *n, pl* **plicae semi·lu·na·res** \-(ˌ)ēz\ : the vertical fold of conjunctiva that occupies the canthus of the eye nearer the nose

pli·ca·tion \pli-'kā-shən\ n 1 : the tightening of stretched or weakened bodily tissues or channels by folding the excess in tucks and suturing 2 : the folding of one part on and the fastening of it to another (as areas of the bowel freed from adhesions and left without normal serosal covering) — **pli·cate** \'plī-ˌkāt\ vb

-ploid \ˌploid\ adj comb form : having or being a chromosome number that bears (such) a relationship to or is (so many) times the basic chromosome number characteristic of a given plant or animal group (polyploid)

ploi·dy \'ploi-dē\ n, pl **ploi·dies** : degree of repetition of the basic number of chromosomes

plom·bage \ˌpläm-'bäzh\ n : sustained compression of the sides of a pulmonary cavity against each other to effect closure by pressure exerted by packing (as of paraffin or plastic sponge)

PLSS abbr portable life-support system

plug \'pləg\ n 1 : an obstructing mass of material in a bodily vessel or the opening of a skin lesion (necrotic ∼) (fibrinous ∼) 2 : a filling for a hollow tooth — **plugged** \'pləgd\ adj

plug·ger \'plə-gər\ n : a dental instrument used for driving and consolidating filling material in a tooth cavity

plum·bism \'pləm-ˌbi-zəm\ n : LEAD POISONING; esp : chronic lead poisoning

Plum·mer–Vin·son syndrome \'plə-mər-'vin-sən-\ n : a condition that is marked esp. by the growth of a mucous membrane across the esophageal lumen, by difficulty in swallowing, and by hypochromic anemia and that is considered to be due to an iron deficiency

    Plummer, Henry Stanley (1874–1936), American physician.
    Vinson, Porter Paisley (1890–1959), American surgeon.

plu·ri·po·ten·cy \ˌplŭr-ə-'pōt-ᵊn-sē\ n, pl **-cies** : PLURIPOTENTIALITY

plu·ri·po·tent \ˌplŭ-'ri-pə-tənt\ adj 1 : not fixed as to developmental potentialities : having developmental plasticity (a ∼ cell) 2 : capable of affecting more than one organ or tissue

plu·ri·po·ten·tial \ˌplŭr-ə-pə-'ten-chəl\ adj : PLURIPOTENT

plu·ri·po·ten·ti·al·i·ty \-pə-ˌten-chē-'a-lə-tē\ n, pl **-ties** : the quality or state of being pluripotent

plu·to·ni·um \plü-'tō-nē-əm\ n : a radioactive metallic element similar chemically to uranium that undergoes slow disintegration with the emission of a helium nucleus to form uranium 235 — symbol Pu; see ELEMENT table

pm abbr premolar

Pm symbol promethium

PM abbr 1 [Latin post meridiem] after noon 2 postmortem

PMN abbr polymorphonuclear neutrophilic white blood cell

PMS n : PREMENSTRUAL SYNDROME

PN abbr psychoneurotic

-pnea \p-nē-ə\ n comb form : breath : breathing (apnea)

pneum- or **pneumo-** comb form 1 : air : gas (pneumothorax) 2 : lung (pneumoconiosis) : pulmonary and (pneumogastric) 3 : respiration (pneumograph) 4 : pneumonia (pneumococcus)

pneumat- or **pneumato-** comb form : air : vapor : gas (pneumatosis)

pneu·mat·ic \nü-'ma-tik, nyü-\ adj : of, relating to, or using gas (as air): as **a** : moved or worked by air pressure **b** : adapted for holding or inflated with compressed air **c** : having air-filled cavities (∼ bone) — **pneu·mat·i·cal·ly** adv

pneu·ma·ti·za·tion \ˌnü-mə-tə-'zā-shən, ˌnyü-\ n : the presence or development of air-filled cavities in a bone (∼ of the temporal bone) — **pneu·ma·tized** \'nü-mə-ˌtīzd, 'nyü-\ adj

pneu·ma·to·cele \'nü-mə-tō-ˌsēl, nyü-; nyü-'ma-tə-, nü-\ n : a gas-filled cavity or sac occurring esp. in the lung

pneu·ma·to·sis \ˌnü-mə-'tō-səs, ˌnyü-\ n, pl **-to·ses** \-ˌsēz\ : the presence of air or gas in abnormal places in the body

pneu·ma·tu·ria \ˌnü-mə-'tŭr-ē-ə, ˌnyü-\ n : passage of gas in the urine

pneu·mo·coc·cae·mia chiefly Brit var of PNEUMOCOCCEMIA

pneu·mo·coc·cal \ˌnü-mə-'kä-kəl, -ər-\ adj : of, relating to, caused by, or derived from pneumococci (∼ pneumonia) (a ∼ vaccine)

pneu·mo·coc·ce·mia \ˌnü-mə-ˌkäk-'sē-mē-ə, ˌnyü-\ n : the presence of pneumococci in the circulating blood

pneu·mo·coc·cus \ˌnü-mə-'kä-kəs, ˌnyü-\ n, pl **-coc·ci** \-'kä-ˌkī, -'käk-ˌsī\ : a bacterium of the genus Streptococcus (S. pneumoniae) that causes an acute pneumonia involving one or more lobes of the lung

pneu·mo·co·lon \ˌnü-mə-'kō-lən, ˌnyü-\ n : the presence of air in the colon

pneu·mo·co·ni·o·sis \ˌnü-mō-ˌkō-nē-'ō-səs, ˌnyü-\ n, pl **-oses** \-ˌsēz\ : a disease of the lungs caused by the habitual inhalation of irritants (as mineral or metallic particles) — called also miner's asthma, pneumonoconiosis; see BLACK LUNG, SILICOSIS

pneu·mo·cys·tic pneumonia \ˌnü-mə-'sis-tik-, ˌnyü-\ n : PNEUMOCYSTIS CARINII PNEUMONIA

Pneu·mo·cys·tis \ˌnü-mə-'sis-təs, ˌnyü-\ n 1 : a genus of microorganisms of uncertain affiliation that are usu. considered protozoans or sometimes fungi and that include one (P. carinii)

causing pneumonia esp. in immuno-compromised individuals 2 : in PNEUMO-CYSTIS CARINII PNEUMONIA

Pneumocystis ca·ri·nii pneumonia \-kə-ˈrī-nē-ˌē-\ *n* : a pneumonia that affects individuals whose immunological defenses have been compromised by malnutrition, by other diseases (as cancer or AIDS), or by artificial immunosuppressive techniques (as after organ transplantation), that is caused by a microorganism of the genus *Pneumocystis* (*P. carinii*) which shows up in specially stained preparations of fresh infected lung tissue as cysts containing six to eight oval bodies, and that attacks esp. the interstitium of the lungs with marked thickening of the alveolar septa and of the alveoli — abbr. *PCP*; called also *pneumocystic pneumonia, Pneumocystis carinii pneumonitis*

pneu·mo·cys·tog·ra·phy \ˌnü-mə-ˌsi-ˈstä-grə-fē, ˌnyü-\ *n, pl* **-phies** : roentgenography of the urinary bladder after it has been injected with air

pneu·mo·cyte \ˈnü-mə-ˌsīt, ˈnyü-\ *n* : any of the specialized cells that occur in the alveoli of the lungs

pneu·mo·en·ceph·a·li·tis \ˌnü-mō-in-ˌse-fə-ˈlī-təs, ˌnyü-\ *n, pl* **-lit·i·des** \-ˈli-tə-ˌdēz\ : NEWCASTLE DISEASE

pneu·mo·en·ceph·a·lo·gram \-in-ˈse-fə-lə-ˌgram\ *n* : a roentgenogram made by pneumoencephalography

pneu·mo·en·ceph·a·lo·graph \-ˌgraf\ *n* : PNEUMOENCEPHALOGRAM

pneu·mo·en·ceph·a·log·ra·phy \-in-ˌse-fə-ˈlä-grə-fē\ *n, pl* **-phies** : roentgenography of the brain after the injection of air into the ventricles — **pneu·mo·en·ceph·a·lo·graph·ic** \-in-ˌse-fə-lə-ˈgra-fik\ *adj*

pneu·mo·en·ter·i·tis \-ˌen-tə-ˈrī-təs\ *n, pl* **-en·ter·it·i·des** \-ˈri-tə-ˌdēz\ *or* **-en·ter·i·tis·es** : pneumonia combined with enteritis

pneu·mo·gas·tric nerve \ˌnü-mə-ˈgas-trik-, ˌnyü-\ *n* : VAGUS NERVE

pneu·mo·gram \ˈnü-mə-ˌgram, ˈnyü-\ *n* : a record of respiratory movements obtained by pneumography

pneu·mo·graph \ˈnü-mə-ˌgraf, ˈnyü-\ *n* : an instrument for recording the thoracic movements or volume change during respiration

pneu·mog·ra·phy \nü-ˈmä-grə-fē, nyü-\ *n, pl* **-phies** 1 : a description of the lungs 2 : roentgenography after the injection of air into a body cavity 3 : the process of making a pneumogram — **pneu·mo·graph·ic** \ˌnü-mə-ˈgra-fik, ˌnyü-\ *adj*

pneu·mol·y·sis \-ˈmä-lə-səs\ *n, pl* **-y·ses** \-ˌsēz\ : PNEUMONOLYSIS

pneu·mo·me·di·as·ti·num \ˌnü-mō-ˌmē-dē-ə-ˈsti-nəm, ˌnyü-\ *n, pl* **-ti·na** \-nə\ 1 : an abnormal state characterized by the presence of gas (as air) in the mediastinum 2 : the induction of

pneumomediastinum as an aid to roentgenography

pneu·mo·my·co·sis \-mī-ˈkō-səs\ *n, pl* **-co·ses** \-ˌsēz\ : a fungus disease of the lungs; *esp* : aspergillosis in poultry

pneumon- *or* **pneumono-** *comb form* : lung ⟨*pneumonectomy*⟩ ⟨*pneumonocentesis*⟩

pneu·mo·nec·to·my \ˌnü-mə-ˈnek-tə-mē, ˌnyü-\ *n, pl* **-mies** : surgical excision of an entire lung or of one or more lobes of a lung — compare SEGMENTAL RESECTION

pneu·mo·nia \nü-ˈmō-nyə, nyü-\ *n* : a disease of the lungs characterized by inflammation and consolidation followed by resolution and caused by infection or irritants — see BRONCHOPNEUMONIA, LOBAR PNEUMONIA, PRIMARY ATYPICAL PNEUMONIA

pneu·mon·ic \nü-ˈmä-nik, nyü-\ *adj* 1 : of, relating to, or affecting the lungs : PULMONARY 2 : of, relating to, or affected with pneumonia

pneumonic plague *n* : plague of an extremely virulent form that is caused by a bacterium of the genus *Pasteurella* (*P. pestis*), involves chiefly the lungs, and usu. is transmitted from person to person by droplet infection — compare BUBONIC PLAGUE

pneu·mo·ni·tis \ˌnü-mə-ˈnī-təs, ˌnyü-\ *n, pl* **-nit·i·des** \-ˈni-tə-ˌdēz\ 1 : a disease characterized by inflammation of the lungs; *esp* : PNEUMONIA 2 : FELINE PNEUMONITIS

pneu·mo·no·cen·te·sis \ˌnü-mə-(ˌ)nō-sen-ˈtē-səs, ˌnyü-\ *n, pl* **-te·ses** \-ˌsēz\ : surgical puncture of a lung for aspiration

pneu·mo·no·co·ni·o·sis \-ˌkō-nē-ˈō-səs\ *n, pl* **-o·ses** \-ˌsēz\ : PNEUMOCONIOSIS

pneu·mo·nol·y·sis \ˌnü-mə-ˈnä-lə-səs, ˌnyü-\ *n, pl* **-y·ses** \-ˌsēz\ : either of two surgical procedures to permit collapse of a lung: **a** : separation of the parietal pleura from the fascia of the chest wall **b** : separation of the visceral and parietal layers of the pleura — called also *intrapleural pneumonolysis*

pneu·mo·nos·to·my \ˌnü-mə-ˈnäs-tə-mē, ˌnyü-\ *n, pl* **-mies** : surgical formation of an artificial opening (as for drainage of an abscess) into a lung

Pneu·mo·nys·sus \ˌnü-mə-ˈni-səs, ˌnyü-\ *n* : a genus of mites (family Halarachnidae) that live in the air passages of mammals and include one (*P. caninum*) found in dogs

pneu·mop·a·thy \nü-ˈmä-pə-thē, nyü-\ *n, pl* **-thies** : any disease of the lungs

pneu·mo·peri·car·di·um \ˌnü-mō-ˌper-ə-ˈkär-dē-əm, ˌnyü-\ *n, pl* **-dia** \-dē-ə\ : an abnormal state characterized by the presence of gas (as air) in the pericardium

pneu·mo·peri·to·ne·um \-ˌper-ə-tə-ˈnē-əm\ *n, pl* **-ne·ums** *or* **-nea** \-ˈnē-ə\ 1 : an abnormal state characterized by the presence of gas (as air) in the peritoneal cavity **2** : the induction of pneumoperitoneum as a therapeutic measure or as an aid to roentgenography

pneu·mo·scle·ro·sis \-sklə-'rō-səs\ *n, pl* **-ro·ses** \-ˌsēz\ : fibrosis of the lungs

pneu·mo·tacho·gram \ˌnü-mō-'tak-ə-ˌgram, ˌnyü-\ *n* : a record of the velocity of the respiratory function obtained by use of a pneumotachograph

pneu·mo·tacho·graph \-ˌgraf\ *n* : a device or apparatus for measuring the rate of the respiratory function

pneu·mo·tax·ic center \ˌnü-mə-'tak-sik-, ˌnyü-\ *n* : a neural center in the upper part of the pons that provides inhibitory impulses on inspiration and thereby prevents overdistension of the lungs and helps to maintain alternately recurrent inspiration and expiration

pneu·mo·tho·rax \-'thōr-ˌaks\ *n, pl* **-tho·rax·es** *or* **-tho·ra·ces** \-'thōr-ə-ˌsēz\ **1** : an abnormal state characterized by the presence of gas (as air) in the pleural cavity — see TENSION PNEUMOTHORAX; compare OLEOTHORAX **2** : the induction of pneumothorax as a therapeutic measure to collapse the lung or as an aid to roentgenography

pneu·mo·tro·pic \-'trō-pik, -'trä-\ *adj* : turning, directed toward, or having an affinity for lung tissues — used esp. of infective agents

-pnoea *chiefly Brit var of* -PNEA

po *abbr* per os — used esp. in writing prescriptions

Po *symbol* polonium

pock \'päk\ *n* : a pustule in an eruptive disease (as smallpox)

pock·et \'pä-kət\ *n* : a small cavity or space; *esp* : an abnormal cavity formed in diseased tissue (a gingival ~) — **pocketing** *n*

pock·mark \'päk-ˌmärk\ *n* : a mark, pit, or depressed scar caused by smallpox or acne — **pock·marked** *adj*

pod- *or* **podo-** *comb form* **1** : foot (*podiatry*) **2** : hoof (*pododermatitis*)

po·dag·ra \pə-'da-grə\ *n* **1** : GOUT **2** : a painful condition of the big toe caused by gout

po·dal·ic \pō-'da-lik\ *adj* : of, relating to, or by means of the feet; *specif* : being an obstetric version in which the fetus is turned so that the feet emerge first in delivery

po·di·a·try \pə-'dī-ə-trē, pō-\ *n, pl* **-tries** : the medical care and treatment of the human foot — called also *chiropody* — **po·di·at·ric** \ˌpō-dē-'a-trik\ *adj* — **po·di·a·trist** \pə-'dī-ə-trist\ *n*

podo·der·ma·ti·tis \ˌpä-dō-ˌdər-mə-'tī-təs\ *n, pl* **-ti·tis·es** *or* **-tit·i·des** \-'ti-tə-ˌdēz\ : a condition (as foot rot) characterized by inflammation of the dermal tissue underlying the horny layers of a hoof

podo·phyl·lin \ˌpä-də-'fi-lən\ *n* : a resin obtained from podophyllum and used in medicine as a caustic

podo·phyl·lo·tox·in \ˌpä-də-ˌfi-lə-'täk-sən\ *n* : a crystalline polycyclic compound $C_{22}H_{22}O_8$ constituting one of the active principles of podophyllum and podophyllin

podo·phyl·lum \-'fi-ləm\ *n* **1** *cap* : a genus of herbs (family Berberidaceae) that have poisonous rootstocks, large palmate leaves, and large fleshy sometimes edible berries **2** *pl* **-phyl·li** \-'fi-ˌlī\ *or* **-phyllums** : the dried rhizome and rootlet of the mayapple (*Podophyllum peltatum*) that is used as a caustic or as a source of the more effective podophyllin

podophyllum resin *n* : PODOPHYLLIN

po·go·ni·on \pə-'gō-nē-ən\ *n* : the most projecting median point on the anterior surface of the chin

-poi·e·sis \(ˌ)pȯi-'ē-səs\ *n comb form, pl* **-poi·e·ses** \-'ē-ˌsēz\ : production : formation (hemopoiesis)

-poi·et·ic \(ˌ)pȯi-'e-tik\ *adj comb form* : productive : formative (hemopoietic)

poi·ki·lo·cyte \'pȯi-ki-lə-ˌsīt, (ˌ)pȯi-'ki-\ *n* : an abnormally formed red blood cell characteristic of various anemias

poi·ki·lo·cy·to·sis \ˌpȯi-ki-lō-sī-'tō-səs\ *n, pl* **-to·ses** \-ˌsēz\ : a condition characterized by the presence of poikilocytes in the blood

poi·ki·lo·der·ma \ˌpȯi-kə-lə-'dər-mə\ *n, pl* **-mas** *or* **-ma·ta** \-mə-tə\ : any of several disorders characterized by patchy discoloration of the skin

poi·ki·lo·ther·mic \-'thər-mik\ *adj* : COLD-BLOODED

¹point \'pȯint\ *n* **1** : a narrowly localized place or area **2** : the terminal usu. sharp or narrowly rounded part of something

²point *vb, of an abscess* : to become distended with pus prior to breaking

pointer — see HIP POINTER

point mutation *n* : mutation due to reorganization within a gene (as by substitution, addition, or deletion of a nucleotide) — called also *gene mutation*

Poiseuille's law \pwä-'zœiz-\ *n* : a statement in physics that relates the velocity of flow of a fluid (as blood) through a narrow tube (as a capillary) to the pressure and viscosity of the fluid and the length and radius of the tube

    Poiseuille, Jean–Léonard–Marie (1797–1869), French physiologist and physician.

¹poi·son \'pȯiz-ən\ *n* **1** : a substance that through its chemical action usu. kills, injures, or impairs an organism **2** : a substance that inhibits the activity of another substance or the course of a reaction or process (a catalyst ~)

²poison *vb* **poi·soned; poi·son·ing 1** : to

injure or kill with poison **2** : to treat, taint, or impregnate with poison

³**poison** *adj* **1** : POISONOUS ⟨a ~ plant⟩ **2** : impregnated with poison ⟨a ~ arrow⟩

poison dog·wood \-'dȯg-ˌwu̇d\ *n* : POISON SUMAC

poison gas *n* : a poisonous gas or a liquid or a solid giving off poisonous vapors designed (as in chemical warfare) to kill, injure, or disable by inhalation or contact

poison hemlock *n* **1** : a large branching biennial poisonous herb (*Conium maculatum*) of the carrot family (Umbelliferae) with finely divided leaves and white flowers **2** : WATER HEMLOCK

poison ivy *n* **1 a** : a climbing plant of the genus *Rhus* (*R. radicans* syn. *Toxicodendron radicans*) that is esp. common in the eastern and central U.S., that has leaves in groups of three, greenish flowers, and white berries, and that produces an acutely irritating oil causing a usu. intensely itching skin rash **b** : any of several plants closely related to poison ivy; *esp* : POISON OAK 1b **2** : a skin rash produced by poison ivy

poison oak *n* **1** : any of several plants included in the genus *Rhus* or sometimes in the genus *Toxicodendron* that produce an irritating oil like that of poison ivy: **a** : a bushy plant (*R. diversiloba* syn. *T. diversilobum*) of the Pacific coast **b** : a bushy plant (*R. toxicodendron* syn. *T. pubescens*) of the southeastern U.S. **2** : POISON IVY 1a **3** : a skin rash produced by poison oak

poi·son·ous \'pȯiz-ᵊn-əs\ *adj* : having the properties or effects of poison : VENOMOUS

poison su·mac \-'shü-ˌmak, -'sü-\ *n* : an American swamp shrub of the genus *Rhus* (*R. vernix* syn. *Toxicodendron vernix*) that has pinnate leaves, greenish flowers, and greenish white berries and produces an irritating oil — called also *poison dogwood*

poison·wood \'pȯiz-ᵊn-ˌwu̇d\ *n* : a caustic or poisonous tree of the genus *Metopium* (*M. toxiferum*) of Florida and the West Indies that has compound leaves, clusters of greenish flowers, and orange-yellow fruits

poke·weed \'pōk-ˌwēd\ *n* : an American perennial herb (*Phytolacca americana* of the family Phytolaccaceae) which has racemose white flowers, dark purple juicy berries, and a poisonous root and from which is obtained a mitogen that has been used to stimulate lymphocyte proliferation

po·lar \'pō-lər\ *adj* **1** : of or relating to one or more poles (as of a spherical body) **2** : exhibiting polarity; *esp* : having a dipole or characterized by molecules having dipoles ⟨a ~ solvent⟩ **3** : being at opposite ends of a spectrum of symptoms or manifestations ⟨~ types of leprosy⟩

polar body *n* : a cell that separates from an oocyte during meiosis: **a** : one containing a nucleus produced in the first meiotic division — called also *first polar body* **b** : one containing a nucleus produced in the second meiotic division — called also *second polar body*

po·lar·i·ty \pō-'lar-ə-tē, pə-\ *n, pl* **-ties 1** : the quality or condition inherent in a body that exhibits contrasting properties or powers in contrasting parts or directions **2** : attraction toward a particular object or in a specific direction **3** : the particular state either positive or negative with reference to the two poles or to electrification

po·lar·ize \'pō-lə-ˌrīz\ *vb* **-ized; -iz·ing 1** : to vibrate or cause (as light waves) to vibrate in a definite pattern **2** : to give physical polarity to — **po·lar·i·za·tion** \ˌpō-lə-rə-'zā-shən\ *n*

polarizing microscope *n* : a microscope equipped to produce polarized light for examination of a specimen

pole \'pōl\ *n* **1 a** : either of the two terminals of an electric cell or battery **b** : one of two or more regions in a magnetized body at which the magnetism is concentrated **2** : either of two morphologically or physiologically differentiated areas at opposite ends of an axis in an organism, organ, or cell

poli- *or* **polio-** *comb form* : of or relating to the gray matter of the brain or spinal cord ⟨*polio*myelitis⟩

pol·i·clin·ic \'päl-ē-ˌkli-nik\ *n* : a dispensary or department of a hospital at which outpatients are treated — compare POLYCLINIC

po·lio \'pō-lē-ˌō\ *n* : POLIOMYELITIS

po·lio·dys·tro·phy \ˌpō-lē-ō-'dis-trə-fē\ *n, pl* **-phies** : atrophy of the gray matter esp. of the cerebrum

po·lio·en·ceph·a·li·tis \ˌpō-lē-(ˌ)ō-in-ˌse-fə-'lī-təs\ *n, pl* **-lit·i·des** \-'li-tə-ˌdēz\ : inflammation of the gray matter of the brain

po·lio·en·ceph·a·lo·my·eli·tis \-in-ˌse-fə-lō-ˌmī-ə-'lī-təs\ *n, pl* **-elit·i·des** \-'li-tə-ˌdēz\ : inflammation of the gray matter of the brain and the spinal cord

po·lio·my·eli·tis \ˌpō-lē-(ˌ)ō-ˌmī-ə-'lī-təs\ *n, pl* **-elit·i·des** \-'li-tə-ˌdēz\ : an acute infectious virus disease characterized by fever, motor paralysis, and atrophy of skeletal muscles often with permanent disability and deformity and marked by inflammation of nerve cells in the ventral horns of the spinal cord — called also *infantile paralysis, polio* — **po·lio·my·elit·ic** \-'li-tik\ *adj*

po·li·o·sis \ˌpō-lē-'ō-səs\ *n, pl* **-o·ses** \-ˌsēz\ : loss of color from the hair

polio vaccine *n* : a vaccine intended to confer immunity to poliomyelitis

po·lio·vi·rus \'pō-lē-(ˌ)ō-ˌvī-rəs\ *n* : an

enterovirus that occurs in several antigenically distinct forms and is the causative agent of human poliomyelitis

po·litz·er bag \\'pō-lit-sər-, -'pä-\ *n* : a soft rubber bulb used to inflate the middle ear by increasing air pressure in the nasopharynx

Politzer, Adam (1835–1920), Austrian otologist.

pol·len \\'pä-lən\ *n* : a mass of male spores in a seed plant appearing usu. as a fine dust

pol·lex \\'pä-ˌleks\ *n, pl* **pol·li·ces** \\'pä-lə-ˌsēz\ : the first digit of the forelimb : THUMB

pollicis — see ABDUCTOR POLLICIS BREVIS, ABDUCTOR POLLICIS LONGUS, ADDUCTOR POLLICIS, EXTENSOR POLLICIS BREVIS, EXTENSOR POLLICIS LONGUS, FLEXOR POLLICIS BREVIS, FLEXOR POLLICIS LONGUS, OPPONENS POLLICIS, PRINCEPS POLLICIS

pol·li·ci·za·tion \\ˌpä-lə-sə-'zā-shən\ *n* : the reconstruction or replacement of the thumb esp. from part of the forefinger

pol·li·no·sis *or* **pol·le·no·sis** \\ˌpä-lə-'nō-səs\ *n, pl* **-no·ses** \\-ˌsēz\ : an acute recurrent catarrhal disorder caused by allergic sensitivity to specific pollens

pol·lut·ant \\pə-'lüt-ᵊnt\ *n* : something that pollutes

pol·lute \\pə-'lüt\ *vb* **pol·lut·ed; pol·lut·ing** : to contaminate (an environment) esp. with man-made waste — **pol·lut·er** *n* — **pol·lut·ive** \\-'lü-tiv\ *adj*

pol·lu·tion \\pə-'lü-shən\ *n* **1** : the action of polluting or the condition of being polluted **2** : POLLUTANT

po·lo·ni·um \\pə-'lō-nē-əm\ *n* : a radioactive metallic element that emits a helium nucleus to form an isotope of lead — symbol *Po;* see ELEMENT table

poly- *comb form* **1** : many : several : much : MULTI- ⟨*poly*arthritis⟩ **2** : excessive : abnormal : HYPER- ⟨*poly*dactyly⟩

poly(A) \\ˌpä-lē-'ā\ *n* : RNA or a segment of RNA that is composed of a polynucleotide chain consisting entirely of adenine-containing nucleotides and that codes for polylysine when functioning as messenger RNA in protein synthesis — called also *polyadenylate, polyadenylic acid*

poly·acryl·amide \\ˌpä-lē-ə-'kri-lə-ˌmīd\ *n* : a polymer $(-CH_2CHCONH_2-)_x$ derived from acrylic acid

polyacrylamide gel *n* : hydrated polyacrylamide that is used esp. to provide a medium for the suspension of a substance to be subjected to gel electrophoresis

poly·ad·en·yl·ate \\ˌpä-lē-ə-ˌad-ᵊn-'i-ˌlāt\ *n* : POLY(A) — **poly·ad·en·yl·at·ed** \\-ˌā-təd\ *adj* — **poly·ad·en·yl·a·tion** \\-i-'lā-shən\ *n*

poly·ad·en·yl·ic acid \\-'l-ilik-\ *n* : POLY(A)

poly·an·dry \\'pä-lē-ˌan-drē\ *n, pl* **-dries** : the state or practice of having more than one husband or male mate at one time — compare POLYGAMY, POLYGYNY — **poly·an·drous** \\ˌpä-lē-'an-drəs\ *adj*

poly·ar·ter·i·tis \\ˌpä-lē-ˌär-tə-'rī-təs\ *n* : POLYARTERITIS NODOSA

polyarteritis nodosa *n* : an acute inflammatory disease that involves all layers of the arterial wall and is characterized by degeneration, necrosis, exudation, and the formation of inflammatory nodules along the outer layer — called also *periarteritis nodosa*

poly·ar·thri·tis \\-är-'thrī-təs\ *n, pl* **-thrit·i·des** \\-'thri-tə-ˌdēz\ : arthritis involving two or more joints

poly·ar·tic·u·lar \\-är-'ti-kyə-lər\ *adj* : having or affecting many joints ⟨∼ arthritis⟩

poly·bro·mi·nat·ed biphenyl \\ˌpä-lē-'brō-mə-ˌnā-təd-\ *n* : any of several compounds that are similar to polychlorinated biphenyls in environmental toxicity and in structure except that various hydrogen atoms are replaced by bromine rather than chlorine — called also *PBB*

poly(C) \\ˌpä-lē-'sē\ *n* : POLYCYTIDYLIC ACID

poly·chlo·ri·nat·ed biphenyl \\ˌpä-lē-'klōr-ə-ˌnā-təd-\ *n* : any of several compounds that are produced by replacing hydrogen atoms in biphenyl with chlorine, have various industrial applications, and are poisonous environmental pollutants which tend to accumulate in animal tissues — called also *PCB*

poly·chro·ma·sia \\-krō-'mā-zhə, -zhē-ə\ *n* : the quality of being polychromatic; *specif* : POLYCHROMATOPHILIA

poly·chro·mat·ic \\-krō-'ma-tik\ *adj* **1** : showing a variety or a change of colors **2** *of a cell or tissue* : exhibiting polychromatophilia

¹poly·chro·ma·to·phil \\-krō-'ma-tə-ˌfil, -ˌkrō-mə-tə-\ *n* : a young or degenerated red blood corpuscle staining with both acid and basic dyes

²polychromatophil *adj* : exhibiting polychromatophilia; *esp* : staining with both acid and basic dyes

poly·chro·mato·phil·ia \\-krō-ˌma-tə-'fi-lē-ə\ *n* : the quality of being stainable with more than one type of stain and esp. with both acid and basic dyes — **poly·chro·mato·phil·ic** \\-krō-ˌma-tə-'fi-lik\ *adj*

poly·clin·ic \\ˌpä-lē-'kli-nik\ *n* : a clinic or hospital treating diseases of many sorts — compare POLICLINIC

poly·clo·nal \\ˌpä-lē-'klōn-ᵊl\ *adj* : produced by or being cells derived from two or more cells of different ancestry or genetic constitution ⟨∼ antibody synthesis⟩

poly·cy·clic \\ˌpä-lē-'sī-klik, -'si-\ *adj* : having more than one cyclic component; *esp* : having two or more usu. fused rings in a molecule

polycyclic aromatic hydrocarbon *n* : any of a class of hydrocarbon molecules with multiple carbon rings that include numerous carcinogenic substances and environmental pollutants — called also *PAH*

poly·cys·tic \-'sis-tik\ *adj* : having or involving more than one cyst

polycystic kidney disease *n* : either of two hereditary diseases characterized by gradually enlarging bilateral cysts of the kidney which lead to reduced renal functioning

polycystic ovary syndrome *n* : a variable disorder that is marked esp. by amenorrhea, hirsutism, obesity, infertility, and ovarian enlargement and is usu. initiated by an elevated level of luteinizing hormone, androgen, or estrogen which results in an abnormal cycle of gonadotropin release by the pituitary gland — called also *polycystic ovarian disease, polycystic ovarian syndrome, polycystic ovary disease, Stein-Leventhal syndrome*

poly·cy·thae·mia,   poly·cy·thae·mic chiefly Brit var of POLYCYTHEMIA, POLYCYTHEMIC

poly·cy·the·mia \-(ˌ)sī-'thē-mē-ə\ *n* : a condition marked by an abnormal increase in the number of circulating red blood cells : HYPERCYTHEMIA; *specif* : POLYCYTHEMIA VERA

polycythemia vera \-'vir-ə\ *n* : polycythemia of unknown cause that is characterized by increase in total blood volume and accompanied by nosebleed, distension of the circulatory vessels, and enlargement of the spleen — called also *erythremia, Vaquez's disease;* compare ERYTHROCYTOSIS

poly·cy·the·mic \ˌpä-lē-(ˌ)sī-'thē-mik\ *adj* : relating to or involving polycythemia or polycythemia vera

poly·cyt·i·dyl·ic acid \-ˌsi-tə-'di-lik-\ *n* : RNA or a segment of RNA that is composed of a polynucleotide chain consisting entirely of cytosine-containing nucleotides and that codes for a polypeptide chain consisting of proline residues when functioning as messenger RNA in protein synthesis — called also *poly(C);* see POLY I:C

poly·dac·tyl \-'dak-təl\ *adj* : characterized by polydactyly; *also* : being a gene that determines polydactyly

poly·dac·tyl·ia \-dak-'ti-lē-ə\ *n* : POLYDACTYLY

poly·dac·tyl·ism \-'dakt-əl-ˌi-zəm\ *n* : POLYDACTYLY

poly·dac·ty·ly \-'dak-tə-lē\ *n, pl* **-lies** : the condition of having more than the normal number of toes or fingers

poly·dip·sia \ˌpä-lē-'dip-sē-ə\ *n* : excessive or abnormal thirst — **poly·dip·sic** \-sik\ *adj*

poly·drug \'pä-lē-ˌdrəg\ *adj* : relating

to or affected by addiction to more than one illicit drug (∼ abuse)

poly·em·bry·o·ny \ˌpä-lē-ˈem-brē-ə-nē, -(ˌ)em-ˈbrī-\ *n, pl* **-nies** : the production of two or more embryos from one ovule or egg

poly·en·do·crine \-ˈen-də-krən, -ˌkrīn, -ˌkrēn\ *adj* : relating to or affecting more than one endocrine gland (a family history of ∼ disorders)

po·lyg·a·my \pə-ˈli-gə-mē\ *n, pl* **-mies** : marriage in which a spouse of either sex may have more than one mate at the same time — compare POLYANDRY, POLYGYNY — **po·lyg·a·mous** \-məs\ *adj*

poly·gene \ˈpä-lē-ˌjēn\ *n* : any of a group of nonallelic genes that collectively control the inheritance of a quantitative character or modify the expression of a qualitative character — called also *multiple factor;* compare QUANTITATIVE INHERITANCE

poly·gen·ic \ˌpä-lē-ˈjē-nik, -ˈje-\ *adj* : of, relating to, or resulting from polygenes : MULTIFACTORIAL

poly·glan·du·lar \ˌpä-lē-ˈglan-jə-lər\ *adj* : of, relating to, or involving several glands (∼ therapy)

poly·graph \ˈpä-lē-ˌgraf\ *n* : an instrument for simultaneously recording variations of several different pulsations (as of the pulse, blood pressure, and respiration); *broadly* : LIE DETECTOR — **poly·graph·ic** \ˌpä-lē-ˈgra-fik\ *adj*

po·lyg·y·ny \pə-ˈli-jə-nē\ *n, pl* **-nies** : the state or practice of having more than one wife or female mate at one time — compare POLYANDRY, POLYGAMY — **po·lyg·y·nous** \-nəs\ *adj*

poly·hy·dram·ni·os \ˌpä-lē-hī-ˈdram-nē-ˌäs\ *n* : HYDRAMNIOS

poly I:C \ˌpä-lē-ˌī-ˈsē\ *n* : a synthetic 2-stranded RNA composed of one strand of polyinosinic acid and one strand of polycytidylic acid that induces interferon formation and has been used experimentally as an anticancer and antiviral agent — called also *poly I·poly C*

poly·ino·sin·ic acid \ˌpä-lē-ˌi-nə-ˈsi-nik-, -ˌī-nə-\ *n* : RNA or a segment of RNA that is composed of a polynucleotide chain consisting entirely of inosinic acid residues — see POLY I:C

poly I·poly C \ˌpä-lē-ˈī-ˌpä-lē-ˈsē\ *n* : POLY I:C

poly·ly·sine \ˌpä-lē-ˈlī-ˌsēn\ *n* : a protein whose polypeptide chain consists entirely of lysine residues

poly·mer \ˈpä-lə-mər\ *n* : a chemical compound or mixture of compounds formed by polymerization and consisting essentially of repeating structural units — **poly·mer·ic** \ˌpä-lə-ˈmer-ik\ *adj* — **po·lym·er·ism** \pə-ˈli-mə-ˌri-zəm, ˈpä-lə-mə-\ *n*

poly·mer·ase \-mə-ˌrās, -ˌrāz\ *n* : any of several enzymes that catalyze the formation of DNA or RNA from precursor substances in the presence of preexisting DNA or RNA acting as a template

po·ly·mer·ase chain reaction n : an in vitro technique for rapidly synthesizing large quantities of a given DNA segment that involves separating the DNA into its two complementary strands, binding a primer to each single strand at the end of the given DNA segment where synthesis will start, using DNA polymerase to synthesize two-stranded DNA from each single strand, and repeating the process — abbr. *PCR*

po·ly·mer·iza·tion \pə-ˌli-mə-rə-ˈzā-shən, ˌpä-lə-mə-rə-\ n : a chemical reaction in which two or more small molecules combine to form larger molecules that contain repeating structural units of the original molecules — compare ASSOCIATION 3 — **po·ly·mer·ize** \pə-ˈli-mə-ˌrīz, ˈpä-lə-mə-\ vb

poly·meth·yl meth·ac·ry·late \ˌpä-lē-ˈme-thəl-me-ˈtha-krə-ˌlāt\ n : a thermoplastic polymeric resin that is used esp. in hard contact lenses and in prostheses to replace bone

poly·mi·cro·bi·al \ˌpä-lē-mī-ˈkrō-bē-əl\ adj : of, relating to, or caused by several types of microorganisms

poly·morph \ˈpä-lē-ˌmorf\ n 1 : a polymorphic organism; *also* : one of the several forms of such an organism 2 : a polymorphonuclear white blood cell

poly·mor·phism \-ˈmor-ˌfi-zəm\ n : the quality or state of being able to assume different forms — **poly·mor·phic** \-ˈmor-fik\ adj

¹**poly·mor·pho·nu·cle·ar** \-ˌmor-fō-ˈnü-klē-ər, -ˈnyü-\ adj, of a white blood cell : having the nucleus complexly lobed; *specif* : being a mature neutrophil with a characteristic distinctly lobed nucleus

²**polymorphonuclear** n : POLYMORPH 2

poly·mor·phous \-ˈmor-fəs\ adj : having, assuming, or occurring in various forms — **poly·mor·phous·ly** adv

polymorphous perverse adj : relating to or exhibiting infantile sexual tendencies in which the genitals are not yet identified as the sole or principal sexual organs nor coitus as the goal of erotic activity

poly·my·al·gia rheu·mat·i·ca \ˌpä-lē-mī-ˈal-jə-rü-ˈma-ti-kə, -jē-ə-\ n : a disorder of the elderly characterized by muscular pain and stiffness in the shoulders and neck and in the pelvic area

poly·myo·si·tis \-ˌmī-ə-ˈsī-təs\ n : inflammation of several muscles at once

poly·myx·in \ˌpä-lē-ˈmik-sən\ n : any of several toxic antibiotics obtained from a soil bacterium of the genus *Bacillus* (*B. polymyxa*) and active against gram-negative bacteria

polymyxin B n : the least toxic of the polymyxins used in the form of its sulfate chiefly in the treatment of some localized, gastrointestinal, or systemic infections

polymyxin E n : COLISTIN

poly·neu·ri·tis \ˌpä-lē-nü-ˈrī-təs, -nyü-\ n, pl **-rit·i·des** \-ˈri-tə-ˌdēz\ or **-ri·tis·es** : neuritis of several peripheral nerves at the same time — **poly·neu·rit·ic** \-ˈri-tik\ adj

poly·neu·rop·a·thy \-nü-ˈrä-pə-thē, -nyü-\ n, pl **-thies** : a disease of nerves; *esp* : a noninflammatory degenerative disease of nerves usu. caused by toxins (as of lead)

poly·nu·clear \-ˈnü-klē-ər, -ˈnyü-\ adj : chemically polycyclic esp. with respect to the benzene ring — used chiefly of certain hydrocarbons that are important as pollutants and possibly as carcinogens

poly·nu·cle·o·tide \-ˈnü-klē-ə-ˌtīd, -ˈnyü-\ n : a polymeric chain of nucleotides

poly·oma virus \ˌpä-lē-ˈō-mə-\ n : a papovavirus of rodents that is associated with various kinds of tumors — called also *polyoma*

poly·opia \ˌpä-lē-ˈō-pē-ə\ n : perception of more than one image of a single object esp. with one eye

poly·os·tot·ic \ˌpä-lē-ä-ˈstä-tik\ adj : involving or relating to many bones

pol·yp \ˈpä-ləp\ n : a projecting mass of swollen and hypertrophied or tumorous membrane

pol·yp·ec·to·my \ˌpä-li-ˈpek-tə-mē\ n, pl **-mies** : the surgical excision of a polyp

poly·pep·tide \ˌpä-lē-ˈpep-ˌtīd\ n : a molecular chain of amino acids — **poly·pep·tid·ic** \-(ˌ)pep-ˈti-dik\ adj

poly·pha·gia \ˌpä-lē-ˈfā-jə, -jē-ə\ n : excessive appetite or eating — compare HYPERPHAGIA

poly·phar·ma·cy \-ˈfär-mə-sē\ n, pl **-cies** : the practice of administering many different medicines esp. concurrently for the treatment of the same disease

poly·pha·sic \-ˈfā-zik\ adj 1 : of, relating to, or having more than one phase (∼ evoked potentials) — compare DIPHASIC b, MONOPHASIC 1 2 : having several periods of activity interrupted by intervening periods of rest in each 24 hours (an infant is essentially ∼)

poly·ploid \ˈpä-lē-ˌploid\ adj : having or being a chromosome number that is a multiple greater than two of the monoploid number — **poly·ploi·dy** \-ˌploi-dē\ n

po·lyp·nea \pä-ˈlip-nē-ə, pə-\ n : rapid or panting respiration — **po·lyp·ne·ic** \-nē-ik\ adj

po·lyp·noea chiefly Brit var of POLYPNEA

pol·yp·oid \ˈpä-lə-ˌpoid\ adj 1 : resembling a polyp (a ∼ intestinal growth) 2 : marked by the formation of lesions suggesting polyps (∼ disease)

pol·yp·o·sis \ˌpä-li-ˈpō-səs\ n, pl **-o·**

ses \-ısēz\ : a condition characterized by the presence of numerous polyps

poly·ri·bo·some \ˌpä-lē-ˈrī-bə-ˌsōm\ n : a cluster of ribosomes linked together by a molecule of messenger RNA and forming the site of protein synthesis — called also *polysome* — **poly·ri·bo·som·al** \-ˌrī-bə-ˈsō-məl\ adj

poly·sac·cha·ride \-ˈsa-kə-ˌrīd\ n : a carbohydrate that can be decomposed by hydrolysis into two or more molecules of monosaccharides; *esp* : one of the more complex carbohydrates (as cellulose, starch, or glycogen) — called also *glycan*

poly·se·ro·si·tis \-ˌsir-ə-ˈsī-təs\ n : inflammation of several serous membranes (as the pleura, pericardium, and peritoneum) at the same time

poly·some \ˈpä-lē-ˌsōm\ n : POLYRIBOSOME

poly·sor·bate \ˌpä-lē-ˈsor-ˌbāt\ n : any of several emulsifiers used in the preparation of some pharmaceuticals and foods — see TWEEN

poly·sper·my \ˈpä-lē-ˌspər-mē\ n, pl **-mies** : the entrance of several spermatozoa into one egg — compare MONOSPERMY — **poly·sper·mic** \ˌpä-lē-ˈspər-mik\ adj

poly·syn·ap·tic \ˌpä-lē-sə-ˈnap-tik\ adj : involving two or more synapses in the central nervous system — **poly·syn·ap·ti·cal·ly** adv

poly·tene \ˈpä-lē-ˌtēn\ adj : relating to, being, or having chromosomes each of which consists of many strands with the corresponding chromomeres in contact — **poly·te·ny** \-ˌtē-nē\ n

poly·tet·ra·fluo·ro·eth·yl·ene \ˌpä-lē-ˌte-trə-ˌflur-ō-ˈe-thə-ˌlēn\ n : a polymer $(CF_2-CF_2)_n$ that is a resin used to fabricate prostheses — abbr. *PTFE;* see TEFLON

poly·the·lia \ˌpä-lē-ˈthē-lē-ə\ n : the condition of having more than the normal number of nipples

poly·thia·zide \-ˈthī-ə-ˌzīd, -zəd\ n : an antihypertensive and diuretic drug $C_{11}H_{13}ClF_3N_3O_4S_3$ — see RENESE

poly(U) \ˌpä-lē-ˈyü\ n : POLYURIDYLIC ACID

poly·un·sat·u·rate \ˌpä-lē-ˌən-ˈsa-chə-rət\ n : a polyunsaturated oil or fatty acid

poly·un·sat·u·rat·ed \-ˌən-ˈsa-chə-ˌrā-təd\ adj, of an oil or fatty acid : having in each molecule many chemical bonds in which two or three pairs of electrons are shared by two atoms — compare MONOUNSATURATED

poly·uria \-ˈyür-ē-ə\ n : excessive secretion of urine

poly·uri·dyl·ic acid \-ˌyür-ə-ˌdi-lik-\ n : RNA or a segment of RNA that is composed of a polynucleotide chain consisting entirely of uracil-containing nucleotides and that codes for a polypeptide chain consisting of phenylalanine residues when functioning

as messenger RNA in protein synthesis — called also *poly(U)*

poly·va·lent \ˌpä-lē-ˈvā-lənt\ adj : effective against, sensitive toward, or counteracting more than one exciting agent (as a toxin or antigen) ⟨a ∼ vaccine⟩ — **poly·va·lence** \-ləns\ n

poly·vi·nyl·pyr·rol·i·done \ˌvīn-əl-pi-ˈrä-lə-ˌdōn\ n : a water-soluble chemically inert solid polymer $(-CH_2CHC_4H_6NO-)_n$ used chiefly in medicine as a vehicle for drugs (as iodine) and esp. formerly as a plasma expander — called also *povidone*

Pompe's disease \ˈpämps-\ n : an often fatal glycogenosis that results from an enzyme deficiency, is characterized by abnormal accumulation of glycogen esp. in the liver, heart, and muscle, and usu. appears during infancy — called also *acid maltase deficiency*

Pompe, J. C. (fl 1932), Dutch physician.

pom·pho·lyx \ˈpäm-fə-ˌliks\ n **1** : FLOWERS OF ZINC **2** : a skin disease marked by an eruption of vesicles esp. on the palms and soles

pon·der·al index \ˈpän-də-rəl-\ n : a measure of relative body mass expressed as the ratio of the cube root of body weight to height multiplied by 100

pons \ˈpänz\ n, pl **pon·tes** \ˈpän-ˌtēz\ : a broad mass of chiefly transverse nerve fibers conspicuous on the ventral surface of the brain at the anterior or end of the medulla oblongata

pons Va·ro·lii \-və-ˈrō-lē-ˌī, -lē-ˌē\ n, pl **pontes Varolii** : PONS

Va·ro·lio \vä-ˈrō-lē-ō\, **Costanzo (1543–1575)**, Italian anatomist.

pon·tic \ˈpän-tik\ n : an artifical tooth on a dental bridge

pon·tile \ˈpän-ˌtīl, -təl\ adj : PONTINE

pon·tine \ˈpän-ˌtīn\ adj : of or relating to the pons ⟨a study of ∼ lesions⟩

pontine flexure n : a flexure of the embryonic hindbrain that serves to delimit the developing cerebellum and medulla oblongata

pontine nucleus n : any of various large groups of nerve cells in the basal part of the pons that receive fibers from the cerebral cortex and send fibers to the cerebellum by way of the middle cerebellar peduncles

pontis — see BRACHIUM PONTIS

Pon·to·caine \ˈpän-tə-ˌkān\ trademark — used for a preparation of tetracaine

¹pool \ˈpül\ vb, of blood : to accumulate or become static (as in the veins of a bodily part) ⟨blood ∼ed in his legs⟩

²pool n : a readily available supply: as **a** : the whole quantity of a particular material present in the body and available for function or the satisfying of metabolic demands — see GENE POOL **b** : a body product (as blood)

collected from many donors and stored for later use

pop·li·te·al \ˌpä-plə-ˈtē-əl, päp-ˈli-tē-\ *adj* : of or relating to the back part of the leg behind the knee joint

popliteal artery *n* : the continuation of the femoral artery that after passing through the thigh crosses the popliteal space and soon divides into the anterior and posterior tibial arteries

popliteal fossa *n* : POPLITEAL SPACE

popliteal ligament — see ARCUATE POPLITEAL LIGAMENT, OBLIQUE POPLITEAL LIGAMENT

popliteal nerve — see COMMON PERONEAL NERVE, TIBIAL NERVE

popliteal space *n* : a lozenge-shaped space at the back of the knee joint — called also *popliteal fossa*

popliteal vein *n* : a vein formed by the union of the anterior and posterior tibial veins and ascending through the popliteal space to the thigh where it becomes the femoral vein

pop·li·te·us \ˌpä-plə-ˈtē-əs, päp-ˈli-tē-əs\ *n, pl* **-li·tei** \-tē-ˌī\ : a flat muscle that originates from the lateral condyle of the femur, forms part of the floor of the popliteal space, and functions to flex the leg and rotate the femur medially

pop·per \ˈpä-pər\ *n, slang* : a vial of amyl nitrite or isobutyl nitrite esp. when used illicitly as an aphrodisiac

pop·py \ˈpä-pē\ *n, pl* **poppies** : any herb of the genus *Papaver* (family Papaveraceae); *esp* : OPIUM POPPY

pop·u·la·tion \ˌpä-pyə-ˈlā-shən\ *n* **1** : the organisms inhabiting a particular locality **2** : a group of individual persons, objects, or items from which samples are taken for statistical measurement

population genetics *n* : a branch of genetics concerned with gene and genotype frequencies in populations — see HARDY-WEINBERG LAW

por·ce·lain \ˈpōr-sə-lən\ *n* : a hard, fine-grained, nonporous, and usu. translucent and white ceramic ware that has many uses in dentistry

por·cine \ˈpōr-ˌsīn\ *adj* : of or derived from swine (∼ heterografts)

pore \ˈpōr\ *n* : a minute opening in an animal or plant; *esp* : one by which matter passes through a membrane

-pore \ˌpōr\ *n comb form* : opening (blasto*pore*)

por·en·ceph·a·ly \ˌpōr-in-ˈse-fə-lē\ *n, pl* **-lies** : the presence of cavities in the brain — **por·en·ce·phal·ic** \-ˌen-sə-ˈfa-lik\ *adj*

pork tapeworm \ˈpōrk-\ *n* : a tapeworm of the genus *Taenia* (*T. solium*) that infests the human intestine as an adult, has a cysticercus larva that typically develops in swine, and is contracted by humans through ingestion of the larva in raw or imperfectly cooked pork

po·ro·ceph·a·li·a·sis \ˌpō-rō-ˌse-fə-ˈlī-ə-

səs\ *n, pl* **-a·ses** \-ˌsēz\ : infestation with or disease caused by a tongue worm of the genus *Porocephalus*

Po·ro·ceph·a·lus \-ˈse-fə-ləs\ *n* : a genus of tongue worms (family Porocephalidae) occurring as adults in the lungs of reptiles and as young in various vertebrates including humans

po·ro·sis \pə-ˈrō-səs\ *n, pl* **po·ro·ses** \-ˌsēz\ *or* **porosises** : a condition (as of a bone) characterized by porosity; *specif* : rarefaction (as of bone) with increased translucency to X rays

po·ros·i·ty \pə-ˈrä-sə-tē, pō-, po-\ *n, pl* **-ties 1 a** : the quality or state of being porous **b** : the ratio of the volume of interstices of a material to the volume of its mass **2** : PORE

po·rot·ic \pə-ˈrä-tik\ *adj* : exhibiting or marked by porous structure or osteoporosis

po·rous \ˈpōr-əs\ *adj* **1** : possessing or full of pores (∼ bones) **2** : permeable to liquids

por·pho·bi·lin·o·gen \ˌpōr-fō-bī-ˈli-nə-jən\ *n* : an acid $C_{10}H_{14}N_2O_4$ having two carboxyl groups per molecule that is derived from pyrrole and is found in the urine in acute porphyria

por·phyr·ia \pōr-ˈfir-ē-ə\ *n* : any of several usu. hereditary abnormalities of porphyrin metabolism characterized by excretion of excess porphyrins in the urine

por·phy·rin \ˈpōr-fə-rən\ *n* : any of various compounds with a structure that consists essentially of four pyrrole rings joined by four =C– groups; *esp* : one (as chlorophyll or hemoglobin) containing a central metal atom and usu. having biological activity

por·phy·rin·uria \ˌpōr-fə-rə-ˈnur-ē-ə, -ˈnyur-\ *n* : the presence of porphyrin in the urine

por·ta \ˈpōr-tə\ *n, pl* **por·tae** \-ˌtē\ : an opening in a bodily part where the blood vessels, nerves, or ducts leave and enter : HILUM

por·ta·ca·val \ˌpōr-tə-ˈkā-vəl\ *adj* : extending from the portal vein to the vena cava (∼ anastomosis)

portacaval shunt *n* : a surgical shunt by which the portal vein is made to empty into the inferior vena cava in order to bypass a damaged liver

porta hep·a·tis \-ˈhe-pə-təs\ *n* : the fissure running transversely on the underside of the liver where most of the vessels enter or leave — called also *transverse fissure*

¹por·tal \ˈpōr-əl\ *n* : a communicating part or area of an organism: as **a** : PORTAL VEIN **b** : the point at which something enters the body (∼s of infection)

²portal *adj* **1** : of or relating to the porta hepatis **2** : of, relating to, or being a portal vein or a portal system

portal cirrhosis *n* : LAENNEC'S CIRRHOSIS

portal hypertension *n* : hypertension in

the hepatic portal system caused by venous obstruction or occlusion that produces splenomegaly and ascites in its later stages

portal system *n* : a system of veins that begins and ends in capillaries — see HEPATIC PORTAL SYSTEM, PITUITARY PORTAL SYSTEM

portal vein *n* : a large vein that is formed by fusion of other veins, that terminates in a capillary network, and that delivers blood to some area of the body other than the heart; *esp* : HEPATIC PORTAL VEIN

por·tio \'pȯr-shē-ˌō, 'pȯr-tē-ˌō\ *n, pl* **-ti·o·nes** \ˌpȯr-shē-'ō-ˌnēz\ : a part, segment, or branch (as of an organ or nerve) ⟨the visible ∼ of the cervix⟩

Por·tu·guese man-of-war \'pȯr-chə-ˌgēz-ˌman-əv-'wȯr\ *n, pl* **Portuguese man-of-wars** *also* **Portuguese men-of-war** : any siphonophore of the genus *Physalia* including large tropical and subtropical oceanic forms having a crested bladderlike float which bears a colony comprised of three types of individuals on the lower surface with one of the three having stinging tentacles

port–wine stain \'pȯrt-ˌwīn-\ *n* : a reddish purple superficial hemangioma of the skin commonly occurring as a birthmark — called also *nevus flammeus*, *port-wine mark*

¹po·si·tion \pə-'zi-shən\ *n* : a particular arrangement or location; *specif* : an arrangement of the parts of the body considered particularly desirable for some medical or surgical procedure ⟨knee-chest ∼⟩ ⟨lithotomy ∼⟩ — **po·si·tion·al** \pə-'zi-shə-nəl\ *adj*

²position *vb* : to put in proper position

pos·i·tive \'pä-zə-tiv\ *adj* 1 : being, relating to, or charged with electricity of which the proton is the elementary unit 2 : affirming the presence of that sought or suspected to be present ⟨a ∼ test for blood⟩ — **pos·i·tive·ly** *adv* — **pos·i·tive·ness** *n*

positive electron *n* : POSITRON

pos·i·tron \'pä-zə-ˌträn\ *n* : a positively charged particle having the same mass and magnitude of charge as the electron

positron–emission tomography *n* : tomography in which an in vivo, noninvasive, cross-sectional image of regional metabolism is obtained by a usu. color-coded CRT representation of the distribution of gamma radiation given off in the collision of electrons in cells with positrons emitted by radionuclides incorporated into metabolic substances — abbr. *PET*

post- *prefix* 1 : after : later than ⟨*post*operative⟩ ⟨*post*coronary⟩ 2 : behind : posterior to ⟨*post*auricular⟩

post·abor·tion \ˌpōst-ə-'bȯr-shən\ *adj* : occurring after an abortion

post·ab·sorp·tive \-əb-'sȯrp-tiv\ *adj* : being in or typical of the period fol-

lowing absorption of nutrients from the alimentary canal

post·ad·o·les·cence \-ˌad-əl-'es-ᵊns\ *n* : the period following adolescence and preceding adulthood — **post·ad·o·les·cent** \-ᵊnt\ *adj or n*

post·an·es·the·sia \-ˌa-nəs-'thē-zhə\ *adj* : POSTANESTHETIC

post·an·es·thet·ic \-'the-tik\ *adj* : occurring in, used in, or being the period following administration of an anesthetic ⟨∼ encephalopathy⟩

post·an·ox·ic \-a-'näk-sik\ *adj* : occurring or being after a period of anoxia

post·au·ric·u·lar \-ō-'ri-kyə-lər\ *adj* : located or occurring behind the auricle of the ear ⟨a ∼ incision⟩

post·ax·i·al \-'ak-sē-əl\ *adj* : of or relating to the ulnar side of the vertebrate forelimb or the fibular side of the hind limb; *also* : of or relating to the side of an animal or side of one of its limbs that is posterior to the axis of its body or limbs

post·cap·il·lary \-'ka-pə-ler-ē\ *adj* : of, relating to, affecting, or being a venule of the circulatory system

post·car·di·ot·o·my \-ˌkär-dē-'ä-tə-mē\ *adj* : occurring or being in the period following open-heart surgery

post·cen·tral \-'sen-trəl\ *adj* : located behind a center or central structure; *esp* : located behind the central sulcus of the cerebral cortex

postcentral gyrus *n* : a gyrus of the parietal lobe located just posterior to the central sulcus, lying parallel to the precentral gyrus of the temporal lobe, and comprising the somesthetic area

post·cho·le·cys·tec·to·my syndrome \-ˌkō-lə-(ˌ)sis-'tek-tə-mē-\ *n* : persistent pain and associated symptoms (as indigestion and nausea) following a cholecystectomy

post·co·i·tal \-'kō-ət-ᵊl, -'ēt-ᵊl; -'kȯit-ᵊl\ *adj* : occurring, existing, or being administered after coitus

post·cor·o·nary \-'kȯr-ə-ˌner-ē, -'kär-\ *adj* 1 : relating to, occurring in, or being the period following a heart attack ⟨∼ exercise⟩ 2 : having suffered a heart attack ⟨a ∼ patient⟩

post·dam \ˌpōst-'dam\ *n* : a posterior extension of a full denture to accomplish a complete seal between denture and tissues

post·en·ceph·a·lit·ic \-in-ˌse-fə-'li-tik\ *adj* : occurring after and presumably as a result of encephalitis ⟨∼ parkinsonism⟩

¹pos·te·ri·or \pō-'stir-ē-ər, pä-\ *adj* : situated behind: **as a** : situated at or toward the hind part of the body : CAUDAL **b** : DORSAL — used of human anatomy in which the upright posture makes dorsal and caudal identical

²pos·te·ri·or \pä-'stir-ē-ər, pō-\ *n* : the posterior bodily parts; *esp* : BUTTOCKS

posterior auricular artery n : a small branch of the external carotid artery that supplies or gives off branches supplying the back of the ear and the adjacent region of the scalp, the middle ear, tympanic membrane, and mastoid cells — called also *posterior auricular*

posterior auricular vein n : a vein formed from venous tributaries in the region behind the ear that joins with the posterior facial vein to form the external jugular vein

posterior brachial cutaneous nerve n : a branch of the radial nerve that arises on the medial side of the arm in the axilla and supplies the skin on the dorsal surface almost to the olecranon

posterior cerebral artery n : CEREBRAL ARTERY c

posterior chamber n : a narrow space in the eye behind the peripheral part of the iris and in front of the suspensory ligament of the lens and the ciliary processes — compare ANTERIOR CHAMBER

posterior column n : DORSAL HORN

posterior commissure n : a bundle of white matter crossing from one side of the brain to the other just rostral to the superior colliculi and above the opening of the aqueduct of Sylvius into the third ventricle

posterior communicating artery n : COMMUNICATING ARTERY b

posterior cord n : a cord of nerve tissue that is formed from the posterior divisions of the three trunks of the brachial plexus and that divides into the axillary and radial nerves — compare LATERAL CORD, MEDIAL CORD

posterior cricoarytenoid n : CRICOARYTENOID 2

posterior cruciate ligament n : CRUCIATE LIGAMENT a(2)

posterior elastic lamina n : DESCEMET'S MEMBRANE

posterior facial vein n : a vein that is formed in the upper part of the parotid gland behind the mandible by the union of several tributaries and joins with the posterior auricular vein to form the external jugular vein

posterior femoral cutaneous nerve n : a nerve that arises from the sacral plexus and is distributed to the skin of the perineum and of the back of the thigh and leg — compare LATERAL FEMORAL CUTANEOUS NERVE

posterior funiculus n : a longitudinal division on each side of the spinal cord comprising white matter between the dorsal root and the posterior median sulcus — compare ANTERIOR FUNICULUS, LATERAL FUNICULUS

posterior gray column n : DORSAL HORN

posterior horn n 1 : DORSAL HORN 2 : the cornu of the lateral ventricle of each cerebral hemisphere that curves backward into the occipital lobe —

compare ANTERIOR HORN 2, INFERIOR HORN

posterior humeral circumflex artery n : an artery that branches from the axillary artery in the shoulder, curves around the back of the humerus, and is distributed esp. to the deltoid muscle and shoulder joint — compare ANTERIOR HUMERAL CIRCUMFLEX ARTERY

posterior inferior cerebellar artery n : an artery that usu. branches from the vertebral artery and supplies much of the medulla oblongata, the inferior portion of the cerebellum, and part of the floor of the fourth ventricle

posterior inferior iliac spine n : a projection on the posterior margin of the ilium that is situated below the posterior superior iliac spine and is separated from it by a notch — called also *posterior inferior spine*

posterior intercostal artery n : INTERCOSTAL ARTERY b

posterior lobe n 1 : NEUROHYPOPHYSIS 2 : the part of the cerebellum between the primary fissure and the flocculonodular lobe

pos•te•ri•or•ly adv : in a posterior direction

posterior median septum n : a sheet of neuroglial tissue in the midsagittal plane of the spinal cord that partitions the posterior part of the spinal cord into right and left halves

posterior median sulcus n : a shallow groove along the midline of the posterior part of the spinal cord that separates the two posterior funiculi

posterior nares n pl : CHOANAE

posterior nasal spine n : the nasal spine that is formed by the union of processes of the two palatine bones

posterior pillar of the fauces n : PALATOPHARYNGEAL ARCH

posterior pituitary n 1 : NEUROHYPOPHYSIS 2 : an extract of the neurohypophysis of domesticated animals for medicinal use — called also *posterior pituitary extract*

posterior pituitary gland n : NEUROHYPOPHYSIS

posterior root n : DORSAL ROOT

posterior sacrococcygeal muscle n : SACROCOCCYGEUS DORSALIS

posterior spinal artery n : SPINAL ARTERY b

posterior spinocerebellar tract n : SPINOCEREBELLAR TRACT a

posterior superior alveolar artery n : a branch of the maxillary artery that supplies the upper molar and bicuspid teeth

posterior superior iliac spine n : a projection at the posterior end of the iliac crest — called also *posterior superior spine*

posterior synechia n : SYNECHIA b

posterior temporal artery n : TEMPORAL ARTERY 3c

posterior tibial artery *n* : TIBIAL ARTERY a

posterior tibial vein *n* : TIBIAL VEIN b

posterior triangle *n* : a triangular region that is a landmark in the neck and has its apex above at the occipital bone — compare ANTERIOR TRIANGLE

posterior ulnar recurrent artery *n* : ULNAR RECURRENT ARTERY b

posterior vein of the left ventricle *n* : a vein that ascends on the surface of the left ventricle facing the diaphragm and that usu. empties into the coronary sinus — called also *posterior vein*

postero- *comb form* : posterior and ⟨*postero*anterior⟩ ⟨*postero*lateral⟩

pos·tero·an·te·ri·or \ˌpäs-tə-rō-an-ˈtir-ē-ər\ *adj* : involving or produced in a direction from the back toward the front (as of the body or an organ)

pos·tero·lat·er·al \ˌpäs-tə-rō-ˈla-tə-rəl\ *adj* : posterior and lateral in position or direction (the ∼ aspect of the leg) — **pos·tero·lat·er·al·ly** *adv*

pos·tero·me·di·al \-ˈmē-dē-əl\ *adj* : located on or near the dorsal midline of the body or a body part

post·ex·po·sure \ˌpōst-ik-ˈspō-zhər\ *adj* : occurring after exposure (as to a virus) ⟨∼ vaccination⟩ — **postexposure** *adv*

post·gan·gli·on·ic \ˌgaŋ-glē-ˈä-nik\ *adj* : distal to a ganglion; *specif* : of, relating to, or being an axon arising from a cell body within an autonomic ganglion — compare PREGANGLIONIC

post·gas·trec·to·my \-ga-ˈstrek-tə-mē\ *adj* : occurring in, being in, or characteristic of the period following a gastrectomy

postgastrectomy syndrome *n* : dumping syndrome following a gastrectomy

post·hem·or·rhag·ic \-ˌhe-mə-ˈra-jik\ *adj* : occurring after and as the result of a hemorrhage ⟨∼ shock⟩

post·he·pat·ic \-hi-ˈpa-tik\ *adj* : occurring or located behind the liver

post·hep·a·tit·ic \-ˌhe-pə-ˈti-tik\ *adj* : occurring after and esp. as a result of hepatitis ⟨∼ cirrhosis⟩

post·her·pet·ic \-hər-ˈpe-tik\ *adj* : occurring after and esp. as a result of herpes ⟨∼ scars⟩

pos·thi·tis \(ˌ)päs-ˈthī-təs\ *n, pl* **pos·thit·i·des** \-ˈthi-tə-ˌdēz\ : inflammation of the prepuce

post·hyp·not·ic \ˌpōst-hip-ˈnä-tik\ *adj* : of, relating to, or characteristic of the period following a hypnotic trance during which the subject will still carry out suggestions made by the operator during the trance state ⟨∼ suggestion⟩

post·ic·tal \-ˈikt-ᵊl\ *adj* : occurring after a sudden attack (as of epilepsy)

posticus — see TIBIALIS POSTICUS

post·in·farc·tion \-in-ˈfärk-shən\ *adj* 1 : occurring after and esp. as a result of myocardial infarction ⟨∼ ventricu-

lar septal defect⟩ 2 : having suffered myocardial infarction

post·in·fec·tion \-in-ˈfek-shən\ *adj* : relating to, occurring in, or being the period following infection — **postinfection** *adv*

post·ir·ra·di·a·tion \-i-ˌrā-dē-ˈā-shən\ *adj* : occurring after irradiation — **postirradiation** *adv*

post·isch·emic \-is-ˈkē-mik\ *adj* : occurring after and esp. as a result of ischemia ⟨∼ renal failure⟩

post·junc·tion·al \-ˈjəŋk-shə-nəl\ *adj* : of, relating to, occurring on, or located on the muscle fiber side of a neuromuscular junction

post·mas·tec·to·my \-ma-ˈstek-tə-mē\ *adj* 1 : occurring after and esp. as a result of a mastectomy 2 : having undergone mastectomy

post·ma·ture \-mə-ˈchúr, -ˈtyúr, -ˈtúr\ *adj* : remaining in the uterus for longer than the normal period of gestation ⟨a ∼ fetus⟩

post·meno·paus·al \ˌpōst-ˌme-nə-ˈpó-zəl\ *adj* 1 : having undergone menopause ⟨∼ women⟩ 2 : occurring after menopause ⟨∼ osteoporosis⟩ — **post·meno·paus·al·ly** *adv*

¹**post·mor·tem** \-ˈmór-təm\ *adj* : done, occurring, or collected after death ⟨∼ tissue specimens⟩

²**postmortem** *n* : AUTOPSY

post–mortem *adv* : after death

postmortem examination *n* : AUTOPSY

post·na·sal \-ˈnä-zəl\ *adj* : lying or occurring posterior to the nose

postnasal drip *n* : flow of mucous secretion from the posterior part of the nasal cavity onto the wall of the pharynx occurring usu. as a chronic accompaniment of an allergic state

post·na·tal \-ˈnāt-ᵊl\ *adj* : occurring or being after birth; *specif* : of or relating to an infant immediately after birth ⟨∼ care⟩ — compare NEONATAL, PRENATAL — **post·na·tal·ly** *adv*

post·ne·crot·ic cirrhosis \-nə-ˈkrä-tik-\ *n* : cirrhosis of the liver following widespread necrosis of liver cells esp. as a result of hepatitis

post·neo·na·tal \-ˌnē-ō-ˈnāt-ᵊl\ *adj* : of, relating to, or affecting the infant usu. from the end of the first month to a year after birth ⟨∼ mortality⟩

post·nor·mal \-ˈnór-məl\ *adj* : having, characterized by, or resulting from a position (as of the mandible) that is distal to the normal position ⟨∼ malocclusion⟩ — compare PRENORMAL — **post·nor·mal·i·ty** \-nór-ˈma-lə-tē\ *n*

post–op \ˈpōst-ˈäp\ *adj* : POSTOPERATIVE — **post–op** *adv*

post·op·er·a·tive \ˌpōst-ˈä-pə-rə-tiv\ *adj* 1 : relating to, occurring in, or being the period following a surgical operation ⟨∼ care⟩ 2 : having undergone a surgical operation ⟨a ∼ patient⟩ — **post·op·er·a·tive·ly** *adv*

post·or·bit·al \-ˈór-bət-ᵊl\ *adj* : situated

or occurring behind the orbit of the eye

post·par·tum \-ˈpär-təm\ adj **1** : occurring in or being the period following parturition ⟨∼ depression⟩ **2** : being in the postpartum period ⟨∼ mothers⟩ — **postpartum** adv

post·phle·bit·ic \-flə-ˈbi-tik\ adj : occurring after and esp. as the result of phlebitis ⟨∼ edema⟩

postphlebitic syndrome n : chronic venous insufficiency with associated pathological manifestations (as pain, edema, stasis dermatitis, varicose veins, and ulceration) following phlebitis of the deep veins of the leg

post·pi·tu·i·tary \-pə-ˈtü-ə-ˌter-ē, -ˈtyü-\ adj : arising in or derived from the posterior lobe of the pituitary gland

post–po·lio \-ˈpō-lē-ˌō\ adj : recovered from poliomyelitis; also : affected with post-polio syndrome

post–polio syndrome n : a condition that affects former poliomyelitis patients long after recovery from the disease and that is characterized by muscle weakness, joint and muscle pain, and fatigue

post·pran·di·al \-ˈpran-dē-əl\ adj : occurring after a meal ⟨∼ hypoglycemia⟩ — **post·pran·di·al·ly** adv

post·pu·ber·tal \-ˈpyü-bərt-ᵊl\ adj : occurring after puberty

post·pu·bes·cent \-pyü-ˈbes-ᵊnt\ adj : occurring or being in the period following puberty : POSTPUBERTAL

post·ra·di·a·tion \-rā-dē-ˈā-shən\ adj : occurring after exposure to radiation

postrema — see AREA POSTREMA

post·sple·nec·to·my \-spli-ˈnek-tə-mē\ adj : occurring after and esp. as a result of a splenectomy ⟨∼ sepsis⟩

post·sur·gi·cal \-ˈsər-ji-kəl\ adj : POSTOPERATIVE ⟨∼ swelling⟩ ⟨∼ patient⟩

post·syn·ap·tic \ˌpōst-sə-ˈnap-tik\ adj **1** : occurring after synapsis ⟨a ∼ chromosome⟩ **2** : relating to, occurring in, or being part of a nerve cell by which a wave of excitation is conveyed away from a synapse — **post·syn·ap·ti·cal·ly** adv

post·tran·scrip·tion·al \-trans-ˈkrip-shə-nəl\ adj : occurring, acting, or existing after genetic transcription — **post·tran·scrip·tion·al·ly** adv

post·trans·fu·sion \-trans-ˈfyü-zhən\ adj **1** : caused by transfused blood ⟨∼ hepatitis⟩ **2** : occurring after blood transfusion

post·trans·la·tion·al \-trans-ˈlā-shə-nəl, -shən-ᵊl\ adj : occurring or existing after genetic translation — **post·trans·la·tion·al·ly** adv

post–trau·mat·ic \ˌpōst-trə-ˈma-tik, -trō-, -trau-\ adj : occurring after or as a result of trauma ⟨∼ epilepsy⟩

post–traumatic stress disorder n : a psychological reaction that occurs after experiencing a highly stressing event (as wartime combat, physical violence, or a natural disaster) outside the range of normal human experience and that is usu. characterized by depression, anxiety, flashbacks, recurrent nightmares, and avoidance of reminders of the event — abbr. PTSD; called also delayed-stress disorder, delayed-stress syndrome, post-traumatic stress syndrome; compare COMBAT FATIGUE

post·treat·ment \-ˈtrēt-mənt\ adj : relating to, typical of, or occurring in the period following treatment ⟨∼ examinations⟩ — **posttreatment** adv

pos·tur·al \ˈpäs-chə-rəl\ adj : of, relating to, or involving posture; also : ORTHOSTATIC ⟨∼ hypotension⟩

postural drainage n : drainage of the lungs by placing the patient in an inverted position so that fluids are drawn by gravity toward the trachea

pos·ture \ˈpäs-chər\ n : the position or bearing of the body whether characteristic or assumed for a special purpose ⟨erect ∼⟩

post·vac·ci·nal \-ˈvak-sən-ᵊl\ adj : occurring after and esp. as a result of vaccination ⟨∼ dermatosis⟩

post·vac·ci·na·tion \-ˌvak-sə-ˈnā-shən\ adj : POSTVACCINAL

post·wean·ing \-ˈwē-niŋ\ adj : relating to, occurring in, or being the period following weaning

pot \ˈpät\ n : MARIJUANA

po·ta·ble \ˈpō-tə-bəl\ adj : suitable for drinking ⟨∼ water⟩

po·tas·si·um \pə-ˈta-sē-əm\ n : a silver-white soft low-melting metallic element that occurs abundantly in nature esp. combined in minerals — symbol K; see ELEMENT table

potassium alum n : ALUM

potassium aluminum sulfate n : ALUM

potassium an·ti·mo·nyl·tar·trate \-ˌan-tə-mə-ˌnil-ˈtär-ˌtrāt, -ˌnēl-\ n : TARTAR EMETIC

potassium bicarbonate n : a crystalline salt $KHCO_3$ that gives a weakly alkaline reaction in aqueous solution and is sometimes used as an antacid and urinary alkalizer

potassium bromide n : a crystalline salt KBr with a saline taste that is used as a sedative

potassium chlorate n : a crystalline salt $KClO_3$ used esp. in veterinary medicine as a mild astringent

potassium chloride n : a crystalline salt KCl that is used esp. in the treatment of potassium deficiency and occasionally as a diuretic

potassium citrate n : a crystalline salt $K_3C_6H_5O_7$ used chiefly as a systemic and urinary alkalizer and in the treatment of hypokalemia

potassium cyanide n : a very poisonous crystalline salt KCN

potassium hydroxide n : a white solid KOH that dissolves in water to form a strongly alkaline liquid and that is used as a powerful caustic and in the making of pharmaceuticals

potassium iodide *n* : a crystalline salt KI that is very soluble in water and is used in medicine chiefly as an expectorant

potassium nitrate *n* : a crystalline salt KNO_3 that is a strong oxidizing agent and is used in medicine chiefly as a diuretic — called also *saltpeter*

potassium perchlorate *n* : a crystalline salt $KClO_4$ that is sometimes used as a thyroid inhibitor

potassium permanganate *n* : a dark purple salt $KMnO_4$ used as a disinfectant

potassium phosphate *n* : any of various phosphates of potassium; *esp* : a salt K_2HPO_4 used as a saline cathartic

potassium sodium tartrate *n* : ROCHELLE SALT

potassium thiocyanate *n* : a crystalline salt KSCN that has been used as an antihypertensive agent

pot-bel-ly \'pät-ˌbe-lē\ *n, pl* **-lies** : an enlarged, swollen, or protruding abdomen; *also* : a condition characterized by such an abdomen that is symptomatic of disease or malnourishment

po-ten-cy \'pōt-ⁿn-sē\ *n, pl* **-cies** : the quality or state of being potent : as **a** : chemical or medicinal strength or efficacy ⟨a drug's ∼⟩ **b** : the ability to copulate — usu. used of the male **c** : initial inherent capacity for development of a particular kind ⟨cells with a ∼ for eye formation⟩

po-tent \'pōt-ⁿnt\ *adj* **1** : having force or power **2** : chemically or medicinally effective ⟨a ∼ vaccine⟩ **3** : able to copulate — usu. used of the male — **po-tent-ly** *adv*

¹**po-ten-tial** \pə-'ten-chəl\ *adj* : existing in possibility : capable of development into actuality — **po-ten-tial-ly** *adv*

²**potential** *n* **1** : something that can develop or become actual **2 a** : any of various functions from which the intensity or the velocity at any point in a field may be readily calculated; *specif* : ELECTRICAL POTENTIAL **b** : POTENTIAL DIFFERENCE

potential difference *n* : the voltage difference between two points that represents the work involved or the energy released in the transfer of a unit quantity of electricity from one point to the other

potential energy *n* : the energy that a piece of matter has because of its position or because of the arrangement of parts

po-ten-ti-ate \pə-'ten-chē-ˌāt\ *vb* **-at-ed; -at-ing** : to make effective or active or more effective or more active; *also* : to augment the activity of (as a drug) synergistically — **po-ten-ti-a-tion** \-ˌten-chē-'ā-shən\ *n* — **po-ten-ti-a-tor** \-'ten-chē-ˌā-tər\ *n*

Pott's disease \'päts-\ *n* : tuberculosis of the spine with destruction of bone resulting in curvature of the spine and occas. in paralysis of the lower extremities

Pott, Percivall (1714–1788), British surgeon.

Pott's fracture *n* : a fracture of the lower part of the fibula often accompanied with injury to the tibial articulation so that the foot is dislocated outward

pouch \'paùch\ *n* : an anatomical structure resembling a bag or pocket

pouch of Doug·las \-'də-gləs\ *n* : a deep peritoneal recess between the uterus and the upper vaginal wall anteriorly and the rectum posteriorly — called also *cul-de-sac, cul-de-sac of Douglas, Douglas's cul-de-sac, Douglas's pouch*

Douglas, James (1675–1742), British anatomist.

poul-tice \'pōl-təs\ *n* : a soft usu. heated and sometimes medicated mass spread on cloth and applied to sores or other lesions to supply moist warmth, relieve pain, or act as a counterirritant or antiseptic — called also *cataplasm* — **poultice** *vb*

pound \'paùnd\ *n, pl* **pounds** *also* **pound** : any of various units of mass and weight: as **a** : a unit of troy weight equal to 12 troy ounces or 5760 grains or 0.3732417216 kilogram — called also *troy pound* **b** : a unit of avoirdupois weight equal to 16 avoirdupois ounces or 7000 grains or 0.45359237 kilogram — called also *avoirdupois pound*

Pou·part's ligament \pü-'pärz-\ *n* : INGUINAL LIGAMENT

Poupart, François (1661–1709), French surgeon and naturalist.

po·vi·done \'pō-və-ˌdōn\ *n* : POLYVINYLPYRROLIDONE

povidone–iodine *n* : a solution of polyvinylpyrrolidone and iodine used as an antibacterial agent in topical application (as in preoperative prepping or a surgical scrub) — see BETADINE

pow·der \'paù-dər\ *n* : a product in the form of discrete usu. fine particles; *specif* : a medicine or medicated preparation in powdered form

pow·er \'paù-ər\ *n* : MAGNIFICATION

pox \'päks\ *n, pl* **pox** *or* **pox·es 1** : a virus disease (as chicken pox) characterized by pustules or eruptions **2** *archaic* : SMALLPOX **3** : SYPHILIS

pox·vi·rus \'päks-ˌvī-rəs\ *n* : any of a group of relatively large round, brick-shaped, or ovoid DNA-containing animal viruses (as the causative agent of smallpox) that have a fluffy appearance caused by a covering of tubules and threads

PPA *abbr* phenylpropanolamine

ppb *abbr* parts per billion

PPD *abbr* purified protein derivative

PPLO \ˌpē-(ˌ)pē-(ˌ)el-'ō\ *n, pl* **PPLO** : MYCOPLASMA

ppm *abbr* parts per million

PPO \ˌpē-(ˌ)pē-ˈō\ *n, pl* **PPOs** : an organization providing health care that gives economic incentives to the individual purchaser of a health-care contract to patronize certain physicians, laboratories, and hospitals which agree to supervision and reduced fees — called also *preferred provider organization*; compare HMO

Pr *symbol* praseodymium

practical nurse *n* : a nurse who cares for the sick professionally without having the training or experience required of a registered nurse; *esp* : LICENSED PRACTICAL NURSE

prac·tice *also* **prac·tise** \ˈprak-təs\ *n* **1** : the continuous exercise of a profession **2** : a professional business; *esp* : one constituting an incorporeal property ⟨the doctor sold his ∼ and retired⟩ — **practice** *or* **practise** *vb*

prac·ti·tion·er \prak-ˈti-shə-nər\ *n* : one who practices a profession and esp. medicine

prac·to·lol \ˈprak-tə-ˌlȯl\ *n* : a beta-blocker $C_{14}H_{22}N_2O_3$ used in the control of arrhythmia

Pra·der–Wil·li syndrome \ˈprä-dər-ˈvil-ē-\ *n* : a genetic disorder characterized by short stature, mental retardation, hypotonia, abnormally small hands and feet, hypogonadism, and uncontrolled appetite leading to extreme obesity

  Prader, Andrea (*b* 1919) and Willi, Heinrich (*fl* 1956), Swiss pediatricians.

praecox — see DEMENTIA PRAECOX, EJACULATIO PRAECOX

pral·i·dox·ime \ˌpra-li-ˈdäk-ˌsēm\ *n* : a substance $C_7H_9ClN_2O$ that restores the reactivity of cholinesterase and is used to counteract phosphorylation (as by an organophosphate pesticide) — called also *2-PAM*; see PROTOPAM

pran·di·al \ˈpran-dē-əl\ *adj* : of or relating to a meal

pra·seo·dym·i·um \ˌprä-zē-ō-ˈdi-mē-əm, ˌprä-sē-\ *n* : a yellowish white trivalent metallic element — symbol *Pr*; see ELEMENT table

Praus·nitz–Küst·ner reaction \ˈpraŭs-nits-ˈkŭest-nər-\ *n* : PASSIVE TRANSFER

  Prausnitz, Carl Willy (*b* 1876), German bacteriologist.

  Küstner, Heinz (*b* 1897), German gynecologist.

-prax·ia \ˈprak-sē-ə\ *n comb form* : performance of movements ⟨apraxia⟩

pra·ze·pam \ˈprä-zə-ˌpam\ *n* : a benzodiazepine derivative $C_{19}H_{17}ClN_2O$ used as a tranquilizer

praz·i·quan·tel \ˌpra-zi-ˈkwän-ˌtel\ *n* : an anthelmintic drug $C_{19}H_{24}N_2O_2$ — see BILTRICIDE

pra·zo·sin \ˈprä-zə-ˌsin\ *n* : an antihypertensive peripheral vasodilator $C_{19}H_{21}N_5O_4$ usu. used in the form of its hydrochloride — see MINIPRESS

pre- *prefix* **1 a** : earlier than : prior to : before ⟨prenatal⟩ **b** : in a formative,

incipient, or preliminary stage ⟨precancerous⟩ **2** : in front of : before ⟨preaxial⟩ ⟨premolar⟩

pre·ad·mis·sion \ˌprē-əd-ˈmi-shən\ *adj* : occurring in or relating to the period prior to admission (as to a hospital) ⟨∼ physical examination⟩

pre·ad·o·les·cence \ˌprē-ˌad-əl-ˈes-əns\ *n* : the period of human development just preceding adolescence; *specif* : the period between the approximate ages of 9 and 12 — **pre·ad·o·les·cent** \-ˌad-əl-ˈes-ənt\ *adj or n*

pre·adult \-ə-ˈdəlt, -ˈa-ˌdəlt\ *adj* : occurring or existing prior to adulthood

pre·al·bu·min \-al-ˈbyü-mən, -ˈal-ˌbyü-\ *n* : TRANSTHYRETIN

¹pre·an·es·thet·ic \-ˌa-nəs-ˈthe-tik\ *adj* : used or occurring before administration of an anesthetic ⟨∼ medication⟩

²preanesthetic *n* : a substance used to induce an initial light state of anesthesia

pre·au·ric·u·lar \-ȯ-ˈri-kyə-lər\ *adj* : situated or occurring anterior to the auricle of the ear ⟨∼ lymph nodes⟩

pre·ax·i·al \-ˈak-sē-əl\ *adj* : situated in front of an axis of the body

pre·can·cer·ous \-ˈkan-sə-rəs\ *adj* : tending to become cancerous

¹pre·cap·il·lary \-ˈka-pə-ˌler-ē\ *adj* : being on the arterial side of and immediately adjacent to a capillary

²precapillary *n, pl* **-lar·ies** : METARTERIOLE

precapillary sphincter *n* : a sphincter of smooth muscle tissue located at the arterial end of a capillary and serving to control the flow of blood to the tissues

pre·cen·tral \-ˈsen-trəl\ *adj* : situated in front of the central sulcus of the brain

precentral gyrus *n* : the gyrus containing the motor area immediately anterior to the central sulcus

pre·cep·tee \ˌprē-ˌsep-ˈtē\ *n* : one that works for and studies under a preceptor ⟨a ∼ in urology⟩

pre·cep·tor \pri-ˈsep-tər, ˈprē-ˌ\ *n* : a practicing physician who gives personal instruction, training, and supervision to a medical student or young physician

pre·cep·tor·ship \pri-ˈsep-tər-ˌship, ˈprē-ˌ\ *n* : the state of being a preceptee : a period of training under a preceptor

¹pre·cip·i·tate \pri-ˈsi-pə-ˌtāt\ *vb* **-tat·ed; -tat·ing 1** : to bring about esp. abruptly **2 a** : to separate or cause to separate from solution or suspension **b** : to cause (vapor) to condense and fall or deposit

²pre·cip·i·tate \pri-ˈsi-pə-tət, -ˌtāt\ *n* : a substance separated from a solution or suspension by chemical or physical change usu. as an insoluble amorphous or crystalline solid

precipitated chalk *n* : precipitated calcium carbonate used esp. as an ingredient of toothpastes and tooth powders for its polishing qualities

pre·cip·i·tat·ed sulfur n : sulfur obtained as a pale yellowish or grayish powder by precipitation and used chiefly in treating skin diseases

pre·cip·i·ta·tion \pri-ˌsi-pə-ˈtā-shən\ n 1 a : the process of forming a precipitate from a solution b : the process of precipitating or removing solid or liquid particles from a smoke or gas by electrical means 2 : PRECIPITATE

pre·cip·i·tin \pri-ˈsi-pə-tən\ n : any of various antibodies which form insoluble precipitates with specific antigens

precipitin test n : a serological test using precipitins to detect the presence of a specific antigen; specif : a test used in criminology for determining the human or other source of a blood stain

pre·clin·i·cal \ˌprē-ˈkli-ni-kəl\ adj 1 : of, relating to, or concerned with the period preceding clinical manifestations ⟨the ∼ stage of a disease of slow onset⟩ 2 : of, relating to, or being the period in medical or dental education preceding the clinical study of medicine or dentistry

pre·co·cious \pri-ˈkō-shəs\ adj 1 : exceptionally early in development or occurrence ⟨∼ puberty⟩ 2 : exhibiting mature qualities at an unusually early age — **pre·co·cious·ly** adv — **pre·co·cious·ness** n — **pre·coc·i·ty** \pri-ˈkä-sə-tē\ n

pre·cog·ni·tion \ˌprē-(ˌ)käg-ˈni-shən\ n : clairvoyance relating to an event or state not yet experienced — compare PSYCHOKINESIS, TELEKINESIS — **pre·cog·ni·tive** \-ˈkäg-nə-tiv\ adj

pre·co·i·tal \-ˈkō-ət-ᵊl, -kō-ˈēt-\ adj : occurring before coitus

pre·co·ma \ˈkō-mə\ n : a stuporous condition preceding coma ⟨diabetic ∼⟩

¹**pre·con·scious** \ˌprē-ˈkän-chəs\ adj : not present in consciousness but capable of being recalled without encountering any inner resistance or repression — **pre·con·scious·ly** adv

²**preconscious** n : the preconscious part of the psyche esp. in psychoanalysis

pre·cor·di·al \-ˈkȯr-dē-əl, -ˈkȯr-jəl\ adj 1 : situated or occurring in front of the heart 2 : of or relating to the precordium

pre·cor·di·um \-ˈkȯr-dē-əm\ n, pl **-dia** \-dē-ə\ : the part of the ventral surface of the body overlying the heart and stomach and comprising the epigastrium and the lower median part of the thorax

pre·cu·ne·us \-ˈkyü-nē-əs\ n, pl **-nei** \-nē-ˌī\ : a somewhat rectangular convolution bounding the mesial aspect of the parietal lobe of the cerebrum and lying immediately in front of the cuneus

pre·cur·sor \pri-ˈkər-sər, ˈprē-ˌ\ n 1 : one that precedes and indicates the onset of another ⟨angina may be the ∼ of a second infarction⟩ 2 : a substance, cell, or cellular component from which another substance, cell, or cellular component is formed esp. by natural processes

pre·den·tin \ˌprē-ˈdent-ᵊn\ or **pre·den·tine** \-ˈden-ˌtēn, -den-ˈ\ n : immature uncalcified dentin consisting chiefly of fibrils

pre·di·a·be·tes \ˌprē-ˌdī-ə-ˈbē-tēz, -ˈbē-təs\ n : an inapparent abnormal state that precedes the development of clinically evident diabetes

¹**pre·di·a·bet·ic** \-ˈbe-tik\ n : a prediabetic individual

²**prediabetic** adj : of, relating to, or affected with prediabetes ⟨∼ patients⟩

pre·dic·tor \pri-ˈdik-tər\ n : a preliminary symptom or indication (as of the development of a disease)

pre·di·ges·tion \ˌprē-dī-ˈjes-chən, -də-\ n : artificial or natural partial digestion of food — **pre·di·gest** \-ˈjest\ vb

pre·dis·pose \ˌprē-di-ˈspōz\ vb **-posed; -pos·ing** : to make susceptible — **pre·dis·po·si·tion** \ˌprē-ˌdis-pə-ˈzi-shən\ n

pred·nis·o·lone \pred-ˈni-sə-ˌlōn\ n : a glucocorticoid $C_{21}H_{28}O_5$ used often in the form of an ester or methyl derivative esp. as an anti-inflammatory drug in the treatment of arthritis — see METICORTELONE

pred·ni·sone \ˈpred-nə-ˌsōn, -ˌzōn\ n : a glucocorticoid $C_{21}H_{26}O_5$ used as an anti-inflammatory agent esp. in the treatment of arthritis, as an antineoplastic agent, and as an immunosuppressant

pre·drug \ˌprē-ˈdrəg\ adj : existing or occurring prior to the administration of a drug ⟨∼ performance level⟩ ⟨∼ temperature⟩

pre·eclamp·sia \ˌprē-i-ˈklamp-sē-ə\ n : a toxic condition developing in late pregnancy that is characterized by a sudden rise in blood pressure, excessive gain in weight, generalized edema, albuminuria, severe headache, and visual disturbances — compare ECLAMPSIA a, TOXEMIA OF PREGNANCY

¹**pre·eclamp·tic** \-tik\ adj : relating to or affected with preeclampsia ⟨a ∼ patient⟩

²**preeclamptic** n : a woman affected with preeclampsia

pree·mie \ˈprē-mē\ n : a baby born prematurely

pre·erup·tive \ˌprē-i-ˈrəp-tiv\ adj : occurring or existing prior to an eruption ⟨∼ tooth position⟩

pre·ex·po·sure \-ik-ˈspō-zhər\ adj : of, relating to, occurring in, or being the period preceding exposure (as to a stimulus or a pathogen)

preferred provider organization n : PPO

pre·fron·tal \ˌprē-ˈfrənt-ᵊl\ adj 1 : situated or occurring anterior to a frontal structure ⟨a ∼ bone⟩ 2 : of, relating to, or constituting the anterior part of the frontal lobe of the brain bounded posteriorly by the ascending frontal convolution

prefrontal lobe *n* : the anterior part of the frontal lobe made up chiefly of association areas and mediating various inhibitory controls

prefrontal lobotomy *n* : lobotomy of the white matter in the frontal lobe of the brain — called also *frontal lobotomy*

pre·gan·gli·on·ic \ˌprē-ˌgaŋ-glē-'ä-nik\ *adj* : anterior or proximal to a ganglion; *specif* : being, affecting, involving, or relating to a usu. myelinated efferent nerve fiber arising from a cell body in the central nervous system and terminating in an autonomic ganglion — compare POSTGANGLIONIC

pre·gen·i·tal \-'jen-ət-ᵊl\ *adj* : of, relating to, or characteristic of the oral, anal, and phallic phases of psychosexual development

preg·nan·cy \'preg-nən-sē\ *n, pl* **-cies 1** : the condition of being pregnant **2** : an instance of being pregnant

pregnancy disease *n* : a form of ketosis affecting pregnant ewes that is marked by dullness, staggering, and collapse and is esp. frequent in ewes carrying twins or triplets

pregnancy test *n* : a physiological test to determine the existence of pregnancy in an individual

preg·nane \'preg-ˌnān\ *n* : a crystalline steroid $C_{21}H_{36}$ that is the parent compound of the corticosteroid and progestational hormones

preg·nane·di·ol \ˌpreg-ˌnān-'dī-ˌòl\ *n* : a crystalline biologically inactive derivative $C_{21}H_{36}O_2$ of pregnane found esp. in the urine of pregnant women

preg·nant \'preg-nənt\ *adj* : containing unborn young within the body : GRAVID

preg·nen·o·lone \preg-'nen-ᵊl-ˌōn\ *n* : a steroid ketone $C_{21}H_{32}O_2$ that is formed by the oxidation of steroids (as cholesterol) and yields progesterone on dehydrogenation

pre·hos·pi·tal \ˌprē-'häs-(ˌ)pit-ᵊl\ *adj* : occurring before or during transportation (as of a trauma victim) to a hospital ⟨~ emergency care⟩

pre·im·plan·ta·tion \-ˌim-ˌplan-'tā-shən\ *adj* : of, involving, or being an embryo before uterine implantation

pre·in·cu·ba·tion \ˌprē-ˌiŋ-kyə-'bā-shən\ *n* : incubation (as of a cell or culture) prior to a treatment or process — **pre·in·cu·bate** \-'iŋ-kyə-ˌbāt\ *vb*

pre·in·va·sive \-in-'vā-siv\ *adj* : not yet having become invasive — used of malignant cells or lesions remaining in their original focus

pre·leu·ke·mia \ˌprē-lü-'kē-mē-ə\ *n* : the stage of leukemia occurring before the disease becomes overt — **pre·leu·ke·mic** \-mik\ *adj*

pre·load \'prē-ˌlōd\ *n* : the stretched condition of the heart muscle at the end of diastole just before contraction

Pre·lu·din \pri-'lüd-ᵊn\ *trademark* — used for a preparation of phenmetrazine

pre·ma·lig·nant \ˌprē-mə-'lig-nənt\ *adj* : PRECANCEROUS

¹pre·ma·ture \ˌprē-mə-'chùr, -'tyùr, -'tùr-\ *adj* : happening, arriving, existing, or performed before the proper, usual, or intended time; *esp* : born after a gestation period of less than 37 weeks ⟨~ babies⟩ — **pre·ma·ture·ly** *adv*

²premature *n* : PREEMIE

premature beat *n* : EXTRASYSTOLE

premature delivery *n* : expulsion of the human fetus after the 28th week of gestation but before the normal time

premature ejaculation *n* : ejaculation of semen that occurs prior to or immediately after penetration of the vagina by the penis — called also *ejaculatio praecox*

premature ejaculator *n* : a man who experiences premature ejaculation

pre·ma·tu·ri·ty \ˌprē-mə-'tùr-ə-tē, -'tyùr-, -'chùr-\ *n, pl* **-ties** : the condition of an infant born viable but before its proper time

pre·max·il·la \ˌprē-mak-'si-lə\ *n, pl* **-lae** \-ˌlē\ : either member of a pair of bones of the upper jaw situated between and in front of the maxillae that in humans form the median anterior part of the superior maxillary bones

pre·max·il·lary \-'mak-sə-ˌler-ē\ *adj* **1** : situated in front of the maxillary bones **2** : relating to or being the premaxillae

¹pre·med \ˌprē-'med\ *n* : a premedical student or course of study

²premed *adj* : PREMEDICAL

pre·med·i·cal \-'me-di-kəl\ *adj* : preceding and preparing for the professional study of medicine

pre·med·i·ca·tion \-ˌme-də-'kā-shən\ *n* : preliminary medication; *esp* : medication to induce a relaxed state preparatory to the administration of an anesthetic — **pre·med·i·cate** \-'me-də-ˌkāt\ *vb*

pre·mei·ot·ic \ˌprē-mī-'ä-tik\ *adj* : of, occurring in, or typical of a stage prior to meiosis ⟨~ DNA synthesis⟩

pre·me·nar·chal \ˌprē-me-'när-kəl\ *or* **pre·me·nar·che·al** \-kē-əl\ *adj* : of, relating to, or being in the period of life of a female before the first menstrual period occurs

pre·meno·paus·al \ˌme-nə-'pò-zəl, -ˌmē-\ *adj* : of, relating to, or being in the period preceding menopause

pre·men·stru·al \-'men-strə-wəl\ *adj* : of, relating to, occurring, or being in the period just preceding menstruation ⟨~ women⟩ — **pre·men·stru·al·ly** *adv*

premenstrual syndrome *n* : a varying constellation of symptoms manifested by some women prior to menstruation that may include emotional instability, irritability, insomnia, fatigue, anxiety, depression, headache, edema, and abdominal pain — abbr. *PMS*

premenstrual tension *n* : tension occurring as a part of the premenstrual syndrome

pre·men·stru·um \-ˈmen-strə-wəm\ *n, pl* **-stru·ums** *or* **-strua** \-strə-wə\ : the period or physiological state that immediately precedes menstruation

pre·mie \ˈprē-mē\ *var of* PREEMIE

¹**pre·mo·lar** \ˌprē-ˈmō-lər\ *adj* : situated in front of or preceding the molar teeth; *esp* : being or relating to those teeth in front of the true molars and behind the canines

²**premolar** *n* : a premolar tooth that in humans is one of two in each side of each jaw — called also *bicuspid*

pre·mon·i·to·ry \pri-ˈmä-nə-ˌtōr-ē\ *adj* : giving warning ⟨a ~ symptom⟩

pre·mor·bid \ˌprē-ˈmor-bəd\ *adj* : occurring or existing before the occurrence of physical disease or emotional illness ⟨~ personality⟩

pre·mor·tem \-ˈmort-ᵊm\ *adj* : existing or taking place immediately before death ⟨~ coronary angiograms⟩

pre·mo·tor \-ˈmō-tər\ *adj* : of, relating to, or being the area of the cortex of the frontal lobe lying immediately in front of the motor area of the precentral gyrus

pre·my·cot·ic \ˌprē-mī-ˈkä-tik\ *adj* : of, relating to, or being the earliest and nonspecific stage of eczematoid eruptions of mycosis fungoides

pre·na·tal \-ˈnāt-ᵊl\ *adj* **1** : occurring, existing, or performed before birth ⟨~ care⟩ ⟨the ~ period⟩ **2** : providing or receiving prenatal medical care ⟨a ~ clinic⟩ ⟨a ~ patient⟩ — compare NEONATAL, POSTNATAL — **pre·na·tal·ly** *adv*

pre·neo·plas·tic \-ˌnē-ə-ˈplas-tik\ *adj* : existing or occurring prior to the formation of a neoplasm ⟨~ cells⟩

pre·nor·mal \-ˈnor-məl\ *adj* : having, characterized by, or resulting from a position (as of the mandible) that is proximal to the normal position ⟨~ malocclusion⟩ — compare POSTNORMAL — **pre·nor·mal·i·ty** \-nor-ˈma-lə-tē\ *n*

preop \ˈprē-ˌäp\ *adj* : PREOPERATIVE

pre·op·er·a·tive \ˌprē-ˈä-pə-rə-tiv, -ˌrāt-\ *adj* : occurring, performed, or administered before a surgical operation ⟨~ care⟩ — **pre·op·er·a·tive·ly** *adv*

pre·op·tic \-ˈäp-tik\ *adj* : situated in front of an optic part or region

preoptic area *n* : a region of the brain that is situated immediately below the anterior commissure, above the optic chiasma, and anterior to the hypothalamus and that regulates certain autonomic activities often with the hypothalamus

preoptic nucleus *n* : any of several groups of nerve cells located in the preoptic area esp. in the lateral and the medial portions

preoptic region *n* : PREOPTIC AREA

pre·ovu·la·to·ry \ˌprē-ˈä-vyə-lə-ˌtōr-ē, -ˈō-\ *adj* : occurring or existing in or typical of the period immediately preceding ovulation ⟨~ oocytes⟩ ⟨a ~ surge of luteinizing hormone⟩

¹**prep** \ˈprep\ *n* : the act or an instance of preparing a patient for a surgical operation

²**prep** *vb* **prepped; prep·ping** : to prepare, for a surgical operation or examination ⟨*prepped* the patient for an appendectomy⟩

prep·a·ra·tion \ˌpre-pə-ˈrā-shən\ *n* : a medicinal substance made ready for use ⟨a ~ for colds⟩

prepared chalk *n* : finely ground calcium carbonate that is freed of most of its impurities and used esp. in dentistry for polishing

pre·par·tum \ˌprē-ˈpär-təm\ *adj* : ANTEPARTUM

pre·pa·tel·lar bursa \-pə-ˈte-lər-\ *n* : a synovial bursa situated between the patella and the skin

pre·pa·tent period \-ˈpāt-ᵊnt-\ *n* : the period between infection with a parasite and the demonstration of the parasite in the body

pre·po·ten·cy \-ˈpōt-ᵊn-sē\ *n, pl* **-cies** : unusual ability of an individual or strain to transmit its characters to offspring because of homozygosity for numerous dominant genes — **pre·po·tent** \-ˈpōt-ᵊnt\ *adj*

pre·pran·di·al \-ˈpran-dē-əl\ *adj* : of, relating to, or suitable for the time just before a meal

pre·preg·nan·cy \-ˈpreg-nən-sē\ *adj* : existing or occurring prior to pregnancy

pre·psy·chot·ic \-sī-ˈkä-tik\ *adj* : preceding or predisposing to psychosis : possessing recognizable features prognostic of psychosis ⟨~ behavior⟩

pre·pu·ber·al \-ˈpyü-bə-rəl\ *adj* : PREPUBERTAL

pre·pu·ber·tal \-ˈpyü-bərt-ᵊl\ *adj* : of, relating to, occurring in, or being in the period immediately preceding puberty — **pre·pu·ber·ty** \-ˈbər-tē\ *n*

pre·pu·bes·cent \-pyü-ˈbes-ᵊnt\ *adj* : PREPUBERTAL

pre·puce \ˈprē-ˌpyüs\ *n* : FORESKIN; *also* : a similar fold investing the clitoris

pre·pu·tial \prē-ˈpyü-shəl\ *adj* : of, relating to, or being a prepuce

preputial gland *n* : GLAND OF TYSON

pre·pu·tium cli·tor·i·dis \prē-ˈpyü-shəm-kli-ˈtor-ə-dəs\ *n* : the prepuce which invests the clitoris

pre·py·lo·ric \ˌprē-pī-ˈlor-ik\ *adj* : situated or occurring anterior to the pylorus ⟨~ ulcers⟩

pre·re·nal \-'rēn-əl\ *adj* : occurring in the circulatory system before the kidney is reached ⟨~ disorders⟩

prerenal azotemia *n* : uremia caused by extrarenal factors

pre·rep·li·ca·tive \ˌprē-'re-pli-ˌkā-tiv\ *adj* : relating to or being the G₁ phase of the cell cycle

pre·ret·i·nal \-'ret-ən-əl\ *adj* : situated or occurring anterior to the retina

pre·sa·cral \-'sa-krəl, -'sā-\ *adj* : done or effected by way of the anterior aspect of the sacrum ⟨~ nerve block⟩

presby- *or* **presbyo-** *comb form* : old age ⟨*presby*opia⟩

pres·by·cu·sis \ˌprez-bi-'kyü-səs, ˌpres-\ *n, pl* **-cu·ses** \-ˌsēz\ : a lessening of hearing acuteness resulting from degenerative changes in the ear that occur esp. in old age

pres·by·ope \'prez-bē-ˌōp\ *n* : one affected with presbyopia

pres·by·opia \ˌprez-bē-'ō-pē-ə, ˌpres-\ *n* : a visual condition which becomes apparent esp. in middle age and in which loss of elasticity of the lens of the eye causes defective accommodation and inability to focus sharply for near vision — **pres·by·opic** \-'ō-pik, -ä-\ *adj*

pre·scribe \pri-'skrīb\ *vb* **pre·scribed; pre·scrib·ing** : to designate the use of as a remedy ⟨~ a drug⟩

pre·scrip·tion \pri-'skrip-shən\ *n* 1 : a written direction for the preparation, compounding, and administration of a medicine 2 : a prescribed remedy 3 : a written formula for the grinding of corrective lenses for eyeglasses 4 : a written direction for the application of physical therapy measures (as directed exercise or electrotherapy) in cases of injury or disability

prescription drug *n* : a drug that can be obtained only by means of a physician's prescription

pre·se·nile \ˌprē-'sē-ˌnīl\ *adj* 1 : of, relating to, occurring in, or being the period immediately preceding the development of senility in an organism or person 2 : prematurely displaying symptoms of senile dementia

presenile dementia *n* : dementia beginning in middle age and progressing rapidly — compare ALZHEIMER'S DISEASE

pres·ent \pri-'zent\ *vb* 1 a : to show or manifest ⟨patients who ~ symptoms of malaria⟩ b : to become manifest ⟨Lyme disease often ~s with erythema chronicum migrans, fatigue, fever, and chills⟩ c : to come forward as a patient ⟨he ~ed with fever and abdominal pain⟩ 2 : to become directed toward the opening of the uterus — used of a fetus or a part of a fetus

pre·sen·ta·tion \ˌprē-ˌzen-'tā-shən, ˌprez-ən-\ *n* 1 : the position in which the fetus lies in the uterus in labor with respect to the mouth of the uterus ⟨face ~⟩ ⟨breech ~⟩ 2 : appearance in conscious experience either as a sensory product or as a memory image 3 : a presenting symptom or group of symptoms 4 : a formal oral report of a patient's medical history

pre·sent·ing *adj* : of, relating to, or being a symptom, condition, or sign which is patent upon initial examination of a patient or which the patient discloses to the physician

pre·ser·va·tive \pri-'zər-və-tiv\ *n* : something that preserves or has the power of preserving; *specif* : an additive used to protect against decay, discoloration, or spoilage ⟨a food ~⟩

pre·sphe·noid \ˌprē-'sfē-ˌnoid\ *n* : a bone or cartilage usu. united with the basisphenoid in the adult and in humans forming the anterior part of the body of the sphenoid — **presphenoid** *also* **pre·sphe·noi·dal** \-sfi-'noid-əl\ *adj*

pres·sor \'pre-ˌsȯr, -sər\ *adj* : raising or tending to raise blood pressure ⟨~ substances⟩; *also* : involving or producing an effect of vasoconstriction

pres·so·re·cep·tor \ˌpre-sō-ri-'sep-tər\ *n* : a proprioceptor that responds to alteration of blood pressure

pres·sure \'pre-shər\ *n* 1 : the application of force to something by something else in direct contact with it : COMPRESSION 2 : ATMOSPHERIC PRESSURE 3 : a touch sensation aroused by moderate compression of the skin

pressure bandage *n* : a thick pad of gauze or other material placed over a wound and attached firmly so that it will exert pressure

pressure dressing *n* : PRESSURE BANDAGE

pressure point *n* 1 : a region of the body in which the distribution of soft and skeletal parts is such that a static position (as of a part in a cast or of a bedridden person) tends to cause circulatory deficiency and necrosis due to local compression of blood vessels — compare BEDSORE 2 : a point where a blood vessel runs near a bone and can be compressed (as to check bleeding) by the application of pressure against the bone

pressure sore *n* : BEDSORE

pressure suit *n* : an inflatable suit for high-altitude or space flight to protect the body from low pressure

pre·sump·tive \pri-'zəmp-tiv\ *adj* 1 : expected to develop in a particular direction under normal conditions 2 : being the embryonic precursor of ⟨~ neural tissue⟩

pre·sur·gi·cal \ˌprē-'sər-ji-kəl\ *adj* : occurring before, performed before, or preliminary to surgery ⟨~ care⟩

pre·symp·to·mat·ic \-ˌsimp-tə-'ma-tik\ *adj* : relating to, being, or occurring before symptoms appear ⟨~ diagnosis of a hereditary disease⟩

pre·syn·ap·tic \-sə-'nap-tik\ *adj* : relating to, occurring in, or being part of a nerve cell by which a wave of excitation is conveyed to a synapse ⟨∼ terminals⟩ ⟨∼ inhibition⟩ ⟨a ∼ membrane⟩ — **pre·syn·ap·ti·cal·ly** *adv*

pre·sys·tol·ic \-sis-ˈtä-lik\ *adj* : of, relating to, or occurring just before cardiac systole ⟨a ∼ murmur⟩

pre·tec·tal \-ˈtekt-əl\ *adj* : occurring in or being the transitional zone of the brain stem between the midbrain and the diencephalon that is associated esp. with the analysis and distribution of light impulses

pre·term \-ˈtərm\ *adj* : of, relating to, being, or born by premature birth ⟨∼ infants⟩ ⟨∼ labor⟩

pre·ter·mi·nal \-ˈtər-mə-nəl\ *adj* **1** : occurring or being in the period prior to death ⟨∼ cancer⟩ ⟨a ∼ patient⟩ **2** : situated or occurring anterior to an end (as of a nerve)

pre·tib·i·al \-ˈti-bē-əl\ *adj* : lying or occurring anterior to the tibia

pretibial fever *n* : a rare infectious disease that is characterized by an eruption in the pretibial region, headache, backache, malaise, chills, and fever and that is caused by a spirochete of the genus *Leptospira* (*L. interrogans autumnalis*)

pretibial myxedema *n* : myxedema characterized primarily by a mucoid edema in the pretibial area

pre·treat·ment \ˈprē-ˈtrēt-mənt\ *n* : preliminary or preparatory treatment — **pre·treat** \-ˈtrēt\ *vb* — **pretreatment** *adj*

prev·a·lence \ˈpre-və-ləns\ *n* : the percentage of a population that is affected with a particular disease at a given time — compare INCIDENCE

pre·ven·ta·tive \pri-ˈven-tə-tiv\ *adj or n* : PREVENTIVE ⟨a ∼ drug⟩

¹**pre·ven·tive** \pri-ˈven-tiv\ *n* : something (as a drug) used to prevent disease

²**preventive** *adj* : devoted to or concerned with the prevention of disease

preventive medicine *n* : a branch of medical science dealing with methods (as vaccination) of preventing the occurrence of disease

pre·ver·te·bral \ˌprē-ˈvər-tə-brəl, -(ˌ)vər-ˈtē-brəl\ *adj* : situated or occurring anterior to a vertebra or the spinal column ⟨∼ muscles⟩

pre·ves·i·cal space \ˌprē-ˈve-si-kəl-\ *n* : RETROPUBIC SPACE

previa — see PLACENTA PREVIA

pre·vi·able \-ˈvī-ə-bəl\ *adj* : not sufficiently developed to survive outside the uterus ⟨a ∼ fetus⟩

pre·vil·lous \-ˈvi-ləs\ *adj* : relating to, being in, or being the stage of embryonic development before the formation of villi ⟨a ∼ human embryo⟩

pri·a·pism \ˈprī-ə-ˌpi-zəm\ *n* : an abnormal, more or less persistent, and often painful erection of the penis; *esp* : one caused by disease rather than sexual desire

Price–Jones curve \ˈprīs-ˈjōnz-\ *n* : a graph of the frequency distribution of the diameters of red blood cells in a sample that has been smeared, stained, and magnified for direct observation and counting

Price–Jones, Cecil (1863–1943), British hematologist.

prick·le cell \ˈpri-kəl-\ *n* : a cell of the stratum spinosum of the skin having numerous intercellular bridges which give the separated cells a prickly appearance in microscopic preparations

prickle cell layer *n* : STRATUM SPINOSUM

prick·ly heat \ˈpri-klē-\ *n* : a noncontagious cutaneous eruption of red pimples with intense itching and tingling caused by inflammation around the sweat ducts — called also *heat rash*; see MILIARIA

pril·o·caine \ˈpri-lə-ˌkān\ *n* : a local anesthetic $C_{13}H_{20}N_2O$ related to lidocaine and used in the form of its hydrochloride as a nerve block for pain esp. in surgery and dentistry

pri·mal scream therapy \ˈprī-məl-\ *n* : psychotherapy in which the patient recalls and reenacts a particularly disturbing past experience usu. occurring early in life and expresses normally repressed anger or frustration esp. through spontaneous and unrestrained screams, hysteria, or violence — called also *primal scream, primal therapy*

pri·ma·quine \ˈprī-mə-ˌkwēn, ˈpri-, -kwin\ *n* : an antimalarial drug $C_{15}H_{21}N_3O$ used in the form of its diphosphate

pri·ma·ry \ˈprī-ˌmer-ē, ˈprī-mə-rē\ *adj* **1 a** (1) : first in order of time or development (2) : relating to or being the deciduous teeth and esp. the 20 deciduous teeth in the human set **b** : arising spontaneously : IDIOPATHIC ⟨∼ tumors⟩ **2** : belonging to the first group or order in successive divisions, combinations, or ramifications ⟨∼ nerves⟩ **3** : of, relating to, or being the amino acid sequence in proteins — compare SECONDARY 3, TERTIARY 2

primary aldosteronism *n* : aldosteronism caused by an adrenal tumor — called also *Conn's syndrome*

primary atypical pneumonia *n* : any of a group of pneumonias (as Q fever and psittacosis) caused esp. by a virus, mycoplasma, rickettsia, or chlamydia

primary care *n* : health care provided by a medical professional (as a general practitioner or a pediatrician) with whom a patient has initial contact and by whom the patient may be referred to a specialist for further treatment — called also *primary health care*

primary fissure *n* : a fissure of the cerebellum that is situated between the culmen and declive and that marks the boundary between the anterior lobe and the posterior lobe

primary health care *n* : PRIMARY CARE

primary host *n* : DEFINITIVE HOST

primary hypertension *n* : ESSENTIAL HYPERTENSION

primary oocyte *n* : a diploid oocyte that has not yet undergone meiosis

primary spermatocyte *n* : a diploid spermatocyte that has not yet undergone meiosis

primary syphilis *n* : the first stage of syphilis that is marked by the development of a chancre and the spread of the causative spirochete in the tissues of the body

primary tooth *n* : MILK TOOTH

pri·mate \'prī-ˌmāt\ *n* : any of an order (Primates) of mammals including humans, apes, monkeys, lemurs, and living and extinct related forms

prime mover \'prīm-\ *n* : AGONIST 1

prim·er \'prī-mər\ *n* : a molecule (as a short strand of RNA or DNA) whose presence is required for formation of another molecule (as a longer chain of DNA)

pri·mi·done \'prī-mə-ˌdōn\ *n* : an anticonvulsant phenobarbital derivative $C_{12}H_{14}N_2O_2$ used esp. to control epileptic seizures

pri·mi·grav·id \ˌprī-mə-'gra-vid\ *adj* : pregnant for the first time

pri·mi·grav·i·da \-'gra-vi-də\ *n, pl* **-i·das** *or* **-i·dae** \-ˌdē\ : an individual pregnant for the first time

pri·mip·a·ra \prī-'mi-pə-rə\ *n, pl* **-ras** *or* **-rae** \-ˌrē\ 1 : an individual bearing a first offspring 2 : an individual that has borne only one offspring

pri·mip·a·rous \-rəs\ *adj* : of, relating to, or being a primipara : bearing young for the first time — compare MULTIPAROUS 2

prim·i·tive \'pri-mə-tiv\ *adj* 1 : closely approximating an early ancestral type : little evolved 2 : belonging to or characteristic of an early stage of development ⟨∼ cells⟩

primitive streak *n* : an elongated band of cells that forms along the axis of an embryo early in gastrulation by the movement of lateral cells toward the axis and that develops a groove along its midline through which cells move to the interior of the embryo to form the mesoderm

pri·mor·di·al \prī-'mȯr-dē-əl\ *adj* : earliest formed in the growth of an individual or organ : PRIMITIVE

pri·mor·di·um \-dē-əm\ *n, pl* **-dia** \-dē-ə\ : the rudiment or commencement of a part or organ : ANLAGE

prin·ceps pol·li·cis \ˌprin-ˌseps-'pä-lə-səs\ *n* : a branch of the radial artery that passes along the ulnar side of the first metacarpal and divides into branches running along the palmar side of the thumb

prin·ci·ple \'prin-sə-pəl\ *n* : an ingredient (as a chemical) that exhibits or imparts a characteristic quality ⟨the active ∼ of a drug⟩

Prin·i·vil \'pri-nə-ˌvil\ *trademark* —

used for a preparation of lisinopril

P–R interval \ˌpē-'är-\ *n* : the interval between the beginning of the P wave and the beginning of the QRS complex of an electrocardiogram that represents the time between the beginning of the contraction of the atria and the beginning of the contraction of the ventricles

pri·on \'prē-ˌän\ *n* : a protein particle that lacks nucleic acid and is sometimes held to be the cause of various infectious diseases of the nervous system (as scrapie and Creutzfeldt≈ Jakob disease)

pri·vate \'prī-vət\ *adj* 1 : of, relating to, or receiving hospital service in which the patient has more privileges than a semiprivate or ward patient 2 : of, relating to, or being private practice ⟨a ∼ practitioner⟩

private–duty *adj* : caring for a single patient either in the home or in a hospital ⟨∼ nurse⟩

private practice *n* 1 : practice of a profession (as medicine) independently and not as an employee 2 : the patients depending on and using the services of a physician in private practice

privileged communication *n* : a communication between parties to a confidential relation (as between physician and patient) such that the recipient cannot be legally compelled to disclose it as a witness

prn *abbr* [Latin *pro re nata*] as needed; as the circumstances require — used in writing prescriptions

pro- *prefix* **1 a** : rudimentary : PROT- ⟨*pro*nucleus⟩ **b** : being a precursor of ⟨*pro*insulin⟩ **2** : front : anterior ⟨*pro*nephros⟩ **3** : projecting ⟨*pro*gnathous⟩

pro·abor·tion \ˌprō-ə-'bȯr-shən\ *adj* : favoring the legalization of abortion — **pro·abor·tion·ist** \-sh-ə-nist\ *n*

pro·ac·cel·er·in \ˌprō-ak-'se-lə-rən\ *n* : FACTOR V

pro·ac·tive \-'ak-tiv\ *adj* : relating to, caused by, or being interference between previous learning and the recall or performance of later learning ⟨∼ inhibition of memory⟩

pro·band \'prō-ˌband\ *n* : an individual actually being studied (as in a genetic investigation) : SUBJECT 1 — called also *propositus*

Pro–Ban·thine \ˌprō-'ban-ˌthēn\ *trademark* — used for a preparation of propantheline bromide

probe \'prōb\ *n* 1 : a surgical instrument that consists typically of a light slender fairly flexible pointed metal instrument like a small rod that is used typically for locating a foreign body, for exploring a wound or suppurative tract by prodding or piercing, or for penetrating and exploring bodily passages and cavities 2 : a device (as an ultrasound generator) or a substance (as DNA used in genetic research) used to obtain specific information for diagnostic or experimental purposes — **probe** *vb*

pro·ben·e·cid \prō-'ben-ə-səd\ *n* : a drug $C_{13}H_{19}NO_4S$ that acts on renal tubular function and is used to increase the concentration of some drugs (as penicillin) in the blood by inhibiting their excretion and to increase the excretion of urates in gout

pro·bos·cis \prə-'bä-səs, -'bäs-kəs\ *n*, *pl* **-bos·cis·es** *also* **-bos·ci·des** \-'bä-sə-ıdēz\ : any of various elongated or extensible tubular processes esp. of the oral region of an invertebrate

pro·cain·amide \prō-'kā-nə-ımīd, -məd; -ıkā-'na-məd\ *n* : a base $C_{13}H_{21}ON_3$ of an amide related to procaine that is used in the form of its crystalline hydrochloride as a cardiac depressant in the treatment of ventricular and atrial arrhythmias — see PRONESTYL

pro·caine \'prō-ıkān\ *n* : a basic ester $C_{13}H_{20}N_2O_2$ of para-aminobenzoic acid or its crystalline hydrochloride used as a local anesthetic — called also *novocaine*; see NOVOCAIN

procaine penicillin G *n* : a mixture of procaine and penicillin G that provides a low but persistent serum level of penicillin G following intramuscular injection

pro·car·ba·zine \prō-'kär-bə-ızēn, -zən\ *n* : an antineoplastic drug $C_{12}H_{19}N_3O$ that is a monoamine oxidase inhibitor and is used in the form of its hydrochloride esp. in the palliative treatment of Hodgkin's disease

Pro·car·dia \prō-'kär-dē-ə\ *trademark* — used for a preparation of nifedipine

pro·cary·ote *var of* PROKARYOTE

pro·ce·dure \prə-'sē-jər\ *n* **1 a** : a particular way of accomplishing something or of acting **b** : a step in a procedure **2** : a series of steps followed in a regular definite order

pro·ce·rus \prō-'sir-əs\ *n*, *pl* **-ri** \-ırī\ *or* **-rus·es** : a facial muscle that arises from the nasal bone and a cartilage in the side of the nose and inserts into the skin of the forehead between the eyebrows

pro·cess \'prä-ıses, 'prō-, -səs\ *n* **1 a** : a natural progressively continuing operation or development marked by a series of gradual changes that succeed one another in a relatively fixed way and lead toward a particular result or end ⟨the $\sim$ of growth⟩ **b** : a natural continuing activity or function ⟨such life $\sim$es as breathing⟩ **2** : a part of the mass of an organism or organic structure that projects outward from the main mass ⟨a bone $\sim$⟩

pro·ces·sus \prō-'se-səs\ *n*, *pl* **processus** : PROCESS 2

processus vag·i·na·lis \-ıva-jə-'nā-ləs\ *n* : a pouch of peritoneum that is carried into the scrotum by the descent

of the testicle and which in the scrotum forms the tunica vaginalis

pro·chlor·per·azine \ıprō-ıklor-'per-ə-ızēn\ *n* : a tranquilizing and antiemetic drug $C_{20}H_{24}ClN_3S$ — see COMPAZINE

pro–choice \ıprō-'chois\ *adj* : favoring the legalization of abortion — **pro-choic·er** \-'choi-sər\ *n*

pro·ci·den·tia \ıprō-sə-'den-chə, ıprä-, -chē-ə\ *n* : PROLAPSE; *esp* : severe prolapse of the uterus in which the cervix projects from the vaginal opening

proc·li·na·tion \ıprä-klə-'nā-shən\ *n* : the condition of being inclined forward ⟨$\sim$ of the upper incisors⟩

¹pro·co·ag·u·lant \ıprō-kō-'a-gyə-lənt\ *n* : procoagulant substance

²procoagulant *adj* : promoting the coagulation of blood ⟨$\sim$ activity⟩

pro·col·la·gen \'kä-lə-jən\ *n* : a molecular precursor of collagen

pro·con·ver·tin \-kən-'vərt-ᵊn\ *n* : FACTOR VII

pro·cre·ate \'prō-krē-ıāt\ *vb* **-at·ed; -at·ing** : to beget or bring forth offspring : PROPAGATE, REPRODUCE — **pro·cre·ation** \ıprō-krē-'ā-shən\ *n* — **pro·cre·ative** \'prō-krē-ıā-tiv\ *adj*

proct- *or* **procto-** *comb form* **1 a** : rectum ⟨*procto*scope⟩ **b** : rectum and ⟨*procto*sigmoidectomy⟩ **2** : anus and rectum ⟨*procto*logy⟩

proct·al·gia fu·gax \ıpräk-'tal-jə-'fyü-gaks, -jē-ə-\ *n* : a condition characterized by the intermittent occurrence of sudden sharp pain in the rectal area

proc·tec·to·my \präk-'tek-tə-mē\ *n*, *pl* **-mies** : surgical excision of the rectum

proc·ti·tis \präk-'tī-təs\ *n* : inflammation of the anus and rectum

proc·toc·ly·sis \präk-'tä-klə-səs\ *n*, *pl* **-ly·ses** \-ısēz\ : slow injection of large quantities of a fluid (as a solution of salt) into the rectum in supplementing the liquid intake of the body

proc·to·co·li·tis \ıpräk-tō-kə-'lī-təs\ *n* : inflammation of the rectum and colon

proc·tol·o·gy \präk-'tä-lə-jē\ *n*, *pl* **-gies** : a branch of medicine dealing with the structure and diseases of the anus, rectum, and sigmoid flexure — **proc·to·log·ic** \ıpräk-tə-'lä-jik\ *or* **proc·to·log·i·cal** \-ji-kəl\ *adj* — **proc·tol·o·gist** \-jist\ *n*

proc·to·pexy \'präk-tə-ıpek-sē\ *n*, *pl* **-pex·ies** : the suturing of the rectum to an adjacent structure (as the sacrum)

proc·to·plas·ty \'präk-tə-ıplas-tē\ *n*, *pl* **-ties** : plastic surgery of the rectum and anus

proc·to·scope \'präk-tə-ıskōp\ *n* : an instrument used for dilating and visually inspecting the rectum — **proc·to·scop·ic** \ıpräk-tə-'skä-pik\ *adj* — **proc·to·scop·i·cal·ly** *adv* — **proc·tos·co·py** \präk-'täs-kə-pē\ *n*

proc·to·sig·moid·ec·to·my \ıpräk-tō-

■sig-moi-ˈdek-tə-mē\ n, pl **-mies** : complete or partial surgical excision of the rectum and sigmoid colon

proc·to·sig·moid·itis \-ˌsig-moi-ˈdī-təs\ n : inflammation of the rectum and sigmoid flexure

proc·to·sig·moid·o·scope \-sig-ˈmoi-də-ˌskōp\ n : SIGMOIDOSCOPE

proc·to·sig·moid·os·co·py \-ˌsig-ˌmoi-ˈdäs-kə-pē\ n, pl **-pies** : SIGMOIDOSCOPY — **proc·to·sig·moid·o·scop·ic** \-ˌmoi-də-ˈskä-pik\ adj

proc·tot·o·my \präk-ˈtä-tə-mē\ n, pl **-mies** : surgical incision into the rectum

prod·ro·ma \ˈprä-drə-mə\ n, pl **-mas** or **-ma·ta** \prō-ˈdrō-mə-tə\ : PRODROME

pro·drome \ˈprō-ˌdrōm\ n : a premonitory symptom of disease — **pro·dro·mal** \ˌprō-ˈdrō-məl\ also **pro·dro·mic** \-mik\ adj

pro·duc·tive \prə-ˈdək-tiv, prō-\ adj : raising mucus or sputum (as from the bronchi) — used of a cough

pro·en·zyme \ˌprō-ˈen-ˌzīm\ n : ZYMOGEN

pro·eryth·ro·blast \-i-ˈri-thrə-ˌblast\ n : a hemocytoblast that gives rise to erythroblasts

pro·es·trus \-ˈes-trəs\ n : a preparatory period immediately preceding estrus and characterized by growth of graafian follicles, increased estrogenic activity, and alteration of uterine and vaginal mucosa

professional corporation n : a corporation organized by one or more licensed individuals (as a doctor or dentist) esp. for the purpose of providing professional services and obtaining tax advantages — abbr. PC

pro·fi·bri·nol·y·sin \ˌprō-ˌfī-brə-nə-ˈlis-ᵊn\ n : PLASMINOGEN

pro·file \ˈprō-ˌfīl\ n **1** : a set of data exhibiting the significant features of something and often obtained by multiple tests **2** : a graphic representation of the extent to which an individual or group exhibits traits as determined by tests or ratings ⟨a personality ∼⟩

pro·fla·vine \ˌprō-ˈflā-ˌvēn\ also **pro·fla·vin** \-vin\ n : a yellow crystalline mutagenic acridine dye $C_{13}H_{11}N_3$; also : the orange to brownish red hygroscopic crystalline sulfate used as an antiseptic esp. for wounds — see ACRIFLAVINE

pro·found·ly \prə-ˈfaund-lē, prō-\ adv **1** : totally or completely ⟨∼ deaf persons⟩ **2** : to the greatest possible degree ⟨∼ retarded persons⟩

pro·fun·da artery \prə-ˈfən-də-\ n **1** : DEEP BRACHIAL ARTERY **2** : DEEP FEMORAL ARTERY

profunda fem·o·ris \-ˈfe-mə-rəs\ n : DEEP FEMORAL ARTERY

profunda femoris artery n : DEEP FEMORAL ARTERY

profundus — see FLEXOR DIGITORUM PROFUNDUS

pro·gen·i·tor \prō-ˈje-nə-tər, prə-\ n **1** : an ancestor of an individual in a direct line of descent along which some or all of the ancestral genes could theoretically have passed **2** : a biologically ancestral form

prog·e·ny \ˈprä-jə-nē\ n, pl **-nies** : offspring of animals or plants

pro·ge·ria \prō-ˈjir-ē-ə\ n : a rare endocrine disorder of childhood characterized by retarded physical growth simultaneous with premature accelerated senility

pro·ges·ta·gen var of PROGESTOGEN

pro·ges·ta·tion·al \ˌprō-jes-ˈtā-shə-nəl\ adj : preceding pregnancy or gestation; esp : of, relating to, inducing, or constituting the modifications of the female mammalian system associated with ovulation and corpus luteum formation ⟨∼ hormones⟩

pro·ges·ter·one \prō-ˈjes-tə-ˌrōn\ n : a female steroid sex hormone $C_{21}H_{30}O_2$ that is secreted by the corpus luteum to prepare the endometrium for implantation and later by the placenta during pregnancy to prevent rejection of the developing embryo or fetus

pro·ges·tin \prō-ˈjes-tən\ n : PROGESTERONE; broadly : PROGESTOGEN

pro·ges·to·gen \-ˈjes-tə-jən\ n : any of several progestational steroids (as progesterone) — **pro·ges·to·gen·ic** \prə-ˌjes-tə-ˈje-nik\ adj

pro·glot·tid \prō-ˈglä-tid\ n : a segment of a tapeworm containing both male and female reproductive organs

pro·glot·tis \-ˈglä-təs\ n, pl **-glot·ti·des** \-ˈglä-tə-ˌdēz\ : PROGLOTTID

prog·na·thic \präg-ˈna-thik, -ˈnā-\ adj : PROGNATHOUS

prog·na·thous \ˈpräg-nə-thəs\ adj : having the jaws projecting beyond the upper part of the face — **prog·na·thism** \ˈpräg-nə-ˌthi-zəm, präg-ˈnā-\ n

prog·no·sis \präg-ˈnō-səs\ n, pl **-no·ses** \-ˌsēz\ **1** : the act or art of foretelling the course of a disease **2** : the prospect of survival and recovery from a disease as anticipated from the usual course of that disease or indicated by special features of the case — **prog·nos·tic** \präg-ˈnäs-tik\ adj

prog·nos·ti·cate \präg-ˈnäs-tə-ˌkāt\ vb **-cat·ed; -cat·ing** : to make a prognosis about the probable outcome of — **prog·nos·ti·ca·tion** \-ˌnäs-tə-ˈkā-shən\ n

pro·gres·sive \prə-ˈgre-siv\ adj : increasing in extent or severity ⟨a ∼ disease⟩ — **pro·gres·sive·ly** adv

progressive multifocal leukoencephalopathy n : a rare progressive and fatal demyelinating disease of the central nervous system that occurs in immunosuppressed individuals prob. due to loss of childhood immunity to a papovavirus ubiquitous in human populations and that is characterized by hemianopia, hemiplegia, alterations in mental state, and eventually coma

pro·guan·il \prō-ˈgwän-ᵊl\ *n* : CHLOROGUANIDE

pro·hor·mone \ˌprō-ˈhȯr-ˌmōn\ *n* : a physiologically inactive precursor of a hormone

pro·in·su·lin \-ˈin-sə-lən\ *n* : a single‑chain pancreatic polypeptide precursor of insulin that gives rise to the double chain of insulin by loss of the middle part of the molecule

pro·ject \prə-ˈjekt\ *vb* 1 : to attribute or assign (something in one's own mind or a personal characteristic) to a person, group, or object 2 : to connect by sending nerve fibers or processes

pro·jec·tile vomiting \prə-ˈjek-təl-, -ˌtil-\ *n* : vomiting that is sudden, usu. without nausea, and so sufficiently vigorous that the vomitus is forcefully projected to a distance

pro·jec·tion \prə-ˈjek-shən\ *n* 1 a : the act of referring a mental image constructed by the brain from bits of data collected by the sense organs to the actual source of stimulation outside the body b : the attribution of one's own ideas, feelings, or attitudes to other people or to objects; *esp* : the externalization of blame, guilt, or responsibility as a defense against anxiety 2 : the functional correspondence and connection of parts of the cerebral cortex with parts of the organism (the ∼ of the retina upon the visual area)

projection area *n* : an area of the cerebral cortex having connection through projection fibers with subcortical centers that in turn are linked with peripheral sense or motor organs

projection fiber *n* : a nerve fiber connecting some part of the cerebral cortex with lower sensory or motor centers — compare ASSOCIATION FIBER

pro·jec·tive \prə-ˈjek-tiv\ *adj* : of, relating to, or being a technique, device, or test (as the Rorschach test) designed to analyze the psychodynamic constitution of an individual by presenting unstructured or ambiguous material (as blots of ink, pictures, and sentence elements) that will elicit interpretive responses revealing personality structure

pro·kary·ote \ˌprō-ˈkar-ē-ˌōt\ *n* : a cellular organism (as a bacterium) that does not have a distinct nucleus — compare EUKARYOTE — **pro·kary·ot·ic** \-ˌkar-ē-ˈä-tik\ *adj*

pro·lac·tin \prō-ˈlak-tən\ *n* : a protein hormone of the anterior lobe of the pituitary gland that induces and maintains lactation in the postpartum mammalian female — called also *luteotropic hormone, luteotropin, mammotropin*

pro·la·min *or* **pro·la·mine** \ˈprō-lə-mən, -ˌmēn\ *n* : any of various simple proteins found esp. in seeds and insoluble in absolute alcohol or water

pro·lapse \prō-ˈlaps, ˈprō-ˌ\ *n* : the falling down or slipping of a body part from its usual position or relations (∼ of the uterus) — **pro·lapse** \prō-ˈlaps\ *vb*

pro-life \prō-ˈlif\ *adj* : ANTIABORTION

pro-lifer \-ˈlī-fər\ *n* : a person who opposes the legalization of abortion

pro·lif·er·a·tion \prə-ˌli-fə-ˈrā-shən\ *n* 1 a : rapid and repeated production of new parts or of offspring (as in a mass of cells by a rapid succession of cell divisions) b : a growth so formed 2 : the action, process, or result of increasing by proliferation — **pro·lif·er·ate** \-ˈli-fə-ˌrāt\ *vb* — **pro·lif·er·a·tive** \-ˈli-fə-ˌrā-tiv\ *adj*

proligerus — see DISCUS PROLIGERUS

pro·line \ˈprō-ˌlēn\ *n* : an amino acid $C_5H_9NO_2$ that can be synthesized by animals from glutamate

Pro·lix·in \prō-ˈlik-sən\ *trademark* — used for a preparation of fluphenazine

pro·mas·ti·gote \prō-ˈmas-ti-ˌgōt\ *n* : a flagellated usu. extracellular stage of some protozoans (family Trypanosomatidae and esp. genus *Leishmania*) characterized by a single anterior flagellum and no undulating membrane; *also* : a protozoan in this stage

pro·ma·zine \ˈprō-mə-ˌzēn\ *n* : a tranquilizer $C_{17}H_{20}N_2S$ derived from phenothiazine and administered in the form of its hydrochloride similarly to chlorpromazine — see SPARINE

pro·mega·kary·o·cyte \ˌprō-ˌme-gə-ˈkar-ē-ō-ˌsīt\ *n* : a cell in an intermediate stage of development between a megakaryoblast and a megakaryocyte

pro·meth·a·zine \prō-ˈme-thə-ˌzēn\ *n* : a crystalline antihistamine drug $C_{17}H_{20}N_2S$ derived from phenothiazine and used chiefly in the form of its hydrochloride — see PHENERGAN

pro·meth·es·trol \-me-ˈthes-ˌtrȯl\ *n* : a synthetic estrogen $C_{20}H_{26}O_2$ — see MEPRANE

pro·me·thi·um \prə-ˈmē-thē-əm\ *n* : a metallic element obtained as a fission product of uranium or from neutron‑irradiated neodymium — symbol *Pm*; called also *illinium*; see ELEMENT table

prom·i·nence \ˈprä-mə-nəns\ *n* : an elevation or projection on an anatomical structure (as a bone)

prominens — see VERTEBRA PROMINENS

pro·mis·cu·ous \prə-ˈmis-kyə-wəs\ *adj* : not restricted to one sexual partner — **pro·mis·cu·i·ty** \ˌprä-məs-ˈkyü-ə-tē, prə-ˌmis-\ *n*

pro·mono·cyte \prə-ˈmä-nə-ˌsīt\ *n* : a cell in an intermediate stage of development between a monoblast and a monocyte

prom·on·to·ry \ˈprä-mən-ˌtōr-ē\ *n, pl*

-ries : a bodily prominence: as **a** : the angle of the ventral side of the sacrum where it joins the vertebra **b** : a prominence on the inner wall of the tympanum of the ear

pro·mot·er \prə-'mō-tər\ *n* **1** : a substance that in very small amounts is able to increase the activity of a catalyst **2** : a binding site in a DNA chain at which RNA polymerase binds to initiate transcription of messenger RNA by one or more nearby structural genes **3** : a chemical believed to promote carcinogenicity or mutagenicity

pro·my·elo·cyte \prō-'mī-ə-lə-ısīt\ *n* : a partially differentiated granulocyte in bone marrow having the characteristic granulations but lacking the specific staining reactions of a mature granulocyte of the blood — **pro·my·elo·cyt·ic** \-ımī-ə-lə-'si-tik\ *adj*

promyelocytic leukemia *n* : a leukemia in which the predominant blood cell type is the promyelocyte

pro·na·tion \prō-'nā-shən\ *n* : rotation of an anatomical part towards the midline: as **a** : rotation of the hand and forearm so that the palm faces backwards or downwards **b** : rotation of the medial bones in the midtarsal region of the foot inward and downward so that in walking the foot tends to come down on its inner margin — **pro·nate** \'prō-ınāt\ *vb*

pro·na·tor \'prō-ınā-tər\ *n* : a muscle that produces pronation

pronator qua·dra·tus \-kwä-'drā-təs\ : a deep muscle of the forearm passing transversely from the ulna to the radius and serving to pronate the forearm

pronator te·res \-'tir-ıēz\ *n* : a muscle of the forearm arising from the medial epicondyle of the humerus and the coronoid process of the ulna, inserting into the lateral surface of the middle third of the radius, and serving to pronate and flex the forearm

prone \'prōn\ *adj* : having the front or ventral surface downward; *esp* : lying facedown — **prone** *adv*

pro·neph·ros \prō-'ne-frəs, -ıfräs\ *n*, *pl* **-neph·roi** \-'ne-ıfroi\ : either member of the first and most anterior pair of the three paired vertebrate renal organs present but nonfunctional in embryos of reptiles, birds, and mammals — compare MESONEPHROS, METANEPHROS — **pro·neph·ric** \prō-'ne-frik\ *adj*

Pro·nes·tyl \prō-'nes-til\ *trademark* — used for a preparation of the hydrochloride of procainamide

pro·neth·a·lol \prō-'ne-thə-ılól, -ılōl\ *n* : a drug $C_{15}H_{19}NO$ that is a beta-adrenergic blocking agent — called also *nethalide*

pron·to·sil \'prän-tə-ısil\ *n* : any of three sulfonamide drugs: **a** : a red azo dye $C_{12}H_{13}N_5O_2S$ that was the first sulfa drug tested clinically — called also *prontosil rubrum* **b** : SULFANILAMIDE **c** : AZOSULFAMIDE

pro·nu·cle·us \prō-'nü-klē-əs, -'nyü-\ *n*, *pl* **-clei** \-klē-ıi\ *also* **-cle·us·es** : the haploid nucleus of a male or female gamete (as an egg or sperm) up to the time of fusion with that of another gamete in fertilization — **pro·nu·cle·ar** \-klē-ər\ *adj*

Pro·pa·drine \'prō-pə-drən, -ıdrēn\ *trademark* — used for a preparation of phenylpropanolamine

prop·a·gate \'prä-pə-ıgāt\ *vb* **-gat·ed; -gat·ing 1** : to reproduce or cause to reproduce sexually or asexually **2** : to cause to spread or to be transmitted — **prop·a·ga·tion** \ıprä-pə-'gā-shən\ *n* — **prop·a·ga·tive** \'prä-pə-ıgā-tiv\ *adj*

pro·pam·i·dine \prō-'pa-mə-ıdēn, -dən\ *n* : an antiseptic drug $C_{17}H_{20}N_4O_2$

pro·pan·o·lol \prō-'pa-nə-ılol, -ılōl\ *n* : PROPRANOLOL

pro·pan·the·line bromide \prō-'pan-thə-ılēn-\ *n* : an anticholinergic drug $C_{23}H_{30}BrNO_3$ used esp. in the treatment of peptic ulcer — called also *propantheline*; see PRO-BANTHINE

pro·par·a·caine \prō-'par-ə-ıkān\ *n* : a drug $C_{16}H_{26}N_2O_3$ used in the form of its hydrochloride as a topical anesthetic

pro·per·din \prō-'pərd-ᵊn\ *n* : a serum protein that participates in destruction of bacteria, neutralization of viruses, and lysis of red blood cells

pro·peri·to·ne·al \prō-ıper-ə-tə-'nē-əl\ *adj* : lying between the parietal peritoneum and the internal musculature of the body cavity ⟨∼ fat⟩

pro·phage \'prō-ıfaj, -ıfazh\ *n* : an intracellular form of a bacteriophage in which it is harmless to the host, is usu. integrated into the hereditary material of the host, and reproduces when the host does

pro·phase \-ıfāz\ *n* **1** : the initial stage of mitosis and of the mitotic division of meiosis characterized by the condensation of chromosomes consisting of two chromatids, disappearance of the nucleolus and nuclear membrane, and formation of the mitotic spindle **2** : the initial stage of the first division of meiosis in which the chromosomes become visible, homologous pairs of chromosomes undergo synapsis and crossing-over, chiasmata appear, chromosomes condense with homologues visible as tetrads, and the nuclear membrane and nucleolus disappear and which is divided into the five consecutive stages leptotene, zygotene, pachytene, diplotene, and diakinesis — **pro·pha·sic** \prō-'fā-zik\ *adj*

¹pro·phy·lac·tic \ıprō-fə-'lak-tik, ıprä-\ *adj* **1** : guarding from or preventing disease ⟨∼ therapy⟩ **2** : tending to prevent or ward off : PREVENTIVE — **pro·phy·lac·ti·cal·ly** *adv*

²**prophylactic** *n* : something (as a medicinal preparation) that is prophylactic; *esp* : a device and esp. a condom for preventing venereal infection or contraception

pro·phy·lax·is \-'lak-səs\ *n, pl* **-lax·es** \-'lak-₁sēz\ : measures designed to preserve health and prevent the spread of disease : protective or preventive treatment

pro·pio·lac·tone \₁prō-pē-ō-'lak-₁tōn\ *or* β-**pro·pio·lac·tone** \₁bā-tə-\ *n* : a liquid disinfectant $C_3H_4O_2$

pro·pio·ma·zine \₁prō-pē-'ō-mə-₁zēn\ *n* : a substituted phenothiazine C_{20}-$H_{24}N_2OS$ used esp. in the form of its hydrochloride as a sedative — see LARGON

pro·pio·nate \'prō-pē-ə-₁nāt\ *n* : a salt or ester of propionic acid

pro·pi·oni·bac·te·ri·um \₁prō-pē-₁ä-nə-bak-'tir-ē-əm\ *n* **1** *cap* : a genus of gram-positive nonmotile usu. anaerobic bacteria (family Propionibacteriaceae) including forms found esp. on human skin and in dairy products **2** *pl* **-ria** \-ē-ə\ : any bacterium of the genus *Propionibacterium*

pro·pi·on·ic acid \₁prō-pē-'ä-nik-\ *n* : a liquid sharp-odored fatty acid C_3-H_6O_2

pro·pos·i·ta \prō-'pä-zə-tə\ *n, pl* **-i·tae** \-₁tē\ : a female proband

pro·pos·i·tus \prō-'pä-zə-təs\ *n, pl* **-i·ti** \-₁tī\ : PROBAND

pro·poxy·phene \prō-'päk-sə-₁fēn\ *n* : an analgesic $C_{22}H_{29}NO_2$ structurally related to methadone but less addicting that is administered in the form of its hydrochloride — called also *dextropropoxyphene*; see DARVON

pro·pran·o·lol \prō-'pra-nə-₁lōl, -₁lōl\ *n* : a beta-blocker $C_{16}H_{21}NO_2$ used in the form of its hydrochloride in the treatment of abnormal heart rhythms and angina pectoris — called also *propanolol*; see INDERAL

propria — see LAMINA PROPRIA, SUBSTANTIA PROPRIA, TUNICA PROPRIA

¹**pro·pri·etary** \prə-'prī-ə-₁ter-ē\ *n, pl* **-tar·ies** : something that is used, produced, or marketed under exclusive legal right of the inventor or maker; *specif* : a drug (as a patent medicine) that is protected by secrecy, patent, or copyright against free competition as to name, product, composition, or process of manufacture

²**proprietary** *adj* **1** : used, made, or marketed by one having the exclusive legal right ⟨a ∼ drug⟩ **2** : privately owned and managed and run as a profit-making organization ⟨a ∼ clinic⟩

pro·prio·cep·tion \₁prō-prē-ō-'sep-shən\ *n* : the reception of stimuli produced within the organism — **pro·prio·cep·tive** \-'sep-tiv\ *adj*

pro·prio·cep·tor \-'sep-tər\ *n* : a sensory receptor located deep in the tissues (as in skeletal or heart muscle) that functions in proprioception

pro·prio·spi·nal \-'spin-ᵊl\ *adj* : distinctively or exclusively spinal ⟨a ∼ neuron⟩

proprius — see EXTENSOR DIGITI QUINTI PROPRIUS, EXTENSOR INDICIS PROPRIUS

pro·pto·sis \präp-'tō-səs, prō-'tō-\ *n, pl* **-pto·ses** \-₁sēz\ : forward projection or displacement esp. of the eyeball

pro·pyl·ene glycol \'prō-pə-₁lēn-\ *n* : a sweet viscous liquid $C_3H_8O_2$ used esp. as an antifreeze and solvent, in brake fluids, and as a food preservative

pro·pyl gallate \'prō-pəl-\ *n* : a white crystalline antioxidant $C_{10}H_{12}O_5$ that is used as a preservative

pro·pyl·hex·e·drine \₁prō-pəl-'hek-sə-₁drēn\ *n* : a sympathomimetic drug $C_{10}H_{21}N$ used chiefly as a nasal decongestant

pro·pyl·par·a·ben \-'par-ə-₁ben\ *n* : a crystalline ester $C_{10}H_{12}O_3$ used as a preservative in pharmaceutical preparations

pro·pyl·thio·ura·cil \-₁thī-ō-'yùr-ə-₁sil\ *n* : a crystalline compound C_7H_{10}-N_2OS used as an antithyroid drug in the treatment of goiter

pro·re·nin \prō-'rē-nən, -'re-\ *n* : the precursor of the kidney enzyme renin

pros- *prefix* : in front ⟨*prosen*cephalon⟩

Pros·car \'präs-₁kär\ *trademark* — used for a preparation of finasteride

pro·sec·tor \prō-'sek-tər\ *n* : one who makes dissections for anatomic demonstrations

pros·en·ceph·a·lon \₁prä-₁sen-'se-fə-₁län, -lən\ *n* : FOREBRAIN

prosop- *or* **prosopo-** *comb form* : face ⟨*prosop*agnosia⟩

pros·op·ag·no·sia \₁prä-sə-pag-'nō-zhə\ *n* : a form of agnosia characterized by an inability to recognize faces

pro·spec·tive \prə-'spek-tiv\ *adj* : relating to or being a study (as of the incidence of disease) that starts with the present condition of a population of individuals and follows them into the future — compare RETROSPECTIVE

pros·ta·cy·clin \₁präs-tə-'sī-klən\ *n* : a prostaglandin that is a metabolite of arachidonic acid, inhibits aggregation of platelets, and dilates blood vessels

pros·ta·glan·din \₁präs-tə-'glan-dən\ *n* : any of various oxygenated unsaturated cyclic fatty acids of animals that have a variety of hormonelike actions (as in controlling blood pressure or smooth muscle contraction)

prostat- *or* **prostato-** *comb form* : prostate gland ⟨*prostat*ectomy⟩ ⟨*prostati*tis⟩

prostatae — see LEVATOR PROSTATAE

pros·tate \'präs-₁tāt\ *n* : PROSTATE GLAND

pros·ta·tec·to·my \₁präs-tə-'tek-tə-mē\

n, pl **-mies :** surgical removal or resection of the prostate gland

prostate gland *n* : a firm partly muscular partly glandular body that is situated about the base of the mammalian male urethra and secretes an alkaline viscid fluid which is a major constituent of the ejaculatory fluid — called also *prostate*

prostate–specific antigen *n* : a protease that is secreted by the epithelial cells of the prostate and is used in the diagnosis of prostate cancer since its concentration in the blood serum tends to be proportional to the clinical stage of the disease — abbr. *PSA*

pros·tat·ic \prä-ˈsta-tik\ *adj* : of, relating to, or affecting the prostate gland ⟨∼ cancer⟩

prostatic urethra *n* : the part of the male urethra from the base of the prostate gland where the urethra begins as the outlet of the bladder to the point where it emerges from the apex of the prostate gland

prostatic utricle *n* : a small blind pouch that projects from the wall of the prostatic urethra into the prostate gland

pros·ta·tism \ˈprä-stə-ˌti-zəm\ *n* : disease of the prostate gland; *esp* : a disorder resulting from obstruction of the bladder neck by an enlarged prostate gland

pros·ta·ti·tis \ˌprä-stə-ˈtī-təs\ *n* : inflammation of the prostate gland

pros·the·sis \präs-ˈthē-səs, ˈpräs-thə-\ *n, pl* **-the·ses** \-ˌsēz\ : an artificial device to replace a missing part of the body ⟨a dental ∼⟩

pros·thet·ic \präs-ˈthe-tik\ *adj* **1** : of, relating to, or being a prosthesis ⟨a ∼ device⟩; *also* : of or relating to prosthetics ⟨∼ research⟩ **2** : of, relating to, or constituting a nonprotein group of a conjugated protein — **pros·thet·i·cal·ly** *adv*

prosthetic dentistry *n* : PROSTHODONTICS

pros·thet·ics \-tiks\ *n sing or pl* : the surgical and dental specialty concerned with the design, construction, and fitting of prostheses

prosthetic valve endocarditis *n* : endocarditis caused by or involving a surgically implanted prosthetic heart valve — abbr. *PVE*

pros·the·tist \ˈpräs-thə-tist\ *n* : a specialist in prosthetics

pros·thi·on \ˈpräs-thē-ˌän\ *n* : a point on the alveolar arch midway between the median upper incisor teeth

prosth·odon·tics \ˌpräs-thə-ˈdän-tiks\ *n sing or pl* : the dental specialty concerned with the making of artificial replacements for missing parts of the mouth and jaw — called also *prosthetic dentistry* — **prosth·odon·tic** \-tik\ *adj*

prosth·odon·tist \-ˈdän-tist\ *n* : a specialist in prosthodontics

Pro·stig·min \prō-ˈstig-mən\ *trademark* — used for a preparation of neostigmine

¹pros·trate \ˈpräs-ˌträt\ *adj* : completely overcome ⟨was ∼ from the heat⟩

²prostrate *vb* **pros·trat·ed; pros·trat·ing** : to put into a state of extreme bodily exhaustion ⟨*prostrated* by fever⟩

pros·tra·tion \prä-ˈstrā-shən\ *n* : complete physical or mental exhaustion — see HEAT EXHAUSTION

prot·ac·tin·i·um \ˌprō-ˌtak-ˈti-nē-əm\ *n* : a shiny metallic radioelement — symbol *Pa*; see ELEMENT table

prot·amine \ˈprō-tə-ˌmēn\ *n* : any of various strongly basic proteins of relatively low molecular weight that are rich in arginine and are found associated esp. with DNA in place of histone in the sperm cells of various animals (as fish)

protamine zinc insulin *n* : a combination of protamine, zinc, and insulin used in suspension in water for subcutaneous injection in place of insulin because of its prolonged effect — abbr. *PZI*

prot·anom·a·ly \ˌprō-tə-ˈnä-mə-lē\ *n, pl* **-lies** : trichromatism in which an abnormally large proportion of red is required to match the spectrum — compare DEUTERANOMALY, TRICHROMAT — **prot·anom·a·lous** \-ləs\ *adj*

pro·ta·nope \ˈprō-tə-ˌnōp\ *n* : an individual affected with protanopia

prot·an·opia \ˌprō-tə-ˈnō-pē-ə\ *n* : a dichromatism in which the spectrum is seen in tones of yellow and blue with confusion of red and green and reduced sensitivity to monochromatic lights from the red end of the spectrum

prote- *or* **proteo-** *comb form* : protein ⟨*proteolysis*⟩

pro·te·ase \ˈprō-tē-ˌās, -ˌāz\ *n* : any of numerous enzymes that hydrolyze proteins and are classified according to the most prominent functional group (as serine or cysteine) at the active site — called also *proteinase*

¹pro·tec·tive \prə-ˈtek-tiv\ *adj* : serving to protect the body or one of its parts from disease or injury

²protective *n* : a protective agent (as a medicine or a dressing)

pro·tein \ˈprō-ˌtēn\ *n, often attrib* **1** : any of numerous naturally occurring extremely complex substances that consist of amino-acid residues joined by peptide bonds, contain the elements carbon, hydrogen, nitrogen, oxygen, usu. sulfur, and occas. other elements (as phosphorus or iron), and include many essential biological compounds (as enzymes, hormones, or immunoglobulins) **2** : the total nitrogenous material in plant or animal substances; *esp* : CRUDE PROTEIN

pro·tein·aceous \ˌprō-tə-ˈnā-shəs, -ˌtē-\ *adj* : of, relating to, resembling, or being protein

pro·tein·ase \'prō-tə-ˌnās, -ˌtē-, -ˌnāz\ n : PROTEASE

protein kinase n : any of a class of allosteric enzymes that are reversibly dissociated in the presence of cyclic AMP yielding a catalytic subunit which catalyzes the phosphorylation of other enzymes by drawing on phosphate from AMP

pro·tein·o·sis \ˌprō-ˌtē-'nō-səs\ n, pl -o·ses \-ˌsēz\ or -o·sis·es : the accumulation of abnormal amounts of protein in bodily tissues — see PULMONARY ALVEOLAR PROTEINOSIS

pro·tein·uria \ˌprō-tə-'nur-ē-ə, -ˌtē-, -'nyur-\ n : the presence of excess protein in the urine — **pro·tein·uric** \-'nur-ik, -'nyur-\ adj

pro·teo·gly·can \ˌprō-tē-ə-'glī-ˌkan\ n : any of a class of glycoproteins of high molecular weight that are found in the extracellular matrix of connective tissue

pro·teo·lip·id \-'li-pəd\ n : any of a class of proteins that contain a considerable percentage of lipid and are soluble in lipids and insoluble in water

pro·te·ol·y·sis \ˌprō-tē-'ä-lə-səs\ n, pl -y·ses \-ˌsēz\ : the hydrolysis of proteins or peptides with formation of simpler and soluble products (as in digestion) — **pro·teo·lyt·ic** \ˌprō-tē-ə-'li-tik\ adj — **pro·teo·lyt·i·cal·ly** adv

pro·te·us \'prō-tē-əs\ n 1 cap : a genus of aerobic usu. motile enterobacteria that are often found in decaying organic matter and include a common causative agent (P. mirabilis) of urinary tract infections 2 pl -tei \-ˌī\ : any bacterium of the genus Proteus

pro·throm·bin \prō-'thräm-bən\ n : a plasma protein produced in the liver in the presence of vitamin K and converted into thrombin by the action of various activators (as thromboplastin) in the clotting of blood — **pro·throm·bic** \-bik\ adj

prothrombin time n : the time required for a particular specimen of prothrombin to induce blood-plasma clotting under standardized conditions in comparison with a time of between 11.5 and 12 seconds for normal human blood

pro·ti·re·lin \prō-'tī-rə-lən\ n : THYROTROPIN-RELEASING HORMONE

pro·tist \'prō-tist\ n : any of a major taxonomic group and usu. a kingdom (Protista) of unicellular, colonial, or multicellular eukaryotic organisms including esp. the protozoans and algae — **pro·tis·tan** \prō-'tis-tən\ adj or n

pro·to·col \'prō-tə-ˌkȯl, -ˌkōl, -ˌkäl\ n 1 : an official account of a proceeding: esp : the notes or records relating to a case, an experiment, or an autopsy 2 : a detailed plan of a scientific or medical experiment or treatment

pro·to·di·as·to·le \ˌprō-tō-dī-'as-tə-lē\ n 1 : the period just before aortic valve closure 2 : the period just after aortic valve closure — **pro·to·di·a·stol·ic** \-ˌdī-ə-'stä-lik\ adj

pro·ton \'prō-ˌtän\ n : an elementary particle that is identical with the nucleus of the hydrogen atom, that along with neutrons is a constituent of all other atomic nuclei, that carries a positive charge numerically equal to the charge of an electron, and that has a mass of 1.673×10^{-24} gram — **pro·ton·ic** \prō-'tä-nik\ adj

pro·to-on·co·gene \ˌprō-tō-'äŋ-kə-ˌjēn\ n : a gene having the potential for change into an active oncogene

Pro·to·pam \'prō-tə-ˌpam\ trademark — used for a preparation of pralidoxime

pro·to·path·ic \ˌprō-tə-'pa-thik\ adj : of, relating to, being, or mediating cutaneous sensory reception that is responsive only to rather gross stimuli — compare EPICRITIC

pro·to·plasm \'prō-tə-ˌpla-zəm\ n 1 : the organized colloidal complex of organic and inorganic substances (as proteins and water) that constitutes esp. the living nucleus, cytoplasm, and mitochondria of the cell 2 : CYTOPLASM — **pro·to·plas·mic** \ˌprō-tə-'plaz-mik\ adj

pro·to·plast \'prō-tə-ˌplast\ n : the nucleus, cytoplasm, and plasma membrane of a cell as distinguished from inert walls and inclusions

pro·to·por·phyr·ia \ˌprō-tō-ˌpȯr-'fir-ē-ə\ n : the presence of protoporphyrin in the blood — see ERYTHROPOIETIC PROTOPORPHYRIA

pro·to·por·phy·rin \ˌprō-tō-'pȯr-fə-rən\ n : a purple porphyrin acid $C_{34}H_{34}N_4O_4$ obtained from hemin or heme by removal of bound iron

Pro·to·stron·gy·lus \-'strän-jə-ləs\ n : a genus of lungworms (family Metastrongylidae) including one (P. rufescens) parasitic esp. in sheep and goats

Pro·to·the·ca \ˌprō-tə-'thē-kə\ n : a genus of microorganisms that include several causing or associated with human infections

pro·to·the·co·sis \-ˌkō-səs\ n, pl -co·ses \-ˌsēz\ : an infection produced by a microorganism of the genus Prototheca

protozoa pl of PROTOZOON

pro·to·zo·a·ci·dal \ˌprō-tə-ˌzō-ə-'sīd-əl\ adj : destroying protozoans

pro·to·zo·al \ˌprō-tə-'zō-əl\ adj : of or relating to protozoans

pro·to·zo·an \-'zō-ən\ n : any of a phylum or subkingdom (Protozoa) of chiefly motile unicellular protists (as amoebas, trypanosomes, sporozoans, and paramecia) that are represented in almost every kind of habitat and include some pathogenic parasites of humans and domestic animals — **protozoan** adj

pro·to·zo·ol·o·gy \-zō-'ä-lə-jē\ n, pl -gies

: a branch of zoology dealing with protozoans — **pro·to·zo·ol·o·gist** \-jist\ *n*

pro·to·zo·on \₁prō-tə-¹zō-₁än\ *n, pl* **pro·to·zoa** : PROTOZOAN

pro·tract \prō-¹trakt\ *vb* : to extend forward or outward — compare RETRACT

pro·trac·tion \-¹trak-shən\ *n* **1** : the act of moving an anatomical part forward **2** : the state of being protracted; *esp* : protrusion of the jaws

pro·trip·ty·line \prō-¹trip-tə-₁lēn\ *n* : a tricyclic antidepressant drug C_{19}-$H_{21}N$ — see VIVACTIL

pro·trude \prō-¹trüd\ *vb* **pro·trud·ed; pro·trud·ing** : to project or cause to project : jut out — **pro·tru·sion** \prō-¹trü-zhən\ *n*

pro·tru·sive \-¹trü-siv, -ziv\ *adj* **1** : thrusting forward **2** : PROTUBERANT

pro·tu·ber·ance \prō-¹tü-bə-rəns, -¹tyü-\ *n* **1** : something that is protuberant (a bony ∼) **2** : the quality or state of being protuberant

protuberans — see DERMATOFIBROSARCOMA PROTUBERANS

pro·tu·ber·ant \-rənt\ *adj* : bulging beyond the surrounding or adjacent surface (a ∼ joint) (∼ eyes)

proud flesh *n* : an excessive growth of granulation tissue (as in an ulcer)

pro·ven·tric·u·lus \₁prō-ven-¹tri-kyə-ləs\ *n, pl* **-li** \-₁lī, -₁lē\ : the glandular or true stomach of a bird that is situated between the crop and gizzard

pro·vi·rus \¹prō-₁vī-rəs\ *n* : a form of a virus that is integrated into the genetic material of a host cell and by replicating with it can be transmitted from one cell generation to the next without causing lysis — **pro·vi·ral** \prō-¹vī-rəl\ *adj*

pro·vi·ta·min \-¹vī-tə-mən\ *n* : a precursor of a vitamin convertible into the vitamin in an organism

provitamin A *n* : a provitamin of vitamin A; *esp* : CAROTENE

pro·voke \prə-¹vōk\ *vb* **pro·voked; pro·vok·ing** : to call forth or induce (a physical reaction) (ipecac ∼s vomiting) — **prov·o·ca·tion** \₁prä-və-¹kā-shən\ *n* — **pro·voc·a·tive** \prə-¹vä-kə-tiv\ *adj*

prox·e·mics \präk-¹sē-miks\ *n sing or pl* : the study of the nature, degree, and effect of the spatial separation individuals naturally maintain (as in various social and interpersonal situations) and of how this separation relates to environmental and cultural factors — **prox·e·mic** \-mik\ *adj*

prox·i·mad \¹präk-sə-₁mad\ *adv* : PROXIMALLY

prox·i·mal \¹präk-sə-məl\ *adj* **1 a** : situated next to or near the point of attachment or origin or a central point; *esp* : located toward the center of the body (the ∼ end of a bone) — compare DISTAL 1a **b** : of, relating to, or being the mesial and distal surfaces of

a tooth **2** : sensory rather than physical or social (∼ stimuli) — compare DISTAL 2 — **prox·i·mal·ly** *adv*

proximal convoluted tubule *n* : the convoluted portion of the vertebrate nephron that lies between Bowman's capsule and the loop of Henle and functions esp. in the resorption of sugar, sodium and chloride ions, and water from the glomerular filtrate — called also *proximal tubule*

proximal radioulnar joint *n* : a pivot joint between the upper end of the radius and the ring formed by the radial notch of the ulna and its annular ligament that permits rotation of the proximal head of the radius

proximal tubule *n* : PROXIMAL CONVOLUTED TUBULE

prox·i·mate cause \¹präk-sə-mət-\ *n* : a cause that directly or with no intervening agency produces an effect

Pro·zac \¹prō-₁zak\ *trademark* — used for a preparation of fluoxetine

pru·rig·i·nous \prü-¹ri-jə-nəs\ *adj* : resembling, caused by, affected with, or being prurigo (∼ dermatosis)

pru·ri·go \prü-¹rī-(₁)gō\ *n* : a chronic inflammatory skin disease marked by a general eruption of small itching papules

pru·rit·ic \prü-¹ri-tik\ *adj* : of, relating to, or marked by itching

pru·ri·tus \prü-¹rī-təs\ *n* : localized or generalized itching due to irritation of sensory nerve endings from organic or psychogenic causes : ITCH

pruritus ani \-¹ā-₁nī\ *n* : pruritus of the anal region

pruritus vul·vae \-¹vəl-vē\ *n* : pruritus of the vulva

Prus·sian blue \¹prə-shən-¹blü\ *n* : a blue iron-containing dye Fe_4-$[Fe(CN)_6]_3 \cdot xH_2O$ used in a test for ferric iron

prus·sic acid \¹prə-sik-\ *n* : HYDROCYANIC ACID

PSA *abbr* prostate-specific antigen

psal·te·ri·um \sol-¹tir-ē-əm\ *n, pl* **-ria** \-ē-ə\ **1** : OMASUM **2** : HIPPOCAMPAL COMMISSURE

psam·mo·ma \sa-¹mō-mə\ *n, pl* **-mas** or **-ma·ta** \-mə-tə\ : a hard fibrous tumor of the meninges of the brain and spinal cord containing calcareous matter — **psam·mo·ma·tous** \sa-¹mō-mə-təs, -¹mä-\ *adj*

pseud- *or* **pseudo-** *comb form* : false : spurious (*pseud*arthrosis) (*pseudo*tumor)

pseud·ar·thro·sis \₁süd-är-¹thrō-səs\ *n, pl* **-thro·ses** \-¹thrō-₁sēz\ : an abnormal union formed by fibrous tissue between parts of a bone that has fractured usu. spontaneously due to congenital weakness — called also *false joint*

pseu·do·an·eu·rysm \₁sü-dō-¹an-yə-₁ri-zəm\ *n* : a vascular abnormality (as an elongation or buckling of the aorta) that resembles an aneurysm in roentgenography

pseu·do·ar·thro·sis *var of* PSEUDAR-THROSIS

pseu·do·bul·bar \-'bəl-bər\ *adj* : simulating that caused by lesions of the medulla oblongata ⟨~ paralysis⟩

pseu·do·cho·lin·es·ter·ase \-,kō-lə-'nes-tə-,rās, -,rāz\ *n* : CHOLINESTERASE 2

pseu·do·cow·pox \-'kau̇-,päks\ *n* : MILKER'S NODULES

pseu·do·cy·e·sis \-sī-'ē-səs\ *n, pl* **-e·ses** \-,sēz\ : a psychosomatic state that occurs without conception and is marked by some of the physical symptoms (as cessation of menses, enlargement of the abdomen, and apparent fetal movements) and changes in hormonal balance of pregnancy

pseu·do·cyst \'sü-dō-,sist\ *n* : a cluster of toxoplasmas in an enucleate host cell

pseu·do·de·men·tia \,sü-dō-di-'men-chə\ *n* : a condition of extreme apathy which outwardly resembles dementia but is not the result of actual mental deterioration

pseu·do·ephed·rine \-i-'fe-drən\ *n* : a crystalline alkaloid $C_{10}H_{15}NO$ that is isomeric with ephedrine and is used for similar purposes esp. in the form of its hydrochloride

pseu·do·gout \-'gau̇t\ *n* : an arthritic condition which resembles gout but is characterized by the deposition of crystalline salts other than urates in and around the joints

pseu·do·her·maph·ro·dite \-(,)hər-'ma-frə-,dīt\ *n* : an individual exhibiting pseudohermaphroditism — **pseu·do·her·maph·ro·dit·ic** \-(,)hər-,ma-frə-'di-tik\ *adj*

pseu·do·her·maph·ro·dit·ism \-rə-,dī-,ti-zəm\ *n* : the condition of having the gonads of one sex and the external genitalia and other sex organs so variably developed that the sex of the individual is uncertain

pseu·do·hy·per·tro·phic \,sü-dō-,hī-pər-'trō-fik\ *adj* : falsely hypertrophic; *specif* : being a form of muscular dystrophy in which the muscles become swollen with deposits of fat and fibrous tissue — **pseu·do·hy·per·tro·phy** \-hī-'pər-trə-fē\ *n*

pseu·do·hy·po·para·thy·roid·ism \-,hī-pō-,par-ə-'thī-,ròi-,di-zəm\ *n* : a usu. inherited disorder that clinically resembles hypoparathyroidism but results from the body's inability to respond normally to parathyroid hormone rather than from a deficiency of the hormone itself

pseu·do·mem·brane \,sü-dō-'mem-,brān\ *n* : FALSE MEMBRANE

pseu·do·mem·bra·nous \-'mem-brə-nəs\ *adj* : characterized by the presence or formation of a false membrane ⟨~ colitis⟩

pseu·do·mo·nad \-'mō-,nad, -,nəd\ *n*

: any bacterium of the genus *Pseudomonas*

pseu·do·mo·nal \-'mō-nəl\ *adj* : of, relating to, or caused by bacteria of the genus *Pseudomonas* ⟨~ infection⟩

pseu·do·mo·nas \,sü-dō-'mō-nəs, sü-'dä-mə-nəs\ *n* 1 *cap* : a genus of gram-negative rod-shaped motile bacteria (family Pseudomonadaceae) including some saprophytes, a few animal pathogens, and numerous important plant pathogens 2 *pl* **pseu·do·mo·na·des** \,sü-dō-'mō-nə-,dēz, -'mä-\ : PSEUDOMONAD

pseu·do·neu·rot·ic \-nu̇-'rä-tik, -nyu̇-\ *adj* : having or characterized by neurotic symptoms which mask an underlying psychosis ⟨~ schizophrenia⟩

pseu·do·pa·ral·y·sis \-pə-'ra-lə-səs\ *n, pl* **-y·ses** \-,sēz\ : apparent lack or loss of muscular power (as that produced by pain) that is not accompanied by true paralysis

pseu·do·par·kin·son·ism \-'pär-kən-sə-,ni-zəm\ *n* : a condition (as one induced by a drug) characterized by symptoms like those of parkinsonism

pseu·do·phyl·lid·ean \,sü-dō-fi-'li-dē-ən\ *n* : any of an order (Pseudophyllidea) of tapeworms (as the fish tapeworm of humans) including numerous parasites of fish-eating vertebrates — **pseudophyllidean** *adj*

pseu·do·pod \'sü-də-,päd\ *n* 1 : PSEUDOPODIUM 2 a : a slender extension from the edge of a wheal at the site of injection of an allergen b : one of the slender processes of some tumor cells extending out from the main mass of a tumor

pseu·do·po·di·um \,sü-də-'pō-dē-əm\ *n, pl* **-dia** \-dē-ə\ : a temporary protrusion or retractile process of the cytoplasm of a cell (as a unicellular organism or a white blood cell of a higher organism) that functions esp. as an organ of locomotion or in taking up food

pseu·do·pol·yp \'sü-dō-,pä-ləp\ *n* : a projecting mass of hypertrophied mucous membrane (as in the stomach or colon) resulting from local inflammation

pseu·do·preg·nan·cy \,sü-dō-'preg-nən-sē\ *n, pl* **-cies** : a condition which resembles pregnancy: as a : PSEUDOCYESIS b : an anestrous state resembling pregnancy that occurs in various mammals usu. after an infertile copulation — **pseu·do·preg·nant** \-nənt\ *adj*

pseu·do·ra·bies \-'rā-bēz\ *n* : an acute febrile virus disease of domestic animals (as cattle and swine) marked by cutaneous irritation and intense itching followed by encephalomyelitis and pharyngeal paralysis and commonly terminating in death within 48 hours — called also *mad itch*

pseu·do·sar·co·ma·tous \,sü-dō-sär-'kō-mə-təs\ *adj* : resembling but not being a true sarcoma (a ~ polyp)

pseu·do·strat·i·fied \-'stra-tə-ˌfīd\ *adj* : of, relating to, or being an epithelium consisting of closely packed cells which appear to be arranged in layers but all of which are in fact attached to the basement membrane — **pseu·do·strat·i·fi·ca·tion** \-ˌstra-tə-fə-'kā-shən\ *n*

pseu·do·tu·ber·cle \-'tü-bər-kəl, -'tyü-\ *n* : a nodule or granuloma resembling a tubercle of tuberculosis but due to other causes

pseu·do·tu·ber·cu·lo·sis \-tü-ˌbər-kyə-'lō-səs, -tyü-\ *n, pl* **-lo·ses** \-ˌsēz\ 1 : any of several diseases that are characterized by the formation of granulomas resembling tubercular nodules but are not caused by the tubercle bacillus 2 : CASEOUS LYMPHADENITIS

pseu·do·tu·mor \-'tü-mər, -'tyü-\ *n* : an abnormality (as a temporary swelling) that resembles a tumor — **pseu·do·tu·mor·al** \-mə-rəl\ *adj*

pseudotumor cer·e·bri \-'ser-ə-ˌbrī\ *n* : an abnormal condition with symptoms (as increased intracranial pressure, headache, and papilledema) which suggest the occurrence of a brain tumor but have a different cause

pseu·do·uri·dine \-'yūr-ə-ˌdēn\ *n* : a nucleoside C₉H₁₂O₆N₂ that is a uracil derivative incorporated as a structural component into transfer RNA

pseu·do·xan·tho·ma elas·ti·cum \ˌsü-dō-zan-'thō-mə-ˌi-'las-ti-kəm\ *n* : a chronic degenerative disease of elastic tissues that is marked by the occurrence of small yellowish papules and plaques on areas of abnormally loose skin

¹psi \'sī\ *adj* : relating to, concerned with, or being parapsychological psychic events or powers (~ phenomena)

²psi *n* : psi events or phenomena

psi·lo·cin \'sī-lə-sən\ *n* : a hallucinogenic tertiary amine C₁₂H₁₆N₂O obtained from a basidiomycetous fungus (*Psilocybe mexicana*)

psi·lo·cy·bin \ˌsī-lə-'sī-bən\ *n* : a hallucinogenic indole C₁₂H₁₇N₂O₄P obtained from a basidiomycetous fungus (*Psilocybe mexicana*)

psit·ta·co·sis \ˌsi-tə-'kō-səs\ *n, pl* **-co·ses** \-ˌsēz\ : an infectious disease of birds caused by a bacterium of the genus *Chlamydia* (*C. psittaci*), marked by diarrhea and wasting, and transmissible to humans in whom it usu. occurs as an atypical pneumonia accompanied by high fever — called also *parrot fever*; compare ORNITHOSIS — **psit·ta·co·tic** \-'kä-tik, -'kō-\ *adj*

pso·as \'sō-əs\ *n, pl* **pso·ai** \'sō-ˌī\ *or* **pso·ae** \-ˌē\ : either of two internal muscles of the loin: **a** : PSOAS MAJOR **b** : PSOAS MINOR

psoas major *n* : the larger of the two psoas muscles that arises from the anterolateral surfaces of the lumbar vertebrae, passes beneath the inguinal ligament to insert with the iliacus into the lesser trochanter of the femur, and serves esp. to flex the thigh

psoas minor *n* : the smaller of the two psoas muscles that arises from the last dorsal and first lumbar vertebrae and inserts into the brim of the pelvis, which functions to flex the trunk and the lumbar spinal column, and which is often absent

psoas muscle *n* : PSOAS

pso·ra·len \'sȯr-ə-lən\ *n* : a substance C₁₁H₆O₃ found in some plants that photosensitizes mammalian skin and has been used in treating psoriasis; *also* : any of various derivatives of psoralen having similar properties

pso·ri·a·si·form \sə-'rī-ə-si-ˌfȯrm\ *adj* : resembling psoriasis or a psoriatic lesion

pso·ri·a·sis \sə-'rī-ə-səs\ *n, pl* **-a·ses** \-ˌsēz\ : a chronic skin disease characterized by circumscribed red patches covered with white scales — **pso·ri·at·ic** \ˌsȯr-ē-'a-tik\ *adj*

psoriatic arthritis *n* : a severe form of arthritis accompanied by psoriasis — called also *psoriatic arthropathy*

Pso·rop·tes \sə-'räp-(ˌ)tēz\ *n* : a genus of mites (family Psoroptidae) living on and irritating the skin of various mammals and resulting in the development of inflammatory skin diseases (as mange)

pso·rop·tic \sə-'räp-tik\ *adj* : of, relating to, caused by, or being mites of the genus *Psoroptes* (~ mange)

PSRO *abbr* professional standards review organization

psych *abbr* psychology

psych- *or* **psycho-** *comb form* 1 : mind : mental processes and activities (*psycho*dynamic) (*psycho*logy) 2 : psychological methods (*psycho*analysis) (*psycho*therapy) 3 : brain (*psycho*surgery) 4 : mental and (*psycho*somatic)

psych·as·the·nia \ˌsī-kəs-'thē-nē-ə\ *n* : a neurotic state characterized esp. by phobias, obsessions, or compulsions that one knows are irrational

psy·che \'sī-(ˌ)kē\ *n* : the specialized cognitive, conative, and affective aspects of a psychosomatic unity : MIND; *specif* : the totality of the id, ego, and superego including both conscious and unconscious components

¹psy·che·del·ic \ˌsī-kə-'de-lik\ *n* : a psychedelic drug (as LSD)

²psychedelic *adj* 1 : of, relating to, or being drugs (as LSD) capable of producing abnormal psychic effects (as hallucinations) and sometimes psychic states resembling mental illness 2 : produced by or associated with the use of psychedelic drugs ⟨a ∼ experience⟩ — **psy·che·del·i·cal·ly** adv

psy·chi·at·ric \ˌsī-kē-'a-trik\ adj 1 : relating to or employed in psychiatry ⟨∼ disorders⟩ 2 : engaged in the practice of psychiatry : dealing with cases of mental disorder ⟨∼ nursing⟩ — **psy·chi·at·ri·cal·ly** adv

psy·chi·a·trist \sə-'kī-ə-trist, sī-\ n : a physician specializing in psychiatry

psy·chi·a·try \-trē\ n, pl **-tries** : a branch of medicine that deals with the science and practice of treating mental, emotional, or behavioral disorders esp. as originating in endogenous causes or resulting from faulty interpersonal relationships

¹**psy·chic** \'sī-kik\ also **psy·chi·cal** \-ki-kəl\ adj 1 : of or relating to the psyche : PSYCHOGENIC 2 : sensitive to nonphysical or supernatural forces and influences — **psy·chi·cal·ly** adv

²**psychic** n : a person apparently sensitive to nonphysical forces

psychic energizer n : ANTIDEPRESSANT

psy·cho \'sī-(ˌ)kō\ n, pl **psychos** : a deranged or psychopathic individual — not used technically — **psycho** adj

psycho- — see PSYCH-

psy·cho·acous·tics \ˌsī-kō-ə-'kü-stiks\ n : a branch of science dealing with hearing, the sensations produced by sounds, and the problems of communication — **psy·cho·acous·tic** \-stik\ adj

psy·cho·ac·tive \ˌsī-kō-'ak-tiv\ adj : affecting the mind or behavior ⟨∼ drugs⟩

psy·cho·anal·y·sis \ˌsī-kō-ə-'na-lə-səs\ n, pl **-y·ses** \-ˌsēz\ 1 : a method of analyzing psychic phenomena and treating emotional disorders that is based on the concepts and theories of Sigmund Freud, that emphasizes the importance of free association, dream analysis, and that involves treatment sessions during which the patient is encouraged to talk freely about personal experiences and esp. about early childhood and dreams 2 : a body of empirical findings and a set of theories on human motivation, behavior, and personality development that developed esp. with the aid of psychoanalysis 3 : a school of psychology, psychiatry, and psychotherapy founded by Sigmund Freud and rooted in applying psychoanalysis — **psy·cho·an·a·lyt·ic** \-ˌan-əl-'i-tik\ also **psy·cho·an·a·lyt·i·cal** \-ti-kəl\ adj — **psy·cho·an·a·lyt·i·cal·ly** adv — **psy·cho·an·a·lyze** \-'an-əl-ˌīz\ vb

psy·cho·an·a·lyst \-'an-əl-ist\ n : one who practices or adheres to the principles of psychoanalysis; specif : a psychotherapist trained at an established psychoanalytic institute

psy·cho·bi·ol·o·gy \-bī-'ä-lə-jē\ n, pl **-gies** : the study of mental functioning and behavior in relation to other biological processes — **psy·cho·bi·o·log·i·cal** \-ˌbī-ə-'lä-ji-kəl\ also **psy·cho·bi**-o·log·ic \-jik\ adj — **psy·cho·bi·ol·o·gist** \-bī-'ä-lə-jist\ n

psy·cho·di·ag·nos·tics \-ˌdī-ig-'näs-tiks\ n : a branch of psychology concerned with the use of tests in the evaluation of personality and the determination of factors underlying human behavior — **psy·cho·di·ag·nos·tic** \-tik\ adj

psy·cho·dra·ma \ˌsī-kō-'drä-mə, -'dra-\ n : an extemporized dramatization designed to afford catharsis and social relearning for one or more of the participants from whose life history the plot is abstracted — **psy·cho·dra·mat·ic** \-ˌkō-drə-'ma-tik\ adj

psy·cho·dy·nam·ics \ˌsī-kō-dī-'na-miks, -də-\ n sing or pl 1 : the psychology of mental or emotional forces or processes developing esp. in early childhood and their effects on behavior and mental states 2 : explanation or interpretation (as of behavior or mental states) in terms of mental or emotional forces or processes 3 : motivational forces acting esp. at the unconscious level — **psy·cho·dy·nam·ic** \-mik\ adj — **psy·cho·dy·nam·i·cal·ly** adv

psy·cho·ed·u·ca·tion·al \-ˌe-jə-'kā-shə-nəl\ adj : of or relating to the psychological aspects of education; specif : relating to or used in the education of children with behavioral disorders or learning disabilities

psy·cho·gal·van·ic reflex \-gal-'va-nik-\ n : a momentary decrease in the apparent electrical resistance of the skin resulting from activity of the sweat glands in response to mental or emotional stimulation — called also psychogalvanic reaction, psychogalvanic response

psy·cho·gen·e·sis \ˌsī-kō-'je-nə-səs\ n, pl **-eses** \-ˌsēz\ 1 : the origin and development of mental functions, traits, or states 2 : development from mental as distinguished from physical origins

psy·cho·gen·ic \-'je-nik\ adj : originating in the mind or in mental or emotional conflict ⟨∼ impotence⟩ ⟨a ∼ disorder⟩ — **psy·cho·gen·i·cal·ly** adv

psy·cho·ge·ri·at·rics \-ˌjer-ē-'a-triks, -ˌjir-\ n : a branch of psychiatry concerned with behavioral and emotional disorders among the elderly — **psy·cho·ge·ri·at·ric** \-trik\ adj

psy·cho·ki·ne·sis \-kə-'nē-səs, -kī-\ n, pl **-neses** \-ˌsēz\ : movement of physical objects by the mind without use of physical means — called also PK; compare PRECOGNITION, TELEKINESIS — **psy·cho·ki·net·ic** \-'ne-tik\ adj

psy·cho·ki·net·ics \-kə-'ne-tiks, -kī-\ n : a branch of parapsychology that deals with psychokinesis

psychol abbr psychologist; psychology

psy·cho·lin·guis·tics \ˌsī-kō-liŋ-'gwis-tiks\ n : the study of the mental faculties involved in the perception, production, and acquisition of language — **psy·cho·lin·guist** \-'liŋ-gwist\

n — **psy·cho·lin·guis·tic** \-liŋ-ˈgwis-tik\ *adj*

psy·cho·log·i·cal \ˌsī-kə-ˈlä-ji-kəl\ *also* **psy·cho·log·ic** \-jik\ *adj* **1 a** : relating to, characteristic of, directed toward, influencing, arising in, or acting through the mind esp. in its affective or cognitive functions ⟨∼ phenomena⟩ **b** : directed toward the will or toward the mind specif. in its conative function ⟨∼ warfare⟩ **2** : relating to, concerned with, deriving from, or used in psychology — **psy·cho·log·i·cal·ly** *adv*

psy·chol·o·gist \sī-ˈkä-lə-jist\ *n* : a specialist in one or more branches of psychology; *esp* : a practitioner of clinical psychology, counseling, or guidance

psy·chol·o·gize \-ˌjīz\ *vb* **-gized; -gizing** : to explain, interpret, or speculate in psychological terms

psy·chol·o·gy \-jē\ *n, pl* **-gies 1** : the science of mind and behavior **2 a** : the mental or behavioral characteristics of an individual or group ⟨mob ∼⟩ **b** : the study of mind and behavior in relation to a particular field of knowledge or activity ⟨the ∼ of learning⟩ **3** : a treatise on or a school, system, or branch of psychology

psy·cho·met·ric \ˌsī-kə-ˈme-trik\ *adj* : of or relating to psychometrics — **psy·cho·met·ri·cal·ly** *adv*

psy·cho·me·tri·cian \-mə-ˈtri-shən\ *n* **1** : a person (as a clinical psychologist) who is skilled in the administration and interpretation of objective psychological tests **2** : a psychologist who devises, constructs, and standardizes psychometric tests

psy·cho·met·rics \-ˈme-triks\ *n* **1** : a branch of clinical or applied psychology dealing with the use and application of mental measurement **2** : the technique of mental measurements : the use of quantitative devices for assessing psychological trends

psy·chom·e·trist \sī-ˈkä-mə-trist\ *n* : PSYCHOMETRICIAN

psy·chom·e·try \sī-ˈkä-mə-trē\ *n, pl* **-tries** : PSYCHOMETRICS

psy·cho·mo·tor \ˌsī-kō-ˈmō-tər\ *adj* **1** : of or relating to motor action directly proceeding from mental activity **2** : of or relating to psychomotor epilepsy ⟨∼ seizures⟩

psychomotor epilepsy *n* : epilepsy characterized by partial rather than generalized seizures that typically originate in the temporal lobe and are marked by impairment of consciousness, automatisms, bizarre changes in behavior, hallucinations (as of odors), and perceptual illusions (as visceral sensations)

psy·cho·neu·ro·im·mu·nol·o·gy \-ˌnùr-ō-ˌi-myū-ˈnä-lə-jē, -nyùr-\ *n* : a field of medicine that deals with the influence of emotional states (as stress) and nervous system activity on immune function esp. in relation to their role in affecting the onset and progression of disease

psy·cho·neu·ro·sis \ˌsī-kō-nù-ˈrō-səs, -nyù-\ *n, pl* **-ro·ses** \-ˌsēz\ : NEUROSIS; *esp* : a neurosis based on emotional conflict in which an impulse that has been blocked seeks expression in a disguised response or symptom

¹psy·cho·neu·rot·ic \-ˈrä-tik\ *adj* : of, relating to, being, or affected with a psychoneurosis ⟨a ∼ disorder⟩ ⟨a ∼ patient⟩

²psychoneurotic *n* : a psychoneurotic individual

psy·cho·path \ˈsī-kō-ˌpath\ *n* : a mentally ill or unstable individual; *esp* : one having a psychopathic personality

psy·cho·path·ic \ˌsī-kō-ˈpa-thik\ *adj* : of, relating to, or characterized by psychopathy or psychopathic personality — **psy·cho·path·i·cal·ly** *adv*

psychopathic personality *n* **1** : an emotionally and behaviorally disordered state characterized by clear perception of reality except for the individual's social and moral obligations and often by the pursuit of immediate personal gratification in criminal acts, drug addiction, or sexual perversion **2** : an individual having a psychopathic personality

psy·cho·pa·thol·o·gist \-pə-ˈthä-lə-jist, -pa-\ *n* : a specialist in psychopathology

psy·cho·pa·thol·o·gy \ˌsī-kō-pə-ˈthä-lə-jē, -pa-\ *n, pl* **-gies 1** : the study of psychological and behavioral dysfunction occurring in mental disorder or in social disorganization **2** : disordered psychological and behavioral functioning (as in mental illness) — **psy·cho·patho·log·i·cal** \-ˌpa-thə-ˈlä-ji-kəl\ *or* **psy·cho·patho·log·ic** \-jik\ *adj* — **psy·cho·patho·log·i·cal·ly** *adv*

psy·chop·a·thy \sī-ˈkä-pə-thē\ *n, pl* **-thies 1** : mental disorder **2** : PSYCHOPATHIC PERSONALITY 1

psy·cho·phar·ma·ceu·ti·cal \ˌsī-kō-ˌfärmə-ˈsü-ti-kəl\ *n* : a drug having an effect on the mental state of the user

psy·cho·phar·ma·col·o·gy \ˌsī-kō-ˌfärmə-ˈkä-lə-jē\ *n, pl* **-gies** : the study of the effect of drugs on the mind and behavior — **psy·cho·phar·ma·co·log·ic** \-ˌfär-mə-kə-ˈlä-jik\ *or* **psy·cho·phar·ma·co·log·i·cal** \-ji-kəl\ *adj* — **psy·cho·phar·ma·col·o·gist** \-ˌfär-mə-ˈkä-lə-jist\ *n*

psy·cho·phys·ics \-ˈfi-ziks\ *n* : a branch of psychology concerned with the effect of physical processes (as intensity of stimulation) on mental processes and esp. sensations of an organism — **psy·cho·phys·i·cal** \ˌsī-kō-ˈfi-zi-kəl\ *adj* — **psy·cho·phys·i·cal·ly** *adv* — **psy·cho·phys·i·cist** \-ˈfi-zə-sist\ *n*

psy·cho·phys·i·o·log·i·cal \ˌsī-kō-ˌfi-zē-ə-ˈlä-ji-kəl\ *also* **psy·cho·phys·i·o·log-**

ic \-jik\ *adj* **1** : of or relating to psychophysiology **2** : combining or involving mental and bodily processes

psy·cho·phys·i·ol·o·gy \-ˌfi-zē-'ä-lə-jē\ *n, pl* **-gies** : a branch of psychology that deals with the effects of normal and pathological physiological processes on mental life — called also *physiological psychology* — **psy·cho·phys·i·ol·o·gist** \-jist\ *n*

psy·cho·sex·u·al \ˌsī-kō-'sek-shə-wəl\ *adj* **1** : of or relating to the mental, emotional, and behavioral aspects of sexual development **2** : of or relating to mental or emotional attitudes concerning sexual activity **3** : of or relating to the psychophysiology of sex

psy·cho·sis \sī-'kō-səs\ *n, pl* **-cho·ses** \-ˌsēz\ : a serious mental disorder (as schizophrenia) characterized by defective or lost contact with reality often with hallucinations or delusions

psy·cho·so·cial \ˌsī-kō-'sō-shəl\ *adj* **1** : involving both psychological and social aspects **2** : relating social conditions to mental health (∼ medicine) — **psy·cho·so·cial·ly** *adv*

psy·cho·so·mat·ic \ˌsī-kō-sə-'ma-tik\ *adj* **1** : of, relating to, concerned with, or involving both mind and body **2 a** : of, relating to, involving, or concerned with bodily symptoms caused by mental or emotional disturbance **b** : exhibiting psychosomatic symptoms — **psy·cho·so·mat·i·cal·ly** *adv*

psy·cho·so·mat·ics \-tiks\ *n* : a branch of medical science dealing with interrelationships between the mind or emotions and the body and esp. with the relation of psychic conflict to somatic symptomatology

psy·cho·sur·geon \-'sər-jən\ *n* : a surgeon specializing in psychosurgery

psy·cho·sur·gery \-'sər-jə-rē\ *n, pl* **-ger·ies** : cerebral surgery employed in treating psychotic symptoms — **psy·cho·sur·gi·cal** \-'sər-ji-kəl\ *adj*

psy·cho·syn·the·sis \ˌsī-kō-'sin-thə-səs\ *n, pl* **-the·ses** \-ˌsēz\ : a form of psychotherapy combining psychoanalytic techniques with meditation and exercise

psy·cho·ther·a·peu·tics \-tiks\ *n sing or pl* : PSYCHOTHERAPY

psy·cho·ther·a·pist \-'ther-ə-pist\ *n* : one (as a psychiatrist, clinical psychologist, or psychiatric social worker) who is a practitioner of psychotherapy

psy·cho·ther·a·py \ˌsī-kō-'ther-ə-pē\ *n, pl* **-pies 1** : treatment of mental or emotional disorder or maladjustment by psychological means esp. involving verbal communication (as in psychoanalysis, nondirective psychotherapy, reeducation, or hypnosis) **2** : any alteration in an individual's interpersonal environment, relationships, or life situation brought about esp. by a qualified therapist and intended to have the effect of alleviating symptoms of mental or emotional disturbance — **psy·cho·ther·a·peu·tic** \-ˌther-ə-'pyü-tik\ *adj* — **psy·cho·ther·a·peu·ti·cal·ly** *adv*

¹psy·chot·ic \sī-'kä-tik\ *adj* : of, relating to, marked by, or affected with psychosis — **psy·chot·i·cal·ly** *adv*

²psychotic *n* : a psychotic individual

¹psy·cho·to·mi·met·ic \ˌsī-ˌkä-tō-mə-'me-tik, -mi-\ *adj* : of, relating to, involving, or inducing psychotic alteration of behavior and personality (∼ drugs) — **psy·cho·to·mi·met·i·cal·ly** *adv*

²psychotomimetic *n* : a psychotomimetic agent (as a drug)

¹psy·cho·tro·pic \ˌsī-kə-'trō-pik\ *adj* : acting on the mind (∼ drugs)

²psychotropic *n* : a psychotropic substance (as a drug)

psyl·li·um \'si-lē-əm\ *n* **1** : FLEAWORT **2** : PSYLLIUM SEED

psyllium seed *n* : the seed of a fleawort (esp. *Plantago psyllium*) that has the property of swelling and becoming gelatinous when moist and is used as a mild laxative — called also *plantago seed, psyllium*; see METAMUCIL

pt *abbr* **1** patient **2** pint

Pt *symbol* platinum

PT *abbr* **1** physical therapist **2** physical therapy

PTA *abbr* plasma thromboplastin antecedent

¹PTC \ˌpē-(ˌ)tē-'sē\ *n* : PHENYLTHIOCARBAMIDE

²PTC *abbr* plasma thromboplastin component

PTCA \ˌpē-(ˌ)tē-(ˌ)sē-'ā\ *n* : PERCUTANEOUS TRANSLUMINAL CORONARY ANGIOPLASTY

pter·o·yl·glu·tam·ic acid \ˌter-ō-il-glü-'ta-mik-\ *n* : FOLIC ACID — abbr. *PGA*

pteryg- or **pterygo-** *comb form* : pterygoid and ⟨*pterygo*maxillary⟩

pte·ryg·i·um \te-'ri-jē-əm\ *n, pl* **-iums** or **-ia** \-jē-ə\ **1** : a triangular fleshy mass of thickened conjunctiva occurring usu. at the inner side of the eyeball, covering part of the cornea, and causing a disturbance of vision **2** : a forward growth of the cuticle over the nail

¹pter·y·goid \'ter-ə-ˌgòid\ *adj* : of, relating to, being, or lying in the region of the inferior part of the sphenoid bone

²pterygoid *n* : a pterygoid part (as a pterygoid muscle or nerve)

pterygoid canal *n* : an anteroposterior canal in the base of each medial pterygoid plate of the sphenoid bone that gives passage to the Vidian artery and the Vidian nerve — called also *Vidian canal*

pter·y·goi·de·us \ˌter-ə-'gòi-dē-əs\ *n, pl* **-dei** \-dē-ˌi\ : PTERYGOID MUSCLE

pterygoid fossa *n* : a V-shaped depression on the posterior part of each pterygoid process that contains the medial pterygoid muscle and the tensor veli palatini

pterygoid hamulus *n* : a hook-shaped

process forming the inferior extremity of each medial pterygoid plate of the sphenoid bone and providing a support around which the tendon of the tensor veli palatini moves

pter·y·goid muscle n : either of two muscles extending from the sphenoid bone to the lower jaw: **a** : a muscle that arises from the greater wing of the sphenoid bone and from the outer surface of the lateral pterygoid plate, is inserted into the condyle of the mandible and the articular disk of the temporomandibular joint, and acts as an antagonist of the masseter, temporalis, and medial pterygoid muscles — called also *external pterygoid muscle, lateral pterygoid muscle* **b** : a muscle that arises from the inner surface of the lateral pterygoid plate and from the palatine and maxillary bones, is inserted into the ramus and the gonial angle, cooperates with the masseter and temporalis in elevating the lower jaw, and controls certain lateral and rotary movements of the jaw — called also *internal pterygoid muscle, medial pterygoid muscle*

pterygoid nerve n : either of two branches of the mandibular nerve: **a** : one that is distributed to the lateral pterygoid muscle — called also *lateral pterygoid nerve* **b** : one that is distributed to the medial pterygoid muscle, tensor tympani, and tensor veli palatini — called also *medial pterygoid nerve*

pterygoid plate n : either of two vertical plates making up a pterygoid process of the sphenoid bone: **a** : a broad thin plate that forms the lateral part of the pterygoid process and gives attachment to the lateral pterygoid muscle on its lateral surface and to the medial pterygoid muscle on its medial surface — called also *lateral pterygoid plate* **b** : a long narrow plate that forms the medial part of the pterygoid process and terminates in the pterygoid hamulus — called also *medial pterygoid plate*

pterygoid plexus n : a plexus of veins draining the region of the pterygoid muscles and emptying chiefly into the facial vein by way of the deep facial vein and into the maxillary vein

pterygoid process n : a process that extends downward from each side of the sphenoid bone, that consists of the medial and lateral pterygoid plates which are fused above anteriorly and separated below by a fissure whose edges articulate with a process of the palatine bone, and that contains on its posterior aspect the pterygoid and scaphoid fossae which give attachment to muscles

pter·y·go·man·dib·u·lar raphe \ˌter-ə-gō-man-ˈdi-byə-lər-\ n : a fibrous seam that descends from the pterygoid hamulus of the medial pterygoid

plate to the mylohyoid line of the mandible and that separates and gives rise to the superior constrictor of the pharynx and the buccinator

pter·y·go·max·il·lary \ˌter-ə-gō-ˈmak-sə-ˌler-ē\ adj : of, relating to, or connecting the pterygoid process of the sphenoid bone and the maxilla

pterygomaxillary fissure n : a vertical gap between the lateral pterygoid plate of the pterygoid process and the maxilla that gives passage to part of the maxillary artery and vein

pter·y·go·pal·a·tine fossa \ˌter-ə-gō-ˈpa-lə-ˌtin-\ n : a small triangular space beneath the apex of the orbit that contains among other structures the pterygopalatine ganglion — called also *pterygomaxillary fossa*

pterygopalatine ganglion n : an autonomic ganglion of the maxillary nerve that is situated in the pterygopalatine fossa and that receives preganglionic parasympathetic fibers from the facial nerve and sends postganglionic fibers to the nasal mucosa, palate, pharynx, and orbit — called also *Meckel's ganglion, sphenopalatine ganglion*

PTFE abbr polytetrafluoroethylene

PTH abbr parathyroid hormone

pto·maine \ˈtō-ˌmān, tō-ˈ\ n : any of various organic bases formed by the action of putrefactive bacteria on nitrogenous matter and including some which are poisonous

ptomaine poisoning n : food poisoning caused by bacteria or bacterial products — not used technically

pto·sis \ˈtō-səs\ n, pl **pto·ses** \-ˌsēz\ : a sagging or prolapse of an organ or part ⟨renal ∼⟩; esp : a drooping of the upper eyelid (as from paralysis of the oculomotor nerve) — **ptot·ic** \ˈtä-tik\ adj

PTSD abbr post-traumatic stress disorder

ptyal- or **ptyalo-** comb form : saliva ⟨ptyalism⟩

pty·a·lin \ˈtī-ə-lən\ n : an amylase found in saliva that converts starch into sugar

pty·a·lism \-ˌli-zəm\ n : an excessive flow of saliva

-p·ty·sis \p-tə-səs\ n comb form, pl **-pty·ses** \p-tə-ˌsēz\ : spewing : expectoration ⟨hemoptysis⟩

Pu symbol plutonium

pub·ar·che \ˈpyü-ˌbär-kē\ n : the beginning of puberty marked by the first growth of pubic hair

pu·ber·al \ˈpyü-bər-əl\ adj : PUBERTAL

pu·ber·tal \ˈpyü-bərt-ᵊl\ adj : of, relating to, or occurring in puberty

pu·ber·ty \ˈpyü-bər-tē\ n, pl **-ties 1** : the condition of being or the period of becoming first capable of reproducing sexually marked by maturing of the genital organs, development of secondary sex characteristics, and in humans and the higher primates by the first occurrence of menstruation in the female **2** : the age at which puberty occurs being typically between 13 and 16 years in boys and 11 and 14 in girls

¹**pu·bes** \'pyü-(ˌ)bēz\ *n, pl* **pubes 1** : the hair that appears on the lower part of the hypogastric region at puberty — called also *pubic hair* **2** : the lower part of the hypogastric region : the pubic region

²**pubes** *pl of* PUBIS

pu·bes·cent \pyü-'bes-ᵊnt\ *adj* **1** : arriving at or having reached puberty **2** : of or relating to puberty

pu·bic \'pyü-bik\ *adj* : of, relating to, or situated in or near the region of the pubes or the pubis

pubic arch *n* : the notch formed by the inferior rami of the two conjoined pubic bones as they diverge from the midline

pubic bone *n* : PUBIS

pubic crest *n* : the border of a pubis between its pubic tubercle and the pubic symphysis

pubic hair *n* : PUBES 1

pubic louse *n* : CRAB LOUSE

pubic symphysis *n* : the rather rigid articulation of the two pubic bones in the midline of the lower anterior part of the abdomen — called also *symphysis pubis*

pubic tubercle *n* : a rounded eminence on the upper margin of each pubis near the pubic symphysis

pu·bis \'pyü-bəs\ *n, pl* **pu·bes** \-(ˌ)bēz\ : the ventral and anterior of the three principal bones composing either half of the pelvis that in humans consists of two rami diverging posteriorly from the region of the pubic symphysis with the superior ramus extending to the acetabulum of which it forms a part and uniting there with the ilium and ischium and the inferior ramus extending below the obturator foramen where it unites with the ischium — called also *pubic bone*

public health *n* : the art and science dealing with the protection and improvement of community health by organized community effort and including preventive medicine and sanitary and social science

public health nurse *n* : VISITING NURSE

pu·bo·cap·su·lar ligament \ˌpyü-bō-'kap-sə-lər-\ *n* : PUBOFEMORAL LIGAMENT

pu·bo·coc·cy·geus \-käk-'si-jəs, -jē-əs\ *n, pl* **-cy·gei** \-'si-jē-ˌī\ : the inferior subdivision of the levator ani that arises from the dorsal surface of the pubis, that inserts esp. into the coccyx, and that acts to help support the pelvic viscera, to draw the lower end of the rectum toward the pubis, and to constrict the rectum and in the female the vagina — compare ILIOCOCCYGEUS — **pu·bo·coc·cy·geal** \ˌpyü-bō-käk-'si-jəl, -jē-əl\ *adj*

pu·bo·fem·o·ral ligament \ˌpyü-bō-'fe-mə-rəl-\ *n* : a ligament of the hip joint that extends from the superior ramus of the pubis to the capsule of the hip joint near the neck of the femur and that acts to prevent excessive extension and abduction of the thigh

pu·bo·pros·tat·ic ligament \ˌpyü-bō-präs-'ta-tik-\ *n* : any of three strands of pelvic fascia in the male that correspond to the pubovesical ligament in the female and that support the prostate gland and indirectly the bladder

pu·bo·rec·ta·lis \ˌpyü-bō-rek-'tā-ləs\ *n* : a band of muscle fibers that is part of the pubococcygeus and acts to hold the rectum and anal canal at right angles to each other except during defecation

pu·bo·vag·i·na·lis \ˌpyü-bō-ˌva-jə-'nā-ləs\ *n* : the most medial and anterior fasciculi of the pubococcygeal part of the levator ani in the female that correspond to the levator prostatae in the male, pass along the sides of the vagina, insert into the coccyx, and act to constrict the vagina

pu·bo·ves·i·cal ligament \ˌpyü-bō-'ve-si-kəl-\ *n* : any of three strands of pelvic fascia in the female that correspond to the puboprostatic ligament in the male and that support the bladder

¹**pu·den·dal** \pyü-'dend-ᵊl\ *adj* : of, relating to, occurring in, or lying in the region of the external genital organs

²**pudendal** *n* : a pudendal anatomical part (as the pudendal nerve)

pudendal artery — see EXTERNAL PUDENDAL ARTERY, INTERNAL PUDENDAL ARTERY

pudendal nerve *n* : a nerve that arises from the second, third, and fourth sacral nerves and that supplies the external genitalia, the skin of the perineum, and the anal sphincters

pudendal vein — see INTERNAL PUDENDAL VEIN

pu·den·dum \pyü-'den-dəm\ *n, pl* **-da** \-də\ : the external genital organs esp. of a woman — usu. used in pl.

pu·er·ile \'pyü-ər-əl, -ˌīl\ *adj* **1** : marked by or suggesting childishness and immaturity **2** : being respiration that is like that of a child in being louder than normal ⟨∼ breathing⟩

pu·er·per·al \pyü-'ər-pə-rəl\ *adj* : of, relating to, or occurring during childbirth or the period immediately following ⟨∼ infection⟩ ⟨∼ depression⟩

puerperal fever *n* : an abnormal condition that results from infection of the placental site following delivery or abortion and is characterized in mild form by fever of not over 100.4°F but may progress to a localized endometritis or spread through the uterine wall and develop into peritonitis or pass into the blood stream and produce septicemia — called also *child-bed fever, puerperal sepsis*

pu·er·pe·ri·um \ˌpyü-ər-ˈpir-ē-əm\ *n, pl* **-ria** \-ē-ə\ : the period between childbirth and the return of the uterus to its normal size

puff·er \ˈpə-fər\ *n* : any of a family (Tetraodontidae) of chiefly tropical marine bony fishes which can distend themselves to a globular form and most of which are highly poisonous — called also *blowfish, globefish, pufferfish*

Pu·lex \ˈpyü-ˌleks\ *n* : a genus of fleas (family Pulicidae) that includes the most common flea (*P. irritans*) that regularly attacks human beings

¹pull \ˈpul\ *vb* **1** : EXTRACT 1 2 : to strain or stretch abnormally ⟨~ a muscle⟩

²pull *n* : an injury resulting from abnormal straining or stretching ⟨a muscle ~⟩ ⟨a groin ~⟩

pul·let disease \ˈpu̇-lət-\ *n* : BLUE COMB

pul·lo·rum disease \pə-ˈlȯr-əm-\ *n* : a destructive typically diarrheic salmonellosis esp. of the domestic chicken caused by a bacterium of the genus *Salmonella* (*S. pullorum*) — called also *pullorum*

pulmon- *also* **pulmoni-** *or* **pulmono-comb form** : lung (*pulmono*logist)

pulmonalia — see CORDIA PULMONALIA

pul·mo·nary \ˈpu̇l-mə-ˌner-ē, ˈpəl-\ *adj* : relating to, functioning like, associated with, or carried on by the lungs

pulmonary alveolar proteinosis *n* : a chronic disease of the lungs characterized by the filling of the alveoli with proteinaceous material and by the progressive loss of lung function

pulmonary artery *n* : an arterial trunk or either of its two main branches that carry blood to the lungs: **a** : a large arterial trunk that arises from the conus arteriosus of the right ventricle and branches into the right and left pulmonary arteries — called also *pulmonary trunk* **b** : a branch of the pulmonary trunk that passes to the right lung where it divides into branches — called also *right pulmonary artery* **c** : a branch of the pulmonary trunk that passes to the left lung where it divides into branches — called also *left pulmonary artery*

pulmonary capillary wedge pressure *n* : WEDGE PRESSURE — abbr. *PCWP*

pulmonary circulation *n* : the passage of venous blood from the right atrium of the heart through the right ventricle and pulmonary arteries to the lungs where it is oxygenated and its return via the pulmonary veins to enter the left auricle and participate in the systemic circulation

pulmonary edema *n* : abnormal accumulation of fluid in the lungs

pulmonary embolism *n* : embolism of a pulmonary artery or one of its branches

pulmonary ligament *n* : a supporting fold of pleura that extends from the lower part of the lung to the pericardium

pulmonary plexus *n* : either of two nerve plexuses associated with each lung that lie on the dorsal and ventral aspects of the bronchi of each lung

pulmonary stenosis *n* : abnormal narrowing of the orifice between the pulmonary artery and the right ventricle

pulmonary trunk *n* : PULMONARY ARTERY a

pulmonary valve *n* : a valve consisting of three semilunar cusps separating the pulmonary trunk from the right ventricle

pulmonary vein *n* : any of usu. four veins comprising two from each lung that return oxygenated blood from the lungs to the superior part of the left atrium

pulmonary wedge pressure *n* : WEDGE PRESSURE

pulmoni- *or* **pulmono-** — see PULMON-

pul·mon·ic \pu̇l-ˈmä-nik, ˌpəl-\ *adj* : PULMONARY ⟨~ lesions⟩

pulmonic stenosis *n* : PULMONARY STENOSIS

pul·mo·nol·o·gist \ˌpu̇l-mə-ˈnä-lə-jist, ˌpəl-\ *n* : a specialist in the anatomy, physiology, and pathology of the lungs

pulp \ˈpəlp\ *n* : a mass of soft tissue: as **a** : DENTAL PULP **b** : the characteristic somewhat spongy tissue of the spleen **c** : the fleshy portion of the fingertip — **pulp·al** \ˈpəl-pəl\ *adj* — **pulp·less** *adj*

pulp canal *n* : ROOT CANAL 1

pulp cavity *n* : the central cavity of a tooth containing the dental pulp and made up of the root canal and the pulp chamber

pulp chamber *n* : the part of the pulp cavity lying in the crown of a tooth

pulp·ec·to·my \ˌpəl-ˈpek-tə-mē\ *n, pl* **-mies** : the removal of the pulp of a tooth

pulp·itis \ˌpəl-ˈpī-təs\ *n, pl* **pulp·it·i·des** \-ˈpi-tə-ˌdēz\ : inflammation of the pulp of a tooth

pulposi, pulposus — see NUCLEUS PULPOSUS

pulp·ot·o·my \ˌpəl-ˈpä-tə-mē\ *n, pl* **-mies** : removal in a dental procedure of the coronal portion of the pulp of a tooth in such a manner that the pulp of the root remains intact and viable

pulp stone *n* : a lump of calcified tissue within the dental pulp — called also *denticle*

pulpy kidney \ˈpəl-pē-\ *n* : a destructive enterotoxemia of lambs caused by a bacterium of the genus *Clostridium* (*C. perfringens*) — called also *pulpy kidney disease*

pul·sate \ˈpəl-ˌsāt\ *vb* **pul·sat·ed; pul·sat·ing** : to exhibit a pulse or pulsation ⟨a *pulsating* artery⟩

pul·sa·tion \ˌpəl-ˈsā-shən\ *n* : rhythmic throbbing or vibrating (as of an artery); *also* : a single beat or throb — **pul·sa·tile** \'pəl-sət-ºl, -sə-ºtīl\ *adj*

pulse \'pəls\ *n* **1 a** : a regularly recurrent wave of distension in arteries that results from the progress through an artery of blood injected into the arterial system at each contraction of the ventricles of the heart **b** : the palpable beat resulting from such pulse as detected in a superficial artery (as the radial artery); *also* : the number of such beats in a specified period of time (as one minute) ⟨a resting ∼ of 70⟩ **2** : PULSATION **3** : a dose of a substance esp. when applied over a short period of time ⟨therapy with intravenous methylprednisolone ∼*s*⟩ — **pulse** *vb* — **pulse·less** \'pəls-ləs\ *adj*

pulse·la·bel \'pəls-ºlā-bəl\ *or* -**la·belled**; **-la·bel·ing** *or* **-la·bel·ling** : to cause a pulse of a radiolabeled atom or substance to become incorporated into (as a molecule or cell component) ⟨∼*ed* DNA⟩

pulse pressure *n* : the pressure that is characteristic of the arterial pulse and represents the difference between diastolic and systolic pressures of the heart cycle

pulse rate *n* : the rate of the arterial pulse usu. observed at the wrist and stated in beats per minute

pul·sus al·ter·nans \'pəl-səs-'ol-tər-ºnanz\ *n* : alternation of strong and weak beats of the arterial pulse due to alternate strong and weak ventricular contractions

pulsus par·a·dox·us \-ºpar-ə-'däk-səs\ : a pulse that weakens abnormally during inspiration and is symptomatic of various abnormalities (as pericarditis)

pulv *abbr* [Latin *pulvis*] powder — used in writing prescriptions

pul·vi·nar \ºpəl-'vī-nər\ *n* : a rounded prominence on the back of the thalamus

¹pump \'pəmp\ *n* **1** : a device that raises, transfers, or compresses fluids or that attenuates gases esp. by suction or pressure or both **2** : HEART **3** : an act or the process of pumping **4** : a mechanism (as the sodium pump) for pumping atoms, ions, or molecules

²pump *vb* **1** : to raise (as water) with a pump **2** : to draw fluid from with a pump **3** : to transport (as ions) against a concentration gradient by the expenditure of energy

punch-drunk \'pənch-ºdrəŋk\ *adj* : suffering cerebral injury from many minute brain hemorrhages as a result of repeated heavy head blows received in boxing

puncta *pl of* PUNCTUM

punctata — see KERATITIS PUNCTATA

punc·tate \'pəŋk-ºtāt\ *adj* : characterized by dots or points ⟨∼ skin lesions⟩

punc·tum \'pəŋk-təm\ *n, pl* **punc·ta** \-tə\ : a small area marked off in any way

from a surrounding surface — see LACRIMAL PUNCTUM

¹punc·ture \'pəŋk-chər\ *n* **1** : an act of puncturing **2** : a hole, wound, or perforation made by puncturing

²puncture *vb* **punc·tured; punc·tur·ing** : to pierce with or as if with a pointed instrument or object

pu·pa \'pyü-pə\ *n, pl* **pu·pae** \-(º)pē, -ºpī\ *or* **pupas** : an intermediate usu. quiescent stage of an insect that occurs between the larva and the adult in forms which undergo complete metamorphosis and that is characterized by internal changes by which larval structures are replaced by those typical of the adult — **pu·pal** \'pyü-pəl\ *adj*

pu·pil \'pyü-pəl\ *n* : the contractile usu. round aperture in the iris of the eye — **pu·pil·lary** *also* **pu·pi·lary** \'pyü-pə-ºler-ē\ *adj*

pupillae — see SPHINCTER PUPILLAE

pupillary reflex *n* : the contraction of the pupil in response to light entering the eye

pupillo- *comb form* : pupil ⟨*pupillo*meter⟩

pu·pil·log·ra·phy \ºpyü-pə-'lä-grə-fē\ *n, pl* **-phies** : the measurement of the reactions of the pupil

pu·pil·lom·e·ter \ºpyü-pə-'lä-mə-tər\ *n* : an instrument for measuring the diameter of the pupil of the eye — **pu·pil·lom·e·try** \-mə-trē\ *n*

pur·ga·tion \ºpər-'gā-shən\ *n* **1** : the act of purging; *specif* : vigorous evacuation of the bowels (as from the action of a cathartic) **2** : administration of or treatment with a purgative

¹pur·ga·tive \'pər-gə-tiv\ *adj* : purging or tending to purge : CATHARTIC — **pur·ga·tive·ly** *adv*

²purgative *n* : a purging medicine : CATHARTIC

¹purge \'pərj\ *vb* **purged; purg·ing** : to have or cause strong and usu. repeated emptying of the bowels

²purge *n* **1** : something that purges; *esp* : PURGATIVE **2** : an act or instance of purging

purified protein derivative *n* : a purified preparation of tuberculin used in a test for tuberculous infection — abbr. **PPD**

pu·rine \'pyür-ºēn\ *n* **1** : a crystalline base $C_5H_4N_4$ that is the parent of compounds of the uric-acid group **2** : a derivative of purine; *esp* : a base (as adenine or guanine) that is a constituent of DNA or RNA

purine base *n* : any of a group of crystalline bases comprising purine and bases derived from it (as adenine) some of which are components of nucleosides and nucleotides

Pur·kin·je cell \pər-'kin-jē\ *n* : any of numerous nerve cells that occupy the middle layer of the cerebellar cortex and are characterized by a large globe-shaped body with massive dendrites directed outward and a single slender axon directed inward

Pur·ky·ně (*or* **Purkinje**) \'pur-kin-ye, -yä\, **Jan Evangelista** (1787–1869), Bohemian physiologist.

Purkinje fiber *n* : any of the modified cardiac muscle fibers with few nuclei, granulated central cytoplasm, and sparse peripheral striations that make up Purkinje's network

Purkinje's network *n* : a network of intracardiac conducting tissue made up of syncytial Purkinje fibers that lie in the myocardium and constitute the bundle of His and other conducting tracts which spread out from the sinoatrial node — called also *Purkinje's system, Purkinje's tissue*

pu·ro·my·cin \ˌpyùr-ə-'mīs-ᵊn\ *n* : an antibiotic $C_{22}H_{29}N_7O_5$ that is obtained from an actinomycete (*Streptomyces alboniger*) and is used esp. as a potent inhibitor of cellular protein synthesis

pur·pu·ra \'pər-pù-rə, -pyù-\ *n* : any of several hemorrhagic states characterized by patches of purplish discoloration resulting from extravasation of blood into the skin and mucous membranes — see THROMBOCYTOPENIC PURPURA — **pur·pu·ric** \ˌpər-'pyùr-ik\ *adj*

purpura hem·or·rhag·i·ca \-ˌhe-mə-'ra-jə-kə\ *n* : THROMBOCYTOPENIC PURPURA

purse–string suture *n* : a surgical suture passed as a running stitch in and out along the edge of a circular wound in such a way that when the ends of the suture are drawn tight the wound is closed like a purse

pu·ru·lence \'pyùr-ə-ləns, 'pyùr-yə-\ *n* : the quality or state of being purulent; *also* : PUS

pu·ru·lent \-lənt\ *adj* **1** : containing, consisting of, or being pus **2** : accompanied by suppuration

pus \'pəs\ *n* : thick opaque usu. yellowish white fluid matter formed by suppuration and composed of exudate containing white blood cells, tissue debris, and microorganisms — **pus·sy** \'pə-sē\ *adj*

pus·tu·lar \'pəs-chə-lər, 'pəs-tyə-\ *adj* **1** : of, relating to, or resembling pustules (~ eruptions) **2** : covered with pustules

pus·tule \'pəs-(ˌ)chül, -(ˌ)tyül, -(ˌ)tül\ *n* **1** : a small circumscribed elevation of the skin containing pus and having an inflamed base **2** : a small often distinctively colored elevation or spot resembling a blister or pimple

pu·ta·men \pyù-'tā-mən\ *n*, *pl* **pu·tam·i·na** \-'ta-mə-nə\ : an outer reddish layer of gray matter in the lentiform nucleus

pu·tre·fac·tion \ˌpyü-trə-'fak-shən\ *n* **1** : the decomposition of organic matter; *esp* : the typically anaerobic splitting of proteins by bacteria and fungi

with the formation of foul-smelling incompletely oxidized products **2** : the state of being putrefied — **pu·tre·fac·tive** \-tiv\ *adj* — **pu·tre·fy** \'pyü-trə-ˌfī\ *vb*

pu·tres·cine \pyü-'tre-ˌsēn\ *n* : a crystalline slightly poisonous ptomaine $C_4H_{12}N_2$ that is formed by decarboxylation of ornithine, occurs widely but in small amounts in living things, and is found esp. in putrid flesh

pu·trid \'pyü-trəd\ *adj* **1** : being in a state of putrefaction **2** : of, relating to, or characteristic of putrefaction

PVD *abbr* peripheral vascular disease

PVE *abbr* prosthetic valve endocarditis

PVP *abbr* polyvinylpyrrolidone

P wave \'pē-ˌwāv\ *n* : a deflection in an electrocardiographic tracing that represents atrial activity of the heart — compare QRS COMPLEX, T WAVE

py- *or* **pyo-** *comb form* : pus ⟨*pyemia*⟩ ⟨*pyorrhea*⟩

py·ae·mia *chiefly Brit var of* PYEMIA

py·ar·thro·sis \ˌpī-är-'thrō-səs\ *n*, *pl* **-thro·ses** \-ˌsēz\ : the formation or presence of pus within a joint

pycn- *or* **pycno-** — see PYKN-

pyc·nic, **pyc·no·dys·os·to·sis**, **pyc·no·sis** *var of* PYKNIC, PYKNODYSOSTOSIS, PYKNOSIS

pyel- *or* **pyelo-** *comb form* : renal pelvis ⟨*pyelography*⟩

py·eli·tis \ˌpī-ə-'lī-təs\ *n* : inflammation of the lining of the renal pelvis

py·elo·gram \'pī-ə-lə-ˌgram\ *n* : a roentgenogram made by pyelography

py·elog·ra·phy \ˌpī-ə-'lä-grə-fē\ *n*, *pl* **-phies** : roentgenographic visualization of the renal pelvis after injection of a radiopaque substance through the ureter or into a vein — see RETROGRADE PYELOGRAPHY — **py·elo·graph·ic** \ˌpī-ə-lə-'gra-fik\ *adj*

py·elo·li·thot·o·my \ˌpī-ə-lō-li-'thä-tə-mē\ *n*, *pl* **-mies** : surgical incision of the pelvis of a kidney for removal of a kidney stone

py·elo·ne·phri·tis \ˌpī-ə-lō-ni-'frī-təs\ *n*, *pl* **-phrit·i·des** \-'fri-tə-ˌdēz\ : inflammation of both the parenchyma of a kidney and the lining of its pelvis esp. due to bacterial infection — **py·elo·ne·phrit·ic** \-'fri-tik\ *adj*

py·elo·plas·ty \'pī-ə-lə-ˌplas-tē\ *n*, *pl* **-ties** : plastic surgery of the pelvis of a kidney

py·emia \pī-'ē-mē-ə\ *n* : septicemia accompanied by multiple abscesses and secondary toxemic symptoms and caused by pus-forming microorganisms (as the bacterium *Staphylococcus aureus*) — **py·emic** \-mik\ *adj*

Py·emo·tes \ˌpī-ə-'mō-tēz\ *n* : a genus of mites that are usu. ectoparasites of insects but that include one (*P. ventricosus*) which causes grain itch in humans

py·gop·a·gus \pī-'gä-pə-gəs\ *n*, *pl* **-gi**

\-₁gī, -₁jī\ : a twin fetus joined in the sacral region

pykn- *or* **pykno-** *also* **pycn-** *or* **pycno-** *comb form* **1** : close : compact : dense : bulky 〈*pykn*ic〉 **2** : marked by short stature or shortness of digits 〈*pykno*dysostosis〉

¹**pyk·nic** \¹pik-nik\ *adj* : characterized by shortness of stature, broadness of girth, and powerful muscularity : ENDOMORPHIC 2

²**pyknic** *n* : a person of pyknic build

pyk·no·dys·os·to·sis \₁pik-nō-₁dis-ä-¹stō-səs\ *n, pl* **-to·ses** \-₁sēz\ : a rare condition inherited as an autosomal recessive trait and characterized esp. by short stature, fragile bones, shortness of the fingers and toes, failure of the anterior fontanel to close properly, and a receding chin

pyk·no·lep·sy \¹pik-nə-₁lep-sē\ *n, pl* **-sies** : a condition marked by epileptiform attacks resembling petit mal

pyk·no·sis \pik-¹nō-səs\ *n* : a degenerative condition of a cell nucleus marked by clumping of the chromosomes, hyperchromatism, and shrinking of the nucleus — **pyk·not·ic** \-¹nä-tik\ *adj*

pyl- *or* **pyle-** *or* **pylo-** *comb form* : portal vein 〈*pyle*phlebitis〉

py·le·phle·bi·tis \₁pī-lə-fli-¹bī-təs\ *n, pl* **-bit·i·des** \-¹bi-tə-₁dēz\ : inflammation of the renal portal vein usu. secondary to intestinal disease and with suppuration

py·lon \¹pī-₁län, -lən\ *n* : a simple temporary artificial leg

pylor- *or* **pyloro-** *comb form* : pylorus 〈*pyloro*plasty〉

py·lor·ic \pī-¹lōr-ik, pə-\ *adj* : of or relating to the pylorus; *also* : of, relating to, or situated in or near the posterior part of the stomach

pyloric glands *n pl* : the short coiled tubular glands of the mucous coat of the stomach occurring chiefly near the pyloric end

pyloric sphincter *n* : the circular fold of mucous membrane containing a ring of muscle fibers that closes the pylorus — called also *pyloric valve*

pyloric stenosis *n* : narrowing of the pyloric opening (as from congenital malformation)

py·lo·ro·my·ot·o·my \₁pī-₁lōr-ō-mī-¹ä-tə-mē, pə-₁lōr-ə-\ *n, pl* **-mies** : surgical incision of the muscle fibers of the pyloric sphincter for relief of stenosis caused by muscular hypertrophy

py·lo·ro·plas·ty \pī-¹lōr-ə-₁plas-tē\ *n, pl* **-ties** : a plastic operation on the pylorus (as to enlarge a stricture)

py·lo·ro·spasm \pī-¹lōr-ə-₁spa-zəm\ *n* : spasm of the pyloric sphincter often associated with other conditions (as an ulcer of the stomach) or occurring in infants and marked by pain and vomiting

py·lo·rus \pī-¹lōr-əs, pə-\ *n, pl* **py·lo·ri** \-¹lōr-₁ī, -₁(₁)ē\ : the opening from the stomach into the intestine — see PYLORIC SPHINCTER

pyo- — see PY-

pyo·der·ma \₁pī-ə-¹dər-mə\ *n* : a bacterial skin inflammation marked by pus-filled lesions

pyo·gen·ic \₁pī-ə-¹je·nik\ *adj* : producing pus 〈~ bacteria〉; *also* : marked by pus production 〈~ meningitis〉

pyo·me·tra \₁pī-ə-¹mē-trə\ *n* : an accumulation of pus in the uterine cavity

pyo·myo·si·tis \₁pī-ō-₁mī-ə-¹sī-təs\ *n* : infiltrative bacterial inflammation of muscles leading to the formation of abscesses

pyo·ne·phro·sis \-ni-¹frō-səs\ *n, pl* **-phro·ses** \-₁sēz\ : a collection of pus in the kidney

py·or·rhea \₁pī-ə-¹rē-ə\ *n* **1** : a discharge of pus **2** : an inflammatory condition of the periodontium that is an advanced form of periodontal disease associated esp. with a discharge of pus from the alveoli and loosening of the teeth in their sockets — **py·or·rhe·ic** \-¹rē-ik\ *adj*

py·or·rhoea *chiefly Brit var of* PYOR-RHEA

pyo·sal·pinx \₁pī-ō-¹sal-(₁)piŋks\ *n, pl* **-sal·pin·ges** \-sal-¹pin-(₁)jēz\ : a collection of pus in an oviduct

pyo·tho·rax \-¹thōr-₁aks\ *n, pl* **-tho·rax·es** *or* **-tho·ra·ces** \-¹thōr-ə-(₁)sēz\ : EMPYEMA

pyr- *or* **pyro-** *comb form* **1** : fire : heat 〈*pyro*mania〉 **2** : fever 〈*pyro*gen〉

pyr·a·mid \¹pir-ə-₁mid\ *n* **1** : a polyhedron having for its base a polygon and for faces triangles with a common vertex **2** : an anatomical structure resembling a pyramid: as **a** : RENAL PYRAMID **b** : either of two large bundles of motor fibers from the cerebral cortex that reach the medulla oblongata and are continuous with the corticospinal tracts of the spinal cord **c** : a conical projection making up the central part of the inferior vermis of the cerebellum — **py·ram·i·dal** \pə-¹ra-məd-²l\ *adj*

pyramidal cell *n* : any of numerous large multipolar pyramid-shaped cells in the cerebral cortex

pyramidal decussation *n* : DECUSSATION OF PYRAMIDS

py·ram·i·da·lis \pə-₁ra-mə-¹dā-ləs\ *n, pl* **-da·les** \-(₁)lēz\ *or* **-dalises** : a small triangular muscle of the lower front part of the abdomen that is situated in front of and in the same sheath with the rectus and functions to tense the linea alba

pyramidal tract *n* : CORTICOSPINAL TRACT

py·ram·i·dot·o·my \pə-₁ra-mə-¹dä-tə-mē\ *n, pl* **-mies** : a surgical procedure in which a corticospinal tract is severed (as for relief of parkinsonism)

pyr·a·mis \¹pir-ə-məs\ *n, pl* **pyram·i·des** \pə-¹ra-mə-₁dēz\ : PYRAMID 2

py·ran·tel \pə-¹ran-₁tel\ *n* : an anthelmintic drug $C_{11}H_{14}N_2S$ administered in the form of its pamoate or tartrate

pyr·a·zin·amide \ˌpir-ə-ˈzi-nə-ˌmīd, -məd\ *n* : a tuberculostatic drug $C_5H_5N_3O$

py·re·thrin \pī-ˈrē-thrən, -ˈre-\ *n* : either of two oily liquid esters $C_{21}H_{28}O_3$ and $C_{22}H_{28}O_5$ that have insecticidal properties and are the active components of pyrethrum

py·re·thrum \pī-ˈrē-thrəm, -ˈre-\ *n* : an insecticide consisting of or derived from the dried heads of any of several Old World chrysanthemums (genus *Chrysanthemum* of the family Compositae)

py·rex·ia \pī-ˈrek-sē-ə\ *n* : abnormal elevation of body temperature : FEVER — **py·rex·i·al** \-sē-əl\ *adj*

py·rex·ic \-sik\ *adj* : PYREXIAL

Pyr·i·ben·za·mine \ˌpir-ə-ˈben-zə-ˌmēn\ *trademark* — used for a preparation of tripelennamine

pyr·i·dine \ˈpir-ə-ˌdēn\ *n* : a toxic water-soluble flammable liquid base C_5H_5N of pungent odor

pyridine nucleotide *n* : a nucleotide characterized by a pyridine derivative as a nitrogen base; *esp* : NAD

pyr·i·do·stig·mine \ˌpir-ə-dō-ˈstig-ˌmēn\ *n* : a cholinergic drug that is administered in the form of its bromide $C_9H_{13}BrN_2O_2$ esp. in the treatment of myasthenia gravis — see MESTINON

pyr·i·dox·al \ˌpir-ə-ˈdäk-ˌsal\ *n* : a crystalline aldehyde $C_8H_9NO_3$ of the vitamin B_6 group that in the form of its phosphate is active as a coenzyme

pyr·i·dox·amine \ˌpir-ə-ˈdäk-sə-ˌmēn\ *n* : a crystalline amine $C_8H_{12}N_2O_2$ of the vitamin B_6 group that in the form of its phosphate is active as a coenzyme

pyr·i·dox·ine \ˌpir-ə-ˈdäk-ˌsēn, -sən\ *n* : a crystalline phenolic alcohol $C_8H_{11}NO_3$ of the vitamin B_6 group found esp. in cereals and convertible in the body into pyridoxal and pyridoxamine

pyridoxine hydrochloride *n* : the hydrochloride salt $C_8H_{11}NO_3·HCl$ of pyridoxine that is used therapeutically (as in the treatment of pyridoxine deficiency)

py·ri·form, py·ri·for·mis *var of* PIRIFORM, PIRIFORMIS

pyr·il·amine \pī-ˈri-lə-ˌmēn\ *n* : an oily liquid base $C_{17}H_{23}N_3O$ or its bitter crystalline maleate $C_{21}H_{27}N_3O_5$ used as an antihistamine drug in the treatment of various allergies — see NEO-ANTERGAN

pyr·i·meth·amine \ˌpī-rə-ˈme-thə-ˌmēn\ *n* : a folic acid antagonist $C_{12}H_{13}ClN_4$ that is used in the treatment of malaria and of toxoplasmosis and as an immunosuppressive drug

py·rim·i·dine \pī-ˈri-mə-ˌdēn, pə-\ *n* **1** : a feeble organic base $C_4H_2N_2$ of penetrating odor that is composed of a single six-membered ring having four carbon atoms with nitrogen atoms in positions one and three **2** : a derivative of pyrimidine having its characteristic ring structure; *esp* : a base (as cytosine, thymine, or uracil) that is a constituent of DNA or RNA

pyrithione zinc *n* : ZINC PYRITHIONE

pyro- — see PYR-

py·ro·gal·lic acid \ˌpī-rō-ˈga-lik-\ *n* : PYROGALLOL

py·ro·gal·lol \-ˈga-ˌlȯl, -ˈgȯ-, -ˌlōl\ *n* : a poisonous bitter crystalline phenol $C_6H_6O_3$ that is used as a topical antimicrobial (as in the treatment of psoriasis)

py·ro·gen \ˈpī-rə-jən\ *n* : a fever-producing substance

py·ro·gen·ic \ˌpī-rō-ˈje-nik\ *adj* : producing or produced by fever — **py·ro·ge·nic·i·ty** \-jə-ˈni-sə-tē\ *n*

py·ro·ma·nia \ˌpī-rō-ˈmā-nē-ə, -nyə\ *n* : an irresistible impulse to start fires — **py·ro·ma·ni·a·cal** \-mə-ˈnī-ə-kəl\ *adj*

py·ro·ma·ni·ac \-nē-ˌak\ *n* : an individual affected with pyromania

py·ro·sis \pī-ˈrō-səs\ *n* : HEARTBURN

py·rox·y·lin \pī-ˈräk-sə-lin\ *n* : a flammable mixture of nitrates of cellulose — see COLLODION

pyr·role \ˈpir-ˌōl\ *n* : a toxic liquid heterocyclic compound C_4H_5N that has a ring consisting of four carbon atoms and one nitrogen atom, and is the parent compound of many biologically important substances (as bile pigments, porphyrins, and chlorophyll); *broadly* : a derivative of pyrrole

py·ru·vate \pī-ˈrü-ˌvāt\ *n* : a salt or ester of pyruvic acid

pyruvate kinase *n* : an enzyme that functions in glycolysis by catalyzing esp. the transfer of phosphate from phosphoenolpyruvate to ADP forming pyruvate and ATP

py·ru·vic acid \pī-ˈrü-vik-\ *n* : a 3-carbon keto acid $C_3H_4O_3$ that is an intermediate in carbohydrate metabolism and can be formed either from glucose after phosphorylation or from glycogen by glycolysis

py·uria \pī-ˈyür-ē-ə\ *n* : the presence of pus in the urine; *also* : a condition (as pyelonephritis) characterized by pus in the urine

PZI *abbr* protamine zinc insulin

Q

qd *abbr* [Latin *quaque die*] every day — used in writing prescriptions

Q fever *n* : a disease that is characterized by high fever, chills, and muscular pains, is caused by a rickettsial bacterium of the genus *Coxiella* (*C. burnetii*), and is transmitted by raw milk, by droplet infection, or by ticks

qh *or* **qhr** *abbr* [Latin *quaque hora*] every hour — used in writing prescriptions often with a number indicating the hours between doses ⟨*q4h* means every 4 hours; *q6h*, every 6 hours⟩

qid *abbr* [Latin *quater in die*] four times a day — used in writing prescriptions

QRS \ˌkyü-(ˌ)är-ˈes\ *n* : QRS COMPLEX

QRS complex *n* : the series of deflections in an electrocardiogram that represent electrical activity generated by ventricular depolarization prior to contraction of the ventricles — compare P WAVE, T WAVE

qt *abbr* quart

Q–T interval \ˌkyü-ˈtē-\ *n* : the interval from the beginning of the QRS complex to the end of the T wave on an electrocardiogram that represents the time during which contraction of the ventricles occurs

Quaa·lude \ˈkwä-ˌlüd\ *trademark* — used for a preparation of methaqualone

quack \ˈkwak\ *n* : a pretender to medical skill : an ignorant or dishonest practitioner — **quack** *adj* — **quackery** \ˈkwa-kə-rē\ *n*

quad·rant \ˈkwä-drənt\ *n* : any of the four more or less equivalent segments into which an anatomic structure may be divided by vertical and horizontal partitioning through its midpoint ⟨pain in the lower right ∼ of the abdomen⟩

quad·rate lobe \ˈkwä-ˌdrāt-\ *n* : a small lobe of the liver on the underside of the right lobe to the left of the fissure for the gallbladder

qua·dra·tus fem·o·ris \kwä-ˈdrā-təs-ˈfe-mə-rəs\ *n* : a small flat muscle of the gluteal region that arises from the ischial tuberosity, inserts into the greater trochanter and adjacent region of the femur, and serves to rotate the thigh laterally

quadratus la·bii su·pe·ri·or·is \-ˈlā-bē-ˌi-sü-ˌpir-ē-ˈor-əs\ *n* : LEVATOR LABII SUPERIORIS

quadratus lum·bor·um \-ləm-ˈbòr-əm\ *n* : a quadrilateral-shaped muscle of the abdomen that arises from the iliac crest and the iliolumbar ligament, inserts into the lowest rib and the upper four lumbar vertebrae, and functions esp. to flex the trunk laterally

quadratus plan·tae \-ˈplan-ˌtē\ *n* : a muscle of the sole of the foot that arises by two heads from the calcaneus, inserts into the lateral side of the tendons of the flexor digitorum longus, and aids in flexing the toes

quad·ri·ceps \ˈkwä-drə-ˌseps\ *n* : a large extensor muscle of the front of the thigh divided above into four parts which include the rectus femoris, vastus lateralis, vastus intermedius, and vastus medialis, and which unite in a single tendon to enclose the patella as a sesamoid bone at the knee and insert as the patellar ligament into the tuberosity of the tibia — called also *quadriceps muscle*

quadriceps fem·o·ris \-ˈfe-mə-rəs\ *n* : QUADRICEPS

quadrigemina — see CORPORA QUADRIGEMINA

quad·ri·ple·gia \ˌkwä-drə-ˈplē-jə, -jē-ə\ *n* : paralysis of both arms and both legs — called also *tetraplegia*

¹quad·ri·ple·gic \ˌkwä-drə-ˈplē-jik\ *adj* : of, relating to, or affected with quadriplegia

²quadriplegic *n* : one affected with paralysis of both arms and both legs

quad·ru·ped \ˈkwä-drə-ˌped\ *n* : an animal having four feet — **qua·dru·pe·dal** \kwä-ˈdrü-pəd-ᵊl, ˌkwä-drə-ˈped-\ *adj*

qua·dru·plet \kwä-ˈdrə-plət, -ˈdrü-; ˈkwä-drə-\ *n* : one of four offspring born at one birth

qual·i·ty \ˈkwä-lə-tē\ *n*, *pl* **-ties** : the character of an X-ray beam that determines its penetrating power and is dependent upon its wavelength distribution

quality assurance *n* : a program for the systematic monitoring and evaluation of the various aspects of a project, service, or facility to ensure that standards of quality are being met

quan·ti·ta·tive analysis \ˈkwän-tə-ˌtā-tiv-\ *n* : chemical analysis designed to determine the amounts or proportions of the components of a substance

quantitative character *n* : an inherited character that is expressed phenotypically in all degrees of variation between one often indefinite extreme and another : a character determined by polygenes — compare QUANTITATIVE INHERITANCE

quantitative inheritance *n* : genic inheritance of a character (as human skin color) controlled by polygenes — compare PARTICULATE INHERITANCE

quan·tum \ˈkwän-təm\ *n*, *pl* **quan·ta** \ˈkwän-tə\ **1** : one of the very small increments or parcels into which many forms of energy are subdivided **2** : one of the small molecular packets of a neurotransmitter (as acetylcholine) released into the synaptic cleft in the transmission of a nerve impulse across a synapse — **quan·tal** \-təl\ adj

quar·an·tine \'kwȯr-ən-₁tēn, 'kwär-\ n **1 a** : a term during which a ship arriving in port and suspected of carrying contagious disease is held in isolation from the shore **b** : a regulation placing a ship in quarantine **c** : a place where a ship is detained during quarantine **2 a** : a restraint upon the activities or communication of persons or the transport of goods that is designed to prevent the spread of disease or pests **b** : a place in which those under quarantine are kept — **quar·an·tin·able** adj — **quarantine** vb

quart \'kwȯrt\ n **1** : a British unit of liquid or dry capacity equal to ¼ gallon or 69.355 cubic inches or 1.136 liters **2** : a U.S. unit of liquid capacity equal to ¼ gallon or 57.75 cubic inches or 0.946 liters

quar·tan \'kwȯrt-ən\ adj : occurring every fourth day; specif : recurring at approximately 72-hour intervals ⟨∼ chills and fever⟩ — compare TERTIAN

quartan malaria n : MALARIAE MALARIA

quartz \'kwȯrts\ n : a silica-containing mineral SiO_2

quas·sia \'kwä-shə, -shē-ə, -sē-ə\ n : a drug consisting of the heartwood of various tropical trees (family Simaroubaceae) used in medicine esp. as a remedy for roundworms

qua·ter·na·ry \'kwä-tər-₁ner-ē, kwə-'tər-nə-rē\ adj : consisting of, containing, or being an atom united by four bonds to carbon atoms

quaternary ammonium compound n : any of numerous strong bases and their salts derived from ammonium by replacement of the hydrogen atoms with organic radicals and important esp. as surface-active agents, disinfectants, and drugs

que·bra·cho \kā-'brä-(₁)chō, ki-\ n : a tree (Aspidosperma quebracho) of the dogbane family (Apocynaceae) which occurs in Argentina and Chile and whose dried bark is used as a respiratory sedative in dyspnea and in asthma

Queck·en·stedt test \'kvek-ən-₁shtet-\ n : a test for spinal blockage of the subarachnoid space in which manual pressure is applied to the jugular vein to elevate venous pressure, which indicates the absence of a block when there is a simultaneous increase in cerebrospinal fluid pressure, and which indicates the presence of a block when cerebrospinal fluid pressure remains the same or almost the same — called also Queckenstedt sign

Queckenstedt, Hans Heinrich Georg (1876–1918), German physician.

quel·lung \'kwe-ləŋ, 'kve-lu̇ŋ\ n, often

cap : swelling of the capsule of a microorganism after reaction with an antibody ⟨the ∼ reaction⟩

quer·ce·tin \'kwȯr-sə-tən\ n : a yellow crystalline pigment $C_{15}H_{10}O_7$ occurring usu. in the form of glycosides in various plants

quick \'kwik\ n : a painfully sensitive spot or area of flesh (as that underlying a fingernail or toenail)

quick·en \'kwi-kən\ vb **quick·ened**; **quick·en·ing** : to reach the stage of gestation at which fetal motion is felt

quickening n : the first motion of a fetus in the uterus felt by the mother usu. somewhat before the middle of the period of gestation

quick·sil·ver \'kwik-₁sil-vər\ n : MERCURY 1

qui·es·cent \kwī-'es-ənt, kwē-\ adj **1** : being in a state of arrest ⟨∼ tuberculosis⟩ **2** : causing no symptoms ⟨∼ gallstones⟩ — **qui·es·cence** \-əns\ n

Qui·lene \'kwi-₁lēn\ trademark — used for a preparation of pentapiperide methylsulfate

quin- or **quino-** comb form **1** : quina : cinchona bark ⟨quinine⟩ ⟨quinoline⟩ **2** : quinoline ⟨quinethazone⟩

qui·na \'kē-nə\ n : CINCHONA 2, 3

quin·a·crine \'kwi-nə-₁krēn\ n : an antimalarial drug derived from acridine and used esp. in the form of its dihydrochloride $C_{23}H_{30}ClN_3O·2HCl·2H_2O$ — called also mepacrine; see ATABRINE

quin·al·bar·bi·tone \₁kwi-nal-'bär-bi-₁tōn\ n, chiefly Brit : SECOBARBITAL

Quin·cke's disease \'kviŋ-kəz-\ n : ANGIOEDEMA

Quincke, Heinrich Irenaeus (1842–1922), German physician.

Quincke's edema n : ANGIOEDEMA

quin·eth·a·zone \₁kwi-'ne-thə-₁zōn\ n : a diuretic $C_{10}H_{12}ClN_3O_3S$ used in the treatment of edema and hypertension

quin·i·dine \'kwi-nə-₁dēn, -dən\ n : a crystalline dextrorotatory stereoisomer of quinine found in some species of cinchona and used sometimes in place of quinine but chiefly in the form of its sulfate in the treatment of cardiac rhythm irregularities

qui·nine \'kwi-₁nīn, 'kwi-, -₁nēn\ n **1** : a bitter crystalline alkaloid $C_{20}H_{24}N_2O_2$ from cinchona bark used in medicine **2** : a salt of quinine used as an antipyretic, antimalarial, antiperiodic, and bitter tonic

quin·o·line \'kwin-əl-₁ēn\ n **1** : a pungent oily nitrogenous base C_9H_7N that is the parent compound of many alkaloids, drugs, and dyes **2** : a derivative of quinoline

qui·none \kwi-'nōn, 'kwi-\ n **1** : either of two isomeric cyclic crystalline compounds $C_6H_4O_2$ that are extremely irritating to the skin and mucous membranes **2** : any of various usu. yellow, orange, or red compounds structurally related to the qui-nones and including several that are biologically important as coenzymes, hydrogen acceptors, or vitamins

quin·sy \'kwin-zē\ *n, pl* **quin·sies** : an abscess in the connective tissue around a tonsil usu. resulting from bacterial infection and often accompanied by fever, pain, and swelling — called also *peritonsillar abscess*

quint \'kwint\ *n* : QUINTUPLET

quinti — see EXTENSOR DIGITI QUINTI PROPRIUS

quin·tu·plet \kwin-'tə-plət, -'tü-, -'tyü-; 'kwin-tə-\ *n* : one of five children or offspring born at one birth

qui·nu·cli·di·nyl ben·zi·late \kwi-'nü-klə-‚dēn-ᵊl-'ben-zə-‚lāt, -'nyü-\ *n* : BZ

quit·tor \'kwi-tər\ *n* : a purulent inflam-mation (as a necrobacillosis) of the feet esp. of horses and donkeys

quo·tid·i·an \kwō-'ti-dē-ən\ *adj* : occur-ring every day ⟨~ fever⟩

quo·tient \'kwō-shənt\ *n* : the numeri-cal ratio usu. multiplied by 100 be-tween a test score and a measurement on which that score might be expect-ed largely to depend — see INTELLI-GENCE QUOTIENT

qv *abbr* [Latin *quantum vis*] as much as you will

Q wave \'kyü-‚\ *n* : the short initial downward stroke of the QRS com-plex in an electrocardiogram formed during the beginning of ventricular depolarization

R

r *abbr* roentgen

Ra *symbol* radium

rabbit fever *n* : TULAREMIA

ra·bies \'rā-bēz\ *n, pl* **rabies** : an acute virus disease of the nervous system of warm-blooded animals that is transmitted with infected saliva usu. through the bite of a rabid animal and is typically characterized by in-creased salivation, abnormal behav-ior, and eventual paralysis and death when untreated — called also *hydro-phobia* — **ra·bid** \'ra-bid, 'rā-\ *adj*

race \'rās\ *n* **1** : a division or group (as a subspecies) within a biological spe-cies **2** : one of the three, four, or five divisions based on inherited physical characteristics into which human be-ings are usu. divided

ra·ce·mic \rā-'sē-mik, rə-\ *adj* : of, re-lating to, or constituting a compound or mixture that is composed of equal amounts of dextrorotatory and levo-rotatory forms of the same compound and is not optically active

ra·ce·mose \'ra-sə-‚mōs; rā-'sē-, rə-\ *adj* : having or growing in a form like that of a cluster of grapes ⟨~ aneu-rysms⟩

rachi- *or* **rachio-** *comb form* : spine ⟨*ra-chischisis*⟩

ra·chis·chi·sis \rə-'kis-kə-səs\ *n, pl* **-chi-ses** \-kə-‚sēz\ : a congenital abnormal-ity (as spina bifida) characterized by a cleft of the vertebral column

ra·chit·ic \rə-'ki-tik\ *adj* : of, relating to, or affected by rickets ⟨~ lesions⟩

rachitic rosary *n* : BEADING

ra·chi·tis \rə-'kī-təs\ *n, pl* **-chit·i·des** \-'ki-tə-‚dēz\ : RICKETS

¹rad \'rad\ *n* : a unit of absorbed dose of ionizing radiation equal to an energy of 100 ergs per gram of irradiated ma-terial

²rad *abbr* [Latin *radix*] root — used in writing prescriptions

radi- — see RADIO-

¹ra·di·al \'rā-dē-əl\ *adj* **1** : arranged or

having parts arranged like rays **2** : of, relating to, or situated near the radius or the thumb side of the hand or fore-arm **3** : developing uniformly around a central axis ⟨~ cleavage of an egg⟩ — **ra·di·al·ly** *adv*

²radial *n* : a body part (as an artery) ly-ing near or following the course of the radius

radial artery *n* : the smaller of the two branches into which the brachial ar-tery divides just below the bend of the elbow and which passes along the radial side of the forearm to the wrist then winds backward around the out-er side of the carpus and enters the palm between the first and second metacarpal bones to form the deep palmar arch

radialis — see EXTENSOR CARPI RADI-ALIS BREVIS, EXTENSOR CARPI RADI-ALIS LONGUS, FLEXOR CARPI RADIAL-IS, NERVUS RADIALIS

radial keratotomy *n* : a surgical opera-tion on the cornea for the correction of myopia that involves flattening it by making a series of incisions in a ra-dial pattern resembling the spokes of a wheel

radial nerve *n* : a large nerve that arises from the posterior cord of the brachi-al plexus and passes spirally down the humerus to the front of the lateral epicondyle where it divides into a su-perficial branch distributed to the skin of the back of the hand and arm and a deep branch to the underlying extensor muscles — called also *nervus radialis*

radial notch *n* : a narrow depression on the lateral side of the coronoid pro-cess of the ulna that articulates with the head of the radius and gives at-tachment to the annular ligament of the radius

radial tuberosity *n* : an oval eminence on the medial side of the radius distal to the neck where the tendon of the biceps brachii muscle inserts

radial vein *n* : any of several deep veins of the forearm that unite at the elbow with the ulnar veins to form the brachial veins

ra·di·ant energy \'rā-dē-ənt-\ *n* : energy traveling as a wave motion; *specif* : the energy of electromagnetic waves

radiata — see CORONA RADIATA

ra·di·ate \'rā-dē-,āt\ *vb* **-at·ed; -at·ing 1** : to issue in or as if in rays : spread from a central point **2** : IRRADIATE

ra·di·ate ligament \'rā-dē-ət-, -,āt-\ *n* : a branching ligament uniting the front of the head of a rib with the bodies of the two vertebrae and the intervertebral disk between them — called also *stellate ligament*

ra·di·a·tion \,rā-dē-'ā-shən\ *n* **1** : energy radiated in the form of waves or particles **2 a** : the action or process of radiating **b** (1) : the process of emitting radiant energy in the form of waves or particles (2) : the combined processes of emission, transmission, and absorption of radiant energy **3** : a tract of nerve fibers within the brain; *esp* : one concerned with the distribution of impulses arising from sensory stimuli to the relevant coordinating centers and nuclei

radiation sickness *n* : sickness that results from exposure to radiation and is commonly marked by fatigue, nausea, vomiting, loss of teeth and hair, and in more severe cases by damage to blood-forming tissue with decrease in red and white blood cells and bleeding

radiation syndrome *n* : RADIATION SICKNESS

radiation therapy *n* : RADIOTHERAPY

¹**rad·i·cal** \'ra-di-kəl\ *adj* : designed to remove the root of a disease or all diseased tissue (~ surgery) — compare CONSERVATIVE — **rad·i·cal·ly** *adv*

²**radical** *n* : FREE RADICAL; *also* : a group of atoms bonded together that is considered an entity in various kinds of reactions

radical mastectomy *n* : a mastectomy in which the breast tissue, associated skin, nipple, areola, axillary lymph nodes, and pectoral muscles are removed — called also *Halsted radical mastectomy*; compare MODIFIED RADICAL MASTECTOMY

ra·dic·u·lar \rə-'di-kyə-lər, ra-\ *adj* **1** : of, relating to, or involving a nerve root **2** : of, relating to, or occurring at the root of a tooth (a ~ cyst)

ra·dic·u·li·tis \rə-,di-kyə-'lī-təs\ *n* : inflammation of a nerve root

ra·dic·u·lop·a·thy \-'lä-pə-thē\ *n, pl* **-thies** : any pathological condition of the nerve roots

radii *pl of* RADIUS

radio- *also* **radi-** *comb form* **1** : radiant energy : radiation ⟨*radio*active⟩ ⟨*radi*opaque⟩ **2** : radioactive ⟨*radio*ele-

ment⟩ **3** : radium : X rays ⟨*radio*therapy⟩ **4** : radioactive isotopes esp. as produced artificially ⟨*radio*cobalt⟩

ra·dio·ac·tiv·i·ty \,rā-dē-ō-ak-'ti-və-tē\ *n, pl* **-ties** : the property possessed by some elements (as uranium) of spontaneously emitting alpha or beta rays and sometimes also gamma rays by the disintegration of the nuclei of atoms — **ra·dio·ac·tive** \-'ak-tiv\ *adj* — **ra·dio·ac·tive·ly** *adv*

ra·dio·al·ler·go·sor·bent \,rā-dē-ō-ə-,lər-gō-'sor-bənt\ *adj* : relating to, involving, or being a radioallergosorbent test (~ testing)

radioallergosorbent test *n* : a radioimmunoassay for specific antibodies of immunoglobulin class IgE in which an insoluble matrix containing allergenic antigens is reacted with a sample of antibody-containing serum and then reacted again with antihuman antibodies against individual IgE antibodies to make specific determinations — abbr. *RAST*

ra·dio·as·say \,rā-dē-ō-'a-,sā, -a-'sā\ *n* : an assay based on examination of the sample in terms of radiation components

ra·dio·au·to·gram \-'o-tə-,gram\ *n* : AUTORADIOGRAPH

ra·dio·au·to·graph \-'o-tə-,graf\ *n* : AUTORADIOGRAPH — **radioautograph** *vb* — **ra·dio·au·to·graph·ic** \-,o-tə-'gra-fik\ *adj* — **ra·dio·au·tog·ra·phy** \-,o-'tä-grə-fē\ *n*

ra·dio·bi·ol·o·gy \,rā-dē-ō-bī-'ä-lə-jē\ *n, pl* **-gies** : a branch of biology dealing with the effects of radiation or radioactive materials on biological systems — **ra·dio·bi·o·log·i·cal** \-,bī-ə-'lä-ji-kəl\ *also* **ra·dio·bi·o·log·ic** \-jik\ *adj* — **ra·dio·bi·o·log·i·cal·ly** *adv* — **ra·dio·bi·ol·o·gist** \-bī-'ä-lə-jist\ *n*

¹**ra·dio·chem·i·cal** \-'ke-mi-kəl\ *adj* : of, relating to, being, or using radiochemicals or the methods of radiochemistry (~ analysis) (~ purity)

²**radiochemical** *n* : a chemical prepared with radioactive elements esp. for medical research or application (as for use as a tracer in renal or heart function studies)

ra·dio·chem·is·try \,rā-dē-ō-'ke-mə-strē\ *n, pl* **-tries** : a branch of chemistry dealing with radioactive substances and phenomena including tracer studies — **ra·dio·chem·ist** \-'ke-mist\ *n*

ra·dio·chro·mato·gram \-krō-'ma-tə-,gram\ *n* : a chromatogram revealing one or more radioactive substances

ra·dio·chro·ma·tog·ra·phy \-,krō-mə-'tä-grə-fē\ *n, pl* **-phies** : the process of making a quantitative or qualitative determination of a radioisotope-labeled substance by measuring the radioactivity of the appropriate zone or spot in the chromatogram — **ra·dio·chro·ma·to·graph·ic** \-krə-,ma-tə-'gra-fik, -,krō-mə-\ *adj*

ra·dio·chro·mi·um \-ˈkrō-mē-əm\ *n* : a radioactive isotope of chromium esp. chromium with mass number 51

ra·dio·co·balt \-ˈkō-ˌbolt\ *n* : radioactive cobalt; *esp* : COBALT 60

ra·dio·den·si·ty \-ˈden-sə-tē\ *n, pl* **-ties** : RADIOPACITY

ra·dio·der·ma·ti·tis \-ˌdər-mə-ˈtī-təs\ *n, pl* **-ti·tis·es** *or* **-tit·i·des** \-ˈti-tə-ˌdēz\ : dermatitis resulting from overexposure to sources of radiant energy (as X rays or radium)

ra·dio·di·ag·no·sis \-ˌdī-ig-ˈnō-səs\ *n, pl* **-no·ses** \-ˌsēz\ : diagnosis by means of radiology — compare RADIOTHERAPY

ra·dio·el·e·ment \ˈē-lə-mənt\ *n* : a radioactive element whether formed naturally or produced artificially — compare RADIOISOTOPE

ra·dio·en·zy·mat·ic \-ˌen-zə-ˈma-tik\ *adj* : of, relating to, or produced by a radioactive enzyme

ra·dio·fre·quen·cy \-ˈfrē-kwən-sē\ *n, pl* **-cies** : any of the electromagnetic wave frequencies that lie in a range extending from below 3000 hertz to about 300 billion hertz and that include the frequencies used in radio and television transmission — **radiofrequency** *adj*

ra·dio·gen·ic \ˌrā-dē-ō-ˈje-nik\ *adj* : produced by radioactivity ⟨~ tumors⟩

ra·dio·gram \ˈrā-dē-ō-ˌgram\ *n* : RADIOGRAPH

ra·dio·graph \-ˌgraf\ *n* : an X-ray or gamma-ray photograph — **radiograph** *vb* — **ra·dio·graph·ic** \ˌrā-dē-ō-ˈgra-fik\ *adj*

ra·di·og·ra·pher \ˌrā-dē-ˈä-grə-fər\ *n* : one who radiographs; *specif* : an X-ray technician

ra·di·og·ra·phy \ˌrā-dē-ˈä-grə-fē\ *n, pl* **-phies** : the art, act, or process of making radiographs

ra·dio·im·mu·no·as·say \ˌrā-dē-ō-i-myə-nō-ˈa-ˌsā, -i-ˌmyü-, -a-ˈsā\ *n* : immunoassay of a substance (as insulin) that has been radioactively labeled — abbr. *RIA* — **ra·dio·im·mu·no·as·say·able** *adj*

ra·dio·im·mu·no·elec·tro·pho·re·sis \-i-ˌlek-trə-fə-ˈrē-səs\ *n, pl* **-re·ses** \-ˌsēs\ : immunoelectrophoresis in which the substances separated in the electrophoretic system are identified by radioactive labels on antigens or antibodies

ra·dio·im·mu·no·log·i·cal \-i-myə-nə-ˈlä-ji-kəl\ *also* **ra·dio·im·mu·no·log·ic** \-ˈlä-jik\ *adj* : of, relating to, or involving a radioimmunoassay

ra·dio·io·dide \-ˈī-ə-ˌdīd\ *n* : an iodide containing radioactive iodine

ra·dio·io·din·ate \-ˈī-ə-də-ˌnāt\ *vb* **-at·ed; -at·ing** : to treat or label with radioactive iodine — **ra·dio·io·din·ation** \-ˌī-ə-də-ˈnā-shən\ *n*

ra·dio·io·dine \-ˈī-ə-ˌdīn, -dən, -ˌdēn\ *n* : radioactive iodine; *esp* : IODINE-131

ra·dio·iron \-ˈī(-ə)rn\ *n* : radioactive

iron; *esp* : a heavy isotope having the mass number 59 produced in nuclear reactors or cyclotrons and used in biochemical tracer studies

ra·dio·iso·tope \ˌrā-dē-ō-ˈī-sə-ˌtōp\ *n* : a radioactive isotope — compare RADIOELEMENT — **ra·dio·iso·to·pic** \-ˌī-sə-ˈtä-pik, -ˈtō-\ *adj*

ra·dio·la·bel \-ˈlā-bəl\ *vb* **-la·beled** *or* **-la·belled; -la·bel·ing** *or* **-la·bel·ling** : to label with a radioactive atom or substance — **radiolabel** *n*

ra·di·ol·o·gist \ˌrā-dē-ˈä-lə-jist\ *n* : a physician specializing in the use of radiant energy for diagnostic and therapeutic purposes

ra·di·ol·o·gy \-jē\ *n, pl* **-gies 1** : the science of radioactive substances and high-energy radiations **2** : a branch of medicine concerned with the use of radiant energy (as X rays and radium) in the diagnosis and treatment of disease — **ra·di·o·log·i·cal** \ˌrā-dē-ə-ˈlä-ji-kəl\ *or* **ra·di·o·log·ic** \-jik\ *adj* — **ra·dio·log·i·cal·ly** *adv*

ra·dio·lu·cent \ˌrā-dē-ō-ˈlüs-ᵊnt\ *adj* : partly or wholly permeable to radiation and esp. X rays — compare RADIOPAQUE — **ra·dio·lu·cen·cy** \-ˈlüs-ᵊn-sē\ *n*

ra·dio·mi·met·ic \-mə-ˈme-tik, -mī-\ *adj* : producing effects similar to those of radiation ⟨~ agents⟩

ra·dio·ne·cro·sis \-nə-ˈkrō-səs, -nē-\ *n, pl* **-cro·ses** \-ˌsēz\ : ulceration or destruction of tissue resulting from irradiation — **ra·dio·ne·crot·ic** \-ˈkrä-tik\ *adj*

ra·dio·nu·clide \-ˈnü-ˌklīd, -ˈnyü-\ *n* : a radioactive nuclide

ra·dio·opac·i·ty \ˌrā-dē-ō-ˈpa-sə-tē\ *n, pl* **-ties** : the quality or state of being radiopaque

ra·dio·opaque \-ō-ˈpāk\ *adj* : being opaque to radiation and esp. X rays — compare RADIOLUCENT

ra·dio·phar·ma·ceu·ti·cal \ˌrā-dē-ō-ˌfär-mə-ˈsü-ti-kəl\ *n* : a radioactive drug used for diagnostic or therapeutic purposes — **radiopharmaceutical** *adj*

ra·dio·phar·ma·cy \-ˈfär-mə-sē\ *n, pl* **-cies** : a branch of pharmacy concerned with radiopharmaceuticals; *also* : a pharmacy that supplies radiopharmaceuticals — **ra·dio·phar·ma·cist** \-sist\ *n*

ra·dio·phos·pho·rus \-ˈfäs-fə-rəs\ *n* : radioactive phosphorus; *esp* : PHOSPHORUS 32

ra·dio·pro·tec·tive \-prə-ˈtek-tiv\ *adj* : serving to protect or aiding in protecting against the injurious effect of radiations ⟨~ drugs⟩ — **ra·dio·pro·tec·tion** \-ˈtek-shən\ *n*

ra·dio·pro·tec·tor \-ˈtek-tər\ *also* **ra·dio·pro·tec·tor·ant** \-ˈtek-tə-rənt\ *n* : a radioprotective chemical agent

ra·dio·re·cep·tor assay \-ri-ˈsep-tər-\ *n* : an assay for a substance and esp. a hormone in which a mixture of the test sample and a known amount of the radiolabeled substance under test is exposed to a measured quantity of receptors for the substance and the amount in the test sample is determined from the proportion of receptors occupied by radiolabeled molecules of the substance under the assumption that labeled and unlabeled molecules bind to the receptor sites at random

ra·dio·re·sis·tant \-ri-ˈzis-tənt\ *adj* : resistant to the effects of radiant energy ⟨∼ cancer cells⟩ — compare RADIOSENSITIVE — **ra·dio·re·sis·tance** \-təns\ *n*

ra·dio·sen·si·tive \ˌrā-dē-ō-ˈsen-sə-tiv\ *adj* : sensitive to the effects of radiant energy ⟨∼ cancer cells⟩ — compare RADIORESISTANT — **ra·dio·sen·si·tiv·i·ty** \-ˌsen-sə-ˈti-və-tē\ *n*

ra·dio·sen·si·tiz·er \-ˈsen-sə-ˌtī-zər\ *n* : a substance or condition capable of increasing the radiosensitivity of a cell or tissue — **ra·dio·sen·si·ti·za·tion** \-ˌsen-sə-tə-ˈzā-shən\ *n* — **ra·dio·sen·si·tiz·ing** \-ˈsen-sə-ˌtī-ziŋ\ *adj*

ra·dio·so·di·um \-ˈsō-dē-əm\ *n* : radioactive sodium; *esp* : a heavy istope having the mass number 24, produced in nuclear reactors, and used in the form of a salt (as sodium chloride) chiefly in biochemical tracer studies

ra·dio·stron·tium \-ˈsträn-chē-əm, -chəm, -tē-əm\ *n* : radioactive strontium; *esp* : STRONTIUM 90

ra·dio·te·lem·e·try \-tə-ˈle-mə-trē\ *n, pl* **-tries 1** : TELEMETRY **2** : BIOTELEMETRY — **ra·dio·tele·met·ric** \-ˌte-lə-ˈme-trik\ *adj*

ra·dio·ther·a·py \ˌrā-dē-ō-ˈther-ə-pē\ *n, pl* **-pies** : the treatment of disease by means of radiation (as X rays) — called also *radiation therapy*; compare RADIODIAGNOSIS — **ra·dio·ther·a·peut·ic** \-ˌther-ə-ˈpyü-tik\ *adj* — **ra·dio·ther·a·pist** \-ˈther-ə-pist\ *n*

ra·dio·tox·ic·i·ty \-täk-ˈsi-sə-tē\ *n, pl* **-ties** : the toxicity of radioactive substances

ra·dio·trac·er \ˈrā-dē-ō-ˌtrā-sər\ *n* : a radioactive tracer

ra·dio·ul·nar \ˌrā-dē-ō-ˈəl-nər\ *adj* : of, relating to, or connecting the radius and ulna

radioulnar joint *n* : any of three joints connecting the radius and ulna at their proximal and distal ends and along their shafts — see INFERIOR RADIOULNAR JOINT

radio wave *n* : an electromagnetic wave having a frequency in the range that extends from about 3000 hertz to about 300 billion hertz and includes the frequencies used for radio and television

ra·di·um \ˈrā-dē-əm\ *n, often attrib* : an intensely radioactive shining white metallic element that emits alpha particles and gamma rays to form radon and is used in the treatment of cancer — symbol *Ra*; see ELEMENT table

ra·di·us \ˈrā-dē-əs\ *n, pl* **ra·dii** \-dē-ˌī\ *also* **ra·di·us·es** : the bone on the thumb side of the forearm that is articulated with the ulna at both ends so as to permit partial rotation about that bone, that bears on its inner aspect somewhat distal to the head a prominence for the insertion of the biceps tendon, and that has the lower end broadened for articulation with the proximal bones of the carpus so that rotation of the radius involves also that of the hand

ra·don \ˈrā-dän\ *n* : a heavy radioactive gaseous element of the group of inert gases formed by disintegration of radium and used similarly to radium in medicine — symbol *Rn*; see ELEMENT table

rag·weed \ˈrag-ˌwēd\ *n* : any of various chiefly No. American weedy herbaceous plants comprising the genus *Ambrosia* and producing highly allergenic pollen: as **a** : an annual weed (*A. artemisiifolia*) with finely divided foliage that is common on open or cultivated ground in much of No. America **b** : a coarse annual (*A. trifida*) with some or all of the leaves usu. deeply 3-cleft or 5-cleft — called also *great ragweed*

Rail·lie·ti·na \ˌrāl-yə-ˈtī-nə\ *n* : a large genus of armed tapeworms (family Davaineidae of the order Cyclophyllidea) having the adults parasitic in birds, rodents, or rarely humans and the larvae in various insects

Rail·liet \rē-ˈyā\, **Louis–Joseph Alcide (1852–1930),** French veterinarian.

rain·bow \ˈrān-ˌbō\ *n, slang* : a drug in a tablet or capsule of several colors; *esp* : a combination of the sodium derivatives of amobarbital and secobarbital in a blue and red capsule

rainbow pill *n, slang* : RAINBOW

rale \ˈral, ˈräl\ *n* : an abnormal sound heard accompanying the normal respiratory sounds on auscultation of the chest — compare RATTLE, RHONCHUS

ram·i·fi·ca·tion \ˌra-mə-fə-ˈkā-shən\ *n* **1** : the act or process of branching; *specif* : the mode of arrangement of branches **2** : a branch or offshoot from a main stock or channel (the ∼ of an artery); *also* : the resulting branched structure — **ram·i·fy** \ˈra-mə-ˌfī\ *vb*

ra·mus \ˈrā-məs\ *n, pl* **ra·mi** \-ˌmī\ : a projecting part, elongated process, or branch: as **a** : the posterior more or less vertical part of the lower jaw on each side which articulates with the skull **b** (1) : the upper more cranial branch of the pubis that extends from the pubic symphysis to the body of the pubis at the acetabulum and forms the cranial part of the obturator foramen — called also *superior ramus* (2) : the thin flat lower branch of the pubis that extends from the pubic symphysis to unite with the ramus of the ischium in forming the inferior rim of the obturator foramen — called also *inferior ramus* **c** : a branch of the ischium that extends down and forward from the ischial tuberosity to unite with the inferior ramus of the pubis in forming the inferior rim of the obturator foramen — called also *inferior ramus* **d** : a branch of a nerve — see RAMUS COMMUNICANS

ramus com·mu·ni·cans \-kə-'myü-nə-ˌkanz\ *n, pl* **rami com·mu·ni·can·tes** \-kə-ˌmyü-nə-'kan-ˌtēz\ : any of the bundles of nerve fibers connecting a sympathetic ganglion with a spinal nerve and being divided into two kinds: **a** : one consisting of myelinated preganglionic fibers — called also *white ramus, white ramus communicans* **b** : one consisting of unmyelinated postganglionic fibers — called also *gray ramus*

ran *past of* RUN

rang *past of* RING

ra·nit·i·dine \ra-'ni-tə-ˌdēn\ *n* : an antihistamine $C_{13}H_{22}N_4O_3S$ that is administered in the form of its hydrochloride to inhibit gastric acid secretion (as in the treatment of duodenal ulcers or Zollinger-Ellison syndrome) — see ZANTAC

ran·u·la \'ran-yə-lə\ *n* : a cyst formed under the tongue by obstruction of a gland duct

rape \'rāp\ *n* **1** : sexual intercourse with a woman by a man without her consent and chiefly by force or deception — see STATUTORY RAPE **2** : unlawful sexual intercourse by force or threat other than by a man with a woman — **rape** *vb*

ra·phe \'rā-fē\ *n* : the seamlike union of the two lateral halves of a part or organ (as of the tongue, perineum, or scrotum) having externally a ridge or furrow and internally usu. a fibrous connective tissue septum

raphe nucleus *n* : any of several groups of nerve cells situated along or near the median plane of the tegmentum of the midbrain

rapid eye movement *n* : a rapid movement of the eyes associated esp. with REM sleep — called also *REM*

rapid eye movement sleep *n* : REM SLEEP

rapid plasma reagin test *n* : a flocculation test for syphilis employing the antigen used in the VDRL test with charcoal particles added so that the flocculation can be seen without the aid of a microscope — called also *RPR card test*

rap·ist \'rā-pist\ *n* : an individual who commits rape

rap·port \ra-'pȯr, rə-\ *n* : confidence of a subject in the operator (as in hypnotism, psychotherapy, or mental testing) with willingness to cooperate

rapture of the deep *n* : NITROGEN NARCOSIS

rap·tus \'rap-təs\ *n* : a pathological paroxysm of activity giving vent to impulse or tension (as in an act of violence)

rar·efy *also* **rar·i·fy** \'rar-ə-ˌfī\ *vb* **-efied** *also* **-ified; -efy·ing** *also* **-ify·ing** : to make or become rare, thin, porous, or less dense : to expand without the addition of matter — **rar·efac·tion** \ˌrar-ə-'fak-shən\ *n*

rash \'rash\ *n* : an eruption on the body typically with little or no elevation above the surface

RAST *abbr* radioallergosorbent test

rat \'rat\ *n* : any of the numerous rodents (family Muridae) of *Rattus* and related genera that include forms (as the brown rat and the black rat) which live in and about human habitations and are destructive pests and vectors of various diseases (as bubonic plague)

rat–bite fever *n* : either of two human febrile diseases usu. transmitted by the bite of a rat: **a** : a septicemia marked by irregular relapsing fever, rashes, muscular pain and arthritis, and great weakness and caused by a bacterium of the genus *Streptobacillus* (*S. moniliformis*) **b** : a disease that is marked by sharp elevation of temperature, swelling of lymph glands, eruption, recurrent inflammation of the bite wound, and muscular pains in the part where the bite wound occurred and that is caused by a bacterium of the genus *Spirillum* (*S. minor* syn. *S. minus*) — called also *sodoku*

rate \'rāt\ *n* **1** : a fixed ratio between two things **2** : a quantity, amount, or degree of something measured per unit of something else — see BASAL METABOLIC RATE, DEATH RATE, HEART RATE

rat flea *n* : any of various fleas that occur on rats: as **a** : NORTHERN RAT FLEA **b** : ORIENTAL RAT FLEA

Rath·ke's pouch \'rät-kəz-\ *n* : a pouch of ectoderm that grows out from the upper surface of the embryonic stomodeum and gives rise to the adenohypophysis of the pituitary gland — called also *Rathke's pocket*

> **Rathke, Martin Heinrich (1793–1860),** German anatomist.

rat·i·cide \'ra-tə-ˌsīd\ *n* : a substance used to kill rats

ra·tio \'rā-(ˌ)shō, -shē-ˌō\ *n, pl* **ra·tios** : the relationship in quantity, amount, or size between two or more things — see SEX RATIO

ra·tion \'ra-shən, 'rā-\ *n* : a food allowance for one day — **ration** *vb*

ra·tio·nal·ize \'ra-shə-nə-ˌliz\ *vb* **-ized; -iz·ing** : to attribute (one's actions) to rational and creditable motives without analysis of true and esp. unconscious motives; *also* : to provide plausible but untrue reasons for conduct — **ra·tio·nal·i·za·tion** \ˌra-shə-nə-lə-ˈzā-shən\ n

rat louse n : a sucking louse (*Polyplax spinulosa*) that is a widely distributed parasite of rats and transmits murine typhus from rat to rat

rat mite n : a widely distributed mite of the genus *Bdellonyssus* (*B. bacoti*) that usu. feeds on rodents but may cause dermatitis and transmit typhus to humans

rat·tle \ˈrat-ᵊl\ n : a throat noise caused by air passing through mucus; *specif* : DEATH RATTLE — compare RALE, RHONCHUS

rat·tle·box \-ˌbäks\ n : CROTALARIA 2; *esp* : one (*Crotalaria spectabilis*) that is highly toxic to farm animals

rat·tle·snake \-ˌsnāk\ n : any of the American pit vipers that have a series of horny interlocking joints at the end of the tail which make a sharp rattling sound when vibrated and that comprise the genera *Sistrurus* and *Crotalus* — see DIAMONDBACK RATTLESNAKE, TIGER RATTLESNAKE, TIMBER RATTLESNAKE

Rat·tus \ˈra-təs\ n : a genus of rodents (family Muridae) that comprise the common rats

Rau·dix·in \raŭ-ˈdiks-ən, rō-\ *trademark* — used for a preparation of reserpine

rau·wol·fia \raŭ-ˈwŭl-fē-ə, rō-\ n **1** a *cap* : a large tropical genus of the dogbane family (Apocynaceae) of somewhat poisonous trees and shrubs yielding emetic and purgative substances **b** : any plant of the genus *Rauwolfia* **2** : a medicinal extract from the root of an Indian rauwolfia (*Rauwolfia serpentina*) used in the treatment of hypertension and mental disorders

Rauwolf, Leonhard (1535–1596), German botanist.

ray·less goldenrod \ˈrā-ləs-\ n : a shrubby or herbaceous plant (*Haplopappus heterophyllus* syn. *Isocoma wrightii*) of the daisy family (Compositae) that occurs esp. on open saline ground from Texas to Arizona and northern Mexico and causes trembles in cattle

Ray·naud's disease \rā-ˈnōz-\ n : a vascular disorder marked by recurrent spasm of the capillaries and esp. those of the fingers and toes upon exposure to cold, characterized by pallor, cyanosis and redness in succession, usu. accompanied by pain, and in severe cases progressing to local gangrene

Raynaud, Maurice (1834–1881), French physician.

Raynaud's phenomenon n : the symptoms associated with Raynaud's disease — called also *Raynaud's syndrome*

Rb *symbol* rubidium

RBC *abbr* **1** red blood cells **2** red blood count

RBE *abbr* relative biological effectiveness

rd *abbr* rutherford

RD *abbr* registered dietitian

RDA *abbr* Recommended Daily Allowance

RDS *abbr* respiratory distress syndrome

Re *symbol* rhenium

re·ab·sorb \ˌrē-əb-ˈsȯrb, -ˈzȯrb\ vb : to take up (something previously secreted or emitted) ⟨sugars ~*ed* in the kidney⟩; *also* : RESORB — **re·ab·sorp·tion** \-ˈsȯrp-shən, -ˈzȯrp-\ n

re·act \rē-ˈakt\ vb **1** : to respond to a stimulus **2** : to undergo or cause to undergo chemical reaction

re·ac·tion \rē-ˈak-shən\ n **1** : the act or process or an instance of reacting **2** : bodily response to or activity aroused by a stimulus: **a** : an action induced by vital resistance to another action; *esp* : the response of tissues to a foreign substance (as an antigen or infective agent) **b** : depression or exhaustion due to excessive exertion or stimulation **c** : heightened activity succeeding depression or shock **d** : a mental or emotional disorder forming an individual's response to his or her life situation **3 a** (1) : chemical transformation or change : the interaction of chemical entities (2) : the state resulting from such a reaction **b** : a process involving change in atomic nuclei

reaction formation n : a psychological defense mechanism in which one form of behavior substitutes for or conceals a diametrically opposed repressed impulse in order to protect against it

reaction time n : the time elapsing between the beginning of the application of a stimulus and the beginning of an organism's reaction to it

re·ac·ti·vate \ˌrē-ˈak-tə-ˌvāt\ vb **-vated; -vat·ing** : to cause to be again active or more active: as **a** : to cause (as a repressed complex) to reappear in consciousness or behavior **b** : to cause (a quiescent disease) to become active again in an individual — **re·ac·ti·va·tion** \-ˌak-tə-ˈvā-shən\ n

re·ac·tive \rē-ˈak-tiv\ adj **1 a** : of, relating to, or marked by reaction ⟨~ symptoms⟩ **b** : capable of reacting chemically **2 a** : readily responsive to a stimulus **b** : occurring as a result of stress or emotional upset esp. from factors outside the organism ⟨~ depression⟩ — **re·ac·tiv·i·ty** \ˌrē-ˌak-ˈti-və-tē\ n

re·ac·tor \rē-ˈak-tər\ n **1** : one that reacts: as **a** : a chemical reagent **b** : an individual reacting to a stimulus **c** : an individual reacting positively to a foreign substance (as in a test for disease) **2** : a device for the controlled release of nuclear energy

re·agent \rē-ˈā-jənt\ n : a substance

used (as in detecting or measuring a component or in preparing a product) because of its chemical or biological activity

re·agin \'rē-ə-jən, -gən\ *n* **1** : a substance in the blood of persons with syphilis responsible for positive serological reactions for syphilis **2** : an antibody in the blood of individuals with some forms of allergy possessing the power of passively sensitizing the skin of normal individuals — **re·agin·ic** \ˌrē-ə-'ji-nik, -'gi-\ *adj*

reality principle *n* : the tendency to defer immediate instinctual gratification so as to achieve longer-range goals or so as to meet external demands — compare PLEASURE PRINCIPLE

reality testing *n* : the psychological process in which acts are explored and their outcomes determined so that the individual will be aware of these consequences when the stimulus to act in a given fashion recurs

ream·er \'rē-mər\ *n* : an instrument used in dentistry to enlarge and clean out a root canal

re·am·pu·ta·tion \ˌrē-ˌam-pyə-'tā-shən\ *n* : the second of two amputations performed upon the same member

re·anas·to·mo·sis \ˌrē-ə-ˌnas-tə-'mō-səs\ *n, pl* **-mo·ses** \-ˌsēz\ : the reuniting (as by surgery or healing) of a divided vessel

re·at·tach \ˌrē-ə-'tach\ *vb* : to attach again (∼ a severed finger) — **re·at·tach·ment** \-mənt\ *n*

re·base \rē-'bās\ *vb* **re·based; re·bas·ing** : to modify the base of (a denture) after an initial period of wear in order to produce a good fit

re·bound \'rē-ˌbau̇nd, ri-'\ *n* : a spontaneous reaction; *esp* : a return to a previous state or condition following removal of a stimulus or cessation of treatment

rebound tenderness *n* : a sensation of pain felt when pressure (as to the abdomen) is suddenly removed

re·breathe \rē-'brēth\ *vb* **re·breathed; re·breath·ing 1** : to breathe (as reconstituted air) again **2** : to inhale previously exhaled air or gases

re·cal·ci·fi·ca·tion \ˌrē-ˌkal-sə-fə-'kā-shən\ *n* : the restoration of calcium or calcium compounds to decalcified tissue (as bone or blood) — **re·cal·ci·fied** \-'kal-sə-ˌfīd\ *adj*

recalcification time *n* : a measure of the time taken for clot formation in recalcified blood

re·cal·ci·trant \ri-'kal-sə-trənt\ *adj* : not responsive to treatment

re·call \ri-'kȯl, 'rē-ˌ\ *n* : remembrance of what has been previously learned or experienced — **re·call** \ri-'kȯl\ *vb*

re·can·a·li·za·tion \ˌrē-ˌkan-əl-ə-'zā-shən\ *n* : the process of restoring flow to or reuniting an interrupted channel of a bodily tube (as a blood vessel or vas deferens) — **re·can·a·lize** \-kə-'na-ˌlīz, -'kan-əl-ˌīz\ *vb*

re·cep·tive \ri-'sep-tiv\ *adj* **1** : open and responsive to ideas, impressions, or suggestions **2 a** *of a sensory end organ* : fit to receive and transmit stimuli **b** : SENSORY 1 — **re·cep·tive·ness** *n* — **re·cep·tiv·i·ty** \ˌrē-ˌsep-'ti-və-tē, ri-\ *n*

re·cep·tor \ri-'sep-tər\ *n* **1** : a cell or group of cells that receives stimuli : SENSE ORGAN **2** : a chemical group or molecule (as a protein) on the cell surface or in the cell interior that has an affinity for a specific chemical group, molecule, or virus **3** : a cellular entity (as a beta-receptor) that is a postulated intermediary between a chemical agent (as a neurohormone) acting on nervous tissue and the physiological or pharmacological response

re·cess \'rē-ˌses, ri-'\ *n* : an anatomical depression or cleft : FOSSA

re·ces·sion \ri-'se-shən\ *n* : pathological withdrawal of tissue from its normal position ⟨gingival ∼⟩

¹re·ces·sive \ri-'se-siv\ *adj* **1** : producing little or no phenotypic effect when occurring in heterozygous condition with a contrasting allele ⟨∼ genes⟩ **2** : expressed only when the determining gene is in the homozygous condition ⟨∼ traits⟩ — **re·ces·sive·ly** *adv* — **re·ces·sive·ness** *n*

²recessive *n* **1** : a recessive character or gene **2** : an organism possessing one or more recessive characters

re·cid·i·vism \ri-'si-də-ˌvi-zəm\ *n* : a tendency to relapse into a previous condition or mode of behavior ⟨∼ among heroin addicts⟩; *esp* : relapse into criminal behavior — **re·cid·i·vist** \-vist\ *n*

rec·i·pe \'re-sə-(ˌ)pē\ *n* : PRESCRIPTION 1

re·cip·i·ent \ri-'si-pē-ənt\ *n* : one who receives biological material (as blood or an organ) from a donor

reciprocal inhibition *n* **1** : RECIPROCAL INNERVATION **2** : behavior therapy in which the patient is exposed to anxiety-producing stimuli while in a controlled state of relaxation so that the anxiety response is gradually inhibited

reciprocal innervation *n* : innervation so that the contraction of a muscle or set of muscles (as of a joint) is accompanied by the simultaneous inhibition of an antagonistic muscle or set of muscles

reciprocal translocation *n* : exchange of parts between nonhomologous chromosomes

Reck·ling·hau·sen's disease \'re-kliŋ-ˌhau̇-zənz-\ *n* : NEUROFIBROMATOSIS
Recklinghausen, Friedrich Daniel von (1833–1910), German pathologist.

rec·og·ni·tion \ˌre-kəg-'ni-shən\ *n* : the form of memory that consists in knowing or feeling that a present object has been met before

¹**re·com·bi·nant** \rē-ˈkäm-bə-nənt\ adj **1** : relating to or exhibiting genetic recombination **2** : relating to or containing recombinant DNA; also : produced by recombinant DNA technology

²**recombinant** n : an individual exhibiting recombination

recombinant DNA n : genetically engineered DNA prepared in vitro by cutting up DNA molecules and splicing together specific DNA fragments usu. from more than one species of organism

re·com·bi·na·tion \ˌrē-ˌkäm-bə-ˈnā-shən\ n : the formation by the processes of crossing-over and independent assortment of new combinations of genes in progeny that did not occur in the parents — **re·com·bi·na·tion·al** adj

Recommended Daily Allowance n : the amount of a substance (as a vitamin or mineral) that is officially recommended for daily consumption by a governmental board of nutrition experts — abbr. RDA

re·com·pres·sion \ˌrē-kəm-ˈpre-shən\ n : a renewed heightening of atmospheric pressure esp. as treatment for decompression sickness

re·con·sti·tute \rē-ˈkän-stə-ˌtüt, -ˌtyüt\ vb **-tut·ed; -tut·ing** : to constitute again or anew; esp : to restore to a former condition by adding liquid ⟨reconstituted blood plasma⟩ — **re·con·sti·tu·tion** \-ˌkän-stə-ˈtü-shən, -ˈtyü-\ n

re·con·struc·tion \ˌrē-kən-ˈstrək-shən\ n : repair of an organ or part by reconstructive surgery (breast ∼) — **re·con·struct** \ˌrē-kən-ˈstrəkt\ vb

re·con·struc·tive \-ˈstrək-tiv\ adj : of, relating to, or being reconstructive surgery

reconstructive surgery n : surgery to restore function or normal appearance by remaking defective organs or parts

re·cov·er \ri-ˈkə-vər\ vb **re·cov·ered; re·cov·er·ing** : to regain a normal position or condition (as of health) — **re·cov·er·able** \ri-ˈkə-və-rə-bəl\ adj

re·cov·ery \ri-ˈkə-və-rē\ n, pl **-er·ies** : the act of regaining or returning toward a normal or healthy state

recovery room n : a hospital room which is equipped with apparatus for meeting postoperative emergencies and in which surgical patients are kept during the immediate postoperative period for care and recovery from anesthesia — abbr. RR

rec·re·a·tion·al therapy \ˌre-krē-ˈā-shə-nəl-\ n : therapy by means of recreational activities engaged in by the patient — compare OCCUPATIONAL THERAPY

re·cru·des·cence \ˌrē-krü-ˈdes-ᵊns\ n : increased severity of a disease after

a remission; also : recurrence of a disease after a brief intermission — compare RELAPSE — **re·cru·desce** \ˌrē-krü-ˈdes\ vb — **re·cru·des·cent** \-ˈdes-ᵊnt\ adj

re·cruit·ment \ri-ˈkrüt-mənt\ n **1** : the increase in intensity of a reflex when the initiating stimulus is prolonged without alteration of intensity due to the activation of increasing numbers of motoneurons **2** : an abnormally rapid increase in the sensation of loudness with increasing sound intensity that occurs in deafness of neural original

rect- or **recto-** comb form **1** : rectum ⟨rectal⟩ **2** : rectal and ⟨rectovaginal⟩

recta pl of RECTUM

rec·tal \ˈrekt-ᵊl\ adj : relating to, affecting, or being near the rectum — **rec·tal·ly** adv

rectal artery n : any of three arteries supplying esp. the rectum: **a** : one arising from the internal pudendal artery and supplying the lower part of the rectum and the perineal region — called also inferior hemorrhoidal artery, inferior rectal artery **b** : one arising from the internal iliac artery and supplying the middle part of the rectum — called also middle hemorrhoidal artery, middle rectal artery **c** : one that is a continuation of the inferior mesenteric artery and that supplies the upper part of the rectum — called also superior hemorrhoidal artery, superior rectal artery

rectal vein n : any of three veins that receive blood from the rectal venous plexus: **a** : one draining the lower part of the rectal venous plexus and emptying into the internal pudendal vein — called also inferior hemorrhoidal vein, inferior rectal vein **b** : one draining the bladder, prostate, and seminal vesicle by way of the middle part of the rectal venous plexus and emptying into the internal iliac vein — called also middle hemorrhoidal vein, middle rectal vein **c** : one draining the upper part of the rectal venous plexus and forming the first part of the inferior mesenteric vein — called also superior hemorrhoidal vein, superior rectal vein

rectal venous plexus n : a plexus of veins that surrounds the rectum and empties esp. into the rectal veins — called also rectal plexus

recti pl of RECTUS

recto- — see RECT-

rec·to·cele \ˈrek-tə-ˌsēl\ n : herniation of the rectum through a defect in the intervening fascia into the vagina

rec·to·sig·moid \ˌrek-tō-ˈsig-ˌmȯid\ n : the distal part of the sigmoid flexure and the proximal part of the rectum

rec·to·uter·ine pouch \ˌrek-tō-ˈyü-tə-ˌrīn-, -rən-\ n : a sac between the rectum and the uterus that is formed by a folding of the peritoneum — compare RECTOVESICAL POUCH

rec·to·vag·i·nal \-'vaj-ən-ᵊl\ *adj* : of, relating to, or connecting the rectum and the vagina (a ~ fistula)

rec·to·ves·i·cal fascia \ˌrek-tō-'ve-si-kəl-\ *n* : a membrane derived from the pelvic fascia and investing the rectum, bladder, and adjacent parts

rectovesical pouch *n* : a sac between the rectum and the urinary bladder in males that is formed by a folding of the peritoneum — compare RECTOUTERINE POUCH

rec·tum \'rek-təm\ *n, pl* **rectums** *or* **rec·ta** \-tə\ : the terminal part of the intestine from the sigmoid flexure to the anus

rec·tus \'rek-təs\ *n, pl* **rec·ti** \-ˌtī\ 1 : any of several straight muscles (as the rectus femoris) 2 : any of four muscles of the eyeball that arise from the border of the optic foramen and run forward to insert into the sclera of the eyeball: **a** : one that inserts into the superior aspect of the sclera — called also *rectus superior, superior rectus* **b** : one that inserts into the lateral aspect of the sclera — called also *lateral rectus, rectus lateralis* **c** : one that inserts into the medial aspect of the sclera — called also *medial rectus, rectus medialis* **d** : one that inserts into the inferior aspect of the sclera — called also *inferior rectus, rectus inferior*

rectus ab·dom·i·nis \-ab-'dä-mə-nəs\ *n* : a long flat muscle on either side of the linea alba extending along the whole length of the front of the abdomen, arising from the pubic crest and symphysis, inserted into the cartilages of the fifth, sixth, and seventh ribs, and acting to flex the spinal column, tense the anterior wall of the abdomen, and assist in compressing the contents of the abdomen

rectus ca·pi·tis posterior major \-'ka-pə-təs-\ *n* : a muscle on each side of the back of the neck that arises from the spinous process of the axis, inserts into the lateral aspect of the inferior nuchal line and the adjacent inferior area of the occipital bone, and acts to extend and rotate the head

rectus capitis posterior minor *n* : a muscle on each side of the back of the neck that arises from the posterior arch of the atlas, inserts esp. into the medial aspect of the inferior nuchal line, and acts to extend the head

rectus fem·o·ris \-'fe-mə-rəs\ *n* : a division of the quadriceps muscle lying in the anterior middle region of the thigh, arising from the ilium by two heads, inserted into the tuberosity of the tibia by a narrow flattened tendon, and acting to flex the thigh at the hip and with the rest of the quadriceps to extend the leg at the knee

rectus inferior *n* : RECTUS 2d

rectus lat·e·ra·lis \-ˌla-tə-'rā-ləs, -'ra-\ *n* : RECTUS 2b

rectus me·di·a·lis \-ˌmē-dē-'ā-ləs, -'a-\ *n* : RECTUS 2c

rectus oc·u·li \-'ä-kyü-ˌlī, -ˌlē\ *n* : RECTUS 2

rectus superior *n* : RECTUS 2a

re·cum·bent \ri-'kəm-bənt\ *adj* : lying down (a patient ~ on a stretcher) — **re·cum·ben·cy** \-bən-sē\ *n*

re·cu·per·a·tion \ri-ˌkü-pə-'rā-shən, -ˌkyü-\ *n* : restoration to health or strength — **re·cu·per·ate** \ri-'kü-pə-ˌrāt\ *vb*

re·cu·per·a·tive \-'kü-pə-ˌrā-tiv, -'kyü-\ *adj* 1 : of or relating to recuperation (~ powers) 2 : aiding in recuperation : RESTORATIVE (strongly ~ remedies)

re·cur·rence \ri-'kər-əns\ *n* 1 : return of symptoms of a disease after a remission 2 : reappearance of a tumor after previous removal — **re·cur** \ri-'kər\ *vb*

re·cur·rent \-'kər-ənt\ *adj* 1 : running or turning back in a direction opposite to a former course — used of various nerves and branches of vessels in the arms and legs 2 : returning or happening time after time (~ complaints) — **re·cur·rent·ly** *adv*

recurrent fever *n* : RELAPSING FEVER

recurrent laryngeal nerve *n* : LARYNGEAL NERVE b — called also *recurrent laryngeal*

red alga \'red-\ *n* : any of a major group (Rhodophyta) of chiefly marine algae that have predominantly red pigmentation — see IRISH MOSS

red–blind *adj* : affected with protanopia

red blindness *n* : PROTANOPIA

red blood cell *n* : any of the hemoglobin-containing cells that carry oxygen to the tissues and are responsible for the red color of blood — called also *erythrocyte, red blood corpuscle, red cell, red corpuscle;* compare WHITE BLOOD CELL

red blood count *n* : a blood count of the red blood cells — abbr. *RBC*

red bone marrow *n* : MARROW 1b

red bug \-ˌbəg\ *n, Southern & Midland* : CHIGGER 2

red cell *n* : RED BLOOD CELL

red corpuscle *n* : RED BLOOD CELL

red devils *n pl, slang* : REDS

red–green blindness *n* : dichromatism in which the spectrum is seen in tones of yellow and blue — called also *red= green color blindness*

re·dia \'rē-dē-ə\ *n, pl* **re·di·ae** \-dē-ˌē\ *also* **re·di·as** : a larva produced within the sporocyst of many trematodes that produces another generation of larvae or develops into a cercaria — **re·di·al** \-dē-əl\ *adj*

red·in·te·gra·tion \ri-ˌdin-tə-'grā-shən, re-\ *n* 1 : revival of the whole of a previous mental state when a phase of it recurs 2 : arousal of any response by a part of the complex of stimuli that orig. aroused that response — **red-in·te·gra·tive** \-'din-tə-ˌgrā-tiv\ *adj*

red marrow *n* : MARROW 1b

red nucleus *n* : a nucleus of gray matter in the tegmentum of the midbrain on each side of the middle line that receives fibers from the cerebellum on the opposite side by way of the superior cerebellar peduncle and gives rise to fibers of the rubrospinal tract of the opposite side

red·out \'red-ˌaut\ *n* : a condition in which centripetal acceleration (as that created when an aircraft abruptly enters a dive) drives blood to the head and causes reddening of the visual field and headache — compare BLACKOUT, GRAYOUT

re·dox \'rē-ˌdäks\ *n* : OXIDATION-REDUCTION — **redox** *adj*

red pulp *n* : a parenchymatous tissue of the spleen that consists of loose plates or cords infiltrated with red blood cells — compare WHITE PULP

reds *n pl, slang* : red drug capsules containing the sodium salt of secobarbital — called also *red devils*

red tide *n* : seawater discolored by the presence of large numbers of dinoflagellates esp. of the genera *Gonyaulax* and *Gymnodinium* which produce a toxin poisonous esp. to many forms of marine vertebrate life and to humans who consume contaminated shellfish — see PARALYTIC SHELLFISH POISONING; compare SAXITOXIN

re·duce \ri-'düs, -'dyüs\ *vb* **re·duced; re·duc·ing 1** : to correct (as a fracture or a herniated mass) by bringing displaced or broken parts back into their normal positions **2 a** : to combine with or subject to the action of hydrogen **b** (1) : to change (an element or ion) from a higher to a lower oxidation state (2) : to add one or more electrons to (an atom or ion or molecule) **3** : to lose weight by dieting — **re·duc·ible** \-'dü-sə-bəl, -'dyü-\ *adj*

reducing *adj* : causing or facilitating reduction

reducing agent *n* : a substance (as hydrogen) that donates electrons or a share in its electrons to another substance — compare OXIDIZING AGENT

reducing sugar *n* : a sugar (as glucose or lactose) that is capable of reducing a mild oxidizing agent (as Fehling solution) — see BENEDICT'S TEST

re·duc·tase \ri-'dək-ˌtās, -ˌtāz\ *n* : an enzyme that catalyzes chemical reduction

re·duc·tion \ri-'dək-shən\ *n* **1** : the replacement or realignment of a body part in normal position or restoration of a bodily condition to normal **2** : the process of reducing by chemical or electrochemical means **3** : MEIOSIS; *specif* : production of the gametic

chromosome number in the first meiotic division

reduction division *n* : the usu. first division of meiosis in which chromosome reduction occurs; *also* : MEIOSIS

re·dun·dant \ri-'dən-dənt\ *adj* : characterized by or containing an excess or superfluous amount

re·du·pli·ca·tion \ri-ˌdü-pli-'kā-shən, ˌrē-, -ˌdyü-\ *n* : an act or instance of doubling ⟨∼ of the chromosomes⟩

red water *n* : any of several cattle diseases characterized by hematuria; *esp* : any of several babesioses (as Texas fever) in which hemoglobin liberated by the destruction of red blood cells appears in the urine

red worm *n* : BLOODWORM

Reed–Stern·berg cell \'rēd-'stərn-bərg-\ *n* : a binucleate or multinucleate acidophilic giant cell found in the tissues in Hodgkin's disease

Reed, Dorothy (1874–1964), American pathologist.

Sternberg, Carl (1872–1935), Austrian pathologist.

re·ed·u·ca·tion \ˌrē-ˌe-jə-'kā-shən\ *n* **1** : training in the use of muscles in new functions or of prosthetic devices in old functions in order to replace or restore lost functions (neuromuscular ∼) **2** : training to develop new behaviors (as attitudes or habits) to replace others that are considered undesirable — **re·ed·u·cate** \-'e-jə-ˌkāt\ *vb*

reef·er \'rē-fər\ *n* : a marijuana cigarette; *also* : MARIJUANA 2

re·en·try \ˌrē-'en-trē\ *n, pl* **-tries** : a cardiac mechanism that is held to explain certain abnormal heart actions (as tachycardia) and that involves the transmission of a wave of depolarization along an alternate pathway when the original pathway is blocked with return of the impulse along the blocked pathway when the alternate pathway is refractory and then transmission along the open pathway resulting in an abnormality

re·ep·i·the·li·al·iza·tion \ˌrē-ˌe-pə-ˌthē-lē-ə-li-'zā-shən\ *n* : restoration of epithelium over a denuded area (as a burn site) by natural growth or plastic surgery

re·fer \ri-'fər\ *vb* **re·ferred; re·fer·ring 1** : to regard as coming from or localized in a certain portion of the body or of space **2** : to send or direct for diagnosis or treatment

re·fer·able \'re-fə-rə-bəl, ri-'fər-ə-\ *adj* : capable of being considered in relation to something else ⟨complaints ∼ to the upper left quadrant of the abdomen⟩

¹ref·er·ence \'re-frəns, -fə-rəns\ *n* — see IDEA OF REFERENCE

²reference *adj* : of known potency and used as a standard in the biological assay of a sample of the same drug of unknown strength

re·fer·rable *var of* REFERABLE

re·fer·ral \ri-ˈfər-əl\ *n* **1** : the process of directing or redirecting (as a medical case or a patient) to an appropriate specialist or agency for definitive treatment **2** : one that is referred

referred pain *n* : a pain subjectively localized in one region though due to irritation in another region

¹**re·fill** \ˈrē-ˈfil\ *vb* : to fill (a prescription) a second or subsequent time — **re·fill·able** *adj*

²**re·fill** \ˈrē-ˌfil\ *n* : a prescription compounded and dispensed for a second or subsequent time without an order from the physician

re·flect \ri-ˈflekt\ *vb* **1** : to bend or fold back : impart a backward curve, bend, or fold to **2** : to push or lay aside (as tissue or an organ) during surgery in order to gain access to the part to be operated on **3** : to throw back light or sound — **re·flec·tion** \ri-ˈflek-shən\ *n*

¹**re·flex** \ˈrē-ˌfleks\ *n* **1** : an automatic and often inborn response to a stimulus that involves a nerve impulse passing inward from a receptor to a nerve center and thence outward to an effector (as a muscle or gland) without reaching the level of consciousness — compare HABIT 2 : the process that culminates in a reflex and comprises reception, transmission, and reaction **3** *pl* : the power of acting or responding with adequate speed

²**reflex** *adj* **1** : bent, turned, or directed back : REFLECTED **2** : of, relating to, or produced by a reflex without intervention of consciousness

reflex arc *n* : the complete nervous path that is involved in a reflex

re·flex·ion *Brit var of* REFLECTION

re·flex·ive \ri-ˈflek-siv\ *adj* : characterized by habitual and unthinking behavior; *also* : relating to or consisting of a reflex

re·flex·ly *adv* : in a reflex manner : by means of reflexes

re·flexo·gen·ic \ˌrē-ˌflek-sə-ˈje-nik\ *adj* **1** : causing or being the point of origin of reflexes (a ~ zone) **2** : originating reflexly

re·flex·ol·o·gy \ˌrē-ˌflek-ˈsä-lə-jē\ *n*, *pl* **-gies** **1** : the study and interpretation of behavior in terms of simple and complex reflexes **2** : massage of the feet or hands based on the belief that pressure applied to specific points on these extremities benefits other parts of the body — **re·flex·ol·o·gist** \-jist\ *n*

re·flux \ˈrē-ˌfləks\ *n* : a flowing back : REGURGITATION (gastroesophageal ~) (mitral valve ~) — **reflux** *adj* — **reflux** *vb*

re·frac·tile \ri-ˈfrak-təl, -ˌtīl\ *adj* : REFRACTIVE (~ cells)

re·frac·tion \ri-ˈfrak-shən\ *n* **1** : the deflection from a straight path undergone by a light ray or a wave of energy in passing obliquely from one medium (as air) into another (as glass) in which its velocity is different **2 a** : the refractive power of the eye **b** : the act or technique of determining ocular refraction and identifying abnormalities as a basis for the prescription of corrective lenses — **re·fract** \ri-ˈfrakt\ *vb*

re·frac·tion·ist \-shə-nist\ *n* : one (as an optometrist) skilled esp. in the determination of errors of refraction in the eye

re·frac·tive \ri-ˈfrak-tiv\ *adj* **1** : having power to refract (~ lens) **2** : relating to or due to refraction — **re·frac·tive·ly** *adv*

refractive index *n* : INDEX OF REFRACTION

re·frac·to·ri·ness \ri-ˈfrak-tə-rē-nəs\ *n* : the insensitivity to further immediate stimulation that develops in irritable and esp. nervous tissue as a result of intense or prolonged stimulation

re·frac·to·ry \ri-ˈfrak-tə-rē\ *adj* **1** : resistant to treatment or cure (a ~ fulminating lesion) **2** : unresponsive to stimulus **3** : resistant or not responding to an infectious agent : IMMUNE

refractory period *n* : the brief period immediately following the response esp. of a muscle or nerve before it recovers the capacity to make a second response — called also *refractory phase;* see ABSOLUTE REFRACTORY PERIOD, RELATIVE REFRACTORY PERIOD

re·frac·ture \ˌrē-ˈfrak-chər\ *vb* **-tured; -tur·ing** : to break along the line of a previous fracture — **refracture** *n*

Ref·sum's disease \ˈref-səmz-\ *n* : an autosomal recessive lipidosis characterized by faulty metabolism of phytanic acid resulting in its accumulation in the blood, retinitis pigmentosa, ataxia, deafness, and mental retardation

Refsum, Sigvold Bernhard (*b* 1907), Norwegian physician.

re·gen·er·a·tion \ri-ˌje-nə-ˈrā-shən, ˌrē-\ *n* : the renewal, regrowth, or restoration of a body or a bodily part, tissue, or substance after injury or as a normal bodily process (continual ~ of epithelial cells) — compare REGULATION 2a — **re·gen·er·ate** \ri-ˈje-nə-ˌrāt\ *vb* — **re·gen·er·a·tive** \ri-ˈje-nə-ˌrā-tiv, -rə-\ *adj*

re·gime \rā-ˈzhēm, ri-ˈjēm\ *n* : REGIMEN

reg·i·men \ˈre-jə-mən\ *n* : a systematic plan (as of diet, therapy, or medication) esp. when designed to improve and maintain the health of a patient

re·gion \ˈrē-jən\ *n* **1** : any of the major subdivisions into which the body or one of its parts is divisible **2** : an indefinite area surrounding a specified body part

re·gion·al \ˈrēj-ən-əl\ *adj* : of, relating to, or affecting a particular bodily region : LOCALIZED

regional anatomy *n* : a branch of anatomy dealing with regions of the body esp. with reference to diagnosis and treatment of disease or injury — called also *topographic anatomy*

regional anesthesia *n* : anesthesia of a region of the body accomplished by a series of encircling injections of an anesthetic — compare BLOCK ANESTHESIA

regional enteritis *n* : CROHN'S DISEASE

regional ileitis *n* : CROHN'S DISEASE

reg·is·tered \'re-ji-stərd\ *adj* : qualified by formal, official, or legal certification or authentication

registered nurse *n* : a graduate trained nurse who has been licensed by a state authority after passing qualifying examinations for registration — called also *RN*

reg·is·trar \'re-ji-ˌsträr\ *n* **1** : an admitting officer at a hospital **2** *Brit* : RESIDENT

reg·is·try \'re-ji-strē\ *n, pl* **-tries 1** : a place where data, records, or laboratory samples are kept and usu. are made available for research or comparative study ⟨a cancer ∼⟩ **2** : an establishment at which nurses available for employment are listed and through which they are hired

Reg·i·tine \'re-ji-ˌtēn\ *trademark* — used for a preparation of phentolamine

re·gres·sion \ri-'gre-shən\ *n* : a trend or shift toward a lower, less severe, or less perfect state: as **a** : progressive decline (as in size or severity) of a manifestation of disease ⟨tumor ∼⟩ **b** (1) : a gradual loss of differentiation and function by a body part esp. as a physiological change accompanying aging ⟨menopausal ∼ of the ovaries⟩ (2) : gradual loss (as in old age) of memories and acquired skills **c** : reversion to an earlier mental or behavioral level or to an earlier stage of psychosexual development in response to organismic stress or to suggestion — **re·gress** \ri-'gres\ *vb* — **re·gres·sive** \ri-'gre-siv\ *adj*

re·grow \rē-'grō\ *vb* **re·grew** \-'grü\; **re·grown** \-'grōn\; **re·grow·ing** \-'grō-iŋ\ : to continue growth after interruption or injury — **re·growth** \-'grōth\ *n*

reg·u·lar \'re-gyə-lər\ *adj* : conforming to what is usual or normal: as **a** : recurring or functioning at fixed or normal intervals ⟨∼ bowel movements⟩ **b** : having menstrual periods or bowel movements at normal intervals — **reg·u·lar·i·ty** \ˌre-gyə-'lar-ə-tē\ *n* — **reg·u·lar·ly** *adv*

reg·u·la·tion \ˌre-gyə-'lā-shən, -gə-\ *n* **1** : the act of fixing or adjusting the time, amount, degree, or rate of something; *also* : the resulting state or condition **2 a** : the process of redistributing material (as in an embryo) to restore a damaged or lost part independent of new tissue growth — compare REGENERATION **b** : the mechanism by which an early em-

bryo maintains normal development **3** : the control of the kind and rate of cellular processes by controlling the activity of individual genes — **reg·u·late** \-ˌlāt\ *vb* — **reg·u·la·to·ry** \-lə-ˌtōr-ē\ *adj*

reg·u·la·tive \'re-gyə-ˌlā-tiv, -lə\ *adj* : INDETERMINATE ⟨∼ eggs⟩

reg·u·la·tor \'re-gyə-ˌlā-tər\ *n* : REGULATORY GENE

regulatory gene *or* **regulator gene** *n* : a gene that regulates the expression of one or more structural genes by controlling the production of a protein (as a genetic repressor) which regulates their rate of transcription

re·gur·gi·tant \rē-'gər-jə-tənt\ *adj* : characterized by, allowing, or being a backward flow (as of blood) ⟨∼ cardiac valves⟩

re·gur·gi·ta·tion \rē-ˌgər-jə-'tā-shən\ *n* **1** : an act of bringing swallowed food back up into the mouth **2** : the backward flow of blood through a defective heart valve — see AORTIC REGURGITATION — **re·gur·gi·tate** \rə-'gər-jə-ˌtāt\ *vb*

re·hab \'rē-ˌhab\ *n, often attrib* : REHABILITATION

re·ha·bil·i·tant \ˌrē-hə-'bi-lə-tənt, ˌrē-ə-\ *n* : an individual undergoing rehabilitation

re·ha·bil·i·ta·tion \ˌrē-hə-ˌbi-lə-'tā-shən, ˌrē-ə-\ *n, often attrib* **1 a** : the physical restoration of a sick or disabled person by therapeutic measures and reeducation ⟨∼ after coronary occlusion⟩ **b** : the process of restoring an individual (as a convict or drug addict) to a useful and constructive place in society through some form of vocational, correctional, or therapeutic retraining **2** : the result of rehabilitation : the state of undergoing or of having undergone rehabilitation — **re·ha·bil·i·tate** \-'bi-lə-ˌtāt\ *vb* — **re·ha·bil·i·ta·tive** \-'bi-lə-ˌtā-tiv\ *adj*

Reh·fuss tube \'rā-fəs-\ *n* : a flexible tube that is used esp. for withdrawing gastric juice from the stomach for analysis and that has a syringe at the upper end and an attachment with a slot at the end passing into the stomach

Rehfuss, Martin Emil (1887–1964), American physician.

re·hy·drate \rē-'hī-ˌdrāt\ *vb* **-drat·ed; -drat·ing** : to restore fluid to (something dehydrated); *esp* : to restore body fluid lost in dehydration to ⟨∼ a patient⟩ — **re·hy·dra·tion** \ˌrē-ˌhī-'drā-shən\ *n*

re·im·plan·ta·tion \ˌrē-ˌim-ˌplan-'tā-shən\ *n* **1** : the restoration of a bodily tissue or part (as a tooth) to the site from which it was removed **2** : the implantation of a fertilized egg in the uterus after it has been removed from the body and fertilized in vitro — **re·im·plant** \-im-'plant\ *vb*

re·in·fec·tion \ˌrē-in-'fek-shən\ *n* : infection following recovery from or superimposed on a previous infection of the same type

re·in·force·ment \ˌrē-ən-ˈfōrs-mənt\ n : the action of causing a subject (as a student or an experimental animal) to learn to give or to increase the frequency of a desired response that in classical conditioning involves the repeated presentation of an unconditioned stimulus (as the sight of food) paired with a conditioned stimulus (as the sound of a bell) and that in operant conditioning involves the use of a reward following a correct response or a punishment following an incorrect response; also : the reward, punishment, or unconditioned stimulus used in reinforcement — **re·in·force** \-ˈfōrs\ vb

re·in·forc·er \-ˈfōr-sər\ n : a stimulus (as a reward or removal of an electric shock) that increases the probability of a desired response in operant conditioning by being applied or removed following the desired response

re·in·ner·va·tion \ˌrē-ˌi-nər-ˈvā-shən, -in-ˌər-\ n : restoration of function e: p. to a denervated muscle by supp,ying it with nerves by regrowth or by grafting — **re·in·ner·vate** \-i-ˈnər-ˌvāt, -ˈi-nər-\ vb

re·in·oc·u·la·tion \ˌrē-i-ˌnä-kyə-ˈlā-shən\ n : inoculation a second or subsequent time with the same organism as the original inoculation — **re·in·oc·u·late** \-ˈnä-kyə-ˌlāt\ vb

re·in·te·gra·tion \ˌrē-ˌin-tə-ˈgrā-shən\ n : repeated and renewed integration (as of the personality and mental activity after mental illness) — **re·in·te·grate** \-ˈin-tə-ˌgrāt\ vb

Reiss·ner's membrane \ˈrīs-nərz-\ n : VESTIBULAR MEMBRANE

Reissner, Ernst (1824–1878), German anatomist.

Rei·ter's syndrome \ˈrī-tərz-\ n : a disease that is usu. initiated by infection in genetically predisposed individuals and is characterized usu. by recurrence of arthritis, conjunctivitis, and urethritis — called also *Reiter's disease*

Reiter, Hans Conrad Julius (1881–1969), German bacteriologist.

re·jec·tion \ri-ˈjek-shən\ n 1 : the action of rebuffing, repelling, refusing to hear, or withholding love from another esp. by communicating negative feelings toward and a wish to be free of the other person 2 : the immunological process of sloughing off foreign tissue or an organ (as a transplant) by the recipient organism — **re·ject** \-ˈjekt\ vb — **re·jec·tive** \-ˈjek-tiv\ adj

re·lapse \ri-ˈlaps, ˈrē-ˌ\ n : a recurrence of illness; *esp* : a recurrence of symptoms of a disease after a period of improvement — compare RECRUDESCENCE — **re·lapse** \ri-ˈlaps\ vb

relapsing febrile nodular non·sup·pu·ra·tive panniculitis \-ˌnän-ˈsə-pyə-rə-tiv-, -ˌrā-\ n : PANNICULITIS 2

relapsing fever n : any of several forms of an acute epidemic infectious disease marked by sudden recurring paroxysms of high fever lasting from five to seven days, articular and muscular pains, and a sudden crisis and caused by a spirochete of the genus *Borrelia* transmitted by the bites of lice and ticks and found in the circulating blood

re·late \ri-ˈlāt\ vb **re·lat·ed; re·lat·ing** : to have meaningful social relationships : interact realistically (an inability to ∼ to other people)

re·la·tion \ri-ˈlā-shən\ n 1 : the attitude or stance which two or more persons or groups assume toward one another (race ∼s) 2 a : the state of being mutually or reciprocally interested (as in social matters) b pl : SEXUAL INTERCOURSE — **re·la·tion·al** \-shə-nəl\ adj

re·la·tion·ship \-shən-ˌship\ n 1 : the state of being related or interrelated (the ∼ between diet, cholesterol, and coronary heart disease) 2 a : a state of affairs existing between those having relations or dealings (the doctor-patient ∼) b : an emotional attachment between individuals

relative biological effectiveness n : the relative capacity of a particular ionizing radiation to produce a response in a biological system — abbr. *RBE*

relative humidity n : the ratio of the amount of water vapor actually present in the air to the greatest amount possible at the same temperature — compare ABSOLUTE HUMIDITY

relative refractory period n : the period shortly after the firing of a nerve fiber when partial repolarization has occurred and a greater than normal stimulus can stimulate a second response — called also *relative refractory phase*; compare ABSOLUTE REFRACTORY PERIOD

re·lax \ri-ˈlaks\ vb 1 : to slacken or make less tense or rigid (alternately contracting and ∼ing their muscles) 2 : to relieve from nervous tension 3 of a muscle or muscle fiber : to become inactive and lengthen 4 : to relieve constipation — **re·lax·ation** \ˌrē-ˌlak-ˈsā-shən, ri-ˌlak\ n

re·lax·ant \ri-ˈlak-sənt\ n : a substance (as a drug) that relaxes; *specif* : one that relieves muscular tension — **re·lax·ant** adj

re·lax·in \ri-ˈlak-sən\ n : a polypeptide sex hormone of the corpus luteum that facilitates birth by causing relaxation of the pelvic ligaments

re·leas·er \ri-ˈlē-sər\ n : a stimulus that serves as the initiator of complex reflex behavior

releasing factor n : HYPOTHALAMIC RELEASING FACTOR

re·li·abil·i·ty \ri-ˌlī-ə-ˈbi-lə-tē\ n, pl **-ties**

: the extent to which an experiment, test, or measuring procedure yields the same results on repeated trials — **re·li·a·ble** \ri-ˈlī-ə-bəl\ *adj*

re·lief \ri-ˈlēf\ *n* : removal or lightening of something oppressive or distressing (~ of pain)

re·lieve \ri-ˈlēv\ *vb* **re·lieved; re·liev·ing 1** : to bring about the removal or alleviation of (pain or discomfort) **2** : to emit the contents of the bladder or bowels of (oneself) — **re·liev·er** *n*

rem \ˈrem\ *n* : the dosage of an ionizing radiation that will cause the same biological effect as one roentgen of X-ray or gamma-ray dosage — compare REP

REM \ˈrem\ *n* : RAPID EYE MOVEMENT

re·me·di·a·ble \ri-ˈmē-dē-ə-bəl\ *adj* : capable of being remedied

re·me·di·al \ri-ˈmē-dē-əl\ *adj* : affording a remedy : intended as a remedy (~ surgery)

re·me·di·a·tion \ri-ˌmē-dē-ˈā-shən\ *n* : the act or process of remedying

rem·e·dy \ˈre-mə-dē\ *n, pl* **-dies** : a medicine, application, or treatment that relieves or cures a disease — **remedy** *vb*

re·min·er·al·i·za·tion \ˌrē-ˌmi-nə-rə-lə-ˈzā-shən\ *n* : the restoring of minerals to demineralized structures or substances (~ of bone) — **re·min·er·al·ize** \-ˈmi-nə-rə-ˌlīz\ *vb*

re·mis·sion \ri-ˈmi-shən\ *n* : a state or period during which the symptoms of a disease are abated — compare INTERMISSION

re·mit \ri-ˈmit\ *vb* **re·mit·ted; re·mit·ting** : to abate symptoms for a period : go into or be in remission

re·mit·tent \ri-ˈmit-ənt\ *adj* : marked by alternating periods of abatement and increase of symptoms (~ fever)

REM sleep *n* : a state of sleep that recurs cyclically several times during a normal period of sleep and that is characterized by increased neuronal activity of the forebrain and midbrain, by depressed muscle tone, and esp. in humans by dreaming, rapid eye movements, and vascular congestion of the sex organs — called also *paradoxical sleep, rapid eye movement sleep;* compare SLOW≠WAVE SLEEP

re·nal \ˈrēn-əl\ *adj* : relating to, involving, affecting, or located in the region of the kidneys : NEPHRITIC

renal artery *n* : either of two branches of the abdominal aorta of which each supplies one of the kidneys and gives off smaller branches to the ureter, adrenal gland, and adjoining structures

renal calculus *n* : KIDNEY STONE

renal cast *n* : a cast of a renal tubule consisting of granular, hyaline, albuminoid, or other material formed in and discharged from the kidney in renal disease

renal clearance *n* : CLEARANCE

renal colic *n* : the severe pain produced by the passage of a calculus from the kidney through the ureter

renal column *n* : any of the masses of cortical tissue extending between the sides of the renal pyramids of the kidney as far as the renal pelvis — called also *Bertin's column, column of Bertin*

renal corpuscle *n* : the part of a nephron that consists of Bowman's capsule with its included glomerulus — called also *Malpighian body, Malpighian corpuscle*

renal glycosuria *n* : excretion of glucose associated with increased permeability of the kidneys without increased sugar concentration in the blood

renal hypertension *n* : hypertension that is associated with disease of the kidneys and is caused by kidney damage or malfunctioning

renal osteodystrophy *n* : a painful rachitic condition of abnormal bone growth that is associated with chronic acidosis, hypocalcemia, hyperplasia of the parathyroid glands, and hyperphosphatemia caused by chronic renal insufficiency — called also *renal rickets*

renal papilla *n* : the apex of a renal pyramid which projects into the lumen of a calyx of the kidney and through which collecting tubules discharge urine

renal pelvis *n* : a funnel-shaped structure in each kidney that is formed at one end by the expanded upper portion of the ureter lying in the renal sinus and at the other end by the union of the calyces of the kidney

renal plexus *n* : a plexus of the autonomic nervous system that arises esp. from the celiac plexus, surrounds the renal artery, and accompanies it into the kidney which it innervates

renal pyramid *n* : any of the conical masses that form the medullary substance of the kidney, project as the renal papillae into the renal pelvis, and are made up of bundles of straight uriniferous tubules opening at the apex of the conical mass — called also *Malpighian pyramid*

renal rickets *n* : RENAL OSTEODYSTROPHY

renal sinus *n* : the main cavity of the kidney that is an expansion behind the hilum and contains the renal pelvis, calyces, and the major renal vessels

renal threshold *n* : the concentration level up to which a substance (as glucose) in the blood is prevented from passing through the kidneys into the urine

renal tubular acidosis *n* : decreased ability of the kidneys to excrete hydrogen ions that is associated with a defect in the renal tubules without a defect in the glomeruli and that results in the production of urine deficient in acidity

renal tubule n : the part of a nephron that leads away from a glomerulus, that is made up of a proximal convoluted tubule, loop of Henle, and distal convoluted tubule, and that empties into a collecting tubule

renal vein n : a short thick vein that is formed in each kidney by the convergence of the interlobar veins, leaves the kidney through the hilum, and empties into the inferior vena cava

Ren·du–Os·ler–Web·er disease \ˌrän-ˈdü-ˈäs-lər-ˈwe-bər-, ˌrän-ˈdyü-\ n : HEREDITARY HEMORRHAGIC TELANGIECTASIA

Ren·du \rän-ˈdue\, **Henry–Jules–Louis–Marie (1844–1902),** French physician.

Osler, Sir William (1849–1919), American physician.

F. P. Weber — see WEBER-CHRISTIAN DISEASE

Ren·ese \ˈre-ˌnēz\ *trademark* — used for a preparation of polythiazide

reni- *or* **reno-** *comb form* **1** : kidney ⟨*reni*form⟩ **2** : renal and ⟨*reno*vascular⟩

re·ni·form \ˈrē-nə-ˌfórm, ˈre-\ *adj* : suggesting a kidney in outline

re·nin \ˈrē-nən, ˈre-\ n : a proteolytic enzyme of the blood that is produced and secreted by the juxtaglomerular cells of the kidney and hydrolyzes angiotensinogen to angiotensin I

ren·nin \ˈre-nən\ n : a crystallizable enzyme that coagulates milk, occurs esp. with pepsin in the gastric juice of young animals, and is used in making cheese

re·no·gram \ˈrē-nə-ˌgram\ n : a photographic depiction of the course of renal excretion of a radioactively labeled substance — **re·no·graph·ic** \ˌrē-nə-ˈgra-fik\ *adj* — **re·nog·ra·phy** \rē-ˈnä-grə-fē\ n

re·no·vas·cu·lar \ˌrē-nō-ˈvas-kyə-lər\ *adj* : of, relating to, or involving the blood vessels of the kidneys ⟨~ hypertension⟩

Ren·shaw cell \ˈren-ˌshó\ n : an internuncial neuron in the ventral horn of gray matter of the spinal cord that has an inhibitory effect on motoneurons

Renshaw, Birdsey (1911–1948), American neurologist.

re·op·er·a·tion \ˌrē-ˌä-pə-ˈrā-shən\ n : an operation to correct a condition not corrected by a previous operation or to correct the complications of a previous operation — **re·op·er·ate** \-ˈä-pə-ˌrāt\ *vb*

reo·vi·rus \ˌrē-ō-ˈvī-rəs\ n : any of a group of double-stranded RNA viruses that lack a lipoprotein envelope, usu. have a capsid consisting of two layers of capsomeres, and include many pathogens of plants or animals

¹rep \ˈrep\ n, *pl* **rep** *or* **reps** : the dosage of any ionizing radiation that will develop the same amount of energy upon absorption in human tissues as one roentgen of X-ray or gamma-ray dosage — compare REM

²rep *abbr* [Latin *repetatur*] let it be repeated — used in writing prescriptions

re·peat \ri-ˈpēt, ˈrē-ˌ\ n : a genetic duplication in which the duplicated parts are adjacent to each other along the chromosome

re·per·fu·sion \ˌrē-pər-ˈfyü-zhən\ n : restoration of the flow of blood to a previously ischemic tissue or organ (as the heart) ⟨~ following myocardial infarction⟩

repetition compulsion n : an irresistible tendency to repeat an emotional experience or to return to a previous psychological state

replacement therapy n : therapy involving the supplying of something (as hormones or blood) lacking from or lost to the system ⟨estrogen *replacement therapy*⟩

re·plan·ta·tion \ˌrē-(ˌ)plan-ˈtā-shən\ n : reattachment or reinsertion of a bodily part (as a limb or tooth) after separation from the body — **re·plant** \rē-ˈplant\ *vb*

rep·li·case \ˈre-pli-ˌkās, -ˌkāz\ n : a polymerase that promotes synthesis of a particular RNA in the presence of a template of RNA — called also *RNA replicase, RNA synthetase*

rep·li·ca·tion \ˌre-plə-ˈkā-shən\ n **1** : the action or process of reproducing or duplicating ⟨~ of DNA⟩ **2** : performance of an experiment or procedure more than once — **rep·li·cate** \ˈre-pli-ˌkāt\ *vb* — **rep·li·cate** \-kət\ n — **rep·li·ca·tive** \ˈre-pli-ˌkā-tiv\ *adj*

rep·li·con \ˈre-pli-ˌkän\ n : a linear or circular section of DNA or RNA which replicates sequentially as a unit

re·po·lar·iza·tion \ˌrē-pō-lə-rə-ˈzā-shən\ n : restoration of the difference in charge between the inside and outside of the plasma membrane of a muscle fiber or cell following depolarization — **re·po·lar·ize** \-ˈpō-lə-ˌrīz\ *vb*

re·port·able \ri-ˈpór-tə-bəl\ *adj* : required by law to be reported ⟨~ diseases⟩

re·po·si·tion \ˌrē-pə-ˈzi-shən\ *vb* : to return to or place in a normal or proper position ⟨~ a dislocated shoulder⟩

re·pos·i·to·ry \ri-ˈpä-zə-ˌtōr-ē\ *adj, of a drug* : designed to act over a prolonged period ⟨~ penicillin⟩

re·press \ri-ˈpres\ *vb* **1** : to exclude from consciousness ⟨~ conflicts⟩ **2** : to inactivate (a gene or formation of a gene product) by allosteric combination at a DNA binding site

re·pressed \ri-ˈprest\ *adj* : subjected to

or marked by repression ⟨a ∼ child⟩ ⟨∼ anger⟩

re·press·ible \ri-ˈpre-sə-bəl\ adj : capable of being repressed

re·pres·sion \ri-ˈpre-shən\ n 1 : the action or process of repressing ⟨gene ∼⟩ 2 a : a process by which unacceptable desires or impulses are excluded from consciousness and left to operate in the unconscious — compare SUPPRESSION c b : an item so excluded

re·pres·sive \ri-ˈpre-siv\ adj : tending to repress or to cause repression

re·pres·sor \ri-ˈpre-sər\ n : one that represses; esp : a protein that is determined by a regulatory gene, binds to a genetic operator, and inhibits the initiation of transcription of messenger RNA

re·pro·duce \ˌrē-prə-ˈdüs, -ˈdyüs\ vb **-duced; -duc·ing 1** : to produce (new individuals of the same kind) by a sexual or asexual process 2 : to achieve (an original result or score) again or anew by repeating an experiment or test

re·pro·duc·tion \ˌrē-prə-ˈdək-shən\ n : the act or process of reproducing; specif : the process by which plants and animals give rise to offspring — **re·pro·duc·tive** \ˌrē-prə-ˈdək-tiv\ adj — **re·pro·duc·tive·ly** adv

reproductive system n : the system of organs and parts which function in reproduction consisting in the male esp. of the testes, penis, seminal vesicles, prostate, and urethra and in the female esp. of the ovaries, fallopian tubes, uterus, vagina, and vulva

RES abbr reticuloendothelial system

res·cin·na·mine \ri-ˈsi-nə-ˌmēn, -ˌmən\ n : an antihypertensive, tranquilizing, and sedative drug $C_{35}H_{42}N_2O_9$ — see MODERIL

re·sect \ri-ˈsekt\ vb : to perform resection on ⟨∼ an ulcer⟩ — **re·sect·abil·i·ty** \ri-ˌsek-tə-ˈbi-lə-tē\ n — **re·sect·able** \ri-ˈsek-tə-bəl\ adj

re·sec·tion \ri-ˈsek-shən\ n : the surgical removal of part of an organ or structure ⟨∼ of the lower bowel⟩ — see WEDGE RESECTION

re·sec·to·scope \ri-ˈsek-tə-ˌskōp\ n : an instrument consisting of a tubular fenestrated sheath with a sliding knife within it that is used for surgery within cavities (as of the prostate through the urethra)

re·ser·pine \ri-ˈsər-ˌpēn, ˈre-sər-pən\ n : an alkaloid $C_{33}H_{40}N_2O_9$ extracted esp. from the root of rauwolfias and used in the treatment of hypertension, mental disorders, and tension states — see RAUDIXIN, SANDRIL, SERPASIL

reservatus see COITUS RESERVATUS

re·serve \ri-ˈzərv\ n 1 : something stored or kept available for future use or need ⟨oxygen ∼⟩ — see CARDIAC RESERVE 2 : the capacity of a solution to neutralize alkali or acid when its reaction is shifted from one hydrogen-ion concentration to another — **reserve** adj

res·er·voir \ˈre-zər-ˌvwär, -ˌvwȯr\ n 1 : a space (as the cavity of a glandular acinus) in which a body fluid is stored 2 : an organism in which a parasite that is pathogenic for some other species lives and multiplies without damaging its host; also : a noneconomic organism within which a pathogen of economic or medical importance flourishes without regard to its pathogenicity for the reservoir ⟨rats are ∼s of plague⟩ — compare CARRIER 1a

reservoir host n : RESERVOIR 2

res·i·den·cy \ˈre-zəd-ən-sē\ n, pl -cies : a period of advanced medical training and education that normally follows graduation from medical school and licensing to practice medicine and that consists of supervised practice of a specialty in a hospital and in its outpatient department and instruction from specialists on the hospital staff

res·i·dent \ˈre-zə-dənt\ n : a physician serving a residency

¹re·sid·u·al \ri-ˈzi-jə-wəl\ adj 1 : of, relating to, or being something that remains: as a : remaining after a disease or operation ⟨∼ paralysis⟩ b : remaining in a body cavity after maximum normal expulsion has occurred ⟨∼ urine⟩ — see RESIDUAL AIR 2 a : leaving a residue that remains effective for some time after application ⟨∼ insecticides⟩ b : of or relating to a residual insecticide ⟨a ∼ spray⟩

²residual n 1 : an internal aftereffect of experience or activity that influences later behavior 2 : a residual abnormality (as a scar or limp)

residual air n : the volume of air still remaining in the lungs after the most forcible expiration possible and amounting usu. to 60 to 100 cubic inches (980 to 1640 cubic centimeters) — called also residual volume; compare SUPPLEMENTAL AIR

residual volume n : RESIDUAL AIR

res·i·due \ˈre-zə-ˌdü, -ˌdyü\ n : something that remains after a part is taken, separated, or designated; specif : a constituent structural unit of a usu. complex molecule ⟨amino acid ∼s in a protein⟩

res·in \ˈrez-ᵊn\ n : any of various substances obtained from the gum or sap of some trees and used esp. in various varnishes and plastics and in medicine; also : a comparable synthetic product — **res·in·ous** \ˈrez-ᵊn-əs\ adj

re·sis·tance \ri-ˈzis-təns\ n 1 : power or capacity to resist; esp : the inherent ability of an organism to resist harmful influences (as disease, toxic agents, or infection) 2 : a mechanism of ego defense wherein a psychoanalysis patient rejects, denies, or otherwise opposes therapeutic efforts by the analyst 3 : the opposition offered by a body to the passage through it of a steady electric current — **re·sis·tant** also **re·sist·ent** \-tənt\ adj

re·so·cial·i·za·tion \ˌrē-ˌsō-shə-lə-ˈzā-shən\ n : readjustment of an individual (as a mentally or physically handicapped person) to life in society

res·o·lu·tion \ˌre-zə-ˈlü-shən\ n 1 : the separating of a chemical compound or mixture into its constituents 2 : the process or capability of making distinguishable the individual parts of an object, closely adjacent optical images, or sources of light 3 : the subsidence of a pathological state (as inflammation) — **re·solve** \ri-ˈzälv, -ˈzolv\ vb

res·o·nance \ˈrez-ᵊn-əns\ n 1 : a quality imparted to voiced sounds by vibration in anatomical resonating chambers or cavities (as the mouth or the nasal cavity) 2 : the sound elicited on percussion of the chest 3 a : the enhancement of an atomic, nuclear, or particle reaction or a scattering event by excitation of internal motion in the system b : MAGNETIC RESONANCE

re·sorb \rē-ˈsorb, -ˈzorb\ vb : to break down and assimilate (something previously differentiated) (~ed bone)

res·or·cin \rə-ˈzors-ᵊn\ n : RESORCINOL

res·or·cin·ol \-ˌol, -ˌōl\ n : a crystalline phenol $C_6H_6O_2$ used in medicine as a fungicidal, bactericidal, and keratolytic agent

resorcinol monoacetate n : a liquid compound $C_8H_8O_3$ that slowly liberates resorcinol and that is used esp. to treat diseases of the scalp

re·sorp·tion \rē-ˈsorp-shən, -ˈzorp-\ n : the action or process of resorbing something (~ of a tooth root) — **re·sorp·tive** \-tiv\ adj

re·spi·ra·ble \ˈres-pə-rə-bəl, ri-ˈspī-rə-\ adj : fit for breathing; also : capable of being taken in by breathing

res·pi·ra·tion \ˌres-pə-ˈrā-shən\ n 1 a : the placing of air or dissolved gases in intimate contact with the circulating medium (as blood) of a multicellular organism (as by breathing) b : a single complete act of breathing (30 ~s per minute) 2 : the physical and chemical processes by which an organism supplies its cells and tissues with the oxygen needed for metabolism and relieves them of the carbon dioxide formed in energy-producing reactions 3 : any of various energy-yielding oxidative reactions in living matter that typically involve transfer of oxygen and production of carbon dioxide and water as end products (cellular ~)

res·pi·ra·tor \ˈres-pə-ˌrā-tər\ n 1 : a device (as a gas mask) worn over the mouth or nose for protecting the respiratory system 2 : a device for maintaining artificial respiration — called also *ventilator*

res·pi·ra·to·ry \ˈres-pə-rə-ˌtōr-ē, ri-

ˈspī-rə-\ adj 1 : of or relating to respiration (~ diseases) 2 : serving for or functioning in respiration (~ organs)

respiratory acidosis n : acidosis caused by excessive retention of carbon dioxide due to a respiratory abnormality (as obstructive lung disease)

respiratory alkalosis n : alkalosis that is caused by excessive elimination of carbon dioxide due to a respiratory abnormality (as hyperventilation)

respiratory center n : a region in the medulla oblongata that regulates respiratory movements

respiratory chain n : the metabolic pathway along which electron transport occurs in cellular respiration; also : the series of enzymes involved in this pathway

respiratory distress syndrome n : HYALINE MEMBRANE DISEASE — abbr. RDS; see ADULT RESPIRATORY DISTRESS SYNDROME

respiratory pigment n : any of various permanently or intermittently colored conjugated proteins and esp. hemoglobin that function in the transfer of oxygen in cellular respiration

respiratory quotient n : the ratio of the volume of carbon dioxide given off in respiration to that of the oxygen consumed — abbr. RQ

respiratory syncytial virus n : a paramyxovirus that forms syncytia in tissue culture and that is responsible for severe respiratory diseases (as bronchopneumonia and bronchiolitis) in children and esp. in infants — abbr. RSV

respiratory system n : a system of organs functioning in respiration and consisting esp. of the nose, nasal passages, nasopharynx, larynx, trachea, bronchi, and lungs — called also *respiratory tract*; see LOWER RESPIRATORY TRACT, UPPER RESPIRATORY TRACT

respiratory therapist n : a specialist in respiratory therapy

respiratory therapy n : the therapeutic treatment of respiratory diseases

respiratory tract n : RESPIRATORY SYSTEM

respiratory tree n : the trachea, bronchi, and bronchioles

re·spire \ri-ˈspīr\ vb **re·spired**; **re·spir·ing** 1 : BREATHE; specif : to inhale and exhale air successively 2 of a cell or tissue : to take up oxygen and produce carbon dioxide through oxidation

res·pi·rom·e·ter \ˌres-pə-ˈrä-mə-tər\ n : an instrument for studying the character and extent of respiration — **res·pi·ro·met·ric** \ˌres-pə-rō-ˈme-trik\ adj — **res·pi·rom·e·try** \ˌres-pə-ˈrä-mə-trē\ n

re·spond \ri-ˈspänd\ vb 1 : to react in response 2 : to show favorable reaction (~ to surgery)

re·spon·dent \ri-ˈspän-dənt\ adj : relating to or being behavior or responses to a stimulus that are followed by a reward ⟨∼ conditioning⟩ — compare OPERANT

re·spond·er \ri-ˈspän-dər\ *n* : one that responds (as to treatment)

re·sponse \ri-ˈspäns\ *n* : the activity or inhibition of previous activity of an organism or any of its parts resulting from stimulation ⟨a conditioned ∼⟩

re·spon·sive \ri-ˈspän-siv\ *adj* : making a response; *esp* : responding to treatment — **re·spon·sive·ness** *n*

rest \ˈrest\ *n* **1** : a state of repose or sleep; *also* : a state of inactivity or motionlessness — see BED REST **2** : the part of a partial denture that rests on an abutment tooth, distributes stresses, and holds the clasp in position **3** : a firm cushion used to raise or support a portion of the body during surgery ⟨a kidney ∼⟩ — **rest** *vb*

rest home *n* : an establishment that provides housing and general care for the aged or the convalescent — compare NURSING HOME

res·ti·form body \ˈres-tə-ˌfȯrm-\ *n* : CEREBELLAR PEDUNCLE c

rest·ing *adj* **1** : not physiologically active **2** : occurring in or performed on a subject at rest ⟨a ∼ EEG⟩ ⟨a ∼ tremor⟩

resting cell *n* : a living cell with a nucleus that is not undergoing division (as by mitosis)

resting potential *n* : the membrane potential of a cell that is not exhibiting the activity resulting from a stimulus — compare ACTION POTENTIAL

resting stage *n* : INTERPHASE

rest·less \ˈrest-ləs\ *adj* **1** : deprived of rest or sleep **2** : providing no rest

res·to·ra·tion \ˌres-tə-ˈrā-shən\ *n* : the act of restoring or the condition of being restored: as **a** : a returning to a normal or healthy condition **b** : the replacing of missing teeth or crowns; *also* : a dental replacement (as a denture) used for restoration — **re·stor·a·tive** \ri-ˈstȯr-ə-tiv\ *adj or n*

re·store \ri-ˈstȯr\ *vb* **re·stored; re·stor·ing** : to bring back to or put back into a former or original state ⟨a tooth *re-stored* with an inlay⟩

Res·to·ril \ˈres-tə-ˌril\ *trademark* — used for a preparation of temazepam

re·straint \ri-ˈstränt\ *n* : a device (as a straitjacket) that restricts movement

re·stric·tion \ri-ˈstrik-shən\ *n*, *often attrib* : the breaking of double-stranded DNA into fragments by restriction enzymes ⟨∼ sites⟩

restriction endonuclease *n* : RESTRICTION ENZYME

restriction enzyme *n* : any of various enzymes that break DNA into fragments at specific sites in the interior of the molecule and are often used as tools in molecular analysis

restriction fragment *n* : a segment of DNA produced by the action of a restriction enzyme on a molecule of DNA

restriction fragment length polymorphism *n* : variation in the length of a restriction fragment produced by a specific restriction enzyme acting on DNA from different individuals that usu. results from a genetic mutation (as an insertion or deletion) and that may be used as a genetic marker — called also *RFLP*

rest seat *n* : an area on the surface of a tooth that is specially prepared (as by grinding) for the attachment of a dental rest

re·sus·ci·ta·tion \ri-ˌsə-sə-ˈtā-shən, rē-\ *n* : the act of reviving from apparent death or from unconsciousness — see CARDIOPULMONARY RESUSCITATION — **re·sus·ci·tate** \-ˈsə-sə-ˌtāt\ *vb* — **re·sus·ci·ta·tive** \ri-ˈsə-sə-ˌtā-tiv\ *adj*

re·sus·ci·ta·tor \ri-ˈsə-sə-ˌtā-tər\ *n* : an apparatus used to restore respiration (as of a partially asphyxiated person)

re·tain·er \ri-ˈtā-nər\ *n* **1** : the part of a dental replacement (as a bridge) by which it is made fast to adjacent natural teeth **2** : a dental appliance used to hold teeth in correct position following orthodontic treatment

re·tar·da·tion \ˌrē-ˌtär-ˈdā-shən, ri-\ *n* **1** : an abnormal slowness of thought or action; *also* : less than normal intellectual competence usu. characterized by an IQ of less than 70 **2** : slowness in development or progress

re·tard·ed \ri-ˈtär-dəd\ *adj* : slow or limited in intellectual or emotional development : characterized by mental retardation

retch \ˈrech\ *vb* : to make an effort to vomit; *also* : VOMIT — **retch** *n*

re·te \ˈrē-tē, ˈrā-\ *n*, *pl* **re·tia** \-tē-ə\ **1** : a network esp. of blood vessels or nerves : PLEXUS **2** : an anatomical part resembling or including a network

re·ten·tion \ri-ˈten-chən\ *n* **1** : the act of retaining: as **a** : abnormal retaining of a fluid or secretion in a body cavity **b** : the holding in place of a tooth or dental replacement by means of a retainer **2** : a preservation of the aftereffects of experience and learning that makes recall or recognition possible

re·ten·tive \ri-ˈten-tiv\ *adj* : tending to retain: as **a** : having a good memory ⟨a ∼ mind⟩ **b** : of, relating to, or being a dental retainer

rete peg *n* : any of the inwardly directed prolongations of the Malpighian layer of the epidermis that mesh with the dermal papillae of the skin

rete testis *n*, *pl* **retia tes·ti·um** \-ˈtes-tē-əm\ : the network of tubules in the mediastinum testis

retia *pl of* RETE

reticul- *or* **reticulo-** *comb form* : reticulum ⟨*reticulo*cyte⟩

reticula • retinal detachment 598

reticula *pl of* RETICULUM

re·tic·u·lar \ri-'ti-kyə-lər\ *adj* : of, relating to, or forming a network

reticular activating system *n* : a part of the reticular formation that extends from the brain stem to the midbrain and thalamus with connections distributed throughout the cerebral cortex and that controls the degree of activity of the central nervous system (as in maintaining sleep and wakefulness)

reticular cell *n* : RETICULUM CELL; *esp* : RETICULOCYTE

reticular fiber *n* : any of the thin branching fibers of connective tissue that form an intricate interstitial network ramifying through other tissues and organs

reticular formation *n* : a mass of nerve cells and fibers situated primarily in the brain stem and functioning upon stimulation esp. in arousal of the organism — called also *reticular substance*

reticularis — see LIVEDO RETICULARIS, ZONA RETICULARIS

reticular layer *n* : the deeper layer of the dermis formed of interlacing fasciculi of white fibrous tissue

reticular tissue *n* : RETICULUM 2a

re·tic·u·late body \ri-'ti-kyə-lət-\ *n* : a chlamydial cell of a spherical intracellular form that is larger than an elementary body and reproduces by binary fission

re·tic·u·lin \ri-'ti-kyə-lən\ *n* : a protein substance similar to collagen that is a constituent of reticular tissue

re·tic·u·lo·cyte \ri-'ti-kyə-lō-₁sīt\ *n* : an immature red blood cell that appears esp. during regeneration of lost blood and has a fine basophilic reticulum formed of the remains of ribosomes — **re·tic·u·lo·cyt·ic** \ri-₁ti-kyə-lō-'si-tik\ *adj*

re·tic·u·lo·cy·to·pe·nia \ri-₁ti-kyə-lō-₁sī-tə-'pē-nē-ə\ *n* : an abnormal decrease in the number of reticulocytes in the blood

re·tic·u·lo·cy·to·sis \-₁sī-'tō-səs\ *n, pl* **-to·ses** \-₁sēz\ : an increase in the number of reticulocytes in the blood

re·tic·u·lo·en·do·the·li·al \ri-₁ti-kyə-lō-₁en-də-'thē-lē-əl\ *adj* : of, relating to, or being the reticuloendothelial system (~ tissue) (~ cells)

reticuloendothelial system *n* : a diffuse system of cells arising from mesenchyme and comprising all the phagocytic cells of the body except the circulating white blood cells — called also *lymphoreticular system*

re·tic·u·lo·en·do·the·li·o·sis \-₁thē-lē-'ō-səs\ *n, pl* **-o·ses** \-₁sēz\ : any of several disorders characterized by proliferation of reticuloendothelial cells or their derivatives — called also *reticulosis*

re·tic·u·lo·sar·co·ma \-sär-'kō-mə\ *n, pl*

-mas *or* **-ma·ta** \-mə-tə\ : RETICULUM CELL SARCOMA

re·tic·u·lo·sis \ri-₁ti-kyə-'lō-səs\ *n, pl* **-lo·ses** \-₁sēz\ : RETICULOENDOTHELIOSIS

re·tic·u·lo·spi·nal tract \ri-₁ti-kyə-lō-'spī-n³l-\ *n* : a tract of nerve fibers that originates in the reticular formation of the pons and medulla oblongata and descends to the spinal cord

re·tic·u·lum \ri-'ti-kyə-ləm\ *n, pl* **-la** \-lə\ **1** : the second compartment of the stomach of a ruminant in which folds of the mucous membrane form hexagonal cells — called also *honeycomb*; compare ABOMASUM, OMASUM, RUMEN **2** : a reticular structure: as **a** : the network of interstitial tissue composed of reticular fibers — called also *reticular tissue* **b** : the network often visible in fixed protoplasm both of the cell body and the nucleus of many cells

reticulum cell *n* : any of the branched anastomosing reticuloendothelial cells that form the reticular fibers

reticulum cell sarcoma *n* : a malignant lymphoma arising from reticulum cells — called also *reticulosarcoma*

retin- *or* **retino-** *comb form* : retina (*retinitis*) (*retinoscopy*)

ret·i·na \'ret-³n-ə\ *n, pl* **retinas** *or* **ret·i·nae** \-³n-₁ē\ : the sensory membrane that lines most of the large posterior chamber of the eye, is composed of several layers including one containing the rods and cones, and functions as the immediate instrument of vision by receiving the image formed by the lens and converting it into chemical and nervous signals which reach the brain by way of the optic nerve

Ret·in-A \₁ret-³n-'ā\ *trademark* — used for a preparation of retinoic acid

ret·i·nac·u·lum \₁ret-³n-'a-kyə-ləm\ *n, pl* **-la** \-lə\ : a connecting or retaining band esp. of fibrous tissue — see EXTENSOR RETINACULUM, FLEXOR RETINACULUM, INFERIOR EXTENSOR RETINACULUM, INFERIOR PERONEAL RETINACULUM, PERONEAL RETINACULUM, SUPERIOR EXTENSOR RETINACULUM, SUPERIOR PERONEAL RETINACULUM

¹ret·i·nal \'ret-³n-əl\ *adj* : of, relating to, involving, or being a retina (a ~ examination) (~ rods)

²ret·i·nal \'ret-³n-₁al, -₁ȯl\ *n* : a yellowish to orange aldehyde $C_{20}H_{28}O$ derived from vitamin A that in combination with proteins forms the visual pigments of the retinal rods and cones — called also *retinene, retinene₁, vitamin A aldehyde*

retinal artery — see CENTRAL ARTERY OF THE RETINA

retinal detachment *n* : a condition of the eye in which the retina has separated from the choroid — called also *detached retina, detachment of the retina*

retinal disparity *n* : the slight difference in the two retinal images due to the angle from which each eye views an object

retinal vein — see CENTRAL VEIN OF THE RETINA

ret·i·nene \'ret-ən-ēn\ *n* : either of two aldehydes derived from vitamin A: **a** : RETINAL **b** : an orange-red crystalline compound $C_{20}H_{26}O$ related to vitamin A_2

retinene₁ \-'wən\ *n* : RETINAL

retinene₂ \-'tü\ *n* : RETINENE b

ret·i·ni·tis \ret-ən-'ī-təs\ *n, pl* **-nit·i·des** \-'i-tə-dēz\ : inflammation of the retina

retinitis pig·men·to·sa \-pig-mən-'tō-sə, -(ˌ)men-, -zə\ *n* : any of several hereditary progressive degenerative diseases of the eye marked by night blindness in the early stages, atrophy and pigment changes in the retina, constriction of the visual field, and eventual blindness — called also *pigmentary retinopathy*

retinitis pro·lif·er·ans \-prə-'li-fə-ranz\ *n* : neovascularization of the retina associated esp. with diabetic retinopathy

retino- — see RETIN-

ret·i·no·blas·to·ma \ret-ən-ō-blas-'tō-mə\ *n, pl* **-mas** *or* **-ma·ta** \-mə-tə\ : a hereditary malignant tumor of the retina that develops during childhood, is derived from retinal germ cells, and is associated with a chromosomal abnormality

ret·i·no·cho·roid·i·tis \-kōr-ˌȯi-'dī-təs\ *n* : inflammation of the retina and the choroid

ret·i·no·ic acid \ret-ən-'ō-ik-\ *n* : an acid $C_{20}H_{28}O_2$ derived from vitamin A and used as a keratolytic esp. in the treatment of acne — called also *tretinoin*; see RETIN-A

ret·i·noid \'ret-ən-ȯid\ *n* : any of various synthetic or naturally occurring analogs of vitamin A — **retinoid** *adj*

ret·i·nol \'ret-ən-ˌȯl, -ˌōl\ *n* : VITAMIN A a

ret·i·nop·a·thy \ret-ən-'ä-pə-thē\ *n, pl* **-thies** : any of various noninflammatory disorders of the retina including some that cause blindness (diabetic ~)

ret·i·no·scope \'ret-ən-ə-ˌskōp\ *n* : an apparatus used in retinoscopy

ret·i·nos·co·py \ret-ən-'äs-kə-pē\ *n, pl* **-pies** : a method of determining the state of refraction of the eye by illuminating the retina with a mirror and observing the direction of movement of the retinal illumination and adjacent shadow when the mirror is turned

ret·i·no·tec·tal \ret-ən-ō-'tek-təl\ *adj* : of, relating to, or being the nerve fibers connecting the retina and the tectum of the midbrain (~ pathways)

re·tract \ri-'trakt\ *vb* **1** : to draw back or in (~ the lower jaw) — compare PROTRACT **2** : to use a retractor

re·trac·tion \ri-'trak-shən\ *n* : an act or instance of retracting; *specif* : backward or inward movement of an organ or part

re·trac·tor \ri-'trak-tər\ *n* : one that retracts: as **a** : any of various surgical instruments for holding tissues away from the field of operation **b** : a muscle that draws in an organ or part

retro- *prefix* **1** : backward : back (*retroflexion*) **2** : situated behind (*retropubic*)

ret·ro·bul·bar \re-trō-'bəl-bər, -bär\ *adj* : situated, occurring, or administered behind the eyeball (a ~ injection)

retrobulbar neuritis *n* : inflammation of the part of the optic nerve lying immediately behind the eyeball

ret·ro·cli·na·tion \-kli-'nā-shən\ *n* : the condition of being inclined backward

ret·ro·flex·ion \re-trō-'flek-shən\ *n* : the state of being bent back; *specif* : the bending back of the body of the uterus upon the cervix — compare RETROVERSION

ret·ro·gnath·ia \-'na-thē-ə\ *n* : RETROGNATHISM

ret·ro·gnath·ism \re-trō-'na-ˌthi-zəm\ *n* : a condition characterized by recession of one or both of the jaws

ret·ro·grade \'re-trō-ˌgrād\ *adj* **1** : characterized by retrogression **2** : affecting a period immediately prior to a precipitating cause (~ amnesia) **3** : occurring or performed in a direction opposite to the usual direction of conduction or flow (~ catheterization); *esp* : occurring along cell processes toward the cell body (~ axonal transport) — compare ANTEROGRADE 2 — **ret·ro·grade·ly** *adv*

retrograde pyelogram *n* : a roentgenogram of the kidney made by retrograde pyelography

retrograde pyelography *n* : pyelography performed by injection of radiopaque material through the ureter

ret·ro·gres·sion \re-trō-'gre-shən\ *n* : a reversal in development or condition: as **a** : return to a former and less complex level of development or organization **b** : subsidence or decline of symptoms or manifestations of a disease — **ret·ro·gres·sive** \-'gre-siv\ *adj*

ret·ro·len·tal fibroplasia \re-trō-'lent-ᵊl-\ *n* : a disease of the retina that occurs esp. in premature infants of low birth weight and that is characterized by the presence of an opaque fibrous membrane behind the lens of the eye

ret·ro·mo·lar \-'mō-lər\ *adj* : situated or occurring behind the last molar

ret·ro·per·i·to·ne·al \-per-ə-tə-'nē-əl\ *adj* : situated or occurring behind the peritoneum (a ~ tumor) — **ret·ro·per·i·to·ne·al·ly** *adv*

retroperitoneal fibrosis *n* : proliferation of fibrous tissue behind the peritoneum often leading to blockage of the ureters — called also *Ormond's disease*

ret·ro·peri·to·ne·um \-ˌper-ə-tə-ˈnē-əm\ *n, pl* **-ne·ums** *or* **-nea** \-ˈnē-ə\ : the space between the peritoneum and the posterior abdominal wall that contains esp. the kidneys and associated structures, the pancreas, and part of the aorta and inferior vena cava

ret·ro·pha·ryn·geal \-ˌfar-ən-ˈjē-əl, -fə-ˈrin-jəl, -jē-əl\ *adj* : situated or occurring behind the pharynx ⟨a ~ abscess⟩

ret·ro·pu·bic \ˌre-trō-ˈpyü-bik\ *adj* **1** : situated or occurring behind the pubis **2** : performed by way of the retropubic space ⟨~ prostatectomy⟩

retropubic space *n* : the potential space occurring between the pubic symphysis and the urinary bladder

ret·ro·rec·tal \-ˈrekt-əl\ *adj* : situated or occurring behind the rectum

ret·ro·spec·tive \-ˈspek-tiv\ *adj* : relating to or being a study (as of a disease) that starts with the present condition of a population of individuals and collects data about their past history to explain their present condition — compare PROSPECTIVE

ret·ro·ster·nal \-ˈstər-nəl\ *adj* : situated or occurring behind the sternum

ret·ro·ver·sion \-ˈvər-zhən, -shən\ *n* : the bending backward of the uterus and cervix out of the normal axis so that the fundus points toward the sacrum and the cervix toward the pubic symphysis — compare RETROFLEXION

Ret·ro·vir \ˈre-trō-ˌvir\ *trademark* — used for a preparation of azidothymidine

ret·ro·vi·rol·o·gy \ˌre-trō-vī-ˈrä-lə-jē\ *n, pl* **-gies** : a branch of science concerned with the study of retroviruses — **ret·ro·vi·rol·o·gist** \-jist\ *n*

ret·ro·vi·rus \ˈre-trō-ˌvī-rəs\ *n* : any of a group of RNA-containing viruses (as HIV and the Rous sarcoma virus) that produce reverse transcriptase by means of which DNA is produced using their RNA as a template and incorporated into the genome of infected cells and that include numerous tumorigenic viruses — called also *RNA tumor virus* — **ret·ro·vi·ral** \-ˈvi-rəl\ *adj*

re·tru·sion \ri-ˈtrü-zhən\ *n* : backward displacement; *specif* : a condition in which a tooth or the jaw is posterior to its proper occlusal position — **re·trude** \-ˈtrüd\ *vb* — **re·tru·sive** \-ˈtrü-siv\ *adj*

reuniens — see DUCTUS REUNIENS

re·up·take \rē-ˈəp-ˌtāk\ *n* : resorption by a neuron of a neurotransmitter following the transmission of a nerve impulse across a synapse

re·vac·ci·na·tion \ˌrē-ˌvak-sə-ˈnā-shən\ *n* : vaccination administered some period after an initial vaccination esp. to strengthen or renew immunity — **re·vac·ci·nate** \-ˈvak-sə-ˌnāt\ *vb*

re·vas·cu·lar·iza·tion \ˌrē-ˌvas-kyə-lə-rə-ˈzā-shən\ *n* : a surgical procedure for the provision of a new, additional, or augmented blood supply to a body part or organ ⟨myocardial ~⟩

reverse tran·scrip·tase \ri-ˈvərs-ˌtran-ˈskrip-(ˌ)tās, -(ˌ)tāz\ *n* : a polymerase esp. of retroviruses that catalyzes the formation of DNA using RNA as a template

reverse transcription *n* : the process of synthesizing double-stranded DNA using RNA as a template and reverse transcriptase as a catalyst

re·vers·ible \ri-ˈvər-sə-bəl\ *adj* **1** : capable of going through a series of actions (as changes) either backward or forward **2** : capable of being corrected or undone : not permanent or irrevocable ⟨~ hypertension⟩ — **re·vers·ibly** *adv*

re·ver·sion \ri-ˈvər-zhən, -shən\ *n* **1** : an act or the process of returning (as to a former condition) **2** : a return toward an ancestral type or condition : reappearance of an ancestral character — **re·vert** \ri-ˈvərt\ *vb*

re·ver·tant \ri-ˈvərt-ᵊnt\ *n* : a mutant gene, individual, or strain that regains a former capability (as the production of a particular protein) by undergoing further mutation ⟨yeast ~s⟩ — **revertant** *adj*

re·vive \ri-ˈvīv\ *vb* **re·vived; re·viv·ing 1** : to return or restore to consciousness or life **2** : to restore from a depressed, inactive, or unused state — **re·viv·able** \-ˈvī-və-bəl\ *adj*

re·ward \ri-ˈwȯrd\ *n* : a stimulus administered to an organism following a correct or desired response that increases the probability of occurrence of the response — **reward** *vb*

Reye's syndrome \ˈrīz-, ˈrāz-\ *also* **Reye syndrome** \ˈrī-, ˈrā-\ *n* : an often fatal encephalopathy esp. of childhood characterized by fever, vomiting, fatty infiltration of the liver, and swelling of the kidneys and brain

Reye, Ralph Douglas Kenneth (1912–1977), Australian pathologist.

RF *abbr* rheumatic fever

R factor \ˈär-\ *n* : a group of genes present in some bacteria that provide a basis for resistance to antibiotics and can be transferred from cell to cell by conjugation

RFLP \ˌär-(ˌ)ef-(ˌ)el-ˈpē\ *n* : RESTRICTION FRAGMENT LENGTH POLYMORPHISM

¹Rh \ˌär-ˈāch\ *adj* : of, relating to, or being an Rh factor ⟨~ antigens⟩

²Rh *symbol* rhodium

rhabd- *or* **rhabdo-** *comb form* : rodlike structure ⟨*rhabdo*virus⟩

rhab·do·my·ol·y·sis \ˌrab-dō-mī-ˈä-lə-səs\ *n, pl* **-y·ses** \-ₜsēz\ : a potentially fatal disease marked by destruction or degeneration of skeletal muscle and often associated with myoglobinuria

rhab·do·myo·o·ma \ₜrab-dō-mī-ˈō-mə\ *n, pl* **-mas** *or* **-ma·ta** \-mə-tə\ : a benign tumor composed of striated muscle fibers (a cardiac ∼)

rhab·do·myo·sar·co·ma \ₜrab-(ₜ)dō-ₜmī-ə-sär-ˈkō-mə\ *n, pl* **-mas** *or* **-ma·ta** \-mə-tə\ : a malignant tumor composed of striated muscle fibers

rhab·do·virus \-ₜvī-rəs\ *n* : any of a group of RNA-containing rod- or bullet-shaped viruses found in plants and animals and including the causative agents of rabies and vesicular stomatitis

rha·chi·tis *var of* RACHITIS

rhag·a·des \ˈra-gə-ₜdēz\ *n pl* : linear cracks or fissures in the skin occurring esp. at the angles of the mouth or about the anus

rha·phe *var of* RAPHE

Rh disease *n* : ERYTHROBLASTOSIS FETALIS

rhe·ni·um \ˈrē-nē-əm\ *n* : a rare heavy metallic element — symbol *Re;* see ELEMENT table

rheo- *comb form* : flow : current ⟨*rheobase*⟩

rheo·base \ˈrē-ō-ₜbās\ *n* : the minimal electrical current required to excite a tissue (as nerve or muscle) given indefinitely long time during which the current is applied — compare CHRONAXIE

rhe·sus factor \ˈrē-səs-\ *n* : RH FACTOR

rheum \ˈrüm\ *n* : a watery discharge from the mucous membranes esp. of the eyes or nose; *also* : a condition (as a cold) marked by such discharge — **rheumy** \ˈrü-mē\ *adj*

¹**rheu·mat·ic** \rü-ˈma-tik\ *adj* : of, relating to, characteristic of, or affected with rheumatism ⟨∼ pain⟩ ⟨a ∼ joint⟩

²**rheumatic** *n* : a person affected with rheumatism

rheumatica — see POLYMYALGIA RHEUMATICA

rheumatic disease *n* : any of several diseases (as rheumatic fever or fibrositis) characterized by inflammation and pain in muscles or joints : RHEUMATISM

rheumatic fever *n* : an acute often recurrent disease occurring chiefly in children and young adults and characterized by fever, inflammation, pain, and swelling in and around the joints, inflammatory involvement of the pericardium and valves of the heart, and often the formation of small nodules chiefly in the subcutaneous tissues and the heart

rheumatic heart disease *n* : active or inactive disease of the heart that results from rheumatic fever and is characterized by inflammatory changes in the myocardium or scar-

ring of the valves causing reduced functional capacity of the heart

rheu·ma·tism \ˈrü-mə-ₜti-zəm, ˈrü-mə-\ *n* **1** : any of various conditions characterized by inflammation or pain in muscles, joints, or fibrous tissue (muscular ∼) **2** : RHEUMATOID ARTHRITIS

rheu·ma·toid \-ₜtȯid\ *adj* : characteristic of or affected with rheumatoid arthritis

rheumatoid arthritis *n* : a usu. chronic disease that is of unknown cause and is characterized esp. by pain, stiffness, inflammation, swelling, and sometimes destruction of joints — compare OSTEOARTHRITIS

rheumatoid factor *n* : an autoantibody of high molecular weight that is usu. present in rheumatoid arthritis

rheumatoid spondylitis *n* : ANKYLOSING SPONDYLITIS

rheu·ma·tol·o·gist \ₜrü-mə-ˈtä-lə-jist, ₜrü-\ *n* : a specialist in rheumatology

rheu·ma·tol·o·gy \-jē\ *n, pl* **-gies** : a medical science dealing with rheumatic diseases

Rh factor \ₜär-ˈāch-\ *n* : any of one or more genetically determined antigens usu. present in the red blood cells of most persons and of higher animals and capable of inducing intense immunogenic reactions — called also *rhesus factor*

rhin- *or* **rhino-** *comb form* **1 a** : nose ⟨*rhinitis*⟩ ⟨*rhinology*⟩ **b** : nose and ⟨*rhinotracheitis*⟩ **2** : nasal ⟨*rhinovirus*⟩

rhi·nal \ˈrīn-ᵊl\ *adj* : of or relating to the nose : NASAL

rhin·en·ceph·a·lon \ₜrī-(ₜ)nen-ˈse-fə-ₜlän, -lən\ *n, pl* **-la** \-lə\ : the anterior inferior part of the forebrain that is chiefly concerned with olfaction and that is considered to include the olfactory bulb together with the forebrain olfactory structures receiving fibers directly from it and often esp. formerly the limbic system which is now known to be concerned with emotional states and affect — called also *smell brain* — **rhin·en·ce·pha·lic** \ₜrī-nen-sə-ˈfa-lik\ *adj*

rhi·ni·tis \rī-ˈnī-təs\ *n, pl* **-nit·i·des** \-ˈni-tə-ₜdēz\ : inflammation of the mucous membrane of the nose (allergic ∼); *also* : any of various conditions characterized by such inflammation

rhi·no·log·ic \ₜrī-nə-ˈlä-jik\ *or* **rhi·no·log·i·cal** \-ji-kəl\ *adj* : of or relating to the nose ⟨∼ disease⟩

rhi·nol·o·gist \rī-ˈnä-lə-jist\ *n* : a physician who specializes in rhinology

rhi·nol·o·gy \-jē\ *n, pl* **-gies** : a branch of medicine that deals with the nose and its diseases

rhi·no·phar·yn·gi·tis \ₜrī-nō-ₜfar-ən-ˈjī-təs\ *n, pl* **-git·i·des** \-ˈji-tə-ₜdēz\ : inflammation of the mucous membrane of the nose and pharynx

rhi·no·phy·ma \-ˈfī-mə\ *n, pl* **-mas** *or* **-ma·ta** \-mə-tə\ : a nodular swelling and congestion of the nose in an advanced stage of acne rosacea

rhi·no·plas·ty \'rī-nō-ˌplas-tē\ n, pl **-ties** : plastic surgery on the nose usu. for cosmetic purposes — called also *nose job* — **rhi·no·plas·tic** \ˌrī-nō-'plas-tik\ adj

rhi·no·pneu·mo·ni·tis \ˌrī-nō-ˌnü-mə-'nī-təs, -ˌnyü-\ n : either of two forms of an acute febrile respiratory disease affecting horses, caused by types of a herpesvirus, characterized esp. by rhinopharyngitis and tracheobronchitis, and sometimes causing abortion in pregnant mares

rhi·nor·rhea \ˌrī-nə-'rē-ə\ n : excessive mucous secretion from the nose

rhi·nor·rhoea chiefly Brit var of RHINORRHEA

rhi·no·scope \'rī-nə-ˌskōp\ n : an instrument for examining the cavities and passages of the nose

rhi·nos·co·py \rī-'näs-kə-pē\ n, pl **-pies** : examination of the nasal passages — **rhi·no·scop·ic** \ˌrī-nə-'skä-pik\ adj

rhi·no·spo·rid·i·o·sis \ˌrī-nō-spə-ˌri-dē-'ō-səs\ n, pl **-o·ses** \-ˌsēz\ : a fungal disease of the external mucous membranes (as of the nose) that is characterized by the formation of pinkish red, friable, sessile, or pedunculated polyps and is caused by an ascomycetous fungus (*Rhinosporidium seeberi*)

rhi·not·o·my \rī-'nä-tə-mē\ n, pl **-mies** : surgical incision of the nose

rhi·no·tra·che·itis \ˌrī-nō-ˌtrā-kē-'ī-təs\ n : inflammation of the nasal cavities and trachea; esp : a disease of the upper respiratory system in cats and esp. young kittens that is characterized by sneezing, conjunctivitis with discharge, and nasal discharges — see INFECTIOUS BOVINE RHINOTRACHEITIS

rhi·no·vi·rus \ˌrī-nō-'vī-rəs\ n : any of a group of picornaviruses that are related to the enteroviruses and are associated with upper respiratory tract disorders (as the common cold)

Rhipi·ceph·a·lus \ˌri-pə-'se-fə-ləs\ n : a genus of ixodid ticks that are parasitic on many mammals and some birds and include vectors of serious diseases (as Rocky Mountain spotted fever and east coast fever)

rhi·zo·me·lic \ˌrī-zə-'mē-lik\ adj : of or relating to the hip and shoulder joints

rhi·zot·o·my \rī-'zä-tə-mē\ n, pl **-mies** : the operation of cutting the anterior or posterior spinal nerve roots

Rh–neg·a·tive \ˌär-ˌāch-'ne-gə-tiv\ adj : lacking Rh factor in the blood

rhod- or **rhodo-** comb form : rose : red (*rhodopsin*)

rho·di·um \'rō-dē-əm\ n : a white hard ductile metallic element — symbol *Rh*; see ELEMENT table

rho·dop·sin \rō-'däp-sən\ n : a red photosensitive pigment in the retinal rods that is important in vision in dim light, is quickly bleached by light to a mixture of opsin and retinal, and is regenerated in the dark — called also *visual purple*

Rho·do·tor·u·la \ˌrō-də-'tòr-yə-lə\ n : a genus of yeasts (family Cryptococcaceae) including one (*R. rubra* syn. *R. mucilaginosa*) sometimes present in the blood or involved in endocarditis prob. as a secondary infection

rhomb·en·ceph·a·lon \ˌräm-(ˌ)ben-'se-fə-ˌlän, -lən\ n, pl **-la** \-lə\ : HINDBRAIN

rhom·boi·de·us \räm-'bói-dē-əs\ n, pl **-dei** \-dē-ˌī\ : either of two muscles that lie beneath the trapezius muscle and connect the spinous processes of various vertebrae with the medial border of the scapula: **a** : RHOMBOIDEUS MINOR **b** : RHOMBOIDEUS MAJOR

rhomboideus major n : a muscle arising from the spinous processes of the second through fifth thoracic vertebrae, inserted into the vertebral border of the scapula, and acting to adduct and laterally rotate the scapula — called also *rhomboid major*

rhomboideus minor n : a muscle arising from the inferior part of the ligamentum nuchae and from the spinous processes of the seventh cervical and first thoracic vertebrae, inserted into the vertebral border of the scapula at the base of the bony process terminating in the acromion, and acting to adduct and laterally rotate the scapula — called also *rhomboid minor*

rhomboid fossa n : the floor of the fourth ventricle of the brain formed by the dorsal surfaces of the pons and medulla oblongata

rhomboid major n : RHOMBOIDEUS MAJOR

rhomboid minor n : RHOMBOIDEUS MINOR

rhon·chus \'rän-kəs\ n, pl **rhon·chi** \'räŋ-ˌkī\ : a whistling or snoring sound heard on auscultation of the chest when the air channels are partly obstructed — compare RALE, RATTLE

rho·ta·cism \'rō-tə-ˌsi-zəm\ n : a defective pronunciation of *r*; esp : substitution of some other sound for that of *r*

Rh–pos·i·tive \ˌär-ˌāch-'pä-zə-tiv\ adj : containing Rh factor in the red blood cells

rhus \'rüs\ n **1** cap : a genus of shrubs and trees of the cashew family (Anacardiaceae) that are native to temperate and warm regions, have compound leaves with three to many leaflets, and include some (as poison ivy, poison oak, and poison sumac) producing irritating oils that cause dermatitis — see TOXICODENDRON **2** pl **rhuses** or **rhus** : any shrub or tree of the genus *Rhus*

rhus dermatitis n : dermatitis caused by contact with various plants of the genus *Rhus* and esp. with the common poison ivy (*R. radicans*)

rhythm \'ri-thəm\ *n* **1** : a regularly recurrent quantitative change in a variable biological process: as **a** : the pattern of recurrence of the cardiac cycle ⟨an irregular ∼⟩ **b** : the recurring pattern of physical and functional changes associated with the mammalian and esp. human sexual cycle **2** : RHYTHM METHOD — **rhythmic** \'rith-mik\ *or* **rhyth·mi·cal** \-mi-kəl\ *adj* — **rhyth·mi·cal·ly** *adv* — **rhyth·mic·i·ty** \rith-'mi-sə-tē\ *n*

rhythm method *n* : a method of birth control involving continence during the period of the sexual cycle in which ovulation is most likely to occur — compare SAFE PERIOD

rhyt·i·dec·to·my \ri-tə-'dek-tə-mē\ *n, pl* **-mies** : FACE-LIFT

RIA *abbr* radioimmunoassay

rib \'rib\ *n* : any of the paired curved bony or partly cartilaginous rods that stiffen the lateral walls of the body and protect the viscera and that in humans normally include 12 pairs of which all are articulated with the spinal column at the dorsal end and the first 10 are connected also at the ventral end with the sternum by costal cartilages — see FALSE RIB, FLOATING RIB, TRUE RIB

rib- *or* **ribo-** *comb form* : related to ribose ⟨*ribo*flavin⟩

ri·ba·vir·in \rī-bə-'vī-rən\ *n* : a synthetic broad-spectrum antiviral drug $C_8H_{12}N_4O_5$ that is a nucleoside resembling guanosine

rib cage *n* : the bony enclosing wall of the chest consisting chiefly of the ribs and the structures connecting them — called also *thoracic cage*

ri·bo·fla·vin \rī-bə-'flā-vən, 'rī-bə-⸳\ *also* **ri·bo·fla·vine** \-⸳vēn\ *n* : a yellow crystalline compound $C_{17}H_{20}N_4O_6$ that is a growth-promoting member of the vitamin B complex and occurs both free (as in milk) and combined (as in liver) — called also *lactoflavin, vitamin B₂*

riboflavin phosphate *or* **riboflavin 5'-phosphate** \-'fiv-'prīm-⸳\ *n* : FMN

ri·bo·nu·cle·ase \rī-bō-'nü-klē-⸳ās, -'nyü-, -⸳āz\ *n* : an enzyme that catalyzes the hydrolysis of RNA — called also *RNase*

ri·bo·nu·cle·ic acid \rī-bō-nü-⸳klē-ik-, -nyü-, -⸳klā-\ *n* : RNA

ri·bo·nu·cleo·pro·tein \-⸳nü-klē-ō-'prō-⸳tēn, -⸳nyü-\ *n* : a nucleoprotein that contains RNA

ri·bo·nu·cleo·side \-'nü-klē-ə-⸳sīd, -'nyü-\ *n* : a nucleoside that contains ribose

ri·bo·nu·cleo·tide \-⸳tīd\ *n* : a nucleotide that contains ribose and occurs esp. as a constituent of RNA

ri·bose \'rī-⸳bōs, -⸳bōz\ *n* : a pentose $C_5H_{10}O_5$ found esp. in the D-form as a constituent of a number of nucleo-

sides (as adenosine, cytidine, and guanosine) esp. in RNA

ribosomal RNA *n* : RNA that is a fundamental structural element of ribosomes — called also *rRNA*

ri·bo·some \'rī-bə-⸳sōm\ *n* : any of the RNA- and protein-rich cytoplasmic organelles that are sites of protein synthesis — **ri·bo·som·al** \rī-bə-'sō-məl\ *adj*

ri·bo·zyme \-⸳zīm\ *n* : a molecule of RNA that functions as an enzyme (as by catalyzing the cleavage of other RNA molecules)

RICE *abbr* rest, ice, compression, elevation — used esp. for the initial treatment of many usu. minor sports⸗related injuries (as sprains)

rice–water stool *n* : a watery stool containing white flecks of mucus, epithelial cells, and bacteria and discharged from the bowels in severe forms of diarrhea (as in Asiatic cholera)

ri·cin \'rīs-ᵊn, 'ris-\ *n* : a poisonous protein in the castor bean

rick·ets \'ri-kəts\ *n* : a deficiency disease that affects the young during the period of skeletal growth, is characterized esp. by soft and deformed bones, and is caused by failure to assimilate and use calcium and phosphorus normally due to inadequate sunlight or vitamin D — called also *rachitis*

rick·etts·ae·mia *chiefly Brit var of* RICK-ETTSEMIA

rick·etts·emia \⸳ri-kət-'sē-mē-ə\ *n* : the abnormal presence of rickettsiae in the blood

Rick·etts, Howard Taylor (1871–1910), American pathologist.

rick·ett·sia \ri-'ket-sē-ə\ *n* **1** *cap* : a genus of rod-shaped, coccoid, or diplococcus-shaped often pleomorphic bacteria (family Rickettsiaceae) that live intracellularly in biting arthropods (as lice or ticks) and when transmitted to humans by the bite of an arthropod host cause a number of serious diseases (as Rocky Mountain spotted fever and typhus) **2** *pl* **-sias** *or* **-si·ae** \-sē-⸳ē\ *also* **-sia** : any of an order (Rickettsiales) and esp. a family (Rickettsiaceae) of rod-shaped, coccoid, or diplococcus-shaped, often pleomorphic bacteria — **rick·ett·si·al** \-sē-əl\ *adj*

rick·ett·si·al·pox \ri-⸳ket-sē-əl-'päks\ *n* : a disease characterized by fever, chills, headache, backache, and a spotty rash and caused by a bacterium of the genus *Rickettsia* (*R. akari*) transmitted to humans by the bite of a mite of the genus *Allodermanyssus* (*A. sanguineus*) living on rodents (as the house mouse)

rick·ett·si·o·sis \ri-⸳ket-sē-'ō-səs\ *n, pl* **-o·ses** \-⸳sēz\ : infection with or disease caused by a rickettsia ⟨a mild ∼⟩

ridge·ling *or* **ridg·ling** \'rij-liŋ\ *n* **1** : a partially castrated male animal **2** : a male animal having one or both testes retained in the inguinal canal

Rie·del's disease \'rēd-ǝlz-\ n : chronic thyroiditis in which the thyroid gland becomes hard and stony and firmly attached to surrounding tissues

Riedel, Bernhard Moritz Karl Ludwig (1846–1916), German surgeon.

Riedel's struma n : RIEDEL'S DISEASE

ri·fam·pin \ri-'fam-pǝn\ or **ri·fam·pi·cin** \ri-'fam-pǝ-sǝn\ n : a semisynthetic antibiotic $C_{43}H_{58}N_4O_{12}$ that acts against some viruses and bacteria esp. by inhibiting RNA synthesis

rif·a·my·cin \ri-fǝ-'mis-ǝn\ n : any of several antibiotics that are derived from a bacterium of the genus *Streptomyces* (*S. mediterranei*)

Rift Valley fever n : a disease of east African sheep and sometimes cattle that is caused by an arbovirus, is characterized by fever and destructive hepatitis, and is occasionally transmitted to humans in a much-attenuated form

right \'rīt\ adj : of, relating to, or being the side of the body which is away from the heart and on which the hand is stronger in most people; also : located nearer to this side than to the left — **right** adv

right atrioventricular valve n : TRICUSPID VALVE

right colic flexure n : HEPATIC FLEXURE

right–eyed adj : using the right eye in preference (as in using a monocular microscope)

right gastric artery n : an artery that arises from the hepatic artery, passes to the left along the lesser curvature of the stomach while giving off a number of branches, and eventually joins a branch of the left gastric artery

right gastroepiploic artery n : GASTROEPIPLOIC ARTERY a

right–hand \'rīt-ˌhand\ adj 1 : situated on the right 2 : RIGHT-HANDED

right hand n 1 : the hand on a person's right side 2 : the right side

right–hand·ed \-'han-dǝd\ adj 1 : using the right hand habitually or more easily than the left 2 : relating to, designed for, or done with the right hand 3 : having the same direction or course as the movement of the hands of a watch viewed from in front 4 : DEXTROROTATORY — **right–handed** adv — **right–hand·ed·ness** n

right heart n : the right atrium and ventricle : the half of the heart that receives blood from the systemic circulation and passes it into the pulmonary arteries

right lymphatic duct n : a short vessel that receives lymph from the right side of the head, neck, and thorax, the right arm, right lung, right side of the heart, and convex surface of the liver and that discharges it into the right subclavian vein at its junction with the right internal jugular vein

right pulmonary artery n : PULMONARY ARTERY a

right subcostal vein n : SUBCOSTAL VEIN a

right–to–life adj : opposed to abortion — **right–to–lif·er** \ˌrīt-tǝ-'lī-fǝr\ n

ri·gid·i·ty \rǝ-'ji-dǝ-tē\ n, pl **-ties** : the quality or state of being stiff or devoid of or deficient in flexibility: as a : abnormal stiffness of muscle b : emotional inflexibility and resistance to change — **rig·id** \'ri-jǝd\ adj

rigidus — see HALLUX RIGIDUS

rig·or \'ri-gǝr\ n 1 a : CHILL 1 b : a tremor caused by a chill 2 a : rigidity or torpor of organs or tissue that prevents response to stimuli b : RIGOR MORTIS

rig·or mor·tis \'ri-gǝr-'mȯr-tǝs\ n : temporary rigidity of muscles occurring after death

ri·ma \'rī-mǝ\ n, pl **ri·mae** \-ˌmē\ : an anatomical fissure or cleft

rima glot·ti·dis \-'glä-tǝ-dǝs\ n : the passage in the glottis between the true vocal cords

rima pal·pe·bra·rum \-ˌpal-pē-'brer-ǝm\ n : PALPEBRAL FISSURE

rin·der·pest \'rin-dǝr-ˌpest\ n : an acute infectious febrile disease of ruminant animals (as cattle) that is caused by a paramyxovirus and is marked by diarrhea and inflammation of mucous membranes

¹**ring** \'riŋ\ n 1 a : a circular band b : an anatomical structure having a circular opening : ANNULUS 2 : an arrangement of atoms represented in formulas or models in a cyclic manner as a closed chain

²**ring** vb **rang** \'raŋ\; **rung** \'rǝŋ\; **ring·ing** : to have the sensation of being filled with a humming sound ⟨his ears *rang*⟩

ring·bone \-ˌbōn\ n : a bony outgrowth on the phalangeal bones of a horse's foot that usu. produces lameness

Ring·er's fluid \'riŋ-ǝrz-\ n : RINGER'S SOLUTION

Ringer, Sidney (1835–1910), British physiologist.

Ring·er's solution \'riŋ-ǝrz-\ also **Ring·er solution** \'riŋ-ǝr-\ n : a balanced aqueous solution that contains chloride, sodium, potassium, calcium, bicarbonate, and phosphate ions and that is used in physiological experiments to provide a medium essentially isosmotic to many animal tissues

ring·hals \'riŋ-ˌhals\ n : a venomous African elapid snake (*Haemachates haemachatus*) that is closely related to the true cobras and that seldom strikes but spits or sprays its venom aiming at the eyes of its victim

ring·worm \'riŋ-ˌwǝrm\ n : any of several contagious diseases of the skin, hair, or nails of humans and domestic animals caused by fungi (as of the genus *Trichophyton*) and characterized by ring-shaped discolored patches on the skin that are covered with vesicles and scales — called also *tinea*

Rin·ne's test \'ri-nəs-\ *or* **Rin·ne test** \'ri-nə-\ *n* : a test for determining a subject's ability to hear a vibrating tuning fork when it is held next to the ear and when it is placed on the mastoid process with diminished hearing acuity through air and somewhat heightened hearing acuity through bone being symptomatic of conduction deafness

Rinne, Heinrich Adolf R. (1819–1868), German otologist.

risk \'risk\ *n* **1** : possibility of loss, injury, disease, or death ⟨hypertension increases the ∼ of stroke⟩ **2** : a person considered in terms of the possible bad effects of a particular course of treatment ⟨a poor surgical ∼⟩ — **at risk** : characterized by high risk or susceptibility ⟨as to disease⟩ ⟨patients *at risk* of developing infections⟩

risk factor *n* : something which increases risk or susceptibility

ri·so·ri·us \ri-'sōr-ē-əs, -'zōr-\ *n, pl* **-rii** \-ē-ī\ : a narrow band of muscle fibers arising from the fascia over the masseter muscle, inserted into the tissues at the corner of the mouth, and acting to retract the angle of the mouth

ris·to·ce·tin \ris-tə-'sēt-ən\ *n* : either of two antibiotics or a mixture of both produced by an actinomycete of the genus *Nocardia* (*N. lurida*)

ri·sus sar·don·i·cus \'rī-səs-ˌsär-'dä-ni-kəs, 'rē-\ *n* : a facial expression characterized by raised eyebrows and grinning distortion of the face resulting from spasm of facial muscles esp. in tetanus

Rit·a·lin \'ri-tə-lən\ *trademark* — used for a preparation of methylphenidate

rit·o·drine \'ri-tə-ˌdrēn, -drən\ *n* : a drug $C_{17}H_{21}NO_3$ used as a smooth muscle relaxant esp. to inhibit premature labor

Rit·ter's disease \'ri-tərz-\ *n* : STAPHYLOCOCCAL SCALDED SKIN SYNDROME

Ritter von Rittershain, Gottfried (1820–1883), German physician.

rit·u·al \'ri-chə-wəl\ *n* : any act or practice regularly repeated in a set precise manner for relief of anxiety ⟨obsessive-compulsive ∼s⟩

river blindness *n* : ONCHOCERCIASIS

RLF *abbr* retrolental fibroplasia

RLQ *abbr* right lower quadrant (abdomen)

Rn *symbol* radon

RN \ˌär-'en\ *n* : REGISTERED NURSE

RNA \ˌär-(ˌ)en-'ā\ *n* : any of various nucleic acids that contain ribose and uracil as structural components and are associated with the control of cellular chemical activities — called also *ribonucleic acid*; see MESSENGER RNA, RIBOSOMAL RNA, TRANSFER RNA

RNAase *var of* RNASE

RNA polymerase *n* : any of a group of enzymes that promote the synthesis of RNA using DNA or RNA as a template

RNA replicase *n* : REPLICASE

RNase \ˌär-ˌen-'ā-ˌās, -'ā-ˌāz\ *n* : RIBONUCLEASE

RNA syn·the·tase \-'sin-thə-ˌtās, -ˌtāz\ *n* : REPLICASE

RNA tumor virus *n* : RETROVIRUS

roach \'rōch\ *n* : COCKROACH

roar·ing \'rōr-iŋ\ *n* : noisy inhalation in a horse caused by nerve paralysis and muscular atrophy and constituting an unsoundness

Rob·ert·so·ni·an \ˌrä-bərt-'sō-nē-ən\ *adj* : relating to or being a reciprocal translocation that takes place between certain types of chromosomes and that yields one nonfunctional chromosome having two short arms and one functional chromosome having two long arms of which one arm is derived from each parent chromosome

Robertson, William Rees Brebner (1881–1941), American biologist.

Ro·bi·nul \'rō-bi-ˌnùl\ *trademark* — used for a preparation of glycopyrrolate

Ro·chelle salt \rō-'shel-\ *n* : a crystalline salt $C_4H_4KNaO_6 \cdot 4H_2O$ that is a mild purgative — called also *potassium sodium tartrate, Seignette salt, sodium potassium tartrate*

rock \'räk\ *n* **1** : a small crystallized mass of crack cocaine **2** : CRACK — called also *rock cocaine*

Rocky Mountain spotted fever *n* : an acute bacterial disease that is characterized by chills, fever, prostration, pains in muscles and joints, and a red purple eruption and that is caused by a bacterium of the genus *Rickettsia* (*R. rickettii*) usu. transmitted by an ixodid tick and esp. by the American dog tick and Rocky Mountain wood tick

Rocky Mountain wood tick *n* : a widely distributed wood tick of the genus *Dermacentor* (*D. andersoni*) of western No. America that is a vector of Rocky Mountain spotted fever and sometimes causes tick paralysis

rod \'räd\ *n* **1** : any of the long rod-shaped photosensitive receptors in the retina responsive to faint light — compare CONE 1 **2** : a bacterium shaped like a rod

ro·dent \'rōd-ənt\ *n* : any of an order (Rodentia) of relatively small mammals (as a mouse or a rat) that have in both jaws a single pair of incisors with a chisel-shaped edge — **rodent** *adj*

ro·den·ti·cide \rō-'den-tə-ˌsīd\ *n* : an agent that kills, repels, or controls rodents

rodent ulcer *n* : a chronic persistent ulcer of the exposed skin and esp. of the face that is destructive locally, spreads slowly, and is usu. a carcinoma derived from basal cells

rod·like \'räd-ˌlīk\ adj : resembling a rod (~ bacteria)

rod of Cor·ti \-'kȯr-tē\ n : any of the minute modified epithelial elements that rise from the basilar membrane of the organ of Corti in two spirally arranged rows so that the free ends of the members incline toward and interlock with corresponding members of the opposite row and enclose the tunnel of Corti

A. G. G. Corti — see ORGAN OF CORTI

¹**roent·gen** \'rent-gən, 'rənt-, -jən, -shən\ adj : of, relating to, or using X rays

Rönt·gen or Roent·gen \'rœnt-gən\, Wilhelm Conrad (1845–1923), German physicist.

²**roentgen** n : the international unit of x-radiation or gamma radiation equal to the amount of radiation that produces in one cubic centimeter of dry air at 0°C (32°F) and standard atmospheric pressure ionization of either sign equal to one electrostatic unit of charge

roent·gen·o·gram \'rent-gə-nə-ˌgram, 'rənt-, -jə-, -shə-\ n : a photograph made with X rays

roent·gen·og·ra·phy \ˌrent-gə-'nä-grə-fē, ˌrənt-, -jə-, -shə-\ n, pl -phies : photography by means of X rays — **roent·gen·o·graph·ic** \-nə-'gra-fik\ adj — **roent·gen·o·graph·i·cal·ly** adv

roent·gen·ol·o·gist \-'nä-lə-jist\ n : a specialist in roentgenology

roent·gen·ol·o·gy \-'nä-lə-jē\ n, pl -gies : a branch of radiology that deals with the use of X rays for diagnosis or treatment of disease — **roent·gen·o·log·ic** \-nə-'lä-jik\ or **roent·gen·o·log·i·cal** \-ji-kəl\ adj — **roent·gen·o·log·i·cal·ly** adv

roent·gen·o·scope \'rent-gə-nə-ˌskōp, 'rənt-, -jə-, -shə-\ n : FLUOROSCOPE — **roent·gen·o·scop·ic** \ˌrent-gə-nə-'skä-pik, ˌrənt-, -jə-, -shə-\ adj — **roent·gen·os·co·py** \-'näs-kə-pē\ n

roentgen ray n : X RAY 1

Ro·gaine \'rō-ˌgān\ trademark — used for a preparation of minoxidil

Rog·er·ian \rä-'jer-ē-ən\ adj : of or relating to the system of therapy or the theory of personality of Carl Rogers

Rog·ers \'rä-jərz\, Carl Ransom (1902–1987), American psychologist.

Ro·lan·dic area \rō-'lan-dik-\ n : the motor area of the cerebral cortex lying just anterior to the central sulcus and comprising part of the precentral gyrus

L. Rolando — see FISSURE OF ROLANDO

Rolandic fissure n : CENTRAL SULCUS

role also **rôle** \'rōl\ n : a socially prescribed pattern of behavior usu. determined by an individual's status in a particular society

role model n : a person whose behavior in a particular role is imitated by others

role–play \'rōl-ˌplā\ vb 1 : ACT OUT 2 : to play a role

rolf \'rȯlf, 'rälf\ vb, often cap : to practice Rolfing on — **rolf·er** n, often cap

Rolf, Ida P. (1896–1979), American biochemist and physiotherapist.

Rolf·ing \'rȯl-fiŋ, 'räl-\ service mark — used for a system of muscle massage intended to serve as both physical and emotional therapy

ro·li·tet·ra·cy·cline \ˌrō-li-ˌte-trə-'sī-ˌklēn\ n : a semisynthetic broad-spectrum tetracycline antibiotic $C_{27}H_{33}N_3O_8$ used esp. for parenteral administration in cases requiring high concentrations or when oral administration is impractical

roll·er \'rō-lər\ — see TONGUE ROLLER

roller bandage n : a long rolled bandage

Rom·berg's sign \'räm-ˌbərgz-\ or **Romberg sign** \-ˌbərg-\ n : a diagnostic sign of tabes dorsalis and other diseases of the nervous system consisting of a swaying of the body when the feet are placed close together and the eyes are closed

Romberg, Moritz Heinrich (1795–1873), German pathologist.

Romberg's test or **Romberg test** n : a test for the presence of Romberg's sign by placing the feet close together and closing the eyes

ron·geur \rōⁿ-'zhər\ n : a heavy-duty forceps for removing small pieces of bone or tough tissue

ron·nel \'rän-əl\ n : an organophosphate $C_8H_8Cl_3O_3PS$ that is used esp. as a systemic insecticide to protect cattle from pests

roent·gen var of ROENTGEN

roof \'rüf, 'rüf\ n, pl roofs \'rüfs, 'rüfs, 'rüvz, 'rüvz\ 1 : the vaulted upper boundary of the mouth supported largely by the palatine bones and limited anteriorly by the dental lamina and posteriorly by the uvula and upper part of the fauces 2 : a covering structure of any of various other parts of the body (~ of the skull)

room·ing–in \'rü-miŋ-'in, 'rü-\ n : an arrangement whereby a newborn infant is kept in the mother's hospital room instead of in a nursery

room temperature n : a temperature of from 59° to 77°F (15° to 25°C) which is suitable for human occupancy

root \'rüt, 'rüt\ n 1 : the part of a tooth within the socket; also : any of the processes into which this part is often divided 2 : the enlarged basal part of a hair within the skin — called also hair root 3 : the proximal end of a nerve; esp : one or more bundles of nerve fibers joining the cranial and spinal nerves with their respective nuclei and columns of gray matter — see DORSAL ROOT, VENTRAL ROOT **4** : the part of an organ or physical structure by which it is attached to the body (the ∼ of the tongue) — **root·less** \-ləs\ *adj*

root canal *n* **1** : the part of the pulp cavity lying in the root of a tooth — called also *pulp canal* **2** : a dental operation to save a tooth by removing the contents of its root canal and filling the cavity with a protective substance

root·ed \'rü-təd, 'rù-\ *adj* **1** : having such or so many roots (single-*rooted* premolars) **2** : having a contracted root nearly closing the pulp cavity and preventing further growth

root·let \'rüt-lət, 'rùt-\ *n* : a small root; *also* : one of the ultimate divisions of a nerve root

root planing *n* : the scraping of a bacteria-impregnated layer of cementum from the surface of a tooth root to prevent or treat periodontitis

Ror·schach \'ror-ˌshäk\ *adj* : of, relating to, used in connection with, or resulting from the Rorschach test

Rorschach test *n* : a personality and intelligence test in which a subject interprets 10 standard black or colored irregular figures (as blots of ink) in terms that reveal intellectual and emotional factors — called also *Rorschach, Rorschach inkblot test*

    Rorschach, Hermann (1884–1922), Swiss psychiatrist.

ro·sa·cea \rō-'zā-shə, -shē-ə\ *n* : ACNE ROSACEA

rosary pea *n* **1** : an East Indian leguminous twining herb (*Abrus precatorius*) that bears jequirity beans and has a root used as a substitute for licorice **2** : JEQUIRITY BEAN 1

rosea — see PITYRIASIS ROSEA

rose ben·gal \-ben-'gȯl, -ben-\ *n* : either of two bluish red acid dyes that are derivatives of fluorescein

rose bengal test *n* : a test of liver function by determining the time taken for an injected quantity of rose bengal to be absorbed from the bloodstream

rose cold *n* : ROSE FEVER

rose fever *n* : hay fever occurring in the spring or early summer

ro·se·o·la \ˌrō-zē-'ō-lə, rō-'zē-ə-lə\ *n* : a rose-colored eruption in spots or a disease marked by such an eruption; *esp* : ROSEOLA INFANTUM — **ro·se·o·lar** \-lər\ *adj*

roseola in·fan·tum \-in-'fan-təm\ *n* : a mild disease of infants and children characterized by fever lasting three days followed by an eruption of rose≠ colored spots

ro·sette \rō-'zet\ *n* : a rose-shaped cluster of cells

ros·tral \'räs-trəl, 'rȯs-\ *adj* **1** : of or relating to a rostrum **2** : situated toward the oral or nasal region: as **a** *of a part of the spinal cord* : SUPERIOR 1 **b** *of a*

part of the brain : anterior or ventral (the ∼ pons) — **ros·tral·ly** *adv*

ros·trum \'räs-trəm, 'rȯs-\ *n, pl* **ros·trums** *or* **ros·tra** \-trə\ : a bodily part or process suggesting a bird's bill: as **a** : the reflected anterior portion of the corpus callosum below the genu **b** : the interior median spine of the body of the basisphenoid bone articulating with the vomer

¹**rot** \'rät\ *vb* **rot·ted; rot·ting** : to undergo decomposition from the action of bacteria or fungi

²**rot** *n* **1** : the process of rotting : the state of being rotten **2** : any of several parasitic diseases esp. of sheep marked by necrosis and wasting

ro·ta·tor \'rō-ˌtā-tər, rō-'\ *n, pl* **rotators** *or* **ro·ta·to·res** \ˌrō-tə-'tōr-ˌēz\ : a muscle that partially rotates a part on its axis; *specif* : any of several small muscles in the dorsal region of the spine arising from the upper and back part of a transverse process and inserted into the lamina of the vertebra above

rotator cuff \-ˌkəf\ *n* : a supporting and strengthening structure of the shoulder joint that is made up of part of its capsule blended with tendons of the subscapularis, infraspinatus, supraspinatus, and teres minor muscles as they pass to the capsule or across it to insert on the humerus — called also *musculotendinous cuff*

ro·ta·vi·rus \'rō-tə-ˌvī-rəs\ *n* : a reovirus that has a double-layered capsid and a wheel-like appearance and that causes diarrhea esp. in infants

ro·te·none \'rōt-ᵊn-ˌōn\ *n* : a crystalline insecticide $C_{23}H_{22}O_6$ that is of low toxicity for warm-blooded animals and is used esp. in home gardens

rotunda — see FENESTRA ROTUNDA

rotundum — see FORAMEN ROTUNDUM

Rou·get cell \rü-'zhā-\ *n* : any of numerous branching cells adhering to the endothelium of capillaries and regarded as a contractile element in the capillary wall

    Rouget, Charles–Marie–Benjamin (1824–1904), French physiologist and anatomist.

rough \'rəf\ *adj* : having a broken, uneven, or bumpy surface; *specif* : forming or being rough colonies usu. made up of organisms that form chains or filaments and tend to marked decrease in capsule formation and virulence — used of dissociated strains of bacteria; compare SMOOTH

rough·age \'rə-fij\ *n* : FIBER 2; *also* : food (as bran) containing much indigestible material acting as fiber

rou·leau \rü-'lō\ *n, pl* **rou·leaux** *same or* -'lōz\ *or* **rouleaus** : a group of red blood corpuscles resembling a stack of coins

round \'raùnd\ *vb* : to go on rounds

round cell *n* : a small lymphocyte or a closely related cell esp. occurring in an area of chronic infection or as the typical cell of some sarcomas

round ligament *n* **1** : a fibrous cord resulting from the obliteration of the umbilical vein of the fetus and passing from the umbilicus to the notch in the anterior border of the liver and along the undersurface of that organ **2** : either of a pair of rounded cords arising from each side of the uterus and traceable through the inguinal canal to the tissue of the labia majora into which they merge

rounds *n pl* : a series of professional calls on hospital patients made by a doctor or nurse — see GRAND ROUNDS

round–shouldered *adj* : having the shoulders stooping or rounded

round window *n* : a round opening between the middle ear and the cochlea that is closed over by a membrane — called also *fenestra cochleae, fenestra rotunda*

round•worm \'raund-ˌwərm\ *n* : NEMATODE; *also* : a related round-bodied unsegmented worm (as an acanthocephalan) as distinguished from a flatworm

roup \'rüp, 'raúp\ *n* : TRICHOMONIASIS c

Rous sarcoma \'raús-\ *n* : a readily transplantable malignant fibrosarcoma of chickens that is caused by a specific carcinogenic retrovirus

Rous, Francis Peyton (1879–1970), American pathologist.

Rous sarcoma virus *n* : the avian retrovirus responsible for Rous sarcoma

route \'rüt, 'raút\ *n* : a method of transmitting a disease or of administering a remedy

RPh *abbr* registered pharmacist

RPR card test \ˌär-ˌpē-ˌär-'kärd-\ *n* : RAPID PLASMA REAGIN TEST

RPT *abbr* registered physical therapist

RQ *abbr* respiratory quotient

RR *abbr* recovery room

RRA *abbr* registered records administrator

-r•rha•gia \'rā-jə, 'rā-, -jē-ə, -zhə, -zhē-ə\ *n comb form* : abnormal or excessive discharge or flow ⟨metror*rhagia*⟩ — **-r•rha•gic** \'ra-jik\ *adj comb form*

-r•rha•phy \r-ə-fē\ *n comb form, pl* **-r•rha•phies** : suture : sewing ⟨nephror*rhaphy*⟩

-r•rhea \'rē-ə\ *n comb form* : flow : discharge ⟨logor*rhea*⟩ ⟨leukor*rhea*⟩

-r•rhex•is \'rek-səs\ *n comb form, pl* **-r•rhex•es** \'rek-ˌsēz\ : rupture ⟨erythrocytor*rhexis*⟩

-r•rhoea *chiefly Brit var of* -RRHEA

RRL *abbr* registered records librarian

rRNA \ˌär-ˌär-ˌen-'ā\ *n* : RIBOSOMAL RNA

RRT *abbr* registered respiratory therapist

RS–T segment \ˌär-ˌes-'tē-\ *n* : ST SEGMENT

RSV *abbr* **1** respiratory syncytial virus **2** Rous sarcoma virus

RT *abbr* **1** reaction time **2** recreational therapy **3** respiratory therapist

Ru *symbol* ruthenium

rub \'rəb\ *n* **1** : the application of friction with pressure ⟨an alcohol ∼⟩ **2** : a sound heard in auscultation that is produced by the friction of one structure moving against another

rub•ber \'rə-bər\ *n* : CONDOM

rubber dam *n* : a thin sheet of rubber that is stretched around a tooth to keep it dry during dental work or is used in strips to provide drainage in surgical wounds

rubbing alcohol *n* : a cooling and soothing liquid for external application that contains approximately 70 percent denatured ethanol or isopropyl alcohol

¹ru•be•fa•cient \ˌrü-bə-'fā-shənt\ *adj* : causing redness of the skin ⟨a ∼ cream⟩

²rubefacient *n* : a substance for external application that produces redness of the skin

ru•bel•la \rü-'be-lə\ *n* : GERMAN MEASLES — see MATERNAL RUBELLA

ru•be•o•la \ˌrü-bē-'ō-lə, rü-'bē-ə-lə\ *n* : MEASLES 1a — **ru•be•o•lar** \-lər\ *adj*

ru•be•o•sis \ˌrü-bē-'ō-səs\ *n, pl* **-o•ses** \-'ō-ˌsēz\ *or* **-osises** : a condition characterized by abnormal redness; *esp* : RUBEOSIS IRIDIS

rubeosis iri•dis \-'ī-rə-dəs\ *n* : abnormal redness of the iris resulting from neovascularization and often associated with diabetes

ru•bid•i•um \rü-'bi-dē-əm\ *n* : a soft silvery metallic element — symbol *Rb*; see ELEMENT table

Ru•bin test \'rü-bən-\ *n* : a test to determine the patency or occlusion of the fallopian tubes by insufflating them with carbon dioxide

Rubin, Isidor Clinton (1883–1958), American gynecologist.

ru•bor \'rü-ˌbor\ *n* : redness of the skin (as from inflammation)

rubra — see PITYRIASIS RUBRA PILARIS

ru•bri•cyte \'rü-bri-ˌsīt\ *n* : an immature red blood cell that has a nucleus, is about half the size of developing red blood cells in preceding stages, and has cytoplasm that stains erratically blue, purplish, and gray due to the presence of hemoglobin : polychromatic normoblast

ru•bro•spi•nal \ˌrü-brō-'spī-nəl\ *adj* **1** : of, relating to, or connecting the red nucleus and the spinal cord **2** : of, relating to, or constituting a tract of crossed nerve fibers passing from the red nucleus to the spinal cord and relaying impulses from the cerebellum and corpora striata to the motoneurons of the spinal cord

ru•di•ment \'rü-də-mənt\ *n* : an incompletely developed organ or part; *esp* : an organ or part just beginning to develop : ANLAGE

ru•di•men•ta•ry \ˌrü-də-'men-tə-rē\ *adj*

: very imperfectly developed or represented only by a vestige

Ruf·fi·ni's corpuscle \rü-'fē-nēz-\ *or* **Ruf·fi·ni corpuscle** \-nē-\ *n* : any of numerous oval sensory end organs occurring in the subcutaneous tissue of the fingers — called also *Ruffini's brush, Ruffini's end organ*

Ruffini, Angelo (1864–1929), Italian histologist and embryologist.

RU 486 \'är-(,)yü-'fōr-,ā-tē-'siks\ *n* : a drug $C_{29}H_{35}NO_2$ taken orally to induce abortion esp. early in pregnancy by blocking the body's use of progesterone — called also *mifepristone*

ru·ga \'rü-gə\ *n, pl* **ru·gae** \-gī, -gē, -jē\ : an anatomical fold or wrinkle esp. of the viscera — usu. used in pl. ⟨*rugae* of an empty stomach⟩

ru·men \'rü-mən\ *n, pl* **ru·mi·na** \-mə-nə\ *or* **rumens** : the large first compartment of the stomach of a ruminant from which food is regurgitated for rumination and in which cellulose is broken down by the action of symbiotic microorganisms — called also *paunch;* compare ABOMASUM, OMASUM, RETICULUM

ru·men·ot·o·my \,rü-mə-'nä-tə-mē\ *n, pl* **-mies** : surgical incision into the rumen

ru·mi·nant \'rü-mə-nənt\ *adj* : of or relating to a suborder (Ruminantia) of even-toed hoofed mammals (as sheep and oxen) that chew the cud and have a complex usu. 4-chambered stomach — **ruminant** *n*

ru·mi·na·tion \,rü-mə-'nā-shən\ *n* : the act or process of regurgitating and chewing again previously swallowed food — **ru·mi·nate** \'rü-mə-,nāt\ *vb*

rump \'rəmp\ *n* **1** : the upper rounded part of the hindquarters of a quadruped mammal **2** : the seat of the body : BUTTOCKS

Rum·pel–Leede test \'rüm-pel-'lēd-\ *n* : a test in which the increased bleeding tendency characteristic of various disorders (as scarlet fever and thrombocytopenia) is indicated by the formation of multiple petechiae on the forearm following application of a tourniquet to the upper arm

Rumpel, Theodor (1862–1923), German physician.

Leede, Carl Stockbridge (b 1882), American physician.

run \'rən\ *vb* **ran** \'ran\; **run; run·ning** : to discharge fluid (as pus or serum)

⟨a *running* sore⟩ — **run a fever** *or* **run a temperature** : to have a fever

rung *past part of* RING

run·ny \'rə-nē\ *adj* : running or tending to run ⟨a ∼ nose⟩

runs \'rənz\ *n sing or pl* : DIARRHEA — used with *the*

ru·pia \'rü-pē-ə\ *n* : an eruption occurring esp. in tertiary syphilis consisting of vesicles having an inflamed base and filled with serous purulent or bloody fluid which dries up and forms large blackish conical crusts — **ru·pi·al** \-əl\ *adj*

rup·ture \'rəp-chər\ *n* **1** : the tearing apart of a tissue ⟨∼ of an intervertebral disk⟩ **2** : HERNIA — **rupture** *vb*

RUQ *abbr* right upper quadrant (abdomen)

rush \'rəsh\ *n* **1** : a rapid and extensive wave of peristalsis along the walls of the intestine ⟨peristaltic ∼⟩ **2** : the immediate pleasurable feeling produced by a drug (as heroin or amphetamine) — called also *flash*

Russian spring–summer encephalitis *n* : a tick-borne encephalitis of Europe and Asia that is transmitted by ticks of the genus *Ixodes* — see LOUPING ILL

¹**rut** \'rət\ *n* **1** : sexual excitement in a mammal (as estrus in the female) esp. when periodic **2** : the period during which rut normally occurs — often used with *the*

²**rut** *vb* **rut·ted; rut·ting** : to be in or enter into a state of rut

ru·the·ni·um \rü-'thē-nē-əm\ *n* : a hard brittle grayish rare metallic element — symbol *Ru;* see ELEMENT table

ruth·er·ford \'rə-thər-fərd\ *n* : a unit strength of a radioactive source corresponding to one million disintegrations per second — abbr. *rd*

Rutherford, Ernest (Baron Rutherford of Nelson) (1871–1937), British physicist.

ru·tin \'rüt-ᵊn\ *n* : a yellow crystalline glycoside $C_{27}H_{30}O_{16}$ that occurs in various plants (as tobacco) and that is used chiefly for strengthening capillary blood vessels (as in cases of hypertension and radiation injury)

R wave \'är-,wāv\ *n* : the positive upward deflection in the QRS complex of an electrocardiogram that follows the Q wave

Rx \,är-'eks\ *n* : a medical prescription

S

¹**S** *abbr* **1** sacral — used esp. with a number from 1 to 5 to indicate a vertebra or segment of the spinal cord in the sacral region **2** signa — used to introduce the signature in writing a prescription **3** subject **4** svedberg

²**S** *symbol* sulfur

sa *abbr* [Latin *secundum artem*] according to art — used in writing prescriptions

S–A *abbr* sinoatrial

sa·ber shin \'sā-bər-\ *n* : a tibia that has

a pronounced anterior convexity resembling the curve of a saber and caused by congenital syphilis

Sa·bin vaccine \\'sā-bin-\ *n* : a polio vaccine that is taken by mouth and contains weakened live virus — called also *Sabin oral vaccine*

Sabin, Albert Bruce (*b* 1906), American immunologist.

sac \\'sak\ *n* : a soft-walled anatomical cavity usu. having a narrow opening or none at all and often containing a special fluid ⟨a synovial ∼⟩ — see AIR SAC, LACRIMAL SAC

sac·cade \sa-'käd\ *n* : a small rapid jerky movement of the eye esp. as it jumps from fixation on one point to another (as in reading) — **sac·cad·ic** \-'kä-dik\ *adj*

sacchar- *or* **sacchari-** *or* **saccharo-** *comb form* : sugar ⟨*sacchar*ide⟩

sac·cha·rase \\'sa-kə-ˌrās, -ˌrāz\ *n* : INVERTASE

sac·cha·ride \\'sa-kə-ˌrīd, -rid\ *n* : a simple sugar, combination of sugars, or polymerized sugar : CARBOHYDRATE — see DISACCHARIDE, MONOSACCHARIDE, POLYSACCHARIDE, TRISACCHARIDE

sac·cha·rin \\'sa-kə-rin\ *n* : a crystalline compound $C_7H_5NO_3S$ that is unrelated to the carbohydrates, is many times sweeter than sucrose, and is used as a calorie-free sweetener

sac·cha·rine \\'sa-kə-rin, -ˌrēn\ *adj* **1 a** : of, relating to, or resembling that of sugar ⟨∼ taste⟩ **b** : yielding or containing sugar ⟨a ∼ fluid⟩ **2** : overly or sickeningly sweet ⟨∼ flavor⟩

sac·cha·ro·my·ces \ˌsa-kə-rō-'mī-(ˌ)sēz\ *n* **1** *cap* : a genus of usu. unicellular yeasts (family Saccharomycetaceae) that are distinguished by their sparse or absent mycelium and by their facility in reproducing asexually by budding **2** *pl* **saccharomyces** : any yeast of the genus *Saccharomyces*

sac·cu·lar \\'sa-kyə-lər\ *adj* : resembling a sac ⟨a ∼ aneurysm⟩

sac·cu·lat·ed \-ˌlā-təd\ *also* **sac·cu·late** \-ˌlāt, -lət\ *adj* : having or formed of a series of saccular expansions

sac·cu·la·tion \ˌsa-kyə-'lā-shən\ *n* **1** : the quality or state of being sacculated **2** : the process of developing or segmenting into sacculated structures **3** : a sac or sacculated structure; *esp* : one of a linear series of such structures ⟨the ∼*s* of the colon⟩

sac·cule \\'sa-(ˌ)kyül\ *n* : a little sac; *specif* : the smaller chamber of the membranous labyrinth of the ear

sac·cu·lus \\'sa-kyə-ləs\ *n*, *pl* **-li** \-ˌlī, -ˌlē\ : SACCULE

sac·like \\'sak-ˌlīk\ *adj* : having the form of or suggesting a sac

sacr- *or* **sacro-** *comb form* **1** : sacrum ⟨*sacral*⟩ **2** : sacral and ⟨*sacro*iliac⟩

sacra *pl of* SACRUM

¹sa·cral \\'sa-krəl, 'sā-\ *adj* : of, relating to, or lying near the sacrum

²sacral *n* : a sacral vertebra or sacral nerve

sacral artery — see LATERAL SACRAL ARTERY, MIDDLE SACRAL ARTERY

sacral canal *n* : the part of the vertebral canal lying in the sacrum

sacral cornu *n* : a rounded process on each side of the fifth sacral vertebra

sacral crest *n* : any of several crests or tubercles on the sacrum: as **a** : one on the midline of the dorsal surface — called also *median sacral crest* **b** : any of a series of tubercles on each side of the dorsal surface lateral to the sacral foramina that represent the transverse processes of the sacral vertebrae and serve as attachments for ligaments — called also *lateral sacral crest*

sacral foramen *n* : any of 16 openings in the sacrum of which there are four on each side of the dorsal surface giving passage to the posterior branches of the sacral nerves and four on each side of the pelvic surface giving passage to the anterior branches of the sacral nerves

sacral hiatus *n* : the opening into the spinal canal in the midline of the dorsal surface of the sacrum between the laminae of the fifth sacral vertebra

sa·cral·iza·tion \ˌsā-krə-lə-'zā-shən\ *n* : a congenital anomaly in which the fifth lumbar vertebra is fused to the sacrum in varying degrees

sacral nerve *n* : any of the spinal nerves of the sacral region of which there are five pairs and which have anterior and posterior branches passing out through the sacral foramina

sacral plexus *n* : a nerve plexus that lies against the posterior and lateral walls of the pelvis, is formed by the union of the lumbosacral trunk and the first, second, and third sacral nerves, and continues onto the thigh as the sciatic nerve

sacral promontory *n* : the inwardly projecting anterior part of the body of the first sacral vertebra

sacral vein — see LATERAL SACRAL VEIN, MEDIAN SACRAL VEIN

sacral vertebra *n* : any of the five fused vertebrae that make up the sacrum

sacro- — see SACR-

sa·cro·coc·cy·geal \ˌsā-krō-käk-'si-jəl, ˌsa-, -jē-əl\ *adj* : of, relating to, affecting, or performed by way of the region of the sacrum and coccyx

sa·cro·coc·cy·geus dor·sa·lis \-käk-'si-jē-əs-ˌdor-'sā-ləs\ *n* : an inconstant muscle that sometimes extends from the dorsal part of the sacrum to the coccyx — called also *posterior sacrococcygeal muscle*

sacrococcygeus ven·tra·lis \-ven-'trā-ləs\ *n* : an inconstant muscle that sometimes extends from the ventral surface of the lower sacral vertebrae to the coccyx — called also *anterior sacrococcygeal muscle*

¹sa·cro·il·i·ac \ˌsa-krō-ˈi-lē-ˌak, ˌsā-\ *adj* : of, relating to, affecting, or being the region of the joint between the sacrum and the ilium (∼ distress)

²sacroiliac *n* : SACROILIAC JOINT

sacroiliac joint *n* : the joint or articulation between the sacrum and ilium — called also *sacroiliac, sacroiliac articulation*

sa·cro·il·i·i·tis \ˌsā-krō-ˌi-lē-ˈī-təs, ˌsā-\ *n* : inflammation of the sacroiliac joint or region

sa·cro·spi·na·lis \ˌsā-krō-spī-ˈnā-ləs, ˌsā-krō-spi-ˈna-ləs\ *n* : a muscle that extends the length of the back and neck, that arises from the iliac crest, the sacrum, and the lumbar and two lower thoracic vertebrae, and that splits in the upper lumbar region into the iliocostalis muscles, the longissimus muscles, and the spinalis muscles — called also *erector spinae*

sa·cro·spi·nous ligament \ˌsā-krō-ˈspī-nəs-, ˌsā-\ *n* : a ligament on each side of the body that is attached by a broad base to the lateral margins of the sacrum and coccyx and passes to the ischial spine and that closes off the greater sciatic notch to form the greater sciatic foramen and with the sacrotuberous ligament closes off the lesser sciatic notch to form the lesser sciatic foramen

sa·cro·tu·ber·ous ligament \ˌsā-krō-ˈtü-bə-rəs-, ˌsā-, -ˈtyü-\ *n* : a thin fan‐shaped ligament on each side of the body that is attached above to the posterior superior and posterior inferior iliac spines and to the sacrum and coccyx, that passes obliquely downward to insert into the inner margin of the ischial tuberosity, and that with the sacrospinous ligament closes off the lesser sciatic notch to form the lesser sciatic foramen

sa·cro·uter·ine ligament \-ˈyü-tə-ˌrīn-, -rən\ *n* : UTEROSACRAL LIGAMENT

sa·crum \ˈsa-krəm, ˈsā-\ *n, pl* **sa·cra** \ˈsa-krə, ˈsā-\ : the part of the spinal column that is directly connected with or forms a part of the pelvis by articulation with the ilia and that in humans forms the dorsal wall of the pelvis and consists of five fused vertebrae diminishing in size to the apex at the lower end which bears the coccyx

SAD *abbr* seasonal affective disorder

sad·dle \ˈsad-ᵊl\ *n* : the part of a partial denture that carries an artificial tooth and has connectors for adjacent teeth attached to its ends

saddle block anesthesia *n* : spinal anesthesia confined to the perineum, the buttocks, and the inner aspect of the thighs — called also *saddle block*

saddle joint *n* : a joint (as the carpometacarpal joint of the thumb) with saddle-shaped articular surfaces that are convex in one direction and concave in another and that permit movements in all directions except axial rotation

sad·dle·nose \ˈsad-ᵊl-ˌnōz\ *n* : a nose marked by depression of the bridge resulting from injury or disease

sa·dism \ˈsā-ˌdiz-əm, ˈsa-\ *n* : a sexual perversion in which gratification is obtained by the infliction of physical or mental pain on others (as on a love object) — compare ALGOLAGNIA, MASOCHISM — **sa·dis·tic** \sə-ˈdis-tik, sā-, sa-\ *adj* — **sa·dis·ti·cal·ly** *adv*

Sade \ˈsäd\, **Marquis de (Comte Donatien–Alphonse–François) (1740–1814),** French soldier and writer.

sa·dist \ˈsā-dist, ˈsa-\ *n* : an individual who practices sadism

sa·do·mas·och·ism \ˌsā-(ˌ)dō-ˈma-sə-ˌki-zəm, ˌsa-, -zə-ˌki-\ *n* : the derivation of pleasure from the infliction of physical or mental pain either on others or on oneself — **sa·do·mas·och·ist·ic** \-ˌma-sə-ˈkist-ik\ *also* **sadomas·ochist** *adj*

L. von Sacher–Masoch — see MASOCHISM

sa·do·mas·och·ist \-kist\ *n* : an individual who practices sadomasochism

safe \ˈsāf\ *adj* **saf·er; saf·est** : not causing harm or injury; *esp* : having a low incidence of adverse reactions and significant side effects when adequate instructions for use are given and having a low potential for harm under conditions of widespread availability — **safe·ty** \ˈsāf-tē\ *n*

safe period *n* : a portion of the menstrual cycle of the human female during which conception is least likely to occur and which usu. includes several days immediately before and after the menstrual period and the period itself — compare RHYTHM METHOD

safe sex *n* : sexual activity and esp. sexual intercourse in which various measures (as the use of latex condoms or the practice of monogamy) are taken to avoid disease (as AIDS) transmitted by sexual contact

saf·flow·er oil \ˈsa-ˌflau̇-ər-\ *n* : an edible oil that is low in saturated fatty acids, is obtained from the seeds of the safflower (*Carthamus tinctorius*) of the daisy family (Compositae), and is often used in diets low in cholesterol

sag·it·tal \ˈsa-jət-ᵊl\ *adj* **1** : of, relating to, or being the sagittal suture of the skull **2** : of, relating to, situated in, or being the median plane of the body or any plane parallel to it — **sag·it·tal·ly** *adv*

sagittal plane *n* : MIDSAGITTAL PLANE; *also* : any plane parallel to a midsagittal plane : a parasagittal plane

sagittal sinus *n* : either of two venous sinuses of the dura mater: **a** : one passing backward in the convex attached superior margin of the falx cerebri and ending at the internal occipital protuberance by fusion with the transverse sinus — called also *superior sagittal sinus* **b** : one lying in the posterior two thirds of the concave free inferior margin of the falx cerebri and ending posteriorly by joining the great cerebral vein to form the straight sinus — called also *inferior sagittal sinus*

sagittal suture *n* : the deeply serrated articulation between the two parietal bones in the median plane of the top of the head

sa·go spleen \'sā-(,)gō-\ *n* : a spleen which is affected with amyloid degeneration and in which the amyloid is deposited in the Malpighian corpuscles which appear in cross section as gray translucent bodies

Saint An·tho·ny's fire \,sānt-'an-thə-nēz-\ *n* : any of several inflammations or gangrenous conditions (as erysipelas or ergotism) of the skin

Anthony, Saint (*ca* 250–350), Egyptian monk.

Saint–John's–wort \,sānt-'jänz-,wərt, -,wort\ *n* : any of a genus (*Hypericum* of the family Guttiferae) of herbs and shrubs with showy yellow flowers; *esp* : one (*H. perforatum*) of dry soil, roadsides, pastures, and ranges that contains a photodynamic pigment causing dermatitis due to photosensitization in sheep, cattle, horses, and goats when ingested

John the Baptist, Saint (*fl first century* A.D.), Jewish prophet.

Saint Lou·is encephalitis \,sānt-'lü-is-\ *n* : a No. American viral encephalitis that is transmitted by several mosquitoes of the genus *Culex*

Saint Vi·tus' dance \-'vī-təs-\ *also* **Saint Vitus's dance** \-'vī-tə-səz-\ *n* : CHOREA; *esp* : SYDENHAM'S CHOREA

Vitus, Saint (*d ca* 300), Italian martyr.

sal·abra·sion \,sa-lə-'brā-zhən\ *n* : a method of removing tattoos from skin in which moist gauze pads saturated with sodium chloride are used to abrade the tattooed area by rubbing

sal am·mo·ni·ac \,sal-ə-'mō-nē-,ak\ *n* : AMMONIUM CHLORIDE

sal·bu·ta·mol \sal-'byü-tə-,mòl, -,mōl\ *n* : a xylene derivative $C_{13}H_{21}NO_3$ used as a bronchodilator

salicyl- *or* **salicylo-** *comb form* : related to salicylic acid (*salicyl*amide)

sal·i·cyl·amide \,sa-lə-'si-lə-,mid\ *n* : the crystalline amide $C_7H_7NO_2$ of salicylic acid that is used chiefly as an analgesic, antipyretic, and antirheumatic

sal·i·cyl·an·il·ide \,sa-lə-sə-'lan-ə-,īd\ *n* : a crystalline compound $C_{13}H_{11}NO_2$ that is used as a fungicidal agent esp. in the external treatment of tinea capitis caused by a fungus of the genus *Microsporum* (*M. audouini*)

sa·lic·y·late \sə-'li-sə-,lāt\ *n* : a salt or ester of salicylic acid; *also* : SALICYLIC ACID

sal·i·cyl·azo·sul·fa·pyr·i·dine \,sa-lə-si-,lā-zō-,səl-fə-'pir-ə-,dēn\ *n* : a sulfonamide $C_{18}H_{14}N_4O_5S$ used in the treatment of chronic ulcerative colitis — called also *sulfasalazine*

sal·i·cyl·ic acid \,sa-lə-'si-lik-\ *n* : a crystalline phenolic acid $C_7H_6O_3$ that is used esp. in making pharmaceuticals and dyes, as an antiseptic and disinfectant esp. in treating skin diseases, and in the form of salts and other derivatives as an analgesic and antipyretic — see ASPIRIN

sal·i·cyl·ism \'sa-lə-si-,li-zəm\ *n* : a toxic condition produced by the excessive intake of salicylic acid or salicylates and marked by ringing in the ears, nausea, and vomiting

¹sa·line \'sā-,lēn, -,līn\ *adj* **1** : consisting of or containing salt (a ~ solution) **2** : of, relating to, or resembling salt : SALTY **3** : consisting of or relating to the salts esp. of lithium, sodium, potassium, and magnesium (a ~ cathartic) **4** : relating to or being abortion induced by the injection of a highly concentrated saline solution into the amniotic sac (~ amniocentesis) — **sa·lin·i·ty** \sā-'lin-ət-ē, sə-\ *n*

²saline *n* **1 a** : a metallic salt; *esp* : a salt of potassium, sodium, or magnesium with a cathartic action **b** : an aqueous solution of one or more such salts **2** : a saline solution used in physiology

sa·li·va \sə-'lī-və\ *n* : a slightly alkaline secretion of water, mucin, protein, salts, and often a starch-splitting enzyme (as ptyalin) that is secreted into the mouth by salivary glands, lubricates ingested food, and often begins the breakdown of starches

saliva ejector *n* : a narrow tubular device providing suction to draw saliva, blood, and debris from the mouth of a dental patient in order to maintain a clear operative field

sal·i·vary \'sa-lə-,ver-ē\ *adj* : of or relating to saliva or the glands that secrete it; *esp* : producing or carrying saliva

salivary gland *n* : any of various glands that discharge a fluid secretion and esp. saliva into the mouth cavity and that in humans comprise large compound racemose glands including the parotid glands, the sublingual glands, and the submandibular glands

sal·i·va·tion \,sa-lə-'vā-shən\ *n* : the act or process of producing a flow of saliva; *esp* : excessive secretion of saliva often accompanied by soreness of the mouth and gums — **sal·i·vate** \'sa-lə-,vāt\ *vb*

sal·i·va·to·ry \'sa-lə-və-,tōr-ē\ *adj* : inducing salivation

Salk vaccine \'sòk-, 'sòlk-\ *n* : a vaccine consisting of three strains of poliomyelitis virus grown on embryonated eggs and treated with formaldehyde for inactivation

Salk, Jonas Edward (*b* 1914), American immunologist.

sal·mo·nel·la \,sal-mə-'ne-lə\ *n* 1 *cap* : a genus of aerobic gram-negative rod-shaped usu. motile enterobacteria that are pathogenic for humans and other warm-blooded animals and cause food poisoning, acute gastrointestinal inflammation, typhoid fever, or septicemia 2 *pl* **-nel·lae** \-'ne-lē\ or **-nellas** or **-nella** : any bacterium of the genus *Salmonella*

Salm·on \'sa-mən\, **Daniel Elmer** (1850–1914), American veterinarian.

sal·mo·nel·lo·sis \,sal-mə-,ne-'lō-səs\ *n*, *pl* **-lo·ses** \-,sēz\ : infection with or disease caused by bacteria of the genus *Salmonella* typically marked by gastroenteritis but often complicated by septicemia, meningitis, endocarditis, and various focal lesions (as in the kidneys)

salmon poisoning *n* : a highly fatal febrile disease of fish-eating dogs and other canine mammals that resembles canine distemper and is caused by a rickettsial bacterium (*Neorickettsia helminthoeca*) transmitted by encysted larvae of a fluke (*Nanophyetus salmincola*) ingested with the raw flesh of infested salmon, trout, or salamanders

sal·ol \'sa-,lȯl, -,ōl\ *n* : PHENYL SALICYLATE

salping- or **salpingo-** *comb form* 1 : fallopian tube ⟨*salpingo*plasty⟩ 2 : eustachian tube ⟨*salpingo*pharyngeus⟩

sal·pin·gec·to·my \,sal-pən-'jek-tə-mē\ *n*, *pl* **-mies** : surgical excision of a fallopian tube

sal·pin·gi·tis \,sal-pən-'jī-təs\ *n* : inflammation of a fallopian or eustachian tube

sal·pin·gog·ra·phy \,sal-piŋ-'gä-grə-fē\ *n*, *pl* **-phies** : visualization of a fallopian tube by roentgenography following injection of an opaque medium

sal·pin·gol·y·sis \,sal-piŋ-'gä-lə-səs\ *n*, *pl* **-y·ses** : surgical correction of adhesions in a fallopian tube

sal·pin·go-oo·pho·rec·to·my \,sal-,piŋ-gō-,ō-ə-fə-'rek-tə-mē\ *n*, *pl* **-mies** : surgical excision of a fallopian tube and an ovary

sal·pin·go-oo·pho·ri·tis \-,ō-ə-fə-'rī-təs\ *n* : inflammation of a fallopian tube and an ovary

sal·pin·go·pha·ryn·ge·us \-fə-'rin-jē-əs\ *n* : a muscle of the pharynx that arises from the inferior part of the eustachian tube near its opening and passes downward to join the posterior part of the palatopharyngeus

sal·pin·go·plas·ty \sal-'piŋ-gə-,plas-tē\ *n*, *pl* **-ties** : plastic surgery of a fallopian tube

sal·pin·gos·to·my \,sal-piŋ-'gäs-tə-mē\ *n*, *pl* **-mies** : a surgical opening of a fallopian tube (as to establish patency or facilitate drainage)

¹salt \'sȯlt\ *n* 1 **a** : a crystalline compound NaCl that is the chloride of sodium, is abundant in nature, and is used esp. to season or preserve food — called also *sodium chloride* **b** : any of numerous compounds that result from replacement of part or all of the acid hydrogen of an acid by a metal or a group acting like a metal : an ionic crystalline compound 2 *pl* **a** : a mineral or saline mixture (as Epsom salts) used as an aperient or cathartic **b** : SMELLING SALTS — **salty** \'sȯl-tē\ *adj*

²salt *adj* 1 : SALINE 2 : being or inducing the one of the four basic taste sensations that is suggestive of seawater — compare BITTER, SOUR, SWEET

sal·ta·to·ry \'sal-tə-,tȯr-ē, 'sȯl-\ *adj* : proceeding by leaps rather than by gradual transitions ⟨~ conduction of nerve impulses⟩

salt·pe·ter \'sȯlt-'pē-tər\ *n* 1 : POTASSIUM NITRATE 2 : SODIUM NITRATE

¹sal·uret·ic \,sal-yə-'re-tik\ *adj* : facilitating the urinary excretion of salt and esp. of sodium ion ⟨a ~ drug⟩

²saluretic *n* : a saluretic agent (as a drug)

Sal·u·ron \'sa-lù-,rän, -,lyü-\ *trademark* — used for a preparation of hydroflumethiazide

sal·vage \'sal-vij\ *vb* **sal·vaged; sal·vag·ing** : to save (an organ, tissue, or patient) by preventive or therapeutic measures ⟨*salvaged* lung tissue⟩ — **salvage** *n*

sal·var·san \'sal-vər-,san\ *n* : ARSPHENAMINE

salve \'sav, 'sȧv, 'salv, 'sȧlv\ *n* : an unctuous adhesive substance for application to wounds or sores

sal vo·la·ti·le \,sal-və-²lat-²l-ē\ *n* 1 : AMMONIUM CARBONATE 2 : SMELLING SALTS

sa·mar·i·um \sə-'mar-ē-əm\ *n* : a pale gray lustrous metallic element — symbol *Sm*; see ELEMENT table

san·a·to·ri·um \,sa-nə-²tȯr-ē-əm\ *n*, *pl* **-riums** or **-ria** \-ē-ə\ 1 : an establishment that provides therapy combined with a regimen (as of diet and exercise) for treatment or rehabilitation 2 **a** : an institution for rest and recuperation (as of convalescents) **b** : an establishment for the treatment of the chronically ill ⟨a tuberculosis ~⟩

sand \'sand\ *n* : gritty particles in various body tissues or fluids

sand crack *n* : a fissure in the wall of a horse's hoof often causing lameness

sand flea *n* : CHIGOE 1

sand fly *n* : any of various small biting dipteran flies (families Psychodidae, Simuliidae, and Ceratopogonidae); *esp* : any fly of the genus *Phlebotomus*

sand·fly fever \'sand-,flī-\ *n* : a virus disease of brief duration that is characterized by fever, headache, pain in the eyes, malaise, and leukopenia and is transmitted by the bite of a sand fly of the genus *Phlebotomus*

(*P. papatasii*) — called also *pappataci fever, phlebotomus fever*

Sand·hoff–Jatz·ke·witz disease \-ˈjats-kə-ˌvits-\ *n* : SANDHOFF'S DISEASE

Sand·hoff's disease \ˈsand-ˌhofs-\ *or* **Sand·hoff disease** \-ˌhof-\ *n* : a variant of Tay-Sachs disease in which both hexosaminidase and hexosaminidase B are present in greatly reduced quantities

Sandhoff, K., An·dreae \än-ˈdrā-e\, U., and Jatzkewitz, H., German medical scientists.

San·dril \ˈsan-ˌdril\ *trademark* — used for a preparation of reserpine

sane \ˈsān\ *adj* **san·er; san·est 1** : free from hurt or disease : HEALTHY **2** : mentally sound; *esp* : able to anticipate and appraise the effect of one's actions **3** : proceeding from a sound mind (~ behavior) — **sane·ly** *adv*

san·guin·eous \saŋ-ˈgwi-nē-əs, san-\ *adj* : of, relating to, or containing blood

san·gui·nous \ˈsaŋ-gwə-nəs\ *adj* : SANGUINEOUS

san·i·tar·i·an \ˌsa-nə-ˈter-ē-ən\ *n* : a specialist in sanitary science and public health (milk ~)

san·i·tar·i·um \ˌsa-nə-ˈter-ē-əm\ *n, pl* **-i·ums** *or* **-ia** \-ē-ə\ : SANATORIUM

san·i·tary \ˈsa-nə-ˌter-ē\ *adj* **1** : of or relating to health (~ measures) **2** : of, relating to, or used in the disposal esp. of domestic waterborne waste (~ sewage) **3** : characterized by or readily kept in cleanliness (~ food handling) — **san·i·tar·i·ly** \ˌsa-nə-ˈter-ə-lē\ *adv*

sanitary napkin *n* : a disposable absorbent pad used (as during menstruation) to absorb the flow from the uterus

san·i·ta·tion \ˌsa-nə-ˈtā-shən\ *n* **1** : the act or process of making sanitary **2** : the promotion of hygiene and prevention of disease by maintenance of sanitary conditions (mouth ~)

san·i·tize \ˈsa-nə-ˌtīz\ *vb* **-tized; -tiz·ing** : to make sanitary (as by cleaning or sterilizing) — **san·i·ti·za·tion** \ˌsa-nə-tə-ˈzā-shən\ *n*

san·i·to·ri·um \ˌsa-nə-ˈtōr-ē-əm\ *n, pl* **-ri·ums** *or* **-ria** \-ē-ə\ : SANATORIUM

san·i·ty \ˈsa-nə-tē\ *n, pl* **-ties** : the quality or state of being sane; *esp* : soundness or health of mind

San Joa·quin fever \ˌsan-wä-ˈkēn-\ *n* : COCCIDIOIDOMYCOSIS

San Joaquin valley fever *n* : COCCIDIOIDOMYCOSIS

S–A node \ˈes-ˈā-\ *n* : SINOATRIAL NODE

santa — see YERBA SANTA

sap \ˈsap\ — see CELL SAP, NUCLEAR SAP

sa·phe·no·fem·o·ral \sə-ˌfē-nō-ˈfe-mə-rəl\ *adj* : of or relating to the saphenous and the femoral veins

sa·phe·nous \sə-ˈfē-nəs, ˈsa-fə-nəs\ *adj* : of, relating to, associated with, or being either of the saphenous veins

saphenous nerve *n* : a nerve that is the

largest and longest branch of the femoral nerve and supplies the skin over the medial side of the leg

saphenous opening *n* : a passage for the great saphenous vein in the fascia lata of the thigh — called also *fossa ovalis*

saphenous vein *n* : either of two chief superficial veins of the leg: **a** : one originating in the foot and passing up the medial side of the leg and through the saphenous opening to join the femoral vein — called also *great saphenous vein, long saphenous vein* **b** : one originating similarly and passing up the back of the leg to join the popliteal vein at the knee — called also *short saphenous vein, small saphenous vein*

sa·pon·i·fi·ca·tion \sə-ˌpä-nə-fə-ˈkā-shən\ *n* **1** : the hydrolysis of a fat by an alkali with the formation of a soap and glycerol **2** : the hydrolysis esp. by an alkali of an ester into the corresponding alcohol and acid; *broadly* : HYDROLYSIS — **sa·pon·i·fy** \sə-ˈpä-nə-ˌfī\ *vb*

sap·phic \ˈsa-fik\ *adj or n* : LESBIAN

Sap·pho \ˈsa-(ˌ)fō\ (*fl ca* 610 BC–*ca* 580 BC), Greek lyric poet.

sap·phism \ˈsa-ˌfi-zəm\ *n* : LESBIANISM

sap·phist \-fist\ *n* : LESBIAN

sapr- *or* **sapro-** *comb form* : dead or decaying organic matter (*saprophyte*)

sap·ro·phyte \ˈsa-prə-ˌfīt\ *n* : a living thing and esp. a plant living on dead or decaying organic matter

sap·ro·phyt·ic \ˌsa-prə-ˈfi-tik\ *adj* : obtaining food by absorbing dissolved organic material; *esp* : obtaining nourishment osmotically from the products of organic breakdown and decay (meningitis caused by ~ bacteria) — **sap·ro·phyt·i·cal·ly** *adv*

sap·ro·zo·ic \-ˈzō-ik\ *adj* : SAPROPHYTIC — used of animals (as protozoans)

sar·al·a·sin \sä-ˈra-lə-sən\ *n* : an antihypertensive polypeptide used esp. in the form of its acetate in the treatment and diagnosis of hypertension

sarc- *or* **sarco-** *comb form* **1** : flesh (*sarcoid*) **2** : striated muscle (*sarcolemma*)

sar·co·cyst \ˈsär-kə-ˌsist\ *n* : the large intramuscular cyst of a protozoan of the genus *Sarcocystis*

Sar·co·cys·tis \ˌsär-kə-ˈsis-təs\ *n* : a genus of sporozoan protozoans (order Sarcosporidia) that form cysts in vertebrate muscle

¹**sar·coid** \ˈsär-ˌkoid\ *adj* : of, relating to, resembling, or being sarcoid or sarcoidosis (~ fibroblastic tissue)

²**sarcoid** *n* **1** : any of various diseases characterized esp. by the formation of nodules in the skin **2** : a nodule characteristic of sarcoid or of sarcoidosis

sar·coid·o·sis \ˌsär-ˌkoi-ˈdō-səs\ *n, pl* **-o·ses** \-ˌsēz\ : a chronic disease of unknown cause that is characterized by the formation of nodules resembling true tubercles esp. in the lymph nodes, lungs, bones, and skin — called also *Boeck's sarcoid*

sar·co·lem·ma \ˌsär-kə-ˈle-mə\ *n* : the thin transparent homogeneous sheath enclosing a striated muscle fiber — **sar·co·lem·mal** \-məl\ *adj*

sar·co·ly·sin \ˌsär-kə-ˈli-sən\ *or* **sar·co·ly·sine** \-sēn\ *also* L-**sar·co·ly·sin** \ˈel-\ *or* L-**sar·co·ly·sine** *n* : MELPHALAN

sar·co·ma \sär-ˈkō-mə\ *n, pl* -**mas** *also* -**ma·ta** \-mə-tə\ : a malignant neoplasm arising in tissue of mesodermal origin (as connective tissue, bone, cartilage, or striated muscle) that spreads by extension into neighboring tissue or by way of the bloodstream — compare CANCER 1, CARCINOMA

sarcoma bot·ry·oi·des \-ˌbä-trē-ˈoi-ˌdēz\ *n* : a malignant tumor of striated muscle that resembles a bunch of grapes and occurs esp. in the urogenital tract of young children

sar·co·ma·to·sis \ˌ(ˌ)sär-ˌkō-mə-ˈtō-səs\ *n, pl* -**to·ses** \-ˌsēz\ : a disease characterized by the presence and spread of sarcomas

sar·co·ma·tous \sär-ˈkō-mə-təs\ *adj* : of, relating to, or resembling sarcoma

sar·co·mere \ˈsär-kə-ˌmir\ *n* : any of the repeating structural units of striated muscle fibrils — **sar·co·mer·ic** \ˌsär-kə-ˈmer-ik\ *adj*

Sar·coph·a·ga \sär-ˈkä-fə-gə\ *n* : a genus of dipteran flies (family Sarcophagidae) comprising typical flesh flies

sar·co·plasm \ˈsär-kə-ˌpla-zəm\ *n* : the cytoplasm of a striated muscle fiber — compare MYOPLASM — **sar·co·plas·mic** \ˌsär-kə-ˈplaz-mik\ *adj*

sarcoplasmic reticulum *n* : the endoplasmic reticulum of cardiac muscle and skeletal striated muscle fiber that functions esp. as a storage and release area for calcium

Sar·cop·tes \sär-ˈkäp-ˌtēz\ *n* : a genus of whitish itch mites (family Sarcoptidae)

sar·cop·tic \sär-ˈkäp-tik\ *adj* : of, relating to, caused by, or being itch mites of the genus *Sarcoptes*

sarcoptic mange *n* : a mange caused by mites of the genus *Sarcoptes* that burrow in the skin esp. of the head and face — compare CHORIOPTIC MANGE, DEMODECTIC MANGE

sar·co·sine \ˈsär-kə-ˌsēn, -sən\ *n* : a sweetish crystalline amino acid $C_3H_7NO_2$ formed by the decomposition of creatine or made synthetically

sar·co·some \ˈsär-kə-ˌsōm\ *n* : a mitochondrion of a striated muscle fiber — **sar·co·som·al** \ˌsär-kə-ˈsō-məl\ *adj*

sar·co·spo·rid·i·o·sis \ˌsär-kō-spə-ˌri-dē-ˈō-səs\ *n, pl* -**o·ses** \-ˌsēz\ : infestation with or disease caused by protozoans of the genus *Sarcocystis*

sardonicus — see RISUS SARDONICUS

sa·rin \ˈsär-ən, zä-ˈrēn\ *n* : an extremely toxic chemical warfare agent $C_4H_{10}FO_2P$ — called also *GB*

sar·to·ri·us \sär-ˈtōr-ē-əs\ *n, pl* -**rii** \-ē-ˌī\ : a muscle that arises from the anterior superior iliac spine, crosses the front of the thigh obliquely to insert on the upper part of the inner surface of the tibia, is the longest muscle in the human body, and acts to flex, abduct, and rotate the thigh laterally at the hip joint and to flex the leg at the knee joint and to rotate it medially in a way that enables one to sit with the heel of one leg on the knee of the opposite leg in a position often attributed to a tailor busy sewing

sas·sa·fras \ˈsa-sə-ˌfras\ *n* **1** : a tall eastern No. American tree (*Sassafras albidum*) of the laurel family (Lauraceae) with mucilaginous twigs and leaves **2** : the dried root bark of the sassafras formerly used as a diaphoretic and flavoring agent but now prohibited for use as a flavoring or food additive because of its carcinogenic properties

sat·el·lite \ˈsat-əl-ˌīt\ *n* **1** : a short segment separated from the main body of a chromosome by a constriction **2** : a bodily structure lying near or associated with another (as a vein accompanying an artery) **3** : a smaller lesion accompanying a main one and situated nearby — **satellite** *adj*

satellite cell *n* : a cell surrounding a ganglion cell

satellite DNA *n* : a fraction of a eukaryotic organism's DNA that differs in density from most of its DNA as determined by centrifugation, that apparently consists of short repetitive nucleotide sequences, that does not undergo transcription, and that in some organisms (as the mouse) is found esp. in centromeric regions

sat·el·lit·o·sis \ˌsat-əl-ī-ˈtō-səs\ *n, pl* -**o·ses** \-ˌsēz\ : a condition characterized by a grouping of satellite cells around ganglion cells in the brain

sa·ti·ety \sə-ˈtī-ə-tē\ *n, pl* -**ties** : the quality or state of being fed or gratified to or beyond capacity

¹**sat·u·rate** \ˈsa-chə-ˌrāt\ *vb* -**rat·ed; -rat·ing** **1** : to treat, furnish, or charge with something to the point where no more can be absorbed, dissolved, or retained **2** : to cause to combine till there is no further tendency to combine

²**sat·u·rate** \-rət\ *n* : a saturated chemical compound

sat·u·rat·ed \ˈsa-chə-ˌrā-təd\ *adj* **1** : being the most concentrated solution that can persist in the presence of an excess of the dissolved substance **2** : being a compound that does not tend to unite directly with another compound — used esp. of organic compounds containing no double or triple bonds

sat·u·ra·tion \ˌsa-chə-ˈrā-shən\ *n* **1** : the act of saturating : the state of being saturated **2** : conversion of an unsaturated to a saturated chemical compound (as by hydrogenation) **3** : a state of maximum impregnation; *esp* : the presence in air of the most water possible under existent pressure and temperature **4** : the one of the three psychological dimensions of color perception that is related to the purity of the color and that decreases as the amount of white present in the stimulus increases — called also *intensity;* compare BRIGHTNESS, HUE

sat·ur·nine \ˈsa-tər-ˌnīn\ *adj* **1** : of or relating to lead **2** : of, relating to, or produced by the absorption of lead into the system (~ poisoning)

sat·urn·ism \ˈsa-tər-ˌni-zəm\ *n* : LEAD POISONING

sa·ty·ri·a·sis \ˌsā-tə-ˈrī-ə-səs, ˌsa-\ *n, pl* **-a·ses** \-ˌsēz\ : excessive or abnormal sexual desire in the male — compare NYMPHOMANIA

sau·cer·ize \ˈsò-sər-ˌīz\ *vb* **-ized; -iz·ing** : to form a shallow depression by excavation of tissue to promote granulation and healing of (a wound) — **sau·cer·iza·tion** \ˌsò-sər-ə-ˈzā-shən\ *n*

sau·na \ˈsau̇-nə, ˈsò-nə\ *n* **1** : a Finnish steam bath in which the steam is provided by water thrown on hot stones; *also* : a bathhouse or room used for such a bath **2** : a dry heat bath; *also* : a room or cabinet used for such a bath

saw \ˈsò\ *n* : a hand or power tool used to cut hard material (as bone) and equipped usu. with a toothed blade or disk

saxi·tox·in \ˌsak-sə-ˈtäk-sən\ *n* : a potent nonprotein neurotoxin $C_{10}H_{17}N_7O_4 \cdot 2HCl$ that originates in dinoflagellates of the genus *Gonyaulax* found in red tides and that sometimes occurs in and renders toxic normally edible mollusks which feed on them

Sb *symbol* [Latin *stibium*] antimony

SBS *abbr* sick building syndrome

Sc *symbol* scandium

scab \ˈskab\ *n* **1** : scabies of domestic animals **2** : a hardened covering of dried secretions as blood, plasma, or pus) that forms over a wound — called also *crust* — **scab** *vb* — **scab·by** \ˈska-bē\ *adj*

scabby mouth *n* : SORE MOUTH 1

sca·bi·cide \ˈskā-bə-ˌsīd\ *n* : a drug that destroys the itch mite causing scabies

sca·bies \ˈskā-bēz\ *n, pl* **scabies** : contagious itch or mange esp. with exudative crusts that is caused by parasitic mites and esp. by a mite of the genus *Sarcoptes* (*S. scabiei*) — **sca·bi·et·ic** \ˌskā-bē-ˈe-tik\ *adj*

scab mite *n* : any of several small mites that cause mange, scabies, or scab; *esp* : one of the genus *Psoroptes*

sca·la \ˈskā-lə\ *n, pl* **sca·lae** \-ˌlē\ : any of the three spirally arranged canals into which the bony canal of the cochlea is partitioned by the vestibular and basilar membranes and which comprise the scala media, scala tympani, and scala vestibuli

scala me·dia \-ˈmē-dē-ə\ *n, pl* **scalae me·di·ae** \-dē-ˌē\ : the spirally arranged canal in the bony canal of the cochlea that contains the organ of Corti, is triangular in cross section, and is bounded by the vestibular membrane above, by the periosteum-lined wall of the cochlea laterally, and by the basilar membrane below — called also *cochlear canal, cochlear duct*

scala tym·pa·ni \-ˈtim-pə-ˌnī, -ˌnē\ *n, pl* **scalae tym·pa·no·rum** \-ˌtim-pə-ˈnòr-əm\ : the lymph-filled spirally arranged canal in the bony canal of the cochlea that is separated from the scala media by the basilar membrane, communicates at its upper end with the scala vestibuli, and abuts at its lower end upon the membrane that separates the round window from the middle ear

scala ves·tib·u·li \-ve-ˈsti-byə-ˌlī\ *n, pl* **scalae ves·tib·u·lo·rum** \-ve-ˌsti-byə-ˈlò-rəm\ : the lymph-filled spirally arranged canal in the bony canal of the cochlea that is separated from the scala media by the vestibular membrane, is connected with the oval window, and receives vibrations from the stapes

¹scald \ˈskòld\ *vb* : to burn with hot liquid or steam (~*ed* skin)

²scald *n* : an injury to the body caused by scalding

scalded–skin syndrome *n* : TOXIC EPIDERMAL NECROLYSIS — see STAPHYLOCOCCAL SCALDED SKIN SYNDROME

¹scale \ˈskāl\ *n* **1** : a small thin dry lamina shed (as in many skin diseases) from the skin **2** : a film of tartar encrusting the teeth

²scale *vb* **scaled; scal·ing 1** : to take off or come off in thin layers or scales (~ tartar from the teeth) **2** : to shed scales or fragmentary surface matter : EXFOLIATE (*scaling* skin)

³scale *n* **1** : a series of marks or points at known intervals used to measure distances (as the height of the mercury in a thermometer) **2** : a graduated series or scheme of rank or order **3** : a graded series of tests or of performances used in rating individual intelligence or achievement

sca·lene \ˈskā-ˌlēn, skā-ˈ\ *n* : SCALENUS — called also *scalene muscle*

sca·le·not·o·my \ˌskā-lə-ˈnä-tə-mē\ *n, pl* **-mies** : surgical severing of one or more scalenus muscles near their insertion on the ribs

sca·le·nus \skā-ˈlē-nəs\ *n, pl* **sca·le·ni** \-ˌnī\ : any of usu. three deeply situated muscles on each side of the neck of which each extends from the transverse processes of two or more cervical vertebrae to the first or second rib: **a** : one arising from the transverse processes of the third to sixth cervical vertebrae, inserting on the scalene tubercle of the first rib, and functioning to bend the neck forward and laterally and to rotate it to the side — called also *scalenus anterior, scalenus anticus* **b** : one arising from the transverse processes of the lower six cervical vertebrae, inserting on the upper surface of the first rib, and functioning similarly to the scalenus anterior — called also *scalenus medius* **c** : one arising from the transverse processes of the fourth to sixth cervical vertebrae, inserting on the outer surface of the second rib, and functioning to raise the second rib and to bend and slightly rotate the neck — called also *scalenus posterior*

scalenus anterior *n* : SCALENUS a

scalenus an·ti·cus \-an-ˈtī-kəs\ *n* : SCALENUS a

scalenus anticus syndrome *n* : a complex of symptoms including pain and numbness in the region of the shoulder, arm, and neck that is caused by compression of the brachial plexus or subclavian artery or both by the scalenus anticus muscle

scalenus me·di·us \-ˈmē-dē-əs\ *n* : SCALENUS b

scalenus posterior *n* : SCALENUS c

scal·er \ˈskā-lər\ *n* : any of various dental instruments for removing tartar from teeth

scalp \ˈskalp\ *n* : the part of the integument of the head usu. covered with hair in both sexes

scal·pel \ˈskal-pəl\ *n* : a small straight thin-bladed knife used esp. in surgery

scaly \ˈskā-lē\ *adj* **scal·i·er; -est** : covered with or composed of scale or scales ⟨∼ skin⟩ — **scal·i·ness** *n*

¹scan \ˈskan\ *vb* **scanned; scan·ning 1 a** : to examine esp. systematically with a sensing device (as a beam of radiation) **b** : to move an electron beam over and convert (an image) into variations of electrical properties (as voltage) that convey information electronically **2** : to make a scan of (as the human body) in order to detect the presence or localization of radioactive material

²scan *n* **1** : the act or process of scanning **2 a** : a depiction (as a photograph) of the distribution of a radioactive material in something (as a bodily organ) **b** : an image of a bodily part produced (as by computer) by combining scan or radiographic data obtained from several angles or sections

scan·di·um \ˈskan-dē-əm\ *n* : a white metallic element — symbol *Sc*; see ELEMENT table

scan·ner \ˈska-nər\ *n* : a device (as a CAT scanner) for making scans of the human body

scanning electron micrograph *n* : a micrograph made by scanning electron microscopy

scanning electron microscope *n* : an electron microscope in which a beam of focused electrons moves across the object with the secondary electrons produced by the object and the electrons scattered by the object being collected to form a three-dimensional image on a cathode-ray tube — called also *scanning microscope;* compare TRANSMISSION ELECTRON MICROSCOPE — **scanning electron microscopy** *n*

scanning speech *n* : speech characterized by regularly recurring pauses between words or syllables

Scan·zo·ni maneuver \skänt-ˈsō-nē-\ *also* **Scan·zo·ni's maneuver** \-nēz-\ *n* : rotation of an abnormally positioned fetus by means of forceps with subsequent reapplication of forceps for delivery

Scanzoni, Friedrich Wilhelm (1821–1891), German obstetrician.

scaph- *or* **scapho-** *comb form* : scaphoid ⟨*scapho*cephaly⟩

sca·pha \ˈska-fə\ *n* : an elongated depression of the ear that separates the helix and antihelix

scaph·o·ceph·a·ly \ˌska-fə-ˈse-fə-lē\ *n, pl* **-lies** : a congenital deformity of the skull in which the vault is narrow, elongated, and boat-shaped because of premature ossification of the sagittal suture

¹scaph·oid \ˈska-ˌfȯid\ *adj* **1** : shaped like a boat : NAVICULAR **2** : characterized by concavity ⟨the ∼ abdomen in some serious diseases⟩

²scaphoid *n* **1** : NAVICULAR a **2** : the largest carpal bone of the proximal row of the wrist that occupies the most lateral position on the thumb side — called also *navicular*

scaphoid bone *n* : SCAPHOID

scaphoid fossa *n* : a shallow oval depression that is situated above the pterygoid fossa on the pterygoid process of the sphenoid bone and that provides attachment for the origin of the tensor veli palatini muscle

scapul- *or* **scapulo-** *comb form* : scapular and ⟨*scapulo*humeral⟩

scap·u·la \ˈska-pyə-lə\ *n, pl* **-lae** \-ˌlē, -ˌlī\ *or* **-las** : either of a pair of large essentially flat and triangular bones lying one in each dorsolateral part of the thorax, being the principal bone of the corresponding half of the pectoral girdle, providing articulation for the humerus, and articulating with the corresponding clavicle — called also *shoulder blade*

scapulae — see LEVATOR SCAPULAE

scap·u·lar \ˈska-pyə-lər\ *adj* : of, relating to, or affecting the shoulder or scapula ⟨a ∼ fracture⟩

scapular notch *n* : a semicircular notch on the superior border of the scapula next to the coracoid process that gives passage to the suprascapular nerve and is converted to a foramen by the suprascapular ligament

scap·u·lo·hu·mer·al \ˌska-pyə-lō-ˈhyü-mə-rəl\ *adj* : of or relating to the scapula and the humerus

scar \ˈskär\ *n* 1 : a mark left (as in the skin) by the healing of injured tissue 2 : a lasting emotional injury — **scar** *vb*

scar·i·fy \ˈskar-ə-ˌfī\ *vb* **-fied; -fy·ing** : to make scratches or small cuts in (as the skin) ⟨∼ an area for vaccination⟩ — **scar·i·fi·ca·tion** \ˌskar-ə-fə-ˈkā-shən\ *n*

scar·la·ti·na \ˌskär-lə-ˈtē-nə\ *n* : SCARLET FEVER — **scar·la·ti·nal** \-ˈtēn-ᵊl\ *adj*

scar·la·ti·ni·form \-ˈtē-nə-ˌförm\ *adj* : resembling the rash of scarlet fever

scar·let fever \ˈskär-lət-\ *n* : an acute contagious febrile disease caused by hemolytic bacteria of the genus *Streptococcus* (esp. various strains of *S. pyogenes*) and characterized by inflammation of the nose, throat, and mouth, generalized toxemia, and a red rash — called also *scarlatina*

scarlet red *n* : SUDAN IV

Scar·pa's fascia \ˈskär-pəz-\ *n* : the deep layer of the superficial fascia of the anterior abdominal wall

Scarpa, Antonio (1752–1832), Italian anatomist and surgeon.

Scarpa's triangle *n* : FEMORAL TRIANGLE

scar tissue *n* : the connective tissue forming a scar and composed chiefly of fibroblasts in recent scars and largely of dense collagenous fibers in old scars

scat·ter·ing \ˈska-tə-riŋ\ *n* : the random change in direction of a beam due to collision of the particles, photons, or waves constituting the radiation with the particles of the medium traversed

ScD *abbr* doctor of science

Schatz·ki ring \ˈshats-kē-\ *or* **Schatzki's ring** \-kēz-\ *n* : a local narrowing in the lower part of the esophagus that may cause dysphagia

Schatzki, Richard (*b* 1901), American radiologist.

sched·ule \ˈske-ˌjül, -jəl; ˈshe-jù-wəl\ *n* 1 : a program or plan that indicates the sequence of each step or procedure; *esp* : REGIMEN 2 *usu cap* : an official list of drugs that are subject to the same legal controls and restrictions — usu. used with a Roman numeral from I to V indicating decreasing potential for abuse or addiction ⟨the Drug Enforcement Administration classifies heroin as a ∼ I drug while the tranquilizer chlordiazepoxide is on ∼ IV⟩

sche·ma \ˈskē-mə\ *n, pl* **sche·ma·ta** \-mə-tə\ *also* **sche·mas** 1 : a nonconscious adjustment of the brain to the afferent impulses indicative of bodily posture that is a prerequisite of appropriate bodily movement and of spatial perception 2 : the organization of experience in the mind or brain that includes a particular organized way of perceiving cognitively and responding to a complex situation or set of stimuli — **sche·mat·ic** \ski-ˈma-tik\ *adj*

scheme \ˈskēm\ *n* : SCHEMA

Scheuer·mann's disease \ˈshöi-ər-ˌmänz-\ *n* : osteochondrosis of the vertebrae associated in the active state with pain and kyphosis

Scheuermann, Holger Werfel (1877–1960), Danish orthopedist.

Schick test \ˈshik-\ *n* : a serological test for susceptibility to diphtheria by cutaneous injection of a diluted diphtheria toxin that causes an area of reddening and induration in susceptible individuals

Schick, Béla (1877–1967), American pediatrician.

Schiff's reagent \ˈshifs-\ *or* **Schiff reagent** \ˈshif-\ *n* : a solution of fuchsin decolorized by treatment with sulfur dioxide that gives a useful test for aldehydes because they restore the reddish violet color of the dye — compare FEULGEN REACTION

Schiff, Hugo Josef (1834–1915), German chemist.

Schil·der's disease \ˈshil-dərz-\ *n* : a demyelinating X-linked recessive disease of the central nervous system that affects males in childhood and is characterized by progressive blindness, deafness, tonic spasms, and mental deterioration — called also *adrenoleukodystrophy, Schilder's encephalitis*

Schilder, Paul Ferdinand (1886–1940), Austrian psychiatrist.

Schil·ler's test \ˈshi-lərz-\ *n* : a preliminary test for cancer of the uterine cervix in which the cervix is painted with an aqueous solution of iodine and potassium iodide and which shows up healthy tissue by staining it brown and possibly cancerous tissue as white or yellow

Schiller, Walter (1887–1960), American pathologist.

Schilling test *n* : a test for gastrointestinal absorption of vitamin B_{12} in which a dose of the radioactive vitamin is taken orally, a dose of the nonradioactive vitamin is given by injection to impede uptake of the absorbed radioactive dose by the liver, and the proportion of the radioactive dose absorbed is determined by measuring the radioactivity of the urine

Schilling, Robert Frederick (*b* 1919), American hematologist.

schin·dy·le·sis \ˌskin-də-ˈlē-səs\ *n, pl* **-le·ses** \-ˌsēz\ : an articulation in which one bone is received into a groove or slit in another

Schiotz tonometer \ˈshyœts-, ˈshyərts-\

n : a tonometer used to measure intra-ocular pressure in millimeters of mercury

Schiötz, Hjalmar (1850–1927), Norwegian physician.

-schi·sis \skə-səs\ *n comb form, pl* **-schi·ses** \skə-₁sēz\ *also* **-schi·sis·es** : breaking up of attachments or adhesions : fissure ⟨gastro*schis*is⟩ ⟨cranio*schisis*⟩

schisto- *comb form* : cleft : divided ⟨*schisto*cyte⟩

schis·to·cyte \'shis-tə-₁sīt, 'skis-\ *n* : a hemoglobin-containing fragment of a red blood cell

schis·to·so·ma \₁shis-tə-'sō-mə, ₁skis-\ *n* **1** *cap* : a genus of elongated digenetic trematode worms (family Schistosomatidae) that parasitize the blood vessels of birds and mammals and cause a destructive human schistosomiasis **2** : any trematode of the genus *Schistosoma* : SCHISTOSOME

schis·to·some \'shis-tə-₁sōm, 'skis-\ *n* : any trematode worm of the genus *Schistosoma* or broadly of the family (Schistosomatidae) to which it belongs — called also *blood fluke* — **schis·to·so·mal** \₁shis-tə-'sō-məl, ₁skis-\ *adj*

schistosome dermatitis *n* : SWIMMER'S ITCH

schis·to·so·mi·a·sis \₁shis-tə-sō-'mī-ə-səs, ₁skis-\ *n, pl* **-a·ses** \-₁sēz\ : infestation with or disease caused by schistosomes; *specif* : a severe endemic disease of humans in much of Asia, Africa, and So. America that is caused by any of three trematode worms of the genus *Schistosoma* (*S. haematobium, S. mansoni,* and *S. japonicum*) which multiply in snail intermediate hosts and are disseminated into freshwaters as cercariae that bore into the body, migrate through the tissues to the visceral venous plexuses (as of the bladder or intestine) where they attain maturity, and cause much of their injury through hemorrhage and damage to tissues resulting from the passage of the usu. spined eggs to the intestine and bladder — called also *snail fever;* compare SWIMMER'S ITCH

schistosomiasis hae·ma·to·bi·um \-₁hē-mə-'tō-bē-əm\ *n* : schistosomiasis caused by a schistosome (*Schistosoma haematobium*) occurring over most of Africa and in Asia Minor and predominantly involving infestation of the veins of the urinary bladder

schistosomiasis ja·pon·i·ca \-jə-'pä-ni-kə\ *n* : schistosomiasis caused by a schistosome (*Schistosoma japonicum*) occurring chiefly in eastern Asia and the Pacific islands and predominantly involving infestation of the portal and mesenteric veins

schistosomiasis man·so·ni \-'man-sə-₁nī\ *n* : schistosomiasis caused by a schistosome (*Schistosoma mansoni*) occurring chiefly in central Africa and eastern So. America and predominantly involving infestation of the mesenteric and portal veins — called also *Manson's disease*

P. Manson — see MANSONELLA

schis·to·som·u·lum \₁shis-tə-'säm-yə-ləm, ₁skis-\ *n, pl* **-la** \-lə\ : an immature schistosome in the body of the definitive host

schiz- *or* **schizo-** *comb form* **1** : characterized by or involving cleavage ⟨*schizo*gony⟩ **2** : schizophrenia ⟨*schiz*oid⟩

schizo \'skit-(₁)sō\ *n, pl* **schiz·os** : SCHIZOPHRENIC

schizo–af·fec·tive \-ə-'fek-tiv\ *adj* : relating to, characterized by, or exhibiting symptoms of both schizophrenia and manic-depressive psychosis

schi·zog·o·ny \ski-'zä-gə-nē, skit-'sä-\ *n, pl* **-nies** : asexual reproduction by multiple segmentation characteristic of sporozoans (as the malaria parasite) — **schizo·gon·ic** \₁skit-sə-'gä-nik\ *or* **schi·zog·o·nous** \ski-'zä-gə-nəs, skit-'sä-\ *adj*

¹schiz·oid \'skit-₁sóid\ *adj* : characterized by, resulting from, tending toward, or suggestive of schizophrenia

²schizoid *n* : a schizoid individual

schizoid personality *n* **1** : a personality disorder characterized by shyness, withdrawal, inhibition of emotional expression, and apparent diminution of affect — called also *schizoid personality disorder* **2** : a person with a schizoid personality

schiz·ont \'skit-₁zänt, 'skit-₁sänt\ *n* : a multinucleate sporozoan (as a malaria parasite) that reproduces by schizogony

schi·zon·ti·cide \ski-'zän-tə-₁sīd, skit-'sän-\ *n* : an agent selectively destructive of the schizont of a sporozoan parasite (as of malaria) — **schi·zon·ti·ci·dal** \ski-₁zän-tə-'sīd-əl, skit-₁sän-\ *adj*

schizo·phrene \'skit-sə-₁frēn\ *n* : SCHIZOPHRENIC

schizo·phre·nia \₁skit-sə-'frē-nē-ə\ *n* : a psychotic disorder characterized by loss of contact with the environment, by noticeable deterioration in the level of functioning in everyday life, and by disintegration of personality expressed as disorder of feeling, thought (as in hallucinations and delusions), and conduct — called also *dementia praecox*

¹schizo·phren·ic \-'fre-nik\ *adj* : relating to, characteristic of, or affected with schizophrenia ⟨∼ behavior⟩

²schizophrenic *n* : a person affected with schizophrenia — called also *schizo, schizophrene*

schizophrenic reaction *n* : SCHIZOPHRENIA

schiz·o·phren·i·form \₁skit-sə-'fre-nə-₁fórm\ *adj* : being similar to schizophrenia in appearance or manifestations but tending to last usu. more than two weeks and less than six months ⟨∼ disorder⟩

schiz•o•phreno•gen•ic \ˌskit-sə-ˌfre-nə-'je-nik\ adj : tending to produce schizophrenia ⟨a ∼ family environment⟩

schizos pl of SCHIZO

schizo•ty•pal \ˌskit-sə-'ti-pəl\ adj : characterized by, exhibiting, or being patterns of thought, perception, communication, and behavior suggestive of schizophrenia but not of sufficient severity to warrant a diagnosis of schizophrenia ⟨∼ personality⟩

Schlemm's canal \'shlemz-\ n : CANAL OF SCHLEMM

Schön•lein–Hen•och \'shœn-līn-'he-nək\ adj : being a form of purpura that is characterized by swelling and pain of the joints in association with gastrointestinal bleeding and pain

Schönlein, Johann Lucas (1793–1864), German physician.

Henoch, Eduard Heinrich (1820–1910), German pediatrician.

Schönlein's disease n : Schönlein–Henoch purpura that is characterized esp. by swelling and pain of the joints — compare HENOCH'S PURPURA

Schuff•ner's dots \'shuf-nərz-\ n pl : punctate granulations present in red blood cells invaded by the tertian malaria parasite

Schüff•ner \'shuef-nər\, **Wilhelm August Paul (1867–1949),** German pathologist.

Schüller–Christian disease n : HAND-SCHÜLLER-CHRISTIAN DISEASE

Schwann cell \'shwän-\ n : a cell that forms spiral layers around a myelinated nerve fiber between two nodes of Ranvier and forms the myelin sheath consisting of the inner spiral layers from which the protoplasm has been squeezed out

Schwann \'shvän\, **Theodor Ambrose Hubert (1810–1882),** German anatomist and physiologist.

schwan•no•ma \shwä-'nō-mə\ n, pl **-mas** \-məz\ or **-ma•ta** \-mə-tə\ : NEURILEMMOMA

Schwann's sheath n : NEURILEMMA

sci•at•ic \sī-'a-tik\ adj 1 : of, relating to, or situated near the hip 2 : of, relating to, or caused by sciatica ⟨∼ pains⟩

sci•at•i•ca \sī-'a-ti-kə\ n : pain along the course of a sciatic nerve esp. in the back of the thigh caused by compression, inflammation, or reflex mechanisms; broadly : pain in the lower back, buttocks, hips, or adjacent parts

sciatic foramen n : either of two foramina on each side of the pelvis that are formed by the hipbone, the sacrospinous ligament, and the sacrotuberous ligament: **a** : one giving passage to the piriformis muscle and to the sciatic, superior and inferior gluteal,

and pudendal nerves together with their associated arteries and veins — called also greater sciatic foramen **b** : one giving passage to the tendon of the obturator internus muscle and its nerve, to the internal pudendal artery and veins, and to the pudendal nerve — called also lesser sciatic foramen

sciatic nerve n : either of the pair of largest nerves in the body that arise one on each side from the sacral plexus and that pass out of the pelvis through the greater sciatic foramen and down the back of the thigh to its lower third where division into the tibial and common peroneal nerves occurs

sciatic notch n : either of two notches on the dorsal border of the hipbone on each side that when closed off by ligaments form the corresponding sciatic foramina: **a** : a relatively large notch just above the ischial spine that is converted into the greater sciatic foramen by the sacrospinous ligament — called also greater sciatic notch **b** : a smaller notch just below the ischial spine that is converted to the lesser sciatic foramen by the sacrospinous ligament and the sacrotuberous ligament — called also lesser sciatic notch

SCID abbr severe combined immunodeficiency

sci•ence \'sī-əns\ n : knowledge or a system of knowledge covering general truths or the operation of general laws esp. as obtained and tested through the scientific method and concerned with the physical world and its phenomena — **sci•en•tif•ic** \ˌsī-ən-'ti-fik\ adj — **sci•en•tif•i•cal•ly** adv

scientific method n : principles and procedures for the systematic pursuit of knowledge involving the recognition and formulation of a problem, the collection of data through observation and experiment, and the formulation and testing of hypotheses

sci•en•tist \'sī-ən-tist\ n : one learned in science and esp. natural science : a scientific investigator

scin•ti•gram \'sin-tə-ˌgram\ n : a picture produced by scintigraphy

scin•tig•ra•phy \sin-'ti-grə-fē\ n, pl **-phies** : a diagnostic technique in which a two-dimensional picture of a bodily radiation source is obtained by the use of radioisotopes ⟨myocardial ∼⟩ — **scin•ti•graph•ic** \ˌsin-tə-'gra-fik\ adj

scin•til•la•tion \ˌsint-ᵊl-'ā-shən\ n, often attrib : a flash of light produced in a phosphorescent substance by an ionizing event — **scin•til•late** \'sint-ᵊl-ˌāt\ vb

scintillation counter n : a device for detecting and registering individual scintillations (as in radioactive emission) — called also scintillometer

scin•til•la•tor \'sint-ᵊl-ˌā-tər\ n 1 : a

phosphorescent substance in which scintillations occur (as in a scintillation counter) **2** : a device for sending out scintillations of light **3** : SCINTILLATION COUNTER

scin·til·lom·e·ter \ˌsint-ᵊl-ˈä-mə-tər\ *n* : SCINTILLATION COUNTER

scin·ti·scan \ˈsin-ti-ˌskan\ *n* : a two-dimensional representation of radioisotope radiation from a bodily organ (as the spleen or kidney)

scirrhi *pl of* SCIRRHUS

scir·rhous \ˈsir-əs, ˈskir-\ *adj* : of, relating to, or being a scirrhous carcinoma

scirrhous carcinoma *n* : a hard slow-growing malignant tumor having a preponderance of fibrous tissue

scir·rhus \ˈsir-əs, ˈskir-\ *n, pl* **scir·rhi** \ˈsir-ˌī, ˈskir-, -ˌē\ : SCIRRHOUS CARCINOMA

scler- *or* **sclero-** *comb form* **1** : hard ⟨*sclero*derma⟩ **2** : sclera ⟨*scler*itis⟩

sclera \ˈskler-ə\ *n* : the dense fibrous opaque white outer coat enclosing the eyeball except the part covered by the cornea — called also *sclerotic, sclerotic coat* — **scler·al** \ˈskler-əl\ *adj*

sclerae — see SINUS VENOSUS SCLERAE

scle·rec·to·my \sklə-ˈrek-tə-mē\ *n, pl* **-mies** : surgical removal of a part of the sclera

scle·re·ma neo·na·to·rum \sklə-ˈrē-mə-ˌnē-ə-nə-ˈtōr-əm\ *n* : hardening of the cutaneous and subcutaneous tissues in newborn infants

scle·ri·tis \sklə-ˈrī-təs\ *n* : inflammation of the sclera

scle·ro·cor·ne·al \ˌskler-ō-ˈkȯr-nē-əl\ *adj* : of or involving both sclera and cornea

scle·ro·dac·ty·ly \-ˈdak-tə-lē\ *n, pl* **-lies** : scleroderma of the fingers and toes

scle·ro·der·ma \skler-ə-ˈdər-mə\ *n, pl* **-mas** *or* **-ma·ta** \-mə-tə\ : a usu. slowly progressive disease marked by the deposition of fibrous connective tissue in the skin and often in internal organs — **scle·ro·der·ma·tous** \-təs\ *adj*

scle·ro·ma \sklə-ˈrō-mə\ *n, pl* **-mas** *or* **-ma·ta** \-mə-tə\ : hardening of tissues

scle·ro·pro·tein \ˌskler-ō-ˈprō-ˌtēn\ *n* : any of a class of fibrous proteins (as collagen and keratin) that are usu. insoluble in aqueous solvents and are resistant to chemical reagents — called also *albuminoid*

scle·rose \sklə-ˈrōs, -ˈrōz\ *vb* **-rosed; -ros·ing 1** : to cause sclerosis in **2** : to undergo or become affected with sclerosis

scle·ros·ing *adj* : causing or characterized by sclerosis ⟨∼ agents⟩ — see SUBACUTE SCLEROSING PANENCEPHALITIS

scle·ro·sis \sklə-ˈrō-səs\ *n, pl* **-ro·ses** \-ˌsēz\ **1** : a pathological condition in which a tissue has become hard and which is produced by overgrowth of fibrous tissue and other changes (as in arteriosclerosis) or by increase in

interstitial tissue and other changes (as in multiple sclerosis) — called also *hardening* **2** : any of various diseases characterized by sclerosis — usu. used in combination; see ARTERIOSCLEROSIS, MULTIPLE SCLEROSIS

scle·ro·stome \ˈskler-ə-ˌstōm\ *n* : STRONGYLE

sclerosus — see LICHEN SCLEROSUS ET ATROPHICUS

scle·ro·ther·a·py \ˌskler-ō-ˈther-ə-pē\ *n, pl* **-pies** : the injection of a sclerosing agent into a varicose vein to create fibrosis which closes the lumen

¹scle·rot·ic \sklə-ˈrä-tik\ *adj* **1** : being or relating to the sclera ⟨the ∼ layer of the eye⟩ **2** : of, relating to, or affected with sclerosis ⟨a ∼ blood vessel⟩

²sclerotic *n* : SCLERA

sclerotic coat *n* : SCLERA

scle·ro·tium \sklə-ˈrō-shəm, -shē-əm\ *n, pl* **-tia** \-shə, -shē-ə\ : a compact mass of hardened mycelium (as in ergot) of a fungus that is stored with reserve food material — **scle·ro·tial** \-shəl\ *adj*

scle·ro·tome \ˈskler-ə-ˌtōm\ *n* : the ventral and mesial portion of a somite that proliferates mesenchyme which migrates about the notochord to form the axial skeleton and ribs — **scle·ro·tom·ic** \ˌskler-ə-ˈtō-mik, -ˈtä-\ *adj*

scle·rot·o·my \sklə-ˈrä-tə-mē\ *n, pl* **-mies** : surgical cutting of the sclera

ScM *abbr* master of science

SCM *abbr* state certified midwife

sco·lex \ˈskō-ˌleks\ *n, pl* **sco·li·ces** \ˈskō-lə-ˌsēz\ *also* **scol·e·ces** \ˈskä-lə-ˌsēz, ˈskō-\ *or* **scolexes** : the head of a tapeworm from which the proglottids are produced by budding

sco·li·o·sis \ˌskō-lē-ˈō-səs\ *n, pl* **-o·ses** \-ˌsēz\ : a lateral curvature of the spine — compare KYPHOSIS, LORDOSIS — **sco·li·ot·ic** \-ˈä-tik\ *adj*

scoop \ˈsküp\ *n* : a spoon-shaped surgical instrument used in extracting various materials (as debris and pus)

scope \ˈskōp\ *n* : any of various instruments for viewing: as **a** : BRONCHOSCOPE **b** : GASTROSCOPE **c** : MICROSCOPE

-scope \ˌskōp\ *n comb form* : means (as an instrument) for viewing or observing ⟨micro*scope*⟩ ⟨laparo*scope*⟩

-scop·ic \ˈskä-pik\ *adj comb form* : viewing or observing ⟨laparo*scopic*⟩

sco·pol·amine \skō-ˈpä-lə-ˌmēn, -mən\ *n* : a poisonous alkaloid $C_{17}H_{21}NO_4$ found in various plants (as jimsonweed) of the nightshade family (Solanaceae) and used chiefly in the form of its crystalline hydrobromide as a sedative in connection with morphine or other analgesics in surgery and obstetrics, in the prevention of motion sickness, and as the truth serum in lie detector tests — called also *hyoscine*

sco·po·phil·ia \ˌskō-pə-ˈfi-lē-ə\ *or* **scop·to·phil·ia** \ˌskäp-tə-ˈfi-lē-ə\ *n* : a desire to look at sexually stimulating scenes esp. as a substitute for actual sexual participation — **sco·po·phil·ic** or **scop·to·phil·ic** \-'fi-lik\ adj

sco·po·phil·i·ac or **scop·to·phil·i·ac** \-'fi-lē-₁ak\ n : a person affected with scopophilia — **scopophiliac** or **scoptophiliac** adj

-s·co·py \s-kə-pē\ n comb form, pl **-s·co·pies** : viewing : observation ⟨laparoscopy⟩

scor·bu·tic \skȯr-'byü-tik\ adj : of, relating to, producing, or affected with scurvy ⟨a ~ diet⟩

scor·pi·on \'skȯr-pē-ən\ n : any of an order (Scorpionida) of arachnids that have an elongated body and a narrow segmented tail bearing a venomous stinger at the tip

sco·to·ma \skə-'tō-mə\ n, pl **-mas** or **-ma·ta** \-mə-tə\ : a blind or dark spot in the visual field

sco·to·pic \skə-'tō-pik, -'tä-\ adj : relating to or being vision in dim light with dark-adapted eyes which involves only the retinal rods as light receptors

¹**scour** \'skau̇r\ vb, of a domestic animal : to suffer from diarrhea or dysentery ⟨a diet causing cattle to ~⟩

²**scour** n sing or pl : diarrhea or dysentery occurring esp. in young domestic animals

scra·pie \'skrā-pē\ n : a usu. fatal disease of the nervous system esp. of sheep that is characterized by twitching, excitability, intense itching, excessive thirst, emaciation, weakness, and finally paralysis and that is caused by a slow virus

scrap·ing \'skrā-piṇ\ n : material scraped esp. from diseased tissue (as infected skin) for microscopic examination

scratch test n : a test for allergic susceptibility made by rubbing an extract of an allergy-producing substance into small breaks or scratches in the skin — compare INTRADERMAL TEST, PATCH TEST

screen — see SUNSCREEN

screen memory n : a recollection of early childhood that may be falsely recalled or magnified in importance and that masks another memory of deep emotional significance

screw·fly \'skrü-₁flī\ n, pl **-flies** : SCREWWORM FLY

screw·worm \'skrü-₁wərm\ n 1 a : a dipteran fly of the genus *Cochliomyia* (*C. hominivorax*) of the warmer parts of America whose larva develops in sores or wounds or in the nostrils of mammals including humans; esp : its larva **b** : SECONDARY SCREWWORM 2 : any of several flies other than the screwworms of the genus *Cochliomyia* and esp. their larvae which parasitize the flesh of mammals

screwworm fly n : the adult of a screwworm — called also *screwfly*

scroful- or **scrofulo-** comb form : scrofula ⟨*scrofulo*derma⟩

scrof·u·la \'skrȯ-fyə-lə, 'skrä-\ n : tuberculosis of lymph nodes esp. in the neck — called also *king's evil*

scrof·u·lo·der·ma \₁skrȯ-fyə-lō-'dər-mə, ₁skrä-\ n : a disease of the skin of tuberculous origin

scrot- or **scroti-** or **scroto-** comb form : scrotum ⟨*scroto*plasty⟩

scro·tal \'skrōt-ᵊl\ adj 1 : of or relating to the scrotum 2 : lying in or having descended into the scrotum ⟨~ testes⟩

scro·to·plas·ty \'skrō-tə-₁plas-tē\ n, pl **-ties** : plastic surgery performed on the scrotum

scro·tum \'skrō-təm\ n, pl **scro·ta** \-tə\ or **scrotums** : the external pouch that in most mammals contains the testes

scrub \'skrəb\ vb **scrubbed; scrub·bing** : to clean and disinfect (the hands and forearms) before participating in surgery — **scrub** n

scrub nurse n : a nurse who assists the surgeon in an operating room

scrub typhus n : TSUTSUGAMUSHI DISEASE

scru·ple \'skrü-pəl\ n : a unit of apothecaries' weight equal to 20 grains or ⅓ dram or 1.296 grams

scurf \'skərf\ n : thin dry scales detached from the epidermis esp. in an abnormal skin condition; specif : DANDRUFF — **scurfy** \'skər-fē\ adj

scur·vy \'skər-vē\ n, pl **scur·vies** : a disease that is characterized by spongy gums, loosening of the teeth, and a bleeding into the skin and mucous membranes and that is caused by a lack of vitamin C

Se symbol selenium

seal·ant \'sē-lənt\ n : material used to seal developmental imperfections in teeth ⟨pit and fissure ~s⟩

seal finger n : a finger rendered swollen and painful by erysipeloid or a similar infection and occurring esp. in individuals handling seals or sealskins

sea·sick·ness \'sē-₁sik-nəs\ n : motion sickness experienced on the water — called also *mal de mer* — **seasick** adj

sea snake n : any of a family (Hydrophidae) of numerous venomous snakes inhabiting the tropical parts of the Pacific and Indian oceans

seasonal affective disorder n : depression that tends to recur as the days grow shorter during the fall and winter — abbr. *SAD*

¹**seat** \'sēt\ n : a part or surface esp. in dentistry on or in which another part or surface rests — see REST SEAT

²**seat** vb : to provide with or position on a dental seat

seat·worm \-₁wərm\ n : a pinworm of the genus *Enterobius* (*E. vermicularis*) that is parasitic in humans

sea wasp n : any of various jellyfishes (order or suborder Cubomedusae of the class Scyphozoa) that sting virulently and sometimes fatally

se·ba·ceous \si-'bā-shəs\ adj 1 : secreting sebum **2** : of, relating to, or being fatty material ⟨a ∼ exudate⟩

sebaceous cyst *n* : a cyst filled with sebaceous matter and formed by distension of a sebaceous gland as a result of obstruction of its excretory duct

sebaceous gland *n* : any of the small sacculated glands lodged in the substance of the derma, usu. opening into the hair follicles, and secreting an oily or greasy material composed in great part of fat which softens and lubricates the hair and skin

sebi- *or* **sebo-** *comb form* : fat : grease : sebum ⟨*seborrhea*⟩

seb·or·rhea \ˌse-bə-ˈrē-ə\ *n* : abnormally increased secretion and discharge of sebum producing an oily appearance of the skin and the formation of greasy scales

seb·or·rhe·al \ˌse-bə-ˈrē-əl\ *adj* : SEBORRHEIC

seb·or·rhe·ic \-ˈrē-ik\ *adj* : of, relating to, or characterized by seborrhea ⟨∼ dermatitis⟩

se·bor·rhoea, se·bor·rhoe·al, se·bor·rhoe·ic *chiefly Brit var of* SEBORRHEA, SEBORRHEAL, SEBORRHEIC

se·bum \ˈsē-bəm\ *n* : fatty lubricant matter secreted by sebaceous glands of the skin

seco·bar·bi·tal \ˌse-kō-ˈbär-bə-ˌtȯl\ *n* : a barbiturate $C_{12}H_{18}N_2O_3$ that is used chiefly in the form of its bitter sodium salt as a hypnotic and sedative — called also *quinalbarbitone;* see SECONAL

Sec·o·nal \ˈse-kə-ˌnȯl, -ˌnal, -nəl\ *trademark* — used for a preparation of secobarbital

sec·ond·ary \ˈse-kən-ˌder-ē\ *adj* **1** : not first in order of occurrence or development: as **a** : dependent or consequent on another disease ⟨∼ hypertension⟩ **b** : occurring or being in the second stage ⟨∼ symptoms of syphilis⟩ **c** : occurring some time after the original injury ⟨a ∼ hemorrhage⟩ **2** : characterized by or resulting from the substitution of two atoms or groups in a molecule ⟨a ∼ salt⟩ **3** : relating to or being the three≈dimensional coiling of the polypeptide chain of a protein esp. in the form of an alpha-helix — compare PRIMARY 3, TERTIARY 2 — **sec·ond·ari·ly** \ˌse-kən-ˈder-ə-lē\ *adv*

secondary amenorrhea *n* : cessation of menstruation in a woman who has previously experienced normal menses

secondary dentin *n* : dentin formed following the loss (as by erosion, abrasion, or disease) of original dentin

secondary gain *n* : a benefit (as sympathetic attention) associated with a mental illness

secondary infection *n* : infection occurring at the site of a preexisting infection

secondary oocyte *n* : an oocyte that is produced by division of a primary oocyte in the first meiotic division

secondary screwworm *n* : a screwworm of the genus *Cochliomyia* (*C. macellaria*)

secondary sex characteristic *n* : a physical characteristic (as the breasts of a female) that appears in members of one sex at puberty or in seasonal breeders at the breeding season and is not directly concerned with reproduction — called also *secondary sex character, secondary sexual characteristic*

secondary spermatocyte *n* : a spermatocyte that is produced by division of a primary spermatocyte in the first meiotic division and that divides in the second meiotic division to give spermatids

secondary syphilis *n* : the second stage of syphilis that appears from 2 to 6 months after primary infection, that is marked by lesions esp. in the skin but also in organs and tissues, and that lasts from 3 to 12 weeks

secondary tympanic membrane *n* : a membrane closing the round window and separating the scala tympani from the middle ear

second cranial nerve *n* : OPTIC NERVE

second-degree burn *n* : a burn marked by pain, blistering, and superficial destruction of dermis with edema and hyperemia of the tissues beneath the burn

second in·ten·tion \-in-ˈten-chən\ *n* : the healing of an incised wound by granulations that bridge the gap between skin edges — compare FIRST INTENTION

second messenger *n* : a cellular substance (as cyclic AMP) that mediates cell activity by relaying a signal from an extracellular molecule (as of a hormone or neurotransmitter) bound to the cell's surface

second polar body *n* : POLAR BODY b

second wind *n* : recovered full power of respiration after the first exhaustion during exertion due to improved heart action

secret- *or* **secreto-** *comb form* : secretion ⟨*secretin*⟩

se·cre·ta·gogue \si-ˈkrē-tə-ˌgäg\ *n* : a substance that stimulates secretion

se·cre·tin \si-ˈkrēt-ᵊn\ *n* : an intestinal proteinaceous hormone capable of stimulating secretion by the pancreas and liver

se·cre·tion \si-ˈkrē-shən\ *n* **1** : the process of segregating, elaborating, and releasing some material either functionally specialized (as saliva) or isolated for excretion (as urine) **2** : a product of secretion formed by an animal or plant; *esp* : one performing a specific useful function in the organism — **se·crete** \si-ˈkrēt\ *vb* — **se·cre·to·ry** \ˈsē-krə-ˌtōr-ē, si-ˈkrē-tə-rē\ *adj*

se·cre·tor \si-ˈkrē-tər\ *n* : an individual

of blood group A, B, or AB who secretes the antigens characteristic of these blood groups in bodily fluids (as saliva)

-sect \ˌsekt\ *vb comb form* : cut : divide 〈hemi*sect*〉 〈tran*sect*〉

sec·tion \ˈsek-shən\ *n* **1** : the action or an instance of cutting or separating by cutting ; *esp* : the action of dividing (as tissues) surgically 〈abdominal ~〉 — see CESAREAN SECTION **2** : a very thin slice (as of tissue) suitable for microscopic examination — **section** *vb*

se·cun·di·grav·id \si-ˌkən-dē-ˈgra-vəd\ *adj* : pregnant for the second time

se·cun·di·grav·i·da \-ˈgra-vi-də\ *n, pl* **-das** : a woman in her second pregnancy

sec·un·dines \ˈse-kən-ˌdēnz, -ˌdinz; se-ˈkən-dənz\ *n pl* : AFTERBIRTH

sec·un·dip·a·ra \ˌse-kən-ˈdi-pə-rə\ *n, pl* **-ras** : a woman who has borne children in two separate pregnancies

security blanket *n* : a blanket carried by a child as a protection against anxiety

se·date \si-ˈdāt\ *vb* **se·dat·ed; se·dat·ing** : to dose with sedatives

se·da·tion \si-ˈdā-shən\ *n* **1** : the inducing of a relaxed easy state esp. by the use of sedatives **2** : a state resulting from sedation

¹**sed·a·tive** \ˈse-də-tiv\ *adj* : tending to calm, moderate, or tranquilize nervousness or excitement

²**sedative** *n* : a sedative agent or drug

¹**sed·i·ment** \ˈse-də-mənt\ *n* : the matter that settles to the bottom of a liquid

²**sed·i·ment** \-ˌment\ *vb* : to deposit as sediment

sed·i·men·ta·tion \ˌse-də-(ˌ)men-ˈtā-shən\ *n* **1** : the action or process of depositing sediment **2** : the depositing esp. by mechanical means of matter suspended in a liquid

sedimentation rate *n* : the speed at which red blood cells settle to the bottom of a column of citrated blood measured in millimeters deposited per hour and which is used esp. in diagnosing the progress of various abnormal conditions

sed rate \ˈsed-\ *n* : SEDIMENTATION RATE

¹**seed** \ˈsēd\ *n, pl* **seed** *or* **seeds 1 a** : the fertilized ripened ovule of a flowering plant **b** : a propagative animal structure ; *esp* : SEMEN **2** : a small usu. glass and gold or platinum capsule used as a container for a radioactive substance (as radium or radon) to be applied usu. interstitially in the treatment of cancer — **seed·ed** \ˈsē-dəd\ *adj*

²**seed** *adj* : selected or used to produce a new crop or stock 〈~ virus〉

Seeing Eye *trademark* — used for a guide dog trained to lead the blind

¹**seg·ment** \ˈseg-mənt\ *n* : one of the constituent parts into which a body, entity, or quantity is divided or marked off by or as if by natural boundaries

〈the affected ~ of the colon was resected〉 — **seg·men·tal** \seg-ˈment-ᵊl\ *adj* — **seg·men·tal·ly** *adv*

²**seg·ment** \ˈseg-ˌment\ *vb* **1** : to cause to undergo segmentation by division or multiplication of cells **2** : to separate into segments

segmental resection *n* : excision of a segment of an organ; *specif* : excision of a portion of a lobe of a lung — called also *segmentectomy*; compare PNEUMONECTOMY

seg·men·ta·tion \ˌseg-(ˌ)men-ˈtā-shən\ *n* **1** : the act or process of dividing into segments ; *esp* : the formation of many cells from a single cell (as in a developing egg) **2** : annular contraction of smooth muscle (as of the intestine) that seems to cut the part affected into segments — compare PERISTALSIS

segmentation cavity *n* : BLASTOCOEL

seg·men·tec·to·my \ˌseg-mən-ˈtek-tə-mē\ *n, pl* **-mies** : SEGMENTAL RESECTION

seg·ment·ed \ˈseg-ˌmen-təd, seg-ˈ\ *adj* **1** : having or made up of segments **2** : being a cell in which the nucleus is divided into lobes connected by a fine filament 〈~ neutrophils〉

seg·re·gant \ˈse-gri-gənt\ *n* : SEGREGATE

¹**seg·re·gate** \ˈse-gri-ˌgāt\ *vb* **-gat·ed; -gat·ing** : to undergo genetic segregation

²**seg·re·gate** \-gət\ *n* : an individual or class of individuals differing in one or more genetic characters from the parental line usu. because of segregation of genes

seg·re·ga·tion \ˌse-gri-ˈgā-shən\ *n* : the separation of allelic genes that occurs typically during meiosis

Seignette salt \sen-ˈyet-\ *or* **Seig·nette's salt** \-ˈyets-\ *n* : ROCHELLE SALT

Seignette, Pierre (1660–1719), French pharmacist.

sei·zure \ˈsē-zhər\ *n* : a sudden attack (as of disease) 〈an epileptic ~〉

Sel·dane \ˈsel-ˌdān\ *trademark* — used for a preparation of terfenadine

se·lec·tion \sə-ˈlek-shən\ *n* : a natural or artificial process that results or tends to result in the survival and propagation of some individuals or organisms but not of others with the result that the inherited traits of the survivors are perpetuated — compare DARWINISM

se·lec·tive \sə-ˈlek-tiv\ *adj* **1** : of, relating to, or characterized by selection : selecting or tending to select **2** : highly specific in activity or effect — **se·lec·tive·ly** *adv* — **se·lec·tiv·i·ty** \sə-ˌlek-ˈti-və-tē, ˌsē-\ *n*

sel·e·nif·er·ous \ˌse-lə-ˈni-fə-rəs\ *adj* : containing or yielding selenium

se·le·ni·um \sə-ˈlē-nē-əm\ *n* : a nonmetallic element that causes poisoning in range animals when ingested by eating some plants growing in soils in which it occurs in quantity — symbol *Se*; see ELEMENT table

se·le·ni·um sulfide *n* : the sulfide SeS$_2$ of selenium usu. in the form of an orange powder that is effective in controlling seborrheic dermatitis and dandruff

sel·e·no·me·thi·o·nine \se-lə-nō-mə-ˈthī-ə-ˌnēn\ *n* : a selenium compound C$_5$H$_{11}$NO$_2$Se that is used as a diagnostic aid in scintigraphy esp. of the pancreas

sel·e·no·sis \se-lə-ˈnō-səs\ *n* : poisoning of livestock by selenium due to ingestion of plants grown in seleniferous soils characterized in the acute phase by diffuse necrosis and hemorrhage resulting from capillary damage and in chronic poisoning by degenerative and fibrotic changes esp. of the liver and of the skin and its derivatives — called also *alkali disease*; see BLIND STAGGERS

self \ˈself\ *n, pl* **selves** \ˈselvz\ **1** : the union of elements (as body, emotions, thoughts, and sensations) that constitute the individuality and identity of a person **2** : material that is part of an individual organism ⟨ability of the immune system to distinguish ∼ from nonself⟩

self–abuse \ˌself-ə-ˈbyüs\ *n* : MASTURBATION

self–ac·tu·al·ize \ˈself-ˈak-chə-wə-ˌlīz\ *vb* **-ized; -iz·ing** : to realize fully one's potential — **self–ac·tu·al·iza·tion** \-ˌak-chə-wə-lə-ˈzā-shən\ *n*

self–ad·min·is·ter \-əd-ˈmi-nə-stər\ *vb* : to administer to oneself ⟨∼*ed* an analgesic⟩ — **self–ad·min·is·tra·tion** \-ˌmi-nə-ˈstrā-shən\ *n*

self–anal·y·sis \-ə-ˈna-lə-səs\ *n, pl* **-y·ses** \-ˌsēz\ *n* : a systematic attempt by an individual to understand his or her own personality without the aid of another person — **self–an·a·lyt·i·cal** \-ˌa-nə-ˈli-ti-kəl\ *or* **self–an·a·lyt·ic** \-ˈtik\ *adj*

self–as·sem·bly \-ə-ˈsem-blē\ *n, pl* **-blies** : the process by which a complex macromolecule (as collagen) or a supramolecular system (as a virus) spontaneously assembles itself from its components — **self–as·sem·ble** \-bəl\ *vb*

self–aware·ness \-ə-ˈwer-nəs\ *n* : an awareness of one's own personality or individuality — **self–aware** *adj*

self–care \-ˈker\ *n* : care for oneself : SELF-TREATMENT

self–con·cept \ˈself-ˈkän-ˌsept\ *n* : the mental image one has of oneself

self–de·struc·tion \-di-ˈstrək-shən\ *n* : destruction of oneself; *esp* : SUICIDE

self–de·struc·tive \-ˈstrək-tiv\ *adj* : acting or tending to harm or destroy oneself ⟨∼ behavior⟩; *also* : SUICIDAL — **self–de·struc·tive·ly** *adv* — **self–de·struc·tive·ness** *n*

self–ex·am·i·na·tion \-ig-ˌza-mə-ˈnā-shən\ *n* : examination of one's body

esp. for evidence of disease ⟨∼ for detection of breast cancer⟩

self–hyp·no·sis \ˌself-hip-ˈnō-səs\ *n, pl* **-no·ses** \-ˌsēz\ : hypnosis of oneself : AUTOHYPNOSIS

self–im·age \-ˈi-mij\ *n* : one's conception of oneself or of one's role

self–in·duced \-in-ˈdüst, -ˈdyüst\ *adj* : induced by oneself ⟨a ∼ abortion⟩

self–in·flict·ed \-in-ˈflik-təd\ *adj* : inflicted by oneself ⟨a ∼ wound⟩

self–lim·it·ed \-ˈli-mə-təd\ *adj* : limited by one's or its own nature; *specif* : running a definite and limited course ⟨a ∼ disease⟩

self–lim·it·ing *adj* : SELF-LIMITED

self–med·i·ca·tion \-ˌme-də-ˈkā-shən\ *n* : medication of oneself esp. without the advice of a physician : SELF-TREATMENT ⟨∼ with nonprescription drugs⟩ — **self–med·i·cate** \-ˈme-də-ˌkāt\ *vb*

self–mu·ti·la·tion \-ˌmyü-tə-ˈlā-shən\ *n* : injury or disfigurement of oneself

self–rec·og·ni·tion \-ˌre-kəg-ˈni-shən\ *n* : the process by which the immune system of an organism distinguishes between the body's own chemicals, cells, and tissues and those of foreign organisms or agents — compare SELF-TOLERANCE

self–rep·li·cat·ing \-ˈre-plə-ˌkā-tiŋ\ *adj* : reproducing itself autonomously ⟨DNA is a ∼ molecule⟩ — **self–rep·li·ca·tion** \-ˌre-plə-ˈkā-shən\ *n*

self–stim·u·la·tion \-ˌstim-yə-ˈlā-shən\ *n* : stimulation of oneself as a result of one's own activity or behavior; *esp* : MASTURBATION — **self–stim·u·la·to·ry** \-ˈstim-yə-lə-ˌtōr-ē\ *adj*

self–tol·er·ance \-ˈtä-lə-rəns\ *n* : the physiological state that exists in a developing organism when its immune system has proceeded far enough in the process of self-recognition to lose the capacity to attack and destroy its own bodily constituents — called also *horror autotoxicus*

self–treat·ment \-ˈtrēt-mənt\ *n* : medication of oneself or treatment of one's own disease without medical supervision or prescription

sel·la \ˈse-lə\ *n, pl* **sellas** *or* **sel·lae** \-lē\ : SELLA TURCICA

sellae see DIAPHRAGMA SELLAE

sel·lar \ˈse-lər, -ˌlär\ *adj* : of, relating to, or involving the sella turcica

sel·la tur·ci·ca \-ˈtər-ki-kə, -si-\ *n, pl* **sel·lae tur·ci·cae** \-ˌki-ˌkī, -si-ˌsē\ : a depression in the middle line of the upper surface of the sphenoid bone in which the pituitary gland is lodged

SEM *abbr* **1** scanning electron microscope **2** scanning electron microscopy

se·men \ˈsē-mən\ *n* : a viscid whitish fluid of the male reproductive tract consisting of spermatozoa suspended in secretions of the accessory glands and esp. of the prostate and Cowper's glands

semi·cir·cu·lar canal \ˌse-mē-ˈsər-kyə-lər-, ˌse-ˌmī-\ n : any of the loop-shaped tubular parts of the labyrinth of the ear that together constitute a sensory organ associated with the maintenance of bodily equilibrium, that consist of an inner membranous canal of the membranous labyrinth and a corresponding outer bony canal of the bony labyrinth, and that form a group of three in each ear usu. in planes nearly at right angles to each other — see SEMICIRCULAR DUCT

semicircular duct n : any of the three loop-shaped membranous inner tubular parts of the semicircular canals that are about one-fourth the diameter of the corresponding outer bony canals, that communicate at each end with the utricle, and that have near one end an expanded ampulla containing an area of sensory epithelium

semi·co·ma \-ˈkō-mə\ n : a semicomatose state from which a person can be aroused

semi·co·ma·tose \-ˈkō-mə-ˌtōs\ adj : lethargic and disoriented but not completely comatose (a ~ patient)

semi·con·scious \-ˈkän-chəs\ adj : incompletely conscious : imperfectly aware or responsive — **semi·con·scious·ness** n

semi·con·ser·va·tive \-kən-ˈsər-və-tiv\ adj : relating to or being genetic replication in which a double-stranded molecule of nucleic acid separates into two single strands each of which serves as a template for the formation of a complementary strand that together with the template forms a complete molecule — **semi·con·ser·va·tive·ly** adv

semi·dom·i·nant \-ˈdä-mi-nənt\ adj : producing an intermediate phenotype in the heterozygous condition

semi·flu·id \-ˈflü-əd\ adj : having the qualities of both a fluid and a solid : VISCOUS — **semifluid** n

semi·lu·nar \-ˈlü-nər\ adj : shaped like a crescent

semilunar bone n : LUNATE BONE

semilunar cartilage n : MENISCUS a(2)

semilunar cusp n : any of the crescentic cusps making up the semilunar valves

semilunares — see LINEA SEMILUNARIS, PLICA SEMILUNARIS

semilunar ganglion n : TRIGEMINAL GANGLION

semilunaris — see HIATUS SEMILUNARIS, LINEA SEMILUNARIS, PLICA SEMILUNARIS

semilunar line n : LINEA SEMILUNARIS

semilunar lobule n : either of a pair of crescent-shaped lobules situated one on each side in the posterior and ventral part of the cerebellum

semilunar notch n : the deep depression in the proximal end of the ulna by which it articulates with the trochlea of the humerus at the elbow

semilunar valve n 1 : either of two valves of which one is situated at the opening between the heart and the aorta and the other at the opening between the heart and the pulmonary artery, which prevent regurgitation of blood into the ventricles, and each of which is made up of three crescent-shaped cusps 2 : SEMILUNAR CUSP

semi·mem·bra·no·sus \ˌse-mē-ˌmem-brə-ˈnō-səs, ˌse-ˌmī-\ n, pl **-no·si** \-ˌsī\ : a large muscle of the inner part and back of the thigh that arises by a thick tendon from the back part of the tuberosity of the ischium, is inserted into the medial condyle of the tibia, and acts to flex the leg and rotate it medially and to extend the thigh

sem·i·nal \ˈse-mən-əl\ adj : of, relating to, or consisting of semen

seminal duct n : a tube or passage serving esp. or exclusively as an efferent duct of the testis and in humans being made up of the tubules of the epididymis, the vas deferens, and the ejaculatory duct

seminal fluid n 1 : SEMEN 2 : the part of the semen that is produced by various accessory glands : semen excepting the spermatozoa

seminal vesicle n : either of a pair of glandular pouches that lie one on either side of the male reproductive tract and that in human males secrete a sugar- and protein-containing fluid into the ejaculatory duct

sem·i·nif·er·ous \ˌse-mə-ˈni-fə-rəs\ adj : producing or bearing semen

seminiferous tubule n : any of the coiled threadlike tubules that make up the bulk of the testis and are lined with a layer of epithelial cells from which the spermatozoa are produced

sem·i·no·ma \ˌse-mi-ˈnō-mə\ n, pl **-mas** or **-ma·ta** \-mə-tə\ : a malignant tumor of the testis

semi·per·me·able \ˌse-mē-ˈpər-mē-ə-bəl, ˌse-ˌmī-\ adj : partially but not freely or wholly permeable; specif : permeable to some usu. small molecules but not to other usu. larger particles (a ~ membrane) — **semi·per·me·abil·i·ty** \-ˌpər-mē-ə-ˈbi-lə-tē\ n

semi·pri·vate \-ˈprī-vət\ adj : of, receiving, or associated with hospital service giving a patient more privileges than a ward patient but fewer than a private patient (a ~ room)

semi·spi·na·lis \ˌse-ˌspī-ˈnä-ləs, -ˌlēz\ : any of three muscles of the cervical and thoracic parts of the spinal column : **a** : SEMISPINALIS THORACIS **b** : SEMISPINALIS CERVICIS **c** : SEMISPINALIS CAPITIS

semispinalis cap·i·tis \-ˈka-pi-təs\ n : a deep longitudinal muscle of the back that arises esp. from the transverse processes of the upper six or seven thoracic and the seventh cervical vertebrae, is inserted on the outer surface of the occipital bone between two ridges behind the foramen magnum, and acts to extend and rotate the head — called also *complexus*

semispinalis cervicis \-'sər-vi-sis\ *n* : a deep longitudinal muscle of the back that arises from the transverse processes of the upper five or six thoracic vertebrae, is inserted into the cervical spinous processes from the axis to the fifth cervical vertebra, and with the semispinalis thoracis acts to extend the spinal column and rotate it toward the opposite side

semispinalis thoracis \-thō-'rā-səs\ *n* : a deep longitudinal muscle of the back that arises from the transverse processes of the lower five thoracic vertebrae, is inserted into the spinous processes of the upper four thoracic and lower two cervical vertebrae, and with the semispinalis cervicis acts to extend the spinal column and rotate it toward the opposite side

semisynthetic \-sin-'the-tik\ *adj* **1** : produced by chemical alteration of a natural starting material ⟨∼ penicillins⟩ **2** : containing both chemically identified and complex natural ingredients ⟨a ∼ diet⟩

semitendinosus \-ten-də-'nō-səs\ *n, pl* **-nosi** \-'sī\ : a fusiform muscle of the posterior and inner part of the thigh that arises from the ischial tuberosity along with the biceps femoris, that is inserted by a long round tendon into the inner surface of the upper part of the shaft of the tibia, and that acts to flex the leg and rotate it medially and to extend the thigh

Semliki Forest virus \'sem-lē-kē-'fōr-əst-\ *n* : an arbovirus isolated from mosquitoes in a Ugandan forest and capable of infecting humans

Sendai virus \'sen-dī-\ *n* : a parainfluenza virus first reported from Japan that infects swine, mice, and humans

senecio \si-'nē-shē-ō, -shō\ *n, pl* **-cios** **1** *cap* : a genus of widely distributed plants of the daisy family (Compositae) including some containing various alkaloids which are poisonous to livestock **2** : any plant of the genus *Senecio*

senecioosis \se-ˌnē-sē-'ō-səs\ *n, pl* **-oses** \-ˌsēz\ : a frequently fatal intoxication esp. of livestock feeding on plants of the genus *Senecio*

senescence \si-'nes-ᵊns\ *n* : the state of being old : the process of becoming old — **senescent** \-ᵊnt\ *adj*

senile \'sē-ˌnīl\ *adj* **1** : of, relating to, exhibiting, or characteristic of old age; *esp* : exhibiting a loss of mental faculties associated with old age **2** : being a cell that cannot undergo mitosis and is in the stage of declining functional capacities prior to the time of death ⟨a ∼ red blood cell⟩

senile cataract *n* : a cataract of a type that occurs in the aged and is characterized by an initial opacity in the lens, subsequent swelling of the lens, and final shrinkage with complete loss of transparency

senile dementia *n* : a mental disorder of old age esp. of the degenerative type associated with Alzheimer's disease — called also *senile psychosis*

senile psychosis *n* : SENILE DEMENTIA

senilis — see ARCUS SENILIS, LENTIGO SENILIS

senility \si-'ni-lə-tē, se-\ *n, pl* **-ties** : the quality or state of being senile; *specif* : the physical and mental infirmity of old age

senium \'sē-nē-əm\ *n* : the final period in the normal life span

senna \'se-nə\ *n* **1** : any of a genus (*Cassia*) of leguminous plants; *esp* : one used medicinally **2** : the dried leaflets or pods of various sennas (esp. *Cassia acutifolia* and *C. angustifolia*) used as a purgative

sensation \sen-'sā-shən, sən-\ *n* **1 a** : a mental process (as hearing or smelling) due to immediate bodily stimulation often as distinguished from awareness of the process — compare PERCEPTION **b** : awareness (as of pain) due to stimulation of a sense organ **c** : a state of consciousness of a kind usu. due to physical objects or internal bodily changes ⟨a burning ∼ in his chest⟩ **2** : something (as a physical object or pain) that causes or is the object of sensation

¹sense \'sens\ *n* **1 a** : the faculty of perceiving by means of sense organs **b** : a specialized animal function or mechanism (as sight, hearing, smell, taste, or touch) basically involving a stimulus and a sense organ **c** : the sensory mechanisms constituting a unit distinct from other functions (as movement or thought) **2** : a particular sensation or kind or quality of sensation ⟨a good ∼ of balance⟩

²sense *vb* **sensed; sensing** : to perceive by the senses

sense-datum \-'dā-təm, -'da-, -'dä-\ *n, pl* **sense-data** \-tə\ : the immediate private perceived object of sensation as distinguished from the objective material object itself

sense organ *n* : a bodily structure that receives a stimulus (as heat or sound waves) and is affected in such a manner as to initiate a wave of excitation in associated sensory nerve fibers : RECEPTOR

sensibility \ˌsen-sə-'bi-lə-tē\ *n, pl* **-ties 1** : ability to receive sensations ⟨tactile ∼⟩ **2** : awareness of and responsiveness toward something

sensible \'sen-sə-bəl\ *adj* **1** : perceptible to the senses or to reason or understanding **2** : capable of receiving sensory impressions ⟨∼ to pain⟩

sensitive \'sen-sə-tiv\ *adj* **1** : SENSORY **2** ⟨∼ nerves⟩ **2 a** : receptive to sense impressions **b** : capable of being stimulated or excited by external agents **3**

: highly responsive or susceptible: as **a** : easily hurt or damaged ⟨∼ skin⟩: *esp* : easily hurt emotionally **b** : excessively or abnormally susceptible : HYPERSENSITIVE **c** : capable of indicating minute differences — **sen·si·tive·ness** *n* — **sen·si·tiv·i·ty** \ˌsen-sə-ˈti-və-tē\ *n*

sensitivity training *n* : training in a small interacting group that is designed to increase each individual's awareness of his or her own feelings and the feelings of others and to enhance interpersonal relations

sen·si·ti·za·tion \ˌsen-sə-tə-ˈzā-shən\ *n* **1** : the action or process of making sensitive or hypersensitive ⟨allergic ∼ of the skin⟩ **2** : the process of becoming sensitive or hypersensitive (as to an antigen); *also* : the resulting state **3** : a form of nonassociative learning characterized by an increase in responsiveness upon repeated exposure to a stimulus — compare HABITUATION 3 — **sen·si·tize** \ˈsen-sə-ˌtīz\ *vb*

sen·si·tiz·er \-ˌtī-zər\ *n* : a substance that sensitizes the skin on first contact so that subsequent contact causes inflammation

sen·sor \ˈsen-ˌsȯr, -sər\ *n* : a device that responds to a physical stimulus (as heat, light, sound, or motion) and transmits a resulting impulse; *also* : SENSE ORGAN

sensori- *also* **senso-** *comb form* : sensory : sensory and ⟨*sensori*motor⟩

sen·so·ri·al \sen-ˈsȯr-ē-əl\ *adj* : SENSORY

sen·so·ri·mo·tor \ˌsen-sə-rē-ˈmō-tər\ *adj* : of, relating to, or functioning in both sensory and motor aspects of bodily activity ⟨∼ disturbances⟩

sen·so·ri·neu·ral \-ˈnur-əl, -ˈnyur-\ *adj* : of, relating to, or involving the aspects of sense perception mediated by nerves ⟨∼ hearing loss⟩

sen·so·ri·um \sen-ˈsȯr-ē-əm\ *n, pl* **-ri·ums** *or* **-ria** \-ē-ə\ **1** : the parts of the brain or the mind concerned with the reception and interpretation of sensory stimuli; *broadly* : the entire sensory apparatus **2 a** : ability of the brain to receive and interpret sensory stimuli **b** : the state of consciousness judged in terms of this ability

sen·so·ry \ˈsen-sə-rē\ *adj* **1** : of or relating to sensation or the senses **2** : conveying nerve impulses from the sense organs to the nerve centers : AFFERENT ⟨∼ nerve fibers⟩

sensory aphasia *n* : inability to understand spoken, written, or tactile speech symbols that results from a brain lesion

sensory area *n* : an area of the cerebral cortex that receives afferent nerve fibers from lower sensory or motor areas

sensory cell *n* **1** : a peripheral nerve cell (as an olfactory cell) located at a sensory receiving surface and being the primary receptor of a sensory impulse **2** : a nerve cell (as a spinal ganglion cell) transmitting sensory impulses

sensory neuron *n* : a neuron that transmits nerve impulses from a sense organ towards the central nervous system — compare ASSOCIATIVE NEURON, MOTONEURON

sen·ti·nel \ˈsent-ᵊn-əl\ *adj* : being an individual or part of a population potentially susceptible to an infection or infestation that is being monitored for the appearance or recurrence of the causative pathogen or parasite

sep·a·ra·tion \ˌse-pə-ˈrā-shən\ *n* **1** : the process of isolating or extracting from or of becoming isolated from a mixture; *also* : the resulting state **2** : DISLOCATION — see SHOULDER SEPARATION — **sep·a·rate** \ˈse-pə-ˌrāt\ *vb*

separation anxiety *n* : a form of anxiety originally caused by separation from a significant nurturant figure (as a mother) and that is duplicated later in life by usu. sudden and involuntary exposure to novel and potentially threatening situations

sep·a·ra·tor \ˈse-pə-ˌrā-tər\ *n* : a dental appliance for separating adjoining teeth to give access to their surfaces

sep·sis \ˈsep-səs\ *n, pl* **sep·ses** \ˈsep-ˌsēz\ : a toxic condition resulting from the spread of bacteria or their products from a focus of infection; *esp* : SEPTICEMIA

sept- *or* **septo-** *also* **septi-** *comb form* : septum ⟨*sept*al⟩ ⟨*septo*plasty⟩

septa *pl of* SEPTUM

sep·tal \ˈsept-ᵊl\ *adj* : of or relating to a septum ⟨∼ defects⟩

septal cartilage *n* : the cartilage of the nasal septum

septa pellucida *pl of* SEPTUM PELLUCIDUM

sep·tate \ˈsep-ˌtāt\ *adj* : divided by or having a septum — **sep·ta·tion** \sep-ˈtā-shən\ *n*

septa transversa *pl of* SEPTUM TRANSVERSUM

sep·tec·to·my \sep-ˈtek-tə-mē\ *n, pl* **-mies** : surgical excision of a septum

sep·tic \ˈsep-tik\ *adj* **1** : of, relating to, or causing putrefaction **2** : relating to, involving, or characteristic of sepsis

septic abortion *n* : abortion caused by or associated with infection by a bacterium esp. of the genus *Clostridium* (*C. perfringens*) or rarely by one of the genus *Mycoplasma* (*M. hominis*)

sep·ti·cae·mia *chiefly Brit var of* SEPTICEMIA

sep·ti·ce·mia \ˌsep-tə-ˈsē-mē-ə\ *n* : invasion of the bloodstream by virulent microorganisms from a focus of infection that is accompanied by chills, fever, and prostration and often by the formation of secondary abscesses in various organs — called also *blood* *poisoning;* see PYEMIA — **sep·ti·ce·mic** \-'sē-mik\ *adj*

septic shock *n* : shock produced by usu. gram-negative bacteria that is characterized by hypoperfusion, hyperpyrexia, rigors, impaired cerebral function, and often by decreased cardiac output

septic sore throat *n* : STREP THROAT

septo- — see SEPT-

sep·to·plas·ty \'sep-tə-ˌplas-tē\ *n, pl* **-ties** : surgical repair of the nasal septum

sep·tos·to·my \sep-'täs-tə-mē\ *n, pl* **-mies** : the surgical creation of an opening through the interatrial septum

sep·tum \'sep-təm\ *n, pl* **sep·ta** \-tə\ : a dividing wall or membrane esp. between bodily spaces or masses of soft tissue; *esp* : NASAL SEPTUM

septum pel·lu·ci·dum \-pə-'lü-sə-dəm\ *n, pl* **septa pel·lu·ci·da** \-də\ : the thin double partition extending vertically from the lower surface of the corpus callosum to the fornix and neighboring parts and separating the lateral ventricles of the brain

septum trans·ver·sum \-tranz-'vər-səm\ *n, pl* **septa trans·ver·sa** \-sə\ : the diaphragm or the embryonic structure from which it in part develops

sep·tup·let \sep-'tə-plət, -'tü-plət, -'tyü-; 'sep-tə-\ *n* **1** : one of seven offspring born at one birth **2** *pl* : a group of seven such offspring

¹se·quel \'sē-kwəl, -ˌkwel\ *n* : SEQUELA

se·quela \si-'kwe-lə\ *n, pl* **se·quel·ae** \-(ˌ)lē\ : an aftereffect of disease, injury, procedure, or treatment

¹se·quence \'sē-kwəns, -ˌkwens\ *n* **1** : a continuous or connected series (as of amino acids in a protein) **2** : a consequence, result, or subsequent development (as of a disease)

²sequence *vb* **se·quenced; se·quenc·ing** : to determine the sequence of chemical constituents (as amino-acid residues) in

se·quenc·er \'sē-kwən-sər, -ˌkwen-\ *n* : any of various devices for arranging (as informational items) into or separating (as amino acids from protein) in a sequence

¹se·quen·tial \si-'kwen-chəl\ *adj* **1** : occurring as a sequela of disease or injury **2** : of, relating to, forming, or taken in a sequence

²sequential *n* : an oral contraceptive in which the pills taken during approximately the first three weeks contain only estrogen and those taken during the rest of the cycle contain both estrogen and progestogen

se·ques·ter \si-'kwes-tər\ *vb* : to hold (as a metallic ion) in solution esp. for the purpose of suppressing undesired chemical or biological activity

se·ques·trant \-trənt\ *n* : a sequestering agent (as citric acid)

se·ques·tra·tion \ˌsē-kwəs-'trā-shən,

se-, si-ˌkwes-\ *n* **1** : the formation of a sequestrum **2** : the process of sequestering or result of being sequestered

se·ques·trec·to·my \ˌsē-ˌkwe-'strek-tə-mē\ *n, pl* **-mies** : the surgical removal of a sequestrum

se·ques·trum \si-'kwes-trəm\ *n, pl* **-trums** *also* **-tra** \-trə\ : a fragment of dead bone detached from adjoining sound bone

sera *pl of* SERUM

serial section *n* : any of a series of sections cut in sequence by a microtome from a prepared specimen (as of tissue) — **serially sectioned** *adj* — **serial sectioning** *n*

ser·ine \'ser-ˌēn\ *n* : a nonessential amino acid $C_3H_7NO_3$ that occurs esp. as a structural part of many proteins and phosphatidylethanolamines

se·ri·ous \'sir-ē-əs\ *adj* : having important or dangerous possible consequences (a ~ injury)

sero- *comb form* **1** : serum (serology) (serodiagnosis) **2** : serous and (seropurulent)

se·ro·con·ver·sion \ˌsir-ō-kən-'vər-zhən, ˌser-\ *n* : the production of antibodies in response to an antigen — **se·ro·con·vert** \-'vərt\ *vb*

se·ro·di·ag·no·sis \-ˌdī-ig-'nō-səs\ *n, pl* **-no·ses** \-ˌsēz\ : diagnosis by the use of serum (as in the Wassermann test) — **se·ro·di·ag·nos·tic** \-'näs-tik\ *adj*

se·ro·epi·de·mi·o·log·ic \-ˌep-ə-ˌdē-mē-ə-'lä-jik\ *or* **se·ro·epi·de·mi·o·log·i·cal** \-ji-kəl\ *adj* : of, relating to, or being epidemiological investigations involving the identification of antibodies to specific antigens in populations of individuals — **se·ro·epi·de·mi·ol·o·gy** \-mē-'ä-lə-jē\ *n*

se·ro·group \'sir-ō-ˌgrüp\ *n* : a group of serotypes having one or more antigens in common

se·rol·o·gist \si-'rä-lə-jist\ *n* : a specialist in serology

se·rol·o·gy \si-'rä-lə-jē\ *n, pl* **-gies** : a science dealing with serums and esp. their reactions and properties — **se·ro·log·i·cal** \ˌsir-ə-'lä-ji-kəl\ *or* **se·ro·log·ic** \-jik\ *adj* — **se·ro·log·i·cal·ly** *adv*

se·ro·neg·a·tive \ˌsir-ō-'ne-gə-tiv, ˌser-ō-\ *adj* : having or being a negative serum reaction esp. in a test for the presence of an antibody (a ~ patient) — **se·ro·neg·a·tiv·i·ty** \-ˌne-gə-'ti-və-tē\ *n*

se·ro·pos·i·tive \-'pä-zə-tiv\ *adj* : having or being a positive serum reaction esp. in a test for the presence of an antibody (a ~ donor) — **se·ro·pos·i·tiv·i·ty** \-ˌpä-zə-'ti-və-tē\ *n*

se·ro·prev·a·lence \-'pre-və-ləns\ *n* : the frequency of individuals in a population that have a particular element (as antibodies to HIV) in their blood serum

se·ro·pu·ru·lent \-'pyùr-ə-lənt, -'pyùr-yə-\ *adj* : consisting of a mixture of serum and pus ⟨a ∼ exudate⟩

se·ro·re·ac·tiv·i·ty \-(ₐ)rē-ₐak-ˈti-və-tē\ *n, pl* **-ties** : reactivity of blood serum — **se·ro·re·ac·tion** \ˌsir-ō-rē-ˈak-shən, ˌser-\ *n*

se·ro·sa \sə-ˈrō-zə\ *n, pl* **-sas** *also* **-sae** \-zē\ : a usu. enclosing serous membrane ⟨the peritoneal ∼⟩ — **se·ro·sal** \-zəl\ *adj*

se·ro·san·guin·e·ous \ˌsir-ō-san-ˈgwi-nē-əs, ˌser-ō-, -sən\ *adj* : containing or consisting of both blood and serous fluid ⟨a ∼ discharge⟩

se·ro·si·tis \ˌsir-ō-ˈsī-təs, ˌser-\ *n* : inflammation of one or more serous membranes ⟨peritoneal ∼⟩

se·ro·sur·vey \ˈsir-ō-ˌsər-ˌvā, ˈser-\ *n* : a test of blood serum from a group of individuals to determine seroprevalence (as of antibodies to HIV)

se·ro·ther·a·py \ˌsir-ō-ˈther-ə-pē, ˌser-ō-\ *n, pl* **-pies** : the treatment of a disease with specific immune serum

se·ro·to·ner·gic \ˌsir-ə-tə-ˈnər-jik\ *or* **se·ro·to·nin·er·gic** \ˌsir-ə-ˌtō-nə-ˈnər-jik\ *adj* : liberating, activated by, or involving serotonin in the transmission of nerve impulses

se·ro·to·nin \ˌsir-ə-ˈtō-nən, ˌser-\ *n* : a phenolic amine neurotransmitter $C_{10}H_{12}N_2O$ that is a powerful vasoconstrictor and is found esp. in the brain, blood serum, and gastric mucous membrane of mammals — called also *5-hydroxytryptamine*

¹se·ro·type \ˈsir-ə-ˌtīp, ˈser-\ *n* **1** : a group of intimately related microorganisms distinguished by a common set of antigens **2** : the set of antigens characteristic of a serotype

²serotype *vb* **-typed; -typ·ing** : to determine the serotype of ⟨∼ streptococci⟩

se·rous \ˈsir-əs\ *adj* : of, relating to, producing, or resembling serum; *esp* : having a thin watery constitution

serous cavity *n* : a cavity (as the peritoneal cavity, pleural cavity, or pericardial cavity) that is lined with a serous membrane

serous cell *n* : a cell (as of the parotid gland) that secretes a serous fluid

serous gland *n* : a gland secreting a serous fluid

serous membrane *n* : any of various thin membranes (as the peritoneum, pericardium, or pleurae) that consist of a single layer of thin flat mesothelial cells resting on a connective tissue stroma, secrete a serous fluid, and usu. line bodily cavities or enclose the organs contained in such cavities — compare MUCOUS MEMBRANE

serous otitis media *n* : a form of otitis media that is characterized by the accumulation of serous exudate in the middle ear

ser·o·var \ˈsir-ə-ˌvär, ˈser-, -ˌvar\ *n* : SEROTYPE 1

Ser·pa·sil \ˈsər-pə-ˌsil\ *trademark* —

used for a preparation of reserpine

ser·pig·i·nous \(ₐ)sər-ˈpi-jə-nəs\ *adj* : slowly spreading; *esp* : healing over in one portion while continuing to advance in another ⟨∼ ulcer⟩

serrata — see ORA SERRATA

ser·rat·ed \ˈser-ˌrā-təd, ˈser-ə-\ *or* **ser·rate** \ˈser-ˌāt, sə-ˈrāt \ *adj* : notched or toothed on the edge ⟨the ∼ sutures of the skull⟩

Ser·ra·tia \se-ˈrā-shə, -shē-ə\ *n* : a genus of aerobic saprophytic flagellated rod-shaped bacteria (family Enterobacteriaceae) that are now usu. considered serotypes of a single species (*S. marcescens*) which has been implicated in some human opportunistic infections

Ser·ra·ti \se-ˈrä-tē\, **Serafino,** Italian boatman.

ser·ra·tus \se-ˈrā-təs\ *n, pl* **ser·ra·ti** \-ˈrā-ˌtī\ : any of three muscles of the thorax that have complex origins but arise chiefly from the ribs or vertebrae: **a** : SERRATUS ANTERIOR **b** : SERRATUS POSTERIOR INFERIOR **c** : SERRATUS POSTERIOR SUPERIOR

serratus anterior *n* : a thin muscular sheet of the thorax that arises from the first eight or nine ribs and from the intercostal muscles between them, is inserted into the ventral side of the medial margin of the scapula, and acts to stabilize the scapula by holding it against the chest wall and to rotate it in raising the arm

serratus posterior inferior *n* : a thin quadrilateral muscle at the junction of the thoracic and lumbar regions that arises chiefly from the spinous processes of the lowest two thoracic and first two or three lumbar vertebrae, is inserted into the lowest four ribs, and acts to counteract the pull of the diaphragm on the ribs to which it is attached

serratus posterior superior *n* : a thin quadrilateral muscle of the upper and dorsal part of the thorax that arises chiefly from the spinous processes of the lowest cervical and the first two or three thoracic vertebrae, is inserted into the second to fifth ribs, and acts to elevate the upper ribs

Ser·to·li cell \ˈser-tə-lē-, ser-ˈtō-lē-\ *also* **Ser·to·li's cell** \-lēz-\ *n* : any of the elongated striated cells in the seminiferous tubules of the testis to which the spermatids become attached and from which they apparently derive nourishment

Sertoli, Enrico (1842–1910), Italian physiologist.

ser·tra·line \ˈsər-trə-ˌlēn\ *n* : an antidepressant drug $C_{17}H_{17}NCl_2$ administered in the form of its hydrochloride and acting to enhance serotonin activity

¹se·rum \ˈsir-əm\ *n, pl* **serums** *or* **se·ra** \-ə\ : the watery portion of an animal fluid remaining after coagulation: **a** (1) : the clear yellowish fluid that remains after suspended material (as blood cells), fibrinogen, and fibrin are removed from blood — called also *blood serum* (2) : ANTISERUM **b** : a normal or pathological serous fluid (as in a blister)

²**serum** *adj* : occurring or found in the serum of the blood ⟨∼ cholesterol⟩ ⟨∼ glutamic-oxaloacetic transaminase⟩

serum albumin *n* : a crystallizable albumin or mixture of albumins that normally constitutes more than half of the protein in blood serum, that serves to maintain the osmotic pressure of the blood, and that is used in transfusions esp. for the treatment of shock

serum globulin *n* : a globulin or mixture of globulins occurring in blood serum and containing most of the antibodies of the blood

serum hepatitis *n* : HEPATITIS B

serum sickness *n* : an allergic reaction to the injection of foreign serum manifested by hives, swelling, eruption, arthritis, and fever

ser·vice \'sər-vis\ *n* : a branch of a hospital medical staff devoted to a particular specialty ⟨pediatric ∼⟩

service mark *n* : a mark or device used to identify a service (as transportation or insurance) offered to customers — compare TRADEMARK

¹**ses·a·moid** \'se-sə-ˌmȯid\ *adj* : of, relating to, or being a nodular mass of bone or cartilage in a tendon esp. at a joint or bony prominence ⟨the patella is the largest ∼ bone in the body⟩

²**sesamoid** *n* : a sesamoid bone or cartilage

ses·a·moid·itis \ˌse-sə-ˌmȯi-'dī-təs\ *n* : inflammation of the navicular bone and adjacent structures in the horse

ses·sile \'se-sil, -səl\ *adj* **1** : attached directly by a broad base : not pedunculated ⟨a ∼ tumor⟩ **2** : firmly attached (as to a cell) : not free to move about

¹**set** \'set\ *vb* **set; set·ting** : to restore to normal position or connection when dislocated or fractured ⟨∼ a broken bone⟩

²**set** *n* : a state of psychological preparedness usu. of limited duration for action in response to an anticipated stimulus or situation

Se·tar·ia \se-'tar-ē-ə\ *n* : a genus of filarial worms parasitic as adults in the body cavity of various ungulate mammals (as cattle and deer)

se·ton \'sēt-ᵊn\ *n* : one or more threads or horsehairs or a strip of linen introduced beneath the skin by a knife or needle to provide drainage

set·tle \'set-ᵊl\ *vb* **set·tled; set·tling** *of an animal* **1** : IMPREGNATE 1a **2** : CONCEIVE

seventh cranial nerve *n* : FACIAL NERVE

seventh nerve *n* : FACIAL NERVE

severe combined immunodeficiency *n*

: a rare congenital disorder of the immune system that is characterized by inability to produce a normal complement of antibodies and T cells and that results usu. in early death — abbr. *SCID;* called also *severe combined immune deficiency*

¹**sex** \'seks\ *n* **1** : either of the two major forms of individuals that occur in many species and that are distinguished respectively as male or female **2** : the sum of the structural, functional, and behavioral characteristics of living things that are involved in reproduction by two interacting parents and that distinguish males and females **3 a** : sexually motivated phenomena or behavior **b** : SEXUAL INTERCOURSE

²**sex** *vb* : to identify the sex of ⟨∼ chicks⟩

sex cell *n* : GAMETE; *also* : its cellular precursor

sex chromatin *n* : BARR BODY

sex chromosome *n* : a chromosome (as the X chromosome or the Y chromosome in humans) that is concerned directly with the inheritance of sex and that is the seat of factors governing the inheritance of various sex-linked and sex-limited characters

sex gland *n* : GONAD

sex hormone *n* : a hormone (as from the gonads or adrenal cortex) that affects the growth or function of the reproductive organs or the development of secondary sex characteristics

sex–limited *adj* : expressed in the phenotype of only one sex ⟨a ∼ character⟩

sex–linked *adj* **1** : located in a sex chromosome ⟨a ∼ gene⟩ **2** : mediated by a sex-linked gene ⟨a ∼ character⟩ — **sex–linkage** *n*

sex object *n* : a person regarded esp. exclusively as an object of sexual interest

sex·ol·o·gy \sek-'sä-lə-jē\ *n, pl* **-gies** : the study of sex or of the interaction of the sexes esp. among human beings — **sex·ol·o·gist** \-jist\ *n*

sex ratio *n* : the proportion of males to females in a population esp. as expressed by the number of males per hundred females

sex·tu·plet \sek-'stə-plət, -'stü-, -'styü-; 'sek-stə-\ *n* : any of six offspring born at one birth

sex·u·al \'sek-shə-wəl\ *adj* **1** : of, relating to, or associated with sex or the sexes ⟨∼ differentiation⟩ ⟨∼ conflict⟩ **2** : having or involving sex ⟨∼ reproduction⟩ — **sex·u·al·ly** *adv*

sexual intercourse *n* **1** : heterosexual intercourse involving penetration of the vagina by the penis : COITUS **2** : intercourse involving genital contact between individuals other than penetration of the vagina by the penis

sex·u·al·i·ty \ˌsek-shə-'wa-lə-tē\ *n, pl* **-ties** : the quality or state of being sexual: **a** : the condition of having sex **b** : sexual activity **c** : expression of sexual receptivity or interest esp. when excessive

sexually transmitted disease *n* : any of various diseases transmitted by direct sexual contact that include the classic venereal diseases (as syphilis, gonorrhea, and chancroid) and other diseases (as hepatitis A, hepatitis B, giardiasis, and AIDS) often or sometimes contracted by other than sexual means — called also *STD*

sexual relations *n pl* : COITUS

Se·za·ry syndrome \ˌsā-zä-ʹrē-\ *or* **Se·za·ry's syndrome** \-ʹrēz-\ *n* : a rare disease that is characterized by the presence in the blood and in the skin of numerous large atypical mononuclear T cells with resultant widespread exfoliation of the skin

Sézary, Albert (1880–1956), French physician.

SGOT *abbr* serum glutamic-oxaloacetic transaminase

SGPT *abbr* serum glutamic pyruvic transaminase

SH *abbr* serum hepatitis

shad·ow \ʹsha-(ˌ)dō\ *n* **1** : a dark outline or image on an X-ray photograph where the X rays have been blocked by a radiopaque mass (as a tumor) **2** : a colorless or scantily pigmented or stained body (as a degenerate cell or empty membrane) only faintly visible under the microscope

shaft \ʹshaft\ *n* : a long slender cylindrical body or part: as **a** : the cylindrical part of a long bone between the enlarged ends **b** : the part of a hair that is visible above the surface of the skin

shaft louse *n* : a biting louse of the genus *Menopon* (*M. gallinae*) that commonly infests domestic fowls

shakes \ʹshāks\ *n sing or pl* **1** : a condition of trembling; *specif* : DELIRIUM TREMENS **2** : MALARIA 1

shaking palsy *n* : PARKINSON'S DISEASE

shal·low \ʹsha-(ˌ)lō\ *adj* : displacing comparatively little air (~ breathing)

shank \ʹshaŋk\ *n* : the part of the leg between the knee and the ankle in humans or a corresponding part in other vertebrates

shape \ʹshāp\ *vb* **shaped; shap·ing** : to modify (behavior) by rewarding changes that tend toward a desired response

Shar·pey's fiber \ʹshär-pēz-\ *n* : any of the thready processes of the periosteum that penetrate the tissue of the superficial lamellae of bones

Sharpey, William (1802–1880), British anatomist and physiologist.

sheath \ʹshēth\ *n, pl* **sheaths** \ʹshēthz, ʹshēths\ **1** : an investing cover or case of a plant or animal body or body part: as **a** : the tubular fold of skin into which the penis of many mammals is retracted **b** : the connective tissue of an organ or part that binds

together its component elements and holds it in place **2** : CONDOM — **sheathed** *adj*

sheath of Schwann \-ʹshwän\ *n* : NEURILEMMA

T. A. H. Schwann — see SCHWANN CELL

shed \ʹshed\ *vb* **shed; shed·ding** : to give off or out: as **a** : to lose as part of a natural process (~ the deciduous teeth) **b** : to discharge usu. gradually from the body (~ a virus in the urine)

Shee·han's syndrome \ʹshē-ənz-\ *n* : necrosis of the pituitary gland with associated hypopituitarism resulting from postpartum hemorrhage

Sheehan, Harold Leeming (b 1900), British pathologist.

sheep botfly *n* : a dipteran fly of the genus *Oestrus* (*O. ovis*) whose larvae parasitize sheep and lodge esp. in the nasal passages, frontal sinuses, and throat

sheep–dip \ʹshēp-ˌdip\ *n* : a liquid preparation of usu. toxic chemicals into which sheep are plunged esp. to destroy parasitic arthropods

sheep ked *n* : a wingless bloodsucking dipteran fly of the genus *Melophagus* (*M. ovinus*) that feeds chiefly on sheep and is a vector of sheep trypanosomiasis — called also *ked, sheep tick*

sheep pox *n* : a disease of sheep and possibly goats that is caused by a poxvirus related to the one causing smallpox and was formerly epizootic in warmer Old World areas

sheep tick *n* : SHEEP KED

shellfish poisoning — see PARALYTIC SHELLFISH POISONING

shell shock *n* : post-traumatic stress disorder in soldiers as a result of combat experience — **shell–shocked** \ʹshel-ˌshäkt\ *adj*

shi·at·su *also* **shi·at·zu** \shē-ʹät-sü\, *often cap* : a massage with the fingers applied to those specific areas of the body used in acupuncture — called also *acupressure*

Shi·ga bacillus \ʹshē-gə-\ *n* : a widely distributed but chiefly tropical bacterium of the genus *Shigella* (*S. dysenteriae*) that causes dysentery

Shiga, Kiyoshi (1870–1957), Japanese bacteriologist.

shi·gel·la \shi-ʹge-lə\ *n* **1** *cap* : a genus of nonmotile aerobic enterobacteria that form acid but no gas on many carbohydrates and that cause dysenteries in animals and esp. humans **2** *pl* **-gel·lae** \-ˌlē\ *also* **-gellas** : any bacterium of the genus *Shigella*

shig·el·lo·sis \ˌshi-gə-ʹlō-səs\ *n, pl* **-lo·ses** \-ʹlō-ˌsēz\ : infection with or dysentery caused by bacteria of the genus *Shigella*

shin \ʹshin\ *n* : the front part of the leg below the knee

shin·bone \ʹshin-ˌbōn\ *n* : TIBIA

shin·er \ʹshī-nər\ *n* : BLACK EYE

shin·gles \'shiŋ-gəlz\ *n* : an acute viral inflammation of the sensory ganglia of spinal and cranial nerves associated with a vesicular eruption and neuralgic pain and caused by reactivation of the herpesvirus causing chicken pox — called also *herpes zoster, zona, zoster*

shin·splints \'shin-ˌsplints\ *n sing or pl* : painful injury to and inflammation of the tibial and toe extensor muscles or their fasciae that is caused by repeated minimal traumas (as by running on a hard surface)

shipping fever *n* : an often fatal febrile disease esp. of young cattle and sheep that occurs under conditions of unusual exposure or exhaustion, is marked by high fever and pneumonia, and is associated with the presence of bacteria (esp. genera *Pasteurella* and *Mycoplasma*) or viruses

shiv·er \'shi-vər\ *vb* : to undergo trembling : experience rapid involuntary muscular twitching esp. in response to cold — **shiver** *n*

shivering *n* **1** : an act or action of one that shivers **2** : a constant abnormal twitching of various muscles in the horse that is prob. due to sensory nerve derangement

shock \'shäk\ *n* **1** : a sudden or violent disturbance in the mental or emotional faculties **2** : a state of profound depression of the vital processes of the body that is characterized by pallor, rapid but weak pulse, rapid and shallow respiration, reduced total blood volume, and low blood pressure and that is caused usu. by severe esp. crushing injuries, hemorrhage, burns, or major surgery **3** : sudden stimulation of the nerves or convulsive contraction of the muscles accompanied by a feeling of concussion that is caused by the discharge of electricity through the body — compare ELECTROSHOCK THERAPY — **shock** *vb*

shock lung *n* : a condition of severe pulmonary edema associated with shock

shock therapy *n* : the treatment of mental disorder by the artificial induction of coma or convulsions through use of drugs or electric current — called also *convulsive therapy, shock treatment;* compare ELECTROSHOCK THERAPY

shock treatment *n* : SHOCK THERAPY

shoot \'shüt\ *vb* **shot** \'shät\; **shooting 1** : to give an injection to **2** : to take or administer (as a drug) by hypodermic needle

shoot·ing *adj* : characterized by sudden sharp piercing sensations ⟨∼ pains⟩

short bone *n* : a bone (as of the tarsus or carpus) that is of approximately equal length in all dimensions

short ciliary nerve *n* : any of 6 to 10 delicate nerve filaments of parasympathetic, sympathetic, and general sensory function that arise in the ciliary ganglion and innervate the smooth muscles and tunics of the eye — compare LONG CILIARY NERVE

shortness of breath *n* : difficulty in drawing sufficient breath : labored breathing

short–nosed cattle louse *n* : a large louse of the genus *Haematopinus* (*H. eurysternus*) that attacks domestic cattle

short posterior ciliary artery *n* : any of 6 to 10 arteries that arise from the ophthalmic artery or its branches and supply the choroid and the ciliary processes — compare LONG POSTERIOR CILIARY ARTERY

short saphenous vein *n* : SAPHENOUS VEIN b

short·sight·ed \'short-'sī-təd\ *adj* : NEARSIGHTED

short·sight·ed·ness *n* : MYOPIA

short–term memory *n* : memory that involves recall of information for a relatively short time (as a few seconds)

shot \'shät\ *n* : an injection of a drug, immunizing substance, nutrient, or medicament ⟨a flu ∼⟩

shoul·der \'shōl-dər\ *n* **1** : the laterally projecting part of the body formed of the bones and joints with their covering tissue by which the arm is connected with the trunk **2** : the two shoulders and the upper part of the back — usu. used in pl.

shoulder blade *n* : SCAPULA

shoulder girdle *n* : PECTORAL GIRDLE

shoulder–hand syndrome *n* : pain in and stiffening of the shoulder followed by swelling and stiffening of the hand and fingers often associated with or following myocardial infarction

shoulder joint *n* : the ball-and-socket joint of the humerus and the scapula

shoulder separation *n* : a dislocation of the shoulder at the acromioclavicular joint

show \'shō\ *n* **1** : a discharge of mucus streaked with blood from the vagina at the onset of labor **2** : the first appearance of blood in a menstrual period

shrink \'shriŋk\ *n* : a clinical psychiatrist or psychologist — called also *headshrinker*

shud·der \'shə-dər\ *vb* **shud·dered; shud·der·ing** : to tremble convulsively : SHIVER — **shudder** *n*

shunt \'shənt\ *n* **1** : a passage by which a bodily fluid (as blood) is diverted from one channel, circulatory path, or part to another; *esp* : such a passage established by surgery or occurring as an abnormality ⟨an arteriovenous ∼⟩ **2 a** : a surgical procedure for the establishment of an artificial shunt — see PORTACAVAL SHUNT **b** : a device (as a narrow tube) used to establish an artificial shunt — **shunt** *vb*

¹shut–in \'shət-ˌin\ *n* : an invalid confined to home, a room, or bed

²**shut–in** \'shət-₁in\ *adj* **1** : confined to one's home or an institution by illness or incapacity **2** : tending to avoid social contact : WITHDRAWN ⟨the ~ personality type⟩

Si *symbol* silicon

SI *abbr* [French *Système International d'Unités*] International System of Units

sial- *or* **sialo-** *comb form* : saliva ⟨*sialo*lith⟩ ⟨*sialo*rrhea⟩

si·al·ad·e·ni·tis \₁sī-ə-₁lad-ᵊn-'ī-təs\ *n* : inflammation of a salivary gland

si·al·a·gogue \sī-'a-lə-₁gäg\ *n* : an agent that promotes the flow of saliva — called also *sialogogue*

si·al·ic acid \sī-'a-lik\ *n* : any of a group of reducing amido acids that are essentially carbohydrates and are found esp. as components of blood glycoproteins and mucoproteins

si·alo·ad·e·nec·to·my \₁sī-ə-lō-₁ad-ᵊn-'ek-tə-mē\ *n, pl* **-mies** : surgical excision of a salivary gland

si·alo·gly·co·pro·tein \-₁gli-kō-'prō-₁tēn\ *n* : a glycoprotein (as of blood) having sialic acid as a component

si·al·o·gogue \sī-'a-lə-₁gäg\ *n* : SIALAGOGUE

si·alo·gram \sī-'a-lə-₁gram\ *n* : a roentgenogram of the salivary tract made by sialography

si·a·log·ra·phy \₁sī-ə-'lä-grə-fē\ *n, pl* **-phies** : roentgenography of the salivary tract after injection of a radiopaque substance

si·al·o·lith \sī-'a-lə-₁lith\ *n* : a calculus occurring in a salivary gland

si·al·o·li·thi·a·sis \₁sī-ə-lō-li-'thī-ə-səs\ *n, pl* **-a·ses** \-₁sēz\ : the formation or presence of a calculus or calculi in a salivary gland

si·al·or·rhea \₁sī-ə-lə-'rē-ə\ *n* : excessive salivation

si·al·or·rhoea *chiefly Brit var of* SIALORRHEA

Si·a·mese twin \'sī-ə-₁mēz-, -₁mēs-\ *n* : one of a pair of congenitally united twins

sib \'sib\ *n* : a brother or sister considered irrespective of sex

sib·i·lant \'si-bə-lənt\ *adj* : characterized by or being a sharp whistling sound ⟨~ breathing⟩ ⟨~ rales⟩

sib·ling \'si-bliŋ\ *n* : SIB; *also* : one of two or more individuals having one common parent

sibling rivalry *n* : competition between siblings esp. for the attention, affection, and approval of their parents

sicca — *see* KERATOCONJUNCTIVITIS SICCA

sic·ca syndrome \'si-kə-\ *n* : SJÖGREN'S SYNDROME

sick \'sik\ *adj* **1 a** : affected with disease or ill health **b** : of, relating to, or intended for use in sickness **c** : affected with nausea : inclined to vomit or being in the act of vomiting **2** : mentally or emotionally unsound or disordered

sick bay *n* : a compartment in a ship used as a dispensary and hospital; *broadly* : a place for the care of the sick or injured

sick·bed \'sik-₁bed\ *n* : the bed upon which one lies sick

sick building syndrome *n* : a set of symptoms (as headache, fatigue, eye irritation, and dizziness) typically affecting workers in modern airtight office buildings that is believed to be caused by indoor pollutants (as formaldehyde fumes, particulate matter, or microorganisms) — *abbr.* SBS

sick call *n* : a scheduled time at which individuals (as soldiers) may report as sick to a medical officer

sick·en \'si-kən\ *vb* : to make or become sick

sick·en·ing *adj* : causing sickness or nausea ⟨a ~ odor⟩

sick headache *n* : MIGRAINE

sick·lae·mia *chiefly Brit var of* SICKLEMIA

¹**sick·le** \'si-kəl\ *n* : a dental scaler with a curved three-sided point

²**sickle** *adj* : of, relating to, or characteristic of sickle-cell anemia or sickle-cell trait ⟨~ hemoglobin⟩

³**sickle** *vb* **sick·led; sick·ling** : to change (a red blood cell) into a sickle cell

sick leave *n* **1** : an absence from work permitted because of illness **2** : the number of days per year for which an employer agrees to pay employees who are sick

sickle cell *n* **1** : an abnormal red blood cell of crescent shape **2** : a condition characterized by sickle cells : SICKLE-CELL ANEMIA, SICKLE-CELL TRAIT

sickle–cell anemia *n* : a chronic anemia that occurs primarily in individuals of African descent who are homozygous for the gene controlling hemoglobin S and that is characterized by destruction of red blood cells and by episodic blocking of blood vessels by the adherence of sickle cells to the vascular endothelium which causes the serious complications of the disease (as organ failure)

sickle–cell disease *n* : SICKLE-CELL ANEMIA

sickle–cell trait *n* : a usu. asymptomatic blood condition in which some red blood cells tend to sickle but usu. not enough to produce anemia and which results from heterozygosity for the gene controlling hemoglobin S

sick·le·mia \si-'klē-mē-ə\ *n* : SICKLE-CELL TRAIT — **sick·le·mic** \-mik\ *adj*

sick·ler \'si-klər\ *n* : a person with sickle-cell trait or sickle-cell anemia

sick·ly \'si-klē\ *adj* **1** : somewhat unwell; *also* : habitually ailing **2** : produced by or associated with sickness **3** : producing or tending to produce disease **4** : tending to produce nausea ⟨a ~ odor⟩

sick·ness \'sik-nəs\ *n* **1** : the condition

of being ill : ill health **2** : a specific disease **3** : NAUSEA

sick·room \'sik-ˌrüm, -ˌrüm\ *n* : a room in which a person is confined by sickness

sick sinus syndrome *n* : a cardiac disorder typically characterized by alternating tachycardia and bradycardia

side \'sīd\ *n* **1** : the right or left part of the wall or trunk of the body ⟨a pain in the ∼⟩ **2** : a lateral half or part of an organ or structure ⟨the right ∼ of one leg⟩

side·bone \-ˌbōn\ *n* **1** *or* **sidebones** : abnormal ossification of the cartilages in the lateral posterior part of a horse's hoof (as of a forefoot) often causing lameness — used with a sing. verb **2** : one of the bony structures characteristic of sidebone

side chain *n* : a branched chain of atoms attached to the principal chain or to a ring in a molecule

side effect *n* : a secondary and usu. adverse effect (as of a drug) — called also *side reaction*

sider- *or* **sidero-** *comb form* : iron ⟨*sideropenia*⟩

sid·ero·blast \'si-də-rə-ˌblast\ *n* : an erythroblast containing cytoplasmic iron granules — **sid·ero·blas·tic** \ˌsi-də-rə-'blas-tik\ *adj*

sid·ero·cyte \'si-də-rə-ˌsīt\ *n* : an atypical red blood cell containing iron not bound in hemoglobin

sid·ero·pe·nia \ˌsi-də-rə-'pē-nē-ə\ *n* : iron deficiency in the blood serum — **sid·ero·pe·nic** \-'pē-nik\ *adj*

sid·er·o·sis \ˌsi-də-'rō-səs\ *n* **1** : pneumoconiosis occurring in iron workers from inhalation of particles of iron **2** : deposit of iron pigment in a bodily tissue — **sid·er·ot·ic** \ˌsi-də-'rä-tik\ *adj*

side·stream \'sīd-ˌstrēm\ *adj* : relating to or being tobacco smoke that is emitted from the lighted end of a cigarette or cigar — compare MAINSTREAM

side·wind·er \'sīd-ˌwīn-dər\ *n* : a small pale-colored rattlesnake of the genus *Crotalus* (*C. cerastes*) of the southwestern U.S. that moves by thrusting its body diagonally forward in a series of S-shaped curves — called also *horned rattlesnake*

SIDS *abbr* sudden infant death syndrome

Sig *abbr* signa — used to introduce the signature in writing a prescription

sight \'sīt\ *n* **1** : something that is seen **2** : the process, power, or function of seeing; *specif* : the sense by which light stimuli received by the eye are interpreted by the brain in the construction of a representation of the position, shape, brightness, and usu. color of objects in the real world **3 a** : a perception of an object by the eye **b** : the range of vision

sight·ed \'sī-təd\ *adj* : having sight : not blind

sight·less \'sīt-ləs\ *adj* : lacking sight : BLIND — **sight·less·ness** *n*

¹sig·moid \'sig-ˌmȯid\ *adj* **1 a** : curved like the letter C **b** : curved in two directions like the letter S **2** : of, relating to, or being the sigmoid flexure of the intestine ⟨∼ lesions⟩

²sigmoid *n* : SIGMOID FLEXURE

sigmoid artery *n* : any of several branches of the inferior mesenteric artery that supply the sigmoid flexure

sigmoid colon *n* : SIGMOID FLEXURE

sig·moid·ec·to·my \ˌsig-mȯi-'dek-tə-mē\ *n, pl* **-mies** : surgical excision of part of the sigmoid flexure

sigmoid flexure *n* : the contracted and crooked part of the colon immediately above the rectum — called also *pelvic colon, sigmoid colon*

sigmoid notch *n* : a curved depression on the upper border of the lower jaw between the coronoid process and the articulatory condyle

sig·moid·o·scope \sig-'mȯi-də-ˌskōp\ *n* : a long hollow tubular instrument designed to be passed through the anus in order to permit inspection, diagnosis, treatment, and photography esp. of the sigmoid flexure — called also *proctosigmoidoscope*

sig·moid·os·co·py \ˌsig-ˌmȯi-'däs-kə-pē\ *n, pl* **-pies** : the process of using a sigmoidoscope — called also *proctosigmoidoscopy* — **sig·moid·o·scop·ic** \-də-'skä-pik\ *adj*

sigmoid sinus *n* : a sinus on each side of the brain that is a continuation of the transverse sinus on the same side, follows an S-shaped course to the jugular foramen, and empties into the internal jugular vein

sigmoid vein *n* : any of several veins that drain the sigmoid flexure and empty into the superior rectal vein

sign \'sīn\ *n* **1** : one of a set of gestures used to represent language **2** : an objective evidence of disease esp. as observed and interpreted by the physician — compare SYMPTOM; PHYSICAL SIGN

sig·na \'sig-nə\ *vb* : write on label — used to introduce the signature in writing a prescription; abbr. *S, Sig*

signal node *n* : a supraclavicular lymph node which when tumorous is often a secondary sign of gastrointestinal cancer — called also *Virchow's node*

sig·na·ture \'sig-nə-ˌchùr, -chər, -ˌtyùr, -ˌtùr\ *n* : the part of a medical prescription which contains the directions to the patient

sign language *n* : a system of communicating by means of conventional chiefly manual gestures that is used esp. by the deaf; *esp* : DACTYLOLOGY

Si·las·tic \sī-'las-tik\ *trademark* — used for a soft pliable plastic

si·lent \'sī-lənt\ *adj* **1** : not exhibiting the usual signs or symptoms of presence ⟨a ∼ infection⟩ **2** : yielding no detectable response to stimulation — used esp. of an association area of the brain ⟨∼ cortex⟩ **3** : having no detectable function or effect ⟨∼ genes⟩ — **si•lent•ly** *adv*

silic- *or* **silico-** *comb form* **1** : relating to or containing silicon or its compounds ⟨*silic*one⟩ **2** : silicosis and ⟨*silic*otuberculosis⟩

sil•i•ca \'si-li-kə\ *n* : the dioxide of silicon SiO_2

silica gel *n* : colloidal silica resembling coarse white sand in appearance but possessing many fine pores and therefore extremely adsorbent

silicate cement *n* : a dental cement used in restorations

sil•i•con \'si-li-kən, -ˌkän\ *n* : a nonmetallic element that occurs combined as the most abundant element next to oxygen in the earth's crust — symbol *Si*; see ELEMENT table

silicon dioxide *n* : SILICA

sil•i•cone \'si-li-ˌkōn\ *n* : any of various polymeric organic silicon compounds some of which have been used as surgical implants

sil•i•co•sis \ˌsi-lə-'kō-səs\ *n*, *pl* **-co•ses** \-ˌsēz\ : pneumoconiosis characterized by massive fibrosis of the lungs resulting in shortness of breath and caused by prolonged inhalation of silica dusts

¹**sil•i•cot•ic** \ˌsi-lə-'kä-tik\ *adj* : relating to, caused by, or affected with silicosis ⟨∼ patients⟩ ⟨∼ lungs⟩

²**silicotic** *n* : an individual affected with silicosis

sil•i•co•tu•ber•cu•lo•sis \ˌsi-li-kō-tü-ˌbər-kyə-'lō-səs, -tyü-\ *n*, *pl* **-lo•ses** \-ˌsēz\ : silicosis and tuberculosis in the same lung

silk \'silk\ *n* **1** : a lustrous tough elastic fiber produced by silkworms **2** : strands of silk thread of various thicknesses used as suture material in surgery ⟨surgical ∼⟩

sil•ver \'sil-vər\ *n* : a white metallic element that has the highest thermal and electric conductivity of any substance — symbol *Ag*; see ELEMENT table

silver iodide *n* : a compound AgI that darkens on exposure to light and is used in medicine as a local antiseptic

silver nitrate *n* : an irritant compound $AgNO_3$ used in medicine esp. as an antiseptic and caustic

silver protein *n* : any of several colloidal light-sensitive preparations of silver and protein used in aqueous solution on mucous membranes as antiseptics and classified by their efficacy and irritant properties: as **a** : a preparation containing 19 to 23 percent of silver — called also *mild silver protein* **b** : a more irritant preparation containing 7.5 to 8.5 percent of silver — called also *strong silver protein*

si•meth•i•cone \si-'me-thi-ˌkōn\ *n* : a liquid mixture of silicone polymers used as an antiflatulent — see MYLICON

Sim•monds' disease \'si-məndz-\ *n* : a disease that is characterized by extreme and progressive emaciation with atrophy of internal organs, loss of body hair, and evidences of premature aging resulting from atrophy or destruction of the anterior lobe of the pituitary gland

   Simmonds, Morris (1855–1925), German physician.

¹**sim•ple** \'sim-pəl\ *adj* **sim•pler; sim•plest 1** : free from complexity or difficulty: as **a** : easily treated or cured **b** : controlled by a single gene ⟨∼ inherited characters⟩ **2** : of, relating to, or being an epithelium in which the cells are arranged in a single layer

²**simple** *n* **1** : a medicinal plant **2** : a vegetable drug having only one ingredient

simple fracture *n* : a bone fracture that does not form an open wound in the skin — compare COMPOUND FRACTURE

simple ointment *n* : WHITE OINTMENT

simple sugar *n* : MONOSACCHARIDE

simplex — see GENITAL HERPES SIMPLEX, HERPES SIMPLEX, PERIODONTITIS SIMPLEX

sim•u•late \'sim-yə-ˌlāt\ *vb* **-lat•ed; -lat•ing** : to have or produce a symptomatic resemblance to ⟨fleas *simulating* leprosy⟩ — **sim•u•la•tion** \ˌsim-yə-'lā-shən\ *n*

Si•mu•li•um \si-'myü-lē-əm\ *n* : a genus of dark-colored bloodsucking dipteran flies (family Simuliidae) of which some are vectors of onchocerciasis or of protozoan diseases of birds — see BLACKFLY

si•nal \'sin-əl\ *adj* : of, relating to, or coming from a sinus ⟨a ∼ discharge⟩

Sind•bis virus \'sind-bis-\ *n* : an RNA-containing spherical arbovirus that is transmitted by mosquitoes and is related to the virus causing western equine encephalomyelitis

Sin•e•quan \'si-nə-ˌkwan\ *trademark* — used for a preparation of doxepin

sin•ew \'sin-yü\ *n* : TENDON

single-blind *adj* : of, relating to, or being an experimental procedure in which while the experiment is actually in progress either the subjects or the experimenters but not both know which individuals are assigned to the test group and which to the control group — compare DOUBLE-BLIND

single bond *n* : a chemical bond consisting of one covalent bond between two atoms in a molecule esp. when the atoms can have more than one bond

single photon emission computed tomography *n* : a medical imaging technique that is used esp. for mapping brain function and that is similar to positron-emission tomography in using the photons emitted by the agency of a radioactive tracer to create an image but that differs in being able to detect only a single photon for each nuclear disintegration and in generating a lower-quality image — abbr. SPECT

sin·gle·ton \'siŋ-gəl-tən\ n : an offspring born singly ⟨∼s are more common than twins⟩

¹**si·nis·tral** \'si-nəs-trəl, sə-'nis-\ adj : of, relating to, or inclined to the left; esp : LEFT-HANDED

²**sinistral** n : a person exhibiting dominance of the left hand and eye : a left-handed person

sin·is·tral·i·ty \ˌsi-nə-'stra-lə-tē\ n, pl **-ties** : the quality or state of having the left side or one or more of its parts (as the hand or eye) different from and usu. more efficient than the right or its corresponding parts; also : LEFT-HANDEDNESS

sino- also **sinu-** comb form : relating to a sinus or sinuses ⟨sinoatrial node⟩

si·no·atri·al \ˌsī-nō-'ā-trē-əl\ adj : of, involving, or being the sinoatrial node

sinoatrial node n : a small mass of tissue that is made up of Purkinje fibers, ganglion cells, and nerve fibers, that is embedded in the musculature of the right atrium, and that originates the impulses stimulating the heartbeat — called also S-A node, sinus node

si·no·au·ric·u·lar \-ō-'ri-kyə-lər\ adj : SINOATRIAL

sin·se·mil·la \ˌsin-sə-'mē-lə, -'mi-, -yə, -lyə\ n : highly potent marijuana from female plants that are specially tended and kept seedless by preventing pollination in order to induce a high resin content; also : a female hemp plant grown to produce sinsemilla

si·no·atri·al \ˌsī-nyü-, -nü-\ var of SINOATRIAL

si·nus \'sī-nəs\ n : a cavity or hollow in the body: as **a** : a narrow elongated tract extending from a focus of suppuration and serving for the discharge of pus ⟨a tuberculous ∼⟩ **b** (1) : a cavity in the substance of a bone of the skull that usu. communicates with the nostrils and contains air (2) : a channel for venous blood (3) : a dilatation in a bodily canal or vessel

sinus bradycardia n : abnormally slow sinus rhythm; specif : sinus rhythm at a rate lower than 60 beats per minute

si·nus·itis \ˌsī-nə-'sī-təs, -nyə-\ n : inflammation of a sinus of the skull

sinus node n : SINOATRIAL NODE

sinus of the dura mater n : any of numerous venous channels (as the sagittal sinuses) that are situated between the two layers of the dura mater and drain blood from the brain and the bones forming the cranium and empty it into the internal jugular vein — called also dural sinus

sinus of Val·sal·va \-väl-'säl-və\ n : any one of the pouches of the aorta and

pulmonary artery which are located behind the flaps of the semilunar valves and into which the blood in its regurgitation toward the heart enters and thereby closes the valves — called also aortic sinus

Valsalva, Antonio Maria (1666–1723), Italian anatomist.

si·nu·soid \'si-nə-ˌsȯid, -nyə-\ n : a minute endothelium-lined space or passage for blood in the tissues of an organ (as the liver) — **si·nu·soi·dal** \ˌsī-nə-'sȯid-əl, -nyə-\ adj — **si·nu·soi·dal·ly** adv

si·nus·ot·o·my \ˌsī-nə-'sä-tə-mē, -nyə-\ n, pl **-mies** : surgical incision into a sinus of the skull

sinus rhythm n : the rhythm of the heart produced by impulses from the sinoatrial node

sinus tachycardia n : abnormally rapid sinus rhythm; specif : sinus rhythm at a rate greater than 100 beats per minute

si·nus ve·no·sus \ˌsī-nəs-vi-'nō-səs\ n : an enlarged pouch that adjoins the heart, is formed by the union of the large systemic veins, and is the passage through which venous blood enters the embryonic heart

sinus venosus scle·rae \-'sklē-rē\ n : CANAL OF SCHLEMM

si·pho·no·phore \sī-'fä-nə-ˌfȯr, 'sī-fə-nə-\ n : any of an order (Siphonophora) of compound free-swimming or floating oceanic coelenterates — see PORTUGUESE MAN-OF-WAR

si·re·no·me·lia \ˌsī-rə-nō-'mē-lē-ə\ n : a congenital malformation in which the lower limbs are fused

sir·up var of SYRUP

sis·ter \'sis-tər\ n, chiefly Brit : a head nurse in a hospital ward or clinic; broadly : NURSE

sister chromatid n : any of the chromatids formed by replication of one chromosome during interphase of the cell cycle esp. while they are still joined by a centromere

Sis·tru·rus \si-'strür-əs\ n : a genus of small rattlesnakes having the top of the head covered with scales

site \'sīt\ n : the place, scene, or point of something ⟨∼ of inflammation⟩

si·tos·ter·ol \sī-'täs-tə-ˌrȯl, sə-, -ˌrȯl\ n : any of several sterols that are widespread esp. in plant products (as wheat germ) and are used in the synthesis of steroid hormones

situ — see IN SITU

sit·u·a·tion·al \ˌsi-chə-'wā-shə-nəl\ adj : of, relating to, or occurring in a particular set of circumstances ⟨∼ impotence⟩ ⟨∼ hypertension⟩

si·tus \'sī-təs\ n : the place where something exists or originates : SITE

situs in·ver·sus \-in-'vər-səs\ n : a congenital abnormality characterized by lateral transposition of the viscera (as of the heart or the liver)

sitz bath \'sits-\ n **1** : a tub in which one

bathes in a sitting posture **2 :** a bath in which the hips and buttocks are immersed in hot water for the therapeutic effect of moist heat in the perineal and anal regions

six–o–six *or* **606** \₁siks-₁ō-ˈsiks\ *n* **:** ARSPHENAMINE

sixth cranial nerve *n* **:**   ABDUCENS NERVE

six–year molar *n* **:** one of the first permanent molar teeth of which there are four including one on each side of the upper and lower jaws and which erupt at about six years of age — called also *sixth-year molar;* compare TWELVE-YEAR MOLAR

Sjö·gren's syndrome \ˈshȫ-₁grenz-\ *also* **Sjögren syndrome** \-₁gren-\ *n* **:** a chronic inflammatory autoimmune disease that affects esp. older women, that is characterized by dryness of mucous membranes esp. of the eyes and mouth and by infiltration of the affected tissues by lymphocytes, and that is often associated with rheumatoid arthritis — called also *sicca syndrome, Sjögren's disease*

Sjögren, Henrik Samuel Conrad (1899–1986), Swedish ophthalmologist.

skelet- *or* **skeleto-** *comb form* **1 :** skeleton ⟨*skelet*al⟩ **2 :** skeletal and ⟨*skeleto*muscular⟩

skel·e·tal \ˈske-lət-ºl\ *adj* **:** of, relating to, forming, attached to, or resembling a skeleton ⟨∼ structures⟩

skeletal muscle *n* **:** striated muscle that is usu. attached to the skeleton and is usu. under voluntary control

skel·e·to·mus·cu·lar \₁ske-lə-tō-ˈməs-kyə-lər\ *adj* **:** constituting, belonging to, or dependent upon the skeleton and the muscles that move it

skel·e·ton \ˈske-lət-ºn\ *n* **:** a usu. rigid supportive or protective structure or framework of an organism; *esp* **:** the bony or more or less cartilaginous framework supporting the soft tissues and protecting the internal organs of a vertebrate

Skene's gland \ˈskēns-\ *n* **:**   PARAURETHRAL GLAND

Skene, Alexander Johnston Chalmers (1838–1900), American gynecologist.

skia·gram \ˈskī-ə-₁gram\ *n* **:**   RADIOGRAPH

skia·graph \-₁graf\ *n* **:**   RADIOGRAPH

skilled nursing facility *n* **:** a health-care institution that meets federal criteria for Medicaid and Medicare reimbursement for nursing care including esp. the supervision of the care of every patient by a physician, the employment full-time of at least one registered nurse, the maintenance of records concerning the care and condition of every patient, the availability of nursing care 24 hours a day, the presence of facilities for storing and dispensing drugs, the implementation

of a utilization review plan, and overall financial planning including an annual operating budget and a three≠year capital expenditures program

skim milk *n* **:** milk from which the cream has been taken — called also *skimmed milk*

¹**skin** \ˈskin\ *n* **:** the 2-layered covering of the body consisting of an outer ectodermal epidermis that is more or less cornified and penetrated by the openings of sweat and sebaceous glands and an inner mesodermal dermis that is composed largely of connective tissue and is richly supplied with blood vessels and nerves

²**skin** *vb* **skinned; skin·ning :** to cut or scrape the skin of ⟨*skinned* his knee⟩

skin graft *n* **:** a piece of skin that is taken from a donor area to replace skin in a defective or denuded area (as one that has been burned)

skinned \ˈskind\ *adj* **:** having skin esp. of a specified kind — usu. used in combination ⟨dark-*skinned*⟩

Skin·ner box \ˈski-nər-₁bäks\ *n* **:** a laboratory apparatus in which an animal is caged for experiments in operant conditioning and which typically contains a lever that must be pressed by the animal to gain reward or avoid punishment

Skinner, Burrhus Frederic (*b* 1904), American psychologist.

Skin·ner·ian \ski-ˈnir-ē-ən, -ˈner-\ *adj* **:** of, relating to, or suggestive of the behavioristic theories of B. F. Skinner ⟨∼ behaviorism⟩

skin tag \-₁tag\ *n* **:** a small soft pendulous growth on the skin esp. around the eyes or on the neck, armpits, or groin — called also *acrochordon*

skin test *n* **:** a test (as a scratch test) performed on the skin and used in detecting allergic hypersensitivity

skull \ˈskəl\ *n* **:** the skeleton of the head forming a bony case that encloses and protects the brain and chief sense organs and supports the jaws

skull·cap \ˈskəl-₁kap\ *n* **:** the upper portion of the skull **:**   CALVARIUM

SLE *abbr* systemic lupus erythematosus

sleep \ˈslēp\ *n* **1 :** the natural periodic suspension of consciousness during which the powers of the body are restored **2 :** a state resembling sleep: as **a :** DEATH 1 ⟨put a pet cat to ∼⟩ **b :** a state marked by a diminution of feeling followed by tingling ⟨his foot went to ∼⟩ — **sleep** *vb* — **sleep·i·ness** \ˈslē-pē-nəs\ *n* — **sleepy** *adj*

sleep apnea *n* **:** intermittent apnea occurring as a sleep disorder

sleeping pill *n* **:** a drug and esp. a barbiturate that is taken as a tablet or capsule to induce sleep — called also *sleeping tablet*

sleeping sickness *n* **1 :** a serious disease that is prevalent in much of tropical Africa, is marked by fever, protracted lethargy, tremors, and loss of weight, is caused by either of two trypanosomes (*Trypanosoma brucei gambiense* and *T. b. rhodesiense*), and is transmitted by tsetse flies — called also *African sleeping sickness* **2** : any of various viral encephalitides or encephalomyelitides of which lethargy or somnolence is a prominent feature; *esp* : EQUINE ENCEPHALOMYELITIS

sleeping tablet *n* : SLEEPING PILL
sleep·less \'slē-pləs\ *adj* : not able to sleep : INSOMNIAC — **sleep·less·ness** *n*
sleep spindle *n* : a burst of synchronous alpha waves that occurs during light sleep
sleep·walk·er \'slēp-ˌwȯ-kər\ *n* : one who is subject to somnambulism : one who walks while sleeping — called also *somnambulist* — **sleep·walk** \-ˌwȯk\ *vb*
sleepy sickness *n, Brit* : ENCEPHALITIS LETHARGICA
slide \'slīd\ *n* : a flat piece of glass on which an object is mounted for microscopic examination
sliding filament hypothesis *n* : a theory in physiology holding that muscle contraction occurs when the actin filaments next to the Z line at each end of a sarcomere are drawn toward each other between the thicker myosin filaments more centrally located in the sarcomere by the projecting globular heads of myosin molecules that form temporary attachments to the actin filaments — called also *sliding filament theory;* see CROSSBRIDGE
slim disease \'slim-\ *n* : AIDS; *also* : severe wasting of the body in the later stages of AIDS
sling \'slin\ *n* : a hanging bandage suspended from the neck to support an arm or hand
slipped disk *n* : a protrusion of an intervertebral disk and its nucleus pulposus that produces pressure on spinal nerves resulting in low-back pain and often sciatic pain
slipped tendon *n* : PEROSIS
slit lamp \'slit-ˌlamp\ *n* : a lamp for projecting a narrow beam of intense light into an eye to facilitate microscopic study (as of the conjunctiva or cornea)
¹slough \'sləf\ *n* : dead tissue separating from living tissue; *esp* : a mass of dead tissue separating from an ulcer
²slough \'sləf\ *vb* : to separate in the form of dead tissue from living tissue ⟨dermal ∼ing⟩
slow infection *n* : a degenerative disease caused by a slow virus
slow–reacting substance of anaphylaxis *n* : a mixture of three leukotrienes produced in anaphylaxis that causes contraction of smooth muscle after minutes in contrast to histamine which acts in seconds and that is prob. responsible for the bronchoconstriction occurring in anaphylaxis —

abbr. *SRS-A;* called also *slow-reacting substance*
slow–twitch \'slō-ˌtwitch\ *adj* : of, relating to, or being muscle fiber that contracts slowly esp. during sustained physical activity requiring endurance — compare FAST-TWITCH
slow virus *n* : any of various viruses with a long incubation period between infection and development of the degenerative disease (as kuru or Creutzfeldt-Jakob disease) associated with it
slow wave *n* : DELTA WAVE
slow–wave sleep *n* : a state of deep dreamless sleep that occurs regularly during a normal period of sleep with intervening periods of REM sleep and that is characterized by delta waves and a low level of autonomic physiological activity — called also *NREM sleep, orthodox sleep, S sleep, synchronized sleep*
slug·gish \'slə-gish\ *adj* : markedly slow in movement, progression, or response ⟨∼ healing⟩ — **slug·gish·ly** *adv* — **slug·gish·ness** *n*
Sm *symbol* samarium
small bowel *n* : SMALL INTESTINE
small calorie *n* : CALORIE 1a
small–cell *adj* : OAT-CELL
small intestine *n* : the part of the intestine that lies between the stomach and colon, consists of duodenum, jejunum, and ileum, secretes digestive enzymes, and is the chief site of the absorption of digested nutrients — called also *small bowel*
small·pox \'smȯl-ˌpäks\ *n* : an acute contagious febrile disease caused by a poxvirus and characterized by skin eruption with pustules, sloughing, and scar formation
small saphenous vein *n* : SAPHENOUS VEIN b
smart \'smärt\ *vb* : to cause or be the cause or seat of a sharp poignant pain; *also* : to feel or have such a pain
smear \'smir\ *n* : material spread on a surface (as of a microscopic slide); *also* : a preparation made by spreading material on a surface ⟨a vaginal ∼⟩ — see PAP SMEAR — **smear** *vb*
smeg·ma \'smeg-mə\ *n* : the secretion of a sebaceous gland; *specif* : the cheesy sebaceous matter that collects between the glans penis and the foreskin or around the clitoris and labia minora
¹smell \'smel\ *vb* **smelled** \'smeld\ *or* **smelt** \'smelt\; **smell·ing** : to perceive the odor or scent of through stimuli affecting the olfactory nerves : get the odor or scent of with the nose
²smell *n* **1** : the property of a thing that affects the olfactory organs : ODOR **2** : the special sense concerned with the perception of odor
smell brain *n* : RHINENCEPHALON
smelling salts *n pl* : a usu. scented aromatic preparation of ammonium

carbonate and ammonia water used as a stimulant and restorative

Smith fracture \\'smith-\ *or* **Smith's fracture** \\'smiths-\ *n* : a fracture of the lower portion of the radius with forward displacement of the lower fragment — compare COLLES' FRACTURE

    Smith, Robert William (1807–1873), British surgeon.

Smith–Pe·ter·sen nail \\'smith-'pē-tər-sən-\ *n* : a metal nail used to fix the femoral head in fractures of the neck of the femur

    Smith–Petersen, Marius Nygaard (1886–1953), American orthopedic surgeon.

smog \\'smäg, 'smog\ *n* : a fog made heavier and darker by smoke and chemical fumes; *also* : a photochemical haze caused by the action of solar ultraviolet radiation on atmosphere polluted with hydrocarbons and oxides of nitrogen from automobile exhaust

smoke \\'smōk\ *vb* **smoked; smok·ing** : to inhale and exhale the fumes of burning plant material and esp. tobacco; *esp* : to smoke tobacco habitually

smok·er \\'smō-kər\ *n* : a person who smokes habitually

smooth \\'smüth\ *adj* : forming or being a colony with a flat shiny surface usu. made up of organisms that form no chains or filaments, show characteristic internal changes, and tend toward marked increase in capsule formation and virulence — used of dissociated strains of bacteria; compare ROUGH

smooth muscle *n* : muscle tissue that lacks cross striations, that is made up of elongated spindle-shaped cells having a central nucleus, and that is found in vertebrate visceral structures (as the stomach and bladder) as thin sheets performing functions not subject to conscious control by the mind and in all or most of the musculature of invertebrates other than arthropods — called also *nonstriated muscle, unstriated muscle*; compare CARDIAC MUSCLE, STRIATED MUSCLE

Sn *symbol* tin

snail \\'snāl\ *n* : any of various gastropod mollusks and esp. those having an external enclosing spiral shell including some which are important in medicine as intermediate hosts of trematodes

snail fever *n* : SCHISTOSOMIASIS

snake \\'snāk\ *n* : any of numerous limbless scaled reptiles (suborder Serpentes syn. Ophidia) with a long tapering body and with salivary glands often modified to produce venom which is injected through grooved or tubular fangs

snake·bite \-·bīt\ *n* : the bite of a snake; *also* : the condition of having been

bitten by a venomous snake characterized by stinging pain in the puncture wound, constitutional symptoms, and injury to blood or nerve tissue

snare \\'snar\ *n* : a surgical instrument consisting usu. of a wire loop constricted by a mechanism in the handle and used for removing tissue masses (as tonsils or polyps)

sneeze \\'snēz\ *vb* **sneezed; sneez·ing** : to make a sudden violent spasmodic audible expiration of breath through the nose and mouth esp. as a reflex act following irritation of the nasal mucous membrane — **sneeze** *n*

Snel·len chart \\'sne-lən-\ *n* : the chart used in the Snellen test with black letters of various sizes against a white background

    Snellen, Hermann (1834–1908), Dutch ophthalmologist.

Snellen test *n* : a test for visual acuity presenting letters of graduated sizes to determine the smallest size that can be read at a standard distance

SNF *abbr* skilled nursing facility

snif·fles \\'sni-fəlz\ *n pl* **1** : a head cold marked by nasal discharge ⟨a case of the ∼⟩ **2** : BULLNOSE — usu. used with a sing. verb

snore \\'snor\ *vb* **snored; snor·ing** : to breathe during sleep with a rough hoarse noise due to vibration of the soft palate — **snore** *n* — **snor·er** *n*

snort \\'snort\ *vb* : to inhale (a narcotic drug in powdered form) through the nostrils ⟨∼ cocaine⟩

snow \\'snō\ *n, slang* **1** : COCAINE **2** : HEROIN

snow blindness *n* : inflammation and photophobia caused by exposure of the eyes to ultraviolet rays reflected from snow or ice — **snow–blind** \-·blīnd\ *or* **snow–blind·ed** \-·blin-dəd\ *adj*

snuff \\'snəf\ *n* : a preparation of pulverized tobacco to be inhaled through the nostrils, chewed, or placed against the gums; *also* : a preparation of a powdered drug to be inhaled through the nostrils

snuf·fles \\'snə-fəlz\ *n pl* **1** : SNIFFLES 1 **2** : a respiratory disorder (as bullnose) in animals marked esp. by catarrhal inflammation and sniffling — usu. used with a sing. verb

soak \\'sōk\ *n* : an often hot medicated solution with which a body part is soaked usu. long or repeatedly esp. to promote healing, relieve pain, or stimulate local circulation

soap \\'sōp\ *n* **1** : a cleansing and emulsifying agent made usu. by action of alkali on fat or fatty acids and consisting essentially of sodium or potassium salts of such acids **2** : a salt of a fatty acid and a metal

SOB *abbr* short of breath

so·cial \\'sō-shəl\ *adj* **1** : tending to form cooperative and interdependent relationships with others of one's kind 2 : of or relating to human society, the interaction of the individual and the group, or the welfare of human beings as members of society ⟨immature ∼ behavior⟩ — **so·cial·ly** adv

social disease n 1 : VENEREAL DISEASE 2 : a disease (as tuberculosis) whose incidence is directly related to social and economic factors

so·cial·i·za·tion \ˌsō-shə-lə-ˈzā-shən\ n : the process by which a human being beginning at infancy acquires the habits, beliefs, and accumulated knowledge of society through education and training for adult status — **so·cial·ize** \ˈsō-shə-ˌlīz\ vb

socialized medicine n : medical and hospital services for the members of a class or population administered by an organized group (as a state agency) and paid for from funds obtained usu. by assessments, philanthropy, or taxation

social psychiatry n 1 : a branch of psychiatry that deals in collaboration with related specialties (as sociology and anthropology) with the influence of social and cultural factors on the causation, course, and outcome of mental illness 2 : the application of psychodynamic principles to the solution of social problems

social psychology n : the study of the manner in which the personality, attitudes, motivations, and behavior of the individual influence and are influenced by social groups — **social psychologist** n

social recovery n : an improvement in a psychiatric patient's clinical status that is not a total recovery but is sufficient to permit the patient's return to his or her former social milieu

social work n : any of various professional services, activities, or methods concretely concerned with the investigation, treatment, and material aid of the economically underprivileged and socially maladjusted — **social worker** n

socio- comb form 1 : society : social ⟨sociopath⟩ 2 : social and ⟨sociopsychological⟩

so·cio·cul·tur·al \ˌsō-sē-ō-ˈkəl-chə-rəl, ˌsō-shē-\ adj : of, relating to, or involving a combination of social and cultural factors — **so·cio·cul·tur·al·ly** adv

so·ci·ol·o·gy \ˌsō-sē-ˈä-lə-jē, ˌsō-shē-\ n, pl -gies : the science of society, social institutions, and social relationships; specif : the systematic study of the development, structure, interaction, and collective behavior of organized groups of human beings — **so·cio·log·i·cal** \ˌsō-sē-ə-ˈlä-ji-kəl, ˌsō-shē-ə-\ also **so·cio·log·ic** \-jik\ adj — **so·cio·log·i·cal·ly** adv — **so·ci·ol·o·gist** \ˌsō-sē-ˈä-lə-jist, -shē-\ n

so·cio·med·i·cal \ˌsō-sē-ō-ˈmed-i-kəl,

ˌsō-shē-\ adj : of or relating to the interrelations of medicine and social welfare

so·cio·path \ˈsō-sē-ə-ˌpath, ˈsō-shē-ə-\ n : a sociopathic person : PSYCHOPATH

so·cio·path·ic \ˌsō-sē-ə-ˈpa-thik, ˌsō-shē-ə-\ adj : of, relating to, or characterized by antisocial behavior or a psychopathic personality — **so·ci·op·a·thy** \ˌsō-sē-ˈä-pə-thē, ˌsō-shē-\ n

so·cio·psy·cho·log·i·cal \ˌsō-sē-ō-ˌsī-kə-ˈlä-ji-kəl, ˌsō-shē-\ adj 1 : of, relating to, or involving a combination of social and psychological factors 2 : of or relating to social psychology

so·cio·sex·u·al \-ˈsek-shə-wəl\ adj : of or relating to the interpersonal aspects of sexuality

sock·et \ˈsä-kət\ n : an opening or hollow that forms a holder for something: as **a** : any of various hollows in body structures in which some other part normally lodges ⟨the bony ∼ of the eye⟩ ⟨an inflamed tooth ∼⟩; esp : the depression in a bone with which the rounded head of another bone fits in a ball-and-socket joint **b** : a cavity terminating an artificial limb into which the bodily stump fits

so·da \ˈsō-də\ n 1 : any of several compounds containing sodium; esp : SODIUM BICARBONATE 2 : SODIUM ⟨∼ alum⟩

soda lime n : a granular mixture of calcium hydroxide with sodium hydroxide or potassium hydroxide or both that is used to absorb moisture and acid gases and esp. carbon dioxide (as in gas masks and in oxygen therapy)

sod disease \ˈsäd-\ n : VESICULAR DERMATITIS

so·di·um \ˈsō-dē-əm\ n : a silver white soft waxy ductile element — symbol Na; see ELEMENT table

sodium ascorbate n : the sodium salt $C_6H_7NaO_6$ of vitamin C

sodium benzoate n : a crystalline or granular salt $C_7H_5O_2Na$ used chiefly as a food preservative

sodium bicarbonate n : a white crystalline weakly alkaline salt $NaHCO_3$ used in medicine esp. as an antacid — called also baking soda, bicarb, bicarbonate of soda

sodium bromide n : a crystalline salt NaBr having a biting saline taste that is used in medicine as a sedative, hypnotic, and anticonvulsant

sodium caprylate n : the sodium salt $C_8H_{15}O_2Na$ of caprylic acid used esp. in the topical treatment of fungal infections

sodium carbonate n : any of several salts (as Na_2CO_3) of carbonic acid

sodium chloride n : SALT 1a

sodium citrate n : a crystalline salt $C_6H_5Na_3O_7$ used chiefly as an expectorant, a systemic and urinary alkalizer, a chelating agent to increase urinary excretion of calcium in hypercalcemia and lead in lead poisoning, and in combination as an anticoagulant (as in stored blood)

sodium cro·mo·gly·cate \-ˌkrō-mō-ˈglī-ˌkāt\ n : CROMOLYN SODIUM

sodium di·hy·dro·gen phosphate \-ˌdī-ˈhī-drə-jən-\ n : SODIUM PHOSPHATE 1

sodium fluoride n : a poisonous crystalline salt NaF that is used in trace amounts in the fluoridation of water, as an antiseptic, and as a pesticide — see LURIDE

sodium glutamate n : MONOSODIUM GLUTAMATE

sodium hydroxide n : a white brittle solid NaOH that dissolves readily in water to form a strongly alkaline and caustic solution and that is used in pharmacy as an alkalizing agent

sodium hypochlorite n : an unstable salt NaOCl produced usu. in aqueous solution and used as a bleaching and disinfecting agent

sodium iodide n : a crystalline salt NaI used as an iodine supplement and expectorant

sodium io·do·hip·pu·rate \-ī-ˌō-dō-ˈhip-yə-ˌrāt\ n : HIPPURAN

sodium lactate n : a hygroscopic syrupy salt C₃H₅NaO₃ used chiefly as an antacid in medicine and as a substitute for glycerol

sodium lau·ryl sulfate \-ˈlȯ-ril-\ n : a crystalline sodium salt C₁₂H₂₅-NaO₄S; also : a mixture of sulfates of sodium consisting principally of this salt and used as a detergent, wetting, and emulsifying agent (as in toothpastes, ointments, and shampoos)

sodium mor·rhu·ate \-ˈmȯr-ü-ˌāt\ n : a pale yellow granular salt administered in solution intravenously as a sclerosing agent esp. in the treatment of varicose veins

sodium nitrate n : a crystalline salt NaNO₃ used in curing meat — called also saltpeter

sodium nitrite n : a colorless or yellowish salt NaNO₂ that is used as a meat preservative and in medicine as a vasodilator and an antidote for cyanide poisoning

sodium ni·tro·prus·side \-ˌnī-trō-ˈprə-ˌsīd\ n : a red crystalline salt C₅Fe-N₆Na₂O administered intravenously as a vasodilator esp. in hypertensive emergencies — see NIPRIDE

sodium pentobarbital n : the sodium salt of pentobarbital

sodium pentobarbitone n, Brit : SODIUM PENTOBARBITAL

sodium per·bor·ate \-pər-ˈbȯr-ˌāt\ n : a white crystalline powder NaBO₃·-4H₂O used as an oral antiseptic

sodium phosphate n 1 : a phosphate NaH₂PO₄ of sodium containing one sodium atom per molecule that with the phosphate containing two sodium atoms per molecule constitutes the principal buffer system of the urine —

called also sodium dihydrogen phosphate 2 : a phosphate Na₂HPO₄ of sodium containing two sodium atoms per molecule that is used in medicine as a laxative and antacid

sodium potassium tartrate n : ROCHELLE SALT

sodium pump n : a molecular mechanism by which sodium ions are actively transported across a cell membrane; esp : the one by which the appropriate internal and external concentrations of sodium and potassium ions are maintained in a nerve fiber and which involves the active transport of sodium ions outward with movement of potassium ions to the interior

sodium salicylate n : a crystalline salt NaC₇H₅O₃ that has a sweetish saline taste and is used chiefly as an analgesic, antipyretic, and antirheumatic

sodium secobarbital n : the sodium salt C₁₂H₁₇N₂NaO₃ of secobarbital

sodium stearate n : a white powdery water-soluble salt C₁₈H₃₅NaO₂ used esp. in glycerin suppositories, cosmetics, and some toothpastes

sodium sulfate n : a bitter salt Na₂SO₄ used in its hydrated form as a cathartic — see GLAUBER'S SALT

sodium thiosulfate n : a hygroscopic crystalline salt Na₂O₃S₂ used in medicine as an antidote in poisoning by cyanides or iodine, in the treatment of tinea versicolor, and to prevent ringworm (as in a footbath)

sodium valproate n : the sodium salt C₈H₁₅NaO₂ of valproic acid used as an anticonvulsant

so·do·ku \ˈsō-dō-ˌkü\ n : RAT-BITE FEVER b

sod·om·ist \ˈsä-də-mist\ n : SODOMITE

sod·om·ite \-ˌmīt\ n : one who practices sodomy

sod·omy \ˈsä-də-mē\ n, pl **-om·ies** 1 : copulation with a member of the same sex or with an animal 2 : noncoital and esp. anal or oral copulation with a member of the opposite sex — **sod·om·it·ic** \ˌsä-də-ˈmi-tik\ or **sod·omit·i·cal** \-ti-kəl\ adj — **sod·om·ize** \ˈsä-də-ˌmīz\ vb

soft \ˈsȯft\ adj 1 : yielding to physical pressure 2 : deficient in or free from substances (as calcium and magnesium salts) that prevent lathering of soap ⟨~ water⟩ 3 : having relatively low energy ⟨~ X rays⟩ 4 : BIODEGRADABLE 5 of a drug : considered less detrimental than a hard narcotic ⟨marijuana is usually regarded as a ~ drug⟩ 6 : being or based on interpretive or speculative data ⟨~ evidence⟩

soft chancre n : CHANCROID

soft contact lens n : a contact lens made of soft water-absorbing plastic that adheres closely and with minimal discomfort to the eye

soft lens n : SOFT CONTACT LENS

soft palate n : the membranous and

muscular fold suspended from the posterior margin of the hard palate and partially separating the mouth cavity from the pharynx

soft spot *n* : a fontanel of a fetal or young skull

sol \'säl, 'sôl\ *n* : a fluid colloidal system; *esp* : one in which the dispersion medium is a liquid

so·la·nine *or* **so·la·nin** \'sō-lə-ˌnēn, -nən\ *n* : a bitter poisonous crystalline alkaloid $C_{45}H_{72}NO_{15}$ from several plants (as some potatoes or tomatoes) of the nightshade family (Solanaceae)

so·la·num \sō-'lā-nəm, -'lä-, -'la-\ *n* **1** *cap* : a genus of chiefly herbs and shrubs of the nightshade family (Solanaceae) that have often prickly-veined leaves, white, purple, or yellow flowers, and a fruit that is a berry **2** : any plant of the genus *Solanum*

so·lar·i·um \sō-'lar-ē-əm, sə-\ *n, pl* **-ia** \-ē-ə\ *also* **-ums** : a room (as in a hospital) used esp. for sunbathing or therapeutic exposure to light

so·lar plex·us \'sō-lər-'plek-səs\ *n* **1** : CELIAC PLEXUS **2** : the part of the abdomen including the stomach and celiac plexus that is particularly vulnerable to the effects of a blow to the body wall in front of it — not used technically

soldier's heart *n* : NEUROCIRCULATORY ASTHENIA

sole \'sōl\ *n* : the undersurface of a foot

So·le·nop·sis \ˌsō-lə-'näp-səs\ *n* : a genus of small stinging ants including several tropical and subtropical forms (as the imported fire ants)

so·le·us \'sō-lē-əs\ *n, pl* **solei** \-lē-ˌī\ *also* **soleuses** : a broad flat muscle of the calf of the leg that lies deep to the gastrocnemius, arises from the back and upper part of the tibia and fibula and from a tendinous arch between them, inserts by a tendon that unites with that of the gastrocnemius to form the Achilles tendon, and acts to flex the foot

¹sol·id \'sä-ləd\ *adj* **1** : not hollow : being without an internal cavity ⟨∼ tumors⟩ **2** : neither gaseous nor liquid

²solid *n* **1** : a substance that does not flow perceptibly under moderate stress **2** : the part of a solution or suspension that when freed from solvent or suspending medium has the qualities of a solid — usu. used in pl. ⟨milk ∼s⟩

solitarius — see TRACTUS SOLITARIUS

sol·i·tary \'sä-lə-ˌter-ē\ *adj* : occurring singly and not as part of a group ⟨a ∼ lesion⟩

sol·u·bil·i·ty \ˌsäl-yə-'bi-lə-tē\ *n, pl* **-ties** **1** : the quality or state of being soluble **2** : the amount of a substance that will dissolve in a given amount of another substance

sol·u·ble \'säl-yə-bəl\ *adj* **1** : susceptible of being dissolved in or as if in a fluid **2** : capable of being emulsified

soluble RNA *n* : TRANSFER RNA

sol·ute \'säl-ˌyüt\ *n* : a dissolved substance; *esp* : a component of a solution present in smaller amount than the solvent

so·lu·tion \sə-'lü-shən\ *n* **1 a** : an act or the process by which a solid, liquid, or gaseous substance is homogeneously mixed with a liquid or sometimes a gas or solid **b** : a homogeneous mixture formed by this process **2 a** : a liquid containing a dissolved substance ⟨an aqueous ∼⟩ **b** : a liquid and usu. aqueous medicinal preparation with the solid ingredients soluble **c** : the condition of being dissolved ⟨a substance in ∼⟩

¹sol·vent \'säl-vənt, 'sôl-\ *adj* : that dissolves or can dissolve ⟨∼ fluids⟩ ⟨∼ action of water⟩

²solvent *n* : a substance capable of or used in dissolving or dispersing one or more other substances; *esp* : a liquid component of a solution present in greater amount than the solute

so·ma \'sō-mə\ *n, pl* **so·ma·ta** \'sō-mə-tə\ *or* **somas 1** : the body of an organism **2** : all of an organism except the germ cells **3** : CELL BODY

som·aes·thet·ic *chiefly Brit var of* SOMESTHETIC

somat- *or* **somato-** *comb form* **1** : body ⟨*somato*sensory⟩ **2** : somatic and ⟨*somato*psychic⟩

so·mat·ic \sō-'ma-tik, sə-\ *adj* **1 a** : of, relating to, or affecting the body esp. as distinguished from the germ plasm or psyche : PHYSICAL **b** : of, relating to, supplying, or involving skeletal muscles ⟨∼ nervous system⟩ **2** : of or relating to the wall of the body as distinguished from the viscera : PARIETAL — **so·mat·i·cal·ly** *adv*

somatic cell *n* : any of the cells of the body that compose the tissues, organs, and parts of that individual other than the germ cells

somatic mutation *n* : a mutation occurring in a somatic cell

so·ma·ti·za·tion disorder \ˌsō-mə-tə-'zā-shən-\ *n* : a somatoform disorder characterized by multiple and recurring physical complaints for which the patient has sought medical treatment over several years without any organic or physiological basis for the symptoms being found

so·ma·to·form \'sō-mə-tə-ˌfôrm, sə-'ma-tə-\ *adj* : relating to or being any of a group of psychological disorders or symptoms involving physical complaints for which no organic or physiological explanation is found and for which there is a strong likelihood that psychological factors are involved ⟨∼ pain disorder⟩

so·ma·to·me·din \sō-ˌma-tə-'mēd-ᵊn, ˌsō-mə-tə-\ *n* : any of several endogenous peptides produced esp. in the liver that are dependent on and prob. mediate growth hormone activity (as in sulfate uptake by epiphyseal cartilage)

so·ma·to·plasm \sō-'ma-tə-ˌpla-zəm, 'sō-mət-ə-ˌ\ n 1 : protoplasm of somatic cells as distinguished from that of germ cells 2 : somatic cells as distinguished from germ cells

so·ma·to·pleure \sō-'ma-tə-ˌplúr, 'sō-mə-tə-\ n : a complex fold of tissue in the embryo consisting of an outer layer of mesoderm together with the ectoderm that sheathes it and giving rise to the amnion and chorion — compare SPLANCHNOPLEURE

so·ma·to·psy·chic \ˌsō-ˌma-tə-'sī-kik, ˌsō-mə-tə-\ adj : of or relating to the body and the mind

so·ma·to·sen·so·ry \ˌsō-ˌma-tə-'sens-ə-rē, ˌsō-mə-tə-\ adj : of, relating to, or being sensory activity having its origin elsewhere than in the special sense organs (as eyes and ears) and conveying information about the state of the body proper and its immediate environment (~ pathways)

so·ma·to·stat·in \ˌsō-mə-tə-'stat-ᵊn\ n : a polypeptide neurohormone that is found esp. in the hypothalamus, is composed of a chain of 14 amino-acid residues, and inhibits the secretion of several other hormones (as growth hormone, insulin, and gastrin)

so·ma·to·ther·a·py \ˌsō-mə-tə-'ther-ə-pē, sō-ˌma-tə-\ n, pl -pies : therapy for psychological problems that uses physiological intervention (as by drugs or surgery) to modify behavior — **so·ma·to·ther·a·peu·tic** \-ˌther-ə-'pyü-tik\ adj

so·ma·to·top·ic \-'tä-pik\ adj : of, relating to, or mediating the orderly and specific relation between particular body regions (as a hand or the tongue) and corresponding motor areas of the brain — **so·ma·to·top·i·cal·ly** adv

so·ma·to·tro·phic \-'trō-fik\, **so·ma·to·tro·phin** \-'trō-fən\ var of SOMATOTROPIC, SOMATOTROPIN

so·ma·to·trop·ic \-'trō-pik, -'trä-\ adj : promoting growth (~ activity)

somatotropic hormone n : GROWTH HORMONE

so·ma·to·tro·pin \-'trō-pən\ n : GROWTH HORMONE

so·ma·to·type \'sō-mə-tə-ˌtīp, sō-'ma-tə-\ n : a body type or physique esp. in a system of classification based on the relative development of ectomorphic, endomorphic, and mesomorphic components — **somatotype** vb

-some \ˌsōm\ n comb form 1 : body ⟨chromosome⟩ 2 : chromosome ⟨monosome⟩

som·es·thet·ic \ˌsō-mes-'the-tik\ adj : of, relating to, or concerned with bodily sensations (a ~ area of the brain)

-so·mia \'sō-mē-ə\ n comb form : condition of having (such) a body ⟨microsomia⟩

-som·ic \ˌsō-mik\ adj comb form : having or being a chromosome complement of which one or more but not all chromosomes or genomes exhibit (such) a degree of reduplication ⟨monosomic⟩

so·mite \'sō-ˌmīt\ n : one of the longitudinal series of segments into which the body of many animals is divided : METAMERE

somnambul- comb form : somnambulism : somnambulist ⟨somnambulant⟩

som·nam·bu·lant \säm-'nam-byə-lənt\ adj : walking or dreaming while asleep

som·nam·bu·late \-ˌlāt\ vb -lat·ed; -lat·ing : to walk while asleep — **som·nam·bu·la·tion** \-ˌnam-byə-'lā-shən\ n

som·nam·bu·lism \säm-'nam-byə-ˌli-zəm\ n 1 : an abnormal condition of sleep in which motor acts (as walking) are performed while asleep 2 : actions characteristic of somnambulism — **som·nam·bu·lis·tic** \-ˌnam-byə-'lis-tik\ adj

som·nam·bu·list \säm-'nam-byə-list\ n : SLEEPWALKER

somni- comb form : sleep ⟨somnifacient⟩

¹som·ni·fa·cient \ˌsäm-nə-'fā-shənt\ adj : inducing sleep : HYPNOTIC (a ~ drug)

²somnifacient n : a somnifacient agent (as a drug) : HYPNOTIC 1

som·nif·er·ous \säm-'ni-fə-rəs\ adj : SOPORIFIC

som·no·lence \'säm-nə-ləns\ n : the quality or state of being drowsy — **som·no·lent** \-lənt\ adj

son- or **sono-** comb form : sound ⟨sonogram⟩

sono·gram \'sä-nə-ˌgram\ n : an image produced by ultrasound

so·nog·ra·pher \sō-'nä-grə-fər\ n : a person trained in the use of ultrasound

so·nog·ra·phy \sō-'nä-grə-fē\ n, pl -phies : ULTRASOUND 2 — **sono·graph·ic** \ˌsä-nə-'gra-fik\ adj

so·po·rif·er·ous \ˌsä-pə-'ri-fə-rəs, ˌsō-\ adj : SOPORIFIC

¹so·po·rif·ic \-'ri-fik\ adj : causing or tending to cause sleep

²soporific n : a soporific agent (as a drug)

sorb \'sórb\ vb : to take up and hold by either adsorption or absorption

sor·bic acid \'sór-bik-\ n : a crystalline acid $C_6H_8O_2$ obtained from the unripe fruits of the mountain ash (genus *Sorbus*) or synthesized and used esp. as a fungicide and food preservative

sor·bi·tol \'sór-bə-ˌtól, -ˌtōl\ n : a faintly sweet alcohol $C_6H_{14}O_6$ that occurs esp. in fruits of the mountain ash (genus *Sorbus*), is made synthetically, and is used esp. as a humectant, a softener, and a sweetener and in making ascorbic acid

sor·des \'sór-(ˌ)dēz\ n, pl **sordes** : the crusts that collect on the teeth and lips in debilitating diseases with protracted low fever

¹**sore** \'sōr\ *adj* **sor•er; sor•est** : causing, characterized by, or affected with pain : PAINFUL ⟨∼ muscles⟩ ⟨a ∼ wound⟩ — **sore•ly** *adv* — **sore•ness** *n*

²**sore** *n* : a localized sore spot on the body; *esp* : one (as an ulcer) with the tissues ruptured or abraded and usu. with infection

sore mouth *n* **1** : a highly contagious disease of sheep and goats that is caused by a poxvirus, occurs esp. in young animals, and is characterized by extensive vesiculation and subsequent ulceration about the lips, gums, and tongue — called also *scabby mouth* **2** : necrobacillosis affecting the mouth; *esp* : CALF DIPHTHERIA

sore•muz•zle \-₁məz-³l\ *n* : BLUETONGUE

sore throat *n* : painful throat due to inflammation of the fauces and pharynx

SOS *abbr* [Latin *si opus sit*] if occasion require; if necessary — used in writing prescriptions

so•ta•lol \'sō-tə-₁lȯl, -₁lōl\ *n* : a beta-adrenergic blocking agent $C_{12}H_{20}$-N_2O_3S administered in the form of its hydrochloride to treat ventricular arrhythmias

souf•fle \'sü-fəl\ *n* : a blowing sound heard on auscultation ⟨the uterine ∼ heard in pregnancy⟩

¹**sound** \'saund\ *adj* **1** : free from injury or disease : exhibiting normal health **2** : deep and undisturbed ⟨a ∼ sleep⟩ — **sound•ness** *n*

²**sound** *n* **1** : a particular auditory impression ⟨heart ∼s heard by auscultation⟩ **2** : the sensation perceived by the sense of hearing **3** : mechanical radiant energy that is transmitted by waves of pressure in a material medium (as air) and is the objective cause of hearing

³**sound** *vb* : to explore or examine (a body cavity) with a sound

⁴**sound** *n* : an elongated instrument for exploring or examining body cavities ⟨a uterine ∼⟩

sound pollution *n* : NOISE POLLUTION

sound wave *n* **1** : SOUND 1 **2** *pl* : waves of pressure esp. when transmitting audible sound

sour \'saur\ *adj* : causing, characterized by, or being the one of the four basic taste sensations that is produced chiefly by acids — compare BITTER, SALT, SWEET — **sour•ness** *n*

South American blastomycosis *n* : blastomycosis caused by a fungus of the genus *Paracoccidioides* (*P. brasiliensis* syn. *Blastomyces brasiliensis*) and characterized by formation of ulcers on the mucosal surfaces of the mouth that spread to lips, nose, and cheeks, by great enlargement of lymph nodes esp. of the throat and chest, and by involvement of the gastrointestinal tract — called also *paracoccidioidomycosis*

South•ern blot \'sə-t̲h̲ərn-\ *n* : a blot

consisting of a sheet of a cellulose derivative that contains spots of DNA for identification by a suitable molecular probe — compare NORTHERN BLOT, WESTERN BLOT — **Southern blotting** *n*

Southern, Edwin M. (*fl* 20th century), British biologist.

spa \'spä, 'spȯ\ *n* **1 a** : a mineral spring **b** : a resort with mineral springs **2** : a commercial establishment with facilities for exercising and bathing; *esp* : HEALTH SPA

space maintainer *n* : a temporary orthodontic appliance used following the loss or extraction of a tooth (as a milk tooth) to prevent the shifting of adjacent teeth into the resulting space — called also *space retainer*

space medicine *n* : a branch of medicine concerned with the physiological and biological effects on the human body of spaceflight

space perception *n* : the perception of the properties and relationships of objects in space esp. with respect to direction, size, distance, and orientation

spac•er \'spā-sər\ *n* : a region of chromosomal DNA between genes that is not transcribed into messenger RNA and is of uncertain function

space retainer *n* : SPACE MAINTAINER

space sickness *n* : sickness and esp. nausea and dizziness that occurs under the conditions of sustained spaceflight — **space•sick** \'spās-₁sik\ *adj*

Spanish fly *n* **1** : a green beetle (*Lytta vesicatoria* of the family Meloidae) of southern Europe that is the source of cantharides **2** : CANTHARIS 2

Spanish influenza *n* : pandemic influenza; *specif* : an outbreak of pandemic influenza which occurred in 1918

spar•ga•no•sis \₁spär-gə-¹nō-səs\ *n*, *pl* **-no•ses** \-₁sēz\ : the condition of being infected with sparganla

spar•ga•num \'spär-gə-nəm\ *n*, *pl* **-na** \-nə\ *also* **-nums** : an intramuscular or subcutaneous vermiform parasite that is the larva of the fish tapeworm (*Diphyllobothrium latum*) or of a related tapeworm

Spar•ine \'spär-₁ēn\ *trademark* — used for a preparation of promazine

spar•te•ine \'spär-tē-ən, 'spär-₁tēn\ *n* : a liquid alkaloid $C_{15}H_{26}N_2$ used in medicine in the form of its sulfate esp. as an oxytocic drug

spasm \'spa-zəm\ *n* **1** : an involuntary and abnormal contraction of muscle or muscle fibers or of a hollow organ (as the esophagus) that consists largely of involuntary muscle fibers **2** : the state or condition of a muscle or organ affected with spasms — **spas•mod•ic** \spaz-¹mä-dik\ *adj* — **spas•mod•i•cal•ly** *adv*

spasmodic dysmenorrhea *n* : dysmenorrhea associated with painful contractions of the uterus

spas·mo·gen·ic \,spaz-mə-'je-nik\ *adj* : inducing spasm ⟨a ~ drug⟩

¹spas·mo·lyt·ic \,spaz-mə-'li-tik\ *adj* : tending or having the power to relieve spasms or convulsions ⟨~ drugs⟩

²spasmolytic *n* : a spasmolytic agent

spas·mo·phil·ia \,spaz-mə-'fi-lē-ə\ *n* : an abnormal tendency to convulsions, tetany, or spasms from even slight mechanical or electrical stimulation ⟨~ associated with rickets⟩

¹spas·tic \'spas-tik\ *adj* : of, relating to, or affected with spasm ⟨a ~ colon⟩ ⟨a ~ patient⟩ — **spas·ti·cal·ly** *adv*

²spastic *n* : an individual affected with spastic paralysis

spastic colon *n* : IRRITABLE BOWEL SYNDROME

spas·tic·i·ty \spa-'sti-sə-tē\ *n, pl* **-ties** : a spastic state or condition; *esp* : muscular hypertonicity with increased tendon reflexes

spastic paralysis *n* : paralysis with tonic spasm of the affected muscles and with increased tendon reflexes

spat *past and past part of* SPIT

spatial summation *n* : sensory summation that involves stimulation of several spatially separated neurons at the same time

spat·u·la \'spa-chə-lə\ *n* : a flat thin instrument used for spreading or mixing soft substances, scooping, lifting, or scraping

spav·in \'spa-vən\ *n* : a bony enlargement of the hock of a horse associated with strain — **spav·ined** \-vənd\ *adj*

spay \'spā\ *vb* **spayed; spay·ing** : to remove the ovaries of (a female animal)

SPCA *abbr* Society for the Prevention of Cruelty to Animals

spe·cial·ist \'spe-shə-list\ *n* : a medical practitioner whose practice is limited to a particular class of patients (as children) or of diseases (as skin diseases) or of technique (as surgery); *esp* : a physician who is qualified by advanced training and certification by a specialty examining board to so limit his or her practice

special sense *n* : any of the senses of sight, hearing, equilibrium, smell, taste, or touch

spe·cial·ty \'spe-shəl-tē\ *n, pl* **-ties** : something (as a branch of medicine) in which one specializes

spe·cies \'spē-(,)shēz, -(,)sēz\ *n, pl* **species** **1 a** : a category of biological classification ranking immediately below the genus or subgenus, comprising related organisms or populations potentially capable of interbreeding, and being designated by a binomial that consists of the name of the genus followed by an uncapitalized noun or adjective that is Latin or has a Latin form and agrees grammatically with the genus name **b** : an individual or kind belonging to a biological species **2** : a particular kind of atomic nucleus, atom, molecule, or ion ⟨a ~ of RNA⟩

¹spe·cif·ic \spi-'si-fik\ *adj* **1 a** : restricted by nature to a particular individual, situation, relation, or effect **b** : exerting a distinctive influence (as on a body part or a disease) ⟨~ antibodies⟩ **2** : of, relating to, or constituting a species and esp. a biological species

²specific *n* : a drug or remedy having a specific mitigating effect on a disease

specific epithet *n* : a noun or adjective that is Latin or has a Latin form and follows the genus name in a taxonomic binomial

specific gravity *n* : the ratio of the density of a substance to the density of some substance (as pure water or hydrogen) taken as a standard when both densities are obtained by weighing in air

spec·i·fic·i·ty \,spe-sə-'fi-sə-tē\ *n, pl* **-ties** : the quality or condition of being specific: as **a** : the condition of being peculiar to a particular individual or group of organisms ⟨host ~ of a parasite⟩ **b** : the condition of participating in or catalyzing only one or a few chemical reactions ⟨enzyme ~⟩

spec·i·men \'spe-sə-mən\ *n* **1** : an individual, item, or part typical of a group, class, or whole **2** : a portion or quantity of material for use in testing, examination, or study ⟨a urine ~⟩

SPECT *abbr* single photon emission computed tomography

spec·ta·cles \'spek-ti-kəlz\ *n pl* : GLASSES

spec·ti·no·my·cin \,spek-tə-nō-'mīs-³n\ *n* : a white crystalline broad-spectrum antibiotic $C_{14}H_{24}N_2O_7$ extracted from a bacterium of the genus *Streptomyces* (*S. spectabilis*) and used clinically esp. in the form of its hydrochloride to treat gonorrhea — called also *actinospectacin*; see TROBICIN

spec·tral \'spek-trəl\ *adj* : of, relating to, or made by a spectrum

spec·trin \'spek-trən\ *n* : a large cytoskeletal protein that is found on the inner cell membrane of red blood cells and that functions esp. in maintaining cell shape

spec·trom·e·ter \spek-'trä-mə-tər\ *n* **1** : an instrument used in determining the index of refraction of a transparent solid in the form of a prism **2** : a spectroscope fitted for measurements of the spectra observed with it — **spec·tro·met·ric** \,spek-trə-'me-trik\ *adj* — **spec·trom·e·try** \spek-'trä-mə-trē\ *n*

spec·tro·pho·tom·e·ter \,spek-trō-fə-'tä-mə-tər\ *n* : a photometer for measuring the relative intensities of the light in different parts of a spectrum — **spec·tro·pho·to·met·ric** \-trə-,fō-tə-'me-trik\ *adj* — **spec·tro·pho·to·met·ri·cal·ly** *adv* — **spec·tro·pho·tom·e·try** \,spek-(,)trō-fə-'tä-mə-trē\ *n*

spec·tro·scope \\'spek-trə-₁skōp\ *n* : an instrument for forming and examining optical spectra — **spec·tro·scop·ic** \₁spek-trə-'skä-pik\ *adj* — **spec·tro·scop·i·cal·ly** *adv* — **spec·tros·co·pist** \spek-'träs-kə-pist\ *n* — **spec·tros·co·py** \spek-'träs-kə-pē\ *n*

spec·trum \'spek-trəm\ *n, pl* **spec·tra** \-trə\ *or* **spectrums 1** : an array of the components of an emission or wave separated and arranged in the order of some varying characteristic (as wavelength, mass, or energy) **2** : a continuous sequence or range; *specif* : a range of effectiveness against pathogenic organisms ⟨an antibiotic with a broad ∼⟩

spec·u·lum \'spe-kyə-ləm\ *n, pl* **-la** \-lə\ *also* **-lums** : any of various instruments for insertion into a body passage to facilitate visual inspection or medication ⟨a vaginal ∼⟩ ⟨a nasal ∼⟩ — **spec·u·lar** \-lər\ *adj*

speech \'spēch\ *n* : the communication or expression of thoughts in spoken words

speech center *n* : a brain center exerting control over speech : BROCA'S AREA

speech therapist *n* : a person specially trained in speech therapy

speech therapy *n* : therapeutic treatment of speech defects (as lisping and stuttering)

speed \'spēd\ *n* : METHAMPHETAMINE; *also* : a related stimulant drug and esp. an amphetamine

spell \'spel\ *n* : a period of bodily or mental distress or disorder ⟨a ∼ of coughing⟩ ⟨fainting ∼s⟩

sperm \'spərm\ *n, pl* **sperm** *or* **sperms 1** : the male impregnating fluid : SEMEN **2** : a male gamete — **sper·mat·ic** \(₁)spər-'ma-tik\ *adj*

sperm- *or* **spermo-** *or* **sperma-** *or* **spermi-** *comb form* : seed : germ : sperm ⟨*spermi*cidal⟩

spermat- *or* **spermato-** *comb form* : seed : spermatozoon ⟨*spermat*id⟩ ⟨*spermato*cyte⟩

spermatic artery — see TESTICULAR ARTERY

spermatic cord *n* : a cord that suspends the testis within the scrotum, contains the vas deferens and vessels and nerves of the testis, and extends from the deep inguinal ring through the inguinal canal and superficial inguinal ring downward into the scrotum

spermatic duct *n* : VAS DEFERENS

spermatic plexus *n* : a nerve plexus that receives fibers from the renal plexus and a plexus associated with the aorta and that passes with the testicular artery to the testis

spermatic vein *n* : TESTICULAR VEIN

sper·ma·tid \'spər-mə-tid\ *n* : one of the haploid cells that are formed by division of the secondary spermatocytes and that differentiate into spermatozoa — compare OOTID

sper·mato·cele \(₁)spər-'ma-tə-₁sēl\ *n*

: a cystic swelling of the ducts in the epididymis or in the rete testis usu. containing spermatozoa

sper·mato·cide \(₁)spər-'ma-tə-₁sīd\ *n* : SPERMICIDE — **sper·mato·cid·al** \-₁ma-tə-'sīd-ºl\ *adj*

sper·mato·cyte \(₁)spər-'ma-tə-₁sīt\ *n* : a cell giving rise to sperm cells; *esp* : a cell that is derived from a spermatogonium and ultimately gives rise to four haploid spermatids

sper·mato·gen·e·sis \₁spər-₁ma-tə-'je-nə-səs\ *n, pl* **-e·ses** \-₁sēz\ : the process of male gamete formation including formation of a primary spermatocyte from a spermatogonium, meiotic division of the spermatocyte, and transformation of the four resulting spermatids into spermatozoa — **sper·mato·gen·ic** \-'je-nik\ *adj*

sper·mato·go·ni·um \-'gō-nē-əm\ *n, pl* **-nia** \-nē-ə\ : a primitive male germ cell — **sper·mato·go·ni·al** \-nē-əl\ *adj*

sper·ma·tor·rhea \₁spər-mə-tə-'rē-ə, (₁)spər-₁ma-\ *n* : abnormally frequent or excessive emission of semen without orgasm

sper·ma·tor·rhoea *chiefly Brit var of* SPERMATORRHEA

spermatozoa *pl of* SPERMATOZOON

sper·ma·to·zo·al \₁spər-mə-tə-'zō-əl, (₁)spər-₁ma-\ *adj* : of or relating to spermatozoa

sper·ma·to·zo·an \(₁)spər-₁ma-tə-'zō-ən, ₁spər-mə-\ *n* : SPERMATOZOON — **spermatozoan** *adj*

sper·ma·to·zo·on \-'zō-₁än, -'zō-ən\ *n, pl* **-zoa** \-'zō-ə\ : a motile male gamete of an animal usu. with rounded or elongate head and a long posterior flagellum

sperm cell *n* : a male gamete : a male germ cell

sperm duct *n* : VAS DEFERENS

spermi- *comb form* — see SPERM-

-sper·mia \'spər-mē-ə\ *n comb form* : condition of having or producing (such) sperm ⟨a*spermia*⟩

-sper·mic \'spər-mik\ *adj comb form* : being the product of (such) a number of spermatozoa : resulting from (such) a multiple fertilization ⟨poly*spermic*⟩

sper·mi·cide \'spər-mə-₁sīd\ *n* : a preparation or substance (as nonoxynol-9) used to kill sperm — called also *spermatocide* — **sper·mi·cid·al** \₁spər-mə-'sid-ºl\ *adj* — **sper·mi·cid·al·ly** *adv*

sper·mio·gen·e·sis \₁spər-mē-ō-'je-nə-səs\ *n, pl* **-e·ses** \-₁sēz\ **1** : SPERMATOGENESIS **2** : transformation of a spermatid into a spermatozoon

-sper·my \₁spər-mē\ *n comb form, pl* **-spermies** : state of exhibiting or resulting from (such) a fertilization ⟨poly*spermy*⟩

SPF \₁es-(₁)pē-'ef\ *abbr* sun protection factor — used for a number assigned to a sunscreen that is the factor by which the time required for unprotected skin to become sunburned is increased when the sunscreen is used

S phase *n* : the period in the cell cycle during which DNA replication takes place — compare G₁ PHASE, G₂ PHASE, M PHASE

sphen- *or* **spheno-** *comb form* : sphenoidal and ⟨*spheno*palatine⟩

sphe·no·eth·moid recess \ˌsfē-nō-ˈeth-ˌmȯid-\ *n* : a small space between the sphenoid bone and the superior nasal concha into which the sphenoidal sinus opens

¹**sphe·noid** \ˈsfē-ˌnȯid\ *or* **sphe·noi·dal** \sfē-ˈnȯid-ᵊl\ *adj* : of, relating to, or being a compound bone of the base of the cranium formed by the fusion of several bony elements with the basisphenoid and in humans consisting of a median body from whose sides extend a pair of broad curved wing-like expansions in front of which is another pair of much smaller triangular lateral processes while ventrally two large deeply cleft processes extend downward — see GREATER WING, LESSER WING

²**sphenoid** *n* : a sphenoid bone

sphenoid sinus *or* **sphenoidal sinus** *n* : either of two irregular cavities in the body of the sphenoid bone that communicate with the nasal cavities

sphe·no·man·dib·u·lar ligament \ˌsfē-nō-man-ˈdib-yə-lər-\ *n* : a flat thin band of fibrous tissue derived from Meckel's cartilage which extends downward from the sphenoid bone to the lingula of the mandibular foramen

sphe·no·max·il·lary fissure \ˌsfē-nō-ˈmak-sə-ˌlər-ē-, -mak-ˈsi-lə-re-\ *n* : ORBITAL FISSURE b

¹**sphe·no·pal·a·tine** \ˌsfē-nō-ˈpa-lə-ˌtīn\ *adj* : of, relating to, lying in, or distributed to the vicinity of the sphenoid and palatine bones

²**sphenopalatine** *n* : a sphenopalatine part; *specif* : PTERYGOPALATINE GANGLION

sphenopalatine foramen *n* : a foramen between the sphenoidal and orbital parts of the vertical plate of the palatine bone; *also* : a deep notch between these parts that by articulation with the sphenoid bone is converted into a foramen

sphenopalatine ganglion *n* : PTERYGOPALATINE GANGLION

sphe·no·pa·ri·etal sinus \ˌsfē-nō-pə-ˈrī-ət-ᵊl-\ *n* : a venous sinus of the dura mater on each side of the cranium arising at the meningeal vein near the apex of the lesser wing of the sphenoid bone and draining into the anterior part of the cavernous sinus

spher- *or* **sphero-** *comb form* : spherical ⟨*sphero*cyte⟩

sphe·ro·cyte \ˈsfir-ə-ˌsīt, ˈsfer-\ *n* : a more or less globular red blood cell that is characteristic of some hemolytic anemias — **sphe·ro·cyt·ic** \ˌsfir-ə-ˈsi-tik, ˌsfer-\ *adj*

sphe·ro·cy·to·sis \ˌsfir-ō-sī-ˈtō-səs, ˌsfer-\ *n* : the presence of spherocytes in the blood; *esp* : HEREDITARY SPHEROCYTOSIS

sphinc·ter \ˈsfiŋk-tər\ *n* : an annular muscle surrounding and able to contract or close a bodily opening — see ANAL SPHINCTER — **sphinc·ter·al** \-tə-rəl\ *adj*

sphincter ani ex·ter·nus \-ˈā-ˌnī-ik-ˈstər-nəs\ *n* : ANAL SPHINCTER a

sphincter ani in·ter·nus \-in-ˈtər-nəs\ *n* : ANAL SPHINCTER b

sphinc·ter·ic \sfiŋk-ˈter-ik\ *adj* : of, relating to, or being a sphincter

sphincter of Od·di \-ˈä-dē\ *n* : a complex sphincter closing the duodenal orifice of the common bile duct

Oddi, Ruggero (1864–1913), Italian physician.

sphinc·tero·plas·ty \ˈsfiŋk-tər-ə-ˌplas-tē\ *n, pl* **-ties** : plastic surgery of a sphincter ⟨anal ∼⟩

sphinc·ter·ot·o·my \ˌsfiŋk-tər-ˈä-tə-mē\ *n, pl* **-mies** : surgical incision of a sphincter

sphincter pu·pil·lae \-pyü-ˈpi-lē\ *n* : a broad flat band of smooth muscle in the iris that surrounds the pupil of the eye

sphincter ure·thrae \-yü-ˈrē-thrē\ *n* : a muscle composed of fibers that arise from the inferior ramus of the ischium and that interdigitate with those from the opposite side of the body to form in the male a narrow ring of muscle around the urethra — called also *urethral sphincter*

sphincter va·gi·nae \-və-ˈjī-nē\ *n* : the bulbocavernosus of the female

sphingo- *comb form* : sphingomyelin ⟨*sphingo*sine⟩

sphin·go·lip·id \ˌsfiŋ-gō-ˈli-pəd\ *n* : any of a group of lipids (as sphingomyelins and cerebrosides) that yield sphingosine or one of its derivatives as one product of hydrolysis

sphin·go·lip·i·do·sis \-ˌli-pə-ˈdō-səs\ *n, pl* **-do·ses** \-ˌsēz\ : any of various usu. hereditary disorders (as Gaucher's disease and Tay-Sachs disease) characterized by abnormal metabolism and storage of sphingolipids

sphin·go·my·elin \ˌsfiŋ-gō-ˈmī-ə-lən\ *n* : any of a group of crystalline phosphatides that are obtained esp. from nerve tissue and that on hydrolysis yield a fatty acid, sphingosine, choline, and phosphoric acid

sphin·go·my·elin·ase \-ˈmī-ə-lə-ˌnās, -ˌnāz\ *n* : any of several enzymes that catalyze the hydrolysis of sphingomyelin and are lacking in some metabolic deficiency diseases (as Niemann-Pick disease)

sphin·go·sine \ˈsfiŋ-gə-ˌsēn, -sən\ *n* : an unsaturated amino compound $C_{18}H_{37}NO_2$ containing two hydroxyl groups and obtained by hydrolysis of various sphingomyelins, cerebrosides, and gangliosides

sphygmo- *comb form* : pulse ⟨*sphygmo-gram*⟩

sphyg·mo·gram \'sfig-mə-ˌgram\ *n* : a tracing made by a sphygmograph and consisting of a series of curves that correspond to the beats of the heart

sphyg·mo·graph \'sfig-mə-ˌgraf\ *n* : an instrument that records graphically the movements or character of the pulse — **sphyg·mo·graph·ic** \ˌsfig-mə-'gra-fik\ *adj*

sphyg·mo·ma·nom·e·ter \ˌsfig-mō-mə-'nä-mə-tər\ *n* : an instrument for measuring blood pressure and esp. arterial blood pressure — **sphyg·mo·ma·nom·e·try** \-mə-trē\ *n*

spi·ca \'spī-kə\ *n, pl* **spi·cae** \-ˌkē\ *or* **spicas** : a bandage that is applied in successive V-shaped crossings and is used to immobilize a limb esp. at a joint; *also* : such a bandage impregnated with plaster of paris

spic·ule \'spi-(ˌ)kyül\ *n* : a minute slender pointed usu. hard body (as of bone)

spi·der \'spī-dər\ *n* **1** : any of an order (Araneae syn. Araneida) of arachnids having a body with two main divisions, four pairs of walking legs, and two or more pairs of abdominal organs for spinning threads of silk used esp. in making webs for catching prey **2** : SPIDER NEVUS (an arterial ∼)

spider nevus *n* : a pigmented area on the skin formed of dilated capillaries or arterioles radiating from a central point like the legs of a spider — called also *spider angioma, spider vein*

Spiel·mey·er–Vogt disease \'shpēl-ˌmī-ər-'fōkt-\ *n* : an inherited progressive fatal disorder of lipid metabolism having an onset at about five years of age and characterized by blindness, paralysis, and dementia — called also *juvenile amaurotic idiocy*

Spielmeyer, Walter (1879–1935), German neurologist.

Vogt, Oskar (1870–1959), German neurologist.

spi·ge·lian hernia \spī-'jē-lē-ən-\ *n, often cap S* : a hernia occurring along the linea semilunaris

Spie·ghel \'spē-gəl\, **Adriaan van den (1578–1625)**, Flemish anatomist.

spigelian lobe *n, often cap S* : CAUDATE LOBE

¹spike \'spīk\ *n* **1** : the pointed element in the wave tracing in an electroencephalogram **2** : a sharp increase in body temperature followed by a rapid fall (a fever with ∼s to 103°) **3** : a momentary sharp increase and fall in the record of an action potential; *also* : ACTION POTENTIAL

²spike *vb* **spiked; spik·ing** : to undergo a sudden sharp increase in (temperature or fever) usu. up to an indicated level

spike potential *n* **1** : SPIKE 3 **2** : ACTION POTENTIAL

spik·ing *adj* : characterized by recurrent sharp rises in body temperature ⟨a ∼ fever⟩; *also* : resulting from a sharp rise in body temperature ⟨a ∼ temperature of 105°⟩

spin- *or* **spini-** *or* **spino-** *comb form* **1** : spinal column : spinal cord ⟨*spinotectal tract*⟩ **2** : of, relating to, or involving the spinal cord and ⟨*spinothalamic*⟩

spi·na \'spī-nə\ *n, pl* **spi·nae** \-ˌnē\ : an anatomical spine or spinelike process

spina bi·fi·da \-'bi-fə-də, -'bī-\ *n* : a congenital cleft of the spinal column with hernial protrusion of the meninges and sometimes the spinal cord

spina bifida oc·cul·ta \-ə-'kəl-tə\ *n* : a congenital cleft of the spinal column without hernial protrusion of the meninges

spinae — see ERECTOR SPINAE

¹spi·nal \'spīn-ᵊl\ *adj* **1** : of, relating to, or situated near the spinal column **2 a** : of, relating to, or affecting the spinal cord ⟨∼ reflexes⟩ **b** : having the spinal cord functionally isolated (as by surgical section) from the brain ⟨experiments on ∼ animals⟩ **c** : used for spinal anesthesia ⟨a ∼ anesthetic⟩ **3** : made for or fitted to the spinal column ⟨a ∼ brace⟩ — **spi·nal·ly** *adv*

²spinal *n* : a spinal anesthetic

spinal accessory nerve *n* : ACCESSORY NERVE

spinal anesthesia *n* : anesthesia produced by injection of an anesthetic into the subarachnoid space of the spine

spinal artery *n* : any of three arteries that supply the spinal cord and its membranes and adjacent structures: **a** : a single unpaired artery that is formed by the anastomosis of a branch of the vertebral artery on each side — called also *anterior spinal artery* **b** : either of two arteries of which one arises from a vertebral artery on each side below the level at which the corresponding branch of the anterior spinal artery arises — called also *posterior spinal artery*

spinal canal *n* : VERTEBRAL CANAL

spinal column *n* : the articulated series of vetebrae connected by ligaments and separated by more or less elastic intervertebral fibrocartilages that forms the supporting axis of the body and a protection for the spinal cord and that extends from the hind end of the skull through the median dorsal part of the body to the coccyx — called also *backbone, spine, vertebral column*

spinal cord *n* : the thick longitudinal cord of nervous tissue that in vertebrates extends along the back dorsal to the bodies of the vertebrae and is enclosed in the vertebral canal formed by their neural arches, is continuous anteriorly with the medulla oblongata, gives off at intervals pairs of spinal nerves to the various parts of the trunk and limbs, serves not only as a pathway for nervous impulses to and from the brain but as a center for carrying out and coordinating many reflex actions independently of the brain, and is composed largely of white matter arranged in columns and tracts of longitudinal fibers about a large central core of gray matter — called also *medulla spinalis*

spinales *pl of* SPINALIS
spinal fluid *n* : CEREBROSPINAL FLUID
spinal fusion *n* : surgical fusion of two or more vertebrae for remedial immobilization of the spine
spinal ganglion *n* : a ganglion on the dorsal root of each spinal nerve that is one of a series of ganglia containing cell bodies of sensory neurons — called also *dorsal root ganglion*
spi·na·lis \spī-'nā-ləs, spi-'na-lis\ *n, pl* **spi·na·les** \-(ₐ)lēz\ : the most medial division of the sacrospinalis situated next to the spinal column and acting to extend it or any of the three muscles making up this division: **a** : SPINALIS THORACIS **b** : SPINALIS CERVICIS **c** : SPINALIS CAPITIS
spinalis ca·pi·tis \-'ka-pə-təs\ *n* : a muscle that arises with, inserts with, and is intimately associated with the semispinalis capitis
spinalis cer·vi·cis \-'sər-və-səs\ *n* : an inconstant muscle that arises esp. from the spinous processes of the lower cervical and upper thoracic vertebrae and inserts esp. into the spinous process of the axis
spinalis tho·ra·cis \-thō-'rā-səs\ *n* : an upward continuation of the sacrospinalis that is situated medially and blends with the longissimus thoracis, arises from the spinous processes of the first two lumbar and last two thoracic vertebrae, and inserts into the spinous processes of the upper thoracic vertebrae
spinal meningitis *n* : inflammation of the meninges of the spinal cord; *also* : CEREBROSPINAL MENINGITIS
spinal nerve *n* : any of the paired nerves which leave the spinal cord, supply muscles of the trunk and limbs, and connect with the nerves of the sympathetic nervous system, which arise by a short motor ventral root and a short sensory dorsal root, and of which there are 31 pairs in humans classified according to the part of the spinal cord from which they arise into 8 pairs of cervical nerves, 12 pairs of thoracic nerves, 5 pairs of lumbar nerves, 5 pairs of sacral nerves, and one pair of coccygeal nerves
spinal puncture *n* : LUMBAR PUNCTURE
spinal shock *n* : a temporary condition following transection of the spinal cord that is characterized by muscular flaccidity and loss of motor reflexes in all parts of the body below the point of transection

spinal tap *n* : LUMBAR PUNCTURE
spin·dle \'spind-ᵊl\ *n* **1** : something shaped like a round stick or pin with tapered ends: as **a** : a network of chiefly microtubular fibers along which the chromosomes are distributed during mitosis and meiosis **b** : MUSCLE SPINDLE **2** : SLEEP SPINDLE
spindle cell *n* : a spindle-shaped cell (as in some tumors)
spindle–cell sarcoma *n* : a sarcoma (as a fibrosarcoma) composed chiefly or entirely of spindle cells
spindle fiber *n* : any of the apparent filaments constituting a mitotic spindle
spine \'spīn\ *n* **1** : SPINAL COLUMN **2** : a pointed prominence or process (as on a bone)
spine of the scapula *n* : a projecting triangular bony process on the dorsal surface of the scapula that divides it obliquely into the area of origin of parts of the supraspinatus and infraspinatus muscles and that terminates in the acromion
spini– *or* **spino–** — see SPIN-
spinn·bar·keit \'spin-ₐbār-ₐkīt, 'shpin-\ *n* : the elastic quality that is characteristic of mucus of the uterine cervix esp. shortly before ovulation
spi·no·cer·e·bel·lar \ₐspi-nō-ₐser-ə-'belər\ *adj* : of or relating to the spinal cord and cerebellum (~ pathways)
spinocerebellar tract *n* : any of four nerve tracts which pass from the spinal cord to the cerebellum and of which two are situated on each side external to the crossed corticospinal tracts: **a** : a posterior tract on each side that begins at the level of the attachments of the second or third lumbar spinal nerves and ascends to the inferior cerebellar peduncle and vermis of the cerebellum — called also *dorsal spinocerebellar tract, posterior spinocerebellar tract* **b** : an anterior tract on each side that arises from cells mostly in the dorsal column of gray matter on the same or opposite side and passes through the medulla oblongata and pons to the superior cerebellar peduncle and vermis — called also *ventral spinocerebellar tract*
spi·no·ol·i·vary \-'ä-lə-ₐver-ē\ *adj* : connecting the spinal cord with the olivary nuclei (~ fibers) (the ~ tract)
spi·nose ear tick \'spi-ₐnōs-\ *n* : an ear tick of the genus *Otobius* (*O. megnini*) of the southwestern U.S. and Mexico that is a serious pest of cattle, horses, sheep, and goats
spinosum — see FORAMEN SPINOSUM, STRATUM SPINOSUM
spi·no·tec·tal tract \ₐspi-nō-'tekt-ᵊl-\ *n* : an ascending tract of nerve fibers in each lateral funiculus of white matter of the spinal cord that passes upward

and terminates in the superior colliculus of the opposite side

spi·no·tha·lam·ic \ˌspī-nō-thə-ˈla-mik\ *adj* : of, relating to, comprising, or associated with the spinothalamic tracts ⟨the ~ system⟩

spinothalamic tract *n* : any of four tracts of nerve fibers of the spinal cord that are arranged in pairs with one member of a pair on each side and that ascend to the thalamus by way of the brain stem: **a** : one on each side of the anterior median fissure that carries nerve impulses relating to the sense of touch — called also *anterior spinothalamic tract*, *ventral spinothalamic tract* **b** : one on each lateral part of the spinal cord that carries nerve impulses relating to the senses of touch, pain, and temperature — called also *lateral spinothalamic tract*

spi·nous \ˈspī-nəs\ *adj* : slender and pointed like a spine

spinous process *n* : SPINE 2; *specif* : the median spinelike or platelike dorsal process of the neural arch of a vertebra

spiny–headed worm *n* : ACANTHOCEPHALAN

spi·ral \ˈspī-rəl\ *adj* **1 a** : winding around a center or pole and gradually receding from or approaching it **b** : HELICAL ⟨the ~ structure of DNA⟩ **2** : being a fracture in which the break is produced by twisting apart the bone ⟨a double ~ break⟩ — **spiral** *n* — **spi·ral·ly** *adv*

spiral ganglion *n* : a mass of bipolar cell bodies occurring in the modiolus of the organ of Corti and giving off axons which comprise the cochlear nerve

spiralis — see LAMINA SPIRALIS

spiral lamina *n* : a twisting shelf of bone which projects from the modiolus into the canal of the cochlea — called also *lamina spiralis*

spiral ligament *n* : the thick periosteum that forms the outer wall of the scala media

spiral organ *n* : ORGAN OF CORTI

spiral valve *n* : a series of crescentic folds of mucous membrane somewhat spirally arranged on the interior of the gallbladder and continuing into the cystic duct

spi·ra·my·cin \ˌspī-rə-ˈmīs-ᵊn\ *n* : a mixture of macrolide antibiotics produced by a soil bacterium of the genus *Streptomyces* (*S. ambofaciens*) and having antibacterial activity

spi·ril·lum \spī-ˈri-ləm\ *n* **1** *cap* : a genus of gram-negative bacteria having tufts of flagella at both poles and usu. living in stagnant water rich in organic matter — see RAT-BITE FEVER b **2** *pl* **-ril·la** \-ˈri-lə\ : any bacterium of the genus *Spirillum*

spir·it \ˈspir-ət\ *n* **1 a** (1) : the liquid containing ethyl alcohol and water that is distilled from an alcoholic liquid or mash — often used in pl. (2) : ALCOHOL 1a **b** : a usu. volatile organic solvent (as an alcohol, ester, or hydrocarbon) **2** : an alcoholic solution of a volatile substance ⟨~ of camphor⟩

spirit of hartshorn *or* **spirits of hartshorn** \-ˈhärts-ˌhórn\ *n* : AMMONIA WATER

spiro- *comb form* : respiration ⟨spirometer⟩

Spi·ro·cer·ca \ˌspī-rō-ˈsər-kə\ *n* : a genus of red filarial worms (family Thelaziidae) forming nodules in the walls of the digestive tract and sometimes the aorta of canines esp. in warm regions

spi·ro·chaet·ae·mia, spi·ro·chaete, spi·ro·chae·ti·ci·dal, spi·ro·chaet·osis *chiefly Brit var of* SPIROCHETEMIA, SPIROCHETE, SPIROCHETICIDAL, SPIROCHETOSIS

spi·ro·chete \ˈspī-rə-ˌkēt\ *n* : any of an order (Spirochaetales) of slender spirally undulating bacteria including those causing syphilis and relapsing fever — **spi·ro·chet·al** \ˌspī-rə-ˈkēt-ᵊl\ *adj*

spi·ro·chet·emia \ˌspī-rə-ˌkē-ˈtē-mē-ə\ *n* : the abnormal presence of spirochetes in the circulating blood

spi·ro·che·ti·ci·dal \ˌspī-rə-ˌkē-tə-ˈsīd-ᵊl\ *adj* : destructive to spirochetes esp. within the body of an animal host ⟨a ~ drug⟩ — **spi·ro·che·ti·cide** \ˌspī-rə-ˈkēt-ə-ˌsīd\ *n*

spi·ro·chet·osis \ˌspī-rə-ˌkē-ˈtō-səs\ *n, pl* **-oses** \-ˌsēz\ : infection with or a disease caused by spirochetes

spi·ro·gram \ˈspī-rə-ˌgram\ *n* : a graphic record of respiratory movements traced on a revolving drum

spi·ro·graph \ˈspī-rə-ˌgraf\ *n* : an instrument for recording respiratory movements — **spi·ro·graph·ic** \ˌspī-rə-ˈgra-fik\ *adj* — **spi·rog·ra·phy** \spī-ˈrä-grə-fē\ *n*

spi·rom·e·ter \spī-ˈrä-mə-tər\ *n* : an instrument for measuring the air entering and leaving the lungs — **spi·ro·met·ric** \ˌspī-rə-ˈme-trik\ *adj* — **spi·rom·e·try** \-ˈrä-mə-trē\ *n*

spi·ro·no·lac·tone \ˌspī-rə-nō-ˈlak-ˌtōn, spī-ˌrō-nə-\ *n* : an aldosterone antagonist $C_{24}H_{32}O_4S$ that promotes diuresis and sodium excretion and is used to treat essential hypertension, edema with congestive heart failure, hepatic cirrhosis with ascites, nephrotic syndrome, and idiopathic edema

¹spit \ˈspit\ *vb* **spit** *or* **spat** \ˈspat\; **spit·ting** : to eject (as saliva) from the mouth

²spit *n* : SALIVA

spitting cobra *n* : either of two African cobras (*Naja nigricollis* and *Hemachatus hemachatus*) that in defense typically eject their venom toward the victim without striking

spit·tle \ˈspit-ᵊl\ *n* : SALIVA

splanch·nic \\'splaŋk-nik\\ *adj* : of or relating to the viscera : VISCERAL

splanch·ni·cec·to·my \\,splaŋk-nə-'sek-tə-mē\\ *n, pl* **-mies** : surgical excision of a segment of one or more splanchnic nerves to relieve hypertension

splanchnic ganglion *n* : a small ganglion on the greater splanchnic nerve that is usually located near the eleventh or twelfth thoracic vertebra

splanchnic nerve *n* : any of three nerves situated on each side of the body and formed by the union of branches from the six or seven lower thoracic and first lumbar ganglia of the sympathetic system: **a** : a superior one ending in the celiac ganglion — called also *greater splanchnic nerve* **b** : a middle one ending in a detached ganglionic mass of the celiac ganglion — called also *lesser splanchnic nerve* **c** : an inferior one ending in the renal plexus — called also *least splanchnic nerve*, *lowest splanchnic nerve*

splanchno- *comb form* : viscera ⟨*splanchno*logy⟩

splanch·nol·o·gy \\,splaŋk-'nä-lə-jē\\ *n, pl* **-gies** : a branch of anatomy concerned with the viscera

splanch·no·pleure \\'splaŋk-nə-,plúr\\ *n* : a layer of tissue that consists of the inner of the two layers into which the unsegmented sheet of mesoderm splits in the embryo together with the endoderm internal to it and that forms most of the walls and substance of the visceral organs — compare SOMATOPLEURE

splay·foot \\'splā-,fút, -'fút\\ *n* : a foot abnormally flattened and spread out: *specif* : FLATFOOT — **splay·foot·ed** \\-'fü-təd\\ *adj*

spleen \\'splēn\\ *n* : a highly vascular ductless organ that is concerned with final destruction of red blood cells, filtration and storage of blood, and production of lymphocytes, and that in humans is a dark purplish flattened oblong object of a soft fragile consistency lying in the upper left part of the abdominal cavity near the cardiac end of the stomach and which is divisible into a loose friable red pulp in intimate connection with the blood supply and with red blood cells free in its interstices and a denser white pulp chiefly of lymphoid tissue condensed in masses about the small arteries

splen- *or* **spleno-** *comb form* : spleen ⟨*splen*ectomy⟩ ⟨*spleno*megaly⟩

sple·nec·to·my \\spli-'nek-tə-mē\\ *n, pl* **-mies** : surgical excision of the spleen — **sple·nec·to·mize** \\spli-'nek-tə-,mīz\\ *vb*

splen·ic \\'sple-nik\\ *adj* : of, relating to, or located in the spleen

splenic artery *n* : the branch of the celiac artery that carries blood to the spleen and sends branches also to the pancreas and the cardiac end of the stomach

splenic fever *n* : ANTHRAX

splenic flexure *n* : the sharp bend of the colon under the spleen where the transverse colon joins the descending colon — called also *left colic flexure*

splenic flexure syndrome *n* : pain in the upper left quadrant of the abdomen that may radiate upward to the left shoulder and inner aspect of the left arm and that sometimes mimics angina pectoris but is caused by bloating and gas in the colon

splenic pulp *n* : the characteristic tissue of the spleen

splenic vein *n* : the vein that carries blood away from the spleen and that joins the superior mesenteric vein to form the portal vein — called also *lienal vein*

sple·ni·um \\'splē-nē-əm\\ *n, pl* **-nia** \\-nē-ə\\ : the thick rounded fold that forms the posterior border of the corpus callosum and is continuous by its undersurface with the fornix

sple·ni·us \\-nē-əs\\ *n, pl* **-nii** \\-nē-,ī\\ : either of two flat oblique muscles on each side of the back of the neck and upper thoracic region: **a** : SPLENIUS CAPITIS **b** : SPLENIUS CERVICIS

splenius cap·i·tis \\-'ka-pi-təs\\ *n* : a flat muscle on each side of the back of the neck and the upper thoracic region that arises from the caudal half of the ligamentum nuchae and the spinous processes of the seventh cervical and the first three or four thoracic vertebrae, that is inserted into the occipital bone and the mastoid process of the temporal bone, and that rotates the head to the side on which it is located and with the help of the muscle on the opposite side extends it

splenius cer·vi·cis \\-'sər-vi-kəs\\ *n* : a flat narrow muscle on each side of the back of the neck and the upper thoracic region that arises from the spinous processes of the third to sixth thoracic vertebrae, is inserted into the transverse processes of the first two or three cervical vertebrae, and acts to rotate the head to the side on which it is located and with the help of the muscle on the opposite side to extend and arch the neck

spleno- — see SPLEN-

sple·no·cyte \\'splē-nə-,sīt, 'sple-\\ *n* : a macrophage of the spleen

spleno·meg·a·ly \\,sple-nō-'me-gə-lē\\ *n, pl* **-lies** : abnormal enlargement of the spleen

spleno·re·nal \\,sple-nō-'rēn-əl\\ *adj* : of, relating to, or joining the splenic and renal veins or arteries

sple·no·sis \\splē-'nō-səs\\ *n, pl* **-no·ses** \\-,sēs\\ *or* **-no·sis·es** : a rare condition in which fragments of tissue from a ruptured spleen become implanted throughout the peritoneal cavity and often undergo regeneration and vascularization

splice \\'splīs\\ *vb* **spliced; splic·ing** : to

combine (genetic information) from either the same organism or different organisms — see GENE-SPLICING

¹splint \'splint\ *n* **1** : material or a device used to protect and immobilize a body part **2** : a bony enlargement on the upper part of the cannon bone of a horse usu. on the inside of the leg

²splint *vb* **1** : to support and immobilize (as a broken bone) with a splint **2** : to protect against pain by reducing the motion of

splin·ter \'splin-tər\ *n* : a thin piece (as of wood) split or rent off lengthwise; *esp* : such a piece embedded in the skin (used tweezers to remove a ~) — **splinter** *vb*

split \'split\ *vb* **split; split·ting** : to divide or break down (a chemical compound) into constituents; *also* : to remove by tooth separation

split–brain \'split-,brān\ *adj* : of, relating to, concerned with, or having undergone separation of the two cerebral hemispheres by surgical division of the optic chiasma and corpus callosum (~ patients)

split personality *n* : SCHIZOPHRENIA; *also* : MULTIPLE PERSONALITY

spondyl- *or* **spondylo-** *comb form* : vertebra : vertebrae ⟨*spondyl*arthritis⟩ ⟨*spondylo*pathy⟩

spon·dyl·ar·thri·tis \,spän-di-lär-'thrī-təs\ *n, pl* **-thrit·i·des** \-'thri-tə-,dēz\ : arthritis of the spine

spon·dy·li·tis \,spän-də-'lī-təs\ *n* : inflammation of the vertebrae (tuberculous ~) — see ANKYLOSING SPONDYLITIS — **spon·dy·lit·ic** \-'li-tik\ *adj*

spon·dy·lo·ar·throp·a·thy \,spän-də-lō-är-'thrä-pə-thē\ *also* **spon·dyl·ar·throp·a·thy** \,spän-də-lär-'thrä-\ *n, pl* **-thies** : any of several diseases (as ankylosing spondylitis) affecting the joints of the spine

spon·dy·lo·lis·the·sis \,spän-də-lō-lis-'thē-səs\ *n* : forward displacement of a lumbar vertebra on the one below it and esp. of the fifth lumbar vertebra on the sacrum producing pain by compression of nerve roots

spon·dy·lol·y·sis \,spän-də-'lä-lə-səs\ *n, pl* **-y·ses** \-,sēz\ : disintegration or dissolution of a vertebra

spon·dy·lop·a·thy \,spän-də-'lä-pə-thē\ *n, pl* **-thies** : any disease or disorder of the vertebrae

spon·dy·lo·sis \,spän-də-'lō-səs\ *n, pl* **-lo·ses** \-,sēz\ *or* **-lo·sis·es** : any of various degenerative diseases of the spine

sponge \'spənj\ *n* **1 a** : a small pad made of multiple folds of gauze or of cotton and gauze used to mop blood from a surgical incision, to carry inhalant medicaments to the nose, or to cover a superficial wound as a dressing **b** : a porous dressing (as of fibrin or gelatin) applied to promote wound healing **c** : a plastic prosthesis used in chest cavities following lung surgery **2** : an absorbent contraceptive device impregnated with spermicide that is inserted into the vagina before sexual intercourse to cover the cervix and act as a barrier to sperm — **sponge** *vb*

sponge bath *n* : a bath in which water is applied to the body without actual immersion

sponge biopsy *n* : biopsy performed on matter collected with a sponge from a lesion

spongi- *or* **spongio-** *comb form* : spongy ⟨*spongio*blast⟩

spon·gi·form \'spən-ji-,form\ *adj* : of, relating to, or being a degenerative disease which causes the brain tissue to have a porous structure like that of a sponge ⟨acute ~ encephalopathies⟩

spon·gi·o·blast \'spän-jē-ō-,blast, 'spän-\ *n* : any of the ectodermal cells of the embryonic spinal cord or other nerve center that are at first columnar but become branched at one end and that give rise to the neuroglia cells

spon·gi·o·blas·to·ma \,spän-jē-ō-(,)bla-'stō-mə, ,spän-\ *n, pl* **-mas** *or* **-ma·ta** \-mə-tə\ : GLIOBLASTOMA

spon·gi·o·cyte \'spän-jē-ō-,sīt, 'spän-\ *n* : any of the cells of the adrenal cortex that have a spongy appearance due to lipid vacuoles the contents of which have been dissolved out

spon·gi·o·sa \,spən-jē-'ō-sə, ,spän-\ *n* : the part of a bone (as much of the epiphyseal area of long bones) made up of spongy cancellous bone

spon·gi·o·sis \,spən-jē-'ō-səs, ,spän-\ *n* : swelling localized in the epidermis and often occurring in eczema

spongiosum — see CORPUS SPONGIO-SUM, STRATUM SPONGIOSUM

spongy \'spən-jē\ *adj* **spong·i·er; -est** : resembling a sponge; *esp* : full of cavities : CANCELLOUS ⟨~ bone⟩

spon·ta·ne·ous \spän-'tā-nē-əs\ *adj* **1** : proceeding from natural feeling or native tendency without external constraint **2** : developing without apparent external influence, force, cause, or treatment ⟨~ nosebleed⟩ — **spon·ta·ne·ous·ly** *adv*

spontaneous abortion *n* : naturally occurring expulsion of a nonviable fetus

spontaneous recovery *n* : reappearance of an extinguished conditioned response without positive reinforcement

spoon nails \'spün-\ *n* : KOILONYCHIA

spor- *or* **spori-** *or* **sporo-** *comb form* : seed : spore ⟨*sporo*cyst⟩

spo·rad·ic \spə-'ra-dik\ *adj* : occurring occasionally, singly, or in scattered instances ⟨~ diseases⟩ — compare ENDEMIC, EPIDEMIC **1** — **spo·rad·i·cal·ly** *adv*

spore \'spōr\ *n* : a primitive usu. unicellular often environmentally resistant dormant or reproductive body produced by plants and some microorganisms and capable of development into a new individual either directly or after fusion with another spore — **spore** *vb*

spo•ro•blast \\'spō-rə-ˌblast\ *n* : a cell of a sporozoan resulting from sexual reproduction and producing spores and sporozoites

spo•ro•cyst \-ˌsist\ *n* **1** : a case or cyst secreted by some sporozoans preliminary to sporogony; *also* : a sporozoan encysted in such a case **2** : a saccular body that is the first asexual reproductive form of a digenetic trematode, develops from a miracidium, and buds off cells from its inner surface which develop into rediae

spo•ro•gen•e•sis \ˌspōr-ə-'je-nə-səs\ *n, pl* **-e•ses** \-ˌsēz\ **1** : reproduction by spores **2** : spore formation — **spo•rog•e•nous** \spə-'rä-jə-nəs, spō-\ *also* **spo•ro•gen•ic** \ˌspōr-ə-'je-nik\ *adj*

spo•rog•o•ny \spə-'rä-gə-nē\ *n, pl* **-nies** : reproduction by spores; *specif* : formation of spores containing sporozoites that is characteristic of some sporozoans and that results from the encystment and subsequent division of a zygote — **spo•ro•gon•ic** \ˌspōr-ə-'gä-nik\ *adj*

spo•ront \\'spōr-ˌänt\ *n* : a sporozoan that engages in sporogony

spo•ro•phore \\'spōr-ə-ˌfōr\ *n* : the spore-producing organ esp. of a fungus

spo•ro•thrix \-ˌthriks\ *n* **1** *cap* : a genus of imperfect fungi (family Moniliaceae) that includes the causative agent (*S. schenckii*) of sporotrichosis **2** : any fungus of the genus *Sporothrix*

spo•ro•tri•cho•sis \ˌspə-rä-tri-'kō-səs, ˌspōr-ə-tri-\ *n, pl* **-cho•ses** \-ˌsēz\ : infection with or disease caused by a fungus of the genus *Sporothrix* (*S. schenckii* syn. *Sporotrichum schenckii*) that is characterized by nodules and abscesses in the superficial lymph nodes, skin, and subcutaneous tissues and that is usu. transmitted by entry of the fungus through a skin abrasion or wound

spo•ro•zo•an \ˌspōr-ə-'zō-ən\ *n* : any of a large class (Sporozoa) of strictly parasitic protozoans that have a complicated life cycle usu. involving both asexual and sexual generations often in different hosts and that include many serious pathogens (as malaria parasites and babesias) — **sporozoan** *adj*

spo•ro•zo•ite \-'zō-ˌīt\ *n* : a usu. motile infective form of some sporozoans (as the malaria parasite) that is a product of sporogony and initiates an asexual cycle in the new host

sport \\'spōrt\ *n* : an individual exhibiting a sudden deviation from type beyond the normal limits of individual variation usu. as a result of mutation esp. of somatic tissue

sports medicine *n* : a medical specialty concerned with the prevention and treatment of injuries and diseases that are related to participation in sports

spor•u•la•tion \ˌspōr-ə-'lā-shən, ˌspōr-yə-\ *n* : the formation of spores; *esp* : division into many small spores (as after encystment) — **spor•u•late** \\'spōr-ə-ˌlāt, 'spōr-yə-\ *vb*

¹spot \\'spät\ *n* : a circumscribed mark or area: as **a** : a circumscribed surface lesion of disease (as measles) **b** : a circumscribed abnormality in an organ seen by means of X rays or an instrument ⟨a ~ on the lung⟩

²spot *vb* **spot•ted; spot•ting** : to experience abnormal and sporadic bleeding in small amounts from the uterus

spot film *n* : a roentgenogram of a restricted area in the body

spotted cow•bane \-'kau-ˌbān\ *n* : a tall biennial No. American herb (*Cicuta maculata*) of the carrot family (Umbelliferae) with clusters of tuberous roots that resemble small sweet potatoes and are extremely poisonous — called also *spotted hemlock*

spotted fever *n* : any of various eruptive fevers; *esp* : ROCKY MOUNTAIN SPOTTED FEVER

sprain \\'sprān\ *n* : a sudden or violent twist or wrench of a joint causing the stretching or tearing of ligaments and often rupture of blood vessels with hemorrhage into the tissues; *also* : the condition resulting from a sprain that is usu. marked by swelling, inflammation, hemorrhage, and discoloration — compare ³STRAIN b — **sprain** *vb*

sprain fracture *n* : the rupture of a tendon or ligament from its point of insertion at a joint with detachment of a splinter of bone

¹spray \\'sprā\ *n* : a jet of vapor or finely divided liquid; *specif* : a jet of fine medicated vapor used as an application to a diseased part or to charge the air of a room with a disinfectant or deodorant

²spray *vb* : to emit a stream or spray of urine ⟨a cat may ~ to mark its territory⟩

spreading factor *n* : HYALURONIDASE

Spren•gel's deformity \\'shpreŋ-əlz-, -gəlz-\ *n* : a congenital elevation of the scapula

Sprengel, Otto Gerhard Karl (1852–1915), German surgeon.

spring \\'spriŋ\ *n* : any of various elastic orthodontic devices used esp. to apply constant pressure to misaligned teeth

spring ligament *n* : PLANTAR CALCANEONAVICULAR LIGAMENT

¹sprout \\'spraut\ *vb* : to send out new growth : produce sprouts

²sprout *n* : a new outgrowth (as of nerve tissue)

sprue \\'sprü\ *n* **1** : CELIAC DISEASE **2** : a disease of tropical regions that is of unknown cause and is characterized by fatty diarrhea and malabsorption of nutrients — called also *tropical sprue*

spud \\'spəd\ *n* : any of various small surgical instruments with a shape resembling that of a spade

spur \\'spər\ *n* : a sharp and esp. bony outgrowth (as on the heel of the foot) — **spurred** \\'spərd\ *adj*

spu·ri·ous \\'spyur-ē-əs\ *adj* : simulating a symptom or condition without being pathologically or morphologically genuine (~ labor pains)

spu·tum \\'spü-təm, 'spyü-\ *n, pl* **spu·ta** \-tə\ : expectorated matter made up of saliva and often discharges from the respiratory passages

squa·ma \\'skwä-mə, 'skwā-\ *n, pl* **squa·mae** \\'skwā-mē, 'skwā-mī\ : a structure resembling a scale or plate: as **a** : the curved platelike posterior portion of the occipital bone **b** : the vertical portion of the frontal bone that forms the forehead **c** : the thin anterior upper portion of the temporal bone

squame \\'skwām\ *n* : a scale or flake (as of skin)

squa·mous \\'skwā-məs\ *adj* **1 a** : covered with or consisting of scales **b** : of, relating to, or being a stratified epithelium that consists at least in its outer layers of small scalelike cells **2** : resembling a scale or plate; *esp* : of, relating to, or being the thin anterior upper portion of the temporal bone

squamous carcinoma *n* : SQUAMOUS CELL CARCINOMA

squamous cell *n* : a cell of or derived from squamous epithelium

squamous cell carcinoma *n* : a carcinoma made up of or arising from squamous cells

squash bite \\'skwäsh-, 'skwȯsh-\ *n* : an impression of the teeth and mouth made by closing the teeth on modeling composition or wax

squill \\'skwil\ *n* **1** : a Mediterranean bulbous herb of the genus *Urginea* (esp. *U. maritima*) **2** : the dried sliced bulb scales of a white-bulbed form of the squill (*Urginea maritima*) of the Mediterranean region used as an expectorant, cardiac stimulant, and diuretic — called also *white squill*

¹squint \\'skwint\ *vb* **1** : to be cross-eyed **2** : to look or peer with eyes partly closed

²squint *n* **1** : STRABISMUS **2** : an instance or habit of squinting

squir·rel corn \\'skwər-əl-\ *n* : a poisonous No. American herb (*Dicentra canadensis* of the family Fumariaceae)

Sr *symbol* strontium

sRNA \\'es-(ˌ)är-(ˌ)en-'ā\ *n* : TRANSFER RNA

SRS–A *abbr* slow-reacting substance of anaphylaxis

ss *abbr* [Latin *semis*] one half — used in writing prescriptions

S sleep *n* : SLOW-WAVE SLEEP

SSPE *abbr* subacute sclerosing panencephalitis

SSSS *abbr* staphylococcal scalded skin syndrome

ST \\'es-'tē\ *n* : ST SEGMENT

stab \\'stab\ *n* : a wound produced by a pointed weapon — **stab** *vb*

stab·bing *adj* : having a sharp piercing quality (~ pain)

stab cell *n* : BAND FORM

sta·bil·i·ty \stə-'bi-lə-tē\ *n, pl* **-ties** : the quality, state, or degree of being stable (emotional ~)

sta·bi·lize \\'stā-bə-ˌlīz\ *vb* **-lized; -lizing** : to make or become stable (~ a patient's condition) — **sta·bi·li·za·tion** \ˌstā-bə-lə-'zā-shən\ *n* — **sta·bi·liz·er** \\'stā-bə-ˌlī-zər\ *n*

sta·ble \\'stā-bəl\ *adj* **sta·bler; sta·blest 1** : not changing or fluctuating (the patient's condition was listed as ~) **2** : not subject to insecurity or emotional illness (a ~ personality) **3 a** : not readily altering in chemical makeup or physical state **b** : not spontaneously radioactive

stable factor *n* : FACTOR VII

stable fly *n* : a biting dipteran fly of the genus *Stomoxys* (*S. calcitrans*) that is abundant about stables and often enters dwellings esp. in autumn

stachy·bot·ryo·tox·i·co·sis \ˌsta-ki-ˌbä-trē-ō-ˌtäk-sə-'kō-səs\ *n, pl* **-co·ses** \-ˌsēz\ : a serious and sometimes fatal intoxication chiefly affecting domestic animals (as horses) that is due to ingestion of a toxic substance elaborated by a mold (*Stachybotrys alternans*)

staff \\'staf\ *n* : the doctors and surgeons regularly attached to a hospital and helping to determine its policies and guide its activities

staff nurse *n* : a registered nurse employed by a medical facility who does not assist in surgery

staff of Aes·cu·la·pi·us \-ˌes-kyə-'lā-pē-əs\ *n* : a conventionalized representation of a staff branched at the top with a single snake twined around it that is used as a symbol of medicine and as the official insignia of the American Medical Association — called also *Aesculapian staff*

stage \\'stāj\ *n* **1** : the small platform of a microscope on which an object is placed for examination **2** : a period or step in a progress, activity, or development: as **a** : one of the distinguishable periods of growth and development of a plant or animal **b** : a period or phase in the course of a disease (the sweating ~ of malaria) **c** : one of two or more operations performed at different times but constituting a single procedure (a two-*stage* thoracoplasty) **d** : any of the four degrees indicating depth of general anesthesia

stag·gers \\'sta-gərz\ *n pl* **1** : any of various abnormal conditions of domestic animals associated with damage to the central nervous system and marked by incoordination and a reeling unsteady gait — used with a sing. or pl. verb; see BLIND STAGGERS; compare GRASS TETANY 2 : vertigo occurring as a symptom of decompression sickness

stag·horn calculus \'stag-ˌhȯrn-\ n : a large renal calculus with multiple irregular branches

stag·ing \'stā-jiŋ\ n : the classification of the severity of a disease in distinct stages on the basis of established symptomatic criteria

¹**stain** \'stān\ vb **1 a** : to cause discoloration of **b** : to color by processes affecting chemically or otherwise the material itself ⟨∼ bacteria with a fluorescent dye⟩ **2** : to receive a stain

²**stain** n **1** : a discolored spot or area (as on the skin or teeth) — see PORT-WINE STAIN **2** : a dye or mixture of dyes used in microscopy to make visible minute and transparent structures, or to differentiate tissue elements, or to produce specific chemical reactions

stair·case effect \'star-ˌkās-\ n : TREPPE

stalk \'stȯk\ n : a slender supporting or connecting part : PEDUNCLE ⟨the pituitary ∼⟩ — **stalked** \'stȯkt\ adj — **stalk·less** adj

stam·i·na \'sta-mi-nə\ n : the strength or vigor of bodily constitution : capacity for standing fatigue or resisting disease

stam·mer \'sta-mər\ vb **stam·mered**; **stam·mer·ing** : to make involuntary stops and repetitions in speaking — **stammer** n — **stam·mer·er** \'sta-mər-ər\ n

stammering n **1** : the act of one who stammers **2** : a defective condition of speech characterized by involuntary stops and repetitions or blocking of utterance — compare STUTTERING 2

stanch \'stȯnch, 'stänch\ vb : to check or stop the flowing of ⟨∼ bleeding⟩; also : to stop the flow of blood from ⟨∼ a wound⟩

stand·still \'stand-ˌstil\ n : a state characterized by absence of motion or of progress : ARREST ⟨cardiac ∼⟩

Stan·ford–Bi·net test \'stan-fərd-bi-'nā-\ n : an intelligence test prepared at Stanford University as a revision of the Binet-Simon scale and commonly employed with children — called also Stanford-Binet

A. Binet — see BINET AGE

stan·nous fluoride \'sta-nəs-\ n : a white compound SnF₂ of tin and fluorine used in toothpaste to combat tooth decay

stan·o·lone \'sta-nə-ˌlōn\ n : an androgen $C_{19}H_{30}O_2$ used esp. in the treatment of breast cancer

stan·o·zo·lol \'sta-nə-zō-ˌlȯl\ n : an anabolic steroid $C_{21}H_{32}N_2O$

sta·pe·dec·to·my \ˌstā-pi-'dek-tə-mē\ n, pl **-mies** : surgical removal and prosthetic replacement of part or all of the stapes to relieve deafness

sta·pe·di·al \stā-'pē-dē-əl, stə-\ adj : of, relating to, or located near the stapes

sta·pe·di·us \stə-'pē-dē-əs\ n, pl **-dii** \-dē-ˌī\ : a small muscle of the middle ear that arises from the wall of the tympanum, is inserted into the neck of the stapes by a tendon that sometimes contains a slender spine of bone, and serves to check and dampen vibration of the stapes — called also stapedius muscle

sta·pes \'stā-(ˌ)pēz\ n, pl **stapes** or **sta·pe·des** \stə-'pē-ˌdēz\ : the innermost of the chain of ossicles of the ear which has the form of a stirrup, a base that occupies the oval window of the tympanum, and a head that is connected with the incus — called also stirrup

staph \'staf\ n : STAPHYLOCOCCUS 2; also : an infection with staphylococci

staphyl- or **staphylo-** comb form : staphylococcal ⟨staphylotoxin⟩

staph·y·lo·coc·cal \ˌsta-fə-lō-'kä-kəl\ also **staph·y·lo·coc·cic** \-'kä-kik, -'käk-sik\ adj : of, relating to, caused by, or being a staphylococcus ⟨∼ infection⟩

staphylococcal scalded skin syndrome n : an acute skin disorder esp. of infants and immunocompromised individuals that is characterized by widespread erythema, peeling, and necrosis of the skin, that is caused by a toxin produced by a bacterium of the genus Staphyloccus (S. aureus), and that exposes the affected individual to serious infections but is rarely fatal if diagnosed and treated promptly — abbr. SSSS; compare TOXIC EPIDERMAL NECROLYSIS

staph·y·lo·coc·co·sis \ˌsta-fə-lō-kä-'kō-səs\ n : infection with or disease caused by staphylococci

staph·y·lo·coc·cus \ˌsta-fə-lō-'kä-kəs\ n **1** cap : a genus of nonmotile gram-positive spherical bacteria (family Micrococcaceae) that occur singly, in pairs of tetrads, or in irregular clusters and include pathogens (as S. aureus) which infect the skin and mucous membranes **2** pl **-coc·ci** \-'käk-ˌsī\ : any bacterium of the genus Staphylococcus; broadly : MICROCOCCUS 2

staph·y·lo·ki·nase \-'kī-ˌnās, -ˌnāz\ n : a proteinase from some pathogenic staphylococci that converts plasminogen to plasmin

staph·y·lo·ma \ˌsta-fə-'lō-mə\ n : a protrusion of the cornea or sclera of the eye

staph·y·lo·tox·in \ˌsta-fə-lō-'täk-sən\ n : a toxin produced by staphylococci

sta·ple \'stā-pəl\ n : a usu. U-shaped and typically metal surgical fastener used to hold layers of tissue together (as in the closure of an incision) — **staple** vb — **sta·pler** \-plər\ n

starch \'stärch\ *n* : a white odorless tasteless granular or powdery complex carbohydrate ($C_6H_{10}O_5$)$_x$ that is the chief storage form of carbohydrate in plants, is an important foodstuff, has demulcent and absorbent properties, and is used in pharmacy esp. as a dusting powder and as a constituent of ointments and pastes — **starchy** \'stär-chē\ *adj*

Star·ling hypothesis \'stär-liŋ-\ *n* : a hypothesis in physiology: the flow of fluids across capillary walls depends on the balance between the force of blood pressure on the walls and the osmotic pressure across the walls so that the declining gradient in blood pressure from the arterial to the venous end of the capillary results in an outflow of fluids at its arterial end with an increasing inflow toward its venous end

E. H. Starling — see FRANK-STARLING LAW

Starling's law of the heart *n* : a statement in physiology: the strength of the heart's systolic contraction is directly proportional to its diastolic expansion with the result that under normal physiological conditions the heart pumps out of the right atrium all the blood returned to it without letting any back up in the veins — called also *Frank-Starling law, Frank≠Starling law of the heart, Starling's law*

starve \'stärv\ *vb* **starved; starv·ing 1 a** : to perish from lack of food **b** : to suffer extreme hunger **2** : to deprive of nourishment — **star·va·tion** \stär-'vā-shən\ *n*

sta·sis \'stā-səs, 'sta-\ *n, pl* **sta·ses** \'stā-ˌsēz, 'sta-\ : a slowing or stoppage of the normal flow of the bodily fluid or semifluid (biliary $\sim$): as **a** : slowing of the current of circulating blood **b** : reduced motility of the intestines with retention of feces

stasis ulcer *n* : an ulcer (as on the lower leg) caused by localized slowing or stoppage of blood flow

stat \'stat\ *adv* : STATIM

-stat \ˌstat\ *n comb form* : agent causing inhibition of growth without destruction (bacterio*stat*)

state \'stāt\ *n* : mode or condition of being: as **a** : condition of mind or temperament (a manic $\sim$) **b** : a condition or stage in the physical being of something (the gaseous $\sim$ of water)

state hospital *n* : a hospital for the mentally ill that is run by a state

stat·im \'sta-tim\ *adv* : without delay or immediately

sta·tion \'stā-shən\ *n* **1** : the place at which someone is positioned or is assigned to remain (the nurse's $\sim$ on a hospital ward) **2** : the act or manner of standing : POSTURE

sta·tion·ary \'stā-shə-ˌner-ē\ *adj* **1** : fixed in position : not moving **2**

: characterized by a lack of change

stato- *comb form* : balance : equilibrium (*stato*lith)

stato·co·nia \ˌsta-tə-'kō-nē-ə\ *n, pl* : OTOCONIA

stato·lith \'stat-ᵊl-ˌith\ *n* : OTOLITH

sta·tus \'stā-təs, 'sta-\ *n, pl* **sta·tus·es** : a particular state or condition

status asth·mat·i·cus \-az-'ma-ti-kəs\ *n* : an attack of asthma of long duration characterized by dyspnea, cyanosis, exhaustion, and sometimes collapse

status ep·i·lep·ti·cus \-ˌe-pə-'lep-ti-kəs\ *n* : a state in epilepsy in which the attacks occur in rapid succession without recovery of consciousness

stat·u·to·ry rape \ˌsta-chə-ˌtōr-ē-\ *n* : sexual intercourse with a person who is below the age of consent as defined by law

staunch *var of* STANCH

STD \ˌes-(ˌ)tē-'dē\ *n* : SEXUALLY TRANSMITTED DISEASE

steady state *n* : a state of physiological equilibrium esp. in connection with a specified metabolic relation or activity

steal \'stēl\ *n* : abnormal circulation characterized by deviation (as through collateral vessels or by backward flow) of blood to tissues where the normal flow of blood has been cut off by occlusion of an artery (coronary $\sim$)

ste·ap·sin \stē-'ap-sən\ *n* : the lipase in pancreatic juice

stea·rate \'stē-ə-ˌrāt, 'stir-ˌāt\ *n* : a salt or ester of stearic acid

stea·ric acid \stē-'ar-ik-, 'stir-ik-\ *n* : a white crystalline fatty acid $C_{18}H_{36}O_2$ obtained from tallow and some other hard fats; *also* : a commercial mixture of stearic and palmitic acids

stea·rin \'stē-ə-rən, 'stir-ən\ *n* : an ester of glycerol and stearic acid $C_3H_5(C_{18}H_{35}O_2)_3$ that is a predominant constituent of many hard fats

steat- *or* **steato-** *comb form* : fat (*steato*ma)

ste·a·ti·tis \ˌstē-ə-'tī-təs\ *n* : inflammation of fatty tissue; *esp* : YELLOW FAT DISEASE

ste·a·to·ma \ˌstē-ə-'tō-mə\ *n, pl* **-mas** *or* **-ma·ta** \-mə-tə\ : SEBACEOUS CYST

ste·ato·py·gia \ˌstē-ə-tə-'pij-ē-ə, stē-ˌa-tō-, -'pī-\ *n* : an accumulation of a large amount of fat on the buttocks that occurs esp. among women of some peoples of African descent — **ste·ato·py·gous** \-'pī-gəs\ *or* **ste·ato·py·gic** \-'pij-ik, -'pī-jik\ *adj*

ste·at·or·rhea \ˌ(ˌ)stē-ˌa-tə-'rē-ə\ *n* : an excess of fat in the stools (idiopathic $\sim$)

ste·at·or·rhoea *chiefly Brit var of* STEATORRHEA

ste·a·to·sis \ˌstē-ə-'tō-səs\ *n, pl* **-to·ses** \-ˌsēz\ : FATTY DEGENERATION

Stein–Lev·en·thal syndrome \'stin-'lev-ᵊn-ˌthäl-\ *n* : POLYCYSTIC OVARY SYNDROME

Stein, Irving Freiler (1887–1976), and **Leventhal, Michael Leo (1901–1971)**, American gynecologists.

Stein·mann pin \'stīn-mən-\ n : a stainless steel spike used for the internal fixation of fractures of long bones

Steinmann, Fritz (1872–1932), Swiss surgeon.

Stel·a·zine \'ste-lə-ˌzēn\ trademark — used for a preparation of trifluoperazine

stel·late \'ste-ˌlāt\ adj : shaped like a star ⟨a ∼ ulcer⟩

stellate cell n : a cell (as a Kupffer cell) with radiating cytoplasmic processes

stellate ganglion n : a composite ganglion formed by fusion of the most inferior of the three cervical ganglia with the first thoracic ganglion of the sympathetic chain

stellate ligament n : RADIATE LIGAMENT

stellate reticulum n : a loosely-connected mass of stellate epithelial cells that in early developmental stages makes up a large portion of the enamel organ

stem cell n : an unspecialized cell that gives rise to differentiated cells ⟨hematopoietic stem cells in bone marrow⟩

ste·nosed \ste-'nōst, -'nōzd\ adj : affected with stenosis : abnormally constricted ⟨a ∼ eustachian tube⟩

ste·nos·ing \ste-'nō-siŋ, -ziŋ\ adj : causing or characterized by stenosis ⟨as of a tendon sheath⟩

ste·no·sis \stə-'nō-səs\ n, pl -no·ses \-ˌsēz\ : a narrowing or constriction of the diameter of a bodily passage or orifice ⟨esophageal ∼⟩

ste·not·ic \stə-'nä-tik\ adj : of, relating to, characterized by, or causing stenosis ⟨∼ lesions⟩

Sten·sen's duct also **Sten·son's duct** \'sten-sənz-\ n : PAROTID DUCT

Sten·sen or **Sten·son** \'stän-sən\, **Niels** (Latin **Nicolaus Steno**) (1638–1686), Danish anatomist and geologist.

stent \'stent\ n : a mold formed from a resinous compound and used for holding a surgical graft in place; also : something (as a pad of gauze immobilized by sutures) used like a stent

Stent, Charles R. (1845–1901), British dentist.

Steph·a·no·fi·lar·ia \ˌste-fə-ˌnō-fi-'lar-ē-ə\ n : a genus of filarial worms parasitic in the skin and subcutaneous tissues of ruminants and horses where they may cause dermatitis and extensive degenerative lesions

Steph·a·nu·rus \ˌste-fə-'nur-əs, -'nyur-\ n : a genus of strongylid nematode worms that includes the kidney worm ⟨S. dentatus⟩ of swine

ster·co·ra·ceous \ˌstər-kə-'rā-shəs\ adj : of, relating to, containing, produced by, or being feces : FECAL

ster·cu·lia gum \stər-'kül-yə-, -'kyül-\ n : KARAYA GUM

stere- or **stereo-** comb form 1 : stereoscopic ⟨stereopsis⟩ 2 : having or dealing with three dimensions of space ⟨stereotaxic⟩

ste·reo·cil·i·um \ˌster-ē-ō-'si-lē-əm, ˌstir-\ n, pl -ia \-lē-ə\ : any of the immobile processes that resemble cilia and occur on the free border of various epithelia — see KINOCILIUM

ste·re·og·no·sis \ˌster-ē-äg-'nō-səs, ˌstir-\ n : ability to perceive or the perception of material qualities (as form and weight) of an object by handling or lifting it : tactile recognition

ste·reo·iso·mer \ˌster-ē-ō-'ī-sə-mər, ˌstir-\ n : any of a group of isomers in which atoms are linked in the same order but differ in their spatial arrangement — **ste·reo·iso·mer·ic** \-ˌī-sə-'mer-ik\ adj — **ste·reo·isom·er·ism** \-ī-'sä-mə-ˌri-zəm\ n

ste·re·op·sis \ˌster-ē-'äp-səs, ˌstir-\ n : stereoscopic vision

ste·reo·scope \'ster-ē-ə-ˌskōp, 'stir-\ n : an optical instrument with two eyepieces for helping the observer to combine the images of two pictures taken from points of view a little way apart and thus to get the effect of solidity or depth

ste·reo·scop·ic \ˌster-ē-ə-'skä-pik, ˌstir-\ adj 1 : of or relating to the stereoscope or the production of three-dimensional images 2 : characterized by the seeing of objects in three dimensions ⟨∼ vision⟩ — **ste·reo·scop·i·cal·ly** adv — **ste·re·os·co·py** \ˌster-ē-'äs-kə-pē, ˌstir-; 'ster-ē-ə-ˌskō-pē, 'stir-\ n

ste·reo·tac·tic \ˌster-ē-ə-'tak-tik, ˌstir-\ adj : STEREOTAXIC — **ste·reo·tac·ti·cal·ly** adv

ste·reo·tax·ic \ˌster-ē-ə-'tak-sik, ˌstir-\ adj : of, relating to, or being a technique or apparatus used in neurological research or surgery for directing the tip of a delicate instrument (as a needle or an electrode) in three planes in attempting to reach a specific locus in the brain — **ste·reo·tax·i·cal·ly** adv

ste·reo·tax·is \-'tak-səs\ n, pl -tax·es \-ˌsēz\ : a stereotaxic technique or procedure

¹**ste·reo·type** \'ster-ē-ə-ˌtīp, 'stir-\ vb **-typed; -typ·ing** 1 : to repeat without variation ⟨stereotyped behavior⟩ 2 : to develop a mental stereotype about

²**stereotype** n : something conforming to a fixed or general pattern; esp : an often oversimplified or biased mental picture held to characterize the typical individual of a group — **ste·reo·typ·i·cal** \ˌster-ē-ə-'ti-pi-kəl\ also **ste·reo·typ·ic** \-pik\ adj

ste·reo·ty·py \'ster-ē-ə-ˌtī-pē, 'stir-\ n, pl -pies : frequent almost mechanical repetition of the same posture, movement, or form of speech (as in schizophrenia)

ster·il·ant \'ster-ə-lənt\ *n* : a sterilizing agent

ster·ile \'ster-əl\ *adj* **1** : failing to produce or incapable of producing offspring ⟨a ~ hybrid⟩ **2** : free from living organisms and esp. microorganisms ⟨a ~ cyst⟩ — **ster·ile·ly** *adv* — **ste·ril·i·ty** \stə-'ri-lə-tē\ *n*

ster·il·ize \'ster-ə-ˌlīz\ *vb* **-ized; -iz·ing** : to make sterile : **a** : to deprive of the power of reproducing **b** : to free from living microorganisms usu. by the use of physical or chemical agents — **ster·il·i·za·tion** \ˌster-ə-lə-'zā-shən\ *n* — **ster·il·iz·er** \'ster-ə-ˌlī-zər\ *n*

stern- *or* **sterno-** *comb form* **1** : breast : sternum : breastbone ⟨*sterno*tomy⟩ **2** : sternal and ⟨*sterno*costal⟩

ster·nal \'stərn-ᵊl\ *adj* : of or relating to the sternum

ster·ne·bra \'stər-nə-brə\ *n, pl* **-brae** \-ˌbrē, -ˌbrī\ : any of the four segments into which the body of the sternum is divided in childhood and which fuse to form the gladiolus

ster·no·cla·vic·u·lar \ˌstər-nō-kla-'vi-kyə-lər\ *adj* : of, relating to, or being articulation of the sternum and the clavicle ⟨the ~ joint⟩ ⟨~ dislocation⟩

ster·no·clei·do·mas·toid \ˌstər-nō-ˌklī-də-'mas-ˌtoid\ *n* : a thick superficial muscle on each side that arises by one head from the first segment of the sternum and by a second from the inner part of the clavicle, that inserts into the mastoid process and occipital bone, flex, and acts esp. to bend, rotate, flex, and extend the head — **sternocleidomastoid** *adj*

ster·no·clei·do·mas·toi·de·us \-ˌmas-'tòi-dē-əs\ *n, pl* **-dei** \-dē-ˌī\ : STERNOCLEIDOMASTOID

ster·no·cos·tal \ˌstər-nō-'käst-ᵊl\ *adj* : of, relating to, or situated between the sternum and ribs

ster·no·hy·oid \ˌstər-nō-'hī-ˌoid\ *n* : an infrahyoid muscle on each side of the midline that arises from the medial end of the clavicle and the first segment of the sternum, inserts into the body of the hyoid bone, and acts to depress the hyoid bone and the larynx — **sternohyoid** *adj*

ster·no·hy·oi·de·us \-hi-'oi-dē-əs\ *n, pl* **-dei** \-dē-ˌī\ : STERNOHYOID

ster·no·mas·toid muscle \-'mas-ˌtoid-\ *n* : STERNOCLEIDOMASTOID

ster·no·thy·roid \ˌstər-nō-'thī-ˌroid\ *n* : an infrahyoid muscle on each side of the body below the sternohyoid that arises from the sternum and from the cartilage of the first and sometimes of the second ribs, inserts into the thyroid cartilage, and acts to draw the larynx downward by depressing the thyroid cartilage — **sternothyroid** *adj*

ster·no·thy·roi·de·us \-'roi-dē-əs\ *n, pl* **-dei** \-dē-ˌī\ : STERNOTHYROID

ster·not·o·my \stər-'nä-tə-mē\ *n, pl* **-mies** : surgical incision through the sternum

ster·num \'stər-nəm\ *n, pl* **-nums** *or* **-na** \-nə\ : a compound ventral bone or cartilage that lies in the median central part of the body of most vertebrates other than fishes and that in humans is about seven inches (18 centimeters) long, consists in the adult of three parts, and connects with the clavicles and the cartilages of the upper seven pairs of ribs — called also **breastbone**

ster·nu·ta·tion \ˌstər-nyə-'tā-shən\ *n* : the act, fact, or noise of sneezing

ster·nu·ta·tor \'stər-nyə-ˌtā-tər\ *n* : an agent that induces sneezing and often lacrimation and vomiting

ste·roid \'ster-ˌoid, 'stir-\ *n* : any of numerous compounds containing a 17-carbon 4-ring system and including the sterols and various hormones and glycosides — **steroid** *or* **ste·roi·dal** \stə-'roid-ᵊl\ *adj*

steroid hormone *n* : any of numerous hormones (as estrogen, testosterone, cortisone, and aldosterone) having the characteristic ring structure of steroids and formed in the body from cholesterol

ste·roi·do·gen·e·sis \stə-ˌroi-də-'je-nə-səs; ˌstir-ˌoi-, ˌster-\ *n, pl* **-e·ses** \-ˌsēz\ : synthesis of steroids ⟨adrenal ~⟩ — **ste·roi·do·gen·ic** \-'je-nik\ *adj*

ste·rol \'stir-ˌol, 'ster-, -ˌōl\ *n* : any of various solid steroid alcohols (as cholesterol) widely distributed in animal and plant lipids

ster·to·rous \'stər-tə-rəs\ *adj* : characterized by a harsh snoring or gasping sound — **ster·to·rous·ly** *adv*

stetho·scope \'ste-thə-ˌskōp\ *n* : an instrument used to detect and study sounds produced in the body that are conveyed to the ears of the listener through rubber tubing connected with a usu. cup-shaped piece placed upon the area to be examined — **stetho·scop·ic** \ˌste-thə-'skä-pik\ *adj* — **stetho·scop·i·cal·ly** *adv*

Ste·vens–John·son syndrome \'stē-vənz-'jän-sən-\ *n* : a severe and sometimes fatal form of erythema multiforme that is characterized esp. by purulent conjunctivitis, Vincent's angina, and ulceration of the genitals and anus and that often results in blindness

Stevens, Albert Mason (1884–1945), and Johnson, Frank Chambliss (1894–1934), American pediatricians.

STH *abbr* somatotropic hormone

sthen·ic \'sthe-nik\ *adj* : notably or excessively vigorous or active ⟨~ fever⟩ ⟨~ emotions⟩ **2** : PYKNIC

stib·o·phen \'sti-bə-ˌfen\ *n* : a crystalline antimony compound $C_{12}H_4Na_5-O_{16}S_4Sb\cdot7H_2O$ used in the treatment of various tropical diseases

stick·tight flea \'stik-ˌtīt-\ *n* : a flea of the genus *Echidnophaga* (*E. gallin-*

acea) that is parasitic esp. on the heads of chickens

sties *pl of* STY

stiff \'stif\ *adj* : lacking in suppleness ⟨∼ muscles⟩ — **stiff·ness** *n*

stiff–lamb disease \'stif-₁lam-\ *n* : white muscle disease occurring in lambs

stiff–man syndrome *n* : a chronic progressive disorder of uncertain etiology that is characterized by painful spasms and increasing stiffness of the muscles

sti·fle \'stī-fəl\ *n* : the joint next above the hock in the hind leg of a quadruped (as a horse) corresponding to the knee in humans

stig·ma \'stig-mə\ *n, pl* **stig·ma·ta** \stig-'mä-tə, 'stig-mə-tə\ *or* **stigmas 1** : an identifying mark or characteristic; *specif* : a specific diagnostic sign of a disease ⟨the *stigmata* of syphilis⟩ **2** : PETECHIA **3** : a small spot, scar, or opening on a plant or animal

stilb·am·i·dine \stil-'ba-mə-₁dēn\ *n* : a drug $C_{16}H_{16}N_4$ used chiefly in the form of one of its salts in treating various fungal infections

stil·bes·trol \stil-'bes-₁tról, -₁tról\ *n* **1** : a crystalline compound $C_{14}H_{12}O_2$ that differs from the related diethylstilbestrol in lack of the ethyl groups and in possession of only slight estrogenic activity **2** : DIETHYLSTILBESTROL

sti·let \'stī-lət\ *or* **sti·lette** \sti-'let\ *n* : STYLET

still–birth \'stil-₁bərth\ *n* : the birth of a dead fetus — compare LIVE BIRTH

still–born \-'bórn\ *adj* : dead at birth — compare LIVE-BORN — **stillborn** *n*

Still's disease \'stilz-\ *n* : rheumatoid arthritis in children

Still, Sir George Frederic (1868–1941), British pediatrician.

stim·u·lant \'stim-yə-lənt\ *n* **1** : an agent (as a drug) that produces a temporary increase of the functional activity or efficiency of an organism or any of its parts **2** : STIMULUS 2

stim·u·late \-₁lāt\ *vb* **-lat·ed; -lat·ing 1** : to excite to activity or growth or to greater activity **2 a** : to function as a physiological stimulus to (as a nerve or muscle) **b** : to arouse or affect by a stimulant (as a drug) — **stim·u·la·tion** \₁stim-yə-'lā-shən\ *n* — **stim·u·la·tive** \'stim-yə-₁lā-tiv\ *adj* — **stim·u·la·to·ry** \-lə-₁tór-ē\ *adj*

stim·u·la·tor \'stim-yə-₁lā-tər\ *n* : one that stimulates; *specif* : an instrument used to provide a stimulus

stim·u·lus \'stim-yə-ləs\ *n, pl* **-li** \-₁lī, -₁lē\ **1** : STIMULANT 1 **2** : an agent (as an environmental change) that directly influences the activity of living protoplasm (as by exciting a sensory organ or evoking muscular contraction or glandular secretion) ⟨a visual ∼⟩

stimulus–response *adj* : of, relating to, or being a reaction to a stimulus; *also*

: representing the activity of an organism as composed of such reactions ⟨∼ psychology⟩

sting \'stiŋ\ *vb* **stung** \'stəŋ\; **sting·ing 1** : to prick painfully: as **a** : to pierce or wound with a poisonous or irritating process **b** : to affect with sharp quick pain **2** : to feel or cause a keen burning pain or smart ⟨the injection *stung*⟩ — **sting** *n*

sting·er \'stiŋ-ər\ *n* : a sharp organ (as of a bee or scorpion) that is usu. connected with a poison gland or otherwise adapted to wound by piercing and injecting a poison

sting·ray \'stiŋ-₁rā\ *n* : any of numerous large flat cartilaginous fishes (order Rajiformes and esp. family Dasyatidae) with one or more large sharp barbed dorsal spines near the base of the whiplike tail capable of inflicting severe wounds

stint *var of* STENT

stip·pling \'stip-liŋ\ *n* : the appearance of spots : a spotted condition (as in basophilic red blood cells)

stir·rup \'stər-əp, 'stir-əp\ *n* **1** : STAPES **2** : an attachment to an examining or operating table designed to raise and spread the legs of a patient

stitch \'stich\ *n* **1** : a local sharp and sudden pain esp. in the side **2 a** : one in-and-out movement of a threaded needle in suturing **b** : a portion of a suture left in the tissue after one stitch ⟨removal of ∼es⟩ — **stitch** *vb*

stock·ing \'stäk-iŋ\ — see ELASTIC STOCKING

Stokes–Ad·ams syndrome \'stōks-'a-dəmz-\ *n* : fainting and convulsions induced by complete heart block with a pulse rate of 40 beats per minute or less — called also *Adams-Stokes syndrome, Stokes-Adams attack, Stokes–Adams disease*

W. Stokes — see CHEYNE-STOKES RESPIRATION

Adams, Robert (1791–1875), British physician.

sto·ma \'stō-mə\ *n, pl* **-mas** : an artificial permanent opening esp. in the abdominal wall made in surgical procedures ⟨a colostomy ∼⟩

stom·ach \'stə-mik\ *n* **1 a** : a dilatation of the alimentary canal communicating anteriorly with the esophagus and posteriorly with the duodenum and being typically a simple often curved sac with an outer serous coat, a strong complex muscular wall that contracts rhythmically, and a mucous lining membrane that contains gastric glands **b** : one of the compartments of a ruminant stomach **2** : the part of the body that contains the stomach : BELLY, ABDOMEN

stom·ach·ache \-₁āk\ *n* : pain in or in the region of the stomach

sto·mach·ic \stə-'ma-kik\ *n* : a stimulant or tonic for the stomach

stomach pump *n* : a suction pump with

a flexible tube for removing liquid from the stomach

stomach tube *n* : a flexible rubber tube to be passed through the esophagus into the stomach for introduction of material or removal of gastric contents

stomach worm *n* : any of various nematode worms parasitic in the stomach of mammals or birds; *esp* : a worm of the genus *Haemonchus* (*H. contortus*) common in domestic ruminants

sto·mal \'stō-məl\ *adj* : of, relating to, or situated near a surgical stoma

stomat- *or* **stomato-** *comb form* : mouth ⟨*stomatitis*⟩ ⟨*stomatology*⟩

sto·ma·ti·tis \ˌstō-mə-'tī-təs\ *n, pl* **-tit·i·des** \-'ti-tə-ˌdēz\ *or* **-ti·tis·es** \ˌti-tə-səz\ : any of numerous inflammatory diseases of the mouth having various causes (as mechanical trauma, irritants, allergy, vitamin deficiency, or infection) ⟨erosive ~⟩

sto·ma·to·gnath·ic \ˌstō-mə-(ˌ)täg-'na-thik\ *adj* : of or relating to the jaws and the mouth

sto·ma·tol·o·gist \ˌstō-mə-'tä-lə-jist\ *n* : a specialist in stomatology

sto·ma·tol·o·gy \ˌstō-mə-'tä-lə-jē\ *n, pl* **-gies** : a branch of medical science dealing with the mouth and its disorders — **sto·ma·to·log·i·cal** \ˌstō-mət-ʔl-'ä-ji-kəl\ *also* **sto·ma·to·log·ic** \-jik\ *adj*

-sto·mia \'stō-mē-ə\ *n comb form* : mouth exhibiting (such) a condition ⟨xero*stomia*⟩

sto·mo·de·um *or* **sto·mo·dae·um** \ˌstō-mə-'dē-əm\ *n, pl* **-dea** *or* **-daea** \-'dē-ə\ *also* **-deums** *or* **-daeums** : the embryonic anterior ectodermal part of the alimentary canal or tract — **sto·mo·de·al** *or* **sto·mo·dae·al** \-'dē-əl\ *adj*

Sto·mox·ys \stə-'mäk-səs\ *n* : a genus of bloodsucking dipteran flies (family Muscidae) that includes the stable fly (*S. calcitrans*)

-sto·my \s-tə-mē\ *n comb form, pl* **-sto·mies** : surgical operation establishing a usu. permanent opening into (such) a part ⟨entero*stomy*⟩

stone \'stōn\ *n* : CALCULUS 1

stone–blind \'stōn-'blīnd\ *adj* : totally blind

stoned \'stōnd\ *adj* : being drunk or under the influence of a drug (as marijuana) taken esp. for pleasure

stone–deaf *adj* : totally deaf

stool \'stül\ *n* : a discharge of fecal matter

storage disease *n* : the abnormal accumulation in the body of one or more specific substances and esp. metabolic substances (as cerebrosides in Gaucher's disease)

sto·rax \'stōr-ˌaks\ *n* **1** : a fragrant balsam obtained from the bark of an Asian tree of the genus *Liquidambar* (*L. orientalis*) that is used as an expectorant — called also *Levant storax* **2** : a balsam similar to storax that is obtained from a No. American

tree of the genus *Liquidambar* (*L. styraciflua*) — called also *liquidambar*

storm \'stȯrm\ *n* : a crisis or sudden increase in the symptoms of a disease — see THYROID STORM

stormy \'stȯr-mē\ *adj* **storm·i·er; -est** : having alternating exacerbations and remissions of symptoms

STP \ˌes-(ˌ)tē-'pē\ *n* : a psychedelic drug chemically related to mescaline and amphetamine — called also *DOM*

stra·bis·mus \strə-'biz-məs\ *n* : inability of one eye to attain binocular vision with the other because of imbalance of the muscles of the eyeball — called also *heterotropia, squint* — **stra·bis·mic** \strə-'biz-mik\ *adj*

straight·jack·et *var of* STRAITJACKET

straight sinus *n* : a venous sinus of the brain that is located along the line of junction of the falx cerebri and tentorium cerebelli and passes posteriorly to terminate in the confluence of sinuses

¹**strain** \'strān\ *n* : a group of presumed common ancestry with clear-cut physiological but usu. not morphological distinctions ⟨a ~ of bacteria⟩

²**strain** *vb* **1 a** : to exert (as oneself) to the utmost **b** : to injure by overuse, misuse, or excessive pressure ⟨~ed his heart by overwork⟩ **2** : to contract the muscles forcefully in attempting to defecate — often used in the phrase *strain at stool*

³**strain** *n* : an act of straining or the condition of being strained: as **a** : excessive physical or mental tension; *also* : a force, influence, or factor causing such tension **b** : bodily injury from excessive tension, effort, or use ⟨heart ~⟩; *esp* : one resulting from a wrench or twist and involving undue stretching of muscles or ligaments ⟨back ~⟩ — compare SPRAIN

strait·jack·et \'strāt-ˌja-kət\ *n* : a cover or garment of strong material (as canvas) used to bind the body and esp. the arms closely in restraining a violent prisoner or patient

stra·mo·ni·um \strə-'mō-nē-əm\ *n* **1** : the dried leaves of the jimsonweed (*Datura stramonium*) or of a related plant of the genus *Datura* that contain toxic alkaloids (as atropine) and are used in medicine similarly to belladonna **2** : JIMSONWEED

strand \'strand\ *n* : something (as a molecular chain) resembling a thread

strand·ed \'strand-dəd\ *adj* : having a strand or strands esp. of a specified kind or number — usu. used in combination ⟨double-*stranded* DNA⟩ — **strand·ed·ness** *n*

stran·gle \'stran-gəl\ *vb* **stran·gled; stran·gling 1** : to choke to death **2** : to obstruct seriously or fatally the normal breathing of

stran·gles \-gəlz\ *n sing or pl* : an infectious febrile disease of horses and other equines that is caused by a bacterium of the genus *Streptococcus* (*S. equi*)

stran·gu·lat·ed hernia \'straŋ-gyə-ˌlā-təd-\ *n* : a hernia in which the blood supply of the herniated viscus is so constricted by swelling and congestion as to arrest its circulation

stran·gu·la·tion \ˌstraŋ-gyə-'lā-shən\ *n* **1** : the action or process of strangling or of becoming constricted so as to stop circulation **2** : the state or condition resulting from strangulation; *esp* : excessive or pathological constriction or compression of a bodily tube (as a blood vessel or a loop of intestine) that interrupts its ability to act as a passage — **stran·gu·late** \'straŋ-gyə-ˌlāt\ *vb*

stran·gu·ry \'straŋ-gyə-rē, -ˌgyùr-ē\ *n, pl* **-ries** : a slow and painful discharge of urine drop by drop produced by spasmodic muscular contraction of the urethra and bladder

¹strap \'strap\ *n* : a flexible band or strip (as of adhesive plaster)

²strap *vb* **strapped; strap·ping 1** : to secure with or attach by means of a strap **2** : to support (as a sprained joint) with overlapping strips of adhesive plaster

strapping *n* : the application of adhesive plaster in overlapping strips upon or around a part (as a sprained ankle) to serve as a splint to reduce motion or to hold surgical dressings in place upon a surgical wound; *also* : material so used

strat·i·fied \'stra-tə-ˌfīd\ *adj* : arranged in layers; *esp* : of, relating to, or being an epithelium consisting of more than one layer of cells — **strat·i·fi·ca·tion** \ˌstra-tə-fə-'kā-shən\ *n*

stra·tum \'strā-təm, 'stra-\ *n, pl* **stra·ta** \'strā-tə, 'stra-\ : a layer of tissue

stratum ba·sa·le \-bā-'sā-lē\ *n, pl* **strata ba·sa·lia** \-lē-ə\ : the layer of stratum germinativum esp. in the endometrium that undergoes mitotic division

stratum com·pac·tum \-kəm-'pak-təm\ *n, pl* **strata com·pac·ta** \-'pak-tə\ : the relatively dense superficial layer of the endometrium

stratum corneum *n, pl* **strata cornea** : the outer more or less horny part of the epidermis

stratum ger·mi·na·ti·vum \-ˌjər-mə-nə-'tī-vəm\ *n, pl* **strata ger·mi·na·ti·va** \-və\ **1** : the innermost layer of the epidermis consisting of a single row of columnar or cuboidal epithelial cells that continually divide and replace the rest of the epidermis — see STRATUM BASALE **2** : MALPIGHIAN LAYER

stratum gran·u·lo·sum \-ˌgran-yə-'lō-səm\ *n, pl* **strata gran·u·lo·sa** \-sə\ : a layer of granular cells lying immediately above the stratum germinativum in most parts of the epidermis

stratum in·ter·me·di·um \-ˌin-tər-'mē-dē-əm\ *n, pl* **strata in·ter·me·dia** \-dē-ə\ : the cell layer of the enamel organ next to the layer of ameloblasts

stratum lu·ci·dum \-'lü-si-dəm\ *n, pl* **strata lu·ci·da** \-də\ : a thin somewhat translucent layer of cells lying under the stratum corneum esp. in thickened epidermis

stratum spi·no·sum \-spi-'nō-səm\ *n, pl* **strata spi·no·sa** \-sə\ : the layers of prickle cells over the layer of the stratum germinativum capable of undergoing mitosis — called also *prickle cell layer*

stratum spon·gi·o·sum \-ˌspən-jē-'ō-səm\ *n, pl* **strata spon·gi·o·sa** \-sə\ : the middle layer of the endometrium between the stratum basale and stratum compactum that contains dilated and tortuous portions of the uterine glands

strawberry gallbladder *n* : an abnormal condition characterized by the deposition of cholesterol in the lining of the gallbladder in a pattern resembling the surface of a strawberry

strawberry mark *n* : a tumor of the skin filled with small blood vessels and appearing usu. as a red and elevated birthmark

strawberry tongue *n* : a tongue that is red from swollen congested papillae and that occurs esp. in scarlet fever and Kawasaki disease

¹streak \'strēk\ *n* **1** : a usu. irregular line or stripe — see PRIMITIVE STREAK **2** : inoculum implanted in a line on a solid medium

²streak *vb* : to implant (inoculum) in a line on a solid medium

stream \'strēm\ *n* : an unbroken current or flow (as of a bodily fluid or a gas) — see BLOODSTREAM, MIDSTREAM

stream of consciousness *n* : the continuous unedited flow of conscious experience through the mind

street virus *n* : a naturally occurring rabies virus as distinguished from virus attenuated in the laboratory

strength \'streŋth, 'strenth\ *n, pl* **strengths 1** : the quality or state of being strong : capacity for exertion or endurance **2** : degree of potency of effect or of concentration **3** : degree of ionization of a solution — used of acids and bases

strep \'strep\ *n, often attrib* : STREPTOCOCCUS (a ~ infection)

strepho·sym·bo·lia \ˌstre-fō-sim-'bō-lē-ə\ *n* : a learning disorder in which symbols and esp. phrases, words, or letters appear to be reversed or transposed in reading

strep throat *n* : an inflammatory sore throat caused by hemolytic streptococci and marked by fever, prostration, and toxemia — called also *septic sore throat, strep sore throat*

strepto- *comb form* **1** : twisted : twisted

chain ⟨*strepto*coccus⟩ 2 : streptococcus ⟨*strepto*kinase⟩

strep·to·ba·cil·lus \ˌstrep-tō-bə-ˈsi-ləs\ *n* 1 *cap* : a genus of facultatively anaerobic gram-negative rod bacteria that includes one (*S. moniliformis*) that is the causative agent of one form of rat-bite fever 2 *pl* **-li** \-ˌlī\ : any of various nonmotile gram-negative bacilli in which the individual cells are joined in a chain; *esp* : one of the genus *Streptobacillus* — **strep·to·ba·cil·la·ry** \-ˈba-sə-ˌler-ē, -bə-ˈsi-lə-rē\ *adj*

strep·to·coc·cal \ˌstrep-tə-ˈkä-kəl\ *also* **strep·to·coc·cic** \-ˈkä-kik, -ˈkäk-sik\ *adj* : of, relating to, caused by, or being streptococci ⟨~ gingivitis⟩

strep·to·coc·cus \-ˈkä-kəs\ *n* 1 *cap* : a genus of spherical or ovoid chiefly nonmotile and parasitic gram-positive bacteria (family Streptococcaceae) that divide only in one plane, occur in pairs or chains, and include important pathogens of humans and domestic animals 2 *pl* **-coc·ci** \-ˈkä-ˌkī, -ˈkäk-ˌsī\ : any bacterium of the genus *Streptococcus*; *broadly* : a coccus occurring in chains

strep·to·dor·nase \ˌstrep-tō-ˈdòr-ˌnās, -ˌnāz\ *n* : a deoxyribonuclease from hemolytic streptococci that dissolves pus and is usu. administered in a mixture with streptokinase — see VARIDASE

strep·to·ki·nase \ˌstrep-tō-ˈkī-ˌnās, -ˌnāz\ *n* : a proteolytic enzyme from hemolytic streptococci active in promoting dissolution of blood clots — see VARIDASE

strep·to·ly·sin \ˌstrep-tə-ˈlīs-ᵊn\ *n* : any of various antigenic hemolysins produced by streptococci

strep·to·my·ces \-ˈmī-ˌsēz\ *n* 1 *cap* : a genus of mostly soil streptomyces including some that form antibiotics as by-products of their metabolism 2 *pl* **streptomyces** : any bacterium of the genus *Streptomyces*

strep·to·my·cete \-ˈmī-ˌsēt, -ˌmī-ˈsēt\ *n* : any of a family (Streptomycetaceae) of actinomycetes (as a streptomyces) that are typically aerobic soil saprophytes but include a few parasites of plants and animals

strep·to·my·cin \-ˈmīs-ᵊn\ *n* : an antibiotic $C_{21}H_{39}N_7O_{12}$ that is produced by a soil actinomycete of the genus *Streptomyces* (*S. griseus*), is active against bacteria, and is used esp. in the treatment of infections (as tuberculosis) by gram-negative bacteria

strep·to·ni·grin \-ˈnī-grən\ *n* : a toxic antibiotic $C_{25}H_{22}N_4O_8$ from an actinomycete of the genus *Streptomyces* (*S. flocculus*) that is used as an antineoplastic agent

strep·to·zo·cin \ˌstrep-tə-ˈzō-sən\ *n* : STREPTOZOTOCIN

strep·to·zot·o·cin \ˌstrep-tə-ˈzä-tə-sən\ *n* : a broad-spectrum antibiotic $C_8H_{15}N_3O_7$ with antineoplastic and diabetogenic properties that has been isolated from a bacterium of the genus *Streptomyces* (*S. achromogenes*)

stress \ˈstres\ *n* 1 **a** : a force exerted when one body or body part presses on, pulls on, pushes against, or tends to compress or twist another body or body part **b** : the deformation caused in a body by such a force 2 **a** : a physical, chemical, or emotional factor that causes bodily or mental tension and may be a factor in disease causation **b** : a state of bodily or mental tension resulting from factors that tend to alter an existent equilibrium 3 : the force exerted between teeth of the upper and lower jaws during mastication — **stress** *vb* — **stress·ful** \ˈstres-fəl\ *adj* — **stress·ful·ly** *adv*

stress breaker *n* : a flexible dental device used to lessen the occlusal forces exerted on teeth to which a partial denture is attached

stress fracture *n* : a usu. hairline fracture of a bone that has been subjected to repeated stress

stress·or \ˈstre-sər, -ˌsòr\ *n* : a stimulus that causes stress

stress test *n* : an electrocardiographic test of heart function before, during, and after a controlled period of increasingly strenuous exercise (as on a treadmill)

¹stretch \ˈstrech\ *vb* 1 : to extend or become extended in length or breadth 2 : to enlarge or distend esp. by force

²stretch *n* : the act of stretching : the state of being stretched

stretch·er \ˈstre-chər\ *n* : a device for carrying a sick, injured, or dead person

stretch·er—bear·er \-ˌbar-ər\ *n* : one who carries one end of a stretcher

stretch marks *n pl* : striae on the skin (as of the hips, abdomen, and breasts) from excessive stretching and rupture of elastic fibers esp. due to pregnancy or obesity

stretch receptor *n* : MUSCLE SPINDLE

stretch reflex *n* : a spinal reflex involving reflex contraction of a muscle in response to stretching — called also *myotatic reflex*

stria \ˈstrī-ə\ *n, pl* **stri·ae** \ˈstrī-ˌē\ 1 : STRIATION 2 2 : a narrow structural band esp. of nerve fibers 3 : a stripe or line (as in the skin) distinguished from surrounding tissue by color, texture, or elevation — see STRETCH MARKS

striata *pl of* STRIATUM

stri·a·tal \strī-ˈāt-ᵊl\ *adj* : of or relating to the corpus striatum ⟨~ neurons⟩

stri·ate cortex \ˈstrī-ət-, -ˌāt-\ *n* : an area of the brain that receives visual impulses, contains a conspicuous band of myelinated fibers, and is located mostly in the walls and along the edges of the calcarine sulcus of the occipital lobe — called also *visual projection area*

stri·at·ed \'strī-ˌā-təd\ *adj* **1** : marked with striae **2** : of, relating to, or being striated muscle

striated muscle *n* : muscle tissue that is marked by transverse dark and light bands, that is made up of elongated multinuclear fibers, and that includes skeletal and cardiac muscle of vertebrates and most muscle of arthropods — compare SMOOTH MUSCLE, VOLUNTARY MUSCLE

stria ter·mi·na·lis \-ˌtər-mə-'nā-ləs\ *n* : a bundle of nerve fibers that passes from the amygdala mostly to the anterior part of the hypothalamus with a few fibers crossing the anterior commissure to the amygdala on the opposite side

stri·a·tion \strī-'ā-shən\ *n* **1** : the fact or state of being striated **2** : a minute groove, scratch, or channel esp. when one of a parallel series **3** : any of the alternate dark and light cross bands of a myofibril of striated muscle

stri·a·to·ni·gral \strī-ˌā-tə-'nī-grəl\ *adj* : connecting the corpus striatum and substantia nigra ⟨~ axons⟩

stri·a·tum \strī-'ā-təm\ *n, pl* **stri·a·ta** \-'ā-tə\ **1** : CORPUS STRIATUM **2** : NEOSTRIATUM

stria vas·cu·la·ris \-ˌvas-kyə-'ler-əs\ *n* : the upper part of the spiral ligament of the scala media that contains numerous small blood vessels

stric·ture \'strik-chər\ *n* : an abnormal narrowing of a bodily passage (as from inflammation or the formation of scar tissue); *also* : the narrowed part

stri·dor \'strī-dər, -ˌdȯr\ *n* : a harsh vibrating sound heard during respiration in cases of obstruction of the air passages (laryngeal ~) — **strid·u·lous** \'strij-ə-ləs\ *adj*

stridulus — see LARYNGISMUS STRIDULUS

strike \'strīk\ *n* : cutaneous myiasis (as of sheep) ⟨body ~⟩ ⟨blowfly ~⟩

string·halt \'striŋ-ˌhȯlt\ *n* : a condition of lameness in the hind legs of a horse caused by muscular spasms — **string·halt·ed** \-ˌhȯl-təd\ *adj*

strip \'strip\ *vb* **stripped** \'stript\ *also* **stript**; **strip·ping** : to remove (a vein) by means of a stripper

strip·per \'stri-pər\ *n* : a surgical instrument used for removal of a vein

stroke \'strōk\ *n* : sudden diminution or loss of consciousness, sensation, and voluntary motion caused by rupture or obstruction (as by a clot) of an artery of the brain — called also *apoplexy*; compare CEREBRAL ACCIDENT

stroke volume *n* : the volume of blood pumped from a ventricle of the heart in one beat

stro·ma \'strō-mə\ *n, pl* **stro·ma·ta** \-mə-tə\ **1** : the supporting framework of an animal organ typically consisting of connective tissue : the spongy protoplasmic framework of some cells (as a red blood cell) — **stro·mal** \-məl\ *adj*

strong silver protein *n* : SILVER PROTEIN b

stron·gyle \'strän-ˌjīl\ *n* : STRONGYLID; *esp* : a worm of the genus *Strongylus* or closely related genera that is parasitic in the alimentary tract and tissues of the horse and may induce severe diarrhea and debility

stron·gy·lid \'strän-jə-lid\ *n* : any of a family (Strongylidae) of nematode worms that are parasites of vertebrates — **strongylid** *adj*

stron·gy·li·do·sis \ˌsträn-jə-lə-'dō-səs\ *n* : STRONGYLOSIS

stron·gy·loid \'strän-jə-ˌlȯid\ *n* : any of a superfamily (Strongyloidea) of nematode worms including the hookworms, strongyles, and related forms — **strongyloid** *adj*

Stron·gy·loi·des \ˌsträn-jə-'lȯi-ˌdēz\ *n* : a genus of nematode worms (family Strongyloididae) having both free-living males and females and parthenogenetic females parasitic in the intestine of various vertebrates and including some medically and economically important pests of humans

stron·gy·loi·di·a·sis \ˌsträn-jə-ˌlȯi-'dī-ə-səs\ *n, pl* **-a·ses** \-ə-ˌsēz\ : infestation with or disease caused by nematodes of the genus *Strongyloides*

stron·gy·loi·do·sis \-'dō-səs\ *n* : STRONGYLOIDIASIS

stron·gy·lo·sis \ˌsträn-jə-'lō-səs\ *n* : infestation with or disease caused by strongyles — called also *strongylidosis*

Stron·gy·lus \'strän-jə-ləs\ *n* : a genus of strongylid nematode worms including gastrointestinal parasites of the horse

stron·tium \'strän-chəm, -chē-əm, -tē-əm\ *n* : a soft malleable ductile bivalent metallic element — symbol *Sr*; see ELEMENT table

strontium 90 *n* : a heavy radioactive isotope of strontium having the mass number 90 that is present in the fallout from nuclear explosions and is hazardous because like calcium it can be assimilated in biological processes and deposited in the bones — called also *radiostrontium*

stro·phan·thin \strō-'fan-thən\ *n* : a bitter toxic glycoside $C_{36}H_{54}O_{14}$ from a woody vine of the genus *Strophanthus* (*S. kombé*) used similarly to digitalis; *also* : a related glycoside (as ouabain)

stro·phan·thus \-thəs\ *n* **1** *cap* : a genus of Asian and African trees, shrubs, or woody vines of the dogbane family (Apocynaceae) including one (*S. kombé*) that furnishes strophanthin **2** : the dried cleaned ripe seeds of any of several plants of the genus *Strophanthus* (as *S. kombé* and *S. hispidus*) that are in moderate doses a cardiac stimulant like digitalis but in larger doses a violent poison and that have strophanthin as their most active constituent

struck \'strək\ *n* : enterotoxemia esp. of adult sheep

struc·tur·al \'strək-chə-rəl\ *adj* **1** : of or relating to the physical makeup of a plant or animal body (~ defects of the heart) — compare FUNCTIONAL 1a **2** : of, relating to, or affecting structure (~ stability) — **struc·tur·al·ly** *adv*

structural formula *n* : an expanded molecular formula (as HOCH₂(CHOH)₄CHO for glucose) showing the arrangement within the molecule of atoms and of bonds

structural gene *n* : a gene that codes for the amino acid sequence of a protein (as an enzyme) or for a ribosomal RNA or transfer RNA

struc·tur·al·ism \'strək-chə-rə-ˌli-zəm\ *n* : psychology concerned esp. with resolution of the mind into structural elements

struc·ture \'strək-chər\ *n* **1** : something (as an anatomical part) arranged in a definite pattern of organization **2 a** : the arrangement of particles or parts in a substance or body (molecular ~) **b** : organization of parts as dominated by the general character of the whole (personality ~) **3** : the aggregate of elements of an entity in their relationships to each other

stru·ma \'strü-mə\ *n, pl* **-mae** \-(ˌ)mē\ *or* **-mas** : GOITER

struma lym·pho·ma·to·sa \-ˌlim-ˌfō-mə-'tō-sə\ *n* : HASHIMOTO'S DISEASE

stru·vite \'strü-ˌvīt\ *n* : a hydrated magnesium-containing mineral Mg(NH₄)(PO₄)·6H₂O which is found in kidney stones associated with bacteria that cleave urea

strych·nine \'strik-ˌnīn, -nən, -ˌnēn\ *n* : a bitter poisonous alkaloid C₂₁H₂₂N₂O₂ that is obtained from nux vomica and related plants of the genus *Strychnos* and is used medicinally as a stimulant of the central nervous system

Strych·nos \'strik-nəs, -ˌnäs\ *n* : a large genus of tropical trees and woody vines (family Loganiaceae) — see CURARE, NUX VOMICA, STRYCHNINE

STS *abbr* serologic test for syphilis

ST segment *or* **S–T segment** \ˌes-'tē-\ *n* : the part of an electrocardiogram between the QRS complex and the T wave

Stu·art–Prow·er factor \'stü-ərt-'prau̇-ər-, -'styü-\ *n* : FACTOR X
  Stuart and **Prower,** 20th century hospital patients.

stuff \'stəf\ *vb* : to choke or block up (as nasal passages) (a ~ed up nose) — **stuff·i·ness** \'stə-fē-nəs\ *n* — **stuffy** \'stə-fē\ *adj*

stump \'stəmp\ *n* **1** : the basal portion of a bodily part (as a limb) remaining

after the rest is removed **2** : a rudimentary or vestigial bodily part

stung *past and past part of* STING

stunt \'stənt\ *vb* : to hinder the normal growth, development, or progress of

stupe \'stüp, 'styüp\ *n* : a hot wet often medicated cloth applied externally (as to stimulate circulation)

stu·pe·fy \'stü-pə-ˌfī, 'styü-\ *vb* **-fied; -fy·ing** : to make stupid, groggy, or insensible — **stu·pe·fac·tion** \ˌstü-pə-'fak-shən, ˌstyü-\ *n*

stu·por \'stü-pər, 'styü-\ *n* : a condition of greatly dulled or completely suspended sense or sensibility (a drunken ~); *specif* : a chiefly mental condition marked by absence of spontaneous movement, greatly diminished responsiveness to stimulation, and usu. impaired consciousness — **stu·por·ous** \'stü-pə-rəs, 'styü-\ *adj*

stur·dy \'stər-dē\ *n, pl* **sturdies** : GID

Sturge–Web·er syndrome \'stərj-'we-bər-\ *n* : a rare congenital condition that is characterized by a port-wine stain affecting the facial skin on one side in the area innervated by the first branch of the trigeminal nerve and by malformed blood vessels in the brain that may cause progressive mental retardation, epilepsy, and glaucoma in the eye on the affected side — called also *Sturge-Weber disease*
  Sturge, William Allen (1850–1919), and **Weber, Frederick Parkes (1863–1962),** British physicians.

¹**stut·ter** \'stə-tər\ *vb* : to speak with involuntary disruption or blocking of speech (as by spasmodic repetition or prolongation of vocal sounds) — **stut·ter·er** \'stə-tər-ər\ *n*

²**stutter** *n* **1** : an act or instance of stuttering **2** : a speech disorder involving stuttering

stuttering *n* **1** : the act of one who stutters **2** : a disorder of vocal communication marked by involuntary disruption or blocking of speech (as by spasmodic repetition or prolongation of vocal sounds), by fear and anxiety, and by a struggle to avoid speech errors — compare STAMMERING 2

sty *or* **stye** \'stī\ *n, pl* **sties** *or* **styes** : an inflamed swelling of a sebaceous gland at the margin of an eyelid — called also *hordeolum*

styl- *or* **stylo-** *comb form* : styloid process (*stylo*glossus)

sty·let \stī-'let, 'stī-lət\ *also* **sty·lette** \stī-'let\ *n* **1** : a slender surgical probe **2** : a thin wire inserted into a catheter to maintain rigidity or into a hollow needle to maintain patency

sty·lo·glos·sus \ˌstī-lō-'glä-səs, -'glò-\ *n, pl* **-glos·si** \-'glä-ˌsī, -'glò-\ : a muscle that arises from the styloid process of the temporal bone, inserts along the side and underpart of the tongue, and functions to draw the tongue upwards

sty·lo·hy·oid \ˌstī-lō-ˈhī-ˌoid\ n : STYLO-
HYOID MUSCLE

sty·lo·hy·oi·de·us \-hī-ˈoi-dē-əs\ n, pl
-dei \-dē-ˌī\ : STYLOHYOID MUSCLE

stylohyoid ligament n : a band of fibrous tissue connecting the tip of the
styloid process of the temporal bone
to the ceratohyal of the hyoid bone

stylohyoid muscle n : a slender muscle
that arises from the posterior surface
of the styloid process of the temporal
bone, inserts into the body of the hyoid bone, and acts to elevate and retract the hyoid bone resulting in
elongation of the floor of the mouth
— called also *stylohyoid, stylohyoi-
deus*

sty·loid \ˈstī-ˌloid\ adj : having a slender pointed shape

styloid process n : any of several long
slender pointed bony processes: as **a**
: a sharp spine that projects downward and forward from the inferior
surface of the temporal bone just in
front of the stylomastoid foramen **b**
: an eminence on the distal extremity
of the ulna giving attachment to a ligament of the wrist joint **c** : a conical
prolongation of the lateral surface of
the distal extremity of the radius that
gives attachment to several tendons
and ligaments

sty·lo·man·dib·u·lar ligament \ˌstī-lō-
man-ˈdi-byə-lər\ n : a band of deep
fascia that connects the styloid process of the temporal bone to the gonial angle

sty·lo·mas·toid foramen \-ˈmas-ˌtoid-\ n
: a foramen that occurs on the lower
surface of the temporal bone between
the styloid and mastoid processes

sty·lo·pha·ryn·ge·us \ˌstī-lō-fə-ˈrin-jē-
əs, -ˌfar-ən-ˈjē-əs\ n, pl **-gei** \-jē-ˌī\ : a
slender muscle that arises from the
base of the styloid process of the temporal bone, inserts into the side of the
pharynx, and acts with the contralateral muscle in swallowing to increase
the transverse diameter of the pharynx by drawing its sides upward and
laterally

¹styp·tic \ˈstip-tik\ adj : tending to check
bleeding; *esp* : having the property of
arresting oozing of blood (as from a
shallow surface injury) when applied
to a bleeding part ⟨∼ agent⟩

²styptic n : an agent (as a drug) having a
styptic effect

styptic pencil n : a cylindrical stick of a
medicated styptic substance used
esp. in shaving to stop the bleeding
from small cuts

sub- *prefix* **1** : under : beneath : below
⟨*sub*coastal⟩ **2** : subordinate portion
of : subdivision of ⟨*sub*species⟩ **3**
: less than completely or perfectly
⟨*sub*normal⟩

sub·acro·mi·al \ˌsəb-ə-ˈkrō-mē-əl\ adj
: of, relating to, or affecting the subacromial bursa ⟨∼ bursitis⟩

subacromial bursa n : a bursa lying between the acromion and the capsule
of the shoulder joint

sub·acute \ˌsəb-ə-ˈkyüt\ adj **1** : falling
between acute and chronic in charac-
ter esp. when closer to acute ⟨∼ en-
docarditis⟩ **2** : less marked in severity
or duration than a corresponding
acute state ⟨∼ pain⟩ — **sub·acute·ly**
adv

subacute sclerosing panencephalitis n
: a central nervous system disease of
children and young adults caused by
infection of the brain by the measles
virus or a closely related virus and
marked by intellectual deterioration,
convulsions, and paralysis — called
SSPE

sub·aor·tic stenosis \ˌsəb-ā-ˈòr-tik-\ n
: aortic stenosis produced by an obstruction in the left ventricle below
the aortic valve

sub·arach·noid \ˌsəb-ə-ˈrak-ˌnòid\ *also*
sub·arach·noid·al \-ˌrak-ˈnòid-ᵊl\ adj **1**
: situated or occurring under the
arachnoid membrane ⟨∼ hemor-
rhage⟩ **2** : of, relating to, or involving
the subarachnoid space and the fluid
within it ⟨∼ meningitis⟩

subarachnoid space n : the space between the arachnoid and the pia mater through which the cerebrospinal
fluid circulates

sub·cal·lo·sal \ˌsəb-ka-ˈlō-səl\ adj : situated below the corpus callosum

subcallosal area n : a small area of cortex in each cerebral hemisphere below the genu of the corpus callosum

sub·cap·su·lar \ˌsəb-ˈkap-sə-lər\ adj
: situated or occurring beneath or
within a capsule ⟨∼ cataracts⟩

subcarbonate n : see BISMUTH SUBCAR-
BONATE

sub·cel·lu·lar \ˌsəb-ˈsel-yə-lər\ adj : IN-
TRACELLULAR

sub·chon·dral \-ˈkän-drəl\ adj : situated
beneath cartilage ⟨∼ bone⟩

sub·cho·roi·dal \ˌsəb-kə-ˈròid-ᵊl\ adj
: situated or occurring between the
choroid and the retina ⟨∼ fluid⟩

sub·class \ˈsəb-ˌklas\ n : a category in
biological classification ranking below a class and above an order

subclavia — see ANSA SUBCLAVIA

¹sub·cla·vi·an \ˌsəb-ˈklā-vē-ən\ adj : of,
relating to, being, or performed on a
part (as an artery or vein) located under the clavicle ⟨∼ angioplasty⟩

²subclavian n : a subclavian part

subclavian artery n : the proximal part
of the main artery of the arm that
arises on the right side from the innominate artery and on the left side
from the arch of the aorta and that
supplies or gives off branches supplying the brain, neck, anterior wall of
the thorax, and shoulder

subclavian trunk n : a large lymphatic
vessel on each side of the body that
receives lymph from the axilla and
arms and that on the right side empties into the right lymphatic duct and

on the left side into the thoracic duct

sub·cla·vian vein *n* : the proximal part of the main vein of the arm that is a continuation of the axillary vein and extends from the level of the first rib to the sternal end of the clavicle where it unites with the internal jugular vein to form the innominate vein

sub·cla·vi·us \səb-ˈklā-vē-əs\ *n, pl* -**vii** \-vē-ˌī\ : a small muscle on each side of the body that arises from the junction of the first rib and its cartilage, inserts into the inferior surface of the clavicle, and acts to stabilize the clavicle by depressing and drawing forward its lateral end during movements of the shoulder joint

sub·clin·i·cal \-ˈkli-ni-kəl\ *adj* : not detectable or producing effects that are not detectable by the usual clinical tests ⟨a ∼ infection⟩ ⟨∼ cancer⟩ — **sub·clin·i·cal·ly** *adv*

sub·con·junc·ti·val \ˌsəb-ˌkän-ˌjəŋk-ˈtī-vəl\ *adj* : situated or occurring beneath the conjunctiva — **sub·con·junc·ti·val·ly** *adv*

¹**sub·con·scious** \ˌsəb-ˈkän-chəs\ *adj* **1** : existing in the mind but not immediately available to consciousness : affecting thought, feeling, and behavior without entering awareness **2** : imperfectly conscious : partially but not fully aware — **sub·con·scious·ly** *adv* — **sub·con·scious·ness** *n*

²**subconscious** *n* : the mental activities just below the threshold of consciousness; *also* : the aspect of the mind concerned with such activities — compare UNCONSCIOUS

sub·cor·a·coid \-ˈkȯr-ə-ˌkȯid\ *adj* : situated or occurring under the coracoid process of the scapula ⟨a ∼ dislocation of the humerus⟩

sub·cor·ti·cal \-ˈkȯr-ti-kəl\ *adj* : of, relating to, involving, or being nerve centers below the cerebral cortex — **sub·cor·ti·cal·ly** *adv*

sub·cos·tal \-ˈkäs-təl, -ˈkȯs-\ *adj* : situated or performed below a rib

subcostal artery *n* : either of a pair of arteries that are the most posterior branches of the thoracic aorta and follow a course beneath the last pair of ribs

sub·cos·ta·lis \-käs-ˈtā-ləs, -ˈkȯs-\ *n, pl* -**ta·les** \-ˌlēz\ : any of a variable number of small muscles that arise on the inner surface of a rib, are inserted into the inner surface of the second or third rib below, and prob. function to draw adjacent ribs together

subcostal vein *n* : either of two veins: **a** : one that arises on the right side of the anterior abdominal wall and joins in the formation of the azygos vein — called also *right subcostal vein* **b** : one on the left side of the body that usually empties into the hemiazygos vein — called also *left subcostal vein*

sub·cul·ture \ˈsəb-ˌkəl-chər\ *n* **1** : a culture (as of bacteria) derived from an-

other culture **2** : an act or instance of producing a subculture — **subculture** *vb*

subcutanea — see TELA SUBCUTANEA

sub·cu·ta·ne·ous \ˌsəb-kyu̇-ˈtā-nē-əs\ *adj* : being, living, used, or made under the skin ⟨∼ parasites⟩ — **sub·cu·ta·ne·ous·ly** *adv*

subcutaneous bursa *n* : a bursa lying between the skin and a bony process or a ligament

subcutaneous emphysema *n* : the presence of a gas and esp. air in the subcutaneous tissue

sub·cu·tic·u·lar \-kyu̇-ˈti-kyə-lər\ *adj* : situated or occurring beneath a cuticle ⟨∼ sutures⟩ ⟨∼ tissues⟩

sub·cu·tis \ˌsəb-ˈkyu̇-təs\ *n* : the deeper part of the dermis

sub·del·toid \ˌsəb-ˈdel-ˌtȯid\ *adj* : situated underneath or inferior to the deltoid muscle ⟨∼ calcareous deposits⟩

subdeltoid bursa *n* : the bursa that lies beneath the deltoid muscle

sub·der·mal \-ˈdər-məl\ *adj* : SUBCUTANEOUS — **sub·der·mal·ly** *adv*

sub·di·a·phrag·ma·tic \ˌsəb-ˌdī-ə-frə-ˈma-tik, -ˌfrag-\ *adj* : situated, occurring, or performed below the diaphragm ⟨a ∼ abscess⟩

subdivision *n* : a category in botanical classification ranking below a division and above a class

sub·du·ral \ˌsəb-ˈdu̇r-əl, -ˈdyu̇r-\ *adj* : situated, occurring, or performed under the dura mater or between the dura mater and the arachnoid ⟨∼ hematoma⟩ — **sub·du·ral·ly** *adv*

subdural space *n* : a fluid-filled space or potential space between the dura mater and the arachnoid

sub·en·do·car·di·al \ˌsəb-ˌen-dō-ˈkär-dē-əl\ *adj* : situated or occurring beneath the endocardium or between the endocardium and myocardium

sub·en·do·the·li·al \-ˌen-dō-ˈthē-lē-əl\ *adj* : situated under an endothelium

sub·ep·en·dy·mal \-e-ˈpen-də-məl\ *adj* : situated under the ependyma

sub·epi·der·mal \ˌsəb-ˌe-pə-ˈdər-məl\ *adj* : lying beneath or constituting the innermost part of the epidermis

sub·epi·the·li·al \-ˌe-pə-ˈthē-lē-əl\ *adj* : situated or occurring beneath an epithelial layer; *also* : SUBCUTANEOUS

sub·fam·i·ly \ˈsəb-ˌfam-lē\ *n* : a category in biological classification ranking below a family and above a genus

sub·fas·cial \-ˈfa-shəl, -shē-əl\ *adj* : situated, occurring, or performed below a fascia ⟨a ∼ tumor⟩ ⟨∼ suturing⟩

sub·fe·brile \-ˈfe-ˌbrīl, -ˈfē-\ *adj* : of, relating to, or constituting a body temperature very slightly above normal but not febrile

sub·fer·til·i·ty \-fər-ˈti-lə-tē\ *n, pl* -**ties** : the condition of being less than normally fertile though still capable of effecting fertilization — **sub·fer·tile** \-ˈfərt-əl\ *adj*

sub·ge·nus \ˈsəb-ˌjē-nəs\ *n, pl* -**gen-**

e·ra \-ˌje-nər-ə\ : a category in biological taxonomy ranking below a genus and above a species

sub·gin·gi·val \ˌsəb-ˈjin-jə-vəl\ *adj* : situated, performed, or occurring beneath the gums and esp. between the gums and the basal part of the crowns of the teeth 〈~ calculus〉 〈~ curettage〉 — **sub·gin·gi·val·ly** *adv*

sub·glot·tic \-ˈglä-tik\ *adj* : situated or occurring below the glottis

su·bic·u·lum \sə-ˈbi-kyə-ləm\ *n, pl* **-la** \-lə\ : a part of the hippocampal gyrus that is a ventral continuation of the hippocampus and is situated ventrally and medially to the dentate gyrus; *also* : a section of this that borders the hippocampal sulcus — **su·bic·u·lar** \-lər\ *adj*

sub·in·tern \-ˈin-ˌtərn\ *n* : a medical student in the last year of medical school who performs work supervised by interns and residents in a hospital

sub·in·ti·mal \-ˈin-tə-məl\ *adj* : situated beneath an intima and esp. between the intima and media of an artery

sub·in·vo·lu·tion \-ˌin-və-ˈlü-shən\ *n* : partial or incomplete involution

sub·ja·cent \ˌsəb-ˈjās-ənt\ *adj* : lying immediately under or below 〈~ tissue〉

sub·ject \ˈsəb-jikt\ *n* **1** : an individual whose reactions or responses are studied **2** : a dead body for anatomical study and dissection

sub·jec·tive \(ˌ)səb-ˈjek-tiv\ *adj* **1 a** : relating to or determined by the mind as the subject of experience 〈~ reality〉 **b** : characteristic of or belonging to reality as perceived rather than as independent of mind **c** : relating to or being experience or knowledge as conditioned by personal mental characteristics or states **2 a** : arising from conditions within the brain or sense organs and not directly caused by external stimuli 〈~ sensations〉 **b** : arising out of or identified by means of one's perception of one's own states and processes and not observable by an examiner 〈a ~ symptom of disease〉 — compare OBJECTIVE 2 — **sub·jec·tive·ly** *adv*

subjective vertigo *n* : vertigo characterized by a sensation that one's body is revolving in space

sub·le·thal \ˌsəb-ˈlē-thəl\ *adj* : less than but usu. only slightly less than lethal 〈a ~ dose〉

sub·li·ma·tion \ˌsə-blə-ˈmā-shən\ *n* : the process of converting and expressing a primitive instinctual desire or impulse to a form that is socially and culturally acceptable — **sub·li·mate** \ˈsə-blə-ˌmāt\ *vb*

sub·lim·i·nal \(ˌ)səb-ˈli-mə-nəl\ *adj* **1** : inadequate to produce a sensation or a perception **2** : existing or functioning below the threshold of consciousness 〈the ~ mind〉 〈~ advertising〉 — **sub·lim·i·nal·ly** *adv*

¹sub·lin·gual \ˌsəb-ˈliŋ-gwəl, -gyə-wəl\ *adj* **1** : situated under or administered under the tongue 〈~ tablets〉 〈~ glands〉 **2** : of or relating to the sublingual glands — **sub·lin·gual·ly** *adv*

²sublingual *n* : SUBLINGUAL GLAND

sublingual gland *n* : a small salivary gland on each side of the mouth lying beneath the mucous membrane in a fossa in the mandible near the symphysis — called also *sublingual salivary gland*

sub·lob·u·lar vein \ˌsəb-ˈlä-byə-lər-\ *n* : one of several veins in the liver into which the central veins empty and which in turn empty into the hepatic veins

sub·lux·a·tion \ˌsəb-ˌlək-ˈsā-shən\ *n* : partial dislocation (as of one of the bones in a joint) — **sub·lux·at·ed** \ˈsəb-ˌlək-ˌsā-təd\ *adj*

¹sub·man·dib·u·lar \ˌsəb-man-ˈdi-byə-lər\ *adj* **1** : of, relating to, situated, or performed in the region below the lower jaw **2** : of, relating to, or associated with the submandibular glands

²submandibular *n* : a submandibular part (as an artery or bone)

submandibular ganglion *n* : an autonomic ganglion that is situated on the hyoglossus muscle above the deep part of the submandibular gland, receives preganglionic fibers from the facial nerve, and sends postganglionic fibers to the submandibular and sublingual glands — called also *submaxillary ganglion*

submandibular gland *n* : a salivary gland inside of and near the lower edge of the mandible on each side and discharging by Wharton's duct into the mouth under the tongue — called also *submandibular salivary gland, submaxillary gland, submaxillary salivary gland*

sub·max·il·lary \ˌsəb-ˈmak-sə-ˌler-ē\ *adj or n* : SUBMANDIBULAR

submaxillary ganglion *n* : SUBMANDIBULAR GANGLION

submaxillary gland *n* : SUBMANDIBULAR GLAND

submaxillary salivary gland *n* : SUBMANDIBULAR GLAND

sub·max·i·mal \ˌsəb-ˈmak-sə-məl\ *adj* : being less than the maximum of which an individual is capable

sub·men·tal \-ˈment-ᵊl\ *adj* : located in, affecting, or performed on the area under the chin

submental artery *n* : a branch of the facial artery that branches off near the submandibular gland and is distributed to the muscles of the jaw

sub·meta·cen·tric \ˌsəb-ˌme-tə-ˈsen-trik\ *adj* : having the centromere situated so that one chromosome arm is somewhat shorter than the other — **submetacentric** *n*

sub·mi·cro·scop·ic \ˌsəb-ˌmī-krə-ˈskä-pik\ *adj* : too small to be seen in an ordinary light microscope 〈~ parti-

cles⟩ — compare MACROSCOPIC, MI-
CROSCOPIC 2, ULTRAMICROSCOPIC 1 —
sub·mi·cro·scop·i·cal·ly *adv*

sub·mis·sion \səb-ʹmi-shən\ *n* : the condition of being submissive

sub·mis·sive \-ʹmi-səv\ *adj* : characterized by tendencies to yield to the will
or authority of others ⟨a ∼ personal-
ity⟩ — **sub·mis·sive·ness** *n*

sub·mu·co·sa \ˌsəb-myü-ʹkō-sə\ *n* : a
supporting layer of loose connective
tissue directly under a mucous membrane — **sub·mu·co·sal** \-zəl\ *adj*

sub·mu·cous \ˌsəb-ʹmyü-kəs\ *adj* : lying under or involving the tissues under a mucous membrane

subnitrate — see BISMUTH SUBNITRATE

sub·nor·mal \ˌsəb-ʹnȯr-məl\ *adj* **1**
: lower or smaller than normal ⟨a ∼
temperature⟩ **2** : having less of something and esp. of intelligence than is
normal — **sub·nor·mal·i·ty** \ˌsəb-nȯr-
ʹma-lə-tē\ *n*

sub·oc·cip·i·tal \-äk-ʹsi-pət-əl\ *adj* **1** : situated or performed below the occip-
ital bone **2** : situated or performed
below the occipital lobe of the brain

suboccipital nerve *n* : the first cervical
nerve that supplies muscles around
the suboccipital triangle and that
sends branches to the rectus capitis
posterior minor and semispinalis capitis

suboccipital triangle *n* : a space of the
suboccipital region on each side of
the dorsal cervical region that is
bounded superiorly and medially by a
muscle arising by a tendon from a spinous process of the axis and inserting
into the inferior nuchal line and the
adjacent inferior region of the occipital bone, that is bounded superiorly
and laterally by the obliquus capitis
superior, and that is bounded inferiorly and laterally by the obliquus capitis inferior

sub·op·ti·mal \ˌsəb-ʹäp-tə-məl\ *adj*
: less than optimal ⟨a ∼ diet⟩ ⟨a ∼
dose of a drug⟩

sub·or·der \ʹsəb-ˌȯr-dər\ *n* : a category
in biological classification ranking below an order and above a family

sub·peri·os·te·al \ˌsəb-ˌper-ē-ʹäs-tē-əl\ *adj*
: situated or occurring beneath the
periosteum ⟨∼ bone deposition⟩ ⟨a ∼
fibroma⟩ — **sub·peri·os·te·al·ly** *adv*

sub·phren·ic \ˌsəb-ʹfre-nik\ *adj* : situated or occurring below the diaphragm

subphrenic space *n* : a space on each
side of the falciform ligament between the underside of the diaphragm
and the upper side of the liver

sub·phy·lum \ʹsəb-ˌfī-ləm\ *n, pl* **-la** \-lə\
: a category in biological classifica-
tion ranking below a phylum and
above a class

sub·pleu·ral \-ʹplu̇r-əl\ *adj* : situated or
occurring between the pleura and the
body wall — **sub·pleu·ral·ly** *adv*

sub·pop·u·la·tion \ˌsəb-ˌpä-pyə-ʹlā-

shən\ *n* : an identifiable fraction or
subdivision of a population

sub·po·tent \ˌsəb-ʹpōt-ᵊnt\ *adj* : less potent than normal ⟨∼ drugs⟩ — **sub-
po·ten·cy** \-ʹpōt-ᵊn-sē\ *n*

sub·pu·bic angle \ˌsəb-ʹpyü-bik-\ *n* : the
angle that is formed just below the
pubic symphysis by the meeting of
the inferior ramus of the pubis on one
side with the corresponding part on
the other side

sub·ret·i·nal \-ʹret-ᵊn-əl\ *adj* : situated
or occurring beneath the retina

sub·scap·u·lar \ˌsəb-ʹska-pyə-lər\ *adj*
: situated under the scapula

subscapular artery *n* : an artery that is
usu. the largest branch of the axillary
artery, that arises opposite the lower
border of the subscapularis muscle,
and that passes down and back to the
lower part of the scapula where it
forms branches and anastomoses
with arteries in that region

subscapular fossa *n* : the concave depression of the anterior surface of the
scapula

sub·scap·u·lar·is \ˌsəb-ˌska-pyə-ʹlar-
əs\ *n* : a large triangular muscle that
fills up the subscapular fossa, that
arises from the surface of the scapula, that is inserted into the lesser tubercle of the humerus, and that
stabilizes the shoulder joint as part of
the rotator cuff and rotates the humerus medially when the arm is held
by the side of the body

sub·scrip·tion \səb-ʹskrip-shən\ *n* : a
part of a prescription that contains directions to the pharmacist

sub·se·rous \ˌsəb-ʹsir-əs\ *or* **sub·se·ro-
sal** \-sə-ʹrō-zəl\ *adj* : situated or occurring under a serous membrane ⟨a
∼ uterine fibroid⟩ ⟨∼ fat⟩

sub·side \səb-ʹsīd\ *vb* **sub·sid·ed; sub-
sid·ing** : to lessen in severity : become
diminished ⟨the fever *subsided*⟩ —
sub·si·dence \səb-ʹsīd-ᵊns, ʹsəb-səd-
əns\ *n*

sub·spe·cial·ty \ˌsəb-ʹspe-shəl-tē\ *n, pl*
-ties : a subordinate field of specialization

sub·spe·cies \ʹsəb-ˌspē-shēz, -sēz\ *n* : a
subdivision of a species: as **a** : a category in biological classification that
ranks immediately below a species
and designates a population of a particular geographical region genetically distinguishable from other such
populations of the same species and
capable of interbreeding successfully
with them where its range overlaps
theirs **b** : a named subdivision (as a
race or variety) of a species — **sub-
spe·cif·ic** \ˌsəb-spi-ʹsi-fik\ *adj*

sub·stage \ʹsəb-ˌstāj\ *n* : an attachment
to a microscope by means of which
accessories (as mirrors, diaphragms,
or condensers) are held in place beneath the stage of the instrument

sub·stance \ʹsəb-stəns\ *n* : something
(as drugs or alcoholic beverages)

deemed harmful and usu. subject to legal restrictions ⟨possession of a controlled ∼⟩

sub·stance abuse *n* : excessive use of a drug (as alcohol, narcotics, or cocaine) : use of a drug without medical justification — **substance abuser** *n*

substance P *n* : a neuropeptide that consists of 11 amino-acid residues, that is widely distributed in the brain, spinal cord, and peripheral nervous system, and that acts across nerve synapses to produce prolonged postsynaptic excitation

sub·stan·tia gel·a·ti·no·sa \səb-ˈstan-chə-ˌje-lə-tə-ˈnō-sə\ *n* : a mass of gelatinous gray matter that lies on the dorsal surface of the dorsal column and extends the entire length of the spinal cord into the medulla oblongata and that functions in the transmission of painful sensory information

substantia in·nom·i·na·ta \-i-ˌnä-mə-ˈnä-tə\ *n* : a band of large cells of indeterminate function that lie just under the surface of the globus pallidus

sub·stan·tia ni·gra \səb-ˈstan-chə-ˈnī-grə, -ˈni-\ *n, pl* **sub·stan·ti·ae ni·grae** \-chē-ˌē-ˈnī-ˌgrē, -ˈni-\ : a layer of deeply pigmented gray matter situated in the midbrain and containing the cell bodies of a tract of dopamine= producing nerve cells whose secretion tends to be deficient in Parkinson's disease

substantia pro·pria \-ˈprō-prē-ə\ *n, pl* **substantiae pro·pri·ae** \-prē-ˌē\ : the layer of lamellated transparent fibrous connective tissue that makes up the bulk of the cornea of the eye

sub·ster·nal \ˌsəb-ˈstər-nəl\ *adj* : situated or perceived behind or below the sternum ⟨∼ pain⟩

sub·stit·u·ent \ˌsəb-ˈsti-chə-wənt\ *n* : an atom or group that replaces another atom or group in a molecule — **substituent** *adj*

sub·sti·tute \ˈsəb-stə-ˌtüt, -ˌtyüt\ *n* : a person or thing that takes the place or function of another ⟨father and mother ∼s⟩ — **substitute** *adj*

sub·sti·tu·tion \ˌsəb-stə-ˈtü-shən, -ˈtyü-\ *n* **1** : the turning from an obstructed desire to another desire whose gratification is socially acceptable **2** : the turning from an obstructed form of behavior to a different and often more primitive expression of the same tendency ⟨a ∼ neurosis⟩

sub·strate \ˈsəb-ˌstrāt\ *n* **1** : the base on which an organism lives **2** : a substance acted upon (as by an enzyme)

sub·stra·tum \ˈsəb-ˌstrā-təm, -ˌstra-\ *n, pl* **-stra·ta** \-tə\ : SUBSTRATE 1

sub·struc·ture \ˈsəb-ˌstrək-chər\ *n* : an underlying or supporting structure — **sub·struc·tur·al** \-chə-rəl\ *adj*

sub·ta·lar \ˌsəb-ˈtā-lər\ *adj* : situated or occurring beneath the talus; *specif* : of, relating to, or being the articula-

tion formed between the posterior facet of the inferior surface of the talus and the posterior facet of the superior surface of the calcaneus

sub·tem·po·ral decompression \-ˈtem-pə-rəl-\ *n* : relief of intracranial pressure by excision of a portion of the temporal bone

sub·tha·lam·ic \ˌsəb-thə-ˈla-mik\ *adj* : of or relating to the subthalamus

subthalamic nucleus *n* : an oval mass of gray matter that is located in the caudal part of the subthalamus and when affected with lesions is associated with hemiballismus of the contralateral side of the body

sub·thal·a·mus \ˌsəb-ˈtha-lə-məs\ *n, pl* **-mi** \-ˌmī\ : the ventral part of the thalamus

sub·ther·a·peu·tic \-ˌther-ə-ˈpyü-tik\ *adj* : not producing a therapeutic effect ⟨∼ doses of penicillin⟩

sub·thresh·old \ˌsəb-ˈthresh-ˌhōld\ *adj* : inadequate to produce a response ⟨∼ dosage⟩ ⟨a ∼ stimulus⟩

sub·to·tal \ˌsəb-ˈtōt-ᵊl\ *adj* : somewhat less than complete : nearly total ⟨∼ thyroidectomy⟩

sub·tro·chan·ter·ic \ˌsəb-ˌtrō-kən-ˈter-ik, -ˌkan-\ *adj* : situated or occurring below a trochanter

sub·un·gual \ˌsəb-ˈəŋ-gwəl, -ˈən-\ *adj* : situated or occurring under a fingernail or toenail ⟨a ∼ abscess⟩

sub·val·vu·lar \ˌsəb-ˈval-vyə-lər\ *adj* : situated or occurring below a valve (as a semilunar valve) ⟨∼ stenosis⟩

sub·vi·ral \ˌsəb-ˈvī-rəl\ *adj* : relating to, being, or caused by a piece or a structural part (as a protein) of a virus

succedaneum — see CAPUT SUCCEDANEUM

suc·ci·nate \ˈsək-sə-ˌnāt\ *n* : a salt or ester of succinic acid

succinate dehydrogenase *n* : an iron= containing flavoprotein enzyme that catalyzes often reversibly the dehydrogenation of succinic acid to fumaric acid — called also *succinic dehydrogenase*

suc·cin·ic acid \(ˌ)sək-ˈsi-nik-\ *n* : a crystalline acid $C_4H_6O_4$ containing two carboxyl groups that is formed in the Krebs cycle and in various fermentation processes

suc·ci·nyl·cho·line \ˌsək-sə-nəl-ˈkō-ˌlēn, -ˌnil-\ *n* : a basic compound that acts similarly to curare and is used intravenously chiefly in the form of a hydrated chloride $C_{14}H_{30}Cl_2N_2O_4\cdot 2H_2O$ as a muscle relaxant in surgery — called also *suxamethonium*; see ANECTINE

suc·ci·nyl·sul·fa·thi·a·zole \ˌsək-sə-nəl-ˌsəl-fə-ˈthī-ə-ˌzōl, -ˌnil-\ *n* : a crystalline sulfa drug $C_{13}H_{13}N_3O_5S_2$ used esp. for treating gastrointestinal infections

suc·cus en·ter·i·cus \ˌsə-kəs-en-ˈter-i-kəs\ *n* : INTESTINAL JUICE

suc·cus·sion \sə-ˈkə-shən\ *n* : the action

or process of shaking or the condition of being shaken esp. with violence: **a** : a shaking of the body to ascertain if fluid is present in a cavity and esp. in the thorax **b** : the splashing sound made by succussion

suck \\ˈsək\\ *vb* **1** : to draw (as liquid) into the mouth through a suction force produced by movements of the lips and tongue **2** : to draw out by suction

suck•er \\ˈsə-kər\\ *n* **1** : an organ in various animals (as a trematode or tapeworm) used for adhering or holding **2** : a mouth (as of a leech) adapted for sucking or adhering

sucking louse *n* : any of an order (Anoplura) of wingless insects comprising the true lice with mouthparts adapted for sucking body fluids

suck•le \\ˈsə-kəl\\ *vb* **suck•led; suck•ling 1** : to give milk to from the breast or udder **2** : to draw milk from the breast or udder of

su•cral•fate \\sü-ˈkral-ˌfāt\\ *n* : an aluminum complex $C_{12}H_mAl_{16}O_nS_8$ where *m* and *n* are approximately 54 and 75 that is used in the treatment of duodenal ulcers

su•crase \\ˈsü-ˌkrās, -ˌkrāz\\ *n* : INVERTASE

su•crose \\ˈsü-ˌkrōs, -ˌkrōz\\ *n* : a sweet crystalline dextrorotatory disaccharide sugar $C_{12}H_{22}O_{11}$ that occurs naturally in most land plants and is the sugar obtained from sugarcane or sugar beets

¹suc•tion \\ˈsək-shən\\ *n* **1** : the act or process of sucking **2 a** : the act or process of exerting a force upon a solid, liquid, or gaseous body by reason of reduced air pressure over part of its surface **b** : force so exerted **3** : the act or process of removing secretions or fluids from hollow or tubular organs or cavities by means of a tube and a device (as a suction pump) that operates on negative pressure

²suction *vb* : to remove (as from a body cavity or passage) by suction

suction pump *n* : a common pump in which the liquid to be raised is pushed by atmospheric pressure into the partial vacuum under a retreating valved piston on the upstroke and reflux is prevented by a valve in the pipe that permits flow in only one direction — see STOMACH PUMP

su•dam•i•na \\sü-ˈda-mə-nə\\ *n pl* : a transient eruption of minute translucent vesicles caused by retention of sweat in the sweat glands and in the corneous layer of the skin and occurring after profuse perspiration — called also *miliaria crystallina* — **su•dam•i•nal** \\-nəl\\ *adj*

Su•dan \\sü-ˈdan\\ *n* : any of several azo solvent dyes including some which have a specific affinity for fatty substances

Sudan IV \\-ˈfōr\\ *n* : a red dye used chiefly as a biological stain and in ointments for promoting (as in the treatment of burns, wounds, or ulcers) the growth of epithelium — called also *scarlet red*

su•dan•o•phil•ia \\sü-ˌda-nə-ˈfi-lē-ə\\ *n* : the quality or state of being sudanophilic

su•dan•o•phil•ic \\sü-ˌda-nə-ˈfi-lik\\ *also* **su•dan•o•phil** \\sü-ˈda-nə-ˌfil\\ *adj* : staining selectively with Sudan dyes; *also* : containing lipids

sudden death *n* : unexpected death that is instantaneous or occurs within minutes from any cause other than violence ⟨*sudden death* following coronary occlusion⟩

sudden infant death syndrome *n* : death of an apparently healthy infant usu. before one year of age that is of unknown cause and occurs esp. during sleep — abbr. *SIDS;* called also *cot death, crib death*

su•do•mo•tor \\ˈsü-də-ˌmō-tər\\ *adj* : of, relating to, or being nerve fibers controlling the activity of sweat glands

su•do•rif•er•ous gland \\ˌsü-də-ˈri-fə-rəs-\\ *n* : SWEAT GLAND

¹su•do•rif•ic \\-ˈri-fik\\ *adj* : causing or inducing sweat : DIAPHORETIC

²sudorific *n* : a sudorific agent or medicine

su•fen•ta•nil \\sü-ˈfen-tə-ˌnil\\ *n* : an opioid analgesic $C_{22}H_{30}N_2O_2S$ that is administered intravenously in the form of its citrate as an anesthetic or an anesthetic adjunct

suf•fo•cate \\ˈsə-fə-ˌkāt\\ *vb* **-cat•ed; -cat•ing 1** : to stop the respiration of (as by strangling or asphyxiation) **2** : to deprive of oxygen **3** : to die from being unable to breathe — **suf•fo•ca•tion** \\ˌsə-fə-ˈkā-shən\\ *n* — **suf•fo•ca•tive** \\ˈsə-fə-ˌkā-tiv\\ *adj*

suf•fuse \\sə-ˈfyüz\\ *vb* **suf•fused; suf•fus•ing** : to flush or spread over or through in the manner of a fluid and esp. blood — **suf•fu•sion** \\sə-ˈfyü-zhən\\ *n*

sug•ar \\ˈshu-gər\\ *n* **1** : a sweet substance that is colorless or white when pure, consists chiefly of sucrose, and is obtained esp. from sugarcane or sugar beets **2** : any of various water-soluble compounds that vary widely in sweetness and comprise the saccharides of smaller molecular size including sucrose

sugar diabetes *n* : DIABETES MELLITUS

su•i•cide \\ˈsü-ə-ˌsīd\\ *n* **1** : the act or an instance of taking one's own life voluntarily and intentionally **2** : a person who commits or attempts suicide — **su•i•cid•al** \\ˌsü-ə-ˈsīd-əl\\ *adj* — **su•i•cid•al•ly** \\-əl-ē\\ *adv* — **suicide** *vb*

su•i•cid•ol•o•gy \\ˌsü-ə-ˌsī-ˈdä-lə-jē\\ *n, pl* **-gies** : the study of suicide and suicide prevention — **su•i•cid•ol•o•gist** \\-jist\\ *n*

suit — see G SUIT, PRESSURE SUIT

suite \\ˈswēt\\ *n* : a group of rooms in a medical facility dedicated to a specified function or specialty ⟨surgical ∼⟩

sul·bac·tam \səl-'bak-ˌtam, -təm\ *n* : a penicillinase inhibitor $C_8H_{11}NO_5S$ that is usu. administered in the form of its sodium salt in combination with a beta-lactam antibiotic (as ampicillin)

sul·cus \'səl-kəs\ *n, pl* **sul·ci** \-ˌkī, -ˌsī\ : FURROW, GROOVE; *esp* : a shallow furrow on the surface of the brain separating adjacent convolutions — compare FISSURE 1c — **sul·cal** \'səl-kəl\ *adj*

sulcus ter·mi·na·lis \-ˌtər-mə-'nā-ləs\ *n, pl* **sulci ter·mi·na·les** \-ˌlēz\ **1** : a V≈ shaped groove separating the anterior two thirds of the tongue from the posterior third and containing the circumvallate papillae **2** : a shallow groove on the outside of the right atrium of the heart

sulf- *or* **sulfo-** *comb form* : sulfur : containing sulfur ⟨*sulf*arsphenamine⟩

¹sul·fa \'səl-fə\ *adj* **1** : related chemically to sulfanilamide **2** : of, relating to, employing, or containing sulfa drugs ⟨∼ therapy⟩

²sulfa *n* : SULFA DRUG

sul·fa·cet·a·mide *also* **sul·fa·cet·i·mide** \ˌsəl-fə-'se-tə-ˌmīd, -məd\ *n* : a sulfa drug $C_8H_{10}N_2O_3S$ that is used chiefly for treating infections of the urinary tract and in the form of its sodium salt derivative for infections of the eye

sul·fa·di·a·zine \ˌsəl-fə-'dī-ə-ˌzēn\ *n* : a sulfa drug $C_{10}H_{10}N_4O_2S$ that is used esp. in the treatment of meningitis, pneumonia, and intestinal infections

sulfa drug *n* : any of various synthetic organic bacteria-inhibiting drugs that are sulfonamides closely related chemically to sulfanilamide — called also *sulfa*

sul·fa·gua·ni·dine \ˌsəl-fə-'gwä-nə-ˌdēn\ *n* : a sulfa drug $C_7H_{10}N_4O_2S$ used esp. in veterinary medicine — called also *sulfanilylguanidine*

sul·fa·mer·a·zine \ˌsəl-fə-'mer-ə-ˌzēn\ *n* : a sulfa drug $C_{11}H_{12}N_4O_2S$ that is a derivative of sulfadiazine and is used similarly

sul·fa·meth·a·zine \-'me-thə-ˌzēn\ *n* : a sulfa drug $C_{12}H_{14}N_4O_2S$ that is a derivative of sulfadiazine and is used similarly

sul·fa·meth·ox·a·zole \-ˌme-'thäk-sə-ˌzōl\ *n* : a sulfonamide $C_{10}H_{11}N_3O_3S$ often combined with trimethoprim and used as an antibacterial esp. in the treatment of urinary tract infections — see BACTRIM

sul·fa·mez·a·thine \-'me-zə-ˌthēn\ *n* : SULFAMETHAZINE

Sul·fa·my·lon \ˌsəl-fə-'mī-ˌlän\ *trademark* — used for a preparation of mafenide

sul·fa·nil·amide \ˌsəl-fə-'ni-lə-ˌmīd, -məd\ *n* : a crystalline sulfonamide $C_6H_8N_2O_2S$ that is the amide of sulfanilic acid and the parent compound of most of the sulfa drugs

sul·fan·i·lyl·gua·ni·dine \səl-ˌfa-ni-ˌlil-'gwä-nə-ˌdēn\ *n* : SULFAGUANIDINE

sul·fa·pyr·i·dine \ˌsəl-fə-'pir-ə-ˌdēn\ *n* : a sulfa drug $C_{11}H_{11}N_3O_2S$ that is derived from pyridine and sulfanilamide and is used in small doses in the treatment of one type of dermatitis and esp. formerly against pneumococcal and gonococcal infections

sul·fa·qui·nox·a·line \-kwi-'näk-sə-ˌlēn\ *n* : a sulfa drug $C_{14}H_{12}N_4O_2S$ used esp. in veterinary medicine

sulf·ars·phen·a·mine \ˌsəl-ˌfärs-'fe-nə-ˌmēn, -mən\ *n* : an orange-yellow powder essentially $C_{12}H_{10}As_2N_2O_2$-$(CH_2SO_3Na_2)$ that is similar to neo-arsphenamine and arsphenamine in structure and uses

sul·fa·sal·a·zine \ˌsəl-fə-'sa-lə-ˌzēn\ *n* : SALICYLAZOSULFAPYRIDINE

¹sul·fate \'səl-ˌfāt\ *n* **1** : a salt or ester of sulfuric acid **2** : a bivalent group or anion SO_4 characteristic of sulfuric acid and the sulfates

²sulfate *vb* **sul·fat·ed; sul·fat·ing 1** : to treat or combine with sulfuric acid or a sulfate **2** : to convert into a sulfate

sul·fa·thi·a·zole \ˌsəl-fə-'thī-ə-ˌzōl\ *n* : a sulfa drug $C_9H_9N_3O_2S_2$ derived from thiazole and sulfanilamide but seldom prescribed because of its toxicity

sul·fa·tide \'səl-fə-ˌtīd\ *n* : any of the sulfates of cerebrosides that often accumulate in the central nervous systems of individuals affected with one form of leukodystrophy

sulf·he·mo·glo·bin \ˌsəlf-'hē-mə-ˌglō-bən\ *n* : a green pigment formed from hemoglobin and found in putrefied organs and cadavers

sulf·he·mo·glo·bi·ne·mia \ˌsəlf-ˌhē-mə-ˌglō-bə-'nē-mē-ə\ *n* : the presence of sulfhemoglobin in the blood

sulf·hy·dryl \ˌsəlf-'hī-drəl\ *n* : THIOL 2 — used chiefly in molecular biology

sul·fide \'səl-ˌfīd\ *n* **1** : any of various organic compounds characterized by a sulfur atom attached to two carbon atoms **2** : a binary compound (as CuS) of sulfur usu. with a more electrically positive element or group

sul·fin·py·ra·zone \ˌsəl-fən-'pi-rə-ˌzōn\ *n* : a uricosuric drug $C_{23}H_{20}N_2O_3S$ used in long-term treatment of chronic gout

sul·fi·sox·a·zole \ˌsəl-fə-'säk-sə-ˌzōl\ *n* : a sulfa drug $C_{11}H_{13}N_3O_3S$ derived from sulfanilamide that is used similarly to other sulfanilamide derivatives but is less likely to produce renal damage because of its greater solubility

sulfo- — see SULF-

sul·fo·bro·mo·phtha·lein \ˌsəl-fō-ˌbrō-mō-'tha-lē-ən, -'thä-ˌlēn\ *n* : a diagnostic material used in the form of its sodium salt $C_{20}H_8Br_4Na_2O_{10}S_2$ in a liver function test

sul·fon·amide \ˌsəl-'fä-nə-ˌmīd, -məd; -'fō-nə-ˌmid\ *n* : any of various amides (as sulfanilamide) of a sulfonic acid; *also* : SULFA DRUG

sul·fon·eth·yl·meth·ane \ˌsəl-ˌfō-ˌne-thəl-ˈme-ˌthän\ *n* : a crystalline hypnotic $C_8H_{18}O_4S_2$ that is an ethyl analog of sulfonmethane

sul·fon·ic acid \ˌsəl-ˈfä-nik-, -ˈfō-\ *n* : any of numerous acids that contain the SO_3H group

sul·fon·meth·ane \ˌsəl-fōn-ˈme-ˌthän\ *n* : a crystalline hypnotic $C_5H_{10}O_4S_2$

sul·fo·nyl·urea \ˌsəl-fə-nil-ˈyur-ē-ə, -ˌni-ˈlur-\ *n* : any of several hypoglycemic compounds related to the sulfonamides and used in the oral treatment of diabetes

sul·fo·sal·i·cyl·ic acid \ˌsəl-fō-ˌsa-lə-ˈsi-lik-\ *n* : a sulfonic acid derivative $C_7H_6O_6S_3$ used esp. to detect and precipitate proteins (as albumin) from urine

sulf·ox·one sodium \ˌsəl-ˈfäk-ˌsōn-\ *n* : a crystalline salt $C_{14}H_{14}N_2Na_2O_6S_3$ used in the treatment of leprosy

sul·fur \ˈsəl-fər\ *n* : a nonmetallic element that occurs either free or combined esp. in sulfides and sulfates — symbol S; see ELEMENT table — **sulfur** *adj*

sul·fu·rat·ed lime solution \ˈsəl-fyə-ˌrā-təd-\ *n* : an orange-colored solution containing sulfides of calcium and used as a topical antiseptic and scabicide

sulfurated potash *n* : a mixture composed principally of sulfurated potassium compounds that is used in treating skin diseases

sulfur dioxide *n* : a heavy pungent toxic gas SO_2 that is a major air pollutant esp. in industrial areas

sul·fu·ric \ˌsəl-ˈfyur-ik\ *adj* : of, relating to, or containing sulfur esp. with a higher valence than sulfurous compounds

sulfuric acid *n* : a heavy corrosive oily strong acid H_2SO_4 having two replaceable hydrogen atoms

sul·fu·rous \ˈsəl-fə-rəs, -fyə-; ˌsəl-ˈfyur-əs\ *adj* **1** : of, relating to, or containing sulfur esp. with a lower valence than sulfuric compounds **2** : resembling or emanating from sulfur and esp. burning sulfur

sulfurous acid *n* : a weak unstable acid H_2SO_3 known in solution and through its salts and used in medicine as an antiseptic

su·lin·dac \sə-ˈlin-ˌdak\ *n* : an antiinflammatory drug $C_{20}H_{17}FO_3S$ used esp. in the treatment of rheumatoid arthritis

sul·i·so·ben·zone \ˌsə-li-sō-ˈben-ˌzōn\ *n* : a sunscreening agent $C_{14}H_{12}O_6S$

sulph- *or* **sulpho-** *chiefly Brit var of* SULF-

sul·pha, sul·phate, sul·phide, sul·phur, sul·phu·ric *chiefly Brit var of* SULFA, SULFATE, SULFIDE, SULFUR, SULFURIC

su·mac *also* **su·mach** \ˈsü-ˌmak, ˈshü-\

n : any of various plants of the genus *Rhus* including several (as poison sumac, *R. vernix*) having foliage poisonous to the touch

su·ma·trip·tan \ˌsü-mə-ˈtrip-ˌtan, -tən\ *n* : a serotonin agonist $C_{14}H_{21}N_3O_2S$ administered by injection in the form of its succinate in the treatment of migraine headaches

sum·ma·tion \(ˌ)sə-ˈmā-shən\ *n* : cumulative action or effect; *esp* : the process by which a sequence of stimuli that are individually inadequate to produce a response are cumulatively able to induce a nerve impulse — see SPATIAL SUMMATION, TEMPORAL SUMMATION

summer complaint *n* : SUMMER DIARRHEA

summer diarrhea *n* : diarrhea esp. of children that is prevalent in hot weather and is usu. caused by ingestion of food contaminated by various microorganisms

summer sores *n sing or pl* : a skin disease of the horse caused by larval roundworms of the genus *Habronema*

sun block *n* : a chemical agent (as zinc oxide or para-aminobenzoic acid) or a preparation of this that is applied to the skin to prevent sunburn by blocking out all or most of the sun's rays — compare SUNSCREEN

sun·burn \ˈsən-ˌbərn\ *n* : inflammation of the skin caused by overexposure to ultraviolet radiation esp. from sunlight — **sunburn** *vb*

sun·glass·es \-ˌgla-səs\ *n pl* : glasses used to protect the eyes from the sun

sun·lamp \ˈsən-ˌlamp\ *n* : an electric lamp designed to emit radiation of wavelengths from ultraviolet to infrared and used esp. for therapeutic purposes or for producing tan artificially

sun·screen \-ˌskrēn\ *n* : a substance (as para-aminobenzoic acid) used in suntan preparations to protect the skin from excessive ultraviolet radiation — **sun·screen·ing** *adj*

sunshine vitamin *n* : VITAMIN D

sun·stroke \-ˌstrōk\ *n* : heatstroke caused by direct exposure to the sun

sun·tan \-ˌtan\ *n* : a browning of the skin from exposure to the rays of the sun — **sun·tanned** \-ˌtand\ *adj*

super- *prefix* **1** : greater than normal : excessive ⟨*super*ovulation⟩ **2** : situated or placed above, on, or at the top of ⟨*super*ciliary⟩; *specif* : situated on the dorsal side of

su·per·cil·i·ary \ˌsü-pər-ˈsi-lē-ˌer-ē\ *adj* : of, relating to, or adjoining the eyebrow : SUPRAORBITAL

superciliary arch *n* : SUPERCILIARY RIDGE

superciliary ridge *n* : a prominence of the frontal bone above the eye caused by the projection of the frontal sinuses — called also *browridge, superciliary arch, supraorbital ridge*

su·per·coil \'sü-pər-ˌkȯil\ n : SUPERHE-LIX — **supercoil** vb

su·per·ego \ˌsü-pər-'ē-(ˌ)gō, 'sü-pər-, -ˌē-(ˌ)gō\ n : the one of the three divisions of the psyche in psychoanalytic theory that is only partly conscious, represents internalization of parental conscience and the rules of society, and functions to reward and punish through a system of moral attitudes, conscience, and a sense of guilt — compare EGO, [1]ID

su·per·fam·i·ly \'sü-pər-ˌfam-lē\ n, pl **-lies** : a category of taxonomic classification ranking next above a family

su·per·fat·ted \'sü-pər-ˌfa-təd\ adj : containing extra oil or fat (~ soap)

su·per·fe·cun·da·tion \ˌsü-pər-ˌfe-kən-'dā-shən, -ˌfē-\ n : successive fertilization of two or more ova from the same ovulation esp. by different mates

su·per·fe·ta·tion \ˌsü-pər-fē-'tā-shən\ n : successive fertilization of two or more ova of different ovulations resulting in the presence of embryos of unlike ages in the same uterus

su·per·fi·cial \ˌsü-pər-'fi-shəl\ adj **1** : of, relating to, or located near the surface (~ blood vessels) **2** : penetrating below or affecting only the surface (~ wounds) — **su·per·fi·cial·ly** adv

superficial external pudendal artery n : EXTERNAL PUDENDAL ARTERY a

superficial fascia n : the thin layer of loose fatty connective tissue underlying the skin and binding it to the parts beneath — called also *hypodermis, tela subcutanea*; compare DEEP FASCIA

superficial inguinal ring n : the inguinal ring that is the external opening of the inguinal canal — called also *external inguinal ring*; compare DEEP INGUINAL RING

superficialis — see FLEXOR DIGITORUM SUPERFICIALIS

superficial palmar arch n : PALMAR ARCH b

superficial peroneal nerve n : a nerve that arises as a branch of the common peroneal nerve and that innervates or supplies branches innervating the muscles of the anterior part of the leg and the skin on the lower anterior part of the leg, on the dorsum of the foot, on the lateral and medial sides of the foot, and between the toes — called also *musculocutaneous nerve*; compare DEEP PERONEAL NERVE

superficial temporal artery n : the one of the two terminal branches of each external carotid artery that arises in the substance of the parotid gland, passes upward over the zygomatic process of the temporal bone, and is distributed by way of branches esp. to the more superficial parts of the side of the face and head

superficial temporal vein n : TEMPORAL VEIN a(1)

superficial transverse metacarpal ligament n : a transverse ligamentous band across the palm of the hand in the superficial fascia at the base of the fingers — called also *superficial transverse ligament*

superficial transverse perineal muscle n : TRANSVERSUS PERINEI SUPERFICIALIS

su·per·fuse \ˌsü-pər-'fyüz\ vb **-fused; -fus·ing** : to maintain the metabolic or physiological activity of (as an isolated organ) by submitting to a continuous flow of a sustaining medium over the outside — **su·per·fu·sion** \-'fyü-zhən\ n

su·per·gene \'sü-pər-ˌjēn\ n : a group of linked genes acting as an allelic unit esp. when due to the suppression of crossing-over

su·per·he·lix \'sü-pər-ˌhē-liks\ n : a helix (as of DNA) which has its axis arranged in a helical coil — called also *supercoil* — **su·per·he·li·cal** \ˌsü-pər-'he-li-kəl, -'hē-\ adj

su·per·in·fec·tion \ˌsü-pər-in-'fek-shən\ n : a second infection superimposed on an earlier one esp. by a different microbial agent of exogenous or endogenous origin that is resistant to the treatment used against the first infection — **su·per·in·fect** \-in-'fekt\ vb

su·pe·ri·or \su-'pir-ē-ər\ adj **1** : situated toward the head and further away from the feet than another and esp. another similar part — compare INFERIOR 1 **2** : situated in a more anterior or dorsal position in the body of a quadruped — compare INFERIOR 2

superior alveolar nerve n : any of the branches of the maxillary nerve or of the infraorbital nerve that supply the teeth and gums of the upper jaw

superior articular process n : ARTICULAR PROCESS a

superior carotid triangle n : a space in each lateral half of the neck that is bounded in back by the sternocleidomastoid muscle, below by the omohyoid muscle, and above by the stylohyoid and digastric muscles

superior cerebellar artery n : an artery that arises from the basilar artery just before it divides to form the posterior cerebral arteries and supplies or gives off branches supplying the superior part of the cerebellum, midbrain, pineal gland, and choroid plexus of the third ventricle

superior cerebellar peduncle n : CEREBELLAR PEDUNCLE a

superior colliculus n : either member of the anterior and higher pair of corpora quadrigemina that together constitute a primitive center for vision — called also *optic lobe, optic tectum*; compare INFERIOR COLLICULUS

superior concha n : NASAL CONCHA c

superior constrictor n : a 4-sided muscle of the pharynx that acts to constrict part of the pharynx in swallowing — called also *constrictor pharyngis superior, superior pharyngeal constrictor muscle;* compare INFERIOR CONSTRICTOR, MIDDLE CONSTRICTOR

superior extensor retinaculum *n* : EXTENSOR RETINACULUM 1b

superior ganglion *n* **1** : the upper and smaller of the two sensory ganglia of the glossopharyngeal nerve that may be absent but when present is situated in a groove in which the nerve passes through the jugular foramen — called also *jugular ganglion;* compare INFERIOR GANGLION 1 **2** : the upper of the two ganglia of the vagus nerve that is situated at the point where it exits through the jugular foramen — called also *jugular ganglion, superior vagal ganglion;* compare INFERIOR GANGLION 2

superior gluteal artery *n* : GLUTEAL ARTERY a

superior gluteal nerve *n* : GLUTEAL NERVE a

superior gluteal vein *n* : any of several veins that accompany the superior gluteal artery and empty into the internal iliac vein

superior hemorrhoidal artery *n* : RECTAL ARTERY c

superior hemorrhoidal vein *n* : RECTAL VEIN c

superior intercostal vein *n* : a vein on each side formed by the union of the veins draining the first two or three intercostal spaces of which the one on the right usu. empties into the azygos vein but sometimes into the right innominate vein and the one on the left empties into the left innominate vein after crossing the arch of the aorta

superioris — see LEVATOR LABII SUPERIORIS, LEVATOR LABII SUPERIORIS ALAEQUE NASI, LEVATOR PALPEBRAE SUPERIORIS, QUADRATUS LABII SUPERIORIS

superiority complex *n* : an excessive striving for or pretense of superiority to compensate for supposed inferiority

superior laryngeal artery *n* : LARYNGEAL ARTERY b

superior laryngeal nerve *n* : LARYNGEAL NERVE a — called also *superior laryngeal*

superior longitudinal fasciculus *n* : a large bundle of association fibers in the white matter of each cerebral hemisphere that extends above the insula from the frontal lobe to the occipital lobe where it curves downward and forward into the temporal lobe

su·pe·ri·or·ly *adv* : in or to a more superior position or direction

superior meatus *n* : a curved relatively short anteroposterior passage on

each side of the nose that occupies the middle third of the lateral wall of a nasal cavity between the superior and middle nasal conchae — compare INFERIOR MEATUS, MIDDLE MEATUS

superior mesenteric artery *n* : MESENTERIC ARTERY b

superior mesenteric ganglion *n* : MESENTERIC GANGLION b

superior mesenteric plexus *n* : MESENTERIC PLEXUS b

superior mesenteric vein *n* : MESENTERIC VEIN b

superior nasal concha *n* : NASAL CONCHA c

superior nuchal line *n* : NUCHAL LINE a

superior oblique *n* : OBLIQUE b(1)

superior olive *n* : a small gray nucleus situated on the dorsolateral aspect of the trapezoid body — called also *superior olivary nucleus;* compare INFERIOR OLIVE

superior ophthalmic vein *n* : OPHTHALMIC VEIN a

superior orbital fissure *n* : ORBITAL FISSURE a

superior pancreaticoduodenal artery *n* : PANCREATICODUODENAL ARTERY b

superior pectoral nerve *n* : PECTORAL NERVE a

superior peroneal retinaculum *n* : PERONEAL RETINACULUM a

superior petrosal sinus *n* : PETROSAL SINUS a

superior pharyngeal constrictor muscle *n* : SUPERIOR CONSTRICTOR

superior phrenic artery *n* : PHRENIC ARTERY a

superior phrenic vein *n* : PHRENIC VEIN a

superior ramus *n* : RAMUS b(1)

superior rectal artery *n* : RECTAL ARTERY c

superior rectal vein *n* : RECTAL VEIN c

superior rectus *n* : RECTUS 2a

superior sagittal sinus *n* : SAGITTAL SINUS a

superior temporal gyrus *n* : TEMPORAL GYRUS a

superior thyroid artery *n* : THYROID ARTERY a

superior turbinate *n* : NASAL CONCHA c

superior turbinate bone *n* : NASAL CONCHA c

superior ulnar collateral artery *n* : a long slender artery that arises from the brachial artery or one of its branches just below the middle of the upper arm, descends to the elbow following the course of the ulnar nerve, and terminates under the flexor carpi ulnaris — compare INFERIOR ULNAR COLLATERAL ARTERY

superior vagal ganglion *n* : SUPERIOR GANGLION 2

superior vena cava *n* : a vein that is the second largest vein in the human body, is formed by the union of the two innominate veins at the level of the space between the first two ribs, and returns blood to the right atrium of the heart from the upper half of the body

superior vena cava syndrome *n* : a condition characterized by elevated venous pressure of the upper extremities with accompanying distension of the affected veins and swelling of the face and neck and caused by blockage (as by a thrombus) or compression (as by a neoplasm) of the superior vena cava

superior vermis *n* : VERMIS 1a

superior vesical *n* : VESICAL ARTERY a

superior vesical artery *n* : VESICAL ARTERY a

superior vestibular nucleus *n* : the one of the four vestibular nuclei on each side of the medulla oblongata that sends ascending fibers to the oculomotor and trochlear nuclei in the cerebrum on the same side of the brain

superior vocal cords *n pl* : FALSE VOCAL CORDS

su·per·na·tant \₁sü-pər-'nāt-ᵊnt\ *n* : the usu. clear liquid overlying material deposited by settling, precipitation, or centrifugation — **supernatant** *adj*

su·per·nu·mer·ary \₁sü-pər-'nü-mə-₁rer-ē, -'nyü-\ *adj* : exceeding the usual or normal number ⟨~ teeth⟩

supero- *comb form* : situated above ⟨superolateral⟩

su·pero·lat·er·al \₁sü-pə-rō-'la-tə-rəl\ *adj* : situated above and toward the side

su·per·ovu·la·tion \-₁ä-vyə-'lā-shən\ *n* : production of exceptional numbers of ova at one time — **su·per·ovu·late** \-'ä-vyə-₁lāt\ *vb*

su·per·ox·ide \-'äk-₁sīd\ *n* : the monovalent anion O^-_2 or a compound containing it ⟨potassium ~ KO_2⟩

superoxide dis·mu·tase \-dis-'myü-₁tās, -₁tāz\ *n* : a metal-containing enzyme that reduces potentially harmful free radicals of oxygen formed during normal metabolic cell processes to oxygen and hydrogen peroxide

su·per·po·tent \₁sü-pər-'pōt-ᵊnt\ *adj* : of greater than normal or acceptable potency — **su·per·po·ten·cy** \-ᵊn-sē\ *n*

su·per·scrip·tion \₁sü-pər-'skrip-shən\ *n* : the part of a pharmaceutical prescription which contains or consists of the Latin word *recipe* or the sign ℞

su·per·son·ic \-'sä-nik\ *adj* 1 : having a frequency above the human ear's audibility limit of about 20,000 cycles per second ⟨~ vibrations⟩ 2 : utilizing, produced by, or relating to supersonic waves or vibrations — **su·per·son·i·cal·ly** *adv*

su·per·vene \₁sü-pər-'vēn\ *vb* **-vened; -ven·ing** : to follow or result as an additional, adventitious, or unlooked= for development or in the course of a disease)

su·pi·na·tion \₁sü-pə-'nā-shən\ *n* 1 : rotation of the forearm and hand so that the palm faces forward or upward and the radius lies parallel to the

ulna; *also* : a corresponding movement of the foot and leg 2 : the position resulting from supination — **su·pi·nate** \'sü-pə-₁nāt\ *vb*

su·pi·na·tor \'sü-pə-₁nā-tər\ *n* : a muscle that produces the motion of supination; *specif* : a deeply situated muscle of the forearm that arises in two layers from the lateral epicondyle of the humerus and adjacent parts of the ligaments and bones of the elbow and that passes over the head of the radius to insert into its neck and the lateral surface of its shaft

supinator crest *n* : a bony ridge on the upper lateral surface of the shaft of the ulna that is the origin for part of the supinator muscle

su·pine \sü-'pīn, 'sü-₁pīn\ *adj* 1 : lying on the back or with the face upward 2 : marked by supination

¹**sup·ple·ment** \'sə-plə-mənt\ *n* : something that completes or makes an addition ⟨dietary ~s⟩

²**sup·ple·ment** \-₁ment\ *vb* : to add a supplement to : serve as a supplement for — **sup·ple·men·ta·tion** \₁sə-plə-₁men-'tā-shən, -mən-\ *n*

sup·ple·men·tal \₁sə-plə-'ment-ᵊl\ *adj* : serving to supplement : SUPPLEMENTARY

supplemental air *n* : the air that can still be expelled from the lungs after an ordinary expiration — compare RESIDUAL AIR

sup·ple·men·ta·ry \₁sə-plə-'men-tə-rē\ *adj* : added or serving as a supplement ⟨~ vitamins⟩

sup·ply \sə-'plī\ *vb* **sup·plied; sup·ply·ing** : to furnish (organs, tissues, or cells) with a vital element (as blood or nerve fibers) — used of nerves and blood vessels

¹**sup·port** \sə-'pōrt\ *vb* 1 : to hold up or serve as a foundation or prop for 2 : to maintain in condition, action, or existence ⟨~ life⟩ — **sup·por·tive** \-'pōr-tiv\ *adj*

²**support** *n* 1 : the act or process of supporting : the condition of being supported ⟨respiratory ~⟩ 2 : SUPPORTER

sup·port·er *n* : a woven or knitted band or elastic device supporting a part; *esp* : ATHLETIC SUPPORTER

support group *n* : a group of people with common experiences and concerns who provide emotional and moral support for one another

support hose *n* : stockings (as elastic stockings) worn to supply mild compression to assist the veins of the legs — usu. used with a pl. verb; called also *support hosiery*

sup·pos·i·to·ry \sə-'pä-zə-₁tōr-ē\ *n, pl* **-ries** : a solid but readily melting cone or cylinder of usu. medicated material for insertion into a bodily passage or cavity (as the rectum)

sup·press \sə-'pres\ *vb* 1 : to exclude from consciousness ⟨~ed anxiety⟩ 2 : to restrain from a usual course or action ⟨∼ a cough⟩ **3** : to inhibit the genetic expression of ⟨∼ a mutation⟩ — **sup·press·ible** \-ʹpre-sə-bəl\ *adj*

¹**sup·press·ant** \sə-ʹpres-ᵊnt\ *adj* : SUPPRESSIVE

²**suppressant** *n* : an agent (as a drug) that tends to suppress or reduce in intensity rather than eliminate something

sup·pres·sion \sə-ʹpre-shən\ *n* : an act or instance of suppressing: as **a** : stoppage of a bodily function or a symptom **b** : the failure of development of a bodily part or organ **c** : the conscious intentional exclusion from consciousness of a thought or feeling — compare REPRESSION 2a

sup·pres·sive \sə-ʹpre-siv\ *adj* : tending or serving to suppress something (as the symptoms of a disease) ⟨∼ drugs⟩

sup·pres·sor \sə-ʹpre-sər\ *n* : one that suppresses; *esp* : a mutant gene that suppresses the expression of another nonallelic mutant gene when both are present

suppressor T cell *n* : a T cell that suppresses the immune response of B cells and other T cells to an antigen — called also *suppressor lymphocyte, suppressor cell, suppressor T lymphocyte*

sup·pu·ra·tion \ˌsə-pyə-ʹrā-shən\ *n* : the formation of, conversion into, or process of discharging pus ⟨∼ in a wound⟩ — **sup·pu·rate** \ʹsə-pyə-ˌrāt\ *vb* — **sup·pu·ra·tive** \ʹsə-pyə-ˌrā-tiv\ *adj*

suppurativa — see HIDRADENITIS SUPPURATIVA

supra- *prefix* **1** : SUPER- 2 ⟨*supra*orbital⟩ **2** : transcending ⟨*supra*molecular⟩

su·pra·cer·vi·cal hysterectomy \ˌsü-prə-ʹsər-vi-kəl\ *n* : a hysterectomy in which the uterine cervix is not removed

su·pra·chi·as·mat·ic \-ˌkī-əz-ʹma-tik\ *adj* : SUPRAOPTIC

suprachiasmatic nucleus *n* : a small group of neurons situated immediately dorsal to the optic chiasma

su·pra·cla·vic·u·lar \-kla-ʹvi-kyə-lər, -klə-\ *adj* : situated or occurring above the clavicle ⟨∼ lymph nodes⟩

supraclavicular nerve *n* : any of three nerves that are descending branches of the cervical plexus arising from the third and fourth cervical nerves and that supply the skin over the upper chest and shoulder

su·pra·clu·sion \ˌsü-prə-ʹklü-zhən\ *n* : SUPRAOCCLUSION

su·pra·con·dy·lar \ˌsü-prə-ʹkän-də-lər, -ˌprä-\ *adj* : of, relating to, affecting, or being the part of a bone situated above a condyle ⟨a ∼ fracture⟩

supracondylar ridge *n* : either of two ridges above the condyle of the humerus of which one is situated laterally and the other medially and which give attachment to muscles

su·pra·gin·gi·val \-ʹjin-jə-vəl\ *adj* : located on the surface of a tooth not

surrounded by gingiva ⟨∼ calculus⟩

su·pra·gle·noid \-ʹgle-ˌnoid, -ʹglē-\ *adj* : situated or occurring superior to the glenoid cavity

su·pra·glot·tic \-ʹglä-tik\ *adj* : situated or occurring above the glottis

su·pra·hy·oid \-ʹhī-ˌoid\ *adj* : situated or occurring superior to the hyoid bone ⟨∼ lymphadenectomy⟩

suprahyoid muscle *n* : any of several muscles (as the mylohyoid and geniohyoid) passing upward to the jaw and face from the hyoid bone

su·pra·mar·gi·nal gyrus \-ˌmär-jən-ᵊl-\ *n* : a gyrus of the inferior part of the parietal lobe that is continuous in front with the postcentral gyrus and posteriorly and inferiorly with the superior temporal gyrus

su·pra·mo·lec·u·lar \-mə-ʹle-kyə-lər\ *adj* : more complex than a molecule; *also* : composed of many molecules

su·pra·nu·cle·ar \-ʹnü-klē-ər, -ʹnyü-\ *adj* : situated, occurring, or produced by a lesion superior or cortical to a nucleus esp. of the brain

su·pra·oc·clu·sion \-ə-ʹklü-zhən\ *n* : the projection of a tooth beyond the plane of occlusion

su·pra·op·tic \-ʹäp-tik\ *adj* : situated or occurring above the optic chiasma

supraoptic nucleus *n* : a small nucleus of closely packed neurons that overlies the optic chiasma and is intimately connected with the neurohypophysis

su·pra·or·bit·al \-ʹor-bət-ᵊl\ *adj* : situated or occurring above the orbit of the eye

supraorbital artery *n* : a branch of the ophthalmic artery supplying the orbit and parts of the forehead

supraorbital fissure *n* : ORBITAL FISSURE a

supraorbital foramen *n* : SUPRAORBITAL NOTCH

supraorbital nerve *n* : a branch of the frontal nerve supplying the forehead, scalp, cranial periosteum, and adjacent parts

supraorbital notch *n* : a notch or foramen in the bony border of the upper inner part of the orbit serving for the passage of the supraorbital nerve, artery, and vein

supraorbital ridge *n* : SUPERCILIARY RIDGE

supraorbital vein *n* : a vein that drains the supraorbital region and unites with the frontal vein to form the angular vein

su·pra·pu·bic \-ʹpyü-bik\ *adj* : situated, occurring, or performed from above the pubis ⟨∼ prostatectomy⟩ — **su·pra·pu·bi·cal·ly** *adv*

¹**su·pra·re·nal** \-ʹrēn-ᵊl\ *adj* : situated above or anterior to the kidneys; *specif* : ADRENAL

²**suprarenal** *n* : a suprarenal part; *esp* : ADRENAL GLAND

suprarenal artery *n* : any of three arteries on each side of the body that supply the adrenal gland located on the same side and that arise from the inferior phrenic artery, the abdominal aorta, or the renal artery

suprarenal gland *n* : ADRENAL GLAND

suprarenal vein *n* : either of two veins of which one arises from the right adrenal gland and empties directly into the inferior vena cava while the other arises from the left adrenal gland, passes behind the pancreas, and empties into the renal vein on the left side

su·pra·scap·u·lar \ˌsü-prə-ˈska-pyə-lər, -ˌprä-\ *adj* : situated or occurring superior to the scapula

suprascapular artery *n* : a branch of the thyrocervical trunk that passes over the suprascapular ligament to the back of the scapula

suprascapular ligament *n* : a thin flat ligament that is attached at one end to the coracoid process and at the other end to the upper margin of the scapula on its dorsal surface

suprascapular nerve *n* : a branch of the brachial plexus that supplies the supraspinatus and infraspinatus muscles

suprascapular notch *n* : a deep notch in the upper border of the scapula at the base of the coracoid process giving passage to the suprascapular nerve

su·pra·sel·lar \-ˈse-lər\ *adj* : situated or rising above the sella turcica — used chiefly of tumors of the hypophysis

su·pra·spi·nal \-ˈspī-nəl\ *adj* : situated or occurring above a spine

supraspinal ligament *n* : a fibrous cord that joins the tips of the spinous processes of the vertebrae from the seventh cervical vertebra to the sacrum and that continues forward to the skull as the ligamentum nuchae — called also *supraspinous ligament*

su·pra·spi·na·tus \-ˌspī-ˈnā-təs\ *n* : a muscle of the back of the shoulder that arises from the supraspinous fossa of the scapula, that inserts into the top of the greater tubercle of the humerus, that is one of the muscles making up the rotator cuff of the shoulder, and that rotates the humerus laterally and helps to abduct the arm

su·pra·spi·nous fossa \ˌsü-prə-ˈspī-nəs-\ *n* : a smooth concavity above the spine on the dorsal surface of the scapula that gives origin to the supraspinatus muscle

supraspinous ligament *n* : SUPRASPINAL LIGAMENT

su·pra·ster·nal \-ˈstərn-əl\ *adj* : situated above or measured from the top of the sternum ⟨∼ height⟩

suprasternal notch *n* : the depression in the top of the sternum between its articulations with the two clavicles

suprasternal space *n* : a long narrow space in the lower part of the deep fascia of the cervical region containing areolar tissue, the sternal part of the sternocleidomastoid muscles, and the lower part of the anterior jugular veins

su·pra·ten·to·ri·al \-ten-ˈtōr-ē-əl\ *adj* : relating to, occurring in, affecting, or being the tissues overlying the tentorium cerebelli ⟨a ∼ glioma⟩

su·pra·thresh·old \-ˈthresh-ˌhōld\ *adj* : of sufficient strength or quantity to produce a perceptible physiological effect

su·pra·troch·le·ar artery \-ˈträ-klē-ər-\ *n* : one of the terminal branches of the ophthalmic artery that ascends upon the forehead from the inner angle of the orbit

supratrochlear nerve *n* : a branch of the frontal nerve supplying the skin of the forehead and the upper eyelid

su·pra·val·vu·lar \-ˈval-vyə-lər\ *adj* : situated or occurring above a valve ⟨∼ aortic stenosis⟩

su·pra·ven·tric·u·lar \-ven-ˈtri-kyə-lər\ *adj* : relating to or being a rhythmic abnormality of the heart caused by impulses originating above the ventricles (as in the atrioventricular node) ⟨∼ tachycardia⟩

su·pra·vi·tal \-ˈvīt-əl\ *adj* : constituting or relating to the staining of living tissues or cells surviving after removal from a living body by dyes that penetrate living substance but induce more or less rapid degenerative changes — compare INTRAVITAL 2 — **su·pra·vi·tal·ly** *adv*

supreme thoracic artery *n* : THORACIC ARTERY 1a

su·ral nerve \ˈsùr-əl-\ *n* : any of several nerves in the region of the calf of the leg; *esp* : one formed by the union of a branch of the tibial nerve with a branch of the common peroneal nerve that supplies branches to the skin of the back of the leg and sends a continuation to the little toe by way of the lateral side of the foot

sur·a·min \ˈsùr-ə-mən\ *n* : a trypanocidal drug $C_{51}H_{34}N_6Na_6O_{23}S_6$ obtained as a white powder and administered intravenously in the early stages of African sleeping sickness — called also *germanin, suramin sodium;* see NAPHURIDE

surface–active *adj* : altering the properties and esp. lowering the tension at the surface of contact between phases (soaps are typical ∼ substances)

surface tension *n* : a condition that exists at the free surface of a body (as a liquid) by reason of molecular forces about the individual surface molecules and is manifested by properties resembling those of an elastic skin under tension

sur·fac·tant \(ˌ)sər-ˈfak-tənt, ˈsər-ˌ\ *n* : a surface-active substance; *specif* : a surface-active lipoprotein mixture which coats the alveoli and which prevents collapse of the lungs by reducing the surface tension of pulmonary fluids — **surfactant** *adj*

surfer's knot *n* : a knobby lump just below a surfer's knee or on the upper surface of the foot caused by friction and pressure between surfboard and skin — called also *surfer's knob, surfer's lump, surfer's nodule*

surg *abbr* **1** surgeon **2** surgery **3** surgical

sur·geon \'sər-jən\ *n* **1** : a medical specialist who performs surgery : a physician qualified to treat those diseases that are amenable to or require surgery — compare INTERNIST **2** : the senior medical officer of a military unit

surgeon general *n, pl* **surgeons general** : the chief medical officer of a branch of the armed services or of a public health service

sur·gery \'sər-jə-rē\ *n, pl* **-ger·ies** **1** : a branch of medicine concerned with diseases and conditions requiring or amenable to operative or manual procedures **2 a** *Brit* : a physician's or dentist's office **b** : a room or area where surgery is performed **3 a** : the work done by a surgeon **b** : OPERATION

sur·gi·cal \'sər-ji-kəl\ *adj* **1** : of, relating to, or concerned with surgeons or surgery **2** : requiring surgical treatment ⟨a ∼ appendix⟩ **3** : resulting from surgery ⟨∼ fever⟩ **4** : done by or used in surgery or surgical conditions — **sur·gi·cal·ly** \'sər-ji-klē, -kə-lē\ *adv* : by means of surgery

surgical neck *n* : a slightly narrowed part of the humerus below the greater and lesser tubercles that is frequently the site of fractures

sur·gi·cen·ter \'sər-jə-ˌsen-tər\ *n* : a medical facility that performs minor surgery on an outpatient basis

sur·ra \'sur-ə\ *n* : a severe febrile and hemorrhagic disease of domestic animals that is caused by a protozoan of the genus *Trypanosoma* (*T. evansi*)

sur·ro·ga·cy \'sər-ə-gə-sē\ *n, pl* **-cies** : the practice of serving as a surrogate mother

sur·ro·gate \-gət\ *n* : one that serves as a substitute: as **a** : a representation of a person substituted through symbolizing (as in a dream) for conscious recognition of the person **b** : a drug substituted for another drug **c** : SURROGATE MOTHER

surrogate mother *n* : a woman who becomes pregnant usu. by artificial insemination or surgical implantation of a fertilized egg for the purpose of carrying the fetus to term for another woman — **surrogate motherhood** *n*

sur·veil·lance \sər-'vā-ləns, -lyəns\ *n* : close and continuous observation or testing ⟨serological ∼⟩ — see IMMUNOLOGICAL SURVEILLANCE

¹sus·cep·ti·ble \sə-'sep-tə-bəl\ *adj* **1** : having little resistance to a specific infectious disease : capable of being infected **2** : predisposed to develop a noninfectious disease ⟨∼ to diabetes⟩ **3** : abnormally reactive to various drugs — **sus·cep·ti·bil·i·ty** \sə-ˌsep-tə-'bil-ə-tē\ *n*

²susceptible *n* : one that is susceptible (as to a disease)

suspended animation *n* : temporary suspension of the vital functions

sus·pen·sion \sə-'spen-chən\ *n* **1 a** : the state of a substance when its particles are mixed with but undissolved in a fluid or solid **b** : a substance in this state **2** : a system consisting of a solid dispersed in a solid, liquid, or gas usu. in particles of larger than colloidal size

¹sus·pen·so·ry \sə-'spen-sə-rē\ *adj* : serving to suspend : providing support

²suspensory *n, pl* **-ries** : something that suspends or holds up; *esp* : a fabric supporter for the scrotum

suspensory ligament *n* : a ligament or fibrous membrane suspending an organ or part: as **a** : a ringlike fibrous membrane connecting the ciliary body and the lens of the eye and holding the lens in place **b** : FALCIFORM LIGAMENT

suspensory ligament of the ovary *n* : a fold of peritoneum that consists of a part of the broad ligament that is attached to the ovary near the end joining the fallopian tube and that contains blood and lymph vessels passing to and from the ovary — called also *infundibulopelvic ligament*; compare LIGAMENT OF THE OVARY

sus·ten·tac·u·lar cell \ˌsəs-tən-'ta-kyə-lər-\ *n* : a supporting epithelial cell (as of the olfactory epithelium) that lacks a specialized function

sustentacular fiber of Müller *n* : FIBER OF MÜLLER

sus·ten·tac·u·lum ta·li \ˌsəs-tən-'ta-kyə-ləm-'tā-ˌlī\ *n* : a medial process of the calcaneus supporting part of the talus

su·ture \'sü-chər\ *n* **1 a** : a stitch made with a suture **b** : a strand or fiber used to sew parts of the living body **c** : the act or process of sewing with sutures **2 a** : the line of union in an immovable articulation (as between the bones of the skull); *also* : such an articulation **b** : a furrow at the junction of adjacent bodily parts — **su·tur·al** \'sü-chə-rəl\ *adj* — **suture** *vb*

sux·a·me·tho·ni·um \ˌsük-sə-mə-'thō-nē-əm\ *n, chiefly Brit* : SUCCINYLCHOLINE

sved·berg \'sfed-ˌbərg, -ˌber-ē\ *n* : a unit of time amounting to 10^{-13} second that is used to measure the sedimentation velocity of a colloidal solution (as of a protein) in an ultracentrifuge and to determine molecular weight by substitution in an equation — called also *svedberg unit*

Svedberg, Theodor (1884–1971), Swedish chemist.

¹swab \'swäb\ n 1 : a wad of absorbent material usu. wound around one end of a small stick and used for applying medication or for removing material from an area 2 : a specimen taken with a swab ⟨a throat ∼⟩

²swab vb **swabbed; swab•bing** : to apply medication to with a swab

swamp fever n : EQUINE INFECTIOUS ANEMIA

Swan–Ganz catheter \'swän-'ganz-\ : a soft catheter with a balloon tip that is used for measuring blood pressure in the pulmonary artery

  Swan, Harold James Charles (b 1922), **and Ganz, William** (b 1919), American cardiologists.

S wave \'es-₁\ n : the negative downward deflection in the QRS complex of an electrocardiogram that follows the R wave

sway•back \'swā-₁bak\ n 1 : an abnormally hollow condition or sagging of the back found esp. in horses; also : a back so shaped 2 : LORDOSIS 3 : a copper-deficiency disease of young or newborn lambs that is marked by demyelination of the brain resulting in weakness, staggering gait, and collapse and is almost universally fatal but is readily preventable by copper supplementation of the diet of the pregnant ewe — **sway•backed** \-₁bakt\ adj

¹sweat \'swet\ vb **sweat** or **sweat•ed; sweat•ing** : to excrete moisture in visible quantities through the opening of the sweat glands : PERSPIRE

²sweat n 1 : the fluid excreted from the sweat glands of the skin : PERSPIRATION 2 : abnormally profuse sweating — often used in pl. ⟨soaking ∼s⟩

sweat duct n : the part of a sweat gland which extends through the dermis to the surface of the skin

sweat gland n : a simple tubular gland of the skin that secretes perspiration and in humans is widely distributed in nearly all parts of the skin — called also sudoriferous gland

sweat test n : a test for cystic fibrosis that involves measuring the subject's sweat for abnormally high sodium chloride content

swee•ny \'swē-nē\ n, pl **sweenies** : an atrophy of the shoulder muscles of a horse; broadly : any muscular atrophy of a horse

sweet \'swēt\ adj : being or inducing the one of the four basic taste sensations that is typically induced by disaccharides and is mediated esp. by receptors in taste buds at the front of the tongue — compare BITTER, SALT 2, SOUR — **sweet•ness** n

sweet clover disease n : a hemorrhagic diathesis of sheep and cattle feeding on sweet clover (genus Melilotus of the family Leguminosae) containing excess quantities of dicumarol

Sweet's syndrome \'swēts-\ n : a disease that occurs esp. in middle-aged women, that is characterized by red raised often painful patches on the skin, fever, and neutrophilia in the peripheral blood, that responds to treatment with corticosteroids but not antibiotics, and that is of unknown cause but is sometimes associated with an underlying malignant disorder — called also acute febrile neutrophilic dermatosis

  Sweet, Robert (fl 1942–64), British dermatologist.

swell \'swel\ vb **swelled; swelled** or **swol•len** \'swō-lən\; **swell•ing** : to become distended or puffed up

swell•ing \'swel-iŋ\ n : an abnormal bodily protuberance or localized enlargement ⟨an inflammatory ∼⟩

Swift's disease \'swifts-\ n : ACRODYNIA

  Swift, H. (fl 1918), Australian physician.

swimmer's itch n : an itching inflammation that is a reaction to the invasion of the skin by schistosomes that are not normally parasites of humans — called also schistosome dermatitis

swine \'swin\ n : any of various stout= bodied short-legged mammals (family Suidae) with a thick bristly skin and a long mobile snout; esp : a domesticated member of a species (Sus scrofa) that occurs wild in the Old World

swine dysentery n : an acute infectious hemorrhagic dysentery of swine

swine erysipelas n : a destructive contagious disease of various mammals and birds that is caused by a bacterium of the genus Erysipelothrix (E. rhusiopathiae) — called also erysipelas

swine fever n : HOG CHOLERA

swineherd's disease n : a form of leptospirosis contracted from swine

swine influenza n : an acute contagious febrile disease of swine caused by interaction of a specific virus introduced by the lungworm (Metastrongylus elongatus) of swine and a bacterium of the genus Haemophilus (H. suis) related to that causing human influenza — called also swine flu

swine pox n : a mild virus disease of young pigs marked by fever, loss of appetite, dullness, and production of skin lesions

swol•len adj : protuberant or abnormally distended (as by injury or disease)

sy•co•sis \si-'kō-səs\ n, pl **sy•co•ses** \-₁sēz\ : a chronic inflammatory disease involving the hair follicles esp. of the bearded part of the face and marked by papules, pustules, and tubercles perforated by hairs with crusting

sycosis bar•bae \-'bär-bē\ n : sycosis of the bearded part of the face

Syd•en•ham's chorea \'sid-ⁿn-əmz-\ n : chorea following infection (as rheumatic fever) and occurring usu. in children and adolescents

Syden·ham, Thomas (1624–1689), British physician.

syl·vat·ic \sil-ˈva-tik\ adj : occurring in, affecting, or transmitted by wild animals (∼ diseases)

sylvatic plague n : a form of plague of which wild rodents and their fleas are the reservoirs and vectors and which is widely distributed in western No. and So. America though rarely affecting humans

Syl·vi·an \ˈsil-vē-ən\ adj : of or relating to the fissure of Sylvius

    F. Dubois or **De Le Boë** — see FISSURE OF SYLVIUS

Sylvian fissure n : FISSURE OF SYLVIUS

sym- — see SYN-

sym·bi·ont \ˈsim-ˌbī-ˌänt, -bē-\ n : an organism living in symbiosis; esp : the smaller member of a symbiotic pair

sym·bi·o·sis \ˌsim-ˌbī-ˈō-səs, -bē-\ n, pl **-bi·o·ses** \-ˌsēz\ 1 : the living together in more or less intimate association or close union of two dissimilar organisms 2 : the intimate living together of two dissimilar organisms in a mutually beneficial relationship — **sym·bi·ot·ic** \ˌsim-ˌbī-ˈä-tik, -bē-\ adj — **sym·bi·ot·i·cal·ly** adv

sym·bi·ote \ˈsim-ˌbī-ˌōt, -bē-\ n : SYMBIONT

sym·bleph·a·ron \sim-ˈble-fə-ˌrän\ n : adhesion between an eyelid and the eyeball

sym·bol \ˈsim-bəl\ n : something that stands for or suggests something else; esp : an object or act representing something in the unconscious mind that has been repressed (phallic ∼s) — **sym·bol·ic** \sim-ˈbä-lik\ adj — **sym·bol·i·cal·ly** adv

Syme's amputation \ˈsīmz-\ or **Syme amputation** \ˈsīm-\ n : amputation of the foot through the articulation of the ankle with removal of the malleoli of the tibia and fibula — compare PIROGOFF'S AMPUTATION

    Syme, James (1799–1870), British surgeon.

Sym·me·trel \ˈsi-mə-ˌtrel\ trademark — used for a preparation of amantadine

sym·me·try \ˈsi-mə-trē\ n, pl **-tries** : correspondence in size, shape, and relative position of parts on opposite sides of a dividing line or median plane or about a center or axis — see BILATERAL SYMMETRY — **sym·met·ri·cal** \sə-ˈme-tri-kəl\ or **sym·met·ric** \-trik\ adj — **sym·met·ri·cal·ly** adv

sympath- or **sympatho-** comb form : sympathetic nerve : sympathetic nervous system (sympatholytic)

sym·pa·thec·to·my \ˌsim-pə-ˈthek-tə-mē\ n, pl **-mies** : surgical interruption of sympathetic nerve pathways — **sym·pa·thec·to·mized** \-ˌmīzd\ adj

¹**sym·pa·thet·ic** \ˌsim-pə-ˈthe-tik\ adj 1 : of or relating to the sympathetic nervous system 2 : mediated by or acting on the sympathetic nerves — **sym·pa·thet·i·cal·ly** adv

²**sympathetic** n : a sympathetic structure; esp : SYMPATHETIC NERVOUS SYSTEM

sympathetic chain n : either of the pair of ganglionated longitudinal cords of the sympathetic nervous system of which one is situated on each side of the spinal column — called also sympathetic trunk; compare VERTEBRAL GANGLION

sympathetic nerve n : a nerve of the sympathetic nervous system

sympathetic nervous system n : the part of the autonomic nervous system that contains chiefly adrenergic fibers and tends to depress secretion, decrease the tone and contractility of smooth muscle, and increase heart rate and that consists essentially of preganglionic fibers arising in the thoracic and upper lumbar parts of the spinal cord and passing through delicate white rami communicantes to ganglia located in a pair of sympathetic chains situated one on each side of the spinal column or to more peripheral ganglia or ganglionated plexuses and postganglionic fibers passing typically through gray rami communicantes to spinal nerves with which they are distributed to various end organs — called also sympathetic system; compare PARASYMPATHETIC NERVOUS SYSTEM

sympathetico- comb form : SYMPATH- (sympatheticomimetic)

sym·pa·thet·i·co·mi·met·ic \ˌsim-pə-ˈthe-ti-kō-mə-ˈme-tik\ adj or n : SYMPATHOMIMETIC

sympathetic ophthalmia n : inflammation in an uninjured eye as a result of injury and inflammation of the other

sym·pa·thet·i·co·to·nia \ˌsim-pə-ˌthe-ti-kə-ˈtō-nē-ə\ n : SYMPATHICOTONIA

sympathetic system n : SYMPATHETIC NERVOUS SYSTEM

sympathetic trunk n : SYMPATHETIC CHAIN

sympathico- comb form : SYMPATH- (sympathicotonia)

sym·path·i·co·lyt·ic \sim-ˌpa-thi-kō-ˈli-tik\ adj or n : SYMPATHOLYTIC

sym·path·i·co·mi·met·ic \-mə-ˈme-tik, -mī-\ adj or n : SYMPATHOMIMETIC

sym·path·i·co·to·nia \sim-ˌpa-thi-kō-ˈtō-nē-ə\ n : a condition produced by relatively great activity or stimulation of the sympathetic nervous system and characterized by goose bumps, vascular spasm, and abnormally high blood pressure — called also sympatheticotonia; compare VAGOTONIA — **sym·path·i·co·ton·ic** \-ˈtä-nik\ adj

sym·pa·thin \sim-pə-thən\ n : a substance (as norepinephrine) that is secreted by sympathetic nerve endings and acts as a chemical mediator

sym·pa·tho·ad·re·nal \ˌsim-pə-thō-ə-ˈdrē-nəl\ adj : relating to or involving the sympathetic nervous system and the adrenal medulla

sym·pa·tho·go·nia \ˌsim-pə-thō-ˈgō-nē-ə\ *n* : precursor cells of the sympathetic nervous system

sym·pa·tho·go·ni·o·ma \-ˌgō-nē-ˈō-mə\ *n, pl* **-ma·ta** \-mə-tə\ *or* **-mas** : a tumor derived from sympathogonia; *also* : NEUROBLASTOMA

¹sym·pa·tho·lyt·ic \ˌsim-pə-thō-ˈli-tik\ *adj* : tending to oppose the physiological results of sympathetic nervous activity or of sympathomimetic drugs — compare PARASYMPATHOLYTIC

²sympatholytic *n* : a sympatholytic agent

¹sym·pa·tho·mi·met·ic \-mə-ˈme-tik, -ˌ(ˌ)mī-\ *adj* : simulating sympathetic nervous action in physiological effect — compare PARASYMPATHOMIMETIC

²sympathomimetic *n* : a sympathomimetic agent

sym·phal·an·gism \(ˌ)sim-ˈfa-lən-ˌji-zəm\ *n* : ankylosis of the joints of one or more digits

sym·phy·se·al \ˌsim-fə-ˈsē-əl\ *adj* : of, relating to, or constituting a symphysis

sym·phy·si·ot·o·my \ˌsim-fə-zē-ˈä-tə-mē, sim-ˌfi-zē-\ *n, pl* **-mies** : the operation of dividing the pubic symphysis

sym·phy·sis \ˈsim-fə-səs\ *n, pl* **-phy·ses** \-ˌsēz\ **1** : an immovable or more or less movable articulation of various bones in the median plane of the body **2** : an articulation (as between the bodies of vertebrae) in which the bony surfaces are connected by pads of fibrous cartilage without a synovial membrane

symphysis pubis *n* : PUBIC SYMPHYSIS

symp·tom \ˈsimp-təm\ *n* : subjective evidence of disease or physical disturbance observed by the patient ⟨headache is a ∼ of many diseases⟩; *broadly* : something that indicates the presence of a physical disorder — compare SIGN 2

symp·tom·at·ic \ˌsimp-tə-ˈma-tik\ *adj* **1 a** : being a symptom of a disease **b** : having the characteristics of a particular disease but arising from another cause ⟨∼ epilepsy resulting from brain damage⟩ **2** : concerned with or affecting symptoms ⟨∼ treatment⟩ **3** : having symptoms ⟨a ∼ patient⟩ — **symp·tom·at·i·cal·ly** *adv*

symp·tom·atol·o·gy \ˌsimp-tə-mə-ˈtä-lə-jē\ *n, pl* **-gies 1** : SYMPTOM COMPLEX **2** : a branch of medical science concerned with symptoms of diseases — **symp·tom·ato·log·i·cal** \-ˌmat-ᵊl-ˈä-ji-kəl\ *or* **symp·tom·ato·log·ic** \-ˈä-jik\ *adj* — **symp·tom·ato·log·i·cal·ly** *adv*

symptom complex *n* : a group of symptoms occurring together and characterizing a particular disease

symp·tom·less \ˈsimp-təm-ləs\ *adj* : exhibiting no symptoms

syn- *or* **sym-** *prefix* **1** : with : along with

: together ⟨symbiosis⟩ **2** : at the same time ⟨synesthesia⟩

syn·aes·the·sia *chiefly Brit var of* SYNESTHESIA

syn·an·throp·ic \ˌsi-nan-ˈthrä-pik\ *adj* : ecologically associated with humans ⟨∼ flies⟩ — **syn·an·thro·py** \si-ˈnan-thrə-pē\ *n*

¹syn·apse \ˈsi-ˌnaps, sə-ˈnaps\ *n* **1** : the place at which a nervous impulse passes from one neuron to another **2** : SYNAPSIS

²synapse *vb* **syn·apsed; syn·aps·ing** : to form a synapse or come together in synapsis

syn·ap·sis \sə-ˈnap-səs\ *n, pl* **-ap·ses** \-ˌsēz\ : the association of homologous chromosomes with chiasma formation that is characteristic of the first meiotic prophase and is held to be the mechanism for genetic crossing-over

syn·ap·tic \si-ˈnap-tik\ *adj* : of or relating to a synapse or to synapsis ⟨∼ transmission⟩ — **syn·ap·ti·cal·ly** *adv*

synaptic cleft *n* : the space between neurons at a nerve synapse across which a nerve impulse is transmitted by a neurotransmitter — called also *synaptic gap*

synaptic vesicle *n* : a small secretory vesicle that contains a neurotransmitter, is found inside an axon near the presynaptic membrane, and releases its contents into the synaptic cleft after fusing with the membrane

syn·ap·to·gen·e·sis \sə-ˌnap-tə-ˈje-nə-səs\ *n, pl* **-e·ses** \-ˌsēz\ : the formation of nerve synapses

syn·ap·tol·o·gy \ˌsi-nap-ˈtä-lə-jē\ *n, pl* **-gies** : the scientific study of nerve synapses

syn·ap·to·some \sə-ˈnap-tə-ˌsōm\ *n* : a nerve ending that is isolated from homogenized nerve tissue — **syn·ap·to·som·al** \-ˌnap-tə-ˈsō-məl\ *adj*

syn·ar·thro·sis \ˌsi-när-ˈthrō-səs\ *n, pl* **-thro·ses** \-ˌsēz\ : an immovable articulation in which the bones are united by intervening fibrous connective tissues

syn·chon·dro·sis \ˌsin-kän-ˈdrō-səs\ *n, pl* **-dro·ses** \-ˌsēz\ : an immovable skeletal articulation in which the union is cartilaginous

syn·cho·ri·al \ˌsin-ˈkōr-ē-əl, siŋ-\ *adj* : having a common placenta — used of multiple fetuses

syn·chro·nized sleep \ˈsiŋ-krə-ˌnīzd-, ˈsin-\ *n* : SLOW-WAVE SLEEP

syn·co·pe \ˈsiŋ-kə-pē, ˈsin-\ *n* : loss of consciousness resulting from insufficient blood flow to the brain : FAINT — **syn·co·pal** \ˈsiŋ-kə-pəl, ˈsin-\ *adj*

syn·cy·tial \sin-ˈsi-shəl, -shē-əl\ *adj* : of, relating to, or constituting syncytium

syn·cy·tio·tro·pho·blast \sin-ˌsi-shē-ō-ˈtrō-fə-ˌblast\ *n* : the outer syncytial layer of the trophoblast that actively invades the uterine wall forming the outermost fetal component of the placenta — called also *syntrophoblast;* compare CYTOTROPHOBLAST

syn·cy·tium \sin-'si-shəm, -shē-ən\ *n, pl* **-tia** \-shə, -shē-ə\ : a multinucleate mass of protoplasm resulting from fusion of cells

syn·dac·tyl \'sin-'dakt-ᵊl\ *adj* : having two or more digits wholly or partly united

syn·dac·ty·lism \sin-'dak-tə-ıli-zəm\ *n* : SYNDACTYLY

syn·dac·ty·lous \sin-'dak-tə-ləs\ *adj* : SYNDACTYL

syn·dac·ty·ly \-lē\ *n, pl* **-lies** : a union of two or more digits that occurs as a human hereditary disorder marked by webbing of two or more fingers or toes

syndesm- *or* **syndesmo-** *comb form* : ligament ⟨*syndesmosis*⟩

syn·des·mo·sis \ısin-ıdez-'mō-səs, -des-\ *n, pl* **-mo·ses** \-ısēz\ : an articulation in which the contiguous surfaces of the bones are rough and are bound together by a ligament

syn·drome \'sin-ıdrōm\ *n* : a group of signs and symptoms that occur together and characterize a particular abnormality

syn·e·chia \si-'ne-kē-ə, -'nē-\ *n, pl* **-chiae** \-kē-ıē, -ıī\ : an adhesion of parts and esp. one involving the iris of the eye: as **a** : adhesion of the iris to the cornea — called also *anterior synechia* **b** : adhesion of the iris to the crystalline lens — called also *posterior synechia*

syn·eph·rine \sə-'ne-frən\ *n* : a crystalline sympathomimetic amine C_9H_{13}-NO_2 isomeric with phenylephrine

syn·er·gic \si-'nər-jik\ *adj* : working together ⟨∼ muscle contraction⟩ — **syn·er·gi·cal·ly** *adv*

syn·er·gism \'si-nər-ıji-zəm\ *n* : interaction of discrete agents (as drugs) such that the total effect is greater than the sum of the individual effects — called also *synergy;* compare ANTAGONISM b — **syn·er·gis·tic** \ısi-nər-'jis-tik\ *adj* — **syn·er·gis·ti·cal·ly** *adv*

syn·er·gist \-jist\ *n* **1** : an agent that increases the effectiveness of another when combined with it; *esp* : a drug that acts in synergism with another **2** : an organ (as a muscle) that acts in concert with another to enhance its effect — compare AGONIST 1, ANTAGONIST a

syn·er·gize \'si-nər-ıjīz\ *vb* **-gized; -gizing 1** : to act as synergists : exhibit synergism **2** : to increase the activity of (a substance)

syn·er·gy \-jē\ *n, pl* **-gies** : SYNERGISM

syn·es·the·sia \ısi-nəs-'thē-zhə, -zhē-ə\ *n* : a subjective sensation or image of a sense (as of color) other than the one (as of sound) being stimulated — **syn·es·thet·ic** \-'the-tik\ *adj*

Syn·ga·mus \'siŋ-gə-məs\ *n* : a genus (family Syngamidae) of nematode worms that are parasitic in the trachea or esophagus of various birds and mammals and include the gapeworm (*S. trachea*)

syn·ga·my \'siŋ-gə-mē\ *n, pl* **-mies** : sexual reproduction by union of gametes

syn·ge·ne·ic \ısin-jə-'nē-ik\ *adj* : genetically identical esp. with respect to antigens or immunological reactions ⟨∼ tumor cells⟩ — compare ALLOGENEIC, XENOGENEIC

syn·kary·on \sin-'kar-ē-ıän, -ē-ən\ *n* : a cell nucleus formed by the fusion of two preexisting nuclei

syn·ki·ne·sia \ısin-kə-'nē-zhə, -ıkī-, -zhē-ə\ *n* : SYNKINESIS

syn·ki·ne·sis \-'nē-səs\ *n, pl* **-ne·ses** \-ısēz\ : involuntary movement in one part when another part is moved : an associated movement — **syn·ki·net·ic** \-'ne-tik\ *adj*

syn·os·to·sis \ısi-ınäs-'tō-səs\ *n, pl* **-to·ses** \-ısēz\ : union of two or more separate bones to form a single bone; *also* : the union so formed (as at an epiphyseal line) — **syn·os·tot·ic** \-'tä-tik\ *adj*

syn·o·vec·to·my \ısi-nə-'vek-tə-mē\ *n, pl* **-mies** : surgical removal of a synovial membrane

sy·no·via \sə-'nō-vē-ə, sī-\ *n* : a transparent viscid lubricating fluid secreted by a membrane of an articulation, bursa, or tendon sheath — called also *synovial fluid*

sy·no·vi·al \-vē-əl\ *adj* : of, relating to, or secreting synovia ⟨∼ effusion⟩; *also* : lined with synovial membrane ⟨a ∼ bursa⟩ ⟨∼ tendon sheaths⟩

synovial fluid *n* : SYNOVIA

synovial joint *n* : DIARTHROSIS

synovial membrane *n* : the dense connective-tissue membrane that secretes synovia and that lines the ligamentous surfaces of articular capsules, tendon sheaths where free movement is necessary, and bursae

sy·no·vi·tis \ısī-nə-'vī-təs\ *n* : inflammation of a synovial membrane usu. with pain and swelling of the joint

sy·no·vi·um \sə-'nō-vē-əm, sī-\ *n* : SYNOVIAL MEMBRANE

syn·the·sis \'sin-thə-səs\ *n, pl* **-the·ses** \-ısēz\ **1** : the composition or combination of parts or elements so as to form a whole **2** : the production of a substance by the union of chemical elements, groups, or simpler compounds or by the degradation of a complex compound ⟨protein ∼⟩ — **syn·the·size** \-ısīz\ *vb*

syn·the·tase \'sin-thə-ıtās, -ıtāz\ *n* : an enzyme that catalyzes the linking together of two molecules esp. by using the energy derived from the concurrent splitting off of a group from a triphosphate (as ATP) — called also *ligase*

¹**syn·thet·ic** \sin-'the-tik\ *adj* : of, relating to, or produced by chemical or biochemical synthesis; *esp* : pro-

duced artificially ⟨∼ drugs⟩ — **syn-thet·i·cal·ly** adv

²**synthetic** n : a product (as a drug) of chemical synthesis

syn·tro·pho·blast \sin-ˈtrō-fə-ˌblast\ n : SYNCYTIOTROPHOBLAST

syphil- or **syphilo-** comb form : syphilis ⟨syphiloma⟩

syph·i·lid \ˈsi-fə-lid\ n : a skin eruption caused by syphilis

syph·i·lis \ˈsi-fə-ləs\ n : a chronic contagious usu. venereal and often congenital disease that is caused by a spirochete of the genus *Treponema* (*T. pallidum*) and if left untreated produces chancres, rashes, and systemic lesions in a clinical course with three stages continued over many years — called also *lues*; see PRIMARY SYPHILIS, SECONDARY SYPHILIS, TERTIARY SYPHILIS

¹**syph·i·lit·ic** \ˌsi-fə-ˈli-tik\ adj : of, relating to, or infected with syphilis — **syph·i·lit·i·cal·ly** adv

²**syphilitic** n : a person infected with syphilis

syph·i·lo·ma \ˌsi-fə-ˈlō-mə\ n, pl **-mas** or **-ma·ta** \-mə-tə\ : a syphilitic tumor : GUMMA (a testicular ∼)

syph·i·lo·ther·a·py \ˌsi-fə-lō-ˈther-ə-pē\ n, pl **-pies** : the treatment of syphilis

Sy·rette \sə-ˈret\ trademark — used for a small collapsible tube fitted with a hypodermic needle for injecting a single dose of a medicinal agent

syring- or **syringo-** comb form : tube : fistula ⟨syringobulbia⟩

sy·ringe \sə-ˈrinj, ˈsir-inj\ n : a device used to inject fluids into or withdraw them from something (as the body or its cavities): as **a** : a device that consists of a nozzle of varying length and a compressible rubber bulb and is used for injection or irrigation (an ear ∼) **b** : an instrument (as for the injection of medicine or the withdrawal of bodily fluids) that consists of a hollow barrel fitted with a plunger and a hollow needle **c** : a gravity device consisting of a reservoir fitted with a long rubber tube ending with an exchangeable nozzle that is used for irrigation of the vagina or bowel — **syringe** vb

sy·rin·go·bul·bia \sə-ˌrin-gō-ˈbəl-bē-ə\ n : the presence of abnormal cavities in the medulla oblongata

sy·rin·go·my·elia \sə-ˌrin-gō-mī-ˈē-lē-ə\ n : a chronic progressive disease of the spinal cord associated with sensory disturbances, muscle atrophy, and spasticity

syr·o·sin·go·pine \ˌsir-ō-ˈsin-gə-ˌpēn, -ˈpin\ n : a white crystalline powder $C_{35}H_{42}N_2O_{11}$ that is closely related to reserpine and is used as an antihypertensive drug

syr·up \ˈsər-əp, ˈsir-əp\ n : a thick sticky liquid consisting of a concentrated solution of sugar and water with or without the addition of a flavoring agent or medicinal substance (∼ of ipecac) — **syr·upy** \-ə-pē\ adj

sys·tem \ˈsis-təm\ n **1** : a group of body organs that together perform one or more vital functions — see CIRCULATORY SYSTEM, NERVOUS SYSTEM, REPRODUCTIVE SYSTEM, RESPIRATORY SYSTEM **2** : the body considered as a functional unit

¹**sys·tem·ic** \sis-ˈte-mik\ adj : of, relating to, or common to a system: as **a** : affecting the body generally — compare LOCAL **b** : supplying those parts of the body that receive blood through the aorta rather than through the pulmonary artery **c** : being a pesticide that as used is harmless to a higher animal or a plant but when absorbed into the bloodstream or the sap makes the whole organism toxic to pests (as cattle grubs) — **sys·tem·i·cal·ly** adv

²**systemic** n : a systemic pesticide

systemic circulation n : the passage of arterial blood from the left atrium of the heart through the left ventricle, the systemic arteries, and the capillaries to the organs and tissues that receive much of its oxygen in exchange for carbon dioxide and the return of the carbon-dioxide carrying blood via the systemic veins to enter the right atrium of the heart and to participate in the pulmonary circulation

systemic lupus erythematosus n : an inflammatory connective tissue disease of unknown cause that occurs chiefly in women and is characterized esp. by fever, skin rash, and arthritis, often by acute hemolytic anemia, by small hemorrhages in the skin and mucous membranes, by inflammation of the pericardium, and in serious cases by involvement of the kidneys and central nervous system

sys·to·le \ˈsis-tə-(ˌ)lē\ n : the contraction of the heart by which the blood is forced onward and the circulation kept up — compare DIASTOLE — **sys·tol·ic** \sis-ˈtä-lik\ adj

systolic pressure n : the highest arterial blood pressure of a cardiac cycle occurring immediately after systole of the left ventricle of the heart — compare DIASTOLIC PRESSURE

T

¹**T** *abbr* **1** thoracic — used with a number from 1 to 12 to indicate a vertebra or segment of the spinal cord ⟨multiple injuries with a fracture of *T-12*⟩ **2** thymine

²**T** *symbol* tritium

2,4,5–T — see entry alphabetized as TWO,FOUR,FIVE-T

Ta *symbol* tantalum

TA *abbr* transactional analysis

tab \'tab\ *n* : TABLET

ta·bar·dil·lo \ˌtä-bär-'dē-yō\ *n* : murine typhus occurring esp. in Mexico

ta·bel·la \tə-'be-lə\ *n, pl* **-lae** \-ˌlē\ : a medicated lozenge or tablet

ta·bes \'tā-(ˌ)bēz\ *n, pl* **tabes 1** : wasting accompanying a chronic disease **2** : TABES DORSALIS

tabes dor·sa·lis \-dor-'sä-ləs, -'sa-\ *n* : a syphilitic disorder that involves the dorsal horns of the spinal cord and the sensory nerve trunks and that is marked by wasting, pain, lack of coordination of voluntary movements and reflexes, and disorders of sensation, nutrition, and vision — called also *locomotor ataxia*

ta·bet·ic \tə-'be-tik\ *adj* : of, relating to, or affected with tabes and esp. tabes dorsalis ⟨~ pains⟩ ⟨a ~ joint⟩

ta·ble·spoon \'tā-bəl-ˌspün\ *n* : a unit of measure equal to 4 fluid drams or ½ fluid ounce or 15 milliliters

ta·ble·spoon·ful \ˌtā-bəl-'spün-ˌfùl, 'tā-bəl-ˌ\ *n, pl* **tablespoonfuls** \-ˌfùlz\ *also* **ta·ble·spoons·ful** \-'spünz-ˌfùl, -ˌspünz-\ : TABLESPOON

tab·let \'ta-blət\ *n* : a small mass of medicated material (as in the shape of a disk) ⟨an aspirin ~⟩

tabo- *comb form* : progressive wasting : tabes ⟨*taboparesis*⟩

ta·bo·pa·re·sis \ˌtā-bō-pə-'rē-səs, -'par-ə-səs\ *n, pl* **-re·ses** \-ˌsēz\ : paresis occurring with tabes and esp. with tabes dorsalis

tache noire \'täsh-'nwär\ *n, pl* **taches noires** *same or* -'nwärz\ : a small dark-centered ulcer that appears at the site of a tick bite and is the primary lesion of boutonneuse fever

ta·chis·to·scope \tə-'kis-tə-ˌskōp-, ta-\ *n* : an apparatus for the brief exposure of visual stimuli that is used in the study of learning, attention, and perception — **ta·chis·to·scop·ic** \-ˌkis-tə-'skä-pik\ *adj* — **ta·chis·to·scop·i·cal·ly** *adv*

tachy- *comb form* : rapid : accelerated ⟨*tachy*cardia⟩

tachy·ar·rhyth·mia \ˌta-kē-ā-'rith-mē-ə\ *n* : arrhythmia characterized by a rapid irregular heartbeat

tachy·car·dia \ˌta-ki-'kär-dē-ə\ *n* : relatively rapid heart action whether physiological (as after exercise) or pathological — see PAROXYSMAL TACHYCARDIA; compare BRADYCARDIA — **tachy·car·di·ac** \-dē-ˌak\ *adj*

tachy·phy·lax·is \ˌta-ki-fi-'lak-səs\ *n, pl* **-lax·es** \-ˌsēz\ : diminished response to later increments in a sequence of applications of a physiologically active substance — **tachy·phy·lac·tic** \-fi-'lak-tik\ *adj*

tachy·pnea \ˌta-kip-'nē-ə\ *n* : increased rate of respiration — **tachy·pne·ic** \-'nē-ik\ *adj*

tachy·pnoea *chiefly Brit var of* TACHYPNEA

tac·rine \'ta-ˌkrēn, -ˌkrīn\ *n* : an anticholinesterase $C_{13}H_{14}N_2$ that crosses the blood-brain barrier and is used esp. in the palliative treatment of cognitive deficits in learning, memory, and mood occurring early in Alzheimer's disease

¹**tac·tile** \'tak-təl, -ˌtīl\ *adj* **1** : of, relating to, mediated by, or affecting the sense of touch **2** : having or being organs or receptors for the sense of touch — **tac·tile·ly** *adv*

²**tactile** *n* : a person whose prevailing mental imagery is tactile rather than visual, auditory, or motor — compare AUDILE, VISUALIZER

tactile corpuscle *n* : one of the numerous minute bodies (as a Meissner's corpuscle) in the skin and some mucous membranes that usu. consist of a group of cells enclosed in a capsule, contain nerve terminations, and are held to be end organs of touch

tactile receptor *n* : an end organ (as a Meissner's corpuscle or a Pacinian corpuscle) that responds to light touch

tac·toid \'tak-ˌtòid\ *n* : an elongated particle (as in a sickle cell) that appears as a spindle-shaped body under a polarizing microscope

tac·tual \'tak-chə-wəl\ *adj* : of or relating to the sense or the organs of touch : derived from or producing the sensation of touch : TACTILE ⟨a ~ sense⟩

taen- *or* **taeni-** *also* **ten-** *or* **teni-** *comb form* : tapeworm ⟨*taeni*asis⟩

tae·nia \'tē-nē-ə\ *n* **1 a** \'tē-nē-ə\ *pl* **tae·nias** : TAPEWORM **b** *cap* : a genus of taeniid tapeworms that comprises forms usu. occurring as adults in the intestines of carnivores and as larvae in various ruminants, and that includes the beef tapeworm (*T. saginata*) and the pork tapeworm (*T. solium*) of humans **2** *pl* **tae·ni·ae** \-nē-ˌē, -ˌī\ *or* **taenias** : a band of nervous tissue or of muscle

taenia co·li \-'kō-ˌlī\ *n, pl* **taeniae coli** : any of three external longitudinal muscle bands of the large intestine

tae·ni·a·sis \tē-'nī-ə-səs\ *n* : infestation with or disease caused by tapeworms

tae·ni·id \'tē-nē-əd\ *n* : any of a family

(Taeniidae) of tapeworms that includes numerous forms of medical or veterinary importance — **taeniid** *adj*

tae·ni·oid \'tē-nē-ˌoid\ *adj* : resembling or related to the taeniid tapeworms

¹**tag** \'tag\ *n* 1 **a** : a shred of flesh or muscle **b** : a small abnormal projecting piece of tissue esp. when potentially or actually neoplastic in character 2 : LABEL

²**tag** *vb* **tagged; tag·ging** : LABEL

Tag·a·met \'ta-gə-ˌmet\ *trademark* — used for a preparation of cimetidine

tail \'tāl\ *n, often attrib* 1 : the rear end or a process or prolongation of the rear end of the body of an animal 2 : any of various parts of bodily structures that are terminal: as **a** : the distal tendon of a muscle **b** : the slender left end of the human pancreas **c** : the common convoluted tube that forms the lower part of the epididymis 3 : the part of a sperm consisting of the middle portion and the terminal flagellum

tail·bone \-ˈbōn\ *n* 1 : a caudal vertebra 2 : COCCYX

tail bud *n* : a knob of embryonic tissue that contributes to the formation of the posterior part of the vertebrate body — called also *end bud*

Ta·ka·ya·su's disease \ˌtä-kə-ˈyä-süz-\ *n* : progressive obliteration of the arteries branching from the arch of the aorta and comprising the innominate artery, left common carotid artery, and left subclavian artery that is marked by diminution or loss of the pulse in and symptoms of ischemia in the head, neck, and arms

Takayasu, Michishige (1872–1938), Japanese physician.

¹**take** \'tāk\ *vb* **took** \'tük\; **tak·en** \'tā-kən\; **tak·ing** 1 : to establish a take esp. by uniting or growing 2 *of a vaccine or vaccination* : to produce a take

²**take** *n* 1 : a local or systemic reaction indicative of successful vaccination 2 : a successful union (as of a graft)

take up *vb* : to absorb or incorporate into itself — **take–up** *n*

tali *pl of* TALUS

tal·i·pes \'ta-lə-ˌpēz\ *n* : CLUBFOOT 1

talipes equi·no·var·us \-ˌe-kwi-nō-ˈvar-əs\ *n* : a congenital deformity of the foot in which both talipes equinus and talipes varus occur so that walking is done on the toes and outer side of the sole

talipes equi·nus \-ˈe-kwi-nəs\ *n* : a congenital deformity of the foot in which the sole is permanently flexed so that walking is done on the toes without touching the heel to the ground

talipes valgus *n* : a congenital deformity of the foot in which it is rotated inward so that walking is done on the inner side of the sole

talipes varus *n* : a congenital deformity of the foot in which it is rotated outward so that walking is done on the outer side of the sole

talo- *comb form* : astragalar and ⟨*talo-tibial*⟩

ta·lo·cru·ral \ˌtā-lō-ˈkrür-əl\ *adj* : relating to or being the ankle joint

ta·lo·na·vic·u·lar \ˌtā-lō-nə-ˈvi-kyə-lər\ *adj* : of or relating to the talus and the navicular of the tarsus

ta·lo·tib·i·al \ˌtā-lō-ˈti-bē-əl\ *adj* : of or relating to the talus and the tibia

ta·lus \'tā-ləs\ *n, pl* **ta·li** \'tā-ˌlī\ 1 : the human astragalus that bears the weight of the body and together with the tibia and fibula forms the ankle joint — called also *anklebone* 2 : the entire ankle

Tal·win \'tal-ˌwin\ *trademark* — used for a preparation of pentazocine

ta·mox·i·fen \ta-ˈmäk-si-ˌfen\ *n* : an estrogen antagonist $C_{26}H_{29}NO$ used esp. to treat postmenopausal breast cancer

¹**tam·pon** \'tam-ˌpän\ *n* : a plug (as of cotton) introduced into a cavity usu. to absorb secretions (as from menstruation) or to arrest hemorrhaging

²**tampon** *vb* : to plug with a tampon

tam·pon·ade \ˌtam-pə-ˈnäd\ *n* 1 : the closure or blockage (as of a wound or body cavity) by or as if by a tampon esp. to stop bleeding 2 : CARDIAC TAMPONADE

tan \'tan\ *n* : a brown color imparted to the skin by exposure to the sun or wind — **tan** *vb*

T and A *abbr* tonsillectomy and adenoidectomy

tan·gle \'taŋ-gəl\ *n* : NEUROFIBRILLARY TANGLE

tan·ta·lum \'tant-ᵊl-əm\ *n* : a hard ductile gray-white acid-resisting metallic element sometimes used in surgical implants and sutures — symbol *Ta;* see ELEMENT table

T antigen \'tē-\ *n* : an antigen occurring in the nuclei of cells transformed into tumor cells or tumorigenic cells by adenoviruses

tap \'tap\ *n* : the procedure of removing fluid (as from a body cavity) — see LUMBAR PUNCTURE — **tap** *vb*

¹**tape** \'tāp\ *n* : a narrow band of woven fabric; *esp* : ADHESIVE TAPE

²**tape** *vb* **taped; tap·ing** : to fasten, tie, bind, cover, or support with tape and esp. adhesive tape

ta·pe·tum \tə-ˈpē-təm\ *n, pl* **ta·pe·ta** \-ˈpē-tə\ 1 : any of various membranous layers or areas esp. of the choroid and retina of the eye 2 : a layer of nerve fibers derived from the corpus callosum and forming part of the roof of each lateral ventricle of the brain — **ta·pe·tal** \-təl\ *adj*

tape·worm \'tāp-ˌwərm\ *n* : any of a class (Cestoda) of platyhelminthic worms that are parasitic as adults in the alimentary tract of vertebrates including humans and as larvae in a great variety of vertebrates and invertebrates and that typically consist of an attachment organ usu. with suckers, grooves, hooks, or other devices for adhering to the host's intestine followed by an undifferentiated growth region from which buds off a chain of segments of which the anterior members are little more than blocks of tissue, the median members have fully developed organs of both sexes, and the posterior members are egg-filled sacs — called also *cestode;* see BEEF TAPEWORM, CAT TAPEWORM, FISH TAPEWORM, PORK TAPEWORM, ECHINOCOCCUS

ta·pote·ment \tə-'pōt-mənt\ *n* : PERCUSSION 2

tar \'tär\ *n* **1** : any of various dark brown or black viscous liquids obtained by distillation of organic material (as wood or coal); *esp* : one used medicinally — see JUNIPER TAR **2** : a substance in some respects resembling tar; *esp* : a residue present in smoke from burning tobacco that contains combustion by-products (as resins and phenols)

ta·ran·tu·la \tə-'ran-chə-lə, -tə-lə\ *n, pl* **ta·ran·tu·las** *also* **ta·ran·tu·lae** \-ˌlē\ : any of a family (Theraphosidae) of large hairy American spiders that are typically rather sluggish and capable of biting sharply though most forms are not significantly poisonous to humans

tarda — see OSTEOGENESIS IMPERFECTA TARDA

tar·dive \'tär-div\ *adj* : tending to or characterized by lateness esp. in development or maturity

tardive dyskinesia *n* : a central nervous system disorder characterized by twitching of the face and tongue and involuntary motor movements of the trunk and limbs and occurring esp. as a side effect of prolonged use of antipsychotic drugs (as phenothiazine) — *abbr. TD*

tar·get \'tär-gət\ *n* **1** : something to be affected by an action or development; *specif* : an organ, part, or tissue that is affected by the action of a hormone **2** : a body, surface, or material bombarded with nuclear particles or electrons **3** : the thought or object that is to be recognized (as by telepathy) or affected (as by psychokinesis) in a parapsychological experiment

target cell *n* : a cell that is acted on preferentially by a specific agent (as a virus, drug, or hormone)

tar·ry stool \'tär-ē-\ *n* : an evacuation from the bowels having the color of tar caused esp. by hemorrhage in the stomach or upper intestines

¹tar·sal \'tär-səl\ *adj* **1** : of or relating to the tarsus **2** : being or relating to plates of dense connective tissue that serve to stiffen the eyelids

²tarsal *n* : a tarsal part (as a bone)

tarsal gland *n* : MEIBOMIAN GLAND

tarsal plate *n* : the plate of strong dense fibrous connective tissue that forms the supporting structure of the eyelid

tarso- *comb form* **1** : tarsus (*tarso-metatarsal*) **2** : tarsal plate (*tarsorrha-phy*)

tar·so·meta·tar·sal \ˌtär-sō-ˌme-tə-'tär-səl\ *adj* : of or relating to the tarsus and metatarsus (~ articulations)

tar·sor·rha·phy \tär-'sôr-ə-fē\ *n, pl* **-phies** : the operation of suturing the eyelids together entirely or in part

tar·sus \'tär-səs\ *n, pl* **tar·si** \-ˌsī, -ˌsē\ **1** : the part of the foot between the metatarsus and the leg; *also* : the small bones that support this part of the limb **2** : TARSAL PLATE

tar·tar \'tär-tər\ *n* : an incrustation on the teeth consisting of salivary secretion, food residue, and various salts (as calcium carbonate)

tartar emetic *n* : a poisonous crystalline salt $KSbOC_4H_4O_6 \cdot \frac{1}{2}H_2O$ of sweetish metallic taste that is used in medicine as an expectorant, in the treatment of amebiasis, and formerly as an emetic — called also *antimony potassium tartrate, potassium antimonyltartrate*

tar·tar·ic acid \(ˌ)tär-'tar-ik-\ *n* : a strong acid $C_4H_6O_6$ of plant origin that contains two carboxyl groups and occurs in three isomeric crystalline forms of which two are optically active

tar·trate \'tär-ˌtrāt\ *n* : a salt or ester of tartaric acid

tar·tra·zine \'tär-trə-ˌzēn, -zən\ *n* : a yellow azo dye used in coloring foods and drugs that sometimes causes bronchoconstriction in individuals with asthma

¹taste \'tāst\ *vb* **tast·ed; tast·ing 1** : to ascertain the flavor of by taking a little into the mouth **2** : to have a specific flavor

²taste *n* **1** : the special sense that is concerned with distinguishing the sweet, sour, bitter, or salty quality of a dissolved substance and is mediated by taste buds on the tongue **2** : the objective sweet, sour, bitter, or salty quality of a dissolved substance as perceived by the sense of taste **3** : a sensation obtained from a substance in the mouth that is typically produced by the stimulation of the sense of taste combined with those of touch and smell

taste bud *n* : an end organ mediating the sensation of taste and lying chiefly in the epithelium of the tongue and esp. in the walls of the circumvallate papillae

taste cell *n* : a neuroepithelial cell that is located in a taste bud and is the actual receptor of the sensation of taste

taste hair *n* : the hairlike free end of a taste cell

tast·er \'tās-tər\ *n* : a person able to

taste the chemical phenylthiocarbamide

TAT *abbr* thematic apperception test

tat·too \ta-'tü\ *n, pl* **tattoos** : an indelible mark or figure fixed upon the body by insertion of pigment under the skin or by production of scars — **tattoo** *vb*

tau·rine \'to·ˌrēn\ *n* : a colorless crystalline cysteine derivative $C_2H_7NO_3S$ found in nerve tissue, in bile, and in the juices of muscle esp. in invertebrates

tau·ro·cho·lic acid \ˌtor-ə-'kō-lik-, -'kä-\ *n* : a deliquescent acid $C_{26}-H_{45}NO_7S$ occurring as the sodium salt in bile

tau·tom·er·ism \'to·'tä-mə-ˌri-zəm\ *n* : isomerism in which the isomers change into one another with great ease so that they ordinarily exist together in equilibrium — **tau·to·mer·ic** \ˌto·tə-'mer-ik\ *adj*

tax·is \'tak-səs\ *n, pl* **tax·es** \-ˌsēz\ **1** : the manual restoration of a displaced body part; *specif* : the reduction of a hernia manually **2 a** : reflex movement of a freely moving and usu. simple organism in relation to a source of stimulation (as a light) **b** : a reflex reaction involving a taxis

tax·ol \'tak-ˌsol\ *n* : an antineoplastic agent $C_{47}H_{51}NO_{14}$ derived esp. from the bark of a yew tree (*Taxus brevifolia* of the family Taxaceae) of the western U.S. and British Columbia and administered intravenously in the treatment of ovarian cancer which has not responded to conventional chemotherapy

tax·on \'tak-ˌsän\ *n, pl* **taxa** \-sə\ *also* **tax·ons 1** : a taxonomic group or entity **2** : the name applied to a taxonomic group in a formal system of nomenclature

tax·on·o·my \tak-'sä-nə-mē\ *n, pl* **-mies 1** : the study of the general principles of scientific classification **2** : orderly classification of plants and animals according to their presumed natural relationships — **tax·o·nom·ic** \ˌtak-sə-'nä-mik\ *adj* — **tax·o·nom·i·cal·ly** *adv* — **tax·on·o·mist** \-mist\ *n*

Tay–Sachs disease \'tā-'saks-\ *n* : a hereditary disorder of lipid metabolism typically affecting individuals of eastern European Jewish ancestry that is characterized by the accumulation of lipids esp. in nervous tissue due to a deficiency of hexosaminidase and causes death in early childhood — called also *Tay-Sachs*; see SANDHOFF'S DISEASE

Tay, Warren (1843–1927), British physician.

Sachs, Bernard (1858–1944), American neurologist.

Tb *symbol* terbium

TB \ˌtē-'bē\ *n* : TUBERCULOSIS

TB *abbr* tubercle bacillus

TBG *abbr* thyroid-binding globulin; thyroxine-binding globulin

Tc *symbol* technetium

TCA *abbr* tricyclic antidepressant

TCDD \ˌtē-(ˌ)sē-(ˌ)dē-'dē\ *n* : a carcinogenic dioxin $C_{12}H_4O_2Cl_4$ found esp. as a contaminant in 2,4,5-T

TCE \ˌtē-(ˌ)sē-'ē\ *n* : TRICHLOROETHYLENE

T cell *n* : any of several lymphocytes (as a helper T cell) that differentiate in the thymus, possess highly specific cell-surface antigen receptors, and include some that control the initiation or suppression of cell-mediated and humoral immunity (as by the regulation of T and B cell maturation and proliferation) and others that lyse antigen-bearing cells — called also *T lymphocyte*; see HELPER T CELL, KILLER CELL, SUPPRESSOR T CELL

TD *abbr* tardive dyskinesia

tds *abbr* [Latin *ter die sumendum*] to be taken three times a day — used in writing prescriptions

Te *symbol* tellurium

TEA *abbr* tetraethylammonium

teaching hospital *n* : a hospital that is affiliated with a medical school and provides the means for medical education to students, interns, residents, and sometimes postgraduates

¹tear \'tir\ *n* **1** : a drop of clear saline fluid secreted by the lacrimal gland and diffused between the eye and eyelids to moisten the parts and facilitate their motion **2** *pl* : a secretion of profuse tears that overflow the eyelids and dampen the face

²tear *vb* : to fill with tears : shed tears

³tear \'tar\ *vb* **tore** \'tōr\; **torn** \'tórn\; **tear·ing** : to wound by or as if by pulling apart by force

⁴tear *n* : a wound made by tearing a bodily part (a muscle ~)

tear duct *n* : LACRIMAL DUCT

tear gas *n* : a solid, liquid, or gaseous substance that on dispersion in the atmosphere blinds the eyes with tears

tear gland *n* : LACRIMAL GLAND

tease \'tēz\ *vb* **teased; teas·ing** : to tear in pieces; *esp* : to shred (a tissue or specimen) for microscopic examination

tea·spoon \'tē-ˌspün\ *n* : a unit of measure equal to ⅙ fluid ounce or ⅓ tablespoon or 5 milliliters

tea·spoon·ful \-ˌfúl\ *n, pl* **teaspoonfuls** \-ˌfúlz\ *also* **tea·spoons·ful** \-ˌspünz-ˌfúl\ : TEASPOON

teat \'tit, 'tēt\ *n* : the protuberance through which milk is drawn from an udder or breast : NIPPLE

tech *abbr* technician

tech·ne·tium \tek-'nē-shəm, -shē-əm\ *n* : a metallic element that is obtained by bombarding molybdenum with deuterons or neutrons and in the fission of uranium and that is used in medicine in the preparation of radiopharmaceuticals — symbol *Tc*; see ELEMENT table

tech·nic \'tek-nik\ *n* : TECHNIQUE

tech·ni·cian \tek-'ni-shən\ *n* : a specialist in the technical details of a subject or occupation ⟨a medical ∼⟩

tech·nique \tek-'nēk\ *n* : a method or body of methods for accomplishing a desired end ⟨new surgical ∼s⟩

tecta *pl of* TECTUM

tec·tal \'tek-təl\ *adj* : of or relating to a tectum

tec·to·ri·al membrane \tek-'tōr-ē-əl-\ *n* : a membrane having the consistency of jelly that covers the surface of the organ of Corti

tec·to·spi·nal \'tek-tō-'spīn-əl\ *adj* : of, relating to, or being a tract of myelinated nerve fibers that mediate various visual and auditory reflexes and that originate in the superior colliculus, cross to the opposite side, and terminate in the ventral horn of gray matter in the cervical region of the spinal cord

tec·tum \'tek-təm\ *n, pl* **tec·ta** \-tə\ 1 : a bodily structure resembling or serving as a roof 2 : the dorsal part of the midbrain including the corpora quadrigemina

teeth *pl of* TOOTH

teethe \'tēth\ *vb* **teethed; teeth·ing** : to cut one's teeth : grow teeth

teeth·ing \'tē-thiŋ\ *n* 1 : the first growth of teeth 2 : the phenomena accompanying the growth of teeth through the gums

Tef·lon \'te-ˌflän\ *trademark* — used for synthetic fluorine-containing resins used esp. for molding articles and for coatings to prevent sticking

teg·men \'teg-mən\ *n, pl* **teg·mi·na** \-mə-nə\ : an anatomical layer or cover; *specif* : TEGMEN TYMPANI

teg·men·tum \teg-'men-təm\ *n, pl* **-men·ta** \-tə\ : an anatomical covering : TEGMEN; *esp* : the part of the ventral midbrain above the substantia nigra — **teg·men·tal** \-təl\ *adj*

tegmen tym·pa·ni \-'tim-pə-ˌnī\ *n* : a thin plate of bone that covers the middle ear

tegmina *pl of* TEGMEN

Teg·o·pen \'te-gə-ˌpen\ *trademark* — used for a preparation of cloxacillin

Teg·re·tol \'te-grə-ˌtōl\ *trademark* — used for a preparation of carbamazepine

tel- *or* **telo-** *also* **tele-** *comb form* : end ⟨*tel*angiectasia⟩

te·la \'tē-lə\ *n, pl* **te·lae** \-ˌlē\ : an anatomical tissue or layer of tissue

tela cho·roi·dea \-kō-'roi-dē-ə\ *n* : a fold of pia mater roofing a ventricle of the brain

tel·an·gi·ec·ta·sia \ˌte-ˌlan-jē-ˌek-'tā-zhə, ˌtē-, tə-, -zhē-ə\ *or* **tel·an·gi·ec·ta·sis** \-'ek-tə-səs\ *n, pl* **-ta·sias** *or* **-ta·ses** \-tə-ˌsēz\ 1 : an abnormal dilatation of capillary vessels and arterioles that often forms an angioma 2

: HEREDITARY HEMORRHAGIC TELANGIECTASIA — **tel·an·gi·ec·tat·ic** \-ˌek-'ta-tik\ *adj*

te·la sub·cu·ta·nea \'tē-lə-ˌsəb-kyü-'tā-nē-ə\ *n* : SUPERFICIAL FASCIA

tele·di·ag·no·sis \ˌte-lə-ˌdī-əg-'nō-səs\ *n, pl* **-no·ses** \-ˌsēz\ : the diagnosis of physical or mental ailments based on data received from a patient by means of telemetry and closed-circuit television

tele·ki·ne·sis \ˌte-lə-kə-'nē-səs, -kī-\ *n, pl* **-ne·ses** \-ˌsēz\ : the apparent production of motion in objects (as by a spiritualistic medium) without contact or other physical means — compare PRECOGNITION, PSYCHOKINESIS — **tele·ki·net·ic** \-'ne-tik\ *adj* — **tele·ki·net·i·cal·ly** *adv*

tele·med·i·cine \-'me-də-sən\ *n* : the practice of medicine when the doctor and patient are widely separated using two-way voice and visual communication esp. by satellite, telemetry, or closed-circuit television

¹tele·me·ter \'te-lə-ˌmē-tər\ *n* : an electrical apparatus for measuring a quantity (as pressure, speed, or temperature), transmitting the result esp. by radio to a distant station, and there indicating or recording the quantity measured

²telemeter *vb* : to transmit (as the measurement of a quantity) by telemeter

te·lem·e·try \tə-'le-mə-trē\ *n, pl* **-tries** 1 : the science or process of telemetering data 2 : data transmitted by telemetry 3 : BIOTELEMETRY — **tele·met·ric** \ˌte-lə-'me-trik\ *adj*

tel·en·ceph·a·lon \ˌte-len-'se-fə-ˌlän, -lən\ *n* : the anterior subdivision of the embryonic forebrain or the corresponding part of the adult forebrain that includes the cerebral hemispheres and associated structures — **tel·en·ce·phal·ic** \-ˌen-sə-'fa-lik\ *adj*

te·lep·a·thy \tə-'le-pə-thē\ *n, pl* **-thies** : apparent communication from one mind to another by extrasensory means — **tele·path·ic** \ˌte-lə-'pa-thik\ *adj* — **tele·path·i·cal·ly** *adv*

tele·ther·a·py \ˌte-lə-'ther-ə-pē\ *n, pl* **-pies** : the treatment of diseased tissue with high-intensity radiation (as gamma rays from radioactive cobalt)

tel·lu·ri·um \tə-'lur-ē-əm, te-\ *n* : a semimetallic element related to selenium and sulfur — symbol *Te*; see ELEMENT table

telo- — see TEL-

telo·cen·tric \ˌte-lə-'sen-trik, ˌtē-\ *adj* : having the centromere terminally situated so that there is only one chromosomal arm — compare ACROCENTRIC, METACENTRIC — **telocentric** *n*

te·lo·gen \'te-lə-ˌjen\ *n* : the resting phase of the hair growth cycle following anagen and preceding shedding

telo·mere \'te-lə-ˌmir, 'tē-\ *n* : the natural end of a chromosome

telo·phase \'te-lə-ˌfāz, 'tē-\ n 1 : the final stage of mitosis and of the second division of meiosis in which the spindle disappears and the nuclear envelope reforms around each set of chromosomes 2 : the final stage in the first division of meiosis that may be missing in some organisms and that is characterized by the gathering at opposite poles of the cell of half the original number of chromosomes including one from each homologous pair

TEM \ˌtē-(ˌ)ē-'em\ n : TRIETHYLENE-MELAMINE

Tem·a·ril \'te-mə-ˌril\ *trademark* — used for a preparation of trimeprazine

te·maz·e·pam \tə-'ma-zə-ˌpam\ n : a benzodiazepine used for its sedative and tranquilizing effects in the treatment of insomnia — see RESTORIL

temp \'temp\ n : TEMPERATURE

tem·per·ate \'tem-pə-rət\ adj : existing as a prophage in infected cells and rarely causing lysis (∼ bacteriophages)

tem·per·a·ture \'tem-pər-ˌchür, -pə-rə-, -ˌchər, -ˌtyür\ n 1 : degree of hotness or coldness measured on a definite scale — see THERMOMETER 2 a : the degree of heat that is natural to a living body b : a condition of abnormally high body heat

tem·plate \'tem-plət\ n : a molecule (as of DNA) that serves as a pattern for the generation of another macromolecule (as messenger RNA)

tem·ple \'tem-pəl\ n 1 : the flattened space on each side of the forehead 2 : one of the side supports of a pair of glasses jointed to the bows and passing on each side of the head

¹tem·po·ral \'tem-pə-rəl\ n : a temporal part (as a bone or muscle)

²temporal adj : of or relating to the temples or the sides of the skull behind the orbits

temporal arteritis n : GIANT CELL ARTERITIS

temporal artery n 1 : either of two branches of the maxillary artery that supply the temporalis and anastomose with the middle temporal artery — called also *deep temporal artery* 2 a : SUPERFICIAL TEMPORAL ARTERY b : a branch of the superficial temporal artery that arises just above the zygomatic arch and sends branches to the temporalis — called also *middle temporal artery* 3 : any of three branches of the middle cerebral artery: a : one that supplies the anterior parts of the superior, middle, and inferior temporal gyri — called also *anterior temporal artery* b : one that supplies the middle parts of the superior and middle temporal gyri — called also *intermediate temporal artery* c : one that supplies the middle and posterior parts of the superior temporal gyrus and the posterior parts of the middle

and inferior temporal gyri — called also *posterior temporal artery*

temporal bone n : a compound bone of the side of the skull that has four principal parts including the squamous, petrous, and tympanic portions, and the mastoid process

temporal fossa n : a broad fossa on the side of the skull behind the orbit that contains muscles for raising the lower jaw and that in humans is occupied by the temporalis muscle

temporal gyrus n : any of three major convolutions of the external surface of the temporal lobe: a : the one that is uppermost and borders the fissure of Sylvius — called also *superior temporal gyrus* b : one lying in the middle between the other two — called also *middle temporal gyrus* c : the lowest of the three — called also *inferior temporal gyrus*

tem·po·ral·is \ˌtem-pə-'rā-ləs\ n : a large muscle in the temporal fossa that serves to raise the lower jaw — called also *temporalis muscle*, *temporal muscle*

temporal line n : either of two nearly parallel ridges or lines on each side of the skull

temporal lobe n : a large lobe of each cerebral hemisphere that is situated in front of the occipital lobe and contains a sensory area associated with the organ of hearing

temporal lobe epilepsy n : PSYCHOMOTOR EPILEPSY

temporal muscle n : TEMPORALIS

temporal nerve — see DEEP TEMPORAL NERVE

temporal process n : a process of the zygomatic bone that forms part of the zygomatic arch

temporal summation n : sensory summation that involves the addition of single stimuli over a short period of time

temporal vein n : any of several veins draining the temporal region: as a (1) : a large vein on each side of the head that unites with the maxillary vein to form a vein that contributes to the formation of the external jugular vein (2) : a vein that drains the lateral orbital region and empties into the superficial temporal vein just above the zygomatic arch — called also *middle temporal vein* b : any of several veins arising from behind the temporalis and emptying into the pterygoid plexus — called also *deep temporal vein*

temporo- *comb form* : temporal and (*temporo*mandibular)

tem·po·ro·man·dib·u·lar \ˌtem-pə-rō-man-'di-byə-lər\ adj : of, relating to, or affecting the temporomandibular joint (∼ dysfunction)

temporomandibular joint n : the synovial joint between the temporal bone and mandible that includes the condyloid process below separated by an articular disk from the glenoid fossa above and that allows for the opening, closing, protrusion, retraction, and lateral movement of the mandible — abbr. *TMJ*

tem·po·ro·pa·ri·etal \-pə-'rī-ət-ªl\ *adj* : of or relating to the temporal and parietal bones or lobes (the ~ region)

ten- — see TAEN-

te·na·cious \tə-'nā-shəs\ *adj* : tending to adhere or cling esp. to another substance : VISCOUS (~ sputum)

te·nac·u·lum \tə-'na-kyə-ləm\ *n, pl* **-la** \-lə\ *or* **-lums** : a slender sharp-pointed hook attached to a handle and used mainly in surgery for seizing and holding parts (as arteries)

ten·der \'ten-dər\ *adj* : sensitive to touch or palpation (a ~ spleen) — **ten·der·ness** *n*

ten·di·ni·tis \ten-də-'nī-təs\ *n* : inflammation of a tendon

ten·di·nous \'ten-də-nəs\ *adj* **1** : consisting of tendons (~ tissue) **2** : of, relating to, or resembling a tendon

tendinous arch *n* : a thickened arch of fascia which gives origin to muscles or ligaments or through which pass vessels or nerves; *esp* : a thickening in the pelvic fascia that gives attachment to supporting ligaments

ten·do cal·ca·ne·us \'ten-dō-kal-'kā-nē-əs\ *n* : ACHILLES TENDON

ten·don \'ten-dən\ *n* : a tough cord or band of dense white fibrous connective tissue that unites a muscle with some other part, transmits the force which the muscle exerts, and is continuous with the connective-tissue epimysium and perimysium of the muscle and when inserted into a bone is continuous with the periosteum of the bone — see APONEUROSIS

ten·do·ni·tis *var of* TENDINITIS

tendon of Achil·les \-ə-'ki-lēz\ *n* : ACHILLES TENDON

tendon of Zinn \-'tsin\ *n* : LIGAMENT OF ZINN

tendon organ *n* : GOLGI TENDON ORGAN

ten·do·nous *var of* TENDINOUS

tendon reflex *n* : a reflex act (as a knee jerk) in which a muscle is made to contract by a blow upon its tendon

tendon sheath *n* : a synovial sheath covering a tendon (as in the hand)

¹-tene \tēn\ *adj comb form* : having (such or so many) chromosomal filaments (poly*tene*) (pachy*tene*)

²-tene *n comb form* : stage of meiotic prophase characterized by (such) chromosomal filaments (diplo*tene*) (pachy*tene*)

tenens, tenentes — see LOCUM TENENS

te·nes·mus \tə-'nez-məs\ *n* : a distressing but ineffectual urge to evacuate the rectum or urinary bladder

teni- — see TAEN-

te·nia, tenia coli, te·ni·a·sis *var of* TAENIA, TAENIA COLI, TAENIASIS

---

tennis elbow *n* : inflammation and pain over the outer side of the elbow involving the lateral epicondyle of the humerus and usu. resulting from excessive strain on and twisting of the forearm

teno- *comb form* : tendon (*teno*synovitis)

te·no·de·sis \te-nə-'dē-səs\ *n, pl* **-de·ses** \-sēz\ : the operation of suturing the end of a tendon to a bone

te·nol·y·sis \te-'nä-lə-səs\ *n, pl* **-y·ses** \-sēz\ : a surgical procedure to free a tendon from surrounding adhesions

teno·my·ot·o·my \te-nō-mī-'ä-tə-mē\ *n, pl* **-mies** : surgical excision of a portion of a tendon and muscle

Te·non's capsule \tə-'nōnz-, 'te-nənz-\ *n* : a thin connective-tissue membrane ensheathing the eyeball behind the conjunctiva

Te·non \tə-'nōⁿ, **Jacques René (1724–1816),** French surgeon.

teno·syn·o·vi·tis \te-nō-sī-nə-'vī-təs\ *n* : inflammation of a tendon sheath

te·not·o·my \te-'nä-tə-mē\ *n, pl* **-mies** : surgical division of a tendon

tense \'tens\ *adj* **tens·er; tens·est 1** : stretched tight : made taut or rigid **2** : feeling or showing nervous tension — **tense** *vb* — **tense·ness** *n*

Ten·si·lon \'ten-si-län\ *trademark* — used for a preparation of edrophonium

ten·sion \'ten-chən\ *n* **1 a** : the act or action of stretching or the condition or degree of being stretched to stiffness (muscular ~) **b** : STRESS 1b **2 a** : either of two balancing forces causing or tending to cause extension **b** : the stress resulting from the elongation of an elastic body **3** : inner striving, unrest, or imbalance often with physiological indication of emotion **4** : PARTIAL PRESSURE (arterial carbon dioxide ~) — **ten·sion·al** \'ten-chə-nəl\ *adj* — **ten·sion·less** *adj*

tension headache *n* : headache due primarily to contraction of the muscles of the neck and scalp

tension pneumothorax *n* : pneumothorax resulting from a wound in the chest wall which acts as a valve that permits air to enter the pleural cavity but prevents its escape

tension–time index *n* : a measure of ventricular work and oxygen demand that is found by multiplying the average pressure in the ventricle during the period in which it ejects blood by the time it takes to do this

ten·sor \'ten(t)-sər, 'ten-sȯ(ə)r\ *n* : a muscle that stretches a part or makes it tense — called also *tensor muscle*

tensor fas·ci·ae la·tae \-'fa-shē-ē-'lä-tē\ *or* **tensor fas·cia la·ta** \-'fa-shē-ə-'lä-tə\ *n* : a muscle that arises esp. from the anterior part of the iliac crest and from the anterior superior iliac spine, is inserted into the iliotibial band of the fascia lata, and acts to flex and abduct the thigh

tensor pa·la·ti \-ˈpa-lə-ˌtī\ n : TENSOR VELI PALATINI

tensor tym·pa·ni \-ˈtim-pə-ˌnī\ n : a small muscle of the middle ear that is located in the bony canal just above the bony part of the eustachian tube and that serves to adjust the tension of the tympanic membrane — called also *tensor tympani muscle*

tensor ve·li pa·la·ti·ni \-ˌvē-ˌlī-ˌpa-lə-ˈtī-ˌnī\ n : a ribbonlike muscle of the palate that acts esp. to tense the soft palate

tent \ˈtent\ n : a canopy or enclosure placed over the head and shoulders to retain vapors or oxygen during medical administration

tenth cranial nerve n : VAGUS NERVE

ten·to·ri·al \ten-ˈtōr-ē-əl\ adj : of, relating to, or involving the tentorium cerebelli

tentorial notch n : an oval opening that is bounded by the anterior border of the tentorium cerebelli, that surrounds the midbrain, and that gives passage to the posterior cerebral arteries — called also *tentorial incisure*

ten·to·ri·um \-ē-əm\ n, pl **-ria** \-ē-ə\ : TENTORIUM CEREBELLI

tentorium ce·re·bel·li \-ˌser-ə-ˈbe-ˌlī\ n : an arched fold of dura mater that covers the upper surface of the cerebellum and supports the occipital lobes of the cerebrum

Ten·u·ate \ˈten-yə-ˌwāt\ trademark — used for a preparation of diethylpropion

te·pa \ˈtē-pə\ n : a soluble crystalline compound $C_6H_{12}N_3OP$ used esp. as a chemical sterilizing agent of insects and in medicine as a palliative in some kinds of cancer — see THIOTEPA

terat- or **terato-** comb form : developmental malformation ⟨*teratogenic*⟩

te·ra·to·car·ci·no·ma \ˌter-ə-tō-ˌkärs-ᵊn-ˈō-mə\ n, pl **-mas** or **-ma·ta** \-mə-tə\ : a malignant teratoma; esp : one involving germinal cells of the testis or ovary

te·ra·to·gen \-ˈra-tə-jən\ n : a teratogenic agent (as a drug or virus)

ter·a·to·gen·e·sis \ˌter-ə-tə-ˈje-nə-səs\ n, pl **-e·ses** \-ˌsēz\ : production of developmental malformations

ter·a·to·gen·ic \-ˈje-nik\ adj : of, relating to, or causing developmental malformations ⟨~ substances⟩ ⟨~ effects⟩ — **ter·a·to·ge·nic·i·ty** \-jə-ˈni-sə-tē\ n

ter·a·to·log·i·cal \ˌter-ət-ᵊl-ˈä-ji-kəl\ or **ter·a·to·log·ic** \-jik\ adj **1** : abnormal in growth or structure **2** : of or relating to teratology

ter·a·tol·o·gy \ˌter-ə-ˈtä-lə-jē\ n, pl **-gies** : the study of malformations or serious deviations from the normal type in organisms — **ter·a·tol·o·gist** \-jist\ n

ter·a·to·ma \ˌter-ə-ˈtō-mə\ n, pl **-mas** or **-ma·ta** \-mə-tə\ : a tumor derived from more than one embryonic layer and made up of a heterogeneous mixture of tissues (as epithelium, bone, cartilage, or muscle)

ter·bi·um \ˈtər-bē-əm\ n : a usu. trivalent metallic element — symbol *Tb*; see ELEMENT table

ter·bu·ta·line \ˌtər-ˈbyü-tə-ˌlēn\ n : a bronchodilator $C_{12}H_{19}NO_3$ used esp. in the form of its sulfate

ter·e·bene \ˈter-ə-ˌbēn\ n : a mixture of terpenes that has been used as an expectorant

teres — see LIGAMENTUM TERES, PRONATOR TERES

te·res major \ˈter-ēz-, ˈtir-\ n : a thick somewhat flattened muscle that arises from the lower axillary border of the scapula, inserts on the medial border of the bicipital groove of the humerus, and functions in opposition to the muscles comprising the rotator cuff by extending the arm when it is in the flexed position and by rotating it medially

teres minor n : a long cylindrical muscle that arises from the upper axillary border of the scapula, inserts chiefly on the greater tubercle of the humerus, contributes to the formation of the rotator cuff of the shoulder, and acts to rotate the arm laterally and draw the humerus toward the glenoid fossa

ter·fen·a·dine \(ˌ)tər-ˈfe-nə-ˌdēn\ n : an antihistamine $C_{32}H_{41}NO_2$ that does not produce the drowsiness associated with many antihistamines — see SELDANE

¹term \ˈtərm\ n : the time at which a pregnancy of normal length terminates ⟨had her baby at full ~⟩

²term adj : carried to, occurring at, or associated with full term

¹ter·mi·nal \ˈtər-mə-nəl\ adj **1** : of, relating to, or being at an end, extremity, boundary, or terminus ⟨the ~ phalanx of a finger⟩ **2 a** : leading ultimately to death : FATAL ⟨~ cancer⟩ **b** : approaching or close to death : being in the final stages of a fatal disease ⟨a ~ patient⟩ **3** : being at or near the end of a chain of atoms making up a molecule — **ter·mi·nal·ly** adv

²terminal n : a part that forms an end; esp : NERVE ENDING

terminal ganglion n : a usu. parasympathetic ganglion situated on or close to an innervated organ and being the site where preganglionic nerve fibers terminate

terminalis — see LAMINA TERMINALIS, STRIA TERMINALIS, SULCUS TERMINALIS

terminal nerve n : NERVUS TERMINALIS

ter·mi·na·tor \ˈtər-mə-ˌnā-tər\ n : a codon that stops protein synthesis since it does not code for a transfer RNA — called also *termination codon*, *terminator codon*; compare INITIATION CODON

ter·pene \ˈtər-ˌpēn\ n : any of various

isomeric hydrocarbons $C_{10}H_{16}$ found in essential oils; *broadly* : any of numerous hydrocarbons $(C_5H_8)_n$ found esp. in essential oils, resins, and balsams

ter·pin hydrate \'tər-pin-\ *n* : a crystalline or powdery compound $C_{10}H_{18}$-$(OH)_2 \cdot H_2O$ used as an expectorant for coughs

Ter·ra·my·cin \₁ter-ə-'mīs-ᵊn\ *trademark* — used for a preparation of oxytetracycline

¹**ter·tian** \'tər-shən\ *adj* : recurring at approximately 48-hour intervals — used chiefly of vivax malaria; compare QUARTAN

²**tertian** *n* : a tertian fever; *specif* : VIVAX MALARIA

ter·tia·ry \'tər-shē-₁er-ē, -shə-rē\ *adj* 1 : of third rank, importance, or value 2 : of, relating to, or being the normal folded structure of the coiled chain of a protein or of a DNA or RNA — compare PRIMARY 3, SECONDARY 3 3 : occurring in or being a third stage ⟨~ lesions of syphilis⟩

tertiary care *n* : highly specialized health care usu. over an extended period of time that involves advanced and complex procedures and treatments performed by medical specialists in state-of-the-art facilities

tertiary syphilis *n* : the third stage of syphilis that develops after the disappearance of the secondary symptoms and is marked by ulcers in and gummas under the skin and commonly by involvement of the skeletal, cardiovascular, and nervous systems

tertius — see PERONEUS TERTIUS

Tesch·en disease \'te-shən-\ *n* : a severe virus encephalomyelitis of swine

test \'test\ *n* 1 : a critical examination, observation, evaluation, or trial 2 : a means of testing: as **a** (1) : a procedure or reaction used to identify or characterize a substance or constituent (2) : a reagent used in such a test **b** : a diagnostic procedure for determining the nature of a condition or disease or for revealing a change in function — see BLOOD TEST, DICK TEST, PATCH TEST, TUBERCULIN TEST, WASSERMANN TEST **c** : something (as a series of questions) for measuring the skill, knowledge, intelligence, capacities, or aptitudes of an individual or group — see INTELLIGENCE TEST, PERSONALITY INVENTORY 3 : a result or value determined by testing — **test** *adj or vb*

test·cross \'test-₁krós\ *n* : a genetic cross between a homozygous recessive individual and a corresponding suspected heterozygote to determine the genotype of the latter — **testcross** *vb*

testes *pl of* TESTIS

tes·ti·cle \'tes-ti-kəl\ *n* : TESTIS; *esp* : one usu. with its enclosing structures

tes·tic·u·lar \tes-'ti-kyə-lər\ *adj* : of, relating to, or derived from the testes

testicular artery *n* : either of a pair of arteries which supply blood to the testes and of which one arises on each side from the front of the aorta a little below the corresponding renal artery and passes downward to the spermatic cord of the same side and along it to the testis — called also *internal spermatic artery*

testicular feminization *n* : a genetic defect characterized by the presence in a phenotypically female individual of the normal X and Y chromosomes of a male, undeveloped and undescended testes, and functional sterility — called also *testicular feminization syndrome*

testicular vein *n* : any of the veins leading from the testes, forming with tributaries from the epididymis the pampiniform plexus in the spermatic cord, and thence accompanying the testicular artery and eventually uniting to form a single trunk which on the right side opens into the vena cava and on the left into the renal vein — called also *spermatic vein*

tes·tis \'tes-təs\ *n, pl* **tes·tes** \'tes-₁tēz\ : a typically paired male reproductive gland that usu. consists largely of seminiferous tubules from the epithelium of which spermatozoa develop and that descends into the scrotum before the attainment of sexual maturity and in many cases before birth

tes·tos·ter·one \te-'stäs-tə-₁rōn\ *n* : a hormone that is a hydroxy steroid ketone $C_{19}H_{28}O_2$ produced by the testes or made synthetically and that is responsible for inducing and maintaining male secondary sex characters

testosterone enan·thate \-ē-'nan-₁thāt\ *n* : a white or whitish crystalline ester $C_{26}H_{40}O_3$ of testosterone that is used esp. in the treatment of eunuchism, eunuchoidism, androgen deficiency after castration, symptoms of the male climacteric, and oligospermia

testosterone propionate *n* : a white or whitish crystalline ester $C_{22}H_{32}O_3$ of testosterone that is used esp. in the treatment of postpubertal cryptorchidism, symptoms of the male climacteric, palliation of inoperable breast cancer, and the prevention of postpartum pain and breast engorgement

test–tube *adj* : produced by fertilization in laboratory apparatus and implantation in the uterus, by fertilization and growth in laboratory apparatus, or sometimes by artificial insemination ⟨~ babies⟩

test tube *n* : a plain or lipped tube usu. of thin glass closed at one end

te·tan·ic \te-'ta-nik\ *adj* : of, relating to, being, or tending to produce tetany or tetanus ⟨a ~ condition⟩

tet·a·nize \'tet-ᵊn-₁īz\ *vb* **-nized; -niz-**

ing : to induce tetanus in ⟨∼ a muscle⟩

tet·a·nus \'tet-ᵊn-əs, 'tet-nəs\ *n* **1 a** : an acute infectious disease characterized by tonic spasm of voluntary muscles and esp. of the muscles of the jaw and caused by the specific toxin produced by the tetanus bacterium which is usu. introduced through a wound — compare LOCK-JAW **b** : TETANUS BACILLUS **2** : prolonged contraction of a muscle resulting from a series of motor impulses following one another too rapidly to permit intervening relaxation of the muscle

tetanus bacillus *n* : a bacterium of the genus *Clostridium* (*C. tetani*) that causes tetanus

tet·a·ny \'tet-ᵊn-ē, 'tet-nē\ *n, pl* **-nies** : a condition of physiological calcium imbalance that is marked by intermittent tonic spasm of the voluntary muscles and is associated with deficiencies of parathyroid secretion or other disturbances (as vitamin D deficiency)

tet·ra·ben·a·zine \ˌte-trə-'be-nə-ˌzēn\ *n* : a serotonin antagonist $C_{19}H_{27}NO_3$ that is used esp. in the treatment of psychosis and anxiety

tet·ra·caine \'te-trə-ˌkān\ *n* : a crystalline basic ester $C_{15}H_{24}N_2O_2$ that is closely related chemically to procaine and is used chiefly in the form of its hydrochloride as a local anesthetic — called also *amethocaine, pantocaine;* see PONTOCAINE

tet·ra·chlo·ride \ˌte-trə-'klōr-ˌid\ *n* : a chloride containing four atoms of chlorine

tet·ra·cy·cline \ˌte-trə-'sī-ˌklēn\ *n* : a yellow crystalline broad-spectrum antibiotic $C_{22}H_{24}N_2O_8$ produced by a soil actinomycete of the genus *Streptomyces* (*S. viridifaciens*) or synthetically; *also* : any of various derivatives of tetracycline

tet·rad \'te-ˌtrad\ *n* : a group or arrangement of four: as **a** : a group of four cells produced by the successive divisions of a mother cell ⟨a ∼ of spores⟩ **b** : a group of four synapsed chromatids that become visibly evident in the pachytene stage of meiotic prophase

tet·ra·eth·yl·am·mo·ni·um \ˌte-trə-ˌe-thə-lə-'mō-nē-əm\ *n* : the quaternary ammonium ion $(C_2H_5)_4N^+$ containing four ethyl groups; *also* : a salt of this ion (as the crystalline chloride used as a ganglionic blocking agent) — abbr. *TEA*

tet·ra·eth·yl·thi·u·ram di·sul·fide \ˌte-trə-ˌe-thəl-'thī-yü-ˌram-ˌdī-'səl-ˌfid\ *n* : DISULFIRAM

tet·ra·hy·dro·can·nab·i·nol \-ˌhī-drə-kə-'na-bə-ˌnȯl, -ˌnōl\ *n* : THC

te·tral·o·gy of Fal·lot \te-'tra-lə-jē-əv-fä-'lō\ *n* : a congenital abnormality of the heart characterized by pulmonary stenosis, an opening in the interventricular septum, malposition of the aorta over both ventricles, and hypertrophy of the right ventricle

Fallot, Étienne–Louis–Arthur (1850–1911), French physician.

tetranitrate — see ERYTHRITYL TETRANITRATE, PENTAERYTHRITOL TETRANITRATE

tet·ra·ple·gia \ˌte-trə-'plē-jə, -jē-ə\ *n* : QUADRIPLEGIA

tet·ra·ploid \'te-trə-ˌplȯid\ *adj* : having or being a chromosome number four times the monoploid number — **tet·ra·ploi·dy** \-ˌplȯi-dē\ *n*

tet·ra·zo·li·um \ˌte-trə-'zō-lē-əm\ *n* : a cation or group CH_3N_4 that is analogous to ammonium; *also* : any of several derivatives used esp. as electron acceptors to test for metabolic activity in living cells

te·tro·do·tox·in \ˌte-ˌtrō-də-'täk-sən\ *n* : a neurotoxin $C_{11}H_{17}N_3O_8$ that is found esp. in puffer fish and that blocks nerve conduction by suppressing permeability of the nerve fiber to sodium ions

te·trox·ide \te-'träk-ˌsīd\ *n* : a compound of an element or group with four atoms of oxygen — see OSMIUM TETROXIDE

Texas fever *n* : an infectious disease of cattle transmitted by the cattle tick and caused by a sporozoan of the genus *Babesia* (*B. bigemina*) that destroys red blood cells — called also *Texas cattle fever*

T–4 \ˌtē-'för\ *n* : THYROXINE

T4 cell *n* : any of the T cells (as a helper T cell) that bear the CD4 molecular marker and become severely depleted in AIDS — called also *T4 lymphocyte*

TGF *abbr* transforming growth factor

T–group \'tē-ˌgrüp\ *n* : a group of people under the leadership of a trainer who seek to develop self-awareness and sensitivity to others by verbalizing feelings uninhibitedly at group sessions — compare ENCOUNTER GROUP

Th *symbol* thorium

thalam- *or* **thalamo-** *comb form* **1** : thalamus ⟨*thalam*otomy⟩ **2** : thalamic and ⟨*thalamo*cortical⟩

tha·lam·ic \thə-'la-mik\ *adj* : of, relating to, or involving the thalamus

thal·a·mo·cor·ti·cal \ˌtha-lə-mō-'kȯr-ti-kəl\ *adj* : of, relating to, or connecting the thalamus and the cerebral cortex

thal·a·mot·o·my \ˌtha-lə-'mä-tə-mē\ *n, pl* **-mies** : a surgical operation involving electrocoagulation of areas of the thalamus to interrupt pathways of nervous transmission through the thalamus for relief of certain mental and psychomotor disorders

thal·a·mus \'tha-lə-məs\ *n, pl* **-mi** \-ˌmī, -ˌmē\ : the largest subdivision of the diencephalon that consists chiefly of an ovoid mass of nuclei in each lateral wall of the third ventricle and serves to relay impulses and esp. sensory impulses to and from the cerebral cortex

thal·as·sae·mia, thal·as·sae·mic *chiefly Brit var of* THALASSEMIA, THALASSEMIC

thal·as·se·mia \ˌtha-lə-ˈsē-mē-ə\ *n* : any of a group of inherited hypochromic anemias and esp. Cooley's anemia controlled by a series of allelic genes that cause reduction in or failure of synthesis of one of the globin chains making up hemoglobin and that tend to occur esp. in individuals of Mediterranean, African, or southeastern Asian ancestry — called also *Mediterranean anemia;* sometimes used with a prefix (as alpha-, beta-, or delta-) to indicate the hemoglobin chain affected; see BETA-THALASSEMIA

thalassemia major *n* : COOLEY'S ANEMIA

thalassemia minor *n* : a mild form of thalassemia associated with the heterozygous condition for the gene involved

¹**thal·as·se·mic** \ˌtha-lə-ˈsē-mik\ *adj* : of, relating to, or affected with thalassemia

²**thalassemic** *n* : a person affected with thalassemia

tha·las·so·ther·a·py \thə-ˌla-sō-ˈther-ə-pē\ *n, pl* **-pies** : the treatment of disease by bathing in sea water, by exposure to sea air, or by taking a sea voyage

tha·lid·o·mide \thə-ˈli-də-ˌmīd, -məd\ *n* : a sedative and hypnotic drug $C_{13}H_{10}N_2O_4$ that has been the cause of malformation in infants born to mothers using it during pregnancy

thal·li·um \ˈtha-lē-əm\ *n* : a sparsely but widely distributed poisonous metallic element — symbol *Tl*; see ELEMENT table

thanat- *or* **thanato-** *comb form* : death ⟨*thanatology*⟩

than·a·tol·o·gy \ˌtha-nə-ˈtä-lə-jē\ *n, pl* **-gies** : the description or study of the phenomena of death and of psychological mechanisms for coping with them — **than·a·to·log·i·cal** \ˌtha-nə-tə-ˈlä-ji-kəl\ *adj* — **than·a·tol·o·gist** \ˌtha-nə-ˈtä-lə-jist\ *n*

than·a·to·phor·ic \ˌtha-nə-tə-ˈfor-ik\ *adj* : relating to, affected with, or being a severe form of congenital dwarfism which results in early death

Than·a·tos \ˈtha-nə-ˌtäs\ *n* : DEATH INSTINCT

THC \ˌtē-(ˌ)āch-ˈsē\ *n* : a physiologically active chemical $C_{21}H_{30}O_2$ from hemp plant resin that is the chief intoxicant in marijuana — called also *tetrahydrocannabinol*

the·ater *or* **the·atre** \ˈthē-ə-tər\ *n* 1 : a room often with rising tiers of seats for assemblies (as for lectures or sur-

gical demonstrations) 2 *usu* theatre, *Brit* : a hospital operating room

the·ba·ine \thə-ˈbā-ˌēn\ *n* : a poisonous crystalline alkaloid $C_{19}H_{21}NO_3$ found in opium in small quantities

The·be·sian vein \thə-ˈbē-zhən-\ *n* : any of the minute veins of the heart wall that drain directly into the cavity of the heart — called also *Thebesian vessel*

The·be·si·us \te-ˈbā-zē-əs\, **Adam Christian (1686–1732),** German anatomist.

the·ca \ˈthē-kə\ *n, pl* **the·cae** \ˈthē-ˌsē, -ˌkē\ : an enveloping case or sheath of an anatomical part — **the·cal** \-kəl\ *adj*

theca cell *n* 1 : an epithelioid cell of the corpus luteum derived from the theca interna — called also *theca lutein cell* 2 : a cell of the columnar epithelium lining the gastric pits of the stomach

theca ex·ter·na \-ek-ˈstər-nə\ *n* : the outer layer of the theca folliculi that is composed of fibrous and muscular tissue

theca fol·lic·u·li \-fə-ˈli-kyə-ˌlī\ *n* : the outer covering of a graafian follicle that is made up of the theca externa and theca interna

theca in·ter·na \-in-ˈtər-nə\ *n* : the inner layer of the theca folliculi that is highly vascular and that contributes theca cells to the formation of the corpus luteum

theca lutein cell *n* : THECA CELL 1

Thee·lin \ˈthē-lən, ˈthē-ə-\ *trademark* — used for a preparation of estrone

thei·le·ria \thī-ˈlir-ē-ə\ *n* 1 *cap* : a genus of parasitic protozoans that includes one (*T. parva*) causing east coast fever of cattle 2 *pl* **-ri·ae** \-ē-ˌē\ *also* **-rias** : any organism of the genus *Theileria* — **thei·le·ri·al** \-ē-əl\ *adj*

Thei·ler \ˈtī-lər\, **Sir Arnold (1867–1936),** South African veterinary bacteriologist.

thei·le·ri·a·sis \ˌthī-lə-ˈrī-ə-səs\ *n, pl* **-a·ses** \-ˌsēz\ : THEILERIOSIS

thei·le·ri·o·sis \thī-ˌlir-ē-ˈō-səs\ *n, pl* **-o·ses** \-ˌsēz\ *or* **-osises** : infection with or disease caused by a protozoan of the genus *Theileria; esp* : EAST COAST FEVER

the·lar·che \thē-ˈlär-kē\ *n* : the beginning of breast development at the onset of puberty ⟨premature ∼⟩

The·la·zia \thə-ˈlā-zē-ə\ *n* : a genus of nematode worms (family Thelaziidae) that includes various eye worms

T–help·er cell \ˌtē-ˈhel-pər-\ *n* : HELPER T CELL

thematic apperception test *n* : a projective technique that is widely used in clinical psychology to make personality, psychodynamic, and diagnostic assessments based on the subject's verbal responses to a series of black and white pictures — abbr. TAT

the·nar \ˈthē-ˌnär, -nər\ *adj* : of, relating to, involving, or constituting the

thenar eminence or the thenar muscles

thenar eminence *n* : the ball of the thumb

thenar muscle *n* : any of the muscles that comprise the intrinsic musculature of the thumb and include the abductor pollicis brevis, adductor pollicis, flexor pollicis brevis, and opponens pollicis

the·o·bro·ma oil \thē-ə-'brō-mə-\ *n* : COCOA BUTTER — used esp. in pharmacy

theo·bro·mine \thē-ə-'brō-ˌmēn, -mən\ *n* : a bitter alkaloid $C_7H_8N_4O_2$ closely related to caffeine that is used as a diuretic, myocardial stimulant, and vasodilator

the·oph·yl·line \thē-'ä-fə-lən\ *n* : a feebly basic bitter crystalline compound $C_7H_8N_4O_2$ that is present in small amounts in tea, is isomeric with theobromine, and is used in medicine esp. as a bronchodilator

theophylline ethylenediamine *n* : AMINOPHYLLINE

the·o·ry \'thir-ē\ *n, pl* **-ries** **1** : the general or abstract principles of a body of fact, a science, or an art **2** : a plausible or scientifically acceptable general principle or body of principles offered to explain natural phenomena — see CELL THEORY, GERM THEORY **3** : a working hypothesis that is considered probable based on experimental evidence of factual or conceptual analysis and is accepted as a basis for experimentation — **the·o·ret·i·cal** \thē-ə-'re-ti-kəl\ *also* **the·o·ret·ic** \-tik\ *adj* — **the·o·ret·i·cal·ly** *adv*

ther·a·peu·sis \ther-ə-'pyü-səs\ *n, pl* **-peu·ses** \-ˌsēz\ : THERAPEUTICS

ther·a·peu·tic \-'pyü-tik\ *adj* **1** : of or relating to the treatment of disease or disorders by remedial agents or methods **2** : CURATIVE, MEDICINAL — **ther·a·peu·ti·cal·ly** *adv*

therapeutic abortion *n* : abortion induced when pregnancy constitutes a threat to the physical or mental health of the mother

therapeutic index *n* : a measure of the relative desirability of a drug for the attaining of a particular medical end that is usu. expressed as the ratio of the largest dose producing no toxic symptoms to the smallest dose routinely producing cures

ther·a·peu·tics \ther-ə-'pyü-tiks\ *n sing or pl* : a branch of medical science dealing with the application of remedies to diseases (cancer ∼) — called also *therapeusis*

ther·a·peu·tist \-'pyü-tist\ *n* : a person skilled in therapeutics

ther·a·py \'ther-ə-pē\ *n, pl* **-pies** : therapeutic treatment esp. of bodily, mental, or behavioral disorder — see ELECTROSHOCK THERAPY, OCCUPATIONAL THERAPY, PHYSICAL THERAPY, PSYCHOTHERAPY, RESPIRATORY THERAPY, SPEECH THERAPY — **ther·a·pist** \'ther-ə-pist\ *n*

the·ri·o·ge·nol·o·gy \thir-ē-ō-jə-'nä-lə-jē\ *n, pl* **-gies** : a branch of veterinary medicine concerned with veterinary obstetrics and with the diseases and physiology of animal reproductive systems — **the·ri·o·gen·o·log·i·cal** \thir-ē-ō-ˌje-nə-'lä-ji-kəl\ *adj* — **the·ri·o·gen·ol·o·gist** \thir-ē-ō-jə-'nä-lə-jist\ *n*

therm- *or* **thermo-** *comb form* : heat ⟨*thermoreceptor*⟩

ther·mal \'thər-məl\ *adj* **1** : of, relating to, or caused by heat **2** : being or involving a state of matter dependent upon temperature ⟨∼ agitation of molecular structure⟩ — **ther·mal·ly** *adv*

-ther·mia \'thər-mē-ə\ *or* **-ther·my** \thər-mē\ *n comb form, pl* **-thermias** *or* **-thermies** : state of heat : generation of heat ⟨dia*thermy*⟩ ⟨hypo*thermia*⟩

ther·mo·co·ag·u·la·tion \thər-mō-kō-ˌa-gyə-'lā-shən\ *n* : surgical coagulation of tissue by the application of heat

ther·mo·di·lu·tion \thər-mō-dī-'lü-shən\ *adj* : relating to or being a method of determining cardiac output by measurement of the change in temperature in the bloodstream after injecting a measured amount of cool fluid (as saline)

ther·mo·gen·e·sis \thər-mō-'je-nə-səs\ *n, pl* **-e·ses** \-ˌsēz\ : the production of heat esp. in the body — **ther·mo·gen·ic** \-'je-nik\ *adj*

ther·mo·gram \'thər-mə-ˌgram\ *n* **1** : the record made by a thermograph **2** : a photographic record made by thermography

ther·mo·graph \-ˌgraf\ *n* **1** : THERMOGRAM **2** : the apparatus used in thermography **3** : a thermometer that produces an automatic record

ther·mog·ra·phy \thər-'mä-grə-fē\ *n, pl* **-phies** : a technique for detecting and measuring variations in the heat emitted by various regions of the body and transforming them into visible signals that can be recorded photographically — **ther·mo·graph·ic** \thər-mə-'gra-fik\ *adj* — **ther·mo·graph·i·cal·ly** *adv*

ther·mo·la·bile \thər-mō-'lā-ˌbīl, -bəl\ *adj* : unstable when heated — **ther·mo·la·bil·i·ty** \-lā-'bi-lə-tē\ *n*

ther·mol·y·sis \(ˌ)thər-'mä-lə-səs\ *n, pl* **-y·ses** \-ˌsēz\ **1** : the dissipation of heat from the living body **2** : decomposition by heat

ther·mom·e·ter \thər-'mä-mə-tər\ *n* : an instrument for determining temperature

ther·mo·met·ric \thər-mə-'me-trik\ *adj* : of or relating to a thermometer or to thermometry

ther·mom·e·try \thər-'mä-mə-trē\ *n, pl* **-tries** : the measurement of temperature

ther·mo·plas·tic \thər-mə-'plas-tik\ *adj*

: capable of softening or fusing when heated and of hardening again when cooled 〈~ synthetic resins〉 — **ther·mo·plastic** *n*

ther·mo·re·cep·tor \ˌthər-mō-ri-ˈsep-tər\ *n* : a sensory end organ that is stimulated by heat or cold

ther·mo·reg·u·la·tion \-ˌre-gyə-ˈlā-shən\ *n* : the maintenance or regulation of temperature; *specif* : the maintenance of a particular temperature of the living body — **ther·mo·reg·u·late** \-ˈre-gyə-ˌlāt\ *vb* — **ther·mo·reg·u·la·to·ry** \-ˈre-gyə-lə-ˌtōr-ē\ *adj*

ther·mo·sta·ble \ˌthər-mō-ˈstā-bəl\ *adj* : stable when heated — **ther·mo·sta·bil·i·ty** \-stə-ˈbi-lə-tē\ *n*

ther·mo·ther·a·py \ˌthər-mō-ˈther-ə-pē\ *n, pl* **-pies** : treatment of disease by heat (as by hot air or hot baths)

-thermy — see **-THERMIA**

the·ta rhythm \ˈthā-tə-ˌrith-əm\ *n* : a relatively high amplitude brain wave pattern between approximately 4 and 9 hertz that is characteristic esp. of the hippocampus but occurs in many regions of the brain including the cortex — called also *theta, theta wave*

thi- *or* **thio-** *comb form* : containing sulfur 〈*thia*mine〉 〈*thio*pental〉

thia·ben·da·zole \ˌthī-ə-ˈben-də-ˌzōl\ *n* : a drug $C_{10}H_7N_3S$ used in the control of parasitic nematodes and in the treatment of fungus infections

thi·acet·azone \ˌthī-ə-ˈse-tə-ˌzōn\ *n* : a bitter pale yellow crystalline tuberculostatic drug $C_{10}H_{12}N_4OS$

thi·am·i·nase \thī-ˈa-mə-ˌnās, ˈthī-ə-mə-, -ˌnāz\ *n* : an enzyme that catalyzes the breakdown of thiamine

thi·a·mine \ˈthī-ə-mən, -ˌmēn\ *also* **thi·a·min** \-mən\ *n* : a vitamin $(C_{12}H_{17}N_4OS)Cl$ of the B complex that is a water-soluble salt occurring widely both in plants and animals and that is essential for conversion of carbohydrate to fat and for normal nerve function — called also *vitamin B₁*

Thi·a·ra \thī-ˈar-ə\ *n* : a genus of freshwater snails (family Thiaridae) that includes several forms (as *T. granifera* of eastern Asia and the western Pacific islands) which are intermediate hosts of medically important trematodes

thi·a·zide \ˈthī-ə-ˌzīd, -zəd\ *n* : any of a group of drugs used as oral diuretics esp. in the control of high blood pressure

thi·a·zine \ˈthī-ə-ˌzēn\ *n* : any of various compounds that are characterized by a ring composed of four carbon atoms, one sulfur atom, and one nitrogen atom — see PHENOTHIAZINE

thi·a·zole \ˈthī-ə-ˌzōl\ *n* **1** : a colorless basic liquid C_3H_3NS; *also* : any of various thiazole derivatives including some used in medicine

thick filament *n* : a myofilament of one

of the two types making up myofibrils that is 100 to 120 angstroms in width and is composed of the protein myosin — compare THIN FILAMENT

Thiersch graft \ˈtirsh-\ *n* : a skin graft that consists of thin strips or sheets of epithelium with the tops of the dermal papillae and that is split off with a sharp knife

Thiersch, Carl (1822–1895), German surgeon.

thigh \ˈthī\ *n* : the proximal segment of the leg extending from the hip to the knee and supported by a single large bone — compare FEMUR

thigh·bone \ˈthī-ˌbōn\ *n* : FEMUR

thi·mer·o·sal \thī-ˈmer-ə-ˌsal\ *n* : a crystalline mercurial antiseptic $C_9H_9HgNaO_2S$ used esp. for its antifungal and bacteriostatic properties — see MERTHIOLATE

thin filament *n* : a myofilament the one of the two types making up myofibrils that is about 50 angstroms in width and is composed chiefly of the protein actin — compare THICK FILAMENT

thin–layer chromatography *n* : chromatography in which the stationary phase is an absorbent medium (as silica gel or alumina) arranged as a thin layer on a rigid support (as a glass plate) — compare COLUMN CHROMATOGRAPHY, PAPER CHROMATOGRAPHY — **thin–layer chromatogram** *n* — **thin–layer chromatographic** *adj*

thio- \ˈthī-ō\ *adj* : relating to or containing sulfur esp. in place of oxygen

thio- — see THI-

thio acid *n* : an acid in which oxygen is partly or wholly replaced by sulfur

thio·amide \ˌthī-ō-ˈa-ˌmīd, -məd\ *n* : amide of a thio acid

thio·car·ba·mide \ˌthī-ō-ˈkär-bə-ˌmīd, -ˌkär-ˈba-ˌmī{d}\ *n* : THIOUREA

thio·ctic acid *also* **6,8–thi·oc·tic acid** \(ˌsiks-ˌāt-)thī-ˈäk-tik-\ *n* : the lipoic acid $C_8H_{14}O_2S_2$ that is held by some to ameliorate the effects of poisoning by mushrooms (as the death cap) of the genus *Amanita*

thio·cy·a·nate \ˌthī-ō-ˈsī-ə-ˌnāt, -nət\ *n* : a compound that consists of the chemical group SCN bonded by the sulfur atom to a group or an atom other than a hydrogen atom

thiocyanoacetate — see ISOBORNYL THIOCYANOACETATE

thio·es·ter \ˌthī-ō-ˈes-tər\ *n* : an ester formed by uniting a carboxyl group of one compound (as acetic acid) with a sulfhydryl group of another (as coenzyme A)

thio·gua·nine \-ˈgwä-ˌnēn\ *n* : a crystalline compound $C_5H_5N_5S$ that is an antimetabolite and has been used in the treatment of leukemia

thi·ol \ˈthī-ˌol, -ōl\ *n* **1** : any of various compounds having the general formula RSH which are analogous to alcohols but in which sulfur replaces the oxygen of the hydroxyl group and which have disagreeable odors **2** : the functional group –SH characteristic of thiols — **thi·o·lic** \thī-ˈō-lik\ *adj*

thio·pen·tal \ˌthī-ō-ˈpen-ˌtal, -ˌtȯl\ *n* : a barbiturate $C_{11}H_{18}N_2O_2S$ used in the form of its sodium salt esp. as an intravenous anesthetic — see PENTOTHAL

thio·pen·tone \-ˌtōn\ *n, Brit* : THIOPENTAL

thio·rid·a·zine \ˌthī-ə-ˈri-də-ˌzēn, -zən\ *n* : a phenothiazine tranquilizer used in the form of its hydrochloride $C_{21}H_{26}N_3S_2 \cdot HCl$ for relief of anxiety states and in the treatment of schizophrenia — see MELLARIL

thio·te·pa \ˌthī-ə-ˈtē-pə\ *n* : a sulfur analog of tepa $C_6H_{12}N_3PS$ that is used esp. as an antineoplastic agent and is less toxic than tepa

thio·thix·ene \ˌthī-ō-ˈthik-ˌsēn\ *n* : an antipsychotic drug $C_{23}H_{29}N_3O_2S_2$ used esp. in the treatment of schizophrenia — see NAVANE

thio·ura·cil \ˌthī-ō-ˈyur-ə-ˌsil\ *n* : a bitter crystalline compound $C_4H_4N_2OS$ that depresses the function of the thyroid gland

thio·urea \-yu̇-ˈrē-ə\ *n* : a colorless bitter crystalline compound $CS(NH_2)_2$ analogous to and resembling urea that is used esp. in medicine as an antithyroid drug — called also *thiocarbamide*

thio·xan·thene \ˌthī-ō-ˈzan-ˌthēn\ *n* : a compound $C_{13}H_{10}S$ that is the parent compound of various antipsychotic drugs (as thiothixene); *also* : a derivative of thioxanthene

third cranial nerve *n* : OCULOMOTOR NERVE

third–degree burn *n* : a severe burn characterized by destruction of the skin through the depth of the dermis and possibly into underlying tissues, loss of fluid, and sometimes shock

third eyelid *n* : NICTITATING MEMBRANE

third ventricle *n* : the median unpaired ventricle of the brain bounded by parts of the telencephalon and diencephalon

thirst \ˈthərst\ *n* : a sensation of dryness in the mouth and throat associated with a desire for liquids; *also* : the bodily condition (as of dehydration) that induces this sensation — **thirsty** \ˈthər-stē\ *adj*

Thom·as splint \ˈtä-məs-\ *n* : a metal splint for fractures of the arm or leg that consists of a ring at one end to fit around the upper arm or leg and two metal shafts extending down the sides of the limb in a long U with a crosspiece at the bottom where traction is applied

Thomas, Hugh Owen (1834–1891), British orthopedic surgeon.

Thom·sen's disease \ˈtȯm-sənz-, ˈtäm-\ *n* : MYOTONIA CONGENITA

Thomsen, Asmus Julius Thomas (1815–1896), Danish physician.

thon·zyl·a·mine \thän-ˈzi-lə-ˌmēn, -mən\ *n* : an antihistaminic drug $C_{16}H_{22}N_4O$ derived from pyrimidine and used in the form of its crystalline hydrochloride — see NEOHETRAMINE

thorac- *or* **thoraci-** *or* **thoraco-** *comb form* **1** : chest : thorax ⟨*thoraco*plasty⟩ **2** : thoracic and ⟨*thoraco*lumbar⟩

tho·ra·cen·te·sis \ˌthō-rə-sen-ˈtē-səs\ *n, pl* **-te·ses** \-ˌsēz\ : aspiration of fluid from the chest (as in empyema) — called also *thoracocentesis*

thoraces *pl of* THORAX

tho·rac·ic \thə-ˈra-sik\ *adj* : of, relating to, located within, or involving the thorax ⟨∼ trauma⟩ ⟨∼ surgery⟩ — **tho·rac·i·cal·ly** *adv*

thoracic aorta *n* : the part of the aorta that lies in the thorax and extends from the arch to the diaphragm

thoracic artery *n* **1** : either of two arteries that branch from the axillary artery or from one of its branches: **a** : a small artery that supplies or sends branches to the two pectoralis muscles and the walls of the chest — called also *supreme thoracic artery* **b** : an artery that supplies both pectoralis muscles and the serratus anterior and sends branches to the lymph nodes of the axilla and to the subscapularis muscle — called also *lateral thoracic artery* **2** — see INTERNAL THORACIC ARTERY

thoracic cage *n* : RIB CAGE

thoracic cavity *n* : the division of the body cavity that lies above the diaphragm, is bounded peripherally by the wall of the chest, and contains the heart and lungs

thoracic duct *n* : the main trunk of the system of lymphatic vessels that lies along the front of the spinal column and receives chyle from the intestine and lymph from the abdomen, the lower limbs, and the entire left side of the body — called also *left lymphatic duct*

thoracic ganglion *n* : any of the ganglia of the sympathetic chain in the thoracic region that occur in 12 or fewer pairs

thoracic nerve *n* : any of the spinal nerves of the thoracic region that consist of 12 pairs of which one pair emerges just below each thoracic vertebra

thoracic vertebra *n* : any of the 12 vertebrae dorsal to the thoracic region and characterized by articulation with the ribs

thoracis — see ILIOCOSTALIS THORACIS, LONGISSIMUS THORACIS, SEMISPINALIS THORACIS, SPINALIS THORACIS, TRANSVERSUS THORACIS

thoraco- — see THORAC-

tho·ra·co·ab·dom·i·nal \ˌthō-rə-ˌkō-ab-ˈdä-mə-nəl\ *also* **tho·rac·i·co·ab·dom·i·nal** \thə-ˌra-si-ˌkō-\ *adj* : of, relating to, involving, or affecting the thorax and the abdomen ⟨a ∼ incision⟩

tho·ra·co·acro·mi·al artery \ˌthō-rə-ˌkō-ə-ˈkrō-mē-əl-\ n : a short branch of the axillary artery that divides into four branches supplying the region of the pectoralis muscles, deltoid, subclavius, and sternoclavicular joint

tho·ra·co·cen·te·sis \-sen-ˈtē-səs\ n, pl **-te·ses** \-ˌsēz\ : THORACENTESIS

tho·ra·co·dor·sal artery \ˌthō-rə-kō-ˈdȯr-səl-\ n : an artery that is continuous with the axillary artery and supplies or gives off branches supplying the subscapularis muscle, latissimus dorsi, serratus anterior, and the intercostal muscles

thoracodorsal nerve n : a branch of the posterior cord of the brachial plexus that supplies the latissimus dorsi

tho·ra·co·lum·bar \-ˈləm-bər, -ˌbär\ adj **1** : of, relating to, arising in, or involving the thoracic and lumbar regions **2** : SYMPATHETIC ⟨∼ nerve fibers⟩

tho·ra·co·plas·ty \ˈthōr-ə-kō-ˌplas-tē\ n, pl **-ties** : the surgical operation of removing or resecting one or more ribs so as to obliterate the pleural cavity and collapse a diseased lung

tho·ra·co·scope \thə-ˈrā-kə-ˌskōp, -ˈra-\ n : an instrument that is designed to permit visual inspection within the chest cavity and is inserted through a puncture in the chest wall in an intercostal space

tho·ra·cos·co·py \ˌthōr-ə-ˈkäs-kə-pē\ n, pl **-pies** : examination of the chest and esp. the pleural cavity by means of a thoracoscope

tho·ra·cos·to·my \ˌthōr-ə-ˈkäs-tə-mē\ n, pl **-mies** : surgical opening of the chest (as for drainage)

tho·ra·cot·o·my \ˌthōr-ə-ˈkä-tə-mē\ n, pl **-mies** : surgical incision of the chest wall

tho·rax \ˈthōr-ˌaks\ n, pl **tho·rax·es** or **tho·ra·ces** \ˈthōr-ə-ˌsēz\ **1** : the part of the body that is situated between the neck and the abdomen and is supported by the ribs, costal cartilages, and sternum; also : THORACIC CAVITY **2** : the middle of the three chief divisions of the body of an insect; also : the corresponding part of a crustacean or an arachnid

Tho·ra·zine \ˈthōr-ə-ˌzēn\ trademark — used for a preparation of chlorpromazine

tho·ri·um \ˈthōr-ē-əm\ n : a radioactive metallic element — symbol Th; see ELEMENT table

thorn–headed worm or **thorny–headed worm** n : ACANTHOCEPHALAN

thor·ough·pin \ˈthər-ō-ˌpin\ n : a synovial swelling just above the hock of a horse that is often associated with lameness

thread lungworm n : a slender nematode worm of the genus Dictyocaulus (D. filaria) that parasitizes the air passages of the lungs of sheep

thread·worm \ˈthred-ˌwərm\ n : any long slender nematode worm

thready pulse \ˈthre-dē-\ n : a scarcely perceptible and commonly rapid pulse that feels like a fine mobile thread under a palpating finger

three–day fever n : a fever or febrile state lasting three days; esp : SANDFLY FEVER

thre·o·nine \ˈthrē-ə-ˌnēn\ n : a colorless crystalline essential amino acid $C_4H_9NO_3$

thresh·old \ˈthresh-ˌhōld\ n : the point at which a physiological or psychological effect begins to be produced (as the degree of stimulation of a nerve which just produces a response) — called also limen

thrill \ˈthril\ n : an abnormal fine tremor or vibration in the respiratory or circulatory systems felt on palpation

throat \ˈthrōt\ n **1** : the part of the neck in front of the spinal column **2** : the passage through the throat to the stomach and lungs containing the pharynx and upper part of the esophagus, the larynx, and the trachea

throat botfly n : a botfly of the genus Gasterophilus (G. nasalis) that lays its eggs on the hairs about the mouth of the horse from where the larvae migrate on hatching and attach themselves to the walls of the stomach and intestine — called also throat fly

¹throb \ˈthräb\ vb **throbbed; throb·bing** : to pulsate or pound esp. with abnormal force or rapidity

²throb n : a single pulse of a pulsating movement or sensation

throe \ˈthrō\ n : PANG, SPASM — usu. used in pl. ⟨death ∼s⟩

thromb- or **thrombo-** comb form **1** : blood clot : clotting of blood ⟨thrombin⟩ ⟨thromboplastic⟩ **2** : marked by or associated with thrombosis ⟨thromboangiitis⟩

throm·base \ˈthräm-ˌbās\ n : THROMBIN

throm·bas·the·nia \ˌthräm-bəs-ˈthē-nē-ə\ n : an inherited abnormality of the blood platelets characterized esp. by defective clot retraction and often prolonged bleeding time

throm·bec·to·my \thräm-ˈbek-tə-mē\ n, pl **-mies** : surgical excision of a thrombus

thrombi pl of THROMBUS

throm·bin \ˈthräm-bən\ n : a proteolytic enzyme formed from prothrombin that facilitates the clotting of blood by catalyzing conversion of fibrinogen to fibrin

throm·bo·an·gi·i·tis \ˌthräm-bō-ˌan-jē-ˈī-təs\ n, pl **-it·i·des** \-ˈi-tə-ˌdēz\ : inflammation of the lining of a blood vessel with thrombus formation

thromboangiitis ob·lit·er·ans \-ə-ˈbli-tə-ˌranz\ n : thromboangiitis of the small arteries and veins of the extremities and esp. the feet resulting in occlusion, ischemia, and gangrene — called also Buerger's disease

throm·bo·cyte \'thräm-bə-ˌsīt\ *n* : BLOOD PLATELET — **throm·bo·cyt·ic** \ˌthräm-bə-'si-tik\ *adj*

throm·bo·cy·top·a·thy \ˌthräm-bə-ˌsī-'tä-pə-thē\ *n, pl* **-thies** : any of various functional disorders of the blood platelets

throm·bo·cy·to·pe·nia \ˌthräm-bə-ˌsī-tə-'pē-nē-ə, -nyə\ *n* : persistent decrease in the number of blood platelets that is often associated with hemorrhagic conditions — called also *thrombopenia* — **throm·bo·cy·to·pe·nic** \-nik\ *adj*

thrombocytopenic purpura *n* : a condition that is characterized by bleeding into the skin with the production of petechiae or ecchymoses and by hemorrhages into mucous membranes and that is associated with a reduction in circulating blood platelets and prolonged bleeding time (idiopathic *thrombocytopenic purpura*) — called also *purpura hemorrhagica*, *Werlhof's disease*

throm·bo·cy·to·sis \ˌthräm-bə-ˌsī-'tō-səs\ *n, pl* **-to·ses** \-'tō-ˌsēz\ : increase and esp. abnormal increase in the number of blood platelets

throm·bo·em·bo·lism \ˌthräm-bō-'em-bə-ˌli-zəm\ *n* : the blocking of a blood vessel by a particle that has broken away from a blood clot at its site of formation — **throm·bo·em·bol·ic** \-em-'bä-lik\ *adj*

throm·bo·end·ar·te·rec·to·my \ˌthräm-bō-ˌen-ˌdär-tə-'rek-tə-mē\ *n, pl* **-mies** : surgical excision of a thrombus and the adjacent arterial lining

throm·bo·gen·ic \ˌthräm-bə-'je-nik\ *adj* : tending to produce a thrombus — **throm·bo·ge·nic·i·ty** \-jə-'ni-sə-tē\ *n*

throm·bo·ki·nase \ˌthräm-bō-'kī-ˌnās, -ˌnāz\ *n* : THROMBOPLASTIN

throm·bo·lyt·ic \ˌthräm-bə-'li-tik\ *adj* : destroying or breaking up a thrombus ⟨a ～ agent⟩ ⟨～ therapy⟩ — **throm·bol·y·sis** \thräm-'bä-lə-səs\ *n*

throm·bo·pe·nia \ˌthräm-bō-'pē-nē-ə\ *n* : THROMBOCYTOPENIA — **throm·bo·pe·nic** \-'pē-nik\ *adj*

throm·bo·phle·bi·tis \-fli-'bī-təs\ *n, pl* **-bit·i·des** \-'bi-tə-ˌdēz\ : inflammation of a vein with formation of a thrombus — compare PHLEBOTHROMBOSIS

throm·bo·plas·tic \ˌthräm-bō-'plas-tik\ *adj* : initiating or accelerating the clotting of blood ⟨a ～ substance⟩

throm·bo·plas·tin \ˌthräm-bō-'plas-tən\ *n* : a complex enzyme that is found esp. in blood platelets and functions in the conversion of prothrombin to thrombin in the clotting of blood — called also *thrombokinase*

throm·bo·plas·tin·o·gen \-ˌplas-'ti-nə-jən\ *n* : FACTOR VIII

throm·bo·sis \thräm-'bō-səs, thrəm-\ *n, pl* **-bo·ses** \-ˌsēz\ : the formation or presence of a blood clot within a blood vessel during life — **throm·bose** \'thräm-ˌbōs, -ˌbōz\ *vb* — **throm·bot·ic** \thräm-'bä-tik\ *adj*

throm·box·ane \thräm-'bäk-ˌsān\ *n* : any of several substances that are formed from endoperoxides, cause constriction of vascular and bronchial smooth muscle, and promote blood coagulation

throm·bus \'thräm-bəs\ *n, pl* **throm·bi** \-ˌbī, -ˌbē\ : a clot of blood formed within a blood vessel and remaining attached to its place of origin — compare EMBOLUS

throw·back \'thrō-ˌbak\ *n* **1** : reversion to an earlier type or phase : ATAVISM **2** : an instance or product of atavistic reversion

throw up *vb* : VOMIT

thrush \'thrəsh\ *n* **1** : a disease that is caused by a fungus of the genus *Candida* (*C. albicans*), occurs esp. in infants and children, and is marked by white patches in the oral cavity; *broadly* : CANDIDIASIS ⟨vaginal ～⟩ **2** : a suppurative disorder of the feet in various animals (as the horse)

thu·li·um \'thü-lē-əm, 'thyü-\ *n* : a metallic element — symbol *Tm*; see ELEMENT table

thumb \'thəm\ *n* : the short and thick first or most preaxial digit of the human hand that differs from the other fingers in having only two phalanges, in having greater freedom of movement, and in being opposable to the other fingers

thumb–suck·ing \-ˌsə-kin\ *n* : the habit of sucking a thumb beyond the period of physiological need — **thumb–suck·er** *n*

thym- or **thymo-** *comb form* : thymus ⟨*thymic*⟩ ⟨*thymocyte*⟩

thy·mec·to·my \thī-'mek-tə-mē\ *n, pl* **-mies** : surgical excision of the thymus — **thy·mec·to·mize** \-ˌmīz\ *vb*

thyme oil \'tīm-, 'thīm-\ *n* : a fragrant essential oil that is obtained from various thymes (genus *Thymus* of the mint family, Labiatae) and is used chiefly as an antiseptic in pharmaceutical and dental preparations

-thy·mia \'thī-mē-ə\ *n comb form* : condition of mind and will ⟨cyclo*thymia*⟩ ⟨dys*thymia*⟩

thy·mic \'thī-mik\ *adj* : of or relating to the thymus ⟨a ～ tumor⟩

thymic corpuscle *n* : HASSALL'S CORPUSCLE

thy·mi·co·lym·phat·ic \ˌthī-mi-(ˌ)kō-lim-'fa-tik\ *adj* : of, relating to, or affecting both the thymus and the lymphatic system ⟨～ involution⟩

thy·mi·dine \'thī-mə-ˌdēn\ *n* : a nucleoside $C_{10}H_{14}N_2O_5$ that is composed of thymine and deoxyribose and occurs as a structural part of DNA

thymidine kinase *n* : an enzyme that is involved in DNA replication and that increases greatly during infection with some viruses (as the herpesvirus causing herpes simplex) and during periods of increased growth rate (as in liver regeneration)

thy·mine \'thī-ˌmēn\ *n* : a pyrimidine base $C_5H_6N_2O_2$ that is one of the four bases coding genetic information in the polynucleotide chain of DNA — compare ADENINE, CYTOSINE, GUANINE, URACIL

thy·mo·cyte \'thī-mə-ˌsīt\ *n* : a cell of the thymus; *esp* : a thymic lymphocyte

thy·mol \'thī-ˌmȯl, -ˌmōl\ *n* : a crystalline phenol $C_{10}H_{14}O$ of aromatic odor and antiseptic properties found esp. in thyme oil or made synthetically and used chiefly as a fungicide and preservative

thy·mo·ma \thī-'mō-mə\ *n, pl* **-mas** or **-ma·ta** \-mə-tə\ : a tumor that arises from the tissue elements of the thymus

thy·mo·sin \'thī-mə-sən\ *n* : a mixture of polypeptides isolated from the thymus; *also* : any of these

thy·mus \'thī-məs\ *n* : a glandular structure of largely lymphoid tissue that functions in cell-mediated immunity by being the site where T cells develop, that is present in the young of most vertebrates typically in the upper anterior chest or at the base of the neck, and that tends to disappear or become rudimentary in the adult — called also *thymus gland*

thyr- *or* **thyro-** *comb form* **1** : thyroid ⟨*thyr*oglobulin⟩ **2** : thyroid and ⟨*thyr*oarytenoid⟩

thy·ro·ac·tive \ˌthī-rō-'ak-tiv\ *adj* **1** : capable of entering into the thyroid metabolism and of being incorporated into the thyroid hormone ⟨~ iodine⟩ **2** : simulating the action of the thyroid hormone ⟨~ iodinated casein⟩

thy·ro·ar·y·te·noid \-ˌar-ə-'tē-ˌnȯid, -ə-'rit-ᵊn-ˌȯid\ *n* : a broad thin muscle that arises esp. from the thyroid cartilage, inserts into the arytenoid cartilage, and that functions to relax and shorten the vocal cords — called also *thyroarytenoid muscle*; see INFERIOR THYROARYTENOID LIGAMENT

thy·ro·ar·y·te·noi·de·us \-ˌar-ə-tə-'nȯi-dē-əs\ *n* : THYROARYTENOID

thy·ro·cal·ci·to·nin \ˌthī-rō-ˌkal-sə-'tō-nən\ *n* : CALCITONIN

thy·ro·cer·vi·cal \-'sər-vi-kəl\ *adj* : of, relating to, or being the thyrocervical trunk ⟨the ~ artery⟩

thyrocervical trunk *n* : a short thick branch of the subclavian artery that divides into the inferior thyroid, suprascapular, and transverse cervical arteries

thy·ro·epi·glot·tic ligament \ˌthī-rō-ˌe-pə-'glä-tik-\ *n* : a long narrow ligamentous cord connecting the thyroid cartilage and epiglottis

thy·ro·glob·u·lin \ˌthī-rō-'glä-byə-lən\ *n* : an iodine-containing protein of the thyroid gland that on proteolysis yields thyroxine and triiodothyronine

relating to, or originating in the thyroglossal duct ⟨~ cysts⟩

thyroglossal duct *n* : a temporary duct connecting the embryonic thyroid gland and the tongue

thy·ro·hy·al \ˌthī-rō-'hī-əl\ *n* : the larger and more lateral of the two lateral projections on each side of the human hyoid bone — called also *greater cornu*; compare CERATOHYAL

¹thy·ro·hy·oid \-'hī-ˌȯid\ *adj* : of, relating to, or supplying the thyrohyoid muscle

²thyrohyoid *n* : a thyrohyoid part; *esp* : THYROHYOID MUSCLE

thyrohyoid membrane *n* : a broad fibroelastic sheet that connects the upper margin of the thyroid cartilage and the upper margin of the back of the hyoid bone

thyrohyoid muscle *n* : a small quadrilateral muscle that arises from the thyroid cartilage, inserts into the thyrohyal of the hyoid bone, and functions to depress the hyoid bone and to elevate the thyroid cartilage — called also *thyrohyoid*

¹thy·roid \'thī-ˌrȯid\ *also* **thy·roi·dal** \thī-'rȯid-ᵊl\ *adj* **1** : of, relating to, or being the thyroid gland ⟨~ cancer⟩ **2** : of, relating to, or being the thyroid cartilage

²thyroid *n* **1** : a large bilobed endocrine gland that arises as a median ventral outgrowth of the pharynx, lies in the anterior base of the neck, and produces esp. the hormones thyroxine and triiodothyronine — called also *thyroid gland* **2** : a preparation of the thyroid gland containing approximately $1/10$ percent of iodine combined in thyroxine and used in treating thyroid disorders — called also *thyroid extract*

thyroid artery *n* : either of two arteries supplying the thyroid gland and nearby structures at the front of the neck: **a** : one that branches from the external carotid artery or sometimes from the common carotid artery — called also *superior thyroid artery* **b** : one that branches from the thyrocervical trunk — called also *inferior thyroid artery*

thyroid–binding globulin *n* : THYROXINE-BINDING GLOBULIN

thyroid cartilage *n* : the chief cartilage of the larynx that consists of two broad lamellae joined at an angle and that forms the Adam's apple

thy·roid·ec·to·my \ˌthī-ˌrȯi-'dek-tə-mē\ *n, pl* **-mies** : surgical excision of thyroid gland tissue — **thy·roid·ec·to·mize** \-ˌmīz\ *vb*

thyroid extract *n* : THYROID 2

thyroid gland *n* : THYROID 1

thyroid hormone *n* : any of several closely related metabolically active compounds (as triiodothyronine) that are stored in the thyroid gland in the form of thyroglobulin or circulate in the blood apparently bound to plasma protein; *esp* : THYROXINE

thy·roid·itis \ˌthī-ˌroi-ˈdī-təs\ *n* : inflammation of the thyroid gland

thyroid–stimulating hormone *n* : THYROTROPIN

thyroid storm *n* : a sudden life=threatening exacerbation of the symptoms (as high fever, tachycardia, weakness, or extreme restlessness) of hyperthyroidism that is brought on by various causes (as in infection, surgery, or stress)

thyroid vein *n* : any of several small veins draining blood from the thyroid gland and nearby structures in the front of the neck

thy·ro·nine \ˈthī-rə-ˌnēn, -nən\ *n* : a phenolic amino acid $C_{15}H_{15}NO_4$ of which thyroxine is a derivative; *also* : any of various derivatives of this iodine-containing derivatives of this

thy·rot·o·my \thī-ˈrä-tə-mē\ *n, pl* **-mies** : surgical incision or division of the thyroid cartilage

thy·ro·tox·ic \ˌthī-rō-ˈtäk-sik\ *adj* : of, relating to, induced by, or affected with hyperthyroidism

thy·ro·tox·i·co·sis \ˈthī-rō-ˌtäk-sə-ˈkō-səs\ *n, pl* **-co·ses** \-ˌsēz\ : HYPERTHYROIDISM

thy·ro·tro·pic \ˌthī-rə-ˈtrō-pik, -ˈträ-\ *also* **thy·ro·tro·phic** \-ˈtrō-fik\ *adj* : exerting or characterized by a direct influence on the secretory activity of the thyroid gland ⟨∼ functions⟩

thyrotropic hormone *n* : THYROTROPIN

thy·ro·tro·pin \ˌthī-rə-ˈtrō-pən\ *also* **thy·ro·tro·phin** \-fən\ *n* : a hormone secreted by the adenohypophysis of the pituitary gland that stimulates the thyroid — called also *thyroid-stimulating hormone, TSH*

thyrotropin–releasing hormone *n* : a tripeptide hormone synthesized in the hypothalamus that stimulates secretion of thyrotropin by the anterior lobe of the pituitary gland — abbr. *TRH;* called also *protirelin, thyrotropin-releasing factor*

thy·rox·ine *or* **thy·rox·in** \thī-ˈräk-ˌsēn, -sən\ *n* : an iodine-containing hormone $C_{15}H_{11}I_4NO_4$ that is an amino acid produced by the thyroid gland as a product of the cleavage of thyroglobulin, increases metabolic rate, and is used to treat thyroid disorders — called also *T-4*

thyroxine–binding globulin *n* : a blood serum glycoprotein that is synthesized in the liver and that binds tightly to thyroxine and less firmly to triiodothyronine preventing their removal from the blood by the kidneys and releasing them as needed at sites of activity — abbr. *TBG;* called also *thyroid-binding globulin*

Thysa·no·so·ma \ˌthī-sə-nō-ˈsō-mə\ *n* : a genus of tapeworms (family Anoplocephalidae) including the common fringed tapeworm of ruminants

Ti *symbol* titanium

TIA *abbr* transient ischemic attack

tib·ia \ˈti-bē-ə\ *n, pl* **-i·ae** \-bē-ˌē, -bē-ˌī\ *also* **-i·as** : the inner and usu. larger of the two bones of the leg between the knee and ankle that articulates above with the femur and below with the talus — called also *shinbone* — **tib·i·al** \-bē-əl\ *adj*

tibial artery *n* : either of the two arteries of the lower leg formed by the bifurcation of the popliteal artery: **a** : a larger posterior artery that divides into the lateral and medial plantar arteries — called also *posterior tibial artery* **b** : a smaller anterior artery that continues beyond the ankle joint into the foot as the dorsalis pedis artery — called also *anterior tibial artery*

tibial collateral ligament *n* : MEDIAL COLLATERAL LIGAMENT

tib·i·a·lis \ˌti-bē-ˈā-ləs\ *n, pl* **tib·i·a·les** \-(ˌ)lēz\ : either of two muscles of the calf of the leg: **a** : a muscle arising chiefly from the lateral condyle and part of the shaft of the tibia, inserting by a long tendon into the first cuneiform and first metatarsal bones, and acting to flex the foot dorsally and to invert it — called also *tibialis anterior, tibialis anticus* **b** : a deeply situated muscle that arises from the tibia and fibula, interosseous membrane, and intermuscular septa, that is inserted by a tendon passing under the medial malleolus into the navicular and first cuneiform bones, and that flexes the foot in the direction of the sole and tends to invert it — called also *tibialis posterior, tibialis posticus*

tibialis anterior *n* : TIBIALIS a

tibialis an·ti·cus \-an-ˈtī-kəs\ *n* : TIBIALIS a

tibialis pos·ti·cus \-pōs-ˈtī-kəs\ *n* : TIBIALIS b

tibial nerve *n* : the large nerve in the back of the leg that is a continuation of the sciatic nerve and terminates at the medial malleolus in the lateral and medial plantar nerves — called also *medial popliteal nerve*

tibial vein *n* : any of several veins that accompany the corresponding tibial arteries and that unite to form the popliteal vein: **a** : one accompanying the posterior tibial artery — called also *posterior tibial vein* **b** : one accompanying the anterior tibial artery — called also *anterior tibial vein*

tibio- *comb form* : tibial and ⟨tibiofemoral⟩

tib·io·fem·o·ral \ˌti-bē-ō-ˈfe-mə-rəl\ *adj* : relating to or being the articulation occurring between the tibia and the femur ⟨the ∼ joint⟩

tib·io·fib·u·lar \-ˈfi-byə-lər\ *adj* : of, relating to, or connecting the tibia and fibula ⟨the proximal ∼ joint⟩

tib·io·tar·sal \-ˈtär-səl\ *adj* : of, relating

to, or affecting the tibia and the tarsus ⟨~ abnormalities⟩

ti·bric acid \'tī-brik-\ *n* : an antihyperlipidemic drug $C_{14}H_{18}ClNO_4S$

tic \'tik\ *n* : local and habitual spasmodic motion of particular muscles esp. of the face — TWITCHING

ti·car·cil·lin \₁tī-kär-'si-lən\ *n* : a semisynthetic antibiotic $C_{15}H_{16}N_2O_6S_2$ used esp. as the disodium salt

tic dou·lou·reux \ₐtik-₁dü-lə-'rü, -'rōō\ *n* : TRIGEMINAL NEURALGIA

tick \'tik\ *n* 1 : any of a superfamily (Ixodoidea) of the order Acarina) of bloodsucking arachnids that are larger than the closely related mites, attach themselves to warm-blooded vertebrates to feed, and include important vectors of various infectious diseases 2 : any of various usu. wingless parasitic dipteran flies (as the sheep ked)

tick–borne *adj* : capable of being transmitted by the bites of ticks ⟨~ encephalitis⟩

tick–borne fever *n* : a mild rickettsial disease of sheep esp. in Great Britain that is transmitted by a tick of the genus *Ixodes; also* : a related disease of cattle

tick fever *n* 1 : TEXAS FEVER 2 : a febrile disease (as Rocky Mountain spotted fever or relapsing fever) transmitted by the bites of ticks

tick paralysis *n* : a progressive spinal paralysis that moves upward toward the brain and is caused by a neurotoxin secreted by some ticks (as *Dermacentor andersoni*)

tick typhus *n* : any of various tick-borne rickettsial spotted fevers or boutonneuse fever)

ti·cryn·a·fen \tī-'kri-nə-₁fen\ *n* : a diuretic, uricosuric, and antihypertensive agent $C_{13}H_8Cl_2O_4S$ recalled from the drug market because of a high incidence of hepatic disorders associated with its use

tid *abbr* [Latin *ter in die*] three times a day — used in writing prescriptions

tid·al \'tīd-ᵊl\ *adj* : of, relating to, or constituting tidal air

tidal air *n* : the air that passes in and out of the lungs in an ordinary breath

tidal volume *n* : the volume of the tidal air

tide \'tīd\ *n* : a temporary increase or decrease in a specified substance or quality in the body or one of its systems ⟨an acid ~ during fasting⟩

tie off *vb* **tied off; ty·ing off** *or* **tie·ing off** : to close by means of an encircling or enveloping ligature ⟨*tie off* a bleeding vessel⟩

Tiet·ze's syndrome \'tēt-səz-\ *n* : a condition of unknown origin that is characterized by inflammation of costochondral cartilage — called also *costochondritis, Tietze's disease*

tiger mosquito *n* : YELLOW-FEVER MOSQUITO

tiger rattlesnake *n* : a rather small rattlesnake of the genus *Crotalus* (*C. tigris*) that occurs in mountainous deserts of western No. America

ti·groid substance \'tī-₁groid-\ *n* : NISSL BODIES

TIL \₁tē-(₁)ī-'el\ *n* : TUMOR-INFILTRATING LYMPHOCYTE

timber rattlesnake *n* : a moderate-sized rattlesnake of the genus *Crotalus* (*C. horridus horridus*) that is widely distributed through the eastern half of the U.S.

time \'tīm\ *n* : the measured or measurable period during which an action, process, or condition exists or continues — see COAGULATION TIME, PROTHROMBIN TIME, REACTION TIME

timed–release *or* **time–release** *adj* : consisting of or containing a drug that is released in small amounts over time (as by dissolution of a coating) usu. in the gastrointestinal tract ⟨*timed-release* capsules⟩

ti·mo·lol \'tī-mə-₁lol\ *n* : a beta-blocker $C_{13}H_{24}N_4O_3S$ used in the form of its maleate salt to treat glaucoma and to reduce the risk of second heart attacks

tin \'tin\ *n* : a soft white crystalline metallic element malleable at ordinary temperatures — symbol *Sn*; see ELEMENT table

tinc·to·ri·al \tiŋk-'tōr-ē-əl\ *adj* : of or relating to dyeing or staining

tinc·tu·ra \tiŋk-'tur-ə, -'tyur-\ *n, pl* **-rae** \-rē\ : TINCTURE

tinc·ture \'tiŋk-chər\ *n* : a solution of a medicinal substance in an alcoholic menstruum — compare LIQUOR

tin·ea \'ti-nē-ə\ *n* : any of several fungal diseases of the skin; *esp* : RINGWORM

tinea ca·pi·tis \-'ka-pə-təs\ *n* : an infection of the scalp caused by fungi of the genera *Trichophyton* and *Microsporum* and characterized by scaly patches penetrated by a few dry brittle hairs

tinea cor·po·ris \-'kor-pə-rəs\ *n* : a fungal infection involving parts of the body not covered with hair

tinea cru·ris \-'krur-əs\ *n* : a fungal infection involving esp. the groin and perineum

tinea pe·dis \-'pe-dəs\ *n* : ATHLETE'S FOOT

tinea ver·si·col·or \-'vər-si-₁kə-lər\ *n* : a chronic noninflammatory infection of the skin esp. of the trunk that is caused by a lipophilic fungus (*Pityrosporum orbiculare* syn. *Melassezia furfur*) and is marked by the formation of irregular macular patches — called also *pityriasis versicolor*

Ti·nel's sign \ti-'nelz-\ *n* : a tingling sensation felt in the distal portion of a limb upon percussion of the skin over a regenerating nerve in the limb

Tinel, Jules (1879–1952), French neurologist.

tine test \'tin-\ n : a tuberculin test in which the tuberculin is introduced subcutaneously by means of four tines on a stainless steel disk

tin·ni·tus \'ti-nə-təs, ti-'nī-təs\ n : a sensation of noise (as a ringing or roaring) that is caused by a bodily condition (as a disturbance of the auditory nerve or wax in the ear) and can usu. be heard only by the one affected

tis·sue \'ti-(₊)shü\ n : an aggregate of cells usu. of a particular kind together with their intercellular substance that form one of the structural materials of a plant or an animal and that in animals include connective tissue, epithelium, muscle tissue, and nerve tissue

tissue culture n : the process or technique of making body tissue grow in a culture medium outside the organism; also : a culture of tissue (as epithelium)

tissue fluid n : a fluid that permeates the spaces between individual cells, that is in osmotic contact with the blood and lymph, and that serves in interstitial transport of nutrients and waste

tissue plasminogen activator n : a clot-dissolving enzyme with an affinity for fibrin that is produced naturally in blood vessel linings and is used in a genetically engineered form to prevent damage to heart muscle following a heart attack — abbr. TPA

tissue typing n : the determination of the degree of compatibility of tissues or organs from different individuals based on the similarity of histocompatibility antigens esp. on lymphocytes and used esp. as a measure of potential rejection in an organ transplant procedure

tis·su·lar \'ti-shyə-lər\ adj : of, relating to, or affecting organismic tissue

ti·ta·ni·um \tī-'tā-nē-əm, -'ta-\ n : a silvery gray metallic element — symbol Ti; see ELEMENT table

titanium dioxide n : an oxide TiO₂ of titanium that is used in sunscreens

ti·ter \'tī-tər\ n 1 : the strength of a solution or the concentration of a substance in solution as determined by titration 2 : the dilution of a serum containing a specific antibody at which the solution just retains a specific activity (as neutralizing or precipitating an antigen) which it loses at any greater dilution — **ti·tered** \-tərd\ adj

ti·tra·tion \tī-'trā-shən\ n : a method or the process of determining the concentration of a dissolved substance in terms of the smallest amount of a reagent of known concentration required to bring about a given effect in reaction with a known volume of the

test solution — **ti·trate** \'tī-₊trāt\ vb

ti·tre chiefly Brit var of TITER

tit·u·ba·tion \₊ti-chə-'bā-shən\ n : a staggering gait observed in some nervous disturbances

Tl symbol thallium

TLC abbr 1 tender loving care 2 thin-layer chromatography

T lym·pho·cyte \'tē-'lim-fə-₊sīt\ n : T CELL

Tm symbol thulium

TMJ abbr temporomandibular joint

TNF abbr tumor necrosis factor

toad·stool \'tōd-₊stül\ n : a fungus having an umbrella-shaped spore-bearing structure : MUSHROOM; esp : a poisonous or inedible one as distinguished from an edible mushroom

to·bac·co \tə-'ba-(₊)kō\ n, pl -cos 1 : any of a genus (*Nicotiana*) of plants of the nightshade family (Solanaceae); esp : an annual So. American herb (*N. tabacum*) cultivated for its leaves 2 : the leaves of cultivated tobacco prepared for use in smoking or chewing or as snuff 3 : manufactured products of tobacco; also : the use of tobacco as a practice

to·bra·my·cin \tō-brə-'mī-sᵊn\ n : a colorless water-soluble antibiotic C₁₈H₃₇N₅O₉ isolated from a soil bacterium of the genus *Streptomyces* (*S. tenebrarius*) and effective esp. against gram-negative bacteria

to·co·dy·na·mom·e·ter var of TOKODY-NAMOMETER

to·coph·er·ol \tō-'kä-fə-₊rȯl, -₊rōl\ n : any of several fat-soluble oily phenolic compounds with varying degrees of antioxidant vitamin E activity; esp : ALPHA-TOCOPHEROL

toe \'tō\ n : one of the terminal members of a foot

toed \'tōd\ adj : having a toe or toes esp. of a specified kind or number — usu. used in combination (five-*toed*)

toe·nail \'tō-₊nāl\ n : a nail of a toe

To·fra·nil \tō-'frä-nil\ trademark — used for a preparation of imipramine

to·ga·vi·rus \'tō-gə-₊vī-rəs\ n : any of a group of medium-sized viruses 50 to 70 nanometers in diameter that are sometimes included in the arboviruses, contain single-stranded RNA, and include the causative agents of encephalitis and rubella

toi·let \'tȯi-lət\ n : cleansing in preparation for or in association with a medical or surgical procedure (a pharyngeal ∼)

toilet training n : the process of training a child to control bladder and bowel movements and to use the toilet — **toilet train** \-₊trān\ vb

to·ko·dy·na·mom·e·ter \₊tō-kō-₊dī-nə-'mä-mə-tər\ n : an instrument by means of which the force of uterine puerperal contractions can be measured

to·laz·amide \tō-'la-zə-₊mīd\ n : a hypoglycemic sulfonamide C₁₄H₂₁N₃-

O_3S used in the treatment of diabetes mellitus — see TOLINASE

to·laz·o·line \tō-ˈla-zə-ˌlēn\ *n* : a weak alpha-adrenergic blocking agent $C_{10}H_{12}N_2$ used in the form of its hydrochloride to produce peripheral vasodilation

tol·bu·ta·mide \täl-ˈbyü-tə-ˌmīd\ *n* : a sulfonylurea $C_{12}H_{18}N_2O_3S$ that lowers blood sugar level and is used in the treatment of diabetes mellitus

Tol·ec·tin \ˈtä-lek-tin\ *trademark* — used for a preparation of tolmetin

tol·er·ance \ˈtä-lə-rəns\ *n* : the capacity of the body to endure or become less responsive to a substance (as a drug) or a physiological insult with repeated use or exposure ⟨immunological ∼ to a virus⟩ ⟨an addict's increasing ∼ for a drug⟩ — **tol·er·ant** \-rənt\ *adj* — **tol·er·ate** \-ˌrāt\ *vb*

tol·er·a·tion \ˌtä-lə-ˈrā-shən\ *n* : TOLERANCE

tol·er·o·gen \ˈtä-lə-rə-jən\ *n* : a tolerogenic antigen

tol·er·o·gen·ic \ˌtä-lə-rə-ˈje-nik\ *adj* : capable of producing immunological tolerance ⟨∼ antigens⟩

To·li·nase \ˈtō-lə-ˌnās, ˈtä-lə-ˌnāz\ *trademark* — used for a preparation of tolazamide

tol·met·in \ˈtäl-mə-tən\ *n* : an antiinflammatory drug $C_{15}H_{15}NO_3$ often administered in the form of its sodium salt — see TOLECTIN

tol·naf·tate \täl-ˈnaf-ˌtāt\ *n* : a topical antifungal drug $C_{19}H_{17}NOS$

to·lu \tə-ˈlü, tō-\ *n* : BALSAM OF TOLU

tolu balsam *n* : BALSAM OF TOLU

tol·u·ene·sul·fon·ic acid \ˌtäl-yə-ˌwēn-səl-ˈfä-nik-\ *n* : any of three isomeric crystalline oily liquid strong acids $CH_3C_6H_4SO_3H$

-tome \ˌtōm\ *n comb form* **1** : part : segment ⟨myo*tome*⟩ **2** : cutting instrument ⟨micro*tome*⟩

Tomes' fiber \ˈtōmz-\ *n* : any of the fibers extending from the odontoblasts into the alveolar canals : a dentinal fiber — called also *Tomes' process*
> **Tomes, Sir John (1815–1895),** British dental surgeon.

to·mo·gram \ˈtō-mə-ˌgram\ *n* : a roentgenogram made by tomography

to·mo·graph \-ˌgraf\ *n* : an X-ray machine used for tomography

to·mog·ra·phy \tō-ˈmä-grə-fē\ *n, pl* **-phies** : a method of producing a three-dimensional image of the internal structures of a solid object (as the human body) by the observation and recording of the differences in the effects on the passage of waves of energy impinging on those structures; see COMPUTED TOMOGRAPHY, POSITRON EMISSION TOMOGRAPHY — **to·mo·graph·ic** \ˌtō-mə-ˈgra-fik\ *adj*

-t·o·my \t-ə-mē\ *n comb form, pl* **-t·o·mies** : incision : section ⟨laparoto*my*⟩

¹tone \ˈtōn\ *n* **1** : a sound of definite

pitch and vibration **2 a** : the state of a living body or of any of its organs or parts in which the functions are healthy and performed with due vigor **b** : normal tension or responsiveness to stimuli; *specif* : TONUS 2

²tone *vb* **toned; ton·ing** : to impart tone to

tone–deaf \ˈtōn-ˌdef\ *adj* : relatively insensitive to differences in musical pitch — **tone deafness** *n*

tongue \ˈtəŋ\ *n* : a process of the floor of the mouth that is attached basally to the hyoid bone, that consists essentially of a mass of extrinsic muscle attaching its base to other parts, intrinsic muscle by which parts of the structure move in relation to each other, and an epithelial covering rich in sensory end organs and small glands, and that functions esp. in taking and swallowing food and as a speech organ

tongue depressor *n* : a thin wooden blade rounded at both ends that is used to depress the tongue to allow for inspection of the mouth and throat — called also *tongue blade*

tongue roll·er \-ˌrō-lər\ *n* : a person who carries a dominant gene which confers the capacity to roll the tongue into the shape of a U

tongue thrust \-ˌthrəst\ *n* : the thrusting of the tongue against or between the incisors during the act of swallowing which if persistent in early childhood can lead to various dental abnormalities

tongue–tie *n* : a congenital defect characterized by limited mobility of the tongue due to shortness of its frenulum — **tongue–tied** *adj*

tongue worm *n* : any of a phylum or arthropod class (Pentastomida) of parasitic invertebrates that live as adults in the respiratory passages of reptiles, birds, or mammals — see HALZOUN

-to·nia \ˈtō-nē-ə\ *n comb form* : condition or degree of tonus ⟨myo*tonia*⟩

¹ton·ic \ˈtä-nik\ *adj* **1 a** : characterized by tonus ⟨∼ contraction of muscle⟩; *also* : marked by or being prolonged muscular contraction ⟨∼ convulsions⟩ **b** : producing or adapted to produce healthy muscular condition and reaction of organs (as muscles) **2 a** : increasing or restoring physical or mental tone **b** : yielding a tonic substance — **ton·i·cal·ly** *adv*

²tonic *n* : an agent (as a drug) that increases body tone

to·nic·i·ty \tō-ˈni-sə-tē\ *n, pl* **-ties 1** : the property of possessing tone; *esp* : healthy vigor of body or mind **2** : TONUS 2

ton·i·co·clon·ic \ˌtä-ni-kō-ˈklä-nik\ *adj* : both tonic and clonic ⟨∼ seizures⟩

tono- *comb form* **1** : tone ⟨*tono*topic⟩ **2** : pressure ⟨*tono*meter⟩

tonoclonic • torpor

tono·clon·ic \ˌtä-nō-ˈklä-nik\ *adj* : TONICOCLONIC

tono·fi·bril \-ˈfī-brəl, -ˈfi-\ *n* : a thin fibril made up of tonofilaments

tono·fil·a·ment \-ˈfi-lə-mənt\ *n* : a slender cytoplasmic organelle found esp. in some epithelial cells

to·nog·ra·phy \tō-ˈnä-grə-fē\ *n, pl* **-phies** : the procedure of recording measurements (as of intraocular pressure) with a tonometer — **to·no·graph·ic** \ˌtō-nə-ˈgra-fik, ˌtä-\ *adj*

to·nom·e·ter \tō-ˈnä-mə-tər\ *n* : an instrument for measuring tension or pressure and esp. intraocular pressure — **to·no·met·ric** \ˌtō-nə-ˈme-trik, ˌtä-\ *adj* — **to·nom·e·try** \tō-ˈnä-mə-trē\ *n*

to·no·top·ic \ˌtō-nə-ˈtä-pik\ *adj* : relating to or being the anatomic organization by which specific sound frequencies are received by specific receptors in the inner ear with nerve impulses traveling along selected pathways to specific sites in the brain

ton·sil \ˈtän-səl\ *n* **1 a** : either of a pair of prominent masses of lymphoid tissue that lie one on each side of the throat between the anterior and posterior pillars of the fauces and are composed of lymph follicles grouped around one or more deep crypts — called also *palatine tonsil* **b** : PHARYNGEAL TONSIL **c** : LINGUAL TONSIL **2** : a rounded prominence situated medially on the lower surface of each lateral hemisphere of the cerebellum (the cerebellar ∼s) — **ton·sil·lar** \ˈtän-sə-lər\ *adj*

tonsill- *or* **tonsillo-** *comb form* : tonsil ⟨*tonsill*ectomy⟩

tonsillar crypt *n* : any of the deep invaginations occurring on the surface of the palatine and pharyngeal tonsils

ton·sil·lec·to·my \ˌtän-sə-ˈlek-tə-mē\ *n, pl* **-mies** : surgical excision of the tonsils

ton·sil·li·tis \ˌtän-sə-ˈlī-təs\ *n* : inflammation of the tonsils of varying degrees of severity and involving simple inflammation associated with acute pharyngitis, streptococcus infection, or formation of an abscess

ton·sil·lo·phar·yn·geal \ˌtän-sə-lō-ˌfar-ən-ˈjē-əl, -fə-ˈrin-jəl, -jē-əl\ *adj* : of, relating to, or involving the tonsils and pharynx (the ∼ area)

ton·sil·lo·phar·yn·gi·tis \-ˌfar-ən-ˈjī-təs\ *n, pl* **-git·i·des** \-ˈji-tə-ˌdēz\ : inflammation of the tonsils and pharynx

to·nus \ˈtō-nəs\ *n* **1** : TONE 2a **2** : a state of partial contraction that is characteristic of normal muscle, is maintained at least in part by a continuous bombardment of motor impulses originating reflexly, and serves to maintain body posture — called also *muscle tone*; compare CLONUS

-to·ny \ˌtō-nē, tən-ē\ *n comb form, pl* **-to·nies** : -TONIA ⟨hypo*tony*⟩

tooth \ˈtüth\ *n, pl* **teeth** \ˈtēth\ : any of

the hard bony appendages that are borne on the jaws and serve esp. for the prehension and mastication of food — see MILK TOOTH, PERMANENT TOOTH

tooth·ache \ˈtüth-ˌāk\ *n* : pain in or about a tooth — called also *odontalgia*

tooth·brush \-ˌbrəsh\ *n* : a brush for cleaning the teeth — **tooth·brush·ing** *n*

tooth bud *n* : a mass of tissue having the potentiality of differentiating into a tooth

tooth germ *n* : TOOTH BUD

tooth·less \ˈtüth-ləs\ *adj* : having no teeth

tooth·paste \ˈtüth-ˌpāst\ *n* : a paste for cleaning the teeth

tooth·pick \-ˌpik\ *n* : a pointed instrument (as a slender tapering piece of wood) used for removing food particles lodged between the teeth

top- *or* **topo-** *comb form* : local ⟨*topec*tomy⟩ ⟨*topo*gnosia⟩

to·pec·to·my \tə-ˈpek-tə-mē\ *n, pl* **-mies** : surgical excision of selected portions of the frontal cortex of the brain for the relief of mental disorders

to·pha·ceous \tə-ˈfā-shəs\ *adj* : relating to, being, or characterized by the occurrence of tophi (∼ gout)

to·phus \ˈtō-fəs\ *n, pl* **to·phi** \ˈtō-ˌfī, -ˌfē\ : a deposit of urates in tissues (as cartilage) characteristic of gout

top·i·cal \ˈtä-pi-kəl\ *adj* : designed for or involving local application to or action on a bodily part (a ∼ remedy) (a ∼ anesthetic) — **top·i·cal·ly** *adv*

top·og·no·sia \ˌtä-ˌpäg-ˈnō-zhə, ˌtō-, -zhē-ə\ *n* : recognition of the location of a stimulus on the skin or elsewhere in the body

topo·graph·i·cal \ˌtä-pə-ˈgra-fi-kəl\ *or* **topo·graph·ic** \-fik\ *adj* **1** : of, relating to, or concerned with topography **2** : of or relating to a mind made up of different strata and esp. of the conscious, preconscious, and unconscious — **topo·graph·i·cal·ly** *adv*

topographic anatomy *n* : REGIONAL ANATOMY

to·pog·ra·phy \tə-ˈpä-grə-fē\ *n, pl* **-phies** **1** : the physical or natural features of an object or entity and their structural relationships (the ∼ of the abdomen) **2** : REGIONAL ANATOMY

tori *pl of* TORUS

to·ric \ˈtōr-ik\ *adj* : of, relating to, or shaped like a torus or segment of a torus; *specif* : being a simple lens having for one of its surfaces a segment of an equilateral zone of a torus and consequently having different refracting power in different meridians

tor·pid \ˈtōr-pəd\ *adj* : sluggish in functioning or acting : characterized by torpor — **tor·pid·i·ty** \tōr-ˈpi-də-tē\ *n*

tor·por \ˈtōr-pər\ *n* : a state of mental and motor inactivity with partial or total insensibility : extreme sluggishness or stagnation of function

¹**torque** \'tȯrk\ *n* : a force that produces or tends to produce rotation or torsion; *also* : a measure of the effectiveness of such a force

²**torque** *vb* **torqued; torqu·ing** : to impart torque to : cause to twist (as a tooth about its long axis)

tor·sion \'tȯr-shən\ *n* **1** : the twisting of a bodily organ or part on its own axis 〈intestinal ∼〉 **2** : the twisting or wrenching of a body by the exertion of forces tending to turn one end or part about a longitudinal axis while the other is held fast or turned in the opposite direction; *also* : the state of being twisted — **tor·sion·al** \'tȯr-shə-nəl\ *adj*

torsion dystonia *n* : DYSTONIA MUSCULORUM DEFORMANS

tor·so \'tȯr-(ˌ)sō\ *n, pl* **torsos** *or* **tor·si** \'tȯr-ˌsē\ : the human trunk

tor·ti·col·lis \ˌtȯr-tə-'kä-ləs\ *n* : a twisting of the neck to one side that results in abnormal carriage of the head and is usu. caused by muscle spasms — called also **wryneck**

tor·tu·ous \'tȯr-chə-wəs\ *adj* : marked by repeated twists, bends, or turns 〈a ∼ blood vessel〉 — **tor·tu·os·i·ty** \ˌtȯr-chə-'wä-sə-tē\ *n*

tor·u·la \'tȯr-yə-lə, 'tär-\ *n* **1** *pl* **-lae** \-ˌlē, -ˌlī\ *also* **-las** : CRYPTOCOCCOSIS **2** *cap, in some classifications* : a genus of yeasts including pathogens (as *T. histolytica* syn. *Cryptococcus neoformans* that causes cryptococcosis) usu. placed in the genus *Cryptococcus*

Tor·u·lop·sis \ˌtȯr-yə-'läp-səs, ˌtär-\ *n* : a genus of round, oval, or cylindrical yeasts that form no spores and no pellicle when growing in a liquid culture medium and that include forms which in other classifications are placed in *Torula* or *Cryptococcus*

tor·u·lo·sis \ˌtȯr-yə-'lō-səs, ˌtär-\ *n* : CRYPTOCOCCOSIS

to·rus \'tȯr-əs\ *n, pl* **to·ri** \'tȯr-ˌī, -ˌē\ : a smooth rounded anatomical protuberance (as a bony ridge on the skull)

torus tu·ba·ri·us \-tü-'ber-ē-əs, -tyü-\ *n* : a protrusion on the lateral wall of the nasopharynx marking the pharyngeal end of the cartilaginous part of the eustachian tube

torus ure·ter·i·cus \-ˌyu̇r-ə-'ter-i-kəs\ *n* : a band of smooth muscle joining the orifices of the ureter and forming the base of the trigone of the bladder

tos·yl·ate \'tä-sə-ˌlāt\ *n* : an ester of or a salt of toluenesulfonic acid

to·ti·po·ten·cy \ˌtō-tə-'pōt-ᵊn-sē\ *n, pl* **-cies** : ability of a cell or bodily part to generate or regenerate the whole organism

to·ti·po·tent \tō-'ti-pə-tənt\ *adj* : capable of developing into a complete organism or differentiating into any of its cells or tissues 〈∼ blastomeres〉

touch \'təch\ *n* **1** : the special sense by which pressure or traction exerted on

the skin or mucous membrane is perceived **2** : a light attack 〈a ∼ of fever〉

Tou·rette's syndrome \tu̇-'rets-\ *also* **Tou·rette syndrome** \-'et-\ *n* : a rare disease characterized by involuntary tics and by uncontrollable verbalizations involving esp. echolalia and coprolalia — called also *Gilles de la Tourette syndrome, Tourette's disease, Tourette's disorder*

    Gilles de la Tourette \'zhēl-də-lä-'tür-et\, **Georges** (1857–1904), French physician.

tour·ni·quet \'tu̇r-ni-kət, 'tər-\ *n* : a device (as a bandage twisted tight with a stick) to check bleeding or blood flow

tower head *n* : OXYCEPHALY

tower skull *n* : OXYCEPHALY

tox- *or* **toxi-** *or* **toxo-** *comb form* **1** : toxic : poisonous 〈*toxin*〉 **2** : toxin : poison 〈*toxigenic*〉

tox·ae·mia *chiefly Brit var of* TOXEMIA

Tox·as·ca·ris \täk-'sas-kə-rəs\ *n* : a genus of ascarid roundworms that infest the small intestine of the dog and cat and related wild animals

tox·e·mia \täk-'sē-mē-ə\ *n* : an abnormal condition associated with the presence of toxic substances in the blood: as **a** : a generalized intoxication due to absorption and systemic dissemination of bacterial toxins from a focus of infection **b** : intoxication due to dissemination of toxic substances (as some by-products of protein metabolism) that cause functional or organic disturbances (as in the kidneys) — **tox·e·mic** \-mik\ *adj*

toxemia of pregnancy *n* : a disorder of unknown cause that is peculiar to pregnancy, is usu. of sudden onset, is marked by hypertension, albuminuria, edema, headache, and visual disturbances, and may or may not be accompanied by convulsions — compare ECLAMPSIA a, PREECLAMPSIA

toxi- — see TOX-

tox·ic \'täk-sik\ *adj* **1** : of, relating to, or caused by a poison or toxin **2 a** : affected by a poison or toxin **b** : affected with toxemia of pregnancy **3** : POISONOUS 〈∼ drugs〉 — **tox·ic·i·ty** \täk-'si-sə-tē\ *n*

²**toxic** *n* : a toxic substance

toxic- *or* **toxico-** *comb form* : poison 〈*toxicology*〉 〈*toxicosis*〉

toxic epidermal necrolysis *n* : a skin disorder characterized by widespread erythema and the formation of flaccid bullae and later by skin that is scalded in appearance and separates from the body in large sheets — called also *epidermal necrolysis, Lyell's syndrome, scalded-skin syndrome;* compare STAPHYLOCOCCAL SCALDED SKIN SYNDROME

Tox·i·co·den·dron \ˌtäk-si-kō-'den-ˌdrän\ *n* : a genus of shrubs and trees (family Anacardiaceae) that includes poison ivy and related plants when they are split off from the genus *Rhus*

tox·i·co·gen·ic \ˌtäk-si-kō-ˈje-nik\ *adj* : producing toxins or poisons

tox·i·co·log·i·cal \ˌtäk-si-kə-ˈlä-ji-kəl\ *or* **tox·i·co·log·ic** \-jik\ *adj* : of or relating to toxicology or toxins — **tox·i·co·log·i·cal·ly** *adv*

tox·i·col·o·gy \ˌtäk-si-ˈkä-lə-jē\ *n, pl* **-gies** : a science that deals with poisons and their effect and with the problems involved (as clinical, industrial, or legal) — **tox·i·col·o·gist** *n*

tox·i·co·sis \ˌtäk-sə-ˈkō-səs\ *n, pl* **-co·ses** \-ˌsēz\ : a pathological condition caused by the action of a poison or toxin

toxic shock *n* : TOXIC SHOCK SYNDROME

toxic shock syndrome *n* : an acute and sometimes fatal disease that is characterized by fever, nausea, diarrhea, diffuse erythema, and shock, that is associated esp. with the presence of a bacterium of the genus *Staphylococcus* (*S. aureus*), and that occurs esp. in menstruating females using tampons — called also *toxic shock*

toxi·gen·ic \ˌtäk-sə-ˈje-nik\ *adj* : producing toxin (∼ bacteria) — **toxi·ge·nic·i·ty** \ˌtäk-si-jə-ˈni-sə-tē\ *n*

tox·in \ˈtäk-sən\ *n* : a poisonous substance that is a specific product of the metabolic activities of a living organism and is usu. very unstable, notably toxic when introduced into the tissues, and typically capable of inducing antibody formation — see ANTITOXIN, ENDOTOXIN, EXOTOXIN

toxin–antitoxin *n* : a mixture of toxin and antitoxin used esp. formerly in immunizing against a disease (as diphtheria) for which they are specific

toxo- — see TOX-

Tox·o·ca·ra \ˌtäk-sə-ˈkar-ə\ *n* : a genus of nematode worms including the common ascarids (*T. canis* and *T. cati*) of the dog and cat

tox·o·ca·ri·a·sis \ˌtäk-sə-kə-ˈrī-ə-səs\ *n, pl* **-a·ses** \-ˌsēz\ : infection with or disease caused by nematode worms of the genus *Toxocara*

tox·oid \ˈtäk-ˌsȯid\ *n* : a toxin of a pathogenic organism treated so as to destroy its toxicity but leave it capable of inducing the formation of antibodies on injection (diphtheria ∼) — called also *anatoxin*

toxo·plas·ma \ˌtäk-sə-ˈplaz-mə\ *n* **1** *cap* : a genus of sporozoans that are typically serious pathogens of vertebrates **2** *pl* **-mas** *or* **-ma·ta** \-mə-tə\ *also* **-ma** : any sporozoan of the genus *Toxoplasma* — **toxo·plas·mic** \-mik\ *adj*

toxo·plas·mo·sis \-ˌplaz-ˈmō-səs\ *n, pl* **-mo·ses** \-ˌsēz\ : infection with or disease caused by a sporozoan of the genus *Toxoplasma* (*T. gondii*) that invades the tissues and may seriously damage the central nervous system esp. of infants

TPA *abbr* tissue plasminogen activator

TPI *abbr* Treponema pallidum immobilization (test)

TPN \ˌtē-(ˌ)pē-ˈen\ *n* : NADP

TPR *abbr* temperature, pulse, respiration

tra·bec·u·la \trə-ˈbe-kyə-lə\ *n, pl* **-lae** \-ˌlē\ *also* **-las 1** : a small bar, rod, bundle of fibers, or septal membrane in the framework of a bodily organ or part (as the spleen) **2** : any of the intersecting osseous bars occurring in cancellous bone — **tra·bec·u·lar** \-lər\ *adj* — **tra·bec·u·la·tion** \trə-ˌbe-kyə-ˈlā-shən\ *n*

tra·bec·u·lec·to·my \trə-ˌbe-kyə-ˈlek-tə-mē\ *n, pl* **-mies** : surgical excision of a small portion of the trabecular tissue lying between the anterior chamber of the eye and the canal of Schlemm in order to facilitate drainage of aqueous humor for the relief of glaucoma

trace \ˈtrās\ *n* **1** : the marking made by a recording instrument (as a kymograph) **2** : an amount of a chemical constituent not always quantitatively determinable because of minuteness **3** : ENGRAM — **trace** *vb* — **trace·able** \ˈtrā-sə-bəl\ *adj*

trace element *n* : a chemical element present in minute quantities; *esp* : one used by organisms and held essential to their physiology — compare MICRONUTRIENT

trac·er \ˈtrā-sər\ *n* : a substance used to trace the course of a process; *specif* : a labeled element or atom that can be traced throughout chemical or biological processes by its radioactivity or its unusual isotopic mass

trache- *or* **tracheo-** *comb form* **1** : trachea (*tracheoscopy*) **2** : tracheal and (*tracheobronchial*)

tra·chea \ˈtrā-kē-ə\ *n, pl* **tra·che·ae** \-kē-ˌē\ *also* **tra·che·as** : the main trunk of the system of tubes by which air passes to and from the lungs that is about four inches (10 centimeters) long and somewhat less than an inch (2.5 centimeters) in diameter, extends down the front of the neck from the larynx, divides in two to form the bronchi, has walls of fibrous and muscular tissue stiffened by incomplete cartilaginous rings which keep it from collapsing, and is lined with mucous membrane whose epithelium is composed of columnar ciliated mucus-secreting cells — called also *windpipe* — **tra·che·al** \-əl\ *adj*

tracheal node *n* : any of a group of lymph nodes arranged along each side of the thoracic part of the trachea

tracheal ring *n* : any of the 16 to 20 C-shaped bands of highly elastic cartilage which are found as incomplete rings in the anterior two thirds of the tracheal wall and of which there are usu. 6 to 8 in the right bronchus and 9 to 12 in the left

tra·che·itis \ˌtrā-kē-ˈī-təs\ *n* : inflammation of the trachea

trachel- *or* **trachelo-** *comb form* **1** : neck ⟨*trachel*omastoid muscle⟩ **2** : uterine cervix ⟨*trachelo*plasty⟩

trach·e·lec·to·my \ˌtra-kə-ˈlek-tə-mē\ *n, pl* **-mies** : CERVICECTOMY

trach·e·lo·mas·toid muscle \ˌtra-kə-lō-ˈmas-ˌtȯid-\ *n* : LONGISSIMUS CAPITIS

trach·e·lo·plas·ty \ˈtra-kə-lō-ˌplas-tē\ *n, pl* **-ties** : a plastic operation on the neck of the uterus

trach·e·lor·rha·phy \ˌtra-kə-ˈlȯr-ə-fē\ *n, pl* **-phies** : the operation of sewing up a laceration of the uterine cervix

tra·cheo·bron·chi·al \ˌtrā-kē-ō-ˈbräŋ-kē-əl\ *adj* : of, relating to, affecting, or produced in the trachea and bronchi ⟨∼ secretion⟩ ⟨∼ lesions⟩

tracheobronchial node *n* : any of the lymph nodes arranged in four or five groups along the trachea and bronchi — called also *tracheobronchial lymph node*

tracheobronchial tree *n* : the trachea and bronchial tree considered together

tra·cheo·bron·chi·tis \ˌtrā-kē-ō-bräŋ-ˈkī-təs\ *n, pl* **-chit·i·des** \-ˈki-tə-ˌdēz\ : inflammation of the trachea and bronchi

tra·cheo·esoph·a·ge·al \-i-ˌsä-fə-ˈjē-əl\ *adj* : relating to or connecting the trachea and the esophagus ⟨a ∼ fistula⟩

tra·cheo·plas·ty \ˈtrā-kē-ə-ˌplas-tē\ *n, pl* **-ties** : a plastic operation on the trachea

tra·che·os·co·py \ˌtrā-kē-ˈäs-kə-pē\ *n, pl* **-pies** : inspection of the interior of the trachea (as by a bronchoscope)

tra·che·os·to·my \ˌtrā-kē-ˈäs-tə-mē\ *n, pl* **-mies** : the surgical formation of an opening into the trachea through the neck esp. to allow the passage of air; *also* : the opening itself

tra·che·ot·o·my \ˌtrā-kē-ˈä-tə-mē\ *n, pl* **-mies 1** : the surgical operation of cutting into the trachea esp. through the skin **2** : the opening created by a tracheotomy

tra·cho·ma \trə-ˈkō-mə\ *n* : a chronic contagious conjunctivitis marked by inflammatory granulations on the conjunctival surfaces, caused by a bacterium of the genus *Chlamydia* (*C. trachomatis*), and commonly resulting in blindness if left untreated — **tra·cho·ma·tous** \trə-ˈkō-mə-təs, -ˈkä-\ *adj*

trac·ing \ˈtrā-siŋ\ *n* : a graphic record made by an instrument (as an electrocardiograph) that registers some movement

tract \ˈtrakt\ *n* **1** : a system of body parts or organs that act together to perform some function ⟨the digestive ∼⟩ — see GASTROINTESTINAL TRACT, LOWER RESPIRATORY TRACT, UPPER RESPIRATORY TRACT **2** : a bundle of nerve fibers having a common origin, termination, and function and esp. one within the spinal cord or brain — called also *fiber tract*; compare FASCICULUS b; see CORTICOSPINAL TRACT, OLFACTORY TRACT, OPTIC TRACT, SPINOTHALAMIC TRACT

trac·tion \ˈtrak-shən\ *n* **1** : the pulling of or tension established in one body part by another **2** : a pulling force exerted on a skeletal structure (as in a fracture) by means of a special device or apparatus ⟨a ∼ splint⟩; *also* : a state of tension created by such a pulling force ⟨a leg in ∼⟩

tract of Burdach *n* : FASCICULUS CUNEATUS

K. F. Burdach — see COLUMN OF BURDACH

tract of Lissauer *n* : DORSOLATERAL TRACT

Lissauer, Heinrich (1861–1891), German neurologist.

trac·tot·o·my \trak-ˈtä-tə-mē\ *n, pl* **-mies** : surgical division of a nerve tract

trac·tus \ˈtrak-təs\ *n, pl* **tractus** : TRACT 2

tractus sol·i·tar·i·us \-sä-li-ˈtar-ē-əs\ *n* : a descending tract of nerve fibers that is situated near the dorsal surface of the medulla oblongata, mediates esp. the sense of taste, and includes fibers from the facial, glossopharyngeal, and vagus nerves

trade·mark \ˈtrād-ˌmärk\ *n* : a device (as a word or mark) that points distinctly to the origin or ownership of merchandise to which it is applied and that is legally reserved for the exclusive use of the owner — compare SERVICE MARK

trag·a·canth \ˈtra-jə-ˌkanth, -gə-, -kənth; ˈtra-gə-ˌsanth\ *n* : a gum obtained from various Asian or East European plants (genus *Astragalus* and esp. *A. gummifer*) of the legume family (Leguminosae) and is used as an emulsifying, suspending, and thickening agent and as a demulcent — called also *gum tragacanth*

tra·gus \ˈtrā-gəs\ *n, pl* **tra·gi** \-ˌgī, -ˌjī\ : a small projection in front of the external opening of the ear

train·able \ˈtrā-nə-bəl\ *adj* : affected with moderate mental retardation and capable of being trained in self-care and in simple social and work skills in a sheltered environment — compare EDUCABLE

trained nurse *n* : GRADUATE NURSE

trait \ˈtrāt\ *n* : an inherited characteristic

Tral \ˈtral\ *trademark* — used for a preparation of hexocyclium methylsulfate

trance \ˈtrans\ *n* **1** : a state of partly suspended animation or inability to function **2** : a somnolent state (as of deep hypnosis) characterized by limited sensory and motor contact with one's surroundings and subsequent lack of recall — **trance·like** \-ˈlīk\ *adj*

tran·ex·am·ic acid \ˌtra-nekˈsa-mik-\ *n* : an antifibrinolytic drug $C_8H_{15}NO_2$

tran·quil·ize *also* **tran·quil·lize** \ˈtraŋ-kwə-ˌlīz, ˈtran-\ *vb* **-ized** *also* **-lized; -iz·ing** *also* **-liz·ing** : to make tranquil or calm; *esp* : to relieve of mental tension and anxiety by means of drugs — **tran·quil·i·za·tion** \ˌtraŋ-kwə-lə-ˈzā-shən, ˌtran-\ *n*

tran·quil·iz·er *also* **tran·quil·liz·er** \-ˌlī-zər\ *n* : a drug used to reduce mental disturbance (as anxiety and tension)

trans·ab·dom·i·nal \ˌtrans-ab-ˈdä-mə-nəl, ˌtranz-\ *adj* : passing through or performed by passing through the abdomen or the abdominal wall ⟨~ amniocentesis⟩

trans·ac·tion·al analysis \-ˌak-shə-nəl-\ *n* : a system of psychotherapy involving analysis of individual episodes of social interaction for insight that will aid communication — abbr. *TA*

trans·am·i·nase \-ˈa-mə-ˌnās, -ˌnāz\ *n* : an enzyme promoting transamination

trans·am·i·na·tion \-ˌa-mə-ˈnā-shən\ *n* : a reversible oxidation-reduction reaction in which an amino group is transferred typically from an alpha-amino acid to an alpha-keto acid

trans·cap·il·lary \-ˈka-pə-ˌler-ē\ *adj* : existing or taking place across the capillary walls

trans·cath·e·ter \-ˈka-thə-tər\ *adj* : performed through the lumen of a catheter ⟨~ embolization⟩

trans·con·dy·lar \-ˈkän-də-lər\ *adj* : passing through a pair of condyles ⟨a ~ fracture of the humerus⟩

trans·cor·ti·cal \-ˈkȯr-ti-kəl\ *adj* : crossing the cortex of the brain; *esp* : passing from the cortex of one hemisphere to that of the other

trans·cor·tin \-ˈkȯrt-ən\ *n* : an alpha globulin produced in the liver that binds with and transports hydrocortisone in the blood

tran·scribe \trans-ˈkrīb\ *vb* **transcribed; tran·scrib·ing** : to cause (as DNA) to undergo genetic transcription

tran·script \ˈtrans-ˌkript\ *n* : a sequence of RNA produced by transcription from a DNA template

tran·scrip·tase \tran-ˈskrip-ˌtās, -ˌtāz\ *n* : RNA POLYMERASE; *also* : REVERSE TRANSCRIPTASE

tran·scrip·tion \trans-ˈkrip-shən\ *n* : the process of constructing a messenger RNA molecule using a DNA molecule as a template with resulting transfer of genetic information to the messenger RNA — compare REVERSE TRANSCRIPTION, TRANSLATION — **tran·scrip·tion·al** \-shə-nəl\ *adj* — **tran·scrip·tion·al·ly** *adv*

tran·scrip·tion·ist \-shə-nist\ *n* : one that transcribes; *esp* : MEDICAL TRANSCRIPTIONIST

trans·cu·ta·ne·ous \ˌtrans-kyü-ˈtā-nē-əs\ *adj* : passing, entering, or made by penetration through the skin

trans·der·mal \trans-ˈdər-məl, ˌtranz-\ *adj* : relating to, being, or supplying a medication in a form for absorption through the skin into the bloodstream ⟨~ drug delivery⟩ ⟨~ nitroglycerin⟩ ⟨~ nicotine patch⟩

trans·dia·phrag·mat·ic \-ˌdī-ə-frəg-ˈma-tik, -ˌfrag-\ *adj* : occurring, passing, or performed through the diaphragm ⟨~ hernia⟩

trans·duce \-ˈdüs, -ˈdyüs\ *vb* **transduced; trans·duc·ing** 1 : to convert (as energy) into another form 2 : to bring about the transfer of (as a gene) from one microorganism to another by means of a viral agent

trans·duc·tion \-ˈdek-shən\ *n* : the action or process of transducing; *esp* : the transfer of genetic material from one microorganism to another by a viral agent (as a bacteriophage) — compare TRANSFORMATION 2 — **trans·duc·tion·al** \-shə-nəl\ *adj*

trans·du·o·de·nal \-ˌdü-ə-ˈdē-nəl, -ˌdyü-; -ˌdü-ˈäd-ən-əl, -dyü-\ *adj* : performed by cutting across or through the duodenum

tran·sect \tran-ˈsekt\ *vb* : to cut transversely — **tran·sec·tion** \-ˈsek-shən\ *n*

trans·epi·the·li·al \ˌtrans-ˌe-pə-ˈthē-lē-əl, ˌtranz-\ *adj* : existing or taking place across an epithelium ⟨~ sodium transport⟩

tran·sep·tal \tran-ˈsep-təl\ *adj* 1 : passing across a septum 2 : passing or performed through a septum ⟨~ cardiac catheterization⟩

trans·esoph·a·ge·al \-i-ˌsä-fə-ˈjē-əl\ *adj* : passing through or performed by way of the esophagus ⟨~ echocardiography⟩

trans·fec·tion \trans-ˈfek-shən\ *n* : infection of a cell with isolated viral nucleic acid followed by production of the complete virus in the cell; *also* : the incorporation of exogenous DNA into a cell — **trans·fect** \-ˈfekt\ *vb*

trans·fer \ˈtrans-fər\ *n* 1 : TRANSFERENCE 2 : the carryover or generalization of learned responses from one type of situation to another — see NEGATIVE TRANSFER

trans·fer·ase \ˈtrans-(ˌ)fər-ˌās, -ˌāz\ *n* : an enzyme that promotes transfer of a group from one molecule to another

trans·fer·ence \trans-ˈfər-əns, ˈtrans-(ˌ)\ *n* : the redirection of feelings and desires and esp. of those unconsciously retained from childhood toward a new object (as a psychoanalyst conducting therapy)

transference neurosis *n* : a neurosis developed in the course of psychoanalytic treatment and manifested by the reliving of infantile experiences in the presence of the analyst

transfer factor *n* : a substance that is

produced and secreted by a lymphocyte functioning in cell-mediated immunity and that upon incorporation into a lymphocyte which has not been sensitized confers on it the same immunological specificity as the sensitized cell

trans·fer·rin \trans-**'**fer-ən\ *n* : a beta globulin in blood plasma capable of combining with ferric ions and transporting iron in the body

transfer RNA *n* : a relatively small RNA that transfers a particular amino acid to a growing polypeptide chain at the ribosomal site of protein synthesis during translation — called also *soluble RNA, tRNA;* compare MESSENGER RNA

trans·fix·ion \trans-**'**fik-shən\ *n* : a piercing of a part of the body (as by a suture or pin) in order to fix it in position — **trans·fix** \-**'**fiks\ *vb*

trans·form \trans-**'**form\ *vb* **1** : to change or become changed in structure, appearance, or character **2** : to cause (a cell) to undergo genetic transformation

trans·for·ma·tion \͵trans-fər-**'**mā-shən, -fȯr-\ *n* **1** : an act, process, or instance of transforming or being transformed ⟨~ of a normal into a malignant cell⟩ **2 a** : genetic modification of a bacterium by incorporation of free DNA from another ruptured bacterial cell — compare TRANSDUCTION **b** : genetic modification of a cell by the uptake and incorporation of exogenous DNA

transforming growth factor *n* : any of a group of polypeptides that are secreted by a variety of cells (as monocytes, T cells, or blood platelets) and have diverse effects (as inducing angiogenesis, stimulating fibroblast proliferation, or inhibiting T cell proliferation) on the division and activity of cells — abbr. *TGF*

trans·fuse \trans-**'**fyüz\ *vb* **trans·fused; trans·fus·ing 1** : to transfer (as blood) into a vein or artery of a human being or an animal **2** : to subject (a patient) to transfusion — **trans·fus·ible** *or* **trans·fus·able** \trans-**'**fyü-zə-bəl\ *adj*

trans·fu·sion \trans-**'**fyü-zhən\ *n* **1** : the process of transfusing fluid into a vein or artery **2** : something transfused — **trans·fu·sion·al** \-zhə-nəl\ *adj*

trans·fu·sion·ist \-zhə-nist\ *n* : one skilled in performing transfusions

trans·gen·ic \͵trans-**'**je-nik, ͵tranz-\ *adj* : having chromosomes into which one or more heterologous genes have been incorporated either artificially or naturally ⟨~ mice⟩

trans·glu·ta·min·ase \-**'**glü-tə-mə-͵nās, -glü-**'**ta-mə-͵nāz\ *n* : a clotting factor that is a variant of factor XIII and that promotes the formation of links between strands of fibrin

trans·he·pat·ic \-hi-**'**pa-tik\ *adj* : involving direct injection (as of a radi-

opaque medium) into the biliary ducts

tran·sient **'**tran-zē-ənt, -shənt, -chənt\ *adj* : passing away in time : existing temporarily ⟨~ symptoms⟩

transient ischemic attack *n* : a brief episode of cerebral ischemia that is usu. characterized by blurring of vision, slurring of speech, numbness, paralysis, or syncope and that is sometimes a forerunner of more serious cerebral accidents — abbr. *TIA*

trans·il·lu·mi·nate \͵trans-ə-**'**lü-mə-͵nāt, ͵tranz-\ *vb* **-nat·ed; -nat·ing** : to pass light through (a body part) for medical examination ⟨~ the sinuses⟩ — **trans·il·lu·mi·na·tion** \-ə-͵lü-mə-**'**nā-shən\ *n*

tran·si·tion·al \tran-**'**si-shə-nəl, -**'**zi-\ *adj* : of, relating to, or being an epithelium (as in the urinary bladder) that consists of several layers of soft cuboidal cells which become flattened when stretched

trans·la·tion \trans-**'**lā-shən, tranz-\ *n* : the process of forming a protein molecule at a ribosomal site of protein synthesis from information contained in messenger RNA — compare TRANSCRIPTION — **trans·late** \-**'**lāt\ *vb* — **trans·la·tion·al** \-**'**lā-shə-nəl\ *adj*

trans·lo·ca·tion \͵trans-lō-**'**kā-shən, ͵tranz-\ *n* **1** : transfer of part of a chromosome to a different position esp. on a nonhomologous chromosome; *esp* : the exchange of parts between nonhomologous chromosomes **2** : a chromosome or part of a chromosome that has undergone translocation — **trans·lo·cate** \-**'**lō-͵kāt\ *vb*

trans·lum·bar \͵trans-**'**ləm-bər, ͵tranz-, -͵bär\ *adj* : passing through or performed by way of the lumbar region; *specif* : involving the injection of a radiopaque medium through the lumbar region

trans·lu·mi·nal \-**'**lü-mə-nəl\ *adj* : passing across or performed by way of a lumen; *specif* : involving the passage of an inflatable catheter along the lumen of a blood vessel ⟨~ angioplasty⟩

trans·mem·brane \-**'**mem-͵brān\ *adj* : taking place, existing, or arranged from one side to the other of a membrane

trans·mis·si·ble \trans-**'**mi-sə-bəl, tranz-\ *adj* : capable of being transmitted ⟨~ diseases⟩ — **trans·mis·si·bil·i·ty** \-͵mi-sə-**'**bi-lə-tē\ *n*

trans·mis·sion \trans-**'**mi-shən, tranz-\ *n* : an act, process, or instance of transmitting ⟨~ of rabies⟩ ⟨~ of a nerve impulse across a synapse⟩

transmission deafness *n* : CONDUCTION DEAFNESS

transmission electron microscope *n* : a conventional electron microscope which produces an image of a cross-sectional slice of a specimen all points of which are illuminated by the electron beam at the same time —

compare SCANNING ELECTRON MICROSCOPE — **transmission electron microscopy** n

trans·mit \trans-ˈmit. tranz-\ vb **transmit·ted; trans·mit·ting** : to pass, transfer, or convey from one person or place to another: as **a** : to pass or convey by heredity (∼ a genetic abnormality) **b** : to convey (infection) abroad or to another ⟨mosquitoes ∼ malaria⟩ **c** : to cause (energy) to be conveyed through space or a medium (substances that ∼ nerve impulses)

trans·mit·ta·ble \-ˈmi-tə-bəl\ adj : TRANSMISSIBLE

trans·mit·ter \-ˈmi-tər\ n : one that transmits; specif : NEUROTRANSMITTER

trans·mu·ral \ˌtrans-ˈmyür-əl, ˌtranz-\ adj : passing or administered through an anatomical wall (∼ stimulation of the ileum); also : involving the whole thickness of a wall (∼ myocardial infarction) — **trans·mu·ral·ly** adv

trans·neu·ro·nal \-nü-ˈrōn-ᵊl, -nyü-; -ˈnür-ən-ᵊl, -ˈnyür-\ adj : TRANSSYNAPTIC (∼ cell atrophy)

trans·or·bit·al \-ˈor-bət-ᵊl\ adj : passing through or performed by way of the eye socket

trans·ovar·i·al \-ō-ˈvar-ē-əl\ adj : relating to or being transmission of a pathogen from an organism (as a tick) to its offspring by infection of eggs in its ovary — **trans·ovar·i·al·ly** adv

trans·ovar·i·an \-ē-ən\ adj : TRANSOVARIAL

trans·par·ent \trans-ˈpar-ənt\ adj **1** : having the property of transmitting light so that bodies lying beyond are entirely visible **2** : pervious to a specified form of radiation (as X rays)

trans·pep·ti·dase \trans-ˈpep-tə-ˌdās, tranz-, -ˌdāz\ n : an enzyme that catalyzes the transfer of an amino acid residue or a peptide residue from one amino compound to another

trans·peri·to·ne·al \-ˌper-ə-tə-ˈnē-əl\ adj : passing or performed through the peritoneum

trans·pla·cen·tal \ˌtrans-plə-ˈsent-ᵊl\ adj : relating to, involving, or being passage (as of an antibody) between mother and fetus through the placenta — **trans·pla·cen·tal·ly** adv

¹**trans·plant** \trans-ˈplant\ vb : to transfer from one place to another; esp : to transfer (an organ or tissue) from one part or individual to another — **trans·plant·abil·i·ty** \-ˌplan-tə-ˈbi-lə-tē\ n — **trans·plant·able** \-ˈplan-tə-bəl\ adj — **trans·plan·ta·tion** \ˌtrans-ˌplan-ˈtā-shən\ n

²**trans·plant** \ˈtrans-ˌplant\ n **1** : something (as an organ or part) that is transplanted **2** : the act or process of transplanting ⟨a liver ∼⟩

trans·pleu·ral \-ˈplür-əl\ adj : passing through or requiring passage through the pleura ⟨a ∼ surgical procedure⟩

¹**trans·port** \trans-ˈpōrt, ˈtrans-ˌ\ vb : to

transfer or convey from one place to another

²**trans·port** \ˈtrans-ˌpōrt\ n : an act or process of transporting; specif : ACTIVE TRANSPORT

transposable element n : a segment of genetic material that is capable of changing its location in the genome or in some bacteria of undergoing transfer between an extrachromosomal plasmid and a chromosome — called also *transposable genetic element*

trans·pose \trans-ˈpōz\ vb **trans·posed; trans·pos·ing** : to transfer from one place or period to another; specif : to subject to or undergo genetic transposition — **trans·pos·able** \-ˈpō-zə-bəl\ adj

trans·po·si·tion \ˌtrans-pə-ˈzi-shən\ n : an act, process, or instance of transposing or being transposed: as **a** : the displacement of a viscus to a side opposite from that which it normally occupies (∼ of the heart) **b** : the transfer of a segment of DNA from one site to another in the genome either between chromosomal sites or between an extrachromosomal site (as on a plasmid) and a chromosome — **trans·po·si·tion·al** \-ˈzi-shə-nəl\ adj

trans·po·son \trans-ˈpō-ˌzän\ n : a transposable element esp. when it contains genetic material controlling functions other than those related to its relocation

trans·py·lor·ic \-pī-ˈlor-ik\ adj : relating to or being the transverse plane or the line marking its intersection with the surface of the abdomen that passes below the rib cage cutting the pylorus of the stomach and the first lumbar vertebra and that is one of the four planes marking off the nine abdominal regions

trans·rec·tal \-ˈrekt-ᵊl\ adj : passing through or performed by way of the rectum (∼ prostatic biopsy)

trans·sep·tal \-ˈsept-ᵊl\ adj : passing through a septum

trans·sex·u·al \-ˈsek-shə-wəl\ n : a person with a psychological urge to belong to the opposite sex that may be carried to the point of undergoing surgery to modify the sex organs to mimic the opposite sex — **transsexual** adj — **trans·sex·u·al·ism** \-wə-ˌli-zəm\ n — **trans·sex·u·al·i·ty** \-ˌsek-shə-ˈwa-lə-tē\ n

trans·sphe·noi·dal \-sfi-ˈnoid-ᵊl\ adj : performed by entry through the sphenoid bone (∼ hypophysectomy)

trans·syn·ap·tic \-sə-ˈnap-tik\ adj : occurring or taking place across nerve synapses (∼ degeneration)

trans·tho·rac·ic \-thə-ˈra-sik\ adj **1** : performed or made by way of the thoracic cavity **2** : crossing or having connections that cross the thoracic cavity ⟨a ∼ pacemaker⟩ — **trans·tho·rac·i·cal·ly** adv

trans·thy·re·tin \-ˈthī-rə-tin\ n : a protein component of blood serum that functions esp. in the transport of thyroxine — called also *prealbumin*

trans·tra·che·al \-'trā-kē-əl\ *adj* : passing through or administered by way of the trachea ⟨∼ anesthesia⟩

tran·su·date \tran-'sü-dət, -'syü-, -'zü-, -'zyü-, -ˌdāt\ *n* : a transuded substance

tran·su·da·tion \ˌtran-sü-'dā-shən, -syü-, -zü-, -zyü-\ *n* **1** : the act or process of transuding or being transuded **2** : TRANSUDATE

tran·sude \tran-'süd, -'syüd, -'züd, -'zyüd\ *vb* **tran·sud·ed; tran·sud·ing** : to pass or permit passage of through a membrane or permeable substance

trans·ure·tero·ure·ter·os·to·my \ˌtrans-yü-ˌrē-tə-ˌrō-yü-ˌrē-tə-'räs-tə-mē\ *n, pl* **-mies** : anastomosis of a ureter to the contralateral ureter

trans·ure·thral \-yü-'rē-thrəl\ *adj* : passing through or performed by way of the urethra ⟨∼ prostatectomy⟩

trans·vag·i·nal \-'va-jən-əl\ *adj* : passing through or performed by way of the vagina ⟨∼ laparoscopy⟩

trans·ve·nous \-'vē-nəs\ *adj* : relating to or involving the use of an intravenous catheter containing an electrode carrying electrical impulses from an extracorporeal source to the heart

trans·ven·tric·u·lar \-ven-'tri-kyə-lər, -vən-\ *adj* : passing through or performed by way of a ventricle

transversa, transversum — see SEPTUM TRANSVERSUM

trans·ver·sa·lis cer·vi·cis \ˌtrans-vər-'sä-ləs-'sər-vi-səs\ *n* : LONGISSIMUS CERVICIS

transversalis fascia *n* : the whole deep layer of fascia lining the abdominal wall; *also* : the part of this covering the inner surface of the transversus abdominis and separating it from the peritoneum

trans·verse \trans-'vərs, tranz-, 'trans-ˌ, 'tranz-ˌ\ *adj* **1** : acting, lying, or being across : set crosswise **2** : made at right angles to the anterior-posterior axis of the body ⟨a ∼ section⟩ — **trans·verse·ly** *adv*

transverse carpal ligament *n* : FLEXOR RETINACULUM 2

transverse cervical artery *n* : an inconstant branch of the thyrocervical trunk or of the subclavian artery that supplies the region at the base of the neck and the muscles of the scapula

transverse colon *n* : the part of the large intestine that extends across the abdominal cavity joining the ascending colon to the descending colon

transverse crural ligament *n* : EXTENSOR RETINACULUM 1b

transverse facial artery *n* : a large branch of the superficial temporal artery that arises in the parotid gland and supplies the parotid gland, masseter muscle, and adjacent parts

transverse fissure *n* : PORTA HEPATIS

transverse foramen *n* : a foramen in each transverse process of a cervical vertebra through which the vertebral artery and vertebral vein pass in each cervical vertebra except the seventh

transverse ligament *n* : any of various ligaments situated transversely with respect to a bodily axis or part: as **a** : the transverse part of the cruciate ligament of the atlas **b** : one in the anterior part of the knee connecting the anterior margins of the lateral and medial menisci

transverse process *n* : a process that projects on the dorsolateral aspect of each side of the neural arch of a vertebra

transverse sinus *n* : either of two large venous sinuses of the cranium that begin at the bony protuberance on the middle of the inner surface of the occipital bone at the intersection of its bony ridges and that terminate at the jugular foramen on either side to become the internal jugular vein

transverse thoracic muscle *n* : TRANSVERSUS THORACIS

transverse tubule *n* : T TUBULE

trans·ver·sion \trans-'vər-zhən, tranz-\ *n* : the eruption of a tooth in an abnormal position on the jaw

trans·ver·sus ab·dom·i·nis \ˌtrans-'vər-səs-ab-'dä-mə-nəs\ *n* : a flat muscle with transverse fibers that forms the innermost layer of the anterolateral wall of the abdomen and that acts to constrict the abdominal viscera and assist in expulsion of the contents of various abdominal organs (as in urination, defecation, vomiting, and parturition)

transversus pe·rin·ei su·per·fi·ci·a·lis \-pe-'ri-nē-ˌī-ˌsü-pər-ˌfi-shē-'ā-ləs\ *n* : a small band of muscle of the urogenital region of the perineum that arises from the ischial tuberosity and that with the contralateral muscle inserts into and acts to stabilize the mass of tissue in the midline between the anus and the penis or vagina — called also *superficial transverse perineal muscle*

transversus tho·ra·cis \-thə-'rā-səs\ *n* : a thin flat sheet of muscle and tendon fibers of the anterior wall of the chest that arises esp. from the xiphoid process and lower third of the sternum, inserts into the costal cartilages of the second to sixth ribs, and acts to draw the ribs downward — called also *transverse thoracic muscle*

trans·ves·i·cal \trans-'ve-si-kəl, tranz-\ *adj* : passing through or performed by way of the urinary bladder

trans·ves·tism \trans-'ves-ˌti-zəm, tranz-\ *n* : adoption of the dress and often the behavior of the opposite sex — called also *eonism*

trans·ves·tite \trans-'ves-ˌtīt, tranz-\ *n* : a person and esp. a male who adopts the dress and often the behavior typical of the opposite sex esp. for purposes of emotional or sexual gratification — **transvestite** *adj*

tran·yl·cy·pro·mine \ˌtran-əl-ˈsī-prə-ˌmēn\ *n* : an antidepressant drug $C_9H_{11}N$ that is an inhibitor of monoamine oxidase and is administered in the form of its sulfate

tra·pe·zi·um \trə-ˈpē-zē-əm, tra-\ *n, pl* **-zi·ums** *or* **-zia** \-zē-ə\ : a bone in the distal row of the carpus at the base of the thumb — called also *greater multangular*

tra·pe·zi·us \trə-ˈpē-zē-əs, tra-\ *n* : a large flat triangular superficial muscle of each side of the upper back that arises from the occipital bone, the ligamentum nuchae, and the spinous processes of the last cervical and all the thoracic vertebrae, is inserted into the outer part of the clavicle, the acromion, and the spine of the scapula, and serves chiefly to rotate the scapula so as to present the glenoid cavity upward

trap·e·zoid \ˈtra-pə-ˌzóid\ *n* : a bone in the distal row of the carpus at the base of the forefinger — called also *lesser multangular, trapezoid bone, trapezoideum*

trapezoid body *n* : a bundle of transverse fibers in the dorsal part of the pons

trap·e·zoi·de·um \ˌtra-pə-ˈzói-dē-əm\ *n* : TRAPEZOID

Tras·en·tine \ˈtra-sən-ˌtīn\ *trademark* — used for a preparation of adiphenine

Tras·y·lol \ˈtra-sə-ˌlól\ *trademark* — used for a preparation of aprotinin

trau·ma \ˈtrau-mə, ˈtró-\ *n, pl* **traumas** *also* **trau·ma·ta** \-mə-tə\ **1 a** : an injury (as a wound) to living tissue caused by an extrinsic agent ⟨surgical ~⟩ **b** : a disordered psychic or behavioral state resulting from mental or emotional stress or physical injury **2** : an agent, force, or mechanism that causes trauma — **trau·mat·ic** \trə-ˈma-tik, tró-, trau-\ *adj* — **trau·mat·i·cal·ly** *adv*

traumat- *or* **traumato-** *comb form* : wound : trauma ⟨*trauma*tism⟩

trau·ma·tism \ˈtrau-mə-ˌti-zəm, ˈtró-\ *n* : the development or occurrence of trauma; *also* : TRAUMA

trau·ma·tize \-ˌtīz\ *vb* **-tized; -tiz·ing** : to inflict a trauma upon — **trau·ma·ti·za·tion** \ˌtrau-mə-tə-ˈzā-shən, ˌtró-\ *n*

trau·ma·tol·o·gy \ˌtrau-mə-ˈtä-lə-jē, ˌtró-\ *n, pl* **-gies** : the surgical treatment of wounds ⟨pediatric ~⟩ — **trau·ma·tol·o·gist** \-ˈtä-lə-jist\ *n*

tra·vail \trə-ˈvāl, ˈtra-ˌvāl\ *n* : LABOR, PARTURITION

traveler's diarrhea *n* : TURISTA

travel sickness *n* : MOTION SICKNESS

tray \ˈtrā\ *n* : an appliance consisting of a rimmed body and a handle for use in holding plastic material against the gums or teeth in making negative impressions for dentures

traz·o·done \ˈtra-zə-ˌdōn\ *n* : an antidepressant drug $C_{19}H_{22}ClN_5O$ that is administered in the form of its hydrochloride and inhibits the uptake of serotonin by the brain

Trea·cher Col·lins syndrome \ˈtrē-chər-ˈkä-lənz-\ *n* : MANDIBULOFACIAL DYSOSTOSIS

Collins, Edward Treacher (1862–1932), British ophthalmologist.

tread·mill \ˈtred-ˌmil\ *n* : a device having an endless belt on which an individual walks or runs in place that is used for exercise and in tests of physiological functions — see STRESS TEST

treat \ˈtrēt\ *vb* : to care for or deal with medically or surgically : deal with by medical or surgical means ⟨~*ed* their diseases⟩ ⟨~*s* a patient⟩ — **treat·abil·i·ty** \ˌtrē-tə-ˈbi-lə-tē\ *n* — **treat·able** \ˈtrē-tə-bəl\ *adj* — **treat·ment** \ˈtrēt-mənt\ *n*

tree \ˈtrē\ *n* : an anatomical system or structure having many branches — see BILIARY TREE, BRONCHIAL TREE, TRACHEOBRONCHIAL TREE

-tre·ma \ˈtrē-mə\ *n comb form, pl* **-tremas** *or* **-tre·ma·ta** \ˈtrē-mə-tə\ : hole : orifice : opening ⟨helico*trema*⟩

trem·a·tode \ˈtre-mə-ˌtōd\ *n* : any of a class (Trematoda) of parasitic platyhelminthic flatworms including the flukes — **trematode** *adj*

trem·bles \ˈtrem-bəlz\ *n* : severe poisoning of livestock and esp. cattle by a toxic alcohol present in several plants (as white snakeroot and rayless goldenrod) of the daisy family (Compositae)

tremens — see DELIRIUM TREMENS

trem·or \ˈtre-mər\ *n* : a trembling or shaking usu. from physical weakness, emotional stress, or disease

trem·u·lous \ˈtrem-yə-ləs\ *adj* : characterized by or affected with trembling or tremors — **trem·u·lous·ness** *n*

trench fever *n* : a disease that is marked by fever and pain in muscles, bones, and joints and that is caused by a bacterium (*Rochalimaea quintana*) transmitted by the human body louse (*Pediculus humanus*)

trench foot *n* : a painful foot disorder resembling frostbite and resulting from exposure to cold and wet

trench mouth *n* **1** : VINCENT'S ANGINA **2** : VINCENT'S INFECTION

Tren·de·len·burg position \ˈtrend-əl-ən-ˌbərg-\ *n* : a position of the body for medical examination or operation in which the patient is placed head down on a table inclined at about 45 degrees from the floor with the knees uppermost and the legs hanging over the end of the table

Trendelenburg, Friedrich (1844–1924), German surgeon.

Tren·tal \ˈtren-ˌtal\ *trademark* — used for a preparation of pentoxifylline

treph·i·na·tion \ˌtre-fə-ˈnā-shən\ *n* : an

act or instance of using a trephine (as to perforate the skull)

tre·phine \'trē-ˌfīn\ n : a surgical instrument for cutting out circular sections (as of bone or corneal tissue) — **trephine** \'trē-ˌfīn, tri-'\ vb

trep·o·ne·ma \ˌtre-pə-'nē-mə\ n 1 cap : a genus of anaerobic spirochetes (family Spirochaetaceae) that are pathogenic in humans and other warm-blooded animals and include one (T. pallidum) causing syphilis and another (T. pertenue) causing yaws 2 pl -ma·ta \-mə-tə\ or -mas : any spirochete of the genus Treponema — **trep·o·ne·mal** \-'nē-məl\ adj

Treponema pal·li·dum immobilization test \-'pa-lə-dəm-\ n : a serological test for syphilis — abbr. TPI

trep·o·ne·ma·to·sis \ˌtre-pə-ˌnē-mə-'tō-səs, -ˌne-\ n, pl -to·ses \-ˌsēz\ : infection with or disease caused by spirochetes of the genus Treponema

trep·o·neme \'tre-pə-ˌnēm\ n : TREPONEMA 2

trep·pe \'tre-pə\ n : the graduated series of increasingly vigorous contractions that results when a corresponding series of identical stimuli is applied to a rested muscle — called also staircase effect

Trest \'trest\ trademark — used for a preparation of methixene

tret·i·no·in \tre-'ti-nō-ən\ n : RETINOIC ACID

TRF abbr thyrotropin-releasing factor

TRH abbr thyrotropin-releasing hormone

tri·ac·e·tyl·ole·an·do·my·cin \(ˌ)trī-ˌa-sət-ᵊl-ˌō-lē-ˌan-dō-'mīs-ᵊn\ n : TROLEANDOMYCIN

tri·ad \'trī-ˌad\ n : a union or group of three ⟨a ~ of symptoms⟩

tri·age \trē-'äzh, 'trē-ˌ\ n 1 : the sorting of and allocation of treatment to patients and esp. battle and disaster victims according to a system of priorities designed to maximize the number of survivors 2 : the sorting of patients (as in an emergency room or an HMO) according to the urgency of their need for care — **triage** vb

tri·al \'trī-əl\ n 1 : a tryout or experiment to test quality, value, or usefulness ⟨a clinical ~ of a drug⟩ 2 : one of a number of repetitions of an experiment

tri·am·cin·o·lone \ˌtrī-am-'sin-ᵊl-ˌōn\ n : a glucocorticoid drug $C_{21}H_{27}FO_6$ used esp. in treating psoriasis and allergic skin and respiratory disorders — see KENACORT

tri·am·ter·ene \trī-'am-tər-ˌēn\ n : a diuretic drug $C_{12}H_{11}N_7$ that promotes potassium retention

tri·an·gle \'trī-ˌaŋ-gəl\ n : a three-sided region or space and esp. an anatomical one — see ANTERIOR TRIANGLE, POSTERIOR TRIANGLE, SCARPA'S TRIANGLE, SUBOCCIPITAL TRIANGLE, SUPERIOR CAROTID TRIANGLE

tri·an·gu·lar \trī-'aŋ-gyə-lər\ n : TRIQUETRAL BONE

triangular bone n : TRIQUETRAL BONE

triangular fossa n : a shallow depression in the anterior part of the top of the ear's auricle between the two crura into which the antihelix divides

tri·an·gu·la·ris \trī-ˌaŋ-gyə-'lar-əs\ n, pl -la·res \-'lar-ˌēz\ : a flat triangular muscle that extends from the base of the mandible to the angle formed by the joining of the upper and lower lips and that acts to depress this angle 2 : TRIQUETRAL BONE

triangular ridge n : a triangular surface that slopes downward from the tip of a cusp of a molar or premolar toward the center of its occlusal surface

tri·at·o·ma \trī-'a-tə-mə\ n 1 cap : a genus of large blood-sucking bugs (family Reduviidae) that feed on mammals and sometimes transmit Chagas' disease to their hosts — see CONENOSE 2 : any bug of the genus Triatoma

¹**tri·at·o·mid** \trī-'a-tə-mid\ adj : belonging to the genus Triatoma

²**triatomid** n : TRIATOMA 2

tri·az·i·quone \trī-'a-zə-ˌkwōn\ n : an antineoplastic drug $C_{12}H_{13}N_3O_2$

tri·az·o·lam \trī-'a-zə-ˌlam\ n : a benzodiazepine $C_{17}H_{12}Cl_2N_4$ used as a sedative in the short-term treatment of insomnia

trib·a·dism \'trī-bə-ˌdi-zəm\ n : a homosexual practice among women which attempts to simulate heterosexual intercourse

tri·bro·mo·eth·a·nol \ˌtrī-ˌbrō-mō-'e-thə-ˌnol, -ˌnōl\ n : a crystalline bromine derivative $C_2H_3Br_3O$ of ethyl alcohol used as a basal anesthetic

trib·u·tary \'tri-byə-ˌter-ē\ n, pl -tar·ies : a vein that empties into a larger vein

tri·car·box·yl·ic acid cycle \ˌtrī-kär-ˌbäk-'si-lik-\ n : KREBS CYCLE

tri·ceps \'trī-ˌseps\ n, pl triceps : a muscle that arises from three heads: **a** : the large extensor muscle that is situated along the back of the upper arm, arises by the long head from the infraglenoid tubercle of the scapula and by two heads from the shaft of the humerus, is inserted into the olecranon at the elbow, and extends the forearm at the elbow joint — called also triceps brachii **b** : the gastrocnemius and soleus muscles viewed as constituting together one muscle

triceps bra·chii \-'brä-kē-ˌī\ n : TRICEPS

trich- or **tricho-** comb form : hair : filament ⟨trichobezoar⟩

-trich·ia \'tri-kē-ə\ n comb form : condition of having (such) hair ⟨atrichia⟩

tri·chi·a·sis \tri-'kī-ə-səs\ n : a turning inward of the eyelashes often causing irritation of the eyeball

tri·chi·na \tri-'kī-nə\ n, pl -nae \-(ˌ)nē\ also -nas : a small slender nematode worm of the genus Trichinella (T. spi-

ralis) that as an adult is a short-lived parasite of the intestines of a flesh-eating mammal where it produces immense numbers of larvae which migrate to the muscles, become encysted, may persist for years, and if consumed by a new host in raw or insufficiently cooked meat are liberated by the digestive processes and rapidly become adult to initiate a new parasitic cycle — see TRICHINOSIS

Trichi•na *n, syn of* TRICHINELLA

trich•i•nel•la \₁tri-kə-'ne-lə\ *n* 1 *cap* : a genus of nematode worms (family Trichinellidae) comprising the trichinae 2 *pl* **-lae** \-lē\ : TRICHINA

trich•i•ni•a•sis \₁tri-kə-'nī-ə-səs\ *n, pl* **-a•ses** \-₁sēz\ : TRICHINOSIS

trich•i•no•sis \₁tri-kə-'nō-səs\ *n, pl* **-no•ses** \-₁sēz\ : infestation with or disease caused by trichinae contracted by eating raw or insufficiently cooked infested food and esp. pork and marked initially by colicky pains, nausea, and diarrhea and later by muscular pain, dyspnea, fever, and edema — called also *trichiniasis*

tri•chlor•ace•tic acid \₁trī-₁klór-ə-'sē-tik-\ *var of* TRICHLOROACETIC ACID

tri•chlor•eth•y•lene \₁trī-₁klór-'e-thə-₁lēn\ *var of* TRICHLOROETHYLENE

tri•chlor•fon \(')trī-'klór-₁fän\ *n* : an organophosphate $C_4H_8Cl_3O_4P$ used as a parasiticide in veterinary medicine

tri•chlor•me•thi•a•zide \₁trī-₁klór-me-'thī-ə-₁zīd\ *n* : a diuretic and antihypertensive drug $C_8H_8Cl_3N_3O_4S_2$ — see METAHYDRIN, NAQUA

tri•chlo•ro•ace•tic acid \₁trī-₁klór-ō-ə-'sē-tik-\ *n* : a strong acid $C_2Cl_3HO_2$ used in medicine as a caustic and astringent

tri•chlo•ro•eth•y•lene \-'e-thə-₁lēn\ *n* : a nonflammable liquid C_2HCl_3 used in medicine as an anesthetic and analgesic

tri•chlo•ro•meth•ane \-'me-₁thān\ *n* : CHLOROFORM

tri•chlo•ro•phe•nol \-'fē-₁nól, -₁nól, -fi-\ *n* : a bactericide and fungicide $C_6H_3Cl_3O$ that is a major constituent of hexachlorophene

tri•chlo•ro•phen•oxy•ace•tic acid \(₁)trī-₁klór-ō-fə-₁näk-sē-ə-'sē-tik-\ *n* : 2,4,-5-T

tri•chlor•phon *var of* TRICHLORFON

tri•cho•be•zoar \₁trī-kō-'bē-₁zór\ *n* : HAIR BALL

Tri•cho•bil•har•zia \₁trī-kō-bil-'här-zē-ə, -'härt-sē-ə\ *n* : a genus of digenetic trematode worms (family Schistosomatidae) including forms that normally parasitize aquatic birds and are leading causes of swimmer's itch in humans

Tri•cho•dec•tes \₁tri-kə-'dek-₁tēz\ *n* : a genus of bird lice (family Trichodectidae) of domesticated mammals

tricho•epi•the•li•o•ma \₁tri-kō-₁e-pə-₁thē-lē-'ō-mə\ *n, pl* **-mas** *or* **-ma•ta** \-mə-tə\ : a benign epithelial tumor developing from the hair follicles esp. on the face

tri•chol•o•gy \tri-'kä-lə-jē\ *n, pl* **-gies** : scientific study of hair and its diseases

tricho•mo•na•cide \₁tri-kə-'mō-nə-₁sīd\ *n* : an agent used to destroy trichomonads — **tricho•mo•na•cid•al** \-₁mō-nə-'sīd-ᵊl\ *adj*

¹tricho•mo•nad \₁tri-kə-'mō-₁nad, -nəd\ *n* : any protozoan of the genus *Trichomonas*

²trichomonad *adj* : TRICHOMONAL

tricho•mo•nal \₁tri-kə-'mō-nəl\ *adj* : of, relating to, or caused by flagellated protozoans of the genus *Trichomonas*

Trich•o•mo•nas \₁tri-kə-'mō-nəs\ *n* : a genus of flagellated protozoans (family Trichomonadidae) that are parasites of the alimentary or genitourinary tracts of numerous vertebrate and invertebrate hosts including one (*T. vaginalis*) causing human vaginitis

tricho•mo•ni•a•sis \₁tri-kə-mə-'nī-ə-səs\ *n, pl* **-a•ses** \-₁sēz\ : infection with or disease caused by trichomonads: as **a** : a human sexually transmitted disease occurring esp. as vaginitis with a persistent discharge and caused by a trichomonad (*Trichomonas vaginalis*) that may also invade the male urethra and bladder **b** : a venereal disease of domestic cattle caused by a trichomonad (*T. foetus*) and marked by abortion and sterility **c** : one or more diseases of various birds apparently caused by trichomonads (as *T. diversa* or *T. gallinorum*) and resembling blackhead — called also *roup*

tricho•phy•ton \₁tri-kə-'fī-₁tän, trī-'kä-fə-₁tän\ *n* 1 *cap* : a genus of ringworm fungi (family Moniliaceae) that are parasitic in the skin and hair follicles — see EPIDERMOPHYTON 2 : any fungus of the genus *Trichophyton*

Tricho•spo•ron \₁trī-kə-'spōr-₁än, trī-'käs-pə-₁rän\ *n* : a genus of parasitic imperfect fungi (order Moniliales) of which some are reputed skin or hair parasites of humans

tricho•stron•gyle \₁tri-kə-'strän-₁jīl\ *n* : any worm of the genus *Trichostrongylus*

tricho•stron•gy•lo•sis \₁tri-kō-₁strän-jə-'lō-səs\ *n* : infestation with or disease caused by roundworms of the genus *Trichostrongylus* chiefly in young sheep and cattle

Tricho•stron•gy•lus \₁tri-kō-'strän-jə-ləs\ *n* : a genus of nematode worms (family Trichostrongylidae) parasitic in birds and mammals including humans that comprises forms formerly placed in the genus *Strongylus*

tricho•til•lo•ma•nia \-₁ti-lə-'mā-nē-ə\ *n* : abnormal desire to pull out one's hair — **tricho•til•lo•man•ic** \-'ma-nik\ *adj*

tri•chro•mat \'trī-krō-₁mat, (₁)trī-'\ *n* : a person with trichromatism

tri•chro•mat•ic \₁trī-krō-'ma-tik\ *adj* **1**

: of, relating to, or consisting of three colors ⟨∼ light⟩ **2 a :** relating to or being the theory that human color vision involves three types of retinal sensory receptors b **:** characterized by trichromatism ⟨∼ vision⟩

tri·chro·ma·tism \(ˌ)trī-ˈkrō-mə-ˌti-zəm\ n : color vision based on the perception of three primary colors and esp. red, green, and blue — compare DEUTERANOMALY, PROTANOMALY

trich·u·ri·a·sis \ˌtri-kyə-ˈrī-ə-səs\ n, pl **-a·ses** \-ˌsēz\ : infestation with or disease caused by nematode worms of the genus *Trichuris*

Trich·u·ris \tri-ˈkyūr-əs\ n : a genus of nematode worms (family Trichuridae) comprising the whipworms

tri·clo·car·ban \ˌtri-ˌklō-ˈkär-ˌban\ n : an antiseptic $C_{13}H_9Cl_3N_2O$ used esp. in soaps

tri·cus·pid \(ˌ)trī-ˈkəs-pəd\ adj **1 :** having three cusps ⟨∼ molars⟩ **2 :** of, relating to, or involving the tricuspid valve of the heart ⟨∼ disease⟩

tricuspid valve n : a valve that is situated at the opening of the right atrium of the heart into the right ventricle and that resembles in structure the bicuspid valve but consists of three triangular membranous flaps — called also *right atrioventricular valve*

¹tri·cy·clic \(ˌ)trī-ˈsī-klik, -ˈsi-\ adj : being a chemical with three usu. fused rings in the molecular structure and esp. a tricyclic antidepressant

²tricyclic n : TRICYCLIC ANTIDEPRESSANT

tricyclic antidepressant n : any of a group of antidepressant drugs (as imipramine, amitriptyline, desipramine, and nortriptyline) that contain three fused benzene rings, potentiate the action of catecholamines, and do not inhibit the action of monoamine oxidase

tri·di·hex·eth·yl chloride \ˌtrī-ˌdī-ˌheks-ˈeth-əl-\ n : a quaternary ammonium compound $C_{21}H_{36}ClNO$ used as an anticholinergic drug — see PATHILON

Tri·di·one \trī-ˈdī-ˌōn\ trademark — used for a preparation of trimethadione

triethiodide — see GALLAMINE TRIETHIODIDE

tri·eth·yl·ene gly·col \(ˌ)trī-ˈe-thə-ˌlēn-ˈglī-ˌkȯl, -ˌkōl\ n : a hygroscopic liquid alcohol $C_6H_{14}O_4$ that is used in medicine as an air disinfectant

tri·eth·yl·ene·mel·amine \(ˌ)trī-ˌe-thə-ˌlēn-ˈme-lə-ˌmēn, -mən\ n : a cytotoxic crystalline compound $C_9H_{12}N_6$ used as an antineoplastic drug — called also *TEM*

tri·fa·cial nerve \ˌtrī-ˈfā-shəl-\ n : TRIGEMINAL NERVE

trifacial neuralgia n : TRIGEMINAL NEURALGIA

tri·fluo·per·a·zine \ˌtrī-ˌflü-ō-ˈper-ə-ˌzēn, -zən\ n : a phenothiazine tranquilizer $C_{21}H_{24}F_3N_3S$ used to treat

psychotic conditions and esp. schizophrenia — see STELAZINE

tri·flu·pro·ma·zine \ˌtrī-ˌflü-ˈprō-mə-ˌzēn, -zən\ n : a phenothiazine tranquilizer $C_{18}H_{19}F_3N_2S$ used esp. in the treatment of psychoses and as an antiemetic — see VESPRIN

¹tri·fo·cal \(ˌ)trī-ˈfō-kəl\ adj, of an eyeglass lens : having one part that corrects for near vision, one for intermediate vision (as at arm's length), and one for distant vision

²tri·fo·cal \ˈtrī-ˌfō-kəl\ n **1 :** a trifocal glass or lens **2** pl : eyeglasses with trifocal lenses

tri·gem·i·nal \trī-ˈje-mə-nəl\ adj : of or relating to the trigeminal nerve

²trigeminal n : TRIGEMINAL NERVE

trigeminal ganglion n : the large flattened sensory root ganglion of the trigeminal nerve that lies within the skull and behind the orbit — called also *gasserian ganglion, semilunar ganglion*

trigeminal nerve n : either of the fifth pair of cranial nerves that are mixed nerves and in humans are the largest of the cranial nerves and that arise by a small motor and a larger sensory root which both emerge from the side of the pons with the sensory root bearing the trigeminal ganglion and dividing into ophthalmic, maxillary, and mandibular nerves and the motor root supplying fibers to the mandibular nerve and through this to the muscles of mastication — called also *fifth cranial nerve, trifacial nerve, trigeminus*

trigeminal neuralgia n : an intense paroxysmal neuralgia involving one or more branches of the trigeminal nerve — called also *tic douloureux*

trigger finger n : an abnormal condition in which flexion or extension of a finger may be momentarily obstructed by spasm followed by a snapping into place

trigger point n : a sensitive area of the body which when stimulated gives rise to reaction elsewhere in the body; esp : a hypersensitive area that evokes referred pain elsewhere when stimulated — called also *trigger zone*

tri·glyc·er·ide \(ˌ)trī-ˈgli-sə-ˌrīd\ n : any of a group of lipids that are esters composed of one molecule of glycerol and three molecules of one or more fatty acids, are widespread in adipose tissue, and commonly circulate in the blood in the form of lipoproteins — called also *neutral fat*

tri·gone \ˈtrī-ˌgōn\ also **tri·gon** \-ˌgän\ n : a triangular body part; specif : a smooth triangular area on the inner surface of the bladder limited by the apertures of the ureters and urethra

tri·go·ni·tis \ˌtrī-gə-ˈnī-təs\ n : inflammation of the trigone of the bladder

tri·go·no·ceph·a·ly \ˌtrī-gə-nə-ˈse-fə-lē, ˌtrī-ˌgō-nō-\ n, pl **-lies** : a congenital

trigonum • trisomic

deformity in which the head is somewhat triangular and flat

tri·go·num \trī-ˈgō-nəm\ *n, pl* **-nums** *or* **-na** \-nə\ : a triangular anatomical part : TRIGONE

trigonum ha·ben·u·lae \-hə-ˈben-yə-ˌlē\ *n* : a triangular area on the dorsomedial surface of the lateral geniculate body rostral to the pineal gland

trigonum ves·i·cae \-ˈve-si-kē\ *n* : the trigone of the urinary bladder

tri·io·do·thy·ro·nine \ˌtrī-ˌī-ə-dō-ˈthī-rə-ˌnēn\ *n* : a crystalline iodine-containing hormone $C_{15}H_{12}I_3NO_4$ that is an amino acid derived from thyroxine, and is used esp. in the form of its soluble sodium salt in the treatment of hypothyroidism and metabolic insufficiency — called also *liothyronine, T_3*

tri·mep·ra·zine \trī-ˈme-prə-ˌzēn\ *n* : a phenothiazine $C_{18}H_{22}N_2S$ used esp. in the form of its tartrate salt as an antipruritic — see TEMARIL

tri·mes·ter \(ˌ)trī-ˈmes-tər, ˈtrī-ˌ\ *n* : a period of three or about three months; *esp* : any of three periods of approximately three months each into which a human pregnancy is divided

tri·metha·di·one \ˌtrī-ˌme-thə-ˈdī-ˌōn\ *n* : a crystalline anticonvulsant $C_6H_9NO_3$ used chiefly in the treatment of petit mal epilepsy — see TRIDIONE

tri·meth·a·phan \trī-ˈme-thə-ˌfan\ *n* : a ganglionic blocking agent used as a salt $C_{32}H_{40}N_2O_5S_2$ to lower blood pressure esp. in hypertensive emergencies

tri·meth·o·ben·za·mide \ˌtrī-ˌme-thə-ˈben-zə-ˌmīd\ *n* : an antiemetic drug $C_{21}H_{28}N_2O_5$ used esp. in the form of its hydrochloride salt

tri·meth·o·prim \trī-ˈme-thə-ˌprim\ *n* : a synthetic antibacterial and antimalarial drug $C_{14}H_{18}N_4O_3$ — see BACTRIM

tri·ni·tro·phe·nol \(ˌ)trī-ˌnī-trō-ˈfē-ˌnōl, -ˌnōl, -fi-ˈnōl\ *or* **2,4,6-trinitrophenol** \ˌtü-ˌfōr-ˌsiks-\ *n* : PICRIC ACID

tri·nu·cle·o·tide \(ˌ)trī-ˈnü-klē-ə-ˌtīd, -ˈnyü-\ *n* : a nucleotide consisting of three mononucleotides in combination : CODON

tri·or·tho·cre·syl phosphate \ˌtrī-ˌor-thō-ˌkre-səl-, -ˌkrē-\ *n* : a usu. colorless, odorless, tasteless neurotoxin $C_{21}H_{21}O_2P$

tri·ox·sa·len \trī-ˈäk-sə-lən\ *n* : a synthetic psoralen $C_{14}H_{12}O_3$ that promotes tanning of the skin

tri·pal·mi·tin \(ˌ)trī-ˈpal-mə-tən, -ˈpäl-, -ˈpä-\ *n* : PALMITIN

tri·par·a·nol \trī-ˈpar-ə-ˌnȯl, -ˌnōl\ *n* : a drug $C_{27}H_{32}ClNO_2$ that inhibits the formation of cholesterol but that has numerous toxic side effects

tri·pel·en·na·mine \ˌtrī-pe-ˈle-nə-ˌmēn, -mən\ *n* : an antihistamine drug $C_{16}H_{21}N_3$ used in the form of its crys-

talline citrate or hydrochloride — see PYRIBENZAMINE

tri·pep·tide \(ˌ)trī-ˈpep-ˌtīd\ *n* : a peptide that yields three amino acid residues on hydrolysis

tri·phe·nyl·meth·ane \ˌtrī-ˌfen-əl-ˈme-ˌthān, -ˌfēn-\ *n* : a crystalline hydrocarbon $CH(C_6H_5)_3$

triphenylmethane dye *n* : any of a group of dyes (as pararosaniline) derived from triphenylmethane

tri·phos·pha·tase \(ˌ)trī-ˈfäs-fə-ˌtās, -ˌtāz\ *n* : an enzyme that catalyzes hydrolysis of a triphosphate — see ATPASE

tri·phos·phate \(ˌ)trī-ˈfäs-ˌfāt\ *n* : a salt or acid that contains three phosphate groups — see ATP, GTP

tri·phos·pho·pyr·i·dine nucleotide \ˌtrī-ˌfäs-fō-ˈpir-ə-ˌdēn-\ *n* : NADP

triple bond *n* : a chemical bond consisting of three covalent bonds between two atoms in a molecule and usu. represented in structural formulas by three lines, three dots, or six dots that denote three pairs of electrons — compare DOUBLE BOND, UNSATURATED b

tri·ple·gia \(ˌ)trī-ˈplē-jə, -jē-ə\ *n* : hemiplegia plus paralysis of a limb on the opposite side

triple point *n* : the condition of temperature and pressure under which the gaseous, liquid, and solid phases of a substance can exist in equilibrium

trip·let \ˈtri-plət\ *n* **1 a** : a combination, set, or group of three **b** : CODON 2 : one of three children or offspring born at one birth

¹trip·loid \ˈtri-ˌplȯid\ *adj* : having or being a chromosome number three times the monoploid number — **triploi·dy** \-ˌplȯi-dē\ *n*

²triploid *n* : a triploid individual

tri·que·tral bone \trī-ˈkwē-trel-\ *n* : the bone in the proximal row of the carpus that is third counting from the thumb side of the wrist, has a pyramidal shape, and is situated between the lunate and pisiform bones — called also *triangular, triangular bone, triangularis, triquetral*

tri·que·trum \trī-ˈkwē-trəm\ *n, pl* **tri·que·tra** \-trə\ : TRIQUETRAL BONE

tris \ˈtris\ *n, often cap* : a white crystalline powder $C_4H_{11}NO_3$ used as a buffer (as in the treatment of acidosis) — called also *tris buffer, tromethamine*

tri·sac·cha·ride \(ˌ)trī-ˈsa-kə-ˌrīd\ *n* : a sugar that yields on complete hydrolysis three monosaccharide molecules

tris buffer *n* : TRIS

tris·kai·deka·pho·bia \ˌtris-ˌkī-ˌde-kə-ˈfō-bē-ə, ˌtris-kə-\ *n* : fear of the number 13

tris·mus \ˈtriz-məs\ *n* : spasm of the muscles of mastication resulting from any of various abnormal conditions or diseases (as tetanus)

¹tri·so·mic \(ˌ)trī-ˈsō-mik\ *adj* : relating

to, caused by, or characterized by trisomy (~ cells)

²trisomic n : a trisomic individual

tri·so·my \\'trī-₁sō-mē\\ n, pl **-mies** : the condition (as in Down's syndrome) of having one or a few chromosomes triploid in an otherwise diploid set

trisomy 21 \\-'twen-tē-'wən\\ n : DOWN'S SYNDROME

trit·an·ope \\'trīt-ⁿn-₁ōp, 'trit-\\ n : a person affected with tritanopia

trit·an·opia \\₁trīt-ⁿn-'ō-pē-ə, ₁trit-\\ n : dichromatism in which the spectrum is seen in tones of red and green — **trit·an·opic** \\₁trīt-ⁿn-'ō-pik, -ⁿn-'ä-\\ adj

tri·ti·um \\'tri-tē-əm, -shəm, -shē-əm\\ n : a radioactive isotope of hydrogen with atoms of three times the mass of ordinary light hydrogen atoms — symbol T

¹trit·u·rate \\'tri-chə-₁rāt\\ vb **-rat·ed; -rat·ing** : to pulverize thoroughly by rubbing or grinding — **trit·u·ra·tion** \\₁tri-chə-'rā-shən\\ n

²trit·u·rate \\-rət\\ n : a triturated substance

tri·va·lent \\(₁)trī-'vā-lənt\\ adj : reacting immunologically with three different combining sites (as of antigens or antibodies)

tRNA \\₁tē-₁är-₁en-'ā\\ n : TRANSFER RNA

Tro·bi·cin \\trō-'bīs-ⁿn\\ trademark — used for a preparation of spectinomycin

tro·car \\'trō-₁kär\\ n : a sharp-pointed surgical instrument fitted with a cannula and used esp. to insert the cannula into a body cavity as a drainage outlet

tro·chan·ter \\trō-'kan-tər\\ n : a rough prominence or process at the upper part of the femur serving usu. for the attachment of muscles and being usu. two on each femur: **a** : a larger one situated on the outer part of the upper end of the shaft at its junction with the neck — called also *greater trochanter* **b** : a smaller one situated at the lower back part of the junction of the shaft and neck — called also *lesser trochanter* — **tro·chan·ter·ic** \\₁trō-kən-'ter-ik, -₁kan-\\ adj

trochanteric fossa n : a depression at the base of the internal surface of the greater trochanter of the femur for the attachment of the tendon of the obturator externus

tro·char var of TROCAR

tro·che \\'trō-kē\\ n : LOZENGE

troch·lea \\'träk-lē-ə\\ n : an anatomical structure held to resemble a pulley: as **a** : the articular surface on the medial condyle of the humerus that articulates with the ulna **b** : the fibrous ring in the inner upper part of the orbit through which the tendon of the superior oblique muscle of the eye passes

troch·le·ar \\-ər\\ adj **1** : of, relating to, or

being a trochlea **2** : of, relating to, or being a trochlear nerve (~ fibers)

trochlear fovea n : a depression that is located in the orbital surface of each bony plate of the frontal bone and that forms a point of attachment for the superior oblique muscle of the eye

trochlear nerve n : either of the 4th pair of cranial nerves that arise from the dorsal aspect of the brainstem just below the inferior colliculus and supply the superior oblique muscle of the eye with motor fibers

trochlear nucleus n : a nucleus that is situated behind the oculomotor nucleus and is the source of the motor fibers of the trochlear nerve

tro·choid \\'trō-₁kȯid\\ n : PIVOT JOINT

tro·land \\'trō-lənd\\ n : PHOTON 2

Troland, Leonard Thompson (1889–1932), American psychologist and physicist.

tro·le·an·do·my·cin \\₁trō-lē-₁an-də-'mīs-ⁿn\\ n : an orally administered antibacterial drug $C_{41}H_{67}NO_{15}$ — called also *triacetyloleandomycin*

trol·ley also **trol·ly** \\'trä-lē\\ n, pl **trolleys** also **trollies** Brit : a stretcher with four wheels used to transport patients in a hospital

trol·ni·trate \\'träl-'nī-₁trāt\\ n : an organic nitrate with vasodilator activity that is used in the form of its diphosphate salt $C_6H_{12}N_4O_9 \cdot 2H_3PO_4$ to prevent or ameliorate attacks of angina pectoris — see METAMINE

Trom·bic·u·la \\träm-'bi-kyə-lə\\ n : a genus of mites (family Trombiculidae) including some forms that in Asia transmit tsutsugamushi disease

tro·meth·amine \\trō-'me-thə-₁mēn\\ n : TRIS

troph- or **tropho-** comb form : nutritive (*trophoblast*)

troph·ec·to·derm \\₁trō-'fek-tə-₁dərm\\ n : TROPHOBLAST; esp : the outer layer of the blastocyst after differentiation of the ectoderm, mesoderm, and endoderm when the outer layer is continuous with the embryonic ectoderm

tro·phic \\'trō-fik\\ adj **1** : of or relating to nutrition : NUTRITIONAL (~ disorders) **2** : TROPIC — **tro·phi·cal·ly** adv

-tro·phic \\'trō-fik\\ adj comb form **1** : of, relating to, or characterized by (such) nutrition or growth (hyper*trophic*) **2** : -TROPIC (gonado*trophic*)

trophic ulcer n : an ulcer (as a bedsore) caused by faulty nutrition in the affected part

tro·pho·blast \\'trō-fə-₁blast\\ n : the outer layer of the blastocyst that supplies nutrition to the embryo, facilitates implantation by eroding away the tissues of the uterus with which it comes in contact, and differentiates into the extraembryonic membranes surrounding the embryo — **tro·pho·blas·tic** \\₁trō-fə-'blas-tik\\ adj

troph·o·derm \'trō-fə-ˌdərm\ *n* : TROPHOBLAST

tro·pho·zo·ite \ˌtrō-fə-'zō-ˌīt\ *n* : a protozoan of a vegetative form as distinguished from one of a reproductive or resting form

-tro·phy \trə-fē\ *n comb form, pl* **-trophies** : nutrition : nurture : growth ⟨hypo*trophy*⟩

tro·pia \'trō-pē-ə\ *n* : deviation of an eye from the normal position with respect to the line of vision when the eyes are open : STRABISMUS — see ESOTROPIA, HYPERTROPIA

tro·pic \'trō-pik\ *adj* **1** : of, relating to, or characteristic of tropism or of a tropism **2** *of a hormone* : influencing the activity of a specified gland

-tro·pic \'trō-pik\ *adj comb form* : attracted to or acting upon (something specified) ⟨neuro*tropic*⟩

tropical medicine *n* : a branch of medicine dealing with tropical diseases and other special medical problems of tropical regions

tropical oil *n* : any of several oils (as coconut oil and palm oil) that are high in saturated fatty acids

tropical sprue *n* : SPRUE 2

tropical ulcer *n* : a chronic sloughing sore of unknown cause occurring usu. on the legs and prevalent in wet tropical regions

tro·pic·amide \trə-'pi-kə-ˌmīd\ *n* : a synthetic anticholinergic $C_{17}H_{20}N_2O_2$ used esp. to dilate pupils in ophthalmological examinations — see MYDRIACYL

-tro·pin \'trō-pən\ *or* **-tro·phin** \-fən\ *n comb form* : hormone (gonado*tropin*) ⟨somato*tropin*⟩

tro·pism \'trō-ˌpi-zəm\ *n* : an automatic movement by an organism in response to a source of stimulation; *also* : a reflex reaction involving a tropism

tro·po·col·la·gen \ˌträ-pə-'kä-lə-jən, ˌtrō-\ *n* : a subunit of collagen fibrils consisting of three polypeptide strands arranged in a helix

tro·po·my·o·sin \ˌträ-pə-'mī-ə-sən, ˌtrō-\ *n* : a protein of muscle that forms a complex with troponin regulating the interaction of actin and myosin in muscular contraction

tro·po·nin \'trō-pə-nən, 'trä-, -ˌnin\ *n* : a protein of muscle that together with tropomyosin forms a regulatory protein complex controlling the interaction of actin and myosin and that when combined with calcium ions permits muscular contraction

trough \'trof\ *n* — see GINGIVAL CREVICE

troy \'troi\ *adj* : expressed in troy weight ⟨a ∼ ounce⟩

troy pound *n* : POUND a

troy weight *n* : a series of units of weight based on a pound of 12 ounces and an ounce of 480 grains or 31.103 grams

true bug \'trü-\ *n* : BUG 1c

true conjugate *n* : CONJUGATE DIAMETER

true pelvis *n* : the lower more contracted part of the pelvic cavity — called also *true pelvic cavity;* compare FALSE PELVIS

true rib *n* : any of the ribs having costal cartilages connected directly with the sternum and in humans constituting the first seven pairs — called also *vertebrosternal rib*

true vocal cords *n pl* : the lower pair of vocal cords each of which encloses a vocal ligament, extends from the inner surface of one side of the thyroid cartilage near the median line to a process of the corresponding arytenoid cartilage on the same side of the larynx, and when drawn taut, approximated to the contralateral member of the pair, and subjected to a flow of breath produces the voice — called also *inferior vocal cords, vocal folds*

trun·cal \'trəŋ-kəl\ *adj* : of or relating to the trunk of the body or of a bodily part (as a nerve) ⟨∼ obesity⟩

trun·cus \'trəŋ-kəs\ *n* : TRUNK 2

truncus bra·chio·ce·phal·i·cus \-ˌbrä-kē-(ˌ)ō-se-'fa-li-kəs\ *n* : BRACHIOCEPHALIC ARTERY

truncus ce·li·a·cus \-se-'lī-ə-kəs\ *n* : CELIAC ARTERY

trunk \'trəŋk\ *n* **1** : the human body apart from the head and appendages : TORSO **2** : the main body of an anatomical part (as a nerve or blood vessel) that divides into branches

truss \'trəs\ *n* : a device worn to reduce a hernia by pressure

truth serum *n* : a hypnotic or anesthetic (as thiopental) held to induce a subject under questioning to talk freely

trypan- *or* **trypano-** *comb form* : trypanosome ⟨*trypano*cidal⟩

try·pano·ci·dal \tri-ˌpa-nə-'sīd-əl\ *adj* : destroying trypanosomes ⟨a ∼ drug⟩ — **try·pano·cide** \tri-'pa-nə-ˌsīd\ *n*

try·pano·so·ma \tri-ˌpa-nə-'sō-mə\ *n* **1** *cap* : a genus of parasitic flagellate protozoans (family Trypanosomatidae) that infest the blood of various vertebrates including humans, are usu. transmitted by the bite of an insect, and include some that cause serious diseases (as Chagas' disease, sleeping sickness, and surra) **2** *pl* **-mas** *or* **-ma·ta** \-mə-tə\ : TRYPANOSOME

try·pano·some \tri-'pa-nə-ˌsōm\ *n* : any flagellate of the genus *Trypanosoma* — **try·pano·so·mal** \-ˌpa-nə-'sō-məl\ *adj*

try·pano·so·mi·a·sis \tri-ˌpa-nə-sə-'mī-ə-səs\ *n, pl* **-a·ses** \-ˌsēz\ : infection with or disease caused by flagellates of the genus *Trypanosoma*

tryp·ars·amide \tri-'pär-sə-ˌmīd\ *n* : an organic arsenical $C_8H_{10}AsN_2O_4Na \cdot \frac{1}{2}H_2O$ used in the treatment of African sleeping sickness and syphilis

tryp·sin \'trip-sən\ *n* **1** : a crystallizable proteolytic enzyme that is produced and secreted in the pancreatic juice in the form of inactive trypsinogen and activated in the intestine — compare CHYMOTRYPSIN **2** : a preparation from the pancreatic juice containing principally proteolytic enzymes and used chiefly as a digestive and lytic agent

tryp·sin·ize \'trip-sə-₁nīz\ *vb* **-ized; -iz·ing** : to subject to the action of trypsin ⟨*trypsinized* tissue cells⟩ — **tryp·sin·i·za·tion** \₁trip-sə-nə-'zā-shən\ *n*

tryp·sin·o·gen \trip-'si-nə-jən\ *n* : the inactive substance released by the pancreas into the duodenum to form trypsin

tryp·tic \'trip-tik\ *adj* : of, relating to, or produced by trypsin or its action

tryp·to·phan \'trip-tə-₁fan\ *also* **tryp·to·phane** \-₁fān\ *n* : a crystalline essential amino acid $C_{11}H_{12}N_2O_2$ that is widely distributed in proteins

tset·se \'tset-sē, 'tsēt-, 'tet-, 'tēt-\ *n, pl* **tsetse** *or* **tsetses** : TSETSE FLY

tsetse fly *n* : any of several dipteran flies of the genus *Glossina* that occur in sub-Saharan Africa and include vectors of human and animal trypanosomes (as those causing sleeping sickness) — called also *tsetse*

TSH \₁tē-(₁)es-'āch\ *n* : THYROTROPIN

TSS *abbr* toxic shock syndrome

tsu·tsu·ga·mu·shi disease \₁tsüt-sə-gə-'mü-shē-, ₁tüt-, ₁süt-, -'gä-mü-shē-\ *n* : an acute febrile bacterial disease that is caused by a rickettsial bacterium (*Rickettsia tsutsugamushi*) transmitted by mite larvae, resembles louse-borne typhus, and is widespread in the western Pacific area — called also *scrub typhus, tsutsugamushi*

T system *n* : the system of T tubules in striated muscle

T₃ *or* **T–3** \₁tē-'thrē\ *n* : TRIIODOTHYRONINE

T–tube *n* : a narrow flexible tube in the form of a T that is used for drainage esp. of the common bile duct

T tubule *n* : any of the small tubules which run transversely through a striated muscle fiber and through which electrical impulses are transmitted from the sarcoplasm to the fiber's interior

tub·al \'tü-bəl, 'tyü-\ *adj* : of, relating to, or involving a tube and esp. a fallopian tube ⟨~ lumens⟩ ⟨a ~ infection⟩

tubal abortion *n* : an aborted tubal pregnancy

tubal ligation *n* : ligation of the fallopian tubes to prevent passage of ova from the ovaries to the uterus used as a method of female sterilization

tubal pregnancy *n* : ectopic pregnancy in a fallopian tube

tubarius — see TORUS TUBARIUS

¹tube \'tüb, 'tyüb\ *n* **1** : a slender channel within a plant or animal body : DUCT — see BRONCHIAL TUBE, EUSTACHIAN TUBE, FALLOPIAN TUBE **2 a** : a piece of laboratory or technical apparatus commonly serving to isolate or convey a product of reaction (a distillation ~) **b** : TEST TUBE **3** : a hollow cylindrical device (as a cannula) used for insertion into bodily passages or hollow organs for removal or injection of materials

²tube *vb* **tubed; tub·ing** : to furnish with, enclose in, or pass through a tube

tube curare *n* : CURARE

tubed *adj* : having the sides sewn together so as to form a tube

tuberalis — see PARS TUBERALIS

tu·ber ci·ne·re·um \'tü-bər-si-'nir-ē-əm, 'tyü-\ *n* : an eminence of gray matter which lies on the lower surface of the brain and of which the upper surface forms part of the floor of the third ventricle and the lower surface bears the infundibulum to which the pituitary gland is attached

tu·ber·cle \'tü-bər-kəl, 'tyü-\ *n* **1** : a small knobby prominence or excrescence: as **a** : a prominence on the crown of a molar tooth **b** : a small rough prominence on a bone usu. being smaller than a tuberosity and serving for the attachment of one or more muscles or ligaments — see GREATER TUBERCLE, LESSER TUBERCLE **c** : an eminence near the head of a rib that articulates with the transverse process of a vertebra **d** : any of several prominences in the central nervous system that mark the nuclei of various nerves **2** : a small discrete lump in the substance of an organ or in the skin; *esp* : the specific lesion of tuberculosis consisting of a packed mass of epithelioid cells, giant cells, disintegration products of leukocytes and bacilli, and usu. a necrotic center

tubercle bacillus *n* : a bacterium of the genus *Mycobacterium* (*M. tuberculosis*) that is a causative agent of tuberculosis

tubercul- *or* **tuberculo-** *comb form* **1** : tubercle ⟨*tubercular*⟩ **2** : tubercle bacillus ⟨*tubercul*in⟩ **3** : tuberculosis ⟨*tuberculoid*⟩

¹tu·ber·cu·lar \tü-'bər-kyə-lər, tyü-\ *adj* **1 a** : of, relating to, or affected with tuberculosis : TUBERCULOUS **b** : caused by the tubercle bacillus ⟨~ meningitis⟩ **2** : characterized by lesions that are or resemble tubercles ⟨~ leprosy⟩ **3** : relating to, resembling, or constituting a tubercle

²tubercular *n* : an individual with tuberculosis

tu·ber·cu·lid \tü-'bər-kyə-lid, tyü-\ *n* : a tuberculous lesion of the skin; *esp* : one that is an id

tu·ber·cu·lin \tü-'bər-kyə-lən, tyü-\ *n* : a sterile liquid containing the growth products of or specific substances extracted from the tubercle bacillus and used in the diagnosis of tuberculosis

tuberculin reaction *n* : TUBERCULIN TEST

tuberculin test *n* : a test for hypersensitivity to tuberculin in which tuberculin is injected usu. into the skin of the individual tested and the appearance of inflammation at the site of injection is construed as indicating past or present tubercular infection — compare MANTOUX TEST

tu·ber·cu·loid \tü-ˈbər-kyə-ˌloid, tyü-\ *adj* **1** : resembling tuberculosis and esp. the tubercles characteristic of it **2** : of, relating to, characterized by, or affected with tuberculoid leprosy

tuberculoid leprosy *n* : the one of the two major forms of leprosy that is characterized by the presence of few or no Hansen's bacilli in the lesions and by the loss of sensation in affected areas of the skin — compare LEPROMATOUS LEPROSY

tu·ber·cu·lo·ma \tü-ˌbər-kyə-ˈlō-mə, tyü-\ *n, pl* **-mas** \-məz\ *also* **-ma·ta** \-mə-tə\ : a large solitary caseous tubercle of tuberculous character occurring esp. in the brain

tu·ber·cu·lo·sis \tü-ˌbər-kyə-ˈlō-səs, tyü-\ *n, pl* **-lo·ses** \-ˌsēz\ : a usu. chronic highly variable disease that is caused by the tubercle bacillus and rarely in the U.S. by a related mycobacterium (*Mycobacterium bovis*), is usu. communicated by inhalation of the airborne causative agent, affects esp. the lungs but may spread to other areas (as the kidney or spinal column) from local lesions or by way of the lymph or blood vessels, and is characterized by fever, cough, difficulty in breathing, inflammatory infiltrations, formation of tubercles, caseation, pleural effusion, and fibrosis — called also *TB*

¹tu·ber·cu·lo·stat·ic \tü-ˌbər-kyə-lō-ˈstatik, tyü-\ *adj* : inhibiting the growth of the tubercle bacillus ⟨a ~ drug⟩

²tuberculostatic *n* : a tuberculostatic agent

tu·ber·cu·lous \tü-ˈbər-kyə-ləs, tyü-\ *adj* **1** : constituting or affected with tuberculosis **2** : caused by or resulting from the presence or products of the tubercle bacillus ⟨~ peritonitis⟩

tu·ber·os·i·ty \ˌtü-bə-ˈrä-sə-tē, ˌtyü-\ *n, pl* **-ties** : a rounded prominence; *esp* : a large prominence on a bone usu. serving for the attachment of muscles or ligaments

tuberous sclerosis *n* : EPILOIA

tu·bo·cu·ra·rine \ˌtü-bō-kyu̇-ˈrär-ən, -ˌēn, tyü-\ *n* : a toxic alkaloid or its crystalline hydrated hydrochloride salt $C_{37}H_{41}ClN_2O_6 \cdot HCl \cdot 5H_2O$ that is obtained chiefly from the bark and stems of a So. American vine (*Chondrodendron tomentosum* of the family Menispermaceae) and in its dextrorotatory form constitutes the chief active constituent of curare and is

used esp. as a skeletal muscle relaxant

tu·bo-ovar·i·an \ˌtü-bō-ō-ˈvar-ē-ən, ˌtyü-\ *adj* : of, relating to, or affecting a fallopian tube and ovary ⟨a ~ abscess⟩

tu·bu·lar \ˈtü-byə-lər, ˈtyü-\ *adj* **1** : having the form of or consisting of a tube **2** : of, relating to, or sounding as if produced through a tube or tubule ⟨~ rales⟩

tu·bule \ˈtü-(ˌ)byül, ˈtyü-\ *n* : a small tube; *esp* : a slender elongated anatomical channel

tu·bu·lin \ˈtü-byə-lən, ˈtyü-\ *n* : a globular protein that polymerizes to form microtubules

tu·bu·lo·ac·i·nar \ˌtü-byə-lō-ˈa-sə-nər, ˌtyü-\ *or* **tu·bu·lo·aci·nous** \-nəs\ *adj* : TUBULOALVEOLAR

tu·bu·lo·al·ve·o·lar \ˌtü-byə-lō-al-ˈvē-ə-lər, ˌtyü-\ *adj* : of, relating to, or being a gland having branching tubules which end in secretory alveoli

tu·bu·lo·in·ter·sti·tial \ˌtü-byə-lō-ˌin-tər-ˈsti-shəl, ˌtyü-\ *adj* : affecting or involving the tubules and interstitial tissue of the kidney ⟨~ disease⟩

tu·bu·lus \ˈtü-byə-ləs, ˈtyü-\ *n, pl* **tu·bu·li** \-ˌlī\ : TUBULE

tuck \ˈtək\ *n* : a cosmetic surgical operation for the removal of excess skin or fat from a body part — see TUMMY TUCK

Tu·i·nal \ˈtü-i-ˌnäl\ *trademark* — used for a preparation of amobarbital and secobarbital

tu·lar·ae·mia *chiefly Brit var of* TULAREMIA

tu·la·re·mia \ˌtü-lə-ˈrē-mē-ə, ˌtyü-\ *n* : an infectious disease esp. of wild rabbits, rodents, humans, and some domestic animals that is caused by a bacterium (*Francisella tularensis*), is transmitted esp. by the bites of insects, and in humans is marked by symptoms (as fever) of toxemia — called also *rabbit fever* — **tu·la·re·mic** \-mik\ *adj*

tulle gras \ˌtül-ˈgrä\ *n* : fine-meshed gauze impregnated with a fatty substance (as soft paraffin)

tu·me·fa·cient \ˌtü-mə-ˈfā-shənt, ˌtyü-\ *adj* : producing swelling

tu·me·fac·tion \-ˈfak-shən\ *n* **1** : an action or process of swelling or becoming tumorous **2** : SWELLING

tu·me·fac·tive \-ˈfak-tiv\ *adj* : producing swelling ⟨~ lesions⟩

tu·mes·cence \tü-ˈmes-əns, tyü-\ *n* : the quality or state of being tumescent; *esp* : readiness for sexual activity marked esp. by vascular congestion of the sex organs

tu·mes·cent \-ˈmes-ənt\ *adj* : somewhat swollen ⟨~ tissue⟩

tummy tuck *n* : a surgical operation for removal of excess skin and fat from the abdominal area

tu·mor \ˈtü-mər, ˈtyü-\ *n* : an abnormal benign or malignant mass of tissue that is not inflammatory, arises without obvious cause from cells of pre-existent tissue, and possesses no physiological function — compare CANCER 1, CARCINOMA, SARCOMA — **tu·mor·al** \-mə-rəl\ adj — **tu·mor·like** \-ˌlīk\ adj

tu·mor·i·cid·al \ˌtü-mə-rə-ˈsīd-ᵊl, ˌtyü-\ adj : destroying tumor cells ⟨∼ activity⟩

tu·mor·i·gen·ic \-ˈje-nik\ adj : producing or tending to produce tumors; also : CARCINOGENIC — **tu·mor·i·gen·e·sis** \-ˈje-nə-səs\ n — **tu·mor·i·ge·nic·i·ty** \-jə-ˈni-sə-tē\ n

tumor–infiltrating lymphocyte n : a T cell that is isolated from a malignant tumor, cultured with interleukin-2, and injected back into the patient as a tumor-killing cell and that has greater cytotoxicity than lymphokine-activated killer cells — called also TIL

tumor necrosis factor n : a protein that is produced by monocytes and macrophages in response esp. to endotoxins and that activates leukocytes and has antitumor activity — abbr. TNF

tu·mor·ous \ˈtü-mə-rəs, ˈtyü-\ adj : of, relating to, or resembling a tumor

tumor virus n : a virus (as Rous sarcoma virus) that causes neoplastic or cancerous growth

tu·mour chiefly Brit var of TUMOR

Tun·ga \ˈtən-gə\ n : a genus of fleas (family Tungidae) that include the chigoe (T. penetrans)

tung·sten \ˈtəŋ-stən\ n : a gray-white high-melting ductile metallic element — called also wolfram; symbol W; see ELEMENT table

tu·nic \ˈtü-nik, ˈtyü-\ n : an enclosing or covering membrane or tissue : TUNICA ⟨the ∼s of the eye⟩

tu·ni·ca \ˈtü-ni-kə, ˈtyü-\ n, pl **tu·ni·cae** \-nə-ˌkē, -ˌkī, -ˌsē\ : an enveloping membrane or layer of body tissue

tunica adventitia n : ADVENTITIA

tunica al·bu·gin·ea \-ˌal-bü-ˈji-nē-ə, -byü-\ n, pl **tunicae al·bu·gin·e·ae** \-ˈji-nē-ˌē, -ˌī\ : a white fibrous capsule esp. of the testis

tunica intima n : INTIMA

tunica media n : MEDIA

tunica mucosa n : mucous membrane and esp. that lining the digestive tract

tunica muscularis n : MUSCULAR COAT

tunica pro·pria \-ˈprō-prē-ə\ n : LAMINA PROPRIA

tunica va·gi·na·lis \-ˌva-jə-ˈnā-ləs, -ˈna-\ n, pl **tunicae va·gi·na·les** \-(ˌ)lēz\ : a pouch of serous membrane covering the testis and derived from the peritoneum

tuning fork n : a 2-pronged metal implement that gives a fixed tone when struck

tun·nel \ˈtən-ᵊl\ n : a bodily channel — see CARPAL TUNNEL

tunnel of Cor·ti \-ˈkȯr-tē\ n : a spiral passage in the organ of Corti

tunnel vision n : constriction of the visual field resulting in loss of peripheral vision

tur·bel·lar·i·an \ˌtər-bə-ˈlar-ē-ən\ n : any of a class (Turbellaria) of mostly aquatic and free-living flatworms — **turbellarian** adj

tur·bid \ˈtər-bəd\ adj : thick or opaque with matter in suspension : cloudy or muddy in appearance ⟨∼ urine⟩ — **tur·bid·i·ty** \ˌtər-ˈbi-də-tē\ n

tur·bi·dim·e·ter \ˌtər-bə-ˈdi-mə-tər\ n 1 : an instrument for measuring and comparing the turbidity of liquids by viewing light through them and determining how much light is cut off 2 : NEPHELOMETER — **tur·bi·di·met·ric** \ˌtər-bə-də-ˈme-trik, ˌtər-ˌbi-\ adj — **tur·bi·dim·e·try** \ˌtər-bə-ˈdi-mə-trē\ n

¹**tur·bi·nate** \ˈtər-bə-nət, -ˌnāt\ adj : of, relating to, or being a nasal concha

²**turbinate** n : NASAL CONCHA

turbinate bone also **tur·bi·nat·ed bone** \ˈtər-bə-ˌnā-təd-\ n : NASAL CONCHA

turcica — see SELLA TURCICA

turf toe n : a minor but painful usu. sports-related injury involving hyperextension of the big toe resulting in sprain of the ligament of the metatarsophalangeal joint

tur·ges·cent \ˌtər-ˈjes-ᵊnt\ adj : becoming turgid, distended, or swollen — **tur·ges·cence** \-ˈjes-ᵊns\ n

tur·gid \ˈtər-jəd\ adj : being in a normal or abnormal state of distension : SWOLLEN ⟨∼ limbs⟩ — **tur·gid·i·ty** \ˌtər-ˈji-də-tē\ n

tur·gor \ˈtər-gər, -ˌgȯr\ n : the normal state of turgidity and tension in living cells

tu·ris·ta \tü-ˈrē-stə\ n : intestinal sickness and diarrhea commonly affecting a tourist in a foreign country; esp : MONTEZUMA'S REVENGE

turn \ˈtərn\ vb : to injure by twisting or wrenching ⟨∼ed his ankle⟩

Tur·ner's syndrome \ˈtər-nərz-\ n : a genetically determined condition that is associated with the presence of only one complete X chromosome and no Y chromosome and that is characterized by a female phenotype with underdeveloped and infertile ovaries

Turner, Henry Hubert (1892–1970), American endocrinologist.

tur·ri·ceph·a·ly \ˌtər-ə-ˈse-fə-lē\ n, pl **-lies** : OXYCEPHALY

tus·sive \ˈtə-siv\ adj : of, relating to, or involved in coughing ⟨∼ force⟩

T wave \ˈtē-ˌwāv\ n : the deflection in an electrocardiogram that represents the electrical activity produced by ventricular repolarization — compare P WAVE, QRS COMPLEX

Tween \ˈtwēn\ trademark — used for any of several preparations of polysorbates

tween–brain \ˈtwēn-ˌbrān\ n : DIENCEPHALON

twee·zers \ˈtwē-zərz\ n sing or pl : any of various small metal instruments that are usu. held between the thumb and forefinger, are used for plucking, holding, or manipulating, and consist of two legs joined at one end

twelfth cranial nerve *n* : HYPOGLOSSAL NERVE

twelve–year molar *n* : any of the second permanent molar teeth which erupt at about 12 years of age and include four of which one is located on each side of the upper and lower jaws — compare SIX-YEAR MOLAR

twen·ty–twen·ty *or* **20/20** *adj* : having the normal visual acuity of the human eye that according to one common scale can distinguish at a distance of 20 feet characters one-third inch in diameter

twig \'twig\ *n* : a minute branch of a nerve or artery

twi·light sleep \'twī-ˌlīt-\ *n* : a state in which awareness of pain is dulled and memory of pain is dimmed or effaced and which is produced by hypodermic injection of morphine and scopolamine and used esp. formerly chiefly in childbirth

twilight state *n* : a dreamy state lacking touch with present reality, occurring in epilepsy, hysteria, and schizophrenia, and sometimes induced with narcotics

¹**twin** \'twin\ *adj* : born with one other or as a pair at one birth ⟨∼ girls⟩

²**twin** *n* : either of two offspring produced at a birth — **twin·ship** \-ˌship\ *n*

twinge \'twinj\ *n* : a sudden sharp stab of pain

twin·ning \'twi-niŋ\ *n* : the bearing of twins

twitch \'twich\ *n* : a short spastic contraction of muscle fibers; *also* : a slight jerk of a body part caused by such a contraction — **twitch** *vb*

two–egg *adj* : DIZYGOTIC ⟨∼ twins⟩

2,4–D \ˌtü-ˌfōr-'dē\ *n* : a white crystalline irritant compound $C_8H_6Cl_2O_3$ used as a weed killer — called also *2,4-dichlorophenoxyacetic acid;* see AGENT ORANGE

2,4,5–T \-ˌfiv-'tē\ *n* : an irritant compound $C_8H_5Cl_3O_3$ used esp. as an herbicide and defoliant — called also *trichlorophenoxyacetic acid;* see AGENT ORANGE

two–winged fly *n* : FLY 2

ty·ba·mate \'tī-bə-ˌmāt\ *n* : a tranquilizing drug $C_{13}H_{26}N_2O_4$

ty·lec·to·my \tī-'lek-tə-mē\ *n, pl* **-mies** : LUMPECTOMY

Ty·le·nol \'tī-lə-ˌnȯl\ *trademark* — used for a preparation of acetaminophen

ty·lo·sin \'tī-lə-sən\ *n* : an antibacterial antibiotic $C_{45}H_{77}NO_{17}$ from an actinomycete of the genus *Streptomyces* (*S. fradiae*) used in veterinary medicine and as a feed additive

ty·lo·sis \tī-'lō-səs\ *n, pl* **ty·lo·ses** \-'lō-sēz\ : a thickening and hardening of the skin : CALLOSITY

tympani — see CHORDA TYMPANI, SCA-LA TYMPANI, TEGMEN TYMPANI, TENSOR TYMPANI

tym·pan·ic \tim-'pa-nik\ *adj* : of, relating to, or being a tympanum

tympanic antrum *n* : a large air-containing cavity in the mastoid process communicating with the tympanum and often being the location of dangerous inflammation — called also *mastoid antrum*

tympanic canal *n* : SCALA TYMPANI

tympanic cavity *n* : MIDDLE EAR

tympanic membrane *n* : a thin membrane that separates the middle ear from the inner part of the external auditory meatus and functions in the mechanical reception of sound waves and in their transmission to the site of sensory reception — called also *eardrum, tympanum*

tympanic nerve *n* : a branch of the glossopharyngeal nerve arising from the petrosal ganglion and entering the middle ear where it takes part in forming the tympanic plexus — called also *Jacobson's nerve*

tympanic plate *n* : a curved platelike bone that is part of the temporal bone and forms the floor and anterior wall of the external auditory meatus

tympanic plexus *n* : a nerve plexus of the middle ear that is formed by the tympanic nerve and two or three filaments from the carotid plexus, sends fibers to the mucous membranes of the middle ear, the eustachian tube, and the mastoid cells, and gives off the lesser petrosal nerve to the otic ganglion

tym·pa·ni·tes \ˌtim-pə-'nī-tēz\ *n* : a distension of the abdomen caused by accumulation of gas in the intestinal tract or peritoneal cavity

tym·pa·nit·ic \ˌtim-pə-'ni-tik\ *adj* **1** : of, relating to, or affected with tympanites ⟨a ∼ abdomen⟩ **2** : resonant on percussion : hollow-sounding

tym·pa·no·plas·ty \'tim-pə-nō-ˌplas-tē\ *n, pl* **-ties** : a reparative surgical operation performed on the middle ear

tym·pa·nos·to·my \ˌtim-pa-'näs-tə-mē\ *n, pl* **-mies** : MYRINGOTOMY

tym·pa·not·o·my \ˌtim-pə-'nä-tə-mē\ *n, pl* **-mies** : MYRINGOTOMY

tym·pa·num \'tim-pə-nəm\ *n, pl* **-na** \-nə\ *also* **-nums 1** : TYMPANIC MEMBRANE **2** : MIDDLE EAR

tym·pa·ny \-nē\ *n, pl* **-nies 1** : TYMPANITES **2** : a resonant sound heard in percussion (as of the abdomen)

¹**type** \'tīp\ *n* : a particular kind, class, or group ⟨personality ∼s⟩; *specif* : a group distinguishable on physiological or serological bases ⟨salmonella ∼s⟩

²**type** *vb* **typed; typ·ing** : to determine the type of (as a sample of blood or a culture of bacteria)

type A *adj* : relating to, characteristic of, having, or being a personality that is marked by impatience, aggressiveness, and competitiveness and that is held to be associated with increased risk of cardiovascular disease

type B *adj* : relating to, characteristic of, having, or being a personality that is marked by a lack of excessive aggressiveness and tension and that is held to be associated with reduced risk of cardiovascular disease

type C *adj* : relating to or being any of the oncornaviruses in which the structure containing the nucleic acid is spherical and centrally located

type I diabetes *n* : INSULIN-DEPENDENT DIABETES MELLITUS — called also *type I diabetes mellitus*

type II diabetes *n* : NON-INSULIN-DEPENDENT DIABETES MELLITUS — called also *type II diabetes mellitus*

¹**ty·phoid** \'tī-ˌfȯid, (ˌ)tī-'-\ *adj* 1 : of, relating to, or suggestive of typhus 2 : of, relating to, affected with, or constituting typhoid fever

²**typhoid** *n* 1 : TYPHOID FEVER 2 : any of several diseases of domestic animals resembling human typhus or typhoid fever

ty·phoi·dal \tī-'fȯid-ᵊl\ *adj* : of, relating to, or resembling typhoid fever

typhoid fever *n* : a communicable disease marked by fever, diarrhea, prostration, headache, splenomegaly, eruption of rose-colored spots, leukopenia, and intestinal inflammation and caused by a bacterium of the genus *Salmonella* (*S. typhi*)

ty·phus \'tī-fəs\ *n* : any of various bacterial diseases caused by rickettsial bacteria: as **a** : a severe human febrile disease that is caused by one (*Rickettsia prowazekii*) transmitted esp. by body lice and is marked by high fever, stupor alternating with delirium, intense headache, and a dark red rash — called also *louse-borne typhus* **b** : MURINE TYPHUS **c** : TSUTSUGAMUSHI DISEASE

typhus fever *n* : TYPHUS

ty·ra·mine \'tī-rə-ˌmēn\ *n* : a phenolic amine $C_8H_{11}NO$ that is found in various foods and beverages (as cheese and red wine), has a sympathomimetic action, and is derived from tyrosine

ty·ro·ci·dine *also* **ty·ro·ci·din** \ˌtī-rə-'sīd-ᵊn\ *n* : a basic polypeptide antibiotic produced by a soil bacterium of the genus *Bacillus* (*B. brevis*) and constituting the major component of tyrothricin

Ty·rode solution \'tī-ˌrōd-\ *or* **Ty·rode's solution** \-ˌrōdz-\ *n* : physiological saline containing sodium chloride 0.8, potassium chloride 0.02, calcium chloride 0.02, magnesium chloride 0.01, sodium bicarbonate 0.1, and sodium dihydrogen phosphate 0.005 percent

Tyrode, Maurice Vejux (1878–1930), American pharmacologist.

ty·ro·sin·ae·mia *chiefly Brit var of* TYROSINEMIA

ty·ro·sine \'tī-rə-ˌsēn\ *n* : a phenolic amino acid $C_9H_{11}NO_3$ that is a precursor of several important substances (as epinephrine and melanin)

tyrosine hydroxylase *n* : an enzyme that catalyzes the first step in the biosynthesis of catecholamines (as dopamine and norepinephrine)

ty·ro·sin·emia \ˌtī-rō-si-'nē-mē-ə\ *n* : a rare inherited disorder of tyrosine metabolism that is characterized by abnormally high concentrations of tyrosine in the blood and urine with associated abnormalities esp. of the liver and kidneys

ty·ro·sin·osis \ˌtī-rō-si-'nō-səs\ *n* : a condition of faulty metabolism of tyrosine marked by the excretion of unusual amounts of tyrosine in the urine

ty·ro·sin·uria \ˌtī-rō-si-'nur-ē-ə, -'nyur-\ *n* : the excretion of tyrosine in the urine

ty·ro·thri·cin \ˌtī-rə-'thrīs-ᵊn\ *n* : an antibiotic mixture that consists chiefly of tyrocidine and gramicidin, is usu. extracted from a soil bacterium of the genus *Bacillus* (*B. brevis*), and is used for local applications esp. for infection caused by gram-positive bacteria

U

¹**U** *abbr* uracil

²**U** *symbol* uranium

ubi·qui·none \yü-'bi-kwə-ˌnōn, ˌyü-bi-kwi-'nōn\ *n* : any of a group of lipid-soluble quinones that function in the part of cellular respiration comprising oxidative phosphorylation

ud·der \'ə-dər\ *n* : a large pendulous organ (as of a cow) consisting of two or more mammary glands enclosed in a common envelope and each provided with a single nipple

¹**ul·cer** \'əl-sər\ *n* : a break in skin or mucous membrane with loss of surface tissue, disintegration and necro-

sis of epithelial tissue, and often pus (a stomach ∼)

²**ulcer** *vb* **ul·cered; ul·cer·ing** : ULCERATE

ul·cer·ate \'əl-sə-ˌrāt\ *vb* **-at·ed; -at·ing** : to become affected with or as if with an ulcer — **ul·cer·ation** \ˌəl-sə-'rā-shən\ *n*

ul·cer·a·tive \'əl-sə-ˌrā-tiv, -rə-\ *adj* : of, relating to, or characterized by an ulcer or by ulceration

ulcerative colitis *n* : a nonspecific inflammatory disease of the colon of unknown cause characterized by diarrhea with discharge of mucus and blood, cramping abdominal pain, and inflammation and edema of the mucous membrane with patches of ulceration

ulcero- *comb form* **1** : ulcer ⟨*ulcero*genic⟩ **2** : ulcerous and ⟨*ulcero*glandular⟩

ul·cero·gen·ic \ˌəl-sə-rō-ˈje-nik\ *adj* : tending to produce or develop into ulcers or ulceration ⟨an ∼ drug⟩

ul·cero·glan·du·lar \ˌəl-sə-rō-ˈglan-jə-lər\ *adj* : being a type of tularemia in which the place of infection is the skin where a papule and then an ulcer develops with enlargement of the lymph nodes in the associated region

ul·cero·mem·bra·nous gingivitis \ˌəl-sə-rō-ˈmem-brə-nəs-\ *n* : VINCENT'S ANGINA

ul·cer·ous \ˈəl-sə-rəs\ *adj* **1** : characterized or caused by ulceration **2** : affected with an ulcer

ul·cus \ˈəl-kəs\ *n, pl* **ul·cera** \ˈəl-sə-rə\ : ULCER

ul·na \ˈəl-nə\ *n, pl* **ul·nae** \-nē\ *or* **ul·nas** : the bone on the little-finger side of the forearm that forms with the humerus the elbow joint and serves as a pivot in rotation of the hand

¹**ul·nar** \ˈəl-nər\ *adj* **1** : of or relating to the ulna **2** : located on the same side of the forearm as the ulna

²**ulnar** *n* : an ulnar anatomical part (as the ulnar nerve or the ulnar artery)

ulnar artery *n* : an artery that is the larger of the two terminal branches of the brachial artery, runs along the ulnar side of the forearm, and gives off near its origin the anterior and posterior ulnar recurrent arteries

ulnar collateral artery — see INFERIOR ULNAR COLLATERAL ARTERY, SUPERIOR ULNAR COLLATERAL ARTERY

ulnaris — see EXTENSOR CARPI ULNARIS, FLEXOR CARPI ULNARIS

ulnar nerve *n* : a large superficial nerve of the arm that is a continuation of the medial cord of the brachial plexus, passes around the elbow superficially in a groove between the olecranon and the medial epicondyle of the humerus, and continues down the inner side of the forearm to supply the skin and muscles of the little-finger side of the forearm and hand — see FUNNY BONE

ulnar notch *n* : the narrow medial concave surface on the lower end of the radius that articulates with the ulna

ulnar recurrent artery *n* : either of the two small branches of the ulnar artery arising from its medial side: **a** : one that arises just below the elbow and supplies the brachialis muscle and the pronator teres — called also *anterior ulnar recurrent artery* **b** : one that is larger, arises lower on the arm, and supplies the elbow and associated muscles — called also *posterior ulnar recurrent artery*

ulnar vein *n* : any of several deep veins of the forearm that accompany the ulnar artery and unite at the elbow with the radial veins to form the brachial veins

ul·tra·cen·tri·fuge \ˌəl-trə-ˈsen-trə-ˌfyüj\ *n* : a high-speed centrifuge able to sediment colloidal and other small particles and used esp. in determining sizes of such particles and molecular weights of large molecules — **ul·tra·cen·trif·u·gal** \-ˌsen-ˈtri-fyə-gəl, -fi-\ *adj* — **ul·tra·cen·tri·fu·ga·tion** \-ˌsen-trə-fyü-ˈgā-shən\ *n* — **ultracentrifuge** *vb*

ul·tra·fil·tra·tion \ˌəl-trə-fil-ˈtrā-shən\ *n* : filtration through a medium (as a semipermeable capillary wall) which allows small molecules (as of water) to pass but holds back larger ones (as of protein) — **ul·tra·fil·tra·ble** \-ˈfil-trə-bəl\ *adj* — **ul·tra·fil·trate** \-ˈfil-ˌtrāt\ *n*

ul·tra·mi·cro·scope \ˌəl-trə-ˈmī-krə-ˌskōp\ *n* : an apparatus for making visible by scattered light particles too small to be perceived by the ordinary microscope — called also *dark-field microscope* — **ul·tra·mi·cros·co·py** \-mī-ˈkräs-kə-pē\ *n*

ul·tra·mi·cro·scop·ic \-ˌmī-krə-ˈskä-pik\ *also* **ul·tra·mi·cro·scop·i·cal** \-pi-kəl\ *adj* **1** : too small to be seen with an ordinary microscope — compare MACROSCOPIC, MICROSCOPIC 2, SUBMICROSCOPIC **2** : of or relating to an ultramicroscope — **ul·tra·mi·cro·scop·i·cal·ly** *adv*

ul·tra·mi·cro·tome \-ˈmī-krə-ˌtōm\ *n* : a microtome for cutting extremely thin sections for electron microscopy — **ul·tra·mi·crot·o·my** \-mī-ˈkrä-tə-mē\ *n*

ul·tra·son·ic \ˈsä-nik\ *adj* **1** : SUPERSONIC: **a** : having a frequency above the human ear's audibility limit of about 20,000 cycles per second — used of waves and vibrations **b** : utilizing, produced by, or relating to ultrasonic waves or vibrations (removal of tartar with an ∼ scaler) **2** : ULTRASOUND — **ul·tra·son·i·cal·ly** *adv*

ul·tra·sono·gram \-ˈsä-nə-ˌgram\ *n* : ECHOGRAM

ul·tra·so·nog·ra·pher \ˌəl-trə-sə-ˈnä-grə-fər\ *n* : a specialist in the use of ultrasound

ul·tra·so·nog·ra·phy \-fē\ *n, pl* **-phies** : ULTRASOUND 2 — **ul·tra·so·no·graph·ic** \ˌsä-nə-ˈgra-fik, -ˌsō-\ *adj*

¹**ul·tra·sound** \ˈəl-trə-ˌsaúnd\ *n* **1** : vibrations of the same physical nature as sound but with frequencies above the range of human hearing **2** : the diagnostic or therapeutic use of ultrasound and esp. a technique involving the formation of a two-dimensional image used for the examination and measurement of internal body structures and the detection of bodily abnormalities — called also *echography, sonography, ultrasonography* **3** : a diagnostic examination using ultrasound

²**ultrasound** *adj* : of, relating to, per-

formed by, using, or expert in ultrasound ⟨an ∼ technician⟩ ⟨∼ imaging⟩

ul·tra·vi·o·let \ˌəl-trə-ˈvī-ə-lət\ *adj* **1** : situated beyond the visible spectrum at its violet end — used of radiation having a wavelength shorter than wavelengths of visible light and longer than those of X rays **2** : relating to, producing, or employing ultraviolet radiation — **ultraviolet** *n*

ultraviolet microscope *n* : a microscope equipped to irradiate material under examination with ultraviolet radiation in order to detect or study fluorescent components — called also *fluorescence microscope*

um·bi·lec·to·my \ˌəm-bi-ˈlek-tə-mē\ *n*, *pl* **-mies** : OMPHALECTOMY

um·bil·i·cal \ˌəm-ˈbi-li-kəl\ *adj* **1** : of, relating to, or used at the umbilicus ⟨∼ infection⟩ **2** : of or relating to the central abdominal region that is situated between the right and left lumbar regions and between the epigastric region above and the hypogastric region below

umbilical artery *n* : either of a pair of arteries that arise from the fetal hypogastric arteries and pass through the umbilical cord to the placenta to which they carry the deoxygenated blood from the fetus

umbilical cord *n* : a cord arising from the navel that connects the fetus with the placenta and contains the two umbilical arteries and the umbilical vein

umbilical hernia *n* : a hernia of abdominal viscera at the umbilicus

umbilical ligament — see MEDIAL UMBILICAL LIGAMENT, MEDIAN UMBILICAL LIGAMENT

umbilical vein *n* : a vein that passes through the umbilical cord to the fetus and returns the oxygenated and nutrient blood from the placenta to the fetus

umbilical vesicle *n* : the yolk sac of a mammalian embryo having a transitory connection with the alimentary canal by way of the omphalomesenteric duct

um·bil·i·cat·ed \ˌəm-ˈbi-lə-ˌkā-təd\ *adj* : having a small depression that resembles an umbilicus ⟨∼ vesicles⟩ — **um·bil·i·cate** \-ˌkāt\ *vb*

um·bi·li·cus \ˌəm-bə-ˈlī-kəs, ˌəm-ˈbi-li-\ *n*, *pl* **um·bi·li·ci** \ˌəm-bə-ˈlī-ˌkī, -ˌsī; ˌəm-ˈbi-lə-ˌkī, -ˌkē\ *or* **um·bi·li·cus·es** : NAVEL

um·bo \ˈəm-(ˌ)bō\ *n*, *pl* **um·bo·nes** \ˌəm-ˈbō-(ˌ)nēz\ *or* **um·bos** : an elevation in the tympanic membrane of the ear

un·anes·the·tized \ˌən-ə-ˈnes-thə-ˌtīzd\ *adj* : not having been subjected to an anesthetic

un·bal·anced \ˌən-ˈba-lənst\ *adj* : mentally disordered or deranged

un·blind·ed \-ˈblin-dəd\ *adj* : made or done with knowledge of significant facts by the participants : not blind ⟨an ∼ study of a drug's effectiveness⟩

un·born \-ˈbȯrn\ *adj* : not yet born : existing in utero ⟨∼ children⟩

un·bro·ken \-ˈbrō-kən\ *adj* : not broken ⟨∼ skin⟩ ⟨an ∼ blister⟩

un·cal \ˈəŋ-kəl\ *adj* : of or relating to the uncus ⟨the ∼ region⟩

un·cal·ci·fied \ˌən-ˈkal-sə-ˌfīd\ *adj* : not calcified ⟨∼ osteoid tissue⟩

uncal herniation *n* : downward displacement of the uncus and adjacent structures into the tentorial notch

unci *pl of* UNCUS

un·ci·form \ˈən-sə-ˌfȯrm\ *n* : HAMATE

unciform bone *n* : HAMATE

Un·ci·nar·ia \ˌən-sə-ˈnar-ē-ə\ *n* : a genus of hookworms (family Ancylostomatidae) now usu. restricted to a few parasites of carnivorous mammals but formerly included most of the common hookworms

un·ci·nate fasciculus \ˈən-sə-ˌnāt-\ *n* : a hook-shaped bundle of long association fibers connecting the frontal lobe with the anterior portion of the temporal lobe

uncinate fit *n* : a psychomotor epileptic seizure that is characterized by hallucinations of taste and odor and disturbances of consciousness that originates in the region of the uncus

un·cir·cum·cised \ˌən-ˈsər-kəm-ˌsīzd\ *adj* : not circumcised

un·com·pen·sat·ed \-ˈkäm-pən-ˌsā-təd, -ˌpen-\ *adj* **1** : accompanied by a change in the pH of the blood ⟨∼ acidosis⟩ ⟨∼ alkalosis⟩ — compare COMPENSATED **2** : not corrected or affected by physiological compensation ⟨∼ congestive heart failure⟩

un·com·pli·cat·ed \ˌən-ˈkäm-plə-ˌkā-təd\ *adj* : not involving or marked by complications ⟨∼ peptic ulcer⟩

un·con·di·tion·al \ˌən-kən-ˈdi-shə-nəl\ *adj* : UNCONDITIONED 2

un·con·di·tioned \-ˈdi-shənd\ *adj* **1** : not dependent on or subjected to conditioning or learning **2** : producing an unconditioned response

¹un·con·scious \ˌən-ˈkän-chəs\ *adj* **1** : not marked by conscious thought, sensation, or feeling ⟨∼ motivation⟩ **2** : of or relating to the unconscious **3** : having lost consciousness ⟨was ∼ for three days⟩ — **un·con·scious·ly** *adv* — **un·con·scious·ness** *n*

²unconscious *n* : the greater part of the psychic apparatus accumulated through life experience that is not ordinarily integrated or available to consciousness yet is manifested as a powerful motive force in overt behavior esp. in neurosis and is often revealed (as through dreams, slips of the tongue, or dissociated acts) — compare SUBCONSCIOUS

un·con·trolled \ˌən-kən-ˈtrōld\ *adj* : not being under control ⟨∼ diabetes⟩

un·co·or·di·nat·ed \-kō-ˈȯrd-ᵊn-ˌā-təd\ *adj* : not coordinated : lacking proper or effective coordination ⟨∼ muscles⟩

un·crossed \-'kròst\ *adj* : not forming a decussation ⟨an ∼ tract of nerve fibers⟩

unc·tu·ous \'ǝŋk-chǝ-wǝs, -shǝ-\ *adj* : rich in oil or fat ⟨FATTY

un·cur·able \ǝn-'kyúr-ǝ-bǝl\ *adj* : IN-CURABLE

un·cus \'ǝŋ-kǝs\ *n, pl* **un·ci** \'ǝn-ˌsī\ : a hooked anatomical part or process; *specif* : the anterior curved end of the hippocampal gyrus

un·de·cyl·en·ic acid \ˌǝn-ˌde-sǝ-'le-nik-, -ˌlē-\ *n* : an acid $C_{11}H_{20}O_2$ used in the treatment of fungal infections (as ringworm) of the skin

¹**un·der** \'ǝn-dǝr\ *adv* : in or into a condition of unconsciousness ⟨put the patient ∼ prior to surgery⟩

²**under** *prep* : receiving or using the action or application of ⟨an operation performed ∼ local anesthesia⟩

³**under** *adj* : being in an induced state of unconsciousness

un·der·achiev·er \ˌǝn-dǝr-ǝ-'chē-vǝr\ *n* : a person and esp. a student who fails to achieve his or her potential or does not do as well as expected — **un·der·achieve** \-'chēv\ *vb* — **un·der·achieve·ment** \-mǝnt\ *n*

un·der·ac·tive \-'ak-tiv\ *adj* : characterized by an abnormally low level of activity ⟨an ∼ thyroid gland⟩ — **un·der·ac·tiv·i·ty** \-ak-'ti-vǝ-tē\ *n*

un·der·arm \'ǝn-dǝr-ˌärm\ *n* : ARMPIT

un·der·cut \'ǝn-dǝr-ˌkǝt\ *n* : the part of a tooth lying between the gum and the points of maximum outward bulge on the tooth's surfaces

un·der·de·vel·oped \ˌǝn-dǝr-di-'ve-lǝpt\ *adj* : not normally or adequately developed ⟨∼ muscles⟩ — **un·der·de·vel·op·ment** \-ǝp-mǝnt\ *n*

un·der·dos·age \-'dō-sij\ *n* : the administration or taking of an insufficient dose ⟨∼ of a drug⟩

un·der·feed \ˌǝn-dǝr-'fēd\ *vb* -**fed** \-'fed\ ; -**feed·ing** : to feed with too little food

un·der·nour·ished \ˌǝn-dǝr-'nǝr-isht\ *adj* : supplied with less than the minimum amount of the foods essential for sound health and growth — **un·der·nour·ish·ment** \-'nǝr-ish-mǝnt\ *n*

un·der·nu·tri·tion \-nü-'tri-shǝn, -nyü-\ *n* : deficient bodily nutrition due to inadequate food intake or faulty assimilation — **un·der·nu·tri·tion·al** \-shǝ-nǝl\ *adj*

un·der·sexed \-'sekst\ *adj* : deficient in sexual desire

un·der·shot \'ǝn-dǝr-ˌshät\ *adj* : having the lower incisor teeth or lower jaw projecting beyond the upper when the mouth is closed — used chiefly of animals

un·der·tak·er \'ǝn-dǝr-ˌtā-kǝr\ *n* : one whose business is to prepare the dead for burial and to arrange and manage funerals — called also *mortician*

un·der·ven·ti·la·tion \ˌǝn-dǝr-ˌven-ti-'lā-shǝn\ *n* : HYPOVENTILATION

un·der·weight \-'wāt\ *adj* : weighing less than the normal amount

un·de·scend·ed \ˌǝn-di-'sen-dǝd\ *adj* : retained within the inguinal region rather than descending into the scrotum ⟨an ∼ testis⟩

un·de·vel·oped \ˌǝn-di-'ve-lǝpt\ *adj* : lacking in development : not developed ⟨physiologically ∼⟩

un·di·ag·nos·able \-di-ig-'nō-sǝ-bǝl\ *adj* : not capable of being diagnosed

un·di·ag·nosed \-'nōst\ *adj* : not diagnosed : eluding diagnosis ⟨∼ disease⟩

un·dif·fer·en·ti·at·ed \-ˌdi-fǝ-'ren-chē-ˌā-tǝd\ *adj* : not differentiated ⟨an ∼ sarcoma⟩

un·di·gest·ed \ˌǝn-dī-'jes-tǝd\ *adj* : not digested ⟨∼ food⟩

un·di·gest·ible \-dī-'jes-tǝ-bǝl\ *adj* : not capable of being digested

un·du·lant fever \'ǝn-jǝ-lǝnt-, -dyǝ-\ *n* : BRUCELLOSIS

un·erupt·ed \ˌǝn-i-'rǝp-tǝd\ *adj, of a tooth* : not yet having emerged through the gum

un·fer·til·ized \-'fǝrt-ᵊl-ˌīzd\ *adj* : not fertilized ⟨an ∼ egg⟩

ung *abbr* [Latin *unguentum*] ointment — used in writing prescriptions

un·gual \'ǝŋ-gwǝl, 'ǝn-\ *adj* : of or relating to a fingernail or toenail

un·guent \'ǝŋ-gwǝnt, 'ǝn-jǝnt\ *n* : a soothing or healing salve : OINTMENT

un·guis \'ǝŋ-gwǝs, 'ǝn-\ *n, pl* **un·gues** \-ˌgwēz\ : a fingernail or toenail

un·gu·late \'ǝŋ-gyǝ-lǝt, 'ǝn-, -ˌlāt\ *n* : a hoofed typically herbivorous quadruped mammal (as a ruminant, swine, camel, or horse) of an evolutionarily diverse group formerly considered a major mammalian taxon (Ungulata) — **ungulate** *adj*

Unh *symbol* unnilhexium

un·healed \ˌǝn-'hēld\ *adj* : not healed

un·health·ful \-'helth-fǝl\ *adj* : detrimental to good health ⟨∼ working conditions⟩ — **un·health·ful·ness** *n*

un·healthy \-'hel-thē\ *adj* **un·health·i·er** ; -**est** **1** : not conducive to health ⟨an ∼ climate⟩ **2** : not in good health : SICKLY — **un·health·i·ness** *n*

un·hy·gi·en·ic \ˌǝn-ˌhī-'je-nik, -'jē-, -jē-'e-\ *adj* : not healthful or sanitary — **un·hy·gi·en·i·cal·ly** \-ni-k(ǝ-)lē\ *adv*

uni·cel·lu·lar \ˌyü-ni-'sel-yǝ-lǝr\ *adj* : having or consisting of a single cell ⟨∼ organisms⟩ — **uni·cel·lu·lar·i·ty** \-ˌsel-yǝ-'lar-ǝ-tē\ *n*

uni·fo·cal \ˌyü-ni-'fō-kǝl\ *adj* : arising from or occurring in a single focus or location ⟨∼ infection⟩

uni·la·mel·lar \ˌyü-ni-lǝ-'me-lǝr\ *adj* : having only one lamella or layer

uni·lat·er·al \ˌyü-ni-'la-tǝ-rǝl\ *adj* : occurring on, performed on, or affecting one side of the body or one of its parts ⟨∼ exophthalmos⟩ — **uni·lat·er·al·ly** *adv*

uni·loc·u·lar \ˌyü-ni-'lä-kyǝ-lǝr\ *adj* : containing a single cavity

un·im·mu·nized \(ˌ)ən-ˈi-myə-ˌnīzd\ *adj* : not immunized

un·in·fect·ed \ˌən-in-ˈfek-təd\ *adj* : free from infection ⟨an ∼ fracture⟩

uni·nu·cle·ate \ˌyü-ni-ˈnü-klē-ət, -ˈnyü-\ *also* **uni·nu·cle·at·ed** \-ˌā-təd\ *adj* : having a single nucleus : MONONUCLEAR

union \ˈyü-nyən\ *n* : an act or instance of uniting or joining two or more things into one: as **a** : the growing together of severed parts ⟨∼ of a fractured bone⟩ **b** : the joining of two germ cells in the process of fertilization

uni·ovu·lar \ˌyü-nē-ˈä-vyə-lər\ *adj* : MONOZYGOTIC ⟨∼ twins⟩

unip·a·ra \yü-ˈni-pə-rə\ *n, pl* **-ras** *or* **-rae** : a woman who has borne one child

uni·pen·nate \ˌyü-ni-ˈpe-ˌnāt\ *adj* : having the fibers arranged obliquely and inserting into a tendon on one side only in the manner of a feather barbed on one side ⟨a ∼ muscle⟩

uni·po·lar \ˌyü-ni-ˈpō-lər\ *adj* **1** : having, produced by, or acting by a single magnetic or electrical pole ⟨a ∼ ECG lead⟩ **2** : having but one process ⟨a ∼ neuron⟩ **3** : relating to or being a manic-depressive disorder in which there is a depressive phase only ⟨∼ depressive illness⟩

un·ir·ra·di·at·ed \ˌun-ir-ˈā-dē-ˌā-təd\ *adj* : not having been exposed to radiation ⟨∼ lymphocytes⟩

unit \ˈyü-nət\ *n* **1** : an amount of a biologically active agent (as a drug or antigen) required to produce a specific result under strictly controlled conditions ⟨a ∼ of penicillin⟩ **2** : a molecule or portion of a molecule esp. as combined in a larger molecule

unit·age \ˈyü-nə-tij\ *n* **1** : specification of the amount constituting a unit (as of a vitamin) **2** : amount in units ⟨a ∼ of 50,000 per capsule⟩

unit membrane *n* : a 3-layered membrane that consists of an inner lipid layer surrounded by a protein layer on each side

¹uni·va·lent \ˌyü-ni-ˈvā-lənt\ *n* : a chromosome that lacks a synaptic mate

²univalent *adj* **1** : MONOVALENT 1 **2** : being a chromosomal univalent **3** *of an antibody* : capable of agglutinating or precipitating but not both : having only one combining group

universal antidote *n* : an antidote for ingested poisons having activated charcoal as its principal ingredient

universal donor *n* **1** : the blood group O characterized by a serum that does not agglutinate the cells of any other ABO blood group **2 a** : a person with blood group O blood **b** : the blood of such a person

universal recipient *n* **1** : the blood group AB characterized by a serum that is not agglutinated by any other ABO blood group **2 a** : a person with blood

group AB blood **b** : the blood of such a person

un·la·beled *or* **un·la·belled** \ˌən-ˈlā-bəld\ *adj* : not labeled esp. with an isotopic label

un·la·bored \ˌən-ˈlā-bərd\ *adj* : produced without exertion, pain, or undue effort ⟨∼ breathing⟩

un·my·elin·at·ed \-ˈmī-ə-lə-ˌnā-təd\ *adj* : lacking a myelin sheath ⟨∼ axons⟩

Un·na's boot \ˈü-nəz-\ *or* **Un·na boot** \-nə-\ *n* : a compression dressing for varicose veins or ulcers consisting of a paste made of zinc oxide, gelatin, glycerin, and water

    Unna, Paul Gerson (1850–1929), German dermatologist.

Unna's paste boot *n* : UNNA'S BOOT

un·nil·hex·i·um \ˌyün-əl-ˈhek-sē-əm\ *n* : the chemical element of atomic number 106 — symbol *Unh;* see ELEMENT table

un·nil·pen·ti·um \ˌyün-əl-ˈpen-tē-əm\ *n* : the chemical element of atomic number 105 — symbol *Unp;* see ELEMENT table

un·nil·qua·di·um \ˌyün-əl-ˈkwä-dē-əm\ *n* : the chemical element of atomic number 104 — symbol *Unq;* see ELEMENT table

un·of·fi·cial \ˌən-ə-ˈfi-shəl\ *adj* : not official; *specif* : of, relating to, or being a drug not described in the *U.S. Pharmacopeia* and *National Formulary* — compare NONOFFICIAL, OFFICIAL

un·os·si·fied \-ˈä-sə-ˌfīd\ *adj* : not ossified

un·ox·y·gen·at·ed \-ˈäk-si-jə-ˌnā-təd, -äk-ˈsi-jə-\ *adj* : not oxygenated ⟨∼ blood⟩

Unp *symbol* unnilpentium

un·paired \-ˈpard\ *adj* **1 a** : not paired; *esp* : not matched or mated **b** : characterized by the absence of pairing ⟨electrons in the ∼ state⟩ **2** : situated in the median plane of the body ⟨an ∼ anatomical part⟩; *also* : not matched by a corresponding part on the opposite side

un·pig·ment·ed \-ˈpig-mən-təd\ *adj* : not pigmented : having no pigment

Unq *symbol* unnilquadium

un·re·ac·tive \-rē-ˈak-tiv\ *adj* : not reactive ⟨pupils ∼ to light⟩

un·re·solved \-ri-ˈzälvd, -ˈzólvd\ *adj* : not resolved : not having undergone resolution ⟨∼ pneumonia⟩

un·re·spon·sive \ˌən-ri-ˈspän-siv\ *adj* : not responsive (as to a stimulus or treatment) — **un·re·spon·sive·ness** *n*

un·san·i·tary \-ˈsa-nə-ˌter-ē\ *adj* : not sanitary : INSANITARY ⟨∼ conditions⟩

un·sat·u·rate \-ˈsa-chə-rət\ *n* : an unsaturated chemical compound

un·sat·u·rat·ed \-ˈsa-chə-ˌrā-təd\ *adj* : not saturated: as **a** : capable of absorbing or dissolving more of something ⟨an ∼ solution⟩ **b** : able to form products by chemical addition; *esp* : containing double or triple bonds between carbon atoms ⟨∼ oils⟩ — **un·sat·u·ra·tion** \-ˌsa-chə-ˈrā-shən\ n

un·seg·ment·ed \-ˈseg-ˌmen-təd\ adj : not divided or made up of segments

un·sound \-ˈsau̇nd\ adj : not sound: as **a** : not healthy or whole ⟨an ∼ limb⟩ **b** : not mentally normal : not wholly sane ⟨of ∼ mind⟩ **c** : not fit to be eaten ⟨∼ food⟩ — **un·sound·ness** n

un·sta·ble \-ˈstā-bəl\ adj : not stable: as **a** : characterized by frequent or unpredictable changes ⟨a patient in ∼ condition⟩ **b** : readily changing in chemical composition or biological activity **c** : characterized by inability to control the emotions

unstable angina n : angina pectoris characterized by sudden changes (as an increase in the severity or length of anginal attacks or a decrease in the exertion required to precipitate an attack) esp. when symptoms were previously stable

un·stri·at·ed muscle \ˌən-ˈstrī-ˌā-təd-\ n : SMOOTH MUSCLE

un·struc·tured \-ˈstrək-chərd\ adj : lacking structure : not formally organized ⟨∼ psychological tests⟩

un·trau·ma·tized \-ˈtrau̇-mə-ˌtīzd, -ˈtrȯ-\ adj : not subjected to trauma ⟨∼ skin⟩

un·treat·ed \-ˈtrē-təd\ adj : not subjected to treatment ⟨an ∼ disease⟩ — **un·treat·able** \-ˈtrē-tə-bəl\ adj

un·vac·ci·nat·ed \-ˈvak-sə-ˌnā-təd\ adj : not vaccinated ⟨∼ children⟩

un·well \-ˈwel\ adj **1** : being in poor health : SICK **2** : undergoing menstruation

¹**up·per** \ˈə-pər\ n : an upper tooth or denture

²**upper** n : a stimulant drug; esp : AMPHETAMINE

upper jaw n : JAW 1a

upper respiratory adj : of, relating to, or affecting the upper respiratory tract ⟨upper respiratory infection⟩

upper respiratory tract n : the part of the respiratory system including the nose, nasal passages, and nasopharynx — compare LOWER RESPIRATORY TRACT

up·set \ˈəp-ˌset\ n **1** : a minor physical disorder ⟨a stomach ∼⟩ **2** : an emotional disturbance — **upset** \ˌ(ˌ)əp-ˈset\ vb — **upset** \ˈəp-ˌset\ adj

up·stream \ˌəp-ˈstrēm\ adv or adj : in a direction along a molecule of DNA or RNA opposite to that in which transcription and translation take place and toward the end having a hydroxyl group attached to the position labeled 5′ in the terminal nucleotide — compare DOWNSTREAM

up·take \ˈəp-ˌtāk\ n : an act or instance of absorbing and incorporating something esp. into a living organism

ur- or **uro-** comb form **1** : urine ⟨uric⟩ **2** : urinary tract ⟨urology⟩ **3** : urinary and ⟨urogenital⟩ **4** : urea ⟨uracil⟩

ura·chal \ˈyu̇r-ə-kəl\ adj : of or relating to the urachus ⟨a ∼ cyst⟩

ura·chus \-kəs\ n : a cord of fibrous tissue extending from the bladder to the umbilicus and constituting the functionless remnant of a part of the duct of the allantois of the embryo

ura·cil \ˈyu̇r-ə-ˌsil, -səl\ n : a pyrimidine base $C_4H_4N_2O_2$ that is one of the four bases coding genetic information in the polynucleotide chain of RNA — compare ADENINE, CYTOSINE, GUANINE, THYMINE

ur·ae·mia chiefly Brit var of UREMIA

ura·ni·um \yu̇-ˈrā-nē-əm\ n : a silvery heavy radioactive metallic element that exists naturally as a mixture of three isotopes of mass number 234, 235, and 238 — symbol U; see ELEMENT table

uranium 235 n : a light isotope of uranium of mass number 235 that is physically separable from natural uranium and that when bombarded with slow neutrons undergoes rapid fission into smaller atoms with the release of neutrons and atomic energy

urate \ˈyu̇r-ˌāt\ n : a salt of uric acid

ure- or **ureo-** comb form : urea ⟨urease⟩

urea \yu̇-ˈrē-ə\ n : a soluble weakly basic nitrogenous compound CH_4N_2O that is the chief solid component of mammalian urine and an end product of protein decomposition and that is administered intravenously as a diuretic drug

urea·plas·ma \yu̇-ˈrē-ə-ˌplaz-mə\ n **1** cap : a genus of mycoplasmas (family Mycoplasmataceae) that are able to hydrolyze urea with the formation of ammonia and that include one (U. urealyticum) found in the human genitourinary tract, oropharynx, and anal canal **2** : a mycoplasma of the genus Ureaplasma

ure·ase \ˈyu̇r-ē-ˌās, -ˌāz\ n : an enzyme that catalyzes the hydrolysis of urea into ammonia and carbon dioxide

Ure·cho·line \ˌyu̇r-ə-ˈkō-ˌlēn\ trademark — used for a preparation of bethanechol

ure·mia \yu̇-ˈrē-mē-ə\ n **1** : accumulation in the blood of constituents normally eliminated in the urine that produces a severe toxic condition and usu. occurs in severe kidney disease associated with uremia — **ure·mic** \-mik\ adj **2** : the toxic bodily condition associated with uremia — **ure·mic** \-mik\ adj

ure·ter \ˈyu̇r-ə-tər, yu̇-ˈrē-tər\ n : either of the paired ducts that carry away urine from a kidney to the bladder or cloaca and that in humans are slender membranous epithelium-lined flat tubes about sixteen inches (41 centimeters) long which open above into the pelvis of a kidney and below into the back part of the same side of the bladder — **ure·ter·al** \yu̇-ˈrē-tə-rəl\ or **ure·ter·ic** \ˌyu̇r-ə-ˈter-ik\ adj

ure·ter·ec·ta·sis \ˌyu̇r-ə-tər-ˈek-tə-səs,

yū-₁rē-tər-\ *n, pl* **-ta·ses** \-₁sēz\ : dilation of a ureter

ure·ter·ec·to·my \₁yùr-ə-tər-'ek-tə-mē, yū-₁rē-tər-\ *n, pl* **-mies** : surgical excision of all or part of a ureter

ure·ter·itis \₁yùr-ə-tər-'ī-təs, yū-₁rē-tər-\ *n* : inflammation of a ureter

uretero- *comb form* **1** : ureter ⟨*ureter-ography*⟩ **2** : ureteral and ⟨*uretero-ileal*⟩

ure·ter·o·cele \yū-'rē-tə-rə-₁sēl\ *n* : cystic dilation of the lower part of a ureter into the bladder

ure·ter·o·en·ter·os·to·my \₁yū-₁rē-tə-rō-₁en-tə-'räs-tə-mē\ *n, pl* **-mies** : surgical formation of an artificial opening between a ureter and the intestine

ure·ter·o·gram \yū-'rē-tə-rə-₁gram\ *n* : an X-ray photograph of the ureters after injection of a radiopaque substance — **ure·ter·og·ra·phy** \yū-₁rē-tə-'rä-grə-fē, ₁yùr-ə-tə-\ *n*

ure·ter·o·il·e·al \yū-₁rē-tə-rō-'i-lē-əl\ *adj* : relating to or connecting a ureter and the ileum

ure·ter·o·lith·ot·o·my \yū-₁rē-tə-rō-li-'thä-tə-mē\ *n, pl* **-mies** : removal of a calculus by incision of a ureter

ure·ter·ol·y·sis \₁yùr-ə-tər-'ä-lə-səs, yū-₁rē-tər-\ *n, pl* **-yses** \-₁sēz\ : a surgical procedure to free a ureter from abnormal adhesions or surrounding tissue (as in retroperitoneal fibrosis)

ure·ter·o·neo·cys·tos·to·my \yū-₁rē-tər-ō-₁nē-ō-sis-'täs-tə-mē\ *n, pl* **-mies** : surgical reimplantation of a ureter into the bladder

ure·ter·o·pel·vic \yū-₁rē-tə-rō-'pel-vik\ *adj* : of, relating to, or involving a ureter and the adjoining renal pelvis ⟨∼ obstruction⟩

ure·ter·o·plas·ty \yū-'rē-tə-rə-₁plas-tē\ *n, pl* **-ties** : a plastic operation performed on a ureter

ure·ter·o·py·elog·ra·phy \yū-₁rē-tə-rō-₁pī-ə-'lä-grə-fē\ *n, pl* **-phies** : X-ray photography of a renal pelvis and a ureter following the injection of a radiopaque medium

ure·ter·o·py·elo·ne·os·to·my \yū-₁rē-tər-ō-₁pī-ə-lō-nē-'äs-tə-mē\ *n, pl* **-mies** : surgical creation of a new channel joining a renal pelvis to a ureter

ure·ter·o·py·e·los·to·my \-₁pī-ə-'läs-tə-mē\ *n, pl* **-mies** : URETEROPYELONEOSTOMY

ure·ter·or·rha·phy \yū-₁rē-tə-'ror-ə-fē, ₁yùr-ə-tə-\ *n, pl* **-phies** : the surgical operation of suturing a ureter

ure·ter·os·co·py \yū-₁rē-tə-'räs-kə-pē, ₁yùr-ə-tə-\ *n, pl* **-pies** : visual examination of the interior of a ureter

ure·ter·o·sig·moid·os·to·my \yū-₁rē-tə-rō-₁sig-₁mȯi-'däs-tə-mē\ *n, pl* **-mies** : surgical implantation of a ureter in the sigmoid flexure

ure·ter·os·to·my \₁yùr-ə-tər-'äs-tə-mē, yū-₁rē-tər-\ *n, pl* **-mies** : surgical creation of an opening on the surface of the body for the ureters

ure·ter·ot·o·my \₁yùr-ə-tər-'ä-tə-mē,

yū-₁rē-tər-\ *n, pl* **-mies** : the operation of cutting into a ureter

ure·tero·ure·ter·os·to·my \yū-₁rē-tə-rō-yū-₁rē-tər-'äs-tə-mē\ *n, pl* **-mies** : surgical establishment of an artificial communication between two ureters or between different parts of the same ureter

ure·tero·ves·i·cal \yū-₁rē-tə-rō-'ve-si-kəl\ *adj* : of or relating to the ureters and the urinary bladder

ure·thane \'yùr-ə-₁thān\ *or* **ure·than** \-₁than\ *n* : a crystalline compound $C_3H_7NO_2$ that is used esp. as a solvent and medicinally as an antineoplastic agent — called also *ethyl carbamate*

urethr- *or* **urethro-** *comb form* : urethra ⟨*urethr*itis⟩ ⟨*urethro*scope⟩

ure·thra \yū-'rē-thrə\ *n, pl* **-thras** *or* **-thrae** \-(₁)thrē\ : the canal that carries off the urine from the bladder and in the male serves also as a genital duct — **ure·thral** \-thrəl\ *adj*

urethral crest *n* : a narrow longitudinal fold or ridge along the posterior wall or floor of the female urethra or the prostatic portion of the male urethra

urethral gland *n* : any of the small mucous glands in the wall of the urethra — see GLAND OF LITTRÉ

urethral intercourse *n* : sexual intercourse in which the penis is inserted into the female urethra

urethral sphincter *n* : SPHINCTER URETHRAE

ure·threc·to·my \₁yùr-i-'threk-tə-mē\ *n, pl* **-mies** : total or partial surgical excision of the urethra

ure·thri·tis \₁yùr-i-'thrī-təs\ *n* : inflammation of the urethra

ure·thro·cele \yə-'rē-thrə-₁sēl\ *n* : a pouched protrusion of urethral mucous membrane in the female

ure·thro·cu·ta·ne·ous \yū-₁rē-thrō-kyū-'tā-nē-əs\ *adj* : of, relating to, or joining the urethra and the skin

ure·thro·cys·tog·ra·phy \yū-₁rē-thrō-sis-'tä-grə-fē\ *n, pl* **-phies** : roentgenography of the urethra and bladder that utilizes a radiopaque substance

ure·throg·ra·phy \₁yùr-i-'thrä-grə-fē\ *n, pl* **-phies** : roentgenography of the urethra after injection of a radiopaque substance

ure·thro·pexy \yū-'rē-thrə-₁pek-sē\ *n, pl* **-pex·ies** : surgical fixation to nearby tissue of a displaced urethra that is causing incontinence by placing stress on the opening from the bladder

ure·thro·plas·ty \yū-'rē-thrə-₁plas-tē\ *n, pl* **-ties** : plastic surgery of the urethra

ure·thro·rec·tal \yū-₁rē-thrō-'rekt-əl\ *adj* : of, relating to, or joining the urethra and the rectum ⟨a ∼ fistula⟩

ure·thror·rha·phy \₁yùr-ə-'thrȯr-ə-fē\ *n, pl* **-phies** : suture of the urethra for an injury or fistula

ure·thro·scope \yū-'rē-thrə-₁skōp\ *n*

: an instrument for viewing the interior of the urethra — **ure·thro·scop·ic** \yü-ˌrē-thrə-ˈskä-pik\ *adj* — **ure·thros·co·py** \ˌyür-ə-ˈthräs-kə-pē\ *n*

ure·thros·to·my \ˌyür-ə-ˈthräs-tə-mē\ *n, pl* **-mies** : the creation of a surgical opening between the perineum and the urethra

ure·throt·o·my \ˌyür-ə-ˈthrä-tə-mē\ *n, pl* **-mies** : surgical incision into the urethra esp. for the relief of stricture

ure·thro·vag·i·nal \yü-ˌrē-thrō-ˈva-jən-ᵊl\ *adj* : of, relating to, or joining the urethra and the vagina ⟨a ~ fistula⟩

ur·gen·cy \ˈər-jən-sē\ *n, pl* **-cies** : a compelling desire to urinate or defecate due to some abnormal stress

ur·gin·ea \ər-ˈji-nē-ə\ *n* **1** *cap* : a genus of bulbous herbs native to the Old World and esp. to the Mediterranean region — see SQUILL 2 *often cap* : squill for medicinal use composed of the sliced young bulbs of the squill (*Urginea indica*) of the Orient — used in the British Pharmacopoeia

URI *abbr* upper respiratory infection

-uria \ˈyür-ē-ə, ˈur-\ *n comb form* **1** : presence of (a specified substance) in urine ⟨albumin*uria*⟩ **2** : condition of having (such) urine ⟨poly*uria*⟩; *esp* : abnormal or diseased condition marked by the presence of (a specified substance) ⟨py*uria*⟩

uric \ˈyür-ik\ *adj* : of, relating to, or found in urine

uric- *or* **urico-** *comb form* : uric acid ⟨*urico*suric⟩

uric acid *n* : a white odorless and tasteless nearly insoluble acid $C_5H_4N_4O_3$ that is present in small quantity in human urine and occurs pathologically in renal calculi and the tophi of gout

uric·ac·id·uria \ˌyür-ik-ˌa-sə-ˈdür-ē-ə, -ˈdyür-\ *n* : the presence of excess uric acid in the urine

uri·cae·mia *chiefly Brit var of* URICEMIA

uri·ce·mia \ˌyür-ə-ˈsē-mē-ə\ *n* : HYPERURICEMIA — **uri·ce·mic** \-mik\ *adj*

uri·co·su·ric \ˌyür-i-kō-ˈsür-ik, -ˈsyür-\ *adj* : relating to or promoting the excretion of uric acid in the urine

uri·dine \ˈyür-ə-ˌdēn\ *n* : a pyrimidine nucleoside $C_9H_{12}N_2O_6$ that is composed of uracil attached to ribose and plays an important role in carbohydrate metabolism

urin- *or* **urino-** *comb form* : UR- ⟨*uri*nary⟩

urinae — see DETRUSOR URINAE

uri·nal \ˈyür-ən-ᵊl\ *n* **1** : a vessel so constructed that it can be used for urination by a bedridden patient **2** : a container worn by a person with urinary incontinence

uri·nal·y·sis \ˌyür-ə-ˈna-lə-səs\ *n, pl* **-y·ses** \-ˌsēz\ : chemical analysis of urine

uri·nary \ˈyür-ə-ˌner-ē\ *adj* **1** : relating to, occurring in, or constituting the organs concerned with the formation and discharge of urine **2** : of, relating to, or for urine **3** : excreted as or in urine

urinary bladder *n* : a distensible membranous sac that serves for the temporary retention of the urine, is situated in the pelvis in front of the rectum, receives the urine from the two ureters, and discharges it at intervals into the urethra through an orifice closed by a sphincter

urinary calculus *n* : a calculus occurring in any portion of the urinary tract and esp. in the pelvis of the kidney — called also *urinary stone, urolith*

urinary system *n* : the organs of the urinary tract comprising the kidneys, ureters, urinary bladder, and urethra

urinary tract *n* : the tract through which urine passes and which consists of the renal tubules and renal pelvis, the ureters, the bladder, and the urethra

uri·nate \ˈyür-ə-ˌnāt\ *vb* **-nat·ed; -nat·ing** : to discharge urine

uri·na·tion \ˌyür-ə-ˈnā-shən\ *n* : the act of urinating — called also *micturition*

urine \ˈyür-ən\ *n* : waste material that is secreted by the kidney, is rich in end products (as urea, uric acid, and creatinine) of protein metabolism together with salts and pigments, and forms a clear amber and usu. slightly acid fluid

uri·nif·er·ous tubule \ˌyür-ə-ˈni-fə-rəs-\ *n* : a tubule of the kidney that collects or conducts urine

uri·no·ma \ˌyür-ə-ˈnō-mə\ *n, pl* **-mas** *or* **-ma·ta** \-mə-tə\ : a cyst that contains urine

uri·nom·e·ter \ˌyür-ə-ˈnä-mə-tər\ *n* : a small hydrometer for determining the specific gravity of urine

uro- — see UR-

uro·bi·lin \ˌyür-ə-ˈbī-lən\ *n* : any of several brown bile pigments formed from urobilinogens and found in normal feces, in normal urine in small amounts, and in pathological urines in larger amounts

uro·bi·lin·o·gen \ˌyür-ə-bī-ˈli-nə-jən, -ˌjen\ *n* : any of several chromogens that are reduction products of bilirubin

uro·ca·nic acid \ˌyür-ə-ˈkä-nik-, -ˈka-\ *n* : a crystalline acid $C_6H_6N_2O_2$ normally present in human skin that is held to act as a screening agent for ultraviolet radiation

uro·dy·nam·ics \ˌyür-ə-dī-ˈna-miks\ *n* : the hydrodynamics of the urinary tract — **uro·dy·nam·ic** \-mik\ *adj*

uro·er·y·thrin \ˌyür-ō-ˈer-ə-thrən\ *n* : a pink or reddish pigment found in many pathological urines and also frequently in normal urine in very small quantity

uro·gas·trone \ˌyür-ə-ˈgas-ˌtrōn\ *n* : a polypeptide that has been isolated from urine and inhibits gastric secretion — compare ENTEROGASTRONE

uro·gen·i·tal \ˌyür-ō-ˈje-nə-tᵊl\ *adj* : of, relating to, affecting, treating, or being the organs or functions of excretion and reproduction

urogenital diaphragm *n* : a double layer of pelvic fascia with its included muscle that is situated between the ischial and pubic rami, supports the prostate in the male, is traversed by the vagina in the female, gives passage to the membranous part of the urethra, and encloses the sphincter urethrae

urogenital sinus *n* : the ventral part of the embryonic mammalian cloaca that eventually forms the neck of the bladder and some of the more distal portions of the genitourinary tract

urogenital system *n* : GENITOURINARY TRACT

urogenital tract *n* : GENITOURINARY TRACT

uro·gram \ˈyür-ə-ˌgram\ *n* : a roentgenogram made by urography

urog·ra·phy \yü-ˈrä-grə-fē\ *n, pl* **-phies** : roentgenography of a part of the urinary tract (as a kidney or ureter) after injection of a radiopaque substance — **uro·graph·ic** \ˌyür-ə-ˈgra-fik\ *adj*

uro·ki·nase \ˌyür-ō-ˈkī-ˌnās, -ˌnāz\ *n* : an enzyme that is produced by the kidney and is found in urine, that activates plasminogen, and that is used therapeutically to dissolve blood clots (as in the heart)

uro·lag·nia \ˌyür-ō-ˈlag-nē-ə\ *n* : sexual excitement associated with urine or with urination

uro·lith \ˈyür-ə-ˌlith\ *n* : URINARY CALCULUS

uro·lith·i·a·sis \ˌyür-ə-li-ˈthī-ə-səs\ *n, pl* **-i·a·ses** \-ˌsēz\ : a condition that is characterized by the formation or presence of calculi in the urinary tract

urol·o·gist \yü-ˈrä-lə-jist\ *n* : a physician who specializes in urology

urol·o·gy \-jē\ *n, pl* **-gies** : a branch of medicine dealing with the urinary or urogenital organs — **uro·log·ic** \ˌyür-ə-ˈlä-jik\ *also* **uro·log·i·cal** \-ji-kəl\ *adj*

urop·a·thy \yü-ˈrä-pə-thē\ *n, pl* **-thies** : a disease of the urinary or urogenital organs — **uro·path·ic** \ˌyür-ə-ˈpa-thik\ *adj*

uro·pep·sin \ˌyür-ō-ˈpep-sən\ *n* : a proteolytic hormone found in urine esp. in cases of peptic ulcers and other disorders of the digestive tract

uro·por·phy·rin \ˌyür-ō-ˈpòr-fə-rən\ *n* : any of four isomeric porphyrins $C_{40}H_{38}N_4O_{16}$ closely related to the coproporphyrins

uro·ra·di·ol·o·gy \ˌyür-ō-ˌrā-dē-ˈä-lə-jē\ *n, pl* **-gies** : radiology of the urinary tract — **uro·ra·dio·log·ic** \-ˌrā-dē-ə-ˈlä-jik\ *adj*

uros·co·py \yür-ˈäs-kə-pē\ *n, pl* **-pies** : examination or analysis of the urine

uro·sep·sis \ˌyür-ō-ˈsep-səs\ *n, pl* **-sep·ses** \-ˌsēz\ : a toxic condition caused by the extravasation of urine into bodily tissues

uros·to·my \yü-ˈräs-tə-mē\ *n, pl* **-mies** : an ostomy for the elimination of urine from the body

Urot·ro·pin \yür-ˈä-trə-pən\ *trademark* — used for a preparation of methenamine

ur·so·de·oxy·cho·lic acid \ˌər-sō-dē-ˌäk-sē-ˈkō-lik-\ *n* : URSODIOL

ur·so·di·ol \ˌər-sō-ˈdī-ˌol, -ˌōl\ *n* : a bile acid $C_{24}H_{40}O_4$ stereoisomeric with chenodeoxycholic acid that is used to dissolve uncalcified radiolucent gallstones — called also *ursodeoxycholic acid*

ur·ti·ca \ˈər-ti-kə\ *n* **1** *cap* : a genus of widely distributed plants of the nettle family (Urticaceae) comprising the nettles with leaves having stinging hairs **2** : NETTLE 1

ur·ti·car·ia \ˌər-tə-ˈkar-ē-ə\ *n* : HIVES — **ur·ti·car·i·al** \-ē-əl\ *adj*

urticata — see ACNE URTICATA

uru·shi·ol \yü-ˈrü-shē-ˌol, -ˌōl\ *n* : an oily toxic irritant mixture present in poison ivy and some related plants of the genus *Rhus*

USAN *abbr* United States Adopted Names — used to designate officially recognized nonproprietary names of drugs as established by a joint committee of medical and pharmaceutical professionals

USP *abbr* United States Pharmacopeia

uta \ˈü-tə\ *n* : a leishmaniasis of the skin occurring in Peru : ESPUNDIA

ut dict *abbr* [Latin *ut dictum*] as directed — used in writing prescriptions

uter- *or* **utero-** \for 2, ˌyü-tə-rō\ *comb form* **1** : uterus (*utero*salpingography) **2** : uterine and (*utero*placental)

uteri *pl of* UTERUS

uter·ine \ˈyü-tə-rən, -ˌrīn\ *adj* : of, relating to, occurring in, or affecting the uterus ⟨∼ tissue⟩ ⟨∼ cancer⟩

uterine artery *n* : an artery that arises from the internal iliac artery and supplies the uterus and adjacent parts and during pregnancy the placenta

uterine gland *n* : any of the branched tubular glands in the mucous membrane of the uterus

uterine plexus *n* : a plexus of veins tributary to the internal iliac vein by which blood is returned from the uterus

uterine tube *n* : FALLOPIAN TUBE

uterine vein *n* : any of the veins that make up the uterine plexus

utero·ovar·ian \ˌyü-tə-rō-(ˌ)rō-ō-ˈvar-ē-ən\ *adj* : of or relating to the uterus and the ovary ⟨∼ blood flow⟩

utero·pla·cen·tal \-plə-ˈsent-ᵊl\ *adj* : of or relating to the uterus and the placenta ⟨∼ circulation⟩

utero·sa·cral ligament \ˌyü-tə-rō-ˈsa-krəl-, -ˈsā-\ n : a fibrous fascial band on each side of the uterus that passes along the lateral wall of the pelvis from the uterine cervix to the sacrum and that serves to support the uterus and hold it in place — called also *sacrouterine ligament*

utero·sal·pin·gog·ra·phy \-ˌsal-ˌpiŋ-ˈgä-grə-fē\ n, pl **-phies** : HYSTEROSALPIN-GOGRAPHY

utero·ton·ic \ˌyü-tə-rō-ˈtä-nik\ adj : stimulating muscular tone in the uterus ⟨a ∼ substance⟩

utero·tub·al \-ˈtü-bəl, -ˈtyü-\ adj : of or relating to the uterus and fallopian tubes

utero·vag·i·nal \-ˈva-jən-ᵊl\ adj : of or relating to the uterus and the vagina

utero·ves·i·cal pouch \-ˈve-si-kəl\ n : a pouch formed by the peritoneum between the uterus and the bladder

uter·us \ˈyü-tə-rəs\ n, pl **uteri** \-ˌrī\ also **uter·us·es** : an organ in female mammals for containing and usu. for nourishing the young during development previous to birth that has thick walls consisting of an external serous coat, a very thick muscular coat of smooth muscle, and a mucous coat containing numerous glands — called also *womb*; see CERVIX 2a, CORPUS UTERI

UTI abbr urinary tract infection

utilization review n : the critical examination of health-care services esp. to detect wasteful practices and unnecessary care

utri·cle \ˈyü-tri-kəl\ n : a small anatomical pouch: as **a** : the part of the membranous labyrinth of the ear into which the semicircular canals open — called also *utriculus* **b** : PROSTATIC UTRICLE — **utric·u·lar** \yü-ˈtri-kyə-lər\ adj

utric·u·lo·sac·cu·lar duct \yü-ˌtri-kyə-lō-ˈsa-kyə-lər-\ n : a narrow tube connecting the utricle to the saccule in

the membranous labyrinth of the ear

utric·u·lus \yü-ˈtri-kyə-ləs\ n, pl **-li** \-ˌlī\ : UTRICLE a

UV abbr ultraviolet

UV–A \ˌyü-ˌvē-ˈā\ n : the region of the ultraviolet spectrum which is nearest to visible light and extends from 320 to 400 nm in wavelength and from which comes the radiation that causes tanning and contributes to aging of the skin

UV–B \ˌyü-ˌvē-ˈbē\ n : the region of the ultraviolet spectrum which extends from 280 to 320 nm in wavelength and from which comes the radiation primarily responsible for sunburn, aging of the skin, and the development of skin cancer

uvea \ˈyü-vē-ə\ n : the middle layer of the eye consisting of the iris and ciliary body together with the choroid coat — called also *vascular tunic* — **uve·al** \ˈyü-vē-əl\ adj

uve·itis \ˌyü-vē-ˈī-təs\ n, pl **uve·it·i·des** \-ˈi-tə-ˌdēz\ : inflammation of the uvea

uveo·pa·rot·id fever \ˌyü-vē-ō-pə-ˈrä-təd-\ n : chronic inflammation of the parotid gland and uvea marked by low-grade fever, lassitude, and bilateral iridocyclitis and sometimes associated with sarcoidosis — called also *Heerfordt's syndrome*

uvu·la \ˈyü-vyə-lə\ n, pl **-las** \-ləz\ or **-lae** \-ˌlē\ **1** : the pendent fleshy lobe in the middle of the posterior border of the soft palate **2** : a lobe of the inferior vermis of the cerebellum located in front of the pyramid — **uvu·lar** \-lər\ adj

uvu·lec·to·my \ˌyü-vyə-ˈlek-tə-mē\ n, pl **-mies** : surgical excision of the uvula

U wave \ˈyü-\ n : a positive wave following the T wave on an electrocardiogram

V

V symbol vanadium

vac·ci·nal \ˈvak-sən-ᵊl, vak-ˈsēn-\ adj : of or relating to vaccine or vaccination ⟨∼ control of a disease⟩

vac·ci·nate \ˈvak-sə-ˌnāt\ vb **-nat·ed; -nat·ing 1** : to inoculate (a person) with cowpox virus in order to produce immunity to smallpox **2** : to administer a vaccine to usu. by injection — **vac·ci·na·tor** \-ˌnā-tər\ n

vac·ci·na·tion \ˌvak-sə-ˈnā-shən\ n **1** : the act of vaccinating **2** : the scar left by vaccinating

vac·cine \vak-ˈsēn, ˈvak-ˌ\ n **1** : matter or a preparation containing the virus of cowpox in a form used for vaccination **2** : a preparation of killed microorganisms, living attenuated organisms, or living fully virulent or-

ganisms that is administered to produce or artificially increase immunity to a particular disease; also : a mixture of several such vaccines

vac·ci·nee \ˌvak-sə-ˈnē\ n : a vaccinated individual

vac·cin·ia \vak-ˈsi-nē-ə\ n **1 a** : COWPOX **b** : the usu. mild systemic reaction of an individual following vaccination against smallpox **2** : the poxvirus that is the causative agent of cowpox and is used for vaccination against smallpox — **vac·cin·i·al** \-nē-əl\ adj

vac·u·o·late \ˈva-kyü-ō-ˌlāt\ or **vac·u·o·lat·ed** \-ˌlā-təd\ adj : containing one or more vacuoles

vac·u·o·la·tion \ˌva-kyü-ō-ˈlā-shən\ n : the development or formation of vacuoles ⟨neuronal ∼⟩

vac·u·ole \'va-kyü-ˌōl\ *n* **1** : a small cavity or space in the tissues of an organism containing air or fluid **2** : a cavity or vesicle in the cytoplasm of a cell usu. containing fluid — **vac·u·o·lar** \ˌva-kyü-'ō-lər, -ˌlär\ *adj*

vac·u·ol·i·za·tion \ˌva-kyü-ˌō-lə-'zā-shən\ *n* : VACUOLATION ⟨∼ of erythroid cells⟩

vac·uum aspiration \'va-(ˌ)kyüm-, -kyəm-\ *n* : abortion in the early stages of pregnancy by aspiration of the contents of the uterus through a narrow tube — **vacuum aspirator** *n*

VAD \ˌvē-(ˌ)ā-'dē\ *n* : an artificial device that is implanted in the chest to assist a damaged or weakened heart in pumping blood — called also *ventricular assist device*

vag- *or* **vago-** *comb form* : vagus nerve ⟨*vagotomy*⟩ ⟨*vagotonia*⟩

va·gal \'vā-gəl\ *adj* : of, relating to, mediated by, or being the vagus nerve — **va·gal·ly** *adv*

vagal escape *n* : resumption of the heartbeat that takes place after stimulation of the vagus nerve has caused it to stop and that occurs despite the continuing of such stimulation

vagal tone *n* : impulses from the vagus nerve producing inhibition of the heartbeat

vagi *pl of* VAGUS

vagin- *also* **vagini-** *comb form* : vagina ⟨*vaginectomy*⟩

va·gi·na \və-'ji-nə\ *n, pl* **-nae** \-(ˌ)nē\ *or* **-nas** : a canal in a female mammal that leads from the uterus to the external orifice opening into the vestibule between the labia minora

vaginae — see SPHINCTER VAGINAE

va·gi·nal \'va-jən-əl, və-'ji-nᵊl\ *adj* **1** : of, relating to, or resembling a vagina : THECAL **2** : of, relating to, or affecting the genital vagina — **va·gi·nal·ly** *adv*

vaginal artery *n* : any of the several arteries that supply the vagina and that usu. arise from the internal iliac artery or the uterine artery

vaginal hysterectomy *n* : a hysterectomy performed through the vagina

vaginal process *n* **1** : a projecting lamina of bone on the inferior surface of the petrous portion of the temporal bone that is continuous with the tympanic plate and surrounds the root of the styloid process **2** : either of a pair of projecting laminae on the inferior surface of the sphenoid that articulate with the alae of the vomer

vaginal smear *n* : a smear taken from the vaginal mucosa for cytological diagnosis

vaginal thrush *n* : candidiasis of the vagina or vulva

vag·i·nec·to·my \ˌva-jə-'nek-tə-mē\ *n, pl* **-mies** : COLPECTOMY

vag·i·nis·mus \ˌva-jə-'niz-məs\ *n* : a painful spasmodic contraction of the vagina

vag·i·ni·tis \ˌva-jə-'nī-təs\ *n, pl* **-nit·i·des** \-'ni-tə-ˌdēz\ : inflammation of the vagina or of a sheath (as a tendon sheath)

vag·i·no·plas·ty \'va-jə-nə-ˌplas-tē\ *n, pl* **-ties** : plastic surgery of the vagina

vago- — see VAG-

va·go·lyt·ic \ˌvā-gə-'li-tik\ *adj* : PARASYMPATHOLYTIC ⟨∼ effects⟩ ⟨∼ drugs⟩

va·got·o·my \vā-'gä-tə-mē\ *n, pl* **-mies** : surgical division of the vagus nerve — **va·got·o·mize** \-ˌmīz\ *vb*

va·go·to·nia \ˌvā-gə-'tō-nē-ə\ *n* : excessive excitability of the vagus nerve resulting typically in vasomotor instability, constipation, and sweating — compare SYMPATHICOTONIA — **va·go·ton·ic** \-'tä-nik\ *adj*

va·go·va·gal \ˌvā-gō-'vā-gəl\ *adj* : relating to or arising from both afferent and efferent impulses of the vagus nerve ⟨a ∼ reflex⟩

va·gus \'vā-gəs\ *n, pl* **va·gi** \'vā-ˌgī, -ˌjī\ : VAGUS NERVE

vagus nerve *n* : either of the tenth pair of cranial nerves that arise from the medulla and supply chiefly the viscera esp. with autonomic sensory and motor fibers — called also *pneumogastric nerve, tenth cranial nerve, vagus*

va·lence \'vā-ləns\ *n* **1** : the degree of combining power of an element or radical as shown by the number of atomic weights of a monovalent element (as hydrogen) with which the atomic weight of the element or the partial molecular weight of the radical will combine or for which it can be substituted or with which it can be compared **2** : relative capacity to unite, react, or interact (as with antigens or a biological substrate)

-va·lent \'vā-lənt\ *adj comb form* : having (so many) chromosomal strands or homologous chromosomes ⟨*bivalent*⟩

valgum — see GENU VALGUM

val·gus \'val-gəs\ *adj* : turned outward; *esp* : of, relating to, or being a deformity in which an anatomical part is turned outward away from the midline of the body to an abnormal degree ⟨∼ deformity of the ankle⟩ — see CUBITUS VALGUS, HALLUX VALGUS, TALIPES VALGUS; compare GENU VALGUM, GENU VARUM, VARUS — **valgus** *n*

va·line \'vā-ˌlēn, 'va-\ *n* : a crystalline essential amino acid $C_5H_{11}NO_2$

val·in·o·my·cin \ˌva-lə-nō-'mīs-ᵊn\ *n* : an antibiotic $C_{54}H_{90}N_6O_{18}$ produced by a bacterium of the genus *Streptomyces* (*S. fulvissimus*)

Val·ium \'va-lē-əm, 'val-yəm\ *trademark* — used for a preparation of diazepam

val·late \'va-ˌlāt\ *adj* : having a raised edge surrounding a depression

vallate papilla *n* : CIRCUMVALLATE PAPILLA

val·lec·u·la \va-'le-kyə-lə\ *n, pl* **-lae**

\-₁lē\ : an anatomical groove, channel, or depression: as **a** : a groove between the base of the tongue and the epiglottis **b** : a fossa on the underside of the cerebellum separating the hemispheres and including the inferior or vermis — **val·lec·u·lar** \-lər\ *adj*

valley fever *n* : COCCIDIOIDOMYCOSIS

val·pro·ate \val-'prō-₁āt\ *n* : a salt or ester of valproic acid

val·pro·ic acid \val-'prō-ik-\ *n* : a valeric-acid derivative $C_8H_{16}O_2$ used as an anticonvulsant esp. in the form of its sodium salt — see SODIUM VALPROATE

Val·sal·va maneuver \val-'sal-və-\ *also* **Val·sal·va's maneuver** \-vəz-\ *n* : a forceful attempt at expiration when the airway is closed at some point; *esp* : a conscious effort made while holding the nostrils closed and keeping the mouth shut for the purpose of testing the patency of the eustachian tubes or of adjusting middle ear pressure — called also *Valsalva*

A. M. Valsalva — see SINUS OF VALSALVA

val·va \'val-və\ *n, pl* **val·vae** \-₁vē\ : VALVE

valve \'valv\ *n* **1** : a structure esp. in a vein or lymphatic that closes temporarily a passage or orifice or permits movement of fluid in one direction only **2** : any of various mechanical devices by which the flow of liquid (as blood) may be started, stopped, or regulated by a movable part that opens, shuts, or partially obstructs one or more ports or passageways; *also* : the movable part of such a device

valve of Kerck·ring *or* **valve of Kerkring** \-'ker-kriŋ\ *n* : PLICAE CIRCULARES

Kerck·ring \'ker-kriŋ\, **Theodor** (1640–1693), Dutch anatomist.

val·vot·o·my \val-'vä-tə-mē\ *n, pl* **-mies** : VALVULOTOMY

valvul- *or* **valvulo-** *comb form* : small valve : fold (*valvulitis*) (*valvulo*tome)

val·vu·la \'val-vyə-lə\ *n, pl* **-lae** \-₁lē, -₁lī\ : a small valve or fold

valvulae con·ni·ven·tes \-₁kä-nə-'ven-₁tēz\ *n pl* : PLICAE CIRCULARES

val·vu·lar \'val-vyə-lər\ *adj* **1** : resembling or functioning as a valve **2** : of, relating to, or affecting a valve esp. of the heart (∼ heart disease)

val·vu·li·tis \₁val-vyə-'lī-təs\ *n* : inflammation of a valve esp. of the heart

val·vu·lo·plas·ty \'val-vyə-lō-₁plas-tē\ *n, pl* **-ties** : a plastic operation performed on a heart valve

val·vu·lo·tome \'val-vyə-lō-₁tōm\ *n* : a surgical blade designed for valvulotomy or commissurotomy

val·vu·lot·o·my \₁val-vyə-'lä-tə-mē\ *n, pl* **-mies** : surgical incision of a valve; *specif* : the operation of enlarging a narrowed heart valve by cutting through the mitral commissures with

a knife or by a finger thrust to relieve the symptoms of mitral stenosis

vampire bat *n* : any of several Central and So. American bats (*Desmodus rotundus*, *Diaemus youngi*, and *Diphylla ecaudata*) that feed on the blood of birds and mammals and esp. domestic animals and that are sometimes vectors of equine trypanosomiasis and of rabies; *also* : any of several other bats that do not feed on blood but are sometimes reputed to do so

va·na·di·um \və-'nā-dē-əm\ *n* : a grayish malleable ductile metallic element — symbol *V*; see ELEMENT table

Van·co·cin \'van-kə-₁sin\ *trademark* — used for a preparation of vancomycin

van·co·my·cin \₁vaŋ-kə-'mīs-ᵊn\ *n* : an antimicrobial agent from an actinomycete of the genus *Streptomyces* (*S. orientalis*) that is used esp. in the form of its hydrochloride salt against staphylococci resistant to other antibiotics — see VANCOCIN

van den Bergh test \'van-dən-₁bərg-\ *also* **van den Bergh's test** \-₁bərgz-\ *n* : a test indicating presence of bilirubin in the blood (as in jaundice)

Van den Bergh, Albert Abraham Hijmans (1869–1943), Dutch physician.

van·il·lyl·man·de·lic acid \₁va-nə-lil-man-'dē-lik-\ *n* : a principal catecholamine metabolite $C_9H_{10}O_5$ whose presence in excess in the urine is used as a test for pheochromocytoma — abbr. *VMA*

van·il·man·de·lic acid \₁van-əl-man-'dē-lik-\ *n* : VANILLYLMANDELIC ACID

va·por \'vā-pər\ *n* : a substance in the gaseous state as distinguished from the liquid or solid state — **va·por·ize** \'vā-pə-₁rīz\ *vb* — **va·por·iz·able** \₁vā-pə-'rī-zə-bəl\ *adj*

va·por·iz·er \'vā-pə-₁rī-zər\ *n* : one that vaporizes: as **a** : ATOMIZER **b** : a device for converting water or a medicated liquid into a vapor for inhalation

va·pour *chiefly Brit var of* VAPOR

Va·quez's disease \vä-'ke-zəz-\ *n* : POLYCYTHEMIA VERA

Vaquez, Louis Henri (1860–1936), French physician.

variable region *n* : the part of the polypeptide chain of a light or heavy chain of an antibody that ends in a free amino group −NH_2, that varies greatly in its sequence of amino-acid residues from one immunoglobulin to another, and that prob. determines the conformation of the combining site which confers the specificity of the antibody for a particular antigen — called also *variable domain*; compare CONSTANT REGION

varic- *or* **varico-** *comb form* : varix (*varic*osis) (*varico*cele)

var·i·ce·al \₁var-ə-'sē-əl, və-'ri-sē-əl\

adj : of, relating to, or caused by varices ⟨∼ hemorrhage⟩

var·i·cel·la \₁var-ə-ˈse-lə\ *n* : CHICKEN POX

varicella zoster *n* : a herpesvirus that causes chicken pox and shingles — called also *varicella-zoster virus*

var·i·cel·li·form \₁var-ə-ˈse-lə-₁fȯrm\ *adj* : resembling chicken pox ⟨a ∼ eruption⟩

varices *pl of* VARIX

var·i·co·cele \ˈvar-i-kō-₁sēl\ *n* : a varicose enlargement of the veins of the spermatic cord producing a soft compressible tumor mass in the scrotum

var·i·co·cel·ec·to·my \₁var-i-kō-sē-ˈlek-tə-mē\ *n, pl* **-mies** : surgical treatment of varicocele by excision of the affected veins often with removal of part of the scrotum

var·i·cose \ˈvar-ə-₁kōs\ *also* **var·i·cosed** \-₁kōst\ *adj* **1** : abnormally swollen or dilated ⟨∼ lymph vessels⟩ **2** : affected with varicose veins ⟨∼ legs⟩

varicose vein *n* : an abnormal swelling and tortuosity esp. of a superficial vein of the legs — usu. used in pl.

var·i·co·sis \₁var-ə-ˈkō-səs\ *n, pl* **-co·ses** \-ˌsēz\ : the condition of being varicose or of having varicose vessels

var·i·cos·i·ty \₁var-ə-ˈkä-sə-tē\ *n, pl* **-ties 1** : the quality or state of being abnormally or markedly swollen or dilated **2** : VARIX

Var·i·dase \ˈvar-ə-₁dās\ *trademark* — used for a preparation containing a mixture of streptodornase and streptokinase

va·ri·e·ty \və-ˈrī-ə-tē\ *n, pl* **-et·ies** : any of various groups of plants or animals ranking below a species : SUBSPECIES

va·ri·o·la \və-ˈrī-ə-lə\ *n* : SMALLPOX

variola major *n* : a severe form of smallpox characterized historically by a death rate up to 40% or more

variola minor *n* : a mild form of smallpox of low mortality — called also *alastrim*

var·i·o·la·tion \₁var-ē-ə-ˈlā-shən\ *n* : the deliberate inoculation of an uninfected person with the smallpox virus (as by contact with pustular matter) that was widely practiced before the era of vaccination as prophylaxis against the severe form of smallpox

variola vac·cin·ia \-vak-ˈsi-nē-ə\ *n* : COWPOX

var·i·ol·i·form \₁var-ē-ˈō-lə-₁fȯrm\ *adj* : resembling smallpox

varioliformis — see PITYRIASIS LICHENOIDES ET VARIOLIFORMIS ACUTA

va·ri·o·loid \ˈvar-ē-ə-₁lȯid, və-ˈrī-ə-₁lȯid\ *n* : a modified mild form of smallpox occurring in persons who have been vaccinated or who have had smallpox

var·ix \ˈvar-iks\ *n, pl* **var·i·ces** \ˈvar-ə-₁sēz\ : an abnormally dilated and lengthened vein, artery, or lymph vessel; *esp* : VARICOSE VEIN

Varolii — see PONS VAROLII

varum — see GENU VARUM

var·us \ˈvar-əs\ *adj* : of, relating to, or being a deformity of a bodily part characterized by bending or turning inward toward the midline of the body to an abnormal degree — see CUBITUS VARUS, TALIPES VARUS; compare GENU VALGUM, GENU VARUM, VALGUS — **varus** *n*

vas \ˈvas\ *n, pl* **va·sa** \ˈvā-zə\ : an anatomical vessel : DUCT

vas- *or* **vaso-** *comb form* **1** : vessel: as **a** : blood vessel ⟨*vaso*motor⟩ **b** : vas deferens ⟨*vas*ectomy⟩ **2** : vascular and ⟨*vaso*vagal⟩

vasa ab·er·ran·tia \-₁a-bə-ˈran-chə, -chē-ə\ *n pl* : slender arteries that are only occas. present and that connect the axillary or brachial artery with an artery (as the radial artery) of the forearm or with its branches

vas ab·er·rans of Hal·ler \-ˈa-bə-₁ranz . . . -ˈhä-lər\, *n pl* **vasa ab·er·ran·tia of Haller** \-₁a-bə-ˈran-chə, -chē-ə\ : a blind tube that is occas. present parallel to the first part of the vas deferens

Haller, Albrecht von (1708–1777), Swiss biologist.

vasa deferentia *pl of* VAS DEFERENS

vasa ef·fer·en·tia \-₁e-fə-ˈren-chə, -chē-ə\ *n pl* : the 12 to 20 ductules that lead from the rete testis to the vas deferens and except near their commencement are greatly convoluted and form the compact head of the epididymis

va·sal \ˈvā-zəl\ *adj* : of, relating to, or constituting an anatomical vessel

vasa rec·ta \-ˈrek-tə\ *n pl* **1** : numerous small vessels that arise from the terminal branches of arteries supplying the intestine, encircle the intestine, and divide into more branches between its layers **2** : hairpin-shaped vessels that arise from the arteriole leading away from a renal glomerulus, descend into the renal pyramids, reunite as they ascend, and play a role in the concentration of urine

vasa va·so·rum \-vā-ˈsȯr-əm\ *n pl* : small blood vessels that supply or drain the walls of the larger arteries and veins and connect with a branch of the same vessel or a neighboring vessel

vascul- *or* **vasculo-** *comb form* : vessel; *esp* : blood vessel ⟨*vasculo*toxic⟩

vas·cu·lar \ˈvas-kyə-lər\ *adj* **1** : of, relating to, constituting, or affecting a tube or a system of tubes for the conveyance of a body fluid (as blood or lymph) **2** : supplied with or containing ducts and esp. blood vessels — **vas·cu·lar·i·ty** \₁vas-kyə-ˈlar-ə-tē\ *n*

vascular bed *n* : an intricate network of minute blood vessels that ramifies through the tissues of the body or of one of its parts

vascularis — see STRIA VASCULARIS

vas·cu·lar·i·za·tion \₁vas-kyə-lə-rə-ˈzā-shən\ *n* : the process of becoming vascular; *also* : abnormal or excessive formation of blood vessels (as in the retina or on the cornea) — **vas·cu·lar·ize** \'vas-kyə-lə-ˌrīz\ *vb*

vascular tunic *n* : UVEA

vas·cu·la·ture \'vas-kyə-lə-ˌchùr, -ˌtyùr, -ˌtùr\ *n* : the arrangement of blood vessels in an organ or part

vas·cu·li·tis \ˌvas-kyə-'lī-təs\ *n, pl* -**lit·i·des** \-'li-tə-ˌdēz\ : inflammation of a blood or lymph vessel — **vas·cu·lit·ic** \-kyə-'li-tik\ *adj*

vas·cu·lo·gen·ic \ˌvas-kyə-lō-'je-nik\ *adj* : caused by disorder or dysfunction of the blood vessels ⟨~ impotence⟩ ⟨~ migraine⟩

vas·cu·lo·tox·ic \ˌvas-kyə-lō-'täk-sik\ *adj* : destructive to blood vessels or the vascular system ⟨~ effects⟩

vas def·er·ens \-'de-fə-rənz, -ˌrenz\ *n, pl* **vasa def·er·en·tia** \-ˌde-fə-'ren-chə, -chē-ə\ : a spermatic duct that is a small but thick-walled tube about two feet (0.61 meter) long that begins at and is continuous with the tail of the epididymis, runs in the spermatic cord through the inguinal canal, and descends into the pelvis where it joins the duct of the seminal vesicle to form the ejaculatory duct — called also *ductus deferens, spermatic duct*

va·sec·to·my \və-'sek-tə-mē, vā-'zek-\ *n, pl* -**mies** : surgical division or resection of all or part of the vas deferens usu. to induce sterility — **va·sec·to·mize** \-ˌmīz\ *vb*

Vas·e·line \ˌva-sə-'lēn\ *trademark* — used for a preparation of petroleum jelly

vaso- — see VAS-

va·so·ac·tive \ˌvā-zō-'ak-tiv\ *adj* : affecting the blood vessels esp. in respect to the degree of their relaxation or contraction — **va·so·ac·tiv·i·ty** \-ak-'ti-və-tē\ *n*

vasoactive intestinal polypeptide *n* : a protein hormone that consists of a chain of 28 amino-acid residues, has been implicated as a neurotransmitter, and has a wide range of physiological activities (as stimulation of secretion by the pancreas and small intestine, vasodilation, and inhibition of gastric juice production) — abbr. *VIP*; called also *vasoactive intestinal peptide*

va·so·con·stric·tion \ˌvā-zō-kən-'strik-shən\ *n* : narrowing of the lumen of blood vessels esp. as a result of vasomotor action — **va·so·con·stric·tive** \-'strik-tiv\ *adj*

va·so·con·stric·tor \ˌvā-zō-kən-'strik-tər\ *n* : an agent (as a sympathetic nerve fiber or a drug) that induces or initiates vasoconstriction — **vasoconstrictor** *adj*

va·so·de·pres·sor \ˌvā-zō-di-'pre-sər\ *adj* : causing or characterized by vasomotor depression resulting in lowering of the blood pressure

va·so·di·la·tion \ˌvā-zo-dī-'lā-shən\ *or*

va·so·di·la·ta·tion \-ˌdī-lə-'tā-shən, -ˌdī-\ *n* : widening of the lumen of blood vessels

va·so·di·la·tor \ˌvā-zō-'dī-ˌlā-tər\ *n* : an agent (as a parasympathetic nerve fiber or a drug) that induces or initiates vasodilation — **vasodilator** *also* **va·so·di·la·to·ry** \-'dī-lə-ˌtōr-ē, -'dī-\ *adj*

va·so·for·ma·tive \ˌvā-zō-'fòr-mə-tiv\ *adj* : functioning in the development and formation of vessels and esp. blood vessels ⟨~ cells⟩

va·sog·ra·phy \ˌvā-'zä-grə-fē\ *n, pl* -**phies** : roentgenography of blood vessels

va·so·li·ga·tion \ˌvā-zō-lī-'gā-shən\ *n* : surgical ligation of a vessel and esp. of the vas deferens

va·so·mo·tion \ˌvā-zō-'mō-shən\ *n* : alteration in the caliber of blood vessels

va·so·mo·tor \ˌvā-zō-'mō-tər\ *adj* : of, relating to, affecting, or being those nerves or the centers (as in the medulla and spinal cord) from which they arise that supply the muscle fibers of the walls of blood vessels, include sympathetic vasoconstrictors and parasympathetic vasodilators, and by their effect on vascular diameter regulate the amount of blood passing to a particular body part or organ

vasomotor rhinitis *n* : rhinitis caused by an allergen : allergic rhinitis

va·so·pres·sin \ˌvā-zō-'pres-ᵊn\ *n* : a polypeptide hormone that is secreted together with oxytocin by the posterior lobe of the pituitary gland, that is also obtained synthetically, and that increases blood pressure and exerts an antidiuretic effect — called also *antidiuretic hormone*; see PITRESSIN

¹**va·so·pres·sor** \-'pre-sər\ *adj* : causing a rise in blood pressure by exerting a vasoconstrictor effect

²**vasopressor** *n* : a vasopressor agent

vasorum — see VASA VASORUM

va·so·spasm \'vā-zō-ˌspa-zəm\ *n* : sharp and often persistent contraction of a blood vessel reducing its caliber and blood flow — **va·so·spas·tic** \ˌvā-zō-'spas-tik\ *adj*

Va·so·tec \'vā-zō-ˌtek\ *trademark* — used for a preparation of enalapril

va·sot·o·my \ˌvā-'zä-tə-mē\ *n, pl* -**mies** : surgical incision of the vas deferens

va·so·va·gal \ˌvā-zō-'vā-gəl\ *adj* : of, relating to, or involving both vascular and vagal factors

vasovagal syncope *n* : a usu. transitory condition that is marked by anxiety, nausea, respiratory distress, and fainting and that is believed to be due to joint vasomotor and vagal disturbances

va·so·va·sos·to·my \ˌvā-zō-vā-'zäs-tə-mē\ *n, pl* -**mies** : surgical anastomosis of a divided vas deferens to reverse a previous vasectomy

Va·sox·yl \vā-'zäk-səl\ *trademark* —

used for a preparation of methoxamine

vas·tus in·ter·me·di·us \'vas-təs-ˌin-tər-'mē-dē-əs\ *n* : the division of the quadriceps muscle that arises from and covers the front of the shaft of the femur

vastus in·ter·nus \-in-'tər-nəs\ *n* : VASTUS MEDIALIS

vastus lat·er·a·lis \-ˌla-tər-'ā-ləs, -'a-\ *n* : the division of the quadriceps muscle that covers the outer anterior aspect of the femur, arises chiefly from the femur, and inserts into the outer border of the patella by a flat tendon — called also *vastus externus*

vastus me·di·a·lis \-ˌmē-dē-'ā-ləs, -'a-\ *n* : the division of the quadriceps muscle that covers the inner anterior aspect of the femur, arises chiefly from the femur and the adjacent intermuscular septum, inserts into the inner border of the patella and into the tendon of the other divisions of the muscle, sends also a tendinous expansion to the capsule of the knee joint, and is closely and in the upper part often inseparably united with the vastus intermedius — called also *vastus internus*

vault \'volt\ *n* : an arched or dome-shaped anatomical structure: as **a** : SKULLCAP, CALVARIUM ⟨the cranial ∼⟩ **b** : FORNIX d

VCG *abbr* vectorcardiogram

VD *abbr* venereal disease

VDRL \ˌvē-(ˌ)dē-(ˌ)är-'el\ *n* : VDRL TEST

VDRL *abbr* venereal disease research laboratory

VDRL slide test *n* : VDRL TEST

VDRL test *n* : a flocculation test for syphilis employing cardiolipin in combination with lecithin and cholesterol

¹vec·tor \'vek-tər\ *n* **1** : a quantity that has magnitude and direction and that is usu. represented by part of a straight line with the given direction and with a length representing the magnitude **2** : an organism (as an insect) that transmits a pathogen from one organism to another ⟨fleas are ∼*s* of plague⟩ — compare CARRIER 1a **3** : a sequence of genetic material (as a transposon or the genome of a bacteriophage) that can be used to introduce specific genes into the genome of an organism — **vec·to·ri·al** \vek-'tōr-ē-əl\ *adj*

²vector *vb* **vec·tored; vec·tor·ing** : to transmit (a pathogen or disease) from one organism to another : act as a vector for ⟨a disease ∼*ed* by flies⟩

vec·tor·car·dio·gram \ˌvek-tər-'kär-dē-ə-ˌgram\ *n* : a graphic record made by vectorcardiography

vec·tor·car·di·og·ra·phy \-ˌkär-dē-'ä-grə-fē\ *n, pl* **-phies** : a method of recording the direction and magnitude of the electrical forces of the heart by means of a continuous series of vectors that form a curving line around a center — **vec·tor·car·dio·graph·ic** \-dē-ə-'gra-fik\ *adj*

veg·an \'ve-jən, -ˌjan; 'vē-gən\ *n* : a strict vegetarian : one that consumes no animal food or dairy products — **veg·an·ism** \-ˌni-zəm, 'vē-gə-\ *n*

veg·e·tar·i·an·ism \ˌve-jə-'ter-ē-ə-ˌni-zəm\ *n* : the theory or practice of living on a diet made up of vegetables, fruits, grains, nuts, and sometimes animal products (as milk and cheese) — **veg·e·tar·i·an** \-'ter-ē-ən\ *n or adj*

veg·e·ta·tion \ˌve-jə-'tā-shən\ *n* : an abnormal outgrowth upon a body part; *specif* : any of the warty excrescences on the valves of the heart that are composed of various tissue elements including fibrin and collagen and that are typical of endocarditis

veg·e·ta·tive \'ve-jə-ˌtā-tiv\ *adj* **1 a** (1) : growing or having the power of growing (2) : of, relating to, or engaged in nutritive and growth functions as contrasted with reproductive functions ⟨a ∼ nucleus⟩ **b** : of, relating to, or involving propagation by nonsexual processes or methods **2** : affecting, arising from, or relating to involuntary bodily functions **3** : characterized by, resulting from, or being a state of severe mental impairment in which only involuntary bodily functions are sustained ⟨a ∼ existence⟩ — **veg·e·ta·tive·ly** *adv*

ve·hi·cle \'vē-i-kəl, -ˌhi-\ *n* **1** : an inert medium in which a medicinally active agent is administered **2** : an agent of transmission

vein \'vān\ *n* : any of the tubular branching vessels that carry blood from the capillaries toward the heart and have thinner walls than the arteries and often valves at intervals to prevent reflux of the blood which flows in a steady stream and is in most cases dark-colored due to the presence of reduced hemoglobin — **veiny** \'vā-nē\ *adj*

vein·ous \'vā-nəs\ *adj* **1** : having veins that are esp. prominent ⟨∼ hands⟩ **2** : VENOUS

vela *pl of* VELUM

veli — see LEVATOR VELI PALATINI, TENSOR VELI PALATINI

ve·lo·pha·ryn·geal \ˌvē-lō-far-ən-'jē-əl, -fə-'rin-jəl, -jē-əl\ *adj* : of or relating to the soft palate and the pharynx

Vel·peau bandage \vel-'pō-\ *or* **Vel·peau's bandage** \-'pōz-\ *n* : a bandage used to support and immobilize the arm when the clavicle is fractured

    Velpeau, Alfred–Armand–Louis–Marie (1795–1867), French surgeon.

ve·lum \'vē-ləm\ *n, pl* **ve·la** \-lə\ : a membrane or membranous part resembling a veil or curtain: as **a** : SOFT PALATE **b** : SEMILUNAR CUSP

ven- *or* **veni-** *or* **veno-** *comb form* : vein ⟨*veni*puncture⟩

ve·na ca·va \ˌvē-nə-ˈkā-və\ *n, pl* **ve·nae ca·vae** \ˌvē-nē-ˈkā-(ˌ)vē\ : either of two large veins by which the blood is returned to the right atrium of the heart: **a** : INFERIOR VENA CAVA **b** : SUPERIOR VENA CAVA — **vena ca·val** \-vəl\ *adj*

vena co·mi·tans \-ˈkō-mə-ˌtanz\ *n, pl* **venae co·mi·tan·tes** \-ˌkō-mə-ˈtan-ˌtēz\ : a vein accompanying an artery

venae cor·dis min·i·mae \-ˈkȯr-dəs-ˈmi-nə-ˌmē\ *n pl* : minute veins in the wall of the heart that empty into the atria or ventricles

vena vor·ti·co·sa \-ˌvȯr-tə-ˈkō-sə\ *n, pl* **venae vor·ti·co·sae** \-(ˌ)sē\ : any of the veins of the outer layer of the choroid of the eye — called also *vorticose vein*

ve·neer \və-ˈnir\ *n* : a plastic or porcelain coating bonded to the surface of a cosmetically imperfect tooth

ve·ne·re·al \və-ˈnir-ē-əl\ *adj* **1** : resulting from or contracted during sexual intercourse (∼ infections) **2** : of, relating to, or affected with venereal disease (a high ∼ rate) **3** : involving the genital organs (∼ sarcoma) — **ve·ne·re·al·ly** *adv*

venereal disease *n* : a contagious disease (as gonorrhea or syphilis) that is typically acquired in sexual intercourse — abbr. *VD*; compare SEXUALLY TRANSMITTED DISEASE

venereal wart *n* : CONDYLOMA ACUMINATUM

ve·ne·re·ol·o·gy \və-ˌnir-ē-ˈä-lə-jē\ *also* **ven·er·ol·o·gy** \ˌve-nə-ˈrä-lə-jē\ *n, pl* **-gies** : a branch of medical science concerned with venereal diseases — **ve·ne·re·o·log·i·cal** \və-ˌnir-ē-ə-ˈlä-ji-kəl\ *adj* — **ve·ne·re·ol·o·gist** \və-ˌnir-ē-ˈä-lə-jist\ *n*

venereum — see LYMPHOGRANULOMA VENEREUM, LYMPHOPATHIA VENEREUM

veneris — see MONS VENERIS

vene·sec·tion \ˈve-nə-ˌsek-shən, ˈvē-\ *n* : PHLEBOTOMY

Venezuelan equine encephalitis *n* : EQUINE ENCEPHALOMYELITIS c

Venezuelan equine encephalomyelitis *n* : EQUINE ENCEPHALOMYELITIS c

veni- — see VEN-

ve·ni·punc·ture \ˈvē-nə-ˌpəŋk-chər, ˈven-ə-\ *n* : surgical puncture of a vein esp. for the withdrawal of blood or for intravenous medication

veni·sec·tion *var of* VENESECTION

veno- — see VEN-

ve·no·ar·te·ri·al \ˌvē-nō-är-ˈtir-ē-əl\ *adj* : relating to or involving an artery and vein

ve·noc·ly·sis \vē-ˈnä-klə-səs\ *n, pl* **-ly·ses** \-ˌsēz\ : clysis into a vein

ve·no·con·stric·tion \ˌvē-nō-kən-ˈstrik-shən\ *n* : constriction of a vein

ve·no·gram \ˈvē-nə-ˌgram\ *n* : a roentgenogram after the injection of an opaque substance into a vein

ve·nog·ra·phy \vi-ˈnä-grə-fē, vā-\ *n, pl*

-phies : roentgenography of a vein after injection of an opaque substance — **ve·no·graph·ic** \ˌvē-nə-ˈgra-fik\ *adj*

ven·om \ˈve-nəm\ *n* : poisonous matter normally secreted by some animals (as snakes, scorpions, or bees) and transmitted to prey or an enemy chiefly by biting or stinging

ven·om·ous \ˈve-nə-məs\ *adj* **1** : POISONOUS **2** : having a venom-producing gland and able to inflict a poisoned wound (∼ snakes)

venosum — see LIGAMENTUM VENOSUM

venosus — see DUCTUS VENOSUS, SINUS VENOSUS, SINUS VENOSUS SCLERAE

ve·not·o·my \vi-ˈnä-tə-mē\ *n, pl* **-mies** : PHLEBOTOMY

ve·nous \ˈvē-nəs\ *adj* **1 a** : full of or characterized by veins **b** : made up of or carried on by veins (the ∼ circulation) **2** : of, relating to, or performing the functions of a vein (a ∼ inflammation) **3** *of blood* : having passed through the capillaries and given up oxygen for the tissues and become charged with carbon dioxide and ready to pass through the respiratory organs to release its carbon dioxide and renew its oxygen supply : dark red from reduced hemoglobin — compare ARTERIAL 2

venous hum *n* : a humming sound sometimes heard during auscultation of the veins of the neck esp. in anemia

venous return *n* : the flow of blood from the venous system into the right atrium of the heart

venous sinus *n* **1** : a large vein or passage (as the canal of Schlemm) for venous blood **2** : SINUS VENOSUS

vent \ˈvent\ *n* : the external opening of the rectum or cloaca : ANUS

vent gleet *n* : CLOACITIS

ven·ti·late \ˈvent-əl-ˌāt\ *vb* **-lat·ed; -lat·ing 1** : to expose to air and esp. to a current of fresh air for purifying or refreshing **2 a** : OXYGENATE, AERATE (∼ blood in the lungs) **b** : to subject the lungs of (an individual) to ventilation **3** : to give verbal expression to (as mental or emotional conflicts)

ven·ti·la·tion \ˌvent-əl-ˈā-shən\ *n* **1** : the act or process of ventilating **2** : the circulation and exchange of gases in the lungs or gills that is basic to respiration — **ven·ti·la·to·ry** \ˈvent-əl-ə-ˌtōr-ē\ *adj*

ven·ti·la·tor \ˈvent-əl-ˌā-tər\ *n* : RESPIRATOR 2

ventr- *or* **ventri-** *or* **ventro-** *comb form* **1** : abdomen (*ventral*) **2** : ventral and (*ventro*medial)

ven·tral \ˈven-trəl\ *adj* **1** : of or relating to the belly : ABDOMINAL **2 a** : being or located near, on, or toward the lower surface of an animal (as a quadruped) opposite the back or dorsal surface **b** : being or located near, on, or toward the front or anterior part of the human body — **ven·tral·ly** *adv*

ventral column *n* : VENTRAL HORN

ventral corticospinal tract *n* : a band of nerve fibers that descends in the ventrolateral part of the spinal cord and consists of fibers arising in the motor cortex of the brain on the same side of the body — called also *anterior corticospinal tract, direct pyramidal tract*

ventral funiculus *n* : ANTERIOR FUNICULUS

ventral gray column *n* : VENTRAL HORN

ventral horn *n* : a longitudinal subdivision of gray matter in the anterior part of each lateral half of the spinal cord that contains neurons giving rise to motor fibers of the ventral roots of the spinal nerves — called also *anterior column, anterior gray column, anterior horn, ventral column, ventral gray column;* compare DORSAL HORN, LATERAL COLUMN 1

ventralis — see SACROCOCCYGEUS VENTRALIS

ventral median fissure *n* : ANTERIOR MEDIAN FISSURE

ventral mesogastrium *n* : MESOGASTRIUM 1

ventral root *n* : the one of the two roots of a spinal nerve that passes anteriorly from the spinal cord separating the anterior and lateral funiculi and that consists of motor fibers — called also *anterior root;* compare DORSAL ROOT

ventral spinocerebellar tract *n* : SPINOCEREBELLAR TRACT b

ventral spinothalamic tract *n* : SPINOTHALAMIC TRACT a

ventri- — see VENTR-

ven·tri·cle \'ven-tri-kəl\ *n* : a cavity of a bodily part or organ: as **a** : a chamber of the heart which receives blood from a corresponding atrium and from which blood is forced into the arteries **b** : one of the communicating cavities in the brain that form a system and are continuous with the central canal of the spinal cord — see LATERAL VENTRICLE, THIRD VENTRICLE, FOURTH VENTRICLE **c** : a fossa or pouch on each side of the larynx between the false vocal cords above and the true vocal cords below

ven·tric·u·lar \ven-'tri-kyə-lər, vən-\ *adj* : of, relating to, or being a ventricle esp. of the heart or brain (∼ tachycardia)

ventricular assist device *n* : VAD

ventricular fibrillation *n* : very rapid uncoordinated fluttering contractions of the ventricles of the heart resulting in loss of synchronization between heartbeat and pulse beat

ventricular folds *n pl* : FALSE VOCAL CORDS

ventricular septal defect *n* : a congenital defect in the interventricular septum — abbr. *VSD*

ven·tric·u·li·tis \ven-ˌtri-kyə-'lī-təs\ *n*

: inflammation of the ventricles of the brain

ven·tric·u·lo·atri·al \ven-ˌtri-kyə-lō-'ā-trē-əl\ *adj* **1** : of, relating to, or being an artificial shunt between a ventricle of the brain and an atrium of the heart esp. to drain cerebrospinal fluid (as in hydrocephalus) **2** : of, relating to, or being conduction from the ventricle to the atrium of the heart

ven·tric·u·lo·atri·os·to·my \-ˌā-trē-'äs-tə-mē\ *n, pl* **-mies** : surgical establishment of a shunt to drain cerebrospinal fluid (as in hydrocephalus) from a ventricle of the brain to the right atrium

ven·tric·u·lo·cis·ter·nos·to·my \-ˌsis-tər-'näs-tə-mē\ *n, pl* **-mies** : the surgical establishment of a communication between a ventricle of the brain and the subarachnoid space and esp. the cisterna magna to drain cerebrospinal fluid esp. in hydrocephalus

ven·tric·u·lo·gram \ven-'tri-kyə-lə-ˌgram\ *n* : an X-ray photograph made by ventriculography

ven·tric·u·log·ra·phy \ven-ˌtri-kyə-'lä-grə-fē\ *n, pl* **-phies** **1** : the act or process of making an X-ray photograph of the ventricles of the brain after withdrawing fluid from the ventricles and replacing it with air or a radiopaque substance **2** : the act or process of making an X-ray photograph of a ventricle of the heart after injecting a radiopaque substance — **ven·tric·u·lo·graph·ic** \-kyə-lō-'gra-fik\ *adj*

ven·tric·u·lo·peri·to·ne·al \ven-ˌtri-kyə-lō-ˌper-ə-tə-'nē-əl\ *adj* : relating to or serving to communicate between a ventricle of the brain and the peritoneal cavity (a plastic ∼ shunt)

ven·tric·u·los·to·my \ven-ˌtri-kyə-'läs-tə-mē\ *n, pl* **-mies** : the surgical establishment of an opening in a ventricle of the brain to drain cerebrospinal fluid esp. in hydrocephalus

ven·tric·u·lot·o·my \ven-ˌtri-kyə-'lä-tə-mē\ *n, pl* **-mies** : surgical incision of a ventricle (as of the heart)

ventro- — see VENTR-

ven·tro·lat·er·al \ˌven-trō-'la-tə-rəl\ *adj* : ventral and lateral — **ven·tro·lat·er·al·ly** *adv*

ven·tro·me·di·al \-'mē-dē-əl\ *adj* : ventral and medial — **ven·tro·me·di·al·ly** *adv*

ventromedial nucleus *n* : a medially located nucleus of the hypothalamus that is situated between the lateral wall of the third ventricle and the fornix

ve·nule \'vēn-(ˌ)yül, 'ven-\ *n* : a small vein; *esp* : any of the minute veins connecting the capillaries with the larger systemic veins — **ven·u·lar** \'ven-yə-lər\ *adj*

vera — see DECIDUA VERA, POLYCYTHEMIA VERA

ve·rap·am·il \və-'ra-pə-ˌmil\ *n* : a calcium channel blocker $C_{27}H_{38}N_2O_4$ with vasodilating properties that is used esp. in the form of its hydrochloride

ver·a·trine \'ver-ə-ˌtrēn\ n : a mixture of alkaloids that is obtained from the seeds of a Mexican plant (*Schoeno-caulon officinalis* of the lily family (Liliaceae) that is an intense local irritant and a powerful muscle and nerve poison, and that has been used as a counterirritant in neuralgia and arthritis

ve·ra·trum \və-'rā-trəm\ n 1 a cap : a genus of herbs having short poisonous rootstocks b : any hellebore of the genus *Veratrum* 2 : HELLEBORE 2b

ver·big·er·a·tion \(ˌ)vər-ˌbi-jə-'rā-shən\ n : continual repetition of stereotyped phrases (as in some forms of mental illness)

verge — see ANAL VERGE

ver·gence \'vər-jəns\ n : a movement of one eye in relation to the other

vermes pl of VERMIS

vermi- comb form : worm ⟨*vermi*cide⟩ ⟨*vermi*form⟩

ver·mi·cide \'vər-mə-ˌsīd\ n : an agent that destroys worms; esp : ANTHELMINTIC

ver·mi·form \'vər-mə-ˌfórm\ adj : resembling a worm in shape

vermiform appendix n : a narrow blind tube usu. about three or four inches (7.6 to 10.2 centimeters) long that extends from the cecum in the lower right-hand part of the abdomen and represents an atrophied terminal part of the cecum

ver·mi·fuge \'vər-mə-ˌfyüj\ n : an agent that serves to destroy or expel parasitic worms : ANTHELMINTIC — **ver·mif·u·gal** \vər-'mi-fyə-gəl, ˌvər-mə-'fyü-gəl\ adj

ver·mil·ion border \vər-'mil-yən-\ n : the exposed pink or reddish margin of a lip

ver·mil·ion·ec·to·my \vər-ˌmil-yə-'nek-tə-mē\ n, pl -mies : surgical excision of the vermilion border

ver·min \'vər-mən\ n, pl vermin : small common harmful or objectionable animals (as lice or fleas) that are difficult to control

ver·min·ous \'vər-mə-nəs\ adj 1 : consisting of, infested with, or being vermin 2 : caused by parasitic worms

ver·mis \'vər-mis\ n, pl ver·mes \-ˌmēz\ 1 : either of two parts of the median lobe of the cerebellum: **a** : one slightly prominent on the upper surface — called also *superior vermis* **b** : one on the lower surface sunk in the vallecula — called also *inferior vermis* 2 : the median lobe or part of the cerebellum

vernal conjunctivitis n : conjunctivitis occurring in warm seasons as a result of exposure to allergens

Ver·ner–Mor·ri·son syndrome \'vər-nər-'mór-ə-sən-, -'mär-\ n : a syndrome characterized esp. by severe watery diarrhea and hypokalemia

that is often due to an excessive secretion of vasoactive intestinal peptide from a vipoma esp. of the pancreas — called also *pancreatic cholera*

Verner, John Victor (b 1927), American physician, and **Morrison, Ashton Byrom** (b 1922), American pathologist.

ver·nix \'vər-niks\ n : VERNIX CASEOSA

vernix ca·se·o·sa \-ˌka-sē-'ō-sə\ n : a pasty covering chiefly of dead cells and sebaceous secretions that protects the skin of the fetus

Ver·o·nal \'ver-ə-ˌnól, -nəl\ trademark — used for a preparation of barbital

ver·ru·ca \və-'rü-kə\ n, pl -cae \-(ˌ)kē\ : a wart or warty skin lesion

verruca acu·mi·na·ta \-ə-ˌkyü-mə-'nā-tə\ n : CONDYLOMA ACUMINATUM

verruca plan·ta·ris \-ˌplan-'tar-əs\ n : PLANTAR WART

verruca vul·ga·ris \-ˌvəl-'gar-əs\ n : WART 2

ver·ru·cose \və-'rü-ˌkōs\ adj 1 : covered with warty elevations 2 : having the form of a wart ⟨a ~ nevus⟩

ver·ru·cous \və-'rü-kəs\ adj 1 : VERRUCOSE 2 : characterized by the formation of warty lesions ⟨~ dermatitis⟩

verrucous endocarditis n : endocarditis marked by the formation or presence of warty nodules of fibrin on the lips of the heart valves

ver·ru·ga \və-'rü-gə\ n 1 : VERRUCA 2 : VERRUGA PERUANA

verruga per·u·a·na \-ˌper-ə-'wä-nə\ also **verruga pe·ru·vi·a·na** \-pə-ˌrü-vē-'a-nə\ n : the second stage of bartonellosis characterized by warty nodules tending to ulcerate and bleed

versicolor — see TINEA VERSICOLOR

ver·sion \'vər-zhən, -shən\ n 1 : a condition in which an organ and esp. the uterus is turned from its normal position 2 : manual turning of a fetus in the uterus to aid delivery

ver·te·bra \'vər-tə-brə\ n, pl -brae \-ˌbrā, -(ˌ)brē\ or -bras : any of the bony or cartilaginous segments that make up the spinal column and that have a short more or less cylindrical body whose ends articulate with pads of elastic or cartilaginous tissue with those of adjacent vertebrae and a bony arch that encloses the spinal cord

¹**ver·te·bral** \(ˌ)vər-'tē-brəl, 'vər-tə-\ adj 1 : of, relating to, or being vertebrae or the spinal column : SPINAL 2 : composed of or having vertebrae

²**vertebral** n : a vertebral part or element (as an artery)

vertebral arch n : NEURAL ARCH

vertebral artery n : a large branch of the subclavian artery that ascends through the foramina in the transverse processes of each of the cervical vertebrae except the last one or two, enters the cranium through the foramen magnum, and unites with the corresponding artery of the opposite side to form the basilar artery

vertebral canal *n* : a canal that contains the spinal cord and is delimited by the neural arches on the dorsal side of the vertebrae — called also *spinal canal*

vertebral column *n* : SPINAL COLUMN

vertebral foramen *n* : the opening formed by a neural arch through which the spinal cord passes

vertebral ganglion *n* : any of a group of sympathetic ganglia which form two chains extending from the base of the skull to the coccyx along the sides of the spinal column — compare SYMPA-THETIC CHAIN

vertebral notch *n* : either of two concave constrictions of which one occurs on the inferior surface and one on the superior surface of the pedicle on each side of a vertebra and which are arranged so that the superior notches of one vertebra and the corresponding inferior notches of a contiguous vertebra combine to form an intervertebral foramen on each side

vertebral plexus *n* : a plexus of veins associated with the spinal column

vertebral vein *n* : a tributary of the brachiocephalic vein that is formed by the union of branches originating in the occipital region and forming a plexus about the vertebral artery in its passage through the foramina of the cervical vertebrae

vertebra prom·i·nens \-'prä-mi-ˌnenz\ *n* : the seventh cervical vertebra characterized by a prominent spinous process which can be felt at the base of the neck

ver·te·brate \'vər-tə-brət, -ˌbrāt\ *n* : any of a subphylum (Vertebrata) of animals with a spinal column including the mammals, birds, reptiles, amphibians, and fishes — **vertebrate** *adj*

ver·te·bro·ba·si·lar \ˌvər-tə-brō-'bā-sə-lər\ *adj* : of, relating to, or being the vertebral and basilar arteries

ver·te·bro·chon·dral rib \ˌvər-tə-brō-'kän-drəl-\ *n* : any of the three false ribs that are located above the floating ribs and that are attached to each other by costal cartilages

ver·te·bro·ster·nal rib \-'stər-nəl-\ : TRUE RIB

ver·tex \'vər-ˌteks\ *n, pl* **ver·ti·ces** \'vər-tə-ˌsēz\ *also* **ver·tex·es** **1** : the top of the head **2** : the highest point of the skull

vertex presentation *n* : normal obstetric presentation in which the fetal occiput lies at the mouth of the uterus

ver·ti·cal \'vər-ti-kəl\ *adj* : relating to or being transmission (as of a disease) by inheritance in contrast to physical contact or proximity — compare HORIZONTAL **2** — **ver·ti·cal·ly** *adv*

vertical dimension *n* : the distance between two arbitrarily chosen points on the face above and below the mouth when the teeth are in occlusion

vertical nystagmus *n* : nystagmus characterized by up-and-down movement of the eyes

ver·tig·i·nous \(ˌ)vər-'ti-jə-nəs\ *adj* : of, relating to, characterized by, or affected with vertigo or dizziness

ver·ti·go \'vər-ti-ˌgō\ *n, pl* **-goes** *or* **-gos** **1** : a disordered state which is associated with various disorders (as of the inner ear) and in which the individual or the individual's surroundings seem to whirl dizzily — see SUBJECTIVE VERTIGO; compare DIZZINESS **2** : disordered vertiginous movement as a symptom of disease in lower animals; *also* : a disease (as gid) causing this

very low–density lipoprotein *n* : VLDL

vesicae — see TRIGONUM VESICAE, UVULA VESICAE

ves·i·ca fel·lea \'ve-si-kə-'fe-lē-ə\ *n* : GALLBLADDER

¹ves·i·cal \'ve-si-kəl\ *adj* : of or relating to a bladder and esp. to the urinary bladder ⟨~ burning⟩

²vesical *n* : VESICAL ARTERY

vesical artery *n* : any of several arteries that arise from the internal iliac artery or one of its branches and that supply the urinary bladder and adjacent parts: as **a** : any of several arteries that arise from the umbilical artery and supply the upper part of the bladder — called also *superior vesical, superior vesical artery* **b** : one that arises from the internal iliac artery or the internal pudendal artery and that supplies the bladder, prostate, and seminal vesicles — called also *inferior vesical, inferior vesical artery*

vesical plexus *n* : a plexus of nerves that comprises preganglionic fibers derived chiefly from the hypogastric plexus and postganglionic neurons whose fibers are distributed to the bladder and adjacent parts

vesical venous plexus *n* : a plexus of veins surrounding the neck of the bladder and the base of the prostate gland

ves·i·cant \'ve-si-kənt\ *adj* : producing or tending to produce blisters ⟨a ~ substance⟩ — **vesicant** *n*

vesica uri·nar·ia \-ˌyür-i-'nar-ē-ə\ *n* : URINARY BLADDER

ves·i·cle \'ve-si-kəl\ *n* **1 a** : a membranous and usu. fluid-filled pouch (as a cyst or cell) in a plant or animal **b** : SYNAPTIC VESICLE **2** : a small abnormal elevation of the outer layer of skin enclosing a watery liquid : BLISTER **3** : a pocket of embryonic tissue that is the beginning of an organ — see BRAIN VESICLE, OPTIC VESICLE

vesico- *comb form* : of or relating to the urinary bladder and ⟨*vesico*uterine⟩

ves·i·co·en·ter·ic \ˌve-si-kō-en-'ter-ik\ *adj* : of, relating to, or connecting the urinary bladder and the intestinal tract ⟨a ∼ fistula⟩

ves·i·cos·to·my \ˌve-si-ˈkäs-tə-mē\ *n, pl* **-mies** : CYSTOSTOMY

ves·i·co·ure·ter·al reflux \ˌve-si-kō-yù-ˈrē-tə-rəl-\ *n* : reflux of urine from the bladder into a ureter

ves·i·co·ure·ter·ic reflux \-ˈter-ik-\ *n* : VESICOURETERAL REFLUX

ves·i·co·uter·ine \ˌve-si-kō-ˈyü-tə-ˌrīn, -rən\ *adj* : of, relating to, or connecting the urinary bladder and the uterus

ves·i·co·vag·i·nal \ˌve-si-kō-ˈva-jən-ᵊl\ *adj* : of, relating to, or connecting the urinary bladder and vagina

vesicul- *or* **vesiculo-** *comb form* **1** : vesicle ⟨*vesicul*ectomy⟩ **2** : vesicular and ⟨*vesiculo*bullous⟩

ve·sic·u·lar \və-ˈsi-kyə-lər, ve-\ *adj* **1** : characterized by the presence or formation of vesicles ⟨a ∼ rash⟩ **2** : having the form of a vesicle

vesicular breathing *n* : normal breathing that is soft and low-pitched when heard in auscultation

vesicular dermatitis *n* : a severe dermatitis esp. of young chickens and turkeys — called also *sod disease*

vesicular exanthema *n* : an acute virus disease of swine that closely resembles foot-and-mouth disease

vesicular ovarian follicle *n* : GRAAFIAN FOLLICLE

vesicular stomatitis *n* : an acute virus disease esp. of horses and mules that is marked by erosive blisters in and about the mouth

ve·sic·u·la·tion \və-ˌsi-kyə-ˈlā-shən\ *n* **1** : the presence or formation of vesicles **2** : the process of becoming vesicular ⟨∼ of a papule⟩

ve·sic·u·lec·to·my \və-ˌsi-kyə-ˈlek-tə-mē\ *n, pl* **-mies** : surgical excision of a seminal vesicle

ve·sic·u·li·tis \və-ˌsi-kyə-ˈlī-təs\ *n* : inflammation of a vesicle and esp. a seminal vesicle

ve·sic·u·lo·bul·lous \və-ˌsi-kyə-lō-ˈbü-ləs\ *adj* : of, relating to, or being both vesicles and bullae ⟨a ∼ rash⟩

ve·sic·u·lo·gram \və-ˈsi-kyə-lə-ˌgram\ *n* : a radiograph produced by vesiculography

ve·sic·u·log·ra·phy \və-ˌsi-kyə-ˈlä-grə-fē\ *n, pl* **-phies** : radiography of the seminal vesicles following the injection of a radiopaque medium

ve·sic·u·lo·pus·tu·lar \və-ˌsi-kyə-lō-ˈpəs-chə-lər\ *adj* : of, relating to, or marked by both vesicles and pustules

ve·sic·u·lot·o·my \və-ˌsi-kyə-ˈlä-tə-mē\ *n, pl* **-mies** : surgical incision of a seminal vesicle

Ves·prin \ˈves-prən\ *trademark* — used for a preparation of triflupromazine

ves·sel \ˈve-səl\ *n* : a tube or canal (as an artery, vein, or lymphatic) in which a body fluid (as blood or lymph) is contained and conveyed or circulated

ves·tib·u·lar \ve-ˈsti-byə-lər\ *adj* **1** : of

or relating to the vestibule of the inner ear, the vestibular apparatus, the vestibular nerve, or the labyrinthine sense **2** : lying within or facing the vestibule of the mouth ⟨the ∼ surface of a tooth⟩ — **ves·tib·u·lar·ly** *adv*

vestibular apparatus *n* : the vestibule of the inner ear together with the end organs and nerve fibers that function in mediating the labyrinthine sense

vestibular folds *n pl* : FALSE VOCAL CORDS

vestibular ganglion *n* : a sensory ganglion in the trunk of the vestibular nerve in the internal auditory meatus that contains cell bodies supplying nerve fibers comprising the vestibular nerve

vestibular gland *n* : any of the glands (as Bartholin's glands) that open into the vestibule of the vagina

vestibular ligament *n* : the narrow band of fibrous tissue contained in each of the false vocal cords and stretching between the thyroid and arytenoid cartilages

vestibular membrane *n* : a thin cellular membrane separating the scala media and scala vestibuli — called also *Reissner's membrane*

vestibular nerve *n* : a branch of the auditory nerve that consists of bipolar neurons with cell bodies collected in the vestibular ganglion, with peripheral processes passing to the semicircular canals, utricle, and saccule, and with central processes passing to the vestibular nuclei of the medulla oblongata

vestibular neuronitis *n* : a disorder of uncertain etiology that is characterized by transitory attacks of severe vertigo

vestibular nucleus *n* : any of four nuclei in the medulla oblongata on each side of the floor of the fourth ventricle of the brain in which fibers of the vestibular nerve terminate — see INFERIOR VESTIBULAR NUCLEUS, LATERAL VESTIBULAR NUCLEUS, MEDIAL VESTIBULAR NUCLEUS, SUPERIOR VESTIBULAR NUCLEUS

vestibular system *n* : VESTIBULAR APPARATUS

ves·ti·bule \ˈves-tə-ˌbyül\ *n* : any of various bodily cavities esp. when serving as or resembling an entrance to some other cavity or space: as **a** (1) : the central cavity of the bony labyrinth of the ear (2) : the parts of the membranous labyrinth comprising the utricle and the saccule and contained in the cavity of the bony labyrinth **b** : the space between the labia minora containing the orifice of the urethra **c** : the part of the left ventricle of the heart immediately below the aortic orifice **d** : the part of the mouth cavity outside the teeth and gums

vestibuli — see FENESTRA VESTIBULI, SCALA VESTIBULI

ves·tib·u·lo·co·chle·ar nerve \ve-ˌsti-byə-lō-ˈkō-klē-ər-, -ˈkä-\ n : AUDITORY NERVE

ves·tib·u·lo·plas·ty \ve-ˈsti-byə-lō-ˌplas-tē\ n, pl **-ties** : plastic surgery of the vestibular region of the mouth

vestibulorum — see SCALA VESTIBULI

ves·tib·u·lo·spi·nal tract \ve-ˌsti-byə-lō-ˈspī-nəl-\ n : a nerve tract on each side of the central nervous system containing nerve fibers that arise from cell bodies in the lateral vestibular nucleus on one side of the medulla oblongata and that descend on the same side in the lateral and anterior funiculi of the spinal cord to synapse with motoneurons in the ventral roots

ves·tige \ˈves-tij\ n : a bodily part or organ that is small and degenerate or imperfectly developed in comparison to one more fully developed in an earlier stage of the individual, in a past generation, or in closely related forms — **ves·tig·ial** \ve-ˈsti-jəl, -jē-əl\ adj

vestigial fold of Mar·shall \-ˈmär-shəl\ n : a fold of endocardium that extends from the left pulmonary artery to the more superior of the two left pulmonary veins

J. Marshall — see OBLIQUE VEIN OF MARSHALL

vet \ˈvet\ n : VETERINARIAN

vet·er·i·nar·i·an \ˌve-tə-rə-ˈner-ē-ən, ˌve-trə-\ n : a person qualified and authorized to practice veterinary medicine

¹**vet·er·i·nary** \ˈve-tə-rə-ˌner-ē, ˈve-trə-\ adj : of, relating to, or being the science and art of prevention, cure, or alleviation of disease and injury in animals and esp. domestic animals ⟨~ medicine⟩

²**veterinary** n, pl **-nar·ies** : VETERINARIAN

veterinary surgeon n, Brit : VETERINARIAN

vi·a·ble \ˈvī-ə-bəl\ adj 1 : capable of living ⟨~ cancer cells⟩; esp : having attained such form and development of organs as to be normally capable of living outside the uterus — often used of a human fetus at seven months but may be interpreted according to the state of the art of medicine ⟨a ~ fetus⟩ 2 : capable of growing or developing ⟨~ eggs⟩ — **vi·a·bil·i·ty** \ˌvī-ə-ˈbi-lə-tē\ n

vi·al \ˈvī-əl, ˈvīl\ n : a small closed or closable vessel esp. for liquids — called also **phial**

Vi antigen \ˈvē-ˈī-\ n : a heat-labile somatic antigen associated with virulence in some bacteria (as of the genus Salmonella) and esp. in the typhoid fever bacterium

Vi·bra·my·cin \ˌvī-brə-ˈmīs-ᵊn\ trademark — used for a preparation of doxycycline

vi·bra·tor \ˈvī-ˌbrā-tər\ n : a vibrating electrical apparatus used in massage or for sexual stimulation

vib·rio \ˈvi-brē-ō\ n 1 cap : a genus of motile gram-negative bacteria (family Vibrionaceae) that are curved rods and include various saprophytes and a few pathogens (as V. cholerae, the cause of cholera in humans) 2 : any bacterium of the genus Vibrio; broadly : a curved rod-shaped bacterium

vib·ri·on·ic abortion \ˌvi-brē-ˈä-nik-\ n : abortion in sheep and cattle caused by a bacterium of the genus Campylobacter (C. fetus syn. Vibrio fetus)

vib·ri·o·sis \ˌvi-brē-ˈō-səs\ n, pl **-oses** \-ˌsēz\ : infestation with or disease caused by bacteria of the genus Vibrio or Campylobacter; specif : VIBRIONIC ABORTION

vi·bris·sa \vī-ˈbri-sə, və-\ n, pl **vi·bris·sae** \vī-ˈbri-(ˌ)sē; və-ˈbri-(ˌ)sē, -ˌsī\ : any of the stiff hairs growing within the nostrils that serve to impede the inhalation of foreign substances

vi·car·i·ous \vī-ˈkar-ē-əs, və-\ adj : occurring in an unexpected or abnormal part of the body instead of the usual one ⟨bleeding from the gums sometimes occurs in the absence of the normal discharge from the uterus in ~ menstruation⟩

vice \ˈvīs\ n : an abnormal behavior pattern in a domestic animal detrimental to its health or usefulness

vid·ar·a·bine \vi-ˈdär-ə-ˌbēn\ n : an antiviral agent $C_{10}H_{13}N_5O_4 \cdot H_2O$ derived from adenine and arabinoside and used esp. to treat keratitis and encephalitis caused by the herpes simplex virus — called also **ara-A, adenine arabinoside**

Vi·dex \ˈvī-ˌdeks\ trademark — used for a preparation of DDI

Vid·i·an artery \ˈvi-dē-ən-\ n : a branch of the maxillary artery passing through the pterygoid canal of the sphenoid bone

Gui·di \ˈgwē-dē\, **Guido** (Latin **Vidus Vidius**) (1508–1569), Italian anatomist and surgeon.

Vidian canal n : PTERYGOID CANAL

Vidian nerve n : a nerve formed by the union of the greater petrosal and the deep petrosal nerves that passes forward through the pterygoid canal in the sphenoid bone and joins the pterygopalatine ganglion

vil·li·ki·nin \ˌvi-lə-ˈki-nən\ n : a hormone postulated to exist in order to explain the activity of intestinal extracts in stimulating the intestinal villi

vil·lo·nod·u·lar \ˌvi-lō-ˈnä-jə-lər\ adj : characterized by villous and nodular thickening (as of a synovial membrane) ⟨~ synovitis⟩

vil·lus \ˈvi-ləs\ n, pl **vil·li** \-ˌlī\ : a small slender vascular process: as **a** : one of the minute fingerlike processes of the mucous membrane of the small intestine that serve in the absorption of nutriment **b** : one of the branching processes of the surface of the chorion of the developing embryo of most mammals that help to form the placenta — **vil·lous** \\'vi-ləs\\ *adj*

vin·blas·tine \\(ˌ)vin-'blas-ˌtēn\\ *n* : an alkaloid $C_{46}H_{58}N_4O_9$ that is obtained from a periwinkle (*Catharanthus roseus*) and that is used esp. in the form of its sulfate to treat human neoplastic diseases (as leukemias and testicular carcinoma) — called also *vincaleukoblastine*

vin·ca \\'viŋ-kə\\ *n* : PERIWINKLE

vin·ca·leu·ko·blas·tine \\ˌviŋ-kə-ˌlü-kə-'blas-ˌtēn\\ *n* : VINBLASTINE

Vin·cent's angina \\'vin-sənts-, (ˌ)van-'sän z-\\ *n* : Vincent's infection in which the ulceration has spread to surrounding tissues (as of the pharynx and tonsils) — called also *trench mouth, ulceromembranous gingivitis*

Vincent, Jean Hyacinthe (1862–1950), French bacteriologist.

Vincent's disease *n* : a disease marked by infection with Vincent's organisms; *esp* : VINCENT'S ANGINA

Vincent's infection *n* : a progressive painful disease of the mouth that is marked esp. by dirty gray ulceration of the mucous membranes, spontaneous hemorrhaging of the gums, and a foul odor to the breath and that is associated with the presence of large numbers of Vincent's organisms — called also *trench mouth*

Vincent's organisms *n pl* : a bacterium of the genus *Fusobacterium* (*F. nucleatum* syn. *F. fusiforme*) and a spirochete of the genus *Treponema* (*T. vincentii* syn. *Borrelia vincentii*) that are part of the normal oral flora and undergo a great increase in numbers in the mucous membrane of the mouth and adjacent parts in Vincent's infection and Vincent's angina

Vincent's stomatitis *n* : VINCENT'S ANGINA

Vincent's ulcer *n* **1** : TROPICAL ULCER **2** : an ulcer of the mucous membranes symptomatic of Vincent's infection or Vincent's angina

vin·cris·tine \\(ˌ)vin-'kris-ˌtēn\\ *n* : an alkaloid $C_{46}H_{56}N_4O_{10}$ that is obtained from a periwinkle (*Catharanthus roseus*) and that is used esp. in the form of its sulfate to treat human neoplastic diseases (as leukemias and Wilms' tumor) — called also *leurocristine*; see ONCOVIN

Vine·berg procedure \\'vīn-ˌbərg-\\ *n* : surgical implantation of an internal thoracic artery into the myocardium

Vineberg, Arthur Martin (1903–1988), Canadian surgeon.

vi·nyl chloride \\'vīn-əl-\\ *n* : a flammable gaseous carcinogenic compound C_2H_3Cl

vinyl ether *n* : a volatile flammable liquid unsaturated ether C_4H_6O that is used as an inhalation anesthetic for short operative procedures

vi·o·my·cin \\ˌvī-ə-'mīs-ən\\ *n* : a polypeptide antibiotic $C_{25}H_{43}N_{13}O_{10}$ that is produced by several soil actinomycetes of the genus *Streptomyces* and is administered intramuscularly in the form of its sulfate in the treatment of tuberculosis esp. in combination with other antituberculous drugs

vi·os·ter·ol \\vī-'äs-tə-ˌrol, -ˌrōl\\ *n* : CALCIFEROL

VIP *abbr* vasoactive intestinal peptide

vi·per \\'vī-pər\\ *n* : a common Eurasian venomous snake of the genus *Vipera* (*V. berus*) whose bite is usu. not fatal to humans; *broadly* : any of a family (Viperidae) of venomous snakes that includes Old World vipers (subfamily Viperinae) and the pit vipers

Vi·pera \\'vī-pə-rə\\ *n* : a genus of Old World venomous snakes (family Viperidae)

vi·po·ma \\vī-'pō-mə, vi-\\ *n* : a tumor of endocrine tissue esp. in the pancreas that secretes vasoactive intestinal polypeptide

vi·rae·mia *chiefly Brit var of* VIREMIA

vi·ral \\'vī-rəl\\ *adj* : of, relating to, or caused by a virus — **vi·ral·ly** \\-rə-lē\\

Vir·chow–Ro·bin space \\'fir-ˌkō-rō-'baⁿ-\\ *n* : any of the spaces that surround blood vessels as they enter the brain and that communicate with the subarachnoid space

Virchow, Rudolf Ludwig Karl (1821–1902), German pathologist, anthropologist, and statesman.

Robin, Charles–Philippe (1821–1885), French anatomist and histologist.

Virchow's node *n* : SIGNAL NODE

vi·re·mia \\vī-'rē-mē-ə\\ *n* : the presence of virus in the blood of a host — **vi·re·mic** \\-mik\\ *adj*

vir·gin \\'vər-jən\\ *n* : a person who has not had sexual intercourse — **vir·gin·i·ty** \\(ˌ)vər-'ji-nə-tē\\ *n*

vir·i·ci·dal \\ˌvī-rə-'sīd-əl\\ *adj* : VIRUCIDAL

vir·i·cide \\'vī-rə-ˌsīd\\ *n* : VIRUCIDE

vir·ile \\'vir-əl, -ˌil\\ *adj* **1** : having the nature, properties, or qualities of an adult male; *specif* : capable of functioning as a male in copulation **2** : characteristic of or associated with men : MASCULINE — **vi·ril·i·ty** \\və-'ri-lə-tē\\ *n*

vir·il·ism \\'vir-ə-ˌli-zəm\\ *n* **1** : precocious development of secondary sex characteristics in the male **2** : the appearance of secondary sex characteristics of the male in a female

vir·il·ize \\'vir-ə-ˌlīz\\ *vb* **-ized; -iz·ing** : to make virile; *esp* : to cause or produce virilism in — **vir·il·i·za·tion** \\ˌvir-ə-lə-'zā-shən\\ *n*

vir·i·on \\'vī-rē-ˌän, 'vir-ē-\\ *n* : a complete virus particle that consists of an RNA or DNA core with a protein coat sometimes with external envelopes and that is the extracellular infective form of a virus

vi·rol·o·gy \vī-'rä-lə-jē\ *n, pl* **-gies** : a branch of science that deals with viruses — **vi·ro·log·i·cal** \ˌvī-rə-'lä-ji-kəl\ *or* **vi·ro·log·ic** \-'jik\ *adj* — **vi·ro·log·i·cal·ly** *adv* — **vi·rol·o·gist** \vī-'rä-lə-jist\ *n*

virtual dead space *n* : PHYSIOLOGICAL DEAD SPACE

vi·ru·cid·al \ˌvī-rə-'sīd-ᵊl\ *adj* : having the capacity to or tending to destroy or inactivate viruses ⟨∼ activity⟩

vi·ru·cide \'vī-rə-ˌsīd\ *n* : an agent having the capacity to destroy or inactivate viruses — called also **viricide**

vir·u·lence \'vir-yə-ləns, 'vir-ə-\ *n* : the quality or state of being virulent: as **a** : relative severity and malignancy **b** : the relative capacity of a pathogen to overcome body defenses — compare INFECTIVITY

vir·u·len·cy \-lən-sē\ *n, pl* **-cies** : VIRULENCE

vir·u·lent \-lənt\ *adj* **1 a** : marked by a rapid, severe, and malignant course ⟨a ∼ infection⟩ **b** : able to overcome bodily defense mechanisms ⟨a ∼ pathogen⟩ **2** : extremely poisonous or venomous : NOXIOUS

vi·rus \'vī-rəs\ *n* **1** : the causative agent of an infectious disease **2** : any of a large group of submicroscopic infective agents that are regarded either as extremely simple microorganisms or as extremely complex molecules, that typically contain a protein coat surrounding an RNA or DNA core of genetic material but no semipermeable membrane, that are capable of growth and multiplication only in living cells, and that cause various important diseases — see FILTERABLE VIRUS **3** : a disease caused by a virus

virus pneumonia *n* : pneumonia caused or thought to be caused by a virus; *esp* : PRIMARY ATYPICAL PNEUMONIA

viscer- *or* **visceri-** *or* **viscero-** *comb form* : visceral : viscera ⟨*viscero*tropic⟩

viscera *pl of* VISCUS

vis·cer·al \'vi-sə-rəl\ *adj* : of, relating to, or located on or among the viscera — compare PARIETAL 1 — **vis·cer·al·ly** *adv*

visceral arch *n* : BRANCHIAL ARCH

visceral leishmaniasis *n* : KALA-AZAR

visceral muscle *n* : smooth muscle esp. in visceral structures

visceral pericardium *n* : EPICARDIUM

visceral peritoneum *n* : the part of the peritoneum that lines the abdominal viscera — compare PARIETAL PERITONEUM

visceral reflex *n* : a reflex mediated by autonomic nerves and initiated in the viscera

vis·cero·mo·tor \ˌvi-sə-rō-'mō-tər\ *adj* : causing or concerned with the functional activity of the viscera ⟨∼ nerves⟩

vis·cer·op·to·sis \ˌvi-sə-räp-'tō-səs\ *n, pl* **-to·ses** \-ˌsēz\ : downward displacement of the abdominal viscera

vis·cer·o·trop·ic \ˌvi-sə-rə-'trä-pik\ *adj* : tending to affect or having an affinity for the viscera — used esp. of a virus — **vis·cer·ot·ro·pism** \ˌvi-sə-'rä-trə-ˌpi-zəm\ *n*

vis·cid \'vi-səd\ *adj* **1** : having an adhesive quality **2** : having a glutinous consistency

vis·com·e·ter \vis-'kä-mə-tər\ *n* : an instrument used to measure viscosity ⟨a blood ∼⟩ — called also **viscosimeter** — **vis·co·met·ric** \ˌvis-kə-'me-trik\ *adj*

vis·cos·i·ty \vis-'kä-sə-tē\ *n, pl* **-ties** : the quality of being viscous; *esp* : the property of resistance to flow in a fluid

vis·cous \'vis-kəs\ *adj* **1** : having a glutinous consistency and the quality of sticking or adhering : VISCID **2** : having or characterized by viscosity

vis·cus \'vis-kəs\ *n, pl* **vis·cera** \'vi-sə-rə\ : an internal organ of the body; *esp* : one (as the heart, liver, or intestine) located in the large cavity of the trunk

vis·i·ble \'vi-zə-bəl\ *adj* **1** : capable of being seen : perceptible to vision **2** : situated in the region of the visible spectrum

visible spectrum *n* : the part of the electromagnetic spectrum to which the human eye is sensitive extending from a wavelength of about 400 nm (3800 angstroms) for violet light to about 700 nm (7600 angstroms) for red light

vi·sion \'vi-zhən\ *n* **1** : the act or power of seeing **2** : the special sense by which the qualities of an object (as color, shape, and size) constituting its appearance are perceived and which is mediated by the eye

vis·it \'vi-zət\ *n* **1** : a professional call (as by a physician to treat a patient) **2** : a call upon a professional person (as a physician or dentist) for consultation or treatment — **visit** *vb*

visiting nurse *n* : a nurse employed (as by a hospital or social-service agency) to perform public health services and esp. to visit sick persons in a community — called also *public health nurse*

vis·na \'vis-nə\ *n* : a chronic retroviral encephalomyelitis of sheep

Vis·ta·ril \'vis-tə-ˌril\ *trademark* — used for a preparation of hydroxyzine

vi·su·al \'vi-zhə-wəl\ *adj* **1** : of, relating to, or used in vision ⟨∼ organs⟩ **2** : attained or maintained by sight ⟨∼ impressions⟩ — **vi·su·al·ly** *adv*

visual acuity *n* : the relative ability of the visual organ to resolve detail

visual area *n* : a sensory area of the occipital lobe of the cerebral cortex receiving afferent projection fibers concerned with the sense of sight — called also *visual cortex*

visual cortex *n* : VISUAL AREA

visual field *n* : the entire expanse of space visible at a given instant without moving the eyes — called also *field of vision*

vi·su·al·i·za·tion \ˌvi-zhə-wə-lə-ˈzā-shən\ *n* **1** : formation of mental visual images **2** : the process of making an internal organ visible by the introduction (as by swallowing, by an injection, or by an enema) of a radiopaque substance followed by roentgenography — **vi·su·al·ize** \ˈvi-zhə-wə-ˌlīz\ *vb*

vi·su·al·iz·er \-ˌlī-zər\ *n* : one that visualizes; *esp* : one whose mental imagery is prevailingly visual — compare AUDILE, TACTILE

visual projection area *n* : STRIATE CORTEX

visual purple *n* : RHODOPSIN

vi·suo·mo·tor \ˌvi-zhə-wō-ˈmō-tər\ *adj* : of or relating to vision and muscular movement ⟨∼ coordination⟩

vi·suo·spa·tial \-ˈspā-shəl\ *adj* : of or relating to thought processes that involve visual and spatial awareness

vi·tal \ˈvīt-ᵊl\ *adj* **1 a** : existing as a manifestation of life **b** : concerned with or necessary to the maintenance of life ⟨∼ organs⟩ **2** : characteristic of life or living beings **3** : recording data relating to lives **4** : of, relating to, or constituting the staining of living tissues — **vi·tal·ly** *adv*

vital capacity *n* : the breathing capacity of the lungs expressed as the number of cubic inches or cubic centimeters of air that can be forcibly exhaled after a full inspiration

vital function *n* : a function of the body (as respiration) on which life is directly dependent

vi·tal·i·ty \vī-ˈta-lə-tē\ *n, pl* **-ties** : capacity to live and develop; *also* : physical or mental vigor esp. when highly developed

Vi·tal·li·um \vī-ˈta-lē-əm\ *trademark* — used for a cobalt-chromium alloy of platinum-white color used esp. for cast dentures and prostheses

vi·tals \ˈvīt-ᵊlz\ *n pl* : vital organs (as the heart, liver, lungs, and brain)

vital signs *n pl* : signs of life; *specif* : the pulse rate, respiratory rate, body temperature, and often blood pressure of a person

vital statistics *n pl* : statistics relating to births, deaths, marriages, health, and disease

vi·ta·min \ˈvī-tə-mən\ *n* : any of various organic substances that are essential in minute quantities to the nutrition of most animals and some plants, act esp. as coenzymes and precursors of coenzymes in the regulation of metabolic processes but do not provide energy or serve as building units, and are present in natural foodstuffs or sometimes produced within the body

vitamin A *n* : any of several fat-soluble vitamins or a mixture of two or more of them whose lack in the animal body causes keratinization of epithelial tissues (as in the eye with result-

ing night blindness and xerophthalmia): as **a** : a pale yellow crystalline alcohol $C_{20}H_{29}OH$ that is found in animal products (as egg yolk, milk, and butter) and esp. in marine fish-liver oils (as of cod, halibut, and shark) — called also *retinol, vitamin A_1* **b** : a yellow viscous liquid alcohol $C_{20}H_{27}OH$ that contains one more double bond in a molecule than vitamin A_1 and is less active biologically in mammals and that occurs esp. in the liver oil of freshwater fish — called also *vitamin A_2*

vitamin A aldehyde *n* : RETINAL

vitamin A_1 \-ā-ˈwən\ *n* : VITAMIN A a

vitamin A_2 \-ā-ˈtü\ *n* : VITAMIN A b

vitamin B *n* **1** : VITAMIN B COMPLEX **2** : any of numerous members of the vitamin B complex; *esp* : THIAMINE

vitamin B_c \-ˌbē-ˈsē\ *n* : FOLIC ACID

vitamin B complex *n* : a group of water-soluble vitamins found esp. in yeast, seed germs, eggs, liver and flesh, and vegetables that have varied metabolic functions and include coenzymes and growth factors — called also *B complex*; see BIOTIN, CHOLINE, NIACIN, PANTOTHENIC ACID

vitamin B_1 \-ˌbē-ˈwən\ *n* : THIAMINE

vitamin B_{17} \-ˌbē-ˌse-vən-ˈtēn\ *n* : LAETRILE

vitamin B_6 \-ˌbē-ˈsiks\ *n* : pyridoxine or a closely related compound found widely in combined form and considered essential to vertebrate nutrition

vitamin B_T \-ˌbē-ˈtē\ *n* : CARNITINE

vitamin B_3 \-ˌbē-ˈthrē\ *n* : NIACIN

vitamin B_{12} \-ˌbē-ˈtwelv\ *n* **1** : a complex cobalt-containing compound $C_{63}H_{88}CoN_{14}O_{14}P$ that occurs esp. in liver, is essential to normal blood formation, neural function, and growth, and is used esp. in treating pernicious and related anemias and in animal feed as a growth factor — called also *cyanocobalamin* **2** : any of several compounds similar to vitamin B_{12} in action but having different chemistry

vitamin B_2 \-ˌbē-ˈtü\ *n* : RIBOFLAVIN

vitamin C *n* : a water-soluble vitamin $C_6H_8O_6$ found in plants and esp. in fruits and leafy vegetables or made synthetically and used in the prevention and treatment of scurvy and as an antioxidant for foods — called also *ascorbic acid*

vitamin D *n* : any or all of several fat-soluble vitamins chemically related to steroids, essential for normal bone and tooth structure, and found esp. in fish-liver oils, egg yolk, and milk or produced by activation (as by ultraviolet irradiation) of sterols: as **a** : CALCIFEROL **b** : CHOLECALCIFEROL — called also *sunshine vitamin*

vitamin D_3 \-ˌdē-ˈthrē\ *n* : CHOLECALCIFEROL

vitamin D_2 \-ˌdē-ˈtü\ *n* : CALCIFEROL

vitamin E *n* : any of several fat-soluble vitamins that are chemically tocopherols, are essential in the nutrition of various vertebrates in which their absence is associated with infertility, degenerative changes in muscle, or vascular abnormalities, are found esp. in leaves and in seed germ oils, and are used chiefly in animal feeds and as antioxidants; *esp* : ALPHA≈ TOCOPHEROL

vitamin G *n* : RIBOFLAVIN

vitamin H *n* : BIOTIN

vitamin K *n* 1 : either of two naturally occurring fat-soluble vitamins that are essential for the clotting of blood because of their role in the production of prothrombin in the liver and that are used in preventing and treating hypoprothrombinemia and hemorrhage: **a** : an oily naphthoquinone $C_{31}H_{46}O_2$ that is obtained esp. from alfalfa or made synthetically and that has a fast, potent, and prolonged biological effect — called also *phylloquinone, phytonadione, vitamin K₁*; see MEPHYTON **b** : a crystalline naphthoquinone $C_{41}H_{56}O_2$ that is obtained esp. from putrefied fish meal and is synthesized by various bacteria (as in the intestines) and that is slightly less active biologically than vitamin K₁ — called also *menaquinone, vitamin K₂* **2** : any of several synthetic compounds that are closely related chemically to vitamins K₁ and K₂ but are simpler in structure; *esp* : MENADIONE

vitamin K₁ \-ˌkā-ˈwən\ *n* : VITAMIN K 1a

vitamin K₃ \-ˌkā-ˈthrē\ *n* : MENADIONE

vitamin K₂ \-ˌkā-ˈtü\ *n* : VITAMIN K 1b

vitamin M *n* : FOLIC ACID

vi·ta·min·ol·o·gy \ˌvī-tə-mə-ˈnä-lə-jē\ *n, pl* **-gies** : a branch of knowledge dealing with vitamins, their nature, action, and use

vitamin PP \-ˌpē-ˈpē\ *n* : NIACIN

vitell- *or* **vitello-** *comb form* : yolk : vitellus (*vitellogenesis*)

vi·tel·lin \vī-ˈte-lən, və-\ *n* : a phosphoprotein in egg yolk — called also *ovovitellin*

vi·tel·line \-ˈte-lən, -ˌlēn, -ˌlīn\ *adj* : of, relating to, or containing yolk

vitelline duct *n* : OMPHALOMESENTERIC DUCT

vitelline membrane *n* : a membrane enclosing the egg proper and corresponding to the plasma membrane of an ordinary cell

vi·tel·lo·gen·e·sis \vī-ˌte-lō-ˈje-nə-səs, və-\ *n, pl* **-e·ses** \-ˌsēz\ : yolk formation — **vi·tel·lo·gen·ic** \-ˈje-nik\ *adj*

vi·tel·lus \vī-ˈte-ləs, və-\ *n* : the egg cell proper including the yolk but excluding any albuminous or membranous envelopes; *also* : YOLK

vit·il·i·go \ˌvi-tə-ˈlī-gō, -ˈlē-\ *n* : a skin disorder manifested by smooth white spots on various parts of the body — compare LEUKODERMA

vit·rec·to·my \və-ˈtrek-tə-mē\ *n, pl*

-mies : surgical removal of all or part of the vitreous humor

¹vit·re·ous \ˈvi-trē-əs\ *adj* : of, relating to, constituting, or affecting the vitreous humor (∼ hemorrhages)

²vitreous *n* : VITREOUS HUMOR

vitreous body *n* : VITREOUS HUMOR

vitreous humor *n* : the clear colorless transparent jelly that fills the eyeball posterior to the lens and is enclosed by a delicate hyaloid membrane

vitro — see IN VITRO

Vi·vac·til \vī-ˈvak-til\ *trademark* — used for a preparation of protriptyline

vi·vax malaria \ˈvī-ˌvaks-\ *n* : malaria caused by a plasmodium (*Plasmodium vivax*) that induces paroxysms at 48-hour intervals — compare FALCIPARUM MALARIA

vivi- *comb form* : alive : living (*vivisection*)

vi·vip·a·rous \vī-ˈvi-pə-rəs, və-\ *adj* : producing living young instead of eggs from within the body in the manner of nearly all mammals, many reptiles, and a few fishes — compare OVIPAROUS, OVOVIVIPAROUS — **vi·vi·par·i·ty** \ˌvī-və-ˈpar-ə-tē, ˌvi-\ *n*

vivi·sec·tion \ˌvi-və-ˈsek-shən, ˈvi-və-ˌ\ *n* : the cutting of or operation on a living animal usu. for physiological or pathological investigation — **vivi·sect** \-ˈsekt\ *vb* — **vivi·sec·tion·ist** \ˌvi-və-ˈsek-sh(ə-)nəst\ *n*

vivo — see IN VIVO

VLDL \ˌvē-(ˌ)el-(ˌ)dē-ˈel\ *n* : a plasma lipoprotein that is produced primarily by the liver with lesser amounts contributed by the intestine, that contains relatively large amounts of triglycerides compared to protein, and that leaves a residue of cholesterol in the tissues during the process of conversion to LDL — called also *very low-density lipoprotein;* compare HDL, LDL

VMA *abbr* vanillylmandelic acid

VMD *abbr* doctor of veterinary medicine

VNA *abbr* Visiting Nurse Association

vo·cal \ˈvō-kəl\ *adj* **1** : uttered by the voice : ORAL **2** : having or exercising the power of producing voice, speech, or sound **3** : of, relating to, or resembling the voice — **vo·cal·ly** *adv*

vocal cord *n* **1** *pl* : either of two pairs of folds of mucous membrane of which each member of each pair stretches from the thyroid cartilage in front to the arytenoid cartilage in back, contains a band of fibrous or elastic tissue, and has a free edge projecting into the cavity of the larynx toward the contralateral member of the same pair forming a cleft which can be opened or closed: **a** : FALSE VOCAL CORDS **b** : TRUE VOCAL CORDS **2** : VOCAL LIGAMENT

vocal folds *n pl* : TRUE VOCAL CORDS

vo·ca·lis \vō-ˈkā-ləs\ *n* : a small muscle that is the medial part of the thyroarytenoid, originates in the lamina of the thyroid cartilage, inserts in the vocal process of the arytenoid cartilage, and modulates the tension of the true vocal cords

vo·cal·iza·tion \ˌvō-kə-lə-ˈzā-shən\ *n* : the act or process of producing sounds with the voice; *also* : a sound thus produced — **vo·cal·ize** *vb*

vocal ligament *n* : the band of yellow elastic tissue contained in each true vocal cord and stretching between the thyroid and arytenoid cartilages — called also *inferior thyroarytenoid ligament*

vocal process *n* : the anterior angle of the arytenoid cartilage on each side of the larynx to which the vocal ligament of the corresponding side is attached

voice \ˈvȯis\ *n* **1** : sound produced esp. by means of lungs or larynx; *esp* : sound so produced by human beings **2** : the faculty of utterance : SPEECH

voice box *n* : LARYNX

void \ˈvȯid\ *vb* : to discharge or emit (as excrement)

vol *abbr* volume

vo·lar \ˈvō-lər, -ˌlär\ *adj* : relating to the palm of the hand or the sole of the foot; *specif* : located on the same side as the palm of the hand

vol·a·tile \ˈvä-lə-təl, -ˌtīl\ *adj* : readily vaporizable at a relatively low temperature — **vol·a·til·i·ty** \ˌvä-lə-ˈti-lə-tē\ *n*

volatile oil *n* : an oil that vaporizes readily; *esp* : ESSENTIAL OIL

volitantes — see MUSCAE VOLITANTES

vo·li·tion \vō-ˈli-shən, və-\ *n* **1** : an act of making a choice or decision; *also* : a choice or decision made **2** : the power of choosing or determining — **vo·li·tion·al** \-ˈli-shə-nəl\ *adj*

Volk·mann's canal \ˈfȯlk-mənz-\ *n* : any of the small channels in bone that transmit blood vessels from the periosteum into the bone and that lie perpendicular to and communicate with the Haversian canals

Volkmann, Alfred Wilhelm (1800–1877), German physiologist.

Volkmann's contracture *or* **Volkmann contracture** *n* : ischemic contracture of an extremity and esp. of a hand

volt \ˈvōlt\ *n* : the practical mks unit of electrical potential difference and electromotive force equal to the difference of potential between two points in a conducting wire carrying a constant current of one ampere when the power dissipated between these two points is equal to one watt

Vol·ta \ˈvōl-tä\, **Alessandro Giuseppe Antonio Anastasio (1745–1827),** Italian physicist.

volt·age \ˈvōl-tij\ *n* : electrical potential or potential difference expressed in volts

voltage clamp *n, often attrib* : stabilization of a membrane potential by de-

polarization and maintenance at a given potential by means of a current from a source outside the living system — **voltage clamp** *vb*

vol·un·tary \ˈvä-lən-ˌter-ē\ *adj* **1** : proceeding from the will or from one's own choice or consent **2** : of, relating to, subject to, or regulated by the will (∼ behavior) — **vol·un·tari·ly** *adv*

voluntary hospital *n* : a hospital that is operated under individual, partnership, or corporation control usu. for little or no profit and provides mainly semiprivate and private care

voluntary muscle *n* : muscle (as most striated muscle) under voluntary control

vol·vu·lus \ˈväl-vyə-ləs\ *n* : a twisting of the intestine upon itself that causes obstruction — compare ILEUS

vo·mer \ˈvō-mər\ *n* : a bone of the skull that in humans forms the posterior and inferior part of the nasal septum comprising a vertical plate pointed in front and expanding at the upper back part into lateral wings

vo·mero·na·sal \ˌvä-mə-rō-ˈnā-zəl, ˌvō-\ *adj* : of or relating to the vomer and the nasal region and esp. to Jacobson's organ or the vomeronasal cartilage

vomeronasal cartilage *n* : a narrow process of cartilage between the vomer and the cartilage of the nasal septum

vomeronasal organ *n* : JACOBSON'S ORGAN

vomica — see NUX VOMICA

¹vom·it \ˈvä-mət\ *n* **1** : VOMITING **2** : stomach contents disgorged through the mouth — called also *vomitus*

²vomit *vb* : to disgorge the contents of the stomach through the mouth

vomiting *n* : an act or instance of disgorging the contents of the stomach through the mouth — called also *emesis*

vomiting center *n* : a nerve center in the medulla oblongata concerned in the act of vomiting

vom·i·tus \ˈvä-mə-təs\ *n* : VOMIT 2

von Grae·fe's sign \ˌvän-ˈgrā-fəz-\ *n* : the failure of the upper eyelid to follow promptly and smoothly the downward movement of the eyeball that is seen in exophthalmic goiter

von Grae·fe \fȯn-ˈgre-fə\, **Albrecht Friedrich Wilhelm Ernst (1828–1870), German ophthalmologist.**

von Hip·pel–Lin·dau disease \vän-ˈhi-pəl-ˈlin-ˌdaů-\ *n* : a rare genetically determined disease that is characterized by angiomatosis of the retina and cerebellum and often by cysts or neoplasms of the liver, pancreas, and kidneys — called also *Lindau's disease*

von Hippel, Eugen (1867–1939), German ophthalmologist.

Lindau, Arvid Vilhelm (1892–1958), Swedish pathologist.

von Reck·ling·hau·sen's disease \-ˈre-**

kliŋ-ˌhaú-zənz-\ *n* : NEUROFIBROMA-
TOSIS

F. D. Recklinghausen — see RECK-
LINGHAUSEN'S DISEASE

von Wil·le·brand's disease \vän-ˈvi-lə-
ˌbränts-\ *n* : a genetic disorder that is
inherited as an autosomal recessive
trait and is characterized by deficiency of a plasma clotting factor and by
mucosal and petechial bleeding due
to abnormal blood vessels

**Willebrand, Erik Adolf von (1870–
1949),** Finnish physician.

vorticosa — see VENA VORTICOSA

vor·ti·cose vein \ˈvȯr-tə-ˌkōs-\ *n* : VENA
VORTICOSA

voy·eur \vȯi-ˈyər, vwä-\ *n* : one obtaining sexual gratification from seeing
sex organs and sexual acts; *broadly*
: one who habitually seeks sexual
stimulation by visual means — **voy·
eur·ism** \-ˌi-zəm\ *n* — **voy·eur·is·tic**
\ˌvwä-(ˌ)yər-ˈis-tik, ˌvȯi-ər-\ *adj*

VS *abbr* vesicular stomatitis

VSD *abbr* ventricular septal defect

vulgaris — see ACNE VULGARIS, ICH-
THYOSIS VULGARIS, LUPUS VULGARIS,
PEMPHIGUS VULGARIS, VERRUCA VUL-
GARIS

vul·ner·a·ble \ˈvəl-nə-rə-bəl\ *adj* : capa-

ble of being hurt : susceptible to injury or disease — **vul·ner·a·bil·i·ty** \ˌvəl-
nə-rə-ˈbi-lə-tē\ *n*

vul·sel·lum \vəl-ˈse-ləm\ *n, pl* **-sel·la**
\-ˈse-lə\ : a surgical forceps with serrated, clawed, or hooked blades

vulv- *or* **vulvo-** *comb form* **1** : vulva
⟨*vulvitis*⟩ **2** : vulvar and ⟨*vulvo*vaginal⟩

vul·va \ˈvəl-və\ *n, pl* **vul·vae** \-ˌvē, -ˌvī\
: the external parts of the female gen-
ital organs comprising the mons pubis, labia majora, labia minora,
clitoris, vestibule of the vagina, bulb
of the vestibule, and Bartholin's
glands — **vul·val** \ˈvəl-vəl\ *or* **vul·var**
\-vər\ *adj*

vulvae — see KRAUROSIS VULVAE, PRU-
RITUS VULVAE

vul·vec·to·my \ˌvəl-ˈvek-tə-mē\ *n, pl*
-mies : surgical excision of the vulva

vul·vi·tis \ˌvəl-ˈvī-təs\ *n* : inflammation
of the vulva

vul·vo·vag·i·nal \ˌvəl-vō-ˈva-jən-ᵊl\ *adj*
: of or relating to the vulva and the
vagina (∼ hematoma)

vul·vo·vag·i·ni·tis \ˌvəl-vō-ˌva-jə-ˈnī-
təs\ *n, pl* **-nit·i·des** \-ˈni-tə-ˌdēz\ : coincident inflammation of the vulva
and vagina

W

W *symbol* [German *wolfram*] tungsten

Waar·den·burg's syndrome \ˈvar-dən-
ˌbergz-\ *n* : a highly variable genetic
disorder inherited as an autosomal
dominant trait and accompanied by
all, any, or none of deafness, a white
forelock, widely spaced eyes, and
heterochromia of the irises

**Waardenburg, Petrus Johannes (b
1886),** Dutch ophthalmologist.

wad·ding \ˈwä-diŋ\ *n* : a soft absorbent
sheet of cotton, wool, or cellulose
used esp. in hospitals for surgical
dressings

WAIS *abbr* Wechsler Adult Intelligence Scale

waist \ˈwāst\ *n* : the narrowed part of
the body between the thorax and hips

waist·line \ˈwāst-ˌlin\ *n* : body circumference at the waist

wake·ful \ˈwāk-fəl\ *adj* : not sleeping or
able to sleep : SLEEPLESS — **wake·
ful·ness** *n*

Wal·den·ström's macroglobulinemia
\ˈväl-dən-ˌstremz-\ *n* : a rare progressive syndrome associated with a high
serum concentration of a monoclonal
antibody of the class IgM and
characterized by adenopathy, hepa-
tomegaly, splenomegaly, anemia, and
lymphocytosis and plasmacytosis of
the bone marrow

Waldenström, Jan Gosta (b 1906),
Swedish physician.

Wal·dey·er's ring \ˈväl-ˌdī-ərz-\ *n* : a
ring of lymphatic tissue formed by the

two palatine tonsils, the pharyngeal
tonsil, the lingual tonsil, and intervening lymphoid tissue

Wal·dey·er–Hartz \ˈväl-ˌdī-ər-
ˈhärts\, **Heinrich Wilhelm Gottfried
von (1836–1921),** German anatomist.

walk·er \ˈwȯ-kər\ *n* : a framework designed to support a baby learning to
walk or an infirm or handicapped person

¹walk–in \ˈwȯk-ˌin\ *adj* : providing
medical services to ambulatory patients without an appointment (a ∼
clinic); *also* : being an individual who
uses such services

²walk–in *n* : a walk-in patient

walk·ing \ˈwȯ-kiŋ\ *adj* : able to walk
: AMBULATORY ⟨the ∼ wounded⟩

walking cast *n* : a cast that is worn on
a patient's leg and has a stirrup with
a heel or other supporting device embedded in the plaster to facilitate
walking

walking pneumonia *n* : a usu. mild
pneumonia caused by a microorganism of the genus *Mycoplasma* (*M.
pneumoniae*) and characterized by
malaise, cough, and often fever

wall \ˈwȯl\ *n* : a structural layer surrounding a cavity, hollow organ, or
mass of material ⟨the intestinal ∼*s*⟩
— **walled** \ˈwȯld\ *adj*

Wal·le·ri·an degeneration \wä-ˈlir-ē-
ən-\ *n* : degeneration of nerve fibers
that occurs following injury or disease and that progresses from the

place of injury along the axon away from the cell body while the part between the place of injury and the cell body remains intact

Wal·ler \'wä-lər\, **Augustus Volney (1816–1870),** British physiologist.

wall·eye \'wȯ-ₗlī\ n **1a :** an eye with a whitish or bluish white iris **b :** an eye with an opaque white cornea **2a :** strabismus in which the eye turns outward away from the nose — called also *exotropia*; compare CROSS-EYE 1 **b** pl **:** eyes affected with divergent strabismus — **wall·eyed** \-ₗlīd\ adj

¹**wan·der·ing** \'wän-də-riŋ\ adj **:** FLOATING ⟨a ~ spleen⟩

²**wandering** n **:** movement of a tooth out of its normal position esp. as a result of periodontal disease

wandering cell n **:** any of various ameboid phagocytic tissue cells

wandering pacemaker n **:** a back and forth shift in the location of cardiac pacemaking esp. from the sinoatrial node to or near the atrioventricular node

Wan·gen·steen apparatus \'waŋ-ən-ₗstēn-, -gən-\ n **:** the apparatus used in Wangensteen suction — called also *Wangensteen appliance*

Wangensteen, Owen Harding (1898–1981), American surgeon.

Wangensteen suction n **:** a method of draining fluid or secretions from body cavities (as the stomach) by means of an apparatus that operates on negative pressure

war·ble \'wȯr-bəl\ n **1 :** a swelling under the hide esp. of the back of cattle, horses, and wild mammals caused by the maggot of a botfly or warble fly **2 :** the maggot of a warble fly — **war·bled** \-bəld\ adj

warble fly n **:** any of various dipteran flies (family Oestridae) whose larvae live under the skin of various mammals and cause warbles

ward \'wȯrd\ n **:** a division in a hospital; esp **:** a large room in a hospital where a number of patients often requiring similar treatment are accommodated ⟨a diabetic ~⟩

war·fa·rin \'wȯr-fə-rən\ n **:** an anticoagulant coumarin-derivative $C_{19}H_{16}$-O_4 related to dicumarol that inhibits the production of prothrombin by vitamin K and is used as a rodent poison and in medicine; also **:** its sodium salt $C_{19}H_{15}N_aO_4$ used esp. in the prevention or treatment of thromboembolic disease — see COUMADIN

war gas n **:** a gas for use in warfare — compare LACRIMATOR, NERVE GAS, STERNUTATOR

warm–blood·ed \'wȯrm-'blə-dəd\ adj **:** having a relatively high and constant body temperature relatively independent of the surroundings — **warm–blood·ed·ness** n

warm up vb **:** to engage in preliminary

exercise (as to stretch the muscles) — **warm–up** \'wȯr-ₗməp\ n

war neurosis n **:** a neurosis (as hysteria or anxiety) occurring in soldiers during war and attributed to their war experiences

wart \'wȯrt\ n **1 :** a horny projection on the skin usu. of the extremities produced by proliferation of the skin papillae and caused by a virus — called also *verruca vulgaris* **2 :** any of numerous verrucous skin lesions — **warty** \'wär-tē\ adj

War·thin–Star·ry stain \'wȯr-thən-'stär-ē-\ n **:** a silver nitrate stain used to show the presence of bacilli

Warthin, Aldred Scott (1866–1931), and **Starry, Allen Chronister (b 1890),** American pathologists.

¹**wash** \'wȯsh, 'wäsh\ vb **1 :** to cleanse by or as if by the action of liquid (as water) **2 :** to flush or moisten (a bodily part or injury) with a liquid **3 :** to pass through a liquid to carry off impurities or soluble components

²**wash** n **:** a liquid medicinal preparation used esp. for cleansing or antisepsis — see EYEWASH, MOUTHWASH

wash·able \'wȯ-shə-bəl, 'wä-\ adj **:** soluble in water ⟨~ ointment bases⟩

washings n pl **:** material collected by the washing of a bodily cavity

wash·out \'wȯsh-ₐaut, 'wäsh-\ n **:** the action or process of progressively reducing the concentration of a substance (as a dye injected into the left ventricle of the heart)

wasp \'wäsp, 'wȯsp\ n **:** any of numerous social or solitary winged hymenopteran insects (esp. families Sphecidae and Vespidae) that usu. have a slender smooth body with the abdomen attached by a narrow stalk, biting mouthparts, and in the females and workers an often formidable sting

Was·ser·mann \'wä-sər-mən, 'vä-\ n **:** WASSERMANN TEST

Wassermann reaction n **:** the complement-fixing reaction that occurs in a positive complement-fixation test for syphilis using the serum of an infected individual

Wassermann, August Paul von (1866–1925), German bacteriologist.

Wassermann test n **:** a test for the detection of syphilitic infection using the Wassermann reaction — called also *Wassermann*

¹**waste** \'wäst\ n **1 :** loss through breaking down of bodily tissue **2** pl **:** bodily waste materials **:** EXCREMENT

²**waste** vb **wast·ed; wast·ing :** to lose or cause to lose weight, strength, or vitality **:** EMACIATE — often used with away

³**waste** adj **:** excreted from or stored in inert form in a living body as a by-product of vital activity ⟨~ materials⟩

¹**wast·ing** \'wäs-tiŋ\ adj **:** undergoing or causing decay or loss of strength

²**wasting** *n* : the process or condition of wasting away : gradual loss of strength or substance : ATROPHY

wa·ter \'wȯ-tər, 'wä-\ *n* **1** : the liquid that descends from the clouds as rain, is a major constituent of all living matter, is an odorless, tasteless, very slightly compressible liquid oxide of hydrogen H_2O, and freezes at 0° C (32° F) and boils at 100° C (212° F) **2** : liquid containing or resembling water: as **a** (1) : a pharmaceutical or cosmetic preparation made with water (2) : a watery solution of a gaseous or readily volatile substance — see AMMONIA WATER **b** : a watery fluid (as tears or urine) formed or circulating in a living body **c** : AMNIOTIC FLUID — often used in pl.; *also* : BAG OF WATERS

water balance *n* : the ratio between the water assimilated into the body and that lost from the body; *also* : the condition of the body when this ratio approximates unity

water blister *n* : a blister with a clear watery content that is not purulent or sanguineous

wa·ter·borne \'wȯ-tər-ˌbōrn, 'wä-\ *adj* : carried or transmitted by water and esp. by drinking water

water brash *n* : regurgitation of an excessive accumulation of saliva from the lower part of the esophagus often with some acid material from the stomach — compare HEARTBURN

water—hammer pulse *n* : CORRIGAN'S PULSE

water hemlock *n* : a Eurasian perennial herb (*Cicuta virosa*) of the carrot family (Umbelliferae) that is highly poisonous; *also* : any of several related plants

Wa·ter·house—Frid·er·ich·sen syndrome \'wȯ-tər-ˌhaus-'fri-də-rik-sən-\ *n* : acute and severe meningococcemia with hemorrhage into the adrenal glands

  Waterhouse, Rupert (1873–1958), British physician, and **Friderichsen, Carl (b 1886),** Danish physician.

wa·ter·logged \-ˌlägd\ *adj* : EDEMATOUS

water moc·ca·sin \-ˈmä-kə-sən\ *n* : a venomous pit viper (*Agkistrodon piscivorus*) of the southern U.S. closely related to the copperhead — called also *cottonmouth, cottonmouth moccasin*

water on the brain *n* : HYDROCEPHALUS

water on the knee *n* : an accumulation of inflammatory exudate in the knee joint often following an injury

water pick \-ˌpik\ *n* : a tooth-cleaning device that cleans by directing a stream of water over and between teeth

water pill *n* : a diuretic pill

water–soluble *adj* : soluble in water ⟨~ vitamin B⟩

wa·tery \'wȯ-tə-rē, 'wä-\ *adj* **1** : consisting of or filled with water **2** : con-

taining, sodden with, or yielding water or a thin liquid ⟨~ stools⟩

Wat·son—Crick \'wät-sən-'krik\ *adj* : of or relating to the Watson-Crick model ⟨*Watson-Crick* helix⟩

  Watson, James Dewey (b 1928), American molecular biologist. **Crick, Francis Harry Compton (b 1916),** British molecular biologist.

Watson—Crick model *n* : a model of DNA structure in which the molecule is a double-stranded helix, each strand is composed of alternating links of phosphate and deoxyribose, and the strands are linked by pairs of purine and pyrimidine bases projecting inward from the deoxyribose sugars and joined by hydrogen bonds with adenine paired with thymine and with cytosine paired with guanine — compare DOUBLE HELIX

watt \'wät\ *n* : the mks unit of power equal to the work done at the rate of one joule per second or to the power produced by a current of one ampere across a potential difference of one volt

  Watt, James (1736–1819), British engineer and inventor.

wave \'wāv\ *n* **1a** : a disturbance or variation that transfers energy progressively from point to point in a medium and that may take the form of an elastic deformation or of a variation of pressure, electric or magnetic intensity, electrical potential, or temperature **b** : one complete cycle of such a disturbance **2** : an undulating or jagged line constituting a graphic representation of an action ⟨an electroencephalographic ~⟩

wave·form \'wāv-ˌfȯrm\ *n* : a usu. graphic representation of the shape of a wave that indicates its characteristics (as frequency and amplitude) — called also *waveshape*

wave·length \-ˌleŋkth\ *n* : the distance in the line of advance of a wave from any one point to the next point of corresponding phase — symbol λ

wax \'waks\ *n* **1** : a substance secreted by bees that is a dull yellow solid plastic when warm — called also *beeswax* **2** : any of various substances resembling beeswax: as **a** : any of numerous substances of plant or animal origin that differ from fats in being less greasy, harder, and more brittle and in containing principally compounds of high molecular weight **b** : a pliable or liquid composition used esp. in uniting surfaces, making patterns or impressions, or producing a polished surface ⟨dental ~es⟩ **3** : EARWAX

wax·ing *n* : the process of removing body hair with a depilatory wax

waxy \'wak-sē\ *adj* **wax·i·er; -est 1** : made of, abounding in, or covered with wax **2** : resembling wax ⟨~ secretions⟩

waxy flexibility *n* : a condition in which a patient's limbs retain any position into which they are manipulated by another person and which occurs esp. in catatonic schizophrenia

WBC *abbr* white blood cell

weal \'wēl\ *n* : WELT

wean \'wēn\ *vb* **1** : to accustom (as a child) to take food otherwise than by nursing **2** : to detach usu. gradually from a cause of dependence or form of treatment

web \'web\ *n* : a tissue or membrane of an animal or plant; *esp* : that uniting fingers or toes at their bases — **webbed** \'webd\ *adj*

Web·er–Chris·tian disease \'we-bər-'kris-chən-\ *also* **Web·er–Chris·tian's disease** \-chənz-\ *n* : PANNICULITIS 2
　　Weber, Frederick Parkes (1863–1962), British physician.
　　H. A. Christian — see HAND-SCHÜLLER-CHRISTIAN DISEASE

We·ber–Fech·ner law \'we-bər-'fek-nər-, 'vā-bər-'fek-nər-\ *n* : an approximately accurate generalization in psychology: the intensity of a sensation is proportional to the logarithm of the intensity of the stimulus causing it — called also *Fechner's law*
　　Weber, Ernst Heinrich (1795–1878), German anatomist and physiologist.
　　Fechner, Gustav Theodor (1801–1887), German physicist and psychologist.

We·ber's law \'we-bərz-, 'vā-bərz-\ *n* : an approximately accurate generalization in psychology: the smallest change in the intensity of a stimulus capable of being perceived is proportional to the intensity of the original stimulus
　　E. H. Weber — see WEBER-FECHNER LAW

We·ber test \'we-bər-, 'vā- *or* **We·ber's test** \-bərz-\ *n* : a test to determine the nature of unilateral hearing loss in which a vibrating tuning fork is held against the forehead at the midline and conduction deafness is indicated if the sound is heard more loudly in the affected ear and nerve deafness is indicated if it is heard more loudly in the normal ear

We·ber–Liel \'vā-bər-'lēl\, **Friedrich Eugen (1832–1891)**, German otologist.

Wechs·ler Adult Intelligence Scale \'weks-lər-\ *n* : an updated version of the Wechsler-Bellevue test having the same structure but standardized against a different population to more accurately reflect the general population — abbr. *WAIS*
　　Wechsler, David (1896–1981), American psychologist.

Wechs·ler–Belle·vue test \-'bel-,vyü-\ *n* : a test of general intelligence and coordination in adults that involves both verbal and performance tests and is now superseded by the

Wechsler Adult Intelligence Scale — called also *Wechsler-Bellevue scale*

wedge pressure \'wej-\ *n* : intravascular pressure that is measured by means of a catheter wedged into the pulmonary artery so as to block the flow of blood and that is equivalent to the pressure in the left atrium — called also *pulmonary capillary wedge pressure, pulmonary wedge pressure*

wedge resection *n* : any of several surgical procedures for removal of a wedge-shaped mass of tissue (as from the ovary or a lung)

WEE *abbr* western equine encephalomyelitis

weep \'wēp\ *vb* **wept** \'wept\; **weeping 1** : to pour forth (tears) from the eyes **2** : to exude (a fluid) slowly

Weg·e·ner's granulomatosis \'ve-gə-nərz-\ *n* : an uncommon disease of unknown cause that is characterized esp. by granuloma formation in the respiratory tract, glomerulonephritis, and necrotizing granulomatous vasculitis
　　Wegener, F. (fl 1936–39), German pathologist.

weigh \'wā\ *vb* **1** : to find the heaviness of **2** : to measure or apportion (a definite quantity) on or as if on a scale **3** : to have weight or a specified weight

weight \'wāt\ *n* **1** : the amount that a thing weighs **2** : a unit of weight or mass

weight·less·ness \'wāt-ləs-nəs\ *n* : the state or condition of having little or no weight due to lack of apparent gravitational pull — **weight·less** *adj*

Weil–Fe·lix reaction \'vīl-'fā-liks-\ *n* : an agglutination test for various rickettsial infections (as typhus and tsutsugamushi disease) using particular strains of bacteria of the genus *Proteus* that have antigens in common with the rickettsias to be identified — called also *Weil-Felix test*
　　Weil, Edmund (1880–1922), and **Felix, Arthur (1887–1956)**, Austrian bacteriologists.

Weil's disease \'vīlz-, 'wīlz-\ *n* : a leptospirosis that is characterized by chills, fever, muscle pain, and hepatitis manifested by more or less severe jaundice and that is caused by a spirochete of the genus *Leptospira* (*L. interrogans* serotype *icterohaemorrhagiae*)
　　Weil, Adolf (1848–1916), German physician.

well \'wel\ *adj* **1** : free or recovered from infirmity or disease : HEALTHY **2** : completely cured or healed

well–adjusted *adj* : WELL-BALANCED 2

well–balanced *adj* **1** : nicely or evenly balanced, arranged, or regulated (a ~ diet) **2** : emotionally or psychologically untroubled

well·ness *n* : the quality or state of being in good health esp. as an actively sought goal

welt \'welt\ *n* : a ridge or lump raised on the body usu. by a blow

wen \'wen\ *n* : SEBACEOUS CYST; *broadly* : an abnormal growth or a cyst protruding from a surface esp. of the skin

Wencke·bach period \'wen-kə-ˌbäk-\ *n* : WENCKEBACH PHENOMENON

Wenckebach, Karel Frederik (1864–1940), Dutch internist.

Wenckebach phenomenon *n* : heart block in which a pulse from the atrium periodically does not reach the ventricle and which is characterized by progressive prolongation of the P-R interval until a pulse is skipped

Werd·nig–Hoff·mann disease \'vert-nik-'hof-ˌmän-\ *n* : muscular atrophy that is caused by degeneration of the ventral horn cells of the spinal cord, is inherited as an autosomal recessive trait, becomes symptomatic during early infancy, is characterized by hypotonia and flaccid paralysis, and is often fatal during childhood — called also *Werdnig-Hoffmann syndrome*

Werdnig, Guido (1844–1919), Austrian neurologist, and **Hoffmann, Johann (1857–1919),** German neurologist.

Werl·hof's disease \'verl-ˌhöfs-\ *n* : THROMBOCYTOPENIC PURPURA

Werlhof, Paul Gottlieb (1699–1767), German physician.

Wer·ner's syndrome \'ver-nərz-\ *n* : a rare hereditary disorder characterized by premature aging with associated abnormalities (as dwarfism, cataracts, osteoporosis, and hypogonadism)

Werner, Otto (b 1879), German physician.

Wer·nick·e's area \'ver-nə-kəs-\ *n* : an area located in the posterior part of the superior temporal gyrus that plays an important role in the comprehension of language

Wernicke, Carl (1848–1905), German neurologist.

Wernicke's encephalopathy *n* : an inflammatory hemorrhagic encephalopathy that is caused by thiamine deficiency, affects esp. chronic alcoholics, and is characterized by nystagmus, diplopia, ataxia, and degenerative mental disorders (as Korsakoff's psychosis)

Wert·heim operation \'vert-ˌhïm-\ *or* **Wert·heim's operation** \-ˌhïmz-\ *n* : radical hysterectomy for cancer of the uterine cervix

Wertheim, Ernst (1864–1920), Austrian gynecologist.

Wes·ter·gren erythrocyte sedimentation rate \'ves-tər-grən-\ *n* : sedimentation rate of red blood cells determined by the Westergren method — called also *Westergren sedimentation rate*

Westergren, Alf Vilhelm (b 1891), Swedish physician.

Westergren method *n* : a method for estimating the sedimentation rate of red blood cells in fluid blood

Western blot *n* : a blot consisting of a sheet of a cellulose derivative that contains spots of protein for identification by a suitable molecular probe and is used esp. for the detection of antibodies — compare NORTHERN BLOT, SOUTHERN BLOT — **Western blotting** *n*

western equine encephalomyelitis *n* : EQUINE ENCEPHALOMYELITIS b

wet dream *n* : an erotic dream culminating in orgasm and in the male accompanied by seminal emission

wet mount *n* : a glass slide holding a specimen suspended in a drop of liquid (as water) for microscopic examination; *also* : a specimen mounted in this way — **wet–mount** *adj*

wet nurse *n* : a woman who cares for and suckles young not her own

wetting agent *n* : any of numerous water-soluble or liquid organic substances that promote spreading of a liquid on a surface or penetration into a material esp. by their oriented adsorption on the surfaces in such a way that the wetting liquid is no longer repelled

Whar·ton's duct \'hwort-ᵊnz-, 'wort-\ *n* : the duct of the submandibular gland that opens into the mouth on a papilla at the side of the frenulum of the tongue

Wharton, Thomas (1614–1673), British anatomist.

Wharton's jelly *n* : a soft connective tissue that occurs in the umbilical cord and consists of large stellate fibroblasts and a few wandering cells and macrophages embedded in a homogeneous jellylike intercellular substance

wheal \'hwēl, 'wēl\ *n* : a suddenly formed elevation of the skin surface: as **a** : WELT **b** : the transient lump occurring at the site of injection of a solution before the solution is normally dispersed **c** : a flat burning or itching eminence on the skin (urticarial ∼s)

wheal·ing *n* : the presence or development of wheals

wheat germ *n* : the embryo of the wheat kernel separated in milling and used esp. as a source of vitamins and protein

wheel·chair \'hwēl-ˌchar, 'wēl-\ *n* : a chair mounted on wheels esp. for the use of disabled persons

¹**wheeze** \'hwēz, 'wēz\ *vb* **wheezed; wheez·ing** : to breathe with difficulty usu. with a whistling sound

²**wheeze** *n* : a sibilant whistling sound caused by difficult or obstructed respiration

whey \'hwā, 'wā\ *n* : the serum or watery part of milk that is separated from the coagulable part or curd, is rich in lactose, minerals, and vitamins. and contains lactalbumin and traces of fat

whip-lash \'hwip-ˌlash. 'wip-\ n : WHIP-LASH INJURY

whiplash injury n : injury resulting from a sudden sharp whipping movement of the neck and head (as of a person in a vehicle that is struck head-on or from the rear by another vehicle)

Whip-ple's disease \'hwi-pəlz-. 'wi-\ n : a rare malabsorption syndrome that is often associated with the presence of an actinomycetous fungus (*Tropheryma whippelli*) in the mucous membrane of the intestine, that affects primarily the small intestine but becomes more generalized affecting esp. the joints, brain, liver, and heart, that is marked by the accumulation of lipid deposits in the intestinal lymphatic tissues, weight loss, joint pain, mental confusion, and generalized lymphadenopathy, and that is diagnosed by the presence of macrophages in the lamina propria of the small intestine which give a positive reaction to a periodic acid-Schiff test — called also *intestinal lipodystrophy*

Whipple, George Hoyt (1878–1976), American pathologist.

whip-worm \'hwip-ˌwərm. 'wip-\ n : a parasitic nematode worm of the genus *Trichuris* having a body that is thickened posteriorly and is very long and slender anteriorly; *esp* : one (*T. trichiura*) that parasitizes the human intestine

whirl-pool bath \'hwərl-ˌpül-. 'wərl-\ n : a therapeutic bath in which all or part of the body is exposed to forceful whirling currents of hot water — called also *whirlpool*

white blood cell n : any of the blood cells that are colorless, lack hemoglobin, contain a nucleus, and include the lymphocytes, monocytes, neutrophils, eosinophils, and basophils — called also *white blood corpuscle, white cell, white corpuscle;* compare RED BLOOD CELL

white count n : the count or the total number of white blood cells in blood usu. stated as the number in one cubic millimeter — compare DIFFERENTIAL BLOOD COUNT

white fat n : normal fat tissue that replaces brown fat in infants during the first year of life

white-head \'hwit-ˌhed. 'wit-\ n : MILIUM

white lotion n : a preparation made of sulfurated potash and zinc sulfate that is applied topically in the treatment of various skin disorders

white matter n : neural tissue that consists largely of myelinated nerve fibers, has a whitish color, and underlies the gray matter of the brain and spinal cord or is gathered into nerves

white muscle disease n : a disease of young domestic animals (as lambs and calves) that is characterized by muscular degeneration — see STIFF-LAMB DISEASE

white noise n : a heterogeneous mixture of sound waves extending over a wide frequency range that has been used to mask out unwanted noise interfering with sleep — called also *white sound*

white ointment n : an ointment consisting of 5 percent white wax and 95 percent white petrolatum — called also *simple ointment*

white petrolatum n : decolorized petroleum jelly — called also *white petroleum jelly*

white piedra n : a form of piedra that affects esp. the facial hairs and is caused by a fungus of the genus *Trichosporan* (*T. beigelii*)

white pulp n : a parenchymatous tissue of the spleen that consists of compact masses of lymphatic cells and that forms the Malpighian corpuscles — compare RED PULP

white ramus n : RAMUS COMMUNICANS a

white ramus communicans n : RAMUS COMMUNICANS a

whites n pl : LEUKORRHEA

white shark n : GREAT WHITE SHARK

white snake-root \-'snāk-ˌrüt. -ˌrút\ n : a poisonous No. American herb (*Eupatorium rugosum*) of the daisy family (Compositae) that is a cause of trembles and milk sickness

white sound n : WHITE NOISE

white squill n : SQUILL 2

Whit-field's ointment \'hwit-ˌfēldz-. 'wit-\ *also* **Whit-field ointment** \-ˈfēld-\ n : an ointment that contains benzoic acid and salicylic acid and is used for its keratolytic effect in treating fungus skin diseases (as ringworm)

Whitfield, Arthur (1868–1947), British dermatologist.

whit-low \'hwit-(ˌ)lō. 'wit-\ n : a deep usu. suppurative inflammation of the finger or toe esp. near the end or around the nail — called also *felon;* compare PARONYCHIA

WHO *abbr* World Health Organization

whole \'hōl\ *adj* : containing all its natural constituents, components, or elements ⟨~ blood⟩

whole–body *adj* : of, relating to, or affecting the entire body ⟨~ radiation⟩ ⟨~ hyperthermia⟩

whoop \'hüp. 'hup. 'hwüp\ n : the crowing intake of breath following a paroxysm in whooping cough — **whoop** vb

whooping cough n : an infectious disease esp. of children caused by a bacterium of the genus *Bordetella* (*B. pertussis*) and marked by a convulsive spasmodic cough sometimes followed by a crowing intake of breath — called also *pertussis*

whorl \'hwórl. 'wórl. 'hwərl. 'wərl\

: a fingerprint in which the central papillary ridges turn through at least one complete turn

Wi·dal reaction \vē-ˈdäl- *also* **Wi·dal's reaction** \-ˈdälz-\ *n* : a specific reaction consisting in agglutination of typhoid bacilli or other salmonellas when mixed with serum from a patient having typhoid fever or other salmonella infection and constituting a test for the disease

　　Widal, Georges–Fernand–Isidore (1862–1929), French physician and bacteriologist.

Widal test *also* **Widal's test** *n* : a test for detecting typhoid fever and other salmonella infections using the Widal reaction

wide–spectrum *adj* : BROAD-SPECTRUM

wild type *n* : a phenotype, genotype, or gene that predominates in a natural population of organisms or strain of organisms in contrast to that of natural or laboratory mutant forms; *also* : an organism or strain displaying the wild type — **wild–type** *adj*

Wilms' tumor \ˈvilmz-\ *also* **Wilms's tumor** \ˈvilm-zəz-\ *n* : a malignant tumor of the kidney that primarily affects children and is made up of embryonic elements — called also *nephroblastoma*

　　Wilms, Max (1867–1918), German surgeon.

Wilson's disease \ˈwil-sənz-\ *n* : a hereditary disease that is determined by an autosomal recessive gene and is marked esp. by cirrhotic changes in the liver and severe mental disorder due to a ceruloplasmin deficiency and resulting inability to metabolize copper — called also *hepatolenticular degeneration;* see KAYSER-FLEISCHER RING

　　Wilson, Samuel Alexander Kinnier (1877–1937), British neurologist.

wind–broken \ˈwind-ˌbrō-kən\ *adj, of a horse* : affected with pulmonary emphysema or with heaves

wind·burn \ˈwind-ˌbərn\ *n* : irritation of the skin caused by wind — **wind-burned** \-ˌbərnd\ *adj*

wind·chill \-ˌchil\ *n* : a still-air temperature that would have the same cooling effect on exposed human flesh as a given combination of temperature and wind speed — called also *chill factor, windchill factor, windchill index*

wind·gall \-ˌgȯl\ *n* : a soft tumor or synovial swelling on a horse's leg in the region of the fetlock joint

win·dow \ˈwin-(ˌ)dō\ *n* **1** : FENESTRA 1 **2** : a small surgically created opening : FENESTRA 2a

wind·pipe \ˈwind-ˌpip\ *n* : TRACHEA

wind puff \-ˌpəf\ *n* : WINDGALL

wing \ˈwiŋ\ *n* **1** : one of the movable feathered or membranous paired appendages by means of which a bird, bat, or insect is able to fly **2** : a wing-

like anatomical part or process : ALA; *esp* : any of the four winglike processes of the sphenoid bone — see GREATER WING, LESSER WING — **winged** \ˈwind, ˈwiŋ-əd\ *adj*

win·ter·green \ˈwin-tər-ˌgrēn\ *n* **1** : any plant of the genus *Gaultheria; esp* : a low evergreen plant (*G. procumbens*) with white flowers and spicy red berries **2** : OIL OF WINTERGREEN

wintergreen oil *n* : OIL OF WINTER-GREEN

winter itch *n* : an itching disorder caused by prolonged exposure to cold dry air

winter tick *n* : an ixodid tick of the genus *Dermacentor* (*D. albipictus*) that is actively parasitic during the winter months on domestic and big-game animals in parts of Canada and northern and western U.S.

wire \ˈwir\ *n* : metal thread or a rod used in surgery to suture soft tissue or transfix fractured bone and in orthodontic dentistry to position teeth — **wire** *vb*

Wir·sung's duct \ˈvir-ˌsuŋz-\ *n* : PANCREATIC DUCT a

　　J. G. Wirsung — see DUCT OF WIRSUNG

wisdom tooth *n* : the third molar that is the last tooth to erupt on each side of the upper and lower jaws

wish–fulfillment *n* : the gratification of a desire esp. symbolically (as in dreams or neurotic symptoms)

Wis·kott–Al·drich syndrome \ˈvis-ˌkät-ˈȯl-ˌdrich-\ *n* : an inherited usu. fatal childhood immunodeficiency disease characterized esp. by thrombocytopenia, leukopenia, recurrent infections, eczema, and abnormal bleeding

　　Wiskott, Alfred (*b* 1898), German pediatrician.

　　Aldrich, Robert Anderson (*b* 1917), American pediatrician.

witch ha·zel \ˈwich-ˌhā-zəl\ *n* **1** : a small tree or shrub (*Hamamelis virginiana* of the family Hamamelidaceae) of eastern No. America that blooms in the fall **2** : an alcoholic solution of a distillate of the bark of the witch hazel used as a soothing and mildly astringent lotion

with·draw·al \with-ˈdrȯ-əl, with-\ *n* **1 a** : a pathological retreat from objective reality (as in some schizophrenic states) **b** : social or emotional detachment **2 a** : the discontinuance of administration or use of a drug **b** : the syndrome of often painful physical and psychological symptoms that follows discontinuance of an addicting drug **3** : COITUS INTERRUPTUS — **withdraw** \-ˈdrȯ\ *vb*

withdrawal symptom *n* : one of a group of symptoms (as nausea, sweating, or depression) produced by deprivation of an addicting drug

with·drawn \with-ˈdrȯn\ *adj* : socially

detached and unresponsive : exhibiting withdrawal : INTROVERTED

with·ers \'wi-thərz\ *n pl* **1** : the ridge between the shoulder bones of a horse **2** : a part corresponding to the withers in a quadruped other than a horse

Wit·zel·sucht \'vit-səl-ˌzükt\ *n* : excessive facetiousness and inappropriate or pointless humor esp. when considered as part of an abnormal condition

wohl·fahr·tia \ˌvōl-ˈfär-tē-ə\ *n* **1** *cap* : a genus of dipteran flies (family Sarcophagidae) that commonly deposit their larvae in wounds or on the intact skin of humans and domestic animals causing severe cutaneous myiasis **2** : any fly of the genus *Wohlfahrtia*

Wol·fart \'vōl-ˌfärt\, **Peter (1675–1726),** German physician.

Wolff·ian body \'wōl-fē-ən-\ *n* : MESONEPHROS

Wolff \'vōlf\, **Caspar Friedrich (1734–1794),** German anatomist and embryologist.

Wolffian duct *n* : the duct of the mesonephros that persists in the female chiefly as part of the epoophoron and in the male as the duct system leaving the testis and including the epididymis, vas deferens, and ejaculatory duct — called also *mesonephric duct*

Wolff–Par·kin·son–White syndrome \'wulf-ˈpär-kən-sən-ˈhwīt-, -ˈwit-\ *n* : an abnormal heart condition characterized by premature activation of the ventricle by atrial impulses and an electrocardiographic tracing with a shortened P-R interval and a widened QRS complex

Wolff, **Louis (*b* 1898),** American cardiologist.

Parkinson, **Sir John (*b* 1885),** British cardiologist.

White, **Paul Dudley (1886–1973),** American cardiologist.

wol·fram \'wul-frəm\ *n* : TUNGSTEN

womb \'wüm\ *n* : UTERUS

wonder drug *n* : MIRACLE DRUG

wood alcohol *n* : METHANOL

wooden tongue *n* : actinobacillosis or actinomycosis of cattle esp. when chiefly affecting the tongue

wood tick *n* : any of several ixodid ticks: as **a** : ROCKY MOUNTAIN WOOD TICK **b** : AMERICAN DOG TICK

wool fat \'wul-\ *n* : wool grease esp. after refining : LANOLIN

wool grease *n* : a fatty slightly sticky wax coating the surface of the fibers of sheep's wool that is used as a source of lanolin

wool·sort·er's disease \'wul-ˌsor-tərz-\ *n* : pulmonary anthrax resulting esp. from inhalation of bacterial spores (*Bacillus anthracis*) from contaminated wool or hair

word–association test *n* : a test of personality and mental function in which the subject is required to respond to each of a series of words with the first

one that comes to mind or with one of a specified class of words

word blindness *n* : ALEXIA

word salad *n* : a jumble of extremely incoherent speech as sometimes observed in schizophrenia

work·up \'wər-ˌkəp\ *n* : an intensive diagnostic study ⟨a gastrointestinal ∼⟩

work up \ˌwər-ˈkəp, ˈwər-ˌ\ *vb* : to perform a diagnostic workup upon ⟨*work up* a patient⟩

¹worm \'wərm\ *n* **1** : any of various relatively small elongated usu. naked and soft-bodied parasitic animals (as a platyhelminth) **2** : HELMINTHIASIS — usu. used in pl. (a dog with ∼*s*) — **worm·like** *adj*

²worm *vb* : to treat (an animal) with a drug to destroy or expel parasitic worms

worm·er \'wər-mər\ *n* : a worming agent used in veterinary medicine

Wor·mi·an bone \'wor-mē-ən-\ *n* : a small irregular inconstant plate of bone interposed in a suture between large cranial bones

Worm \'worm\, **Ole (1588–1654),** Danish physician.

worm·seed \'wərm-ˌsēd\ *n* **1** : any of various plants (as of the genera *Artemisia* or *Chenopodium*) whose seeds possess anthelmintic properties

worm·wood \'wərm-ˌwud\ *n* : any of various aromatic shrubs and herbs (genus *Artemisia* and esp. *A. absinthium*) of the daisy family (Compositae)

wound \'wünd\ *n* **1a** : an injury to the body consisting of a laceration or breaking of the skin or mucous membrane usu. by a hard or sharp instrument forcefully driven or applied **b** : an opening made in the skin or a membrane of the body incidental to a surgical operation or procedure **2** : a mental or emotional hurt or blow — **wound** *vb*

wrench \'rench\ *n* : a sharp twist or sudden jerk straining muscles or ligaments; *also* : the resultant injury (as of a joint) — **wrench** *vb*

Wright's stain \'rīts-\ *n* : a stain used in staining blood and parasites living in blood

Wright, **James Homer (1869–1928),** American pathologist.

wrin·kle \'riŋ-kəl\ *n* : a small ridge or furrow in the skin esp. when due to age, care, or fatigue — **wrinkle** *vb*

wrist \'rist\ *n* : the joint or the region of the joint between the human hand and the arm

wrist·bone \-ˌbōn\ *n* **1** : a carpal bone **2** : the styloid process of the human radius that forms a prominence on the outer side of the wrist above the thumb

wrist–drop \-ˌdräp\ *n* : paralysis of the extensor muscles of the hand causing the hand to hang down at the wrist

wrist joint *n* : the articulation at the wrist

writer's cramp *n* : a painful spasmodic cramp of muscles of the hand or fingers brought on by excessive writing — called also **graphospasm**

wry·neck \'rī-₁nek\ *n* : TORTICOLLIS

wt *abbr* weight

Wuch·er·e·ria \₁wü-kə-'rir-ē-ə\ *n* : a genus of filarial worms (family Dipetalonematidae) including a parasite (*W. bancrofti*) that causes elephantiasis

Wu·cher·er \'vü-kər-ər\, **Otto Eduard Heinrich (1820–1873),** German physician.

X

x \'eks\ *n, pl* **x's** *or* **xs** \'ek-səz\ : the basic or haploid number of chromosomes of a polyploid series : the number contained in a single genome — compare N 1

x *symbol* power of magnification

Xan·ax \'za-₁naks\ *trademark* — used for a preparation of alprazolam

xanth- *or* **xantho-** *comb form* : yellow ⟨*xanthoma*⟩

xan·than gum \'zan-thən-\ *n* : a polysaccharide that is produced by fermentation of carbohydrates by a bacterium (*Xanthomonas campestris*) and is a thickening and suspending agent used esp. in pharmaceuticals and prepared foods — called also **xanthan**

xan·the·las·ma \₁zan-thə-'laz-mə\ *n* : xanthoma of the eyelid

xanthelasma pal·pe·bra·rum \-₁pal-₁pē-'brar-əm\, *n* : XANTHELASMA

xan·thene dye \'zan-₁thēn-\ *n* : any of various brilliant fluorescent yellow to pink to bluish red dyes

xan·thine \'zan-₁thēn\ *n* : a feebly basic compound $C_5H_4N_4O_2$ that occurs esp. in animal or plant tissue, is derived from guanine and hypoxanthine, and yields uric acid on oxidation; *also* : any of various derivatives of this

xan·tho·chro·mia \₁zan-thə-'krō-mē-ə\ *n* : xanthochromic discoloration

xan·tho·chro·mic \-'krō-mik\ *adj* : having a yellowish discoloration (~ cerebrospinal fluid)

xan·tho·ma \zan-'thō-mə\ *n, pl* **-mas** *or* **-ma·ta** \-mə-tə\ : a fatty irregular yellow patch or nodule on the skin (as of the eyelids, neck, or back) that is associated esp. with disturbances of cholesterol metabolism

xan·tho·ma·to·sis \(₁)zan-₁thō-mə-'tō-səs\ *n, pl* **-to·ses** \-₁sēz\ : any of several metabolic disorders characterized by the accumulation of yellow fatty deposits in the skin and in internal tissues

xan·tho·ma·tous \zan-'thō-mə-təs\ *adj* : of, relating to, marked by, or characteristic of a xanthoma or xanthomatosis

xan·tho·phyll \'zan-thə-₁fil\ *n* : any of several neutral yellow to orange carotenoid pigments that are oxygen-derivatives of carotenes; *esp* : LUTEIN

xan·thop·sia \zan-'thäp-sē-ə\ *n* : a visual disturbance in which objects appear yellow

xan·tho·tox·in \'zan-thə-₁täk-sən\ *n* : METHOXSALEN

xanth·uren·ic acid \₁zanth-yə-'re-nik-\ *n* : a yellow crystalline phenolic acid $C_{10}H_7NO_4$ excreted in the urine when tryptophan is added to the diet of experimental animals deficient in pyridoxine

X chromosome *n* : a sex chromosome that usu. occurs paired in each female cell and single in each male cell in species in which the male typically has two unlike sex chromosomes — compare Y CHROMOSOME

X–disease *n* : any of various usu. virus diseases of obscure etiology and relationships; *esp* : a viral encephalitis of humans first detected in Australia

Xe *symbol* xenon

xen- *or* **xeno-** *comb form* **1** : strange : foreign ⟨*xenobiotic*⟩ **2** : HETER- ⟨*xenograft*⟩

xe·no·bi·ot·ic \₁ze-nō-bī-'ä-tik, ₁zē-, -bē-\ *n* : a chemical compound (as a drug, pesticide, or carcinogen) that is foreign to a living organism — **xenobiotic** *adj*

xe·no·di·ag·no·sis \₁ze-nō-₁dī-ig-'nō-səs, ₁zē-\ *n, pl* **-no·ses** \-₁sēz\ : the detection of a parasite by feeding test material (as blood) from a suspected host (as a human) to a suitable intermediate host (as an insect) and later examining the intermediate host for the parasite — **xe·no·di·ag·nos·tic** \-'näs-tik\ *adj*

xe·no·ge·ne·ic \₁ze-nō-jə-'nē-ik, ₁zē-\ *also* **xe·no·gen·ic** \-'je-nik\ *adj* : derived from, originating in, or being a member of another species — compare ALLOGENEIC, SYNGENEIC

xe·no·graft \'ze-nə-₁graft, 'zē-\ *n* : a graft of tissue taken from a donor of one species and grafted into a recipient of another species — called also *heterograft, heterotransplant*; compare HOMOGRAFT

xe·non \'zē-₁nän, 'zē-\ *n* : a heavy, colorless, and relatively inert gaseous element — symbol *Xe*; see ELEMENT table

xe·no·phobe \'ze-nə-₁fōb, 'zē-\ *n* : one unduly fearful of what is foreign and esp. of people of foreign origin — **xe·no·pho·bic** \₁ze-nə-'fō-bik, ₁zē-\ *adj*

xe·no·pho·bia \₁ze-nə-'fō-bē-ə, ₁zē-\

: fear and hatred of strangers or for-
eigners or of anything that is strange
or foreign

Xen·op·syl·la \,ze-näp-'si-lə\ *n* : a genus
of fleas (family Pulicidae) including
several (as the oriental rat flea) that
are important as vectors of plague

xe·no·tro·pic \,ze-nə-'trä-pik, ,zē-nə-
'trō-pik\ *adj* : replicating or reproducing only in cells other than those of
the host species ⟨∼ viruses⟩

xer- *or* **xero-** *comb form* : dry : arid
⟨*xeroderma*⟩

xe·ro·der·ma \,zir-ə-'dər-mə\ *n* : a disease of the skin characterized by dryness and roughness and a fine scaly
desquamation

xeroderma pig·men·to·sum \-,pig-mən-
'tō-səm, -,men-\ *n* : a genetic condition inherited as a recessive autosomal trait that is caused by a defect in
mechanisms that repair DNA muta-
tions and is characterized by the development of pigment abnormalities
and multiple skin cancers in body areas exposed to the sun — abbr. *XP*

xe·rog·ra·phy \zə-'rä-grə-fē, zir-'ä-\ *n*,
pl **-phies 1** : a process for copying
graphic matter by the action of light
on an electrically charged surface in
which the latent image is developed
with a resinous powder **2** : XERORA-
DIOGRAPHY — **xe·ro·graph·ic** \,zir-ə-
'gra-fik\ *adj* — **xe·ro·graph·i·cal·ly** *adv*

xe·ro·mam·mog·ra·phy \,zir-ō-ma-'mä-
grə-fē\ *n*, *pl* **-phies** : xeroradiography
of the breast — **xe·ro·mam·mo·gram**
\-'ma-mə-,gram\ *n*

xe·roph·thal·mia \,zir-,äf-'thal-mē-ə,
-,äp-'thal-\ *n* : a dry thickened luster-
less condition of the eyeball resulting
esp. from a severe systemic deficiency of vitamin A — compare KERA-
TOMALACIA — **xe·roph·thal·mic** \-mik\
adj

xe·ro·ra·di·og·ra·phy \,zir-ō-,rā-dē-'ä-
grə-fē\ *n*, *pl* **-phies** : radiography used
esp. in mammography for breast can-
cer that produces an image using X
rays in a manner similar to the way an
image is produced by light in xerogra-
phy — **xe·ro·ra·dio·graph·ic** \-,rā-dē-
ō-'gra-fik\ *adj*

xe·ro·sis \zi-'rō-səs\ *n*, *pl* **xe·ro·ses**
\-,sēz\ : abnormal dryness of a body
part or tissue (as the skin)

xe·ro·sto·mia \,zir-ə-'stō-mē-ə\ *n* : abnormal dryness of the mouth due to
insufficient secretions — called also
dry mouth

xiph- *or* **xiphi-** *or* **xipho-** *comb form*
: sword-shaped ⟨*xiphi*sternum⟩

xi·phi·ster·num \,zi-fə-'stər-nəm, ,zī-\
n, *pl* **-na** \-nə\ : XIPHOID PROCESS

xi·phoid \'zī-,foid, 'zi-\ *n* : XIPHOID
PROCESS — **xiphoid** *adj*

xiphoid process *n* : the smallest and
lowest division of the human sternum
that is cartilaginous early in life but
becomes more or less ossified during
adulthood — called also *ensiform
cartilage, ensiform process*

x–ir·ra·di·a·tion \'eks-\ *n*, *often cap X*
: X-RADIATION 1 — **x–ir·ra·di·ate** *vb,
often cap X*

X–linked *adj* : located in an X chromosome ⟨an ∼ gene⟩; *also* : transmitted
by an X-linked gene ⟨an ∼ mutation⟩

XP *abbr* xeroderma pigmentosum

x–ra·di·a·tion *n*, *often cap X* **1** : exposure to X rays **2** : radiation composed
of X rays

x–ra·di·og·ra·phy *n*, *often cap X*, *pl*
-phies : radiography by means of X
rays : ROENTGENOGRAPHY

x–ray \'eks-,rā\ *vb*, *often cap X* : to examine, treat, or photograph with X
rays

X ray *n* **1** : any of the electromagnetic
radiations of the same nature as visible radiation but of an extremely
short wavelength that has the properties of ionizing a gas upon passage
through it, of penetrating various
thicknesses of all solids, of producing
secondary radiations by impinging on
material bodies, of acting on photographic films and plates as light does,
and of causing fluorescent screens to
emit light — called also *roentgen ray*
2 : a photograph obtained by use of X
rays ⟨a chest *X ray*⟩ — **X–ray** *adj*

X–ray therapy *n* : medical treatment
(as of cancer) by controlled application of X rays

xy·lene \'zī-,lēn\ *n* : any of three toxic
flammable oily isomeric aromatic hydrocarbons C_8H_{10}

xy·li·tol \'zī-lə-,tol, -,tōl\ *n* : a crystalline alcohol $C_5H_{12}O_5$ that is a derivative of xylose and is used as a
sweetener

Xy·lo·caine \'zī-lə-,kān\ *trademark* —
used for a preparation of lidocaine

xy·lose \'zī-,lōs, -,lōz\ *n* : a crystalline
aldose sugar $C_5H_{10}O_5$

xy·lu·lose \'zil-yü-,lōs, 'zī-,lə-,lōz\ *n*
: a ketose sugar $C_5H_{10}O_5$ of the pentose class that plays a role in carbohydrate metabolism and is found in
the urine in cases of pentosuria

Y

Y *symbol* yttrium

yaw \'yȯ\ *n* : one of the lesions characteristic of yaws

yawn \'yȯn, 'yän\ *n* : a deep usu. involuntary intake of breath through the wide open mouth often as an involuntary reaction to fatigue or boredom — **yawn** *vb*

yaws \'yȯz\ *n sing or pl* : an infectious contagious tropical disease that is caused by a spirochete of the genus *Treponema* (*T. pertenue*) and that is characterized by a primary ulcerating lesion on the skin followed by a secondary stage in which ulcers develop all over the body and by a third stage in which the bones are involved — called also *frambesia, pian*

Yb *symbol* ytterbium

Y chromosome \'wī-\ *n* : a sex chromosome that is characteristic of male cells in species in which the male typically has two unlike sex chromosomes — compare X CHROMOSOME

yeast \'yēst\ *n* **1 a** : a yellowish surface froth or sediment that occurs esp. in saccharine liquids (as fruit juices) in which it promotes alcoholic fermentation, consists largely of cells of a fungus (family Saccharomycetaceae), and is used esp. in the making of alcoholic liquors and as a leaven in baking **b** : a commercial product containing yeast plants in a moist or dry medium **2 a** : a minute fungus (esp. *Saccharomyces cerevisiae*) that is present and functionally active in yeast, usu. has little or no mycelium, and reproduces by budding **b** : any of various similar fungi (esp. orders Endomycetales and Moniliales) — **yeast-like** \-ₗlīk\ *adj*

yeast infection *n* : an infection of the female genital tract by a yeast of the genus *Candida* (*C. albicans*) and characterized by vaginal discharge and vulvovaginitis; *broadly* : an infection (as thrush or tinea versicolor) caused by a yeast fungus

yellow body *n* : CORPUS LUTEUM

yellow fat disease *n* : a disease esp. of swine, cats, and ranch-raised mink that is associated with a deficiency of vitamin E and is marked by inflammation of the fatty tissue, subcutaneous edema, and varied visceral lesions — called also *steatitis, yellow fat*

yellow fever *n* : an acute destructive disease of warm regions marked by sudden onset, prostration, fever, albuminuria, jaundice, and often hemorrhage and caused by a flavivirus transmitted esp. by a mosquito of the genus *Aedes* (*A. aegypti*)

yellow–fever mosquito *n* : a small dark= colored mosquito of the genus *Aedes* (*A. aegypti*) that is the usual vector of yellow fever — called also *tiger mosquito*

yellow jacket *n* **1** : any of various yellow-marked social wasps (esp. genus *Vespula* of the family Vespidae) that usu. nest in the ground and can sting repeatedly and painfully **2** : a yellow capsule containing a preparation of pentobarbital — usu. used in pl.

yellow marrow *n* : MARROW 1a

yellow petrolatum *n* : petrolatum that has not been wholly or mostly decolorized

yel-lows \'ye-(ₗ)lōz\ *n sing or pl* : any of several diseases of domestic animals (as sheep) that are characterized by jaundice

yellow wax *n* : a wax obtained as a yellow to brown solid by melting a honeycomb with boiling water, straining, and cooling — called also *beeswax*

yer-ba san-ta \'yer-bə-'sän-tə, 'yȯr-, -'san-\ *n* **1** : an evergreen shrub (*Eriodictyon californicum* of the family Hydrophyllaceae) of California with aromatic leaves **2** : ERIODICTYON

Yer-sin-ia \yər-'si-nē-ə\ *n* : a genus of enterobacteria that includes several important pathogens (as the plague bacterium, *Y. pestis*) formerly included in the genus *Pasteurella* — see PLAGUE 2

Yer-sin \yer-'seⁿ\, **Alexandre–Émile-John (1863–1943),** French bacteriologist.

Y ligament *n* : ILIOFEMORAL LIGAMENT

yo-gurt *also* **yo-ghurt** \'yō-gərt\ *n* : a fermented slightly acid often flavored semisolid food made of whole or skimmed cow's milk and milk solids to which cultures of bacteria of the genus *Lactobacillus* (*L. bulgarius*) and *Streptococcus* (*S. thermophilus*) have been added

yo-him-bine \yō-'him-ₗbēn, -bən\ *n* : an alkaloid $C_{21}H_{26}N_2O_3$ that is a weak blocker of alpha-adrenergic receptors and has been used as an aphrodisiac

yolk \'yōk\ *n* : material stored in an ovum that supplies food to the developing embryo and consists chiefly of proteins, lecithin, and cholesterol

yolk sac *n* : a membranous sac that is attached to an embryo and encloses food yolk, that is continuous in most forms through the omphalomesenteric duct with the intestinal cavity of the embryo, that being abundantly supplied with blood vessels is throughout embryonic life and in some forms later the chief organ of nutrition, and that in the mammals having a placenta is nearly vestigial and functions chiefly prior to the formation of the placenta

yolk stalk *n* : OMPHALOMESENTERIC DUCT

Young–Helm·holtz theory \\'yəŋ-'helm-ˌhōlts-\ *n* : a theory in color vision: the eye has three separate elements each of which is stimulated by a different primary color

> **Young, Thomas (1773–1829),** British physician, physicist, and archeologist.

> **Helmholtz, Hermann Ludwig Ferdi-**

nand von **(1821–1894),** German physicist and physiologist.

yt·ter·bi·um \i-'tər-bē-əm\ *n* : a bivalent or trivalent metallic element — symbol *Yb*; see ELEMENT table

yt·tri·um \\'i-trē-əm\ *n* : a trivalent metallic element — symbol *Y*; see ELEMENT table

yup·pie flu \\'yə-pē-\ *n* : CHRONIC FATIGUE SYNDROME

Z

zal·cit·a·bine \zal-'si-tə-ˌbēn, -ˌbīn\ *n* : DDC

Zan·tac \\'zan-ˌtak\ *trademark* — used for a preparation of the hydrochloride of ranitidine

Z–DNA \\'zē-\ *n* : a section of DNA that spirals to the left rather than to the right and that may exert some control over the activity of adjacent genes

Zei·gar·nik effect \zī-'gär-nik-\ *n* : the psychological tendency to remember an uncompleted task rather than a completed one

> **Zeigarnik, Bluma (*b* 1900),** Russian psychologist.

Zen·ker's diverticulum \\'zen-kərz-, 'tseŋ-\ *n* : an abnormal pouch in the upper part of the esophagus in which food may become trapped causing bad breath, irritation, difficulty in swallowing, and regurgitation — called also *pharyngoesophageal diverticulum*

> **Zenker, Friedrich Albert von (1825–1898),** German pathologist and anatomist.

Zeph·i·ran \\'ze-fə-ˌran\ *trademark* — used for a preparation of benzalkonium chloride

Zes·tril \\'zes-tril\ *trademark* — used for a preparation of lisinopril

zi·do·vu·dine \zī-'dō-vü-ˌdēn, -vyü-\ *n* : AZIDOTHYMIDINE

Ziehl–Neel·sen stain \\'tsēl-'nāl-sən-\ *n* : a stain used esp. for detecting the tubercle bacillus

> **Ziehl, Franz (1857–1926),** German bacteriologist.

> **Neelsen, Friedrich Carl Adolf (1854–1894),** German pathologist.

zi·mel·i·dine \zi-'me-lə-ˌdēn\ *n* : a bicyclic antidepressant drug $C_{16}H_{17}BrN_2$

zinc \\'ziŋk\ *n* : a bluish white crystalline bivalent metallic element that is an essential micronutrient for both plants and animals — symbol *Zn*; see ELEMENT table

zinc carbonate *n* : a crystalline salt $ZnCO_3$ having astringent and antiseptic properties

zinc chloride *n* : a poisonous caustic salt $ZnCl_2$ that is used as a disinfectant and astringent

zinc ointment *n* : ZINC OXIDE OINTMENT

zinc oxide *n* : a white solid ZnO used in

pharmaceutical and cosmetic preparations (as ointments and powders)

zinc oxide ointment *n* : an ointment that contains about 20 percent of zinc oxide and is used in treating skin disorders

zinc peroxide *n* : any of various white to yellowish white powders that have the peroxide ZnO_2 of zinc as their chief ingredient and are used chiefly as disinfectants, astringents, and deodorants

zinc pyr·i·thi·one \-ˌpir-i-'thī-ˌōn\ *n* : a powder $C_{10}H_8N_2O_2S_2Zn$ that is nearly insoluble in water, possesses cytostatic activity against epidermal cells, and is the active ingredient in various shampoos used to control dandruff and seborrheic dermatitis — called also *pyrithione zinc*

zinc stearate *n* : an insoluble salt usu. of commercial stearic acid and usu. containing some zinc oxide that has astringent and antiseptic properties and is used as a constituent of ointments and powders

zinc sulfate *n* : a crystalline salt $ZnSO_4$ used in medicine as an astringent, emetic, and weak antiseptic

zinc un·dec·y·len·ate \-ˌən-de-si-'le-ˌnāt\ *n* : a fine white powder $C_{22}H_{38}$-O_4Zn that is used as a fungistatic agent

zinc white *n* : ZINC OXIDE

zir·co·ni·um \ˌzər-'kō-nē-əm\ *n* : a strong ductile metallic element — symbol *Zr*; see ELEMENT table

zit \\'zit\ *n* : PIMPLE 1

Z line *n* : any of the dark thin lines across a striated muscle fiber that mark the boundaries between adjacent sarcomeres

Zn *symbol* zinc

zo- *or* **zoo-** *comb form* : animal ⟨*zoo*-nosis⟩

-zo·ic \\'zō-ik\ *adj comb form* : having a (specified) animal mode of existence ⟨sapro*zoic*⟩

Zol·ling·er–El·li·son syndrome \\'zä-liŋ-ər-'e-li-sən-\ *n* : a syndrome consisting of fulminating intractable peptic ulcers, gastric hypersecretion and hyperacidity, and the occurrence of gastrinomas of the pancreatic cells of the islets of Langerhans

Zollinger, Robert Milton (1903–1992), American surgeon.

Ellison, Edwin Homer (1918–1970), American surgeon.

Zo•max \'zō-ˌmaks\ *trademark* — used for a preparation of zomepirac

zo•me•pir•ac \ˌzō-mə-'pir-ˌak\ *n* : an anti-inflammatory and analgesic drug administered in the form of the sodium salt $C_{15}H_{13}ClNNaO_3 \cdot 2H_2O$ — see ZOMAX

zo•na \'zō-nə\ *n, pl* **zo•nae** \-ˌnē, -ˌnī\ *or* **zonas** 1 : an anatomical zone or layer; *esp* : ZONA PELLUCIDA 2 : SHINGLES

zona fas•cic•u•la•ta \-fa-ˌsi-kyə-'lā-tə\ *n* : the middle of the three layers of the adrenal cortex that consists of radially arranged columnar epithelial cells

zona glo•mer•u•lo•sa \-glō-ˌmer-yə-'lō-sə\ *n* : the outermost of the three layers of the adrenal cortex that consists of round masses of granular epithelial cells that stain deeply — called also *glomerulosa*

zona pel•lu•ci•da \-pə-'lü-sə-də\ *n* : the transparent more or less elastic outer layer or envelope of a mammalian ovum often traversed by numerous radiating striae

zona re•tic•u•lar•is \-re-ˌti-kyə-'lar-əs\ *n* : the innermost of the three layers of the adrenal cortex that consists of irregularly arranged cylindrical masses of epithelial cells

zone \'zōn\ *n* 1 : an encircling anatomical structure 2 : a region or area set off as distinct

zo•nu•la \'zōn-yə-lə\ *n, pl* **-lae** \-ˌlē\ *or* **-las** : ZONULE OF ZINN

zonula cil•i•ar•is \-ˌsi-lē-'ar-əs\ *n* : ZONULE OF ZINN

zo•nu•lar \'zōn-yə-lər\ *adj* : of or relating to the zonule of Zinn ⟨~ attachments⟩

zon•ule \'zōn-ˌyül\ *n* : ZONULE OF ZINN

zonule of Zinn \-'tsin\ *n* : the suspensory ligament of the crystalline lens of the eye — called also *zonula, zonula ciliaris*

J. G. Zinn — see LIGAMENT OF ZINN

zoo- — see ZO-

zo•ol•o•gy \zō-'äl-ə-jē\ *n, pl* **-gies** 1 : a branch of biology that deals with the classification and the properties and vital phenomena of animals 2 : the properties and vital phenomena exhibited by an animal, animal type, or group — **zoo•log•i•cal** \ˌzō-ə-'läj-i-kəl\ *also* **zoo•log•ic** \-ik\ *adj* — **zo•ol•o•gist** \zō-'äl-ə-jəst\ *n*

-zo•on \'zō-ˌän, -ən\ *n comb form* : animal ⟨spermato*zoon*⟩

zoo•no•sis \ˌzō-ə-'nō-səs, zō-'ä-nə-səs\ *n, pl* **-no•ses** \-ˌsēz\ : a disease communicable from animals to humans under natural conditions — **zoo•not•ic** \ˌzō-ə-'nä-tik\ *adj*

zoo•par•a•site \ˌzō-ə-'par-ə-ˌsīt\ *n* : a parasitic animal

zoo•phil•ia \ˌzō-ə-'fil-ē-ə\ *n* : an erotic fixation on animals that may result in sexual excitement through real or fancied contact

zoo•pho•bia \ˌzō-ə-'fō-bē-ə\ *n* : abnormal fear of animals

zos•ter \'zäs-tər\ *n* : SHINGLES

Zo•vi•rax \zō-'vī-ˌraks\ *trademark* — used for a preparation of acyclovir

zox•a•zol•amine \ˌzäk-sə-'zä-lə-ˌmēn\ *n* : a drug $C_7H_5ClN_2O$ used esp. formerly as a skeletal muscle relaxant and uricosuric agent

ZPG *abbr* zero population growth

Zr *symbol* zirconium

Z-plas•ty \'zē-ˌplas-tē\ *n, pl* **-ties** : a surgical procedure for the repair of constricted scar tissue in which a Z-shaped incision is made in the skin and the two resulting flaps are interposed

zyg- *or* **zygo-** *comb form* 1 : pair ⟨*zyg*apophysis⟩ 2 : union : fusion ⟨*zygo*genesis⟩

zyg•apoph•y•sis \ˌzī-gə-'pä-fə-səs\ *n, pl* **-y•ses** \-ˌsēz\ : any of the articular processes of the neural arch of a vertebra of which there are usu. two anterior and two posterior

zy•go•gen•e•sis \ˌzī-gō-'je-nə-səs\ *n, pl* **-e•ses** \-ˌsēz\ : reproduction by means of specialized germ cells or gametes : sexual reproduction

zy•go•ma \zī-'gō-mə\ *n, pl* **-ma•ta** \-mə-tə\ *also* **-mas** 1 : ZYGOMATIC ARCH 2 : ZYGOMATIC BONE

¹**zy•go•mat•ic** \ˌzī-gə-'ma-tik\ *adj* : of, relating to, constituting, or situated in the region of the zygomatic bone and the zygomatic arch

²**zygomatic** *n* : ZYGOMATIC BONE

zygomatic arch *n* : the arch of bone that extends along the front or side of the skull beneath the orbit and that is formed by the union of the temporal process of the zygomatic bone in front with the zygomatic process of the temporal bone behind

zygomatic bone *n* : a bone of the side of the face below the eye that forms part of the zygomatic arch and part of the orbit and articulates with the temporal, sphenoid, and frontal bones and with the maxilla of the upper jaw — called also *cheekbone, jugal, malar bone, zygoma*

zygomatic nerve *n* : a branch of the maxillary nerve that divides into a facial branch supplying the skin of the prominent part of the cheek and a temporal branch supplying the skin of the anterior temporal region

zygomatico- *comb form* : zygomatic and ⟨*zygomatico*facial⟩

zy•go•mat•i•co•fa•cial \ˌzī-gə-ˌma-ti-kō-'fā-shəl\ *adj* 1 : of, relating to, or being the branch of the zygomatic nerve that supplies the skin of the prominent part of the cheek 2 : of, relating to, or being a foramen in the zygomatic bone that gives passage to the zygomaticofacial branch of the zygomatic nerve

zy·go·mat·i·co·max·il·lary \-ˈmak-sə-ˌler-ē\ adj : of, relating to, or uniting the zygomatic bone and the maxilla of the upper jaw ⟨the ~ suture⟩

zy·go·mat·i·co·tem·po·ral \-ˈtem-pə-rəl\ adj **1** : of, relating to, or uniting the zygomatic arch and the temporal bone ⟨the ~ suture⟩ **2 a** : of, relating to, or being the branch of the zygomatic nerve that supplies the skin of the anterior temporal region **b** : of, relating to, or being a foramen in the zygomatic bone that gives passage to the zygomaticotemporal branch of the zygomatic nerve

zygomatic process n : any of several bony processes that articulate with the zygomatic bone: as **a** : a long slender process of the temporal bone helping to form the zygomatic arch **b** : a narrow process of the frontal bone articulating with the zygomatic bone **c** : a rough triangular eminence of the maxilla of the upper jaw articulating with the zygomatic bone

zy·go·mat·i·cus \ˌzī-gə-ˈma-ti-kəs\ n **1** : ZYGOMATICUS MAJOR **2** : ZYGOMATICUS MINOR

zygomaticus major n : a slender band of muscle on each side of the face that arises from the zygomatic bone, inserts into the orbicularis oris and skin at the corner of the mouth, and acts to pull the corner of the mouth upward and backward when smiling or laughing

zygomaticus minor n : a slender band of muscle on each side of the face that arises from the zygomatic bone, inserts into the upper lip between the zygomaticus major and the levator labii superioris, and acts to raise the upper lip upward and laterally

zy·gos·i·ty \zī-ˈgä-sə-tē\ n, pl **-ties** : the makeup or characteristics of a particular zygote

zy·gote \ˈzī-ˌgōt\ n : a cell formed by the union of two gametes; broadly : the developing individual produced from such a cell — **zy·got·ic** \zī-ˈgä-tik\ adj — **zy·got·i·cal·ly** adv

zy·go·tene \ˈzī-gə-ˌtēn\ n : the stage of meiotic prophase which immediately follows the leptotene and during which synapsis of homologous chromosomes occurs — **zygotene** adj

-zy·gous \ˈzī-gəs\ adj comb form : having (such) a zygotic constitution ⟨heterozygous⟩

zym- or **zymo-** comb form : enzyme ⟨zymogen⟩

-zyme \ˌzīm\ n comb form : enzyme ⟨lysozyme⟩

zy·mo·gen \ˈzī-mə-jən\ n : a protein that is an inactive precursor of an enzyme, is secreted by living cells, and is activated by catalysis (as by a kinase or an acid) — called also proenzyme

zy·mo·gram \ˈzī-mə-ˌgram\ n : an electrophoretic strip (as of starch gel) or a representation of it exhibiting the pattern of separated enzymes and esp. isoenzymes after electrophoresis

zy·mo·san \ˈzī-mə-ˌsan\ n : an insoluble largely polysaccharide fraction of yeast cell walls

Signs and Symbols

Biology

○	an individual, specif., a female—used chiefly in inheritance charts
□	an individual, specif., a male—used chiefly in inheritance charts
♀	female
♂ *or* ♂	male
×	crossed with;
	hybrid
+	wild type
F_1	offspring of the first generation
F_2	offspring of the second generation
F_3, F_4, F_5, etc.	offspring of the third, fourth, fifth, etc. generation

Chemistry and Physics

(for element symbols see ELEMENT table)

α	alpha particle
β	beta particle, beta ray
λ	wavelength
+	signifies "plus", "and", "together with" and is used between the symbols of substances brought together for, or produced by, a reaction;

signifies a unit charge of positive electricity when placed to the right of a symbol as a superscript: Ca^{++} denotes the ion of calcium, which carries two positive charges;

signifies a dextrorotatory compound when preceding in parentheses a compound name, as in (+) tartaric acid

− signifies a unit charge of negative electricity when placed to the right of a symbol as a superscript: Cl^- denotes a chlorine ion carrying a negative charge;

signifies a levorotatory compound when preceding in parentheses a compound name, as in $(-)$ quinine;

signifies removal or loss of a part from a compound during a reaction (as $-CO_2$)

− signifies a single bond and is used between the symbols of elements or groups which unite to form a compound: H–Cl for HCl, H–O–H for H_2O

\> signifies separate single bonds from an atom to two other atoms or groups (as in the grouping >C=NNHR characteristic of hydrazone)

· used to separate parts of a substance regarded as loosely joined (as $CuSO_4 \cdot 5H_2O$);

also used to denote the presence of a single unpaired electron (as H·)

= indicates a double bond;

signifies two unit charges of negative electricity when placed to the right of a symbol as a superscript (as $SO_4^=$, the negative ion of sulfuric acid)

≡ signifies a triple bond or a triple negative charge

: signifies a pair of electrons belonging to an atom that is not shared with another atom (as in : NH_3);

sometimes signifies a double bond (as in $CH_2 : CH_2$)

( ) marks groups within a compound, as in $C_6H_4(CH_3)_2$, the formula for xylene which contains two methyl groups (CH_3)

━ or ▬ joins attached atoms or groups in structural formulas for cyclic compounds, as that for glucose

$$\overline{\qquad O \qquad}$$
$$CH_2OHCH(CHOH)_3CHOH$$

1-, 2-, etc. used initially in names, referring to the positions of substituting groups, attached to the first, second, etc., of the numbered atoms of the parent compound

x, m, n used as subscripts following an atom or group in a chemical formula to indicate that the number of times the atom or group occurs is indefinite, as in $(C_6H_{10}O_5)_x$ for glycogen, or approximate, as in

$C_{12}H_mAl_{16}O_nS_8$ for sucralfate where m and n are approximately 54 and 75

R   group—used esp. of an organic group

′   used to distinguish between different substituents of the same kind (as R′, R″, R‴ to indicate different organic groups)

Medicine

℞   take—used on prescriptions; prescription; treatment

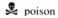 poison

APOTHECARIES' MEASURES

℥   ounce

ƒ℥   fluid ounce

ƒʒ   fluid dram

min *or* ♍   minim

APOTHECARIES' WEIGHTS

℔   pound

℥   ounce: as

    ℥ i or ℥ j, one ounce;

    ℥ ss, half an ounce;

    ℥ iss or ℥ jss, one ounce and a half;

    ℥ ij, two ounces

ʒ   dram

℈   scruple

Notes

Notes